DAVIDSON'S
Principles and Practice of
MEDICINE

The Editors

Christopher Haslett BSc (Hons) FRCPE FRCP
Professor of Respiratory Medicine, University of Edinburgh
Chairman of the Division of Clinical and Community Science, University of Edinburgh
Honorary Consultant Physician, Royal Infirmary of Edinburgh

Edwin R. Chilvers BMedSci BMBS PhD FRCPE
Professor of Respiratory Medicine, University of Cambridge School of Clinical Medicine
Honorary Consultant Physician, Addenbrooke's and Papworth Hospitals, Cambridge

John A.A. Hunter *OBE* BA MD FRCPE
Professor of Dermatology, University of Edinburgh
Honorary Consultant Dermatologist, Royal Infirmary of Edinburgh

Nicholas A. Boon MA MD FRCPE
Consultant Cardiologist, Royal Infirmary of Edinburgh
Honorary Senior Lecturer, Department of Medicine, University of Edinburgh

Illustrated by
Robert Britton

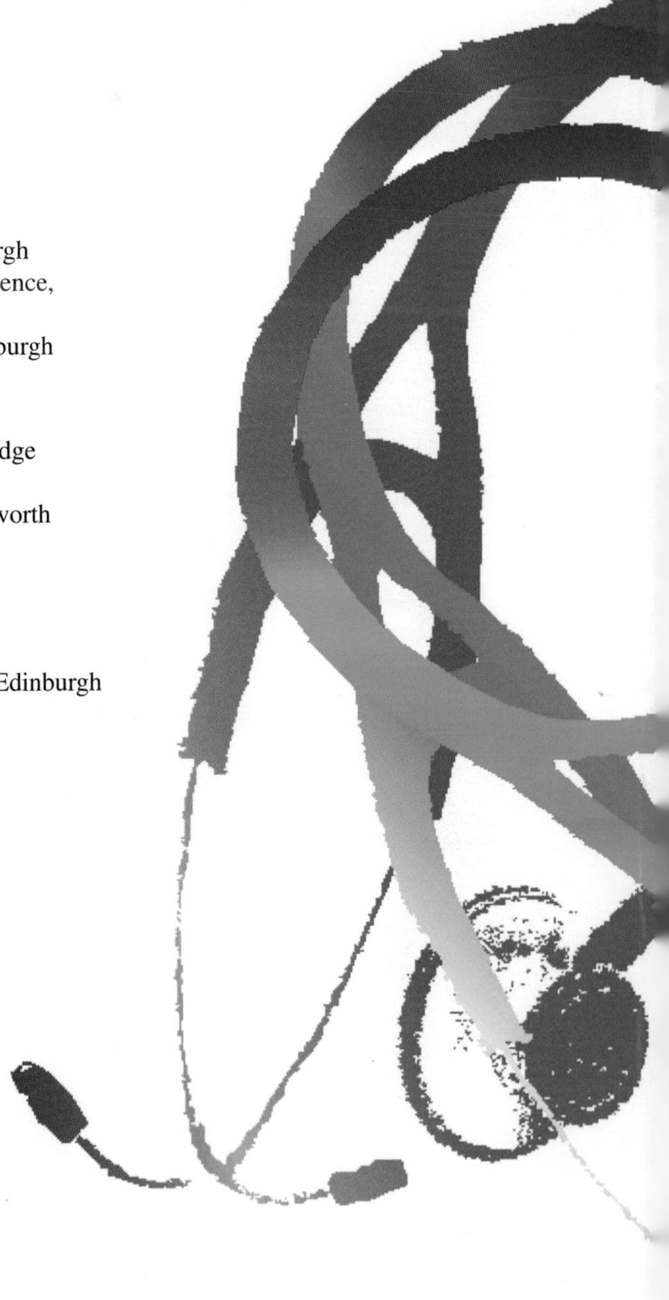

CHURCHILL LIVINGSTONE

EDINBURGH LONDON NEW YORK PHILADELPHIA
SYDNEY TORONTO 1999

EIGHTEENTH EDITION

DAVIDSON'S Principles and Practice of MEDICINE

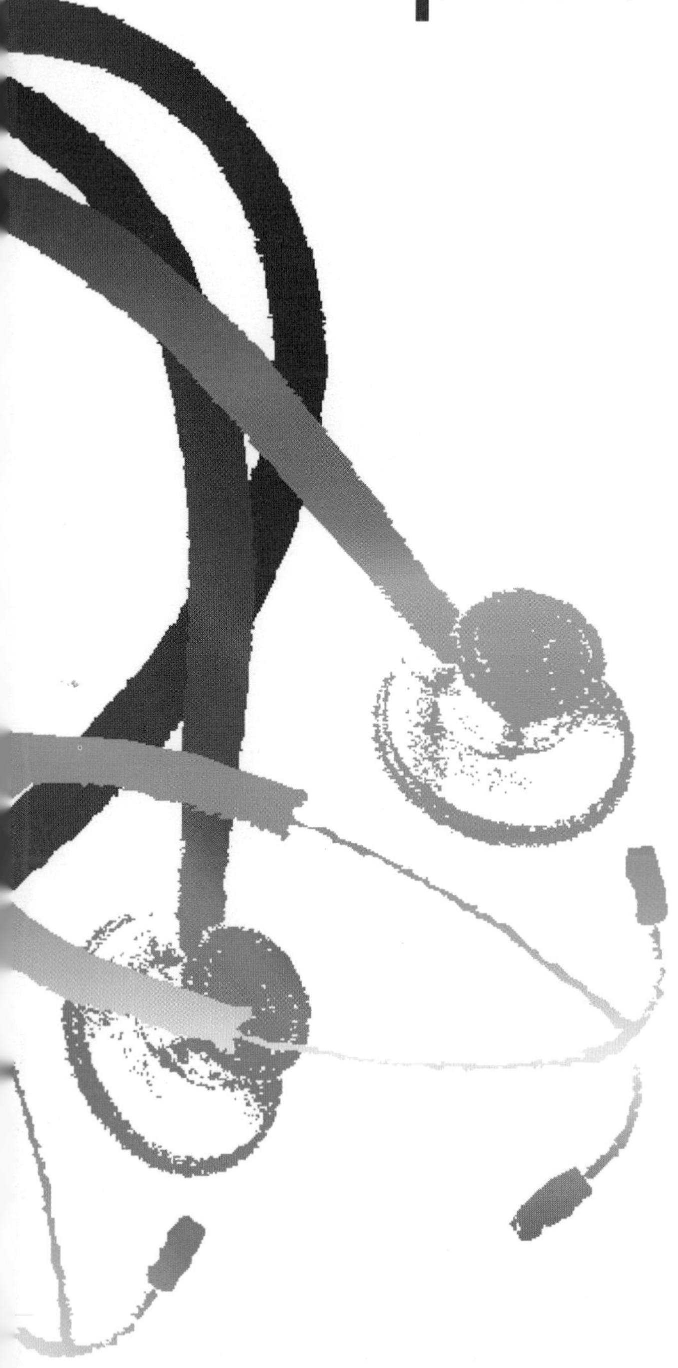

CHURCHILL LIVINGSTONE
An imprint of Harcourt Brace and Company Limited

First edition 1952
Second edition 1954
Third edition 1956
Fourth edition 1958
Fifth edition 1960
Sixth edition 1962
Seventh edition 1964
Eighth edition 1966
Ninth edition 1968
Tenth edition 1971
Eleventh edition 1974
Twelfth edition 1977
Thirteenth edition 1981
Fourteenth edition 1984
Fifteenth edition 1987
Sixteenth edition 1991
Seventeenth edition 1995
Eighteenth edition 1999

ISBN 0443 059446

International edition ISBN 0443 060002

British Library Cataloguing in Publication Data
A catalogue record for this book is available from the British Library

Library of Congress Cataloging in Publication Data
A catalog record for this book is available from the Library of Congress

Note
Medical knowledge is constantly changing. As new information becomes available, changes in treatment, procedures, equipment and the use of drugs become necessary. The editors, contributors and the publishers have, as far as it is possible, taken care to ensure that the information given in this text is accurate and up to date. However, readers are strongly advised to confirm that the information, especially with regard to drug usage, complies with the latest legislation and standards of practice.

Printed in the UK

For Churchill Livingstone

Commissioning Editor: Laurence Hunter
Project Manager: Wendy Lee
Project Controller: Nancy Arnott
Designer: Erik Bigland

Preface

Medicine is the most dynamic of biological disciplines; while the basic principles remain unaltered, current practice is undergoing exponential change. With this new edition of *Davidson's Principles and Practice of Medicine*, the central aim of the editors and contributors has been to reflect this transformation, whilst at the same time continuing our tradition of providing a concise yet up-to-date and comprehensive text on clinical medicine which meets the requirements of medical students preparing for their final examinations. Many doctors preparing for postgraduate qualifications such as the MRCP use 'Davidson' as a core text, together with *Macleod's Clinical Examination*, which focuses on clinical methods. Response from our readers reveals that a large number of general practitioners, nurses, pharmacists and other health-care professionals also value 'Davidson' as an easy-to-use reference source.

This truly international textbook has a large following of medical students and doctors all around the globe; their numerous comments have helped shape the development of this latest edition. Increased travel to the tropics only serves to reinforce our desire to continue to provide full and accurate coverage of infectious and tropical diseases.

The previous edition, which featured the introduction of colour, represented a new milestone in the long history of this textbook. This and other changes have been very well received and we thank the retiring editors, Professors Christopher Edwards and Ian Bouchier, for their work. Nevertheless, the content and presentation of this, the eighteenth, edition have been completely reworked and new chapters introduced without adding to the overall length (and weight!) of the book. This has been achieved by optimising the mix of text, information boxes, tables and illustrations. Popular innovations from the last edition have been reinforced. For example, the recognition that patients do not present with a 'disease' but with certain symptoms, or a constellation of symptoms, has led us to develop the 'major manifestations' sections in most chapters; indeed the neurology chapter is now almost entirely based on this approach.

Most of the chapters have new or additional contributors, all of whom are leading figures in the teaching of medicine in their specialties. One of the purposes of this edition is to link recent scientific advances to disease pathogenesis and therapeutic innovations; many of our contributors pursue basic research in the diseases they describe and are able to give an exciting appreciation — 'from the gene to the bedside'. The boundaries between such topics as genetics, immunology and inflammation have become blurred, if not entirely removed, by the recent explosion of knowledge in molecular and cell biology. As a consequence, the eighteenth edition begins with a new chapter devoted to the molecular and cellular basis of disease which gives an up-to-date account of the basic machinery of life, taking the reader from DNA and intracellular processes through the biology of orchestrated cellular responses in inflammation and immunology to human genetics. Other major changes include a new chapter on the management of patients in the intensive care unit; the dermatology chapter has been extended and enhanced to provide coverage which is sufficient to meet the requirements of final examinations; the gastrointestinal chapter has been completely rewritten and contains more than 50 new illustrations; and the chapters on diabetes, nutrition and metabolic diseases, psychiatry, and oncology and palliative care have been focused to concentrate on important principles as they relate to medical practice.

'Davidson' has one of the longest pedigrees of any textbook designed for medical students, and this edition represents a further transformation. We hope that these changes considerably improve its value without losing its much-loved qualities of 'approachability and readability'. The editors believe that the eighteenth edition, in terms of content and presentation, is indeed a medical text which meets the needs of tomorrow's doctors.

Edinburgh and Cambridge 1999

C.H.
E.R.C.
J.A.A.H.
N.A.B.

Sir Stanley Davidson (1894–1981)

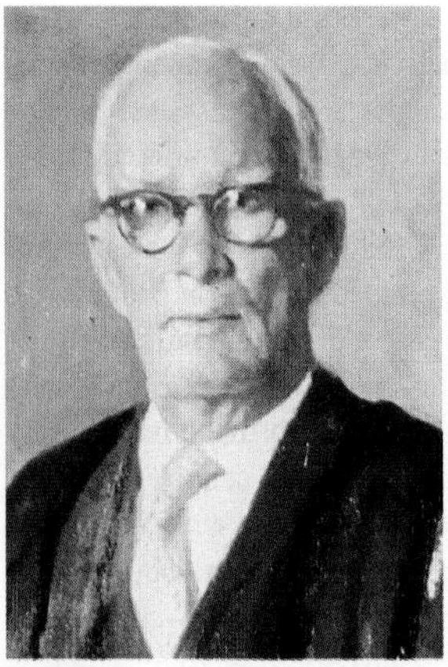

This famous textbook was inspired by one of the great Professors of Medicine of the present century. Stanley, as he was known by all, began his medical undergraduate training at Trinity College, Cambridge, but this was interrupted by World War I and later resumed in Edinburgh. He served in the Gordon Highlanders until he was seriously wounded in Belgium. That this period had a profound effect on his subsequent attitudes and values was clear from his emotional recollection, in later years, of the carnage and useless wastage of young life.

In the 1920s he favoured appointments in bacteriology, and this is reflected in his early interests. However, he soon decided to dedicate his life to clinical medicine and clinical research. Exciting contemporary discoveries led to an affection for haematology which he always retained and which was transmitted to many of his disciples.

In 1930 Stanley was appointed Professor of Medicine at the University of Aberdeen. This was one of the first full-time Chairs of Medicine anywhere, and the first in Scotland. The period in Aberdeen was marked by several developing qualities of academic leadership: toughness, fairness and integrity which quickly earned respect; finding and attracting young talent; recognition of the need for decent facilities and accommodation for teaching and research; and research emphasis on the needs of the community.

Appointment to the Chair of Medicine at his Alma Mater, Edinburgh, came in 1938 and he was to remain in this post until retirement in 1959. World War II was to inhibit and delay Stanley's aspirations for the Edinburgh Medical School, but those of us who were privileged to be undergraduate students at the time have much to remember. He was a splendid educator and a particularly gifted bedside teacher where everything had to be questioned and explained. He seemed to be totally at ease with everyone, and would stop and talk with students, nurses, domestic staff and frequently with a complete stranger. He had endless time to listen to and communicate with his patients, who quickly seemed at ease with him. His main thesis was that if you could take a good history and do a careful physical examination, the rest might not be too difficult or expensive. He gave most of the systematic lectures in Medicine himself, the substance of which was made available in typewritten notes; these were marked by an emphasis on essentials and far surpassed any textbook available at the time.

When the war ended Stanley's first priority was to develop the old municipal hospitals in the north of Edinburgh, to extend the teaching capacity of the Medical School and to recognise and establish units for the specialist branches of medicine that were beginning to emerge. These units were to be headed by the best physicians and teachers that could be found and were to retain commitment to general internal medicine. Within a few years Stanley's far-sightedness became reality.

But Stanley will be best remembered for this textbook, *The Principles and Practice of Medicine*. He conceived the idea in the late 1940s. It was to be of modest size and price and yet sufficiently comprehensive and up to date to provide the good student with the main elements of sound medical practice.

The origins of the book were Stanley's lecture notes. Each of the senior members of Stanley's now extended departmental family was given a chapter to write. In the early days there was occasional annoyance when a carefully drafted manuscript was massacred by Stanley's editorial pencil; but no offence was taken because none was intended. The book was to be readable without ambiguity, uncertainty or wordiness. The result, a masterpiece of clarity and uniformity of style, is the basis from which this eighteenth edition has evolved. Although the format and presentation have seen many changes, Stanley's original vision and objectives remain.

It is an honour to salute the memory of a great physician and teacher and, for a fortunate few, a great mentor and friend.

Edinburgh 1999 Professor John Richmond

Portrait reproduced by courtesy of the Royal College of Physicians of Edinburgh

Acknowledgements

Since the last edition of *Davidson's Principles and Practice of Medicine* Professor John Hunter and Dr Nick Boon have joined the Editorial Board and a total of 24 new authors have written or contributed new chapter material. While these changes have increased the breadth and depth of expertise necessary in any major revision, we are indebted for the invaluable past contributions from Dr Joyce D. Baird, Professor David J.H. Brock, Dr Anthony D.M. Bryceson, Dr Roger E. Cull, Professor Anne Ferguson, Professor Alasdair M. Geddes, Dr Alexander A.H. Lawson, Professor William J. MacLennan, Professor David J.C. Shearman, Dr Colin A. Soutar, Dr Roger N. Thin, Professor Robert G. Will and, in particular, Professor Ian A.D. Bouchier and Professor Christopher R.W. Edwards as previous senior editors.

We are also grateful for the critical reviews provided by a large number of consultant and specialist registrar colleagues and Drs A. Boyd, K. Brunt, K. Elliot, A. Marsland, A. Ryding and S. Forbes. Dr Jean-Michel Sallenave, Dr David A. Lomas, Dr David Gilligan and Dr Chris Summerton also provided advice at the page-proof stage. We would like to extend special thanks to Dr Simon Walker, Department of Clinical Biochemistry, University of Edinburgh, for his careful revision of the Appendices.

Once again we have had to beg, borrow and steal many of the new illustrations from our colleagues and we are grateful for their forbearance and support. These individuals are acknowledged on pages 1141–1142.

Finally, we are especially grateful to all those working for Churchill Livingstone, in particular Laurence Hunter, Wendy Lee and Robert Britton, for their expertise in the shaping, collation and illustration of this edition.

Edinburgh and Cambridge 1999

C.H.
E.R.C.
J.A.A.H.
N.A.B.

Contributors

C.M.C. Allen MA MD FRCP
Consultant Neurologist, Addenbrooke's Hospital, Cambridge; Clinical Dean, University of Cambridge School of Clinical Medicine

J.K. Aronson MA DPhil FRCP
Clinical Reader in Clinical Pharmacology and Honorary Consultant Physician, University of Oxford

Peter Bloomfield MD FRCP FACC
Consultant Cardiologist, Royal Infirmary of Edinburgh

Nicholas A. Boon MA MD FRCPE FESC
Consultant Cardiologist, Royal Infirmary of Edinburgh; Honorary Senior Lecturer, Department of Medicine, University of Edinburgh

Edwin R. Chilvers BMedSci BMBS PhD FRCPE
Professor of Respiratory Medicine, University of Cambridge School of Clinical Medicine; Honorary Consultant Physician, Addenbrooke's and Papworth Hospitals, Cambridge

Peter L. Chiodini BSc PhD FRCP FRCPath
Consultant Parasitologist, Hospital for Tropical Diseases, London; Honorary Senior Lecturer, London School of Hygiene and Tropical Medicine

Nicki R. Colledge BSc (Hons) MB ChB FRCPE
Consultant Geriatrician, Liberton Hospital, Edinburgh and Royal Infirmary of Edinburgh; Honorary Senior Lecturer, Department of Medicine, University of Edinburgh

Graham K. Crompton MB ChB FRCPE
Consultant Physician, Respiratory Unit, Western General Hospital; Part-time Senior Lecturer, Department of Medicine, University of Edinburgh

Allan D. Cumming MB ChB MD FRCPE
Senior Lecturer, Department of Medicine, University of Edinburgh; Honorary Consultant Physician, Department of Renal Medicine, Royal Infirmary of Edinburgh

Alex M. Davison MD FRCPE FRCP
Professor of Renal Medicine, University of Leeds; Consultant Renal Physician, St James's University Hospital, Leeds

Christopher R.W. Edwards MD FRCP FRCPE FRSE
Principal, Imperial College School of Medicine, London; Professor of Medicine, University of London

Niall D.C. Finlayson *OBE* PhD FRCP FRCPE
Consultant Physician, Royal Infirmary of Edinburgh; Honorary Senior Lecturer in Medicine, University of Edinburgh

Keith A.A. Fox BSc (Hons) MB ChB FRCP FESC
Duke of Edinburgh Professor of Cardiology and Honorary Consultant Cardiologist, University of Edinburgh and Royal Infirmary of Edinburgh

Brian M. Frier BSc (Hons) MD FRCPE FRCPG
Consultant Physician, Department of Diabetes, Royal Infirmary of Edinburgh; Part-time Reader in Medicine, University of Edinburgh

George E. Griffin BSc PhD FRCP FRCPE FRCPath
Professor of Infectious Diseases and Medicine, St George's Hospital Medical School (University of London), London; Honorary Consultant Physician, St George's Hospital, London

Christopher Haslett BSc (Hons) FRCPE FRCP
Professor of Respiratory Medicine, University of Edinburgh; Chairman of the Division of Clinical and Community Science, University of Edinburgh; Honorary Consultant Physician, Royal Infirmary of Edinburgh

Peter C. Hayes BMedSci MBChB MD PhD FRCPE
Professor of Hepatology, Department of Medicine, Royal Infirmary of Edinburgh

Andrew Haynes MA (Cantab) MRCP MRCPath DM
Leukaemia Research Fund Senior Lecturer in Haematological Oncology, City Hospital, Nottingham

John A.A. Hunter *OBE* BA MD FRCPE
Professor of Dermatology, University of Edinburgh; Honorary Consultant Dermatologist, Royal Infirmary of Edinburgh

Roland Jung MA MD FRCPE FRCP
Consultant Physician and Honorary Professor of Medicine;

Director of Research and Development, Ninewells Hospital and Medical School, Dundee

Jonathan R. Lamb BDS MA PhD FRCPath
Glaxo–Wellcome/British Lung Foundation Professor of Respiratory Science, Respiratory Medical Unit, University of Edinburgh

G.G. Lloyd MA MD MPhil FRCPE FRCP FRCPsych
Consultant Psychiatrist, Royal Free Hospital, London

Anne de Looy PhD PGDipDiet SRD
Professor of Dietetics and Head of Department, Department of Dietetics and Nutrition, Queen Margaret College, Edinburgh

Christopher A. Ludlam PhD FRCP FRCPath
Director, Haemophilia and Thrombosis Centre, Royal Infirmary of Edinburgh; Part-time Reader, Department of Medicine, University of Edinburgh

C.J. Lueck PhD FRCPE
Consultant Neurologist, Department of Clinical Neuroscience, Western General Hospital, Edinburgh

Raashid Luqmani DM FRCPE
Consultant Rheumatologist and Part-time Senior Lecturer in Rheumatology, Western General Hospital, Edinburgh

Michael J. Mackie BMedBiol MD FRCPath FRCPE
Consultant Haematologist, Western General Hospital, Edinburgh; Part-time Senior Lecturer, University of Edinburgh

David M. Mitchell MA MD MBA FRCP
Consultant Physician and Honorary Senior Lecturer in Medicine, St Mary's Hospital, Paddington and Imperial College School of Medicine, London

George Nuki FRCP FRCPE
Arthritis Research Campaign Professor of Rheumatology, University of Edinburgh; Honorary Consultant Rheumatologist, Western General Hospital and Royal Infirmary of Edinburgh

Kelvin R. Palmer MD FRCPE
Consultant Gastroenterologist, Western General Hospital, Edinburgh

I.D. Penman BSc MD MRCP
Consultant Gastroenterologist, Western General Hospital, Edinburgh; Part-time Senior Lecturer, Department of Medicine, University of Edinburgh

Alex T. Proudfoot BSc (Hons) FRCPE FRCP
Former Consultant Physician, Royal Infirmary of Edinburgh; Director, Scottish Poisons Information Bureau, Edinburgh

Stuart H. Ralston MB ChB MD FRCPG FRCPE
Professor of Medicine, Department of Medicine and Therapeutics, University of Aberdeen; Honorary Consultant Physician, Aberdeen Royal Hospitals, Aberdeen

Olivia M.V. Schofield MB MRCP
Consultant Dermatologist, Royal Infirmary of Edinburgh

James Shepherd MB PhD FRCPath FRCP FRSE
Clinical Director, Laboratory Medicine, GRI University NHS Trust, Glasgow

Claire L. Shovlin PhD MA MRCP
Wellcome Advanced Fellow, University of Edinburgh; Honorary Consultant Physician, Royal Infirmary of Edinburgh

Kenneth J. Simpson MD PhD MRCP
Consultant Physician, Scottish Liver Transplant Unit, Royal Infirmary of Edinburgh; Part-time Senior Lecturer, University of Edinburgh

J.G.P. Sissons MD FRCP FRCPath
Professor of Medicine, Department of Medicine, School of Clinical Medicine, University of Cambridge

J.F. Smyth MA MD(Cantab) MSc FRCPE FRCP FRCSE FRCR FRSE
Imperial Cancer Research Fund Professor of Medical Oncology, University of Edinburgh; Honorary Consultant Physician, Western General Hospital, Edinburgh

Charles P. Swainson MB FRCPE
Consultant Renal Physician, Royal Infirmary of Edinburgh; Senior Lecturer, University of Edinburgh

A.D. Toft *CBE* BSc MD FRCP FRCPE FRCPG FRCPI FRCSE
Consultant Physician, Royal Infirmary of Edinburgh; Honorary Senior Lecturer, Department of Medicine, University of Edinburgh

D.F. Treacher MA FRCP
Consultant Physician and Director of Intensive Care, St Thomas's Hospital, London

A. Stewart Truswell MD DSc FRCP FRACP FFPHM
Professor of Human Nutrition, University of Sydney

A. Neil Turner PhD FRCP
Professor of Nephrology, Renal Medicine, University of Edinburgh, Royal Infirmary of Edinburgh

Brian R. Walker BSc MB ChB MD MRCP
British Heart Foundation Senior Research Fellow, University of Edinburgh; Honorary Consultant Physician, Western General Hospital, Edinburgh

Contents

The molecular and cellular basis of disease

1

C.L. SHOVLIN • J.R. LAMB • C. HASLETT

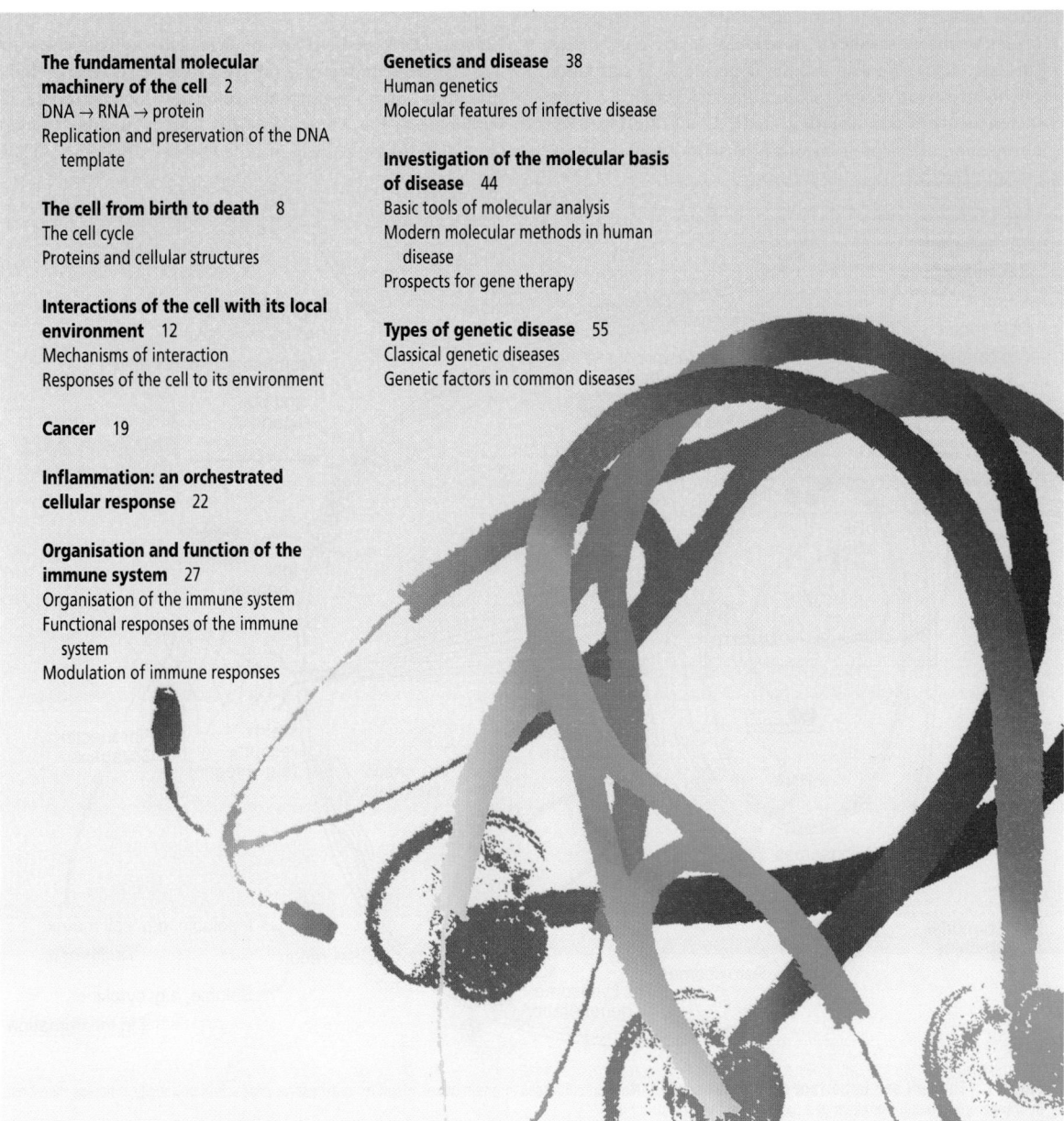

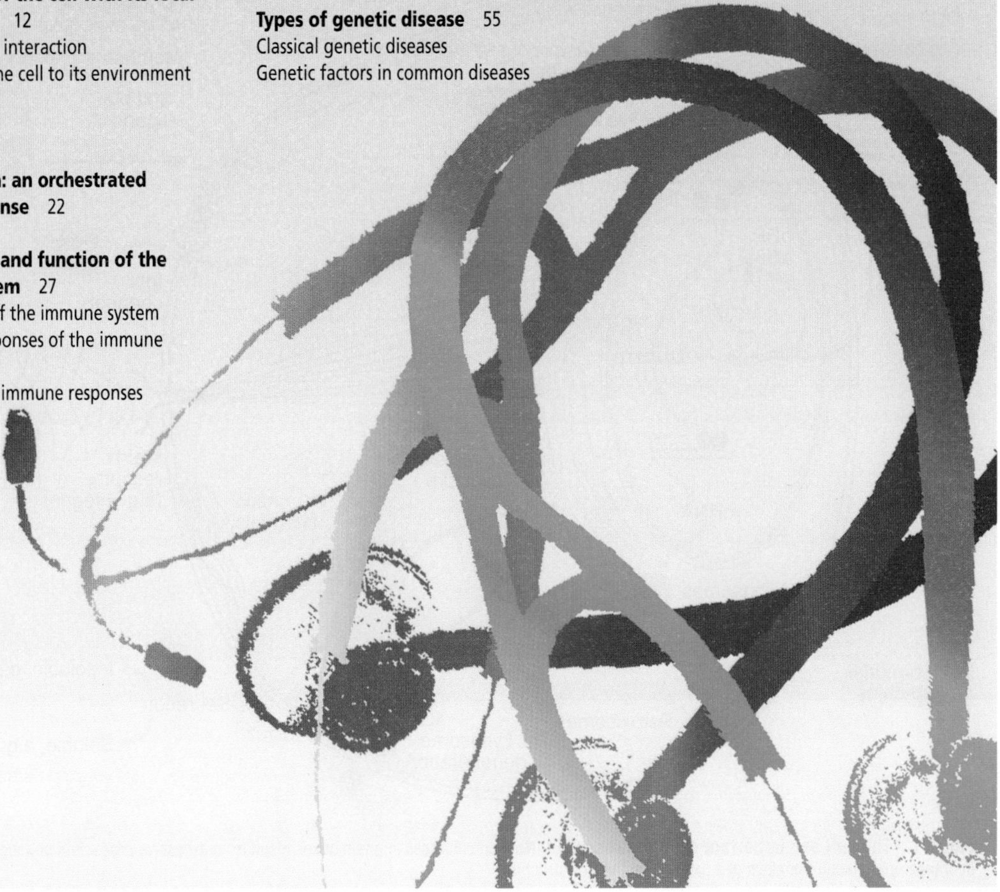

This chapter progresses through the essentials of molecular and cellular biology, from the sequence whereby DNA synthetic information is used to synthesise RNA then protein, to the means by which this generates the cell and extracellular structures, coordinates cellular interactions with each other, and regulates the more complex responses in a multicellular environment. In a sense, the chapter follows an evolutionary theme, as increasing levels of complexity are reached. Unfortunately, this necessitates starting with some of the most difficult material in the chapter. The reader may need to revisit the first section and should not be deterred from following the chapter through. We aim to review pre-clinical material with a particular emphasis on processes relevant to clinical medicine, providing selective examples of disease states. We also use the opportunity to introduce tools of investigative analysis in a manner which we hope will render them less daunting, and provide the basis for interpretation of scientific medical journals. Supplementary information useful for reference is given in Chapter 20. Figure 1.1 gives an overview of the sorts of processes which will be described in detail later in the chapter.

THE FUNDAMENTAL MOLECULAR MACHINERY OF THE CELL

DNA → RNA → PROTEIN

DNA

Cellular DNA (deoxyribose nucleic acid) contains all of the information required to synthesise cellular and extracellular structures, and to regulate the cell's development in the environment of the whole organism. This is possible because strict and orderly pairing of bases between two nucleic acid

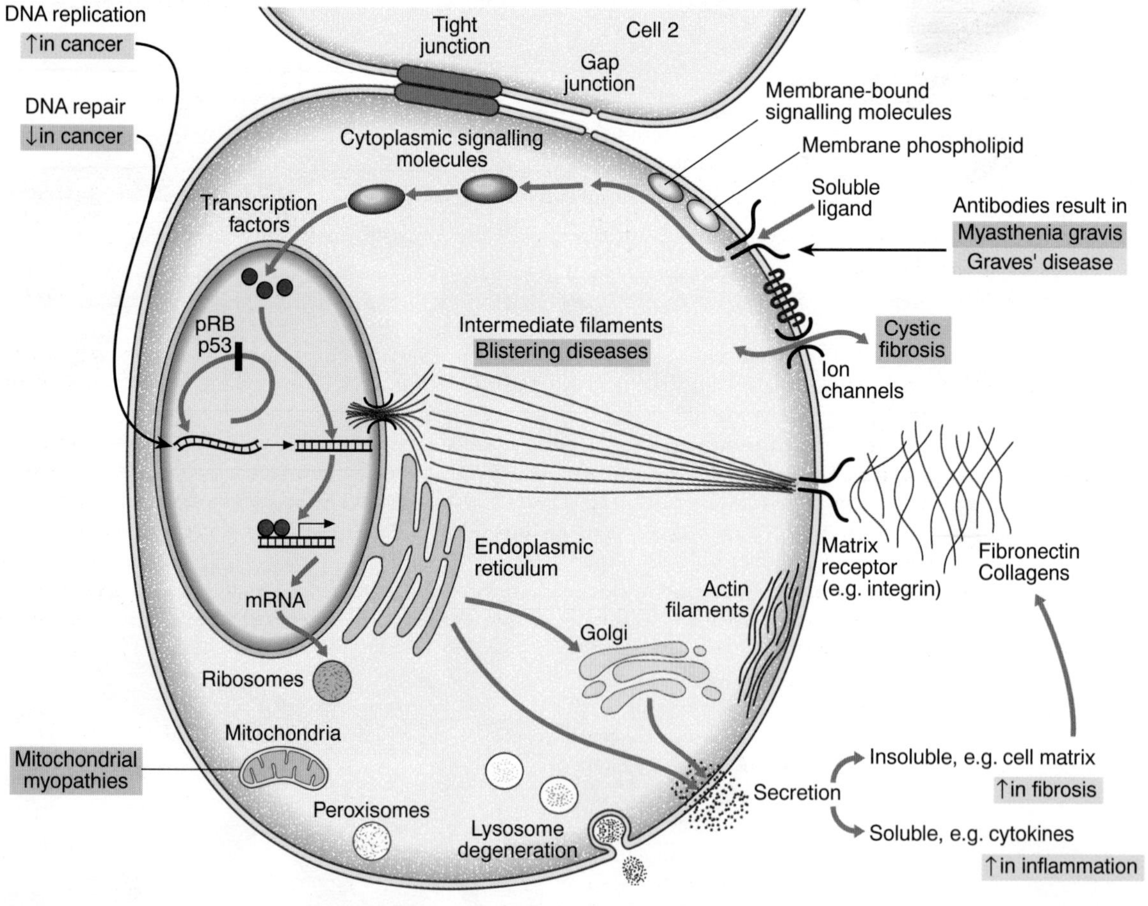

Fig. 1.1 The cell and important cellular processes. Note that diseases in green boxes result from excessive production or activity, whereas diseases in orange boxes result from loss of a particular activity or structure.

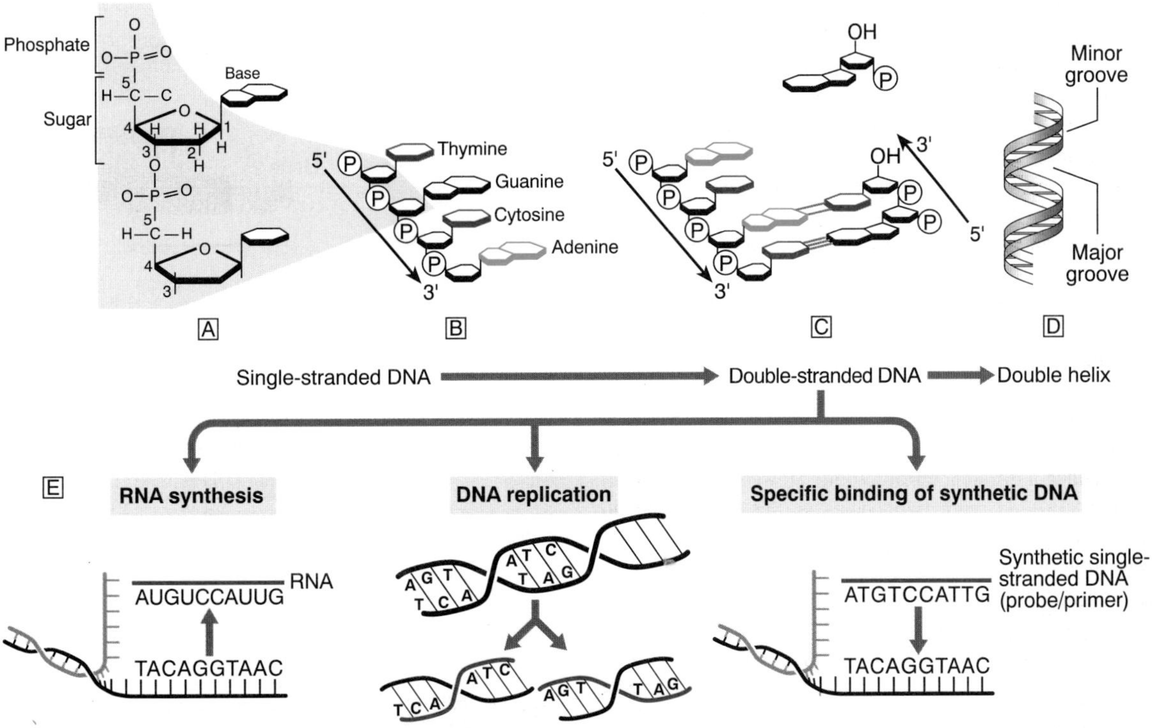

Fig. 1.2 DNA structure. A Biochemical structure of DNA indicating relationship of base, sugar and phosphate in two adjacent nucleotide units. B Cartoon illustrating single-stranded DNA with bases colour-coded. Note the base ring structures. C The formation of double-stranded DNA. Base ring structures and hydrogen bonding generate strict pairings between T–A and C–G. D Spiralling of the double-stranded DNA molecule creates the double helix. E Three consequences of base-pairing: RNA synthesis (see p. 4), DNA replication (see p. 6) and use of synthetic DNA in laboratory applications (see p. 46 and following section).

strands provides both coding potential and the capacity to be replicated faithfully from generation to generation.

As illustrated in Figure 1.2, a single strand of DNA is a linear polymer of *nucleotide* units, each consisting of a pentose sugar (deoxyribose) linked via its 5 prime (5') carbon to a phosphate group, and via its 1' carbon to one of four bases. Nucleotide units polymerise in a single strand by the formation of a sugar-phosphate-sugar-phosphate backbone, in which the orientation of the sugar carbons designates the direction of the strand 5' to 3'. The accompanying four bases can occur in any order, and comprise purines (guanine *(G)* and adenine *(A)*, which consist of two rings) and pyrimidines (cytosine *(C)* and thymine *(T)*, which consist of only one ring).

The critical feature of DNA is its ability to direct the sequential association of incoming nucleotide units which polymerise running in the opposite direction to the parent strand (see Fig. 1.2C). If these are deoxyribonucleotides, the second polymer will also be DNA and the two polymers will form a double-stranded structure through hydrogen bonding. Only two base-pairings are possible: G–C and A–T (see Table 1.1). This is because a stable structure requires three rings between the sugar-phosphate backbones, and optimal hydrogen bonding between bases on opposite strands. The double-stranded DNA unit of two nucleotides is referred to as a *base pair* (bp).

In turn, the most stable three-dimensional structure for the double-stranded DNA polymer to adopt is a helix, in which the sugar-phosphate backbones spiral around, with 10 base pairs per turn, the bases protected in the centre (see Fig. 1.2D). Since this is a spiralling duplex, two different grooves are generated in the structure—a narrow *minor groove* spanning the base-paired strands, and a wider *major groove* between consecutive spirals. Base pairs create specific

Table 1.1 Principles of Watson–Crick base-pairing

Base	Base type	Number of rings	Hydrogen bonds	Base pair
Guanine	Purine	2	3	G–C
Cytosine	Pyrimidine	1	3	
Adenine	Purine	2	2	A–T
Thymine	Pyrimidine	1	2	

patterns within the major groove, allowing their recognition by DNA binding proteins without breaking the helix. The helix is disrupted when DNA is required to act as a template, as in the natural and experimental situations illustrated in Figure 1.2E. DNA helicases catalyse the unwinding of DNA and separation of the hydrogen bonds between bases using energy derived from adenosine triphosphate (ATP) hydrolysis. Inherited defects in genes encoding helicases are responsible for a number of diseases characterised by premature age-related defects and malignancy, such as Werner's syndrome.

The genome

In humans, one copy of the entire double-stranded DNA content is referred to as the *haploid* genome and consists of approximately 3×10^9 base pairs in 23 separate molecules, each part of a different chromosome. However, virtually all cells are *diploid*, with two copies of this genome in 46 chromosomes: 22 pairs of autosomes (numbered 1 to 22, generally in order of size), and two sex chromosomes (X and X for women; X and Y for men). In addition to DNA, the chromosomes contain a chromatin scaffold which packages DNA with histones and other small chromosomal proteins. This is subjected to different orders of higher packing according to need. For example, DNA which is not required by the cell as a template at a given time is kept in a particularly inert state, tightly packaged within the chromatin scaffold of the chromosomes, as exemplified by the structure of inactive chromosomes segregating to daughter cells during cell division.

The genetic code, genes and loci

The genetic code by which DNA directs the synthesis of the protein constituents of the cell is a series of words running 5' to 3' along the linear coding strand of DNA. Each word is a three-nucleotide unit (triplet) which specifies a particular amino acid to be incorporated into the mature protein. There are 4^3 (64) different triplets: 61 specify one of the 20 amino acids. Three, TAA, TAG and TGA, are nonsense codons which do not specify an amino acid and instead terminate the growing polypeptide chain.

Only about 1% of human DNA is decoded into protein sequences; these discrete areas within the genome are referred to as *genes*. By contrast, a *locus* can be any area of the genome. Not all of the DNA within a gene codes for the eventual protein: sequences within the gene include coding regions (exons), non-coding regions (introns) and regulatory sequences (see Fig. 1.3). DNA is not decoded directly into protein, since during transcription, chromosomal DNA remains in the nucleus whereas protein synthesis requires metabolic apparatus associated with ribosomes in the cytoplasm. Instead, a mobile molecule (messenger RNA, *mRNA*) carries the DNA sequence from nucleus to cytoplasm.

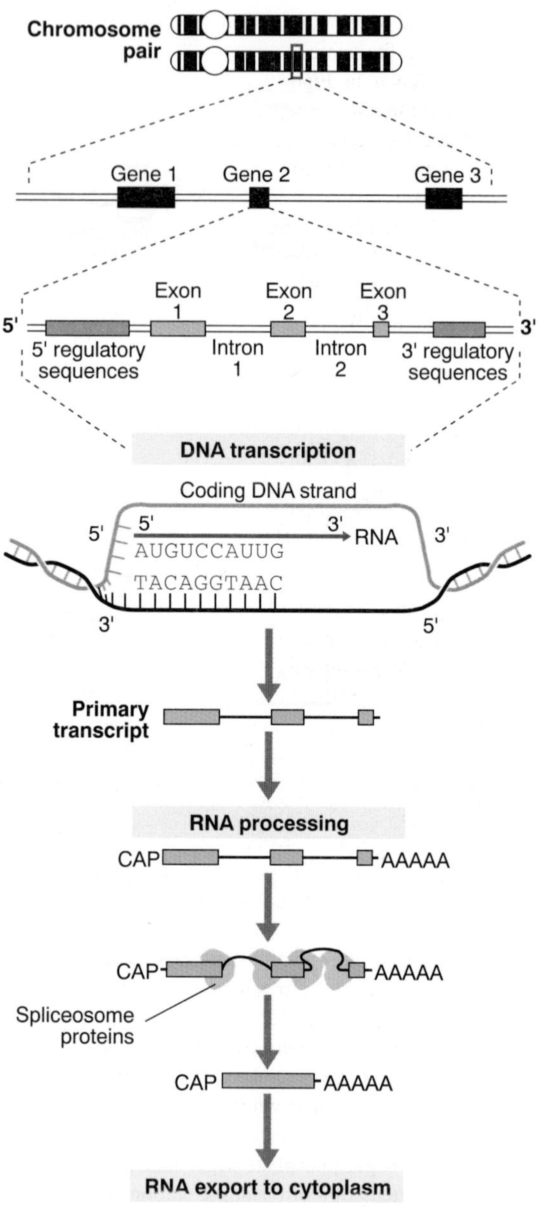

Fig. 1.3 RNA synthesis.

DNA → RNA

RNA synthesis and processing

To synthesise RNA in the process of DNA transcription, the enzyme RNA polymerase II and associated enzymes distort the chromatin structure to expose the underlying DNA, unwind a section of the double-stranded DNA helix, and disrupt the hydrogen bonds between the bases. As a result, a section of DNA can serve as a template for a new polymer, based on incoming ribonucleotide triphosphate units (in which the pentose sugars are ribose with a 2' -OH group), as shown in Figures 1.2E and 1.3. Note that in RNA the base uracil (U) replaces thymine (T) to base-pair with adenine (A), and since the transcribed RNA has the same sequence as the coding parental DNA strand, the template strand for RNA synthesis is actually the non-coding or complementary strand.

Immediately after synthesis of the primary mRNA transcript, nuclear proteins associate with the newly transcribed polymer which, as it is complementary to the parent DNA, includes introns. As illustrated in Figure 1.3, the primary RNA transcript is modified first by addition of a 5' CAP structure, and a 3' polyadenine (polyA) tail, which stabilise the ends of the short single-stranded molecule to protect it against intracellular breakdown. Secondly, highly accurate splicing machinery removes introns, joins adjacent exons, and creates an exon-only complement. The reagents involved include *s*mall *n*uclear *RNA*s complexed to *p*roteins such as snRNPs U1 and U2. These assemble in a spliceosome complex which coordinates the recognition of splice site consensus sequences demarcating the exon-intron boundaries, and catalyses the requisite biochemical reactions. Splicing usually occurs exclusively between adjacent donor and receptor sites to excise a single intron accurately, although many genes have alternative splicing patterns, which may be exhibited in different tissues, at specific developmental stages or in response to exogenous stimuli.

The processed mRNA is then exported to the cytoplasm for translation into protein. Additional modifications may occur in specific tissues, and include mRNA editing, by which the actual coding sequence of the mRNA changes. For example, in apolipoprotein B, a C to U editing change produces a new termination codon resulting in a truncated apoB48 rather than apoB100 protein (see p. 535). In other settings, prior to the translation process, precise signals can induce the premature decay of mRNA, including progressive shortening of the polyA tail, decapping and enzymatic cleavage.

Regulation and initiation of DNA transcription

Transcription of individual genes is regulated and finely tuned to the requirements of the cell and its environment. Before initiating the RNA synthetic process outlined above, RNA polymerase II identifies a gene to be transcribed by the recognition of upstream DNA regulatory sequences to which it binds (see Fig. 1.4). Additional transcription factors also bind to the promoter and enhancers to increase or decrease the rate of transcription of the gene at specific times. The means by which transcription factors interact with DNA is illustrated in Figure 1.4. Structural features distinguish different families of transcription factors such as helix-turn-helix, zinc finger, leucine zipper and helix-loop-helix motifs. Examples of transcription factors which will be discussed in later sections are the family which consists of homo- or heterodimers of c-Jun, c-Fos, bZIP and other proteins interacting at the common activating protein-1 (AP-1) DNA binding site.

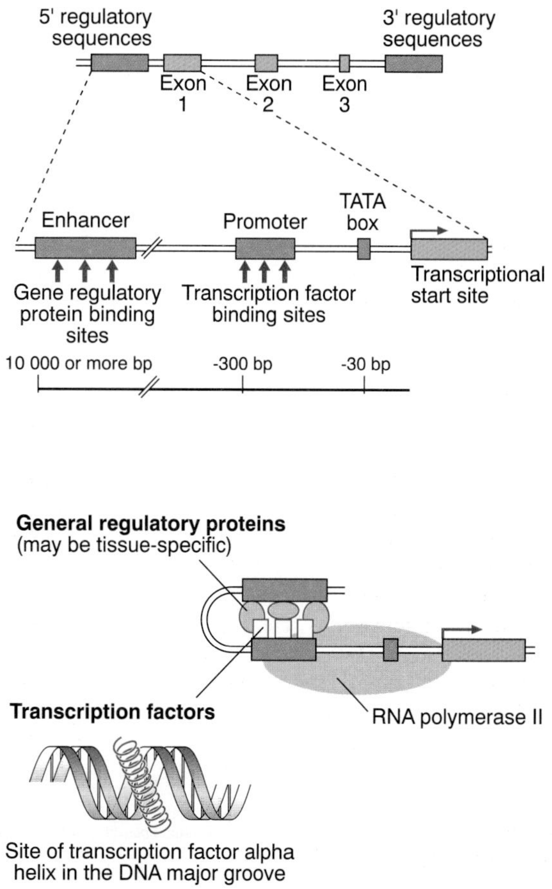

Fig. 1.4 Initiation and regulation of DNA transcription.

PROTEIN SYNTHESIS (RNA TRANSCRIPTION)

Proteins are synthesised from mRNA in cytoplasmic RNA-protein complexes known as ribosomes. These contain synthetic enzymes, and bind small single-stranded transfer RNAs. Each *tRNA* carries one of the 20 amino acids and the complementary sequence to the corresponding triplet codon, known as the anticodon. To commence protein synthesis (see Fig. 1.5), an mRNA molecule binds via its 5' CAP structure to the small 40S ribosomal subunit, which scans along the mRNA for the start codon AUG. The ribosome-bound initiator $tRNA^{Met}$ molecule carrying the AUG anticodon (UAC) base-pairs to the mRNA, when it activates the methionine which it carries. The activated methionine can then form a peptide bond with the amino

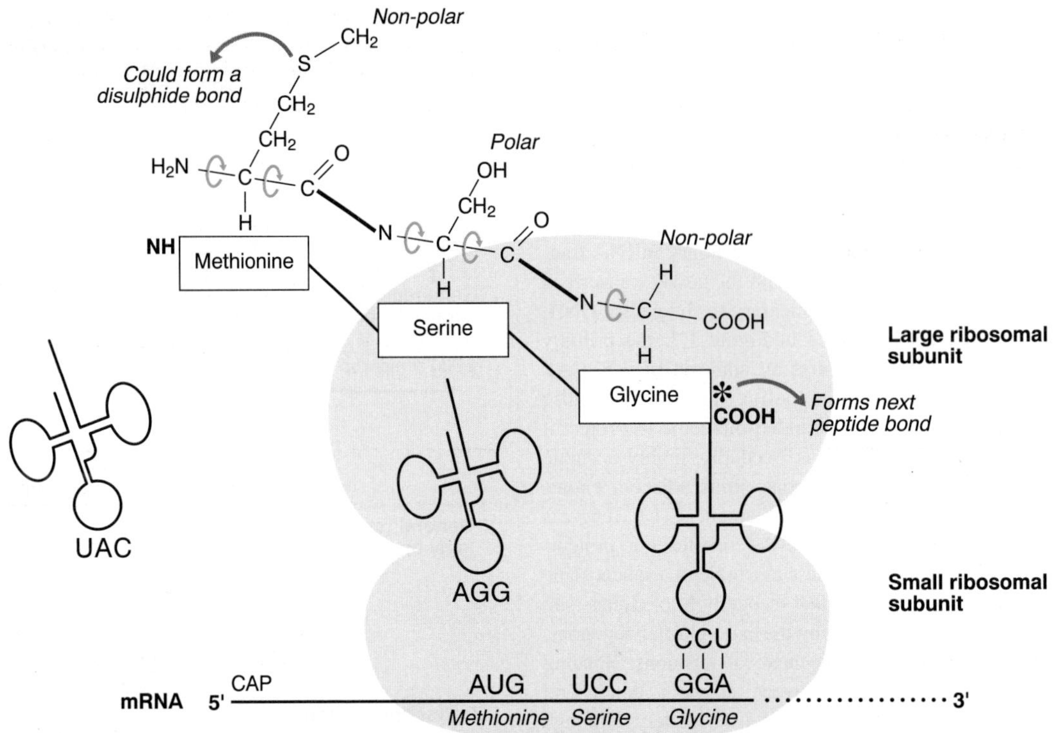

Fig. 1.5 Protein synthesis. Note that the 5′ to 3′ designation of mRNA corresponds to the amino-carboxyl orientation of the mature peptide. The secondary structure of the mature protein is determined by the degree of rotational freedom in the polymerising non-peptide bonds (indicated in green) and the nature of any side-chains such as their bulk, polarity or other features which may permit additional bonding—for example, between neighbouring sulphur atoms.

acid brought in by the next aminoacyl tRNA, before the ribosome releases the now-empty initiator tRNA. The polymerisation of the amino acids to form a peptide chain is catalysed by peptidyl transferase in the large 60S ribosomal subunit, and proceeds rapidly with about 1000 amino acids polymerised per minute. The stop codons UAA, UAG and UGA are not recognised by tRNAs, but by other proteins termed release factors, which lead to peptidyltransferase adding a water molecule rather than an amino acid to the activated peptide bond.

The mRNA, peptide chain and ribosomes then disassemble, leaving the ribosomes free to associate with another mRNA molecule. However, one of the signals which promotes mRNA decay is impaired translation—for example, failure to initiate translation, incorrect site of initiation, or arrest at a premature stop codon (a common pattern of human mutation—see Fig. 1.31, p. 39). If the mRNA does not decay, at any one time, it may be associated with multiple ribosomes transcribing different sections of the code. The limiting event in this setting is the rate of initiation of synthesis, which depends upon the supply of ribosome-bound initiator $tRNA^{Met}$ and adequate ribosomal initiation factors.

Nomenclature

Genes and the proteins which they encode are often designated by the same name. Common means of distinguishing the two include referring to the gene in italics (*c-abl*: c-abl) or adding a small ‘p’ to designate the protein (RB: pRB). In addition, many proteins are designated by their molecular weight in kDaltons (e.g. p53). Sometimes the name of the same protein described in a different organism is given as a superscript (e.g. $p34^{CDC2}$).

REPLICATION AND PRESERVATION OF THE DNA TEMPLATE

DNA REPLICATION AND RECOMBINATION

The principle of heredity is the ability of the sequence of DNA bases to be copied faithfully to new daughter DNA polymers to preserve the genetic code in the next generation. In a manner somewhat analogous to RNA transcription, the enzyme DNA polymerase separates the double strands, and initiates two daughter strands, each copied from one of the

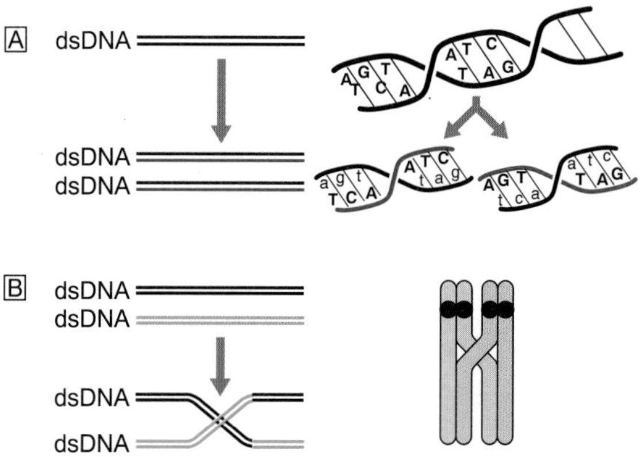

parental strands (see Fig. 1.6A). However, during meiosis, homologous DNA strands from different polymers exchange material at specialised crossover structures termed chiasmata (see Fig. 1.6B and p. 16). This process of DNA recombination also occurs in non-germ line cells during the rearrangement of immunoglobulin genes (see p. 30).

DNA REPAIR

DNA is not an inert molecule, since the sequence of a

Fig. 1.6 DNA processes relevant to inheritance. A Replication. B Recombination.

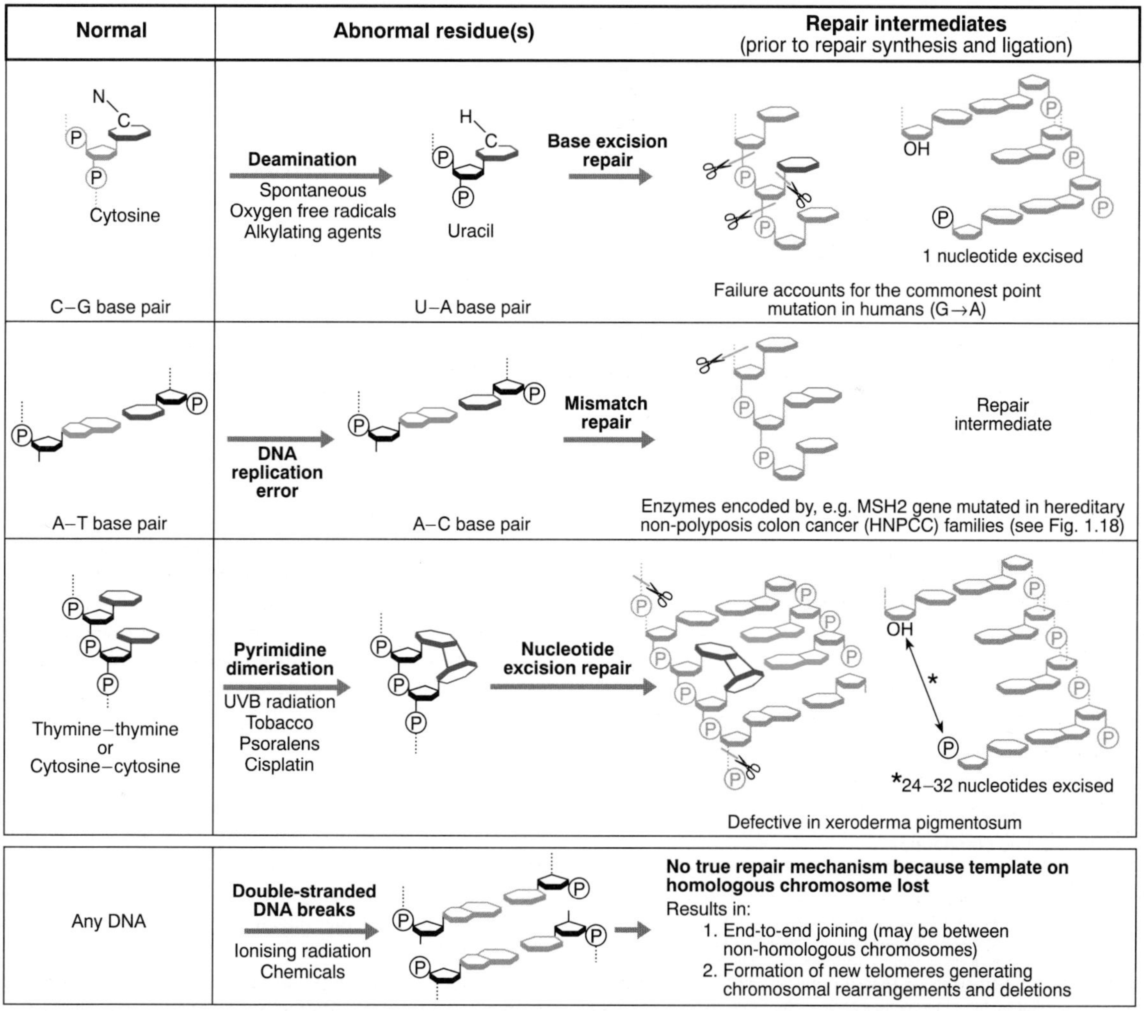

Fig. 1.7 DNA repair. Examples of DNA damage, important precipitants and repair mechanisms are illustrated. To facilitate DNA repair, single-stranded repair intermediates induce the transcription of a repertoire of genes including p53 to arrest the cell cycle and, in some instances, directly stimulate DNA repair enzymes to allow the repair processes to complete. However, there are no effective repair mechanisms for double-stranded DNA breaks; loss or rearrangement of chromosomal material is common.

single strand can alter after its synthesis—for example, as a result of spontaneous chemical changes, particularly if DNA is exposed to external radiation or chemical carcinogens (see Fig. 1.7). It is critical that such coding errors are not transmitted to the daughter strands when the DNA is replicated. The base-pairing of DNA provides an opportunity to recognise such events, since they will result in abnormal or mismatched base-pairings. If repair mechanisms fail, or if the mispaired daughter strands are immediately separated into single strands to be replicated themselves, such errors may persist, leading to a *mutation*. The mutation rate in genomic DNA (which is protected by the nucleus and chromatin) is as low as 10^{-9} to 10^{-12}. The most frequent single-base mutation in humans is a C to T substitution, resulting from failure to correct deaminated cytosine. If mutations occur in cells contributing to the germ line, this coding error will be transmitted to the next generation. More commonly, a new mutation will arise in a somatic cell, when transmission to the progeny of the particular cell only affects a proportion of cells in a given individual. Cells have complex detection and regulatory mechanisms to optimise DNA repair prior to DNA replication; these mechanisms will be described on page 16.

Although some initiators of DNA damage are naturally occurring, are unavoidable or carry a potential therapeutic benefit (e.g. cancer chemotherapy), others may be minimised. For example, the international efforts to reduce depletion of the ozone layer may reduce the consequences of terrestrial ultraviolet (UV) light exposure (see Fig. 1.8).

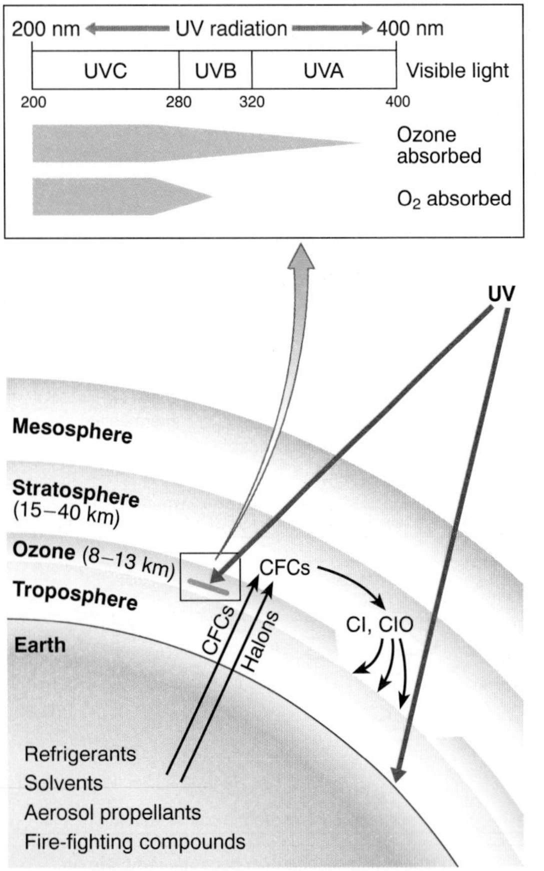

Fig. 1.8 UV and the ozone layer. Ozone (O_3) normally absorbs high-energy UV irradiation. Chlorinated fluorocarbons (CFCs) emitted from the Earth remain stable (atmospheric lifetimes may exceed 50 years) until reaching the stratosphere, where the stronger solar radiation leads to their breakdown to simple chlorine compounds. These react with O_3, resulting in the formation of O_2 and dissolution of the ozone layer. This permits increased terrestrial UVB which, as it may be absorbed by macromolecules, may lead to increased sunburn, photodermatoses and skin cancer. The 1989 Montreal protocol and its amendments aim to reduce the emission of long-lifespan halogenated fluorocarbons.

FURTHER INFORMATION ON THE FUNDAMENTAL MOLECULAR MACHINERY OF THE CELL

Alberts B, Bray D, Lewis J, Raff M, Roberts K, Watson J D 1994 Molecular biology of the cell, 3rd edn. Garland, New York
See recent reviews in Cell, Nature and other specialised journals

THE CELL FROM BIRTH TO DEATH

THE CELL CYCLE

CHROMOSOMES AND THE CELL CYCLE

The processes of DNA replication, cellular growth and cell division are strictly regulated to ensure that cells divide at periods appropriate to cellular size and DNA status (see Fig. 1.9). A resting cell replicates its DNA during a discrete synthetic period (S phase) once it has sufficient nutrients and cellular mass. A further cellular growth phase (G2) is required before the cell can divide into daughter cells, except in early embryonic divisions. As *mitosis* (M phase) commences, chromatin is remodelled to allow the chromosomes to condense; since they have replicated, they appear as a doublet structure of two daughter chromatids joined at the centromere. In the next stage, the nuclear envelope disassembles, and a new subcellular structure, the mitotic spindle, forms by the polymerisation of microtubules around γ-tubulin. Chromosomes attach to the spindle by their centromeres, and migrate to the centre of the spindle. A series of spindle motors then move the microtubules to opposite ends of the cell, carrying with them the centromeres which divide to ensure chromatid segregation. At the end of mitosis, the nuclear membrane reforms around the two daughter cells, the chromosomes decondense, and a further period of cellular growth (G1) ensues.

The process of *meiosis* which generates the gametes is fundamentally different from mitosis in two respects. To ensure that after fertilisation a diploid (2n) cell is created, a second round of chromatid segregation occurs to reduce the DNA content of each gamete to haploid (n). Secondly, at the outset of meiosis, genetic material is exchanged between the paired chromosomes which form crossover structures known as chiasmata (see Fig. 1.6, p. 7). Several chiasmata can be present per chromosomal pair. This process of *DNA recombination* is critical in generating the variation that enables species to adapt to their environment. Should such exchange of genetic material barely alter the DNA sequence on the resulting chromosomes—for example, in progeny derived from a single parental pair after generations of inbreeding—the species risks extinction if exposed to environmental stresses, and is more likely to suffer from autosomal recessive diseases (see p. 39 and Fig. 1.32).

SENESCENCE, TELOMERES AND TELOMERASE

Normal mammalian cells are only able to undergo a finite number of cell divisions. Partial explanations of this phenomenon include failure to repair exogenous damage and defective processing of key macromolecules such as DNA.

A further process appears to be of particular importance in limiting the general number of cell divisions, yet rendering

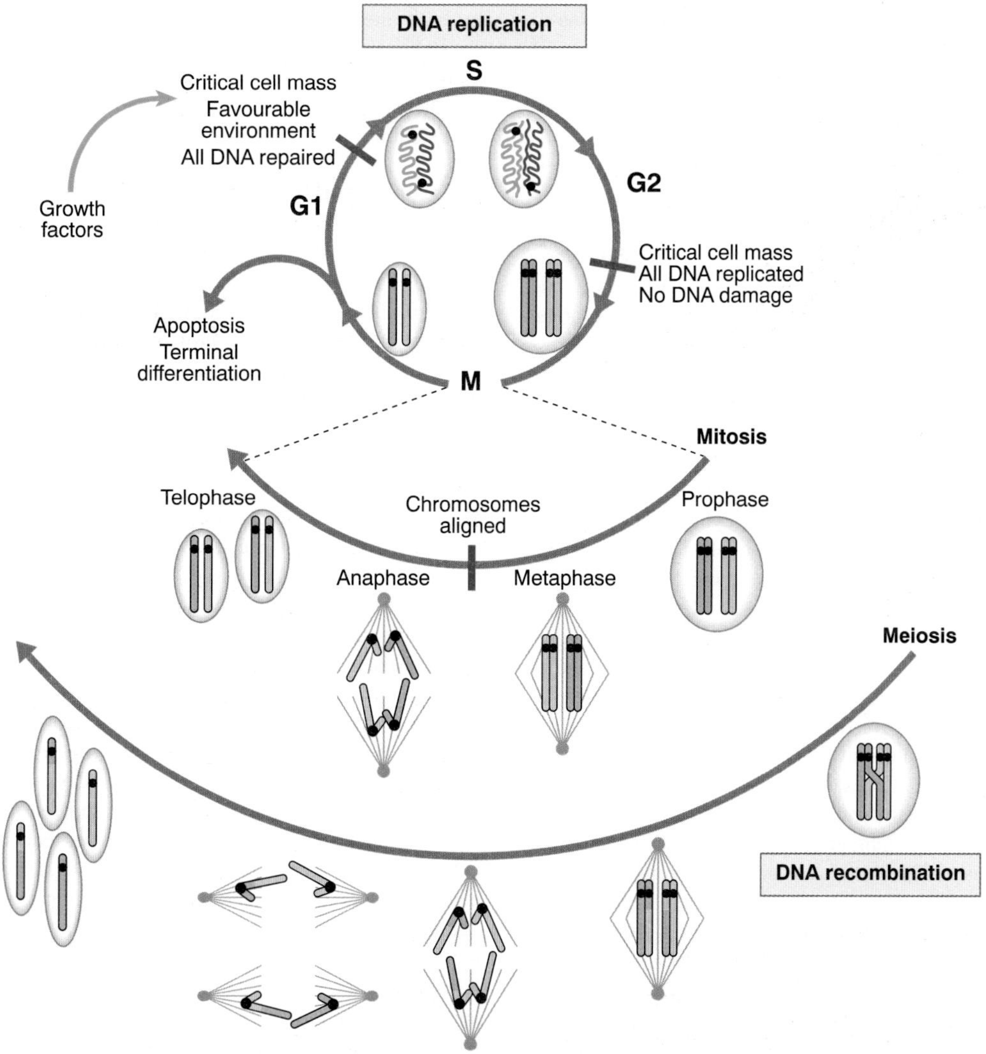

Fig. 1.9 The cell cycle. A single homologous chromosomal pair from chromosomes 1–22 or X is illustrated. The cell cycle can complete in as little as 16–20 hours. Red lines indicate major checkpoints (see p. 17).

specific cells capable of dividing an extended number of times, as required to generate a renewing stem cell, a germ-line cell and particularly cancerous cells. The ends of chromosomes, termed *telomeres*, are specialised structures that confer stability on the chromosome by coordinating and positioning chromosomes during mitosis, preventing aberrant chromosomal fusion events and enabling the cell to replicate chromosomal ends. Telomeres consist of a linear array of a G-rich sequence, but the number of these repeats is reduced at each cell division since DNA polymerases cannot fully replicate blunt-ended DNA. Progressive shortening of the telomere is thought to be responsible for cellular senescence, though a relationship to the lifespan of an individual is not clear. Cells can counteract the loss of telomeric repeat units during cell division by adding them using the enzyme *telomerase*, and cells which express telomerase are able to undergo more divisions before becoming senescent.

PROTEINS AND CELLULAR STRUCTURES

SUBCELLULAR COMPARTMENTS

As illustrated in Figures 1.1 (see p. 2) and 1.10, eukaryotic cells are divided into subcellular compartments. The presence of a nuclear membrane separating the genome from the cytoplasm is the key feature which distinguishes eukaryotic ('having a true nucleus') cells from bacteria and other prokaryotic ('pre-nuclear') cells, as discussed further on page 42. The nuclear membrane consists of two lipid bilayers, the inner of which is lined by a filamentous meshwork of the protein laminin. Both bilayers are traversed by nuclear pores which are cylindrical complexes of nucleoporin proteins that exhibit eight-fold symmetry, permit passive transport, and facilitate regulated passage of molecules in and out of the nucleus by interacting with a family of nuclear import and export receptors. Nuclear pores connect to short fibres extending into the cytoplasm and to longer fibres extending into the nucleus, to which molecules may 'dock' before traversing the pore. The nucleus itself is heterogeneous, with different components modulating distinct functions—for example, the nucleolus involved in generating the protein-synthesising ribosomes.

The nuclear membrane separates the nucleus from the cytoplasm. The latter contains numerous additional organelles, and filamentous biopolymers ranging in diameter from 7 nm actin filaments, through 10 nm intermediate filaments (e.g. keratin, vimentin, desmin), to 24 nm microtubules. These cytoskeletal proteins confer rigidity upon a cell, and provide tracks by which organelles can be transported around the cell. In addition, rapid and carefully regulated polymerisation and depolymerisation of filaments are responsible for processes such as cell shape changes, pseudopodia in phagocytosis, and cellular migration. Perhaps the best known of these are the specialised actin- and myosin-based microfilaments in muscle cells which are responsible for myocyte contraction (see Fig. 3.2, p. 194).

Endoplasmic reticulum (ER) and Golgi apparatus

The ER and Golgi play critical roles in the export of secreted proteins to the extracellular environment, essentially acting as a control station to permit only mature protein to reach the cell surface. The ER is an extensive membrane-bound organelle continuous with the outer nuclear membrane, forming networks through the cytoplasm. Rough ER has associated ribosomes; ribosome-free smooth ER is particularly evident in cholesterol-synthesising cells. The Golgi apparatus consists of flattened cisternae which receive proteins from the ER and sort them for their subsequent destination. In both the ER and Golgi apparatus, extensive post-translational modification, folding, oligomerisation and translocation of proteins occur. In addition, the ER has specific roles in lipid biosynthesis and maintenance of the ER calcium store.

Endosomes and lysosomes

Endosomes transport proteins between cellular compartments, and are particularly involved in the recycling of proteins internalised from the cell surface. In contrast, the acidic pH and enzymes within the similarly structured lysosomes provide a major source of protein degradation within the cell. Lysosomal storage diseases stem from inherited defects in lysosomal enzymes, resulting in the failure to degrade intracellular toxic substances.

Mitochondria

Mitochondria are intracellular organelles essential for aerobic metabolism since they generate ATP by oxidative phosphorylation via the passage of electrons down an ionic gradient across the inner mitochondrial membrane. Although some of its structural and enzymatic components are encoded by chromosomal genes, the mitochondrion possesses its own small genome in which the DNA displays important differences to chromosomal DNA. In keeping with an organelle which is believed to have arisen from the symbiotic association of a prokaryotic bacterium, the DNA is a double-stranded circular form of 16,569 bp (compared to 3×10^9 for the haploid genome), with 2–12 copies per mitochondrion. Other key differences to chromosomal DNA include inheritance from the maternal line (as zygotic cytoplasmic structures are derived predominantly from the oocyte), replication independent of the proliferation of the cell, and a high mutational rate due to a different DNA polymerase and lack of DNA protection by chromatin as in the nucleus. As a result, the mitochondrial DNA of somatic cells may change as the cells age, generating a heteroplasmic state with wild type and mutant DNA in the same cell. Mitochondria are most numerous in cells with high metabolic demands, as reflected in the high incidence of myopathies amongst mitochondrial disease states (see Table 20.7, p. 1131, and p. 998).

Peroxisomes

These cytoplasmic organelles contain numerous enzymes involved in the metabolism of fatty and bile acids, cholesterol, purines and amino acids. All enzymes are encoded by nuclear genes and need to be transported into peroxisomes. The inability to import proteins into peroxisomes due to perturbed peroxisome transport signals results in general peroxisomal diseases such as Zellweger's syndrome and rhizomelic dwarfism. Specific enzyme deficiencies also occur (see p. 532).

PROTEINS

Protein trafficking

Proteins are transported from their site of synthesis on ribosomes to their eventual destination (see Fig. 1.10) which may be in the cytoplasm, in subcellular compartments, membrane-bound or in the extracellular space.

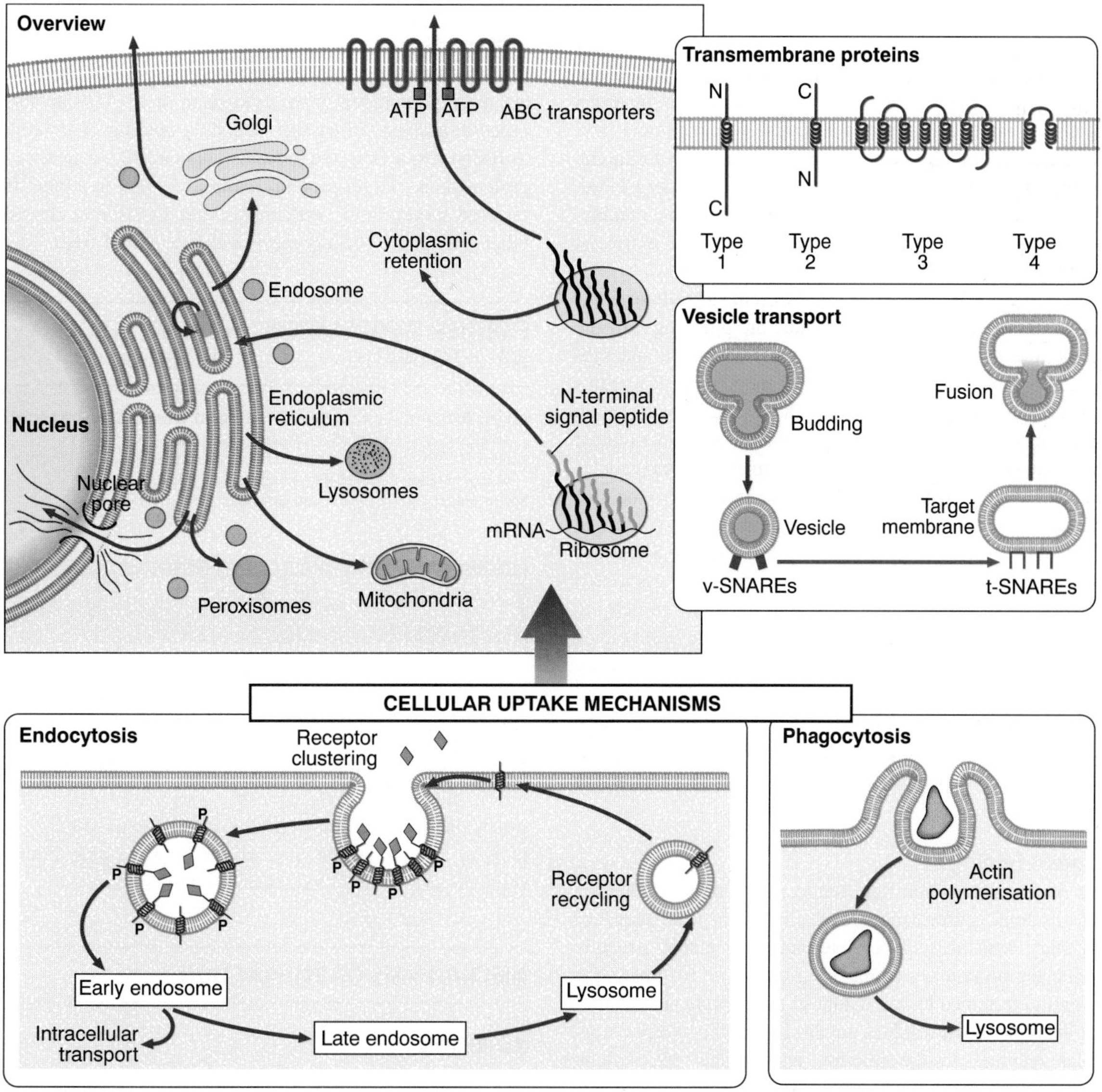

Fig. 1.10 Routes and mechanisms of protein transport between cellular and extracellular compartments.

Accurate protein sorting is critical not only to generate the structure of the cell and its environment, but also to enable the cell to carry out biochemical reactions efficiently. Most proteins, as they leave their site of synthesis on the large ribosomal subunit, are targeted to the rough endoplasmic reticulum by means of specific sequences at their N-terminus. In some cases, transport commences while the polypeptide chain is still being synthesised on the ribosome. Proteins are either integrated into the ER membrane or transported through, sorted by an assembly of integral proteins. Lack of a signal sequence may result in the protein being retained in the cytoplasm by default, although there are other mechanisms to secrete proteins without a signal. For example, up-regulation of cell surface ATPase binding cassettes (which couple the hydrolysis of ATP with the secretion of such proteins) is responsible for cancer cells acquiring resistance to multiple cytotoxic drugs (via the multidrug resistance (MDR) transporter) and *Plasmodium falciparum* becoming resistant to chloroquine (see pp. 1058 and 153). Reduced activity of another ATPase binding cassette, the cystic fibrosis transmembrane conductance regulator (CFTR) which regulates cellular extrusion of chloride, results in cystic fibrosis (see p. 337).

Exchange of proteins between different subcellular compartments (see Fig. 1.10) depends on pinching off the membrane of one compartment, vesicle formation and subsequent vesicle fusion with the target membrane. It remains a puzzle how the individual organelles manage to retain their individual compositions in the face of acquisition of vesicular contents from other compartments. Such vesicles may be 'coated' with proteins derived from the cytoplasm (clathrin for endocytosed vesicles; coatamers for internal vesicles). A series of proteins on the vesicle (v-SNAREs) and target membranes (t-SNAREs), together with associated soluble molecules, allow recognition of the vesicle to initiate fusion. In viral infections (of which the best studied are *Haemophilus influenzae* and human immunodeficiency virus—HIV), specific virus-encoded proteins undergo conformational changes to allow them to function in a fusion molecule complex and permit viral DNA entry through the lipid bilayer. Further details are provided on page 42 and in Chapter 2.

Protein folding

All of the information required to fold a protein correctly into its final conformation resides in the peptide sequence (primary structure) which determines the stable structure which the protein can adopt (see Fig. 1.5, p. 6). Folding is in part determined by the nature of the peptide side-chains; for example, polar residues are directed to the exterior, non-polar residues to the interior, and in the extracellular environment sulphur-containing side-chains form stable disulphide bonds. In addition, the flexible bonds flanking the peptide bonds direct two predictable patterns of folding of adjacent peptide chains: the α-helix, whereby a single peptide spirals around in a stable structure, critical in binding to DNA (e.g. transcription factors, see Fig. 1.4, p. 5) and forming the hydrophobic internal residues in membranes; and the β-pleated sheet between neighbouring peptides of opposite orientation. The combination of α-helices, β-pleated sheets and additional forms of protein secondary structure results in its final three-dimensional conformation, which currently cannot be predicted from sequence alone, but requires determination by X-ray diffraction studies. To increase the efficiency of such folding, the process is facilitated by additional proteins or chaperones, such as members of the heat shock protein family.

Protein degradation

Proteins with short half-lives, or incorrectly folded proteins, are usually degraded in the cytoplasm in an ATP-mediated process, accelerated by the reversible binding of ubiquitin to lysine residues in the protein. This targets the protein to proteosomes, large protein complexes that degrade the targeted moiety into smaller peptides. Lysosomes degrade other proteins, especially those with longer half-lives.

FURTHER INFORMATION ON THE CELL FROM BIRTH TO DEATH

Alberts B, Bray D, Lewis J, Raff M, Roberts K, Watson J D 1994 Molecular biology of the cell, 3rd edn. Garland, New York

Alberts B 1998 The cell as a collection of protein machines: preparing the next generation of molecular biologists. Cell 92: 291–294

See recent reviews in Cell, Nature and other specialised journals

INTERACTIONS OF THE CELL WITH ITS LOCAL ENVIRONMENT

Cells do not exist in isolation. All cells are supported and regulated by mesenchymal-derived connective tissue, an important element of which is the cell-secreted extracellular matrix consisting of polymeric proteins including collagens, elastic fibres and proteoglycans. Specialised cell surface molecules mediate cell–cell and cellular–extracellular contacts to allow constant interactions between neighbouring cells, the extracellular matrix and soluble molecules.

MECHANISMS OF INTERACTION

ADHESION

The intercellular space is bridged by a series of transmembrane proteins connecting to cytoplasmic filamentous networks. These cell–cell junctional complexes have different properties according to the nature and requirements of the cell. For example, tight junctions closely oppose neighbouring cells, providing a barrier of high electrical resistance, whereas gap junctions, formed by the connexin family of proteins, function not as barriers but as intercellular passages for ions and small molecules.

Cell-matrix binding uses adhesion molecules as anchors between the cell surface and matrix molecules. The predominant extracellular matrix receptors on cells are integrins, which are transmembrane glycoproteins requiring cations for ligand binding (see p. 890). Precise adhesion molecules are often specific to the matrix component.

Numerous molecules are involved in particular processes, each mediating specific functions. As an example, adhesion molecules involved in the interactions between leucocytes and the endothelium are illustrated in Table 1.3, page 26 and Figures 1.22 and 1.29, pages 25 and 32.

EXTRACELLULAR SECRETION AND TRANSMEMBRANE PROTEINS

Proteins are generally secreted from the cell by exocytosis, a process whereby vesicles containing material destined for the cell exterior detach from the Golgi apparatus and are guided by microtubules to the plasma membrane, from which they may be discharged, often requiring an additional specific stimulus. Transmembrane proteins are retained within membranes due to the presence of stretches of approximately 25 hydrophobic amino acid residues which anchor the protein in the non-polar interior, initially of the endoplasmic reticulum membrane, and subsequently the plasma membrane. The major groups of transmembrane proteins are illustrated in Figure 1.10, page 11. Once in the plasma membrane, proteins diffuse laterally and may cluster, either spontaneously or in response to specific stimuli.

OUTSIDE-IN COMMUNICATION

A cell needs to be able to internalise substances from its exterior—for example, for nutrient uptake, recycling or protein degradation. In addition, the cell needs to recognise changes in its environment and initiate suitable responses, which may be immediate (such as the reorganisation of existing protein structures leading to processes such as contraction or depolarisation), or which may depend on the synthesis of new proteins, initiated by transcription of a specific repertoire of genes.

Internalisation processes

Direct cellular entry

The fastest way for small extracellular molecules to enter the cell is by passive diffusion along osmotic gradients, directly through the lipid bilayer if lipid-soluble, through an aqueous channel if highly charged or, in the case of water itself, through aquaporin channel-forming proteins (see Fig. 1.11A, p. 14). Alternatively, carrier proteins may be required to facilitate passive transport by conformational change, randomly opening first to the exterior and then to the interior of the cell, allowing different ions to diffuse along their concentration gradients. In a limited number of cases, transport against concentration gradients is possible by the synchronous transport of another molecule down its concentration gradient (see Fig. 1.11B, p. 14).

Endocytosis and associated mechanisms are used for internalising larger particles (< 0.2 μm in diameter). These mechanisms, some of which are illustrated in Figure 1.10, include the invagination of simple plasma membrane pits (caveolae), or engulfment, particularly of larger particles, by pseudopodia which extend from the plasma membrane due to the polymerisation of filamentous F-actin. Such phagocytosis, which is particularly observed in macrophages and neutrophils, may invaginate up to 50% of the membrane surface area. On a smaller scale, membrane ruffling (also an F-actin-dependent process) may lead to occasional fusion and the invagination of small particles in a process known as micropinocytosis. Vesicles formed by these processes fuse rapidly with endosomes and subsequently lysosomes. However, not all noxious substances are subsequently degraded—for example, mycobacteria modify the endosome/lysosome system and remain viable in the altered vacuoles (see p. 347).

Receptor-regulated cellular entry

The processes described above would not allow for specific regulation of membrane transfer to permit the transient flux of ions such as K^+, Na^+, Ca^{++} or Cl^- at designated times to alter intracellular environments, or initiate membrane depolarisation. Many ion channels open only after a specific signal has been received. This may be from within the cell, such as an alteration in voltage, intracellular volume or Ca^{++} concentrations, or from the extracellular environment, often mediated by G-protein coupled receptors which are examples of type 3 transmembrane proteins (see Fig. 1.10). Such events may be relatively simple receptor-mediated events. For example, acetylcholine induces membrane depolarisation by binding to the nicotinic cholinergic receptor which undergoes a conformational change to permit Na^+ influx. Other ion channels depend on signals generated by more complex intracellular pathways (see below).

Analogous receptor-mediated mechanisms operate to allow the internalisation of moderate-sized particles using clathrin-coated pits. The low-density lipoprotein (LDL) receptor operates in this way; hereditary defects lead to a failure in uptake of cholesterol from the plasma, and the consequences of familial hypercholesterolaemia.

Cells use energy to set up concentration gradients which can be subsequently exploited by the rapid and regulated opening

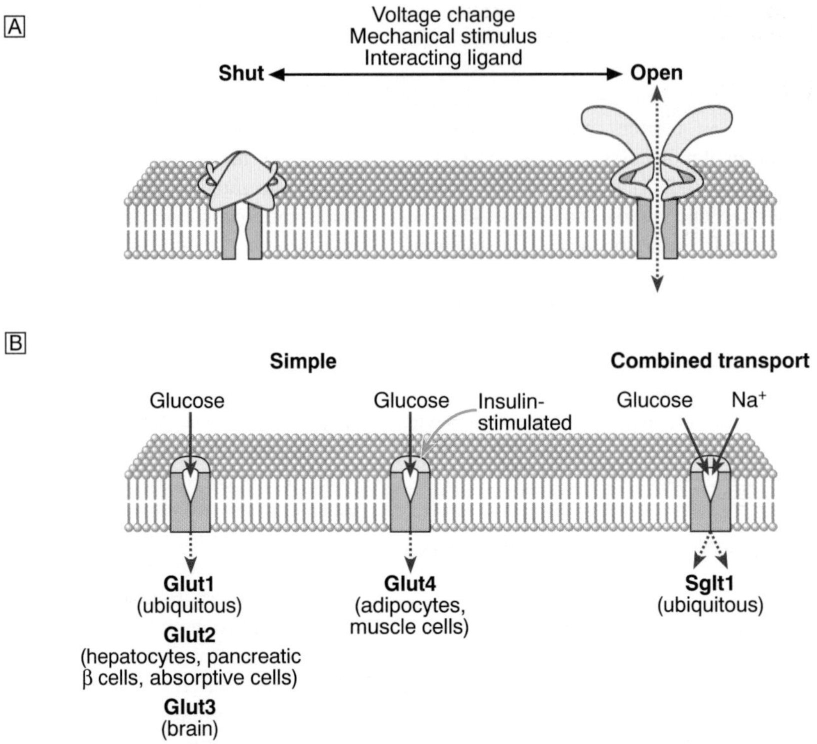

Fig. 1.11 Membrane transport mechanisms. A Gated ion channels are often formed from multiple subunits which generate a pore-like structure with a hydrophilic surface in the lipid bilayer. B Glucose transporters exchange glucose between the blood, extracellular fluid, and cellular sites of uptake (most cells) or synthesis (hepatocytes). The Glut transporters contain 12 membrane-spanning domains, creating pores as indicated. They differ in their biochemical characteristics, site of expression, and regulation. For example, Glut2 is a low-affinity high-capacity transporter expressed on specific cells as indicated to enable 'sensing' of ambient glucose concentrations and high rates of membrane transport.

of specific ion channels. For example, the cytosolic Ca^{++} concentration is maintained at 10^{-7} M, compared to an extracellular concentration in the order of 10^{-3} M by two calcium transporter pumps, one driven by ATPase, the other by the coupled transport of sodium ions in the opposite direction. Similarly, ATP is hydrolysed to provide the energy for the Na^+/K^+ ATPase to transport sodium ions into and potassium ions out of the cell, maintaining osmotic homeostasis.

Signal transduction

As noted with acetylcholine, a molecule does not have to enter a cell in order to alter the cellular environment. Instead, molecules may be recognised at the cell surface by a specific receptor. Binding of the extracellular ligand activates the receptor, which then initiates events which may alter the cellular structure directly (e.g. by depolarisation).

In more complex reactions, the signal is propagated downstream via a number of intermediate signalling moieties. Ligand binding generally leads to receptor activation, and the activated receptor then stimulates a series of other membrane-bound or cytoplasmic signalling molecules, which in the final stages may translocate to the nucleus to alter nuclear transcription, or interact with other cytoplasmic and membrane components. Key features of such cascades are to allow for substantial amplification of the initial signal, and to permit a coordinated cellular response, since more than one series of downstream events may be triggered. This results in the components of these pathways being numerous and potentially confusing. Several different types of signalling cascade are illustrated in a simplified form in Figure 1.12, showing how the cell responds to major families of ligands—for example, hormones, inflammatory cytokines and growth factors.

Second messengers

Phospholipase cascades. Many receptors trigger the hydrolysis of phospholipids within the plasma membrane to generate a series of specific second messengers. For example, phospholipase C (PLC) cleaves phosphatidylinositol 4,5-bisphosphate (PIP_2) into two short-lived messengers, diacylglycerol (DAG) and inositol 1,4,5-trisphosphate (IP_3). DAG activates protein kinase C and

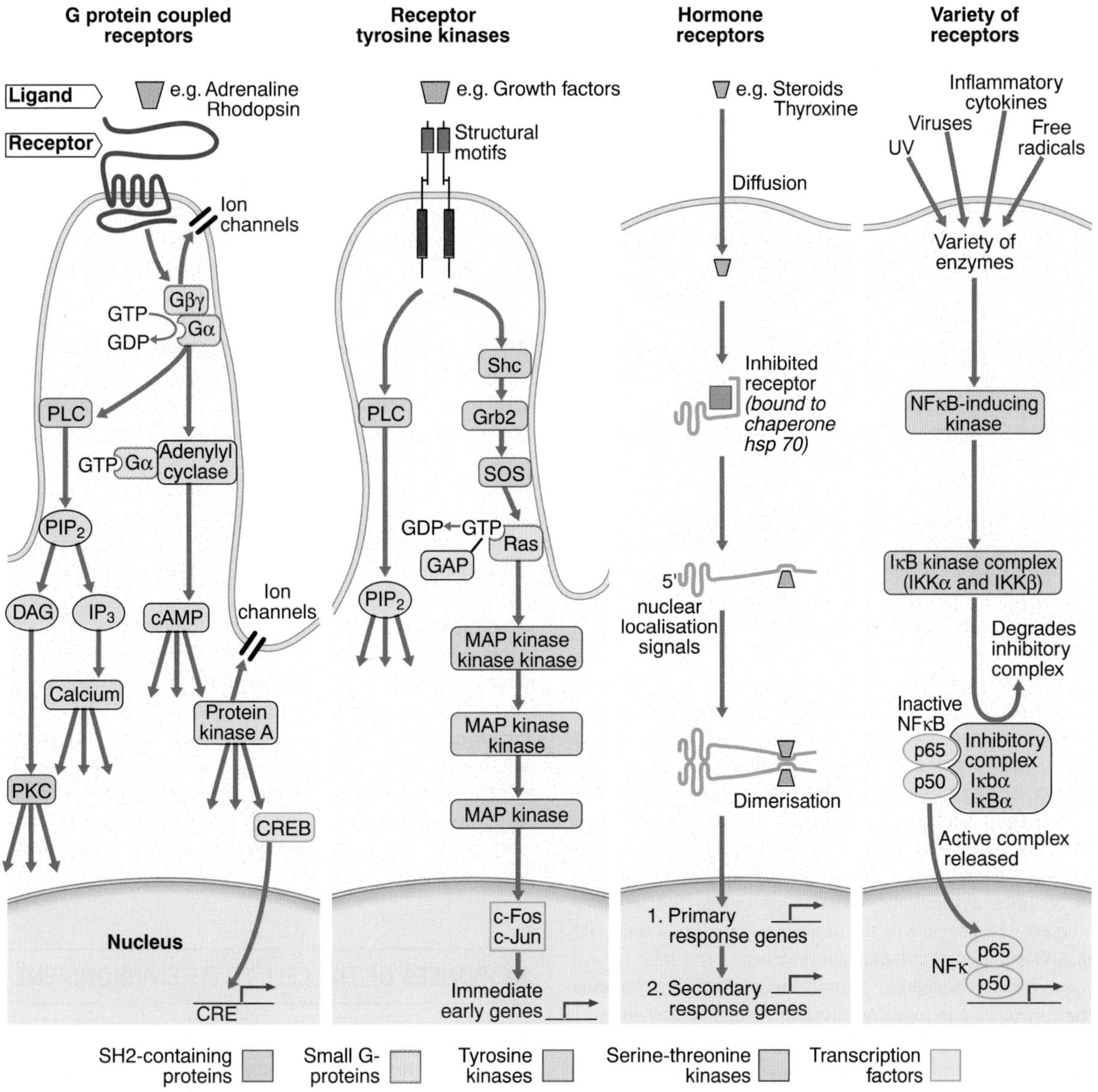

Fig. 1.12 Selection of simplified signal transduction mechanisms. Note that while the first three pathways highlight a cascade based upon activation of substrates, the NFκB mechanism depends upon deactivation of an inhibitory complex to allow release of an activated transcription factor which translocates to the nucleus.

initiates further downstream activation of signalling proteins. IP_3 causes the rapid release of calcium from intracellular stores by opening calcium channels in the endoplasmic reticulum (and sarcoplasmic reticulum in smooth muscle cells). Calcium is a particularly good messenger for rapid release since, as mentioned above, extrusion of calcium maintains tightly controlled low intracellular concentrations allowing rapid re-uptake of the molecule for signalling purposes. Intracellular calcium ions can then interact with a number of proteins which contain calcium recognition motifs, such as a helix-loop-helix motif known as an EF hand, initiating further downstream events. Examples include the activation of protein kinase C (DAG increases its affinity for calcium) and calmodulin which, when activated by calcium binding, stimulates mutifunctional kinases such as calmodulin-dependent protein kinase II which regulates neurotransmitter release and ionic permeabilities. Receptor-mediated activation of other phospholipases, including phospholipase D and phospholipase A_2, operates by similar principles, generating the second messengers DAG and arachidonic acid respectively.

Cyclic nucleotide cascades. Numerous signalling pathways stimulate transmembrane adenylyl cyclase to convert ATP to adenosine 3',5'-cyclic monophosphate (cAMP), or guanylyl cyclase to convert guanosine triphosphate (GTP) to guanosine 3',5'-cyclic monophosphate (cGMP). These pathways include hormonal signalling via G-protein coupled receptors (e.g. β_2-adrenoceptor causing accumulation of cAMP), and nitric oxide which stimulates a cytosolic guanylyl cyclase to produce cGMP, initiating a cascade which in appropriate cell types culminates in vasodilatation. Responses to these cyclic nucleotides often depend upon activation of downstream enzymes. For example, cAMP activates the enzyme protein kinase A, which can open ion channels directly, alter cellular metabolic pathways, or alter nuclear transcription by binding to a cAMP-response element binding protein (CREB), which binds to calcium/cAMP-response elements in promoters of genes such as *c-fos*.

Phosphorylation cascades

Many signalling cascades involve the transfer of phosphate groups to molecules to render the phosphorylated product enzymatically active as a kinase, enabling the subsequent transfer of phosphate groups in further catalytic reactions downstream. Such cascades often commence with the activation of a receptor following ligand binding, by phosphorylating tyrosine or serine and threonine residues on receptor cytoplasmic tails, according to the receptor subtype. The progress of the cascade usually involves serial phosphorylation of cytoplasmic proteins.

Recognition domains. Intracellular signalling proteins often have motifs to allow them to recognise and interact with activated (phosphorylated) molecules in signalling cascades. Several families of recognition motifs are recognised and designated by their homologies to key signalling molecules, e.g. *Src* homology (SH2 and SH3) and plextrin homology (PH) domains. Most signalling proteins have at least two of these motifs, which effectively create 'docking sites' to allow correct orientation of a series of proteins.

Phosphorylation switches. The phosphate groups involved in the immediate phosphorylation of these receptors are often derived from the γ-P of ATP, whereas the phosphate groups used to phosphorylate cytoplasmic signalling proteins are generally derived from GTP, bound to a series of guanine-nucleotide binding proteins (G-proteins). The cytoplasmic provision of GTP is regulated by proteins of the Ras family which carry guanosine diphosphate (GDP) that is converted to GTP by activated upstream signalling molecules. The 'deactivation' of Ras proteins is accelerated by GTPase-activating (GAP) proteins which may be inhibited by growth factor–receptor interactions. These series of effector molecules are conserved signalling molecules from yeast to humans. Aberrant activation of Ras-GTP molecules provides a continuous signal for cell replication in many cancers (see p. 19). Other examples include the Rab family of Ras-like GTPases which provide the energy for vesicle transport (see Fig. 1.10, p. 11), and neurofibromin, a Ras-regulating GAP, the gene for which is mutated in neurofibromatosis (see pp. 916 and 1020).

Mechanisms of retaining a specific cellular response

At first sight it may appear that despite specificity at the level of the ligand–receptor interaction, the signalling cascades converge on common pathways and will be able to generate only a limited number of cellular responses. Specificity therefore relies on the repertoire of receptors and signalling proteins expressed by individual cells, the precise magnitude and timing of the signalling events, and the functional responses available to a particular cell type.

Mechanisms of desensitisation and tolerance

Most signalling pathways are controlled by activated components with short half-lives, and negative feedback loops. In addition, a number of them can become resistant to continued ligand stimulation, a process critical in the repeated administration of drugs. Mechanisms inducing such down-regulation include receptor desensitisation, up-regulation of downstream signalling moieties and up-regulation of transporters to displace intracellular molecules from sites of activity (see Fig. 1.13).

RESPONSES OF THE CELL TO ITS ENVIRONMENT

In its simplest form, an environmental signal may result in a specific cellular result—for example, the opening of an ion channel or the alteration of a cell's synthetic repertoire by altered transcription of a particular gene, or altered protein stability. Complex cellular responses depend on the integration of signals from several sources, as illustrated in the following key examples determining the overall fate of a cell.

Regulation of the cell cycle

A series of mechanisms operate to ensure that progression to the next stage of the cell cycle (see Fig. 1.9, p. 9) should only occur if the cell is in the appropriate environment, and if the preceding stage of the cell cycle has been completed successfully. The understanding of this sequential series of controls has stemmed from two observations made in lower organisms:

- Yeast mutants which did not complete the cell cycle stopped at discrete periods, particularly before S phase *(G1-S phase arrest)* and before mitosis *(G2-M phase arrest)*.
- In frogs, the concentrations of certain proteins were shown to vary through the cell cycle *(cyclins)*.

The cyclins subsequently were shown to be the regulatory subunits for a series of enzymes (cyclin-dependent kinases, Cdks). When activated, Cdks phosphorylate downstream proteins to enable the cell cycle to progress (see Fig. 1.14). Regulation of Cdk activity after cellular assessment of environmental signals and intracellular events such as the status of DNA or cellular mass permits transient arrest of the cycle at a series of 'checkpoints', as observed in yeast. The same mechanisms have since been shown to operate through all eukaryotic organisms including humans (see Fig. 1.15). They facilitate physiological control of cell replication in the appropriate tissue environment or in response to external stimuli. Particularly important is their

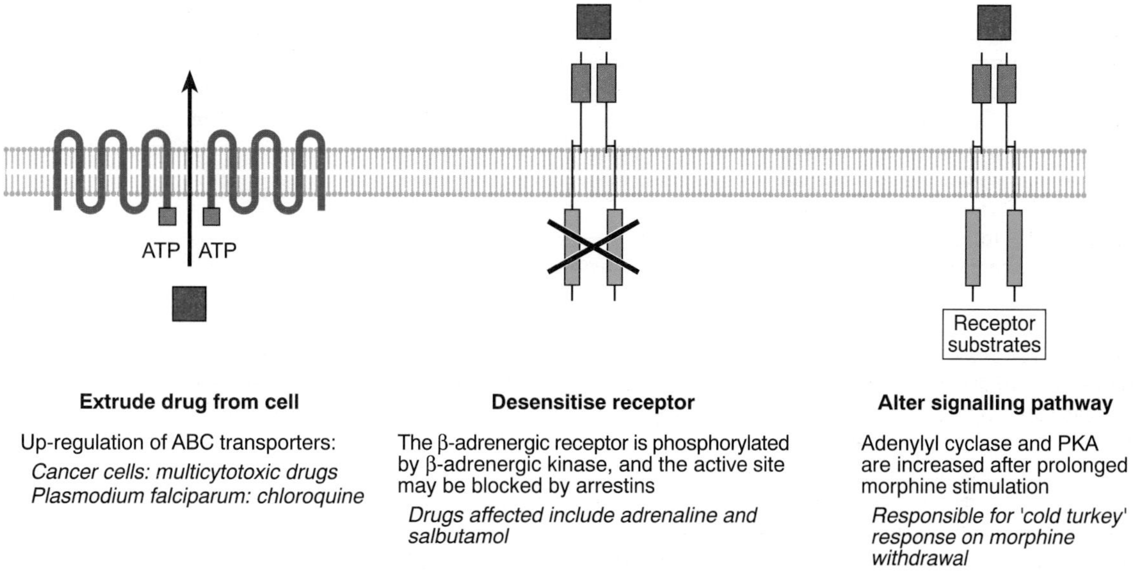
ATP
ATP
Receptor substrates
Extrude drug from cell
Up-regulation of ABC transporters:
Cancer cells: multicytotoxic drugs
Plasmodium falciparum: chloroquine
Desensitise receptor
The β-adrenergic receptor is phosphorylated by β-adrenergic kinase, and the active site may be blocked by arrestins
Drugs affected include adrenaline and salbutamol
Alter signalling pathway
Adenylyl cyclase and PKA are increased after prolonged morphine stimulation
Responsible for 'cold turkey' response on morphine withdrawal

Fig. 1.13 Mechanisms of signalling pathway desensitisation with clinically relevant examples. (ABC = ATPase binding cassettes)

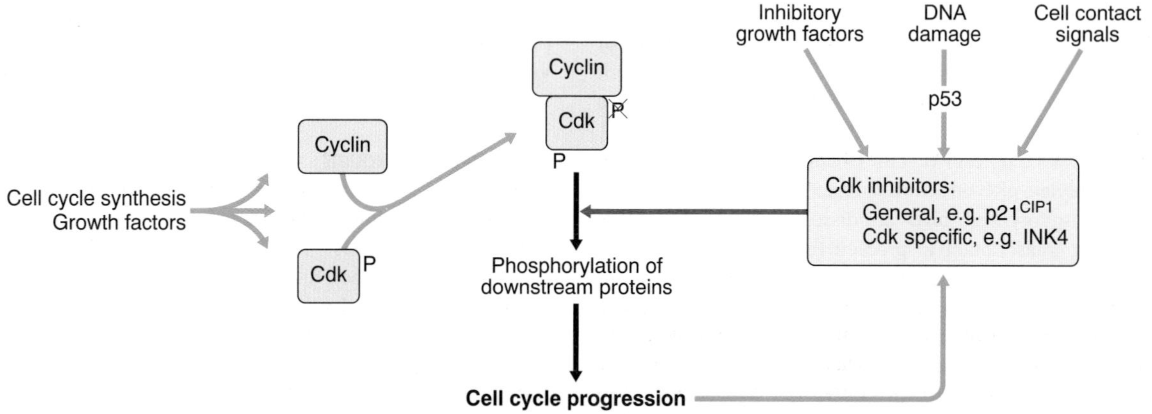

Fig. 1.14 Activation and inhibition of cyclin-Cdk complexes. Most complexes have a regulated synthetic period, and the appropriate cyclin and Cdk are further activated by phosphorylation and dephosphorylation. Inactivation occurs by degradation of the active cyclin-Cdk complex, or by regulated inhibition by a number of Cdk inhibitors which are often cell type-specific, and synthesised in response to a number of further signals as illustrated.

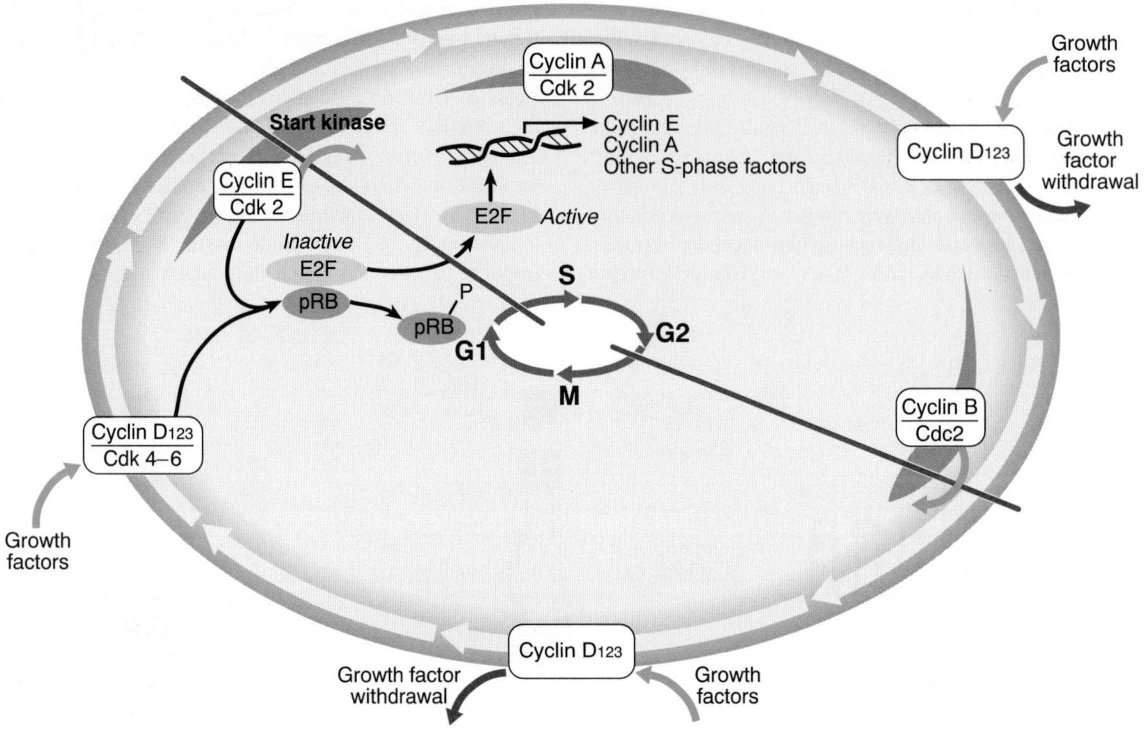

Fig. 1.15 Control of the cell cycle. Simplified view of the mammalian cell cycle illustrating two major checkpoints, and the approximate times of synthesis of the important cyclin-Cdk complexes. Note that in contrast to cyclins A, B and E, cyclins D1, D2 and D3 are synthesised throughout the cell cycle and are particularly involved in sensing growth factor stimulation.

'damage limitation' function which allows pauses in the cell cycle to facilitate DNA repair (see Fig. 1.7, p. 7) before DNA replication transmits any uncorrected errors.

G1-S phase checkpoint

DNA synthesis in S phase requires the transcription of S-phase factors by members of the E2F transcription factor family. The active transcription factor is inhibited by the normal product of the retinoblastoma gene (pRB). The G1 cyclin-Cdk complexes (cyclin D-Cdk4 and cyclin D-Cdk6) phosphorylate pRB on serine and threonine residues, allowing the phosphorylated pRB to dissociate from E2F-DP1, enabling transcription to proceed (in a manner similar to the control of NFκB, see Fig. 1.12, p. 15). The mRNAs for a variety of S-phase-specific proteins are then synthesised. Cyclin D complexes are activated by growth factors, but this can be overridden by a number of other signals, including inhibitory growth factors and signals indicating DNA damage (e.g. from p53), or that cell–cell contact has been achieved. If these negative signals are present, the cell suspends progression until, for example, DNA damage is repaired.

Escape from these regulatory mechanisms allows cells to pass through the G1-S phase checkpoint and synthesise DNA irrespective of their environment, a cardinal feature of malignancy. This can occur, for example, in the absence of pRB (due to deletion or other mutations in retinoblastomas and other tumours), or by inappropriate pRB phosphorylation—for example, by the human papillomavirus E7 protein in cervical carcinoma.

G2-M phase checkpoint

The complex series of cellular changes during mitosis are mediated by the phosphorylation of certain macromolecules at the onset of mitosis—for example, laminin (to dissolve the nuclear membrane), histones (involved in chromosomal condensation) and microtubules (leading to the formation of the mitotic spindle). The phosphorylation of these molecules is regulated by another cyclin-Cdk complex (cyclin B-Cdc2^{p34}, itself regulated by signals derived from DNA damage and DNA synthesis. This complex is also thought to arrest membrane trafficking, allowing approximately equal redistribution of organelles to daughter cells at the end of mitosis.

Withdrawal from the cell cycle

Differentiation

The process of differentiation requires a cell to exit the cell cycle, a path which occurs when some cells are deprived of growth factor stimulation. Integration of signals in different cells—some maintained as self-renewing stem cells, others undergoing terminal differentiation—is the essence of development, in which the lineage of a particular cell, as well as the environmental signals which it receives, plays a crucial role in shaping its ultimate fate.

For example, in undifferentiated cells two sets of transcription factors, the MyoD gene family (including myogenin and MyoD itself) and the myocyte enhancer factor (MEF) 2 family, are inhibited by a large number of proteins including helix-loop-helix proteins, regulators of cell cycle progression, and regulators promoting non-muscle cell fates. Myocyte differentiation requires the activation of the MyoD and MEF2 proteins to establish the cell as a muscle cell precursor, ultimately inducing the transcription of muscle-specific genes such as myosin and actin.

Programmed cell death (apoptosis)

Apoptosis refers to the morphological characteristics of cells undergoing programmed cell death, an alternative result of withdrawal from the cell cycle. Cell types which depend upon continued growth factor stimulation for survival will undergo apoptosis if they are deprived of growth factors, a process again mediated in part by regulation of cyclin-Cdk complexes. Usually this occurs at the critical G1-S phase transition, but some cells such as thymocytes can undergo apoptosis anywhere in the cell cycle. Additional causes of apoptosis include signals of continued DNA damage, or inflammatory-related stimuli, to be discussed on page 24.

Programmed cell death occurs in three molecular phases: an initiation event (which is cell-type and stimulus specific), an effector stage when molecules of the Bcl-2 family act as opposing death agonists (e.g. Bax) and antagonists (e.g. Bcl-2) to interact with other apoptosis factors, ultimately activating a cascade of caspases leading to the degradation phase. Apoptosis is of crucial importance in regulating cell numbers without subjecting local tissues to damaging cellular enzymes and contents, since apoptotic cells are engulfed by local macrophages and do not discharge their contents to the exterior.

FURTHER INFORMATION ON INTERACTIONS OF THE CELL WITH ITS LOCAL ENVIRONMENT

Nurse P 1997 Checkpoint pathways come of age. Cell 91: 865–867

Paulovich A G, Toczyski D, Hartwell L H 1997 When checkpoints fail. Cell 88: 315–321

See recent reviews in Cell, Nature and other specialised journals

CANCER

Cancer arises because certain cells within a given tissue escape from normal growth controls, replicate more frequently, and migrate to sites distant from the parent tissue where further uncontrolled replication occurs. Such escape is facilitated by the accumulation of mutations within a cancerous cell as a result of the innate and environmental carcinogens to which cellular DNA is subjected. If errors generated in coding DNA are not repaired, these will be transmitted to the daughter strands as the cell divides. Clearly, mutations will arise more rapidly if external mutagenic stimuli are increased, or if the cell is defective in DNA repair systems.

ONCOGENES

This term refers to a gene which has been mutated to facilitate neoplastic growth. The normal function of such genes may be the synthesis of factors involved in growth control, the cell cycle or apoptosis. Oncogenes can be broadly divided into two groups, according to whether their oncogenic effect results from overactivity of a 'proto-oncogene' or the loss of a 'tumour suppressor' function.

Proto-oncogenes

The majority of known oncogenes are components of signal transduction pathways in which mutations or the presence of increased copies of a gene result in overactivity, mimicking persistent growth factor stimulation. These include genes encoding receptors (e.g. *erbB* in breast carcinoma), cytoplasmic signalling moieties such as *K-ras*, and transcription factors such as *c-myc* (important in gastrointestinal tumours and leukaemias). A recently described class encode mitotic spindle binding proteins; mutations in these genes promote premature exit from anaphase, leading to incorrect chromosome segregation to daughter cells, and anaploidy. In animals, a number of tumours are caused by retroviruses which carry activated oncogenes, but to date this has not been shown to be a common mechanism in human cancer. Nevertheless, several human cancers are undoubtedly caused by infectious agents. Important examples include human papillomavirus E7 (which inappropriately phosphorylates pRB), leading to cervical carcinoma; herpesvirus 8 (which encodes a cyclin that drives the host cell through the G1-S checkpoint); and Epstein–Barr virus, responsible for Burkitt's lymphoma and nasopharyngeal carcinoma.

Tumour suppressors and the two-hit model of tumorigenesis

Tumour suppressor genes tend to encode proteins whose

normal function is to inhibit the cell cycle or to induce apoptosis to prevent transmission of uncorrectable DNA defects. Direct inhibitors of the cell cycle include pRB, illustrated in Figure 1.15. Other tumour suppressor genes encode components of inhibitory growth factor-signalling pathways, particularly those of transforming growth factor (TGF)-β and its associated cytoplasmic signalling molecules such as *Smad2* and *Smad4* (which is the *DPC4* '*d*eleted in *p*ancreatic *c*arcinoma' gene). As noted in the previous section, *neurofibromin* encodes a Ras inhibitor which is mutated in neurofibromatosis. *APC*, the gene mutated in familial adenomatous polyposis and 60% of sporadic colon adenomas and carcinomas, is thought to operate as an oncogene by rendering cells less susceptible to apoptosis. P53, a key tumour suppressor gene, normally uses both mechanisms to override other signals which would otherwise stimulate cell proliferation; details of p53 activity are highlighted in Figure 1.16. The importance of p53 is illustrated by the fact that it is inactivated in over 50% of human tumours, including breast and colon carcinomas, and childhood leukaemias.

When an oncogene results from a mutation reducing the activity of a tumour suppressor, a single mutation usually is insufficient to generate oncogenic activity unless an additional mutation inactivates the second copy of the gene. This 'two-hit' model of tumorigenesis, developed by Knudson, is illustrated in Figure 1.17. If, on the other hand, an oncogene results from overactivity of a proto-oncogene, a mutation in only one of the two copies may be sufficient to promote tumorigenesis. This is also true in an important exception to the two-hit rule, in the case of the tumour suppressor gene p53, since mutations in only one allele may be sufficient to result in a biological effect. This reflects the operation of the protein as a tetramer, so abnormalities in any one of the subunits may derange its function.

MULTISTEP CARCINOGENESIS

The cell's complex self-regulating machinery means that more than one mutation is often required to produce a malignant, metastasising tumour, such as a carcinoma, derived from epithelial cells. For example, if a cell mutates to produce a growth factor to which it already expresses the receptor (paracrine stimulation), that cell will replicate more frequently but will still be subject to cell cycle checkpoints to promote DNA integrity in its progeny. If an additional mutation overriding a cell cycle checkpoint occurs, that cell and its progeny may go on to accumulate further mutations, some of which may allow it to replicate an unlimited number of times by synthesis of telomerase, or to separate from its matrix and cellular attachments without undergoing apoptosis. As deregulated growth continues, cancer cells become increasingly unable to differentiate, fail to respond to local signals as in the normal tissue, and cease to ensure appropriate chromosomal segregation pre-division, generating the classical malignant pathological appearances of disorganised growth, variable levels of differentiation, and polyploidy. This sequence is illustrated for colon carcinomas in Figure 1.18.

Since DNA mutations occur so infrequently, only an occasional cell will go on to acquire a further mutation, but this will be transmitted to the progeny of that cell which, due to their faster replication rates, are likely to constitute an increasing fraction of the tumour. It is likely that the morphological premalignant appearances of cancers reflect the underlying number of mutations, particularly as pathological evidence of increased malignancy can be seen arising within premalignant lesions.

INHERITED BASIS

It is important to recognise that most of the mutations described above arise in a somatic cell and are not transmitted to the patient's offspring. Nevertheless, some human families are genetically prone to cancer. One group of cancer patients, exemplified by xeroderma pigmentosum (XP) and the hereditary non-polyposis colon cancer (HNPCC) families, have defects in DNA repair enzymes (see Fig. 1.7, p. 7) so that they accumulate mutations at a faster rate. More commonly, individuals in cancer-prone families inherit a mutation in a particular oncogene, essentially reducing the

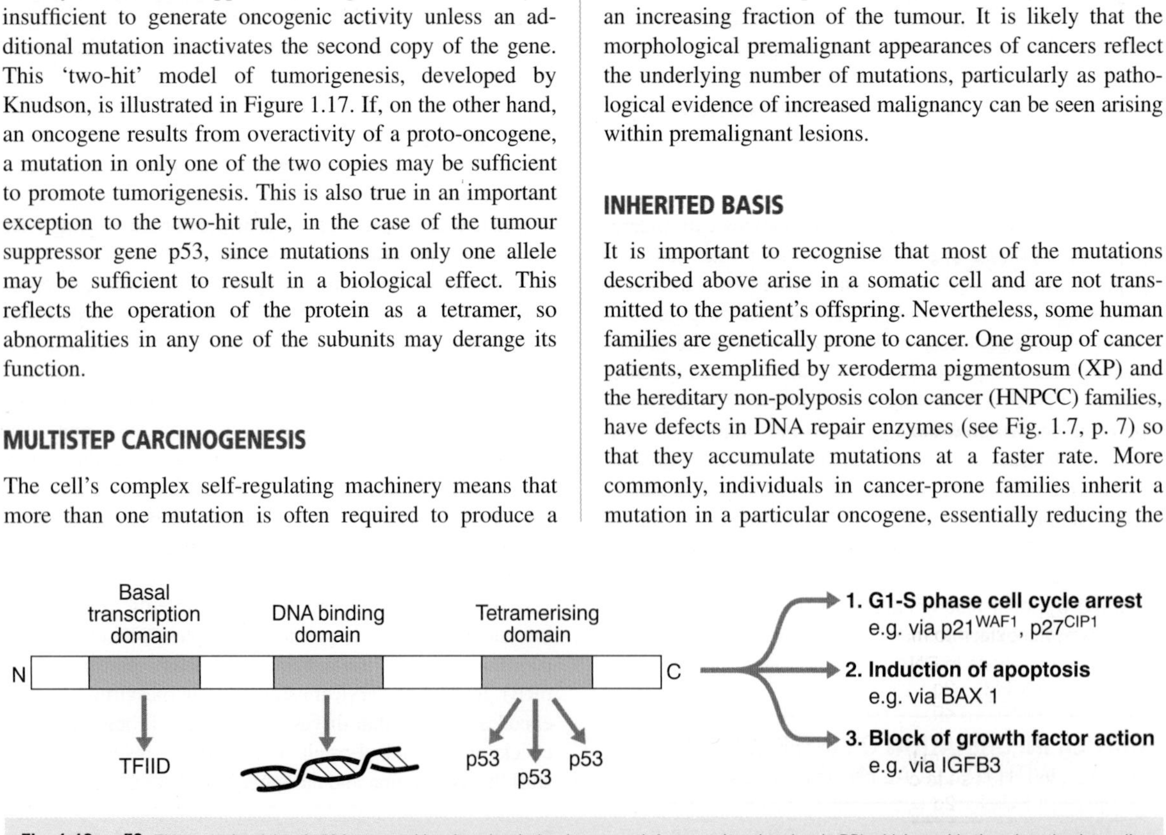

Fig. 1.16 p53. The normal activity of p53 is to override other signals (such as growth factors, phosphorylated pRB) which would otherwise stimulate cell proliferation. The nuclear concentration is held at low levels due to a short half-life (20 minutes, ubiquitin-mediated), but the concentrations are increased on recognition of DNA damage or an unfavourable environment for DNA replication.

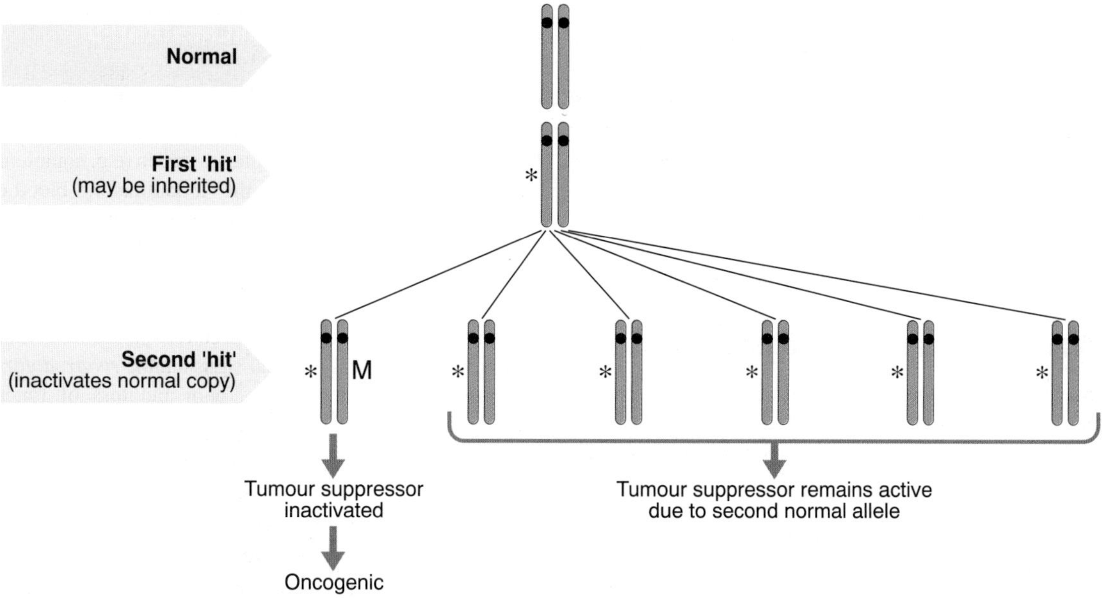

Fig. 1.17 The 'two-hit' hypothesis. The first mutation is marked by an asterisk, the second by an M.

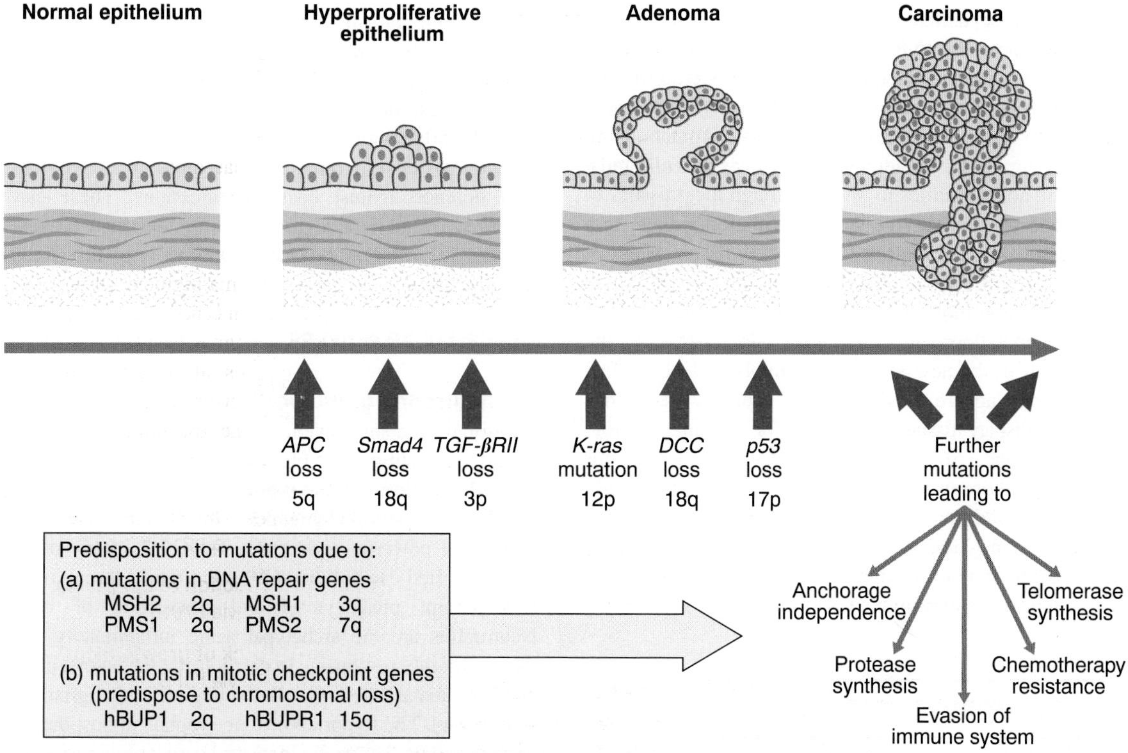

Fig. 1.18 The multistep origin of cancer: molecular events implicated in colorectal carcinogenesis.

number of additional mutations a cell from that person requires to become neoplastic. The two-hit model explains why even in these cancer-prone families, tumours may require many years to develop. The inherited oncogene may be particularly relevant for a certain cell type, predisposing to a particular form of tumour (e.g. *N-Ras* and neurological tumours), or be able to deregulate growth in a variety of different cell types (e.g. *p53* mutations in Li–Fraumeni families which are particularly prone to early-onset leukaemias, sarcomas, and breast and brain malignancies).

ADDITIONAL FEATURES OF SOLID TUMOURS

Haematological malignancies occur in cells which are already anchorage-independent and circulating. However, additional features are required for a solid tumour to grow and metastasise. The acquisition of additional mutations means that the secondary tumour cells may replicate faster than the primary, or be unable to differentiate as fully.

The blood supply to the enlarging mass of cells is initially rate-limiting, as evidenced by the ischaemic centres to solid tumours. Some tumours may acquire mutations to enhance the secretion of factors to stimulate neovascularisation (angiogenesis), but in many instances physiology suffices since hypoxia is a potent stimulus of the angiogenic factor VEGF (vascular endothelial cell growth factor).

Metastasis, the cardinal feature of most malignant tumours, requires a cancer cell to have the ability to detach from its surroundings without undergoing apoptosis. Certain mutations result in nuclei receiving signals *as if* they were anchored to local structures—for example, mutations in *APC* (see Fig. 1.18). In addition, metastasising cells must acquire the novel abilities to invade through local tissues to reach blood vessels, survive in the circulation, adhere to a blood vessel wall and migrate into the new tissue. Many of these features are facilitated by the synthesis of novel cellular adhesion molecules or tissue-degradative enzymes such as metalloproteinases. The adherence to the endothelium in the new site cannot simply reflect the fact that the cells adhere to the nearest capillary bed, since metastases display tissue specificity—for example, thyroid cancer to bone. Specific cellular adhesion mechanisms analogous to those used by inflammatory cells are thought to operate. In addition, to escape destruction by cells of the immune system, tumour cells may down-regulate cell-surface expression of recognition molecules or induce a general depression of immune responses (see p. 36).

FURTHER INFORMATION ON CANCER

Hanahan D, Folkman J 1996 Patterns and emerging mechanisms of the angiogenic switch during tumorigenesis. Cell 86: 353–364

Weinberg R A Sept 1996 How cancer arises. Scientific American 32–40

INFLAMMATION: AN ORCHESTRATED CELLULAR RESPONSE

The inflammatory response results from a complex interplay between different mediator cascades (e.g. complement, cytokines and chemokines), the 'inflammatory' blood cells (neutrophils, eosinophils and monocytes) that are recruited to the site, and 'resident' tissue cells, particularly the microvascular cells of the organ or tissue involved. The beneficial nature of the inflammatory response, particularly in host defence against infection, has been recognised for centuries, as have the classical external signs: *calor*, *rubor*, *dolor* and *functio laesa*—heat, redness, pain and loss of function. However, it has only comparatively recently become clear that these identical processes may, under circumstances that are not fully understood, be centrally involved in the pathogenesis of a wide range of common and important diseases (see the information box, p. 24). The *acute* inflammatory response is often restricted to recruitment of neutrophil granulocytes and inflammatory macrophages yet its effectiveness is clearly exemplified in streptococcal lobar pneumonia (see below and p. 341). In more complex situations (e.g. some viral diseases), a *chronic* inflammatory response causes additional local recruitment of lymphocytes, sometimes leading to a fibrotic response; or against some parasites (e.g. in schistosomiasis, see p. 165) there may be local recruitment of large numbers of eosinophil granulocytes in addition to neutrophils and lymphocytes, thus completing the cellular picture typical of *allergic* inflammation. Defects in the cellular or mediator components of inflammation can lead to major problems in host defence against bacterial infections. These can be inherited (e.g. leucocyte adhesion deficiency—LAD—see the information box) or acquired (e.g. drug-induced neutropenia).

THE CELLULAR PLAYERS

The neutrophil granulocyte

Neutrophils are short-lived, bone marrow-derived (half-life 6 hours), circulating white blood cells with a diameter of about 5.5 μM. On ultrastructure (see Fig. 1.20) they contain a large number of cytoplasmic granules, which in turn contain a large number of powerful agents (see Table 1.2), many of which when secreted can aid the cell's rapid transit through tissues, and prompt phagocytosis and destruction of bacteria. Neutrophils are the archetypal acute inflammatory cells—they are highly responsive to chemotactic mediators, e.g. IL-8 and C5a, and are the first cells to emigrate to the inflamed site (see below). The importance of neutrophils in host defence is emphasised by the greatly increased susceptibility to infection found in patients with neutropenia or inherited disorders of neutrophil function. A number of diseases have been linked

LEUCOCYTE ADHESION DEFICIENCY (LAD)
See Figure 1.19
Mechanism
• Inherited defect of β_2 integrins on the neutrophil surface
Clinical features
• Destructive skin ulceration without pus formation (no neutrophil emigration) • Chronic neutrophilia • Poor wound-healing with dystrophic scars • Delayed umbilical cord separation in the neonate • Recurrent septicaemia and life-threatening infections

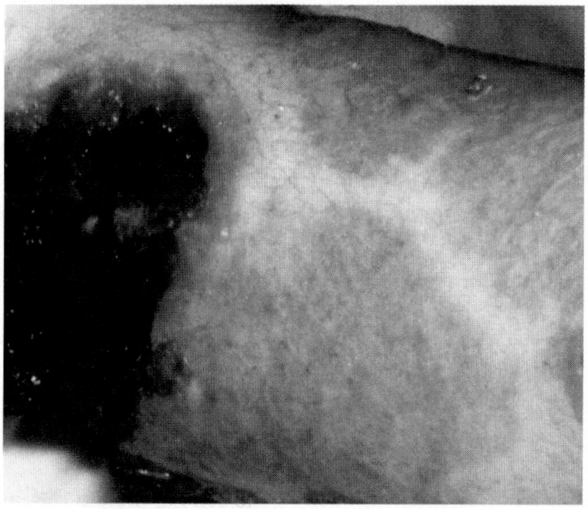

Fig. 1.19 Necrotic skin ulcers and dystrophic scars in leucocyte adhesion deficiency.

with rare inherited abnormalities in neutrophil granules. Most of these are characterised by repeated bacterial infections. Chronic granulomatous disease due to a defect in NADPH oxidase is perhaps the best-recognised example.

The macrophage

Resident tissue macrophages, e.g. Kupffer cells in the liver, alveolar macrophages in the lung, mesangial cells in the kidney, microglial cells in the brain and resident macrophages in the peritoneum and lymph nodes, derive from circulating monocytes which originate in the bone marrow. Tissue macrophages have a number of important functions (see the information box) and via a range of surface receptors are able to respond in different ways to a wide range of external stimuli. Like neutrophils, resident macrophages can ingest and kill bacteria, but perhaps their major role in acute inflammation is to initiate and orchestrate the inflammatory response by the secretion of important cytokines (see Table 1.4, p. 33) and chemokines. For example, they can secrete large quantities of the neutrophil chemokine IL-8 and other chemokines that specifically attract monocytes to the inflamed site. These monocytes rapidly mature into *inflammatory macrophages*, which have huge phagocytic and bacterial killing capacity and which also have

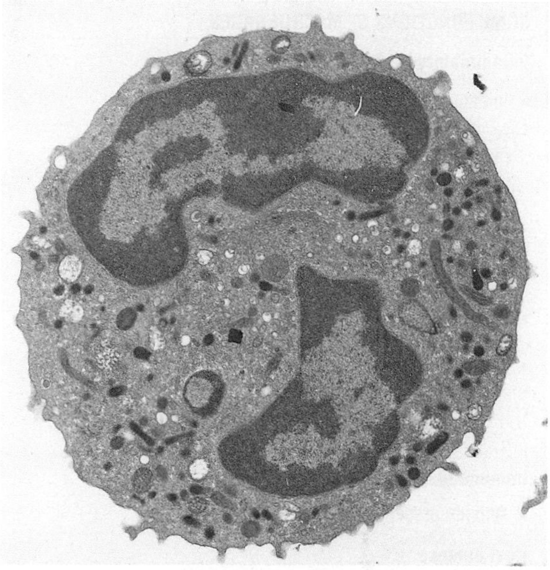

Fig. 1.20 The neutrophil granulocyte. Electron micrograph demonstrating the multilobed nucleus and cytoplasmic granules.

Table 1.2 Constituents of human neutrophil granules

	Azurophil granules	**Specific granules**
Microbicidal enzymes	Lysozyme Myeloperoxidase	Lysozyme
Neutral proteinases	Elastase Collagenases Cathepsin G	Collagenase
Acid hydrolases	Phosphatases Lipases Sulphatases Histonase Cathepsin D B glycerophosphatase Esterase Neuraminidase 5' nucleotidase	Phosphatases
Others	Bactericidal/ Permeability-inducing protein Defensins Cationic proteins Glycosaminoglycans Chondroitin sulphate Heparin sulphate	Lactoferrin Vitamin B_{12} binding protein C3bi receptor Cytochrome B Flavoproteins

SOME FUNCTIONS OF MACROPHAGES
Inflammatory response
• Initiation Generation of neutrophil chemokines (e.g. IL-8) Generation of monocyte chemokines (e.g. MIP-1α) Generation of agents (IL-1, TNF-α) that activate endothelial cells Generation of acute phase response (IL-1, TNF, IL-6) • Amplification Secretion of agents that stimulate bone marrow generation of leucocytes (IL-1, TNF-α) • Resolution Scavenging of necrotic and apoptotic cells and debris • Repair/fibrosis Remodelling—elastase, collagenase Scar formation—IL-1, platelet-derived growth factor (PDGF), fibroblast growth factor (FGF)
Immune response
• Antigen presentation—lymphocyte activation
Host defence
• Phagocytosis and killing of microorganisms by oxygen radicals, nitric oxide-dependent mechanisms and enzymes
Antitumour effects
• Lysis of tumour cells by TNF-α and nitric oxide-dependent mechanisms

important scavenging function for damaged microorganisms and proteins and for aged and damaged host cells in the 'clearing up' processes during the resolution of the inflammatory response. Finally, resident and inflammatory macrophages can secrete a range of cytokines that are responsible for tissue repair processes, but clearly ineffective control of these processes may underlie the excessive fibroproliferative response that characterises chronic inflammatory diseases such as pyelonephritis and fibrosing alveolitis (see the information box bottom left).

SOME EXAMPLES OF DISEASES FEATURING AN INAPPROPRIATE OR EXCESSIVE INFLAMMATORY RESPONSE
Acute inflammatory tissue injury (neutrophil dominant)
• Acute respiratory distress syndrome (ARDS) • Acute gout • Myocardial infarction/reperfusion injury • Acute glomerulonephritis
Chronic inflammation (lymphocyte/macrophage dominant ± fibrosis)
• Fibrosing alveolitis • Chronic bronchitis and emphysema • Chronic pyelonephritis • Atherogenesis • Rheumatoid arthritis • Psoriasis • Multiple sclerosis
Chronic allergic inflammation (lymphocytes and eosinophil dominant)
• Bronchial asthma • Eczema

The eosinophil granulocyte

Like the neutrophil, the eosinophil is a bone marrow-derived, blood-borne polymorphonuclear leucocyte, but unlike the neutrophil its cytoplasm stains pink on haemotoxylin/eosin staining, and electron microscopy (see Fig. 1.21) shows the large angular granules that characterise this cell. Eosinophils appear to be selectively attracted to tissues as the result of specific chemotaxins (e.g. IL-5 and the chemokines RANTES and eotaxin that are secreted by macrophages and T lymphocytes). Most of the granule contents are common to the neutrophil, although some agents, e.g. eosinophil peroxidase (EPO) and major basic protein (MBP), are specific for the eosinophil. Eosinophils have probably evolved to aid human host defences against parasites such as schistosomes and worms (see Ch. 2), but they are also implicated in allergic diseases such as asthma.

THE ACUTE INFLAMMATORY RESPONSE

In a classical acute anti-inflammatory response, such as occurs as a result of streptococcal invasion of the lung airspaces in the evolution of lobar streptococcal pneumonia (see p. 341), a stereotyped sequence of cellular and mediator events is usually provoked (see Fig. 1.22):

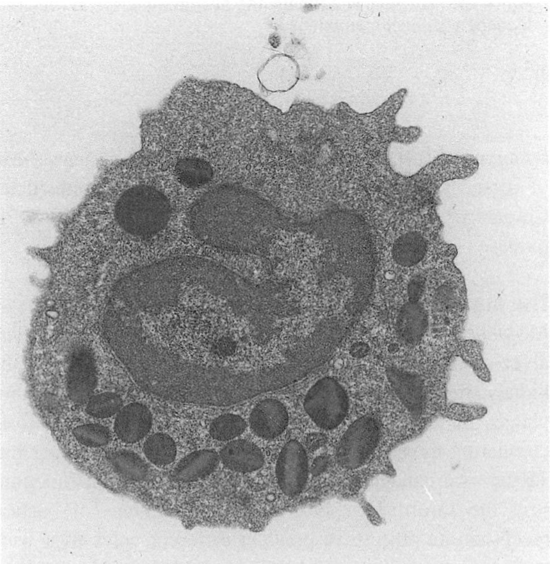

Fig. 1.21 The human eosinophil granulocyte. Electron micrograph illustrating the characteristic angular granules.

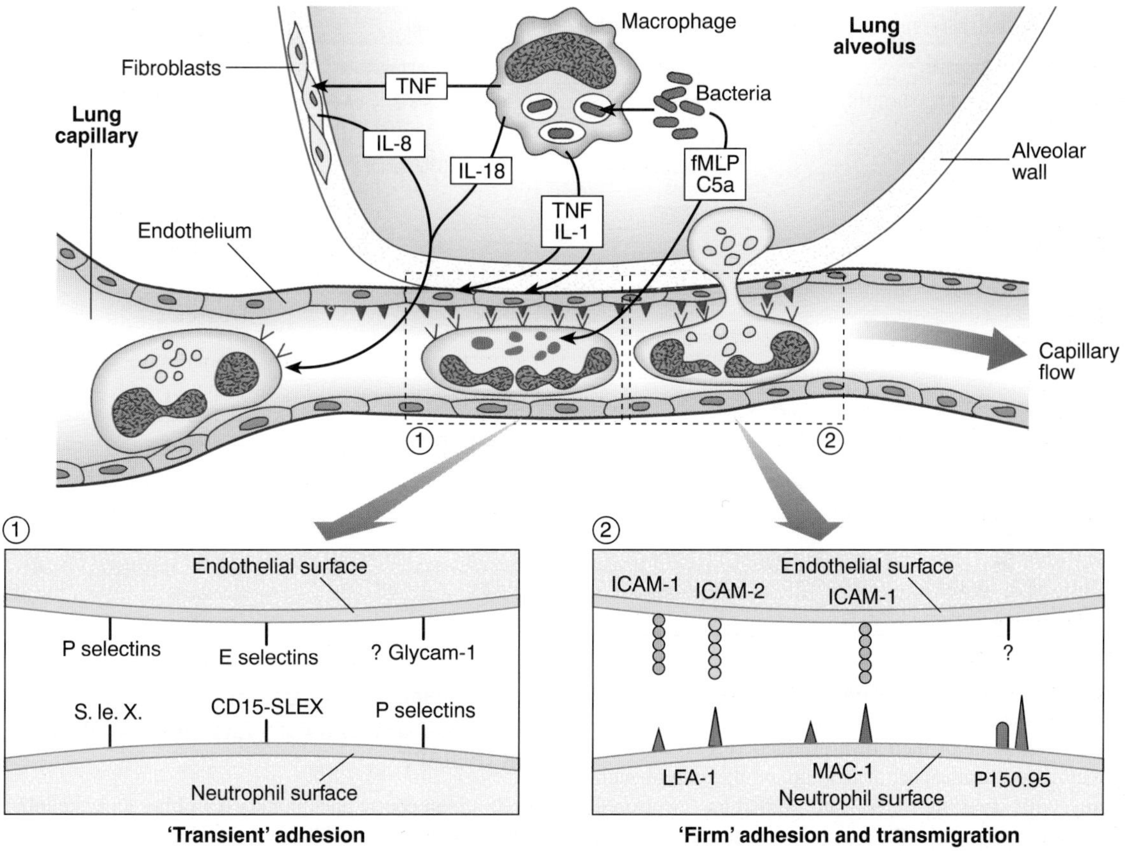

Fig. 1.22 Initiation of the acute inflammatory response: neutrophil emigration. (1) Transient adhesion mediated by selectin molecules. (2) Tight adhesion and transendothelial emigration—mediated by adhesion molecules of the integrin family. See Table 1.3.

- Neutrophils sequester in the local lung capillaries, emigrate through the vascular endothelium, the basement membrane and the alveolar epithelial layer, and begin to appear in the alveolar spaces within 2 hours, with a peak of emigration at 4–6 hours.
- Neutrophils become activated, phagocytose and destroy opsonised bacteria by secreting reactive oxygen species (ROS) and granule enzymes into the phagosome.
- Monocytes begin to emigrate from capillaries into tissues at about 6 hours, reaching a peak at 18–24 hours. Monocytes rapidly mature into inflammatory macrophages which kill and scavenge dead organisms and debris.

In most inflammatory reactions there is vascular dilatation and leakage of fluid and proteins during the early stage of neutrophil emigration. This exudate contains an array of proteins and other mediators, e.g. members of the complement and coagulation cascades, immunoglobulins and other factors that may aid host defence and later repair. In a 'successful' beneficial inflammatory response, such as occurs in most cases of lobar pneumonia, the inflammatory cells rapidly disappear as the lesion resolves. It is likely that extravasated granulocytes undergo apoptosis locally and are phagocytosed by macrophages; tissue numbers of macrophages then return to normal. Even in 'beneficial inflammation' like lobar pneumonia, there is often 'bystander' injury to local endothelial cells and epithelial cells; these must be repaired/replaced before tissue homeostasis is re-established.

Much has been learned about the cellular and mediator events involved in the initiation of acute inflammation; some of these mechanisms may provide new targets for therapy in inflammatory disease. Local tissue perturbation, e.g. bacterial invasion, causes the release of inflammatory mediators. Some of these act as chemotaxins, attracting neutrophils then monocytes to the site; others (e.g. TNF-α, IL-1) act on local vascular endothelial cells to promote their

Table 1.3 Important receptors in leucocyte-endothelial adhesion and transmigration

Family	Receptor	Distribution	Ligand/counter-receptor	Promotes adhesion to
Integrin family	LFA-1 (CD11a/CD18)	All leucocytes	ICAM-1, ICAM-2, ICAM-3	Endothelial cells
	MAC-1/CR3 (CD11b/CD18)	Granulocytes Monocytes Lymphocytes	ICAM-1, C3bi, factor X	Endothelial cells Opsonised particles
	P150.95 (CD11c/CD18)	Granulocytes Monocytes	?	Endothelial cells
Selectin family	L-selectin (CD)	Neutrophils Monocytes Lymphocytes	?	Endothelial cells
	P-selectin (CD62)	Endothelium	Sialyl Lewis X (CD15)	Neutrophils
Immunoglobulin superfamily	ICAM-1 (CD54)	Endothelium Epithelium	LFA-1 (CD11a/CD18) MAC-1 (CD11b/CD18)	All leucocytes
	ICAM-2	Monocytes Lymphocytes Endothelium	LFA-1 (CD11a/CD18)	All leucocytes
	VCAM-1	Activated endothelium	VLA-4	Monocytes Eosinophils

adhesion to the surface of activated inflammatory cells (see Table 1.3). Bacteria can generate neutrophil chemotaxins in several ways; some of their own products (e.g. formylated peptides) are chemotactic; activation of the complement system will generate C5a, an important neutrophil chemotaxin; but perhaps the most important mechanism is the induction of chemokine generation by resident macrophages and other tissue cells. The chemokines (e.g. IL-8, RANTES and eotaxin) are a large family of small, but potent, peptides which attract and activate different inflammatory cells via specific surface receptors. The arrest of neutrophils in local microvessels is a necessary prelude to their transmigration through the endothelial and epithelial layers and it involves a two-step process. The first phase is one of transient adhesion which is mediated by adhesion molecules of the *selectin* family; the second phase of tight adhesion and transmigration is mediated by adhesion molecules of the *integrin* family (see Table 1.3). It is now clear that just as there are many neutrophil chemotaxins, there are also many adhesion molecules that can mediate neutrophil adhesion to microvascular endothelial cells. The importance of the integrin mechanism in host defence is well illustrated by LAD (see p. 23), which is caused by an inherited defect in the β chain of the leucocyte integrins.

Although eosinophils and monocytes sequester and emigrate by very similar mechanisms, it is likely that selective accumulation is achieved by differential secretion and expression of the different members of the chemokine and adhesion molecule repertoire (e.g. IL-8 is chemotactic specifically for neutrophils, whereas RANTES and eotaxin specifically attract eosinophils).

MORE COMPLEX INFLAMMATORY RESPONSES, INFLAMMATORY DISEASES AND NEW PROSPECTS FOR THERAPY

While streptococcal pneumonia exemplifies an acute inflammatory response in which the recruited cells are virtually restricted to neutrophil granulocytes and cells of the monocyte/macrophage lineage, in other situations, e.g. some viral infections, large numbers of lymphocytes are recruited. This more persistent tissue picture results from a combination of the inflammatory and classical immune responses (see p. 30). The further recruitment of eosinophils in a chronic inflammatory response is a feature of *allergic* inflammation, e.g. in filariasis and schistosomiasis.

However, these patterns of cellular responses can also be 'turned against us' in various diseases if they occur inappropriately or in an uncontrolled fashion. For example, an excessive or inappropriate acute inflammatory response is responsible for many acute tissue injury syndromes, acute gout (see p. 831) and acute glomerulonephritis (see p. 442). A chronic inflammatory response and chronic tissue destruction or an excessive fibrogenic response are key features of rheumatoid arthritis (see p. 835), chronic pyelonephritis (see p. 461), fibrosing alveolitis (see p. 369) and chronic bronchitis and emphysema. An allergic inflammatory response characterises asthma (see p. 326) and eczema (see p. 896). The vast redundancy of mechanisms displayed in various aspects of the inflammatory response may be advantageous in antibacterial host defence but it poses problems for the development of specific therapy in inflammatory diseases.

FURTHER INFORMATION ON INFLAMMATION: AN ORCHESTRATED CELLULAR RESPONSE

Gallin J I, Goldstein I M, Snyderman R 1992 Inflammation: basic principles and clinical correlates. Raven, New York

ORGANISATION AND FUNCTION OF THE IMMUNE SYSTEM

The immune system has evolved to recognise and eliminate foreign molecules through an integrated network of cellular and molecular interactions and thus provides the defence mechanism against pathogens. Defining the molecular basis and functional consequences of these molecular interactions may offer an opportunity both to diagnose and regulate qualitative and quantitative aspects of immune responses and, therefore, contribute to the prevention and treatment of immunologically based disorders.

INNATE AND ADAPTIVE IMMUNITY

As discussed above, the cellular and mediator events of the acute inflammatory response play a key role in the 'first-line' or *innate* immunity against infection. If, however, innate immunity fails to provide effective protection then induction of the adaptive immune system occurs. This response develops after a period of days and is mediated by lymphocytes which express antigen-specific receptors. When recirculating naive T cells recognise antigen processed by antigen presenting cells (APCs) in lymphoid organs, the population expands and differentiates into effector or regulatory cells. The latter contribute to the development of humoral responses by stimulating B cells that have bound specific antigen to secrete antibodies. The adaptive immune response invariably eliminates the pathogen, as a result of which T cell activity and serum antibody levels decline. However, immunological memory remains, such that re-exposure to the same antigen induces a more rapid response of greater magnitude (see the information box).

CHARACTERISTIC FEATURES OF ADAPTIVE IMMUNITY
Specificity
• Distinct antigens generate specific responses
Diversity
• Antigens are recognised by different lymphocytes
Memory
• Re-exposure to antigen induces more rapid and effective response
Self-regulation
• Normal immune responses decrease with time
Self-/non-self-discrimination
• During development lymphocytes learn to distinguish between self and foreign antigens

ORGANISATION OF THE IMMUNE SYSTEM

The immune system must provide protection against an extensive array of pathogens and achieve this within a relatively short period of time. In order to meet these requirements, B and T lymphocytes have evolved selective biological properties, which are reflected in their unique characteristics of specificity, diversity, memory, self-regulation and self-/non-self-discrimination. At the organisational level the immune system needs to provide different environments to allow the development of clonally diverse lymphocytes and then to bring together antigen and specific mature lymphocytes as required to facilitate clonal expansion and differentiation. Mechanisms must also exist which allow effector/memory lymphocytes to traffic to sites of disease.

MIGRATION OF LYMPHOCYTES

The primary lymphoid organs (thymus and bone marrow), where stem cells develop into T and B cells, are linked by lymphatic vessels to the secondary lymphoid organs. It is in the latter, which include lymph nodes, spleen, and mucosa-associated lymphoid tissue, that lymphocytes encounter antigen and become sensitised, converting from naive to memory/effector cells. Antigen carried by APCs or retained from afferent lymph by specialised cells is presented to recirculating lymphocytes. Naive T and B cells migrate through the high endothelial venules (HEVs) in the cortex, with T and B cells locating to the paracortical area and follicles, respectively (see Fig. 1.23). This process of migration through the HEVs is regulated by differential expression of cell surface adhesion molecules and is initiated by the binding of lymphocytes to the endothelium. Adhesion molecules also contribute to the activation and effector function of lymphocytes. Once activated, plasma cells leave via the efferent lymphatics and migrate to the bone marrow, while memory B cells either recirculate or remain in residual follicles. The retention of antigen in selected sites such as lymphoid follicles may be important in the maintenance of immunological memory. Memory/effector T cells recirculate through the lymphatic system or migrate to 'tertiary' lymphoid organs. These may be anywhere in the body but are principally in the skin and mucosa of the pulmonary, genitourinary and gastrointestinal tracts.

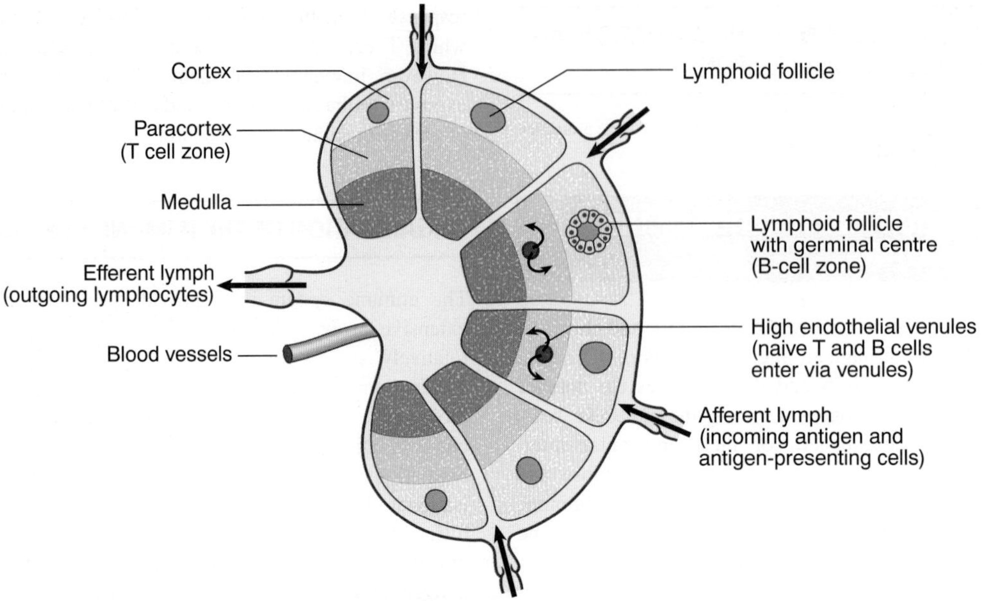

Fig. 1.23 Cartoon of lymph node indicating lymphocyte trafficking.

LYMPHOCYTE POPULATIONS

The expression of clonally distributed receptors for the recognition of antigen is characteristic of both B and T lymphocytes and underlies their vast range of specificities. They also display extensive heterogeneity in function. While the properties of B cells are, in general, restricted to immunoglobulin (Ig) synthesis and antigen presentation, functional differences are reflected in the various antibody isotypes. From their expression of either the CD4 or CD8 coreceptors, T cells can be segregated broadly into regulatory (CD4+) and effector/cytotoxic (CD8+) T cells. T cells can also be categorised by their receptor complement (αβ and γδ). αβ cells play a key role in the adaptive immune response whereas γδ cells have an additional response in epithelial defence.

RECEPTORS

Antigen-specific receptors

As regards B cells, cell-surface Ig functions as the antigen receptor. On activation, mediated by the binding of native antigen together with signals derived from helper T (T_H) cells, B cells differentiate into plasma cells producing antibody with the same specificity as their initial surface receptor. In contrast to B cells which bind native antigen, T cell antigen receptors (TCR), expressed on both T_H and cytotoxic (T_C) cells, recognise antigen as peptide fragments associated with products encoded by the major histocompatibility gene complex (MHC; see Fig. 1.24) which, together with costimulatory signals, results in cytokine production and clonal expansion.

Immunoglobulin

There are five distinct classes of Ig molecule (IgM, IgD, IgG, IgA and IgE), made up of four polypeptide chains, each with two identical light (L) and heavy (H) chains. Each L chain pairs with an H chain, and the two H chains are joined together by disulphide bonds. This allows the formation of two identical antigen-binding sites, which consist of variable regions located at the amino termini (see Fig. 1.25). For different Igs the variable regions have different sequences, with three regions of hypervariability, which confer their unique specificity. The constant regions of the H chains, termed the Fc fragment, determine the functional properties of the different Ig isotypes. Membrane Ig forms a complex with two other chains, CD79α and CD79β, that are required for intracellular signalling through their association with protein tyrosine kinases (PTKs).

T cell antigen receptors (TCRs)

Each TCR consists of two paired polypeptide chains (α and β or γ and δ) containing a variable region, which forms the antigen binding site, and a constant domain located towards the membrane region of the molecule. The αβ and γδ heterodimers are expressed on the T cell surface associated

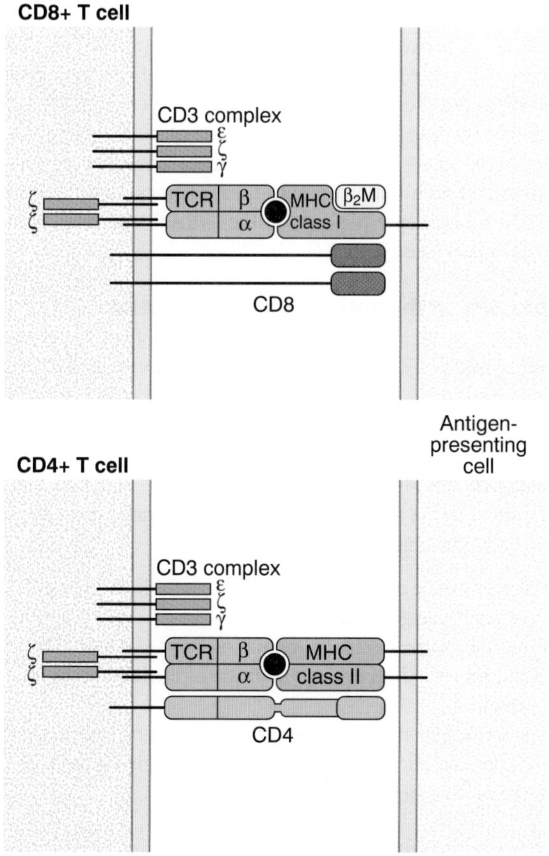

Fig. 1.24 CD8+ and CD4+ T cells recognise peptide fragments of antigen bound to gene products of the major histocompatibility gene complex (MHC).

with chains of the CD3 complex (CD3 γ, δ, ε and dimers of ζ:ζ or ζ:η; see Figs 1.24 and 1.25). Ligation of the TCR results in phosphorylation of CD3ζ and the subsequent activation of intracellular signalling pathways.

Coreceptors

CD19, CD21 and CD81 together form the coreceptor on B cells that binds to CD23 expressed on follicular dendritic cells and acts to amplify the signal delivered by antigen-binding.

The respective coreceptors for T_H and T_C cells are CD4 and CD8. CD4 is a single-chain molecule, which binds to an invariant region of the MHC class II molecule located away from the TCR binding site. The cytoplasmic domain of CD4 is associated with a PTK. CD8 has similar functions and synergises with TCR-mediated signalling, but unlike CD4 this molecule is heterodimeric and interacts with the invariant α3 domain of MHC class I molecules.

Major histocompatibility gene complex (MHC) encoded molecules

The principal function of MHC class I and II molecules is to bind and present antigenic peptides to the immune system. MHC class I (human leucocyte antigen (HLA)-A, -B and -C) molecules present antigenic peptides to CD8+ cells. Since the peptides are derived from proteins synthesised and processed in the cytoplasm, such as viral and tumour antigens, this is termed the endogenous pathway of antigen processing. In contrast, the peptides that MHC class II (HLA-DR, -DQ and -DP) molecules (see Fig. 1.26) present to CD4+ T cells are generated by the exogenous pathway of antigen presentation, namely from antigens internalised and degraded in acidified intracellular vesicles. The overall structure of the peptide-binding site for both MHC class I

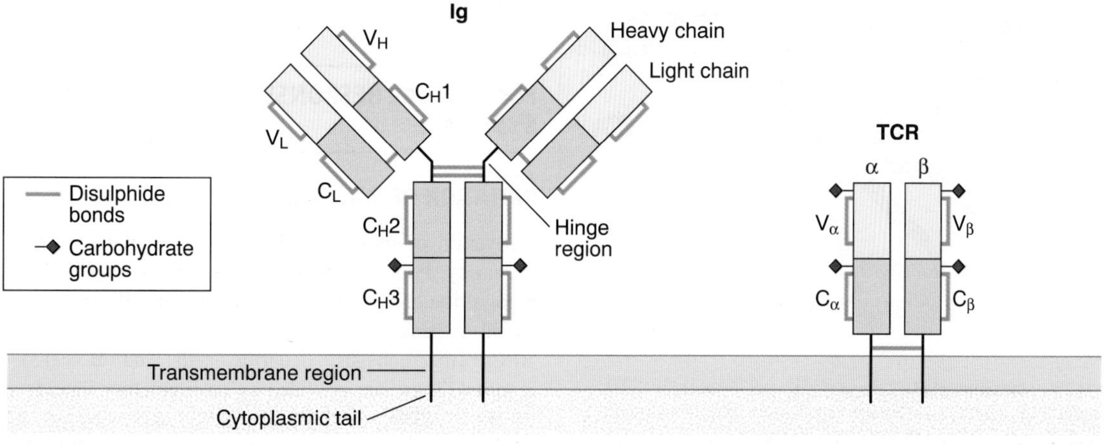

Fig. 1.25 Schematic diagram of the structures of B cell (Ig) and T cell (TCR) antigen receptors. (V = variable domain; C = constant domain)

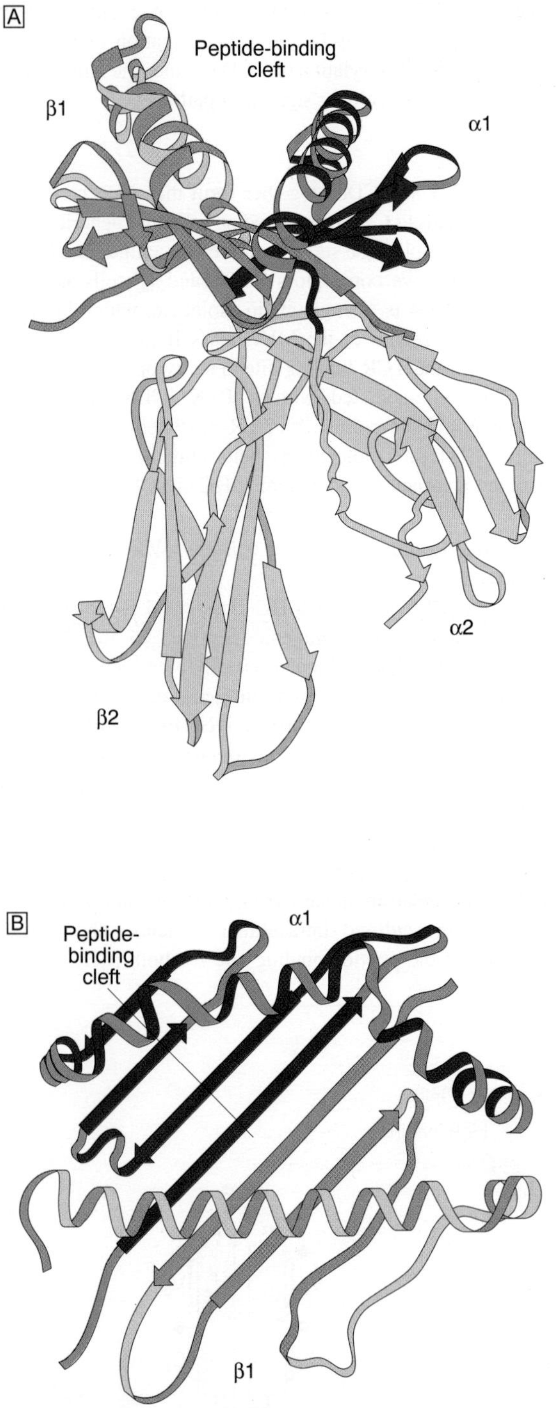

Fig. 1.26 Structure of MHC class II. A The α chain is associated with a β chain, and the α_1 and β_1 domains form the antigen binding site. B Aerial view of the antigen binding site.

and class II is similar. Each comprises a cleft formed by helical walls overlaying a floor of β sheets (e.g. MHC class II; see Fig. 1.26). Variability in amino acid residues located in both the floor and the walls of the cleft influences peptide binding and arises as a result of polymorphism in the MHC class I and II genes. Genes encoding proteins associated with the processing (proteasomes) and transport (TAP) of antigenic peptides in the cytosol also map in the MHC locus (see Fig. 1.27).

Diversity in the antigen-specific receptors

In order to recognise the vast array of potentially pathogenic microbes, B and T cells both express a broad repertoire of antigen-specific receptors that are clonally distributed and, thus, unique to each lymphocyte.

Antibody diversity

Diversity in the antibody repertoire is generated through the following mechanisms (see Fig. 1.28):

- the presence of multiple copies of variable (V) region genes in the germ line
- random somatic recombination of the V, diversity (D) and joining (J) genes and addition of nucleotides at the junctions
- somatic hypermutation: antigen restimulation selects for V region mutations that give the antibody higher affinity
- the pairing of heavy and light chains.

Diversity in TCRs

With the notable exception of somatic hypermutation, similar mechanisms operate to generate diversity in the TCR repertoire. Rearrangement occurs between the V, D and J gene segments for TCR-β chains and V and J for α chains; additional J and D segments allow greater diversity in the TCR antigen binding site. Thus the overall degree of diversity of the Ig and TCR repertoires is comparable.

FUNCTIONAL RESPONSES OF THE IMMUNE SYSTEM

INITIATION OF IMMUNE RESPONSES

Activation of naive T cells by APCs initiates productive immunity. Following adhesion between T cells and APCs, recognition of specific antigen alone is insufficient to induce clonal expansion. Additional costimulatory signals from APCs (macrophages, dendritic cells and B cells) are required. These are provided by costimulatory ligands such as B7.1 (CD80) and B7.2 (CD86) expressed on APCs binding to their counter-receptors on T cells (CD28 and CTLA-4) (see Fig. 1.29). Subsequent clonal expansion of T cells is driven by up-regulation of specific cytokines and

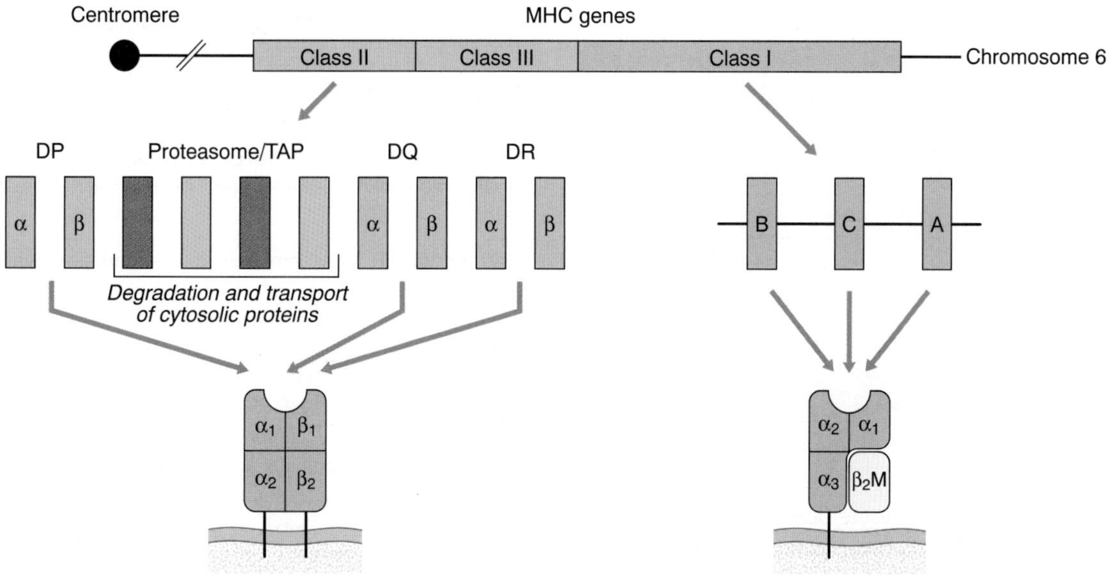

Fig. 1.27 The human major histocompatibility complex (HLA). Genes within the class III locus encode TNF-α, complement and other molecules of immunological interest. (TAP = transporters associated with antigen processing)

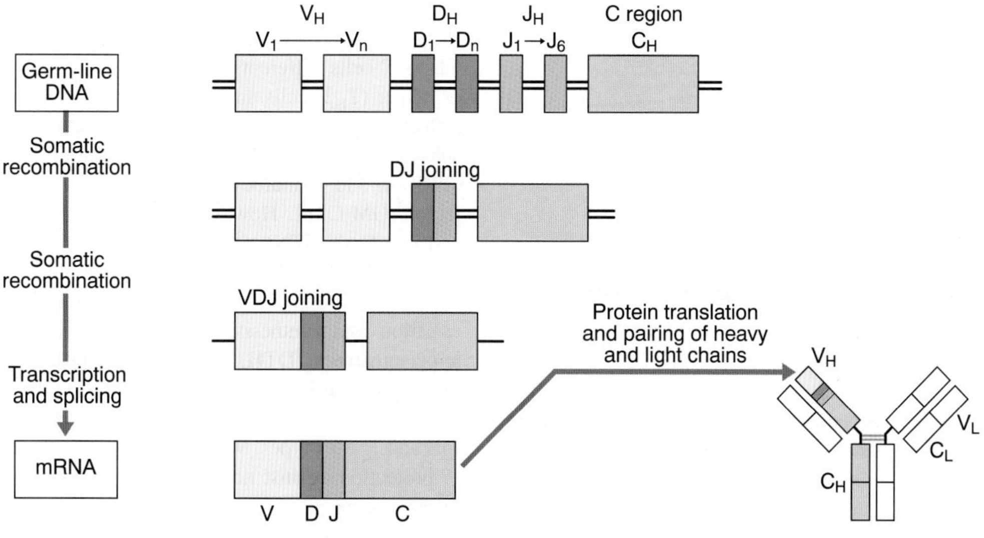

Fig. 1.28 Generation of diversity in the antibody repertoire. The example given is for the Ig heavy chain.

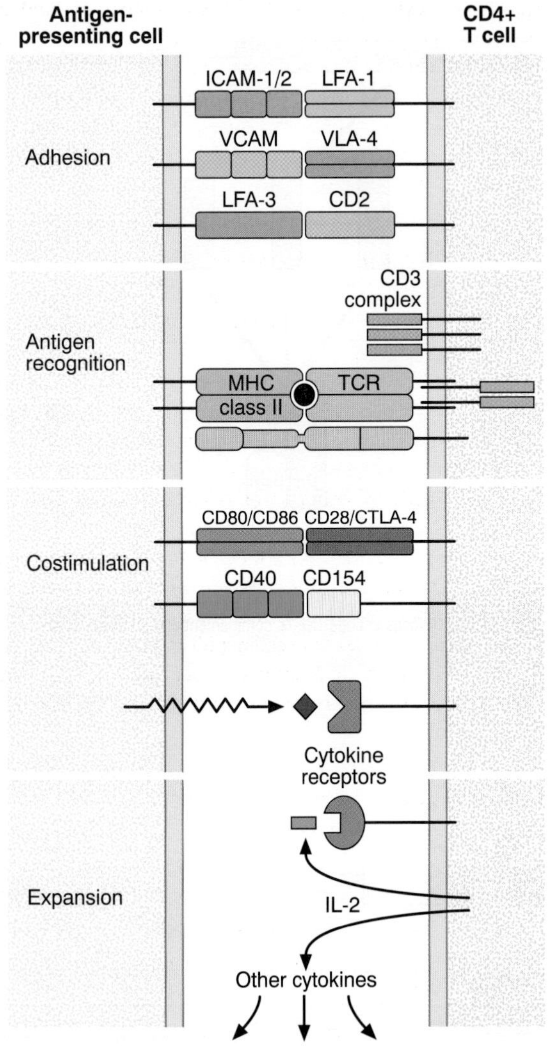

Fig. 1.29 CD4+ T cell activation and the initiation of the immune response.

their receptors. Recognition of MHC class II/peptide complexes in the absence of costimulation leads to functional inactivation of the T cells, which is termed anergy.

HUMORAL IMMUNITY

The principal components of humoral immunity are antibodies and the complement system. Antibody synthesis in response to most foreign antigens requires both the binding of antigen to surface Ig and the action of T_H cells. The activated B cells expand and differentiate, resulting in the production of high-affinity antibody and isotype switching. The interaction between CD40 ligand on T_H cells and CD40 on the B cells provides a costimulation which, together with cytokines, induces Ig isotype switching. Ig isotypes differ in their functions and tissue distribution (see the information box).

FUNCTION AND DISTRIBUTION OF THE MAIN HUMAN Ig ISOTYPES

- **IgM** Complement activation *(serum)*
- **IgG** Neutralisation, opsonisation and complement activation *(serum and extracellular fluid)*
- **IgA** Neutralisation *(secretions and mucosal surfaces)*
- **IgE** Sensitisation of mast cells *(skin and mucosa)*

Antibodies can neutralise pathogens both directly, by binding to specific surface structures, and indirectly through enhanced Fc receptor-mediated uptake by phagocytosis and complement activation. Components of the complement cascade contribute to the destruction of microbes in several ways. C3b binds to membrane receptors and opsonises bacteria, allowing them to be ingested by phagocytes. Pathogens may be lysed by creating pores in the membrane via the membrane attack complex. Other components of complement (C4a, C3a and C5a) act to recruit phagocytic cells to the site of infection.

T CELL-MEDIATED IMMUNITY

Helper (CD4+) T cells

CD4+ T cells differentiate into either inflammatory (T_H1) or helper (T_H2) cells and their distinct functional activities reflect differences in their cytokine secretion profiles. Both subsets produce interleukin (IL)-3, tumour necrosis factor (TNF)-α and granulocyte-macrophage colony stimulating factor (GM-CSF). However, T_H1 cells also produce IL-2 and interferon (IFN)-γ. These cytokines promote induction of cytotoxic T cells, the activation of macrophages and antibody (natural killer—NK) cells, and B cell differentiation and synthesis. They also mediate delayed-type hypersensitivity (DTH) responses and promote the killing of intracellular bacteria. In contrast, T_H2 cells secrete IL-4, IL-5 and IL-13, activate B cells and switch Ig synthesis to IgE and IgA isotypes. While T_H2-type cytokines contribute to protection against helminths, they also mediate allergic inflammation.

Cytotoxic (CD8+) T cells

CD8+ T cells produce cytotoxins (fragmentins and perforin) with which they eliminate tumour cells and target cells infected with viruses and other intracellular microorganisms. In addition, ligation of Fas and TNF receptors by CD8+ T cells may also induce apoptosis in the target cells. CD8+ cells secrete IFN-γ, which has antiviral activity, and in some instances TNF. Recent evidence suggests that some CD8+ T cells may display polarity in their cytokine profiles similar to T_H1 or T_H2 and are, therefore, termed T_C1 or T_C2 cells.

Cytokines and chemokines

Some of the cytokines associated with the different T cell subsets have been described above; however, with the exception of IL-2, cytokines are often made by several different cell types (see Table 1.4). They have shared characteristics in that they are antigen non-specific, synthesised and rapidly secreted and, in general, have short half-lives. Different cytokines may have overlapping activities. Their primary function is to regulate immune responses.

Cytokine receptors can be categorised into four families, namely:

- the Ig superfamily (e.g. IL-1)
- the haemopoietic receptor family (e.g. IL-2, erythropoietin and GM-CSF)
- the TNF receptor family (TNF receptors I and II)
- the chemokine receptor family (see below).

Chemokines are secreted proteins that regulate the host defence systems to inflammation. They can be divided into major families based on the presence of conserved cysteine residues. The CXC family (e.g. interferon-γ-inducible protein 10 (IP-10) and IL-8) are chemoattractants for neutrophils, while the CC chemokines (e.g. RANTES, macrophage inflammatory protein (MIP)-1α, MIP-1β and monocyte chemoattractant protein (MCP)-1, MCP-2 and MCP-3) attract monocytes and T cells. Most chemokines bind to more than one receptor; receptors are seven transmembrane molecules linked to G-proteins. Several subtypes of receptor have been identified and form two major families, termed CXCR and CCR, which are differentially expressed on leucocytes and display distinct patterns of chemokine binding.

IMMUNE-MEDIATED MECHANISMS OF DISEASE

Type I hypersensitivity reactions—antibody-mediated

Type I anaphylactic reactions are mediated by IgE antibodies, the production of which is dependent on T_H2 cytokines, that bind to high-affinity receptors (FcεRI) on mast cells and basophils (see Table 1.5). Subsequent cross-linking of FcεRI by antigen triggers degranulation and the release of a range of mediators (e.g. histamine, prostaglandins and leucotrienes), which produce the immediate symptoms typical of this response—namely, increased vascular permeability and smooth muscle constriction. The release of cytokines leads to eosinophil recruitment. The site of mast cell activation determines whether there is a local response (such as allergic rhinitis) or systemic anaphylaxis.

Type II hypersensitivity reactions—antibody-mediated cytotoxicity

In type II hypersensitivity reactions, specific antibodies

Table 1.4 Some of the major cytokines and their functions

Cytokine	Produced by	Actions
IL-1	Macrophages and other cell types	Fever, T cell and macrophage activation
IL-2	T cells (T_H1)	T cell growth factor and NK cell activation
IL-3	T cells	Growth of haemopoietic and mast cells
IL-4	T cells (T_H2) and mast cells	Growth of B and T cells and IgE isotype switching
IL-5	T cells (T_H2) and mast cells	Growth of B cells, IgA isotype switching and differentiation of eosinophils
IL-6	T cells, macrophages and other cell types	B, T and haemopoietic cell growth and differentiation
IL-7	Stromal cells	Growth of pre-B and T cells
IL-8	Many cell types	Chemotactic for neutrophils and T cells
IL-9	T cells	Mast cell activation
IL-10	T cells (T_H2) and macrophages	Inhibits immune function
IL-12	B cells and macrophages	Activates NK cells and promotes differentiation of T_H1 cells
IL-13	T cells (T_H2)	Growth of B cells and IgE isotype switch
IL-15	Macrophages and other cell types	Growth of T cells
IFN-γ	T cells, NK cells and other cell types	Antiviral activity and activation of NK cells, CD8+ T cells and macrophages
TGF-β	T cells, monocytes and other cell types	Anti-inflammatory activity, inhibits differentiation of T_H1 cells
TNF-α	Macrophages, monocytes and T cells	Pro-inflammatory
GM-CSF	T cells and monocytes	Growth of precursors for mast cells, granulocytes, monocytes and macrophages

See also Figure 11.2, page 739.

Table 1.5 Types of immune-mediated tissue injury

	Immediate			Delayed
	Type I	**Type II**	**Type III**	**Type IV**
Immune mechanism	IgE, T_H2 cells	IgG and IgM antibodies reactive with cell surface molecules or receptors	Immune complexes	T cells T_H1, CD4+ and CD8+ cells
Mechanism of tissue injury	Mast cell activation and release of mediators—vasoactive amines, prostaglandins, leucotrienes and cytokines	Complement activation, recruitment and activation of phagocytic and NK cells	Complement activation, recruitment and activation of phagocytic cells	Macrophage activation, T cell-derived cytokines and CD8+ T cell-mediated cytotoxicity
Examples	Systemic anaphylaxis and atopic disease	Transfusion and drug-induced reactions	Serum sickness, farmers' lung	Graft rejection, contact dermatitis and tuberculoid leprosy

bind to cell-surface or extracellular matrix molecules. Cell lysis results from complement activation or Fc or C3b receptor-mediated opsonisation, leading to phagocytosis and destruction of the cell by macrophages and neutrophils. Cells with a lower capacity for complement regulation, such as red blood cells and platelets, are particularly susceptible.

Antibodies directed against cell-surface receptor molecules can also result either in loss of function (e.g. anti-acetylcholine receptors in myasthenia gravis) or in increased function (e.g. anti-thyroid-stimulating hormone antibodies in Graves' disease).

Type III hypersensitivity reactions—immune complex-mediated disease

Should the antigen be soluble, circulating aggregates of antibody and antigen (immune complexes) may arise. The deposition of immune complexes in tissues such as blood vessel walls may directly cause inflammation and tissue damage. In addition, immune complexes resulting from repeated exposure to antigen in the presence of pre-existing anti-IgG antibodies may activate complement (C3a and C5a), leading to increased vascular permeability and the recruitment of polymorphonuclear leucocytes, termed the Arthus reaction. Immune complex disease can also occur in response to a single immunisation with a pre-formed antibody. The recipient develops an antibody response against the foreign immunoglobulin, and immune complexes formed result in the picture of acute serum sickness until the foreign serum proteins are cleared.

Type IV hypersensitivity reactions—delayed-type hypersensitivity

Type IV delayed-type hypersensitivity (DTH) reactions are mediated by antigen-specific T cells with the appearance of a local inflammatory reaction 24–48 hours after a sensitised individual is challenged with antigen. Inflammatory T_H1 cells migrate to the site of injection, recognise peptide/MHC class II complexes on APCs and release cytokines such as IL-2, IFN-γ, TNF and other chemoattractants. The cytokines and chemokines lead to increased vascular permeability and the recruitment and activation of macrophages and CD8+ cytotoxic T cells.

IMMUNODEFICIENCY DISEASES

Primary immunodeficiency diseases

Primary or inherited immunodeficiency diseases may affect one or multiple components of the immune system, including B cells, T cells, macrophages, NK cells and complement (see Table 1.6). They are characterised by increased susceptibility to infection and often an increased incidence of autoimmunity, malignancy and elevated levels of IgE. The definition of the molecular basis of primary immunodeficiency diseases has proven valuable in diagnosis, and has potential in gene therapy (see p. 54). Currently, disorders resulting in severe combined immunodeficiency (SCID) rely on conventional treatments such as bone marrow transplantation or enzyme replacement therapy.

Acquired immunodeficiency diseases

A variety of agents, such as drugs, irradiation, ultraviolet light and certain pathogens, may cause acquired immunodeficiency disorders. However, of these diseases chronic infection with human immunodeficiency virus (HIV), which causes acquired immune deficiency syndrome (AIDS), is a health-care problem of catastrophic proportions. During the initial acute infectious phase, which has influenza-like symptoms, the immune response controls but does not clear the infection. The expression of CD4 allows binding of HIV by the surface glycoprotein gp120 (see Fig. 1.33, p. 43), but entry into the cell is mediated by chemokine receptors such as CCR5 and CCR2. Persistent infection follows and, through the deletion of CD4+ T cells and accompanying reduction in antibody and cytotoxic T-cell (CTL) responses, immunity decreases and the host becomes more susceptible to opportunistic infections. In addition, loss

Table 1.6 Inherited immunodeficiency diseases

Defects affecting	Disorder	Immune deficiency	Susceptibility
B cells	X-linked agammaglobulinaemia	No antibody; loss of B cell-specific tyrosine kinase	Extracellular bacteria
	X-linked hyper-IgM	No IgG, IgA; defect in CD40 ligand; no Ig isotype switching	Extracellular bacteria
	Selective IgA deficiency	No IgA	Respiratory infections
	Selective Ig subclass deficiencies	Ig heavy or light chain deletions	Various infections
	Common variable immunodeficiency	Defective antibody production	Extracellular bacteria
	Wiskott–Aldrich syndrome	No antibody responses to polysaccharides	Encapsulated extracellular bacteria
T cells	Di George's syndrome	No T cells; thymic aplasia	Bacteria and viruses
	X-linked lymphoproliferative syndrome	Abnormal response to Epstein–Barr virus (EBV) infection	
B and T cells	Severe combined immunodeficiency	Defective cytokines, e.g. X-linked SCID (IL-2 Rγ deficiency) IL-2 or Jak3 deficiency (autosomal recessive) Defective TCR, e.g. CD3 mutations (autosomal recessive) Recombinase deficiency (autosomal recessive) Other Adenosine deaminase (ADA) deficiency Purine nucleotide phosphorylase (PNP) deficiency (autosomal recessive)	Bacteria, viruses and other pathogens
HLA	HLA class I	No surface expression of HLA class I; no CD8+ T cells; mutations in TAP genes	Viruses
	Bare lymphocyte syndrome (HLA class II)	No surface expression of HLA class II; no CD4+ T cells; defective antibody production	Bacteria and viruses
Phagocytes	Integrins	Prevent cell adhesion and migration	Extracellular bacteria
	G6PD deficiency	Defect in respiratory burst	
	Myeloperoxidase deficiency		
NK cells	Associated with SCID and X-linked lymphoproliferative syndrome	Impairs allograft rejection	Viruses
Complement	Different components (C1–C8, factor D and factor P)	Defect in specific complement components	Pyogenic bacteria *Neisseria* spp. infection

of effective immunity may occur from the generation of viral escape mutants and modification of the amino-acid sequence of critical T cell epitopes which fail to be presented or shift the immune response to the non-protective T_H2 pathway.

AUTOIMMUNITY

Autoimmune diseases arise when immune responses, either antibodies or T cells directed against self-antigens, cause tissue damage. The aetiology of these diseases is multifactorial, involving both environmental and genetic influences (see Fig. 1.30, p. 38). Susceptibility to many autoimmune diseases is linked to specific HLA genotypes and is more commonly associated with HLA class II rather than class I expression (see Table 1.7).

Both humoral and cell-mediated immunity may contribute to the tissue damage that occurs in autoimmune diseases but to varying degrees, as illustrated in the following examples.

Rheumatoid arthritis is characterised by local inflammation and destruction of the joint. The synovial membrane is infiltrated by CD4+ T cells, activated B cells, polymorphonuclear leucocytes and macrophages. Cytokines, including IL-1, IL-15, TNF-α and IFN-γ, can be detected in synovial fluid. In clinical trials treatment with anti-TNF-α antibody has been reported to have transient therapeutic effects. In addition to T cell activity, antibodies, predominantly IgM anti-IgG autoantibodies, are generated and form immune complexes, which lead to complement activation and further tissue damage. In rheumatoid arthritis, as with many other autoimmune diseases, the target antigens remain ill-defined.

Systemic lupus erythematosus (SLE) is a systemic autoimmune disease, in which immune complexes are formed

Table 1.7 HLA association and susceptibility to autoimmune diseases

Disease	HLA association	Relative risk
Myasthenia gravis	DR3	~ 5
Graves' disease	DR3	~ 5
Systemic lupus erythematosus	DR3	~ 5
Insulin-dependent (type 1) diabetes mellitus	DR3 and DR4	~ 20
Rheumatoid arthritis	DR4	~ 5
Ankylosing spondylitis	B27	~ 90

Note With the exception of ankylosing spondylitis these display female predominance (ranging from 2 x to 10 x female:male ratio).

between antinuclear (IgG) antibodies and their target antigens (DNA, ribonucleoprotein, histones and ribosomes). These may become trapped in arteriolar walls and induce inflammatory responses such as glomerulonephritis, arthritis and vasculitis affecting small arteries throughout the body.

Insulin-dependent diabetes mellitus (type 1, IDDM) is an organ-specific autoimmune disease and appears to be caused by autoreactive T cells, both CD4+ and CD8+ T cells, which together with macrophages infiltrate and destroy the β cells of the islets of Langerhans. Autoantibodies against islet cells are also detectable and may be present years before the onset of disease. Autoimmune haemolytic anaemia is caused by antibodies reactive with Rh or I antigens on the surface of red blood cells. The autoantibodies adhere to the red blood cells, which are then lysed by complement or destroyed through Fc receptor- and complement-mediated phagocytosis.

Myasthenia gravis is also an example of antibody-mediated autoimmunity in which antibodies reactive with the α chain of the acetylcholine receptor inhibit reception of the nerve impulse through enhanced internalisation and degradation of the receptors at the neuromuscular junction.

Mechanisms of autoimmunity

Tolerance to self-antigens occurs by deletion of self-reactive B and T cells during their maturation in the bone marrow and thymic environments. Recognition of peptide/MHC complexes by peripheral T cells in the absence of costimulatory signals elicits anergy and, therefore, may prevent the activation of potentially self-reactive T cells in the periphery. Similarly, clonal expansion of autoreactive cells may be inhibited by regulatory (suppressor) T cells, which produce immunosuppressive cytokines, such as TGF-β, IL-10 and IL-4. In addition, some tissues (for example, the eye and the brain) are termed immunologically privileged sites, since they do not normally encounter immunocompetent cells. In these situations self-antigen may be inaccessible or present in such low quantities as to trigger an immune response.

If these mechanisms fail then autoimmune disease may occur. The events that trigger autoimmune disease in many instances are not known. However, it is thought that infection may induce autoimmune disease in those individuals who are genetically susceptible. This may lead to increased or aberrant expression of costimulatory molecules and so change the antigenicity of the infected tissue, such that it now becomes a target of the immune response. In addition, or alternatively, T cells and antibodies generated in response to the infectious agent may cross-react with self-antigens, a mechanism termed molecular mimicry. A good example is rheumatic fever where streptococcal cell wall antigen-induced antibodies cross-react with cardiac muscle. It is also possible that superantigens, such as bacterial toxins which stimulate families of T cells expressing a particular TCR-Vβ segment, may induce autoreactive T cells that are normally present but in too few numbers to cause disease. Thus, possible associations between TCR-Vβ-specific T cells and autoimmune diseases have been investigated.

TRANSPLANTATION

The transplantation of organs to replace those that are terminally diseased has become commonplace. Invariably (unless between monozygotic twins), the HLA type of the graft and recipient are mismatched (termed allograft), which induces a vigorous immune response estimated at up to 5% of the T cell repertoire, with both HLA class I and II molecules acting as targets. Although compatibility of HLA loci improves graft survival, immunosuppression with drugs is nevertheless still required. Otherwise, an allograft, though initially accepted, will be rejected during the next 2 weeks (first set rejection). If tissue from the same donor is regrafted into the recipient, rejection is accelerated and occurs within 2–3 days (second set rejection). Rejection is mediated by both CD4+ and CD8+ T cells. In some instances, hyperacute graft rejection may occur (within a few hours) and is mediated by pre-existing antibodies which bind to vascular endothelial cells and activate complement.

In order to address the problem of the shortage of human organs for transplantation, the use of animal organs (xenografts) is under consideration. Attention has focused on the pig because of the similarities in the anatomy and physiology of some organs to their human counterparts. Although T cell responses to xenografts may be less vigorous than allografts, the presence of antibodies that react with endothelial cells on the graft results in the activation of the complement system and hyperacute graft rejection ensues. Since complement regulatory proteins are species-specific, they fail to protect xenogeneic endothelial cells from attack by human complement. The application of transgenesis (see Fig. 1.44, p. 53) may allow this and other problems of xenotransplantation to be resolved by genetically modifying antigens.

TUMOUR IMMUNOLOGY

The concept of immune surveillance—namely, that the immune system detects and destroys tumours that arise continually in the normal host as the result of somatic mutation—remains in dispute. Nevertheless, in some instances, recognition of tumour-specific transplantation antigens (TSTA), which are specific to tumours of a particular type, can induce immune responses and subsequent rejection of the tumour. These should be distinguished from tumour-associated antigens (TAAs), which arise from over-expression of gene products present in normal cells. The antitumour activity of humoral immune responses in vivo is unclear. CD8+ T_C cells, NK cells, lymphokine-activated killer (LAK) cells and activated macrophages may play a more important role.

Certain tumours continue to grow despite the presence of a competent immune system. There are several possible mechanisms by which they may avoid or resist destruction by the immune system. Some tumours may fail to generate and present the appropriate antigens or costimulatory ligands for T cell recognition and activation. Tumour cells may become less immunogenic by losing their antigens through gene mutation and down-regulating expression of MHC molecules. Other means of inhibiting immune responses could include induction of suppressor T cells or secretion of immunosuppressive mediators.

To date, immunotherapy has not made a major impact on the treatment of human tumours. Antibody-based approaches, such as the administration of anti-idiotypic antibodies in the treatment of B lymphomas, or antibodies specific to tumour or tumour vasculature antigens have been tested in clinical trials with variable success. Other approaches focus on increasing the immunogenicity of tumours by the transfection of genes for costimulatory ligands or cytokines. This may facilitate the induction of protective immunity.

MODULATION OF IMMUNE RESPONSES

IMMUNOSUPPRESSION BY DRUGS OR ANTIBODIES

In diseases generated by an excessive or inappropriate immune response, immunosuppressive drugs provide the basis of current treatment regimens. However, drugs such as cyclophosphamide, methotrexate and corticosteroids have broad-spectrum activity, and therefore disrupt the function of many cell types. Furthermore, prolonged treatment with many of these drugs is associated with an increased incidence in B cell lymphomas and other malignant disease.

Cyclosporin, which is derived from a soil fungus, and the structurally dissimilar drug FK506 are now used to suppress the rejection of allografts. They both act by binding to calcineurin and inhibiting signalling pathways leading to IL-2 synthesis.

Antilymphocyte serum has beneficial effects in acute graft rejection but, due to its lack of specificity for only alloreactive cells, has limited value. The role of antibodies reactive with TCR, coreceptors (CD4 and CD8), costimulatory molecules (CD80 and CD86) and adhesion molecules in modulating autoimmune disease and graft rejection are being investigated in experimental models. In clinical trials the therapeutic effects of anti-CD4 antibodies have been generally limited.

VACCINE DEVELOPMENT

The potential to prevent disease by inducing immunity through vaccination remains an important area of research in medicine. There is a need both to generate vaccines for those diseases where at present none exists, such as AIDS, and to improve the efficacy of other vaccines that are currently in use, e.g. for influenza.

Of the different features required for an ideal vaccine (see the first information box), safety and protection are perhaps the most important elements.

The design of potential vaccines is greatly influenced by the qualitative nature of the immune response (cell-mediated or humoral immunity) required to mediate protection. To meet these specific needs, different approaches have been adopted (see the second information box). Furthermore, the route of administration may also be important and, where down-regulation of the immune response is required, delivery via the mucosal surfaces of the gastrointestinal and respiratory tracts is an effective way of inducing immunological tolerance.

CHARACTERISTICS OF EFFECTIVE VACCINES
Safety
• No disease must be caused by the vaccine itself
Protection
• Protection must be at the population level and prevent disease when the infectious agent is encountered
Long-lasting effects
• Protection must be long-lasting, i.e. induce T and B cell memory
Cost
• Inexpensive to produce and deliver
Administration
• Easy to deliver with no side-effects

APPROACHES TO VACCINE DESIGN
Intact pathogen
• Heat-killed or chemically denatured • Attenuated by growth conditions or genetic manipulation
Subunit vaccines
• Recombinant proteins • Synthetic peptides
Vaccine vehicles
• Live vectors: viral (e.g. adenovirus) and bacteria (e.g. mycobacteria)
Adjuvants
• Conjugated to lipid or protein carrier molecules • Microencapsulated in lipids
DNA immunisation
• Injection of plasmid DNA

FURTHER INFORMATION ON ORGANISATION AND FUNCTION OF THE IMMUNE SYSTEM

See Current Opinions in Immunology, Annual Review of Immunology, Immunology Today

GENETICS AND DISEASE

HUMAN GENETICS

OVERVIEW

Individuals inherit a unique pattern of DNA sequences. Much of the variation in DNA occurs in non-coding regions and is of no direct relevance to development and function. Other variants occur within genes leading to a different protein product. If a particular variation results in sufficient impairment of protein function to bring about a deleterious effect, a genetic disease may result. We can only recognise diseases in which the genetic abnormality has been sufficiently 'mild' to permit early development; other genetic abnormalities may impair such vital processes that embryogenesis cannot proceed. The *genotype* of individuals refers to their genetic make-up, i.e. the sequence of their genes. The *phenotype* describes any aspect of structure, development or pathophysiology in an individual. Diseases may result from purely genetic, purely environmental factors or, more frequently, a combination of the two (see Fig. 1.30).

MUTATIONS AND POLYMORPHISMS

Definitions

These terms cause much confusion in the medical literature, as they can be defined in more than one way. Each refers to the different forms of a gene *(alleles)* which can be present in a population. As described on page 8, the term 'mutation' has been used to describe any permanent variation between template and daughter sequences in DNA polymerisation. The strict definition of a 'polymorphism' is that at least 1% of the population must have a different allele from the usual form. However, in the study of human disease, the same terms are used to distinguish two types of DNA variation, and have slightly different connotations. By convention, a *mutation* is recognised as a disease-causing DNA variation, whereas sequence changes which do not result in a disease state are referred to as *polymorphisms*, even if they occur in less than 1% of individuals.

Mutations

A disease-causing mutation is a variation in DNA sequence which alters the protein product in such a way as to contribute to a disease process. In the simplest sense, these mutations may be divided into two subgroups (see Fig. 1.31). Alteration of the genetic code accounts for most mutations and may result from the deletion of all or part of a gene, or a specific alteration of the genetic code. As a result, the encoded protein may be unable to function sufficiently due to lack of intrinsic activity or inefficient cellular

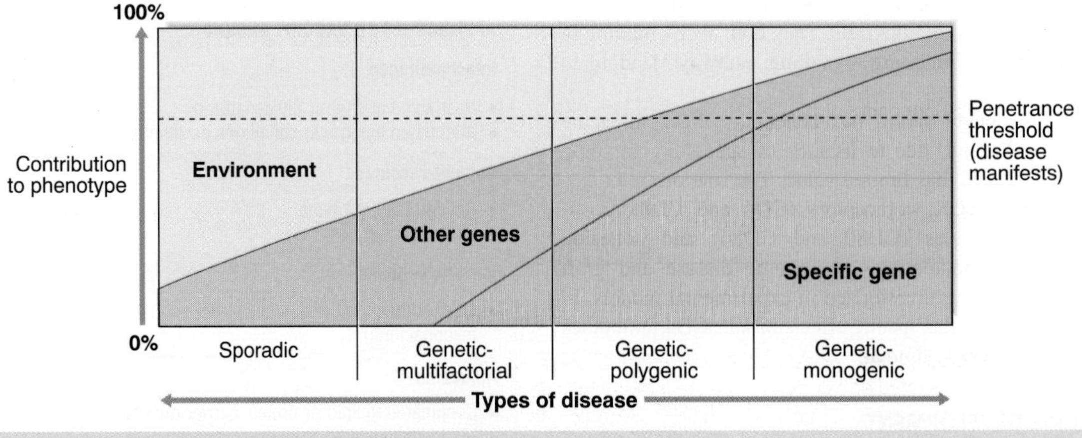

Fig. 1.30 The spectrum of genetic disease: how the genotype influences the phenotype. A particular characteristic or disease in an individual may be due to a specific genetic abnormality (monogenic disease), or may reflect several predisposing genes (polygenic disease). In each case, environmental factors may further influence the phenotype, and in their absence, genetic factors alone may be insufficient to allow the disease to develop, resulting in non-penetrance (see p. 41).

processing and transport mechanisms. Sometimes, the mutated protein may have a novel effect which means the normal copy is unable to function normally, the so-called 'dominant-negative' effect. Alternatively, a mutation may result in less RNA being available for translation into protein, either due to promoter region mutations reducing gene transcription, or to mutations in introns altering RNA stability.

Polymorphisms

Small DNA sequence changes may be functionally silent if they:

- are located in non-coding DNA (which constitutes the majority of the genome)
- do not alter the amino acid inserted in a given protein (for example, there are six serine codons)
- result in a novel amino acid which is able to perform the same function as the original, even if the two are distinguishable (e.g. polymorphisms at the ABO blood group and major histocompatibility loci).

INHERITANCE PATTERNS

Site of mutated gene and inheritance pattern

Dominant and recessive traits

The manner in which a mutated gene behaves is determined in the first instance by its chromosomal site. As alluded to in the section on cancer, the critical question is whether there is a second 'normal' copy of the gene which can compensate for the abnormal. This varies between genes according to their function and position; for example, there is no second copy of X or Y chromosome genes in men. Figure 1.32 illustrates the essential features of inheritance, the patterns of inheritance and the terminology used in describing family pedigrees. It shows the processes involving a single gene in a monogenic trait. However, the same principles of genotype inheritance, if not phenotypic manifestations, apply to genes involved in polygenic and multifactorial traits where the effects of more than one gene are required to generate disease.

It should be remembered that there is always the 'first'

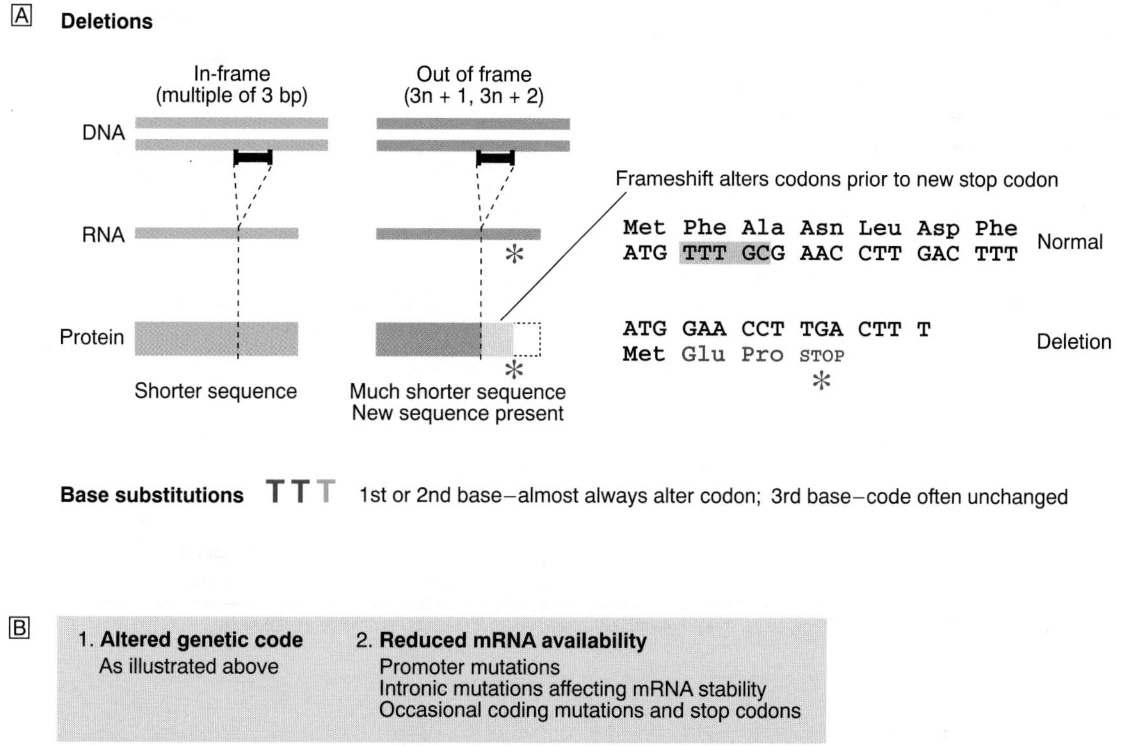

Fig. 1.31 Mutations. A Important types of mutation, illustrating molecular mechanism (deletions and base substitutions). B The effects of mutations on encoded proteins.

A

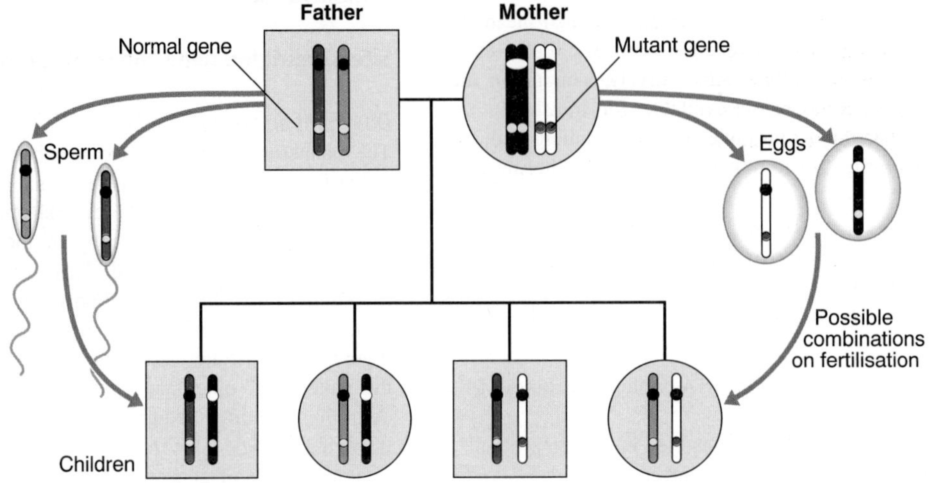

B

Autosomal inheritance (gene on chromosome 1–22)

X-linked inheritance (X chromosome gene)

Non-germline cytoplasmic inheritance (e.g. gene on mitochondrial DNA)

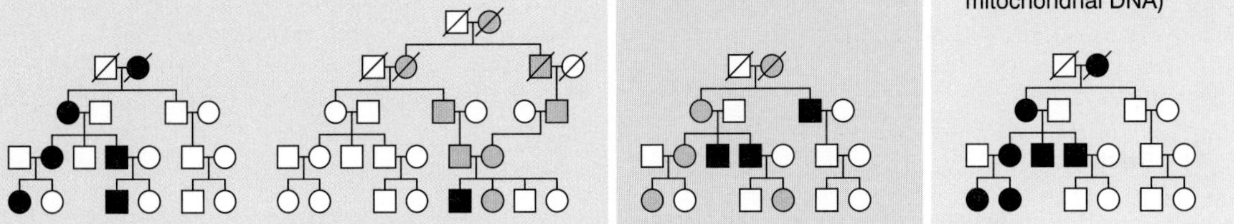

Dominant inheritance

The second copy of the gene on the homologous chromosome cannot compensate for the mutated copy:

- Consecutive generations affected
- Half of offspring affected, male = female
- Unaffected individual cannot transmit disease

Assuming full penetrance; see text

Recessive inheritance

The second copy of the gene on the homologous chromosome compensates for the mutated copy:

- Unaffected carrier individuals transmit disease
- If both parents are carriers, then one-quarter of their offspring are affected, and one-half are carriers
- Usually only one generation is affected

Affected individuals may have two identical mutant copies arising from a common ancestor as shown, or different in 'compound heterozygotes'

A second copy of the gene is only present in females. In X-linked recessive disease:

- Males only affected
- Unaffected female carriers transmit the disease
- All of carrier female's offspring inherit mutation —males are affected, and females are carriers
- Affected males cannot transmit the disease to their sons, but all of their daughters are carriers

X-linked diseases are occasionally dominant

- Males and females are affected
- No males transmit disease
- Variable proportion of offspring from female are affected

Fig. 1.32 Principles of inheritance. A Mendelian transmission of a single pair of autosomes, where the mother has a single mutant gene (red circle) on the chromosome drawn in white. B Inheritance of a mutant gene using conventional symbol designation (male: square; female: circle; unaffected: white; affected: black; unaffected carrier: stippled; deceased: strike-through), with characteristic features of resulting genetic diseases.

mutation in a particular family. If this is in a somatic cell in an individual, it will be passed on to a proportion of the tissues (generating a mosaic), but not to the offspring. If, however, the mutation arises in a germ-line cell which will generate sperm or oocytes, then the offspring of that individual may be affected even though no grandparent had the mutated gene.

Variations in the effects of mutations between different individuals and throughout successive generations

Penetrance

Individuals who inherit a particular mutation rarely demonstrate identical consequences, since they may not have the other genetic or environmental predisposition to unmask the full effect of the mutation in question. The mutation is said to be fully penetrant if all individuals who inherit the abnormality display a result (an altered phenotype). If additional environmental factors are needed, the gene may display late-onset penetrance, or may even be non-penetrant, if the individual is never exposed to sufficient additional factors (see Fig. 1.30, p. 38).

Epigenetics and imprinting

These are processes which alter the effect of a gene according to whether it lies on one or other of a chromosomal pair, and may result in a mutated gene resulting in different effects according to whether it was inherited from the mother or the father (see Table 20.5, p. 1131).

One example is the mechanism which inactivates one of the two X chromosomes in female cells to prevent the cell from having twice as much protein product of an X-linked gene as male cells. The X-inactivation centre recognises if more than one X chromosome is present, and after 15 days of embryogenesis, in each cell of the embryo, one of the X chromosomes is randomly selected to be condensed and inactivated. During subsequent cell divisions, X-chromosomes replicated from the inactivated chromosome are also inactivated. Both X chromosomes are active only in the female germ cells.

On other chromosomes, shorter stretches of DNA may be inactivated according to whether the chromosomal region was inherited from the individual's mother or father. The section of DNA is usually inactivated by the addition of a methyl group to cytosine on both DNA strands of the chromosome. Following DNA replication, the newly synthesised daughter strand is also methylated, hence all DNA derived from the methylated template will be 'imprinted'. Imprinted DNA leads to a modification of the chromatin scaffold, restricting the transcriptional activity of the imprinted gene. If an imprinted gene carries a mutation, then the manifestation of any resultant disease will vary according to which parent transmitted the mutation. For example, a critical region on chromosome 15 contains several genes in which only the paternal allele is transcriptionally active. Mutations in one or more of these genes are likely to contribute to the Prader–Willi syndrome, which results from a lack of a normal paternal contribution to the chromosome 15 region (see Table 20.5, p. 1131).

Trinucleotide repeats and genetic anticipation

An unusual genetic phenomenon was observed in a number of inherited neurological diseases, and was described as genetic anticipation, since the disease demonstrated increasing severity (as shown by earlier age of onset, or disease severity) during transmission through the generations. The mutation in these cases was shown to reside in a stretch of repetitive DNA sequence, altered not in sequence but in the number of repeat units present. Repeat sequences occur throughout the human genome and are key tools in gene mapping (see p. 50). Variation in their length may cause disease if they alter the sequence of the mature peptide—for example, by expansion of the [CAG] codon for glutamine, or if repeats (triplet and non-triplet) expand in non-coding regions, disturbing mRNA stability or DNA replication. The basis of the anticipation phenomenon is that the replication machinery tends to increase the number of repeats in offspring, with alleles inherited from a father expanding further. Examples are given in Table 20.6, page 1131.

POPULATION GENETICS

The basis of population genetics follows from simple statistical principles. If only two forms of an autosomal gene are possible, say the red and yellow circles in Figure 1.32, then all individuals will have either identical alleles and be homozygous (YY or RR), or two different alleles in a heterozygote (Y and R). Heterozygotes will be twice as common as homozygotes, since if a yellow- and red-sided coin were to be tossed twice, there would be twice as many chances of getting a heterozygote (Y then R, or R then Y) as a homozygote. This would be true, no matter how heavily the coin were 'weighted'. In population genetics terms, the coin is weighted by how common the particular allele is in the population. This is best understood by considering the Hardy–Weinberg equilibrium, in this case describing the situation if the yellow normal allele is found on 99% of chromosomes (gene frequency p = 0.99), and the red mutant allele on 1% (gene frequency q = 0.01):

All individuals will be	=	YY	or	RR	or	(YR)	or	(RY)
at a frequency of		*0.99 × 0.99*		*0.01 × 0.01*		*0.99 × 0.01*		*0.01 × 0.99*
i.e.	**1 =**	p^2	+	q^2	+	2(pq)		

A disease gene is virtually always less common in the population than the normal gene, so heterozygotes are more common than homozygotes. For example, as approximately 1 in 25 of the Caucasian population carries a mutant gene for cystic fibrosis, the gene frequency q is 0.04, hetero-

Table 1.8 Distribution of ABO blood groups as an illustration of a three-allele system

Phenotype	Genotype	Frequency	Combined frequency
Group O	OO	0.7^2	$0.7^2 = 0.49$
Group A	AA AO OA	0.2^2 0.2×0.7 0.7×0.2	$0.2^2 + 2(0.2 \times 0.7) = 0.32$
Group B	BB BO OB	0.1^2 0.1×0.7 0.7×0.1	$0.1^2 + 2(0.1 \times 0.7) = 0.15$
Group AB	AB BA	0.1×0.2 0.2×0.1	$2(0.1 \times 0.2) = 0.04$
All groups			$= 1$

zygote carriers will occur at a frequency of 8% (from $2 \times 0.04 \times [1 - 0.04]$), and homozygotes who have the disease, at a frequency of 0.16% $(0.04)^2$.

If there are three alleles, a three-sided dice tossed twice analogy is more appropriate, but the same principles apply: $1 = p^2 + q^2 + r^2 + 2(pq) + 2(pr) + 2(qr)$. An example of such a system is the ABO group, which is more complicated since blood group O is recessive to A and B, although it is the most common gene. If the gene frequencies are 0.7 (p, group O), 0.2 (q, group A) and 0.1 (r, group B), the incidences of particular blood groups in the population are as shown in Table 1.8.

Selection pressures and heterozygote advantage

Since polymorphisms do not result in major functional consequences, there are virtually no controls on the spread of a particular allele throughout the population. In contrast, the disease produced by a mutant gene may prevent the affected individual from reproducing and transmitting the gene. Thus dominant disease genes can only persist in the population if the disease phenotype is mild during the reproductive period of an individual, or by virtue of new mutations. In contrast, recessive genes can persist in the population, no matter how severe the phenotype in homozygotes, by virtue of the pool of normal carriers. Furthermore, there may be instances in which it is advantageous to have one copy of a recessive disease gene, so-called *heterozygous advantage*. The best-known example of this is the protection sickle-cell heterozygotes have against malaria, accounting for the high incidence of the mutated genes in malaria-endemic, but not malaria-free areas.

MOLECULAR FEATURES OF INFECTIVE DISEASE

OVERVIEW OF PROKARYOTES

Infectious agents demonstrate a vast repertoire of successful molecular strategies profoundly different from the mammalian (or to be precise, human) regulation which has been discussed so far. Prokaryotic cells do not possess a nucleus, and generally have smaller genomes than humans. For example, bacterial genomes are around 1/1000 to 1/10 000 the size of the human genome, and viral genomes a further two to three orders of magnitude smaller. However, the organisation of their genes is more elaborate than in humans, with the same stretch of bases coding for several genes reading in different directions, or in different frames. Instead of organisation into linear chromosomes, the DNA in many bacteria such as *Escherichia coli* is organised in a circular form. Different viral species use either DNA or RNA as their nucleic acid, and these may be linear or circular.

Although prokaryotes will be discussed in detail in Chapter 2, this section will be used to introduce two of the different mechanisms.

HIV—A RETROVIRUS WITH AN RNA GENOME

HIV, a member of the Lentivirinae subgroup of retroviruses, has an RNA genome, with each mature spherical HIV-1 particle containing two positive strands of viral RNA. These linear strands encode critical viral genes, as highlighted in Figure 1.33. In addition to RNA, the viral core contains reverse transcriptase, structural proteins derived from the *gag* gene, and additional regulatory proteins. The core is surrounded by a matrix and the entire structure enveloped by an outer lipid-bilayer membrane. Embedded in the membrane are proteins derived from the viral *env* gene (gp120 and gp41), and various immune molecules, especially MHC class II molecules derived on budding from a human cell. In part due to the high replication error rate of the reverse transcriptase, HIV-1 displays marked genetic variability, especially in the gp120 region, rendering vaccine development more difficult.

The virus recognises susceptible host cells via its high-affinity receptor, the CD4+ antigen, but fusion of viral and host cell membranes requires a co-receptor, such as CCR5 in initial infections. The virus then injects its RNA, gag and pol proteins, and DNA reverse-transcribed from the RNA template. The resultant double-stranded proviral DNA migrates to the nucleus where it uses the long terminal repeat sequences to integrate into the host chromosomes, particularly of replicating cells. According to the state of the cell and supply of factors activating the HIV promoter, the viral sequences may remain latent or be transcribed to produce viral proteins which assemble into new virions and bud from the cell surface. The consequences of such infection are discussed in Chapter 2.

The susceptibility of a particular individual to infection by HIV is in part determined by sequence variations in HIV co-receptors such as CCR5. Some accelerate and others delay disease progression. For example, some individuals (≈ 1% in Western Europe) who appear relatively resistant to HIV infection are homozygous for a 32 bp deletion

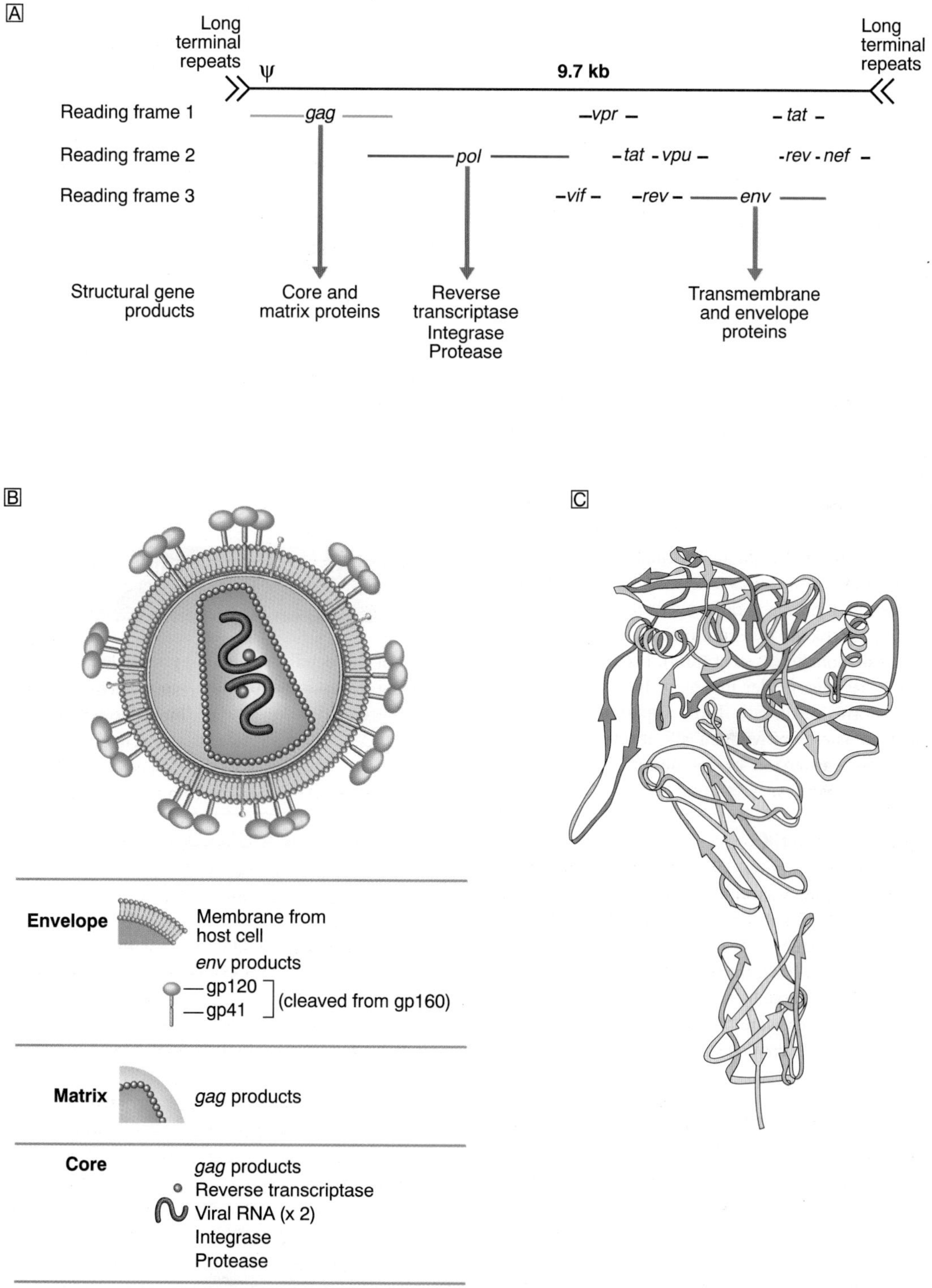

Fig. 1.33 The human immunodeficiency virus. A HIV genome ψ provides a signal for packaging DNA into a new virion. B HIV structure illustrating gene derivation of components. C Ribbon diagram of gp120 (blue) binding to CD4 (yellow).

(CCR5Δ32) and do not express a functioning CCR5 receptor. There appear to be no ill effects for European homozygotes, probably reflecting the fact that other receptors may compensate or that functioning CCR5 is only required for immunity against infections that are not endemic in temperate zones. In contrast to previous examples, this 'mutation' would therefore appear to be beneficial.

PRION DISEASES—THE RESULT OF AN INFECTIOUS PROTEIN SPECIES?

A group of inexorably progressive neurodegenerative conditions affecting several species are transmissible from affected individuals, though a long incubation period (averaging over 10 years in humans) is characteristic. In humans, the best-known forms are Creutzfeldt–Jakob disease (CJD) and kuru, the clinical consequences of which are discussed on page 1016. Further examples are given in Table 1.9.

The predominant if not sole component of the infectious particle is a protein, termed PrP. This is expressed in all mammalian brains as the soluble *c*ellular PrP^{C}, which becomes infectious if it acquires a new conformation rendering it insoluble, as in the *sc*rapie agent (PrP^{Sc}). Normally, PrP^{C} only rarely adopts this conformation (accounting for the occasional sporadic cases of CJD), but inherited mutations in the PrP gene render this more likely and result in the familial forms of disease. Most importantly, once one PrP^{Sc} molecule is present within a cell, it acts as a template to enhance the conversion of the normal PrP^{C} to PrP^{Sc}, resulting in pathogenesis.

The BSE story in the UK

Prior to 1980, the prion disease bovine spongiform encephalopathy (BSE) was virtually unknown in UK cattle populations, although scrapie, a similar disease affecting sheep, had been endemic for over 30 years and cattle were fed sheep derivatives. By 1987, there was a significant incidence of BSE, which was thought to be due to an alteration in feeding practices which were banned in 1988. Nevertheless, the incidence of BSE continued to rise, peaking in 1992. Currently, the disease persists, particularly in older cattle.

Initially, based on the scrapie experience, it was believed that a 'species barrier' prevented transmission of animal forms of prion disease to humans. However, since 1995 a surprising number of cases of CJD have been described in young adults in the UK, displaying atypical pathological features. The temporal association with the BSE outbreak led to speculation that humans may be infected with the BSE prion by eating infected beef. Such speculation is now increasingly supported by epidemiological, biochemical and molecular evidence of shared properties between the early-onset CJD cases and BSE.

FURTHER INFORMATION ON GENETICS AND DISEASE

See recent reviews in Cell, Nature, Nature Genetics and other specialised journals

INVESTIGATION OF THE MOLECULAR BASIS OF DISEASE

Much of the detailed technology involved in isolating and studying genes is beyond the scope of this chapter, but a basic introduction to some of the techniques used is given below.

BASIC TOOLS OF MOLECULAR ANALYSIS

KARYOTYPING

The earliest genetic methods studied morphological appearances of chromosomes associated with inherited disease. Human chromosomes are most conveniently studied in mitogen-stimulated peripheral blood lymphocytes in which cell division is arrested in metaphase when the chromosomes

Table 1.9 Examples of prion diseases

Species	Disease	Transmission	Cases
Humans	Kuru	Infectious (ritual cannibalism, New Guinea 1957–82)	≈ 2500
	Creutzfeldt–Jakob (CJD)	(a) Sporadic	1 in 10^6
		(b) Familial *(autosomal dominant)*	1 in 10^7
		(c) Infectious—from humans (e.g. pituitary growth hormone, dural grafts)	≈ 100
		—?from cows (atypical form, BSE association)	> 15
	Gerstmann–Sträussler–Scheinker	Familial *(autosomal dominant)*	Rare
	Fatal familial insomnia	Familial *(autosomal dominant)*	Rare
Sheep	Scrapie		
Cattle	Bovine spongiform encephalopathy (BSE)		

are condensed. The cells are swollen with a hypotonic solution, spread on microscope slides to separate the individual chromosomes and stained.

A classical favourite dye is Giemsa which preferentially binds to A-T base pairs resulting in the G-banded appearances visible in the metaphase spread (see Fig. 1.34). More recently, methods using fluorescent probes have been used (fluorescence in situ hybridisation, FISH), particularly to identify chromosomal translocations and locate the site of new genes (see Fig. 1.35). With the advent of chromosomal 'painting', where colour probes specific to each chromosome are used, it is likely that this will become a more routine method of analysis.

PREPARATION AND DETECTION OF DNA

DNA can be obtained readily from any nucleated cell by breaking open the cell with proteinases and detergents, removing non-DNA components using specific enzymes or lipid solvents such as phenol, and precipitating the DNA.

When suspended in solution, pure DNA is colourless and invisible, although the presence and concentration of DNA can be deduced by the absorption of light at a wavelength

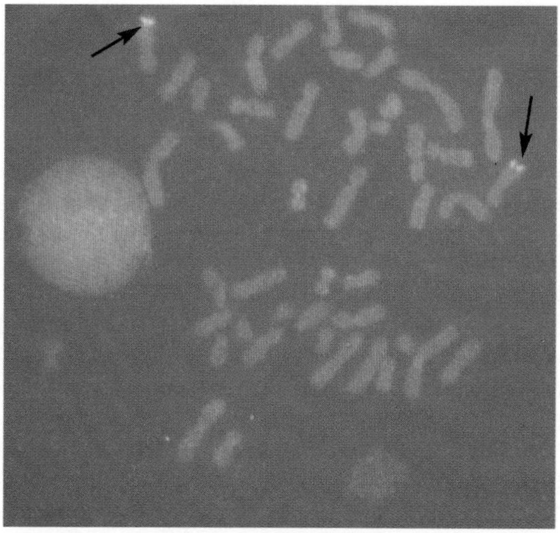

Fig. 1.35 Fluorescence in situ hybridisation (FISH). Fluorescent molecular probes hybridising to the tips of a chromosomal pair (arrows).

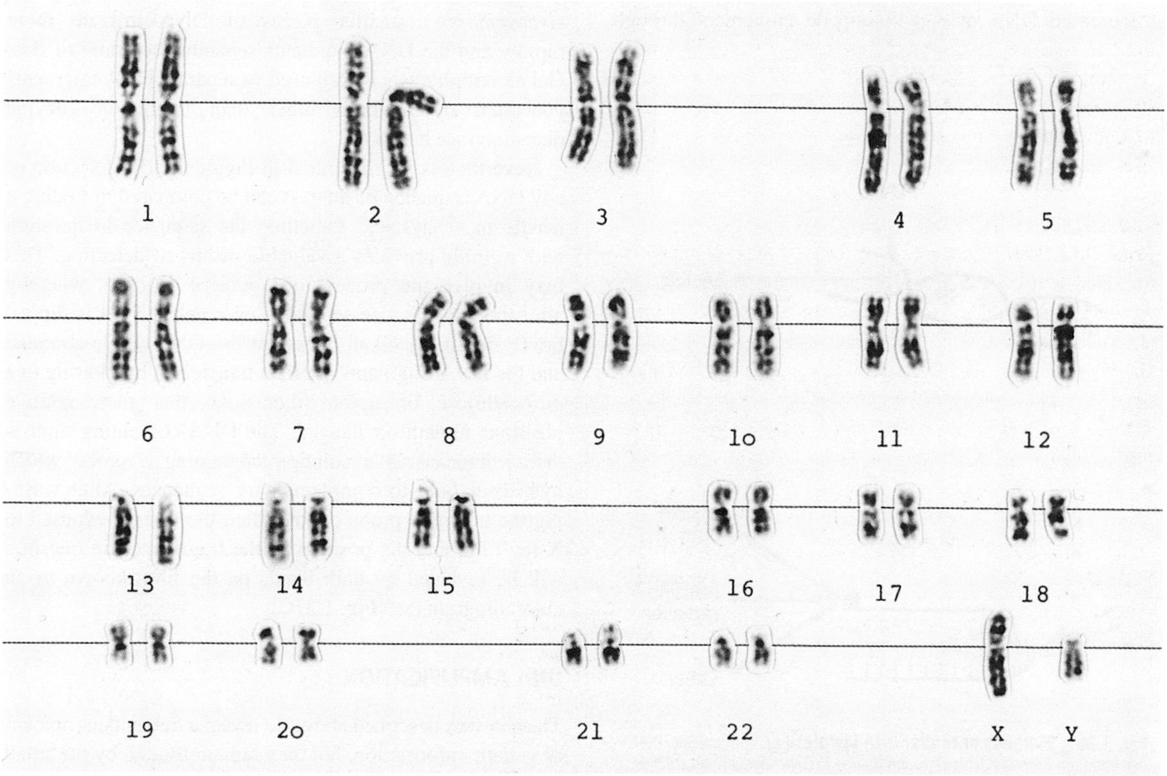

Fig. 1.34 Karyotype of a normal male on Giemsa banding (G-banding).

of 260 nm. However, it is usually more convenient to view DNA directly (see Fig. 1.36). Some methods are non-specific, such as ethidium bromide labelling. Most exploit the specific base-pair binding discussed on page 3 by use of a short stretch of DNA which is single-stranded and complementary to the DNA sequence under analysis. Such short single-stranded DNA molecules are referred to as 'probes' and are usually labelled to emit ionising radiation or fluorescent light.

Generation and analysis of short DNA fragments

Analysis of naturally occurring DNA is made difficult because DNA consists of a series of large molecules which are difficult to handle, and each cell provides only two copies of the sequence of interest in 6×10^9 base pairs.

To facilitate handling, DNA can be cut into smaller fragments using restriction endonucleases (see Fig. 1.37A). These enzymes cleave double-stranded DNA at a specific recognition site usually made up of a four or six base-pair sequence. Any change in the recognition site abolishes the ability of the restriction enzyme to cut the DNA. As these cleavage sites are specific, characteristic 'restriction fragment' sizes should result. This would still be of little benefit were it not for the fact that fragments of DNA can be separated easily. Since DNA is negatively charged, it will move towards the anode in an electric field, and as increased DNA mass will impede movement through gel solids such as agarose or acrylamide, during *gel electrophoresis* smaller pieces of DNA migrate more rapidly and the DNA fragments separate according to size. Gel electrophoresis is also used to separate DNA fragments generated by methods other than restriction enzyme digestion (see below).

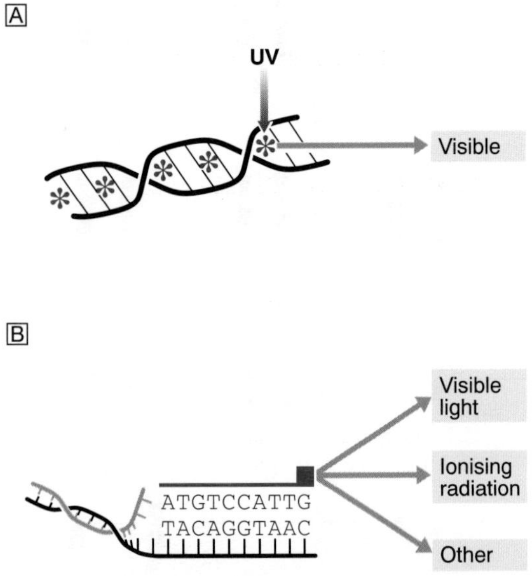

Fig. 1.36 Methods to render DNA visible. A Non-specific: the dye ethidium bromide binds non-specifically to DNA between the stacked bases, and fluoresces on exposure to UV light. B Specific labelling: short single-stranded DNA probes (modified to allow them to be traced) exploit specific base-pairing by binding to complementary sequences.

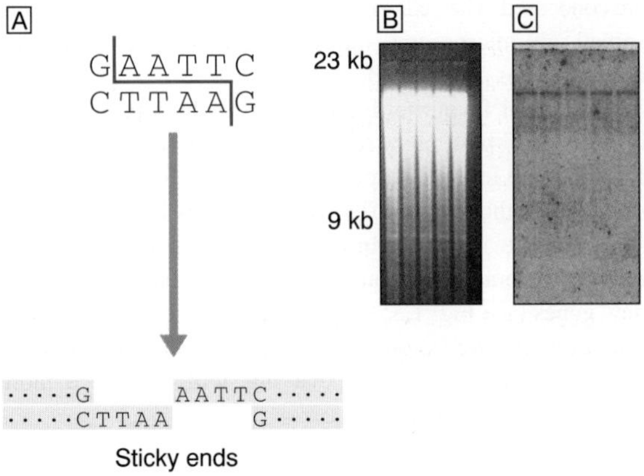

Fig. 1.37 Southern blotting (see text for method). A Digestion of genomic DNA with restriction enzyme *ECoRI*, which cleaves at the indicated site to generate homologous sticky ends. B *ECoRI* digestion of genomic DNA—huge numbers of different products, each of the same length, generate the blurred appearance on gel electrophoresis. C A radioactive probe hybridised to the DNA transferred to a filter identifies the same fragment of interest in each individual.

Nevertheless, as illustrated in Figure 1.37B, detection of any DNA sequence of interest can be compared to finding a needle in a haystack. Labelling the sequence in question with a *probe* provides a valuable means of detection. This may involve the process of *Southern blotting*, whereby after the DNA is size-separated on a gel, the gel is dipped briefly in strong alkali to render the DNA single-stranded and the DNA fragments are then transferred by blotting to a nitrocellulose or nylon filter such that their relative positions remain unchanged. The DNA-containing filter is then immersed in a solution containing a probe which hybridises only to complementary sequences. After washing the unbound probe off the filter, the filter is exposed to X-ray film, and the position of the fragment(s) in question will be revealed by dark bands on the film, known as an autoradiogram (see Fig. 1.37C).

DNA AMPLIFICATION

The analyses described above do reveal a tremendous amount of genetic information, but they remain limited by the small number of available DNA molecules. The following section describes the two main methods to amplify the specific sequence of DNA in which the investigator is interested.

Cloning

Microorganisms can take up exogenous DNA by a process known as transformation, but unless this DNA is incorporated into the host genome, it will tend to be lost during the process of cell division. However, the same microorganisms can also take up DNA which has been digested with restriction enzymes and incorporated (by joining together sticky ends) into a self-replicating unit, or *vector* (see Fig. 1.38). In this case, the vector and the exogenous DNA which it contains will be replicated within each cell, and bacterial cell division will result in large numbers of infected cells from which the vector-associated DNA can be prepared separately to the host DNA. Every cell derived from the founder cell should contain the same vector DNA, providing a means to amplify and purify DNA. In routine genetic manipulation experiments, the host microorganism is usually *E. coli* bacteria, and the vector an infecting virus (bacteriophage), or a plasmid analogous to mitochondria. Other synthetic vectors such as yeast artificial chromosomes (YACs) have been developed to allow host bacteria to propagate larger stretches of exogenous DNA and are particularly important in gene mapping.

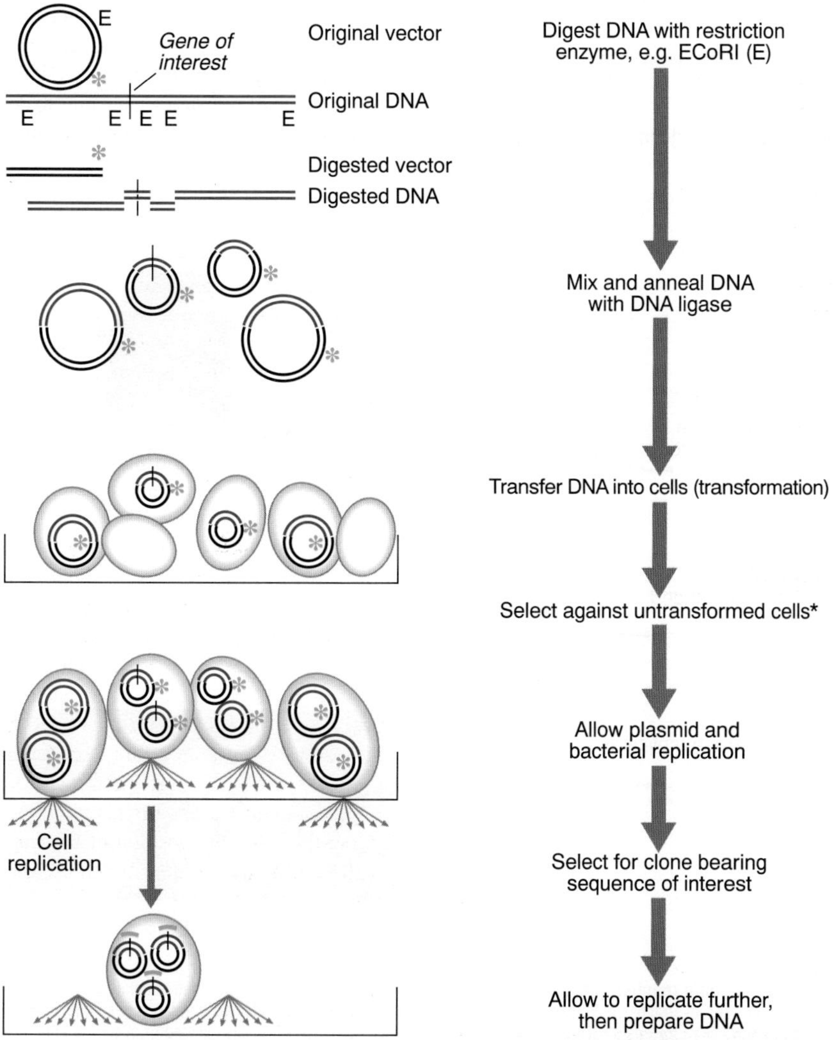

Fig. 1.38 Cloning. In negative selection against untransformed cells, all cells are grown in the presence of an antibiotic. Only cells containing the vector with a gene for antibiotic resistance (asterisked) are resistant and able to grow. Positive selection for the clone of interest may use the polymerase chain reaction (PCR) or a probe to detect inserted DNA sequences.

The polymerase chain reaction (PCR)

The development of polymerase chain reaction technique in the mid-1980s revolutionised molecular biology, and again is based upon the base-pairing principle discussed on page 3. It allows specific amplification of up to 10^{10} copies of a particular stretch of DNA from a single DNA template. The essence is very simple (see Fig. 1.39). Short stretches (around 20–25 nucleotides) of single-stranded DNA are added to the template DNA. These are complementary to the sequence to be amplified, and under the correct conditions, will anneal to single-stranded template DNA and 'prime' DNA replication. The products from each round of replication can serve as the template for the next cycle of amplification and, over a number of cycles, exponential amplification ensues.

DNA SEQUENCING AND THE HUMAN GENOME PROJECT

Molecular methods allow the deciphering of the genetic code by determining the sequence of bases along a stretch of prepared DNA. Sequencing methods are based on the DNA synthetic process, either carried out in a single synthetic step or in PCR-based cycles. Many of these methods exploit the ability of dideoxynucleotide triphosphates (ddNTPs) to prevent elongation of the newly synthesised strand if they are incorporated at the 3' end to the daughter strand of DNA instead of the relevant deoxynucleotide triphosphate (dNTP) (see Fig. 1.40). The products from four separate reactions, each containing all four dNTPs but a different ddNTP, are size-separated on a gel in separate tracks. As the fragments migrate proportional to their length, a ladder pattern is generated in each lane in which each band represents a specific termination event, and the sequence can be read from the shortest fragment at intervals of one nucleotide across all four lanes. Again, this process can be highly automated, with sequences read by computer rather than the eye.

The Human Genome Project (HGP) is an international programme of research which aims to determine the sequence and structure of all functional human genes (and important

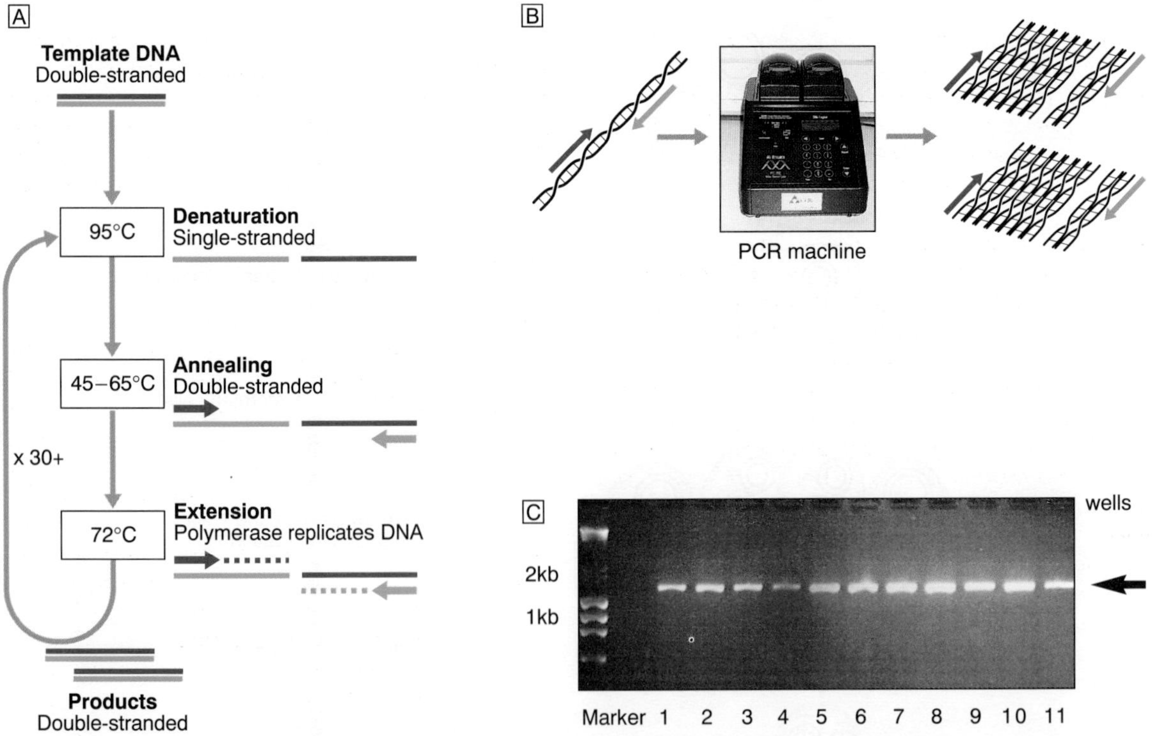

Fig. 1.39 The polymerase chain reaction (PCR). A The process. *Denaturation*: the double-stranded template DNA is rendered single-stranded by heating. *Annealing*: on cooling, the two strands could reanneal, but because of the short size and relative abundance of synthetic single-stranded primers, primer-template hybrids are more likely. *Extension*: the temperature is increased to allow DNA synthesis initiated from each primer, reading off a single-stranded DNA template. *End result*: at the end of these three stages, the number of copies of the sequence of interest will have been doubled. (Note that only the sequence between the two primers is amplified.) The three steps are usually repeated between 25 and 40 times to allow exponential amplification. B Automated temperature variation in PCR machines simplifies the process. C Gel electrophoresis of a PCR product amplified from genomic DNA. Note the specificity of the reaction; only a single product has been amplified from the 3×10^9 bp of the human genome in each of the 11 different reactions.

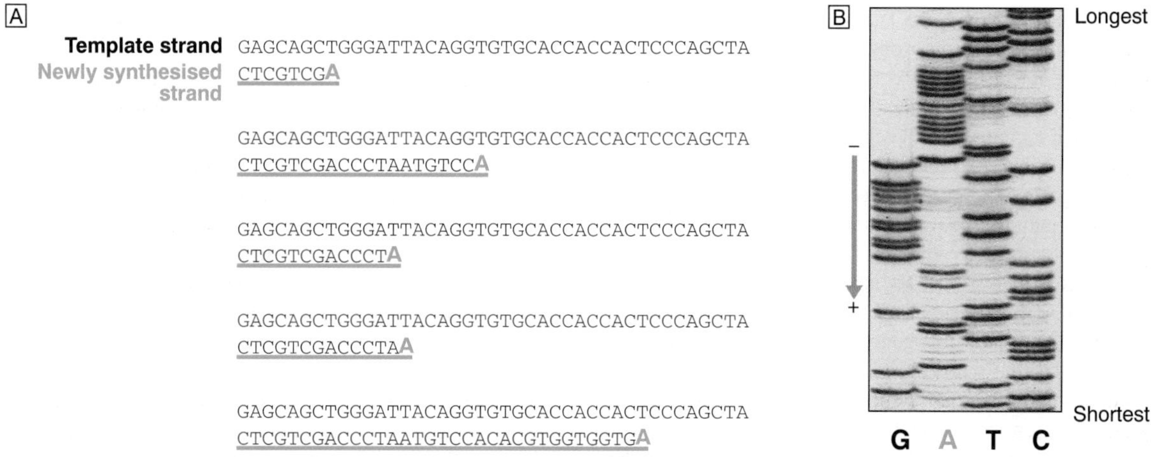

Fig. 1.40 DNA sequencing. A Generation of A track due to random incorporation of a labelled ddATP chain terminator instead of dATP in DNA synthesis. (Unlabelled dCTP, dGTP and dTTP are incorporated as normal.) B The result of acrylamide gel electrophoresis of all four reactions, separating the fragments according to size, and autoradiography. Only the newly synthesised strands are detectable, and allow the sequence to be read from bottom to top (sequence commences CTCGTCGACCC…).

microorganisms). Although driven by molecular geneticists with an aim to improving our fundamental knowledge of biological processes, the HGP has enormous implications for all types of human disease. The biological questions which will be addressed should improve our therapeutic options, and the methods used to assist the HGP's sequencing efforts have generated resources and sequence which are facilitating the detection of abnormal sequences associated with disease states. However, a major issue for science and medicine to address is what to do with this information. The identification of a genetic susceptibility state in an individual may allow the institution of preventive and therapeutic measures to slow or prevent the development of a disease, but such information carries huge implications for individuals, ranging from the psychological impact of knowing that they are likely to develop a particular disease, to interference with their position in society—for example, in terms of health insurance. Similarly, knowing that some individuals are relatively resistant to disease (e.g. HIV infection) may hamper efforts to improve society's response to a major health risk. Medicine and society have not yet formulated safeguards to ensure that the recent molecular advances result in predominantly beneficial results.

MODERN MOLECULAR METHODS IN HUMAN DISEASE

Studies and treatments of human disease have already been transformed by applications of new molecular techniques. Cloning has proved invaluable not only in the detection and amplification of DNA, as described in the previous section, but also in the safe generation of large amounts of purified proteins encoded by the DNA—for example, recombinant clotting factor VIII. The next section highlights three specific areas at the forefront of current medical research.

IDENTIFYING DISEASE GENES

Historical overview

The earliest disease genes to be identified were analysed because insights into the pathological biochemical defects allowed analysis of the implicated gene, e.g. the globin genes in haemoglobinopathies. Such an approach would now be known as *candidate gene* analysis. The advances in molecular technologies have also allowed us to explore human diseases that had previously yielded few clues as to their cause. Instead, the disease endpoint can be correlated with inheritance of a particular chromosomal region, as a means of identifying the precise location of a disease gene before proceeding to its ultimate identification and isolation. Since this type of mapping approach leads to the characterisation of genes of unknown function, the process was originally referred to by Frank Ruddle as 'reverse genetics'.

Identifying the site of a disease gene

The most efficient method of detecting the chromosomal segment bearing a disease gene is to identify a causative structural disruption which can be observed microscopically by karyotype analysis (see p. 44). Identification of numerous disease genes has been facilitated in this way. For example, the chromosomal locations of many tumour suppressor oncogenes were identified because a common mechanism for loss of the 'normal' second copy is by deletion of a chromosomal segment sufficiently large to be recognised by chromosomal analysis (the 'loss of heterozygosity' approach). A second approach is to identify a co-segregating genetic disease for which the disease gene position is already known. Usually, neither of these approaches is possible, so inheritance of the disease is compared to the inheritance patterns of anonymous markers of DNA for which the genetic location has been determined. These markers exploit *polymorphisms* that distinguish alleles on different chromosomes. Early markers were based on restriction fragment length polymorphisms (RFLPs), but these have been superseded by short tandem repeat polymorphisms in which repeats of 2–5 bp such as (CA)n and (AGAT)n occur, with the number of repeat units varying between different chromosomes (see Fig. 1.41). Allele-sharing by individuals with the disease may then be assessed in:

- large families (linkage studies)
- family subsections such as affected siblings (sib-pair analyses)
- isolated populations with a small pool of genes (and often a shared environment)
- laboratory animal populations which transmit a disease similar to that of humans.

Linkage studies and other approaches in polygenic diseases

To date, the most consistently successful approach has been linkage analysis in monogenic diseases, exploiting Mendelian inheritance principles through large families. The principles of linkage analysis are illustrated in Figure 1.42.

Linkage studies are less useful in polygenic and multifactorial diseases when the contribution of each mutation to the disease is small. In this case, allele-sharing may be assessed between affected individuals who do not belong to the same family. A discussion of the advantages and limitations of these methods is beyond the scope of this text. However, their strengths may be illustrated by successes such as asthma, in which susceptibility loci have been determined using many of the approaches listed above—allele-sharing between siblings, in a geographically remote population (Tristan da Cunha), and in mouse models.

Positional cloning and candidate genes

The methods outlined above identify the sites of novel disease genes. Two complementary approaches can then be used to identify the disease gene from the identified region, and are illustrated in Figure 1.43.

Positional cloning strategies characterise the disease gene interval in detail by defining distances between genetic markers in the region. The approaches have been assisted by the availability of a number of libraries containing segments of human genomic DNA cloned into a variety of

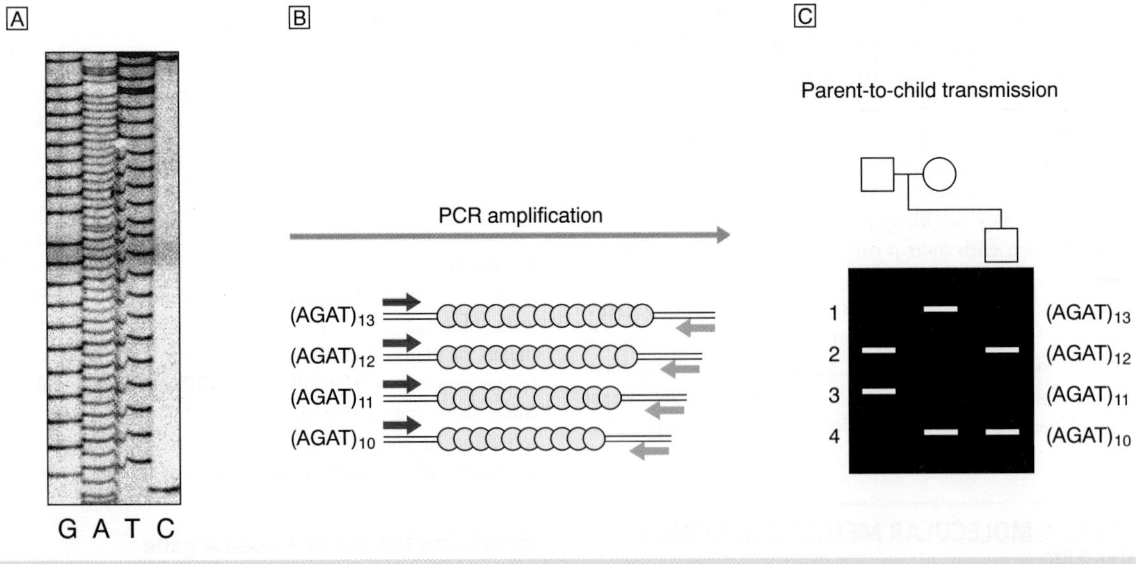

Fig. 1.41 Polymorphic markers. A Sequence of a polymorphic short tandem repeat (AGAT)n sequence suitable for use as a marker. B The repeat sequence is PCR-amplified between flanking primers of unique sequence. As the number of repeat units varies between alleles on different chromosomes, this results in different-sized products. C PCR products from family members are size-separated by gel electrophoresis. This can distinguish both sets of parental alleles.

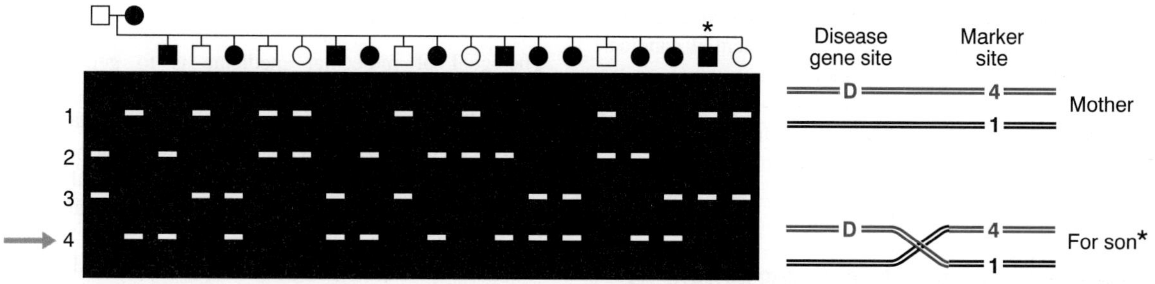

Fig. 1.42 Linkage analysis. A polymorphic marker is PCR-amplified in a large family with an autosomal dominant trait. In this example, almost all affected individuals but no unaffected individuals have inherited allele 4, arrowed, from their affected mother. (Inheritance of the father's alleles can be ignored.) This suggests that the gene for the marker lies close to the disease gene (D), or is 'linked', on one of the mother's chromosomes (though in small families, this could easily occur due to chance alone). The asterisk displays a recombination event because a crossover has occurred between the two maternal chromosomes, between the disease gene and marker M genes.

Linkage is tested mathematically by assessing the likelihood of the allele inheritance in affected and unaffected individuals due to chance, and the likelihood that the allele inheritance has occurred because the disease gene and marker lie close together on the same chromosome. The LOD score is the logarithm (base 10) of the ratio:

$$\frac{\text{Likelihood due to linkage at a specific genetic distance}}{\text{Likelihood due to chance alone}}$$

A score of +3.6 or more indicates linkage at a significance level of 0.05; a score of −2 or less excludes linkage in a genome wide search.

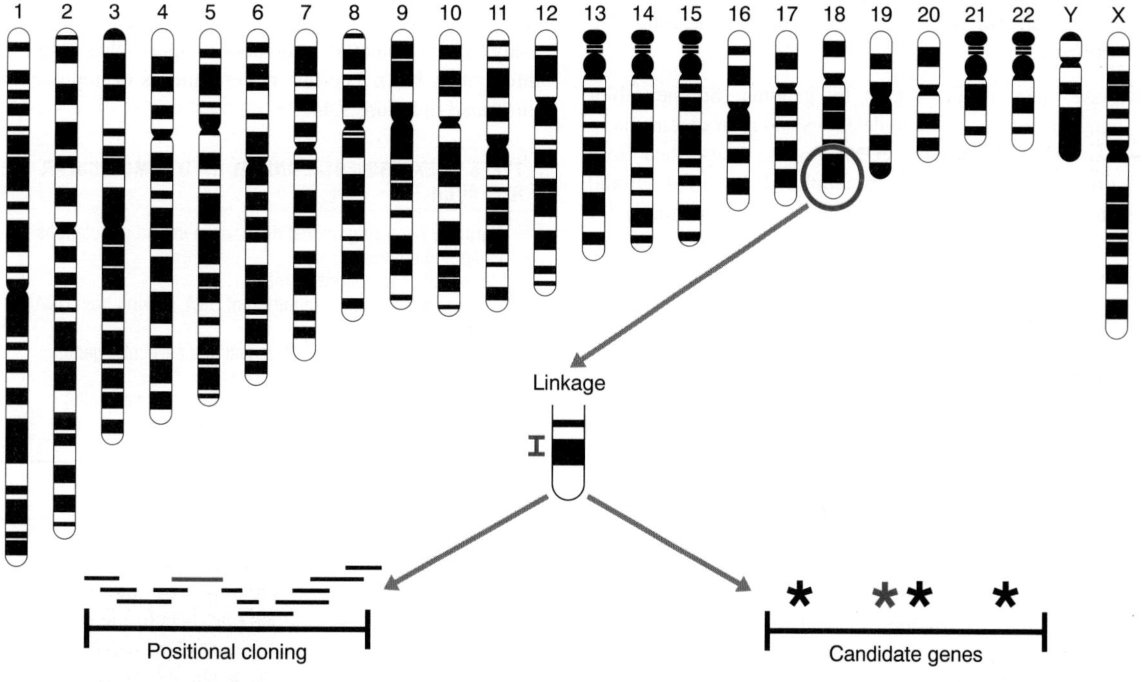

Fig. 1.43 Molecular methods to locate a disease gene.

viral, bacterial or yeast-based vectors. These clones may be required to isolate genes in the region; alternatively, they may aid the fine placement of genes already known to map to the general area. Finally, a suitable gene located within the disease interval can be analysed for mutations in individuals with the disease.

Particularly with the advances of the HGP, once a disease gene region has been identified, it is often found to encompass the map placement of previously identified genes, some of which may be considered as potential candidate disease genes by virtue of their molecular structure, or data concerning the encoded protein. Such a *'positional candidate'* approach, combining mapping and functional data, has become the most frequent means of identification of inherited disease genes.

ANALYSIS OF CANDIDATE GENES FOR MUTATIONS

Essentially, the sequence of the suspected gene in affected individuals needs to be determined and compared to the normal sequence. However, even with advances in automated sequencing technologies, this can still be a daunting task, particularly for large genes with numerous exons, and genes for which limited sequence information is available at the outset. Disease-causing mutations often occur in coding DNA sequence or intron-exon boundaries, but may reside in the promoter region or within introns, or may have deleted the mutant gene entirely so that in autosomal genes only the normal allele is detected. The exact methods used vary according to the nature of the suspected disease gene, but usually include the following elements:

- Assessment of the region by genomic Southern blot analysis to exclude large deletions and rearrangements.
- Sequence of DNA (or cDNA reverse transcribed from mRNA) which has been amplified by PCR. Initial strategies are likely to include screening methods for mutations such as altered gel mobility or mismatch-generated susceptibility to digesting enzymes.

In the course of these studies, a number of variations are likely to be found in the DNA sequence in affected individuals. All will have been co-inherited with the disease-causing mutation—that is, the variation and disease gene will be in *linkage disequilibrium*. Distinguishing between incidental variations in sequence and disease-causing mutations in that gene, or an adjacent gene, is not always easy. Definition of a disease-causing mutation should be based on evidence that:

- The variation is genuine, and not due to artefact generated by a single method of analysis. This is helpfully addressed by supporting data from at least two of genomic DNA, mRNA or protein.
- There is no other potential causative variation within the gene, i.e. the gene should usually be sequenced entirely.
- Only individuals with the abnormality have the disease or disease predisposition, and all affected individuals within the family share the same abnormality. This is relatively simple for a monogenic disease but more difficult in polygenic diseases.

MODELLING DISEASE

The goal of molecular medicine is to generate new therapies for disease to accompany the goals of basic molecular biology directed towards the understanding of biological processes and disease. Unfortunately, to date molecular techniques have tended to generate information about disease susceptibility in the absence of any therapeutic advances.

However, several approaches are likely to lead to better understanding of disease pathogenesis and the generation of new therapies. This is particularly true of attempts to create a 'model' of a human disease in a system which can be manipulated. Biochemical effects can be studied in an individual cell type by in vitro culture experiments, either studying cells derived at biopsy from affected individuals or transforming cells with abnormal DNA to mimic the human disease state. While crucial, the potential of such studies is limited to selected conditions and devoid of the types of cellular, hormonal and immune-mediated responses critical in the whole organism.

A particularly powerful technique is to recapitulate the disease state in a laboratory animal, allowing assessment of the natural history of disease, effects of risk factors, and analysis of potential therapeutic approaches (see the information box). The two major patterns of approach are illustrated in Figure 1.44.

TYPES OF EXPERIMENTAL ANIMAL USED IN MOLECULAR RESEARCH

- Naturally occurring animal diseases in inbred populations (mapping studies)
- Genetically engineered animals
  Transgenic animals (addition of DNA, leaving host DNA intact)
  Knock-out technology (removal of a particular gene, currently only feasible in mice)
  Cloned animals (preliminary stages only, e.g. Dolly)

PROSPECTS FOR GENE THERAPY

Gene therapy refers to the transfer of exogenous DNA into cells in order to combat disease by modifying gene expression. Such modifications may benefit the cell directly, or may modulate disease activity elsewhere by altering protein secretion by that cell. It should be noted that for ethical purposes, the principle of gene therapy into cells contributing to the germ line has not been accepted; instead, the aim is to offer specific treatment to each individual (and not their descendants by default) by transferring DNA into non-germ line 'somatic' cells.

Monogenic diseases such as adenosine deaminase (ADA) deficiency (see below) and cystic fibrosis were the first to be tackled, providing an active gene where both copies of

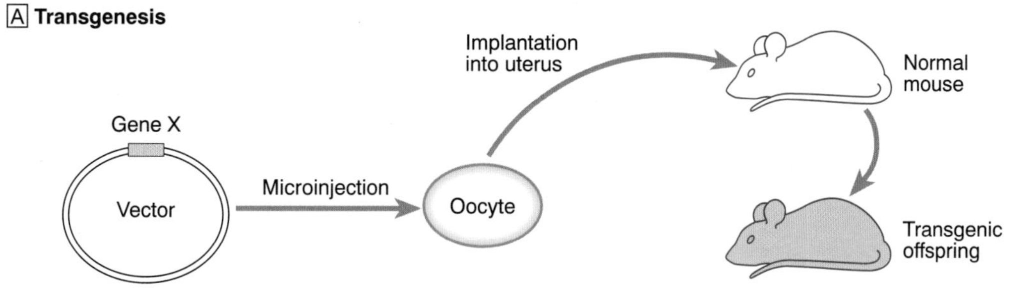

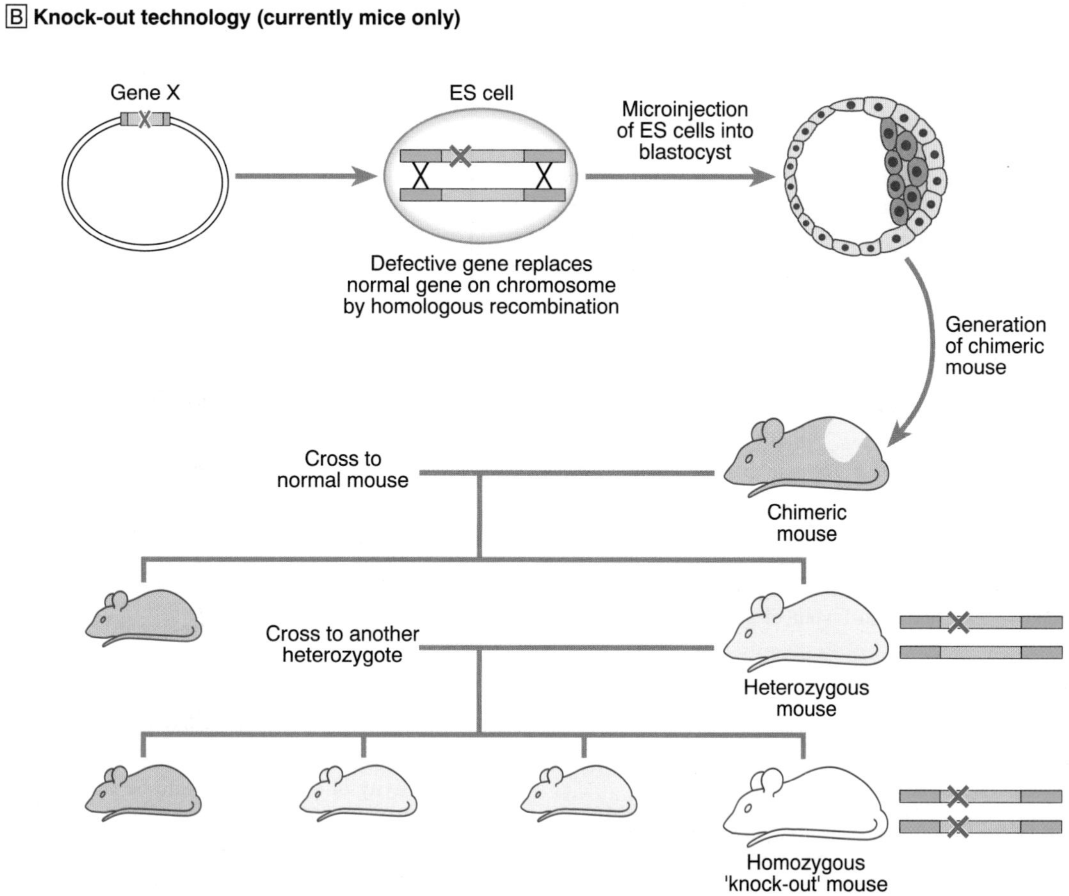

Fig. 1.44 Genetically engineered animals. A Transgenesis. The gene of interest (with suitable regulatory elements) is placed in a vector and microinjected into oocytes. The DNA integrates into the host chromosomes, usually at random, and at more than one site. It is hoped that the gene will be expressed *in addition* to the full complement of normal genes. The oocyte is then implanted into the uterus of a foster mother. B Knock-out technology (currently mice only). DNA encoding part of the gene of interest is modified (e.g. by deletion), and cloned into a vector. The vector is incorporated into embryonal stem cells *(ES cells).* Random integration will occur, but in around 1 in a million cells, the vector DNA will replace the equivalent part of the normal gene by *homologous recombination* between the flanking sequences. The two events, homologous recombination and specific integration, are selected for by markers incorporated in the original vector. ES cells are pluripotential and able to generate mature mice. The selected cells are injected into fertilised early embryos. Chimeric animals which contain the 'knock-out' gene in their germ line are used to generate heterozygous mice which are interbred to produce homozygotes in which the gene activity has been abolished.

the endogenous genes had been inactivated by inherited mutations. The current trend is aimed at polygenic disease. Cancer is a major target for gene therapy, with the aim, for example, of transferring 'suicide genes' into cancer cells. The earlier discussions catalogued the ability of molecular techniques to cut and reanneal adjacent pieces of DNA, and to alter DNA sequence, and the use of such modified nucleic acids to produce genetically engineered animals. Such descriptions might make it appear that the concept of gene therapy will be realised easily. Unfortunately, this is not the case. Of more than 200 gene therapy trials to date, there has not been one unqualified success, possibly reflecting an over-eagerness to rush to clinical trials.

Figure 1.45 outlines current gene therapy strategies. Naked DNA may be transferred to a cell, but successful delivery is rare. Some improvement is obtained by transferring the DNA in a liposome with a lipid coat, but viral-based vectors, either non-integrative such as adeno- and herpes simplex viruses, or integrative such as retro- and lentiviruses, lead to marked improvements in delivery. Furthermore, a virus which selectively infects a particular cell type may be chosen. However, the use of viruses generates additional problems. For example, adenoviral vectors are more likely to stimulate a significant immune response, and integrative viruses carry the risk of insertional mutagenesis. The development of new and improved naturally occurring or synthetic vectors is a current priority for research, and the field is advancing rapidly.

The paradigm of adenosine deaminase (ADA) deficiency

This was the first disease for which gene therapy was attempted. In ADA deficiency, inheritance of mutations in both copies of the gene resulting in ADA activity of less than 5% of normal leads to severe combined immunodeficiency (SCID, see Table 1.6, p. 35) due to lack of ADA in lymphocytes. Factors in favour of gene therapy success were that lymphocytes were readily accessible, and that it was known that for clinical effectiveness, improvement of enzyme activity of even 1–2% could be sufficient to delay immunodeficiency for months or even years. However, current gene therapy approaches, while well tolerated, have yet to result in a sufficient increase in ADA activity to allow withdrawal of enzyme replacement therapy.

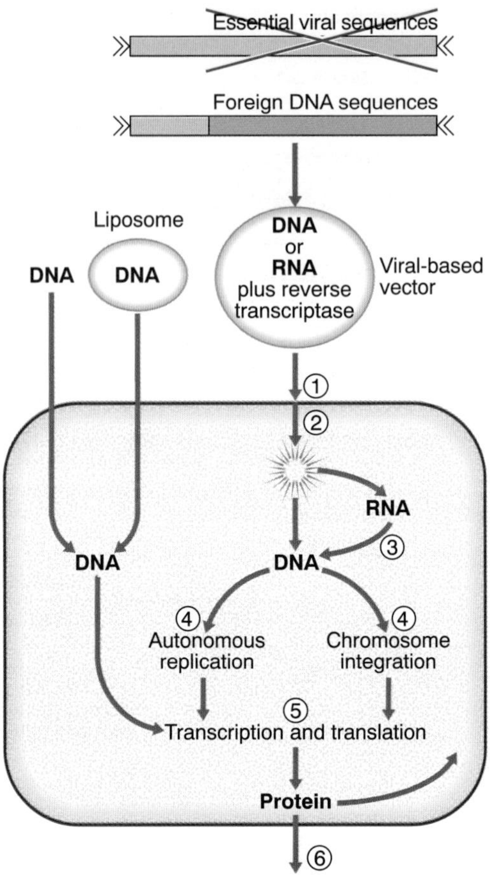

Fig. 1.45 Gene therapy. Cellular uptake of exogenous DNA is enhanced by packing the DNA, for example, in a viral genome from which crucial genes have been deleted. Steps in direct cellular entry: (1) Binding to surface receptors. (2) Entry of virus into cell. (3) +/– reverse transcription. (4) DNA replication (if viral-based). (5) Transcription and translation of protein (but, if viral vector, reassembly of infective viruses prevented). (6) Export of protein but not mature virus particle from cell.

GENE THERAPY
Requirements
• Efficient DNA delivery into cells • Persistent and sufficient DNA expression • Persistence of the infected cell and its progeny in the face of cellular lifespan and host immune responses • Efficacy of transferred genetic material in correcting disease • Safety in view of: Unknown effects of long-term expression of foreign genes Irreversible integration of foreign DNA (retroviruses)
Some current and future targets
• Replacement of defective inherited gene Adenosine deaminase (ADA) deficiency Cystic fibrosis • Local transfer for acquired disease Angioplasty-associated re-stenosis (VEGF) Cancer cells (e.g. p53 transfer)

FURTHER INFORMATION ON INVESTIGATION OF THE MOLECULAR BASIS OF DISEASE

Collins F S 1995 Positional cloning moves from perditional to traditional. Nature Genetics 9: 347–350
Old R W, Primrose S B 1994 Principles of gene manipulation: an

introduction to genetic engineering, 5th edn. Blackwell Scientific, Oxford
Supplement 1998 Therapeutic horizons. Nature 392
Verma I M, Somia N 1997 Gene therapy—promises, problems and prospects. Nature 389: 239–242

TYPES OF GENETIC DISEASE

CLASSICAL GENETIC DISEASES

The term 'genetic disease' generally conjures up an image of a chromosomal aberration often incompatible with life, or monogenic disorders inherited by classical Mendelian principles (see Fig. 1.32, p. 40). These conditions are generally rare, but are considerably more common in exam situations. Examples of important diseases are provided in the tables in Chapter 20, as follows:

- chromosomal disorders: Table 20.1
- single gene disorders
  —autosomal dominant: Table 20.2
  —autosomal recessive: Table 20.3
  —X-linked: Table 20.4
- non-Mendelian inheritance
  —imprinted genes: Table 20.5
  —triplet and repeat sequences: Table 20.6
  —mitochondrial inheritance: Table 20.7.

It will be noted that there is considerable overlap between diseases in Tables 20.2–20.4, as molecular techniques have often identified more than one gene defect which can result in an almost indistinguishable phenotype. This is not surprising if one considers the number of regulatory and biochemical pathways converging on a final outcome reflected in a limited number of disease end-points. In the tables, we have tried to illustrate the most common forms of inheritance and the most frequently implicated genes.

GENETIC FACTORS IN COMMON DISEASES

It is becoming increasingly difficult to propose any disease that is wholly non-genetic. In addition to the 2–3% of pregnancies that result in the birth of a child with a condition that can be attributed to defective or absent genes, the frequency of adult diseases with a strong genetic component may be as high as 50%, and even infectious diseases such as HIV and toxin insults as in Wernicke–Korsakoff syndrome, are now known to be modified by host susceptibility factors.

To conclude the chapter, we would like to highlight genetic influences on two common disorders, asthma and diabetes. In these, as in other polygenic diseases, a number of genes provide the individual with an overall susceptibility to disease which may be unmasked by additional mutations in other genes, or environmental triggers. In each, genetic studies have identified a number of genes or chromosomal regions at which variants appear to provoke the disease in some (but not all) individuals. There are, however, many ways to recapitulate the disease phenotypes, and for both diseases studies have indicated key environmental precipitants which may be responsible for the increasing prevalence of these diseases in affluent societies.

ASTHMA

The reversible bronchoconstriction which defines asthma (see p. 326) is provoked by numerous inflammatory events, often occurring on a background of atopy (see Table 1.5, p. 34). A number of candidate genes and regions identified as predisposing to an asthmatic phenotype have been identified and are illustrated in Table 1.10.

DIABETES MELLITUS

The normal products of many genes are required to coordinate the exquisite regulation of insulin secretion within a few minutes of a hyperglycaemic stimulus. In insulin-dependent (type 1) diabetes mellitus, insulin secretion is impaired due to destruction of the islet beta cells; the major contributing gene is in the HLA complex, with sequence variations in HLA-DQB influencing both susceptibility and resistance to type 1 diabetes. Non-insulin-dependent (type 2) diabetes mellitus is a much more heterogeneous disease, resulting from numerous mechanisms of peripheral insulin resistance and beta cell dysfunction. Specific genetic defects are responsible for certain well-defined type 2 diabetes subtypes (see Table 1.11) in which diabetes presents earlier in life than is usual for type 2 diabetes, e.g. maturity-onset diabetes in the young (MODY) and mitochondrial diabetes.

Table 1.10 Genes currently implicated in asthma

Pathological process	Candidate region	Candidate gene(s)	Normal function of gene product(s)
Atopic responses			
IgE generation	6p21	HLA complex	Antigen presentation
	12q14	Interferon-γ	Inhibition of T_H2 cells and IgE switching
	14q11	TCR α/δ complex	T-cell activation
	16p12–p11	IL-4 receptor	Regulates IgE production
Mast cell response	11q13	FcεRI-β	High-affinity IgE receptor
	12q24	Mast cell growth factor	Mast cell growth
Eosinophil recruitment	5q31	IL-3, 4, 5, 9, 13 and GM-CSF	Cytokines up-regulating IgE responses
Inflammatory mediator release	6p21.3	TNF-α	Inflammatory cytokine
	12q	Nitric oxide synthase 1	Inflammatory mediator
Bronchial hyper-responsiveness and bronchoconstriction			
	5q31	Corticosteroid receptor	Mediates inflammation
	5q35	Leucotriene C4 synthase	Inflammatory mediator
	5q32–q34	β_2-adrenoceptor	Bronchodilatation
Unknown			
	?	Wheeze 1	Two asthma loci identified in Tristan da Cunha population, $p < 0.0001$:
	?	Wheeze 2	*details not available* (> 10 loci also identified for atopy)

Individual polymorphisms are not shown as it is not clear which, if any, are causative rather than merely in linkage disequilibrium with the disease-causing mutation.

Table 1.11 Some of the genes currently implicated in diabetes mellitus (DM)

Mechanism of disease	Chromosomal region	Gene	Proportion of cases of subset (if known)
Insulin-dependent DM (IDDM, type 1)			
Reduced insulin production by islet cells, e.g. T cell-mediated destruction, defective synthesis	6p21	*IDDM 1 (HLA)*	~ 35%
	11p15	*IDDM2 (insulin gene)*	
	Numerous other regions including IDDM 4–10		Contribution probably differs between different populations leading to current discrepancies between genetic studies
Non-insulin-dependent DM (NIDDM, type 2)			
A. Well-characterised genetic defects			
	20q12	*MODY1 (hepatocyte nuclear factor)*	
	7p15	*MODY2 (glucokinase)*	40% of MODY, 1% of type 2 diabetes
	12q24	*MODY3 (hepatocyte nuclear factor 1α)*	
	Mitochondrial DNA	*tRNA-Leu*	
B. Other genes implicated			
1. Insulin secretion genes influencing	11p15	*Insulin gene*	
glucose sensing	3q26	*Glut2 transporter*	
glucose transport	5q15	*Proprotein convertase*	
intracellular signalling	8p12	*β_3 adrenoceptor*	
insulin exocytosis	19q13	*Glycogen synthase*	
	21q22	*ATP-dependent K^+ channel*	
2. Insulin resistance genes	2q36	*Insulin receptor substrate-1*	15%, especially in Mexican Americas
	19p13	*Insulin receptor*	1%
	17q25	*Glucagon receptor*	1–5%
	6q22–q23	*PC-1 (phosphodiesterase-1)*	
	16q22	*Ras-related protein*	
	17p13	Glut4 transporter	
3. HLA and	6p21	*HLA-DR4*	
cytokine genes		*TNF-α (tumour necrosis factor-α)*	
4. Obesity genes	4q	*Intestinal fatty acid binding proteins*	

Evolutionarily, NIDDM genes would have been beneficial to store energy during periods of starvation, but no longer advantageous, are now deleterious in the sedentary, well-fed lifestyle of the Western world. In addition, numerous further genes influence susceptibility to complications such as retinopathy and nephropathy, and other well-characterised genetic diseases have a significant incidence of diabetes (e.g. cystic fibrosis).

Diseases due to infection

G.E. GRIFFIN • J.G.P. SISSONS • P.L. CHIODINI • D.M. MITCHELL

2

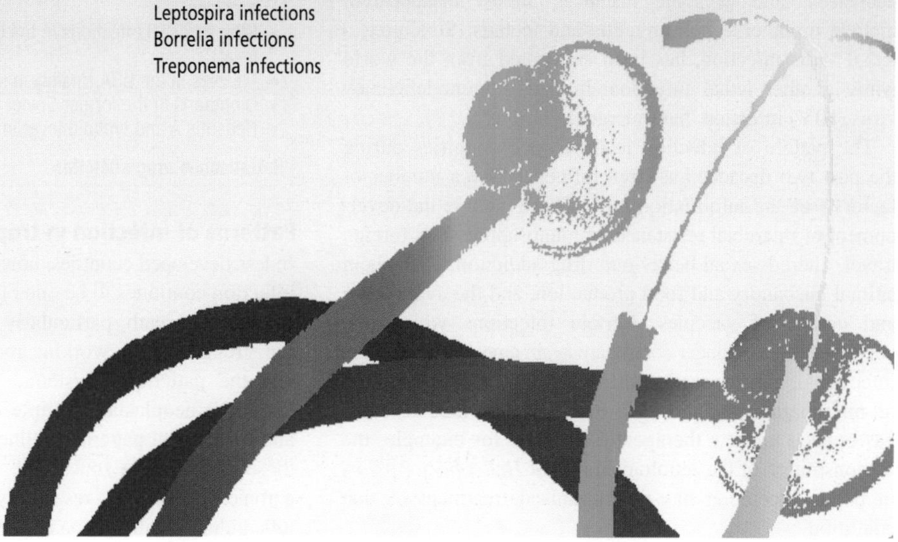

CONCEPTS OF INFECTION

Infection can involve any organ or system of the body and thus embraces all medical disciplines. In this chapter an introduction is given to the general aspects, epidemiology, diagnosis, prevention and treatment of infection as well as descriptions of individual infectious diseases. Infections involving specific organs or systems are described in the appropriate chapters.

Infection differs from other diseases in a number of aspects. The most important is that it is caused by living microorganisms which can usually be identified, thus establishing the aetiology early in the illness. Many of these organisms, including all bacteria, are sensitive to antibiotics and most infections are potentially curable, unlike many non-infectious diseases which are degenerative and frequently become chronic. Communicability is another factor which differentiates infections from non-infectious diseases. Transmission of pathogenic organisms to other people, directly or indirectly, may lead to an epidemic. Finally, many infections are preventable by hygienic measures, by vaccines or by the judicious use of drugs (chemoprophylaxis).

PATTERNS OF INFECTION

Pattern of infection in developed countries

In the 20th century there has been a dramatic fall in the incidence of communicable diseases in developed countries. This is due to factors such as immunisation, antimicrobial chemotherapy, improved nutrition, and better sanitation and housing. Infectious diseases which have decreased, and in some instances almost disappeared, include diphtheria, poliomyelitis and tetanus. Smallpox, a lethal virus infection, has been eradicated from the world while another lethal infection, human immunodeficiency virus (HIV) infection, has emerged.

The pattern of infection in developed countries during the past two decades has been influenced by a number of factors (see the information box). These include the development of microbial resistance, immunosuppression, foreign travel, altered sexual behaviour, drug addiction, changes in animal husbandry and food production, and the availability and uptake of vaccines. Certain infections which had decreased or come under control are again emerging (resurgent infections), e.g. tuberculosis. In addition, the identification of microorganisms causing previously described diseases has opened up new therapeutic avenues; for example, the demonstration of the aetiological role of *Helicobacter pylori* in peptic ulceration has revolutionised treatment of that condition.

INFLUENCES ON PATTERNS OF INFECTION IN DEVELOPED COUNTRIES
Vaccines
• Improved uptake of vaccines • New vaccines, e.g. *Haemophilus influenzae* type B and hepatitis A
Animal husbandry and preparation of food
• *Salmonella* and *Campylobacter* infections originating in poultry and eggs • *Escherichia coli* type 0157 causing haemorrhagic colitis associated with beef • *Listeria* infections from soft cheeses
Microbial resistance
• Increased resistance in common bacterial pathogens including *Staphylococcus aureus* (MRSA), Gram-negative bacilli, *Streptococcus pneumoniae*, vancomycin-resistant enterococci (VRE) and *Mycobacterium tuberculosis*
Sexual behaviour
• Increase in HIV infection and other sexually transmitted diseases
International travel
• Importation of malaria (in 1996 there were 2500 cases in the UK, 2117 cases in continental France and 1021 cases in Germany) • Legionnaires' disease from holiday hotels • HIV infection
Immunosuppression
• Advances in the treatment of malignant disease and in organ transplantation leading to infections with opportunistic organisms
Resurgence of infections
• Tuberculosis—world-wide, especially in association with HIV infection • Poliomyelitis in the Netherlands (in a religious sect refusing vaccines) • Streptococcal infections in the USA (including rheumatic fever) • Measles in the USA (mainly in immigrants in inner cities) • Diphtheria in the former Soviet Union • Hepatitis A and typhoid fever in the former Yugoslavia
Intravenous drug addiction

Patterns of infection in tropical countries

In less developed countries, however, especially in the tropics, infection continues to be one of the most common causes of disease and death, particularly in children, and determines the strength of the working man, the health of the mother and the pattern of systemic disease in the community, including neoplasia. Multiple disease entities are the rule and the clinical patterns of illness differ in many ways from those in temperate zones. The complex interaction between chronic parasitism, respiratory and diarrhoeal diseases, tuberculosis, malnutrition and its immunosuppressive effects, and HIV infection, poses special problems for the health of children. Up to 40% of children may die before they reach 5 years of age in such undeveloped countries.

Chronic infections do serious damage to important organs, such as liver and kidneys in schistosomiasis, the heart in trypanosomiasis cruzi, the lungs, bones and lymph nodes in tuberculosis, the bone marrow reserves in malaria and hookworm infections, the gut in tropical sprue and the nerves in leprosy. These organs may then fail if the demand upon them is increased through work, growth, pregnancy or additional disease. Such diseases impose chronic ill health on millions of children and adults in the tropics.

Many of the decimating diseases of the past are controllable by vaccination (yellow fever), vector control (malaria and sleeping sickness) and general improvement in living standards (plague and relapsing fever), but control is imperfect and the diseases reappear. Other epidemic diseases such as cholera in Asia and meningococcal meningitis in Africa remain largely uncontrolled, and kill hundreds of thousands of people annually. Efficient vaccines exist for many diseases such as poliomyelitis, measles, rubella, meningitis and tetanus, but in many countries they have made little impact because of cost and the practical difficulty in delivering them.

Development, especially in the form of dams and irrigation, has often encouraged the spread of vector-borne disease such as malaria and schistosomiasis, while the exploitation of the Amazonian forests has resulted in mutilating outbreaks of mucocutaneous leishmaniasis. Migration to urban slums increases the risk of gastrointestinal disease and tuberculosis and of 'Western' diseases such as hypertension, and has contributed materially to the AIDS epidemic which is wreaking havoc in developing countries, especially in Africa, the Indian subcontinent and South-east Asia.

Finally, in developing countries infectious diseases are frequently associated with natural disasters such as drought, flooding and earthquakes as well as with war and revolution.

The information box illustrates patterns of infection in tropical countries.

PATTERNS OF INFECTION IN TROPICAL COUNTRIES

Killers of children, preventable but variably prevalent

- Measles
- Diphtheria
- Pertussis
- Poliomyelitis
- Tetanus
- Hepatitis B
- Gastroenteritis
- Malaria
- Meningococcal disease

Chronic disabling infections, widely prevalent

- Leprosy
- Tuberculosis
- Trachoma
- Malaria
- Trypanosomiasis cruzi
- Amoebiasis
- Intestinal helminths
- Schistosomiasis
- Filarial infection

Epidemic diseases, actual (marked *) and potential

- Louse-borne typhus and relapsing fever
- Cholera*
- Malaria
- Visceral leishmaniasis*
- Human immunodeficiency virus infection*
- Tuberculosis*, in association with HIV epidemic
- Influenza

Infections liable to focal outbreaks (zoonotic or vector-borne)

- Dengue fever, e.g. Thailand
- Plague, e.g. Vietnam
- Cutaneous leishmaniasis, e.g. Sudan
- African trypanosomiasis, e.g. Zambia
- Yellow fever, e.g. Kenya, Nigeria
- Anthrax

MICROORGANISM–HOST INTERACTIONS

Effects of infection on the body

Infection has many effects on the body. These are summarised in the first information box on page 60 and may be acute, chronic or allergic. Chronic effects are seen especially in children in tropical countries.

Pathology of infection

Disease due to infection is the result of interaction between a microorganism and the defence mechanisms of the body. The outcome of this interaction can range from no demonstrable effect to death, and will depend on the number and virulence of the organisms, physiological and anatomical effects that they induce, and the effectiveness of the natural defences. It is now demonstrated that there are strong genetic influences which determine the response to infection. A clear example of this is the genetic polymorphism in expression of cytokine release (tumour necrosis factor-α, TNF-α) and cytokine receptor expression (interferon γ).

The mechanisms by which microorganisms cause disease are summarised in the second information box on page 60 and discussed in other sections of this book. Organisms act directly and/or through their toxins. Many of these effects are general, but some act at specific anatomical sites—for example, poliomyelitis virus in anterior horn cells, hepatitis virus in hepatocytes, pneumococcus in the lung alveoli, and tetanus and diphtheria toxins at nerve terminals.

Shock is an especial problem in severe infections. Its aetiology is complex and results from reduced systemic vascular resistance brought about by dilated small vessels

CLINICAL EFFECTS OF INFECTION ON THE BODY
Acute
• Fever; anorexia, protein catabolism, negative nitrogen balance, acute-phase protein response, hypoalbuminaemia, low serum iron, sequestration of iron, anaemia, neutrophilia • Inflammation; pain, dysfunction, tissue damage • Convulsions; especially in children • Shock; sustained fall in circulating blood volume associated with lowered systemic vascular resistance • Haemorrhage; haemolytic anaemia, intravascular coagulation • Organ failure; kidneys, liver, lung, heart, brain, necrosis of skin
Chronic
• Weight loss and muscle-wasting • Malnutrition; especially associated with diarrhoea • Retardation of growth and intellect in children • Anaemia; iron sequestration, maturation arrest in marrow, folate deficiency • Tissue destruction; e.g. lung in pneumonia or tuberculosis, nerves in leprosy, liver in hepatitis B • Post-infective syndromes; e.g. lactose intolerance, malabsorption, irritable colon, depression, post-viral fatigue syndrome
Allergic
• Rash; e.g. erythema with streptococci, urticaria with helminths, maculo-papular in typhoid and endocarditis, erythema nodosum in tuberculosis • Arthritis; e.g. in rheumatic fever, Reiter's syndrome • Pericarditis; e.g. in meningococcal infection • Encephalitis; e.g. in measles or following vaccines • Peripheral neuropathy; e.g. in post-infective polyneuritis • Haemolytic anaemia; e.g. in infectious mononucleosis • Nephritis; e.g. in streptococcal infection

PATHOLOGY OF INFECTION	
Microbe-mediated	**Host-mediated**
• Direct cell destruction, e.g. poliomyelitis, rabies, hepatitis • Exotoxin, e.g. tetanus, cholera, botulism, diphtheria • Endotoxin, e.g. typhoid, Gram-negative septicaemia, meningococcal infection	• Neutrophils and macrophages • Complement activation • Activation of clotting cascade • Immune mechanisms • Secondary autoimmune mechanisms

and leaky capillaries under the influence of several mediators, which include kinins, complement components, histamine, cytokines and endogenous opiates (see Ch. 1). Endotoxin from Gram-negative bacteria is one of the known mediators causing release of these agents. However, Gram-positive shock is caused by other cell wall components and by lipoteichoic acid, and is clinically indistinguishable from Gram-negative shock. The cycle of shock, tissue anoxia and organ failure is difficult to break and may kill the patient within hours.

Host response to infection

Non-specific defences

The body has a number of 'natural' antimicrobial defences, especially on the skin and at mucosal surfaces (e.g. lysozyme secretion, gastric acid, intestinal enzymes, vaginal secretions). However, these non-specific systems are not entirely adequate and pathogenic microorganisms can breach them under conditions such as trauma and intense exposure to pathogens. The colonisation of host tissues by pathogens is then counteracted by the body's immune response. Host immunity is expressed through several different mechanisms which depend upon antigen-specific lymphocytes and their products. Polymorphs and macrophages play an important part in defence against microorganisms, especially bacteria (see Ch. 1).

Immune response

The immune system has evolved largely to block the access of pathogenic organisms to host tissues and, where this fails, to limit their colonisation and spread. Microorganisms carry molecules which are foreign to the host, and some bacteria secrete toxins. Both antibody and cell-mediated immune mechanisms may be directed against these antigens (see p. 30). T lymphocytes can kill virus-infected cells, and they also secrete a variety of cytokines which attract and promote the antibacterial and antiviral activity of other inflammatory and immune cells (see p. 33), particularly macrophages. Eosinophil granulocytes are important in host defence against parasites, e.g. worm infestations. Antibodies can neutralise bacterial toxins and bind to the surface of microorganisms, where they inhibit spread and initiate complement fixation which promotes phagocytosis of micro-

Table 2.1 Source and spread of infection

Source/route of transmission	Method of spread	Examples of infection
Contact		
Person to person	Skin or mucous membrane contact	Impetigo, scabies, wound infection, infectious mononucleosis Sexually transmitted diseases (including HIV and hepatitis B)
Soil	Via wounds and abrasions	Tetanus, Buruli ulcer, hookworm, mycetoma
Water	Penetration of skin	Schistosomiasis, leptospirosis
Air-borne spread	Respiratory droplets or dust	Measles, rubella, whooping cough, scarlet fever, mumps, meningococcal infection Upper respiratory tract infection, influenza
	Water aerosols	Legionellosis
Faecal/oral spread	Faecal contamination of food or drink	Salmonella infection, bacillary and amoebic dysentery, enteroviral infections, cholera, giardiasis, hepatitis A, *Campylobacter* infection
Transplacental	Maternal blood	Rubella, cytomegalovirus (CMV) infection, toxoplasmosis, syphilis, malaria, HIV infection
Medical and nursing procedures	Needles, ventilators, infusion fluid	Hepatitis B, staphylococcal infection, *Pseudomonas* infection
Zoonoses (Animal, fish or bird to humans)	Beef or pork	Tapeworms, toxoplasmosis, *Trichinella* infection
	Poultry or eggs	Salmonellosis
	Milk	Tuberculosis, *Campylobacter* infection, brucellosis
	Cheese	Listeriosis, brucellosis
	Rats' or dogs' urine	Leptospirosis, Lassa fever
	Dogs' faeces	*Toxocara* infection, hydatid disease
	Dog bite	Rabies
	Birds	Psittacosis
	Fish	Tapeworms, mycobacterial infections
Arthropods (see Table 2.39, p. 182)		

organisms. The complement membrane attack complex may destroy certain bacteria, especially Gram-negative organisms.

Source and spread of infection

Infection may originate from the patient (autogenous), usually from skin, nasopharynx or bowel, or from outside sources (exogenous), often another person who may either be suffering from an infection or carrying a pathogenic microorganism. Carriers are usually healthy and may harbour the organism in the throat (for example, diphtheria), bowel (salmonella) or blood (hepatitis B or HIV). Non-human sources of infection include water (cholera), milk (tuberculosis), food (botulism), animals (rabies), birds (psittacosis) and also the soil (legionnaires' disease).

Microorganisms may be transmitted by several routes. Autogenous infection may develop as a result of local spread, e.g. from bowel to peritoneum, or by the blood stream. An example of the latter type is endocarditis caused by *Streptococcus sanguis* originating in the patient's mouth and entering the blood during dental procedures. Exogenous infection may be acquired directly or indirectly by one of the routes shown in Table 2.1.

Incubation period is the period between the invasion of the tissues by pathogens and the appearance of clinical features of infection. *Period of infectivity* is the time that the patient is infectious to others. Details of the incubation periods of major infections and periods of infectivity in childhood infectious diseases are summarised in Tables 20.8 and 20.10, page 1132.

MAJOR MANIFESTATIONS OF INFECTION

A knowledge of infections prevailing in the geographical locality is an essential guide to diagnosis, especially with imported infections, as is a knowledge of where and how to find the relevant organism. Enquiry should be made about contacts among family, friends and workmates. Persons following certain occupations may be exposed to infection, e.g. leptospirosis occurs in abattoir and farm workers and anthrax in handlers of hides and bone meal.

Recent surgical history may give a clue as to the origin of abscess as a cause of unexplained fever.

Residence or travel abroad raises the possibility of malaria, amoebic abscess of the liver or other exotic disease. In many infections a diagnosis can often be made on clinical features, e.g. measles or chickenpox. In others, a diagnosis may require confirmation by microbiological, immunological, haematological, histopathological or radiological investigations; see the information box.

METHODS USED TO DIAGNOSE INFECTION
MICROBIOLOGICAL
A. Recognition of causative agent • In stained or fresh preparations, usually a smear: malaria in blood slide, *Vibrio cholerae* in stool, diphtheria in throat swab, bacilli in urine, staphylococci in pus smear, *Entamoeba* in rectal scrape, plague bacilli in bubo aspirate, schistosome ova in rectal snip, rickettsia in rash aspirate*, fungi in skin scrapings, pneumococci in purulent sputum, spirochaetes in condylomata (dark ground microscopy), leprosy bacilli and leishmania in slit skin smear • By electron microscopy: viruses in stool; herpesviruses from skin • By histology of biopsy specimen: acid-fast bacilli in leprosy and tuberculosis, *Pneumocystis* in pneumonia, hepatitis B in liver*, rabies virus in brain*
B. Culture of causative organism • From blood: typhoid, brucellosis, Gram-negative septicaemia, pneumococcal pneumonia, HIV • From bone marrow: tuberculosis, brucellosis, leishmaniasis, histoplasmosis • From other body fluids, faeces or tissues: urinary tract infection, bacillary dysentery, sputum in pneumonia, liver in tuberculosis
IMMUNOLOGICAL
A. Detection of microbial antigen • Meningococcal and pneumococcal disease (blood, cerebrospinal fluid, sputum, urine)
B. Detection of antibody of IgM class • Toxoplasmosis, hepatitis A, rubella, parvovirus
C. Demonstration of antibody • Rising titre: typhoid, brucellosis, HIV infection • Closely linked to clinical syndrome: amoebic abscess, visceral leishmaniasis • Screening for latent disease: syphilis, schistosomiasis, trypanosomiasis cruzi
D. Delayed hypersensitivity skin testing • Tuberculosis, histoplasmosis, leishmaniasis
NON-SPECIFIC
A. Tissue biopsy • Characteristic histology: hepatitis, leprosy • Suggestive histology: tuberculosis, toxoplasmosis
B. Radiology • Association of site and pattern with infection: lobar pneumonia, renal tuberculosis, muscular cysticercosis
C. Scanning • Isotope: detection of abscess, osteomyelitis (polymorph scan) • Ultrasound: abscess, hydatid cyst • Computed tomography (CT) or magnetic resonance imaging (MRI): intracranial infection, visceral abscesses, mediastinal lymph node enlargement
* Usually performed using immunofluorescent staining.

BACTERAEMIA AND SEPTICAEMIA

Bacteraemia, the presence of living organisms in the blood, can occur in healthy people without causing symptoms. For example, viridans streptococci may transiently enter the blood during dental procedures or even when teeth are cleaned vigorously. Unless there is a focus on which they can settle and multiply, e.g. an abnormal heart valve, these organisms are normally cleared very rapidly from the blood. Other organisms invading the blood stream, such as *Staphylococcus aureus* or *Escherichia coli*, are less likely to be dealt with by the immune system and more likely to cause disease; this is referred to as septicaemia.

The organisms causing septicaemia may originate from one of the areas of the body which are normally colonised by microorganisms, such as skin, large bowel or genital tract. Alternatively, the source may be infection in a major organ such as kidney or liver.

Septicaemia can be complicated by metastatic septic lesions in organs or tissues. Examples include staphylococcal osteomyelitis, pneumococcal pneumonia and meningococcal meningitis. Figure 2.1 outlines common sources of bacteria causing septicaemia, the causative organisms and examples of metastatic lesions.

Circulatory failure—the septic shock syndrome—is the most dangerous complication of septicaemia and is caused by Gram-positive, Gram-negative or fungal organisms. In HIV infection a septic shock syndrome has been described in response to mycobacteria in the blood. Septic shock is dealt with on page 1033.

Blood cultures are the most important initial investigation in septicaemia but if shock develops, tests of hepatic, renal and cardiopulmonary function and of coagulation must be performed and monitored.

The treatment of septicaemia involves prompt administration of a broad-spectrum antibiotic or a combination of antibiotics. The choice usually has to be made on an empirical basis before the results of cultures are available. Examples of initial therapy include ceftazidime alone or an aminoglycoside such as gentamicin plus a β-lactam antibiotic, e.g. azlocillin. Shock is managed as described on page 1034.

INFECTION IN IMMUNOCOMPROMISED PATIENTS

The term 'immunocompromised' refers to individuals whose resistance to infection has been reduced by disease (congenital or acquired) or by therapeutic measures such as the treatment of malignant disease or organ transplantation. Increased susceptibility to infection may result from a defect in the immune system and/or neutropenia.

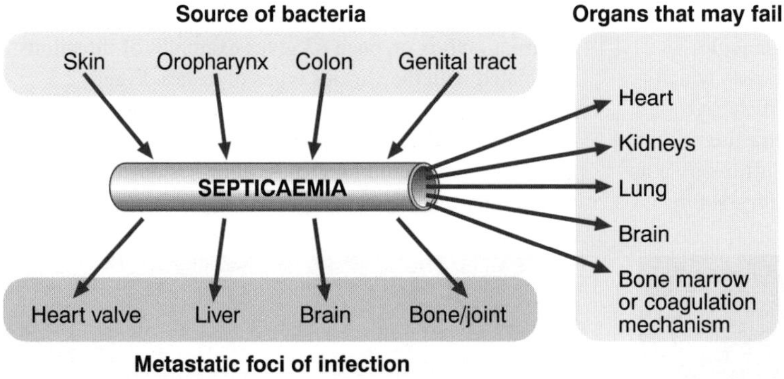

Fig. 2.1 Septicaemia. Source of infection, metastatic lesions and complications.

The infection may be endogenous, i.e. arising from within the patient, or exogenous. Endogenous infection may be due to invasion of tissues or organs by bacteria, e.g. *E. coli*, by fungi such as *Candida albicans* which are present in health in the patient's gastrointestinal tract, or by reactivation of organisms which have remained dormant since primary infection earlier in life. Examples of latent organisms which can cause infection in immunocompromised patients include the herpesviruses (varicella zoster, Herpes simplex, Epstein–Barr virus and cytomegalovirus), mycobacteria, *Toxoplasma gondii* and leishmania.

Infection is a common cause of death in immunocompromised patients, in whom it may have a fulminating onset or be refractory to therapy. Diagnosis can be difficult as the infections may present atypically, sometimes with very few signs and symptoms until well advanced. Due to the body's reduced defences against infection, treatment should be started on clinical suspicion, modified according to the results of investigations.

Table 2.2 lists the important organisms causing infections in immunocompromised patients.

Table 2.2 Microorganisms causing infections in immunocompromised patients

Defect in host response	Microorganism	Infections (examples)
Phagocytic abnormalities (Polymorphs, macrophages)	*Staph. aureus*	Skin, soft tissue
	Strep. pneumoniae	Pneumonia
	Legionella pneumophila	Pneumonia
	Strep. pyogenes	Septicaemia
	H. influenzae	Meningitis
	Gram-negative bacilli	Septicaemia
	Candida albicans	Fungaemia
Cell-mediated defects (T cells)	Herpesviruses	Shingles
	Parvovirus	Bone marrow infection
	Candida albicans	Pneumonia
	Cryptococcus	CNS infections
	Mycobacteria	Tuberculosis
	Listeria monocytogenes	Meningitis
	Pneumocystis carinii	Pneumonia
	Toxoplasma gondii	Encephalitis
	Leishmania	Leishmaniasis
	Cryptosporidium	Enteritis
Humoral defects (Immunoglobulins)	*Strep. pneumoniae*	Pneumonia
	Strep. pyogenes	Septicaemia
	Pseudomonas aeruginosa	Septicaemia
	Neisseria meningitidis	Meningitis
	H. influenzae	Pneumonia
	Mycoplasma spp.	Arthritis

RASHES

PATTERNS OF RASH ASSOCIATED WITH INFECTION

Macular or maculo-papular
- Measles*
- Rubella
- Enteroviral infections
- Herpesvirus type 6 infections
- Infectious mononucleosis
- Toxoplasmosis
- Cytomegalovirus infections
- HIV seroconversion illness
- Typhoid and paratyphoid fevers
- Rickettsial infections
- Dengue fever
- Secondary syphilis
- Drug rashes

Haemorrhagic
- Meningococcal infection*
- Viral haemorrhagic fevers
- Leptospirosis
- Septicaemia with disseminated intravascular coagulation
- Rickettsial infections
- Trypanosomiasis

Urticarial
- Toxocariasis
- Hydatidosis
- Fascioliasis
- Strongyloidiasis
- Schistosomiasis

Vesicular
- Chickenpox*
- Shingles
- Herpes simplex infections
- Hand, foot and mouth disease
- Herpangina (mouth)
- Poxviruses (monkeypox)

Nodular
- Erythema nodosum (primary TB and leprosy)

Erythematous
- Scarlet fever*
- Toxic shock syndrome
- Lyme disease
- Drug rashes
- Dengue fever

Chancres (ulcerating nodules)
- Syphilis
- Trypanosomiasis
- Typhus (tick and mite)
- Anthrax
- Rat-bite fever

* Rash is illustrated in Figure 2.2, page 64.

Rashes are common clinical features of many systemic infectious diseases. They can be classified as maculopapular (discrete or sometimes confluent red spots which can be elevated), nodular, erythematous (a diffuse red eruption which blanches on finger pressure), haemorrhagic, vesicular (associated with blister formation), urticarial or as chancres. Certain infections are associated with specific skin lesions which are characteristic of that infection. The information box on page 63 gives examples of infections associated with the various types of rashes. Figure 2.2 illustrates the common types of eruption (measles, scarlet fever, chickenpox, meningococcaemia). Drugs, including antibiotics, are a common cause of rashes during infection, particularly the β-lactams.

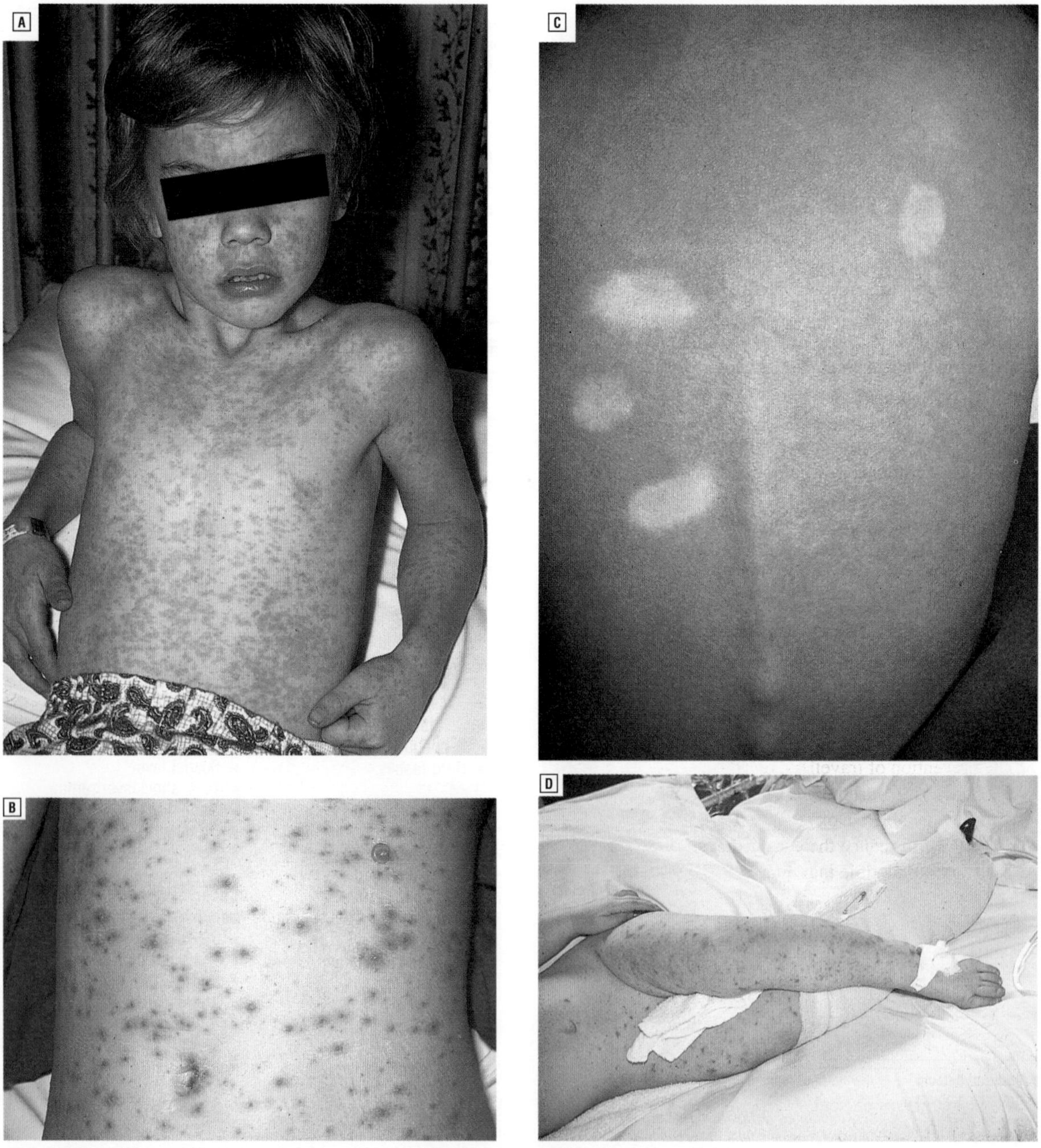

Fig. 2.2 Childhood rashes: skin eruptions. A Measles. B Chickenpox. C Scarlet fever (note blanching on pressure). D Meningococcal infection.

TRAVELLERS' DIARRHOEA

Pathogens which may be responsible for travellers' diarrhoea are shown in the information box. Commonly, however, no organism is identified (around 60–70% of patients).

SOME MICROBIAL CAUSES OF TRAVELLERS' DIARRHOEA

- Enterotoxigenic *Escherichia coli*
- *Vibrio parahaemolyticus*
- Salmonellae
- *Campylobacter jejuni*
- Shigellae
- *Giardia lamblia*
- *Vibrio cholerae*
- Rotaviruses and Norwalk viruses

An attack of diarrhoea lasting 2–5 days commonly affects travellers, particularly when visiting developing countries. The onset is usually abrupt and the stool is watery. Abdominal cramps, anorexia and vomiting are common and there may be fever. Examination of the abdomen usually shows no abnormality but there may be diffuse tenderness.

The disorder usually resolves spontaneously. Antidiarrhoeal agents are best avoided, especially in children, as they may occasionally cause toxic dilatation of the bowel. Loperamide 4 mg will stop the diarrhoea if prolonged or very severe. Antibiotics are not necessary for mild attacks, especially as they may induce antibiotic resistance. Severe attacks can be aborted in most cases with two doses of 500 mg of ciprofloxacin 12 hours apart. Dehydration should be prevented by drinking of non-alcoholic fluids and the use of oral rehydration supplements in children, and in adults if the diarrhoea is severe.

The prevention of travellers' diarrhoea involves good hygienic practices, drinking clean water and avoiding uncooked vegetables. Doxycycline 100 mg or trimethoprim 80 mg daily will reduce the attack rate but these are best reserved for susceptible individuals. Boiling water is the safest decontamination method since cysts of *Giardia* and *Cryptosporidium* are highly chemically resistant.

Table 2.3 Causes of fever imported into the UK

Frequency	Cause
Common	Malaria Presumed viral
Frequent	Bacterial: dysentery, upper respiratory tract including diphtheria, pneumonia; urinary tract, typhoid Proven viral: hepatitis A, HIV, Epstein–Barr virus, aseptic meningitis, dengue
Occasional	Tuberculosis, toxoplasmosis, rickettsial
Rare	Brucellosis, amoebic abscess, visceral leishmaniasis

INVESTIGATION AND MANAGEMENT OF FEVER FROM THE TROPICS

On admission

- Thick and thin blood films for malaria; repeat if negative
- Full blood count (neutrophilia, eosinophilia, thrombocytopenia, atypical lymphocytes)
- Cultures of blood × 3 (or bone marrow × 1 if the patient has had an antibiotic), urine, throat swab and stool if diarrhoea
- Liver function tests
- Dip-stick urine for blood, protein, bile
- Store serum for possible serology later
- Consider lumbar puncture for neck stiffness
- Treat clinically diagnosed infection for which there is no rapid confirmatory test (e.g. tick-typhus) or where delay is unjustified (e.g. malaria)

Over the next 3 days

- Re-examine the patient and look for new signs
- Treat infection diagnosed
- Consider Lassa fever if from endemic area

After 3 days

- Reassess. If getting better, wait. If not:
- Repeat initial tests
- Consider chest radiograph, abdominal ultrasound scan
- Consider serology for Epstein–Barr virus, HIV, dengue, *Rickettsia, Toxoplasma, Entamoeba, Schistosoma*, according to clinical and epidemiological situation
- Consider treatment on clinical grounds alone (e.g. getting worse and clinical features suggest typhoid)

After 10 days

- Consider more chronic infections (e.g. tuberculosis, brucellosis, HIV, leishmaniasis)
- Consider non-infectious diseases
- Obtain a second opinion

FEVER IN A PATIENT FROM THE TROPICS

Fever is a common presentation in people who have recently arrived in Britain from tropical countries. The most common diagnoses are listed in Table 2.3. The most important is malaria, because untreated *Plasmodium falciparum* infection in a non-immune patient (including expatriates and immigrants of over 3 years' duration) may become rapidly fatal. *P. falciparum* malaria usually presents within 2 months of arrival but occasionally up to 6 months later, rarely longer. The clinical features of malaria are given on pages 150–152; they may include fever, cough and diarrhoea. The pattern of fever does not distinguish malaria from other imported or domestic fevers such as influenza, but splenomegaly, thrombocytopenia and hyperbilirubinaemia strongly suggest the diagnosis. Asian immigrants are at especial risk of tuberculosis and Africans of HIV infection. Physical examination should be directed especially towards:

- the skin (rashes in meningococcaemia, dengue, rickettsioses, typhoid)
- the chest (bronchitis and pneumonitis are features of malaria and typhoid)
- the lymph glands (toxoplasmosis and seroconversion illness of infectious mononucleosis and HIV infection)
- the spleen (malaria, typhoid, acute schistosomiasis, leishmaniasis)
- the liver (hepatitis, amoebic abscess)
- neck stiffness (meningitis).

The investigation and management of fever from the tropics are shown in the information box.

PYREXIA OF UNKNOWN ORIGIN

Patients commonly develop transient febrile illnesses, often caused by viruses, which subside spontaneously and a definitive diagnosis is never made. Other fevers persist but a diagnosis is reached rapidly and treatment started. In a few patients fever persists and defies diagnosis.

The best definition of pyrexia or fever of unknown origin (PUO or FUO) was given by Petersdorf and Beeson in the United States in 1951 in a paper describing the results of a study which they carried out in 100 patients. They defined PUO as a temperature of 38.3°C or above persisting or recurring during a period of 3 weeks which included 7 days' investigation in hospital. Principal causes of PUO are illustrated in the first information box.

Petersdorf and Beeson found that only one-third of their patients eventually proved to have an infection (the most common being tuberculosis). Another third had malignant disease (the most common being a reticulosis), and one-fifth diseases of connective tissue. The remainder had various less common disorders including factitious fever. This is a condition (factitious pyrexia) where an individual, who often has medical or nursing training, mimics pyrexia—for example, by placing the thermometer on a radiator; there is usually an underlying psychiatric disorder in these cases. The second information box illustrates the investigation of PUO. Repeated examination for the development of new signs is most important.

PRINCIPAL CAUSES OF PYREXIA OF UNKNOWN ORIGIN

Malignant disease

- Reticuloses (e.g. Hodgkin's disease)
- Hypernephroma

Diseases of connective tissue

- Polyarteritis nodosa
- Still's disease
- Lupus erythematosus

Infections

- Tuberculosis (esp. lymph gland)
- Endocarditis (e.g. Q fever)
- Abscesses (liver, paraspinal, pelvic)
- Malaria (esp. if suppressed by prophylaxis)
- Visceral leishmaniasis

Other causes

- Drug fever (esp. β-lactam antibiotics)
- Factitious fever (self-induced)
- Thrombophlebitis
- Familial Mediterranean fever
- Granulomatous diseases

INVESTIGATION OF PYREXIA OF UNKNOWN ORIGIN

Retake the history

- Contact with infection (tuberculosis) or animals (brucellosis)
- Sexual contacts (HIV)
- Travel abroad (malaria)
- Drug therapy (penicillins)
- Occupation (leptospirosis)
- Recent operations or dental treatment (abscess or endocarditis)

Repeat the examination

- Heart murmurs (endocarditis)
- Splenomegaly (visceral leishmaniasis)
- Lymph glands (reticulosis, HIV)
- Retinal changes (tuberculosis, CMV infection and disseminated candidiasis)

Review results of investigations (and repeat if indicated)

- Re-examine chest radiograph (minimal lesion)
- Biochemical results abnormal (liver involvement)
- Haematology results abnormal (haematological malignancy)
- Microbiology results abnormal (pyuria)

Consider further investigations

- Serological investigations (brucellosis)
- CT/MRI scanning (abdominal lymph glands, tumours)
- Tissue biopsies (histology, culture and gene rearrangement studies—tuberculosis, malignancy)

Consider therapeutic trial (generally as a last resort)

- Antimicrobial therapy (cryptic miliary tuberculosis)
- Corticosteroid therapy (connective tissue disease)
- Cytotoxic therapy (lymphoma)

PRINCIPLES OF MANAGEMENT OF INFECTION

The management of infection depends on non-specific and specific therapeutic measures (see the information box) and also on techniques of prevention of infection.

THERAPEUTIC MEASURES IN MANAGEMENT OF INFECTION
Non-specific management
• This includes the treatment of general symptoms such as fever, myalgia, headache and thirst, and complications such as dehydration, hypovolaemia, organ failure, haemorrhage and hyperpyrexia
Specific management
• This involves the use of antimicrobial agents to kill or inhibit the growth of microorganisms

The ability of one microorganism to interfere with the growth of another is called antibiosis and is due to specific diffusible metabolic products termed *antibiotics*. Since the introduction of penicillin in 1940, research has produced a wide range of antibiotics. In addition, a variety of other chemotherapeutic agents such as metronidazole, trimethoprim, ciprofloxacin and isoniazid followed the demonstration of the therapeutic effects of sulphanilamide in 1935. A general term for all of these substances is *antimicrobial agents*. Those that kill microorganisms are referred to as bactericidal while agents that inhibit their growth are called bacteriostatic. Table 2.4 illustrates the sites and modes of action on bacteria of selected antimicrobial agents.

Effective therapy is available against all known bacteria, rickettsiae, mycoplasmas and chlamydiae. However, the evolution of antimicrobial resistance is seriously restricting treatment, and reports of total antibiotic resistance in *Staph. aureus* and enterococci are causing great concern. Specific antiprotozoal compounds are used in the treatment of diseases such as sleeping sickness, leishmaniasis, malaria and amoebic dysentery. An increasing number of drugs are available for the treatment of fungal infection. Antimicrobial agents active against viruses are now receiving great attention and use of antiherpes drugs is common and highly effective. Similarly, antiretroviral drugs have revolutionised the management of HIV.

ANTIBACTERIAL DRUGS

Antimicrobial agents have been one of the most important, and successful, groups of therapeutic agent introduced. Initially these agents were discovered and developed empirically (for example, sulphonamides and penicillin). The search for new antibiotics then involved screening of biological materials such as sewage and soil specimens to look for antimicrobial substances produced by organisms. Cephalosporins were discovered as agents produced from a sewage sample from Sardinia. Such screening processes are now largely regarded as dated and most screening takes place using a highly mechanised combinatorial approach in which vast numbers of organic molecules are tested for antimicrobial activity. Promising compounds are then identified and chemically modified to produce higher antimicrobial activity and the desired antimicrobial spectrum of activity. Agents discovered and refined in this way are already in phase III testing and will reach clinical use in the near future, e.g. oxazaladines.

THE β-LACTAM ANTIBIOTICS

These are the *penicillins* and *cephalosporins* whose basic structure includes a four-membered β-lactam ring (see Fig. 2.3). Resistance is commonly due to bacterial enzymes called β-lactamases (penicillinases and cephalosporinases) which can cleave the ring and inactivate the antibiotic. The plasmids which code for these enzymes are transmissible between bacteria. Resistance may also be due to other mechanisms

Table 2.4 Mechanisms of action of antimicrobial agents

Site of action in bacteria	Mode of action	Antibiotic
Nucleic acid synthesis	Interrupts folate synthesis Inhibits DNA supercoiling Breaks DNA strands Inhibits RNA polymerase	Sulphonamides/trimethoprim 4-quinolones Nitrofurantoin Rifampicin
Protein synthesis	Binds to 30S ribosome and causes RNA code misreading Binds to 50S ribosome subunit and blocks translocation Inhibits transfer of amino acids to ribosome Binds to 30S ribosome and blocks RNA attachment	Aminoglycosides Macrolides Chloramphenicol Tetracycline
Cell membrane function	Disrupts cell membrane Inhibits sterol synthesis	Polymyxins Amphotericin
Cell wall synthesis	Inhibits carriage of subunits from cell membrane to cell wall Inhibits final cross-linkage of peptidoglycan	Vancomycin Cephalosporins/penicillins

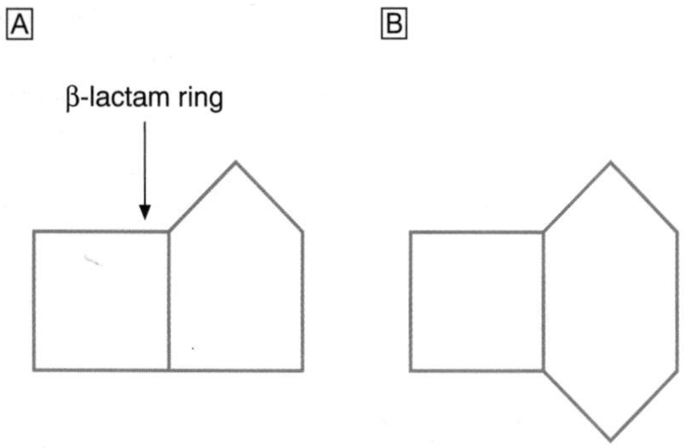

Fig. 2.3 The β-lactam antibiotics: nuclei. A Penicillin. B Cephalosporin.

such as inability of the antibiotics to penetrate the bacterial cell wall. Penicillin-resistant pneumococci and meningococci and methicillin-resistant staphylococci (MRSA), which are also resistant to cloxacillin, are increasing problems in many countries.

The penicillins

All penicillins are bactericidal, killing bacteria by interfering with their cell wall synthetic processes. The range of their activity is wide, as both Gram-positive and certain Gram-negative organisms are sensitive to individual penicillins (see Table 2.5). Their most important adverse effect is hypersensitivity (see the information box). This may take the form of urticaria and pyrexia or an acute anaphylactic reaction which may occasionally prove fatal.

ADVERSE EFFECTS OF THE PENICILLINS

Hypersensitivity	Dose-related
• Skin rash (urticaria or maculo-papular) • Anaphylaxis • Drug fever • Interstitial nephritis	• Encephalopathy • Neutropenia (reversible) • Haemolysis

Although penicillin is otherwise a safe antibiotic, its accumulation in patients with renal failure may lead to encephalopathy. In these patients dosage must be modified and guided by blood levels. In severe infections penicillin should be given intravenously; it should never be given intrathecally due to risk of seizure.

Benzylpenicillin

This is rapidly absorbed following intramuscular injection and is excreted by the kidneys within a few hours. Probenecid, 2 g daily by mouth, will raise the blood level of penicillin by delaying its excretion by the kidney and thus

Table 2.5 The penicillins

	β-lactamase stable	Route of administration	Average adult dose (mg given 6-hourly)	Indications
Benzylpenicillin	–	Parenteral	600–2400	Streptococcal and meningococcal infections, anthrax, diphtheria, gas gangrene, syphilis, yaws, gonorrhoea, actinomycosis
Procaine penicillin	–	Parenteral	300 (daily)	As for benzylpenicillin
Phenoxymethylpenicillin	–	Oral	500	Mild streptococcal infections
Cloxacillin/flucloxacillin	+	Parenteral/oral	500–2000	Staphylococcal infections
Ampicillin/amoxycillin	–	Parenteral/oral	250–1000	Infections caused by aerobic Gram-negative bacilli, streptococci, salmonellae and shigellae
Amoxycillin plus clavulanic acid (Augmentin)	+	Parenteral/oral	250–1000 (amoxycillin dose)	As for amoxycillin plus staphylococci and bacteroides
Ampicillin plus sulbactam (sultamicillin)	+	Oral	375 (12-hourly)	Infections caused by susceptible organisms and surgical prophylaxis where β-lactamase inhibition is required
Carbenicillin	–	Parenteral	1000–5000	*Pseudomonas* infections
Ticarcillin	–	Parenteral	1000–5000	*Pseudomonas* infections
Ticarcillin plus clavulanic acid (Timentin)	+	Parenteral	3200 (6–8-hourly)	*Pseudomonas* and *Proteus* infections
Azlocillin	–	Parenteral	1000–5000	*Pseudomonas* infections
Mezlocillin	–	Parenteral	1000–5000	Infections caused by aerobic Gram-negative bacilli and surgical prophylaxis (bowel and pelvic surgery)
Piperacillin	–	Parenteral	1000–5000	Infections caused by aerobic Gram-negative bacilli
Temocillin	+	Parenteral	1000–2000 (12-hourly)	Infections caused by Gram-negative bacilli

allow smaller doses or less frequent administration. Penicillin is also used prophylactically to prevent endocarditis, tetanus and gas gangrene.

Phenoxymethylpenicillin
This is incompletely absorbed from the stomach and is only used for less serious infections such as tonsillitis.

Cloxacillin and flucloxacillin
These are semi-synthetic penicillins which are stable to staphylococcal β-lactamases. For oral therapy, flucloxacillin is superior to cloxacillin as it is almost twice as well absorbed from the gut.

Temocillin
This is active against penicillinase-producing Gram-negative bacilli.

Ampicillin
This is a semi-synthetic penicillin which has a bactericidal action against both Gram-positive and certain Gram-negative organisms. It is susceptible to degradation by β-lactamases and not well absorbed with food. Maculo-papular rashes occur in approximately 5% of all patients given ampicillin and in over 90% of patients given it for infectious mononucleosis; this antibiotic should not therefore be prescribed for sore throats which may be due to infectious mononucleosis. There are a number of ampicillin esters including bacampicillin and pivampicillin. These are better absorbed and produce higher blood levels of ampicillin.

Amoxycillin
This is an analogue of ampicillin which has a similar antibacterial spectrum but is more reliably absorbed from the gastrointestinal tract. Clavulanic acid is a β-lactam agent with only weak antibacterial activity. It is, however, a potent inhibitor of many β-lactamases and can protect β-lactamase-susceptible antibiotics, such as amoxycillin, from inactivation by these enzymes. A combination of amoxycillin plus sodium clavulanate (ratio 1:2 oral and 1:5 i.v.) is available (Augmentin). There is also a combination of ampicillin and another β-lactamase inhibitor called sulbactam (Unasyn).

Ticarcillin
Carbenicillin was initially the only penicillin with activity against *Pseudomonas aeruginosa*. This organism, however, is only moderately sensitive to carbenicillin, which has been replaced by its more active analogue ticarcillin. There is a preparation containing ticarcillin plus clavulanic acid (Timentin).

Mezlocillin, azlocillin and piperacillin
These acylureidopenicillins have a wider range of activity than ampicillin and are also more effective against many Gram-negative bacilli. They are used in combination with other antibiotics for the treatment of undiagnosed infections in immunocompromised patients. Azlocillin is more active than ticarcillin against *Ps. aeruginosa*, and is usually used in combination with an aminoglycoside for *Pseudomonas* infections. Piperacillin also has anti-anaerobic activity.

The cephalosporins
The cephalosporins have a wide range of activity against many important Gram-positive and Gram-negative bacteria and are therefore of value for the treatment of serious infections and for the initial empirical therapy of undiagnosed infections. The information box lists the cephalosporins available in 1998. They have been developed over the past 30 years and the historical classification by 'generations', although helpful, is not ideal. A more systematic approach based on groupings according to antimicrobial activity and β-lactamase production has been suggested and categorises cephalosporins into seven groups (see O'Grady et al, Further information, p. 78). The first-generation agents developed in the 1960s have generally been replaced by the newer compounds. The second-generation drugs are more stable to β-lactamases. The third-generation agents are more active than the second against Gram-negative bacilli; however, they are less active

CEPHALOSPORINS

Injectable

First generation • Cephradine (also oral) • Cephazolin **Second generation** • Cefamandole • Cefuroxime (also oral)	**Third generation** • Cefotaxime • Ceftazidime • Ceftizoxime • Cefodizime • Cefpirome • Cefsulodin (*Pseudomonas* infections only) • Ceftriaxone (long serum half-life) **Fourth generation** • Cefepime • Cefpirome

Oral

First generation • Cephalexin • Cephradine • Cefadroxil **Second generation** • Cefaclor • Cefixime • Ceftibuten • Cefuroxime axetil	**Third generation** • Cefpodoxime proxetil

against Gram-positive bacteria, especially *Staph. aureus*. The third-generation agents are very expensive.

Cefoxitin, a broad-spectrum cephamycin antibiotic, has activity against *Bacteroides fragilis*, an anaerobic bacillus which is a common cause of intra-abdominal sepsis, and is used for such infections.

The orally active cephalosporins are principally used for the treatment of lower respiratory tract, ear and urinary tract infections. They all have a similar spectrum but the newer agents are more resistant to β-lactamases.

The dose of the cephalosporins ranges from 250–2000 mg 6–8-hourly, depending on the weight of the patient, renal function and severity of infection. Ceftazidime is the most active against Gram-negative bacilli and is specifically useful in *Pseudomonas* infection. It is used for the treatment of septicaemia and infections in the immunocompromised. Ceftriaxone has a much longer serum half-life (10 hours) than the other cephalosporins (1 hour) and need only be given once daily. Agents such as cefotaxime and ceftriaxone are now used extensively for the treatment of meningitis.

Adverse reactions are similar to those of the penicillins. A small number (around 10%) of penicillin-sensitive patients may also be allergic to the cephalosporins, which should be avoided if there is a history of significant hypersensitivity to the penicillins.

Other β-lactam agents

Imipenem

This is a β-lactam antibiotic with a very broad spectrum which includes aerobic and anaerobic Gram-positive and Gram-negative organisms. It is partially inactivated by a renal enzyme and is therefore given along with an inhibitor of this enzyme called *cilastatin*. Side-effects are similar to other β-lactam antibiotics.

Aztreonam

This is a monocyclic β-lactam antibiotic, the efficacy of which is limited to Gram-negative aerobic bacteria including *Ps. aeruginosa* and *Haemophilus influenzae*. Side-effects are similar to those of other β-lactam antibiotics.

THE MACROLIDE ANTIBIOTICS

These are erythromycin, clarithromycin, azithromycin and spiramycin.

Erythromycin

This has a similar although not identical spectrum to penicillin and is commonly used to treat infections caused by Gram-positive organisms in penicillin-allergic patients in combination with fusidic acid. It is also effective in whooping cough, *Campylobacter* enteritis and legionnaires' disease, provided it is given early enough in the course of these illnesses. Many physicians now use erythromycin as first-line treatment for community-acquired pneumonia in view of its wider spectrum of activity than penicillin. It has activity against mycoplasmas and chlamydiae and is an effective antibiotic for the treatment of many acute respiratory infections. Erythromycin is prescribed in a dosage of 250–500 mg by mouth 6-hourly. There is a preparation for intravenous injection which is highly thrombophlebitic. Diarrhoea, vomiting and abdominal pain are the principal side-effects. Cholestatic jaundice may rarely develop if the course of treatment exceeds 10 days.

Clarithromycin

This has slightly greater activity than erythromycin, and achieves higher concentrations in tissues. The dose is 200–500 mg 12-hourly.

Azithromycin

This has more activity than erythromycin against certain Gram-negative organisms, including *H. influenzae*, but is less active against Gram-positive bacteria. As with clarithromycin, tissue levels are high but plasma levels are low. The serum half-life is long, allowing once-daily administration (500 mg). Due to their greater activity against *H. influenzae* and also against the organisms causing atypical pneumonia (mycoplasma, chlamydia and *Legionella*), clarithromycin and azithromycin may replace erythromycin for the treatment of lower respiratory tract infections.

Spiramycin

This is a macrolide used as second-line treatment for toxoplasmosis.

THE TETRACYCLINE ANTIBIOTICS

Tetracycline, oxytetracycline, chlortetracycline and *minocycline* are closely related bacteriostatic agents which, for practical purposes, have an identical range of activity. The adult dose is 250–500 mg 6-hourly before meals because the absorption of most tetracyclines is reduced by chelation with calcium (e.g. in milk). *Doxycycline* is an exception and also has the advantage that it is given only once daily, 200 mg on the first day and 100 mg thereafter.

The tetracyclines inhibit the growth of a wide range of Gram-positive and Gram-negative bacteria although in the context of treating lower respiratory tract infections their value is limited by the emergence of tetracycline-resistant pneumococci and *H. influenzae*. The tetracyclines are also active against rickettsiae (typhus fevers), *Coxiella burnetii* (Q fever), *Mycoplasma pneumoniae* and chlamydiae (lymphogranuloma venereum, psittacosis and non-gonococcal urethritis) and are effective in brucellosis. They are also employed systemically in acne vulgaris and rosacea (see pp. 904 and 906) where their beneficial effect is not due solely to their antibacterial action. Chlortetracycline is used for the local treatment of skin infections as it does not cause cutaneous sensitisation.

The tetracyclines are generally safe antibiotics, with few side-effects. The most common is diarrhoea, which usually stops when the antibiotic is discontinued. Tetracyclines chelate with calcium and are deposited in developing bone and teeth, causing a brown discoloration. They should not therefore be given to children or pregnant women. With the exception of doxycycline and minocycline, the tetracyclines can exacerbate renal failure and should not be given to patients with impaired renal function.

THE AMINOGLYCOSIDE ANTIBIOTICS

Streptomycin, gentamicin, tobramycin, netilmicin, amikacin and neomycin have similar chemical structures and adverse effects. They are not absorbed and for systemic treatment must be given by injection (except neomycin).

Streptomycin

This has the important property that it is bactericidal against the tubercle bacillus (see p. 347). It is given with two other antituberculous drugs and this triple therapy prevents the emergence of resistant strains. For long-term therapy the daily dose of streptomycin should not exceed 1 g. It is also useful in the treatment of brucellosis.

Gentamicin

This is active against most Gram-negative bacilli, including *Ps. aeruginosa.* It is also active against penicillin-resistant staphylococci but inactive against anaerobes and streptococci with the exception of *Enterococcus faecalis*; in serious infections caused by this organism gentamicin is combined with ampicillin. The dose of gentamicin depends on renal function and the age and weight of the patient (see Table 2.6); 5 mg/kg body weight per 24 hours in divided doses (usually given 8-hourly) is indicated for most infections. Recent evidence shows that single daily dosing is effective. A loading dose of gentamicin is required in all patients to ensure therapeutic levels are rapidly achieved. Up to 7.5 mg/kg may be required for serious infections and in neonates, but 2 mg/kg is sufficient for uncomplicated urinary tract infections and for synergistic therapy with penicillin for the treatment of streptococcal endocarditis. Serum concentrations of gentamicin must be measured during therapy to ensure efficacy and also to prevent toxicity due to unduly high levels, especially in renal failure and in the elderly. These measurements are usually carried out on two specimens of blood, the first taken 1 hour after a dose (peak) and the second just before the next dose (trough concentration). One-hour levels should be between 4 and 10 mg/l and trough levels less than 2 mg/l.

Table 2.6 The aminoglycosides: dosages

Aminoglycoside	Max. daily dose (mg/kg/24 hrs)	Maximum plasma levels: Peak level	Maximum plasma levels: Pre-dose level
Gentamicin	5	10 mg/l	2 mg/l
Tobramycin	5	10 mg/l	2 mg/l
Netilmicin	6	12 mg/l	2 mg/l
Amikacin	15	30 mg/l	10 mg/l

Notes
1. Plasma levels should be monitored in all patients if possible and MUST be measured in the elderly, in infants, and if high doses are given or IF RENAL FUNCTION IS IMPAIRED.
2. Gentamicin, tobramycin and netilmicin are usually given 8- or 12-hourly if renal function is normal. Single daily dosage is also effective.
3. 60–80 mg 12-hourly of gentamicin is recommended for streptococcal endocarditis.

Tobramycin

This is more active than gentamicin against *Ps. aeruginosa* but has no other advantage.

Netilmicin

A gentamicin derivative, netilmicin is stable to three of nine aminoglycoside-inactivating enzymes, and should be reserved for infection caused by gentamicin-resistant organisms. Netilmicin is slightly less nephrotoxic than gentamicin, to which it is preferred in the elderly and if renal function is impaired.

Amikacin

This has less intrinsic antibacterial activity than gentamicin, but has the advantage of being stable to eight of the nine aminoglycoside-inactivating enzymes, in contrast to gentamicin which is susceptible to six of the nine. For this reason amikacin is active against many gentamicin-resistant Gram-negative bacilli and should be reserved for the treatment of infections caused by these organisms.

Neomycin

This is too toxic to be given parenterally but local applications containing neomycin are used in infections of the skin and eye. Neomycin may be used orally in hepatic encephalopathy to reduce the numbers of colonic bacteria.

The aminoglycosides are all nephrotoxic and ototoxic. The most common adverse effect of the aminoglycosides is on the 8th cranial nerve. Aminoglycosides, especially gentamicin, should not be administered together with the diuretic frusemide, as additive ototoxicity may result from the combination.

The toxicity of the aminoglycosides is related to the age of the patient, the serum level of the antibiotic and the duration of administration. The aminoglycosides are principally excreted from the body by the kidneys and the risk of toxicity is increased when there is impairment of renal function. Serum levels of the aminoglycosides must be measured in all patients to prevent toxicity and also to ensure therapeutic blood levels.

OTHER ANTIBIOTICS AND CHEMOTHERAPEUTIC AGENTS

Chloramphenicol

This has a range of activity similar to that of the tetracyclines, with the important difference that it is effective in enteric fever. It is more active than the tetracyclines against *H. influenzae* and is an antibiotic of choice in meningitis due to this organism, particularly in developing countries where cefotaxime may not be available. The daily oral dose for an adult is 1–3 g. Preparations for parenteral administration are also available and are particularly useful in severe infection in developing countries. Plasma levels resulting from intramuscular injections are equivalent to those resulting from intravenous route administration. Chloramphenicol eye drops and ointment are useful for purulent conjunctivitis.

Chloramphenicol has in its chemical structure a benzene ring of the type known to cause bone marrow aplasia. Although pancytopenia due to chloramphenicol is very uncommon, it is almost invariably a serious complication; this antibiotic should be used systemically only if there is no adequate alternative therapy. It is inexpensive and therefore used widely in developing countries. Chloramphenicol should never be given to premature infants or to the newborn because of the risk of the development of the frequently fatal 'grey baby syndrome'. This is a state of acute circulatory failure caused by the very high blood levels of chloramphenicol due to its inadequate conjugation in the liver at this age.

Clindamycin (7-chlorolincomycin)

This has a similar antibacterial spectrum to penicillin against most Gram-positive organisms, including penicillin-resistant staphylococci. It penetrates well into bone and is therefore useful for osteomyelitis caused by *Staph. aureus*. The other principal indications are for the treatment of infections caused by *B. fragilis* and for lung abscess. The dose is 300 mg 6-hourly, orally or by injection.

Clindamycin is a common cause of *antibiotic-associated colitis*. This adverse reaction, which can also complicate treatment with other antibiotics, especially ampicillin, is due to selective overgrowth of *Clostridium difficile* which produces toxins detectable in faeces and are the direct cause of the disease. Treatment is with oral vancomycin or metronidazole, the latter being less costly.

Sodium fusidate

This is bactericidal against *Staph. aureus* and is useful in infections caused by penicillin-resistant staphylococci. The dose is 250–500 mg 8-hourly by mouth. Nausea and vomiting are common. An intravenous preparation is available; cholestatic jaundice has occasionally been associated with its use. It is expensive and is indicated only for serious infections due to staphylococci, especially osteomyelitis and endocarditis. The drug is very well absorbed and the oral route can be used instead of the parenteral route.

Spectinomycin

This is an aminocyclitol compound with a certain structural similarity to streptomycin, although it is not an aminoglycoside. Its only clinical use is for the treatment of gonorrhoea if penicillin is contraindicated because of allergy or bacterial resistance.

Vancomycin and teicoplanin

These are glycopeptide bactericidal antibiotics. Indications for their use are limited to serious infections such as endocarditis (treatment and prophylaxis) or septicaemia caused by *Staph. aureus* and *Staph. epidermidis*, including methicillin-resistant strains (MRSA and MRSE). Oral vancomycin (125 mg 6-hourly) is used for antibiotic-associated colitis. Teicoplanin has a longer serum half-life than vancomycin and can therefore be given once daily.

Parenteral administration of vancomycin is by slow intravenous infusion of 500–1000 mg over 60 minutes 12-hourly if renal function is normal. Plasma levels must be monitored—peak (1-hour) levels should not exceed 30 mg/l and pre-dose levels must not exceed 10 mg/l. Side-effects include fever, rash and, if plasma levels exceed recommended concentrations, nephrotoxicity and ototoxicity. The daily dose must be reduced in renal failure.

Sulphonamides

These have largely been superseded by antibiotics although their usefulness was extended by the discovery of their synergistic action with trimethoprim, dapsone and pyrimethamine. Co-trimoxazole, a preparation containing sulphamethoxazole and trimethoprim, is, however, active against a wide range of bacteria. Dapsone-sulphamethoxazole is used to treat malaria, and pyrimethamine-sulphamethoxazole to treat toxoplasmosis.

The sulphonamides most suitable for clinical use are short-acting preparations such as sulphadimidine, which is rapidly absorbed and quickly excreted in the urine in a soluble form. One of the few remaining indications for the

ADVERSE EFFECTS OF THE SULPHONAMIDES

- Skin rash, including Stevens–Johnson syndrome (erythema multiforme and mucous membrane ulceration)
- Drug fever
- Blood dyscrasias including haemolysis in glucose-6-phosphate deficiency
- Nephritis
- Photosensitivity (topical use)
- Interaction with warfarin and sulphonylurea drugs

sulphonamides is cystitis (see p. 460). However, the use of double-dose co-trimoxazole is a first-line treatment for *Pneumocystis carinii* pneumonia in immunocompromised hosts, e.g. HIV. Sulphonamides have a wide range of potential hazards (see the information box).

Co-trimoxazole

This consists of trimethoprim and sulphamethoxazole, which act by inhibiting enzymes at two successive stages in the synthesis of para-aminobenzoic acid to folic acid and DNA. Co-trimoxazole is used for treatment of exacerbations of chronic bronchitis (see p. 322) and urinary tract infections (see p. 460). It is also effective in the treatment of invasive salmonella infections (see p. 123). The adult dose is two tablets (each containing 80 mg of trimethoprim and 400 mg of sulphamethoxazole) given 12-hourly by mouth. There is also a preparation for injection.

The adverse effects are those of the sulphonamides (see the information box on p. 72). Stevens–Johnson syndrome has been reported in association with co-trimoxazole. In addition, haematological reactions to trimethoprim, including thrombocytopenia and megaloblastic anaemia, may occur due to folate deficiency. Side-effects are most common in the elderly, in whom co-trimoxazole should be avoided.

Trimethoprim

On its own this is used for the treatment of urinary tract infection in a dose of 200 mg 12-hourly, or 100 mg each evening for long-term chemoprophylaxis. It is also used for the treatment of respiratory tract infections. Side-effects are fewer than with co-trimoxazole, especially in the elderly.

Nalidixic acid

This was the first 4-quinolone to be introduced, 30 years ago. These agents are inhibitors of DNA gyrase, the enzyme responsible for supercoiling of bacterial DNA. While nalidixic acid has only modest antibacterial activity and is poorly absorbed from the gut, several new 4-quinolones have been developed with significantly greater activity and improved absorption.

Ciprofloxacin

This is the most important of the new 4-quinolones. It has a relatively broad spectrum with particularly high activity against aerobic Gram-negative bacilli including salmonellae, shigellae, *Campylobacter* and *Pseudomonas* species. It is also active against chlamydiae and mycoplasmas but not against anaerobic bacteria. Although many Gram-positive organisms are sensitive to ciprofloxacin, the activity is only moderate, especially against pneumococci. Ciprofloxacin diffuses readily into infected tissues and cells. The oral dose is 250–750 mg 12-hourly and for intravenous infusion 200 mg 12-hourly.

Ciprofloxacin has a wide range of indications including gastrointestinal, urinary tract and lower respiratory tract infections (not pneumococcal), septicaemia and gonorrhoea.

Indications for the other available 4-quinolones are listed in the first information box. With the exception of ciprofloxacin which has an oral and intravenous formulation, they are given orally. The adverse reactions encountered with the 4-quinolones are summarised in the second information box. Newer quinolones will be available with a wider antimicrobial spectrum.

INDICATIONS FOR THE USE OF THE 4-QUINOLONE ANTIBIOTICS

Treatment of gonorrhoea

- Acrosoxacin (300 mg single dose)

Treatment of urinary tract infections

- Nalidixic acid (1 g 6-hourly)
- Norfloxacin (400 mg 12-hourly)
- Cinoxacin (500 mg 12-hourly)

Broad-spectrum

- Ofloxacin (UTI, LRTI, STD) (200–400 mg daily)
- Ciprofloxacin (UTI, LRTI, STD, GI infections, typhoid fever, septicaemia, meningococcal prophylaxis) (see text for dose)

All given orally; ciprofloxacin also available for i.v. injection (UTI = urinary tract infection; LRTI = lower respiratory tract infection but not pneumococcal; STD = sexually transmitted disease; GI = gastrointestinal)

ADVERSE EFFECTS OF 4-QUINOLONES

Gastrointestinal

- Nausea
- Vomiting
- Diarrhoea

Rashes

- Maculo-papular
- Photosensitivity
- Urticaria

Neurotoxicity

- Insomnia
- Dizziness
- Headache
- Convulsions (rare)

Drug interactions

- NSAIDs
- Theophylline
- Peptic ulcer drugs

Note 4-quinolones are contraindicated in children and pregnancy (arthropathy in young animals).

Metronidazole

This imidazole compound has high activity against anaerobic bacteria and intestinal protozoa but none against aerobic bacteria. It is effective against infection due to *Trichomonas vaginalis*, *Giardia lamblia* and *Entamoeba histolytica*, and is widely used for the treatment and prophylaxis of infections caused by anaerobic bacteria, notably *B. fragilis*. It is active against *Clostridium tetani* and *Cl. difficile*. Side-effects of metronidazole are usually limited to headache and nausea but it should not be given to women during the first trimester of pregnancy as fetal abnormalities have been reported in animals given high doses for prolonged periods. Alcohol should be avoided during therapy with metronidazole, which has a similar action to disulfiram and has an Antabuse-like effect (nausea, lightheadedness). The oral dose varies from 200–400 mg 8-hourly; 800 mg 8-hourly is required for intestinal amoebic infections. There are preparations for intravenous infusion and rectal use.

Tinidazole

This is similar to metronidazole but has a longer serum half-life (12 hours as compared to 7 hours), allowing less frequent administration, and is less toxic.

Mupirocin

This is not related to any other antibiotic and is only indicated for application to the skin or anterior nose for the treatment of skin infection or eradication of staphylococcal carriage.

ANTITUBERCULOUS DRUGS

These are discussed on page 352.

ANTIFUNGAL DRUGS

For therapeutic purposes, fungal infections are classified either as superficial (skin or mucous membranes) or systemic. The former usually respond readily to topical application of an antifungal agent (see Table 2.7). Systemic fungal infections usually occur in compromised hosts and can be extremely difficult to cure. Relatively high doses of antifungal agents given for prolonged periods of time may be required for these infections and expert advice should be sought for their management.

Nystatin

This is the most commonly prescribed agent for the treatment of *Candida* infections of skin and mucous membranes. It is not absorbed when given by mouth and cannot be administered parenterally because of its low solubility and toxicity. A suspension, tablets and pessaries are available for the treatment of oral, intestinal and vaginal thrush.

Table 2.7 Antifungal drugs

Drug	Dose
For topical application	
Nystatin	
Clotrimazole	
Econazole	
Amphotericin	
For oral administration	
Miconazole	250 mg 6-hourly
Ketoconazole	200 mg daily
Fluconazole	50–200 mg daily (max. 14 days)*
Itraconazole	100–200 mg daily
Flucytosine	200 mg/kg daily
Griseofulvin	500 mg daily
Terbinafine	250 mg daily
For intravenous infusion	
Amphotericin (also a liposomal preparation)	Initially 1 mg/kg/day (consult expert)
Miconazole	600 mg 8-hourly
Flucytosine	200 mg/kg daily
Fluconazole	200–400 mg daily

* Up to 400 mg daily for several weeks may be necessary in severely immunocompromised patients with invasive fungal infections.
Invasive fungal infections requiring high doses and prolonged therapy should be treated by physicians with experience of these diseases. In an immunocompromised host (HIV) chronic antifungal secondary prophylaxis may be required.

Clotrimazole, econazole, miconazole, isoconazole, sulconazole, tioconazole and ketoconazole

All these belong to the imidazole group of antifungal agents. They are effective against a wide range of fungi. The first two agents are used for the topical therapy of superficial fungal infections. Miconazole and ketoconazole are absorbed from the gut and have been successfully used for the treatment of systemic fungal infections as well as for superficial mycoses. There is also an intravenous formulation of miconazole. Hepatotoxicity (occasionally fatal) has been reported during ketoconazole therapy. Liver function tests should be performed during long-term therapy and ketoconazole should NOT be used for superficial infections.

Fluconazole and itraconazole

Fluconazole is an oral triazole antifungal drug indicated for mucocutaneous and systemic candidiasis and for cryptococcal infections. Itraconazole, also a triazole, is indicated for oropharyngeal and genital candidiasis and for tinea infections. It is contraindicated in liver disease. It has some efficacy in aspergillus infections.

Amphotericin

This is an important antibiotic for the treatment of systemic fungal infections. It is a moderately toxic drug and side-effects are relatively common. These include fever, vomiting, thrombophlebitis, anaemia and nephrotoxicity. The antibiotic is given by intravenous infusion in increasing daily doses, usually commencing with 1 mg. A liposomal preparation of amphotericin (AmBisome) is more effective and less toxic, but is very much more expensive; it should only be used in renal failure or in patients who have previously suffered nephrotoxicity with conventional amphotericin.

Flucytosine

This is well absorbed from the gut and side-effects are relatively uncommon, although bone-marrow depression can occur. It is active only against yeasts and has been used for the treatment of systemic candidiasis, sometimes in combination with amphotericin. *C. albicans* can develop resistance to flucytosine.

Griseofulvin

This is concentrated in keratin and is a drug of choice for widespread or chronic dermatophyte infections such as ringworm. It is well absorbed from the gut and is given in a daily dose of 250 mg (child) or 500 mg (adult). Skin lesions respond quickly but infection of the nails requires several months of therapy. Localised and minor ringworm lesions usually respond to topical application of Whitfield's ointment or miconazole.

Terbinafine

The newer agent terbinafine, an allylamine antifungal given in an adult dose of 250 mg daily, is as effective for ringworm when given for 2–4 weeks.

ANTIVIRAL DRUGS

The challenge with antiviral chemotherapy is to find an agent which will arrest the replication of viruses without interfering with the metabolism of mammalian cells. Great advances have been made recently in antiviral chemotherapy. A further problem is that by the time a viral infection has been diagnosed using laboratory tests, much of the damage has been done to the host tissues. Table 2.8 provides information on currently available antiviral drugs. Their doses are given with the descriptions of individual viral diseases.

Aciclovir is an effective agent for herpes simplex and varicella zoster infections, particularly in the immunosuppressed. It does not, however, eradicate the viruses from the body. The use of this agent has been advocated in childhood chickenpox since it reduces the length of illness without reducing the immune response. Cost of this treatment is, however, likely to be prohibitive in many countries. Aciclovir is a useful agent in treating genital herpes, as both primary and prophylactic treatment. Resistance to aciclovir has now been regularly reported. *Famciclovir* is a newer antiherpes agent which is given as prodrug requiring metabolism first pass to produce the active form penciclovir. Famciclovir has some activity against Epstein–Barr (EB) virus and hepatitis B virus.

Ganciclovir is an antiherpes agent with activity against cytomegalovirus (CMV). Again, resistance to this agent is acquired rapidly on treatment, being detected in 8% of patients on this drug for >3 months. Currently, ganciclovir is only indicated for life-threatening CMV infection. There is considerable toxicity to monitor when using the drug, principally involving myelosuppression. *Ribovirine* is active against RNA viruses and good activity has been found against influenza, parainfluenza, mumps, measles and respiratory syncytial virus (RSV). The only clinical use of this drug is in the aerosolised form for RSV infection.

The antiretroviral agents are discussed later (see p. 92).

Table 2.8 Antiviral drugs

Drug (doses are given in text)	Routes of administration	Indications	Side-effects
Aciclovir	Topical Oral Intravenous	Herpes zoster Chickenpox (esp. in immunosuppressed) Herpes simplex infection: encephalitis, genital tract, eye	Rash, headache, gastrointestinal toxicity, neurotoxicity (i.v. only) Increase in urea and creatinine
Famciclovir	Oral	Herpes zoster and genital H. simplex infection	Rash, headache
Idoxuridine	Topical	Herpes zoster H. simplex keratitis	Local irritation
Amantadine	Oral	Prophylaxis of influenza A	CNS symptoms Nausea
Ribovirine	Oral	Lassa fever Respiratory syncytial virus infection in infants (inhalation)	Reticulocytosis Respiratory depression
Ganciclovir	Intravenous/oral	Cytomegalovirus infection in immunosuppressed	Leucopenia, thrombocytopenia
Zidovudine	Oral	HIV infection (incl. AIDS)	CNS symptoms, anaemia, neutropenia, thrombocytopenia

ANTIPARASITIC DRUGS

Few of the antibacterial antibiotics work against protozoa or helminths.

Amphotericin inhibits the production of ergosterol, which is the major sterol of cell membranes of the yeast stages of fungi and the amastigote stages of leishmania. Conventional preparations are too toxic for routine use, as a first choice. The liposomal preparations are more efficient and less toxic but extremely expensive. *Ivermectin* is an antibiotic widely used against helminths in veterinary medicine and is valuable in human filarial infections.

Many antiparasitic drugs are derived from traditional remedies (quinine comes from cinchona bark), ancient pharmacopoeias (stibogluconate and melarsen B contain toxic heavy metals), or from random screening (mepacrine and chloroquine). Recently, the pharmaceutical industry has taken a more serious interest in tropical parasitic infections and logical derivatives are being developed. Among the most useful are those based on the imidazole ring. The nitroimidazoles, metronidazole and tinidazole, are effective against intestinal protozoa, as well as anaerobic bacteria, while the benzimidazoles, such as mebendazole and albendazole, are effective against a wide range of helminthic infections. Other azoles such as ketoconazole inhibit enzymes in the ergosterol pathway and have some action against leishmania as well as fungi. Praziquantel is an important agent in the management of schistosome infection. Atovaquone, a hydroxynaphthoquinone, has been developed as an antimalarial and is marketed in combination with proguanil.

The indications and dosages are given in individual sections dealing with specific infections.

SELECTION OF ANTIMICROBIAL AGENT

The choice of effective chemotherapy involves the nature and site of the infection, the known or suspected causative organism, the characteristics of the patient, the available antibiotics, their pharmacokinetic profiles and their cost.

The nature and site of the infection

When the nature of the infection (and the likely causative organism) can be predicted from the clinical features of the illness, treatment can proceed without isolation of the causative organism, as in the prescription of penicillin for acute follicular tonsillitis or lobar pneumonia. In exacerbations of chronic bronchitis the causative organisms are almost always pneumococci and *H. influenzae*, and ampicillin or co-trimoxazole is, therefore, indicated without specific laboratory diagnosis.

If the patient is seriously ill, antibiotic therapy must be started on a 'best guess' (empirical) basis. The presentation of the illness may assist in the selection of the most appropriate agent. If there are no clues as to the nature of the infection, treatment should be started with a combination of antibiotics such as gentamicin plus a penicillin, or with a cephalosporin such as cefotaxime.

The known or suspected causative organism

When there is uncertainty about the nature of the infection a bacteriological diagnosis should be made, whenever possible, so that the appropriate antibiotic can be given. If the organism is one such as *Streptococcus pyogenes*, which has a predictable susceptibility to the generally used antimicrobial agents, it is still wise to obtain an antibiotic sensitivity profile in view of emerging resistance.

Sensitivity tests will be required for bacteria known to vary in their susceptibility to antimicrobial agents (an increasing problem). The acquisition of resistance occurs particularly with staphylococci, Gram-negative bacilli and mycobacteria. Once the sensitivity of the organism has been determined, it is relatively rare for this to change during the course of treatment.

The patient

The age and sex of the patient, together with a knowledge of previous adverse reactions, and immune, renal and liver function must all be considered before a final selection of the antibiotic or antibiotics is made.

Children and pregnant women should not be given tetracyclines or 4-quinolones. Co-trimoxazole is also best avoided in pregnancy and the elderly, and this compound, together with other sulphonamides, must not be given to patients with glucose-6-phosphate dehydrogenase deficiency as haemolysis may be precipitated. Chloramphenicol should be prescribed only in the circumstances described on page 72 and is contraindicated in the neonate. Ampicillin must not be given to patients suffering from infectious mononucleosis and the aminoglycoside antibiotics should be used with caution in patients with renal disease and in the elderly. Clindamycin should not be used for trivial infection because of the risk of colitis.

The available antibiotics

Having considered the above factors, the clinician selects an appropriate antibiotic with reference to its microbiological and pharmacological properties, adverse reactions and cost. The *British National Formulary* published in the UK is a valuable guide.

More than one antibiotic (but rarely more than two) may be required for the initial treatment of septicaemia or for serious infections in the immunosuppressed. The use of two or more antibacterial drugs is only occasionally of proven value in other than the seriously ill. Thus, in tuberculosis, three agents are prescribed, at least initially, to reduce the emergence of resistant strains. Two drugs with different modes of action may also be used when it has been shown that the combination is synergistic.

Antimicrobial agents are often very expensive. In general, new agents are more expensive than older compounds, while parenteral preparations are always much more costly than the oral formulation. Unusual or new antibiotics should not be prescribed without good reason as the difference in cost compared with other agents can be over a hundred-fold. Particularly expensive agents include vancomycin, imipenem, the newer cephalosporins, aciclovir, zidovudine and the liposomal formulation of amphotericin.

PREVENTION OF INFECTION

Non-specific

Non-specific methods used to prevent the spread of infection include health education, good hygiene (especially hand-washing), safe disposal of excreta, clean water supplies, the use of antiseptics, disinfectants and disposable equipment and of sterilisation facilities, mosquito nets, vector control (insects and rodents), and the isolation of infectious patients (source isolation) and of those especially susceptible to infection such as the immunocompromised (protective isolation).

Specific

This involves the use of prophylactic immunisation and/or chemoprophylaxis.

IMMUNISATION AGAINST INFECTIOUS DISEASE

Immunisation may be active or passive.

Active immunisation

Vaccines are either live attenuated organisms, inactivated organisms or toxoids (inactivated toxins) (see Table 2.9). In the UK parents are advised to have their children immunised against whooping cough, diphtheria, tetanus, measles, mumps, rubella, poliomyelitis, *Haemophilus influenzae* type B and tuberculosis (see Table 20.11, p. 1133). The World Health Organization (WHO) has provided guidelines for immunisation of children in developing countries; these appear on page 1133. Indications for immunisation against influenza, hepatitis A and B, typhoid fever, cholera, plague, typhus, yellow fever, Japanese encephalitis and rabies depend upon the likelihood of exposure or upon current international health regulations. Acute demyelinating encephalomyelitis and polyneuropathy are the most important, but fortunately very rare, complications of immunisation.

General guidelines for immunisation are given in the information box.

HIV-infected persons should be immunised in the same way as other individuals but adults must not be given BCG (bacille Calmette–Guérin), live poliomyelitis or yellow fever vaccines, as disseminated infection with the vaccine strain may occur. Vaccination of HIV-infected children is currently being determined in terms of safety.

Passive immunisation

An injection of immunoglobulin will give temporary protection (usually) for 2–6 months against certain infectious diseases (see Table 20.13, p. 1133) by providing pre-formed antibodies against those infections. The immunoglobulin preparation may be pooled (prepared from blood collected from many donors) or hyperimmune (extracted from the blood of an individual recovering from an infection or from an immunised animal). Concerns about possible contami-

Table 2.9 Vaccines and toxoids

Live attenuated vaccines	Inactivated vaccines	Toxoid (inactivated toxin)
Childhood immunisation		
Measles	Pertussis	Diphtheria
Mumps	*H. influenzae* type B	Tetanus
Rubella		
Poliomyelitis*		
BCG (tuberculosis)		
Travel		
Yellow fever	Typhoid*	
Typhoid*	Cholera	
	Rabies	
	Japanese encephalitis	
	Hepatitis A	
Special risk groups		
Influenza*	Pneumococcal	
Varicella	Hepatitis B	
	Influenza*	
	Meningococcal (types A and C only)	
	Plague	
	Poliomyelitis*	

* Both live and inactivated vaccines available. Vaccinated groups are not exclusive.

GUIDELINES FOR IMMUNISATION AGAINST INFECTIOUS DISEASE

- The principal contraindication to inactivated vaccines is a significant reaction to a previous dose
- Live vaccines should not be given to pregnant women or to the immunosuppressed, or in the presence of an acute infection
- If two live vaccines are required they should either be given simultaneously in opposite arms or 3 weeks apart
- Live vaccines should not be given for 3 months after an injection of human normal immunoglobulin (HNI)
- HNI should not be given for 2 weeks after a live vaccine
- Hay fever, asthma, eczema, sickle-cell disease, topical steroid therapy, antibiotic therapy, prematurity and chronic heart and lung diseases, including tuberculosis, are *not* contra-indications to immunisation

nation of immunoglobulin preparations by hepatitis viruses, cytomegalovirus and HIV are often expressed. Safety procedures in donor selection and screening, together with virus inactivation during manufacture of the products, minimise this risk. Nevertheless, a slight risk remains and blood or its products should never be given unless absolutely necessary.

CHEMOPROPHYLAXIS

The use of antimicrobial agents to prevent infection is known as chemoprophylaxis. The indications for this are limited, and are listed on page 1133.

NOTIFICATION OF INFECTIOUS DISEASES

Clinicians in Britain have a statutory obligation to notify certain infectious diseases to the appropriate Public Health Authority. This provides epidemiological information which assists in the control of infection. The notifiable infectious diseases for the UK are listed on page 1132.

FURTHER INFORMATION ON PRINCIPLES OF MANAGEMENT OF INFECTION

British National Formulary (published annually). Pharmaceutical Press, Oxford

Frontiers in Medicine: vaccines. Science 1994 265: 1333–1496

Griffin G E 1997 Cytokines involved in septic shock: the paradigm of Jarisch–Herxheimer reaction. Journal of Antimicrobial and Chemotherapy 40: 212–216

Naber S P 1994 Molecular pathology—diagnosis of infectious diseases. New England Journal of Medicine 331: 1212–1215

O'Grady F, Lambert H P, Finch R, Greenwood D 1997 Antibiotic and chemotherapy: anti-infective agents and their use in therapy. Churchill Livingstone, Edinburgh

Salisbury D, Begg N 1996 Immunisation against infectious diseases. HMSO, London

Tomasz A 1994 Multiple-antibiotic-resistant bacteria—a report on the Rockefeller University Workshop. New England Journal of Medicine 330: 1247–1251

Tomasz A 1995 The pneumococcus at the gates. New England Journal of Medicine 331: 514–515

Tompkins L S, Tenover F, Arvin A 1994 New technology in the clinical microbiology laboratory: what you always wanted to know but were afraid to ask. Journal of Infectious Diseases 170: 1068–1074

DISEASES DUE TO VIRUSES

Viruses are the smallest microorganisms causing human disease. Their genome is composed of either DNA or RNA; the complete base sequence of nearly all human virus genomes is now known and genome structure is used as the basis of virus classification. The virus genome is enclosed in a protein shell, and in some cases a lipid envelope. Unlike bacteria which can grow in cell-free medium, all viruses are obligate intracellular pathogens. Glycoproteins on the virus surface recognise specific cellular receptors, whose distribution is often a major determinant of which cells the virus infects (its tropism), and hence of the type of disease produced. Table 2.10 presents the current classification of the viruses which cause human disease. This section covers the major viral diseases not dealt with elsewhere in the book; they are presented here by virus family, and are complemented by the discussion of infective syndromes due to viruses in other sections—see particularly those on meningitis and encephalitis (Ch. 14), respiratory infections (Ch. 4), hepatitis (Ch. 10) and enteric infections (Ch. 9).

Table 2.10 Viruses causing human disease

Family	Genus or type
RNA VIRUSES	
Arenaviruses	Lassa fever virus
Astroviruses	Five serotypes
Bunyaviruses	Hantaviruses
Caliciviruses	Calicivirus
Coronaviruses	Coronavirus
Filoviruses	Marburg and Ebola viruses
Flaviviruses	Hepatitis C virus
	Yellow fever virus
Orthomyxoviruses	Influenza viruses
Paramyxoviruses	Parainfluenza viruses
	Mumps virus
	Measles virus
	Respiratory syncytial virus
Picornaviruses	Enteroviruses
	Poliovirus, 3 types
	Echovirus, 31 types
	Coxsackie A virus, 24 types
	Coxsackie B virus, 6 types
	Enterovirus types 68–71
	Hepatitis A virus
	Rhinoviruses
Reoviruses	Rotaviruses
Retroviruses	HIV 1 and 2
	HTLV 1 and 2
Rhabdoviruses	Rabies virus
Togaviruses	Rubella virus
	Alphaviruses
DNA VIRUSES	
Adenoviruses	Numerous serotypes
Hepadnaviruses	Hepatitis B viruses
Herpesviruses	Herpes simplex viruses 1 and 2
	Epstein–Barr virus
	Cytomegalovirus
	Varicella zoster virus
	Human herpesviruses 6, 7 and 8
Papovaviruses	Papillomaviruses
Parvoviruses	B19 virus
Poxviruses	Variola, vaccinia
	Molluscum contagiosum virus
	Orf

RNA VIRUSES

ARBOVIRUSES

The arboviruses were previously grouped as a family because

of their common mode of transmission by arthropods (*ar*thropod-*bo*rne viruses). They produce viraemia in their vertebrate hosts, and infect blood-sucking arthropod hosts (mosquitoes, ticks, sandflies and biting midges) during feeding; after replication in the arthropod they are transmitted in the saliva injected during feeding. Many of these virus infections are zoonoses transmitted primarily between vectors and animals. Transovarial transmission in ticks, sandflies and mosquitoes, and transtadial transmission in ticks, are probably important maintenance mechanisms. However, most of the former arboviruses were taxonomically unrelated, and have now been regrouped in related families:

- *Togaviridae* Alphaviruses (former group A arboviruses) are the principal genus—see p. 107.
- *Flaviridae* Flaviviruses (former group B arboviruses) are the principal genus (type virus yellow fever)—see p. 81.
- *Bunyaviridae*—see p. 80.
- *Reoviridae*—see p. 87.
- *Rhabdoviridae*—see p. 107.

Many of the viruses produce encephalitis, haemorrhagic fever or arthritis in various combinations, which also provided some clinical justification for their former grouping. However, there is no close correlation between taxonomically related viruses and the particular clinical syndromes they produce, and the diseases associated with a particular virus are thus now described under the appropriate individual virus headings.

ARENAVIRUSES

Arenaviruses are single-stranded RNA viruses which are carried principally in rodents, from which they may be transmitted to humans. One group of New World arenaviruses (the Tacaribe complex) is responsible for South American haemorrhagic fevers. Lymphocytic choriomeningitis virus occasionally produces viral meningitis in humans. Lassa is an Old World arenavirus.

LASSA FEVER

Since the first report in 1969, the disease has so far been limited to sub-Saharan West Africa, where serological studies have shown that past infection is widespread in rural areas. Isolated cases and small rural outbreaks are most common, but unlike other arenaviruses Lassa can spread person to person, and nosocomial outbreaks in hospital have also occurred (see Table 2.11).

Clinical features

The disease has the general features of a viral infection, high fever, intercostal myalgia, bradycardia, low blood pressure and leucopenia. Adherent yellow exudates on the pharynx are particularly characteristic. The fever lasts between 7 and 17 days. In severe cases liver and renal failure, electrolyte imbalance, haemorrhage and acute circulatory failure develop, hence the classification of Lassa fever as a viral haemor-

Table 2.11 Common viral haemorrhagic fevers

Disease	Viral agent	Reservoir	Transmission	Geography	Case mortality
Lassa fever	Arenavirus	Multimammate rat (*Mastomys natalensis*) Patient	Urine Body fluids	West Africa	Up to 50% (responds to tribavirin)
Marburg/Ebola virus disease	Filovirus	? Patient	Via monkeys' body fluids	Central Africa	25–90%
Yellow fever	Flavivirus	Monkeys	Mosquitoes	Tropical Africa, South and Central America	10–60%
Dengue	Flavivirus (dengue types 1–4)	Humans	*Aedes aegypti* et al	Tropical and sub-tropical coasts	Nil–10%*
Omsk	Togavirus	Musk rat	Ticks	Siberia	2%
Crimean-Congo	Bunyavirus	*Ixodes* tick	*Ixodes* tick	Africa, Asia, Eastern Europe	15–70%
Bolivian and Argentinian	Arenavirus (Machupa and Junin)	Rodents (*Calomys* spp.)	Urine	South America	?
Haemorrhagic fever with renal syndrome	Hantavirus	Rodents	Faeces	Northern Asia, northern Europe	30%

* Mortality of uncomplicated and haemorrhagic dengue fever, respectively.

rhagic fever (see Table 2.11). Case mortality is high, but mild and subclinical infections also occur.

The virus may be isolated, or antigen-detected, in maximum security laboratories from serum, pharynx, pleural exudate and urine, but diagnosis will usually be established from 'paired sera', the later specimen being taken 6–8 weeks after the onset of infection. The diagnosis should be considered in the UK and other non-endemic areas in patients presenting with fever within 21 days of leaving West Africa, particularly if they have organ failure or haemorrhagic features (although most patients initially suspected of having viral haemorrhagic fevers in the UK turn out to have malaria).

Management

Strict isolation and general supportive measures, preferably in a special unit, are required. Tribavirin (ribavirin) is given intravenously (100 mg/kg, then 25 mg/kg daily for 3 days and 12.5 mg/kg daily for 4 days).

Prevention

The administration of convalescent immune plasma has been followed by recovery and is therefore recommended for prophylaxis after accidental exposure to infection.

BUNYAVIRUSES

Most bunyaviruses are transmitted by arthropods. They comprise the genera *Bunyavirus*, *Phlebovirus*, *Nairovirus* and *Hantavirus*.

The genus *Bunyavirus* (type virus *Bunyamwera*)

This group contains 138 viruses in 18 antigenic groups. Most important are the California encephalitis group viruses such as LaCrosse virus, which are transmitted by mosquitoes. In the Simbu antigenic group Oropouche virus is one of the few midge-transmitted viruses that cause human epidemics (in Brazil).

The genus *Phlebovirus*

This genus has 37 members. The most important phlebovirus is probably Rift Valley fever virus, which has caused large-scale epizootics and human epidemics of febrile illness, sometimes with haemorrhagic fever, in sub-Saharan Africa; it is transmitted to humans by *Aedes* mosquitoes, in which (like California encephalitis virus) it can be maintained by transovarial transmission (in the eggs). Most other viruses in the group are associated with phlebotomine sandflies. The Uukuniemi group viruses are tick-associated.

The genus *Nairovirus*

This includes Crimean-Congo haemorrhagic fever virus, which is transmitted from animals to humans by ticks, in the republics of the former Soviet Union, the Middle East and Africa, and causes severe haemorrhagic fever.

The genus *Hantavirus*

Hantaviruses differ from other bunyaviruses in being parasites of rodents. Hantaan virus and related viruses cause haemorrhagic fever with renal syndrome, which has occurred in outbreaks in Korea (hence its alternative name, Korean haemorrhagic fever), Manchuria and Eastern Europe. The infection causes severe capillary congestion, leakage and haemorrhage, especially in the renal medulla, so that oedema and acute renal failure develop, with oliguria and the passage of cells and protein in the urine. If the infection is left untreated, mortality is high, but with proper treatment for acute renal failure (see p. 429) and blood transfusion if necessary, patients should recover. A less severe form of the disease, nephropathia epidemica, is found in Scandinavia.

Another hantavirus disease, hantavirus pulmonary syndrome, was first recognised in an outbreak in the south-west United States in 1993; a hantavirus transmitted from the deer mouse caused an outbreak of severe respiratory illness with features of acute respiratory distress syndrome.

FILOVIRUSES

MARBURG AND EBOLA VIRAL DISEASE

In 1967 a severe infectious illness broke out among laboratory workers in Marburg, West Germany, who had handled tissues from a batch of vervet monkeys imported from Uganda. In 1976 outbreaks of the disease occurred in Sudan and Zaire from a focus on the Ebola River. The viruses causing these two outbreaks were structurally identical but antigenically distinct. In 1995 a further outbreak of Ebola disease occurred in Zaire with a 77% mortality. It is believed there is an unknown animal reservoir from which virus can be transmitted to primates and humans. Sporadic cases have occurred elsewhere in Africa. In person-to-person outbreaks the mortality is high, but successive human passage seems to reduce virulence. The incubation period is 5–9 days.

The illness presents suddenly with fever, severe myalgia and diarrhoea, followed by pharyngitis, generalised erythematous rash and lymphadenopathy. Fatal complications include haemorrhage, secondary infection, encephalitis, renal failure and pneumonia.

Management consists of supportive measures alone.

OTHER HAEMORRHAGIC FEVERS

The term 'haemorrhagic fevers', while popular, covers too broad a field of diseases to be of great value. Hence, in addition to the different families of viruses which cause haemorrhagic fever, covered in this chapter and listed in Table 2.11, other non-viral infections are associated with haemorrhagic features, as listed in the information box.

CAUSES OF HAEMORRHAGIC FEVERS
Viruses
• See Table 2.10
Rickettsiae
• Rocky Mountain spotted fever
Bacteria
• Meningococcaemia, plague • Gram-negative septicaemia
Spirochaetes
• Relapsing fever
Protozoa
• African trypanosomiasis

FLAVIVIRUSES

This family contains 68 members. Yellow fever virus is the prototype virus. Uncomplicated dengue fever and the severe dengue haemorrhagic fever/dengue shock syndrome (DHF/DSS) are the most important flavivirus diseases transmitted pan-tropically to humans by peridomestic urban breeding mosquitoes. The hepatitis C viruses are also classified as flaviviruses but are covered on page 706. Significant tick-borne viruses are tick-borne encephalitis and Kyasanur forest disease. Important mosquito-borne viruses are Japanese, St Louis and Murray Valley encephalitis viruses and West Nile virus (in addition to yellow fever and dengue viruses).

YELLOW FEVER

Yellow fever, caused by a flavivirus, is normally a zoonosis of monkeys that inhabit tropical rainforests in West and Central Africa and South and Central America, among whom it may cause devastating epidemics (see Fig. 2.4). It is transmitted by mosquitoes living in tree-tops (see Fig. 2.5). *Aedes africanus* in Africa and the *Haemagogus* species in America are the vectors. The infection is brought down to humans either by infected mosquitoes when trees are felled, or by monkeys raiding human plantations. In the latter case *Aedes simpsoni*, which breeds in the axils of banana plants, may transmit the disease to humans. In towns yellow fever may be transmitted between humans by *Aedes aegypti* which breeds efficiently in small collections of water. The distribution of this mosquito is far wider than that of yellow fever and poses a continual risk of spread.

Humans are infectious during the viraemic phase, which starts 3–6 days after the bite of the infected mosquito and lasts for 4–5 days. Mosquitoes become infectious 8–12 days after biting a patient and remain so for the rest of their 6–8-week lifespan. They may pass on the virus transovarially. The incubation period is 3–6 days.

Pathology

In the liver, acute mid-zonal necrosis leads to deposits of hyalin called Councilman bodies, and intranuclear eosinophilic

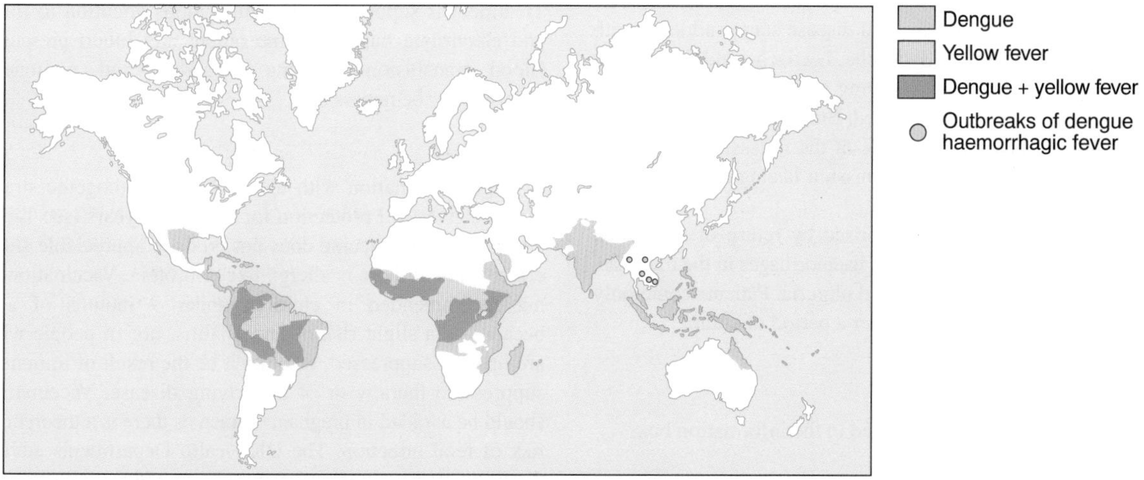

Fig. 2.4 Endemic zones of yellow fever and dengue.

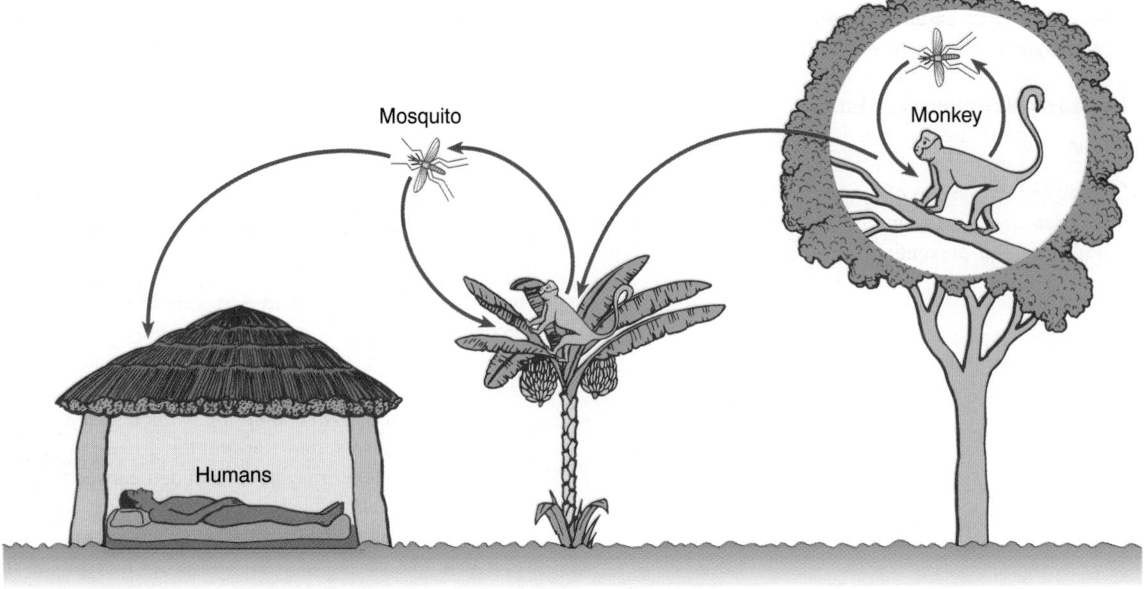

Fig. 2.5 Transmission of yellow fever. From tree-top cycle, via peridomestic cycle, to humans.

inclusions called Torres bodies; another characteristic feature is the absence of inflammatory infiltrate. The kidneys show tubular degeneration, which may partly be due to reduced blood flow. Widespread petechial haemorrhages are most marked in the stomach and duodenum. Haemorrhage is due to liver damage and disseminated intravascular coagulation.

Clinical features

Yellow fever is often a mild febrile illness lasting less than a week. However, the classical disease starts suddenly with rigors and high fever. Backache, headache and bone pains are severe. Nausea and vomiting start. The face is flushed and the conjunctivae are infected. Bradycardia and leucopenia are characteristic of this phase of the illness, which lasts 3 days and is followed by a remission lasting a few hours or days.

The third stage is characterised by return of fever, and the onset of jaundice, petechial haemorrhages in the mucosae, ecchymoses, haematemesis and oliguria. Patients commonly die in the third stage, often after a period of coma.

Investigations

Diagnostic procedures are listed in the information box.

Management

Patients should be nursed under a mosquito net (where the vector is present) until the viraemic stage has passed. Treatment is supportive, with meticulous attention to fluid and electrolyte balance, urine output and blood pressure. Blood transfusions, plasma expanders and peritoneal dialysis may be necessary.

DIAGNOSIS OF YELLOW FEVER

- Clinical features in endemic area
- Virus isolation from blood in first 4 days
- Four-fold rise in antibody titre
- Post-mortem liver biopsy
- Differentiate from viral hepatitis, haemorrhagic fevers, malaria, typhoid, leptospirosis, aflatoxin poisoning

Prevention

A single vaccination with the 17 D non-pathogenic strain of virus gives full protection for at least 10 years (see Table 2.9, p. 77). The vaccine does not produce appreciable side-effects, unless there is allergy to egg protein. Vaccination is not recommended in children under 9 months of age because of a slight risk of encephalitis, nor in people who are immunosuppressed, whether it be the result of immunosuppressive therapy or of underlying disease. Vaccination should be avoided in pregnant women as there is a theoretical risk of fetal infection. The UK Health Departments advise that if a pregnant woman must travel to a high-risk area she should be immunised, since the risk from yellow fever outweighs that of immunisation.

Only travellers possessing valid certificates of vaccination against yellow fever are allowed to proceed from an endemic area to 'receptive areas', by which is meant countries free from the disease but in which the potential exists.

In this way the disease has been kept out of Asia. Mosquito control of airports should be maintained. The urban disease can be eradicated by the abolition of the breeding places of *Aedes aegypti* by the use of residual insecticides in houses and by mass vaccination in endemic areas. Vaccination is the only means of preventing humans from being infected from forest reservoirs.

DENGUE

This disease is the most common flavivirus infection of humans and is a risk in many tropical and subtropical countries (see Fig. 2.4), especially in coastal areas during the hot season when mosquitoes are numerous. The principal vector is *Aedes aegypti*. It is endemic in South-east Asia but there are increasingly frequent large epidemics in the Caribbean and Americas; it should be considered in the differential diagnosis of fever in the returning traveller in the UK. There are four serotypes of dengue virus, all of which produce a similar clinical syndrome; homotypic immunity is life-long but heterotypic immunity between serotypes lasts only a few months. The incubation period from being bitten by an infected mosquito is usually 2–7 days.

Clinical features

The disease varies in severity. The clinical features are listed in the information box. Subclinical infections are common.

CLINICAL FEATURES OF DENGUE FEVER
Prodrome
• 2 days' malaise and headache
Acute onset
• Fever, backache, arthralgias, headache, generalised pains ('breakbone fever'), pain on eye movement, lacrimation, anorexia, nausea, vomiting, relative bradycardia, prostration, depression, lymphadenopathy, scleral injection
Fever
• Continuous or 'saddle-back', with break on fourth or fifth day; usually lasts 7–8 days
Rash
• Transient macular in first 1–2 days. Maculo-papular, scarlet morbilliform from days 3–5 on trunk, spreading centrifugally sparing palms and soles. May desquamate on resolution
Convalescence
• Slow

Dengue haemorrhagic fever or dengue shock syndrome

This occurs mainly in children in South-east Asia, but is sometimes seen in adults in epidemics elsewhere. In mild forms there is thrombocytopenia and haemoconcentration. In the most severe form, after 3–4 days of fever, hypotension and circulatory failure develop with features of a capillary leak syndrome. Minor (petechiae, ecchymoses, epistaxis) or major (gastrointestinal bleeding) haemorrhagic signs may occur. The pathogenesis is unclear but pre-existing immunity to a dengue virus serotype heterotypic to the one causing the current infection predisposes to the syndrome. In vitro such heterotypic antibody causes enhanced virus entry and replication in monocytes; it is believed that enhancing antibody from previous dengue infection with a different serotype, or from acquired maternal antibody in infants, facilitates development of a very heavy viral load. Disseminated intravascular coagulation, complement activation and release of vasoactive mediators may contribute to the pathogenesis of the syndrome, possibly triggered by immunopathological mechanisms. Cytokine release is thought to be the cause of vascular damage at the site of post-capillary endothelial junctions. Even with treatment the case fatality may be up to 10%.

Investigations

Diagnosis of dengue is usually easy in an endemic area when a patient has the characteristic symptoms and signs. However, mild cases may resemble other viral disease. Leucopenia is usual, and thrombocytopenia common. The virus can be recovered from the blood and there are tests for viral antigen. Antibody titres rise but serological tests may detect cross-reacting antibodies from other flaviviruses, including yellow fever vaccine.

Management and prevention

There is no specific treatment. The severe pains can be relieved by paracetamol, but occasionally opiates are required. Aspirin should be avoided. Volume replacement, blood transfusions and management of capillary leak are indicated in shock syndrome. Corticosteroids have not been shown to help. No existing antivirals are effective.

Patients are nursed under a mosquito net. Breeding places of *Aedes* mosquitoes should be abolished and the adults destroyed by insecticides. There is as yet no vaccine but a tetravalent live attenuated version is at an advanced stage of development.

ORTHOMYXOVIRUSES

INFLUENZA (see also Table 4.10, p. 339)

There are three distinct types of influenza virus: A, B and

C. The haemagglutinin (HA) and neuraminidase (NA) surface proteins are critical for protective immunity. Influenza A also infects many other animals (including birds, pigs and horses), unlike B and C, and also shows much greater antigenic variation. Antigenic variation occurs by antigenic drift (due to point mutations in the HA gene) or antigenic shift (due to acquisition of completely new HA or NA genes—possibly from animal influenza viruses by re-assortment of the segmented RNA genome between viruses). Antigenic shift can produce a virus new to humans, and in the absence of pre-existing immunity this can result in influenza pandemics; there have been four in the 20th century and the first and greatest of these in 1918 caused 20 million deaths world-wide. Epidemics occur in the winter months in temperate climates, beginning abruptly, peaking after 2–3 weeks and lasting 6–10 weeks; attack rates may be 10–20% in the community and hospital admissions rise.

Clinical features

The virus is transmitted in respiratory secretions. The incubation period until onset of illness and virus shedding is 1–3 days and virus is shed for 3–7 days. Influenza A and B infection is characterised by the sudden onset of fever, rigors, headache, malaise and myalgias and arthralgias, with dry cough and nasal discharge. Influenza C usually only causes upper respiratory infection.

Complications

Respiratory complications include primary influenza viral pneumonia (particularly in patients with underlying lung or heart disease or immunodeficiency), secondary bacterial pneumonia (particularly due to *Staph. aureus*) and mixed pneumonia. Asthma and chronic bronchitis may be exacerbated. Reye's syndrome is a recognised complication in children. (Aspirin should be avoided in patients under 16 because of its association with this syndrome.) Myocarditis, pericarditis, aseptic meningitis and post-influenzal encephalitis are rare.

Management

Diagnosis can be made by detecting virus in throat and nasal secretions and retrospectively by a rise in antibody titres.

Amantadine and rimantadine are active only against influenza A and shorten illness if given early. They may cause side-effects in the central nervous system and are rarely used in the UK. Treatment is otherwise symptomatic.

Prevention

Inactivated influenza vaccines are prepared annually; they contain the most recently circulating strains of influenza A and B, and provide 60–90% protection against these strains. Vaccine should be given annually to patients over 65, and those with chronic lung, heart and renal disease, diabetes and immunodeficiency. Amantadine and rimantadine can be used to prevent influenza A.

PARAMYXOVIRUSES

MEASLES (RUBEOLA)

Measles is caused by a paramyxovirus which spreads by droplet infection. One attack confers a high degree of immunity. Most people suffer from measles in childhood, and a mother who has had the disease confers passive immunity on her infant for the first 6 months of life. In tropical countries and on a background of malnutrition measles can be very severe, with a high mortality. The incubation period is about 10 days to the commencement of the catarrhal stage.

Clinical features (see the information box)

CLINICAL FEATURES OF MEASLES
Catarrhal stage
• Days 1–2: Fever, running nose, red, watery eyes • Day 2+: Cough, photophobia, Koplik's spots
Exanthematous stage
• Days 3–4: Maculo-papular rash • Days 6–7: Fever settles and rash begins to fade

Catarrhal stage

There is a febrile onset, with nasal catarrh, sneezing, redness of the conjunctivae and watering of the eyes. In addition, cough, hoarseness of the voice and photophobia usually appear by the second day.

At this stage, a diagnosis of measles may be made from the presence of Koplik's spots on the mucous membrane of the mouth. These are small white spots surrounded by a narrow zone of inflammation. The disease is highly infectious during the catarrhal stage and the child is miserable and irritable.

Exanthematous stage

After 3 or 4 days Koplik's spots disappear and the red macular or maculo-papular rash develops, first at the back of the ears and at the junction of the forehead and the hair. Within a few hours there is invasion of the whole skin and as the spots rapidly become more numerous they fuse to form the characteristic blotchy appearance of measles (see Fig. 2.2, p. 64). The rash fades after several days into a faint brown staining followed by a fine desquamation. The malaise and the fever subside as the rash fades. As with most infectious diseases, measles is more severe in older children and adults.

Complications

These are listed in the information box.

COMPLICATIONS OF MEASLES
Effects of measles virus
• Stomatitis • Enteritis • Pneumonia • Keratitis
Secondary bacterial infection
• Otitis media • Bronchopneumonia • Conjunctivitis
Neurological complications
• Post-viral encephalitis • Subacute sclerosing panencephalitis (persistent measles virus infection of the brain)
Nutritional
• Severe weight loss • Kwashiorkor (tropics) • Corneal ulceration (tropics—vitamin A deficiency)

Management

The patient should be isolated if possible and excluded from school for 10 days from the appearance of the rash. Most patients, in spite of the high temperature, remain uncomplicated and antibiotics should be prescribed only for bacterial complications.

Prevention

Active immunisation

There is a highly effective live attenuated measles vaccine (usually given in association with mumps and rubella vaccines, as 'MMR' vaccine). In the UK it is recommended that children should receive two doses: shortly after their first birthday and prior to school entry. In countries where measles is epidemic there may be a case for earlier immunisation, but if it is given too early, residual maternal antibody may diminish vaccine efficacy.

Passive immunisation

Human normal immunoglobulin, given intramuscularly, is used for the prevention or attenuation of measles in contacts under 18 months of age and for non-immune debilitated children, especially those with malignant disease. The dose is 250 mg for children under 1 year old, 500 mg for those 1–2 years old, and 750 mg over 3 years.

MUMPS

Mumps is spread by droplet infection and affects mainly children of school age and young adults. The infectivity rate is not high and there is serological evidence that 30–40% of infections are clinically unapparent. The incubation period is about 18 days.

Clinical features

Malaise, fever, trismus and pain near the angle of the jaw are soon followed by tender swelling of one or both parotid glands. Parotid swelling alone is often the first feature. The submandibular salivary glands may also be involved. The swollen glands subside in a few days, and may be succeeded by swelling of a previously unaffected gland. Acute lymphocytic meningitis is another mode of presentation and is the most common form of extra-salivary gland involvement; encephalomyelitis is rare. Orchitis occurs in about 1 in 4 males who develop mumps after puberty; it is usually on one side only, but if it is bilateral, sterility may be a sequel. Obscure abdominal pain may be due to pancreatitis or oophoritis.

Investigations

Most cases of mumps can be diagnosed on clinical grounds alone but, if in doubt, the diagnosis can be confirmed by the demonstration of specific antibodies; alternatively, the virus may be cultured from the saliva, or from the cerebrospinal fluid in meningitis. Differential diagnosis is from salivary calculus, which is unilateral, and sarcoidosis, which causes bilateral chronic parotitis.

Management

Apart from the relief of symptoms, no other treatment is necessary. Orchitis can be relieved by prednisolone (40 mg orally daily for 4 days).

Prevention

Mumps vaccine is given in two doses with measles and rubella vaccines (MMR) shortly after the first birthday and prior to school entry.

RESPIRATORY SYNCYTIAL VIRUS

Respiratory syncytial virus (RSV) is the major cause of lower respiratory tract infection in infants and young children. It produces yearly epidemics and during these RSV can be isolated from nearly 90% of children admitted to hospital with lower respiratory tract disease. Most children are infected within their first 2–3 years. (By age 2, 95% are seropositive.)

Clinical features

RSV produces upper respiratory tract infection (nasal congestion, pharyngitis) which, particularly with primary infection in infants (in 30–80%), progresses to lower respiratory tract infection with bronchiolitis and pneumonia.

Cough, often paroxysmal, is a prominent symptom. Bronchiolitis is characterised by wheezing and hyperinflation of the lungs. Infection in older children and adults is frequently symptomatic, including secondary and repeated infections; upper respiratory tract infection and tracheobronchitis are common but lower respiratory tract illness is uncommon in these groups.

Management

There are several rapid diagnostic techniques—for instance, those based on immunofluorescence of throat washings or swabs; serology is unhelpful for hospital diagnosis. For young children admitted to hospital with lower respiratory tract infection supportive respiratory care is important. Ribavirin given as a small-particle aerosol (by tent, mask or ventilator for 12–18 hours a day for 3–7 days) has been shown to improve arterial oxygen saturation and clinical outcome in severe RSV bronchiolitis.

Prevention

Maternal antibody does not protect infants and repeated infection occurs in older children and adults despite previous infection. A killed vaccine introduced in the 1960s was associated with worse disease when the recipients encountered natural infection. This has suggested that the immune response may somehow contribute to the pathogenesis of natural RSV infection, and there is still no vaccine for RSV.

PARAINFLUENZA VIRUSES

These are associated with upper respiratory tract infections—colds, croup, otitis media—and conjunctivitis, and with lower respiratory tract infections—tracheobronchitis, bronchiolitis and pneumonia (see Tables 4.10 and 4.11, pp. 339 and 340).

PICORNAVIRUSES

This group of viruses comprises the rhinoviruses, enteroviruses (whose members are listed in the information box) and hepatitis A virus (see p. 706). Two other groups of picornaviruses only cause diseases in animals, including foot and mouth disease.

RHINOVIRUSES

Rhinoviruses are the major known cause of the common cold, being responsible for 30–50% of colds in adults (although many other viruses also cause colds). They may also cause sinusitis, and may contribute to exacerbations of chronic bronchitis and asthma. There are over 100 serotypes. There are no effective antivirals or vaccines and treatment is symptomatic.

ENTEROVIRUSES

Enteroviruses are so called because they enter the body via the intestinal tract. They cause a wide spectrum of disease (see the information box). They are excreted in the stool and also, if there is respiratory infection, from the nasopharynx.

INFECTIONS CAUSED BY ENTEROVIRUSES
Echoviruses (approximately 40 strains)
• Meningitis • Encephalitis • Conjunctivitis • Gastroenteritis • Pharyngitis • Fever and rash • Neonatal infection
Coxsackie viruses (24 type A strains, 6 type B strains)
• Myocarditis • Pericarditis • Meningitis • Herpangina • Bornholm disease • Hand, foot and mouth disease • Gastroenteritis • Pharyngitis • Neonatal infection
Polioviruses (3 strains)
• Poliomyelitis (see p. 1011)

Most of the infections caused by enteroviruses are described elsewhere in this book, with some exceptions. Two syndromes usually caused by group A Coxsackie viruses are herpangina, which produces a vesicular rash on the fauces and soft palate, and hand, foot and mouth disease, a highly infectious but benign disease of childhood characterised by vesicles on hands, feet and mouth. Bornholm disease (so called for the island where it was first described, and also called epidemic pleurodynia) is usually associated with group B Coxsackie viruses; it is characterised by the abrupt onset of spasmodic and paroxysmal pain in the muscles of the thorax and/or upper abdomen, with fever and tenderness of the affected muscles. It may mimic other causes of pleuritic pain or of upper abdominal pain.

Coxsackie viruses (particularly group B) and echoviruses together account for the majority (about 90%) of cases of viral ('aseptic') meningitis (see Ch. 14, p. 1006 for further details of this and poliovirus).

Diagnosis of enterovirus infection may be based on virus isolation by tissue culture (especially from cerebrospinal fluid, CSF), and by detection of enterovirus IgM antibody in blood. Virus detection by the polymerase chain reaction (PCR) is becoming increasingly used, again particularly for detection of enteroviruses in CSF in suspected viral meningitis.

REOVIRUSES

This family includes the genera *Coltivirus* (causing Colorado tick fever in humans) and *Orbivirus* (only a few members of which are implicated in isolated cases of human disease). Other genera are *Orthoreovirus* (a rare cause of enteritis and upper respiratory infection in humans) and *Rotavirus* (a very important cause of viral gastroenteritis).

ROTAVIRUSES

Viral gastroenteritis is a major cause of illness and death, particularly in developing countries where 5–10 million deaths from gastroenteritis, most in young children, occur annually. Rotaviruses (mainly group A) are the major cause of diarrhoeal illness in young children, accounting for 30–50% of cases admitted to hospital in developed countries, and 10–20% of deaths due to gastroenteritis in developing countries. Although infection protects against subsequent severe disease, it does not prevent reinfection. Rotavirus vaccines are urgently needed and some are in trials.

Other causes of viral gastroenteritis are enteric adenoviruses (the second most frequent cause) and Norwalk virus, caliciviruses, astroviruses and small, round, non-structured viruses (which may all cause sporadic cases or outbreaks).

The most important aspect of treatment for viral gastroenteritis is adequate fluid and electrolyte replacement, if possible by oral replacement using glucose–electrolyte solution. (The WHO recommended solution is widely used and effective.) See the section on gastroenteritis, p. 124, for further details.

RETROVIRUSES

HUMAN IMMUNODEFICIENCY VIRUS INFECTION AND THE ACQUIRED HUMAN IMMUNODEFICIENCY SYNDROME

During 1981, cases of a rare neoplasm, Kaposi's sarcoma, and *Pneumocystis carinii* pneumonia (an unusual opportunist infection only seen in severely immunocompromised patients—for example, chemotherapy patients and those with severe malnutrition) were reported in the USA in previously healthy homosexual men. This was the beginning of an epidemic eventually termed the acquired immunodeficiency syndrome (AIDS). In 1984 the association between infection with the human immunodeficiency virus (HIV) and the development of AIDS was established. The subsequent global AIDS pandemic has stimulated an unprecedented biomedical research effort which has resulted in a major expansion of knowledge in many aspects of this infection, and in recent years the understanding of the pathogenesis, management and control of the disease has greatly expanded.

Epidemiology

The World Health Organization estimated that by the year 2000 there would be 26 million persons infected with HIV, the cumulative total since the beginning of the epidemic being 40 million. Around 90% of cases are in developing countries unable to afford the expensive medical care required to control progress of the disease. The current global pandemic of HIV consists of many different regional epidemics in different countries, each with its own dynamics and different clinical pattern of evolution. HIV probably originated from remote rural areas where it was endemic at low levels but then spread amongst sexually active populations in cities, initially in the early 1980s amongst homosexual men in the developed countries of Europe, North America and Australia. Recent serological tests have demonstrated HIV seropositivity in an African male in a blood sample taken in 1947. This series of epidemics was then followed by a further wave with predominant heterosexual spread in sub-Saharan Africa and South America and, more recently, the Indian subcontinent and South-east Asia, where the epidemics were late in developing but are accelerating at an alarming rate. The early dissemination of HIV was facilitated by travel and migration. Later epidemics have been facilitated by female sex workers and their clients, whereas intravenous drug use and use of HIV-infected blood and blood products have been important risk factors for spread throughout. The epidemics in Europe, North America and Australia have now apparently stabilised, although cases contracted heterosexually and through vertical transmission continue to increase. So far, sub-Saharan Africa has been hardest hit in clinical and sociological terms by the HIV epidemic and rapid spread continues in South-east Asia. The economic and demographic impact of HIV infection is profound as the disease is prevalent between 15 and 50 years of age, the most economically productive age group in most countries, and indeed HIV is now the most common cause of death in this age group in some parts of the world. A consequence of heterosexual transmission of HIV is the increase in the number of paediatric cases, which will greatly influence the expectation of life in many regions.

The characteristics of HIV disease in each region are determined by many different microbiological, cultural, social and behavioural aspects. For example, HIV infection in many parts of the USA remains rare, the highest density being seen in the major cities amongst homosexual men and intravenous drug users, whereas in Uganda, where heterosexual spread is predominant, it is estimated that 10% of the general population are now infected. Such relatively high seroprevalence figures are seen in rural areas and may be more than double in the cities.

Modes of transmission of HIV

There are three possible modes of transmission:

- sexual } mucosal routes
- perinatal } mucosal routes
- parenteral.

Infection with HIV essentially requires exchange of semen, vaginal or other body secretions, milk, or blood or blood products infected by the virus. The main mode of transmission world-wide is via the heterosexual route, accounting for over 75% of global cases. In the early 1980s, homosexual transmission was predominant but this has now been eclipsed by heterosexual transmission. The risk of HIV transmission is greatest with vaginal and anal intercourse and greater for the recipient of penetrative sex. The risk of transmission during intercourse is considerably increased if there is concomitant presence of sexually transmitted diseases, particularly if genital ulceration is present. As a control measure for the spread of HIV it has been shown that if sexually transmitted diseases can be controlled and reduced in incidence this is accompanied by a fall in HIV transmission rates.

Perinatal transmission is of increasing importance globally as a direct result of the increase in numbers of women with HIV infection who are of childbearing age. HIV infection may occur in utero, during delivery or postnatally as a result of breastfeeding. There is now good evidence that acquisition of HIV during parturition on contact with HIV-containing fluids in the vagina accounts for around 80% of vertical transmission. Neonates of HIV-infected women have a 13–52% chance of acquiring HIV from the mother. There is a wide regional variation in the risk. The risk is increased if the mother has advanced HIV disease with high viral titres. In utero the virus may infect the fetus by crossing the placenta. During delivery infection may result from feto-maternal blood interchange or transmission of HIV across fetal mucous membranes and finally, the virus may be present in breast milk so that breastfed babies have an additional risk of between 10 and 20%. This is a major problem in developing countries where switching to bottle-feeding carries high risks of infection due to poor sanitation. Use of pre-partum and postnatal antiretroviral agents (zidovudine) has been shown to reduce the risk of transmission to the fetus, in one series from 26% to 8%, a 68% reduction in risk. This emphasises the importance of prenatal screening of mothers for HIV infection.

Intravenous drug users (IVDUs) are at risk of HIV infection as a result of the practice of needle sharing, which allows transmission of HIV-infected blood from one individual to another. Transfusion of HIV-infected blood or blood products is an extremely efficient way of transmitting the virus and resulted in many haemophiliac patients acquiring the infection in the 1980s. Transmission via blood and blood products has now been virtually eliminated in many parts of the world following the introduction of routine screening for HIV, and needle exchange programmes for IVDUs have helped to reduce transmission in this group. It is estimated that with screening of donated blood using serodiagnosis the risk of a single unit of blood transmitting HIV is 1 in 10^6. The screening test will not pick up blood in patients incubating HIV prior to seroconversion.

Transmission to health-care workers

Studies of many thousands of health-care workers have shown that transmission of HIV following occupational exposure is a rare event. In these cases the major risk factor is needlestick injury with HIV-contaminated blood from an infected patient. Overall, the risk of transmission following needlestick injury has been calculated to be 0.3% (1 case per 300 needlestick incidents). Generally, the greater the size and depth of the blood inoculum, the greater the risk. Transmission of HIV has also been postulated through the conjunctiva and open lesions on the skin when in contact with HIV-containing body fluids. (See p. 93 for management of occupational exposure.)

Virology

HIV belongs to the Lentivirinae subfamily of retroviruses which have an RNA genome. The viral enzyme reverse transcriptase has the property of transcribing a DNA copy of the RNA genome following viral penetration of the host cell (see Fig. 2.6). This DNA copy then randomly integrates into the host cell genome for a variable and sometimes long period of time. This DNA copy can then be used as a template to transcribe new RNA viral copies and this can occur under a number of circumstances, including activation of the host cell. This process thus led to the term 'retrovirus'. Following production of new viral RNA copies in the host cell, translation results in the production of viral proteins. These precursor polyproteins are then cleaved by the viral protease enzyme to form new viral structural proteins and viral enzymes such as the viral reverse transcriptase and protease. (There are currently two classes of antiretroviral drug in clinical practice: the reverse transcriptase inhibitors and the protease inhibitors, both of which block viral replication.) Lentiviruses, including HIV, cause brisk T cell and cellular responses but cause persistent infections which are not naturally eliminated in a number of species. HIV has a core consisting of the RNA genome and core protein surrounded by an envelope with high lipid content, rendering it sensitive to organic solvents. HIV gains entry to host cells by binding to the CD4 receptor using the viral surface membrane glycoprotein gp120. Host target cells of preference, therefore, carry the CD4 molecule which is recognised by the virus, but in addition other cell surface molecules act as receptors and coreceptors for the virus. Many of these are chemokine receptors—for example, the CCR5 receptor. Following productive HIV infection new virions bud from

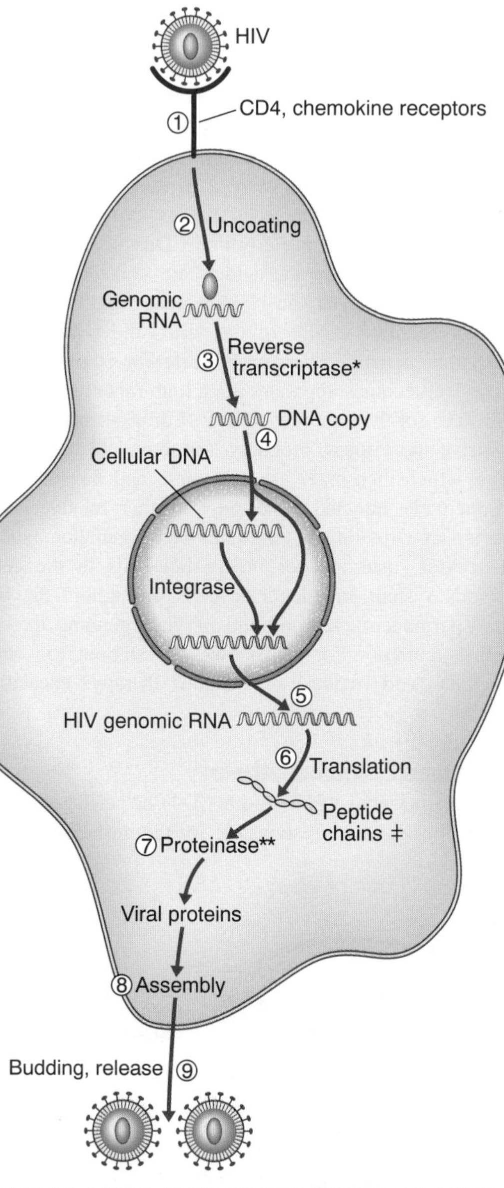

Fig. 2.6 Schematic representation of HIV entry, disassembly, replication and release from susceptible cell (lymphocyte or macrophage). (1) HIV binds to cell surface via receptors (CD4 molecule and coreceptors). (2) Viral uncoating in cytoplasm. (3) RNA viral genome transcribed to DNA copy–reverse transcriptase (RT) enzyme.* (4) DNA copy integrates into host cell genome in cell nucleus via integrase enzyme. (5) Following cell activation viral DNA is translated to RNA copies in cytoplasm. (6) Viral peptide chains translated from cytoplasmic viral RNA. (7) HIV proteinase cleaves functional viral proteins from polypeptides.** (8) Virion assembly. (9) Viral release from cell surface—cell lysis.
* RT inhibitors act here.
** Proteinase inhibitors act here.

the cell surface incorporating the host cell membrane as their own lipid bilayer coat (see Fig. 2.7) and cell lysis occurs. New virions are then available to infect new uninfected cells and repeat the process.

There is a huge diversity amongst HIVs, which occur in two main types: HIV 1 and HIV 2. Disease caused by HIV 2 is similar to disease caused by HIV 1 but is generally milder, slower to progress and poorly transmitted vertically. HIV 1 is responsible for most of the disease seen world-wide. Until recently, HIV 2 was confined to West Africa but it is now being detected in India. HIV 1 is divided into several subtypes (see Fig. 2.8); there are at least five subtypes of HIV 2. HIV 1 subtype B is predominant in Europe and North America, whereas subtype E predominates in Central Africa. Now mixed patterns are being seen. For example, in India HIV 1 subtypes A, B, C and E have been identified along with HIV 2. Within each subtype there are huge strain variations and indeed many different strains may be identified within one individual.

Recently, the dynamics of viral replication have become better defined using indirect studies in humans which employ potent combinations of antiretroviral agents to determine the change in viral populations within different cell compartments and plasma. These studies have also been made possible following the advent of the polymerase chain reaction to make quantitative measures of viral load (copies of viral RNA per ml of plasma). The half-life of free HIV in plasma is only 6 hours (see Fig. 2.9). Such free virus

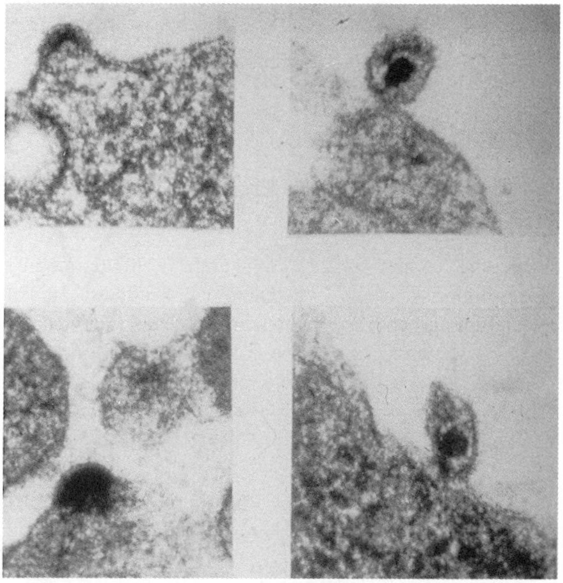

Fig. 2.7 Human immunodeficiency virus. Transmission electron micrograph of the virus budding from the surface of an infected CD4 lymphocyte.

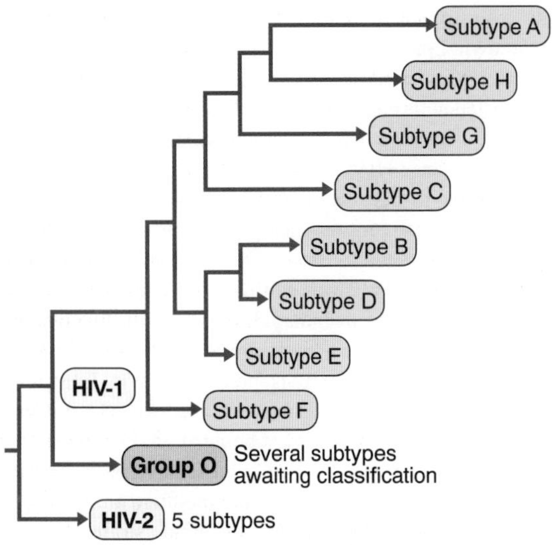

Fig. 2.8 Simplified phylogenetic tree of human immunodeficiency virus. The tree was constructed using sequence data from the *env* gene. This tree will undoubtedly expand as new isolates are identified. The complexity of the tree is a result of immense genetic diversity resulting from high transcription rates of HIV. The resulting phenotypic diversity of HIV-1 gives major problems for vaccine design, diagnostic kits and natural immunity. HIV-2 is genetically more similar to simian immunodeficiency virus (SIV) than HIV-1 and is subdivided into five subtypes.

then infects predominantly uninfected CD4+ T-helper lymphocytes, the majority of which become productively infected with a half-life of about 1.6 days, resulting in the release of more free virus which is then available to infect another cohort of uninfected cells. Each generation of virus has been estimated to take 2.6 days, allowing approximately 140 generations of virus per year within one individual. It has been calculated that each day as many as 10 billion virions are produced and 2 billion CD4+ cells are infected and destroyed. When these facts are considered together with the infidelity of the reverse transcriptase enzyme in making accurate copies of the virus, the reason for the enormous genetic diversity of different strains of virus produced becomes apparent. Such high mutation rates have relevance for the rapid generation of drug-resistant mutants. Some of the viruses, probably less than 1%, infect CD4+ cells, which then enter a latent phase and do not become productively infected, whereas a further relatively small amount of virus infects long-lived cell populations such as monocytes, macrophages, microglial cells in the central nervous system and dendritic cells throughout the body. Such permanent incorporation of viral genome into host cells is common for retroviruses throughout the animal kingdom and makes eradication therapy exceedingly difficult.

HIV-induced immunopathology

As mentioned above, HIV infects CD4+ helper T lymphocytes (T_H cells) which are responsible for the initiation of nearly

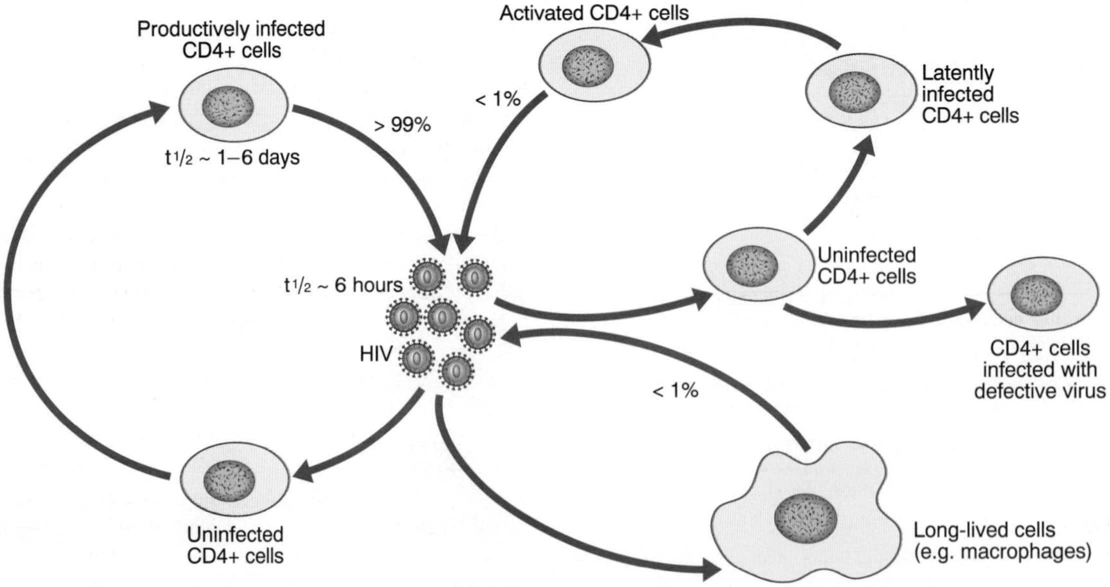

Fig. 2.9 Viral dynamics.

all immunological responses to pathogens. Following infection by HIV there is gradual attrition of the CD4 cell population, resulting in gradual and increasing failure of most aspects of immune function but particularly cell-mediated immunity. The predominant opportunist infections seen in HIV disease are intracellular parasites (e.g. *Mycobacterium tuberculosis*) or are pathogens susceptible to cell-mediated rather than antibody-mediated immune responses. HIV infects other cell lineages, including cells of the monocyte/macrophage lineage, microglial cells in the central nervous system and dendritic cells. The main immunological abnormalities in HIV infection are listed in the information box. Much of the damage done to the immune system is a result of primary damage inflicted by HIV 1 replication within these cells. However, the exact mechanism of immunopathology remains undetermined; direct infection and damage by HIV to T_H cells is not sufficient as only 1:10 000 of T_H cells is actually infected by HIV at any one time, whereas HIV can impair the function of other cell types, such as monocytes, macrophages, dendritic cells and B lymphocytes. During progression of HIV infection very small numbers of infected lymphocytes and macrophages are detected in peripheral blood during the asymptomatic period. It was originally thought that this represented viral latency with little viral production until activation occurred late in the disease and AIDS developed. We now know that this is not the case and even in the asymptomatic period there is large production of HIV in lymphoid tissue kept under control by the immune system.

IMMUNOLOGICAL ABNORMALITIES IN AIDS
T-helper (CD4) lymphocytes
• Decreased in number (low CD4 count in peripheral blood) • Abnormal function Reduced responses to antigen/mitogen Reduced responses to interleukin-2 Reduced production of interleukin-2 and interferon gamma
B lymphocytes
• Abnormal function Reduced responses to specific antigen or mitogen Polyclonal activation leading to increases in immunoglobulins
Monocytes/macrophages and dendritic cells
• Defective antigen presentation • Defective cytokine secretion • Defective phagocytosis/killing

During the course of HIV disease there is a gradual reduction in the number of CD4 cells circulating in peripheral blood. Routine clinical measurement of the CD4 cell count is used in patients as a measure of disease progression. HIV load can be measured using the polymerase chain reaction. HIV copy number in plasma is regarded as a measure of disease progression and is useful in monitoring therapy. The various complications of HIV disease and survival correlate well with the HIV copy number and to a lesser extent with the CD4 count. Both these measures are used as a guide as to when to institute antiretroviral therapy.

The major abnormality of immune function caused by HIV is in cell-mediated immunity, which particularly protects against intracellular parasites (e.g. viruses, protozoa and mycobacteria), whereas failure of appropriate neo and recall antibody responses also occurs, resulting in infection with encapsulated bacteria. HIV also indirectly affects cells of the central nervous system. This is probably due to migration of HIV-infected monocytes to the brain, where they become microglial cells, resulting in damage to the central nervous system. Most disease induced by HIV infection is, however, a consequence of immune system failure resulting in opportunist infections and secondary neoplasms. It is now clear that following infection with HIV in addition to antibody responses to various viral components, CD8+ cytotoxic T lymphocytes are generated; it is thought that these have a protective role in containing infection in the initial stages.

Testing for HIV and counselling

Although HIV infection may be suspected on clinical grounds, HIV infection is confirmed by demonstrating the presence of antibodies to HIV in serum. The current enzyme-linked immunosorbent assay (ELISA) test used for detecting such antibodies is simple and cheap and has the advantage of a very low false negative rate so that infected cases are unlikely to be missed. However, all positive results are normally confirmed by the more precise immunoblot (western blot) test, which also detects the presence of anti-HIV antibodies. Following HIV infection, seroconversion—that is, the production of detectable antibodies to various components of the virus, including antibody to the gag protein, integrase and reverse transcriptase—may not occur for 6–12 weeks and sometimes much longer. This means that serial testing may be required following a high risk of exposure to HIV to exclude infection. In special circumstances—for example, in neonates who may be infected—antibody detection tests are unhelpful or misleading because of the presence of transplacentally acquired maternal antibody. The polymerase chain reaction can be used in this situation to detect the presence of viral genome in peripheral blood lymphocytes. In special circumstances direct viral culture from peripheral blood lymphocytes can confirm infection. However, ELISA remains the routine screening test and is used by centres offering rapid (same-day) testing services.

The diagnosis of HIV infection depends on being clinically astute, having a clear knowledge of the clinical manifestations of HIV disease, asking the patient about relevant risk factors and maintaining a high index of suspicion. The importance of HIV testing for the patient is related to the serious consequences, both social and medical, of having a positive test. Before a test is performed it is important that adequate counselling of the patient is undertaken, including a discussion of the way in which the virus is spread, the effects of the virus, the psychological stress that a positive test will exert, and the effects on the individual's social, work and medical life. Issues relating to confidentiality need to be discussed in the event of the test being positive. Other disadvantages of a positive test for the patient, apart from the medical consequences, include feelings of guilt, social stigma and the fact that some countries will not admit HIV-positive persons. However, the advantages of knowing that an individual is HIV-seropositive include appropriate medical care and prophylactic measures which will benefit health, prolong life and avoid infection of others. When an HIV test is negative the patient should be advised to practise safe sex and to abstain from other avoidable risk factors, such as sharing needles for intravenous drug use. When giving a positive HIV test result, clinicians should remember that this is a major event for the patient. Adequate time must be set aside for this without interruption and, if possible, a partner, close friend or family member should be available to provide immediate support once the news has been broken.

Therapeutic approaches to HIV infection

Many programmes in different parts of the world have been implemented in an attempt to prevent the spread of HIV infection since early in the epidemic (see the information box). The overall success of these programmes is difficult to estimate but the fact that currently reported numbers of AIDS cases and HIV-infected individuals in many countries fall far short of epidemiological predictions of a few years ago must be attributed in part to success of these strategies. However, there is an urgent need for major education campaigns and implementation of other measures in parts of the world where the epidemic is proceeding unchecked.

Hopes for an effective vaccine remain high but elusive at the moment despite an enormous research effort. Reasons for the failure of vaccine programmes include our incomplete understanding of the components of the immunological response to HIV which are protective, the inability of antibody to neutralise the virus, and the enormous ability of the virus to mutate rapidly and produce new strains capable of evading the immune response.

The major therapeutic effort at present is directed at individuals already infected with HIV. There are now numerous agents in regular clinical use which interfere with HIV replication (see Table 2.12), and more agents will be available soon following further trials. Reverse transcriptase inhibitors prevent the spread of infectious virus into uninfected cells but do not affect replication of the HIV genome once integrated into the host cell. Protease inhibitors prevent post-translational cleavage of polypeptides into functional virus proteins. The first agent to be used clinically was the reverse transcriptase inhibitor, zidovudine. In a large controlled study, it was shown to prolong survival of patients with advanced HIV disease. It has, however, subsequently been shown that zidovudine given in early HIV disease has little benefit in delaying the onset of AIDS or in improving survival (Concorde trial). It is now known that zidovudine quickly loses its efficacy as an anti-HIV agent due to the emergence of drug-resistant strains of the virus. Controlled studies have now shown improved survival with combinations of two or three antiretroviral agents taken together. Many different combinations of drugs are effective and monotherapy is no longer used. In mild disease two-drug combinations (e.g. zidovudine and

PREVENTION MEASURES FOR HIV TRANSMISSION

Sexual

- Public awareness campaigns for HIV
- Safe sex practices
  - Avoidance of penetrative intercourse
  - Use of condoms
- Targeting safe sex methods at sex industry workers
- Control of sexually transmitted diseases

Parenteral

- Routine screening of blood/blood products for HIV
- Needle exchange programmes for IVDUs

Perinatal

- Routine HIV testing in antenatal clinics
- Avoidance of pregnancy if HIV-seropositive
- Antiretroviral therapy during pregnancy/delivery/postnatally
- Avoidance of breastfeeding

Table 2.12 Antiretroviral agents

Drug	Adverse effects
Nucleoside analogue reverse transcriptase inhibitors	
AZT/ZDV (**zidovudine**)	Marrow suppression, myopathy, nausea, vomiting
ddI (**didanosine**)	Peripheral neuropathy, pancreatitis
ddC (**zalcitabine**)	Peripheral neuropathy, pancreatitis
3Tc (**lamivudine**)	Peripheral neuropathy, pancreatitis, nausea, vomiting, headache
d4T (**stavudine**)	Pancreatitis, marrow suppression, peripheral neuropathy
Protease inhibitors*	
Saquinavir	Rash, headache, peripheral neuropathy
Ritonavir	Nausea, vomiting, abdominal pain, diarrhoea, headache
Indinavir	Hyperbilirubinaemia, renal stones
Non-nucleoside reverse transcriptase inhibitors	
Nevirapine	
Delavirdine	
Loviride	

* Multiple drug interactions as metabolised by hepatic cytochrome P450 system.

Table 2.13 Indications for antiretroviral drug treatment of HIV disease

	USA	UK
HIV copy number (PCR plasma measurement)	5000–30 000/ml	10 000–50 000/ml
CD4+ (T_H count in peripheral blood)	< 500/mm^3	< 300/mm^3
Stage/severity of HIV infection		
Mild disease	Two drugs (e.g. zidovudine + lamivudine)	
Moderate/severe disease	Three drugs (e.g. zidovudine + lamivudine + indinavir)	

lamivudine, or lamivudine and stavudine) are used, whereas in more severe HIV disease triple therapy, a combination of two nucleoside reverse transcriptase inhibitors together with a protease inhibitor, is effective. These new combination drug therapies (HAART; highly active antiretroviral therapy) have been highly effective in delaying the progress of HIV disease and have brought about major changes to clinical practice where these drugs are available. Unfortunately, due to cost this is not the case for the vast majority of HIV-infected individuals in developing countries. The indications for starting antiretroviral therapy are listed in Table 2.13. Some authorities advocate early intervention on the grounds that this will prevent or delay extensive damage to the immune system, whereas others advocate starting much later in the natural history of HIV disease on the grounds that many patients have a long asymptomatic phase of many years during which treatment is unnecessary and expensive, and will induce morbidity through drug toxicity, raising problems with compliance, and through increasing drug resistance. Even with potent combinations of three antiretroviral drugs, drug resistance inevitably develops and following a period of clinical improvement HIV disease will relapse. This raises further problems relating to the sequence in which the antiretroviral drugs are used in an individual. All antiretroviral drugs are toxic; for example, side-effects of zidovudine include nausea, vomiting, headaches and myalgia, anaemia, macrocytosis, neutropenia and occasionally leucopenia and thrombocytopenia.

Prophylactic use of anti-HIV drugs is recommended for health-care workers who have had percutaneous exposure to HIV-infected blood following needlestick injury or injury with surgical instruments. Such an injury carries the risk of HIV transmission of around 0.3%. The risk of percutaneous injury can be reduced by adopting universal precautions and taking care in handling sharps—for example, by not resheathing needles. A case control study demonstrated that zidovudine administered shortly after exposure reduced the risk of seroconversion by 80%. However, protection is not absolute and health-care workers have been reported to seroconvert despite taking zidovudine. The risk of seroconversion is raised with the increase in size of blood inoculum and the disease stage of the patient from which the infected blood was taken. Following needlestick injury, a rapid decision must be taken as to whether prophylaxis is desired or not. The drugs must be readily available as, to be effective, they must be started within an hour or two. Current recommendations are that zidovudine, lamivudine and indinavir should be taken for a 4-week period. In developed countries HIV seroconversion due to occupational exposure may be subject to industrial compensation and many health-care workers store their serum at regular intervals for subsequent HIV testing.

Clinical features of HIV disease

Following infection with HIV there is a latent period of a few (classically 8–12) weeks during which there may be intense viraemia. This period is followed by seroconversion when detectable antibodies to HIV and HIV-specific cytotoxic T lymphocytes appear in serum (see Fig. 2.10). At this time there is a rapid fall in viraemia, suggesting that the immunological response has contained the infection. At this stage approximately one-third of individuals have a brief illness lasting about 2 weeks. Symptoms include fever, malaise, headache, fleeting arthralgia, maculo-papular rash, tender lymphadenopathy, and occasionally encephalitis, diarrhoea and mouth ulcers. There then follows an asymptomatic phase of variable duration. Some individuals have quite rapid progression to symptomatic disease over a year or two, whereas others remain asymptomatic and completely well for many years. An early study from San Francisco of patients infected with HIV 11 years previously showed that 50% had died of AIDS; of the survivors, 20% had AIDS and 40% had symptoms attributable to HIV infection, whereas 40% remained completely free of symptoms. AIDS is thus the long-term consequence of chronic infection with HIV. The average time to developing AIDS from infection in most developed countries is 10–11 years but there is a considerable variation. Some will develop AIDS in less than 5 years but it is thought that eventually all HIV-infected individuals will develop AIDS in due course.

Some, but not all, HIV-infected patients develop persistent generalised lymphadenopathy (PGL), which is defined as the presence of enlarged lymph nodes greater than 1 cm in diameter in two anatomically distinct sites for more than 3 months in the absence of other detectable causes of lymphadenopathy. Most of these patients are asymptomatic although a few have fever and weight loss. The diagnosis of PGL is usually made clinically; biopsy of lymph nodes shows reactive hyperplasia. The prognosis for patients who develop PGL is the same as for those who do not. Asymmetric lymphadenopathy suggests alternative diagnoses such as lymphoma or tuberculosis. Percutaneous fine-needle aspiration of lymph nodes is a very useful test

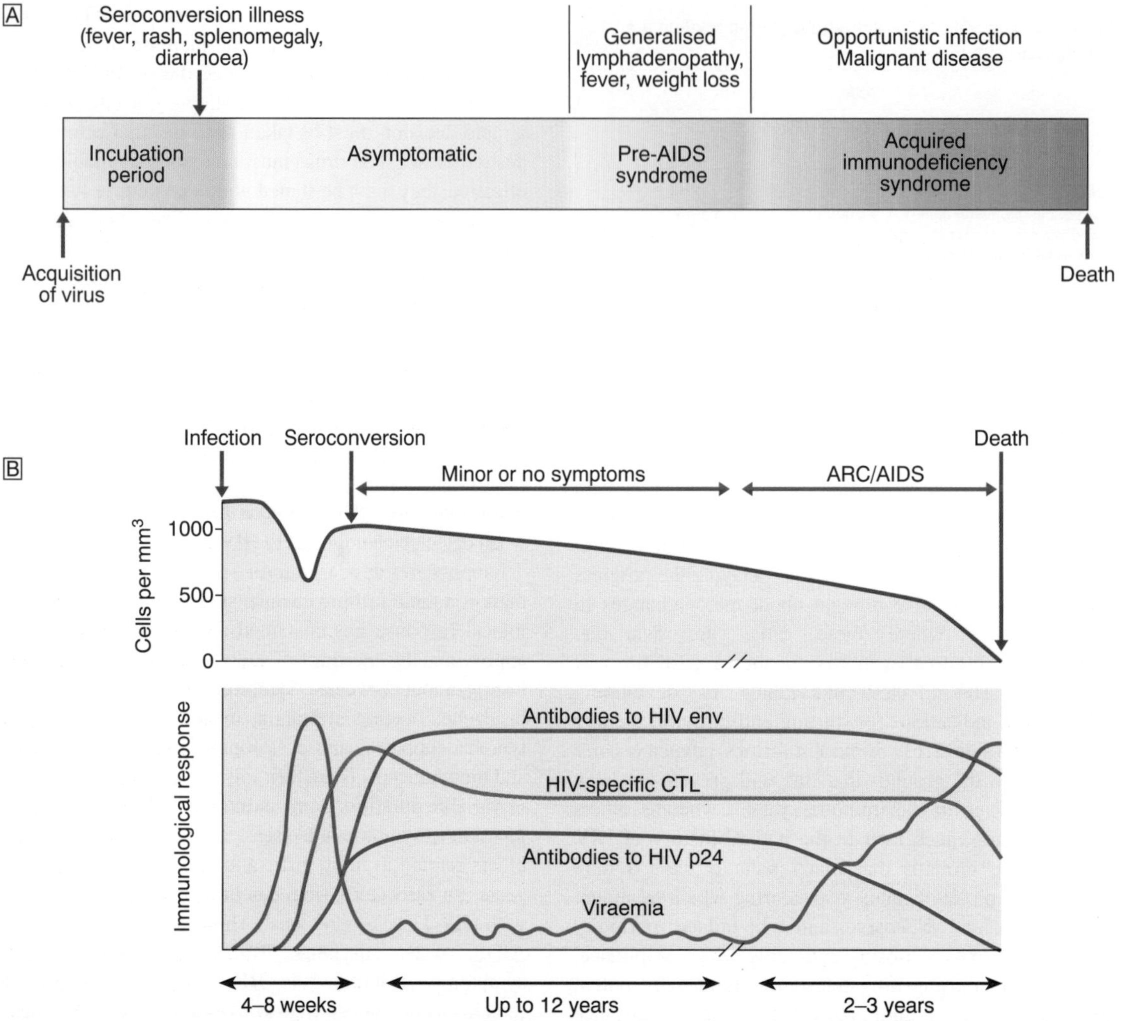

Fig. 2.10 Clinical stages and progression of HIV infection. A The development of AIDS was originally on clinical grounds; however, in the USA a CD4 count of < 200 is now recognised as AIDS-defining. The pattern of opportunistic infection varies between countries and has been altered significantly by the use of antibiotic prophylaxis (for example, Kaposi's sarcoma being common in male homosexuals). B Schematic virological and immunological progression of HIV infection. (env = viral envelope protein; CTL = cytolytic lymphocyte)

to differentiate causes of lymphadenopathy under these conditions.

Classification of HIV-associated conditions

Patients with acute HIV infection, or who are asymptomatic, fall into group A of the Centers for Disease Control (CDC) classification of HIV-associated conditions. Group B patients have symptoms but do not have an AIDS-defining condition. This group is sometimes referred to as the AIDS-related complex (ARC) and is characterised by conditions not exclusively confined to immunocompromised individuals (see the information box). As these patients are relatively immunosuppressed, they are also more prone to develop ordinary infections such as herpes zoster and bacterial pneumonia. Group C includes patients who have AIDS and therefore have one of the conditions meeting the CDC case

CLINICAL FEATURES OF SYMPTOMATIC HIV DISEASE

General symptoms	General signs
• Fatigue • Fever • Malaise • Weight loss • Diarrhoea	• Lymphadenopathy • Wasting • Oral *Candida* • Oral hairy leucoplakia • Perianal herpes • Splenomegaly

CONDITIONS THAT MEET THE 1987 CDC/WHO* CASE DEFINITION FOR AIDS

- Disseminated clinical cytomegalovirus infection (not liver, spleen or lymph node)
- Chronic (> 1 month) mucocutaneous disseminated herpes simplex infection
- Progressive multifocal leucoencephalopathy (papova (JC) virus)
- Extra-pulmonary tuberculosis or pulmonary tuberculosis with CD4 count < $200/mm^3$
- Disseminated *Mycobacterium avium intracellulare* or *Mycobacterium kansasii* infection
- *Pneumocystis carinii* pneumonia
- Candidiasis of oesophagus, bronchi or pulmonary tree
- Chronic (> 1 month) cryptosporidiosis
- Toxoplasmosis of brain
- Isosporiasis
- Disseminated histoplasmosis or coccidioidomycosis
- Cryptococcosis
- Extraintestinal strongyloidiasis

Secondary neoplasms

- Kaposi's sarcoma
- Primary lymphoma of brain
- Non-Hodgkin's (immunoblastic) lymphoma

Other

- Lymphocytic interstitial pneumonia (mainly children)

* CDC = Centers for Disease Control, Atlanta, Georgia; WHO = World Health Organization

definition for AIDS (see the information box above). As HIV disease progresses and patients become symptomatic, the peripheral blood CD4 count declines and the viral load increases. These two measures now offer the opportunity of precise clinical staging of HIV disease and are important in deciding when to commence antiretroviral chemotherapy (see Table 2.13). Taken together, they are useful surrogate markers for clinical progression. The lower the CD4 count and the higher the viral load, the greater the likelihood of opportunist infections and secondary neoplasms. Survival for patients once AIDS is established used to be poor, with only 50% of patients still alive by 18 months. However, the situation has improved since the introduction of combination antiretroviral therapy, more intense clinical surveillance with rapid diagnosis and treatment of opportunist infections, and effective antimicrobial prophylaxis for many recurrent and relapsing opportunist infections. The major opportunist infections and other conditions that characterise AIDS will be described in the rest of this chapter.

Disseminated disease in AIDS

A logical approach to describing opportunist infections and neoplasms of AIDS is not straightforward as many affect more than one organ or site. These will be described first, whereas conditions that have a particular organ predilection will be described under appropriate organ headings. Conditions seen in AIDS which tend to be disseminated at presentation are listed in the information box.

DISSEMINATED DISEASE IN AIDS

Infections	Secondary neoplasms
• Cytomegalovirus (CMV) infection • Bacterial septicaemia (e.g. pneumococcal, salmonella) • *M. tuberculosis* infection • *M. avium intracellulare* infection • Toxoplasmosis • Cryptococcosis • Histoplasmosis	• Kaposi's sarcoma • Non-Hodgkin's lymphoma

Cytomegalovirus (CMV)

CMV is a herpesvirus, and infection is extremely common in HIV disease. Approximately 50% of the general population and 90% of homosexual men are seropositive and harbour the virus. Clinical disease results from reactivation of latent CMV infection in the face of severe immunosuppression. This is seen when the CD4 count is normally below $50/mm^3$ and the HIV load is high. Diagnosis of CMV disease is based on the clinical picture and histology. Many organs can be involved including eyes, central nervous system, liver, gut, adrenals, mouth, oesophagus and lung. The most common and dramatic problem is CMV choroidoretinitis (see Fig. 2.11), which can lead very rapidly to blindness and is characterised by fundal perivascular haemorrhages and exudates. Overt adrenal involvement is uncommon but can occasionally present with lassitude, postural hypotension, dehydration and hyponatraemia which respond to corticosteroid therapy. CMV encephalitis usually presents subacutely in contrast to the more gradual progression of HIV-related encephalopathy, with personality change, poor concentration,

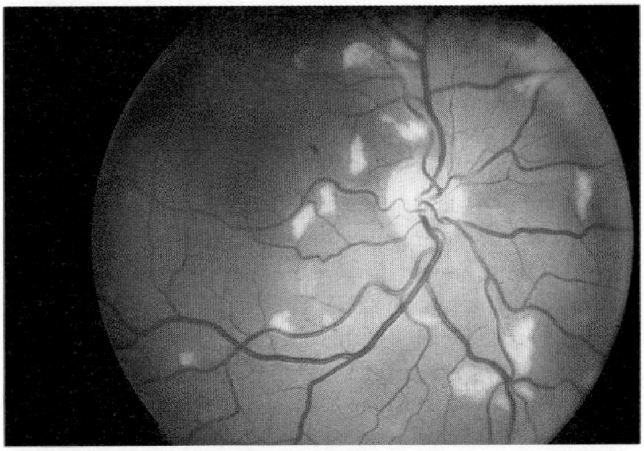

Fig. 2.11 CMV retinitis. Characteristic perivascular exudates often accompanied by haemorrhages in more severe cases.

headaches and insomnia. CMV may also cause transverse myelitis and polyradiculopathy. It can also cause colitis presenting with diarrhoea, weight loss, anorexia and fever, but is a less common cause of colitis than other pathogens which include cryptosporidia, microsporidia and *Mycobacterium avium intracellulare*, *Shigella* and *Campylobacter*. Sigmoidoscopy reveals diffuse submucosal haemorrhages and ulcerations. CMV may also cause oesophagitis. Unlike the other sites where CMV undoubtedly does cause disease, in the lungs CMV is a rare cause of pneumonia although it is frequently isolated from the lung of AIDS patients. Treatment of CMV is with ganciclovir or, alternatively, foscarnet. Originally, both drugs had to be given intravenously and permanent venous access via a Hickman line or similar device was normally required. However, ganciclovir can now be given orally and intra-ocular implants are available for localised eye disease. A favourable clinical response is normally obtained but maintenance therapy at lower dose may be required. Drug resistance may develop, necessitating a switch to alternative therapy, and occasionally dual therapy is required.

Other herpesviruses

Herpes zoster infection, usually in the form of multi-dermatomal shingles, is seen in HIV-infected patients, usually belonging to group B of the CDC classification. Rarely, herpes zoster may cause pneumonitis or encephalitis in AIDS patients. Chronic mucocutaneous herpes simplex infection is an AIDS-defining diagnosis and infection may be extensive but disseminated infection is rare. In addition, both Kaposi's sarcoma and B-cell lymphomas associated with AIDS are now known to result from herpesvirus 8 infection and will be discussed later.

Bacterial infections in HIV

Although many of the serious opportunist infections in AIDS are due to viruses, fungi or protozoa, bacterial infections are very common in these patients. It is important to recognise that such infections are often not contained within a particular organ and septicaemia is common. These infections will be discussed further in later sections. Neurosyphilis should be considered in the differential diagnosis of neurological disease in AIDS and, conversely, HIV infection should be considered in patients presenting with syphilis.

Mycobacterium tuberculosis. Tuberculosis (TB) is probably the most important opportunist infection related to HIV in global terms and HIV is now regarded as the most important risk factor for the development of TB (see the information box). The relationship between HIV and TB is closely determined by the prevalence of the two separate infections, which geographically is extremely variable. If TB is prevalent in a community, the incidence of clinical TB is greatly increased by the presence of HIV infection within that population. This is particularly the case in developing countries such as those in sub-Saharan Africa, where both infections are very common. In Uganda, for example, it is estimated that 10% of the population are now infected with HIV. As a result, the incidence of TB since the early 1980s has increased dramatically. In the USA, the annual decline in TB that had been occurring since the beginning of the century ceased in 1986 and numbers began to increase. This increase was directly related to cases of HIV disease in major American cities such as New York, Miami and San Francisco, whereas the decline overall continues in the general (HIV-negative) population in the USA. In the countries of Europe, increases in the number of TB cases have been observed since the beginning of the HIV epidemic in HIV-infected individuals. In sub-Saharan Africa TB is the most common opportunist infection seen in HIV disease.

MAIN FEATURES OF TUBERCULOSIS IN HIV INFECTION

- Incidence of TB reflects background prevalence in community
- Can be due to reactivation or new infection
- TB can occur at any stage of HIV disease
- Atypical features and extra-pulmonary disease are common
- Diagnosis may be difficult
- Treatment response generally is good
- Overall prognosis is poor; TB accelerates HIV disease
- Multidrug-resistant TB is an increasing problem

The association between HIV and TB relates to the decline in cell-mediated immunity, allowing reactivation to occur in previously infected individuals. It has been estimated that people previously infected with TB who do not develop clinical disease at the time of infection have a 5% lifetime chance of developing clinical disease as a result of reactivation at some later stage in their lives. In HIV-infected individuals this risk is increased to 8% per year. TB in HIV-infected individuals generally follows a more rapid clinical course with a higher mortality than in individuals with TB who are not HIV-infected. This is because the TB itself accelerates HIV disease by increasing HIV production in macrophages. It has now been determined that recent infection with TB is as important as, if not more important than, reactivation, and TB is unique amongst opportunist infections in HIV disease in being pathogenic to normal individuals. Tuberculosis may occur at any stage of HIV infection. When immunity is still relatively well preserved, pulmonary disease alone is seen, often resembling post-primary disease in normal individuals. When severe immunosuppression is present, extra-pulmonary disease involving lymph nodes, bone, pericardium, peritoneum, central nervous system, liver and marrow may occur, as well as miliary TB. Overall, 60–70% of TB cases with HIV infection have extra-pulmonary disease, compared to about 15% in those who are HIV-negative. Non-specific features of fever, weight loss and fatigue may also be present. In overwhelming mycobacterial infection HIV-infected patients may present with a classical septicaemia and mycobacteria can be cultured directly from blood.

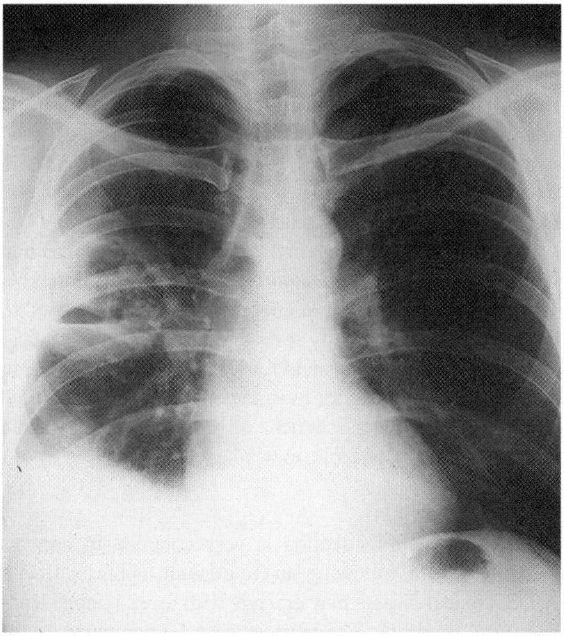

Fig. 2.12 Chest radiograph of pulmonary tuberculosis in HIV infection. Appearances are often atypical but in this case there is a typical large cavity accompanied by a pleural effusion.

The diagnosis of TB classically relies on sputum examination and culture, tuberculin testing and the chest radiograph. However, in HIV infection the tuberculin test is often negative because of the defect in cell-mediated immunity. As TB may be disseminated, pulmonary disease may be minimal and there may be no sputum for examination. If there is, this is frequently negative on smear and culture. Thirdly, the chest radiograph appearances may be atypical (see Fig. 2.12). Diagnosis therefore relies on a high index of clinical suspicion and remembering that the clinical presentation may be unusual.

Clinical response to standard treatment with isoniazid, rifampicin, pyrazinamide and ethambutol is generally good, with rapid improvement in symptoms. However, overall survival is poor due to acceleration of HIV disease. Drug reactions are generally more common in HIV-infected individuals than in HIV-seronegative individuals and this may be a particular problem in the treatment of TB. For example, thioacetazone, a drug used in developing countries for TB, can cause life-threatening side-effects and is now generally contraindicated. Also, numerous drug interactions can occur. Due to these features, compliance may be a problem and in some cases supervised or directly observed therapy may be appropriate to ensure compliance. To prevent TB developing in HIV disease due to reactivation, chemoprophylaxis with isoniazid for a period of 1 year is effective, particularly in individuals who are tuberculin-positive and who either live in or have come from areas of the world with a high prevalence of TB. Not only does chemoprophylaxis prevent development of TB but it has also been shown to delay progress to AIDS and death.

Over the last few years there has been increasing concern following the emergence of multidrug-resistant TB (MDR-TB). These strains of tuberculosis are resistant to both isoniazid and rifampicin and may also be resistant to other first- and second-line drugs. MDR-TB is at best extremely difficult to treat and at worst may be resistant to all anti-tuberculosis drugs. The prognosis is generally very poor. The development of MDR-TB relates to poor compliance, and inappropriate and incomplete treatment. The prevention of the development of MDR-TB is a strong argument in favour of supervised or directly observed therapy. A further hazard is that MDR-TB can be transmitted to health-care workers and fatalities have been described. There is great concern regarding outbreaks of MDR-TB in hospitals and other health-care facilities. The technique of restriction fragment length polymorphism analysis (DNA fingerprinting) has confirmed that MDR-TB can be spread rapidly amongst HIV-positive patients and health-care workers.

Atypical mycobacteria. Of the non-tuberculous mycobacteria *Mycobacterium avium intracellulare* (MAI) is the most common to cause disease in AIDS patients. *M. kansasii* can also produce disseminated infection. Unlike TB, MAI is a pathogen of very low virulence and is commonly found in the environment, being present in soil, water and food. MAI usually causes clinical disease when the CD4 count is very low (less than 50/mm^3). The portal of entry is thought to be the gut. The most common presenting features are persistent fever, night sweats, anaemia and weight loss, in addition to non-specific symptoms of malaise, anorexia, diarrhoea, myalgia and occasional painful lymphadenopathy.

On examination hepatomegaly is frequently present, and the chest radiograph and CT scan often reveal widespread intrathoracic and intra-abdominal lymphadenopathy. The diagnosis is generally easy, provided it is considered, as clinical specimens from affected organs contain numerous acid-fast bacilli. Unlike TB, MAI is universally resistant to most first-line antituberculosis drugs. It has now been shown in several clinical trials that clarithromycin, azithromycin, rifabutin, ethambutol and amikacin are effective and these drugs are used in combination. Clarithromycin, rifabutin and ethambutol in combination are probably the most effective. Toxicity may be a problem but this is outweighed by clinical benefits in most cases. Monotherapy, usually with clarithromycin, is now used for prophylaxis.

Fungal infections

Candidiasis. Oral candidiasis is almost universal at some stage of HIV infection (see Fig. 2.13), and if seen unexpectedly in the mouth of a young patient should prompt consideration of significant immunodeficiency and HIV infection. Lesions

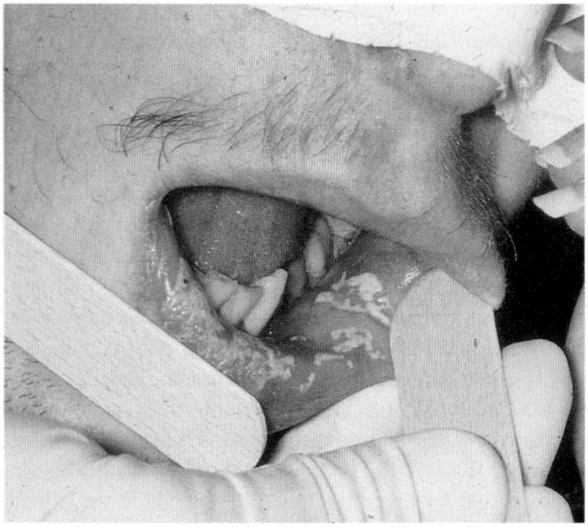

Fig. 2.13 Oral candidiasis. A careful examination of the mouth is important as plaques may initially be quite small.

in the mouth may initially respond to topical antifungal agents such as nystatin or amphotericin but when more advanced, systemic therapy is required, normally with ketoconazole or fluconazole. When *Candida* spreads beyond the mouth to the oesophagus or, more rarely, the lung it becomes an AIDS-defining diagnosis with oesophageal involvement; painful dysphagia is frequent and barium swallow may reveal a ragged-looking mucosal surface. Once *Candida* infection is firmly established, antifungal therapy often needs to be continuous and liver function tests should be closely monitored if ketoconazole is used. Fluconazole has now replaced ketoconazole as it is much less hepatotoxic. Continuous use of azole drugs in the long term often leads to resistance developing. Widely disseminated disease is generally rare but can become a problem in patients with neutropenia, intravenous drug users and patients with in-dwelling central venous lines.

Cryptococcal infection. *Cryptococcus neoformans* is the most common cause of meningitis in AIDS patients and may also cause pulmonary disease. Although clinically disseminated infection is rare, the organism may be cultured from blood, urine, gut or bone marrow. Initial symptoms of cryptococcal meningitis are fatigue, fever and weight loss, followed by headache, nausea, vomiting and photophobia. Diagnosis may be delayed because the poor inflammatory response often masks the classic symptoms and signs of meningitis. Diagnosis is made by Indian ink staining of CSF to identify the organism, and culture and measurement of cryptococcal antigen both in serum and CSF. The CT scan of the brain is usually normal and CSF examination may show a monocytosis and raised protein. Standard therapy has traditionally been amphotericin with or without flucytosine. However, because of the toxicity associated with amphotericin use, fluconazole or liposomal amphotericin is now often used, with satisfactory clinical responses. Relapse is common, so long-term suppressive therapy is required with high-dose oral fluconazole. Commonly such treatment merely arrests the meningitis and after several months clinical escape occurs, resulting in papilloedema, blindness and severe headache.

Endemic fungal infection in AIDS. Disseminated infection with *Histoplasma capsulatum* and *Coccidioidomyces immitis* is seen in AIDS patients who have been exposed to these fungi in endemically restricted areas such as occur in certain parts of the USA and Africa. It is therefore vital to take a good travel history from anyone with HIV infection. Amphotericin is the treatment of choice, although azole drugs, such as fluconazole, may be useful.

Protozoal infections

Toxoplasma gondii infection is very common in humans (see p. 163) and, following severe immunosuppression with AIDS, clinical disease may emerge, with fever, lymphadenopathy and headache. The brain is the most common site for lesions, which usually present with focal neurological symptoms, convulsions, cognitive impairment, confusion, lethargy or coma. Other organs including the retina may be involved. Diagnosis is usually made by cranial CT scan which shows characteristic ring-enhancing lesions surrounded by cerebral oedema (see Fig. 2.14). Magnetic resonance imaging is more sensitive. Serological tests may be unreliable in this context and definitive diagnosis requires demonstration of

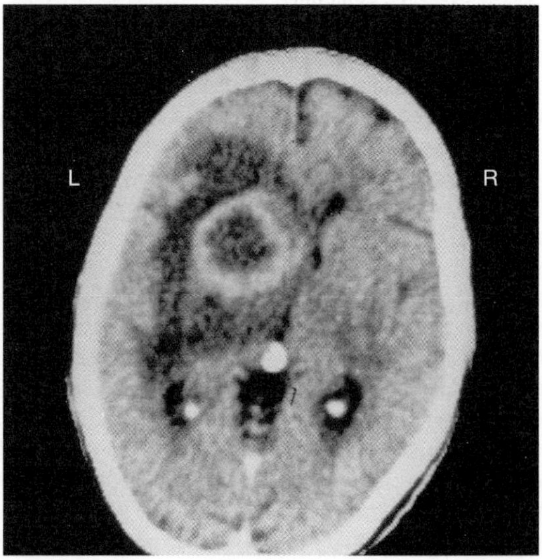

Fig. 2.14 ***Toxoplasma* brain abscess.** Characteristic ring-enhancing lesion following contrast with surrounding cerebral oedema (low-attenuation area).

the organism in brain biopsy material. However, such biopsy is hardly ever necessary, the diagnosis being made on clinical grounds and radiological and clinical response to treatment in 2–4 weeks. If *Toxoplasma* serology is completely negative, a space-occupying lesion in the brain of an AIDS patient is unlikely to be due to toxoplasmosis. Treatment of toxoplasmosis employs folate antagonists, usually pyrimethamine and sulphadiazine given with folinic acid. A combination of clindamycin and pyrimethamine is also effective. Pyrimethamine plus either clarithromycin or azithromycin are alternatives. Dexamethasone may be necessary to relieve cerebral oedema and anticonvulsants to control convulsions. Relapse is likely to occur if treatment is stopped completely and therefore maintenance is recommended with lower doses of similar drug combinations taken twice weekly. Routine prophylaxis of patients with co-trimoxazole (three times weekly) when the peripheral blood CD4 count falls below 200 offers good protection against toxoplasmosis and *Pneumocystis carinii* (see p. 103).

Nematode infections

Strongyloides stercoralis is acquired as an endemic infection in certain parts of the world (see p. 172), normally resulting in latent infection which very rarely becomes disseminated in AIDS patients. The diagnosis is made by identifying larvae in the faeces and treatment is with ivermectin. Albendazole or thiabendazole are alternatives.

Neoplasms associated with AIDS

Kaposi's sarcoma

Kaposi's sarcoma is an unusual neoplastic condition which was rare before AIDS. It is the most common secondary neoplasm seen in North American and European AIDS cases. It is unusual in that although it has many features of malignant disease it invariably arises at multiple sites within a short space of time, the cell of origin being the venular capillary endothelium. AIDS-associated Kaposi's sarcoma is closely linked with a new herpesvirus, human herpesvirus 8 (HHV 8). Kaposi's sarcoma is most common in homosexual male AIDS patients in Europe and North America (up to 25% of cases) and also occurs in sexually transmitted HIV infection in sub-Saharan African patients; it is rare in AIDS patients with haemophilia who acquired HIV from blood products. Histologically, the tumour consists of spindle cells and small blood vessels. Some authorities regard it as a hyperplastic rather than a true neoplastic condition. The most common site of involvement is the skin. The mouth, hard palate, tip of the nose, penis and lower legs are favoured sites (see Fig. 2.15). Lesions are red or violaceous, well circumscribed, and flat or raised. In dark-skinned individuals lesions may appear brown or even black. When multiple skin lesions are present they tend to develop along skin flexures. The prognosis for skin disease

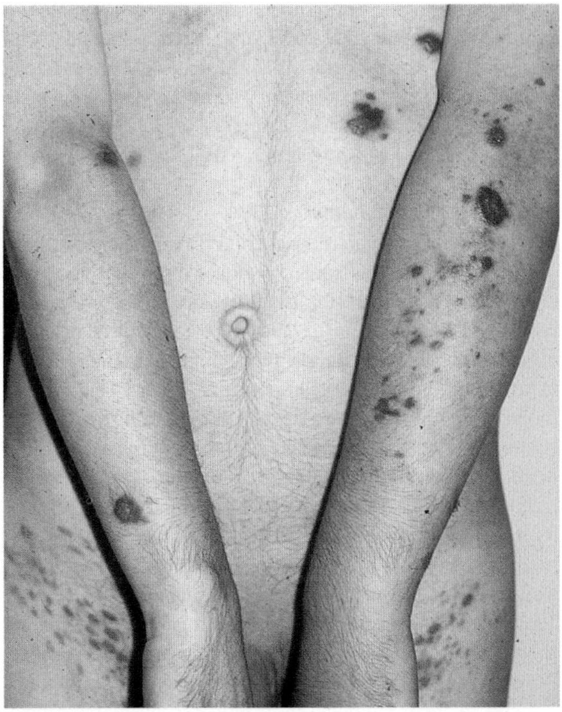

Fig. 2.15 Widespread cutaneous Kaposi's sarcoma. Lesions tend to be pleomorphic and slightly raised.

is very variable, although as the CD4 count falls, Kaposi's sarcoma tends to become more aggressive. Lymph nodes are the second most common site and, along with extranodal visceral disease, lymph node involvement indicates a poor prognosis compared to isolated skin disease. The gastrointestinal tract may be involved at any point and such patients may present with abdominal pain, bleeding or obstruction. Liver and spleen involvement causes hepatosplenomegaly, and pulmonary involvement may result in cough and breathlessness due to bronchial and parenchymal involvement or the development of pleural effusions. Patients with visceral involvement nearly all have mucocutaneous or lymph node involvement. In patients with a few skin lesions the disease may follow an indolent course, whereas extensive disease tends to be more aggressive. Skin lesions, particularly on the face, are unsightly and single lesions can be treated by local radiotherapy. Satisfactory palliation of disseminated disease can be achieved by combination chemotherapy with vincristine or vinblastine and bleomycin, often with the addition of doxorubicin. More recently, treatment with a single agent, with liposome encapsulated daunorubicin or doxorubicin, has produced good results comparable to combination therapy, with far lower drug toxicity. Treatment reduces morbidity but does not improve survival. It is noteworthy that Kaposi's sarcoma virtually never involves the brain. Restoration of immune function with combination antiretroviral therapy (HAART) has been associated with regression of Kaposi's sarcoma. The mechanism is not yet clearly elucidated but is thought to involve enhanced immune recognition associated with restoration of immune function and destruction of cells expressing HHV 8 antigens.

Non-Hodgkin's lymphoma

This group of lymphomas arises from B lymphocytes in 80% of cases, with the remainder arising from T lymphocytes. Of the B-cell tumours the majority are high-grade B-cell lymphomas of various histological types, including immunoblastic lymphoma and Burkitt-type lymphoma. The development of one of these lymphomas in an HIV-positive individual constitutes an AIDS-defining diagnosis and, in contrast to their development in normal individuals, these tumours tend to arise largely at extranodal sites, most frequently the CNS, bone marrow, gastrointestinal tract and liver. They are often advanced at the time of diagnosis, producing B symptoms (fever, constitutional symptoms and weight loss). Diagnosis is by tissue biopsy of affected sites and histological examination. Treatment is with combination chemotherapy and various regimens produce useful response. Primary lymphoma of the brain, however, is particularly difficult to treat, although short-term responses have been reported following cranial irradiation. Overall survival, irrespective of location or initial response to therapy, is poor and usually less than 1 year.

Carcinoma

There is an increased incidence of cervical dysplasia and neoplasia in HIV-infected women and of anal carcinoma, particularly in HIV-infected homosexual men. Women with HIV infection should have regular cervical smears. The association between these carcinomas and HIV is thought to be due to a greater incidence of infection by the human papillomavirus in HIV-infected patients rather than a consequence of immunodeficiency.

Organ-specific HIV disease

In this section infections and other conditions which tend to be more organ-specific than the conditions already discussed will be described.

Skin

Skin disease is extremely common in HIV-infected patients. Some of these diseases are also seen in the normal population but less frequently and less severely (e.g. molluscum contagiosum (see Fig. 2.16) and seborrhoeic dermatitis), whereas others are specific to HIV infection (e.g. Kaposi's sarcoma). The common skin diseases seen in HIV-infected patients are listed in the information box. In Africa, Slim disease consists of weight loss, diarrhoea (due to either HIV itself or enteric tuberculosis) and dermatitis, and is an AIDS-defining diagnosis. Management of the various skin infections observed in these patients is identical to the treatment given to non-HIV-infected patients. Pruritus is the most common skin problem in African patients and is exceedingly difficult to treat.

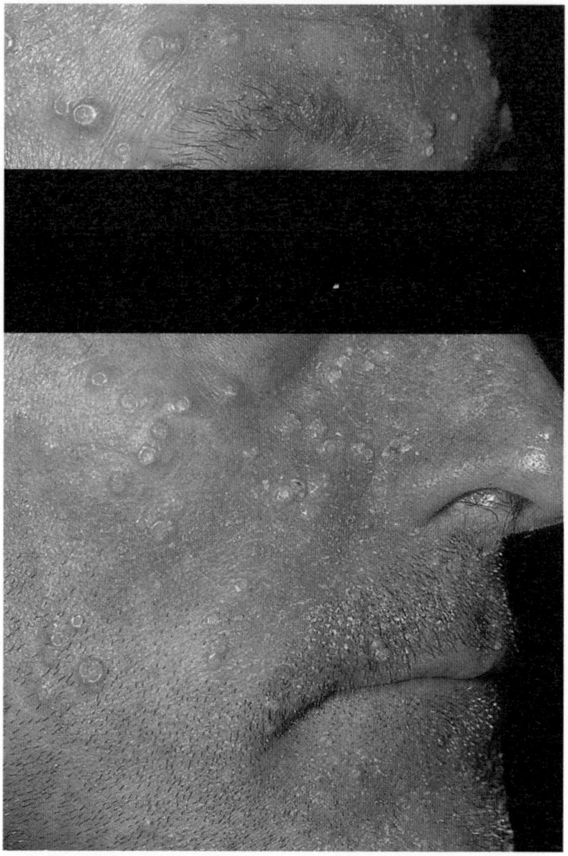

Fig. 2.16 Molluscum contagiosum. Extensive and disfiguring involvement of the face may occur.

COMMON SKIN DISEASES IN HIV INFECTION

- Seborrhoeic dermatitis
- Folliculitis/impetigo/cellulitis
- Secondary syphilis
- Herpes simplex/herpes zoster
- Molluscum contagiosum
- Fungal infections
- Kaposi's sarcoma
- Drug eruptions

Drug eruptions

Drug-induced skin eruptions are very common and more severe in HIV disease than in the general population. This is thought to be as a result of the immune dysregulation

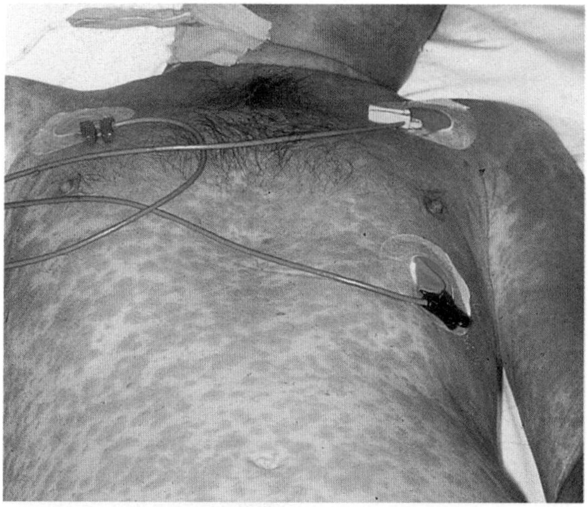

Fig. 2.17 Drug-induced skin eruption. Hypersensitivity drug reactions are common, in this case due to co-trimoxazole.

induced by HIV. Drug eruptions are a very important aspect of the care of AIDS patients, as the majority will develop a major drug eruption at some stage. Many drugs produce these reactions but particular culprits are co-trimoxazole, which frequently induces a widespread, intensely itchy, maculopapular rash (see Fig. 2.17) and Fansidar (pyrimethamine, sulfadoxine combination), sometimes used in prophylaxis against *Pneumocystis* pneumonia, which may induce erythema multiforme and the Stevens–Johnson syndrome. The drugs used to treat tuberculosis may result in skin eruptions, as may dapsone. Itchy drug reactions may respond to antihistamines such as chlorpheniramine, although it may be necessary to stop the drug.

Oral disease

Oral disease is prominent in HIV infection (see Table 2.14) and maintenance of good dental and oral hygiene is hence very important in these patients. As mouth lesions are so common in HIV and may be present early in HIV disease, a very careful inspection of the mouth during clinical examination is mandatory. Oral disease may cause disabling symptoms but most conditions are responsive to appropriate therapy. The most common condition is oral candidiasis and initially local therapy with amphotericin lozenges, nystatin pastilles or clotrimazole may control the infection. More extensive disease will require a systemic azole (fluconazole, itraconazole or ketoconazole); however, resistance to azoles may occur. Oral hairy leucoplakia (see Fig. 2.18) may occur in HIV infection and presents as serrated white areas, normally along the sides of the tongue. These plaques are adherent and cannot be pushed off with a spatula like *Candida*. They are usually painless, are due to the Epstein–Barr virus and

Table 2.14 Oral diseases in HIV

Disease	Treatment
Candidiasis	Nystatin/amphotericin/azoles
Angular stomatitis	Antifungals/antibiotics
Bacterial periodontal disease **Gingivitis** **Hairy leucoplakia**	Dental hygiene Penicillin/metronidazole Aciclovir
CMV/herpes simplex/herpes zoster stomatitis	Ganciclovir/aciclovir
Aphthous ulcers	Orabase triamcinolone Benzocaine lozenges Thalidomide
Warts	Cryotherapy/podophyllin
Kaposi's sarcoma	Local radiotherapy/chemotherapy

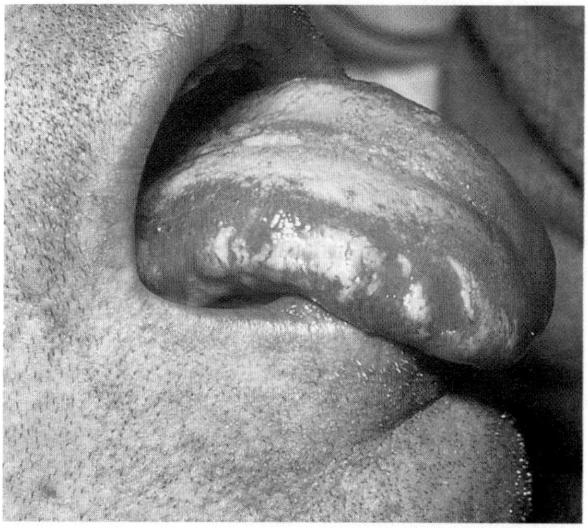

Fig. 2.18 Oral hairy leucoplakia. This tends to occur along the edge of the tongue.

usually respond to aciclovir or ganciclovir. It should be noted from Table 2.14 that for refractory aphthous ulceration thalidomide produces useful relief, but if used, the dose should be kept to a minimum to prevent the development of peripheral neuropathy; it is vital that female patients take contraceptive measures while on thalidomide.

Gastrointestinal disease

Weight loss is a marked feature of AIDS and much morbidity and death in late AIDS is due to gastrointestinal disease. Many of the pathogens which cause diarrhoea and marked weight loss in advanced AIDS are essentially untreatable. For example, microsporidia and cryptosporidia cannot be eradicated; they cause damage to the small bowel villous architecture, leading to malabsorption, maldigestion, diarrhoea and weight loss. Weight loss is a major contributor to cause of death in many AIDS patients and is commonly due to protozoal gut infection with microsporidia and cryptosporidia, producing a picture of starvation clinically which can be ameliorated with additional calories by the enteral route. This is in distinction to the weight loss and cachexia seen in systemic infections such as MAI and CMV which do not respond to simple refeeding. Parenteral nutrition has been successfully used in severe intestinal failure of AIDS but is very expensive. Salmonellosis with septicaemia is often seen in AIDS and is a particular problem requiring antibiotic treatment and constant surveillance of the patient after recovery, as return of bacteraemia is common.

The oesophagus. Painful dysphagia is common in HIV disease due to oesophagitis. The most common cause is candidiasis and the majority of patients also have oral candidiasis. Barium swallow appearances are characteristic but endoscopy provides definitive diagnosis. Initial response to a systemic azole such as fluconazole is normally good and rapid. CMV is a quite common cause of oesophagitis, either causing diffuse disease or discrete ulcers. Pain on swallowing and intermittent retrosternal pain may be present. Mucosal biopsy reveals characteristic inclusion bodies, confirming the diagnosis. Response to ganciclovir or foscarnet is normally satisfactory but maintenance therapy is normally required to prevent relapse. In up to 10% of cases no specific diagnosis of oesophageal ulceration is made. Some of these respond to thalidomide. Occasionally, primary lymphoma and Kaposi's sarcoma are found in HIV patients with dysphagia. Finally, HIV patients are not immune from ordinary diseases and gastro-oesophageal reflux may result in oesophagitis and ulceration. Tablet-induced ulceration may be seen. In view of the wide differential diagnosis, all AIDS patients with dysphagia refractory to antifungal agents should be considered for endoscopy.

Gastric disease. Nausea and vomiting are very common in AIDS and are frequently the result of drug therapy, in particular, high-dose co-trimoxazole in the treatment of *Pneumocystis* pneumonia. Alternatively, they may result from intrinsic gastric disease due to Kaposi's sarcoma, lymphoma or gastric ulcer. Mallory–Weiss tears and variceal bleeding are also seen as many AIDS patients belonging to the homosexual IVDU risk group have high alcohol intake, and hepatitis B and C are also common in this group. Nausea and vomiting in AIDS, from whatever cause, can be a major management problem but usually respond to either metoclopramide, domperidone, prochlorperazine or ondansetron.

Small bowel disease. Weight loss, high-volume diarrhoea and colicky para-umbilical pain are suggestive of small bowel disease which may be due to a wide range of infections (see the information box). Diagnosis depends on microscopic examination and culture of stools to allow for specific therapy with appropriate antimicrobial agents. Three sequential stool examinations and cultures will result in a diagnosis in 80% of cases. Small bowel biopsy is sometimes required, which may demonstrate subtotal villous atrophy in addition to specific pathogens. HIV itself produces minor changes in the small gut, termed HIV enteropathy, and this damage may be immunologically mediated. It is thought not to be severe enough of itself to cause diarrhoea. Similarly, bacterial overgrowth and hypochlorhydria are found quite commonly in advanced AIDS but are not thought to have an important role in villous atrophy. Overall, the most common causes of diarrhoea in AIDS are protozoal gut infections with cryptosporidia and microsporidia, leading to malabsorption, maldigestion and malnutrition, resulting in diarrhoea which can present a major management problem in AIDS. Fluid and electrolyte replacement, nutritional supplements and antidiarrhoeal agents such as loperamide, diphenoxylate and codeine are first steps in management. Some patients with secretory diarrhoea will respond to the somatostatin analogues, octreotide and vapreotide.

SMALL BOWEL DISEASE IN HIV

- *Cryptosporidium*
- *Salmonella* species
- *Entamoeba histolytica*
- *Giardia lamblia*
- *Campylobacter*
- CMV
- *Microsporidium*
- *Clostridium difficile*
- *Strongyloides stercoralis*
- MAI
- Kaposi's sarcoma

Cryptosporidiosis, which is an AIDS-defining diagnosis if chronic, is a parasitic infection which affects the brush border of the gastrointestinal tract and normally presents with profuse watery diarrhoea accompanied by abdominal pain, fever, anorexia, malaise, malabsorption and wasting. In one-third of cases spontaneous resolution occurs. Prophylactic measures involve boiling tap water before drinking; for established infection, paromomycin may be weakly effective. Cryptosporidiosis may also involve the biliary tract, causing biliary tract pain, the pancreatic duct and gallbladder. Microsporidium may respond to albendazole, whereas *Isospora belli* sometimes responds to co-trimoxazole. Bacterial gut infections such as salmonella and shigella are often accompanied by signs of disseminated infection and septicaemia. Response is normally good to appropriate antibiotics.

Colorectal disease. Colonic disease normally results in frequent small-volume stools, left lower quadrant and suprapubic colicky pain, tenesmus and pain on defaecation. A number of infectious causes are seen, two important ones being cryptosporidiosis and CMV. In homosexual patients a sexual history should be taken and proctoscopy performed, swabs being taken for chlamydia and gonorrhoea. Warts and herpes simplex are common in this group and syphilis serology should be performed.

Hepatobiliary disease

Abnormal liver function tests, right upper quadrant pain and hepatomegaly are extremely common findings in AIDS patients, as hepatic disease is extremely common. The main causes of hepatic disease in HIV-infected patients are: hepatitis A, B or C, hepatotoxic drugs, and CMV and MAI infections. Investigations should include hepatitis and syphilis serology, ultrasound or CT of the upper abdomen, and liver biopsy if indicated. MAI and CMV are particularly common causes of hepatitis as part of disseminated disease and CMV, *Candida*, cryptosporidia and microsporidia are recognised causes of acalculous sclerosing cholangitis. The liver may be involved in Kaposi's sarcoma and lymphoma.

Respiratory disease

Respiratory disease is very common in AIDS and the spectrum of causes is listed in the information box. One of the most serious common opportunist infections in the lung is due to the atypical fungus *Pneumocystis carinii* in Europe and North America. Before the introduction of chemoprophylaxis, up to 80% of all patients with AIDS had one or more episodes of *Pneumocystis* pneumonia. In Africa, however, *Pneumocystis* pneumonia is unusual whereas tuberculosis is very common. *Pneumocystis* infection is largely confined to the lung, where the air spaces fill with foamy exudate containing cysts and trophozoites of the organism. *Pneumocystis* pneumonia usually starts insidiously with an irritating dry cough and breathlessness. There is often a background of fatigue, weight loss and fever as well as other signs of HIV infection. Sputum production is unusual, and audible crackles in the chest are rare. An increased respiratory rate is common, with cyanosis indicative of severe disease (see the information box). Since the introduction of chemoprophylaxis, the incidence of *Pneumocystis* pneumonia has fallen dramatically; however, the infection remains common in individuals unaware of their HIV status, or individuals who are HIV-seropositive but are not taking prophylaxis. Risk factors for *Pneumocystis* pneumonia are: a low CD4 count—95% of cases occur when the CD4 count is $< 200/mm^3$; or if symptoms such as fever, weight loss or oral *Candida* are present and the CD4 count is $> 200/mm^3$; or failure of antibiotic prophylaxis. Typically the chest radiograph shows diffuse bilateral interstitial perihilar shadowing (see Fig. 2.19), although 10% of cases have a normal chest radiograph and 10% have atypical features such as focal consolidation or nodular shadows. A pleural effusion and mediastinal adenopathy are both rare in *Pneumocystis* pneumonia and suggest alternative diagnoses such as mycobacterial infection or Kaposi's sarcoma. Non-invasive investigations, such as arterial oxygen desaturation on exercise

SPECTRUM OF LUNG DISEASE IN AIDS

Common	Rare
• *Pneumocystis* pneumonia	• Herpes simplex/varicella zoster
• *M. tuberculosis*	• Adenovirus
• *M. avium intracellulare*	• *Nocardia*
• *Strep. pneumoniae*	• *M. xenopi/kansasii* etc.
• *Haemophilus influenzae*	• *Candida/Aspergillus* spp.
• *Staph. aureus*	• Cryptococcus/*Histoplasma*
• *Moraxella catarrhalis*	• *Strongyloides stercoralis*
• Gram-negative bacteria	• *Toxoplasma gondii*
• Mycoplasma	• Cryptosporidia
• Cytomegalovirus	• Lymphoma
• Kaposi's sarcoma	• Non-specific interstitial pneumonitis
	• Lymphocytic interstitial pneumonitis
	• Pulmonary drug reactions

***PNEUMOCYSTIS CARINII* PNEUMONIA**

- Most common opportunist infection in AIDS prior to chemoprophylaxis usage
- Commonly the AIDS-defining diagnosis
- 60–80% of all AIDS patients will have an episode if not taking prophylaxis
- Mortality 5–15%
- Annual incidence in AIDS (without prophylaxis) 30%
- Relapse rate (without prophylaxis) 35% by 6 months, 50–60% by 1 year

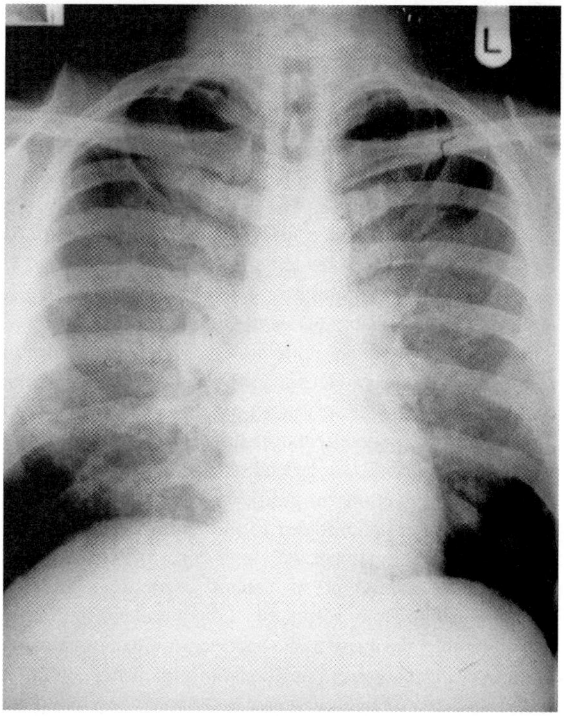

Fig. 2.19 ***Pneumocystis* pneumonia.** Typical chest radiograph appearance. Note the sparing at the apex and base of both lungs.

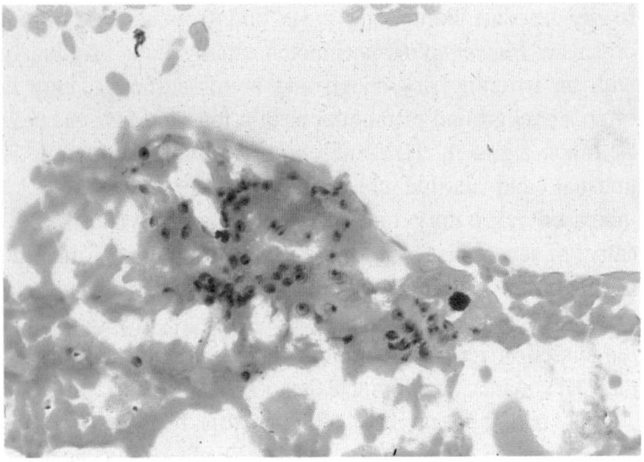

Fig. 2.20 *Pneumocystis carinii*. Broncho-alveolar lavage sample obtained at fibreoptic bronchoscopy. Methenamine-silver stain demonstrating black *Pneumocystis* cysts.

determined by a pulse oximeter or pulmonary function testing, lack diagnostic specificity but are helpful at a stage when the chest radiograph may be normal, to confirm that organic pulmonary disease is present. As *Pneumocystis carinii* does not grow in vitro and sputum production is rare, diagnosis usually requires bronchoscopy and broncho-alveolar lavage or nebulised hypertonic saline-induced sputum. The lung washings reveal cysts of *Pneumocystis carinii* with silver stain (see Fig. 2.20). Giemsa stain can be used to provide rapid provisional diagnosis whereas immunofluorescent techniques with specific monoclonal antibodies have improved sensitivity and specificity. Use of the polymerase chain reaction (PCR) to detect specific genomic sequences of *Pneumocystis* has extremely high diagnostic sensitivity and specificity but is expensive.

The treatment of choice for *Pneumocystis* pneumonia is high-dose co-trimoxazole, initially given intravenously. If the patient improves significantly a switch to oral therapy is appropriate and treatment should continue for 3 weeks. Alternative therapies are with dapsone and trimethoprim in combination or clindamycin and primaquine in combination. Intravenous pentamidine is also effective but is not used because of toxic side-effects. At least 90% of patients will respond to treatment. As a general rule, admission to intensive care units and intermittent positive pressure ventilation are avoided in these patients due to the high mortality. It has been shown that treatment with high-dose corticosteroids at the time of admission in patients with *Pneumocystis* pneumonia who are in respiratory failure reduces morbidity and mortality. Like many of the opportunist infections already discussed, *Pneumocystis* pneumonia is a relapsing condition and secondary prophylaxis should be offered. Oral treatment with co-trimoxazole or dapsone and pyrimethamine provides good protection against further attacks. Co-trimoxazole is the most effective agent, and primary prophylaxis to prevent first episodes should be offered to all HIV-seropositive patients with a CD4 count below 200/mm^3 and all patients with AIDS. Dapsone and pyrimethamine in combination and co-trimoxazole have the added advantage of providing some protection against toxoplasmosis. It is increasingly recognised that respiratory tract infections generally are more common in HIV-seropositive individuals than seronegative, with an increased incidence of colds, sore throats, sinusitis and acute bronchitis. The incidence of bacterial pneumonia is also increased over and above the incidence in a normal population. Illness tends to be more severe but response to appropriate antibiotics is usually good. TB and MAI have been discussed in a previous section, as has CMV. Although frequently isolated from the lung, CMV does not seem to cause pneumonia very frequently.

It is important to make a specific microbiological diagnosis of serious respiratory disease in HIV to allow specific therapy. Attention to which HIV risk group the patient belongs to is important; for example, IVDUs have an increased incidence of pneumococcal infection, whereas homosexual men are at risk from Kaposi's sarcoma. A travel history is also important, particularly if the patient is from high-prevalence areas for TB, pathogenic fungi and *Strongyloides*. A chest radiograph may show characteristic appearances of *Pneumocystis* pneumonia but these appearances can be seen with other pathologies. If the CD4 lymphocyte count and HIV viral load measurements are available, these are helpful as, generally speaking, the lower the CD4 count and the higher the viral load, the wider the differential diagnosis.

Non-invasive tests, such as simple lung function tests, are of value in excluding the presence of serious organic pulmonary disease where the chest radiograph is normal, but if these are abnormal then bronchoscopy is frequently indicated.

Neurological disease

HIV infects the central nervous system at an early stage in the disease and inflicts damage resulting in clinical disease. HIV can be readily isolated from brain tissue and CSF in a high proportion of patients with HIV infection, and at post-mortem pathological changes are present in the brain in about three-quarters of patients with AIDS. Neurological symptoms in HIV infection require careful investigation, which often includes CT or MRI, lumbar puncture and electrophysiological studies. Very occasionally, brain biopsy is required. Causes of nervous system disease are listed in Table 2.15.

Direct effects of HIV infection. During seroconversion following HIV infection, encephalitis may occur with mood change, convulsions or altered level of consciousness. Meningitis may also occur. In late HIV disease, HIV itself can cause aseptic meningitis but, more importantly, causes a diffuse encephalopathy referred to as the AIDS dementia complex (ADC), characterised by cognitive, motor and

Table 2.15 Diseases of the nervous system in HIV infection and their presentation

Organism/disease	Clinical manifestation
HIV	
Seroconversion illness	Encephalitis, meningitis (uncommon)
Chronic disease	AIDS dementia complex (ADC)
	Encephalopathy
	Meningitis
	Myelopathy
	Peripheral neuropathy
Other infections	
Toxoplasmosis	Brain abscess
Cryptococcosis	Meningitis
Papova (JC) virus infection	Progressive multifocal leucoencephalopathy
CMV	Retinitis, encephalitis
Herpes zoster	Meningitis
Tuberculosis	Brain abscess/meningitis
Syphilis	Neurosyphilis
Tumours	
Secondary neoplasms	Space-occupying lesion
Primary lymphoma	

behavioural dysfunction. This is the most common neurological complication of HIV infection and affects the majority of AIDS patients to varying degrees. In late AIDS the majority of patients have some degree of dementia even if it is mild. Zidovudine has been shown to be effective in reducing the prevalence of AIDS dementia complex. Onset is usually insidious with increasing forgetfulness, loss of concentration and loss of cognitive skills, leading to confusion, apathy, agitation and social withdrawal with behavioural disturbance. Motor dysfunction normally starts with unsteadiness of gait, weakness of the legs and lack of coordination. Steady decline leads to global dementia with limb weakness and pyramidal tract signs, ataxia and incontinence. Convulsions may occur in late disease. Investigations often show cortical atrophy on CT scan and increased protein and lymphocyte count in the CSF. HIV can also cause myelopathy, contributing to the motor disturbance seen in the AIDS dementia complex. A variety of peripheral neuropathies occur in HIV infection, with the most common being a sensory neuropathy, probably directly due to HIV.

Other neurological diseases. The most common cause of meningitis is cryptococcal infection; other causes include bacterial infection, tuberculosis, syphilis, other fungal infections and HIV itself. A diffuse encephalopathy may be caused by metabolic disturbance, herpes zoster or simplex, and CMV. Toxoplasmosis is the most common cause of a space-occupying lesion in HIV disease (see p. 163). Less common causes of space-occupying lesions are primary cerebral lymphoma and tuberculosis. CMV most commonly causes choroidoretinitis, presenting with blurring and then loss of vision, which is often unilateral at first. Less commonly, CMV causes encephalitis or radiculopathy. Progressive multifocal leucoencephalopathy (PML) is relatively uncommon and is an opportunist infection caused by the JC papovavirus. This results in damage predominantly to the white matter; the clinical course is more protracted than that seen in toxoplasmosis or lymphoma and a definitive diagnosis can only be made by brain biopsy or at autopsy although specific appearances on gadolinium-enhanced MRI scans are reported. There is no effective treatment. Peripheral neuropathies of various types in addition to those caused by HIV may occur, including autonomic neuropathy. These may be secondary to herpes zoster or CMV infection, or drug-induced—in particular as a result of the use of antiretroviral agents. Finally, myopathy, polymyositis and a dermatomyositis-like illness of undetermined aetiology are seen. Myopathy may also be caused by zidovudine. Autonomic neuropathy is also well recognised in AIDS and may be manifest by postural hypotension and abnormal Valsalva manoeuvre.

The eye. Non-specific conjunctivitis is common in HIV disease. CMV is the most common cause of retinal disease in AIDS. CMV choroidoretinitis can rapidly lead to blindness. Treatment with ganciclovir or foscarnet is successful but maintenance therapy is usually required to prevent relapse. The exudates of CMV retinitis may be confused with the cotton wool spot exudates due to HIV itself. Other causes of retinal disease in AIDS include toxoplasmosis, candidiasis and syphilis.

Psychiatric problems

A positive HIV test result can lead to a variety of psychological reactions ranging from anger, guilt and anxiety with panic attacks, through to depression. Patients with HIV infection may present with symptoms of organic brain syndrome due to HIV infection itself. The stress of having HIV infection or AIDS in terms of relationships, work and social life is likely to result in a wide range of affective disorders, with depression being common. Acute psychosis is relatively rare but does occur. More common are mood change, behaviour change and cognitive disorders that herald the AIDS dementia complex.

Haematological complications

Idiopathic thrombocytopenic purpura (ITP) can complicate early HIV disease. This is thought to be related to HIV itself and is associated with antiplatelet antibodies. It is usually relatively mild and tends to resolve with the onset of AIDS. Treatment may be required and initially involves high-dose prednisolone or intravenous gammaglobulin. Progressive lymphopenia, in particular a progressive fall in the CD4 count, is the hallmark of HIV infection. Anaemia with or without other cytopenias is extremely common with the onset of AIDS and represents direct bone marrow suppression; it may arise from a wide variety of causes relating to both the infectious and neoplastic complications of AIDS. For example, anaemia may be associated with marrow infiltration due to MAI, *M. tuberculosis* or lymphoma, chronic blood loss from Kaposi's sarcoma of the stomach or B_{12} deficiency due to malabsorption as a result of chronic gastrointestinal infections. Finally, many drugs commonly used in AIDS are myelosuppressive—for example, antiretroviral agents, co-trimoxazole and ganciclovir.

Renal, cardiac and endocrine disease

HIV-induced nephropathy characterised by glomerulonephritis has been described, but this is relatively uncommon. It is more common in AIDS patients who are intravenous drug users or Afro-Caribbean patients with intrinsic renal disease. However, a large number of nephrotoxic drugs (e.g. amphotericin B, foscarnet, pentamidine) are commonly used in AIDS patients. A variety of cardiac pathologies have been described from post-mortem studies but the most consistent finding is of myocarditis. Clinical cardiac disease is relatively rare in AIDS patients and usually presents as congestive cardiomyopathy or pericardial effusion. Diffuse endocrine gland pathology has been reported from autopsy studies and clinical endocrine abnormalities have been described; these are generally rare but adrenal insufficiency is extremely important to diagnose. CMV frequently causes adrenalitis but clinical adrenal insufficiency, although reported, is rare.

Paediatric HIV

Paediatric infection is a direct consequence of heterosexual spread of HIV and of HIV-seropositive mothers. There are three routes of transmission from mother to fetus:

- In utero transmission can occur as early as the first trimester and this transplacental spread accounts for around 25% of the total transmission events.
- During labour and delivery the fetus may become infected as a result of materno-fetal blood exchange during contractions or mucous membrane spread as a result of trauma or fetal swallowing of HIV-infected blood or maternal secretions in the birth canal. It is of note that in twin births the first-born has twice the risk of HIV infection compared with the second-born.
- The third route of transmission is via breastfeeding. This accounts for an additional 14% of paediatric infections. HIV is present in breast milk, and fetal gut cells are susceptible to HIV infection.

Overall, the risk of materno-fetal transmission of HIV is between 13% and 42% and is twice as common in Africa as in Europe. The risk of infection is increased if the mother has advanced HIV disease, or a low CD4 count and a high viral load, as may be the case if maternal seroconversion occurs during pregnancy or breastfeeding.

As the number of women with HIV infection increases, so will the number of children infected, and prevention is therefore crucial. Universal screening for HIV infection in antenatal clinics is one approach to identifying HIV-infected mothers-to-be. The risk of fetal infection from infected mothers can be reduced with zidovudine during pregnancy, labour and delivery and for the neonate after delivery. This reduces the overall risk of infection from (in one series) 25% to 8%, a reduction of nearly 70% overall. Caesarean section also reduces the risk by a surprisingly small factor and further reductions can be achieved by avoiding breastfeeding. However, in the developing world this raises problems with the risk of bottle feeding-associated infections.

Early diagnosis of HIV infection in the neonate is complicated by the presence of maternal IgG antibodies which cross the placenta. These antibodies can persist for up to 18 months, making standard antibody tests unreliable. Definitive diagnosis therefore relies on viral culture techniques or use of PCR. Generally, a diagnosis before 3 months of age is difficult but a firm diagnosis can usually be made at this time. Transient HIV infection in the neonate has been described and it appears that the virus can, in some rare situations, be cleared. Of infected neonates, about one-quarter develop rapid HIV disease and onset of AIDS within 1 year. The remainder progress more slowly and some children remain well until the age of 8–10 years. However, most have some signs of HIV disease by 6 months of age, and by 1 year 80% have evidence of disease. Age at onset of symptoms predicts for survival and there is a wide spectrum of clinical manifestations. Non-specific features may be present: hepatosplenomegaly, failure to thrive, fever without obvious cause and recurrent gastroenteritis. Between 30 and 50% have early opportunist infections, of which *Pneumocystis* pneumonia is the most common, and prophylaxis for this infection is therefore important. Other opportunist infections commonly seen in children are oral *Candida*, CMV, cryptosporidiosis, TB, MAI, toxoplasmosis and serious bacterial infections. Lymphoid interstitial pneumonitis is relatively common in children but rare in adults; this is due to lymphoid proliferation in the lung interstitium. Presentation is with tachypnoea, hypoxaemia and clubbing; the chest radiograph shows diffuse reticular nodular shadows with hilar adenopathy.

Drug interactions

Many of the drugs used to treat AIDS patients are toxic in their own right and this must always be considered. Furthermore, many of these patients require large numbers of different drugs with complex interactions. Since small intestinal disease is relatively common, malabsorption of drugs has been demonstrated and this must be borne in mind.

Terminal care

Despite all available treatment, AIDS remains a fatal disease and good support from a partner, family and friends can be of great help during this distressing time. During this phase, good symptom relief is vital and attention to the control of anorexia, nausea, vomiting, dry mouth, dysphagia, pressure areas and diarrhoea is important, as well as effective pain control if necessary. Many patients are anxious or depressed. Dysphagia can be a particular problem and some medications can be given rectally. Intramuscular injections should be avoided as, in addition to being painful, they are difficult to administer; these patients are often wasted with little muscle mass. Syringe drivers for subcutaneous or intravenous delivery of antiemetics and opiates can be extremely useful.

HUMAN T-CELL LYMPHOTROPIC VIRUS (HTLV) INFECTIONS

There are two other retroviruses, HTLV 1 and HTLV 2, associated with disease in humans.

HTLV 1 is endemic in Japan, the Caribbean and certain areas of West Africa. It is transmitted by blood transfusion, by drug users sharing needles and from mother to child, principally through breastfeeding. It can also be transmitted by sexual intercourse, especially from male to female.

HTLV 1 is associated with adult T-cell leukaemia/lymphoma and with a degenerative neurological disease characterised by demyelination of the long motor neurons in the spinal cord, known as tropical spastic paraparesis in the Caribbean and HTLV 1-associated myelopathy in Japan. These diseases also occur in Europe and in North America in immigrants from areas of the world where HTLV 1 infection is endemic.

HTLV 2, a much more rarely isolated virus than HTLV 1, has been isolated from Native Americans and in Africa, and also from intravenous drug users in the USA. Its role in human disease is uncertain; although it was first isolated from a case of hairy cell leukaemia, it is infrequently associated with this disease.

RHABDOVIRUSES

Vesicular stomatitis virus and related vesiculoviruses produce vesicular exanthems in domestic and wild animals, but are occasionally transmitted to humans and produce an influenza-like illness. Rabies virus is the principal rhabdovirus infecting humans.

RABIES

This is described on page 1010.

TOGAVIRUSES

This family contains the genera *Alphavirus* (former group A arboviruses) and *Rubivirus* (rubella virus).

ALPHAVIRUSES

The *Alphavirus* genus contains 27 viruses, all mosquito-borne. The most important viruses are the 'New World' alphaviruses, eastern, western and Venezuelan equine encephalitis viruses that have caused epizootics in horses and human epidemics of encephalitis in the Americas; and the 'Old World' alphaviruses chikungunya and O'nyong-nyong virus in Africa, Ross River virus in Australia and the Pacific islands, and Sindbis virus in Africa, Scandinavia, the former Soviet Union and Asia. These cause epidemic disease characterised by fever, rash and polyarthritis. The arthropathy may be severe and can last for months, or up to 3 years in the case of Ross River virus.

RUBELLA (GERMAN MEASLES)

Rubella is caused by a togavirus (genus *Rubivirus*) which spreads by droplet infection. One attack confers a high degree of immunity. It tends to affect older children, adolescents and young adults and spreads less readily than measles. The incubation period is usually about 18 days. The disease in children is trivial. In adults the illness may be more severe, but is of short duration and little importance except when it develops in a woman during the first 4 months of pregnancy. In such cases the child may be born with one or more congenital malformations (see the information box).

RUBELLA AND THE FETUS
Risk of congenital abnormality
• 1st 4 weeks of pregnancy—80% • 16th week of pregnancy and onwards—less than 5%
Causes of congenital abnormalities
• Heart (septal defect) • Eye (cataract) • Brain (mental retardation) • Ear (deafness)

Clinical features

In children the constitutional symptoms are so slight that the illness is rarely suspected until the rash is seen. The spots are pink macules which appear first behind the ears and on the forehead. The rash spreads rapidly, first to the trunk and then to the limbs. Tender enlargement of the suboccipital lymph nodes is usual. In adolescents and adults the onset may be acute, with fever and generalised aches, but even then the illness lasts for only 2 or 3 days. Polyarthritis is the most common complication and may occur in up to one-third of adult women. Encephalomyelitis and thrombocytopenic purpura are very rare. Complete recovery from all of these complications is the rule.

The rash of rubella is very similar to that due to certain drugs, enteroviruses and also parvovirus B19 which causes erythema infectiosum (fifth disease). Serological tests are necessary for a definitive diagnosis of rubella.

Management

No treatment is available. If infection is known to have occurred during the first 16 weeks of pregnancy there is such a high chance of fetal abnormality that termination should be discussed.

Prevention

Rubella vaccine should be given to all children at the age of 12–15 months, and again at about 4 years, with measles and mumps vaccine (as MMR vaccine). Rubella vaccine should also be offered to adolescents who have not previously been immunised. Women of childbearing age who are found to be serologically negative should also be offered vaccine, provided that they are not pregnant and are willing to avoid pregnancy for 12 weeks after vaccination. (A history of prior rubella is unreliable and only serological testing reliably detects immunity.)

DNA VIRUSES

ADENOVIRUSES

Adenoviruses cause disease by infecting epithelial cells in a variety of tissues and organs. Specific syndromes tend to be associated with particular adenovirus serotypes, of which there are nearly 50.

In immunocompetent patients they cause epidemics of pharyngoconjunctival fever (serotypes 3, 7), keratoconjunctivitis (serotypes 8, 19) and lower respiratory infection (in military recruits). They also cause endemic upper respiratory tract infection (serotypes 1, 2, 5), a small proportion of pneumonia (about 10% in children), sporadic gastroenteritis (serotypes 40, 41) and haemorrhagic cystitis (serotypes 7, 11, 21, 35).

In immunosuppressed patients they may cause disseminated infection involving the lung, liver, gut and urinary tract. Haemorrhagic cystitis and pneumonia are the most frequent adenovirus syndromes in transplant recipients.

There is no effective antiviral therapy and no vaccines available for general use.

HERPESVIRUSES

There are eight herpesviruses which cause infection in humans (see Table 2.16).

Table 2.16 Herpesvirus infections

Virus	Infection
Herpesvirus hominis (Herpes simplex)	
Type 1	Herpes labialis ('cold sores') Keratoconjunctivitis Finger infections ('whitlows') Encephalitis Primary stomatitis Genital infections
Type 2	Genital infections Neonatal infection (acquired during vaginal delivery)
Cytomegalovirus (CMV)	Congenital infection Disease in immunocompromised patients Pneumonitis Retinitis Enteritis Generalised infection
Epstein–Barr virus (EBV)	Infectious mononucleosis Burkitt's lymphoma Nasopharyngeal carcinoma Oral hairy leucoplakia (AIDS patients)
Varicella zoster virus (VZV)	Chickenpox Shingles (herpes zoster)
Human herpesvirus 6 (HHV 6) and 7 (HHV 7)	Exanthem subitum ? Disease in immunocompromised patients
Human herpesvirus 8 (HHV 8)	Associated with Kaposi's sarcoma

Herpes simplex virus (HSV) type 1, human cytomegalovirus (CMV) and Epstein–Barr virus (EBV) are ubiquitous agents which commonly cause asymptomatic infection in early life—hence many adults have serological evidence of infection with these agents. Varicella zoster virus (VZV) usually causes clinical infection (chickenpox) in childhood and 80% of adults will have antibodies to the virus in their blood. Following primary infection all herpesviruses establish latent infection and persist in the body for life; they may subsequently reactivate from latency. In normal people VZV may reactivate to cause herpes zoster (shingles) in later life and HSV may reactivate to produce recurrent lesions on the face (eye and lips) or external genitalia. However, reactivation of CMV and EBV usually only causes disease if the patient has become immunosuppressed. HHV 6 and HHV 8 have only been isolated in the last decade.

HERPES SIMPLEX VIRUS INFECTIONS

Herpes simplex virus (HSV) is a common virus which frequently causes asymptomatic infection, often in childhood; hence many people have serum antibodies to the organism. It has assumed greater importance as a cause of serious, and sometimes fatal, infections in immunocompromised patients. There are two strains of HSV, type 1 and type 2,

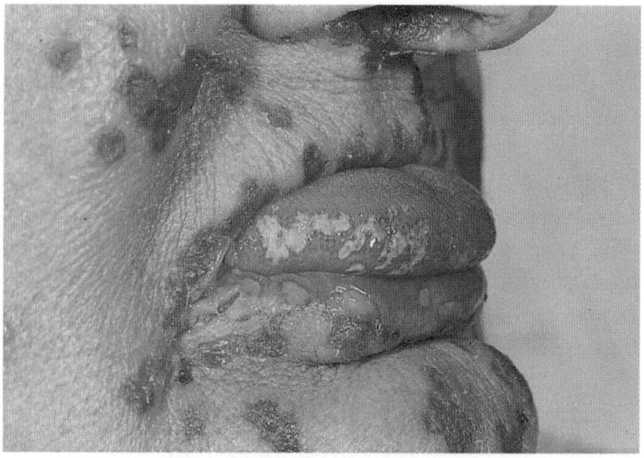

Fig. 2.21 Herpes simplex virus. Ulcerative stomatitis.

the latter being principally responsible for sexually transmitted anogenital infections. Infections caused by these viruses can be categorised as primary or recurrent.

Clinical features

Primary infection

This may produce gingivostomatitis and pharyngitis (see Fig. 2.21) (most common in infants), keratitis (dendritic ulcer), finger infections (whitlows), vulvovaginitis, balanitis and encephalitis.

Recurrent infection

HSV becomes latent in sensory ganglia, from where it may reactivate. HSV recurrent infections are most common on the lips and adjoining skin (herpes labialis or 'cold sore'). The lesions start as macules, and become vesicular and then pustular (see Fig. 2.21). Attacks of herpes labialis may be precipitated by various stimuli including sunlight, menstruation and viral and bacterial infections. Genital lesions (usually due to HSV 2) also commonly recur.

Complications

In neonates HSV infection may be disseminated, involving many organs and tissues, and can be fatal. In the immunosuppressed (patients with lymphoma, leukaemia or AIDS) progressive mucocutaneous, and occasionally disseminated, infection may occur. The newborn may contract the infection from the mother's genital tract during birth and active genital HSV infection may be an indication for Caesarean section, although aciclovir treatment may now be an alternative.

HSV encephalitis is the most serious complication of HSV infection; it may occur with primary or recurrent infection and is characterised by a necrotising haemorrhagic encephalitis, mainly affecting the temporal lobes. Although not common, it is one of the most common causes of acute viral encephalitis in the UK and it is striking that most cases are seen in apparently normal immunocompetent patients. Untreated, it carries a high mortality (around 80%) and, if suspected, is an indication for immediate high-dose intravenous aciclovir. (See p. 1009 for encephalitis.)

Investigations

The virus can be cultured from lesions, or identified by electron microscopy. Detection by PCR from cerebrospinal fluid is increasingly used, and shows good specificity for HSV encephalitis. Serology is of limited use except in primary infection.

Management

HSV is sensitive to aciclovir and the newer related nucleoside analogues, famciclovir and valaciclovir (a prodrug of aciclovir), although most infections in the immunocompetent resolve spontaneously. Drops containing aciclovir are effective in eye infections. Intravenous aciclovir is indicated for disseminated infections in immunocompromised patients and also for HSV encephalitis. The adult dose for intravenous infusion is from 5–10 mg/kg 8-hourly, the higher dose being indicated for encephalitis and the immunosuppressed. Oral aciclovir is available for infections of the skin and mucous membranes; the dose is 200–400 mg 4–5 times daily. Aciclovir will not eradicate latent HSV from posterior root ganglia, but recurrent attacks can usually be prevented by giving continuous aciclovir 200–400 mg 12-hourly, with a drug-free period every 6–12 months. Resistance of HSV to aciclovir has only been seen in immunosuppressed patients who have been given the drug for long periods.

VARICELLA ZOSTER VIRUS INFECTIONS

Chickenpox (varicella) is caused by the varicella zoster virus (VZV) which spreads by droplets from the upper respiratory tract, or from the discharge from ruptured lesions on the skin, or through contact with herpes zoster. Herpes zoster is due to reactivation of VZV from a dorsal root ganglion. Although it can occur at all ages it is increasingly common with age and will eventually affect about 20% of the population.

Chickenpox is highly infectious and chiefly affects children under 10 years of age. Most children tolerate this disease well but, as often happens with viral infections, adults may develop a more severe illness. In patients who are immunocompromised, the disease may be severe or even fatal. The incubation period is 14–21 days.

Clinical features

Chickenpox

Constitutional symptoms are usually brief and mild in children but can be severe in adults. Lesions are sometimes present on the palate before the characteristic rash (see Fig. 2.2) appears on the trunk on the second day of the illness. Then the face and finally the limbs are involved. The spots reach their maximum density upon the trunk, and are more sparse on the periphery of the limbs. Macules appear first, and within a few hours the lesions become papular, then vesicular and, within 24 hours, pustular. Damage from scratching is frequent, since itching may be troublesome. Whether or not the pustules rupture, they dry up in a few days to form scabs. The spots appear in crops, so that lesions at all stages of development are seen in any area at the same time.

Herpes zoster

This is characterised first by pain and then by a vesicular rash in a dermatomal distribution; it may be accompanied by a scanty varicelliform rash in the immunocompetent. (See p. 1012 for further details.)

Complications

The course of chickenpox is usually uneventful but complications occasionally occur (see the information box) and are more common in adults. Pneumonia may be severe in adults, especially in pregnant women, patients who smoke and the immunosuppressed; it is not always accompanied by clinical chickenpox.

COMPLICATIONS OF CHICKENPOX
Viral effects
• Pneumonitis (usually adults or immunosuppressed) • Diffuse encephalitis (within first week) • Cerebellar syndrome (usually in second week) • Transverse myelitis, optic neuritis • Myocarditis (usually adults or immunosuppressed) • Glomerulonephritis
Secondary bacterial infection
• Skin • Septicaemia
Intrauterine infection
• Congenital limb defects (varicella embryopathy—rare)

Management

No specific treatment is required for chickenpox in the majority of patients. Aciclovir is indicated for the immunocompromised (10 mg/kg 8-hourly by intravenous infusion) and (orally or intravenously) for chickenpox in adults and older adolescents in whom the infection can be more severe than in children. If there is secondary infection a local antiseptic should be applied to the skin, e.g. chlorhexidine. If bacterial infection progresses, an antibiotic such as flucloxacillin 500 mg 6-hourly should be prescribed.

For herpes zoster aciclovir, famciclovir and valaciclovir are all licensed; they shorten the disease if given early in the normal adult and are required to limit dissemination in the immunosuppressed.

Prevention

Immunosuppressed patients, neonates and pregnant women who have no antibody to VZV and have had significant contact with chickenpox should be given an injection of human varicella zoster immunoglobulin. A live attenuated vaccine is available but is not yet licensed in the UK.

EPSTEIN–BARR VIRUS AND INFECTIOUS MONONUCLEOSIS (GLANDULAR FEVER)

Infectious mononucleosis (glandular fever) is an acute infectious disease caused by primary infection with Epstein–Barr virus. It principally occurs in teenagers and young adults, although occasionally other age groups may be affected. The age at which primary infection occurs influences the likelihood of symptoms; seroconversion in young children is usually asymptomatic. The virus infects, and replicates primarily in, B lymphocytes and is shed in the throat following the acute disease. Transmission is, therefore, usually by oral contact, with exchange of saliva. The incubation period is probably between 7 and 10 days.

Clinical features

The infection usually presents with malaise, tiredness, headache, abdominal discomfort, anorexia and fever. The clinical features can be variable (see the information box). The rash is especially common if ampicillin or amoxycillin has been given, occurring in around 90% of patients. Conditions to be excluded in the differential diagnosis include

CLINICAL FEATURES OF INFECTIOUS MONONUCLEOSIS
Acute illness
• Exudative tonsillitis • Petechial rash on palate • Lymphadenopathy • Splenomegaly • Maculo-papular rash
Abnormal laboratory test
• Atypical lymphocytosis • Positive Monospot test • Raised liver enzymes
Complications
• Chronic fatigue (common) • Hepatitis (rare) • Haemolytic anaemia (rare) • Thrombocytopenia (rare) • Rupture of spleen (rare) • Meningoencephalitis (rare)

cytomegalovirus infection, toxoplasmosis and acute HIV infection, which can all present with lymphadenopathy, splenomegaly and fever with an atypical lymphocytosis (but not usually sore throat).

Investigations

The diagnosis is suspected by the finding of a predominance of atypical lymphocytes in the peripheral blood and confirmed by a positive Monospot or Paul–Bunnell test; these detect the presence of heterophile antibody (able to agglutinate ox or horse red cells). Specific virus serological tests are also available for diagnosis but are not required in most cases; IgM antibody to virus capsid antigen (VCA) indicates primary infection, whilst EBV carriers have IgG antibodies to VCA and EBV nuclear antigen (EBNA).

Complications

These are listed in the information box. Chronic fatigue with prolonged debility, inability to concentrate, depression, tiredness and low-grade fever may follow infectious mononucleosis. However, in most cases the chronic fatigue syndrome, sometimes referred to as myalgic encephalomyelitis (ME), develops without preceding EBV mononucleosis, or indeed any other defined virus infection; it is believed there is frequently an underlying psychological component.

Management

This is entirely symptomatic. Rest is important during the acute illness. A 48-hour course of corticosteroids (e.g. intravenous hydrocortisone 200 mg 6-hourly or prednisolone 10 mg 6-hourly if the patient can swallow) is indicated for severe tonsillar enlargement causing dysphagia or difficulty in breathing.

EBV-associated lymphomas and immunosuppression

EBV is associated with African Burkitt's lymphoma and with B-cell lymphomas in immunosuppressed patients (transplant recipients and AIDS patients). However, these tumours are also characterised by chromosomal translocations which result in increased expression of the *c-myc* oncogene, indicating that other factors besides EBV are involved in malignant transformation. Before this translocation and consequent clonal proliferation occur, some EBV-associated post-transplant lymphomas are initially polyclonal and may regress with cessation of immunosuppressive therapy alone, without requiring chemotherapy. This indicates the important role of antiviral T-cell responses in controlling the oncogenic potential of EBV in normal virus carriers.

EBV is associated with the proliferative epithelial lesion seen on the tongue of patients with AIDS—oral hairy leucoplakia. EBV DNA is also found in the cells of nasopharyngeal carcinoma, an epithelial malignancy with which it is believed to be causally associated, although the mechanism is unknown.

CYTOMEGALOVIRUS INFECTION

CMV is present in more than 50% of normal adults, and its seroprevalence increases with age. Primary infection may be asymptomatic or associated with a mononucleosis syndrome. CMV then becomes latent, probably mainly in monocytes, and symptomatic reactivation only occurs in the context of immunosuppression. It is shed in saliva and urine and from the genital tract; transmission is thus from contact with infected saliva or urine, or by sexual contact.

Clinical features

The various features of CMV infection are listed in the information box. CMV mononucleosis is similar to EBV mononucleosis without the prominent pharyngitis seen with the latter. Cytomegalovirus is a particularly important pathogen in immunosuppressed patients (organ and bone marrow allograft recipients and especially those with AIDS); primary infection and reactivation of latent infection cause much morbidity and mortality in these patients. CMV (along with rubella, toxoplasmosis and syphilis) is an important although rare (less than 0.5% of live births) cause of congenital infection which is acquired during a pregnancy in which the mother develops symptomatic or asymptomatic CMV infection—particularly primary infection. The child may be stillborn, or have features listed in the information box, although only about 20% of congenital CMV infection is symptomatic in the infant.

Investigations

CMV may be cultured from blood and urine of infected

CYTOMEGALOVIRUS INFECTION

Congenital infection

- Hepatosplenomegaly
- Purpura
- Encephalitis
- Mental retardation
- Deafness

Acquired infection

In immunocompetent
- Asymptomatic infection
- Mononucleosis-like illness
- Retinitis (rare)
- Hepatitis (rare)
- Association with Guillain–Barré syndrome

In immunosuppressed
- Retinitis (esp. in AIDS)
- Pneumonitis
- Enteritis
- Generalised infection

patients—viraemia is usually associated with disease due to CMV. The DEAFF (detection of early antigen fluorescent foci) test allows quicker detection of virus in blood, and PCR-based methods are now becoming quite widely used to detect CMV in plasma. Rapid diagnosis is important in immunosuppressed patients. Diagnosis may also be confirmed by biopsy of infected tissue (e.g. lung or bowel). IgM antibody to CMV usually indicates primary infection but serology is less useful in immunosuppressed patients.

Management

Two main drugs are currently used to treat CMV disease in immunosuppressed patients (infection in normal people requires no treatment). Ganciclovir (a nucleoside analogue) is given by intravenous infusion over 1 hour, initially in a dose of 5 mg/kg 12-hourly for 14–21 days; it is myelotoxic and expensive. Foscarnet (trisodium phosphonoformate, a non-nucleoside inhibitor of the virus DNA polymerase) is generally just as effective as ganciclovir and also has to be given intravenously. An oral preparation of ganciclovir is available but is only appropriate for prevention of recurrent CMV disease in the immunosuppressed. Aciclovir is not effective for treatment of CMV. Patients with advanced AIDS usually require life-long prophylaxis after CMV disease, particularly retinitis, usually with ganciclovir. (See also the section on HIV, p. 95.)

HHV 6, HHV 7 AND HHV 8 INFECTION

Human herpesvirus 6 (HHV 6) is a relatively recently discovered virus which is the cause of *exanthem subitum (roseola infantum)*, a benign febrile illness of children, associated with a maculo-papular rash. It has also been associated with lymphadenopathy and may cause disease in the immunosuppressed. *HHV 7* is a distinct but closely related herpesvirus to HHV 6 which probably produces a similar spectrum of disease.

Human herpesvirus 8 (HHV 8) has recently been isolated from patients with Kaposi's sarcoma (KS) associated with AIDS. It is present in the KS tumour cells (in AIDS and non-AIDS-associated forms of KS) and postulated, but not proven, to have a causal association. The seroepidemiology of this newly discovered virus is still being defined; present evidence suggests it is acquired mainly by sexual transmission in those populations at risk of KS, and is less widely prevalent than other herpesviruses.

PAPOVAVIRUSES

PAPILLOMAVIRUSES AND VIRAL WARTS

Most people have warts at some time in their life, usually before the age of 20. Genital warts occur during the sexually active years. Warts result from infection with the DNA human papillomavirus (HPV), of which over 60 subtypes are now recognised. Different subtypes are responsible for several clinical variants. Transmission is by contact with the virus, either in living skin or in fragments of shed skin, and is encouraged by trauma and moisture (e.g. at swimming pools, amongst butchers, fishmongers etc.). Genital warts are frequently spread by intercourse and perianal warts may reflect homosexual activity. There appears to be a close, if not causative, relationship between human papillomaviruses, especially HPV types 16 and 18, and carcinoma of the cervix. Other types of HPV may act as tumour promoters and, with ultraviolet radiation, cause skin cancer in immunosuppressed individuals.

Clinical features

Common warts appear initially as smooth, skin-coloured papules. As they enlarge, their surfaces become irregular and hyperkeratotic, producing the typical 'warty' appearance. They usually occur on the hands but may also often be seen on the face and genitalia; multiple warts are common. Plantar warts ('verrucae') are characterised by a rough surface, protruding only slightly from the skin and surrounded by a horny collar. On paring, oozing capillary loops distinguish plantar warts from corns. Often multiple, plantar warts may be painful. Other variants of warts include mosaic warts (mosaic-like plaques of tightly packed individual warts), plane warts (smooth, flat-topped papules seen most commonly on the face and backs of hands), facial warts (often filiform and hyperkeratotic) and anogenital warts (may be papillomatous and even cauliflower-like).

Most viral warts in the healthy will eventually resolve spontaneously but this may take years. In immunocompromised patients warts persist and spread (see Fig. 2.22); 70% of renal allograft recipients will have warts 5 years after transplantation, and there is also an increased risk of cervical cancer.

Management

Warts may be treated in many different ways. Common warts in children should be managed with wart paints containing salicylic acid. Stubborn lesions should be treated with liquid nitrogen cryotherapy or removed by curettage. Anogenital warts are treated with either cryotherapy or podophyllin paint (applied initially for only 2 hours and avoided in pregnancy). Facial warts are most easily treated with cryotherapy or electrodesiccation. Plane warts are best left alone.

HUMAN POLYOMAVIRUSES JC AND BK

The two human polyomaviruses known as JC and BK are widely prevalent in normal people and are only associated with disease in immunosuppressed patients. JC virus is the

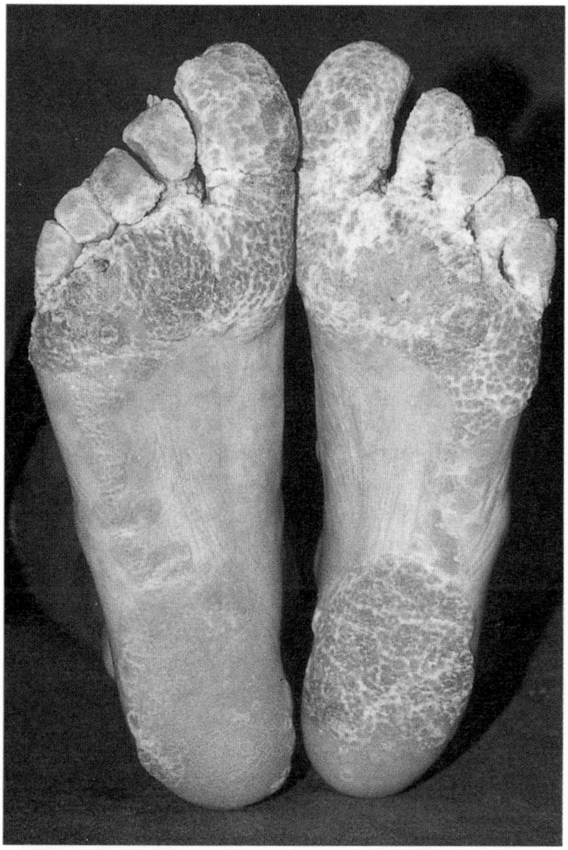

Fig. 2.22 Extensive plantar warts in a patient receiving immunosuppressive treatment.

cause of progressive multifocal leucoencephalopathy, seen most often in patients with AIDS (see section on HIV for details). BK and JC are excreted in the urine of immunosuppressed patients; an association between BK virus and ureteric stenosis in renal transplant recipients, and haemorrhagic cystitis in marrow transplant recipients has been suggested.

PARVOVIRUSES

Parvovirus B19 is the cause of erythema infectiosum (fifth disease) in young children. The infection is characterised by fever and rash with erythema of the cheeks ('slapped cheek' appearance); there is usually a lacy pink or morbilliform rash on the limbs and trunk. Parvovirus is particularly associated with the production of arthropathy; this is much more frequent in adults, especially women, in whom primary parvovirus B19 infection can produce polyarthritis, in about half of cases without erythema infectiosum. Parvovirus B19 is tropic for erythroid progenitor cells (the erythrocyte P antigen is the virus receptor). Infection causes erythroid arrest, which can result in aplastic crises in individuals with sickle-cell disease, and other diseases with high red-cell turnover. Intrauterine infection from infection in pregnancy can result in hydrops fetalis, due to fetal anaemia from infection of fetal erythroid progenitors. Infection in immunodeficient subjects can cause chronic anaemia associated with persistent B19 infection; the virus can be cleared in these patients by administration of intravenous immunoglobulin (which contains neutralising antibody). Diagnosis is by detection of IgM antibody to B19, or of virus DNA in blood.

POXVIRUSES

SMALLPOX (VARIOLA) AND VACCINIA

As a result of the WHO programme of case detection and vaccination, it is confidently believed that smallpox has been eradicated world-wide. Apart from two laboratory-acquired infections in 1978, the last known case occurred in Somalia in 1977.

Major smallpox produced a severe constitutional illness associated with a peripherally distributed rash with lesions which, in any one area, progressed in unison from macules through papules, and vesicles, to pustules. The mortality rate was as high as 40%.

A similar virus causes *monkeypox* in primates in jungle areas of Central Africa, with lesions resembling those of smallpox. Some human cases have occurred in those in contact with infected primates but interhuman spread is exceptional.

The virus of smallpox is maintained in two designated laboratories, one in the USA and the other in Russia, in order to be able to differentiate such diseases as monkeypox from smallpox. Only staff employed in these designated laboratories now require to be vaccinated against smallpox. Limited stocks of smallpox vaccine are available for this purpose, and in case the disease should reappear.

Vaccinia virus is derived from cowpox virus (originally shown by Jenner to prevent smallpox) and is a distinct poxvirus. It is used as the live vaccine for smallpox, as it elicits cross-protective immunity to smallpox virus. Complications of vaccination include progressive vaccinia in immunodeficient subjects due to dissemination from the vaccine site, eczema vaccinatum in patients with eczema, and fetal vaccinia in pregnant women given vaccine. Generalised vaccinia refers to self-limiting blood-borne spread of vaccinia in normal recipients. Post-vaccinial encephalitis was very rare.

MOLLUSCUM CONTAGIOSUM ('WATER WARTS')

This common and easily recognised poxvirus infection usually affects children and atopic or immunocompromised adults. Spread is by direct contact or by infected towelling, clothing etc. The incubation period is 2–6 weeks.

Clinical features

Individual lesions are shiny, white and hemispherical and grow slowly up to about 0.5 cm in diameter. Their characteristic umbilicated look is due to a central punctum which may contain a cheesy core. Multiple lesions are common (see Fig. 2.16). Like warts, many lesions will clear spontaneously, often after brief local inflammation.

Management

No treatment may be best in some children but cryotherapy or rapid expression is tolerated well by others, especially if performed by an experienced operator.

FURTHER INFORMATION ON DISEASES DUE TO VIRUSES

Fields B N, Knipe D M, Howley P M (eds) 1996 Virology. Lippincott Raven, Philadelphia
Mandell G L, Bennett J E, Dolin R (eds) 1995 Principles and practice of infectious disease, 4th edn. Churchill Livingstone, Edinburgh
Salisbury D M, Begg N T (eds) 1996 Immunisation against infectious disease. HMSO, London

DISEASES DUE TO CHLAMYDIAE

Chlamydiae are small Gram-negative organisms which, like viruses, only grow inside cells. However, they differ from viruses in that they have both RNA and DNA in their structure. They also have a cell wall and divide by binary fission. There are three species of chlamydia:

- *Chlamydia trachomatis*, which causes trachoma, non-gonococcal urethritis and cervicitis (leading to pelvic inflammatory disease)
- *Chlamydia psittaci*, which causes psittacosis
- *Chlamydia pneumoniae*, which causes atypical pneumonia.

TRACHOMA

Trachoma is a specific communicable keratoconjunctivitis caused by *Chlamydia trachomatis*, and is the most common cause of avoidable blindness in the world. Transmission is usually by contact or from fomites in unhygienic surroundings. Some infections occur during birth from infected genital passages.

Vast numbers of people suffer from trachoma in the hot, dry, dusty areas of the subtropics and tropics but it is also present in southern Europe and among immigrants in Britain. The disease varies markedly in incidence and in severity in different geographical regions. In endemic areas the disease is most common in children.

Pathology

The infection lasts for years, may be latent over long periods and may recrudesce. The conjunctiva of the upper lid is first affected with vascularisation and cellular infiltration. Scarring causes inversion of the lids (entropion) so that the lashes rub against the cornea (trichiasis). The cornea becomes vascularised and opaque.

Clinical features

The onset is usually insidious and infection may not be apparent to the patient. Early symptoms include conjunctival irritation and blepharospasm, but the problem may not be detected until vision begins to fail. Trachoma may also present as an acute ophthalmia neonatorum.

The early follicles of trachoma are characteristic (see Fig. 2.23), but clinical differentiation from conjunctivitis due to other viruses may be difficult.

Investigations

Intracellular inclusions may be demonstrated in conjunctival scrapings by staining with iodine or immunofluorescence. Chlamydia may be isolated in chick embryo or cell culture.

Management

Ophthalmic ointment or oily drops of 1–3% tetracycline should be applied twice daily for 3 months. In mass therapy in endemic areas topical application twice daily for 3–6 consecutive days each month for 6 months has given good

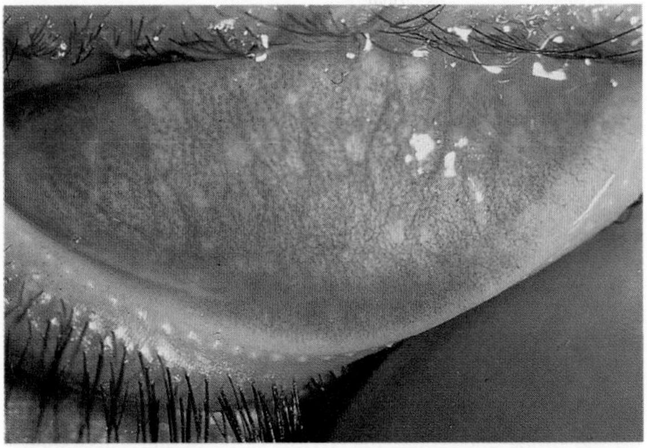

Fig. 2.23 Trachoma. Trachoma is characterised by hyperaemia and numerous pale follicles.

results. Oral tetracycline (15 mg/kg daily), doxycycline (15 mg/kg daily) or sulphonamide (30 mg/kg daily) given for 2 weeks is just as effective. Deformity and scarring of the lids, corneal opacities, ulceration and scarring require surgical treatment after control of local infection.

Prevention

Personal and family cleanliness should be improved. Proper care of the eyes of newborn and young children is essential. Family contacts should be examined. Population surveys lead to discovery and treatment of asymptomatic infections. Trachoma clinics are required in areas of high endemicity.

FURTHER INFORMATION ON DISEASES DUE TO CHLAMYDIAE

Centers for Disease Control and Prevention (CDC) 1993 Morbidity and mortality weekly report: Recommendations for the prevention and management of *Chlamydia trachomatis* infections. MMWR 42 (RR-12): 1–39

DISEASES DUE TO RICKETTSIAE

Rickettsiae are rod-shaped, spherical or pleomorphic Gram-negative organisms which are smaller than the true bacteria but still visible using the light microscope. Most are intracellular pathogens which grow only in living cells.

These organisms are natural parasites of the cells of the intestinal canal of arthropods, although some species may parasitise higher mammals including humans. Infection is usually conveyed to humans through the skin from excreta of arthropods but the saliva of some biting vectors is infected. Essential features of rickettsial infections are compared in Table 2.17. Transovarian infection to the next generation occurs in ticks and mites, which serve as reservoirs as well as vectors of infection.

Pathology and clinical features

In humans rickettsiae multiply in vascular endothelial cells especially of capillaries, producing lesions in the skin, central nervous system, heart, lungs, kidneys and skeletal muscles. Endothelial proliferation, associated with a perivascular reaction (nodules of Fraenkel) may cause thromboses and small haemorrhages. In epidemic typhus the brain and in scrub typhus the cardiovascular system and lungs are particularly attacked.

The common clinical findings are fever, severe prostration, mental disturbance and often a rash.

An eschar is often found in tick- and mite-borne typhus. An eschar is a necrotic sore, often scabbed, at the site of the bite and is due to vasculitis following immunological recognition of the inoculated organism. Regional lymph nodes often enlarge. There are epidemic, endemic, tick and scrub typhus fevers.

The investigation, management and prevention of rickettsial infections are discussed on page 117.

EPIDEMIC TYPHUS FEVER

Louse-borne or epidemic typhus is caused by *Rickettsia prowazekii* and is transmitted by infected faeces of the human body louse, *Pediculus humanus*, usually through scratching the skin, or sometimes by inhalation. Patients suffering from epidemic typhus infect the lice, which leave when the patient is febrile. In conditions of overcrowding the disease spreads

Table 2.17 Essential features of rickettsial infections

Disease	Reservoir	Vector	Primary-complex[1]	Rash	Gangrene	Target organs	Mortality
Epidemic typhus	Humans	Louse	—	Morbilliform Haemorrhagic	Often	Brain, skin, bronchi, myocardium	Up to 40%
Endemic typhus	Rats	Flea	—	Slight	—	—	Rare[2]
Rocky Mountain spotted fever	Rodents, dogs, ticks	Ixodid tick	Often	Morbilliform Haemorrhagic	Often	Bronchi, myocardium, brain, skin	2–12%[3]
Other tick-borne typhus	Rodents, dogs, ticks	Ixodid tick	Usual	Maculo-papular	—	Skin, meninges	Rare[2]
Scrub typhus	Rodents, mites	Trombiculid mite	Often	Maculo-papular	Unusual	Bronchi, myocardium, brain, skin	Rare[2]
Rickettsialpox	Domestic mice	Mite	Usual	Maculo-papular	—	—	Rare[2]
Trench fever	Humans	Louse	—	Maculo-papular	—	—	Rare[2]

[1] Eschar at bite site and local lymphadenopathy. [2] Except in infants, elderly and debilitated. [3] Highest in adult males.

rapidly. During interepidemic periods the disease may be maintained by unapparent or latent cases or perhaps by infected fleas and rats. The disease is prevalent in parts of Africa, especially Ethiopia and Rwanda, the South American Andes and Afghanistan. Large epidemics have occurred in Europe, usually as a sequel to war. The incubation period is usually 12–14 days.

There may be a few days of malaise but the onset is more often sudden with rigors, fever, frontal headaches, pains in the back and limbs, constipation and bronchitis. The face is flushed and cyanotic, the eyes are congested, and the patient soon becomes dull and confused.

The rash appears on the fourth to the sixth day and often resembles measles. In its early stages it disappears on pressure but soon becomes petechial with subcutaneous mottling. It appears first on the anterior folds of the axillae, sides of the abdomen or back of hands, then on the trunk and forearms. The neck and face are seldom affected.

During the second week symptoms increase in severity. Sores collect on the lips. The tongue becomes dry, brown, shrunken and tremulous. The spleen is palpable, the pulse feeble and the patient stuporous and delirious. The temperature falls rapidly at the end of the second week and the patient recovers gradually. In fatal cases the patient usually dies in the second week from toxaemia, cardiac or renal failure or pneumonia.

Common complications are listed in the information box.

COMPLICATIONS OF LOUSE-BORNE TYPHUS
Vascular
• Venous thrombosis, gangrene of fingers, toes, nose and genitalia
Infective
• Parotitis, bronchopneumonia
Brill's disease
• A mild relapse many years later

ENDEMIC TYPHUS FEVER

Flea-borne or 'endemic' typhus caused by *R. mooseri* is endemic world-wide. Humans are infected when, by scratching, they introduce the faeces or contents of a crushed flea which has fed on an infected rat. The incubation period is 8–14 days. The symptoms resemble those of a mild louse-borne typhus. The rash may be scanty and transient. Laboratory aids to diagnosis are discussed on page 117, together with treatment.

ROCKY MOUNTAIN SPOTTED FEVER

The organism *R. rickettsii* is transmitted by the bite of hard (ixodid) ticks which carry the infection to rodents and dogs and on occasion to humans. It is widely distributed and increasing in western and south-eastern states of the USA and also in South America. The pathological changes are similar to those in epidemic typhus. The incubation period is about 7 days.

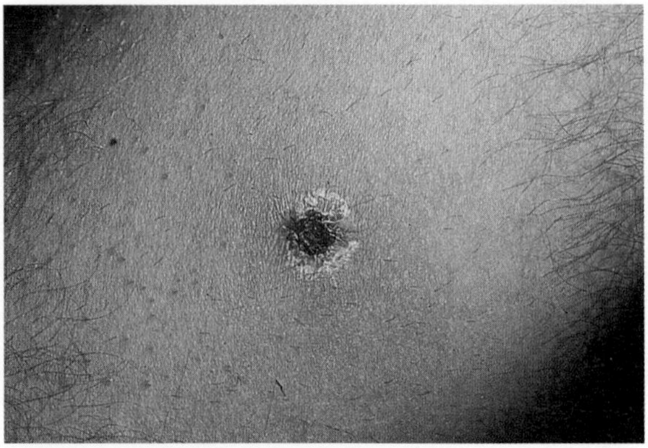

Fig. 2.24 Tick-borne typhus fever. Eschar at the site of the tick-bite.

There may be an eschar at the site of the bite (see Fig. 2.24) with enlargement of the regional lymph nodes. Symptoms closely resemble those of louse-borne typhus. The rash appears on about the third or fourth day, and is at first like measles, but in a few hours the typical maculo-papular eruption develops. Each day it becomes more distinct and papular and finally petechial. The rash first appears on the wrists, forearms and ankles, and spreads in 24–48 hours to the back, limbs and chest and lastly to the abdomen where it is least pronounced. The fully developed rash often also affects the palms, soles and face. Petechiae may appear in crops. Larger cutaneous and subcutaneous haemorrhages may appear in severe cases. The liver and spleen become palpable. Complications are as in louse-borne typhus, but gangrene is more common. Untreated, the course of the disease may be mild or rapidly fatal.

Other forms of tick-borne typhus fever

The causal agents of African tick-borne typhus in South and East Africa are *R. conorii* and a substrain *R. conorii pijperi*, the reservoir hosts being dogs and rodents. *'Fièvre boutonneuse'* of the Mediterranean is similar, as is also the infection *R. australis* in Queensland. Infected hard ticks may be picked up by walking on grasslands or dogs may bring the ticks into the house. Tourists may acquire tick typhus and import it into Britain. A careful search is needed to find the tell-tale eschar, and maculo-papular rash on the trunk, limbs, palms and soles. There may be delirium and meningeal signs in severe infections but recovery is the rule.

SCRUB TYPHUS FEVER

Mite-borne or 'scrub' typhus is caused by *R. tsutsugamushi*, transmitted by the bite of infective larval trombiculid mites. It occurs in the Far East, Myanmar (formerly Burma), Pakistan, Bangladesh, India, Indonesia, the South Pacific Islands and Queensland, particularly where patches of forest cleared for plantations have attracted rats and attendant mites.

The pathology is similar to that of louse-borne typhus, but lesions in the lungs are more prominent. In many patients one eschar or more develops, surrounded by an area of cellulitis and enlargement of regional lymph nodes. The incubation period is about 9 days.

Mild or subclinical cases are common. The onset of symptoms is usually sudden with headache, often retro-orbital, fever, malaise, weakness and cough. In severe illness the general symptoms increase, with apathy and prostration. An erythematous maculo-papular rash often appears on about the fifth to the seventh day and spreads to the trunk, face and limbs including the palms and soles, with generalised painless lymphadenopathy. The rash fades by the fourteenth day. The temperature rises rapidly and continues as a remittent fever with sweating until it falls by lysis about the twelfth to the eighteenth day. In severe infection the patient is prostrate with cough, pneumonia, confusion and deafness. Cardiac failure, renal failure and haemorrhage may develop. Convalescence is often slow and tachycardia may persist for some weeks.

RICKETTSIALPOX

This is due to *R. akari*, transmitted from the domestic mouse by a mite. It appears to be restricted to New York and Philadelphia, where mice are now adapted to live in communal rubbish chutes of apartment houses.

The illness starts with a papule, which develops into an eschar, and is followed a week later by the sudden onset of fever, sweating, backache and a rash, maculo-papular at first but which soon vesiculates and crusts, healing without scarring.

TRENCH FEVER

This is caused by *R. quintana* and is spread to humans by louse faeces. It was prevalent in the First World War in Europe among troops in the trenches and again in the Second World War in the USSR. The disease is otherwise rare. The incubation period is 10–20 days.

The onset is sudden, with headache and severe pains in trunk and limbs. The temperature rises sharply and remains raised for 5–7 days. The initial illness is like a mild case of typhus fever but febrile relapses are common, usually at intervals of 5–6 days, and may be debilitating.

Investigation of rickettsial infections

The Weil–Felix reaction is the non-specific agglutination of the somatic antigens of non-motile *Proteus* species by the patient's serum. A four-fold rise in titre is diagnostic.

Species-specific antibodies may be detected by complement fixation, microagglutination and fluorescence in specialised laboratories. Rickettsiae may be isolated from the blood in the first week of illness by intraperitoneal inoculation into male guinea-pigs or mice.

Management of the rickettsial diseases

The various fevers due to rickettsiae vary greatly in severity but all respond to tetracycline or chloramphenicol. Tetracycline is administered in a dose of 500 mg 6-hourly. The fever usually settles within 2 or 3 days. Tetracycline should be continued for 2–3 days after the patient is afebrile as there is a tendency otherwise to relapse. In endemic areas good results have been obtained in louse-borne typhus and scrub typhus by a single dose of 100 mg doxycycline.

Nursing care is important, especially in epidemic typhus. Sedation may be required for delirium and blood transfusion for haemorrhage. Relapsing fever and typhoid are common intercurrent infections in epidemic typhus, and pneumonia in scrub typhus. They must be sought and treated. Convalescence is usually protracted, especially in older people.

Prevention of rickettsial infections

Vector and reservoir control

See the information box.

VECTOR AND RESERVOIR CONTROL OF RICKETTSIAL INFECTIONS
Louse control
• Insufflate 5% carbaryl or 0.5% malathion powder into clothing of population at risk • Delouse patient's clothing by insecticide or heat (e.g. domestic tumble dryer)
Flea control
• Vacuum-clean floors. Treat floors and rodent burrows with residual insecticide powder • Control rodents
Tick control
• Remove ticks from dogs, mechanically or with insecticide shampoo • Inspect oneself twice daily for ticks and remove them before they have fed • Creosote floors of log cabins in USA
Mite control
• Impregnate trousers and socks with insect repellent (e.g. 2% dimethyl phthalate) and use insect repellent creams on skin • Clear campsites of all vegetation and spray ground with oily residual insecticide

Active immunisation
Vaccines can be prepared from killed *R. prowazekii*, *R. mooseri* or *R. rickettsii* cultured in eggs, but they are not generally available.

Chemoprophylaxis
It is likely that doxycycline 100 mg weekly will protect those at risk.

Q FEVER

Q (Query) fever is caused by *Coxiella burnetii*, a rickettsia-like organism, which is widespread in nature and highly resistant to drying. It is carried by ticks among animals, including cattle and sheep. Transmission to humans is airborne through aerosols from animal birth products and contaminated dust. Unpasteurised milk is another source of infection. The incubation period of Q fever is from 7 to 14 days.

Clinical features

The clinical features of the illness are protean, ranging from subclinical infection to fatal encephalitis or endocarditis (see p. 286). Acute Q fever usually starts like influenza with pyrexia followed by myalgia, headache and sweating. Many cases resolve without specific therapy. Some patients have a cough, and radiological examination may reveal a pneumonitis. Less common features of Q fever include hepatitis, myocarditis, epididymo-orchitis, iritis and osteomyelitis.

Investigations

The diagnosis of Q fever should be considered in patients living in rural areas, especially if there is occupational contact work with livestock. *C. burnetii* does not grow in the media used for routine blood cultures and it is therefore important to consider Q fever as a possible cause in patients with clinical evidence of endocarditis who have sterile blood cultures. The diagnosis of Q fever is confirmed by the detection of serum antibodies to the two polysaccharide antigens of *C. burnetii*; acute infection is confirmed by a four-fold rise in phase II antibody titre in paired specimens of blood taken at intervals of between 10 and 14 days. Phase I antibody titres rise more slowly than phase II and the persistence of both suggests chronic infection.

Management

C. burnetii is sensitive to the tetracyclines, clindamycin, chloramphenicol and rifampicin. Acute infections respond within a few days to tetracycline in a dose of 500 mg 6-hourly for 2 weeks, or doxycycline 200 mg daily for 2 weeks. The treatment of chronic infections, especially if there is endocarditis, requires prolonged therapy with tetracycline plus clindamycin or rifampicin.

FURTHER INFORMATION ON DISEASES DUE TO RICKETTSIAE

Kirkland K B, Marcom P K, Sexton D J 1993 Rocky Mountain spotted fever complicated by gangrene: report of six cases and review. Clinical Infectious Diseases 16: 629–634

DISEASES DUE TO BACTERIA

Bacteria are classified according to several properties; these include their shape, growth requirements and reaction to Gram staining. Most are either round (cocci) or elongated (bacilli). Vibrios and campylobacters are comma-shaped, spirochaetes are thin spiral filaments, and all three are motile when seen under the light microscope.

The main growth characteristic used in classification is their ability to grow in either aerobic or anaerobic environments. Some bacteria possess toxins which are responsible for producing pathological changes in tissues and organs. Examples include endotoxins produced by Gram-negative organisms such as *Escherichia coli* and exotoxins by *Corynebacterium diphtheriae*.

Certain bacteria exist in the environment in durable vegetative forms called spores.

STREPTOCOCCAL INFECTIONS

Streptococci produce a wide variety of infections (see the information box). All species can cause septicaemia.

STREPTOCOCCUS PYOGENES INFECTIONS

Infections caused by *Strep. pyogenes* result in features which vary with the invasiveness of the organism, its capacity to produce toxins, the site involved and the reaction of the host. If resistance is low and the invasive properties of the streptococcus are high, a rapidly spreading erysipelas, cellulitis, lymphangitis or bacteraemia may result. The organism may produce a specific exotoxin causing a widespread punctate erythema. When the infection is associated with such a rash the syndrome is known as scarlet fever. The same type of streptococcus may produce acute tonsillitis in one person, in another scarlet fever and in a third erysipelas. *Necrotising fasciitis* caused by *Strep. pyogenes* causes great tissue destruction and has a high mortality.

SCARLET FEVER

Although scarlet fever is at present a mild disease, it may not necessarily remain so, as fluctuations in its severity have been recorded for the past 300 years. The primary site of

STREPTOCOCCAL INFECTIONS

Streptococcus pyogenes

- Skin and soft tissue infection (incl. erysipelas, impetigo, necrotising fasciitis)
- Bone and joint infection
- Tonsillitis
- Scarlet fever
- Glomerulonephritis
- Rheumatic fever
- Puerperal sepsis

Enterococcus faecalis

- Endocarditis
- Urinary tract infection

Viridans streptococci *(Strep. mitior, sanguis, mutans, salivarius)*

- Endocarditis
- Septicaemia in immunosuppressed

Group B streptococci

- Neonatal infections
- Female pelvic infections

Anaerobic streptococci

- Peritonitis
- Dental infections
- Liver abscess
- Pelvic inflammatory disease

N.B. All streptococci can cause septicaemia.

infection in scarlet fever is usually the pharynx or tonsils but the disease can be associated with streptococcal infection in other sites, e.g. in the genital tract after childbirth or in wounds. It is transmitted by air-borne infection, or more rarely by milk or ice cream contaminated by streptococci. The incubation period is 2–4 days.

Clinical features

Scarlet fever occurs most commonly in children. It has a sudden onset and the more severe cases present with a sore throat, shivering, pyrexia, headache and vomiting. There is inflammation of the fauces; the tonsils are enlarged and may be covered with a follicular exudate. The exudate can be distinguished from the membrane seen in diphtheria by its yellow appearance and by being more easily wiped off. There is tender enlargement of the tonsillar lymph nodes. The rash, which usually appears first behind the ears on the second day, rapidly becomes a generalised punctate erythema (see Fig. 2.2, p. 64), most intense in the flexures of the arms and legs. The face is not affected by the rash, though it is usually flushed due to fever, and the region round the mouth is pale. The tongue is initially furred but shows prominent red papillae. The rash fades in about 1 week and is succeeded by desquamation. A profuse growth of *Strep. pyogenes* can usually be obtained from a throat swab.

Complications

The complications are less common than formerly because of the mild form of the disease and effective chemotherapy. Otitis media, cervical adenitis and sinusitis may occur. Rheumatic fever and glomerulonephritis are rare sequelae which develop 2 or 3 weeks after the onset of any haemolytic streptococcal infection.

Management

The treatment of scarlet fever is the same as for streptococcal sore throat. Most patients respond rapidly to phenoxymethylpenicillin (250 mg for children and 500 mg for adults 6-hourly for 7 days). Nasopharyngeal carriage of the organism should be treated with the same course of phenoxymethylpenicillin.

ERYSIPELAS

Erysipelas is an acute streptococcal infection of the skin, more common in the elderly.

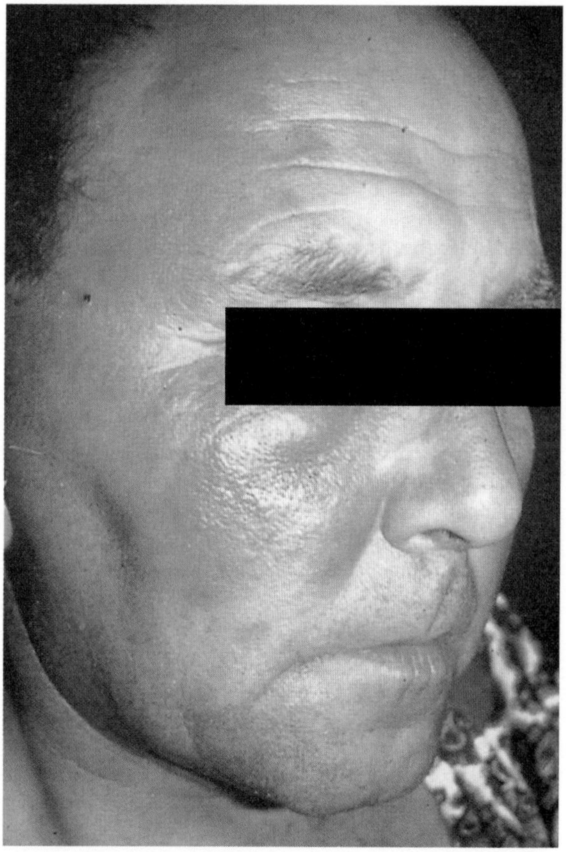

Fig. 2.25 Erysipelas. There is an area of clearly defined erythema with oedema of the subcutaneous tissues causing an 'orange-skin' appearance.

Clinical features

The onset is abrupt, with heat and pain in the infected skin and systemic upset. There is a rapidly spreading red patch of inflamed skin with underlying oedema of the subcutaneous tissues (see Fig. 2.25). The edge of the patch is palpably raised and clearly defined and the lymph nodes draining the area become enlarged and tender. As the oedema subsides, vesicles and bullae appear in the central part of the affected area. The face is involved in at least 80% of all cases of erysipelas because of the spread of streptococci from the nose.

Management

Erysipelas is usually brought under control within 48 hours with penicillin; hence the prognosis is excellent for a disease which used to be very serious. Recurrent infections are common.

STAPHYLOCOCCAL INFECTIONS

Staph. aureus is responsible for a wide variety of suppurative conditions (see Fig. 2.26). Many infections, particularly boils, carbuncles and abscesses, are due to autogenous infection, as the organisms can be grown from nasopharynx and skin of up to 30% of healthy persons. The staphylococcus is readily spread from these sites and from clothing to contaminate the dust in which it survives in the dry state for weeks or months. In hospital this organism is an important cause of wound infection, pneumonia and neonatal sepsis. Under suitable conditions it multiplies freely in food and milk to produce a heat-stable toxin which is a cause of food poisoning.

Staphylococcal endocarditis (see p. 286)

This condition may occur as a complication of staphylococcal bacteraemia in the presence of an abnormal heart valve. In addition, it occurs in IVDUs, in whom it usually causes right-sided heart valve lesions, and as a complication of septic thrombophlebitis associated with intravenous cannulae and lines. *Staph. aureus* infection of the aortic valve frequently causes fulminant valve destruction requiring surgical valve replacement.

Toxic shock syndrome

This is caused by the toxins of certain *Staph. aureus* strains and occurs in women using some types of tampon, the infection originating in the vagina and presenting with fever, rash and shock. The syndrome has also been described in men and women as a complication of staphylococcal infections of the skin, lungs and breasts. Onset is with fever, followed by the development of a punctate erythematous rash as in scarlet fever. There is hypotension with shock. Renal failure may develop and death can occur if treatment is not started immediately.

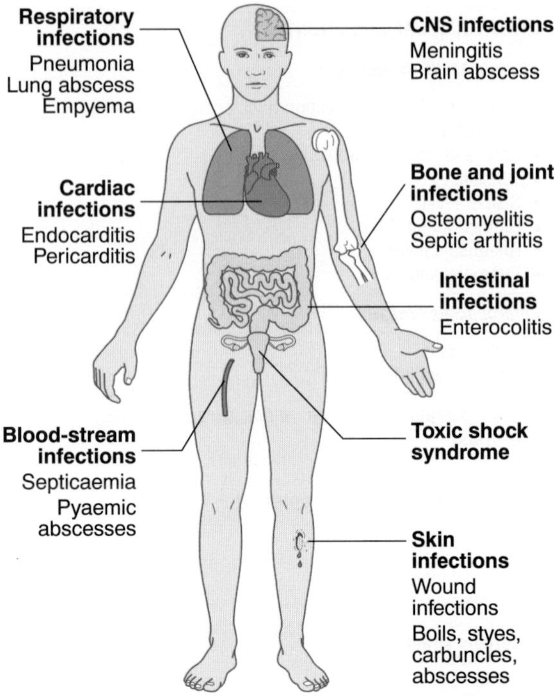

Fig. 2.26 Infections caused by *Staphylococcus aureus*.

Management

Approximately 90% of *Staph. aureus* strains are now resistant to penicillin, which should be used only if the organism is shown to be sensitive. If the illness is severe, treatment should be commenced with flucloxacillin 500 mg 6-hourly, unless the patient is known to be allergic to the penicillins, when erythromycin 500 mg 6-hourly, fusidic acid 500 mg 6-hourly or clindamycin 300 mg 6-hourly should be given. Nasal carriage of staphylococci can be eradicated by topical application of neomycin plus chlorhexidine or mupirocin.

Staph. aureus strains resistant to all antibiotics except vancomycin are causing outbreaks of hospital infection in many countries. Known as methicillin- (or multiply) resistant *Staph. aureus* (MRSA), these organisms can cause serious and often fatal infections. Patients colonised by MRSA should ideally be placed in isolation but since the infection is so common this is now unpracticable.

Staph. epidermidis is a skin commensal organism which can cause serious infections in the immunosuppressed and in those with prosthetic heart valves and joint implants. Endocarditis due to this organism is indolent and particularly difficult to cure. Methicillin-resistant *Staph. epidermidis* strains (MRSE) have now emerged as pathogens and are spread throughout the world. These organisms pose specific cross-infection problems on intensive care units.

CORYNEBACTERIAL INFECTIONS

DIPHTHERIA

In many parts of the developing world diphtheria is an important cause of illness. Recent outbreaks have occurred in the former Soviet Union. It is now very rare in Britain.

Pathology

Infection with *Corynebacterium diphtheriae* occurs most commonly in the upper respiratory tract, and sore throat is frequently the presenting feature. The disease is usually spread by droplet infection from cases or carriers. The organisms remain localised at the site of infection and the serious consequences result from the absorption of a soluble exotoxin which damages the heart muscle and the nervous system. The infection may occur rarely on the conjunctiva or in the genital tract, or it may complicate wounds, abrasions or diseases of the skin.

The average incubation period is 2–4 days. Cases are isolated until cultures from six daily nose and throat swabs are negative.

Clinical features

These are summarised in the information box. The disease begins insidiously. The temperature is seldom much raised although tachycardia is usually marked. The diagnostic feature is the 'wash-leather' elevated greyish-green membrane on the tonsils, with a well-defined edge and surrounded by a zone of inflammation. The membrane is firm and adherent. There may be swelling of the neck ('bull-neck') and tender enlargement of the lymph nodes. In the mildest infections, especially in the presence of a high degree of immunity, a membrane may never appear and the throat is merely slightly injected.

CLINICAL FEATURES OF DIPHTHERIA

Acute infection

- Membranous tonsillitis
- *or* Nasal infection
- *or* Laryngeal infection
- *or* Skin/wound/conjunctival infection (rare)

Complications

- Laryngeal obstruction or paralysis
- Myocarditis
- Peripheral neuropathy

With anterior nasal infection there is nasal discharge, often tinged with blood. In laryngeal diphtheria there is a husky voice, a high-pitched cough, and a danger of respiratory obstruction which can be fatal if tracheostomy is not carried out. When the infection spreads towards the uvula, to the fauces and then to the nasopharynx, the patient is often gravely ill. The pulse is rapid and of poor volume and the blood pressure low. Death from acute circulatory failure may occur within the first 10 days. Those who survive the earlier toxaemia may later develop arrhythmias or cardiac failure. ECG changes are common due to myocarditis. These are reversible and there is no permanent damage to the heart in those who survive.

Involvement of the nervous system sometimes occurs, and after tonsillar or pharyngeal diphtheria it usually commences with palatal palsy on about the tenth day of the illness. Paralysis of accommodation often follows and may be inferred from difficulty in reading small print. A week or two later, though somewhat rarely, weakness and paraesthesia in the limbs due to polyneuritis may develop. Recovery from such neuritis is always ultimately complete.

Management

Upon making a clinical diagnosis of diphtheria, the case should be notified to the public health authorities and sent urgently to a hospital for infectious diseases. If the clinician considers that diphtheria is likely to be the cause of the illness (see the information box) antitoxin must be injected intramuscularly without awaiting the result of a throat swab. Delay increases the danger to the patient because toxin, once fixed to the tissues, can no longer be neutralised by antitoxin. However, horse serum, in which antitoxin is contained, is liable to cause undesirable reactions as it is a foreign protein. There may be an immediate anaphylactic reaction with dyspnoea, pallor and collapse or even death. Serum sickness, with fever, urticaria and joint pains may occur 7–12 days later. If there is a previous history of inoculation of horse serum, the symptoms commonly appear in 3–4 days. As anaphylaxis is potentially lethal, all patients must be asked whether they have ever had antiserum before and whether they suffer from any allergic disorder. A small test injection of serum should be given half an hour before the full dose in every patient. 1/1000 adrenaline solution must be available to deal with any immediate type of reaction (0.5–1.0 ml intramuscularly). An antihistamine is also given.

In a severely ill patient the risk of anaphylactic shock is outweighed by the mortal danger of diphtheritic toxaemia and

MANAGEMENT OF DIPHTHERIA

- Admit to isolation facility
- Administer antitoxin (4000–32 000 units i.m.—test dose first)
- Give benzylpenicillin 600 mg 6-hourly i.v. for 7 days
- Notify public health authorities
- Treat complications
  - Tracheostomy for respiratory obstruction
  - Monitor for, and treat, arrhythmias due to myocarditis
- Protect close contacts
  - Erythromycin prophylaxis
  - Immunisation

up to 100 000 units of antitoxin are injected intravenously if the test dose has not given rise to symptoms. For disease of moderate severity, 16 000–32 000 units i.m. will suffice, and for mild cases 4000–8000 units.

Penicillin 1200 mg 6-hourly intravenously or amoxycillin 500 mg 8-hourly should be administered for 1 week to eliminate *C. diphtheriae*. Patients allergic to penicillin can be given erythromycin.

Prevention

Active immunisation should be given to all children.

If diphtheria occurs in a closed community, contacts should be given erythromycin, which is more effective than penicillin in eradicating the organism in carriers. All contacts should also be immunised or given a booster dose of toxoid. Adults should be given a dilute preparation of vaccine to avoid severe reactions.

BACILLUS INFECTIONS

ANTHRAX

Anthrax is a disease of domestic animals which become infected by inhaling or ingesting spores of *Bacillus anthracis* passed in faeces. Grazing lands remain infective for years. In humans anthrax is an occupational disease of farmers, butchers and dealers in hides, hair, wool and bone meal from endemic areas. Anthrax is endemic in communities where skins are used as sleeping mats, for clothing or for carrying water, and where diseased cattle are eaten. Inoculation of spores subcutaneously is more common than their spread by inhalation or ingestion. The incubation period is usually 1–3 days. The organism is potentially important in biological warfare.

Clinical features

A cutaneous lesion begins as an itching papule which enlarges and forms a vesicle filled with serosanguineous fluid surrounded by gross oedema—the 'malignant pustule'. The lesion is relatively painless and accompanied by slight enlargement of regional lymph nodes. The vesicle dries to form a thick black eschar surrounded by blebs. Occasionally there are multiple lesions. In endemic areas patients may exhibit only slight constitutional symptoms and little oedema but in non-immune persons high fever, toxaemia and fatal septicaemia may develop.

When infected meat has been eaten an ulcer with surrounding oedema may develop in the pharynx or, more commonly, the infection causes a severe, fatal gastroenteritis.

Those who acquire the infection by inhalation may develop an acute laryngitis or a virulent haemorrhagic bronchopneumonia (wool-sorters' disease). Anthrax may also present as meningitis.

Investigations

A stained smear of fluid taken from the edge of a lesion demonstrates the organism, which can be confirmed by culture. *B. anthracis* is also recoverable from laryngeal and pulmonary anthrax and from the CSF in meningitis. Anthrax should be suspected if a group of people who have feasted on an animal which has sickened and died are taken abruptly ill with fulminating gastroenteritis. *B. anthracis* may be cultured from the faeces.

Management

Treatment is with penicillin 1200 mg 6-hourly. The organism is also sensitive to erythromycin, tetracycline, chloramphenicol and streptomycin.

Prevention

The disease is controlled in cattle by slaughter and deep burial of the diseased animal and by vaccination of healthy animals at risk. Potentially infected imports from endemic areas must be subject to strict control. Persons at risk through their occupation should be vaccinated. A vaccine is available for those at specific risk.

BORDETELLA INFECTIONS

WHOOPING COUGH

Whooping cough (pertussis) is a highly infectious disease caused by *Bordetella pertussis*. It is spread by droplet infection and while it occurs at all ages, approximately 90% of cases are in children under 5 years of age. The incubation period is 7–14 days. Recent studies have shown that evidence of *B. pertussis* infection can be detected in North American college students complaining of cough of over 5 days' duration.

Clinical features

The first stage consists of a highly infectious upper respiratory infection lasting about 1 week, during which conjunctivitis, rhinitis and an unproductive cough are present. The distinctive paroxysmal stage follows and is characterised by severe bouts of coughing. The number of such paroxysms in 24 hours varies from an occasional attack to 40 or 50, and they are more severe at night. Each paroxysm consists of a succession of short sharp coughs, gathering in speed and duration and ending in a deep inspiration during which the characteristic whoop may be heard. It may be absent in older children and in adults because the air passages are so much wider. The last paroxysm of a series frequently ends with vomiting. The paroxysmal stage lasts from 1 to several weeks.

Complications

The complications of whooping cough are listed in the information box.

COMPLICATIONS OF WHOOPING COUGH

Respiratory	Other
• Bronchopneumonia • Atelectasis • Bronchiectasis	• Convulsions • Conjunctival haemorrhage • Ulceration of frenum • Prolapse of rectum

Investigations

Diagnosis can be difficult in the catarrhal stage when the disease is most infectious. It can be confirmed in the laboratory by the isolation of *B. pertussis* taken from the posterior wall of the nasopharynx on small swabs passed along the floor of the nose. Examination of the blood shows a lymphocytosis which, however, may not develop until the disease is well established. The diagnosis is easy in the paroxysmal stage when the whoop has developed.

Management

Erythromycin 125–250 mg 6-hourly may reduce the severity of the infection if given during the initial stage. A cough suppressant such as methadone may be helpful in controlling the severity of paroxysms. When the illness is of long duration and vomiting is frequent, skilled nursing will be required to maintain nutrition, especially in infants and young children. Feeds are usually accepted and retained if they are given immediately after the vomiting which frequently follows a paroxysm of coughing.

Prevention

Active immunisation should be given to all children except where there is a history of severe local or general reaction to a preceding dose or where there is evidence of an evolving neurological abnormality. Personal or family history of febrile convulsions or epilepsy, or a stable neurological condition, is not a contraindication to immunisation. Seizures or neurological damage resulting from active immunisation are exceedingly rare (1:310 000 injections). Neurological complications after whooping cough itself are considerably more common than after the vaccine. Infants of less than 3 months (who are too young to be immunised) can develop severe and occasionally fatal attacks; those who are exposed should be given prophylactic erythromycin. The original vaccine consisting of whole killed *B. pertussis* organisms works well, but newer vaccines consisting of up to five specific proteins (acellular pertussis vaccine) work as well but are not as reactigenic on parenteral administration.

SALMONELLA INFECTIONS

There are approaching 2000 salmonella serotypes, most of which originate in animals, especially poultry, and are transmitted to humans either directly or in food. The exception is *S. typhi,* which invariably has a human source. There are six clinical syndromes caused by salmonellae (see the information box).

SALMONELLA INFECTIONS

- Typhoid and paratyphoid fever (enteric fever)
- Gastroenteritis (food poisoning)
- Enterocolitis
- Septicaemia
- Metastatic lesions (complicating septicaemia)
  Osteomyelitis/septic arthritis
  Liver abscess
  Brain abscess
- Asymptomatic carrier state

TYPHOID AND PARATYPHOID (ENTERIC) FEVERS

In many countries where sanitation is primitive, typhoid and paratyphoid fevers, which are transmitted by the faecal-oral route, are important causes of illness. Elsewhere they are relatively rare. Nevertheless, outbreaks occur from time to time in developed countries and the infection may be contracted from returned travellers, especially if they are symptomless carriers of the infecting organism.

Aetiology

The enteric fevers are caused by infection with *S. typhi* and *S. paratyphi A* and *B*. In Britain spread is usually by carriers, often food-handlers, through the contamination of food, milk or water; infected shellfish are occasionally responsible for an outbreak. The bacilli may live in the gallbladder of carriers for months or years after clinical recovery and pass intermittently in the stool and less commonly in the urine. The incubation period of typhoid fever is about 10–14 days; that of paratyphoid is somewhat shorter.

Pathology

After a few days of bacteraemia, the bacilli localise mainly in the lymphoid tissue of the small intestine. The typical lesion is in the Peyer's patches and follicles. These swell at first, then ulcerate and ultimately heal, but during this sequence they may perforate or bleed.

Clinical features

Typhoid fever

Clinical features are outlined in the information box. The

CLINICAL FEATURES OF TYPHOID FEVER
First week
• Fever, headache, myalgia, bradycardia, constipation (diarrhoea and vomiting)
End of first week
• Rose spots on trunk, splenomegaly, cough, abdominal distension, diarrhoea
End of second week
• Delirium, complications, then coma and death (if untreated)

onset may be insidious. The temperature rises in a stepladder fashion for 4 or 5 days. There is malaise, with increasing headache, drowsiness and aching in the limbs. Cough and epistaxis occur. Constipation may be present, although in children diarrhoea and vomiting may be prominent early in the illness. The pulse is often slower than would be expected from the height of the temperature.

At the end of the first week a rash may appear on the upper abdomen and on the back as sparse, slightly raised, rose-red spots which fade on pressure. It is usually visible only on white skin. Around the seventh to tenth day the spleen becomes palpable. Constipation is then succeeded by diarrhoea and abdominal distension with tenderness. Bronchitis and delirium may develop. By the end of the second week the patient may be profoundly ill unless the disease is modified by antibiotic treatment. In the third week toxaemia increases and the patient may pass into coma and die. Such extreme cases are rare in countries with developed health services.

Following recovery, up to 5% of patients become chronic carriers of *S. typhi* and classically such patients have gallbladder disease.

Paratyphoid fever

The most common variety in Britain is due to *S. paratyphi B*. The course tends to be shorter and milder than that of typhoid fever and the onset is often more abrupt with acute enteritis. The rash may be more abundant and the intestinal complications less frequent.

Complications

These are given in the information box. Haemorrhage from, or a perforation of, the ulcerated Peyer's patches may occur at the end of the second week or during the third week of the illness. Additional complications may involve almost any viscus or system because of the septicaemia present during the first week; these include cholecystitis, pneumonia, myocarditis, arthritis, osteomyelitis and meningitis. Bone and joint infection is seen, especially in children with sickle-cell disease.

COMPLICATIONS OF TYPHOID FEVER
Bowel
• Perforation, haemorrhage
Septicaemic foci
• Bone and joint infection, meningitis, cholecystitis
Toxic phenomena
• Myocarditis, nephritis

Investigations

In the first week the diagnosis may be difficult because in this invasive stage with bacteraemia the symptoms are those of a generalised infection without localising features. A white blood count may be helpful as there is typically a leucopenia. Blood culture is the most important diagnostic method in a suspected case. The faeces will contain the organism more frequently during the second and third weeks. The Widal reaction detects antibodies to the causative organisms. However, it is not a reliable diagnostic test and should be interpreted with caution, particularly in typhoid-vaccinated patients.

Management

Several antibiotics are effective in enteric fever. Ciprofloxacin in a dose of 500 mg 12-hourly is the drug of choice. Alternatives include co-trimoxazole (two tablets or intravenous equivalent 12-hourly), amoxycillin (750 mg 6-hourly) and chloramphenicol (500 mg 6-hourly). However, an increasing number of salmonellae, including *S. typhi*, are now resistant to many antibiotics and some are only sensitive to ciprofloxacin. Treatment should be continued for 14 days. Pyrexia may persist for up to 5 days after the start of specific therapy. Even with effective chemotherapy there is still a danger of complications, of recrudescence of the disease and of the development of a carrier state. The chronic carrier should be treated for 4 weeks with ciprofloxacin; cholecystectomy may be necessary in some cases.

Prevention

Those who propose to travel to or live in countries where enteric infections are endemic should be inoculated with one of the three available typhoid vaccines (two inactivated injectable and one oral live attenuated).

FOOD POISONING

Food poisoning (gastroenteritis) can be due to many causes, infective and non-infective (see the information box). It presents with vomiting, diarrhoea, or both, usually between 1 and 48 hours after consumption of the contaminated food

CAUSES OF FOOD POISONING
Infective
Non-toxin-mediated • *Salmonella* species • *Campylobacter jejuni* • *Bacillus cereus* • Viruses, e.g. Norwalk viruses • *Listeria monocytogenes* (causing meningitis) • *Bacillus anthracis* (anthrax)
Toxin-mediated • *Staphylococcus aureus* • *Clostridium perfringens* • *Clostridium botulinum* (botulism) • *E. coli* 0157 (verocytotoxin-producing)
Non-infective
Allergic • Shellfish, strawberries
Non-allergic • Scrombotoxin (fish) • Ciguatoxin (tropical fish) • Fungi (e.g. *Amanita phalloides*) • Chemicals, metals (e.g. in cooking-pots)

or drink. Outbreaks are common, especially in institutions and restaurants. Non-infective causes and bacterial toxins, which are pre-formed in the infected food, produce symptoms within minutes or hours of a meal, whereas the other infections may not produce illness for up to 48 hours. Infective gastroenteritis can be classified as *non-toxin type* and *toxin type*.

Non-toxin-mediated food poisoning

Salmonella species (other than *S. typhi*) are very common causes of food poisoning. *Campylobacter*, *S. typhimurium* and *S. enteritidis* are the most frequently isolated in Britain at present. The domestic fowl is the most common source of infection, which may be contracted from inadequately defrosted and undercooked chicken or from undercooked or raw eggs. Intensive rearing, infected poultry food and deep-freezing of carcasses all contribute to the high level of human salmonella infection. Symptomless faecal carriers of salmonella who are food-handlers are also a source of infection. The size of the infecting dose of bacteria bears a close relationship to the speed of onset of symptoms and to the severity of the illness. This indicates the dangers of bacterial multiplication which may take place when food is contaminated and thereafter remains warm for many hours or days.

Campylobacter jejuni is now the most common bacterial cause of food poisoning in Britain. Sources of infection include poultry, dogs, water and unpasteurised milk.

Bacillus cereus infection is a hazard of eating rice which has been cooked and then reheated and eaten at a later date.

Listeria monocytogenes is an environmental bacterium which can contaminate food, including poultry and cheese. It does not usually cause intestinal symptoms but is a cause of septicaemia and meningitis, especially in pregnancy, the neonate, the immunosuppressed, diabetics and alcoholics.

Certain viruses (commonly referred to as small round structured viruses because of their morphology) such as Norwalk viruses, coronaviruses and rotaviruses, which can be identified only by electron microscopy of stool and are not yet culturable, commonly cause outbreaks of food poisoning, especially in institutions and catering establishments. Agglutination tests are now available for diagnosis of rotavirus on stool.

The protozoal organisms *Giardia lamblia* and *Cryptosporidium* species can also cause food poisoning or water-borne outbreaks of diarrhoeal disease (see pp. 155–156).

Toxin-mediated food poisoning

Such poisoning is most commonly caused by the enterotoxin of *Staph. aureus*, frequently from a food-handler with a septic lesion on the hand. Incubation at a suitable temperature leads to growth of the organism and production of toxin which is relatively heat-resistant and may not be destroyed by cooking.

Strains of clostridia, many of them relatively resistant to heat, can also contaminate certain foods, particularly meat. Pre-cooking of stews and pies may not destroy all the spores, and the keeping of such food will lead to the formation of heat-stable toxins which can give rise to gastroenteritis, sometimes severe.

A verocytotoxin produced by a strain of *E. coli* (enterohaemorrhagic *E. coli* type 0157) is an important cause of food poisoning in the UK and USA. The clinical syndrome may present with features of haemorrhagic colitis. The syndrome has also been associated with the development of the haemolytic-uraemic syndrome (see p. 441). The organism is destroyed by adequate cooking.

Botulism is a rare form of bacterial food poisoning due to the ingestion of the toxin produced by *Clostridium botulinum* in imperfectly treated tinned food or preserved fish contaminated with the organism. The clinical features differ from all other types of bacterial food poisoning and consist chiefly of vomiting and pareses of skeletal, ocular, pharyngeal and respiratory muscles. Mortality can be high.

Clinical features

The simultaneous occurrence of symptoms in more than one member of a household or institution simplifies diagnosis. However, isolated cases are very common. The incubation period is a useful pointer to the aetiology (see Table 2.18).

In severe cases there may be prostration, collapse and dehydration. In the chemical and toxin types of food poisoning the onset tends to be sudden and severe and the patient may rapidly become shocked. Recovery, however, usually occurs within 24 hours. In the infective type, symptoms develop more slowly and there is usually pyrexia and toxicity. The

Table 2.18 Initial clinical features of food poisoning

Aetiology	Incubation	Symptoms
Chemical poison	30 minutes	Vomiting
Staphylococcal or clostridial toxin	2–6 hours	Vomiting initially—may be diarrhoea and abdominal pain later
***Salmonella* or *Campylobacter* infection**	12–48 hours	Diarrhoea (bloody with *Campylobacter*), abdominal pain, vomiting Septicaemia can occur with *Salmonella* infection
Haemorrhagic colitis (*E. coli* 0157)	12–48 hours	Bloody diarrhoea predominates—may be abdominal pain

stools are watery and offensive, and may contain blood and some mucus, in contrast to bacillary dysentery where there is also pus. Salmonella septicaemia may be associated with osteomyelitis and septic arthritis, and is a specific problem in HIV infection, with a very high incidence of recurrence and failure to eradicate the organism from stool. Antibiotic treatment is always indicated in salmonella gastroenteritis in HIV infection in contrast to immunocompetent patients.

Severe abdominal pain and blood in the stool are common in *Campylobacter* infections. Rarely, septicaemia may complicate *Campylobacter* gastroenteritis, and endocarditis has been reported. *Campylobacter* enteritis may be confused with ulcerative colitis and rectal biopsies can appear similar in both diseases. Bloody diarrhoea should suggest the possibility of haemorrhagic colitis due to *E. coli* 0157.

Investigations

A specimen of the patient's stool or vomit, together with the suspected food, if available, should be sent for culture. *Campylobacter* and organisms of the *Salmonella* group can usually be readily isolated. In more severe cases blood should be sent for culture. Notification of salmonella infection and other types of food poisoning is compulsory in Britain.

Management

This is summarised in the information box. Most cases are mild and symptoms subside in a few days. Solid food should be withheld and the patient instructed to take fluids only. Fluid and electrolytes can usually be replaced orally. Patients who are ill or dehydrated require intravenous fluid therapy. When acute symptoms cease, a semi-fluid low-roughage diet may be taken. Codeine phosphate or loperamide is useful in controlling diarrhoea. Lactose should be avoided during the recovery phase because of temporary lactase deficiency.

Antibiotics should not be given routinely for acute diarrhoea and vomiting as they are usually ineffective and frequently exacerbate symptoms. If salmonella bacteraemia is suspected or confirmed or if diarrhoea is severe or prolonged, ciprofloxacin 500 mg 12-hourly or trimethoprim 200 mg 12-hourly should be given. *Campylobacter* enteritis is treated with erythromycin 500 mg 6-hourly or ciprofloxacin 500 mg 12-hourly. *Listeria monocytogenes* is susceptible to amoxycillin; gentamicin is given in addition in the immunosuppressed and for the treatment of meningitis.

MANAGEMENT OF FOOD POISONING

Supportive

- Fluid and electrolyte replacement—oral or i.v.
- Bowel sedation—not for mild cases or until at least 24 hours after onset of diarrhoea. Not in children. Codeine phosphate or loperamide useful

Specific

- Majority of cases—none required
- *Salmonella* infections, suspected septicaemia or severe or prolonged symptoms—ciprofloxacin or trimethoprim
- *Campylobacter* infections—erythromycin or ciprofloxacin (although efficacy not fully proven)

If the poisoning is thought to be due to a chemical or a poisonous food, the patient's stomach should be washed out with tepid water (see p. 1111), and the stomach contents kept for analysis. Such a situation is rare in clinical practice.

Prevention

A reduction in the high incidence of food poisoning can best be achieved by improving the standards of personal hygiene, especially in those handling food, and by stressing the importance of *hand-washing* after using the lavatory. Low-temperature storage is required for food which has to be kept for some hours or days before being consumed. It is essential to keep frozen poultry at room temperature long enough to ensure adequate defrosting before cooking or pathogens at the centre may survive unharmed. Improvements in poultry-rearing methods are urgently required.

DYSENTERY

Dysentery is an acute inflammation of the large intestine characterised by diarrhoea with blood and mucus in the stools. Its causes are bacillary or amoebic infection. The latter condition is described on page 154.

BACILLARY DYSENTERY (SHIGELLOSIS)

The bacilli belong to the genus *Shigella*, of which there are four main pathogenic groups, *dysenteriae*, *flexneri*, *boydii* and *sonnei*, the first two having numerous serotypes. In Britain the majority of cases of bacillary dysentery are caused by *Sh. sonnei*, although in recent years there has been a significant increase in imported infections caused by *Sh. flexneri* while indigenous *sonnei* dysentery has decreased. Shigella strains, especially in tropical countries, are now commonly resistant to many antibiotics. These multiresistant organisms have been responsible for epidemics of bacillary dysentery in Bangladesh and other tropical countries. The organism only infects humans and its spread is facilitated by its potency in that only around 10 organisms constitute an infectious dose.

Epidemiology

Bacillary dysentery is endemic all over the world. It occurs in epidemic form wherever there is a crowded population with poor sanitation, and has been a constant accompaniment of wars and natural catastrophes. Spread may occur by contaminated food or by flies, but contact through unwashed hands after defaecation is by far the most important factor. Outbreaks occur in mental hospitals, residential schools and other closed institutions.

Pathology

There is inflammation of the large bowel which may involve the lower part of the small intestine. Sigmoidoscopy shows that the mucosa is red and swollen, the submucous veins are obscured and mucopus is seen on the surface. Bleeding points appear readily at the touch of the endoscope. Ulcers may form.

Clinical features

There is great variation in disease severity (see the information box). *Sh. sonnei* infections may be so mild as to escape detection and the patient remains ambulant with a few loose stools and perhaps some colic, fever and headache. *Sh. flexneri* infections are usually more severe, while those due to *Sh. dysenteriae* may be fulminating and cause death within 48 hours.

CLINICAL FEATURES OF BACILLARY DYSENTERY
Shigella sonnei
• Usually mild diarrhoea in children. Most common type in UK
Shigella flexneri
• More severe diarrhoea, often blood in stool. Second most common type in UK
Shigella boydii
• Rarest type. Similar clinical features to *Sh. flexneri*
Shigella dysenteriae
• Causes severe infections with profuse bloody diarrhoea and prostration. Haemolytic uraemic syndrome may cause renal failure. Can be fatal. Multiresistant strains common in South-east Asia

In a moderately severe illness, the patient complains of diarrhoea, colicky abdominal pain and tenesmus. The stools are usually small, and after the first few evacuations, contain blood and purulent exudate with little faecal material. There is frequently fever, with dehydration and weakness if the diarrhoea persists. There is usually tenderness over the colon. Arthritis or iritis may occasionally complicate bacillary dysentery (Reiter's syndrome, see p. 850), and may be associated with HLA-B27. Shigella infection may spread rapidly amongst promiscuous homosexuals.

Investigations

Diagnosis depends on faecal culture.

Management

A fluid or semi-fluid low-roughage diet should be given, depending on severity of symptoms. Oral rehydration therapy is a mainstay of treatment. If diarrhoea is severe, intravenous replacement of water and electrolyte loss will be necessary (see p. 131). The use of antidiarrhoeal medication should be avoided in all but the mildest cases, in which codeine 30 mg 8-hourly, or loperamide 4 mg initially, followed by 2 mg after each loose stool (maximum 16 mg daily), may be given. *Sonnei* dysentery is usually self-limiting and antibiotics are not indicated in most cases. In infections caused by *dysenteriae* or *flexneri* strains, ciprofloxacin (500 mg 12-hourly) should be given.

Prevention

The prevention of faecal contamination of food and milk and the isolation of patients are methods which are theoretically important but may be difficult to apply except in limited outbreaks. Hand-washing is very important.

OTHER TRUE BACTERIAL INFECTIONS

BRUCELLOSIS

Brucellosis (undulant fever, Malta fever, abortus fever) is caused in northern Europe by infection with *Brucella abortus*, which is usually spread to humans by the ingestion of raw milk from infected cattle. It is an occupational hazard of veterinary surgeons, laboratory personnel and slaughterhouse workers. The infection has now been virtually eradicated from cattle in Britain. In Malta and other Mediterranean and Middle Eastern countries the disease is frequently due to *B. melitensis* and is transmitted by infected goats or sheep. In the USA and the Far East *B. suis* acquired from pigs may be the causative organism. The incubation period is about 3 weeks. Subclinical infections are common in farmers and veterinarians.

Clinical features

The disease has features of both a blood-stream infection and an intracellular infection. These are listed in the information box. Untreated, the disease may last for a few days or for many months. Neutropenia and lymphocytosis occur in the more severely affected.

CLINICAL FEATURES OF BRUCELLOSIS
Onset
• Acute with high continuous fever *or* insidious with fever undulating over 7–10-day periods
Symptoms
• Fever, sweating, weakness, headache, anorexia, pain in limbs and back, rigors, joint pains
Signs
• Fever and splenomegaly
Complications
• Relapse within 2 years of recovery • Localised disease causing suppurative or granulomatous lesions including arthritis, spondylitis, bursitis, osteomyelitis, meningoencephalitis, endocarditis, epididymo-orchitis, pneumonia, hepatitis • Chronic brucellosis: low-grade fever and neuropsychiatric symptoms

Investigations

Blood, and especially bone marrow, cultured under special conditions usually yield the organism in acutely ill patients. Brucella serology is unreliable; a four-fold rise in titre of agglutinating antibody, which detects IgM antibody, may be diagnostic but cross-reactions are common. Complement fixation and anti-human globulin tests are more useful in chronic infections.

Management

Tetracycline 500 mg 6-hourly, plus rifampicin 600 mg daily for 4 weeks is curative and relapses are unusual. Streptomycin 1 g daily may be used instead of rifampicin. Tetracycline alone or co-trimoxazole, two tablets twice daily, is usually effective, but the disease may relapse.

Prevention

Infected herds of cattle can be identified and destroyed. The spread of brucellosis by milk is prevented by pasteurisation or boiling. Veterinary surgeons and others handling infected animals need to exercise scrupulous hygiene.

PLAGUE

Epidemics of plague, such as the 'Black Death', have attacked humans since ancient times. Now, the disease is limited to rodents in the wild with sporadic human cases or local outbreaks, predominantly in Vietnam and East Africa with occasional cases in the USA and elsewhere (see Fig. 2.27). The causative organism, *Yersinia pestis*, is a small Gram-negative bacillus. It is spread between rodents by their fleas. If domestic rats become infected, infected fleas may bite humans. In the late stages of human plague, *Y. pestis* may be expectorated and spread between humans by droplets. 'Pneumonic plague' may follow. Hunters and trappers can contract plague from handling rodents.

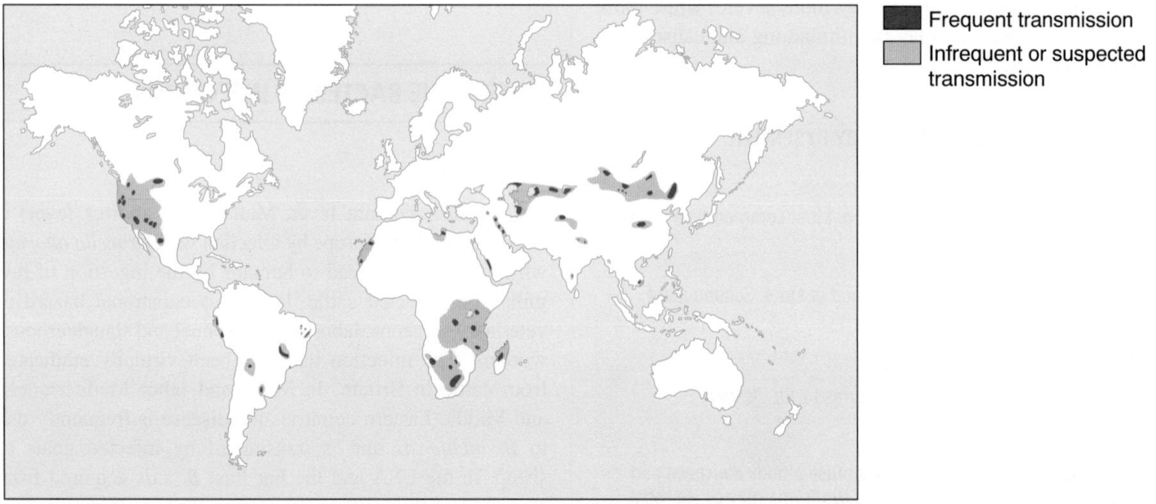

Fig. 2.27 Foci of the transmission of plague.

Pathology

Organisms inoculated through the skin are taken rapidly to the draining lymph nodes where they elicit a severe inflammatory response that may be haemorrhagic. If the infection is not contained, septicaemia ensues and necrotic, purulent or haemorrhagic lesions develop in many organs. Oliguria and shock follow, and disseminated intravascular coagulation may result in widespread haemorrhage. Inhalation of *Y. pestis* causes alveolitis. The incubation period is 3–6 days, but less in pneumonic plague.

Bubonic plague

In this, the most common form of the disease, the onset is usually sudden with a rigor, high fever, dry skin and severe headache. Soon, aching and swelling at the site of the affected lymph nodes begin. The most common site of the bubo, made up of the swollen lymph nodes and surrounding tissue, is one groin. Some infections are relatively mild but in the majority of patients toxaemia quickly increases with a rapid pulse, hypotension and mental confusion. The spleen is usually palpable.

Septicaemic plague

Those not exhibiting a bubo usually deteriorate rapidly. Meningitis, pneumonia and expectoration of blood-stained sputum containing *Y. pestis* may complicate bubonic or septicaemic plague.

Pneumonic plague

The onset is very sudden with cough and dyspnoea. The patient soon expectorates copious blood-stained, frothy, highly infective sputum, becomes cyanosed and dies. Radiographs of the lung show a lobar opacity.

Investigations

Reports of death among rats should alert suspicion of an outbreak. Early diagnosis is urgent. An aspirate from a bubo, sputum, or the buffy coat (leucocyte fraction) of blood is used to show the characteristic organism by staining with methylene blue or by immunofluorescence. Blood, sputum and aspirate should be cultured. Plague is notifiable under the International Health Regulations.

Management

If the diagnosis is suspected on clinical and epidemiological grounds, treatment must be started as soon as, or even before, samples have been collected for laboratory diagnosis. Streptomycin is given by intramuscular injection every 6 or 12 hours, at a daily dose of 30 mg/kg for 10 days, or tetracycline 10 mg/kg 6-hourly orally or intravenously for 10 days. Treatment may also be needed for acute circulatory failure, disseminated intravascular coagulation or hypoxia.

Prevention

Rats and fleas should be controlled (see the information box on p. 117). In endemic areas people should avoid handling and skinning wild animals.

A formalin-killed vaccine is available for those at occupational risk. Patients are isolated and attendants must wear gowns, masks and gloves. Contacts should be protected by tetracycline 2 g daily, or co-trimoxazole one tablet daily for a week. Post-mortem examination is dangerous.

TULARAEMIA

Tularaemia is an infection due to *Francisella tularensis*, transmitted to mammals and birds by the bites of infected blood-sucking flies and ticks. Humans may be infected by ticks or while skinning infected wild rabbits or hares. The microorganisms enter through dermal abrasions, the conjunctiva or mouth. The disease is found in the Americas, Japan, the former Soviet Union and most European countries excluding Britain.

Pathology

Focal areas of necrosis occur, especially in lymph nodes, spleen, liver, kidneys and lungs. There may be cutaneous, oral or ophthalmic lesions when infection is by these routes.

Clinical features

The most common presentation is of a skin ulcer, with painful regional lymphadenopathy. There may be a systemic illness with fever, often prolonged. Sometimes the conjunctiva or throat is the site of entry, and is inflamed. Occasionally, the presentation is only with lymphadenopathy.

Septicaemia is the rarest but most severe form of the disease. There is a sudden onset of high fever, prostration, aching limbs, vomiting, diarrhoea and mental confusion. Pneumonia, pleurisy and pericarditis are serious complications.

Investigations

The organism may be isolated with difficulty and danger by culture or guinea-pig inoculation. Agglutination and complement-fixation tests become positive after 10–12 days.

Management

Streptomycin, as for plague (see above), or gentamicin is the treatment of choice. Tetracycline (500 mg 6-hourly for 2 weeks) is less effective.

Prevention

Masks should be worn in the laboratory and gloves used when skinning rabbits and hares in endemic areas. Adequate cooking renders infected meat safe for eating.

MELIOIDOSIS

Melioidosis is caused by *Burkholderia (Pseudomonas) pseudomallei*, which is a saprophyte found in soil and water (paddy fields). Infection is through abrasions of the skin. Diabetics and patients with severe burns are particularly susceptible. In addition, aerosol spread is thought to be possible and is reported from helicopter downdraught. The disease is most common in the Far East, South-east Asia and Australia, and occurs rarely in India, Africa and the USA.

Pathology

A bacteraemia is followed by the formation of abscesses in the lungs, liver and spleen.

Clinical features

There is high fever, prostration and sometimes diarrhoea, with signs of pneumonia and enlargement of the liver and spleen. A chest radiograph resembles that of acute caseous tuberculosis. In more chronic forms multiple abscesses recur in subcutaneous tissue and bone.

Investigations

Culture of blood, sputum or pus may yield *B. pseudomallei*. Except in fulminating infections, antibodies may be detected by indirect haemagglutination, direct agglutination, and complement-fixation tests.

Management

In acute illness prompt treatment, without waiting for confirmation by culture, may be life-saving. Ceftazidime 120 mg/kg plus tetracycline 3 g daily are given in divided doses for about 2–3 weeks, followed by doxycycline 200 mg daily for 2–3 months, until pulmonary cavities have healed. Abscesses should be drained surgically. In chronic cases profound wasting is a major clinical problem.

CHOLERA

Cholera is a severe acute gastrointestinal infection, caused by *Vibrio cholerae* serotype 01. Its home is in the valleys of the Ganges and other great rivers of the Far East where high humidity and population density have maintained the disease. In these valleys devastating epidemics have occurred, often following large religious festivals, and pandemics have spread throughout Asia and Europe and even to North America. The seventh pandemic began in 1961. Good hygiene has prevented its spread to Europe, but cholera is present in the Near East and Africa, where it has for the first time become endemic. In 1990 it reached Peru and has spread throughout South and Central America. The biotype of *V. cholerae*, El Tor, that is responsible for the pandemic, is more resistant than the classical vibrio, and amenable to more prolonged carriage following infection. In 1982 the classical vibrio began to re-establish itself in Bangladesh where, in 1992, a new pandemic began, with a new serotype 0139. Currently, cholera is endemic in many South American countries.

The organism is passed in stools or vomit of patients with cholera and the very much larger number of subclinical cases, who excrete it for a few days. Chronic carriage is rare. The organism survives for up to 2 weeks in fresh water and 8 weeks in salt water. Transmission is normally through infected drinking water. Shellfish, and food contaminated by flies or hands, also transmit the infection.

Pathology

Cholera vibrios multiply in the lumen of the small bowel and are non-invasive. They adhere to the mucosal surface and secrete a powerful exotoxin (enterotoxin) which stimulates the adenylyl cyclase-adenosine monophosphate pathway of the mucosa, resulting in an outpouring of small bowel fluid. In addition, several other toxins are now known to be secreted by the organism which can alter gut motility. There is no inflammatory infiltrate into the affected intestinal mucosa during infection. Severe dehydration follows rapidly even though absorption of fluid by the bowel is hardly impaired. Up to 15 litres of watery diarrhoea may be passed in a day.

There may be acidosis and depletion of sodium and potassium with attendant complications, of which renal failure is the most important. The incubation period is a few hours to 5 days.

Clinical features

Severe diarrhoea without pain or colic, followed by vomiting, begins suddenly. After the faecal contents of the gut have been evacuated the typical 'rice-water' material is passed which consists of clear fluid with flecks of mucus. The enormous loss of fluid and electrolytes leads to intense dehydration with muscular cramps. The skin becomes cold, clammy and wrinkled and the eyes sunken. The blood pressure falls, the pulse becomes imperceptible and the urine output diminishes. The patient usually remains mentally clear. Death from acute circulatory failure may occur within a few hours unless fluid and electrolytes are replaced. Improvement is rapid, however, with proper treatment.

Although this is the classical picture of cholera, the majority of infections cause only mild illness, with slight diarrhoea. Occasionally, a very intense illness, 'cholera sicca', occurs, in which the loss of fluid into the dilated bowel kills the

COMPLICATIONS OF CHOLERA IN CHILDREN

- Electrolyte imbalance with hypocalcaemia, tetany, hypoglycaemia, hypernatraemia, acidosis
- Febrile convulsions
- Risk of over-treatment causing pulmonary oedema
- High mortality—15% compared to 5% in adults

patient before typical gastrointestinal symptoms appear. The disease is more dangerous in children. The complications are listed in the information box.

Investigations

Clinical diagnosis is usually easy during an epidemic but in other situations it is important to confirm the diagnosis bacteriologically so that an outbreak may be brought rapidly under control. *V. cholerae* has a characteristic movement that can be seen under the microscope. Culture of the stool or a rectal swab is used to isolate the organism. Other diseases such as acute bacillary dysentery, viral enteritis, *P. falciparum* malaria, food poisoning, including *Vibrio parahaemolyticus* infections from eating infected shellfish, and certain chemical poisons may produce symptoms like those of cholera. Cholera is notifiable under the International Health Regulations.

Management

The chief aim is to maintain the circulation by replacement of water and electrolytes; the earlier this is started, the better the prognosis. A quick clinical assessment of the state of dehydration is made from the appearance of the patient, the pulse, blood pressure and skin turgor. Fluids are given intravenously in severe cases or when there is vomiting. A large needle is inserted into a large vein (the femoral, for example) and fluid is run in as fast as possible until pulse and blood pressure return. The rest of the estimated deficit is replaced more slowly. If intravenous fluids or drip apparatus are unavailable, fluid is administered via a nasogastric tube.

Vomiting usually stops once the patient is rehydrated, and fluid should then be given orally every hour. Patients are made to drink up to 500 ml hourly. The quantity of fluid required is calculated every 8 hours from the output of urine, stool, vomit, and estimated insensible loss, which may be as much as 5 litres in 24 hours in a hot humid climate.

Total fluid requirements can be in excess of 50 litres over a period of 2–5 days. Accurate records are essential and are greatly facilitated by the use of a 'cholera cot' which has a reinforced hole under the patient's buttocks beneath which a graded bucket is placed.

The ideal fluid replacements are shown in Table 2.19. Other satisfactory fluids include Ringer lactate (BP), Hartman's solution or Darrow's solution, in which event supplements of potassium are given as 10 mmol/l of intravenous fluid or 2–4 g potassium chloride or citrate 3 times daily by mouth. Isotonic saline is better than nothing but every 2 litres should be alternated with 1 litre of isotonic sodium lactate (18.7 g/l) or bicarbonate (14 g/l) and added potassium. Acetate is a satisfactory substitute for bicarbonate, and more stable. The presence of glucose or rice flour in the oral fluid has been shown to promote electrolyte absorption. Chlorpromazine 50 mg 6-hourly reduces intestinal secretion and fluid loss.

Table 2.19 Recommended fluid replacement for treatment of cholera

Intravenous	g/l	mmol/l	Oral	g/l
Sodium chloride	5	Na 133 Cl 98	Commercial salt (NaCl)	3.5
Potassium chloride	1	K 13	Potassium chloride *or* citrate	1.5 2.7
Sodium bicarbonate ***or* acetate**	4 6.5	HCO_3 48	Sodium bicarbonate Glucose*	2.5 20

* Rice flour (50 g) is more effective and cheaper than glucose.

The use of correct fluids for replacement has eliminated the need for the estimation of plasma electrolytes. In children, the elderly, the anaemic and those with underlying heart disease, over-vigorous intravenous rehydration may cause pulmonary oedema. Children require most careful attention to fluid balance; Ringer lactate is the fluid of choice. They are also prone to hypoglycaemia. Any deterioration despite adequate rehydration is an indication for a bolus infusion of 25% glucose 4 ml/kg and maintenance with 10 mg/kg per hour. The management of renal failure is given on page 430.

Three days' treatment with tetracycline 250 mg 6-hourly or co-trimoxazole one tablet daily reduces the duration of excretion of vibrios and the total volume of fluid needed for replacement.

Prevention

Personal prophylaxis means strict personal hygiene. Water for drinking should come from a clean piped supply or be boiled. Flies must not be allowed access to food. Parenteral vaccination with a killed suspension of *V. cholerae* may provide limited protection. Oral vaccines containing killed *V. cholerae* and the B subunit of cholera toxin are available but of limited efficacy.

Control of water sources and of population movement and public education are most important in an epidemic. Mass vaccination with a single dose of vaccine and mass treatment with tetracycline are valuable. Disinfection of infective discharges and soiled clothing, and scrupulous hand-washing by medical attendants reduce the danger of spread from treatment centres.

MYCOBACTERIAL INFECTIONS

TUBERCULOSIS

See page 347.

LEPROSY

Leprosy is the most common cause of peripheral neuritis in

the world. It is a chronic granulomatous disease caused by *Mycobacterium leprae*, an acid- and alcohol-fast bacillus that has a very slow multiplication time of 12–14 days. Leprosy is one of the most seriously disabling and economically important diseases of the world and it is estimated that 20 million people are affected. *M. leprae* will grow in mice and the armadillo, but not in artificial media. Local multiplication of the organism in the footpads of mice is a useful technique for demonstrating the identity and viability of *M. leprae*, and the existence of drug-resistant strains for the screening of drugs, and for studying vaccines. The most important mode of spread of *M. leprae* is by droplets from the sneezes of lepromatous patients whose nasal mucosa is heavily infected. The organism may enter the body through the nasal mucosa or by inoculation through the skin.

The disease is common in tropical Asia, the Far East, tropical Africa, Central and South America, and in some Pacific islands. It is still endemic in southern Europe, North Africa and the Middle East.

Pathology

The organisms show a predilection for peripheral nerves, skin and mucosa of the upper respiratory tract. The pathology is determined by, and reflects, the balance between the patient's cell-mediated immune response and bacillary multiplication, thus creating a spectrum of disease (see Fig. 2.28).

Tuberculoid leprosy

In tuberculoid leprosy, disease is confined to a few sites in

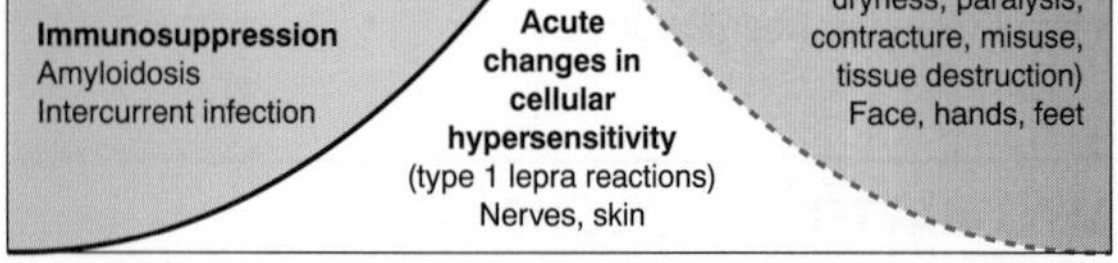

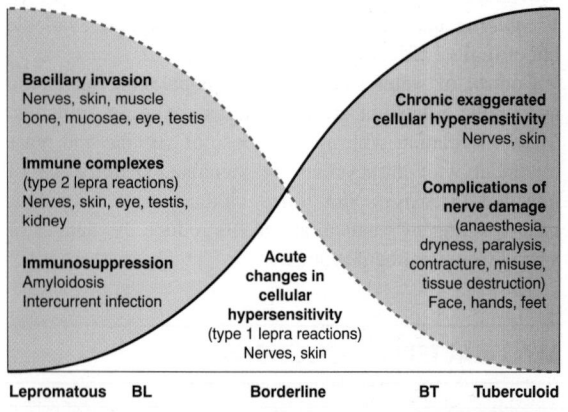

Fig. 2.28 Leprosy: mechanisms of damage and tissue affected. Mechanisms under the broken line are characteristic of disease near the lepromatous end of the spectrum and those under the solid line of the tuberculoid end. They overlap in the centre where, in addition, instability predisposes to type 1 lepra reactions. At the peak in the centre neither bacillary growth nor cell-mediated immunity has the upper hand. (BL = borderline lepromatous; BT = borderline tuberculoid)

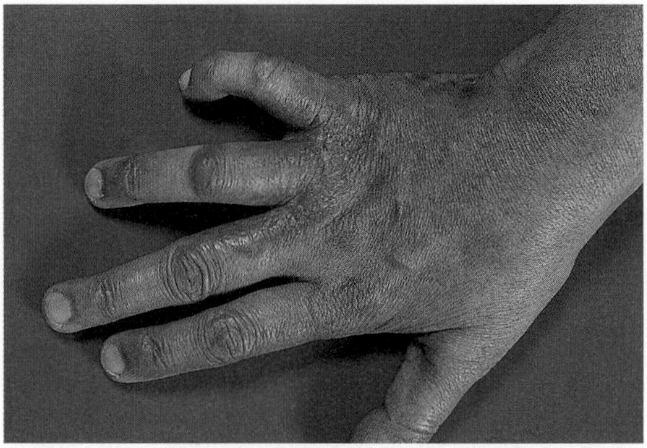

Fig. 2.29 Tuberculoid leprosy. Skin lesions.

skin or peripheral nerves. In skin lesions a vigorous cell-mediated immune response surrounds nerves, sweat glands and hair follicles, which are quickly destroyed. In peripheral nerves, lesions are restricted to one or more of the 'sites of predilection' (see Fig. 2.29) but the presence of the sheath permits the inflammation to create lethal pressure on the axons. Caseation is rare. Organisms are scanty and difficult to demonstrate histologically.

Lepromatous leprosy

In the infective form of this disease, there is no cell-mediated immune response to *M. leprae*. Organisms are present in great abundance in the dermis, in histiocytes, Schwann cells, erectores pilorum muscles and endothelial cells of blood vessels. Organisms are carried in the blood stream to the peripheral nerves, eye and mucosa of the nose and upper respiratory tract, the testes and small muscles and bones of the hands, feet and face, in which they multiply. Tissue damage is slow but widespread. Nephritis and amyloidosis (see p. 541) are common late complications.

Borderline or dimorphous leprosy

Between these two 'polar' types of leprosy, there is a spectrum of manifestations grouped under the terms 'borderline' or 'dimorphous'. The host reaction varies from the near-lepromatous (see Fig. 2.30) to the near-tuberculoid. *M. leprae* is histologically demonstrable in varying numbers. In the centre of the spectrum the disease is unstable. Immunity may diminish (downgrading) in untreated patients, especially in pregnancy or at other times of stress, and the disease becomes more lepromatous. Alternatively, immunity may increase (upgrading or reversal), especially in response to successful chemotherapy, and the disease becomes more tuberculoid. Such upgrading is mediated by local pro-inflammatory cytokine release initiated by T cell-macrophage interaction.

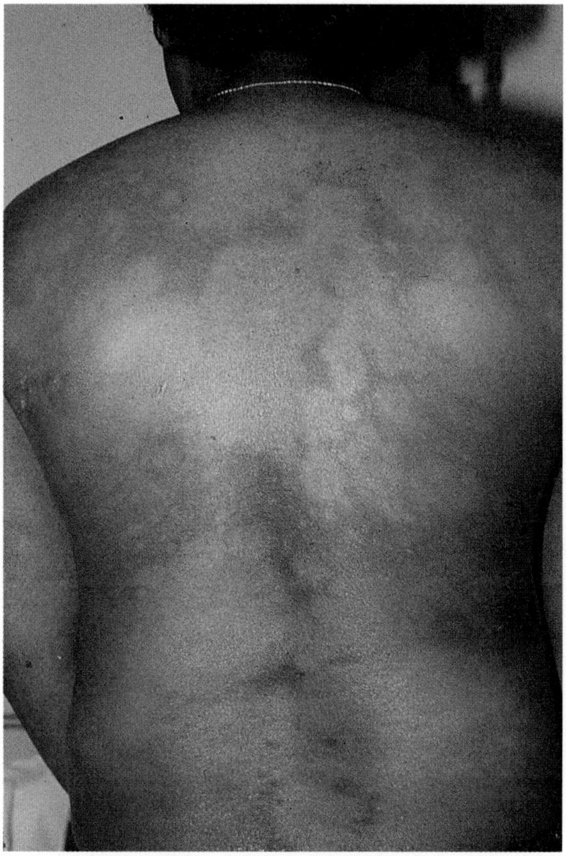

Fig. 2.30 'Borderline' or 'dimorphous' leprosy. Host reaction in this case is near-lepromatous.

Lepra reactions

Any form of leprosy may undergo an acute exacerbation or reaction which is caused by an episode of acute inflammation. In lepromatous disease the reaction, lepra reaction type 2, is due to immune complex-mediated vasculitis. In borderline and tuberculoid disease the reaction, lepra reaction type 1, is due to sudden increase in cellular hypersensitivity. Borderline reactions are often associated with upgrading or downgrading. Lepra reactions may be insidious or rapid, sometimes destroying affected tissues within hours (see Table 2.20).

Leprosy damages the body in three main ways:

- *Peripheral neuritis.* This leads to loss of sensory, motor and autonomic functions. Sensory loss permits trauma from pressure, friction, burns and cuts, the effects of which are intensified if there are abnormal pressures from the contractures following muscular paralysis. Autonomic neuropathy also contributes to skin changes with cracking and slow healing. Secondary bacterial infection in an anaesthetic, unprotected limb leads to cellulitis, osteomyelitis and gross tissue destruction, which produces the deformities with which the disease is still, so unnecessarily, associated. Paralyses result in claw hand and dropped foot from damage respectively to the ulnar and peroneal nerves. A combination of 5th and 7th cranial nerve damage exposes an anaesthetic cornea to trauma and sepsis, so the eye is easily blinded.
- *Bacillary infiltration.* In lepromatous leprosy bacillary growth insidiously damages infiltrated organs and renders them liable to type 2 lepra reactions.
- *Acute lepra reactions.* In children, the incubation period is 2–5 years, but post-primary disease is common in young adults, as in tuberculosis (see p. 347). The disease may also appear in old people as immunity declines.

Clinical features

The onset is usually gradual. The most common first symptom is a small but persistent area of impaired sensation or numbness. In other patients the first noticeable feature may be macules, which are usually hypopigmented and erythematous. The disease may also present acutely, in a lepra

Table 2.20 Reactions in leprosy

	Lepra reaction type 1	Lepra reaction type 2
Mechanism	Cell-mediated hypersensitivity	Immune complexes Arthus phenomenon
Clinical features	Painful tender nerves, loss of function Swollen skin lesions New skin lesions Rarely fever	Tender roseolar papules, may ulcerate Painful tender nerves, loss of function Iritis, orchitis, myositis, lymphadenitis Fever, oedema
Management	Mild: aspirin 600 mg 6-hourly Severe[1]: prednisolone 40–80 mg, reducing over 3–9 months	Mild: aspirin 600 mg 6-hourly Severe[1]: thalidomide[2] or prednisolone 20–40 mg, reducing over 1–6 months Local if eye involved[3]

[1] Includes any threat to nerve or eye function.
[2] See text for details.
[3] 1% hydrocortisone drops or ointment and 1% atropine drops.

Table 2.21 Clinical characteristics of the polar forms of leprosy

Clinical and tissue-specific features	Lepromatous	Tuberculoid
Skin and nerves		
Number and distribution	Widely disseminated	One or a few sites, asymmetrical
Skin lesions		
Definition		
Clarity of margin	Poor	Good
Elevation of margin	Never	Common
Colour		
Dark skin	Slight hypopigmentation	Marked hypopigmentation
Light skin	Slight erythema	Coppery or red
Surface	Smooth, shiny	Dry, scaly
Central healing	None	Common
Sweat and hair growth	Impaired late	Impaired early
Loss of sensation	Late	Early and marked
Nerve enlargement and damage	Late	Early and marked
Bacilli (Bacterial Index)	Many (5 or 6 +)	Absent (0)
Natural outcome	Progression	Healing
Other tissues	Upper respiratory mucosa, eye, testes, bones, muscle	None
Reactions	Immune complexes	Cell-mediated

reaction, with neuritis, iritis or erythema nodosum leprosum (see Table 2.21).

Often the first and only lesion is the inconspicuous macule of *indeterminate leprosy*. It is situated anywhere on the body, exhibiting slight pigmentary and sensory changes. It usually heals spontaneously.

Tuberculoid leprosy

This is characterised by one or a few solitary lesions in skin and peripheral nerves. Skin lesions are macular or raised as plaques or as rings whose flat centres indicate central healing. The lesion is hypopigmented in dark skins and coppery in pale skins, with a well-defined margin. Its surface is dry, often scaly, and usually anaesthetic unless the lesion is on the face. Lesions are of almost any size and occur anywhere on the body (see Fig. 2.29). The nerve supplying the skin lesion or a large peripheral nerve at one of the sites of predilection may be enlarged—for example, the ulnar nerve above the elbow, the median above the elbow or at the wrist, radical at the wrist, common peroneal in the popliteal fossa, posterior tibial around the medial malleolus, and great auricular across the sternomastoid muscle.

Tuberculoid leprosy tends spontaneously to heal slowly, often without residual disability. Sometimes its course is punctuated by a reaction and occasionally it downgrades into the borderline part of the spectrum.

Lepromatous leprosy

Early skin lesions are macular (see Table 2.21). They are numerous, hypopigmented and erythematous. They differ from tuberculoid macules in that they are small, inconspicuous, widely scattered on the body, usually symmetrically, and with margins that merge imperceptibly with normal skin. Overlying sensation is not impaired. As disease advances, the macular lesions become infiltrated and raised; in advanced lepromatous leprosy nodular lesions appear, especially on the ears and face, and eyebrows are lost. Diffuse symmetrical thickening of the skin causes thickened brow and lobes of the ear, producing the 'leonine facies'.

Clinical evidence of nerve damage appears relatively late in lepromatous leprosy. Anaesthesia and anhidrosis are first

THE EFFECTS OF BACILLARY INFILTRATION IN LEPROMATOUS LEPROSY

Skin and nerves
- See text

Muscles of hands, feet and face
- Weakness and wasting

Testes
- Atrophy, impotence, gynaecomastia

Mucosa of nose, mouth, pharynx and larynx
- Rhinitis, hoarseness, perforation of nasal septum and palate, laryngeal obstruction

Bones of hands, feet and face
- Cystic lesions of phalanges permitting fractures, loss of upper incisor teeth and nasal spine leading to nasal collapse

Eye
- Keratitis iridocyclitis, corneal anaesthesia leading to blindness

detected in the distal aspects of the forearms and lower legs, later in a 'glove and stocking' distribution and eventually over the trunk and face, although the palms, soles, axillae and groins may be spared. The effects on other organs are summarised in the information box. Untreated lepromatous leprosy gradually gets worse.

Borderline or dimorphous leprosy

This may present with lesions intermediate in character between lepromatous and tuberculoid or as a mixture of them. Skin lesions are often bizarre. The eyes and nose are spared. Nerve lesions are more numerous than in tuberculoid disease. In Asia, the majority of patients have borderline lepromatous leprosy. In Africa the majority have borderline tuberculoid leprosy. If the disease upgrades, nerve damage may increase, with severe residual disability. If it downgrades, the complications of extensive bacillary multiplication are added to those of widespread nerve damage. In either event the patient is liable to undergo reactions.

Lepra reactions

These may be defined as episodes of inflammation in pre-existing lesions of leprosy (see Table 2.20). Sometimes a reaction is the first clinical manifestation of the disease. One-half of patients with lepromatous leprosy and one-quarter with borderline lepromatous disease will suffer *type 2 lepra reactions* at some time during the course of their disease, most commonly in their second year of treatment. These reactions are characterised by fever and the appearance of crops of painful red papules or nodules called *erythema nodosum leprosum*, which may necrose and discharge sterile pus before subsiding.

Type 1 lepra reactions are especially common in borderline tuberculoid patients. They occur spontaneously or may be precipitated by treatment. Nerve function is rapidly lost, irretrievably so unless the reaction is promptly treated.

Investigations

Lepromatous and borderline lepromatous disease ('multi-bacillary leprosy') is diagnosed by demonstration of *M. leprae* in material obtained by a slit skin smear. The skin is pinched between finger and thumb to expel blood, incised with the point of a scalpel and the exposed dermis scraped with the flat of the blade. The tissue fluid so obtained is smeared on a microscope slide and stained by a modified Ziehl–Neelsen method. Smears are made from skin lesions, earlobes and dorsum of the ring or middle finger—sites in which bacilli multiply readily and persist. Nasal mucus may also contain the organisms in lepromatous leprosy and this is a good indication of infectivity. *M. leprae* is less readily demonstrable in skin smears in borderline disease and is undetectable in tuberculoid disease.

In borderline and especially tuberculoid disease ('paucibacillary leprosy'), the cardinal signs of leprosy are enlarged nerves and anaesthesia. Nerves are usually enlarged at sites of predilection asymmetrically and irregularly; they may be tender.

Loss or diminution of sensation, or misreference (the inability to locate accurately the site stimulated), may be detected in a skin lesion or in the distribution of a large peripheral nerve. Biopsy of skin or nerve is seldom necessary except for accurate classification.

The lepromin test

Lepromin is a suspension of dead *M. leprae*. The test is performed like the tuberculin test, but is read after 4 weeks. The result indicates the degree of cellular immunity that an individual can mount against the organism. This test is of no value in establishing the diagnosis of leprosy, but it is useful in helping to classify the disease, and so determine treatment and prognosis.

Management

Treatment of leprosy is long and often complicated. The patient must understand the disease and its complications, comply and persevere in the treatment and learn to look after anaesthetic limbs, control fear and cope with any stigma that exists in the community. Admission to hospital for a few days is useful to establish rapport and start education.

Specific chemotherapy

The essential features of the available antibiotics are given in Table 2.22.

Patients with multibacillary disease (lepromatous and borderline lepromatous). These are preferably isolated until they are rendered non-infectious, which takes only a few days with rifampicin. Ideally, treatment should be with three drugs, rifampicin, clofazimine and dapsone, to prevent the emergence of drug resistance. Rifampicin, the most expensive but most efficient bactericidal drug, need only be given monthly because of the long generation time of *M. leprae*. It is most effective if given for 2 consecutive days in a daily dose of 600 mg, or 450 mg for patients under 35 kg in weight. Clofazimine is given in a dose of 50 mg daily, or 100 mg three times in the week (totalling 6 mg/kg per week for children). Dapsone is given in a dose of 2 mg/kg daily, not

Table 2.22 Main features of drugs available to treat leprosy

Drugs	Dose (mg)	Peak serum level/MIC*	Duration of MIC (days)	Bactericidal activity
Dapsone	100	100–500	4–12	+
Rifampicin	600	30	1	+++
Clofazimine	100	(Stored in macrophage cells, possible depot)		?
Minocycline	100	10–20	1	++
Ofloxacin	400	—	1	++

* MIC = minimum inhibitory concentration.

PROBLEMS WITH THE CHEMOTHERAPY OF LEPROSY
Compliance
Side-effects of drugs
• Dapsone: dermatitis, psychosis, haemolytic anaemia • Clofazimine: red, brown or blue-black discoloration, abdominal pain • Ethionamide: hepatitis, especially in Asians, notably Chinese • Rifampicin: influenza-like syndrome after each dose, red urine
Drug resistance
• Dapsone: secondary resistance common, when given alone for lepromatous leprosy • Rifampicin: rapid onset if given alone • Thiacetazone: rapid onset if given alone, cross-resistance with ethionamide

exceeding 100 mg. For mass treatment campaigns when compliance is often poor, WHO recommends that rifampicin be given in a single supervised monthly dose of 600 mg, and that a supervised monthly dose of clofazimine 300 mg be given in addition to the self-administered daily dose of clofazimine and dapsone. Patients are treated for 2 years and followed for a further 5 years.

Patients with paucibacillary disease (intermediate, tuberculoid and borderline tuberculoid). These are treated with rifampicin once monthly and dapsone daily for 1 year, and are followed for a further 2 years.

Side-effects of dapsone are rare. They include psychosis, dermatitis and haemolytic anaemia. Minocycline and ofloxacin are the most useful second-line drugs, less toxic but more expensive than ethionamide and thiacetazone (see Table 2.22).

Treatment of lepra reactions

Chemotherapy for leprosy is maintained and appropriate anti-inflammatory drugs used (see Table 2.20). Reactional neuritis is a medical emergency as irreversible paralysis may occur overnight.

Type 2 reactions in lepromatous patients respond rapidly to thalidomide in a dose of 100 mg 6-hourly. The dose is reduced slowly over weeks or months. This drug must never be given to pre-menopausal women because of its disastrous teratogenic effects. Care is also needed in the use of thalidomide because of somnolence. If thalidomide is contra-indicated or unavailable, prednisolone is used. Increasing the dose of clofazimine to 200 mg or 300 mg daily for a few weeks will help control the reaction and permit prednisolone to be reduced or withdrawn. Iritis is a dangerous complication but can usually be managed by local measures.

Type 1 reactions in borderline patients are controlled with corticosteroids. Prednisolone is given in a dose of 40–60 mg daily and reduced gradually over 2–6 months for patients with borderline tuberculoid disease, and 6–9 months for patients with borderline lepromatous disease.

Management of nerve damage

In the event of acute paralysis complicating reactional neuritis, the affected limb is splinted and exercised passively each day until function begins to return, when active exercises can be added. A patient with an anaesthetic limb must be taught to accept the limitations it imposes, to adjust life accordingly, to inspect the limb daily for trauma or infection and to learn how not to damage it.

Tarsorrhaphy helps protect an exposed anaesthetic cornea. Secondary sepsis is treated with antibiotics; osteomyelitis and its sequelae are managed as conservatively as possible. Patients with plantar ulcers are confined to bed, or given crutches or a walking-plaster until healing is complete. Shoes must fit and protect anaesthetic feet against trauma and must be made specially if there is added deformity.

Prevention

In endemic areas the disease is most common among intimate contacts of patients, and children and young adults are especially susceptible. *M. leprae* is easily spread and two-thirds of contacts undergo subclinical immunising infections within 2 years of regular exposure. Of the small proportion of contacts (about 1%) that develop clinical disease, only about 2% will be lepromatous. Identification of this small group at risk and logical prophylaxis are at present impossible. No specific vaccine is available. Bacille Calmette–Guérin (BCG) is of some value, especially in Africa, and should be given to all child contacts of lepromatous patients. Dapsone and rifampicin may be given as for paucibacillary disease (above) for 6 months to child contacts of lepromatous patients. Neither measure is a substitute for 6-monthly examination of contacts. Surprisingly, leprosy does not appear to accelerate HIV infection, in contrast to coincident HIV and tuberculosis.

Mass prophylaxis is impossible, but treatment and follow-up of all cases identified during a population survey reduce deformity and lower the incidence of leprosy. With improvement of socio-economic conditions the disease tends to disappear. The rapid spread of dapsone resistance poses a great problem to existing control schemes.

FURTHER INFORMATION ON DISEASES DUE TO BACTERIA

Butler T 1994 Yersinia infections: centennial of the discovery of the plague bacillus. Clinical Infectious Diseases 19: 655–663
Crook L D, Tempest B 1992 Plague. A clinical review of 27 cases. Archives of Internal Medicine 152: 1253–1256
Dance D A B 1991 Melioidosis: the tip of the iceberg. Clinical Microbiology Reviews 4: 52–60
Drasar B S 1992 Pathogenesis and ecology: the case of cholera. Journal of Tropical Medicine and Hygiene 95: 365–372
Lienhardt C, Fine P E M 1992 Controlling leprosy: multidrug treatment is not enough alone. Lancet 305: 206–207
O'Grady F, Lambert H P, Finch R, Greenwood D 1997 Antibiotic and chemotherapy: anti-infective agents and their use in therapy. Churchill Livingstone, Edinburgh

DISEASES DUE TO SPIROCHAETES

The classification of spirochaetal infections is outlined in the information box.

SPIROCHAETAL INFECTIONS: CLASSIFICATION
Leptospira infections
• Leptospirosis *(L. icterohaemorrhagiae, L. hardjo, L. canicola)*
Borrelia infections
• Lyme disease *(B. burgdorferi)* • Louse-borne relapsing fever *(B. recurrentis)* • Tick-borne relapsing fever *(B. duttoni)* • Tropical ulcer *(B. vincenti)* • Cancrum oris *(B. vincenti)*
Treponema infections
• Syphilis *(T. pallidum)* • Yaws *(T. pertenue)* • Pinta *(T. carateum)* • Bejel *(T. pallidum)*

LEPTOSPIRA INFECTIONS

LEPTOSPIROSIS

Although over 100 serotypes of *Leptospira* have been identified, only *L. icterohaemorrhagiae*, *L. hardjo* and *L. canicola* have been shown to cause human disease in Britain (see Table 2.23).

The natural host of *Weil's disease*, caused by *L. icterohaemorrhagiae*, is the rat and other rodents. Infected urine contains spirochaetes which can penetrate the skin or mucosa of humans. Abattoir and farm workers and water sports enthusiasts are most at risk.

Table 2.23 Leptospiral infections in the UK

Organism	Source
Leptospira icterohaemorrhagiae (Weil's disease) Hepatitis Renal tubular necrosis Myocarditis Purpura Haemorrhagic conjunctivitis	Water contaminated by rats' urine
Leptospira canicola Non-specific febrile illness Aseptic meningitis	Dogs and pigs
Leptospira hardjo Non-specific febrile illness Chronic ill health Aseptic meningitis	Cattle

L. canicola infection, which is contracted from dogs and pigs, usually presents as aseptic meningitis. It is not often associated with jaundice and is less severe than Weil's disease.

L. hardjo infection occurs in farm workers in contact with cattle, in whom it can cause ill health resembling chronic brucellosis. It can also cause aseptic meningitis.

The average incubation period of leptospirosis is 10 days, the range being 4–21 days.

Clinical features of Weil's disease

Weil's disease usually begins abruptly with headache, severe myalgia, pyrexia, conjunctival suffusion, anorexia and vomiting. A rash may develop with petechiae, and enlargement of the liver and spleen occurs.

The temperature falls by lysis and is usually normal in 2 or 3 days. In the majority of patients, there is further pyrexia for a few days and transient meningism followed by recovery. In severe infections hepatitis, renal tubular necrosis, myocarditis and meningitis may occur during this phase. The condition may progress to acute liver necrosis. Renal tubular necrosis may lead to acute renal failure. Myocarditis is suggested by tachycardia, fall in blood pressure, arrhythmias and cardiac failure.

The majority of patients enter the convalescent phase by the third and fourth week of the illness. When there has been serious involvement of the liver, kidneys and heart, mortality in Weil's disease is in the region of 15–20%. Those who recover do so completely.

Investigations

A rising titre of specific leptospiral antibodies is found from the second week onwards. When there is liver involvement, liver function tests indicate hepatocellular damage with an intrahepatic obstructive element. The urine contains protein, red blood cells and cellular and granular casts in patients with renal failure.

Management

Benzylpenicillin 1.2 g i.v. or i.m. 6-hourly is the drug of choice. Alternatives are doxycycline 100 mg 12-hourly p.o. or erythromycin 500 mg 12-hourly p.o. Supportive treatment is needed for anaemia secondary to bleeding and for renal failure.

BORRELIA INFECTIONS

The world-wide distribution of the major diseases caused by *Borrelia* infection is shown in Figure 2.31.

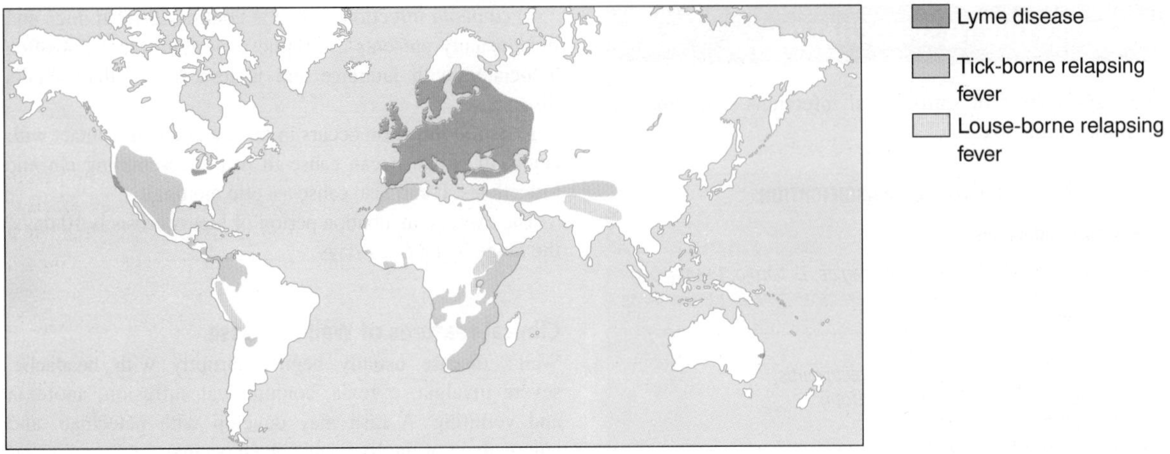

Fig. 2.31 Distribution of diseases due to *Borrelia*.

LYME DISEASE

Lyme disease is caused by *Borrelia burgdorferi*, a spirochaetal organism transmitted by the *Ixodes* tick. The disease was first identified in the New England county of Lyme where a cluster of cases of arthritis of unknown aetiology occurred in the early 1980s.

Epidemiology

In the UK the vector for *B. burgdorferi* is *Ixodes ricinus*, a tick which infests dogs, sheep and deer. It is probable that deer are the principal source of infection for humans, and in the New Forest area of southern England approximately one-quarter of forestry workers are seropositive for the organism.

The infection is particularly common in the eastern states of North America, especially in New England, but also occurs in Europe, particularly Sweden, and the countries of Eastern Europe.

Clinical features

The information box lists the clinical features of Lyme disease. The primary infection, which occurs 2–3 weeks after the initial tick bite, is often asymptomatic, although it may present with influenza-like symptoms and a characteristic rash known as erythema chronicum migrans, an annular red lesion surrounding a paler area of skin. Neurological and cardiac manifestations usually occur within 3–6 weeks of the primary infection. Large-joint arthritis is a later manifestation, while the chronic skin lesion, acrodermatitis chronica atrophica, can occur several years after the primary infection. Arthritis and cardiac involvement are seen more often in the USA, whereas neurological illness and acrodermatitis are more common in Europe.

CLINICAL FEATURES OF LYME DISEASE
Early clinical manifestations
• Rash (erythema chronicum migrans) with or without febrile illness
Early complications
• Neurological—cranial nerve palsies, meningitis or radiculopathy • Cardiac—conduction disorders (most common), myocarditis, pericarditis or cardiomyopathy
Late complications
• Large-joint arthritis • Acrodermatitis chronica atrophica • Chronic neurological—polyneuropathy, encephalopathy

Investigations

The diagnosis of Lyme disease is made on the clinical history together with a positive serum antibody test. This is usually an ELISA test confirmed by immunoblot. However, serological tests are unreliable. Around 30% of acute cases are seronegative; positive tests may reflect past rather than current infection. More sophisticated immunological tests are being developed.

Management

B. burgdorferi is sensitive to the β-lactam antibiotics (penicillins and cephalosporins) and to the tetracyclines. Therapeutic options include oral doxycycline or amoxycillin given for 3 weeks. For more severe cases, intravenous benzylpenicillin or ceftriaxone is indicated. Relapses may occur, especially if treatment is delayed.

TROPICAL ULCER

Tropical ulcer is a specific infection with *Borrelia vincenti* and anaerobic bacteria. Minor injury in the presence of undernourishment, poor hygiene and debilitating disease are predisposing factors. It is most common in adolescent males, on the lower third of thc leg.

Clinical features

The initial lesion is a bleb filled with sanguineous fluid. The bleb ruptures and a green-grey slough is exposed which spreads, rapidly and painfully, in the skin and subcutaneous tissue up to a diameter of 5 cm or more. In a few days these tissues slough and liquefy, releasing an offensive discharge. After about a week there is usually no further spread and the necrotic tissue separates, exposing an ulcer.

In a chronic ulcer the edges are raised and slope sharply. The damage may be limited to the skin and superficial fascia, but in severe cases deep structures, including tendons and periosteum, may be invaded. The ulcer is usually solitary and heals slowly with a tissue-paper-like scar which breaks down easily. Big ulcers fail to heal and may undergo malignant changes after many years.

Management

Local treatment consists in thorough cleaning of the ulcer with hypertonic saline or magnesium sulphate. Acute ulcers heal in response to procaine penicillin 300 mg intramuscularly, metronidazole 400 mg 8-hourly, or tetracycline 2 g daily for 7 days. Ulcers over 5 cm in diameter need grafting. Chronic ulcers are excised and grafted.

Prevention

Where tropical ulcers are a risk, abrasions should be cleaned and covered. The provision of a good diet, washing facilities and adequate first aid of minor skin injuries significantly reduces incidence of this disease.

CANCRUM ORIS

Cancrum oris is rare, except in poorly nourished children in the tropics. It is characteristically preceded by an infective illness, especially measles. The manifestation is that of a rapidly developing gangrene, beginning inside the mouth and penetrating through the lips and cheek. Gangrene becomes demarcated and ulceration follows, resulting in severe disfigurement. Untreated, it frequently causes death. *B. vincenti* and an anaerobic bacterium are frequently found in the ulcer. Penicillin (see Table 2.5, p. 68) arrests the infection but does not prevent gangrene of already diseased tissue. Coexistent malnutrition, anaemia or dehydration should be corrected. Subsequently, skilled plastic surgery may do much to overcome the hideous defects.

Prevention depends on improved nutrition and hygiene in the community and on control of acute infectious diseases.

THE RELAPSING FEVERS

The relapsing fevers are a group of diseases due to infections by spirochaetes of the genus *Borrelia* transmitted by body lice or soft (argasid) ticks. Sodoku, due to *Spirillum minus*, also relapses (see Table 2.24). The louse-borne *Borrelia recurrentis* infects only humans and is not transmitted from a louse to its progeny. This disease appears in epidemics, particularly during wars or famine when refugees are crowded together in conditions under which infestation with the human body louse *Pediculus humanus* is frequent. It may accompany louse-borne typhus. The disease is endemic in Ethiopia and Bolivia.

Table 2.24 Comparative features of the 'relapsing fevers' due to *Borrelia* and *Spirillum*

	Louse-borne relapsing fever (LBRF)	Tick-borne relapsing fever (TBRF)	Sodoku	Haverhill	Lyme disease
Incubation	2–12 days	2–12 days	5–21 days	1–5 days	4 days to months
Fever	4–10 days	3–5 days	7 days	3 days	Weeks
Remission	7 days	3–5 days	3–5 days	—	No consistent pattern
Relapses	0–3	Up to 10	Numerous	None	—
Jarisch–Herxheimer reaction	Severe	Mild	Mild/none	None	None
Mortality	Up to 40%	Under 10%	None	None	Rare
Major complications	Hepatitis Myocarditis Meningitis Shock Bleeding	Similar to LBRF but less severe Neurological in relapses	Chancre Adenitis Rash	Arthritis	Rash Arthritis Carditis Meningitis

Species of *Borrelia* that cause tick-borne relapsing fever are transmitted by various species of the genus *Ornithodoros*. Ticks live for years and once infected remain so for life and may convey the infection to the offspring. Tick-borne relapsing fever is thus an endemic disease.

LOUSE-BORNE RELAPSING FEVER

Lice cause itching. Borreliae are liberated from the infected louse when it is crushed during scratching, which also inoculates the borreliae into the skin.

Pathology

The borreliae multiply in the blood, where they are abundant in the febrile phases, and invade most tissues, especially the liver, spleen and meninges. Hepatitis causing jaundice is frequent in severe infections and there may be petechial haemorrhages in the skin, mucous membranes and serous surfaces of internal organs. Thrombocytopenia is marked.

Clinical features

Onset is sudden with fever. The temperature rises to 39.5–40.5°C and is accompanied by a rapid pulse, headache, generalised aching, injected conjunctivae and frequently a petechial rash (see Fig. 2.32), epistaxis and herpes labialis. As the disease progresses, the liver and spleen frequently become tender and palpable and jaundice is common. There may be severe serosal and intestinal haemorrhage. Mental confusion and meningism may occur. The fever ends by crisis between the fourth and tenth days, often associated with profuse sweating, hypotension, circulatory and cardiac failure (see Table 2.24). There may be no further fever but in a proportion of patients, after an afebrile period of about 7 days, there may be one or more relapses which are usually milder and less prolonged. In the absence of specific treatment the mortality rate may be as high as 40%, especially among the elderly and malnourished.

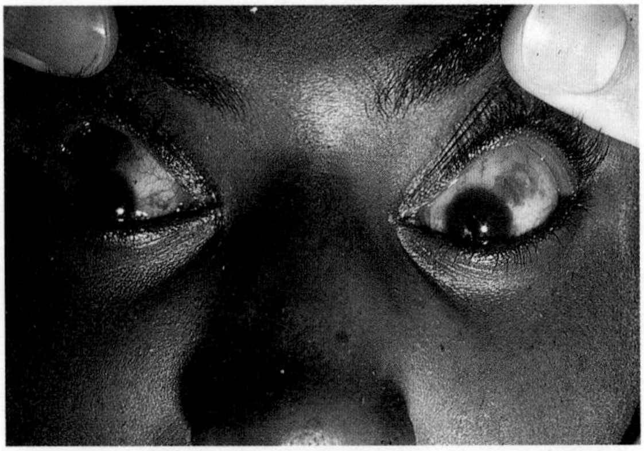

Fig. 2.32 Louse-borne relapsing fever. Injected conjunctivae.

Investigations

The organisms are demonstrated in the blood during fever either by dark ground illumination of a wet film or by staining thick and thin films.

Management

The problems of treatment are to eradicate the organism, to minimise the severe Jarisch–Herxheimer reaction (JHR) (see below) which inevitably follows successful chemotherapy, and to prevent relapses. The safest treatment is procaine penicillin 300 mg intramuscularly, followed the next day by 0.5 g tetracycline. Tetracycline alone is effective and prevents relapse, but may give rise to a worse reaction. Doxycycline, 200 mg once by mouth as an alternative to tetracycline, has the advantage of being curative also for typhus, which often accompanies epidemics of relapsing fever.

Treatment is followed within half an hour to 3 hours by a chill or rigor, a brisk rise of temperature to 40–42°C, tachypnoea, tachycardia and often cough, confusion, distress, delirium and, occasionally, convulsions and coma. This phase is rapidly followed by profound hypotension and vasodilatation which may last from 8–12 hours and may be complicated by cardiac failure. The patient must be confined strictly to bed for 48 hours after treatment, carefully observed and managed as complications demand. Tepid sponging for fever over 41°C, careful attention to hydration, preferably by oral fluids, and prompt treatment of cardiac failure are required.

The aetiology of JHR is now well recognised to be due to a sudden and massive release of pro-inflammatory cytokines (TNF, IL-6) into the circulation. Glucocorticoids do not ameliorate JHR.

Prevention

The patient, clothing and all contacts must be freed from lice as in epidemic typhus (see p. 117).

TICK-BORNE RELAPSING FEVER

This disease is conveyed by a variety of soft ticks, and its endemicity is governed by presence of this vector. In the Mediterranean area *Ornithodoros tholozani* is responsible; in the Middle East, Iran, Afghanistan and India and in the New World there are other vectors. These ticks can become infected from rodents or bats as well as by congenital transmission, and humans are only an incidental host. In Central and East Africa, however, where *O. moubata* is the vector of *Borrelia duttoni*, humans are probably the only important mammalian host. The disease in these areas is thus confined to old campsites, old houses and their surroundings, where *O. moubata* lives in dried mud floors and walls.

The pathological changes resemble those of louse-borne relapsing fever but with late neurological lesions.

Clinical features

These are similar to those of louse-borne relapsing fever (see Table 2.24). The febrile bouts, although severe, usually last only for 3–5 days, and the apyrexial periods may also be shorter. Relapses are, however, more frequent. Iritis and neurological complications, including cranial nerve palsies, optic atrophy, localised palsies and spastic paraplegia, may develop during these later relapses.

Investigations

The methods used in diagnosis are similar to those for louse-borne relapsing fever. *B. duttoni* is, however, scantier in the peripheral blood but young mice are readily infected.

Management

As many strains are resistant to penicillin, tetracycline 1 g daily for 7 days is given and the course repeated after an interval of a week. Good results may follow a single dose of 200 mg doxycycline.

Prevention

Ticks can be killed by lindane applied to the inside of the walls, to floors and across the entrance to houses.

RAT-BITE FEVERS

There are two rat-bite fevers, one caused by *Spirillum minus*, the other by *Streptobacillus moniliformis*. The latter, in addition to being transmitted by a rat bite, has also occurred as an epidemic due to infected milk (Haverhill fever); in other cases there has been no known contact with rats or mice. Both infections are world-wide. The incubation period of *Streptobacillus* fever is 1–5 days; with *S. minus* it is 1–4 weeks.

The main features are summarised in Table 2.24. Diagnosis is by demonstration of spirochaete in fluid from chancre, lymph node or joint effusion, by dark ground microscopy or mouse inoculation. *S. minus* infections cross-react serologically with syphilis. The infections are cured by penicillin or tetracycline.

TREPONEMA INFECTIONS

SYPHILIS

See page 184.

YAWS

Yaws is a granulomatous disease mainly involving the skin and bones and caused by *Treponema pertenue*, morphologically indistinguishable from the causative organisms of syphilis and pinta (see Table 2.25). The three infections induce similar serological changes and possibly some degree of cross-immunity. Organisms are transmitted by bodily contact from a patient with infectious yaws through minor abrasions of the skin of another patient, usually a child. The mass campaigns by WHO between 1950 and 1960 treated over 60 million people and eradicated yaws from many areas, but the disease has persisted patchily throughout the tropics and there has been a resurgence in the 1980s and 1990s in West and Central Africa and the South Pacific.

Pathology

A proliferative granuloma containing numerous treponemes develops at the site of the inoculation. This primary lesion is followed by secondary eruptions. In addition, there may be hypertrophic periosteal lesions of many bones, with underlying cortical rarefaction. Lesions of late yaws are characterised by destructive changes which closely resemble the osteitis and gummas of tertiary syphilis and which heal with much scarring and deformity. The incubation period is 3–4 weeks.

Table 2.25 Comparison of the major treponemal diseases

					Lesions		
Disease	**Organism**	**Source**	**Transmission**	**At risk**	**Primary**	**Early***	**Late***
Yaws	*T. pertenue*	Skin	Contact	Children	Ulcer or nodule	Skin, bones	Skin, bones, palms and soles
Pinta	*T. carateum*	Skin	Contact	Family	Papule	Skin	Skin
Bejel	*T. pallidum*	Mouth utensils	Contact	Family	Rare	Skin, mucosae, bones	Skin, mucosae, bones, palms and soles
Venereal syphilis	*T. pallidum*	Genital sores, mouth	Sexual, placenta	Sexual partners, fetus	Genital ulcer, lymphadenopathy	Skin, mucosae, bones, meninges	Cardiovascular, CNS, bones etc.

* Early and late correspond with secondary and tertiary lesions.

Clinical features

Early yaws

The primary lesion or 'mother yaw' is usually on the leg or buttocks. The secondary eruption usually follows a few weeks or months later, as crops of papillomas covered with a whitish-yellow exudate, especially in the flexures and around the mouth. Sometimes a lesion erupts through the palm or sole, when walking becomes painful ('wet crab yaws'). Phalanges, nasal bones and tibiae swell and become distorted. Most of the lesions of early yaws will eventually subside, even if untreated.

Latent yaws

Following the spontaneous resolution of 'early yaws' serological changes may persist, to be followed by further manifestations of 'early yaws' or, after an interval of as much as 5–10 years, by the tertiary lesions or 'late yaws'.

Late yaws

Solitary or multiple lesions appear as nodules or ulcers in the skin, hyperkeratotic lesions of palms or soles ('dry crab yaws') and gummatous lesions of bone. They heal with scarring. Lesions of the facial and palatal bones cause terrible disfigurement (gangosa).

Investigations and management

See the information box.

DIAGNOSIS AND TREATMENT OF YAWS, PINTA AND BEJEL
Diagnosis of early stages
• Detection of spirochaetes in exudate of lesions by dark ground microscopy
Diagnosis of latent and early stages
• Positive serological tests, as for syphilis (see p. 186)
Treatment of all stages
• Single intramuscular injection of 1.2 g long-acting (e.g. benzathine) penicillin G

Prevention

The disease disappears with improved housing and cleanliness. In few fields of medicine have chemotherapy and improved hygiene achieved such dramatic success as in the control of yaws.

PINTA AND BEJEL

These two treponemal infections occur in poor rural populations with low standards of domestic hygiene, but in separate parts of the world. They have features in common, notably that they are transmitted by contact, usually within the family and not sexually; and in the case of bejel, through common eating and drinking utensils (see Table 2.25). Their diagnosis and management is as for yaws (see the information box).

Pinta

Pinta is probably the oldest of the treponemal infections of humans and *T. carateum* the parent of the organism that came to Europe with the return of Christopher Columbus's sailors in 1493, starting the epidemic of venereal syphilis known as the 'Great Pox'. It is found only in South and Central America, where its incidence is declining. The early lesions are scaly papules or dyschromic patches on the skin. The late lesions are often depigmented and disfiguring. The infection is confined to the skin.

Bejel

Bejel is the Middle Eastern name for non-venereal syphilis, which has a patchy distribution across sub-Saharan Africa, the Middle East, Central Asia and Australia. It has been eradicated from Eastern Europe. Transmission is most commonly from the mouth of the mother or child and the primary mucosal lesion is seldom seen. The early and late lesions resemble those of secondary and tertiary syphilis (see pp. 185–186) but cardiovascular and neurological disease is rare.

FURTHER INFORMATION ON DISEASES DUE TO SPIROCHAETES

Barclay A J G, Coulter J B S 1990 Tick-borne relapsing fever in Central Tanzania. Transactions of the Royal Society of Tropical Medicine and Hygiene 84: 852–856

Mehens A, Antal G M 1992 The endemic treponematoses not yet eradicated. World Health Statistics Quarterly 45: 228–237

Steere A C 1989 Lyme disease. New England Journal of Medicine 321: 586–596

DISEASES DUE TO FUNGI (MYCOSES)

There are three groups of fungi which cause human disease—multinucleate branched filamentous forms (moulds), round or ovoid single cells known as yeasts, and dimorphic fungi which have certain of the growth characteristics of both. *Trichophyton*, a fungus which causes foot infections, is an example of a filamentous fungus while *Cryptococcus neoformans*, which causes meningitis, is a yeast. *Candida albicans*, the cause of thrush, is a dimorphic fungus.

Certain fungi cause only superficial infections while others can cause invasive disease. *Candida* can cause both superficial and deep infections. Fungal infections are often referred to as mycoses. These diseases are listed in the information box. Pathogenic fungi are ubiquitous; their importance varies between different parts of the world. Some fungi are opportunistic and will not normally invade unless the defence mechanisms are impaired, as in the immunocompromised host. Fungal infections are transmitted by spores or hyphae and normally enter the body through the lungs or skin, where they may cause disease or from where they may disseminate to other parts of the body. Fungal infections tend to be chronic and often require prolonged chemotherapy. For some infections there is still no effective treatment. Fungi also cause disease through allergy and from toxins such as ergot, muscarine and aflatoxin.

Fungal infections commonly present as skin disease, as subcutaneous swellings or as systemic infections.

FUNGAL DISEASE IN HUMANS

Cutaneous infections	Systemic infections
• Dermatophytes • Candidiasis • Pityriasis versicolor **Subcutaneous infections** • Mycetoma (see Table 2.26, p. 145) • Other soft tissue infections (see Table 2.27, p. 146)	• Histoplasmosis • Aspergillosis • Coccidioidomycosis • Paracoccidioidomycosis • Blastomycosis • Cryptococcosis • Candidiasis

CUTANEOUS FUNGAL INFECTIONS

An intact healthy skin is especially important in the tropics, where fungal infections are common. Extensive infections may impair sweating and heat loss, and cause distress through irritation. Scratching leads to secondary pyogenic infection.

RINGWORM (TINEA INFECTIONS)

Ringworm is due to infection by dermatophyte fungi. There are three main genera: *Trichophyton* (skin, hair and nail infections), *Microsporum* (skin and hair) and *Epidermophyton* (skin and nails).

Dermatophytes invade keratin only and in general zoophilic fungi (those transmitted to humans from animals) cause a more severe but short-lived inflammatory response than anthropophilic ones (spread from person to person).

Clinical features

These depend upon the site and the species of fungus involved.

Tinea pedis ('athlete's foot')

This is the most common type of fungal infection in humans. It is encouraged by the sharing of wash places and swimming pools. Infrequent washing of socks and the use of occlusive footwear encourage relapses. It may present in three main ways: soggy interdigital scaling, diffuse powdery scaling of the soles (which is often unilateral and which picks out skin creases), and recurrent bouts of vesiculation of the soles. The organisms involved are usually *T. rubrum*, *T. mentagrophytes var. interdigitale* and *E. floccosum*.

Tinea unguium (tinea of the nails)

Toe nail infection is more common than finger nail infection and is often accompanied by tinea pedis. Usually only a few nails are infected. The first changes occur at the free edge of the nail, which becomes yellow and crumbly. Thickening of the nail and separation of the nail from the nail bed may follow. *T. rubrum* is a frequent cause.

Tinea manuum (tinea of the hands)

This is usually asymmetrical and involves the palms (dry, powdery scaling picking out the creases) more often than the backs of the hands.

Tinea cruris (tinea of the groin)

This affects men more than women and causes well-demarcated redness and peripheral scaling of the groins and upper thighs. A few vesicles or pustules are usually seen within the lesions. The eruption is often unilateral or asymmetrical, and itchy.

Tinea corporis (tinea of the trunk)

This is the archetypal 'ringworm' eruption. Erythematous scaly plaques expand slowly and clear in the centre, leaving a ring-like pattern (see Fig. 2.33). Peripheral scaling, a few vesicles and pustules are characteristic.

Tinea imbricata (due to *T. concentricum*), common in southern Asia, islands of the South Pacific and in some South American countries, is characterised by multiple concentric scaly rings. If untreated, the eruption becomes widespread and is often intensely itchy.

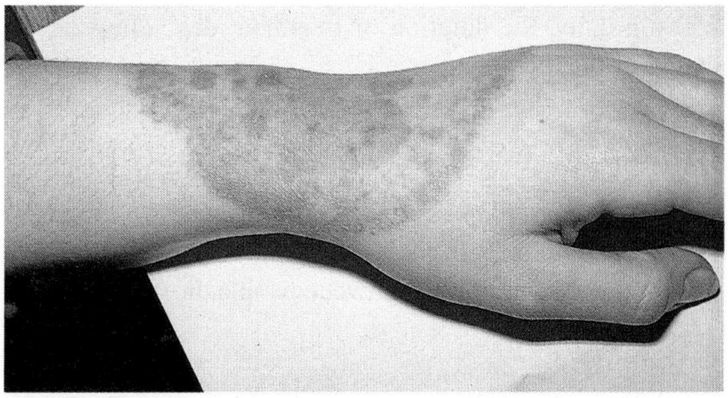

Fig. 2.33 Tinea infection of the arm and wrist.

Tinea capitis (tinea of the scalp)

The causative organism varies from country to country. Adults rarely develop scalp infections with anthropophilic fungi.

Anthropophilic species cause bald, slightly scaly patches with the hairs broken off a few millimetres from the scalp; inflammation is minimal. Some species, especially *Microsporum*, fluoresce green under Wood's ultraviolet light, so schoolchildren may be screened in epidemics. Better hygiene and more effective therapy have made such outbreaks rare in the UK. Favus due to *T. schoenleinii* is characterised by foul-smelling, shield-like crusts and may cause permanent scarring with hair loss.

Zoophilic species (e.g. those causing cattle ringworm) induce considerable inflammation, with boggy swelling and pustulation ('kerion' reaction) leading to scarring. Tinea of the beard, usually due to a zoophilic organism, shows the same features.

Complications

These include permanent alopecia due to scarring and an allergic vesicular reaction on the sides of the fingers and palms from which no fungus can be isolated (the 'ide' eruption). Atypical presentations of tinea occur in the immunosuppressed and when the rash is mistreated with topical steroids ('tinea incognito').

Investigations

Microscopic examination of skin scrapings, nail clippings or hair pluckings, cleared in potassium hydroxide, is the easiest way to check for fungi. Cultures may be carried out if facilities are available. Wood's ultraviolet light examination of the scalp is useful for screening those in institutions where outbreaks of tinea capitis occur, but some fungi do not fluoresce.

Management

Mild infections are treated with topical ointments containing imidazoles or terbinafine. Stubborn, extensive scalp and nail infections should be treated with systemic drugs such as griseofulvin (fine particle) 500 mg daily or terbinafine 250 mg daily, the duration of treatment depending on the nature of the infection.

CANDIDIASIS (MONILIASIS)

A yeast, *Candida albicans*, is the most common fungus of medical importance. It is ubiquitous in the environment but it may also be transmitted between people directly.

Pathology

Candidiasis is usually a superficial infection of skin, nails or mucous membrane with the yeast form of the fungus, causing mild inflammation. However, these tissues are rarely affected if they are entirely healthy. Factors that predispose to candidiasis are listed in the information box. A congenital immune deficiency of T lymphocytes predisposes to the syndrome of chronic mucocutaneous candidiasis, while more severe, often iatrogenic, forms of immune suppression may permit systemic infection in which mycelia, as well as yeasts, invade tissue and form microabscesses.

FACTORS THAT PREDISPOSE TO CANDIDIASIS
Loss of integrity of skin and mucosae
• Maceration of skin due to climate or obesity • Eczema • Dentures
Encouragement of local multiplication of *Candida*
• Alteration of mucosal flora: antibiotic treatment • Hormonal: diabetes, pregnancy
Suppression of inflammatory and immune responses
• Specific congenital T lymphocyte defect • Leucopenia of any cause • Immunosuppressive drugs, including topical corticosteroids • Malignancy • Human immunodeficiency virus infection

Clinical features

Infections of the skin may resemble those caused by other dermatophytes but are most common where the skin is moist and in contact with itself, e.g. groins, perineum, breasts, axillae. Nail infections start at the base, forming ridges, often accompanied by paronychia. In the mouth, white curd-like patches are seen, which can be scraped away leaving a bleeding base. Atrophy of the gums and angular stomatitis are common in the elderly. Vaginitis causes intense pruritus and a thick creamy discharge. In children affected by mucocutaneous candidiasis, there is widespread involvement of skin, nails, hair and mucosae, which is troublesome, disfiguring and responds poorly to treatment. Systemic candidiasis may present as septicaemia or with the features of an infection of oesophagus, gastrointestinal tract, heart, lungs, urinary tract or brain meninges.

Investigations

The yeast may be identified microscopically or by culture from swabs or scrapings from the lesions and be cultured from the blood in systemic disease. Underlying local or systemic defects should be sought.

Management

Most important is to correct or control the underlying predisposition. Cutaneous candidiasis is treated with a topical azole ointment (see Table 2.7, p. 74). Mucosal infection usually responds well to lozenges or suspension of nystatin or amphotericin. Persistent infections and nail infections require oral fluconazole or itraconazole. Systemic infections should be treated with intravenous amphotericin or with amphotericin plus flucytosine.

PITYRIASIS VERSICOLOR

This trivial but often unsightly condition is due to an overgrowth of the normally commensal yeast, *Pityrosporum orbiculare*. It is especially prevalent in hot humid climates.

Clinical features

Pityriasis versicolor mainly affects young adults. The term 'versicolor' refers to the process whereby asymptomatic fawn, scaly and slightly wrinkled macules become depigmented and non-scaly after sun exposure. The rash is most common on the upper trunk. The depigmented lesions should not be mistaken for patches of vitiligo (see p. 589).

Investigations

The diagnosis can be confirmed by microscopic examination of skin scrapings cleared with potassium hydroxide.

Management

2.5% selenium sulphide in a detergent base (Selsun shampoo) is useful and relatively cheap. It is lathered on to affected areas, allowed to dry and left overnight before washing off the next morning. Applications once weekly for a month are usually adequate. Topical imidazole preparations are an effective alternative, though treatment for 1 month is usually required. Stubborn or widespread infections are best treated with a short course of itraconazole (200 mg daily for 7 days).

SUBCUTANEOUS FUNGAL INFECTIONS

MYCETOMA (MADURA FOOT)

Mycetoma, in this restricted sense, is a chronic fungal infection of the deep soft tissues and bones, most commonly of the limbs, but also of the abdominal or chest wall or head. It is produced by members of two groups of organisms classified as *Eumycetes* and aerobic *Actinomycetes*. A feature common to both groups is the formation of grains, which are colonies of matted organisms with characteristic colours, ranging from 60 microns to 3 mm in diameter. The incidence appears to be related to climate, being especially high when an arid hot season ends in rains. The more common species of fungi causing mycetoma are shown in Table 2.26.

Table 2.26 Fungi causing mycetoma

Species	Type of grain
Eumycetoma	
Madurella mycetomatis	Brown or black (big)
Madurella grisea	Black or brown (big)
Exophiala jeanselmei	Black
Pseudallescheria boydii	White or yellow (big)
Acremonium spp.	White or yellow
Actinomycetoma	
Actinomadura madurae	White, yellow or red (big)
Actinomadura pelletieri	Red (small)
Streptomyces somaliensis	White or yellow (big)
Nocardia brasiliensis	White or yellow (microscopic)

Pathology

The histology is that of a chronic granuloma with a fibrous stroma and cyst-like spaces in which lie the characteristic grains.

Clinical features

The fungus is usually introduced by a thorn and the infection is most common in the foot. The mycetoma begins as a painless swelling at the site of implantation, which grows and spreads steadily within the soft tissues causing further swelling, and eventually penetrates bones. Nodules develop under the epidermis and these rupture revealing sinuses through which grains are discharged. Some sinuses may heal with scarring while fresh sinuses appear elsewhere.

There is little pain and usually no fever nor lymphadenopathy, but there is progressive disability. When the lesion is in the scalp, the skull may be affected but the dura mater appears to be an effective barrier. *Nocardia brasiliensis* often affects the skin of the back. It is seldom localised and may spread widely.

Investigations

Diagnosis is confirmed by demonstration of fungal grains in pus or tissue biopsy. Culture is usually necessary for species identification. Specific antibodies can usually be detected by precipitation.

Management

The difference between *Eumycetes* and *Actinomycetes* is crucial because there is no drug of proven efficacy for the former. Sporadic successes against *Eumycetes* have been reported with griseofulvin, ketoconazole or itraconazole, but the results have been mostly disappointing and eumycetoma requires to be excised. It has a tendency to recur. Treatment with liposomal amphotericin or long-term oral terbinafine is currently being evaluated.

The treatment of actinomycetoma is more helpful. It consists of rifampicin (4 mg/kg daily by mouth) or streptomycin (14 mg/kg daily i.m.) for 3 months plus oral dapsone (1.5 mg/kg 12-hourly) or oral co-trimoxazole for 4–24 months. *Nocardia* infection may respond to dapsone alone. Precipitating antibodies disappear if treatment is successful.

Table 2.27 Subcutaneous fungal infections, other than mycetoma

	Zygomycosis	Chromoblastomycosis	Rhinosporidiosis	Sporotrichosis
Agent	Several	Several	*Rhinosporidium seeberi*	*Sporothrix schenckii*
Geography	Tropics	Tropics	Widespread, e.g. South America, India, East Africa	Central and South Africa
Site	Face, limbs, systemic in immunocompromised or diabetic	Feet, others	Nose, cheeks	Limbs, rarely systemic
Presentation	Subcutaneous swellings	Mossy foot	Nasal polyps, subcutaneous nodules	Subcutaneous swellings, ulcer, lymphatic spread, rare cases of meningitis
Management	Potassium iodide 1.5–3.5 g daily, amphotericin B or itraconazole	Flucytosine and/or itraconazole	Surgery	Potassium iodide 10 g daily, itraconazole or terbinafine

OTHER SUBCUTANEOUS MYCOSES

These are summarised in Table 2.27.

SYSTEMIC FUNGAL INFECTIONS

HISTOPLASMOSIS

Histoplasmosis is caused by *Histoplasma capsulatum* (Darling) which is a yeast in its parasitic phase but is a filamentous fungus of soil at other times. A variant, *Histoplasma duboisii*, is found in parts of tropical Africa.

H. capsulatum multiplies in soil enriched by the droppings of birds and bats, and the spores remain viable for years. Natural infections are found in several species of small mammal, including bats. Infection is by inhalation of infected dust. The infection is an especial hazard for explorers of caves and people who clear out bird (including chicken) roosts.

H. capsulatum is found in all parts of the USA, especially in the east central states, and less commonly in Latin America from Mexico to Argentina, in Europe, North, South and East Africa, Nigeria, Malaysia, Indonesia and Australia.

Pathology

The parasite in its yeast phase multiplies mainly in monocytes and macrophages and produces areas of necrosis in which the parasites may abound. From these foci the blood stream may be invaded, producing metastatic lesions in the liver, spleen and lymph nodes. Pulmonary histoplasmosis may cause pathological changes similar to those of tuberculosis, including the production of a primary complex with enlarged regional lymph nodes, multiple small discrete lesions and occasionally cavitation. Healed lesions may calcify.

Clinical features

These are listed in the information box.

CLINICAL SYNDROMES ASSOCIATED WITH INFECTIONS WITH *HISTOPLASMA CAPSULATUM*

Infection by inhalation

- Subclinical disease: the majority of infections
- Self-limiting fever, chills, cough, chest pain, fatigue, dyspnoea. Occasionally fatal pulmonary insufficiency due to heavy infection causing severe alveolitis

Inoculation

- Solitary lesion of skin or mucosa

Disseminated histoplasmosis

Pattern depends on age and immunity
- *Acute* in children: severe, with fever, hepatosplenomegaly, cough, pancytopenia
- *Subacute* in the majority: fever, lymphadenopathy, hepatosplenomegaly, focal lesions of oropharynx, gut, adrenals, endocardium, meninges, brain
- *Chronic* in adults: low-grade fever with fatigue. Various focal lesions possible

Chronic localised infection

- Notably pulmonary bullae resembling cavitating tuberculosis

Investigations

In an area where the disease occurs, histoplasmosis should be suspected in every obscure infection in which there are pulmonary signs or where there are enlarged lymph nodes or hepatosplenomegaly. Tissue is obtained by biopsy for an impression smear, histology and culture. Radiological examination in long-standing cases may show calcified lesions in the lungs, spleen or other organs. In the more acute phases of the disease single or multiple soft pulmonary shadows with enlarged tracheobronchial nodes are seen.

Delayed hypersensitivity to the intradermal injection of histoplasmin develops in patients with either active or healed infections but is usually negative in acute disseminated disease. Complement-fixing antibodies are detected within 3 weeks of the onset of an acute primary infection and increase in titre as the disease progresses. Precipitating antibodies may also be detected.

Management

Specific treatment with amphotericin is indicated only in severe infections; the dosage (0.5 mg/kg in 500 ml of 5% glucose) is given intravenously over a 6-hour period, gradually increasing to a maximum of 1.0 mg/kg. Treatment is given on alternate days to a total adult dose of 2 g. If badly tolerated, the dose may have to be reduced. Side-effects are anorexia, nausea, fever, headache, and venous thrombosis which may be controlled by the addition of 10 mg prednisolone to the intravenous solution. Plasma urea rises and haemoglobin falls during treatment but later they return to normal. Amphotericin may have to be continued for up to 3 months or longer, depending on the clinical response. Severe dyspnoea in histoplasmosis should be treated with prednisolone 20–40 mg daily for a few days. Itraconazole 200–400 mg daily can be used in chronic pulmonary histoplasmosis and chronic disseminated histoplasmosis.

HISTOPLASMA DUBOISII

Histoplasma duboisii, the fungus of African histoplasmosis, is larger than the classical *H. capsulatum*. It is found throughout East, Central and West Africa.

This disease differs in several ways from *H. capsulatum* infection. The bones, skin, lymph nodes and liver develop granulomatous lesions or cold abscesses resembling tuberculosis, but the lungs are seldom involved. The visceral form with liver and splenic invasion is often fatal, while ulcerative skin lesions and bone abscesses follow a more benign course.

Radiological examination may show rounded foci of bone destruction, sometimes associated with abscess formation. Multiple lesions of the ribs are common and the bones of the limbs may be involved. Systemic disease is treated in the same way as *H. capsulatum* infections. A solitary lesion in bone may require only local surgical treatment.

ASPERGILLOSIS

This is the most common respiratory mycosis in Britain and is discussed on page 354.

COCCIDIOIDOMYCOSIS

This is caused by *Coccidioides immitis* and found in the southern USA, and Central and South America. The disease is acquired by inhalation. The infection behaves like tuberculosis or histoplasmosis. In 60% of cases it is asymptomatic. In 40% of cases it affects the lungs, lymph nodes and skin. Rarely, it may be carried by the blood stream to the bones, adrenals, meninges and other organs. Pulmonary coccidioidomycosis has two forms: primary and progressive. Primary coccidioidomycosis behaves like primary tuberculosis or histoplasmosis and is often asymptomatic. The progressive form of the disease is associated with marked systemic upset and features of lobar pneumonia. In more chronic cases it may resemble chronic tuberculosis. Infections, including subclinical attacks, are followed by immunity.

The fungi grow readily on culture media but as they are highly infective, diagnostic investigations are usually limited to intradermal, complement fixation and precipitin tests.

Amphotericin (as for histoplasmosis), itraconazole, ketoconazole or fluconazole may be helpful but relapse is common. Some localised pulmonary lesions can be treated by surgery.

PARACOCCIDIOIDOMYCOSIS

This is caused by *Paracoccidioides brasiliensis* and occurs in South America. Mucocutaneous lesions occur early. Involvement of lymphatic nodes and the lungs is prominent and the gastrointestinal tract may also be attacked. Most patients respond to ketoconazole 200 mg/day for at least 6 months; itraconazole 100–200 mg daily is an alternative. Liver function must be monitored for either agent. For those who do not respond, amphotericin (as for histoplasmosis) may be used.

BLASTOMYCOSIS

North American blastomycosis is caused by *Blastomyces dermatitidis*. It also occurs in Africa. Systemic infection begins in the lungs and mediastinal lymph nodes and resembles pulmonary tuberculosis. Bones, skin and the genitourinary tract may also be affected. Treatment is with itraconazole 200–400 mg daily, ketoconazole 200–400 mg daily or amphotericin (see above).

CRYPTOCOCCOSIS

This is caused by *Cryptococcus neoformans*. Its distribution is world-wide. It causes local gumma-like tumours and granulomatous lesions of the lung, bones, brain and meninges. The CSF often contains the fungus when the nervous system is affected. Immunocompromised individuals are at special risk, including those with human immunodeficiency virus infection.

The diagnosis is made by culture or recognition of spores in the CSF biopsy and serological detection of antigen.

Amphotericin should be given intravenously (see above) and flucytosine orally (see p. 75). Surgical removal of local pulmonary lesions may be necessary. Recovery may be monitored by fall in antigen titre. Cryptococcal meningitis is particularly important in HIV infection.

CANDIDIASIS

Candida albicans is a cause of systemic fungal infection in the immunosuppressed (see pp. 97 and 144).

FURTHER INFORMATION ON DISEASES DUE TO FUNGI (MYCOSES)

Hay R J 1996 Yeast infections. Dermatologic Clinics 14: 113–124
McGinnis M R 1996 Mycetoma. Dermatologic Clinics 14: 97–104
Rex J H, Walsh T J, Anaissie E J 1998 Fungal infections in iatrogenically compromised hosts. Advances in Internal Medicine 43: 321–371
Rinaldi M G 1997 Controversies in medical mycology. Dermatology 194, suppl. 1: 45–47

DISEASES DUE TO PROTOZOA

Protozoa are unicellular eukaryotic organisms and belong to the animal kingdom. They are more complex than bacteria and often motile. Many are free-living and do not infect humans or other animals. Others have become specialised and have acquired precise biological niches as parasites of animals, including humans. In the well-defined anatomical and biochemical microclimate of each niche, from which they seldom stray, the protozoa can multiply freely, until contained by the immune response. In order to survive transmission to another host, they must either transform into strong-walled cysts that can resist harsh external conditions (e.g. *Entamoeba*, *Giardia*), or pass through a vector insect or bug (e.g. *Plasmodium* in the mosquito), in which a second cycle of multiplication takes place. The vector also acts as a reservoir of infection, of variable efficiency. Some protozoa have acquired an intermediate host, in which the organism may persist in a dormant state for many years (e.g. *Toxoplasma* in the muscles of herbivores) and humans may only be incidental hosts.

Protozoal diseases are of especial importance among livestock in the tropics. Epidemics of Ngama (cattle trypanosomiasis) and East Coast fever (theileriosis) have given rise to famine. The important human diseases due to protozoa are listed in the information box.

PROTOZOAL DISEASES OF HUMANS
In the blood
• Malaria, trypanosomiasis
In the gut
• Giardiasis, amoebiasis, cyclosporiasis
In the tissues
• Toxoplasmosis, leishmaniasis

MALARIA

Human malaria is caused by *Plasmodium falciparum*, *P. vivax*, *P. ovale* and *P. malariae*. It is transmitted by the bite of anopheline mosquitoes, in which the parasite undergoes a temperature-dependent cycle of development. Malaria is therefore predominantly a disease of hot, wet climates, but it used to occur in Europe as far north as England and Denmark. Malaria may also be transmitted by blood transfusion or injection. Transplacental infection may occur.

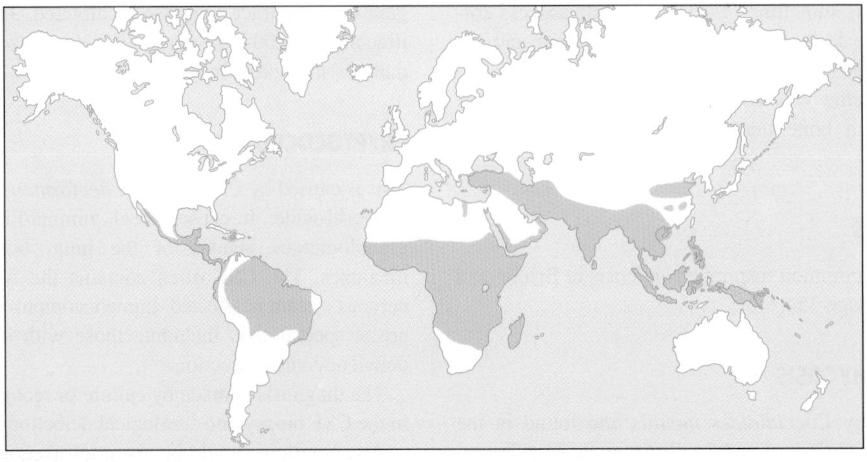

Fig. 2.34 Distribution of malaria.

Malaria is endemic or sporadic throughout most of the tropics and subtropics below an altitude of 1500 m, excluding the Mediterranean littoral, the USA and Australia (see Fig. 2.34). One hundred million people are attacked annually, of whom 1% die, mainly children. Following WHO-sponsored campaigns of prevention and more effective treatment, the incidence of malaria was greatly reduced in 1950–60 but since 1970 there has been a resurgence. In the 1980s *P. falciparum* became resistant to chloroquine over a steadily increasing area (see Table 2.29, p. 153). Most serious was the emergence of resistance in Africa, where it is now widespread. Malaria due to this parasite is more severe than that due to the sensitive parasites.

Due to increased travel and neglect of chemoprophylaxis, over 2000 cases are imported annually into Britain. Most are due to *P. falciparum*, usually from Africa, and of these 1% die because of late diagnosis. A few people living near airports in Europe have acquired malaria from accidentally imported mosquitoes.

Pathogenesis

Life cycle of parasite (see Figs 2.35 and 2.36)

The female anopheline mosquito becomes infected when it feeds on human blood containing gametocytes, the sexual forms of the malarial parasite. The development in the mosquito takes from 7–20 days. Sporozoites inoculated by an infected mosquito disappear from human blood within half an hour and enter the liver. After some days (see Table 2.28) merozoites leave the liver and invade red blood cells, where further asexual cycles of multiplication take place, producing schizonts. Rupture of the schizont releases more merozoites into the blood and causes fever, whose periodicity depends on the species of parasite.

P. vivax and *P. ovale* may persist in liver cells as dormant forms, hypnozoites, capable of developing into merozoites months or years later. Thus the first attack of clinical malaria may occur long after the patient has left the endemic area, and the disease may relapse after treatment with drugs that kill only the erythrocytic stage of the parasite.

P. falciparum and *P. malariae* have no persistent exoerythrocytic phase but recrudescences of fever may result from multiplication in the red cells of parasites which have not been eliminated by treatment and immune processes.

Effects on red blood cells and capillaries

Malaria is always accompanied by haemolysis and in a

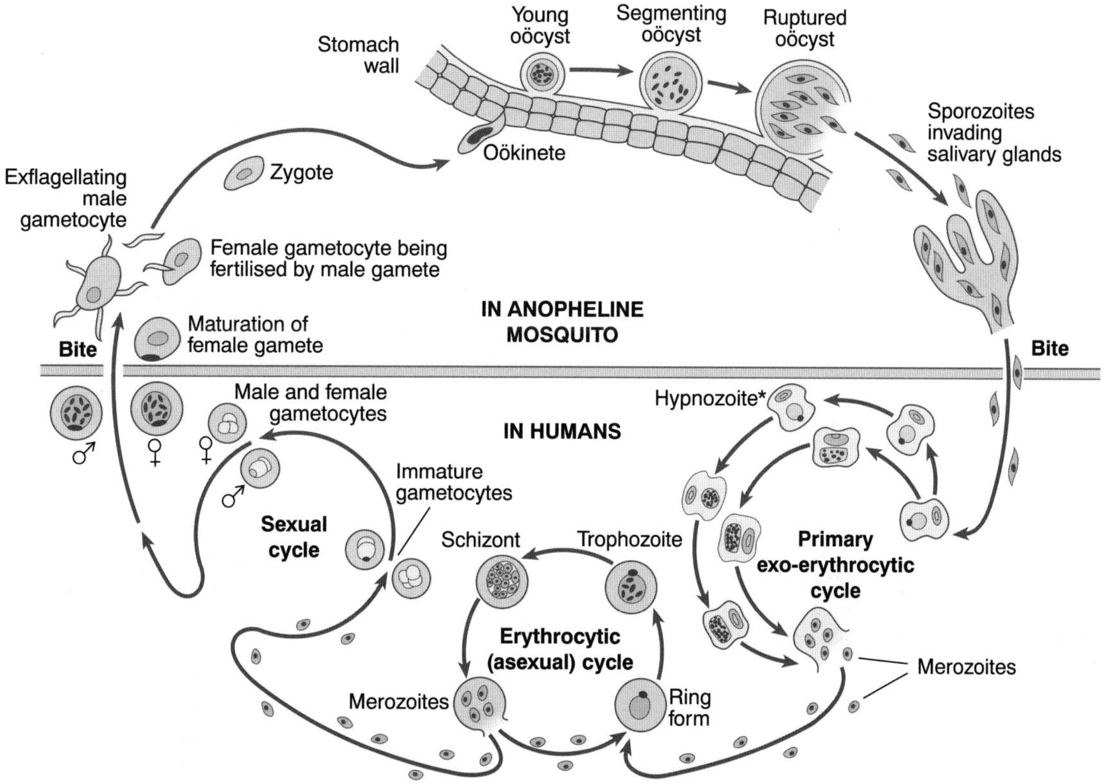

Fig. 2.35 Malarial parasites. Life cycle. Hypnozoites(*) are present only in *P. vivax* and *P. ovale* infections.

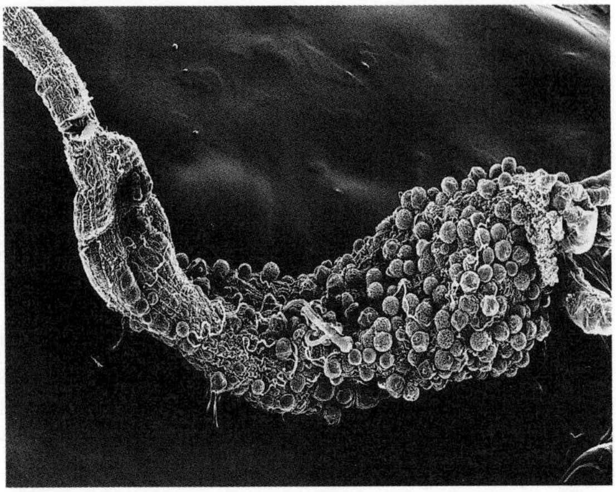

A

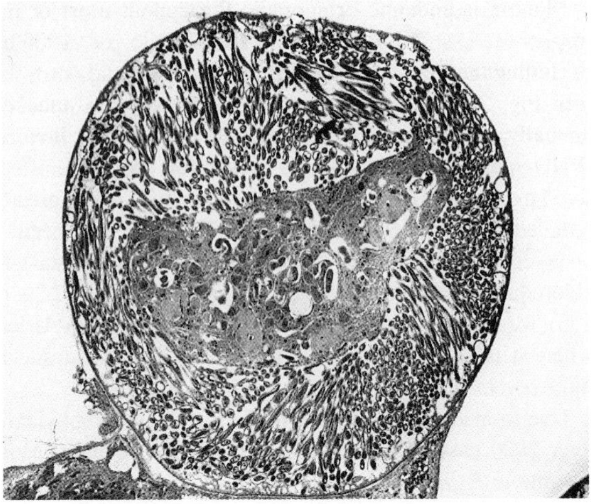

B

Fig. 2.36 Electron microscopic appearance of oöcysts and sporozoites in the anopheline mosquito phase of the life cycle of *Plasmodium falciparum*. A Oöcysts lining the mosquito's stomach (scanning electron micrograph). B Sporozoites within an oöcyst (transmission electron micrograph).

Table 2.28 Relationships between life cycle of parasite and clinical features of malaria

Cycle/feature	*P. vivax, P. ovale*	*P. malariae*	*P. falciparum*
Pre-patent period (minimum incubation)	8–25 days	15–30 days	8–25 days
Asexual cycle	48 hrs synchronous	72 hrs synchronous	< 48 hrs asynchronous
Periodicity of fever	'Tertian'	'Quartan'	Aperiodic
Exo-erythrocytic cycle	Persistent as hypnozoites	Pre-erythrocytic only	Pre-erythrocytic only
Delayed onset	Common	Rare	Rare
Relapses	Common up to 2 years	Recrudescence many years later	Recrudescence up to 1 year

severe or prolonged attack anaemia may be profound. The causes of anaemia are listed in the information box.

Haemolysis is most severe with *P. falciparum*, which invades red cells of all ages but especially young cells. *P. vivax* and *P. ovale* invade reticulocytes, and *P. malariae* normoblasts, so that infections remain lighter.

In *P. falciparum* malaria, red cells containing schizonts adhere to the lining of capillaries in brain, kidney, liver, lungs and gut. The vessels become congested and the organs anoxic. Rupture of schizonts liberates toxic and antigenic substances which may cause further damage.

CAUSES OF ANAEMIA IN MALARIA

- Haemolysis of infected erythrocytes
- Haemolysis of uninfected erythrocytes
- Dyserythropoiesis
- Splenomegaly causing erythrocyte sequestration and haemodilution
- Depletion of folate stores

Thus the main effects of malaria are haemolytic anaemia and, with *P. falciparum*, widespread organ damage.

P. falciparum does not grow well in red cells that contain haemoglobin F, C or especially S. Haemoglobin S heterozygotes (AS) are protected against the lethal complications of malaria. *P. vivax* cannot enter red cells that lack the Duffy blood group. West African and American Black people are protected.

Clinical features

Malaria in the non-immune

This is the pattern in children in an endemic area once they have lost the protection conferred by maternal antibodies, or in visitors of any age from a non-endemic area. The incubation period is often longer than the pre-erythrocytic cycle and may be up to several weeks for *P. falciparum* or months for *P. vivax*.

P. vivax and P. ovale malaria. In many cases the illness starts with a period of several days of continued fever before the development of classical bouts of fever on alternate days. Fever starts with a rigor. The patient feels cold and the temperature rises to about 40°C. After half an hour to an hour the hot or flush phase begins. It lasts several hours and gives way to profuse perspiration and gradual fall in temperature. The cycle is repeated 48 hours later. Gradually the spleen and liver enlarge and may become tender. Anaemia develops slowly. Herpes simplex is common. Relapses are common in the first 2 years of leaving the malarious area.

P. malariae infection. This is usually associated with mild symptoms and bouts of fever every third day. Parasitaemia may persist for many years with the occasional recrudescence of fever, or without producing any symptoms. *P. malariae* causes glomerulonephritis and the nephrotic syndrome in children.

P. falciparum infections. These are more dangerous than other forms of malaria. The onset, especially of primary attacks, is often insidious, with malaise, headache and vomiting. Cough and mild diarrhoea are common, suggesting influenza. The fever has no particular pattern and does not usually rise quite so high as in the other forms. The cold, hot and sweating stages are seldom found. Jaundice is common due to haemolysis and hepatic dysfunction. The liver and spleen enlarge and become tender. Anaemia develops rapidly.

A patient with *falciparum* malaria, apparently not seriously ill, may develop serious complications. Children die rapidly without any special symptoms other than fever. Immunity is impaired in pregnancy, and abortion from parasitisation of the maternal side of the placenta is frequent. Splenectomy increases the risk of severe malaria.

Mixed infections with more than one species of malaria parasite may occur.

The complications of *falciparum* malaria are listed in the information box.

Cerebral malaria. This is the most urgent complication and is manifested either by confusion or coma, usually without localising signs.

Blackwater fever. This is associated with chronic *falciparum* malaria, most commonly in those who have taken antimalarial treatment irregularly, or are deficient in glucose-6-phosphate dehydrogenase. Haemolysis is unpredictable and severe, destroying uninfected as well as parasitised red cells. The urine is dark or black.

Endemic malaria

The manifestations of malaria in people who grow up in an endemic area vary with the degree of endemicity, the age of the patient and the development of immunity.

In hypoendemic areas little immunity is acquired, epidemics of malaria are liable to occur and the disease does not differ materially from that in non-immunes.

COMPLICATIONS OF MALARIA DUE TO *PLASMODIUM FALCIPARUM*

Severe anaemia

Organ damage due to anoxia
- Brain: confusion, coma
- Kidneys: oliguria, uraemia (acute tubular necrosis)
- Lungs: cough, pulmonary oedema
- Intestine: diarrhoea, congestion, possibly leaky to bacteria
- Liver: jaundice, encephalopathy (rare)

Intravascular haemolysis
- Blackwater fever

Hypoglycaemia, especially with quinine treatment

Shock secondary to septicaemia

Hypotensive shock

Metabolic acidosis

Splenic rupture

In pregnancy
- Maternal death, abortion, stillbirth, low birth weight

In mesoendemic areas malaria is frequent but only seasonal. Repeated infections lead to anaemia, considerable enlargement of the spleen, which is in danger of rupture, and chronic ill health with bouts of fever. The growth and development of children may be retarded.

In hyperendemic areas malaria transmission takes place throughout the year but with seasonal increases. Adults develop considerable immunity; although affected individuals may have palpable spleens and parasitaemia, malaria causes only occasional short bouts of fever.

In holoendemic areas malarial transmission is intense throughout the year and adults do not suffer from the infection although they support a low parasitaemia and the spleen becomes impalpable.

In hyperendemic and in holoendemic areas malaria may kill up to 15–20% of children below the age of 5 years. Pregnancy lowers resistance to malaria. The risks are greatest in the first pregnancy (see the information box above).

Hyperreactive malarial splenomegaly (tropical splenomegaly syndrome)

In some hyperendemic areas gross splenomegaly is associated with an exaggerated immune response to malaria and is seen, unexpectedly, in adults who have high antibody titres to malaria and low parasitaemias. The condition, which is more common in females and in certain racial and family groups, is characterised by enormous overproduction of IgM, levels reaching 3–20 times the local mean value. Much of the IgM is aggregated with other immunoglobulin or complement and precipitates in the cold, in vitro. IgM aggregates are phagocytosed by reticulo-endothelial cells in the spleen and liver, and the demonstration of this by immunofluorescence in a liver biopsy section is diagnostic. Light microscopy of the liver usually shows sinusoidal lymphocytosis. Anaemia and lymphocytosis can be confused with leukaemia. Portal hypertension may develop.

Investigations

Malaria should be considered if a febrile patient is in, or has recently left, a malarious locality. Besides malaria there are many causes for acute febrile splenomegaly in the tropics. Gross enlargement of the spleen may also result from tuberculosis, visceral leishmaniasis, schistosomiasis and chronic brucellosis as well as leukaemia and lymphoma. Well-stained blood films, thick and thin, should be repeated if necessary. *P. falciparum* parasites may be very scanty, especially in patients who have been partially treated. With *P. falciparum* only ring forms are normally seen in the early stages. With the other species all stages of the erythrocytic cycle may be found. Gametocytes appear after about 2 weeks. They persist despite treatment and are harmless. Immunochromatographic 'dip-stick' tests for *P. falciparum* antigen are now marketed and provide a useful non-microscopic means of diagnosing this infection. They should be used in parallel with blood film examination. Malaria may coexist with other diseases and not be the cause of the illness in semi-immune persons in endemic areas.

Management

Chemotherapy of the acute attack

For all infections with *P. vivax*, *P. ovale* and *P. malariae*, the drug of choice is chloroquine. The usual course of treatment is 600 mg of the effective *base* followed by 300 mg *base* in 6 hours then 150 mg *base* twice daily for 2 more days.

In most areas of the world *P. falciparum* is now resistant to chloroquine, so this agent should not be used to treat *falciparum* malaria unless it is certain the infection was acquired in an area of chloroquine sensitivity. Infections with *P. falciparum* from a chloroquine-resistant area should be treated with quinine dihydrochloride or sulphate 600 mg *salt* (10 mg/kg) 8-hourly by mouth until better and the blood is free of parasites (usually 3–5 days). This regimen should be followed by a single dose of sulfadoxine 1.5 g combined with pyrimethamine 75 mg, i.e. 3 tablets of Fansidar. The dose is reduced to 12-hourly if quinine toxicity develops. In pregnancy a 7-day course of quinine alone should be given. If sulphonamide sensitivity is suspected, quinine may be followed by tetracycline 250 mg 6-hourly for 7 days. Alternatives to quinine plus Fansidar are mefloquine 20 mg/kg *base* up to a maximum 1.5 g, in two divided doses 8 hours apart; Malarone (atovaquone 250 mg plus proguanil 100 mg) 4 tablets once daily for 3 days, or halofantrine 500 mg every 6 hours for 3 doses. Mefloquine may occasionally cause alarming neuropsychiatric side-effects which can persist for several days due to its plasma half-life of 14 days. Halofantrine is now rarely used due to its potential to induce hazardous cardiac arrhythmias in susceptible individuals.

Management of complicated P. falciparum *malaria*

Patients with 'cerebral malaria' or other severe manifestations, or those who are non-immune with more than 1% of red cells infected, are medical emergencies. Quinine is indicated if a chloroquine-resistant infection is at all likely. Quinine is given as an intravenous infusion over 4 hours. The dose is 10 mg/kg of quinine *salt* up to a maximum 700 mg. The dose should be repeated at intervals of 8–12 hours until the patient can take drugs orally. In severely ill patients a loading dose infusion of 20 mg/kg quinine *salt* up to a maximum 1.4 g can be given over 4 hours, then after 8–12 hours maintenance dosage at 10 mg/kg quinine *salt* as above. The loading dose should *not* be given if the patient has received quinine, quinidine or mefloquine during the previous 24 hours. Quinine may instead be given intramuscularly but may cause necrosis of muscle; the hydrochloride is less irritant than the dihydrochloride. In a comatose patient lumbar puncture may be indicated to exclude coexisting bacterial meningitis.

Severe anaemia requires transfusion with packed red cells. Careful attention to fluid balance is essential; underhydration or overhydration is dangerous. If oliguria develops, frusemide or an infusion of mannitol may forestall renal failure. Intravenous fluid, if necessary, should be monitored by the central venous pressure because pulmonary oedema is more likely to develop if the patient is overinfused. Exchange blood transfusion is life-saving in complicated very heavy infections (over 10% of red cells infected). Hypoglycaemia, especially in children or in pregnancy, or septicaemia may be the cause of failure to respond to treatment. Dialysis may be needed if renal failure develops.

Management of tropical splenomegaly syndrome

Splenomegaly and anaemia usually resolve over a period of months of continuous treatment with proguanil 100 mg daily, which should be continued for life to prevent relapse. Complicating folate deficiency is treated with folic acid 5 mg daily.

Radical cure of malaria due to P. vivax *and* P. ovale

Relapses can be prevented by taking one of the antimalarial drugs in suppressive doses. Radical cure is achieved in most patients by a course of primaquine (15 mg per day for 14 days) which destroys the hypnozoite phase in the liver. Haemolysis may develop in those who are glucose-6-phosphate dehydrogenase (G6PD)-deficient. Cyanosis due to the formation of methaemoglobin in the red cells is more common but not dangerous.

Prevention

Chemoprophylaxis

Clinical attacks of malaria may be preventable by drugs such as proguanil which attack the pre-erythrocytic form ('causal prophylaxis'), or by drugs such as chloroquine or mefloquine after it has entered the erythrocyte ('suppression'). Table 2.29 gives the recommended doses for protection of the non-immune. Expert advice is required for individuals unable to tolerate the first-line agents listed, or in whom they are contraindicated. Doses for children vary, depending on age and body weight. Reference should be made according to standard dosage recommendations (*British National Formulary* in the UK). Chemoprophylaxis is begun 1 week before entering the malarious area and is continued until 4 weeks after leaving it. Resistance to the cheap and well-tolerated drug proguanil is increasing, and frequently coincides with the much more serious spread of chloroquine resistance. Chloroquine should not be taken continuously as prophylactic for over 5 years without regular ophthalmic examination, as it may cause irreversible retinopathy. Pregnant and lactating women may take proguanil or chloroquine safely. Mefloquine is contraindicated in the first trimester of pregnancy. Fansidar should not be used for chemoprophylaxis, as deaths have occurred from agranulocytosis or Stevens–Johnson syndrome. Mefloquine is useful in areas of multiple drug resistance, such as East and Central Africa and Papua New Guinea. Experience shows it to be safe for at least 2 years. There are several contraindications to its use (see Table 2.29).

Chemoprophylaxis alone may not be sufficient to prevent malaria. It is also important to avoid anopheline mosquitoes, which bite at night. Long sleeves and trousers should be worn outside the house. Repellent creams and sprays can be used. Screened windows, the use of a mosquito net and burning repellent coils or tablets also reduce the risk.

AMOEBIASIS

Amoebiasis is usually caused by *Entamoeba histolytica*, a pathogenic intestinal amoeba that is spread between humans by its cysts. It is common throughout the tropics and occasionally acquired in Britain. The parasite formerly termed *E. histolytica* is now known to consist of two separate species, *E. dispar*, which is *non*-pathogenic and *E. histolytica*, which *is* pathogenic. Cysts of these two species are morphologically identical, but can be distinguished by molecular techniques, isoenzyme studies, or monoclonal antibody typing after culture of the trophozoites. Only *E. histolytica* can give rise to amoebic dysentery or extraintestinal amoebiasis, e.g. amoebic liver abscess. In addition, two amoebae of genera *Naegleria* and *Acanthamoeba*, which inhabit polluted surface water and swimming pools all over the world, are occasional causes respectively of fulminating meningitis and granulomatous encephalitis.

Pathology

Cysts of *E. histolytica* survive well outside the body and are ingested in water or uncooked food which has been contaminated by human faeces. Lettuce is a common vehicle of infection.

In the colon the vegetative trophozoite forms emerge from the cysts (see Fig. 2.37). While these remain free in the colon the condition is symptomless but the parasite may invade the mucous membrane of the large bowel. The lesions, which are usually maximal in the caecum but may be found as far down as the anal canal, are flask-shaped ulcers varying greatly in size and surrounded by healthy mucosa. A localised granuloma (amoeboma), presenting as a palpable mass in the rectum or causing a filling defect in

Table 2.29 Chemoprophylaxis of malaria

Area	Antimalarial tablets	Adult prophylactic dose	
Chloroquine resistance present[1]	Chloroquine[2]	150 mg base	Two tablets weekly
	PLUS Proguanil	100 mg	Two tablets daily
	OR Mefloquine[3]	250 mg	One tablet weekly
Chloroquine resistance absent	Chloroquine	150 mg base	Two tablets weekly
	OR Proguanil	100 mg	One or two tablets daily

[1] Choice of regimen is determined by area to be visited, length of stay, level of malaria transmission, level of drug resistance, presence of underlying disease in the traveller and concomitant medication taken.
[2] British preparations of chloroquine usually contain 150 mg base, French preparations 100 mg base and American preparations 300 mg base.
[3] Contraindicated with the first trimester of pregnancy, lactation, cardiac conduction disorders, epilepsy, psychiatric disorders. May cause neuropsychiatric disorders.

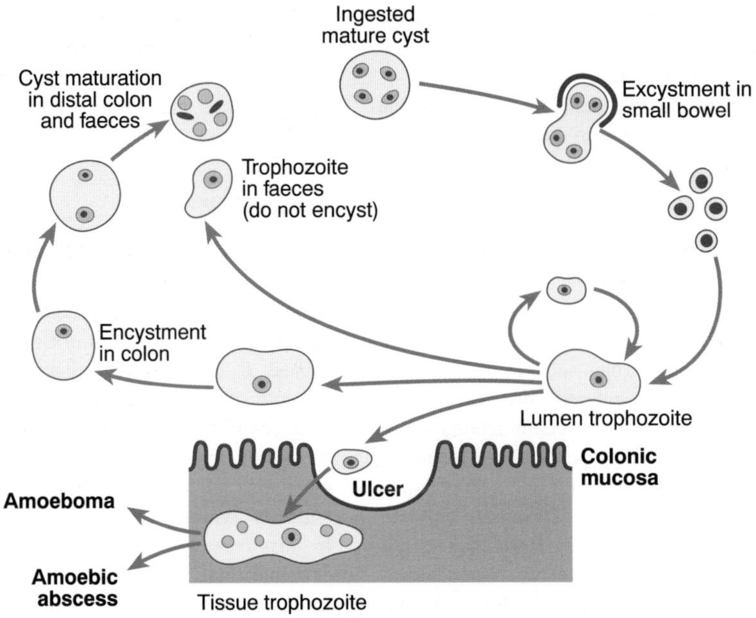

Fig. 2.37 Amoebiasis. Life cycle of *Entamoeba histolytica.*

the colon on radiography, is a rare complication. Since an amoeboma responds well to anti-amoebic treatment it is important that it is not mistaken for a colonic carcinoma.

Amoebae may enter a portal venous radicle and be carried to the liver where they multiply rapidly and destroy the parenchyma, causing an amoebic abscess. The liquid contents at first have a characteristic pinkish colour which later may change to chocolate brown.

Amoebic ulcers may cause severe haemorrhage but rarely perforate the bowel wall. Cutaneous amoebiasis presents as progressive genital or perianal ulceration or around abdominal surgical wounds. The incubation period of amoebiasis ranges from 2 weeks to many years.

Clinical features

Intestinal amoebiasis or amoebic dysentery

This usually runs a chronic course with grumbling abdominal pains and two or more unformed stools a day. Periods of diarrhoea alternating with constipation are common. Mucus is usually passed, sometimes with streaks of blood, and the stools often have an offensive odour. There may be tenderness along the line of the colon, usually more marked over the caecum and pelvic colon. The right iliac pain may simulate acute appendicitis. There may be more acute bowel symptoms, with very frequent motions and the passage of much blood and mucus, simulating bacillary dysentery or ulcerative colitis. This occurs particularly in the aged, in the puerperium and with superadded pyogenic infection of the ulcers.

Hepatic amoebiasis

This often occurs without a history of recent diarrhoea. It is common in the tropics and an important cause of imported fever in Britain. The abscess is usually found in the right hepatic lobe. Early symptoms may be local discomfort only and malaise; later, a swinging temperature and sweating may develop. An enlarged, tender liver, cough, and pain in the right shoulder are characteristic, but symptoms may remain vague and signs minimal. In particular, the less common abscess in the left lobe is difficult to diagnose. There is usually neutrophil leucocytosis and a raised diaphragm, with diminished movement on the right side. A large abscess may penetrate the diaphragm and rupture into the lung, from where its contents may be coughed up. Rupture into the pleural cavity, the peritoneal cavity or pericardial sac is less common but more serious.

Investigations

A careful naked-eye inspection of a freshly passed stool should be made. Any exudate is examined at once under the microscope for motile trophozoites, which are about 30 microns in diameter with a clear ectoplasm and a granular endoplasm, and usually contain red blood cells. Movements cease rapidly as the stool preparation cools. Sigmoidoscopy may reveal typical flask-shaped ulcers, and a scraping should be examined immediately for *E. histolytica*. Several stools may need to be examined in chronic amoebiasis before cysts are found. The presence of cysts in the faeces does not equate with invasive amoebiasis; in endemic areas one-third of the population are symptomless passers of amoebic cysts.

An amoebic abscess of the liver is suspected from the clinical and radiographic appearances and confirmed by ultrasonic scanning. Aspirated pus from an amoebic abscess has the characteristic appearance described above but only rarely contains free amoebae.

Antibodies are detectable by immunofluorescence in over 95% of patients with hepatic amoebiasis and intestinal amoeboma but in only about 60% of dysenteric amoebiasis.

Management

Invasive intestinal amoebiasis responds quickly to oral metronidazole (800 mg 8-hourly for 5 days) or tinidazole (single doses of 2 g daily for 3 days). Diloxanide furoate 500 mg should be given orally 8-hourly for 10 days after treatment to eliminate luminal cysts. Stools are re-examined 4 weeks later.

Early hepatic amoebiasis responds promptly to treatment with metronidazole or tinidazole as above, or to chloroquine 150 mg base 6-hourly for 2 days, followed by 150 mg 12-hourly for 19 days. Diloxanide furoate is given to eliminate the intestinal infection. If the abscess is large or threatens to burst, or if the response to chemotherapy is not prompt, aspiration is required and repeated if necessary. Rupture of an abscess into the pleural cavity, pericardial sac or peritoneal cavity necessitates immediate aspiration or surgical drainage. Small serous effusions resolve without drainage.

Prevention

Personal precautions against contracting amoebiasis in the tropics and subtropics consist of not eating fresh uncooked vegetables nor drinking unboiled water.

GIARDIASIS

Infection with the flagellate *Giardia intestinalis*, known also as *G. lamblia*, is world-wide but common in the tropics. It particularly affects children in endemic areas, tourists and immunosuppressed individuals and may be a commensal in some individuals. It is the parasite most commonly imported into Britain. The cysts remain viable in water for up to 3 months and infection usually occurs by ingesting contaminated water. The flagellates attach to the mucosa of the duodenum and jejunum and cause inflammation (see Fig. 2.38).

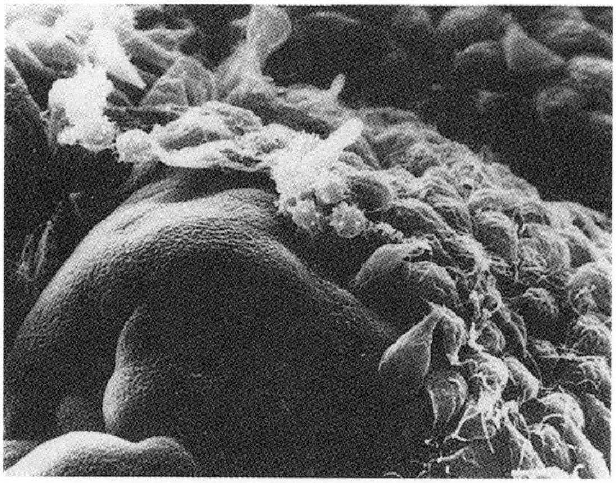

Fig. 2.38 Trophozoites of *Giardia lamblia* swarming over jejunal mucosa. Electron micrograph.

Clinical features

After an incubation period of 1–3 weeks, there is diarrhoea, abdominal pain, weakness, anorexia, nausea and vomiting. On examination there may be abdominal distension and tenderness. These features usually last for only a few days but in some individuals they continue for weeks or months. Such patients become lethargic and flatulent and lose weight. Investigation may reveal steatorrhoea, malabsorption of xylose and vitamin B_{12}, lactose intolerance and partial villous atrophy. Thus in persons returning from the tropics with diarrhoea, giardiasis may be confused with tropical sprue, and in residents of Western communities it must be considered in the differential diagnosis of other causes of malabsorption such as coeliac disease or Crohn's disease of the small intestine.

Investigations

Stools are obtained at 2–3-day intervals on three separate occasions and examined for cysts. The diagnostic yield is improved by examination of duodenal or jejunal fluid. Thus if endoscopy is being performed for upper gastrointestinal symptoms, it is important to remember the possibility of giardiasis and to aspirate juice for microscopic examination. If a jejunal biopsy is obtained, the mucus should be examined fresh. Histology shows *Giardia* on the surface of the epithelium. Jejunal mucus may be obtained with a string test (Enterotest capsule).

Management

Treatment is with a single dose of tinidazole 40 mg/kg in the range 0.5–2 g, or metronidazole 2 g once daily for 3 days. Albendazole 400 mg daily for 5 days is an effective alternative, but does not have a UK product licence for use in giardiasis.

CRYPTOSPORIDIOSIS

Cryptosporidium parvum is a coccidian protozoan of humans and domestic animals. Infection is acquired by the faecal-oral route. Contaminated water supplies have led to large outbreaks of human infection. The incubation period is approximately 7–10 days, followed by watery diarrhoea and abdominal cramps. The illness is usually self-limiting, but in immunocompromised patients, especially those with AIDS, the illness can be devastating, with persistent severe diarrhoea and substantial weight loss. In such cases *Cryptosporidium* can affect the biliary tree, leading to acalculous cholecystitis or sclerosing cholangitis. Pancreatitis and infection of the respiratory tract can also occur. Diagnosis is by demonstrating the oöcysts on faecal microscopy. In those with normal immunity no specific treatment is necessary. In immunocompromised patients, where possible, attempts should be made to correct the underlying immunodeficiency. Resolution of cryptosporidiosis in HIV-infected patients appears to correlate with the presence of a CD4 count of greater than 180 cells per cubic millimetre. Combination antiretroviral therapy that includes a protease inhibitor has restored immunity to *Cryptosporidium parvum* in HIV 1-infected individuals with good clinical and parasitological response. At present there is no highly effective anticryptosporidial drug, though paromomycin has been reported effective in a double-blind, placebo-controlled trial. Azithromycin and hyperimmune bovine colostrum have also been used. The possible effectiveness of clarithromycin and rifabutin for cryptosporidiosis chemoprophylaxis in HIV 1 disease is under evaluation.

CYCLOSPORIASIS

Cyclospora cayetanensis is a newly recognised coccidian protozoan parasite of humans which was given its scientific name only as recently as 1992. Its precise geographical distribution is still being documented but potentially it has a world-wide distribution. It has been particularly reported from Nepal and the Indian subcontinent, and from South America. Infection is acquired by ingestion of contaminated water. Ingestion of raspberries imported from Guatemala was associated with a large outbreak of cyclosporiasis in the United States. The incubation period is approximately 2–11 days and is followed by acute onset of diarrhoea with abdominal cramps. The disease can remit and relapse. Although the illness is usually self-limited, the mean duration of diarrhoea has lasted as long as 43 days with significant associated weight loss. Malabsorption can occur. The disease is more severe in immunocompromised individuals. Diagnosis is by detection of oöcysts on faecal microscopy. Treatment may be necessary in a few cases, and the agent of choice is co-trimoxazole 960 mg 12-hourly for 7 days.

MICROSPORIDIOSIS

Microsporidia are obligate intracellular spore-forming protozoa. Intestinal microsporidiosis is a cause of diarrhoea in AIDS patients. The causative organisms are *Enterocytozoon bieneusi* or *Encephalitozoon* (formerly *Septata*) *intestinalis*. Diagnosis by faecal microscopy is difficult and time-consuming and speciation often depends upon electro-microscopy on faecal specimens or intestinal biopsies. Polymerase chain reaction is being brought into use. The treatment of choice is albendazole, although this drug appears to be less effective on *Enterocytozoon bieneusi*.

LEISHMANIASIS

This group of diseases is caused by protozoa of the genus *Leishmania*, conveyed to humans by female phlebotomine sandflies in which the flagellate (promastigote) forms of leishmania develop. In humans the leishmaniae are found in cells of the monocyte/macrophage system as oval forms known as amastigotes or Leishman–Donovan bodies (see Fig. 2.39). Leishmaniasis may take the form of a generalised visceral infection, kala-azar, or of a purely cutaneous infection, known in the Old World as oriental sore. In South America cutaneous leishmaniasis may remain confined to the skin or metastasise to the nose and mouth.

VISCERAL LEISHMANIASIS (KALA-AZAR)

Visceral leishmaniasis is caused by *Leishmania donovani* and is prevalent in the Mediterranean and Red Sea littorals, Sudan, parts of East Africa, Asia Minor, mountainous regions of southern Arabia, eastern parts of India, China and South America. In India, where the disease is epidemic, humans appear to be the chief hosts. In most other areas, including the Mediterranean, dogs and foxes are the main reservoirs of infection. Here the disease is endemic and occurs chiefly in young children or tourists. In Africa various wild rodents provide the reservoir, and the disease is rural, occurring in older children and visiting hunters and soldiers. Transmission has also been reported to follow blood transfusion in northern Europe. The disease has presented unexpectedly in immunosuppressed patients—for example, after renal transplantation and in AIDS.

Pathology

Multiplication of leishmaniae takes place by simple fission in monocytes and macrophages in various organs, especially in the liver and spleen which become greatly enlarged, the bone marrow, lymphoid tissue and the small intestinal submucosa. The disease is accompanied by malnutrition and immunosuppression which is both specific to *Leishmania* and non-specific. Acute intercurrent pneumococcal infection or tuberculosis is a common complication. Granulo-

A

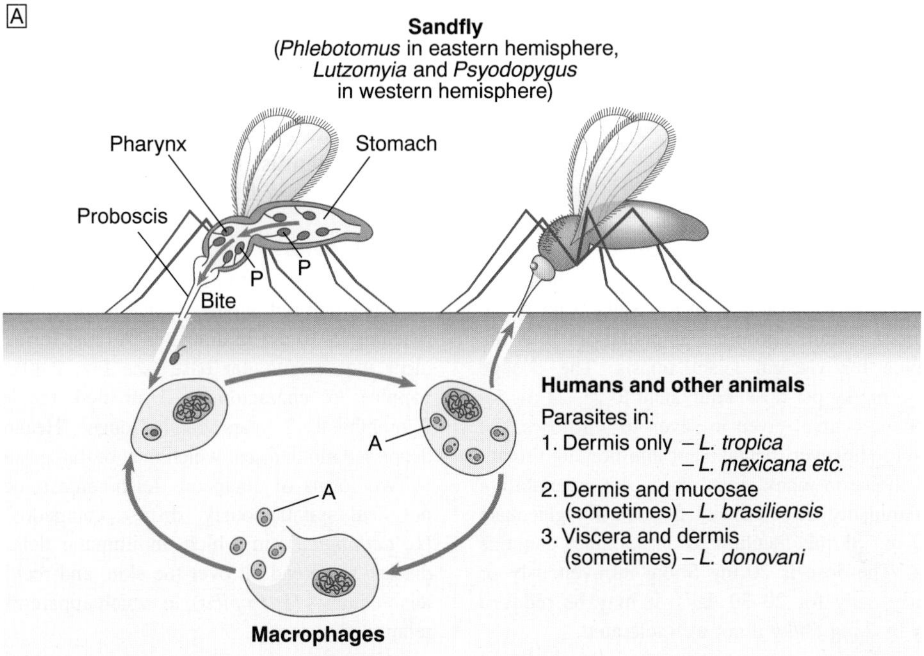

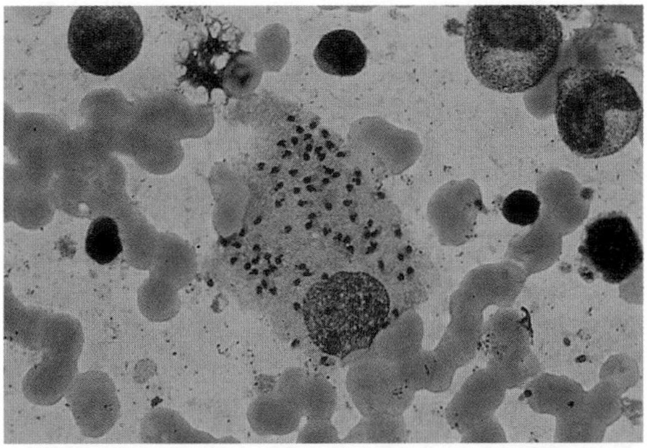

B

Fig. 2.39 Leishmaniasis. A Life cycle of leishmania. (A = amastigote (Leishman–Donovan body); P = promastigote) B Bone marrow smear showing numerous intracellular, and a few extracellular, amastigotes.

cytopenia and thrombocytopenia occur. Anaemia is due to haemolysis, hypersplenism and ineffective erythropoiesis. Serum albumin is low and globulin, mainly IgG, high. Hepatocellular damage and bleeding are late complications.

Clinical features

The incubation period is usually about 1 or 2 months but may be up to 10 years. The onset is usually insidious with a low-grade fever, the patient remaining ambulant, or it may be abrupt with sweating and high intermittent fever, sometimes showing a double rise of temperature in 24 hours. The spleen soon becomes enlarged, often massively; hepatomegaly is less marked. If not treated, the patient will become anaemic and wasted, frequently with increased pigmentation especially on the face. Cough and diarrhoea develop. In Africa lymphadenopathy is common, and rarely the only clinical finding.

After recovery post-kala-azar dermal leishmaniasis sometimes develops. It may present first as hypopigmented or erythematous macules on any part of the body or as a nodular eruption especially on the face.

Investigations

Diagnosis is established by demonstrating the parasite in stained smears of aspirates of bone marrow, lymph node, spleen or liver, or by culture of these aspirates. Polymerase chain reaction is also available for diagnosis. Amastigotes are scanty in skin biopsies from post-kala-azar dermal leishmaniasis. Antibody is detected by immunofluorescence or the direct agglutination test early in the disease. The leishmanin skin test is negative; it is performed and read in the same way as the tuberculin test, using a suspension of killed promastigotes as antigen.

Management

The response to treatment varies with the geographic area in which the disease has been acquired. In Europe the disease is readily cured but resistance to antimonials has become a problem—for example, in the Sudan and India. Where resources permit, liposomal amphotericin B is the drug of choice for visceral leishmaniasis. The dosage regimen is 2–3 mg/kg per dose, equivalent to 21–24 mg/kg total dose for the course, given in seven to ten doses, the last on day ten. However, pentavalent antimonials remain the drugs of choice in many areas when cost, availability, efficacy and familiarity are considered. Sodium stibogluconate contains 100 mg Sb/ml; meglumine antimoniate contains 85 mg Sb/ml. The dose is 20 mg Sb/kg intravenously or intramuscularly daily for 20–30 days. It may be reduced progressively by 2 mg Sb/kg if not well tolerated.

Intercurrent infection is sought and treated. Rarely, blood transfusion is needed for anaemia or bleeding. Measurement of spleen size, haemoglobin and serum albumin are useful in assessing progress. A small proportion of patients relapse, and should be retreated for 2 months with a full 20 mg Sb/kg daily. Second-line drugs for patients who fail to respond to antimonials include pentamidine 3–4 mg/kg once or twice weekly, and liposomal or conventional amphotericin (see p. 147).

Prevention

Infected or stray dogs should be destroyed in an endemic area, where they are the reservoir. Sandflies should be combated. They are extremely sensitive to insecticides. Mosquito nets treated with permethrin will keep out the tiny sandfly. Insect repellent creams may be helpful.

Early diagnosis and treatment of human infections reduces the reservoir and controls epidemic kala-azar in India. Serology is useful for case detection in the field. There is no vaccine.

CUTANEOUS LEISHMANIASIS OF THE OLD WORLD (ORIENTAL SORE)

Cutaneous leishmaniasis is found around the Mediterranean littoral, throughout the Middle East and Central Asia as far as Pakistan, and in sub-Saharan West Africa and Sudan. It is caused either by zoonotic *L. major*, a parasite of gerbils and other desert rodents, or by the anthroponotic *L. tropica* in towns. In the highlands of Ethiopia and Kenya a third parasite, of hyraxes, *L. aethiopica*, is the cause. The disease is commonly imported into Britain. On inoculation the parasites are taken up by dermal histiocytes, in which they multiply and around which lymphocytes and plasma cells accumulate. With time, the histological appearance becomes more tuberculoid and the overlying epidermis crusts and may ulcerate centrally. Healing is accompanied by subepidermal fibrosis. The incubation period is from 2 weeks to 5 years or more but usually is from 2 to 3 months.

Clinical features

Lesions, single or multiple, on exposed parts of the body, start as small red papules which increase gradually in size, reaching 2–10 cm in diameter. A crust forms, overlying an ulcer with a granular base (see Fig. 2.40). Tiny satellite papules are characteristic. Untreated, the lesion heals in 3 months to 3 years, rarely longer. Healing produces a depressed mottled scar which may be disfiguring or disabling.

Two forms of cutaneous leishmaniasis occur which do not heal spontaneously: diffuse cutaneous leishmaniasis *(L. aethiopica)*, in which an immune defect permits the disease to spread all over the skin, and recidivans (lupoid) leishmaniasis *(L. tropica)*, in which apparently healed sores relapse persistently.

Investigations

The appearance of a typical lesion in a patient from an endemic area suggests the diagnosis. Amastigotes can be demonstrated by making a slit skin smear (see p. 135) and staining the material obtained with Giemsa stain or culturing it. Cultured parasites may be speciated by isoenzyme or DNA studies. The leishmanin skin test is positive except in diffuse cutaneous leishmaniasis. Serology is unhelpful.

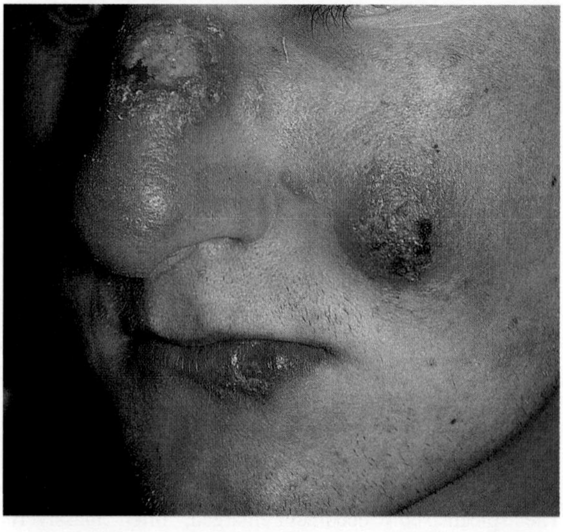

Fig. 2.40 Cutaneous leishmaniasis.

Management
Small lesions may be treated by freezing with liquid carbon dioxide, curettage or infiltration with 1–2 ml sodium stibogluconate. When the lesions are multiple or in a disfiguring site it is better to treat the patient by parenteral injections of pentavalent antimonials as outlined under visceral leishmaniasis above, but *L. aethiopica* is not sensitive to antimonials. Diffuse cutaneous leishmaniasis is treated with aminosidine plus sodium stibogluconate daily or with pentamidine once weekly.

Prevention
In addition to those prophylactic measures against animals and sandflies described under visceral leishmaniasis, a lasting immunity can be achieved by deliberate inoculation of a living culture of *L. major* on the upper arm, which produces a typical sore but protects against a subsequent, possibly disfiguring, lesion with the same species of parasite.

CUTANEOUS AND MUCOSAL LEISHMANIASIS OF THE NEW WORLD

In South and Central America, cutaneous leishmaniasis is endemic and mostly caused by *L. mexicana, L. amazonensis* and *L. brasiliensis*, which occur in hot, moist forest regions and are conveyed to humans from a variety of animals by several species of sandfly (see Fig. 2.39A). *L. mexicana* is responsible for chiclero's ulcer, the self-healing sores of Mexico, Guatemala and Honduras, and for some of the sores in the north of South America, including diffuse cutaneous leishmaniasis *(L. amazonensis)*. *L. brasiliensis* extends widely from the Amazon basin as far as Paraguay and Costa Rica and is responsible for self-healing sores and for mucosal leishmaniasis. A third variety of the disease occurring in the Peruvian Andes is known as 'uta' and is caused by *L. peruviana*, dogs providing the reservoir.

Pathology
The microscopic appearances of the skin lesions may be similar to oriental sore. Mucosal lesions begin as a perivascular infiltration; later endarteritis may cause destruction of the surrounding tissues.

Clinical features
Clinically, lesions of *L. mexicana* and *L. peruviana* closely resemble those seen in the Old World but lesions on the pinna of the ear are common and are chronic and destructive. The primary lesions of *L. brasiliensis* are similar but in some areas up to 80% of infected persons develop 'espundia', metastatic lesions in the mucosa of the nose or mouth. Mucosal lesions usually occur 1–2 years after the skin lesions but may appear many years later. The nasal mucosa becomes congested and ulcerates; later, all soft tissues of the nose may be destroyed. The lips, soft palate, fauces and larynx may also be invaded and destroyed, leading to considerable suffering and deformity. Secondary bacterial infection is common. Two related species, *L. guyanensis* and *L. panamensis*, rarely cause espundia.

Investigations
Diagnosis depends on the history and clinical appearance, confirmed by demonstration of the parasites in smears, culture or histological section. Polymerase chain reaction is available and can be used on histological sections as well as on material from culture. As parasites are not easily found, the leishmanin test is of value. Serology may be useful in mucosal leishmaniasis.

Management
Purely cutaneous disease may be successfully treated by sodium stibogluconate given as recommended for visceral leishmaniasis above, but in established espundia amphotericin is sometimes necessary.

AFRICAN TRYPANOSOMIASIS (SLEEPING SICKNESS)

African sleeping sickness is caused by trypanosomes conveyed to humans by the bites of infected tsetse flies of either sex. The disease is naturally acquired only in Africa between 12°N and 25°S. Two trypanosomes affect humans: *Trypanosoma brucei gambiense* conveyed by *Glossina palpalis* and *G. tachinoides*; and *T. rhodesiense* transmitted by *G. morsitans, G. pallidipes, G. swynnertoni* and *G. palpalis*.

Gambiense trypanosomiasis has a wide distribution in West and Central Africa reaching to Uganda and Kenya; *rhodesiense* trypanosomiasis is found in parts of East and Central Africa, where it is currently on the increase (see Fig. 2.41). In West Africa transmission is mainly at the riverside, where the fly rests in the shade of trees. Animal reservoirs of *T. gambiense* have not been identified, although pigs may carry it. *T. rhodesiense* has a large reservoir in numerous wild animals and transmission takes place in the shade of woods bordering grasslands (see Fig. 2.42). Devastating epidemics of both types have occurred. Trypanosomiasis of cattle, caused mainly by *T. brucei*, is also widespread and seriously limits grazing land and the production of meat and milk. Only a low percentage of tsetse flies are infected.

Clinical features
A bite by a tsetse fly is painful and commonly becomes inflamed, but if trypanosomes are introduced, the site may again become painful and swollen about 10 days later ('trypanosomal chancre') and the regional lymph nodes enlarge. Within 2–3 weeks of infection the trypanosomes invade the blood stream (see Table 2.30).

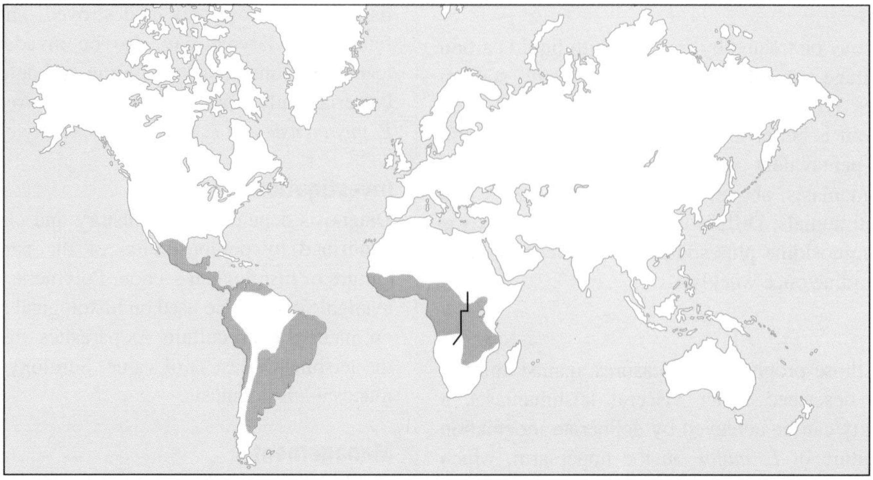

Fig. 2.41 Endemic zones of African and American trypanosomiasis. Within these zones, the actual distribution may be patchy and variable. The vertical line in central Africa separates the distribution of *T. gambiense* (left) from *T. rhodesiense* (right).

Gambiense *infections*

In these infections the disease usually runs a slow course over months or years, with irregular bouts of fever and enlargement of lymph nodes. These are characteristically firm, discrete, rubbery and painless and are particularly prominent in the posterior triangle of the neck. The spleen and liver may become palpable. After some months, in the absence of treatment, the central nervous system is invaded. This is shown clinically by headache and changed behaviour, insomnia by night and sleepiness by day, mental confusion and eventually tremors, pareses, wasting, coma and death. The histological changes in the brain are similar to those found in viral encephalitis but trypanosomes are scattered in the substance of the brain and large mononuclear (morula) cells are found whose cytoplasm contains globules of IgM.

Table 2.30 Comparison of the clinical and laboratory features of trypanosomiasis due to *T. rhodesiense* and *T. gambiense*

Feature	*T. rhodesiense*	*T. gambiense*
Incubation	7–14 days	Weeks to months
Onset	Abrupt	Insidious
Primary complex	Usual	Rare
Fever	High, swinging	Low-grade
Early features	Effusions, hepatitis, myocarditis	Lymphadenopathy
Rash	Macular, petechial	Erythematous, circinate
Late features	Drowsiness, tremors, coma, death	Headache, insomnia, behavioural, tremors, paresis, wasting, coma
Duration of illness	Weeks or months	Months or years
Trypanosomes	Numerous in blood	Numerous in lymph node aspirate
Cerebrospinal fluid	Protein, cells, trypanosomes	Protein, cells, trypanosomes

Rhodesiense *infections*

In these infections the disease is altogether more acute and severe than in *gambiense* infections, so that within days or a few weeks the patient is usually severely ill and may have developed pleural effusions and signs of myocarditis or hepatitis. There may be a petechial rash. The patient may die before there are signs of involvement of the central nervous system. If the illness is less acute, drowsiness, tremors and coma develop.

Investigations

Trypanosomiasis should be considered in any febrile patient from an endemic area. In *rhodesiense* infections thick and thin blood films, stained as for the detection of malaria, will reveal trypanosomes. The trypanosomes may be seen in the blood or from puncture of the primary lesion in the earliest stages of *gambiense* infections, but it is usually easier to demonstrate them by puncture of a lymph node. Concentration methods include buffy coat microscopy and miniature anion exchange chromatography. Animal inoculation is sometimes used for the detection of

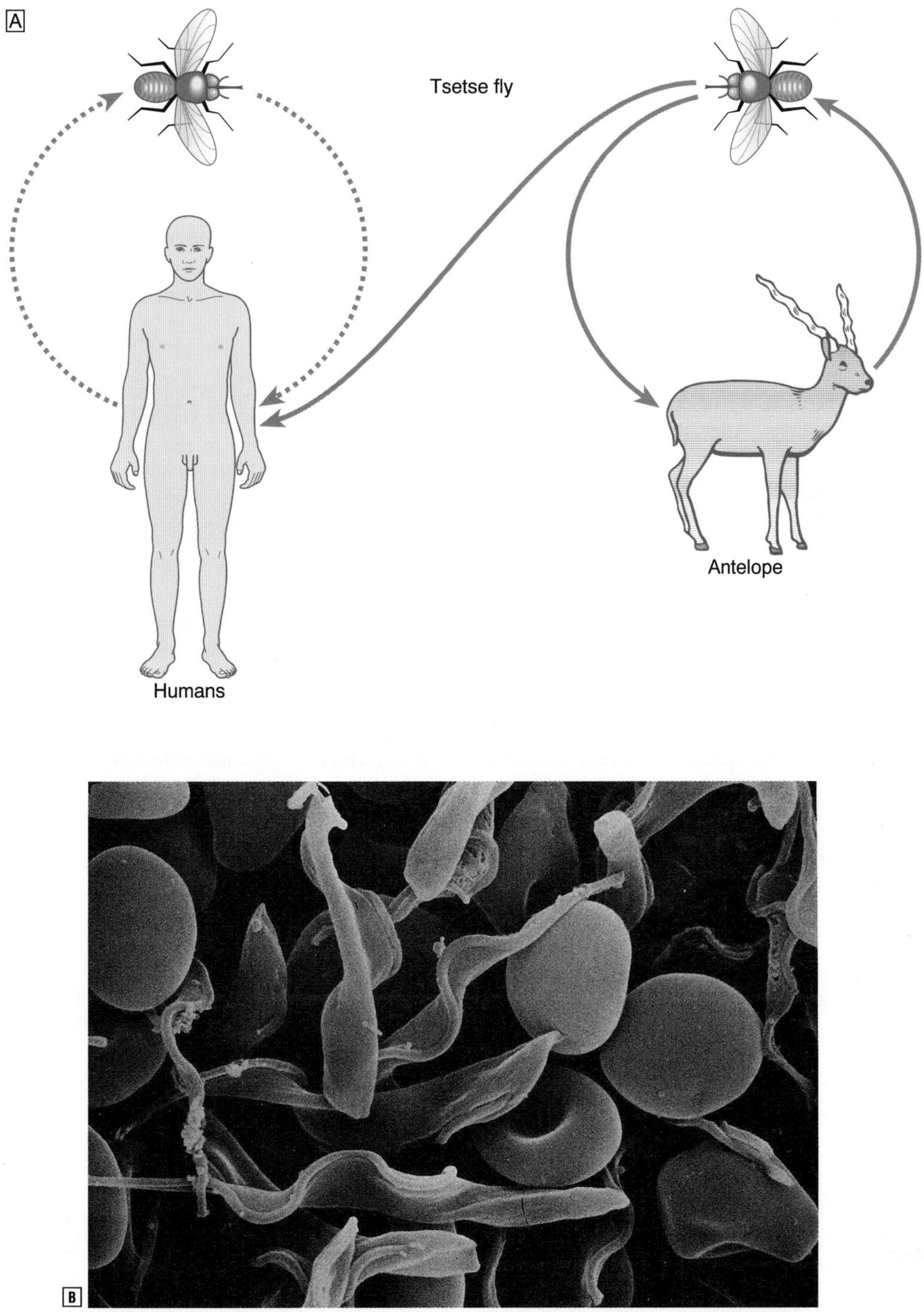

Fig. 2.42 Trypanosomiasis. [A] Transmission of *T. gambiense* (left) and *T. rhodesiense* (right). [B] Scanning electron micrograph showing trypanosomes swimming among erythrocytes.

rhodesiense infections. Serological tests are useful in the diagnosis of chronic infection and are employed in field work.

If the central nervous system is affected the cell count and protein content of the CSF are increased and the glucose is diminished. Sometimes trypanosomes may be found by centrifugation. Very high levels of serum IgM or the presence of IgM in the CSF are suggestive of trypanosomiasis. Antibody detection assays can be used on CSF in parallel to serum samples.

Management

The prognosis is good if treatment is begun early before the brain has been invaded. At this stage either suramin or pentamidine may be used, the latter being employed only for *gambiense* infections. After the nervous system is affected an arsenical or difluoromethyl ornithine will be required. Details are given in Table 2.31.

Prevention

A single intramuscular injection of 250 mg pentamidine gives protection against *T. gambiense* for 6 months because of the slow excretion of the drug. As the protection against *T. rhodesiense* is less sure and shorter in duration, chemoprophylaxis is not advised in *rhodesiense* areas. In endemic *gambiense* areas various measures may be taken against tsetse flies and field teams detect and treat early human infection. In *rhodesiense* areas control is difficult.

AMERICAN TRYPANOSOMIASIS (CHAGAS DISEASE)

Chagas disease occurs widely in South and Central America. The cause is *Trypanosoma cruzi*, transmitted to humans from the faeces of a reduviid bug in which the trypanosomes have a cycle of development before becoming infective to humans. Bugs live in the mud and wattle walls and thatch roofs of simple rural houses, and emerge at night to feed on the sleeping occupants. While feeding they defaecate. Infected faeces are rubbed in through the conjunctiva, mucosa of mouth or nose or abrasions of the skin. Over 100 species of mammals, domestic, peridomestic and wild, may serve as reservoirs of infection. In some areas blood transfusion accounts for about 5% of cases. Congenital transmission occurs occasionally.

Pathology

The trypanosomes migrate via the blood stream and develop into amastigote forms in the tissues. These multiply in many sites, especially in the myocardium causing pseudocysts, in smooth muscle fibres, and also in the ganglion cells of the autonomic nervous system.

Clinical features

The entrance of *T. cruzi* through an abrasion produces a dusky-red firm swelling and enlargement of regional lymph nodes. A conjunctival lesion, though less common, is more characteristic; the unilateral firm reddish swelling of the lids may close the eye and constitutes 'Romaña's sign'. Young children are most commonly affected. In a few patients an acute generalised infection soon appears, with fever, lymphadenopathy and enlargement of the spleen and liver. Neurological features include personality changes and signs of meningoencephalitis. The acute infection may be fatal to infants. In many patients the early infection is silent.

Table 2.31 Chemotherapy of trypanosomiasis

Drug	Route of administration	Dosage	Toxicity	Indications
Suramin	Intravenous	Test dose 200 mg then 1 g in 10 ml water every 5 days, to total dose 5–6 g	Mild: proteinuria, arthralgia Severe: dermatitis, diarrhoea, nephritis (red cells and casts)	*Rhodesiense* and *gambiense* infection before CNS involvement
Pentamidine	As base intramuscular	4 mg/kg, max. 250 mg/dose alternate days for 10 doses	Collapse if injected intravenously, hypoglycaemia, nephritis, diabetes mellitus, injection abscess	*Gambiense* infection before CNS involvement
Melarsoprol (Mel B)	3.6% in propylene glycol, intravenous	3 consecutive days/week for 4 weeks wk 1: 0.5 ml, 1 ml, 1 ml wk 2: 2.5 ml × 3 wk 3: 3.5 ml × 3 wk 4: 5 ml × 3	Jarisch–Herxheimer reaction, arsenical encephalopathy, mortality up to 10%*	*Rhodesiense* and *gambiense* disease after CNS involvement
Difluoromethyl ornithine	Intravenous	200–400 mg/kg daily × 4 weeks	Diarrhoea, abdominal pain	Cerebral *gambiense* infections
Nitrofurazone	Oral	10 mg/kg 8-hourly × 10 days	Haemolysis, neuropathy	Resistance to arsenicals

* Toxicity is greatly reduced if the blood has been cleared of trypanosomes with suramin (test dose plus 1 g) a few days previously.

After a latent period of several years features of the chronic infection appear, notably damage to Auerbach's plexus with resulting dilatation of various parts of the alimentary canal, especially the colon and oesophagus, so-called 'mega' disease. Dilatation of the bile ducts and bronchi are also recognised sequelae. Chronic low-grade myocarditis and damage to conducting fibres cause a cardiomyopathy characterised by cardiac dilatation, arrhythmias, partial or complete heart block and sudden death. Autoimmune processes may be responsible for much of the damage. There are geographical variations of the basic pattern of disease.

Investigations

T. cruzi may be seen in a blood film in the acute illness. In chronic disease it may be recovered in up to 50% of cases by xenodiagnosis in which infection-free, laboratory-bred reduviid bugs are fed on the patient; subsequently the hind gut or faeces of the bug are examined for parasites. Complement fixation, direct agglutination and fluorescent antibody tests are positive in 95% of cases.

Management

Nifurtimox is given orally. The dose, which has to be carefully supervised to minimise toxicity while preserving parasiticidal activity, is 10 mg/kg divided into three equal doses, daily by mouth for 60–90 days. The paediatric dose is 15 mg/kg daily. Cure rates of 80% in acute disease are obtained. Benznidazole is an alternative drug at a dose of 5–10 mg/kg daily by mouth, in two divided doses for 60 days; children receive 10 mg/kg daily. Both nifurtimox and benznidazole are toxic, with adverse reaction rates of 30–55%. Specific drug treatment of chronic Chagas disease is not usually undertaken and does not reverse established tissue damage. Surgery may be needed for 'mega' disease.

Prevention

Preventive measures include improving housing and destruction of reduviid bugs by spraying of houses with chlorinated hydrocarbon insecticides. Blood taken for transfusion in endemic areas which is potentially infected with *T. cruzi* and cannot be discarded is treated with gentian violet. Long-term resolution requires better housing.

TOXOPLASMOSIS

Toxoplasmosis is a world-wide infection caused by *Toxoplasma gondii*. Transmission from a mother infected during pregnancy to the fetus causes congenital toxoplasmosis. Infection after birth occurs from the ingestion of cysts excreted in the faeces of infected cats or from eating undercooked beef or lamb. Immunocompromised patients are particularly at risk.

Pathology

In the congenital form of the disease the organism is widespread in the central nervous system, eyes, heart, lungs and adrenals. If the infant survives, the parasite soon disappears from most organs except the central nervous system and retina. The brain shows areas of necrosis with cyst formation and patchy calcification; the spinal cord may be similarly affected. The organism commonly invades lymph nodes and spleen in the acquired disease, and less commonly liver and myocardium.

Clinical features

The manifestations in congenital infections are mainly cerebral. There may be hydrocephalus or microcephaly associated with convulsions, tremors or paralysis. Radiological examination may show patches of calcification in the brain. Microphthalmos, nystagmus and choroidoretinitis are common. The CSF is often xanthochromic, with increased protein and mononuclear cells. An enlarged liver, jaundice, thrombocytopenia and purpura may also occur. Severe congenital infections are usually fatal, and if the child survives it is frequently disabled and blind but milder cases may show only signs of choroidoretinitis.

Many acquired infections are symptomless. In the acute form there may be pneumonia with fever, cough, generalised aches and pains, profound malaise, a maculopapular rash and, rarely, jaundice and myocarditis. More chronic infections are often afebrile and there may be only enlargement of the lymph nodes with a lymphocytosis showing atypical mononuclear cells similar to those present in infectious mononucleosis. Toxoplasmosis is a cause of choroidoretinitis and uveitis in adults.

Latent toxoplasmosis may reactivate and cause encephalitis and necrosis of brain in immunocompromised patients, especially in AIDS (see p. 105). Seronegative recipients of organ grafts may acquire the disease from seropositive donors.

Investigations

Serological tests are of value. Antibodies detectable by the dye test appear early in the disease and persist for years. Enzyme-linked immunoassay is also helpful. A rise in the titre of IgM antibodies indicates acute infection. Antibodies may not be detectable in adult ocular toxoplasmosis. Antibodies persisting in an infant beyond 6 months of age imply congenital toxoplasmosis. Biopsy material from a lymph node may be tested by polymerase chain reaction, inoculated into mice, or show characteristic histological changes. *Toxoplasma* may be found in the CSF of immunocompromised patients.

Management

Most patients with acquired toxoplasmosis do not require specific therapy as the infection usually resolves spontaneously. Patients for whom treatment is essential include infants, the immunosuppressed and those with eye involvement. For non-pregnant, immunologically intact individuals a combination of sulphadiazine 2 g daily and pyrimethamine 25 mg daily, both for 4 weeks, is given together with folinic acid 15 mg daily. Blood count is monitored weekly.

Toxoplasmosis and pregnancy

A seronegative woman who acquires toxoplasmosis during pregnancy is at risk of producing a damaged fetus, especially if infection takes place in the first trimester. Management requires expert assessment in a reference centre. The outlook for toxoplasmosis acquired in pregnancy has improved in recent years as a result of better diagnosis and treatment, though termination of pregnancy is sometimes necessary. Those who are seropositive before becoming pregnant do not risk fetal damage.

FURTHER INFORMATION ON DISEASES DUE TO PROTOZOA

Berrebi A, Kobuch W E, Bessieres M H et al 1994 Termination of pregnancy for maternal toxoplasmosis. Lancet 344: 36–39

Bradley D J, Warhurst D C 1997 Guidelines for the prevention of malaria in travellers from the United Kingdom. Communicable Disease Review 7: R137–R152

Davidson R N, di Martino L, Gradoni L et al 1994 Liposomal amphotericin B (AmBisome) in Mediterranean visceral leishmaniasis: a multi-centre trial. Quarterly Journal of Medicine 87: 75–81

Pépin J, Milord F 1994 The treatment of human African trypanosomiasis. Advances in Parasitology 33: 1–47

Ravdin J I 1995 Amebiasis. Clinical Infectious Diseases 20: 1453–1466

Tanowicz H B, Kirkhoff C V, Simon D 1992 Chagas' disease. Clinical Microbiological Reviews 5: 400–419

Thompson R C A, Reynoldson J A, Lymbery A J (eds) 1994 Giardia: from molecules to disease. CAB International, Wallingford

White N J 1996 The treatment of malaria. New England Journal of Medicine 335: 800–806

DISEASES DUE TO HELMINTHS

Helminths cause much disease among humans and domestic animals in the tropics and are a common cause of imported disease in temperate countries. Infections caused by the more common helminths or worms are listed in the information box.

The most common parasitic helminth of humans in Britain is the nematode *Enterobius (Oxyuris) vermicularis* or threadworm. Other worms which may be acquired in Britain include *Toxocara canis, Echinococcus granulosus* causing hydatid disease, and *Fasciola hepatica*, the endemic fluke of sheep.

Helminths are the largest of human parasites. They contain an efficient reproductive system that generates millions of eggs and may occupy most of the adult female or hermaphroditic worm. Nematodes and trematodes also have a mouth and intestinal tract but cestodes absorb food through the tegument. Worms that live in the gut often have suckers or hooklets at the head end for attachment to the mucosa. They are all motile and this is essential for certain phases of their developmental cycle: e.g. the migration on grass of segments of *Taenia*, the emigration of threadworms through the anus to lay eggs, the penetration of human skin by infective hookworm larvae and the initial migratory phase of many helminths in humans. Once established in their definitive site, however, adult worms are usually sedentary. All this is regulated by nervous and hormonal systems. A given species of helminth will only parasitise one genus or a small range of genera of higher animal hosts. It is not known what determines this selectivity, nor the worm's ability to migrate to its correct definitive site. Worms may be long-lived: *Onchocerca* up to 15 years and *Schistosoma* over 30 years.

Many helminths have a complicated life cycle, often involving one or more intermediate host. Disease may be caused by invasive larval stages (e.g. Loeffler's syndrome), adult worms (e.g. hookworms) or their progeny, either eggs (e.g. schistosomiasis) or microfilariae (e.g. onchocerciasis). Adult worms may be present in the body for many years

ZOOLOGICAL CLASSES OF HELMINTH WHICH PARASITISE HUMANS

Trematodes or flukes

- Blood flukes: *Schistosoma haematobium, S. mansoni, S. japonicum*
- Lung flukes: *Paragonimus* species
- Hepatobiliary flukes: *Clonorchis sinensis, Opisthorchis felineus, Fasciola hepatica*
- Intestinal flukes: *Fasciolopsis buski*

Cestodes or tapeworms

- Intestinal tapeworms (adult stages): *Taenia saginata, Taenia solium, Diphyllobothrium latum, Dipylidium caninum, Hymenolepis nana*
- Tissue-dwelling cysts or worms (larval stages): *Taenia solium* (cysticercosis), *Echinococcus granulosus* (hydatid disease), *Multiceps multiceps* (coenurus), *Spirometra mansoni* (sparganosis)

Nematodes or roundworms

- Intestinal human nematodes: *Enterobius vermicularis, Ascaris lumbricoides, Trichuris trichiura, Necator americanus, Ancylostoma duodenale, Strongyloides stercoralis, Capillaria philippinensis*
- Tissue-dwelling human nematodes: *Wuchereria bancrofti, Brugia malayi, Loa loa, Onchocerca volvulus* (all filarial worms), *Dracunculus medinensis* (guinea worm)
- Zoonotic nematodes: *Toxocara canis, Ancylostoma braziliense, Oesophagostomum* species, *Angiostrongylus cantonensis, Trichinella spiralis, Gnathostoma spinigerum, Anisakis marina*

before, or without, producing disease. Sometimes larval stages that normally develop in intermediate hosts cause cystic disease in humans (e.g. cysticercosis). Humans may also suffer from invasion by larval stages of worms that normally only infect other animals (e.g. hydatid disease).

Eosinophilia is a characteristic feature of helmintic infections. The eosinophilic syndromes associated with them are summarised in the information box on page 181.

TREMATODE (FLUKE) INFECTIONS

Flukes are flat, usually oval-shaped worms, like a small thick leaf, although schistosomes are elongated. They attach with suckers. Adult worms produce eggs that are passed from the body in faeces, urine or sputum, according to the site of infection, which depends upon the species of fluke. The life cycles are complex and involve fresh-water snails and sometimes an intermediate host that humans must eat. Disease is caused by the inflammatory response, either to worms or to eggs in tissues.

SCHISTOSOMIASIS

Schistosomiasis (bilharziasis) is one of the most important causes of morbidity in the tropics and is being spread by irrigation schemes. Schistosome eggs have been found in Egyptian mummies dated 1250 BC.

There are three species of the genus *Schistosoma* which commonly cause disease in humans: *S. haematobium*, *S. mansoni* and *S. japonicum*. *S. haematobium* was discovered by Theodor Bilharz in Cairo in 1861 and the genus is sometimes called *Bilharzia* and the disease bilharziasis. The ovum is passed in the urine or faeces of infected individuals and gains access to fresh water where the ciliated miracidium inside it is liberated and enters its intermediate host, a species of fresh-water snail, in which it multiplies. Large numbers of fork-tailed cercariae are then liberated into the water, where they may survive for 2–3 days. Cercariae can penetrate the skin or the mucous membrane of the mouth of their definitive host, humans. They transform into schistosomulae and moult as they pass through the lungs and are carried by the blood stream to the liver and so to the portal vein where they mature (see Fig. 2.43). The male worm is up to 20 mm in length and the

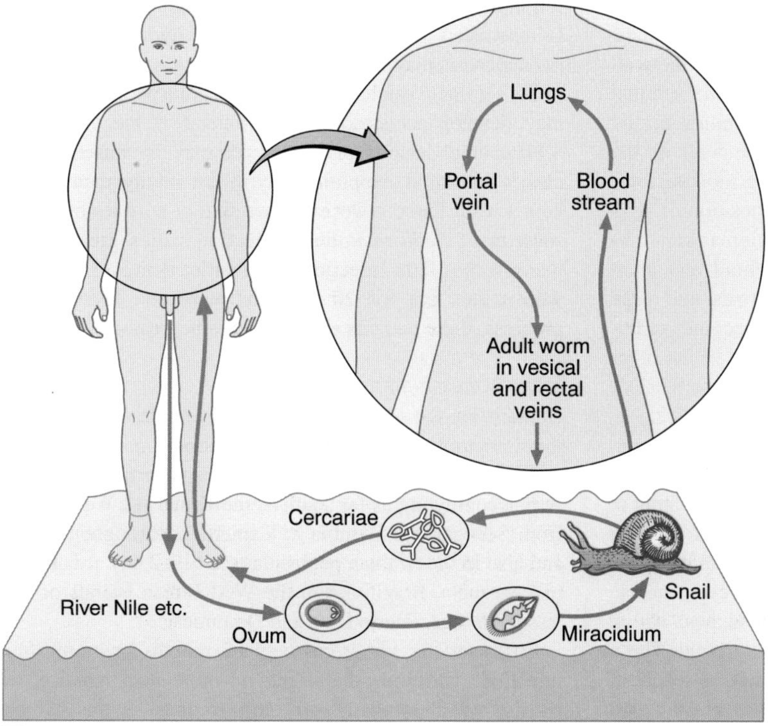

A

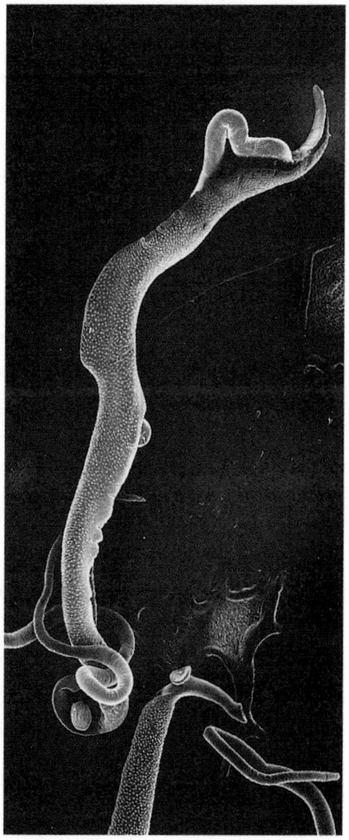

B

Fig. 2.43 ***Schistosoma.*** A Life cycle. B Scanning electron micrograph of adult schistosome worms showing the larger male worm embracing the thinner female.

Table 2.32 Pathogenesis of schistosomiasis

Stage	Time	*S. haematobium*	*S. mansoni* and *S. japonicum*
Cercarial penetration	Days	Papular dermatitis at site of penetration	As for *S. haematobium*
Larval migration and maturation	Weeks	Pneumonitis, myositis, hepatitis, fever, 'serum sickness', eosinophilia, seroconversion	As for *S. haematobium*
Early egg deposition	Months	Cystitis, haematuria Ectopic granulomatous lesions: skin, CNS etc. Immune complex glomerulonephritis	Colitis, granulomatous hepatitis, acute portal hypertension As for *S. haematobium*
Late egg deposition	Years	Fibrosis and calcification of ureters, bladder; bacterial infection, calculi, hydronephrosis, carcinoma Pulmonary granulomas and pulmonary hypertension	Colonic polyposis and strictures, periportal fibrosis, portal hypertension As for *S. haematobium*

more slender cylindrical female, usually enfolded longitudinally by the male, is rather longer. Within 4–6 weeks of infection they migrate to the venules draining the pelvic viscera, where the females deposit ova.

Pathology

The pathological changes and symptoms depend on species and stage of infection (see Table 2.32). Penetration of the skin by schistosomes not pathogenic in humans in, for example, Scotland can produce a similar rash. Most of the disease is due to the passage of eggs through mucosa and to the granulomatous reaction to eggs deposited in tissues. The eggs of *S. haematobium* pass mainly through the wall of the bladder, but may also involve rectum, seminal vesicles, vagina, cervix and uterine tubes. *S. mansoni* and *S. japonicum* eggs pass mainly through the wall of the lower bowel, or are carried to the liver. The most serious, though rare, consequence of the ectopic deposition of eggs is transverse myelitis and paraplegia. Granulomas are composed of macrophages, eosinophils, epithelioid and giant cells around an ovum. Later there is fibrosis and eggs calcify, often in sufficient numbers to become radiologically visible. Eggs of *S. haematobium*, and of the other two species after the development of portal hypertension, may reach the lungs.

Clinical features

During the early stages of infection there may be itching at the site of cercarial penetration lasting 1–2 days. After a symptom-free period of 3–5 weeks allergic manifestations may develop, such as urticaria, eosinophilia, fever, muscle aches, abdominal pain, splenomegaly, headaches, cough and sweating. Patches of pneumonia may be present. These allergic phenomena (Katayama syndrome) may be severe in infections with *S. mansoni* and *S. japonicum* but are rare with *S. haematobium*. The features subside after 1–2 weeks and it may be 2 or 3 months before further symptoms are seen. These depend upon the deposition of eggs, the intensity of infection and the species of infecting schistosome.

Schistosomiasis haematobium

Humans are the only natural hosts of *S. haematobium*, which is highly endemic in Egypt, the east coast of Africa and the adjacent islands and occurs throughout most of Africa and in Iran, Iraq, Syria, Yemen and Lebanon. It also occurs in a solitary focus in the Maharashtra state of India (see Fig. 2.44).

Painless terminal haematuria is usually the first and most common symptom. Frequency of micturition follows, due to the contracted fibrosed or calcified bladder. Pain is often felt in the iliac fossa or in the loin and radiates to the groin. In advanced disease, pyelonephritis, hydronephrosis or pyonephrosis may lead to hypertension or uraemia. Disease of the seminal vesicles may lead to haemospermia. Females may develop schistosomal papillomata of the vulva and schistosomal lesions of the cervix may be mistaken for cancer. Intestinal symptoms may follow involvement of the bowel wall. Ectopic worms cause skin or cord lesions. The severity of *S. haematobium* infection varies greatly, and many with a light infection suffer little. However, as adult worms can live for 20 years or more and lesions may progress, these patients should always be treated.

Schistosomiasis mansoni

Humans are the only natural hosts of importance, although the infection is also found in baboons. *S. mansoni* is endemic in the Nile delta and Libya, southern Sudan, East Africa continuing as far south as the Transvaal, West Africa from Senegal and Gambia to Cameroon, throughout Zaire and also in the Arabian peninsula (see Fig. 2.44). It is found in Venezuela, Brazil and in the West Indian islands of the lesser Antilles, Puerto Rico and Dominica.

Characteristic symptoms begin 2 months or more after infection. They may be slight, no more than malaise, or consist of abdominal pain and frequent stools which contain blood-stained mucus. With severe advanced disease increased discomfort from rectal polypi may be experienced. The early hepatomegaly is reversible but portal hypertension may cause massive splenomegaly, fatal

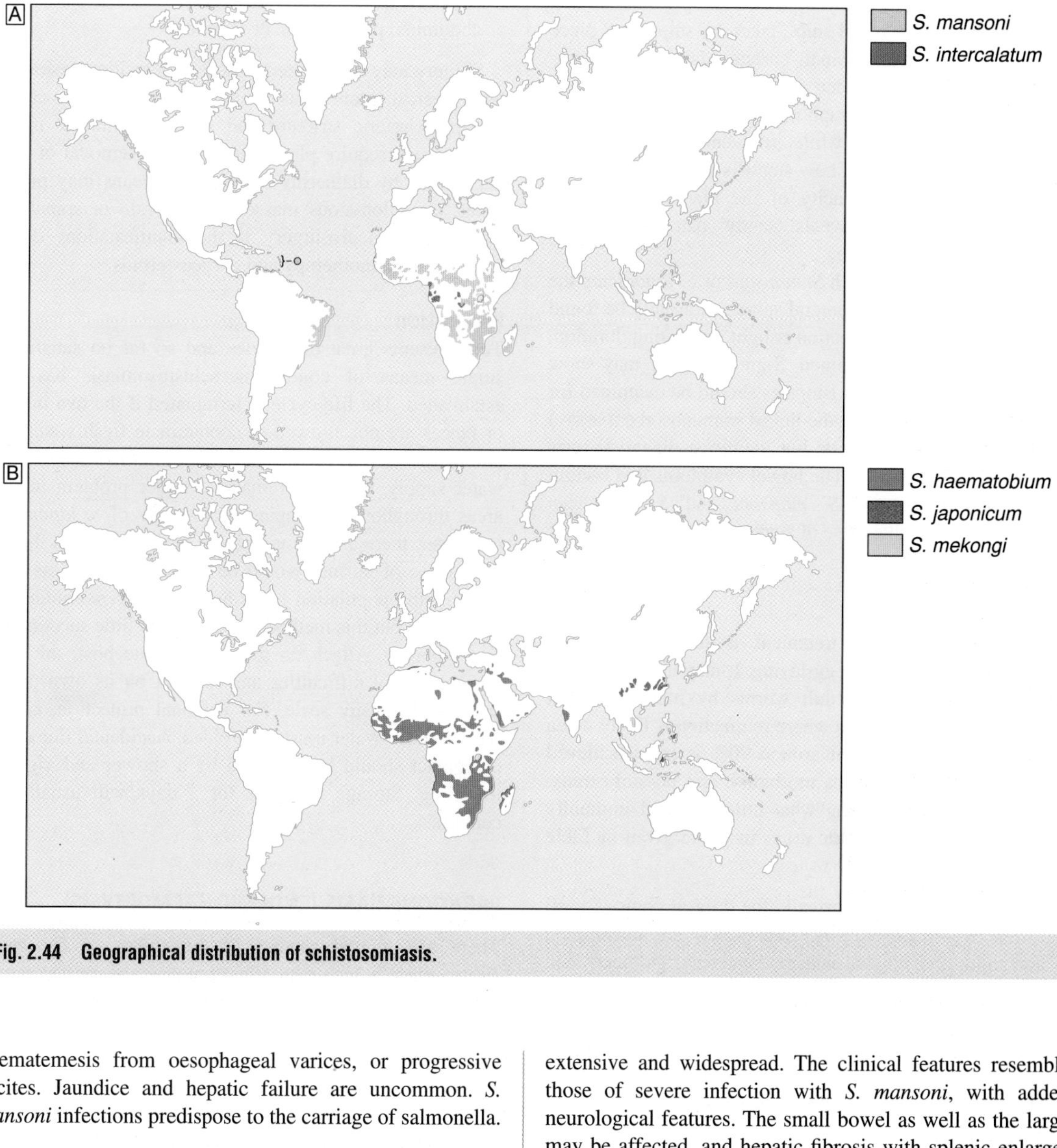

Fig. 2.44 Geographical distribution of schistosomiasis.

haematemesis from oesophageal varices, or progressive ascites. Jaundice and hepatic failure are uncommon. *S. mansoni* infections predispose to the carriage of salmonella.

Schistosomiasis japonicum

In addition to humans the adult worm infects the dog, rat, field mouse, water buffalo, ox, cat, pig, horse and sheep. *S. japonicum* is prevalent in the Yellow River and Yangtze-Jiang basins in China, where the infection is a major public health problem. It also has a focal distribution in the Philippines, Indonesia and Thailand. There is now no human transmission of this parasite in Japan. A related parasite, *S. mekongi*, occurs in Laos, Thailand and the Shan States of Myanmar, formerly Burma. The pathology of *S. japonicum* is similar to that of *S. mansoni*, but as this worm produces more eggs, the lesions tend to be more extensive and widespread. The clinical features resemble those of severe infection with *S. mansoni*, with added neurological features. The small bowel as well as the large may be affected, and hepatic fibrosis with splenic enlargement is usual. Deposition of eggs or worms in the central nervous system, especially in the brain, causes symptoms in about 5% of infections, notably epilepsy, hemiplegia, blindness and paraplegia.

Investigations

A history of residence in an endemic area, with characteristic symptoms, will indicate the need for investigation. In *S. haematobium* infection, dip-stick urine testing shows blood and albumin. The terminal spined eggs can usually be found by microscopic examination of the centrifuged deposit of terminal stream urine, especially after exercise.

The eggs may also be found by a microscopic examination of the stools or of a 'rectal snip', taken by snipping a piece of rectal mucosa with a small curette against the proctoscope. The snip is examined fresh; live and dead ova are easily identified. A radiograph may indicate calcification of the wall of the bladder while intravenous urography or ultrasound scanning may show stenosis or dilatation of the ureters, reduction in capacity of the bladder, or hydronephrosis. Cystoscopy reveals 'sandy' patches, bleeding mucosa and later distortion.

In a heavy infection with *S. mansoni* or *S. japonicum* the characteristic egg with its lateral spine can usually be found in the stool. When the infection is light, or of long duration, a rectal snip can be examined. Sigmoidoscopy may show inflammation or bleeding. Biopsies should be examined for ova. Serological tests (enzyme-linked immunosorbent assay) are useful as screening tests but definitive diagnosis rests on demonstration of ova. The bowel symptoms and barium enema appearances of *S. mansoni* and *S. japonicum* infection may resemble those of amoebiasis or a neoplasm of the large bowel.

Management

The object of specific treatment is to kill the adult schistosomes and so stop egg-laying. It may not be possible or desirable to kill all adult worms by mass treatment campaigns in communities where reinfection is likely, but a reduction in egg output of around 90% is often achieved which significantly reduces morbidity, and possibly transmission, without impairing what little acquired immunity there may be. Details of the drugs used are given in Table 2.33.

- *Praziquantel.* This is normally the drug of choice for all forms of schistosomiasis. Side-effects are uncommon and mild, and include nausea, headache, giddiness and drowsiness.
- *Oxamniquine.* This is safe in the chronic hepatic forms of the disease though it may cause fever for a few days.
- *Metrifonate.* This is an organophosphorus inhibitor of cholinesterase, and paralyses the worm. Higher or more frequent doses than those given in the table cause abdominal pain, nausea or vomiting.

Table 2.33 Drugs used in the treatment of schistosomiasis

Infection	Praziquantel*	Oxamniquine	Metrifonate
S. mansoni	40 mg/kg once	15 mg/kg 12-hourly for 2 days	Not useful
S. japonicum	30 mg/kg twice in one day	Not useful	Not useful
S. haematobium	40 mg/kg once	Not useful	7.5 mg/kg every 2 weeks × 3

* Doses quoted give cure rates of about 90% and reduce egg excretion by over 99%, and are used in mass campaigns and in primary health-care centres.

Surgery may be required to deal with residual lesions but large vesical granulomas usually respond well to chemotherapy. Ureteric stricture and the small fibrotic urinary bladder may require plastic procedures. Removal of rectal papillomas by diathermy or by other means may provide relief. Granulomatous masses in the brain or spinal cord may require neurosurgery if the manifestations do not respond to chemotherapy and corticosteroids.

Prevention

This presents great difficulties and so far no satisfactory single means of controlling schistosomiasis has been established. The life cycle is terminated if the ova in urine or faeces are not allowed to contaminate fresh water containing the snail host. The provision of latrines and of a safe water supply, however, remains a major problem in rural areas throughout the tropics. In the case of *S. japonicum*, moreover, there are so many hosts besides humans that the proper use of latrines would be of little avail. Mass treatment of the population helps against *S. haematobium* and *S. mansoni* but this method has so far had little success with *S. japonicum*. Attack on the intermediate host, the snail, presents many difficulties and has not on its own proved successful on any scale. For personal protection, contact with infected water must be avoided. Accidental immersion or contact should be followed by a shower and vigorous towelling. Storage of water for 3 days will usually kill cercariae.

PARAGONIMIASIS (ENDEMIC HAEMOPTYSIS)

There are several species of the flukes of the genus *Paragonimus* which may affect humans, the most common being *P. westermani*. The adult flukes measuring 10 × 6 mm live in small 'nests' in the lung and elsewhere. The sputum contains ova, which may be expectorated or swallowed and passed in the faeces. Miracidia emerge in water from these eggs and seek the first intermediate host, a fresh-water snail. Larvae emerging from the snail encyst as metacercariae in fresh-water crabs or crayfish. Humans or certain other mammals become infected if they eat these crustacea raw or inadequately cooked. Human infections are most frequent in the Far East but there are also endemic foci in South America, West Africa, Somalia and India.

Pathology

The adults lie in cysts up to 1 cm in diameter, situated chiefly in the lung and containing reddish-brown fluid. There are seldom more than 20 such cysts present. In heavy infections, cysts may also be present in the pleural or peritoneal cavities, in the brain, muscles, skin or elsewhere.

Clinical features

The first symptoms are slight fever, cough and the expectoration of brown or black sputum. Occasionally, there are bouts of frank haemoptysis with severe pain in the chest. Increasing clinical signs in the chest may simulate pneumonia or pulmonary tuberculosis, which may coexist. When the parasites lodge in the abdomen there may be symptoms of enteritis or hepatitis. If they settle in the abdominal wall they may produce sinuses which discharge through the skin. Cysts in the central nervous system may cause signs of cerebral irritation, encephalitis or myelitis. The disease may be extremely chronic as the adult worms may survive for 20 years.

Investigations

Ova may be found on microscopic examination of the faeces, sputum or a discharge. The radiological appearances of affected lungs are variable but the lesions are usually situated close to the pleural surfaces. Extra-pulmonary lesions are diagnosed by biopsy.

Management

Praziquantel is given orally in a dose of 25 mg/kg 12-hourly for 2 days. Lesions localised to or maximal in one lobe of a lung may be treated surgically.

Prevention

In an endemic area crab or crayfish should not be eaten unless adequately cooked. Immersion of crustaceans in wine, vinegar or brine does not kill the parasites.

LIVER FLUKES

Table 2.34 sets out the main features of the diseases caused by flukes which infect the bile ducts of humans. In the Far East and South-east Asia, liver flukes are an important cause of ill health.

CESTODE (TAPEWORM) INFECTIONS

Cestodes are ribbon-shaped worms which inhabit the intestinal tract. They have no alimentary system and absorb nutrients through the tegumental surface. The anterior end, or scolex, is provided with suckers for attachment to the host. From the scolex arises a series of progressively developing segments, the proglottides, which when shed may continue to show active movements. Cross-fertilisation takes place between segments. Ova, present in large numbers in mature proglottides, remain viable for weeks and during this period they may be consumed by the intermediate host. Larvae liberated from the ingested ova pass into the tissues.

Humans acquire tapeworm by eating undercooked beef infected with *Cysticercus bovis*, the larval stage of *Taenia saginata* (beef tapeworm), undercooked pork containing *Cysticercus cellulosae*, the larval stage of *T. solium* (pork tapeworm), or undercooked fresh-water fish containing larvae of *Diphyllobothrium latum* (fish tapeworm). Usually only one adult tapeworm is present in the gut but up to 10 have been reported. The life cycles of *Spirometra mansoni*,

Table 2.34 Diseases caused by flukes in the bile duct

	Clonorchiasis	Opisthorchiasis	Fascioliasis
Parasite	*Clonorchis sinensis*	*Opisthorchis felineus*	*Fasciola hepatica*
Other mammalian hosts	Dogs, cats, pigs	Dogs, cats, foxes, pigs	Sheep, cattle
Mode of spread	Ova in faeces, water	As for *C. sinensis*	Ova in faeces on to wet pasture
1st intermediate host	Snails	Snails	Snails
2nd intermediate host	Fresh-water fish	Fresh-water fish	Encysts on vegetation
Geographical distribution	Far East, esp. S. China	Far East, esp. N.E. Thailand	Cosmopolitan incl. UK
Pathology	*E. coli* cholangitis, abscesses, biliary carcinoma	As for *C. sinensis*	Toxaemia, cholangitis, eosinophilia
Symptoms	Often symptom-free, recurrent jaundice	As for *C. sinensis*	Obscure fever, tender liver, may be ectopic, e.g. subcutaneous fluke
Diagnosis	Ova in stool or duodenal aspirate	As for *C. sinensis*	As for *C. sinensis*, also serology
Prevention	Cook fish	Cook fish	Avoid contaminated watercress
Treatment	Praziquantel 25 mg/kg 8-hourly for 2 days	As for *C. sinensis* but 1 day only	Triclabendazole 10 mg/kg single dose; repeat treatment may be required*

* In UK available from the Hospital for Tropical Diseases, London.

Table 2.35 Essential features of the less common tapeworm infections of humans

Species	Geography	Definitive host	Intermediate host(s)	Stage and site in humans	Clinical features
Multiceps multiceps	E. and S. Africa	Dog	Sheep	Larval cysts/brain	CNS
Diphyllobothrium latum	Scandinavia Asia	Fish-eating mammals	*Cyclops* Fish *Diaptomus*	Adult worm/gut	Nil *or* megaloblastic anaemia
Spirometra mansoni	Africa Far East	Cats and dogs	*Cyclops*, frogs, snakes	Sparganum/various	Subcutaneous swellings
Dipylidium caninum	World-wide	Dogs and cats	Flea	Adult worm/gut	Ova in faeces
Hymenolepis nana	World-wide	Humans	None	Adult worm/gut	Ova in faeces

Treatment of intestinal tapeworms is with praziquantel 20 mg/kg once, or niclosamide (1 g repeated after 2 hours). Treatment of larval cysts and sparganosis is surgical.

Dipylidium caninum and *Hymenolepis nana* are different (see Table 2.35). *Echinococcus granulosus* is a tapeworm of dogs.

TAENIA SAGINATA

This worm may be several metres long. The scolex, the size of a pinhead, has four suckers; mature segments, 1.3 cm × 1 cm, contain a central stemmed uterus with lateral branches which are easily seen if the segments are left in water for 24 hours. The ova of both *T. saginata* and *T. solium* are indistinguishable microscopically. Infection with *T. saginata* occurs in all parts of the world. The adult worm produces little or no intestinal upset in human beings, but knowledge of its presence, by noting segments in the faeces or on underclothing, may distress the patient. Ova may be found in the stool.

Praziquantel is the drug of choice (see Table 2.35), and prevention depends on efficient meat inspection and the thorough cooking of beef.

TAENIA SOLIUM AND CYSTICERCOSIS

T. solium, the pork tapeworm, is common in central Europe, South Africa, South America and parts of Asia. It is not as large as *T. saginata*. The scolex has, in addition to suckers, two circular rows of hooklets anterior to the suckers. The adult worm is found only in humans following the eating of undercooked pork containing cysticerci.

Human cysticercosis

This results from ova usually being swallowed or possibly gaining access to the human stomach by regurgitation from the person's own adult worm (see Fig. 2.45). The larvae are liberated from eggs in the stomach, penetrate the intestinal mucosa and are carried to many parts of the body where they develop and form cysticerci, 0.5–1 cm cysts that contain the head of a young worm. They do not grow further or migrate. Common locations are the subcutaneous tissue, skeletal muscles and brain.

Clinical features

When superficially placed, cysts can be palpated under the skin or mucosa as pea-like ovoid bodies. Here they cause few or no symptoms, and will eventually die and become calcified.

Heavy brain infections, especially in children, may cause features of encephalitis. More commonly, however, cerebral signs do not occur until the larvae die, 5–20 years later. Epilepsy, personality changes, staggering gait or signs of internal hydrocephalus are the most common features.

Investigations

Calcified cysts in muscles can be recognised radiologically. In the brain, however, less calcification takes place and larvae are only occasionally demonstrated radiologically but usually by computed tomography or magnetic resonance imaging. Epileptic fits starting in adult life should suggest the possibility of cysticercosis if the patient has lived or travelled in an endemic area. The subcutaneous tissue should be palpated and any nodule excised for histology. Radiological examination of the skeletal muscles may be helpful. Antibody detection by fluorescent antibody test, ELISA or immunoblotting is available for serodiagnosis.

Management

Praziquantel (see Table 2.35) improves the prognosis of cerebral cysticercosis; the dose is 50 mg/kg in three divided doses daily for 10 days. Albendazole, 15 mg/kg daily for a minimum of 8 days, has now become the drug of choice for parenchymal neurocysticercosis. Prednisolone, 10 mg every 8 hours, is also given for 14 days, starting 1 day before the albendazole or praziquantel. In addition, anti-epileptic drugs should be given until the reaction in the

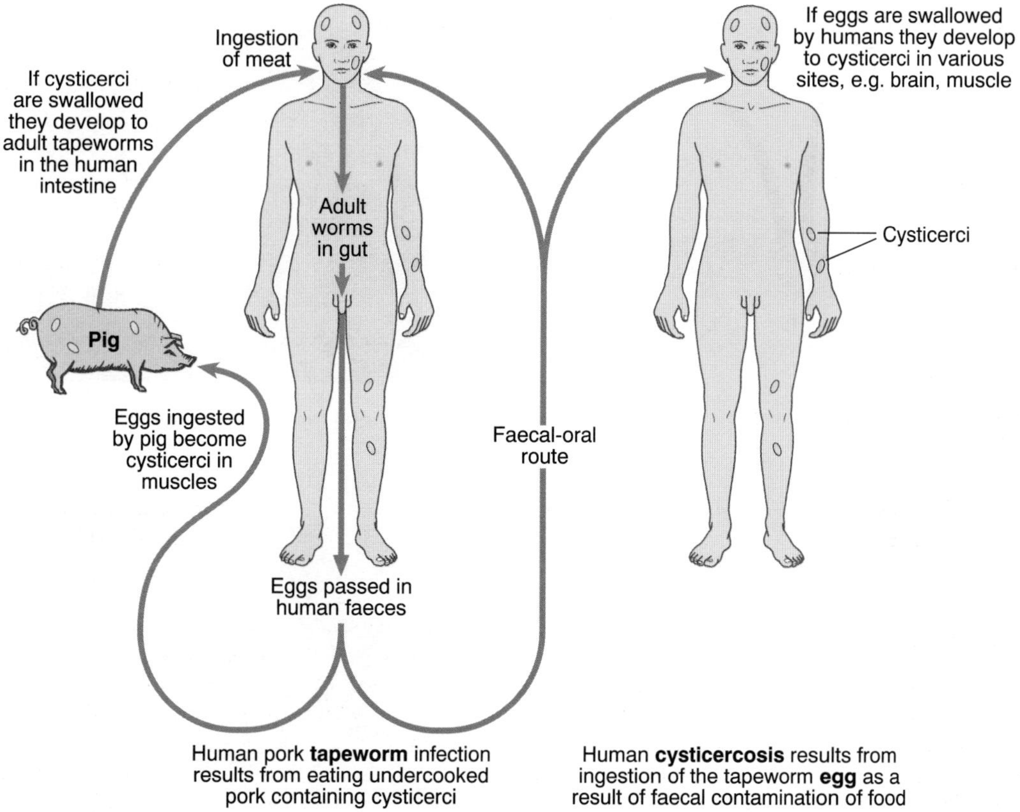
Ingestion of meat
If cysticerci are swallowed they develop to adult tapeworms in the human intestine
Adult worms in gut
Pig
Eggs ingested by pig become cysticerci in muscles
Eggs passed in human faeces
Faecal-oral route
If eggs are swallowed by humans they develop to cysticerci in various sites, e.g. brain, muscle
Cysticerci
Human pork **tapeworm** infection results from eating undercooked pork containing cysticerci
Human **cysticercosis** results from ingestion of the tapeworm **egg** as a result of faecal contamination of food

Fig. 2.45 Cysticercosis. Life cycle of *Taenia solium.*

brain has subsided. Operative intervention is indicated for hydrocephalus.

Prevention

Prevention of adult *T. solium* infection consists in cooking pork well. Cysticercosis is avoided if food is not contaminated by ova or segments. Patients with pork tapeworm probably acquire cysticercosis by ingesting food subjected to faecal contamination or ingesting ova from contaminated fingers, rather than from regurgitation of segments. Great care must be taken by nurses and other adults while attending a patient harbouring an adult worm.

ECHINOCOCCUS GRANULOSUS (TAENIA ECHINOCOCCUS) AND HYDATID DISEASE

The dog and certain wild canines are the definitive host of the tiny tapeworm *E. granulosus*. The larval stage, a hydatid cyst, normally occurs in sheep, cattle, camels and other animals that are infected from contaminated pastures or water. By handling a dog or drinking contaminated water, humans may ingest eggs (see Fig. 2.46). The embryo is liberated from the ovum in the small intestine and gains access to the blood stream and thus to the liver. The resultant cyst grows very slowly, sometimes intermittently, and may outlive the patient. It may calcify or may rupture giving rise to multiple cysts. The disease is common in the Middle East and North and East Africa, Australia and Argentina. Foci of infection persist in rural Wales and Scotland. A variant, *E. multilocularis*, which has a cycle between foxes and voles, causes a similar but more severe infection, 'alveolar hydatid disease', which invades the liver like cancer.

Clinical features

A hydatid cyst is typically acquired in childhood and it may, after growing for some years, cause pressure symptoms. These vary, depending on the organ or tissue involved. In nearly 75% of patients with hydatid disease the right lobe of the liver is invaded and contains a single cyst. In others a cyst may be found in lung, bone, brain or elsewhere.

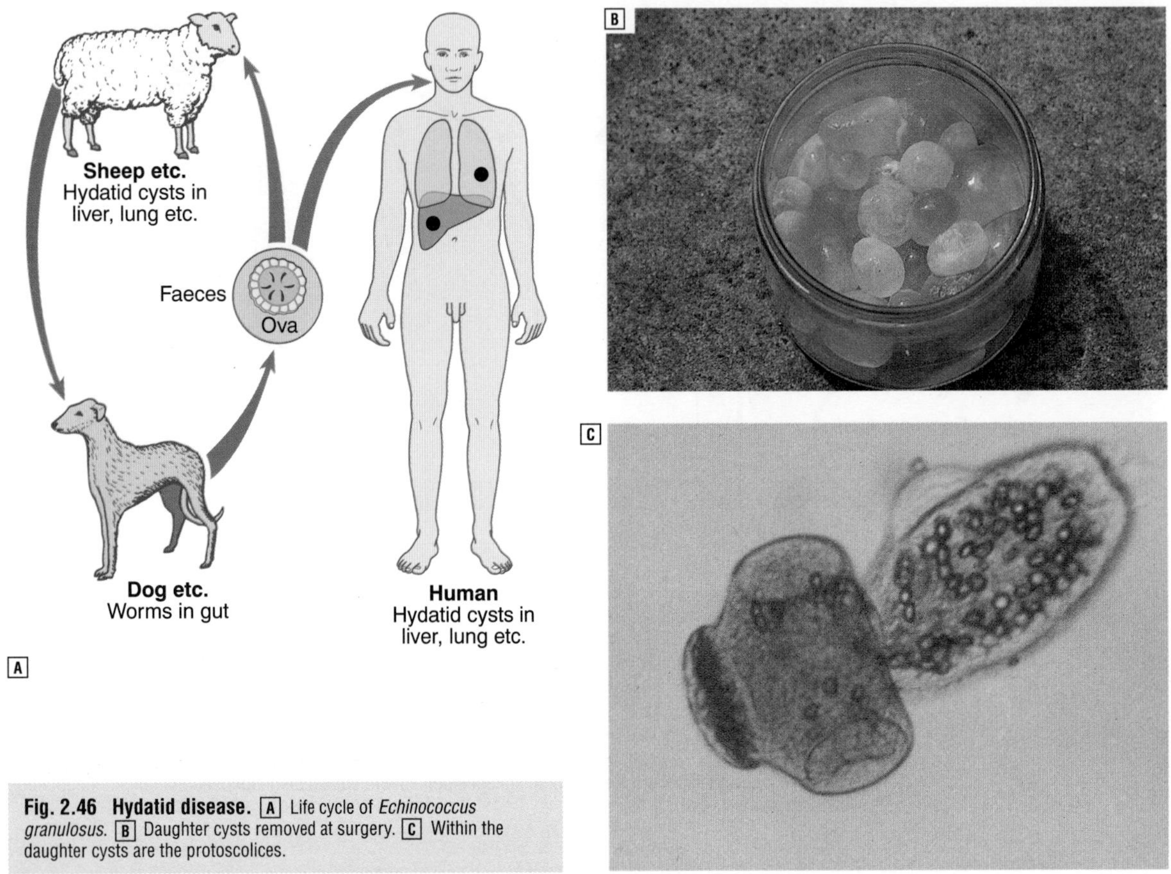

Fig. 2.46 Hydatid disease. [A] Life cycle of *Echinococcus granulosus.* [B] Daughter cysts removed at surgery. [C] Within the daughter cysts are the protoscolices.

Investigations

The diagnosis depends on the clinical, radiological and ultrasound findings in a patient who has lived in close contact with dogs in an endemic area. Complement fixation and enzyme-linked immunosorbent assay are positive in 70–90% of patients.

Management

Hydatid cysts should be excised wherever possible. Great care is taken to avoid spillage and cavities are sterilised with 0.5% silver nitrate or 2.7% sodium chloride. Albendazole (400 mg 12-hourly for 3 months) is used for inoperable disease, and to reduce the infectivity of cysts pre-operatively. Praziquantel 20 mg/kg 12-hourly for 14 days kills protoscolices perioperatively.

Prevention

Prevention is difficult in situations where there is a close association with dogs and sheep. Personal hygiene, satisfactory disposal of carcasses, meat inspection and deworming of dogs can greatly reduce the prevalence of disease.

OTHER TAPEWORMS

There are many other cestodes whose adult or larval stages may infect humans, the most common of which are summarised in Table 2.35. Sparganosis is a condition in which an immature worm develops in humans, usually subcutaneously, as a result of eating or applying to the skin the secondary or tertiary intermediate host.

NEMATODE (ROUNDWORM) INFECTIONS

Nematode infections of humans may be divided into three groups (see the information box on page 164).

Intestinal nematodes

The most common that cause disease are listed in the information box.

Adult male and female worms live in the lumen of the gut and do not normally invade tissues. They often have complex life cycles and may cause a syndrome of fever, cough and eosinophilia during the stage of larval invasion. Eggs or larvae are passed in the faeces and the worm does not normally complete its life cycle in humans. *Strongyloides*, however, behaves differently and is potentially very dangerous.

Tissue-dwelling human nematodes

These are the filarial worms and the guinea worm *Dracunculus medinensis*.

These worms have complex life cycles, with an intermediate host that is also a vector. Depending on the species, disease may be due to the presence of the adult worms or to their progeny, the microfilariae, which migrate in the blood or tissues, provoking a massive eosinophilia; but often the infection is long-lived and well tolerated.

Zoonotic nematodes

Nematodes that normally infect other animals may cause serious incidental infections in humans.

The infective larvae of these worms are unable to 'home' to their normal site for development into adults, in their abnormal host. They may wander or may become trapped in a particular organ. They tend to provoke severe inflammatory reactions characterised by eosinophilic granulomas.

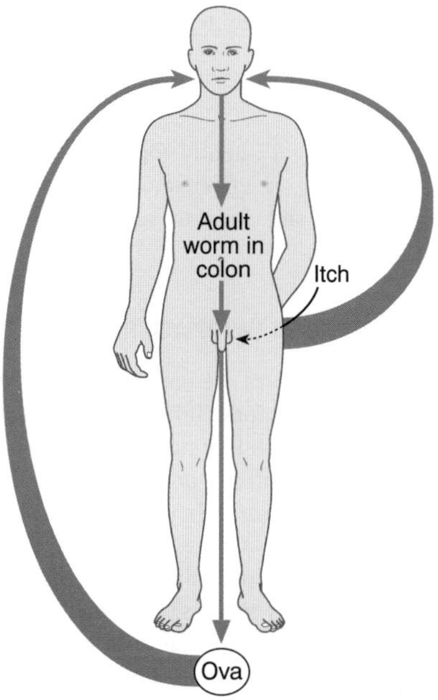

Fig. 2.47 Threadworm. Life cycle of *Enterobius vermicularis.*

ENTEROBIUS VERMICULARIS (THREADWORM)

This helminth is common throughout the world. It affects children especially. The male worm is 2–5 mm long and the female 8–13 mm. After the ova are swallowed, development takes place in the small intestine, but the adult worms are found chiefly in the colon.

Clinical features

The gravid female worm lays ova around the anus, and causes intense itching, especially at night. The ova are often carried to the mouth on the fingers and so reinfection takes place (see Fig. 2.47). In females the genitalia may be involved. The adult worms may be seen moving on the buttocks or in the stool.

Investigations

Ova are detected by applying the adhesive surface of cellophane tape to the perianal skin in the morning. This is then examined on a glass slide under the microscope. A perianal swab, moistened with saline, is an alternative method for diagnosis.

Management

A single dose of mebendazole 100 mg or pyrantel pamoate 10 mg base/kg or piperazine 4 g is given and may be repeated after 2 weeks to control auto-reinfection. Where infection constantly recurs in a family, each member should be treated as above. During this period all night clothes and bed linen are laundered. Finger nails must be kept short and hands washed carefully before meals. Subsequent therapy is reserved for those family members who develop recurrent infection.

ASCARIS LUMBRICOIDES (ROUNDWORM)

This pale yellow worm is 20–35 cm long. Humans are infected by eating food contaminated with mature ova. These hatch in the duodenum and the larvae migrate through the lungs, where they moult, ascend the bronchial tree and are swallowed. They mature in the small intestine. In heavy infections, larvae in the lung may cause pneumonitis and eosinophilia.

Clinical features

Adult worms commonly cause abdominal discomfort or colic and may be vomited or passed per rectum. A tangled mass of worms may cause intestinal obstruction and a heavy infestation will compete for nourishment and contribute to malnutrition. Other complications include blockage of the bile or pancreatic duct and obstruction of the appendix by adult worms.

Investigations

The diagnosis is made microscopically by finding ova in the faeces or by observing an adult worm. A solely male infection is usually revealed only after the giving of an antihelmintic to a patient with an unexplained eosinophilia.

Occasionally the worms are demonstrated radiographically by a barium examination.

Management

Mebendazole 100 mg 12-hourly for 3 days, or piperazine 4 g as a single dose, is effective. Surgery is required if obstruction occurs and fails to respond to nasogastric suction and sedation.

TRICHURIS TRICHIURA (WHIPWORM)

Infections with whipworm are common all over the world under unhygienic conditions. Infection takes place by the ingestion of earth or food contaminated with ova which have become infective after lying for 3 weeks or more in moist soil. The adult worm is 3–5 cm long and has a coiled anterior end resembling a whip. Whipworms inhabit the caecum, lower ileum, appendix, colon and anal canal. There are usually no symptoms, but intense infections in children may cause persistent diarrhoea or rectal prolapse, and stunting. The diagnosis is readily made by identifying ova in faeces. Treatment is with mebendazole in doses of 100 mg 12-hourly for 3–5 days or a single dose of oxantel (see Table 2.36).

ANCYLOSTOMIASIS (HOOKWORM)

Ancylostomiasis is caused by parasitisation of the small intestine with *Ancylostoma duodenale* or *Necator americanus*. It is one of the main causes of anaemia in the tropics. The adult hookworm is a greyish-white nematode about 1 cm long which lives, often in large numbers, in the duodenum and upper jejunum. Eggs are passed in the faeces. In warm, moist, shady soil the larvae develop and reach the filariform infective stage; they then penetrate human skin and are carried to the lungs (see Fig. 2.48). After entering the alveoli they ascend the bronchi, are swallowed and develop in the small intestine, reaching maturity 4–7 weeks after infection.

Hookworm infection is widespread under insanitary conditions in the tropics and subtropics and used to be common in mines in Europe. *A. duodenale* is endemic in the Far East and Mediterranean coastal regions and is also present in Africa, while *N. americanus* is endemic in West, East and Central Africa and Central and South America as well as in the Far East.

Pathology

The larvae may cause allergic inflammation at the site of entry through the skin. When infection is heavy, the passage through the lungs may cause pulmonary eosinophilia. The worms attach themselves to the mucosa of the small intestine by their buccal capsule (see Fig. 2.49) and withdraw blood. The mean daily loss of blood from one *A. duodenale* is 0.15 ml and for *N. americanus* 0.03 ml. The degree of iron and protein deficiency which develops depends not only on the load of worms but also on the nutrition of the patient and especially on the iron stores. Thus in a light infection there may be no anaemia. In the early stages of infection eosinophilia is common.

Clinical features

Dermatitis usually on the feet (ground itch) may be experienced at the time of infection. The passage of the larvae through the lungs in a heavy infection causes a paroxysmal cough with blood-stained sputum, associated

Table 2.36 Relative activity of drugs used for the common gut nematodes

	Ascaris	Hookworm	*Enterobius*	*Trichuris*	*Strongyloides*
Piperazine salts 75 mg/kg	+++	+	+++	–	–
Pyrantel pamoate 10 mg/kg	+++	++	+++	–	–
Oxantel pamoate 10 mg/kg	–	–	–	+++	–
Mebendazole 100 mg (any age)	++	++	+++	++	+
Albendazole 400 mg	++	++	+	+	++
Thiabendazole 25 mg/kg	(++)	(++)	(++)	(+)	+++
Levamisole 5 mg/kg	+++	+	+	–	–
Pyrvinium 5 mg/kg	+	–	+++	–	–

Size of a single dose is given. (+ = quite effective therapy; ++ = effective; +++ = very effective; – = ineffective) Activities given in parentheses indicate that the drug is not used for that species. Piperazine is cheap and safe, but with a limited range. Mebendazole given twice daily for 3 days is completely safe and eradicates most infections. Thiabendazole has a wide spectrum; it is absorbed and effective against many tissue-dwelling nematodes, but toxic, causing dizziness, headaches, anorexia, vomiting and drowsiness. A single-dose antihelmintic is ideal for mass treatment and control schemes. Levamisole is the first choice for roundworms, and has a useful action against hookworms. A single dose of pyrantel pamoate and oxantel pamoate or of albendazole is used for multiple infections.

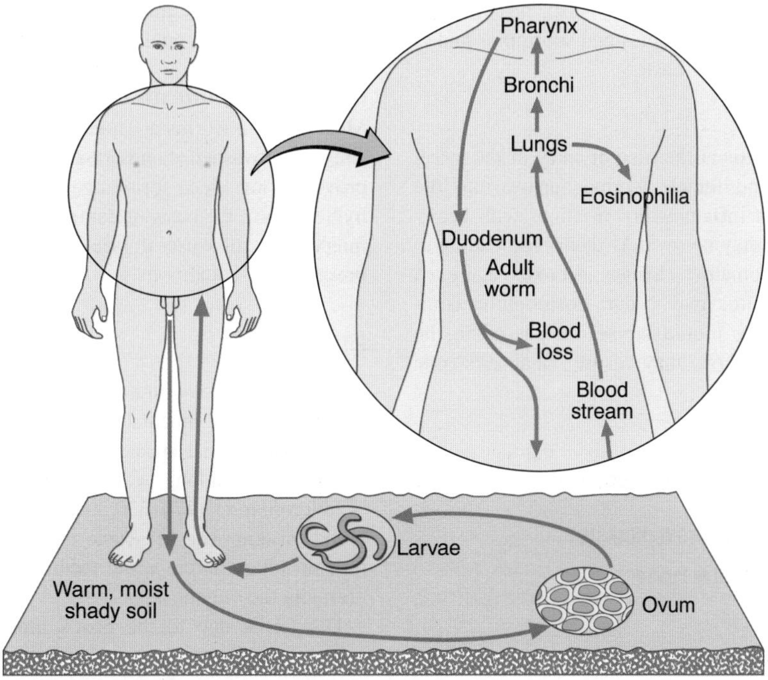

Fig. 2.48 Ancylostomiasis. Life cycle.

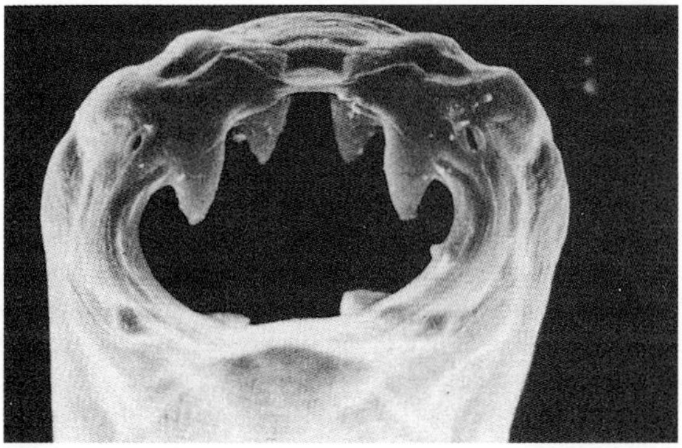

Fig. 2.49 *Ancylostoma duodenale*. Electron micrograph showing the ventral teeth.

with patchy pulmonary consolidation. When the worms have reached the small intestine, vomiting and epigastric pain resembling peptic ulcer disease may ensue. Sometimes frequent loose stools are passed, the condition then resembling early sprue or giardiasis. Anaemia and hypoproteinaemia may develop in the undernourished. The mental and physical development of children may be retarded. There may be no symptoms in a well-nourished person with a light infection.

Investigations

The characteristic ovum can be recognised in the stool. If hookworms are present in numbers sufficient to cause anaemia, tests of the stool for occult blood will be positive and ova will be present in large numbers.

Management

This is listed in Table 2.36. Mebendazole twice daily for 3 days is preferred, but for single-dose treatment pyrantel is the best choice. Anaemia associated with hookworm infection responds well to oral iron. When anaemia is severe enough to cause heart failure, blood should be transfused slowly, giving frusemide in a dose of 20 mg for each unit.

STRONGYLOIDIASIS

Strongyloides stercoralis is a very small nematode (2 mm × 0.4 mm) which parasitises the mucosa of the upper part of the small intestine, often in large numbers. The eggs hatch in the bowel but only larvae are passed in the faeces. In moist soil they moult and become the infective filariform larvae. After penetrating human skin they undergo a development cycle similar to that of hookworms but the female worms burrow into the mucosa and submucosa. Some larvae in the intestine may develop into filariform larvae which may then penetrate the mucosa or the perianal skin and lead to autoinfection and a very persistent infection. Humans are the natural hosts but dogs may also be infected. Strongyloidiasis occurs in the tropics and subtropics and is especially prevalent in the Far East.

Pathology

There may be a dermatitis at the time of entry of the larval worms. In the intestine female worms burrow into the mucosa and induce an inflammatory reaction; with heavy infections the mucosa may be severely damaged, leading to malabsorption. Granulomatous changes, necrosis, and even perforation and peritonitis may occur. Eosinophilia commonly persists. Actively motile larvae are passed in the faeces. Immunosuppression may cause fatal systemic strongyloidiasis.

Clinical features

These are shown in the information box.

CLINICAL FEATURES OF STRONGYLOIDIASIS
Penetration of skin by infective larvae
• Itchy rash
Presence of worms in gut
• Abdominal pain, diarrhoea, steatorrhoea, weight loss
Allergic phenomena
• Urticarial plaques and papules, wheezing, arthralgia
Autoinfection
• Transient itchy linear urticarial wheals across abdomen and buttocks (larva currens)
Systemic (super-)infection
• Diarrhoea, pneumonia, meningoencephalitis, death

Systemic strongyloidiasis (the strongyloides hyperinfestation syndrome) occurs in association with immune suppression (intercurrent disease, HTLV1 infection, corticosteroid treatment) and is rapidly fatal unless diagnosed and promptly treated.

Investigations

Motile larvae can be seen on microscopic examination of the faeces and occasionally in the sputum. Excretion is intermittent so repeated examinations or jejunal aspiration or a string test (see p. 155) may be necessary. Serology (ELISA) is helpful, but definitive diagnosis depends upon finding the larvae.

Management

Ivermectin 200 μg/kg as a single dose, or two doses of 200 μg/kg on successive days, is effective. Albendazole is given orally in a dose of 15 mg/kg body weight twice daily for 3 days. A second course may be required. For the strongyloides hyperinfestation syndrome, ivermectin is given at 200 μg/kg on days 1 and 2, 15 and 16.

Prevention of intestinal nematode infections

Most of these worms are transmitted through contaminated soil or unwashed hands. Safe disposal of faeces, the provision of clean drinking water and strict personal hygiene form the basis of control. Mass treatment at yearly intervals is also useful (see Table 2.36). Capillariasis is prevented by cooking fish.

FILARIASES

Several nematodes of the family *Filarioidea* infect humans. Larval stages are inoculated by biting flies, each specific to a particular filarial species. The larvae develop into adult worms (2–50 cm long) which, after mating, produce millions of microfilariae (170–320 microns long) that migrate in blood or skin. The life cycle is completed when the flies take up microfilariae while feeding on humans, which are normally the only host.

Disease is due to the host's immune response to the worms, particularly dying worms, and its pattern and severity vary with the site and stage of each species (see Table 2.37). The worms are long-lived; microfilariae survive 2–3 years and adult worms 10–15 years. The infections are chronic and worst in individuals constantly exposed to reinfection. Filarial infections cause the highest eosinophilia of all helmintic infections, and are normally diagnosed by the morphology of the microfilariae.

LYMPHATIC FILARIASIS

Wuchereria bancrofti is conveyed to humans by the bites of infected mosquitoes of a number of different species, the most common being *Culex fatigans*. The adult worms, 4–10 cm in length, live in the lymphatics, and the females produce microfilariae which at night circulate in large numbers in the peripheral blood. In the mosquito, ingested microfilariae develop into infective larvae. As *Culex*

Table 2.37 Pathology of filarial infections depending upon the site and stage of worms

Worm species	Adult worm	Microfilariae
Wuchereria bancrofti* and *Brugia malayi	Lymphatic vessels^{+++}	Blood^{-} Pulmonary capillaries^{++}
Loa loa	Subcutaneous^{+}	Blood^{+}
Onchocerca volvulus	Subcutaneous^{+}	Skin^{+++} Eye^{+++}
Mansonella perstans	Retroperitoneal^{-}	Blood^{-}
Mansonella streptocerca	Skin^{+}	Skin^{++}

($^{+++}$ = severe; $^{++}$ = moderate; $^{+}$ = mild; $^{-}$ = rarely pathogenic) *fatigans* bites at night the nocturnal periodicity of the microfilariae facilitates the spread of the infection. There is a non-periodic strain of *W. bancrofti* in some of the Pacific islands, maintained by mosquitoes which bite in the daytime. The microfilariae are chiefly in the capillaries in the lungs when not circulating in the peripheral blood. The infection is widespread in tropical Africa, the North African coast, coastal areas of Asia, Indonesia and northern Australia, South Pacific islands, the West Indies and also in North and South America.

Brugia malayi resembles *W. bancrofti* closely. The microfilariae usually exhibit nocturnal periodicity. The vectors are mosquitoes mostly belonging to the genus *Mansonia*. *B. malayi* is found in Indonesia, Borneo, Malaysia, Vietnam, South China, South India and Sri Lanka. A distinct, closely related species, *B. timori*, occurs in Timor.

Pathology

The presence of adult worms in the lymphatics causes allergic lymphangitis (see Table 2.37). Recurrent episodes may lead to intermittent lymphatic obstruction and transient lymphoedema, which may later become permanent in the leg, arm, genitalia or breast, and to hydrocele. Obstructed lymphatics become dilated and tortuous and may rupture. Rupture into tissues leads to cellulitis, fibrosis and elephantiasis. Increased lymphatic pressure may cause retrograde flow or rupture, in turn causing chyluria, chylous ascites and chylous pleural effusions (see Fig. 2.50). The incubation period is not less than 3 months.

Clinical features

There are bouts of fever accompanied by pain, tenderness and erythema along the course of inflamed lymphatic vessels. Inflammation of the spermatic cord, epididymitis and orchitis are common. The fever abates after a few days and the symptoms and signs subside.

Further attacks follow, temporary oedema becomes more persistent, and regional lymph nodes enlarge. Progressive enlargement, coarsening, corrugation and fissuring of the skin and subcutaneous tissue with warty superficial excrescences develop gradually, causing irreversible 'elephantiasis'. The scrotum may reach an enormous size. Chyluria and chylous effusions are milky and opalescent; on standing, fat globules rise to the top. Eventually, the adult worms may die but the lymphatics remain obstructed. The interval between infection and the onset of elephantiasis is usually not less than 10 years and elephantiasis develops only in association with repeated infections in highly endemic areas.

Tropical pulmonary eosinophilia

Occasionally, and especially in Indians, microfilariae become trapped in the pulmonary capillaries and are destroyed by allergic inflammation. The resulting pneumonitis causes persistent cough, fever, weight loss and radiological changes suggestive of miliary tuberculosis.

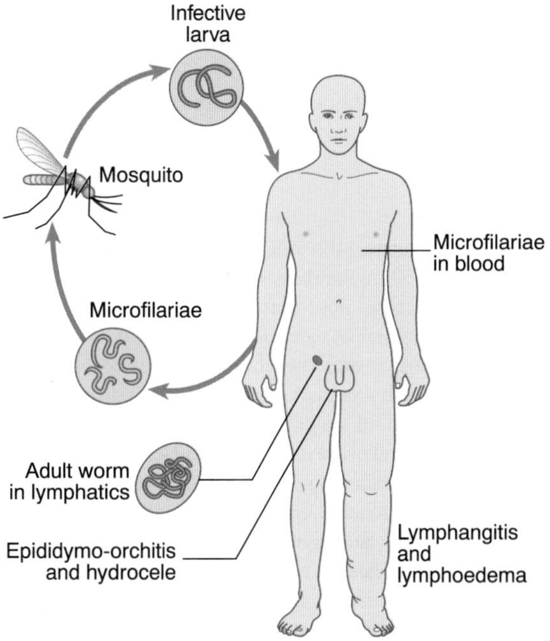

Fig. 2.50 *Wuchereria bancrofti* and *Brugia malayi*. Life cycle and pathogenesis of lymphatic filariasis.

Non-filarial elephantiasis

Usually affecting one or both legs, this occurs in certain geographical areas which are free from filariasis. It is attributable to damage to lymphatics by silicates absorbed from soil derived from volcanic rocks.

Investigations

In the earliest stages of lymphangitis the diagnosis is made on clinical grounds, supported by eosinophilia and sometimes by positive serology. Microfilariae appear in the blood at night after about a year from the time of infection and can be seen moving in a wet blood film or by microfiltration of a sample of lysed blood. They are usually present in hydrocele fluid which may occasionally yield an adult filaria. By the time elephantiasis develops, microfilariae become difficult to find. Calcified filariae may sometimes be demonstrable by radiography. An initial exaggeration of symptoms following the administration of diethylcarbamazine suggests a filarial infection.

Immunodiagnosis

Indirect fluorescence and enzyme-linked immunosorbent assay detect antibodies in over 95% of active cases and 70% of established elephantiasis. Cross-reactions occur in

15% of cases of *Strongyloides* and 5% of other intestinal nematodes. The test becomes negative 1–2 years after cure. None of these tests distinguishes between the different filarial infections. In tropical pulmonary eosinophilia, serology is strongly positive but circulating microfilariae are not found.

Management

Diethylcarbamazine kills microfilariae and adult worms. The dose is 9–12 mg/kg daily orally in three divided doses for 14 days. The full dose must be reached slowly, starting with 50 mg (one tablet) and doubling daily unless serious allergic reactions ensue. This course may be repeated twice at intervals of 4–6 weeks. Antihistamines or corticosteroids may be required to control allergic phenomena. Plastic surgery may be indicated in established elephantiasis. Great relief can be obtained by removal of excess tissue but recurrences are probable unless new lymphatic drainage is established. Tight bandaging, bed rest with suspension or raising of the affected part, or the nightly use of pneumatic stockings may control the swelling to some extent. Assiduous skin care is essential in established elephantiasis to prevent secondary bacterial infection. Prompt diagnosis and antibiotic therapy of bacterial cellulitis are important in preventing further lymphatic damage and worsening of existing elephantiasis.

Prevention

Treatment of the whole population in endemic areas with diethylcarbamazine, 100 mg for adults (50 mg for children) three times daily for 7 days, has reduced but not eliminated the infection. Children are given such a course on starting and before leaving school. Ivermectin, alone or in combination with albendazole, is under evaluation as an alternative to diethylcarbamazine. This mass treatment should be combined with control of the vector by insecticides. Early chemotherapy prevents later elephantiasis. Individuals should avoid being bitten by mosquitoes (see p. 153).

LOIASIS

Loiasis is caused by infection with the filaria *Loa loa*. The adults, 3–7 cm × 4 mm, parasitise chiefly the subcutaneous tissue of humans. The larval microfilariae circulate harmlessly in the peripheral blood in the daytime. The vector is *Chrysops*, a forest-dwelling fly which bites by day.

Pathology

The adult worms move harmlessly about in the subcutaneous tissues and other interstitial planes (see Table 2.37). From time to time a short-lived, inflammatory, oedematous swelling (a *Calabar swelling*) is produced, presumably around an adult worm. Heavy infections, especially when treated, may cause encephalitis. The incubation period is commonly over a year but may be as short as 3 months.

Clinical features

The infection is often symptomless. The first sign is usually a Calabar swelling, which is an irritating, tense, localised swelling that may be painful, especially if it is near a joint. The swelling is generally on a limb; it measures a few centimetres in diameter but sometimes is more diffuse and extensive. It usually disappears after a few days but may persist for 2 or 3 weeks. A succession of such swellings may appear at irregular intervals, often in adjacent sites. Sometimes there is urticaria and pruritus elsewhere. Occasionally a worm may be seen wriggling under the skin, especially of an eyelid, and may cross the eye under the conjunctiva, taking many minutes to do so. Severe unilateral headaches resembling migraine may be experienced when an adult worm moves in the retro-orbital tissues.

Investigations

The diagnosis is made by demonstrating microfilariae in the blood, but they may not always be found in patients with Calabar swellings. Antifilarial antibodies are positive in 95% of patients and there is massive eosinophilia. Occasionally, a calcified worm may be seen on a radiograph.

Management

Diethylcarbamazine (see above) is curative, gradually increased to a dose of 9–12 mg/kg daily which is continued for 21 days. Treatment may precipitate a severe reaction in patients with a heavy microfilaraemia characterised by fever, joint and muscle pain and encephalitis; microfilaraemic patients should be given steroid cover (see p. 180).

Prevention

Protection is afforded by siting houses away from trees and by having dwellings wire-screened against the fly. Protective clothing and repellents are also useful. Diethylcarbamazine in a dose of 5 mg/kg daily for 3 days each month is partially protective.

ONCHOCERCIASIS (RIVER BLINDNESS)

Onchocerciasis is the result of infection by *Onchocerca volvulus*. Although only about 0.3 mm in diameter, the adult female may be as long as 50 cm; the male is 13 cm. The infection is conveyed by flies of the genus *Simulium* which inflict a painful bite. In West Africa the vector is *S. damnosum*, in northern Nigeria also *S. bovis* and in East Africa and Zaire *S. neavei*. The flies breed in rapidly flowing, well-aerated water, the larvae being attached to submerged vegetation, rocks or crabs. Adult flies bite during the daytime both inside and outside houses. Humans are the only known definitive hosts.

Onchocerciasis is endemic in well-defined areas throughout tropical Africa, in southern Arabia and Yemen and also in South Mexico, Guatemala, Colombia, Venezuela and Brazil. It is estimated that over 20 million people are infected. In parts of West and Central Africa it affects the whole adult population and blindness rates of 10% are common, reaching 35% in some parts of Ghana. Due to onchocerciasis huge tracts of fertile land lie virtually untilled, and individuals and communities are impoverished.

Pathology

Infective larvae of *O. volvulus* are introduced into the skin by the bite of an infected *Simulium* fly (see Fig. 2.51). The worms mature in 2–4 months and live for up to 17 years in small colonies in subcutaneous and connective tissues (see Table 2.37). At sites of trauma, over bony prominences and around joints, fibrosis may form nodules around adult worms which otherwise cause no direct damage. Innumerable microfilariae, discharged by the female *O. volvulus*, move actively in these nodules and in the adjacent tissues, are widely distributed in the skin, and may invade the eye.

Live microfilariae elicit little tissue reaction, but dead microfilariae may cause severe allergic inflammation leading to hyaline necrosis and loss of collagen and elastin. Death of microfilariae in the eye causes conjunctivitis, sclerosing keratitis with pannus formation, uveitis which may lead to glaucoma and cataract and, less commonly, choroidoretinitis and optic neuritis.

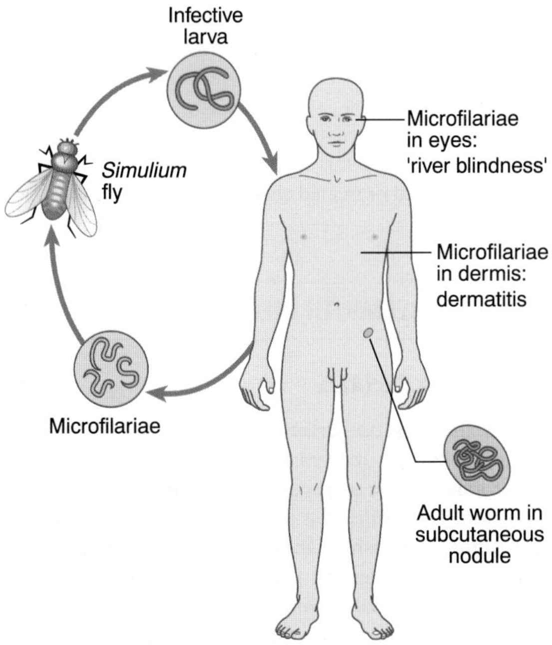

Fig. 2.51 ***Onchocerca volvulus.*** Life cycle and pathogenesis of onchocerciasis.

Clinical features

The infection may remain symptomless for months or years. The first symptom is usually itching, localised to one quadrant of the body and later becoming generalised and involving the eyes. Evanescent oedema of part or all of a limb in Europeans is an early sign, followed by papular urticaria spreading gradually from the site of infection. This is difficult to see on dark skins, in which the most common signs are papules excoriated by scratching, spotty hyperpigmentation from resolving inflammation and more chronic changes of a rough, thickened skin or inelastic wrinkled skin. Superficial lymph nodes enlarge and may hang down in folds of loose skin at the groins. Hydrocele, femoral hernias and scrotal elephantiasis occur. Firm subcutaneous nodules occur in chronic infection (onchocercomas), which are palpable, 1 cm or more in diameter.

Eye disease is most common in highly endemic areas and is associated with chronic heavy infections and nodules on the head. Early manifestations include itching, lacrimation, conjunctival injection and evidence of the features listed under Pathology. Classically, 'snowflake' deposits are seen in the edges of the cornea.

Investigations

The finding of nodules or characteristic lesions of the skin or eyes in a patient from an endemic area, associated with eosinophilia, is suggestive. Skin snips or shavings, taken with a corneoscleral punch or scalpel blade from calf, buttock and shoulder are placed in saline under a cover slip on a microscope slide and examined after 4 hours. Microfilariae are seen wriggling free in all but the lightest infections. If negative, a test dose of diethylcarbamazine is given to see if it aggravates the rash. Slit-lamp examination of the eye may reveal microfilariae moving in the anterior chamber of the eye, or trapped in the cornea. A nodule may be removed and incised, showing the coiled thread-like adult worm. Filarial antibodies may be detected in up to 95% of patients, but antibody positivity can be much lower in lightly infected expatriates.

Management

Ivermectin, in a single dose of 100–200 μg/kg, kills microfilariae and prevents their return for 9 months. It is non-toxic and does not trigger severe reactions, in contrast to diethylcarbamazine which is no longer used for this infection.

In the rare event of a severe reaction causing oedema or postural hypotension, prednisolone 20–30 mg may be given daily for 2 or 3 days.

Adult worms are killed by suramin (1 g intravenously, weekly for 5–6 doses), but a repeated dose of ivermectin every 6–12 months is preferred to the potential significant toxicity of suramin (see Table 2.31, p. 162). Palpable nodules should be excised.

Prevention

Mass treatment with ivermectin is in use. It reduces morbidity in the community and prevents eye disease from getting worse. *Simulium* can be destroyed in its larval stage by the application of insecticide to streams. Dimethyl phthalate applied to skin or clothing will repel the fly for several hours. Long trousers, skirts and sleeves discourage the fly from biting.

OTHER FILARIASES

Mansonella perstans

This filarial worm is transmitted by the midges *Culicoides austeni* and *C. grahami*. It is common throughout equatorial Africa as far south as Zambia, and also in Trinidad and parts of northern and eastern South America.

M. perstans has never been shown to cause disease but it may be responsible for a persistent eosinophilia and occasional allergic manifestations (see Table 2.37, p. 176). *M. perstans* is resistant to ivermectin and diethylcarbamazine and the infection may persist for many years.

Mansonella ozzardi

This is non-pathogenic and is found in the West Indies and South America.

DRACONTIASIS (GUINEA WORM)

The female *Dracunculus medinensis*, which measures over a metre in length and 0.9–1.7 mm in diameter, lives in the interstitial and subcutaneous tissues of humans. The male worm, which is rarely seen, is only 2.5 cm long. Humans are infected by ingesting a small crustacean, *Cyclops*, which inhabits wells and ponds and which contains the infective larval stage of the worm.

Pathology

Ingested larvae mature, penetrate the intestinal wall and migrate through the connective tissues of the host. After 9–18 months the fully mature female surfaces under the skin, usually on the leg, where a vesicle is raised, ruptures and exposes the anterior end of the worm. The worm's distended uterus ruptures and discharges its larvae externally. The worm is attracted to the surface by cooling, hence the larvae are likely to be expelled into water, where they complete the life cycle.

The disease can be extremely disabling and is especially liable to affect those who collect water at water-holes, or farmers at the beginning of the rains, and thus seriously interferes with planting. It is found in sub-Saharan Africa, Egypt, the Arabian peninsula, Iran, Afghanistan and in parts of Pakistan and India.

Clinical features

The adult worm may sometimes be felt beneath the skin. Some hours before the head of the worm emerges from the skin there is painful, hot, local inflammation which vesiculates. It takes 3–4 weeks for the larvae to be discharged, during which time the ulcer persists and there is pain and cellulitis, especially if it is close to an ankle or knee. There will be a marked allergic inflammation if the worm dies or is broken during extraction. Secondary infection is common and may cause cellulitis, arthritis or septicaemia. Tetanus is a well-recognised complication. Multiple infections may occur and reactions around aberrant worms may cause serious lesions.

Diagnosis

This is usually clinical. Discharge fluid may contain larvae. A radiograph may show calcified worms.

Management

Traditionally, the protruding worm is extracted by winding it out gently over several days on a matchstick. *The worm must never be broken.* Niridazole 25 mg/kg daily in two divided doses for 10 days, or mebendazole 100 mg 12-hourly for 7 days, may reduce inflammation and aid the extraction of the worm. Antibiotics for secondary infection and prophylaxis of tetanus are also required.

Prevention

The provision of a satisfactory water supply will eradicate the infection. Where this is impracticable, wells and ponds may be protected or treated chemically to kill *Cyclops*.

ZOONOTIC HELMINTH INFECTIONS

TRICHINELLA SPIRALIS

This is the most important zoonotic nematode to cause disease in humans. Others are given in Table 2.38 and in the information box on page 164.

Trichinella spiralis is a parasite of rats and pigs and is transmitted to humans if they eat partially cooked infected pork, usually as sausage or ham. Symptoms result from invasion of intestinal submucosa by ingested larvae, which develop into adult worms, and the secondary invasion of tissues by fresh larvae produced by these adult worms. The main tissue invaded is striated muscle, in which the larvae encyst. Outbreaks have occurred in Britain as well as in

Table 2.38 Zoonotic helminths that commonly cause incidental infections in humans

	Toxocara canis	*Ancylostoma braziliense*	*Angiostrongylus cantonensis*	*Gnathostoma spinigerum*
Distribution	World-wide	Tropics and subtropics	Far East, Pacific	Bangladesh, South-east Asia, Far East
Vector/reservoir	Adult roundworms in dog intestine. Ova on contaminated fur and soil	Adult hookworms in dog intestine. Infective larvae on soil	Adults in lungs of rodents. Larvae in snails, slugs, crustacea	Adults in dog and cat intestine. Larvae in *Cyclops*, fish, frogs and snakes
Transmission	Geophagia; handling dogs, especially puppies	Larvae penetrate skin on contact with soil	Eating undercooked snails etc.	Drinking *Cyclops* in water, eating undercooked frogs etc.
Site of parasite in humans	Larval worms migrate and die in tissues	Larval worms migrate in skin	Larval worms in brain, meninges	Larval worms migrate subcutaneously
Clinical features	Visceral larva migrans. Febrile hepatomegaly, rarely blindness	Cutaneous larva migrans. Slowly moving inflamed irritating tracts on buttocks, feet	Eosinophilic meningitis	Recurrent migratory subcutaneous swellings
Laboratory diagnosis	Eosinophilia, serology	May be eosinophilia	Eosinophilia in CSF and blood, serology	Eosinophilia, serology
Treatment	Albendazole 400 mg daily for 7 days	Topical 10% thiabendazole; oral albendazole 400 mg daily for 2 days	Albendazole 400 mg 12-hourly for 14 days Prednisolone (dose varies with age)	Albendazole 400 mg 12-hourly for 14 days

other countries where pork is eaten. Bear meat is another source.

Clinical features

The clinical features of trichinosis depend largely on the number of larvae. There may be no symptoms if there are only a few worms present, but many worms may cause nausea and diarrhoea 24–48 hours after the infected meal. A few days later, these symptoms are overshadowed by those associated with the larval invasion, namely fever and oedema of the face, eyelids and conjunctivae. Invasion of the diaphragm may cause pain, cough and dyspnoea; involvement of the muscles of the limbs, chest and mouth causes stiffness, pain and tenderness in the affected muscle groups. Fever may reach 40°C with daily remissions. Larval migration may cause acute myocarditis and encephalitis. An eosinophilia is usually found after the second week. An intense infection may prove fatal but those who survive recover completely.

Investigations

Commonly, a group of people who have eaten infected pork from a common source develop symptoms at about the same time. Biopsy from the deltoid or gastrocnemius after the third week of symptoms in suspected cases may reveal encysted larvae. Serological tests are also helpful.

Management

Treatment is with albendazole 20 mg/kg daily for 7 days. Given early in the infection it may kill newly formed adult worms in the submucosa and thus reduce the number of larvae reaching the muscles. Corticosteroids are necessary to control the serious effects of acute inflammation.

EOSINOPHILIC SYNDROMES ASSOCIATED WITH HELMINTIC INFECTIONS

Urticarial rashes
- Strongyloidiasis, onchocerciasis, fascioliasis, hydatid disease, trichinosis

Cutaneous larva migrans
- *Ancylostoma braziliense*

Dermatitis
- Onchocerciasis

Migratory subcutaneous swellings
- Loiasis, gnathostomiasis

Lymphangitis, orchitis
- Lymphatic filariasis

Myositis
- Trichinosis, cysticercosis

Febrile hepatosplenomegaly
- Schistosomiasis, toxocariasis

Pneumonitis
- Migratory stage of larval helminths (Loeffler's syndrome), lymphatic filariasis (tropical pulmonary eosinophilia), systemic strongyloidiasis

Enteritis and colitis
- Strongyloidiasis, capillariasis, trichinosis, rarely other intestinal worms

Meningitis
- Angiostrongyliasis, strongyloidiasis

FURTHER INFORMATION ON DISEASES DUE TO HELMINTHS

Arjona R, Riancho J A, Aguado J M, Salesa R, Gonzalez-Macias J 1995 Fascioliasis in developed countries: a review of classic and aberrant forms of the disease. Medicine (Baltimore) 74: 13–23

Cui J, Wang Z Q, Wu F, Jin X X 1997 Epidemiological and clinical studies on an outbreak of trichinosis in central China. Annals of Tropical Medicine and Parasitology 91: 481–488

Del Brutto O H 1997 Neurocysticercosis. Current Opinion in Neurology 10: 268–272

De Silva N R, Guyatt H L, Bundy D A 1997 Morbidity and mortality due to Ascaris-induced intestinal obstruction. Transactions of the Royal Society of Tropical Medicine and Hygiene 91: 31–36

Horton R J 1997 Albendazole in treatment of human cystic echinococcosis: 12 years of experience. Acta Tropica 64: 79–93

Jordan P, Webbe G, Sturrock R F 1993 Human schistosomiasis. CAB International, Wallingford

Mahmoud A A 1996 Strongyloidiasis. Clinical Infectious Diseases 23: 949–952

Van Laethem Y, Lopes C 1996 Treatment of onchocerciasis. Drugs 52: 861–869

Wolfe M S 1992 Eosinophilia in the returning traveller. Infectious Disease Clinics of North America 6: 489–502

DISEASES DUE TO ARTHROPODS

Arthropods may be responsible for disease in four ways:

- They may act as vectors of infectious agents (see Table 2.39).
- They may envenomate through stings or bites.
- They may infest or even infect the human body directly.
- They may cause allergic dermatitis.

LICE

As well as transmitting serious disease, the body louse *Pediculus humanus* causes dermatitis and sleeplessness through itching, especially in poor crowded communities in cold countries (for control see p. 117).

The head louse, *Pediculus capitis*, is cosmopolitan and increasing in prevalence in British schools. It makes the child itch and alarms parents and teachers. Tiny white oval eggs, 'nits', are seen attached to the base of hairs on the scalp. Malathion, carbaryl and the pyrethroids are effective. Resistance is evident in some districts of Britain. Wet combing with a plastic detection comb for 30 minutes provides an alternative but there are no published trials of its efficacy. The crab louse, *Pthirus pubis*, is transmitted in shared beds. Treatment is with malathion or carbaryl.

Table 2.39 Infections conveyed by arthropods

Name	Genus	Disease
House fly	*Musca*	Dysenteries, enteric fevers, salmonelloses; and possibly cholera, trachoma, tropical ulcer
Horse fly	*Tabanus*	Tularaemia, ? anthrax
Oscinid fly	*Hippelates*	Streptococcal dermatitis, conjunctivitis, ? yaws
Tsetse fly	*Glossina*	African trypanosomiasis
Tumbu fly	*Cordylobia*	Myiasis
Mosquito	*Anopheles* *Aedes* *Culex*	Malaria, some arboviruses, Bancroftian and Brugian filariasis Yellow fever, dengue and other arboviruses Bancroftian and Brugian filariasis, Japanese encephalitis and other arboviruses
Black fly	*Simulium*	Onchocerciasis
Midge	*Culicoides*	*Mansonella perstans, M. streptocerca, M. ozzardi*
Soft tick	*Ornithodoros*	Tick-borne relapsing fever, Lyme disease
Hard tick (ixodidae)	*Rhipicephalus* etc.	Some typhus fevers, Kyasanur forest disease, tularaemia, ? Q fever
Sandfly	*Phlebotomus* etc.	Leishmaniasis, sandfly fever, bartonellosis
Louse	*Pediculus*	Epidemic typhus fever, louse-borne relapsing fever, trench fever, *Dipylidium caninum*
Mite	*Leptotrombidium* *Sarcoptres* *Allodermanyssus*	Scrub typhus fever Scabies Rickettsialpox
Winged bug	*Triatoma*	Chagas disease
Flea	*Xenopsylla* *Ctenocephalides* *Tunga*	Plague, endemic typhus fever *Dipylidium caninum* Jiggers

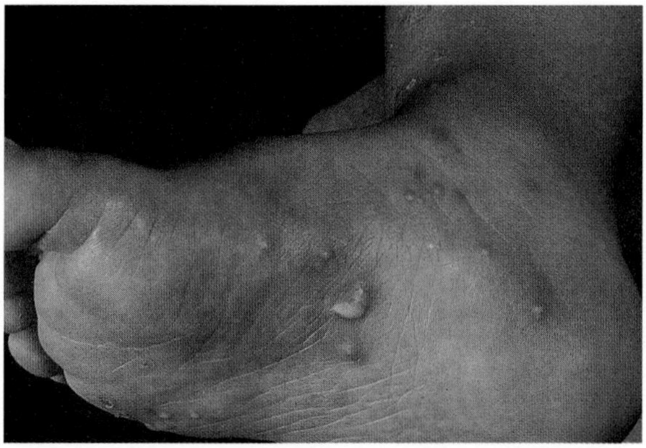

Fig. 2.52 Scabies. Tracks and papules on the soft foot skin of a child.

SCABIES

This disease is due to the mite *Sarcoptes scabiei*; it is common all over the world. There is itching, initially between the fingers or on the buttocks or genitals where the mite burrows, and later all over the body (see Fig. 2.52). Secondary streptococcal infection is an important cause of glomerulonephritis in the tropics. Severe widespread ('Norwegian') scabies occurs in the debilitated or immunosuppressed. The diagnosis of scabies is confirmed by scraping the mite out of a burrow. Scabies is treated by malathion or permethrin. Benzyl benzoate is no longer a first choice. Ivermectin 200 μg/kg single dose by mouth, in combination with topical drugs, is used for 'Norwegian' scabies, which does not respond to topical treatment alone.

JIGGERS (TUNGIASIS)

This is due to infestation with *Tunga penetrans* (the chigoe or jigger flea). It is widespread in tropical America and Africa. Humans and pigs are important hosts. The pregnant female flea burrows into the skin about the toes and soles and grows as large as a pea, packed with eggs which are subsequently discharged on to the surface. The burrows irritate and become inflamed but the chief danger is from secondary pyogenic infection or tetanus.

The chigoe or egg sac should be removed with a sterile needle and a mild antiseptic ointment applied. Massive infestations, such as may be seen in neglected children and in senile persons, may be treated by immersing the feet in an aqueous solution containing benzene hexachloride 5% and cetrimide 0.8%.

MYIASIS

This is an infestation of various tissues of humans by the larvae of flies.

Cutaneous myiasis

A common cause of cutaneous myiasis is *Cordylobia anthropophaga* (Tumbu fly), which lays its eggs on laundry spread on grass. The larvae penetrate the skin and produce lesions like boils with central orifices through which the larvae breathe. On reaching maturity they emerge. A drop of thick oil or petroleum jelly usually brings a larva out in search of air and facilitates its removal. Occasionally, the common warble fly *Hypoderma bovis* may infest humans.

Myiasis of wounds, sores and cavities

The larvae of many flies may infest necrotic tissues in open wounds or ulcers and occasionally invade living tissue. *Chrysomyia bezziana* is found in Africa, India and South Vietnam. It may penetrate the nasal sinuses and cause great destruction. The application of 10% chloroform in a light vegetable oil is the treatment of choice for infested wounds.

Intestinal myiasis

In the tropics especially, vague digestive disturbances or abdominal cramps with diarrhoea and vomiting may be caused by fly larvae in the intestinal canal, the eggs having been ingested with food.

FURTHER INFORMATION ON DISEASES DUE TO ARTHROPODS

Taplin D, Meinking T L 1997 Treatment of HIV-related scabies with emphasis on the efficacy of ivermectin. Seminars in Cutaneous Medicine and Surgery 16: 235–240

SEXUALLY TRANSMITTED DISEASES

Most sexually transmitted diseases (STDs) are increasing in all countries throughout the world. They include syphilis, gonorrhoea, human immunodeficiency virus (HIV) infection, genital herpes simplex virus (HSV) infection, genital warts, chlamydial infection, trichomoniasis and genital candidiasis.

The approach to the patient with suspected STD

Patients who suspect an STD are anxious; staff must be friendly, sympathetic and reassuring, and doctors must put patients at ease and explain that treatment is confidential. The history focuses on genital symptoms. In both sexes this covers genital ulceration, rash, itch, pain or swelling and urinary symptoms, especially burning on micturition. In men the clinician should ask about urethral discharge and in women vaginal discharge and pelvic pain/dyspareunia. General health must be recorded, including menstruation and recent medication, especially with antimicrobial or antiviral agents. The sexual history should cover number of

Table 2.40 Investigations in sexually transmitted disease

Patient and focus	Investigation
FEMALES	
Cervical os	Gram stain and culture for gonococci *Chlamydia* test Smear for cytological examination
Urethral meatus	Gram stain and culture for gonococci
Vagina	Wet (saline) mount and Gram stain for *Candida*, *Trichomonas* and bacterial vaginosis Culture for *Candida* and *Trichomonas*
MALES	
Urethra	Gram stain and culture for gonococci *Chlamydia* test
ALL PATIENTS	Blood for syphilis serology (e.g. Venereal Disease Research Laboratory test—VDRL—(cardiolipin) and fluorescent treponemal antibody absorbed test—FTA-abs) Urinalysis dip-stick, including glucose, protein, blood, leucocyte esterase and nitrite
Genital ulcers	Swab for herpes simplex virus culture Scraping for dark ground microscopy for *T. pallidum* Swab for bacterial culture if secondarily infected
Contacts of gonorrhoea	Rectal Gram stain and culture for gonococci Throat culture for gonococci
Drug abusers and homosexual or bisexual men plus others at risk	Blood for serum markers for hepatitis B and C Blood for HIV antibodies (with informed consent)

sexual partners, dates, casual or regular relationship, symptoms, and genital to genital, anogenital and orogenital contact. Contraception should be recorded, especially condom use. Past history should include treatment for STD, and the family and obstetric history should be recorded.

The genitals must always be examined and in females this includes passing a bivalve vaginal speculum. The history will indicate other systems requiring examination; ideally, all patients should have a complete examination.

Several genital tract infections may be present at the same time; all patients should therefore have the investigations in Table 2.40 at their first visit. Positive investigations must be repeated after treatment to ensure cure.

Spread and control of STDs

Spread

The fundamental factors in spread are the acquisition of infection from one partner and its transmission to another. These depend on the availability of partners, which increases with population movement including migration from rural to urban areas and world-wide travel. Social factors which promote spread include poverty, alcohol, leisure, personal freedom, prostitution and ignorance. Additional factors are asymptomatic infection, antimicrobial resistance and contraception. Unlike condoms and to a lesser extent the cap, oral contraceptives and the intrauterine device provide no barrier to infection. All socio-economic groups acquire STDs; people at special risk are shown in the information box.

THOSE AT PARTICULAR RISK OF STDs

- Men aged 18–34 years
- Women aged 16–24 years
- Frequent travellers
- Commercial sex workers
- Armed services personnel
- Merchant seamen
- Entertainers
- Homosexual men with multiple partners

Control

Good control of STDs is based on a number of important principles:

- good clinical practice, including accurate diagnosis, effective treatment and close follow-up to ensure cure
- partner notification—the identification of potentially infected partners and their treatment
- education on STDs
- screening—certain groups of at-risk patients (see the information box) should be screened, and routine blood donor and antenatal serological testing should continue.

SEXUALLY TRANSMITTED BACTERIAL DISEASES

SYPHILIS

Syphilis is due to infection with *Treponema pallidum*. It is systemic from the beginning, infectious and chronic. There are florid features at some times but there may be long periods of latency at others. It can be transmitted transplacentally to the fetus, but it responds to penicillin, which is the drug of choice. The classification of syphilis is shown in the information box.

The division between early and late syphilis is 2 years.

CLASSIFICATION OF SYPHILIS

Acquired	Congenital
Early • Primary • Secondary • Latent **Late** • Latent • Tertiary (benign gummatous) • Quarternary (cardiovascular, neurosyphilis)	**Early** • Clinical and latent **Late** • Clinical and latent, stigmata (or scars)

Table 2.41 Management of syphilis

Medication	Regimen
Primary stage	
Procaine penicillin	600–1200 mg i.m. once daily for 12 days
Oxytetracycline	500 mg orally 6-hourly for 15 days
Doxycycline	100 mg orally 8-hourly for 15 days
Secondary stage	
Procaine penicillin	600–1200 mg i.m. once daily for 15 days
Tertiary stage	
Oxytetracycline	500 mg orally 6-hourly for 15 days
Latent stage	
Doxycycline	100 mg orally 8-hourly for 15 days
Cardiovascular and central nervous systems	
Procaine penicillin	900–1200 mg i.m. once daily for 21 days
Oxytetracycline	500 mg orally 6-hourly for 28 days
Doxycycline	100 mg orally 8-hourly for 28 days

The course is variable and may be latent throughout, but clinical features may develop at any time, so all cases must be treated (see Table 2.41).

Acquired syphilis

Early stage

The incubation period is commonly 14–28 days, with extremes of 9–90 days.

Primary syphilis. The primary lesion or chancre (see Fig. 2.53) develops at the site of infection, usually on the genitals. It is nearly always painless. A small pink macule appears, becomes papular and ulcerates. The regional lymph nodes are moderately enlarged, mobile, discrete, rubbery, painless and non-tender. Primary syphilis must be included in the differential diagnosis of all genital ulcers—see the information box.

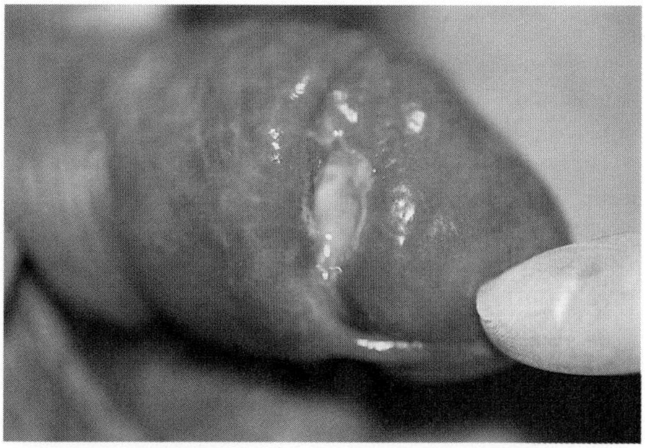

Fig. 2.53 Primary syphilis. A painless ulcer is shown in the coronal sulcus of the penis. This is usually associated with inguinal lymphadenopathy.

CAUSES OF GENITAL ULCERS, NON-SYPHILITIC

Common	Uncommon
• Herpes simplex (see pp. 108 and 189) • Erosive balanitis (see p. 190) • Trauma with secondary infection	• Secondary syphilis • Scabies (see p. 183) • Reiter's disease (see p. 850) • Stevens–Johnson syndrome (see p. 918) • Behçet's syndrome (see p. 868)

Secondary syphilis. This starts 6–8 weeks after the chancre with mild fever, malaise and headache. The features are shown in the information box and Figure 2.54.

DIFFERENTIAL DIAGNOSIS OF SECONDARY SYPHILIS

Macular rash
- Drug eruption
- Rubella
- Pityriasis rosea

Mouth ulcers
- Herpes simplex
- Aphthous ulcers
- Ulcerative stomatitis
- Agranulocytosis

Papular rash
- Drug eruption
- Scabies
- Acne vulgaris
- Chickenpox

Genital ulcers
- Herpes simplex
- Erosive balanitis

Condylomata lata
- Viral warts

Lymphadenopathy
- Infectious mononucleosis
- Lymphoma
- HIV infection

The rash varies from faint macules on the trunk, or a scaly eruption through to widespread papules. It is symmetrical and not itchy. Characteristically, the palms and soles are affected. Condylomata lata are flat papules in warm, moist areas such as at the anus. Lymphadenopathy may be generalised with nodes like those in primary syphilis. Mucosal ulcers affect the genitals, mouth, pharynx and larynx. Early lesions are superficial; later, they develop a white base and a red margin, and coalesce to form 'snail track ulcers'.

After several weeks without treatment, resolution occurs and the disease enters the latent phase, but may relapse during the first 2 years.

Many cases are identified in this stage following serological testing. Antimicrobial therapy (see Table 2.41) gives cure rates of over 95%.

The differential diagnosis of secondary syphilis is summarised in the information box. Syphilis must be distinguished clinically from yaws (see p. 141), endemic (non-venereal) syphilis and pinta (see p. 142). These diseases are caused by treponemes morphologically indistinguishable from *T. pallidum* of syphilis.

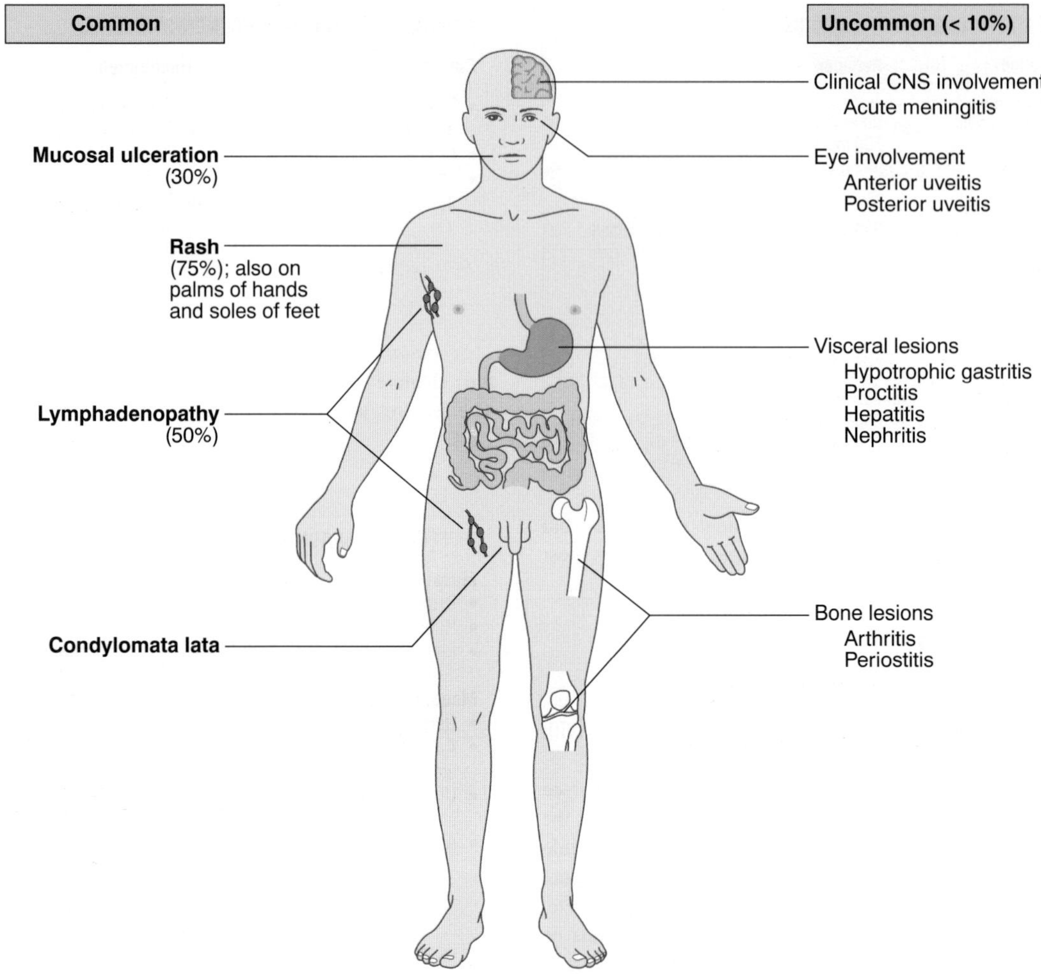

Fig. 2.54 Features of secondary acquired syphilis.

Late stage

Latency may persist for many years.

Tertiary stage. This stage (rare) takes at least 2 years to develop and affects skin, mucosa and bones. The characteristic feature is a granuloma called a gumma.

Quaternary stage. Cardiovascular syphilis and neurosyphilis take longer to develop and may lead to the patient's death.

Congenital syphilis

The fetus may contract syphilis from a mother with early acquired syphilis. With severe disease the child is born dead. A less severely affected baby has vesicles, bullae and mucosal ulcers at birth. Multisystem disease is often manifest by hepatosplenomegaly and CNS involvement. In a third group the disease remains latent for years. Congenital syphilis is rare where antenatal serological screening is practised. Antibiotic treatment during pregnancy usually produces a healthy baby but may not prevent the stigmata of late congenital syphilis (interstitial keratitis, Hutchinson's teeth, sensorineural deafness) if administered after 20 weeks' gestation.

Investigations

T. pallidum is found in early acquired and congenital syphilis (see Table 2.40). Serological tests for syphilis are listed in the information box.

Serological tests are positive from the fourth week of acquired syphilis and at birth in congenital syphilis. False positive results occur occasionally, most often to the VDRL and RPR tests in other infections and also in connective tissue diseases; therefore results must be confirmed with

SEROLOGICAL TESTS FOR SYPHILIS
Non-specific or lipoidal antigen tests
• Venereal Disease Research Laboratory (VDRL) test • Rapid plasma reagin (RPR)
Specific treponemal antigen tests
• *Treponema pallidum* haemagglutination assay (TPHA) • Fluorescent treponemal antibody absorbed (FTA-abs) test • Treponemal enzyme-linked immunosorbent assay (ELISA)

specific tests. When syphilis is suspected lipoidal antigen and specific tests are used together.

In the latent stages the CSF is examined to exclude or confirm neurological disease and chest radiographs or echocardiograms are taken to assess the presence of thoracic aortic aneurysm.

Management

Antimicrobial treatment for syphilis is summarised in Table 2.41. Tetracyclines are indicated for patients hypersensitive to penicillin, except pregnant women who are given erythromycin stearate in the same dosage; erythromycin crosses the placenta poorly so the newborn baby needs careful management. All patients must be followed to ensure cure; partner notification is important.

NEUROSYPHILIS

See page 1015.

GONORRHOEA

Gonorrhoea is caused by the Gram-negative diplococcus *Neisseria gonorrhoeae* which infects columnar epithelium in the lower genital tract, rectum, pharynx and eyes. The incubation period in men with gonococcal urethritis is 2–10 days.

Clinical features

In males the anterior urethra is the common site for infection. Anterior urethritis causes dysuria and purulent discharge but these may be mild or absent in 5–10%. The lower cervical canal is infected in 80% of women, with the urethra and rectum involved in 50%. There may be vaginal discharge and dysuria, but 60% of women with uncomplicated infection are symptom-free. Homosexual men may have asymptomatic rectal infection. Symptomless pharyngeal gonorrhoea occasionally affects males and females.

Differential diagnosis in uncomplicated gonorrhoea is given in the information box.

DIFFERENTIAL DIAGNOSIS OF UNCOMPLICATED GONORRHOEA
Males
• Non-gonococcal urethritis
Females
• Urinary infection, trichomoniasis, candidiasis, bacterial vaginosis
Both sexes
• Proctitis, pharyngitis

Investigations

Gram-negative intracellular diplococci may be seen on microscopy (see Fig. 2.55) of infected secretions but must be confirmed by culture (see Table 2.40, p. 184).

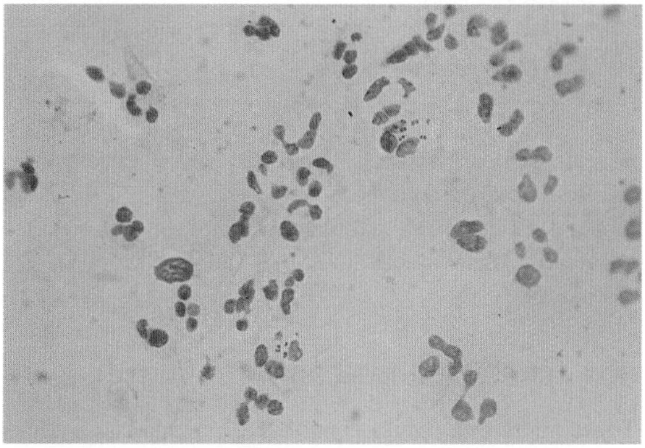

Fig. 2.55 A Gram-stained urethral smear from a man with gonococcal urethritis. Gram-negative diplococci are seen with polymorphonuclear leucocytes.

Management

Uncomplicated gonorrhoea responds to a single adequate dose of a suitable antimicrobial. In Britain infections are usually sensitive to penicillin. Elsewhere, such as the Far East and West Africa, up to 50% of infections are totally resistant to penicillin. Occasional strains of *N. gonorrhoeae* isolated in Europe and more in the Far East have diminished sensitivity to ciprofloxacin. Antimicrobial regimens are shown in Table 2.42. Partners should be notified as soon as possible.

Prognosis

Symptoms gradually resolve without treatment but it is not known how long the patient remains infectious. Delay in treatment leads to complications, which include:

- epididymo-orchitis
- salpingitis and pelvic infection
- perihepatitis—characterised by right hypochondrial pain and tenderness
- bacteraemia—rare but causes fever, joint pains and sparse peripheral pustular rash

Table 2.42 Treatment of uncomplicated anogenital gonorrhoea

Drug	Route	Regimen
Penicillin-sensitive		
Ampicillin *AND*	Oral	2–3.5 g
Probenecid	Oral	1 g single dose
Co-trimoxazole dispersible tablets	Oral	8 × 480 mg single dose *OR* 5 × 480 mg 12-hourly × 3 doses
Penicillin-resistant		
Ciprofloxacin	Oral	250–500 mg single dose
Cefotaxime	I.m.	0.5–1.0 g single dose
Spectinomycin	I.m.	2–4 g single dose
Pharyngeal gonorrhoea		
Co-trimoxazole dispersible tablets	Oral	5 × 480 mg 12-hourly × 3 doses
Ciprofloxacin	Oral	500 mg single dose

- acute gonococcal arthritis (see p. 854) and septicaemia—rare in developed countries
- acute purulent conjunctivitis (ophthalmia neonatorum) in infants born to infected mothers—rare in developed countries.

NON-GONOCOCCAL INFECTION

This clinically resembles gonorrhoea, but gonococci cannot be identified; a cause is recognised in only 50% (about half may be due to *Chlamydia trachomatis*—see Table 2.43) and the aetiology is obscure in the remainder (see the information box).

Non-gonococcal urethritis (NGU) in men

Urethritis in men is much more commonly non-gonococcal than gonococcal in origin. NGU also occurs in Reiter's disease (see p. 850). Clinically, NGU resembles gonococcal urethritis but is milder. The incubation period varies from a few days to a few weeks. Urethritis is confirmed by finding polymorphonuclear leucocytes in a Gram stain of urethral secretions obtained by meatal swab; gonorrhoea is excluded by absence of organisms on Gram stain and culture. An additional urethral swab should be taken for chlamydiae. A wet preparation will show *Trichomonas vaginalis*.

Untreated NGU runs a prolonged low-grade course and may be complicated by epididymo-orchitis. In Britain and some other countries epididymo-orchitis is more common with NGU than with gonorrhoea.

A satisfactory response to a single course of therapy (see the information box) is achieved in up to 80%. Non-responders should be retreated with an alternative regimen. Epididymo-orchitis should be treated with oxytetracycline or erythromycin 500 mg 6-hourly for 14 days. Whether or not a causative agent is identified, partner notification is important because untreated female partners may develop pelvic inflammatory disease.

CAUSES OF NON-GONOCOCCAL URETHRITIS (NGU) IN MEN

Common

- *Chlamydia trachomatis* (approx. 50%)
- *Mycoplasma genitalium*

Rare

- *Ureaplasma urealyticum*
- *Trichomonas vaginalis*
- Herpes simplex virus
- Upper urinary tract infection
- Trauma

Remainder

- Obscure

Table 2.43 Salient features of lymphogranuloma venereum (LGV), chancroid and granuloma inguinale (donovanosis)

Condition and distribution	Organism	Incubation period	Genital lesion	Lymph nodes	Diagnosis	Management
LGV World-wide, especially E. and W. Africa, India, S.E. Asia, S. America, Caribbean	*Chlamydia trachomatis* types LI, II, III	1–5 weeks	Small transient, often not recognised	Tender, unilateral, matted, adherent, suppurative, multilocular	Culture or antigen identification, circulating (micro IF) antibodies	Oxytetracycline 500 mg 6-hourly for 14 days; increase and prolong if severe
Chancroid Africa, S.E. Asia	*Haemophilus ducreyi* (small Gram-negative rod)	1–8 days	Multiple, irregular, tender ulcers	Tender, unilateral, matted, adherent, suppurative	Microscopy and culture of scrapings	Erythromycin 500 mg 6-hourly for 7 days or co-trimoxazole 2 (80/400 mg) 12-hourly for 7 days
Granuloma inguinale S. India, S.E. Asia, Central and W. Africa, Caribbean, S. America, Central Australia among Aborigines	*Calymmatobacterium granulomatis* (bipolar rods)	Few days to 3 months	Spreading granulomas, pink and red velvety appearance	Only if secondarily infected	Microscopy of scrapings	Streptomycin 1 g 12-hourly i.m. for 10–20 days or oxytetracycline 500 mg 6-hourly for 14–21 days

TREATMENT OF NON-GONOCOCCAL URETHRITIS (NGU)

(All regimens for 14 days by mouth. Presence or absence of *Chlamydia* on culture does not influence antibiotic choice)

- Oxytetracycline 250 mg 6-hourly or 500 mg 12-hourly
- Doxycycline 100 mg 12-hourly
- Erythromycin 250 mg 6-hourly or 500 mg 12-hourly
- Azithromycin 1 g as a single dose

Non-gonococcal infection in women

This is principally due to *C. trachomatis* in 50% of cases and no other cause has yet been identified. *C. trachomatis* infects the lower cervical canal and the urethra. Many women have additional infections; therefore all require full investigation (see Table 2.40, p. 184).

Uncomplicated lower genital tract chlamydia-positive or negative infection may cause no symptoms or signs, but it may also progress to pelvic inflammatory disease which may recur, become chronic, and lead to tubal pregnancy or infertility. A woman with cervical infection may infect her baby's eyes at birth (ophthalmia neonatorum). Investigations for NGU in women are outlined in Table 2.40.

The antimicrobial treatment of uncomplicated and complicated chlamydia-positive and negative infection is the same as that for men (see the information box). Swabbing of newborn babies' eyes with antiseptic solution has been shown to be highly effective in reducing ophthalmia neonatorum.

SEXUALLY TRANSMITTED VIRAL DISEASES

Until recently, viral infections of the genital tract have been difficult to treat. However, the introduction of specific antiviral agents has revolutionised management of these conditions. This is particularly true for herpesvirus infections and great progress has been made for human immunodeficiency virus (HIV) infection, which is covered in detail on pages 87–107.

ANOGENITAL HERPES SIMPLEX

This is due to herpes simplex virus (see p. 108) spread by sexual contact. There is a severe first attack followed by milder recurrences which resemble labial herpes simplex (cold sores). Classically, HSV 2 causes anogenital disease but HSV 1 currently accounts for up to 50% of such infections in the UK.

First attack

This starts with malaise, fever and local irritation, followed by widespread painful tender vesicles affecting the genitals and, rarely, the anorectum. The vesicles rupture, leaving erosions followed by further crops of lesions. Regional lymph nodes swell. There may be nerve root pains in the 2nd and 3rd sacral dermatomes and, rarely, retention of urine. First attacks heal in 2–4 weeks and are followed by painful recurrence.

Recurrent attacks

These resemble first attacks but there is one cluster of lesions covering an area of about 1 cm^2, which heal in 3–10 days.

The virus is identified by electron microscopy or culture from vesicular fluid or scrapings from fresh erosions. Lesions always heal and local saline bathing may be all that is necessary. Aciclovir, 200 mg five times daily for 5 days by mouth, inhibits viral replication so if given early shortens first attacks. Aciclovir is not prescribed for mild or infrequent recurrences. A few patients suffer frequent recurrence, which may be suppressed by continuous oral aciclovir 400 mg twice daily.

GENITAL WARTS

Warts are due to the human papillomavirus (HPV—see p. 112) and are common on the genitals and anus. Infection with certain strains of HPV, particularly types 16 or 18, predisposes to carcinoma of the cervix.

Exophytic warts can be recognised from their appearance. Flat warts are more difficult to diagnose. Atypical and persistent lesions should be biopsied. Treatment is with 10–25% podophyllin applied weekly, or 0.5% podophyllotoxin applied 12-hourly for 3 consecutive days per week for a maximum of 5 weeks. Alternative methods are destruction by cryotherapy, electrocautery or laser. Warts tend to recur so all patients must be followed to ensure cure. Partners must be notified.

MOLLUSCUM CONTAGIOSUM

Molluscum contagiosum virus (see p. 114) produces small, shiny, pink papules, with a central depression which allows differentiation from warts. Treatment is by destruction with cryotherapy or electrocautery.

HEPATITIS

Hepatitis B (see p. 709) is transmitted readily between homosexual men but rarely between heterosexuals. This is in contrast to hepatitis A and C, as these are rarely sexually transmitted. Hepatitis B vaccination policy should target patients attending STD clinics.

Table 2.44 Treatment of balanitis and vulvovaginal conditions

Cause	Vulvovaginal condition	Balanitis
Candidiasis	Clotrimazole 500 mg pessary once *OR* Clotrimazole 200 mg pessary at night × 3 *AND* Clotrimazole cream twice daily	Clotrimazole cream twice daily
Trichomoniasis, bacterial vaginosis and anaerobic infection	Metronidazole 200 mg 8-hourly for 7 days *OR* 400 mg 12-hourly for 5 days	Metronidazole 200 mg 8-hourly for 7 days *OR* 400 mg 12-hourly for 5 days
Streptococcal infection	Amoxycillin 250 mg 8-hourly for 5 days	Amoxycillin 250 mg 8-hourly for 5 days

Table 2.45 Causes and features of vulvovaginal conditions

Condition	Cause	Features
Non-infective vulvovaginitis	Chemicals, e.g. antiseptics; trauma	Soreness, redness and variable discharge
Atrophic vaginitis	Oestrogen deficiency	Soreness, itch and pale atrophic appearance
Infective candidiasis	*Candida albicans*	Itch, vulval oedema, thick white discharge
Trichomoniasis	*T. vaginalis*	Painful irritation, smell, erythema, thin yellow discharge
Bacterial vaginosis	*Gardenerella vaginalis* and anaerobes	Smell and off-white discharge

MISCELLANEOUS CONDITIONS

BALANITIS AND BALANOPOSTHITIS

Balanitis is inflammation of the glans penis; balanoposthitis involves the glans and undersurface of the prepuce. These conditions are common in men with a long tight prepuce and poor hygiene. Causal agents include *Candida* species, *T. vaginalis*, some streptococci and anaerobes, but sometimes no cause is identified. Dermatoses such as eczema may underlie recurrent balanitis. Immune deficiency, diabetes mellitus (see p. 472), broad-spectrum antimicrobials, corticosteroids and antimitotic drugs predispose to candidiasis.

Clinical features

There is general or patchy erythema with erosions when severe and a white or purulent exudate. Circinate balanitis occurs in Reiter's disease (see p. 850) with round erosions which coalesce. Balanitis xerotica obliterans (BXO) is the genital manifestation of lichen sclerosus et atrophicus; initial patchy erythema progresses to atrophy with a white appearance, meatal stenosis and phimosis. Diagnosis is from the clinical appearance. Swabs are taken to identify possible causes.

Management

Specific treatment should be given as in Table 2.44. Local saline bathing is always advised and is sufficient when no cause is found. Saline may suffice for circinate balanitis and BXO but hydrocortisone cream 1% or a more potent steroid is recommended in severe cases. Partner notification is indicated in candidiasis and trichomoniasis.

VULVOVAGINAL CONDITIONS

Vaginal discharge is common, may be associated with vulval inflammation, and is due to a variety of causes summarised with the clinical features in Table 2.45. All of the infections may occur without symptoms but treatment is indicated as clinical disease may develop. Investigate as in Table 2.40, page 184. Saline bathing is indicated for vulval involvement and specific treatment prescribed as in Table 2.44. Partner notification is required in trichomoniasis and recurrent candidiasis.

Scabies (see p. 183) and pediculosis (see p. 182) can be sexually transmitted and this must be considered in their management.

FURTHER INFORMATION ON SEXUALLY TRANSMITTED DISEASES

Holmes K K, Mardh P-A, Sparling P F, Wiesner P J 1989 Sexually transmitted diseases, 2nd edn. McGraw-Hill, New York

Diseases of the cardiovascular system

3

N.A. BOON • K.A.A. FOX • P. BLOOMFIELD

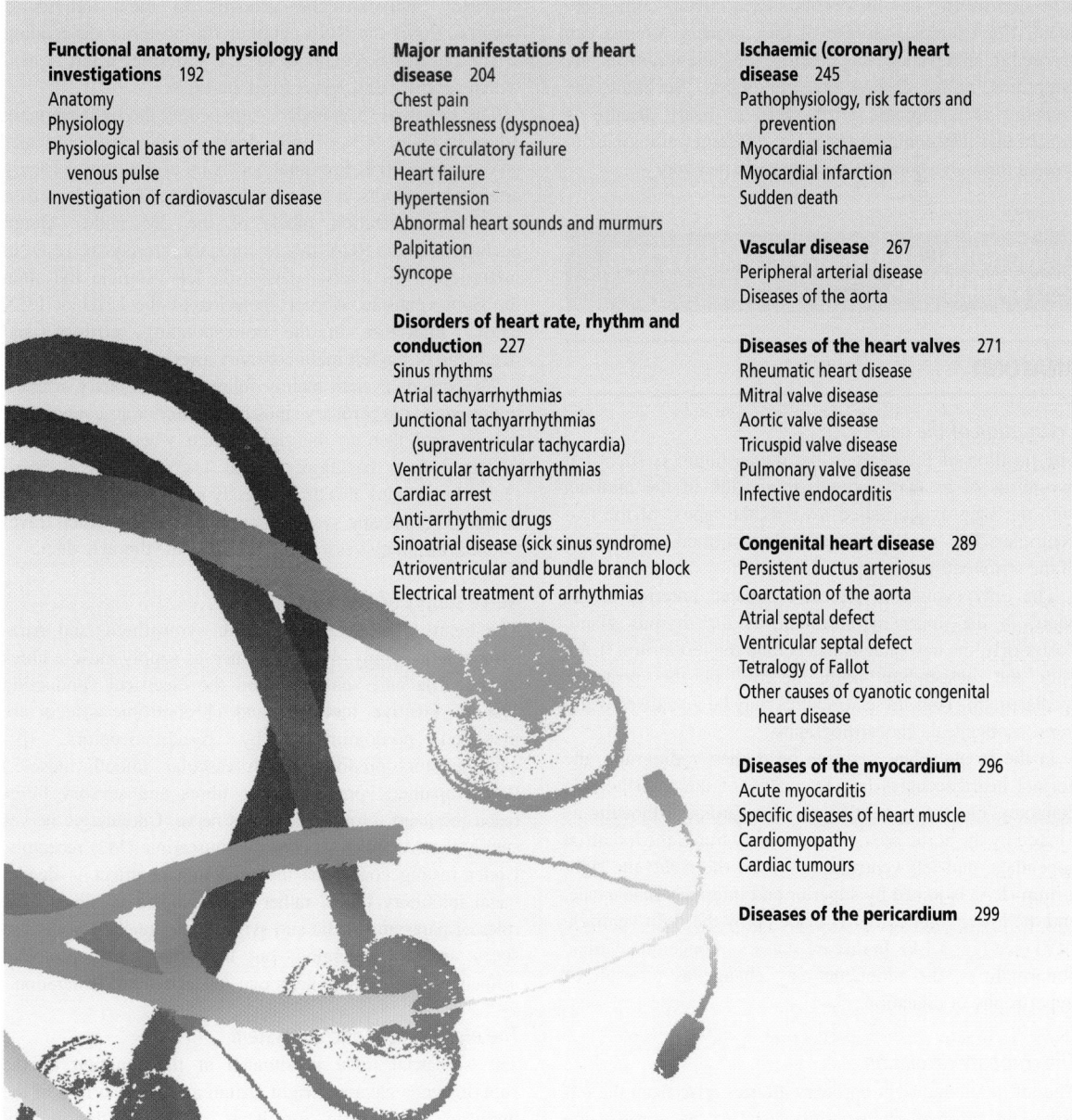

Cardiovascular disease is the most frequent cause of adult death in industrialised societies, and is increasingly important in developing countries. In early life minor congenital abnormalities affect 1 in 100 live births and more serious abnormalities approximately 1 in 500.

Since the 1960s, mortality from cardiac disease has steadily declined in the United States of America, and more recently in Australia, Europe and certain other countries. This probably reflects changing lifestyles, improved diagnosis and management, and other factors as yet unrecognised.

Prompt recognition of the development of heart disease is limited by two key factors. Firstly, it is very commonly latent. For example, disease of the coronary arteries can proceed to an advanced stage before the patient notices any symptoms, unlike disease of other organs. Secondly, the diversity of symptoms attributable to heart disease is limited and it is common for many different pathologies to present through a common symptomatic pathway.

FUNCTIONAL ANATOMY, PHYSIOLOGY AND INVESTIGATIONS

ANATOMY

Orientation of the heart

The position of the heart in the mediastinum is such that two-thirds of its mass extends to the left of the midline, with the long axis oriented towards the 'apex' of the two ventricles. The 'base' of this triangle is formed by the plane of the atrioventricular groove.

The only significant structure situated anterior to the heart, in the upper mediastinum, is the thymus gland. Posteriorly, the oesophagus lies behind the left atrium (LA), with the descending aorta nearby, in the posterior mediastinum. Thus these structures may be visualised using transoesophageal echocardiography.

In the frontal plane, as seen on a chest radiograph, the normal heart occupies less than 50% of the transthoracic diameter. On the patient's left, the cardiac silhouette is formed by the aortic arch, the pulmonary trunk, the left atrial appendage and left ventricle (LV). On the right, the right atrium (RA) is joined by superior and inferior venae cavae, and the lower right border is made up by the right ventricle (RV) (see Fig. 3.1A). In disease states, or congenital cardiac abnormalities, the silhouette may change as a result of hypertrophy or dilatation.

The coronary circulation

The left main and right coronary arteries arise from the left and right coronary sinuses, just distal to the aortic valve (see Fig. 3.1B). Within 2.5 cm of its origin the left main coronary divides into the left anterior descending artery (LAD), which runs in the anterior interventricular groove, and the circumflex artery (LCX) which runs posteriorly in the atrioventricular groove. The LAD gives branches to supply the anterior left ventricle, the apex, and the anterior part of the septum. The LCX gives marginal branches to supply the posterior left ventricle and inferior surface. The right coronary artery (RCA) runs in the right atrioventricular groove, giving branches to supply the right atrium, right ventricle and infero-posterior aspects of the left ventricle (as the posterior descending vessel, in the posterior interventricular groove). In most individuals (approx. 90%) the RCA supplies the posterior descending artery, but in the remainder there is a dominant left system which supplies this vessel from the LCX.

The sinoatrial (SA) node is supplied by the right coronary artery in about 60% of individuals and the atrioventricular (AV) node in 90%. Proximal occlusion of the right coronary artery often results in sinus bradycardia, and may also cause electrical conduction block of the AV node. Abrupt occlusions in the RCA, due to coronary thrombosis, result in infarction of the inferior part of the left ventricle and often the right ventricle. Abrupt occlusion of the LAD or LCX causes infarction in the corresponding territory, and occlusion of the left main coronary artery is usually fatal.

The venous system mainly follows the coronary arteries, but drains to the coronary sinus in the inferior atrioventricular groove, and then to the right atrium where its orifice is protected from backflow by the Thebesian valve. Small (eustachian) veins also drain directly into the right atrium. An extensive lymphatic system drains into vessels which travel with the coronary vessels and then into the thoracic duct.

Nerve supply of the heart

The heart is innervated by both sympathetic and parasympathetic supply. Adrenergic nerves supply muscle fibres in the atria and ventricles and the electrical conducting system. Positive inotropic and chronotropic effects are mediated predominantly by β_1-adrenoceptors. (β_2-adrenoceptors predominate in vascular smooth muscle.) Parasympathetic pre-ganglionic fibres and sensory fibres reach the heart through the vagus nerve. Cholinergic nerves supply the AV and SA nodes via muscarinic (M2) receptors. Under resting conditions the predominant effect is due to vagal inhibitory fibres, rather than sympathetic fibres. The roles of parasympathetic and sympathetic function in disease states are still emerging, but they may exert profound influences on control of heart rate and arrhythmia generation.

The electrical conduction system

The sinoatrial node is situated at the junction of the superior vena cava and right atrium and is the origin of the impulses responsible for heart rhythm under normal

A

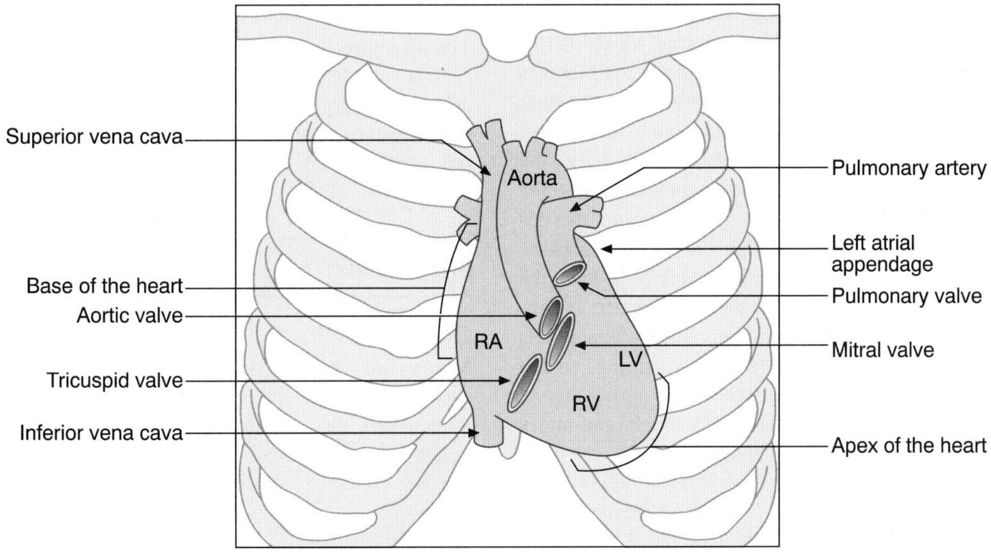

B

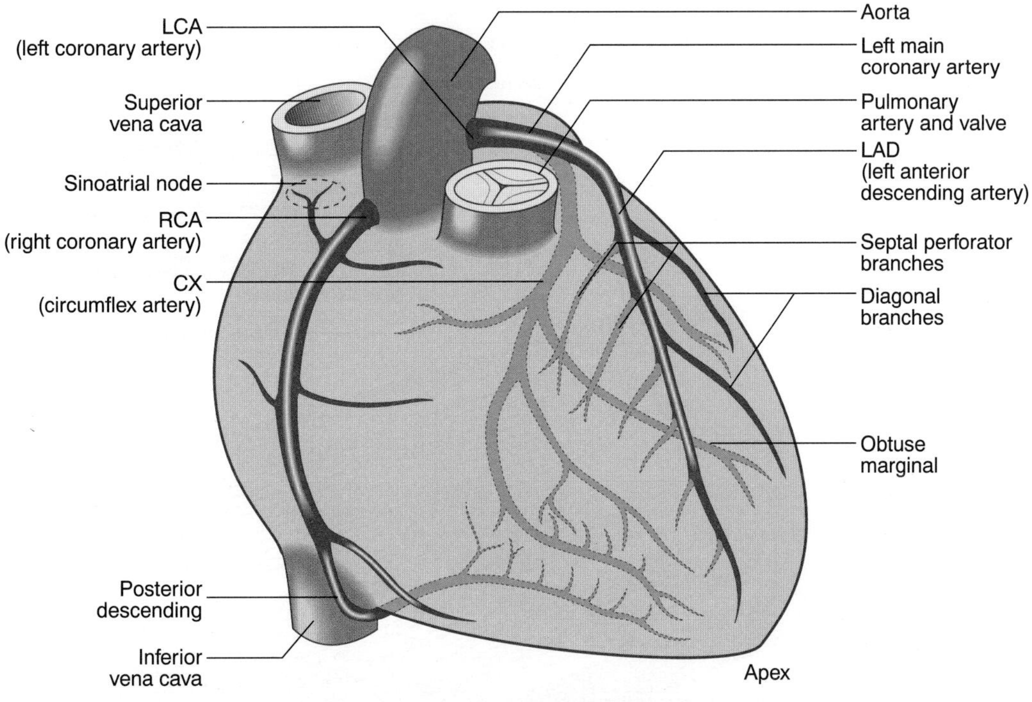

Fig. 3.1 A **Radiological outline of the heart.** The positions of the major cardiac chambers and heart valves are shown. B **The coronary arteries of the heart** (anterior view). The left (LCA) and right (RCA) coronary arteries arise in the respective sinuses just distal to the aortic valve. The left main coronary artery divides into a left anterior descending branch (LAD) which supplies the front wall and apex of the heart, and a circumflex (CX) branch which supplies the posterior wall of the heart and a variable proportion of the inferior wall. The right coronary artery gives off right ventricular branches and may give rise to the posterior descending vessel which runs in the posterior interventricular groove. The sinoatrial node (sinus node) is situated at the junction of the superior vena cava and right atrium, and the atrioventricular (AV) node is situated beneath the right atrial endocardium at the lower end of the interatrial septum.

conditions ('sinus rhythm'). Depolarisation of the sinus node triggers a wave front of depolarisation which travels through the atrium. Conduction directly to the ventricles is prevented by the annulus fibrosus, which insulates the atria from the ventricles. The atrioventricular node is situated beneath the right atrial endocardium at the lower end of the interatrial septum. It conducts slowly and regulates the frequency of conduction to the ventricles. From the AV node the His bundle passes through the annulus fibrosus and divides into right and left bundles which pass down the respective sides of the ventricular septum. The left is subdivided into anterior and posterior hemibundles, and all His fibres radiate out as the Purkinje network. Injury to the right or left bundle is evident on the electrocardiogram as the respective right or left bundle branch block, and injury to a hemibundle as a deviation in electrical axis.

The valves of the heart

The structure and function of the atrioventricular valves (mitral and tricuspid) and ventricular outflow valves (aortic and pulmonary) are considered in relation to cardiac investigations (see p. 201) and to disorders of the valves (see p. 271).

PHYSIOLOGY

Myocardial contraction

Myocardial cells (myocytes) are about 100 μm long and each cell branches and interdigitates with adjacent cells. An intercalated disc permits electrical conduction (via gap junctions) and force conduction (via the fascia adherens) to

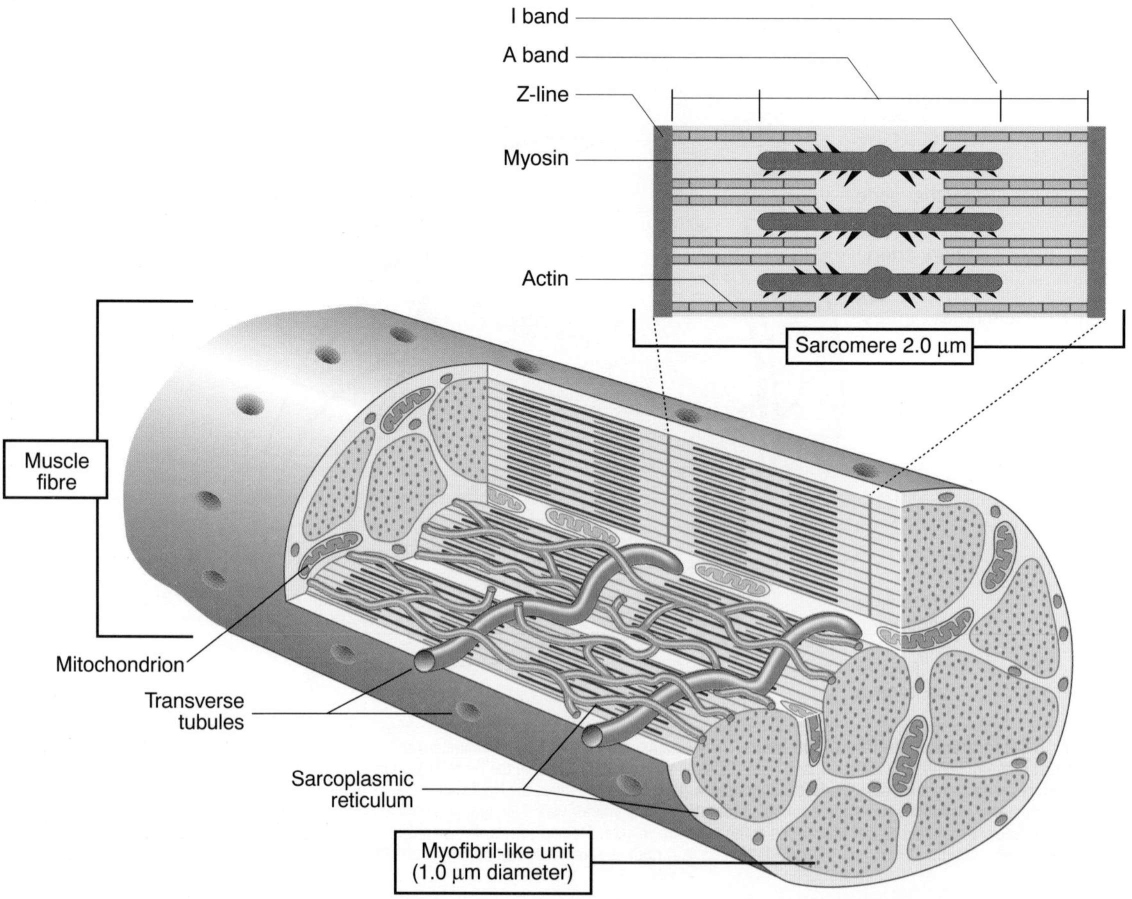

Fig. 3.2 Schematic of a muscle fibre. The arrangement of myofibrils, and longitudinal and transverse tubules extending from the sarcoplasmic reticulum are shown. Expanded section shows schematic of an individual sarcomere with thick filaments composed of myosin and thin filaments composed primarily of actin.

adjacent cells. The basic unit of contraction is the sarcomere (2 μm length), which is aligned to those of adjacent myofibrils, giving a striated appearance due to the Z-lines (see Fig. 3.2). Actin filaments (molecular weight 47 000) are attached at right angles to the Z-lines, and interdigitate with thicker parallel myosin filaments (molecular weight 500 000). The cross-links between actin and myosin molecules contain myofibrillar ATPase, which breaks down adenosine triphosphate (ATP) to provide the energy for contraction. Two chains of actin molecules form a helical structure, with a second molecule, tropomyosin, in the grooves of the actin helix, and a further molecule, troponin, attached to every seventh actin molecule (see Fig. 3.3).

During contraction, shortening of the sarcomere results from the actin and myosin molecules interdigitating, without altering the length of either molecule. Contraction is initiated when calcium is made available during the plateau phase of the action potential by calcium ions entering the cell and being mobilised from the sarcolemma. As its concentration rises calcium binds to troponin C, precipitating contraction. The force of cardiac muscle contraction, or inotropic state, is regulated by the influx of calcium ions through 'slow calcium channels'. The extent to which the sarcomere can shorten determines stroke volume of the ventricle. It is maximally shortened in response to powerful inotropic drugs or severe exercise. However, the enlargement of the heart seen in heart failure is due to slippage of the myofibrils and adjacent cells, rather than lengthening of the sarcomere.

Factors influencing cardiac output

Cardiac output is determined by the product of stroke volume and heart rate. Stroke volume is dependent upon end-diastolic pressure (preload) and peripheral vascular resistance (afterload).

Stretch of cardiac muscle (as indicated by an increment in end-diastolic volume) results in increased force of contraction (measured as increased stroke volume). This relationship is known as Starling's Law of the heart. Afterload falls as blood pressure is reduced and this allows greater shortening of the muscle fibres and hence increased stroke volume.

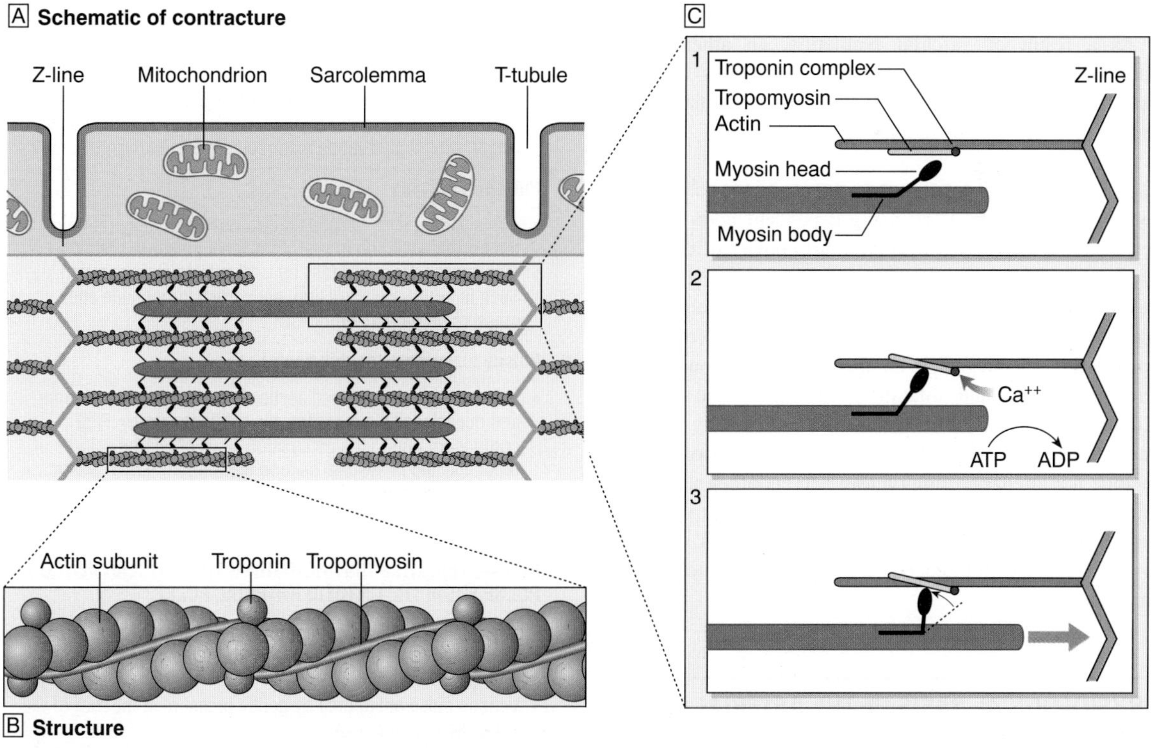

Fig. 3.3 A **Schematic of a sarcomere** showing overlapping of actin and myosin filaments. B **Enlarged diagram of the structure of an actin filament.** C **The three stages of contraction** resulting in shortening of the sarcomere. *Top:* The actin binding site is blocked by tropomyosin. *Centre:* ATP-dependent release of calcium ions which bind to troponin C, displacing tropomyosin. The binding site is exposed. *Bottom:* Tilting of the angle of attachment of the myosin head, resulting in fibre shortening.

The contractile state of the myocardium is controlled, in part, by the neuro-endocrine system, including, for example, sympathetic tone and reflexes. It is influenced by various inotropic drugs and their antagonists.

Determination of the response to a physiological change, or a drug, can be predicted on the basis of the combined influence on preload, afterload and contractility.

Factors influencing resistance to coronary blood flow

Coronary blood vessels receive sympathetic and parasympathetic innervation. Stimulation of α-receptors causes vasoconstriction and β_2-adrenoceptors vasodilatation, but the predominant effect of sympathetic stimulation in coronary arteries is vasodilatation. Parasympathetic stimulation also causes a modest dilatation of normal coronary arteries. Intracoronary acetylcholine stimulates the release of nitric oxide from endothelium ('endothelial-derived relaxing factor') and this causes vasodilatation. In the presence of endothelial damage or atheroma, acetylcholine acts directly on vascular smooth muscle, causing constriction. Systemic hormones, neuropeptides and other locally derived factors such as endothelins, which are the most potent vasoconstrictors identified, also influence arterial tone and coronary flow. A similar balance exists in the systemic circulation influencing blood pressure.

As a result of vascular regulation, an atheromatous narrowing (stenosis) in a coronary artery does not limit flow, even during exercise, until the cross-sectional area of the vessel is reduced by at least 70%.

Factors influencing resistance to systemic blood flow

Systemic blood flow is critically dependent upon vascular resistance, which varies with the fourth power of the radius of the resistance vessel. Thus small changes in calibre have a marked influence on blood flow. Metabolic and mechanical factors control arteriolar tone. Neurogenic constriction operates via α-adrenergic receptors on vascular smooth muscle, and dilatation via muscarinic and β_2-adrenoceptors. In addition, systemic and locally released vasoactive substances influence tone; vasoconstrictors include noradrenaline, angiotensin and endothelin, whereas adenosine, bradykinin, prostaglandins and nitric oxide are vasodilators. Resistance to blood flow rises with viscosity, and is mainly influenced by red cell concentration (haematocrit).

PHYSIOLOGICAL BASIS OF THE ARTERIAL AND VENOUS PULSE

Detailed techniques for physical examination are beyond the scope of this book but recommendations for further reading can be found on page 204.

The arterial pulse

Normal variations in pulse volume reflect physiological changes in stroke volume and arterial resistance and may be influenced by many factors such as age, fitness level, arousal and pregnancy. A wide range of disease states can also affect pulse volume (see the information box).

Abnormalities of pulse rate and rhythm are discussed in the section on disorders of heart rate, rhythm and conduction (see pp. 227–245).

The jugular venous pulse

The jugular venous pulse (JVP) provides a convenient bedside means of measuring right atrial pressure. *The jugular venous pressure is the vertical height between the manubriosternal angle and the top of the venous wave*

ARTERIAL PULSE VOLUME
Depends on cardiac stroke volume and arterial compliance
Small pulse volume (pulsus parvus)
• Occurs in cardiac failure, hypovolaemia, vasoconstriction and any cause of reduced cardiac output
Large pulse volume
• Occurs in vasodilatation, pyrexia, anaemia, aortic regurgitation and arteriovenous shunting
Pulsus alternans
• Describes an alternating pattern of large and small volume beats, despite a regular rhythm, and is seen in cardiac failure. Uncommon and must be distinguished from coupled ectopics
Pulsus paradoxus
• A misleading term because it describes an exaggeration of the normal variation in systolic arterial pressure seen with respiration. (Normally falls by < 10 mmHg on inspiration.) Seen in airways obstruction, pericardial tamponade and massive pulmonary embolism
Pulsus bisferiens ('double peak')
• May be seen in combined aortic stenosis and regurgitation, and occasionally in hypertrophic cardiomyopathy. First component due to the percussion wave of a large volume of blood ejected in systole; second component due to elastic recoil in the arteries

CHARACTERISTICS DISTINGUISHING THE JUGULAR VENOUS PULSE FROM THE CAROTID ARTERIAL PULSE
• Venous pulse visible but not palpable • Two peaks in each cycle of the venous pulse, one in the arterial • Venous pulse obliterated by gentle pressure at the root of the neck; arterial pulse not • Venous pulse rises and falls with respiration and position of the patient • Abdominal compression causes the venous pulse to rise—'hepato-jugular reflux'

(normally 3–4 cm). The mid right atrium lies approximately 5 cm below the manubriosternal angle, with an average diastolic pressure of less than 8 mmHg.

Abnormally low venous pressure occurs in hypovolaemia (e.g. haemorrhage). Elevated jugular venous pressure occurs in any form of cardiac failure involving the right heart; pericardial constriction or tamponade; expanded circulating volume or obstruction of the superior vena cava.

The jugular venous pressure wave is illustrated in Figure 3.4. The *a* wave is produced by atrial systole and the *v* wave by venous filling during ventricular systole. The *x* descent is produced by atrial relaxation and downward displacement of the tricuspid valve ring in ventricular systole, and the *y* descent by the fall in pressure as the tricuspid valve opens. After the *a* wave there is a small positive pressure wave during early atrial relaxation, the *c* wave, possibly due to recoil or transmission from the carotid pulse. The *c* wave can seldom be distinguished at the bedside.

The *a* wave is abolished in atrial fibrillation. Large *a* waves occur in pulmonary hypertension, right ventricular

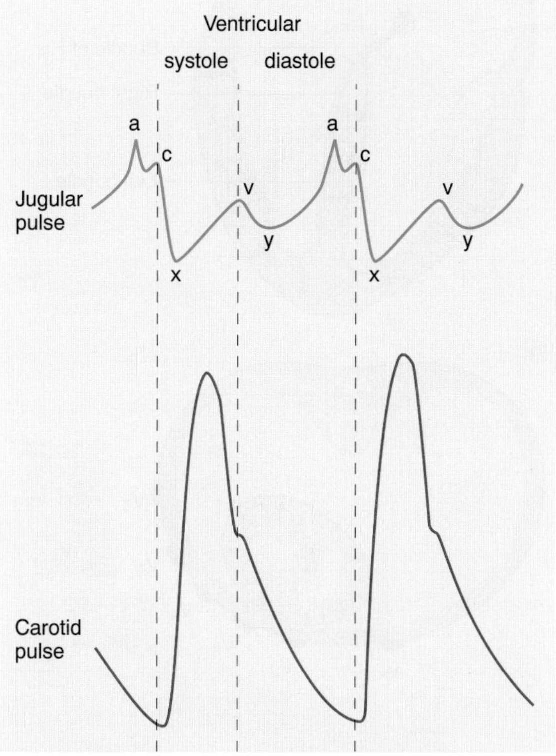

Fig. 3.4 Carotid and jugular pulses. Simultaneous central arterial and venous pulses to demonstrate carotid and jugular pulse waveform. (a = atrial contraction; c = onset of ventricular contraction; v = pressure peak immediately prior to opening of the tricuspid valve; c to x = the x descent; v to y = the y descent)

hypertrophy and tricuspid stenosis (unless the patient is in atrial fibrillation). In the presence of atrioventricular dissociation the atrium sometimes contracts against a closed tricuspid valve (for example, in complete heart block or ventricular tachycardia), and the blood regurgitates into the venae cavae giving rise to a very large *a* wave, the *cannon wave*. Cannon waves are almost always intermittent. In junctional rhythms regular cannon waves may occasionally be produced due to simultaneous atrial and ventricular contractions.

Tricuspid regurgitation produces giant *v* waves with each ventricular contraction, and hence the waves are visible in time with systole and with every beat.

Steep *y* descent due to an abrupt fall in diastolic pressure occurs in constrictive pericarditis, tricuspid regurgitation, and to a lesser extent in right ventricular failure.

INVESTIGATION OF CARDIOVASCULAR DISEASE

Investigations can be considered in two categories: non-invasive tests conveniently performed at the bedside such as electrocardiography (ECG), chest radiograph and echocardiography, and more complex procedures usually performed in a specialised facility such as cardiac catheterisation, nuclear scanning, computed tomography (CT) and magnetic resonance imaging (MRI).

ELECTROCARDIOGRAPHY (ECG)

Electrocardiography is used to elucidate cardiac arrhythmias and conduction defects, and to diagnose and localise myocardial hypertrophy, ischaemia or infarction. It may also give information about electrolyte imbalance and the toxicity of certain drugs.

The fundamental basis for electrocardiography is that the electrical activation of a heart muscle cell causes a depolarisation of its membrane. The depolarisation is propagated along the length of a cell or fibre, and transmitted to adjoining cells. The result is a moving wavefront of depolarisation, which passes through the heart and sets up electrical currents; these are detected by surface electrodes, and amplified and displayed as the electrocardiogram. For each lead of the ECG the electrocardiogram represents summation of depolarisation and repolarisation, as seen from that position in the vertical or frontal plane.

The standard 12-lead ECG

Components of the ECG complex are illustrated in Figure 3.5. Leads I, II, III, AVR, AVL and AVF are orientated in the frontal plane and are referred to as limb leads (see Fig.

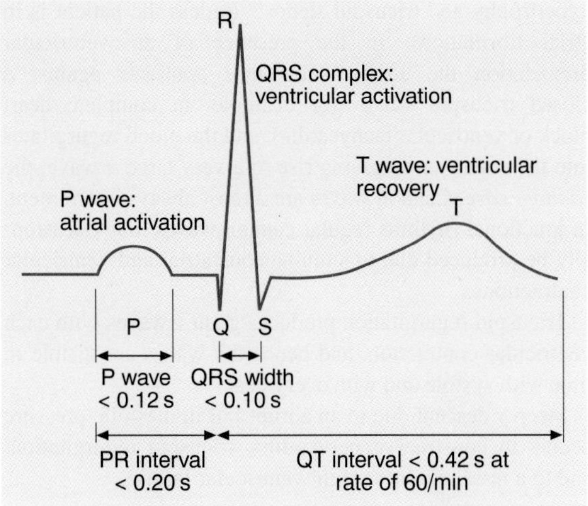

Fig. 3.5 The components of an ECG complex. (P wave = atrial depolarisation; QRS complex = ventricular activation; QT interval = repolarisation; R-R interval = interval between successive R waves in the ECG)

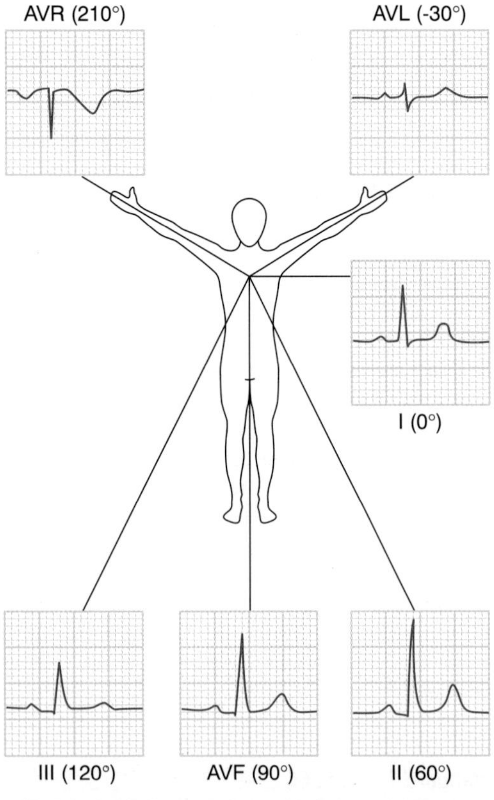

Fig. 3.6 The appearance of the ECG from various recording positions in the frontal plane.

3.6). Leads V_1–V_6 are orientated in the horizontal plane and are called chest leads (see Fig. 3.7). V_1–V_2 mainly reflect the right ventricle, V_3–V_4 the interventricular septum, and V_5–V_6 the left ventricle.

The axis of depolarisation and amplitude of complexes are influenced by patient build. In an obese patient, with an elevated diaphragm, the axis is more horizontal and the complexes are smaller. In a very slim patient there is less attenuation of the signal and the amplitude of the chest leads is increased. In babies and young children the ECG reflects a more prominent right ventricular contribution to the complexes.

Normally, cardiac activation starts in the sinoatrial (SA) node, but this cannot be detected on the ECG. The depolari-

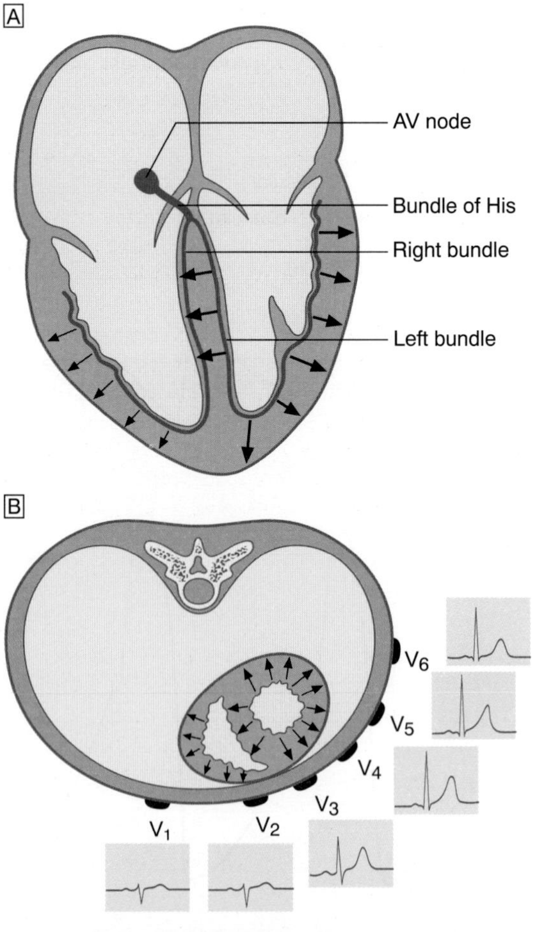

Fig. 3.7 Activation of the septum. A Activation is from left to right followed by spreading of the impulse through both ventricles. B Electrocardiographic complexes from various positions in the horizontal plane and the sequence of activation from the atrium to ventricles.

ECG CONVENTIONS AND INTERVALS

- Depolarisation towards electrode: positive deflection
- Depolarisation away from electrode: negative deflection
- Sensitivity: 10 mm = 1 mV
- Paper speed: 25 mm per second
- Each large (5 mm) square = 0.2 s
- Each small (1 mm) square = 0.04 s
- Heart rate = 1500/R-R interval (mm)
- If R-R interval = 10 mm, heart rate = 150/min
- If R-R interval = 25 mm, heart rate = 60/min

sation then spreads through the atria, producing an upright P wave in all leads except AVR. (The net vector is towards all leads except AVR.) The only point at which the impulse can be transmitted to the ventricles is via the atrioventricular (AV) node, through which conduction is relatively slow (the PR interval). It then goes rapidly through the left and right branches of the bundle of His to ventricular muscle, triggering ventricular activation. The QRS complex represents ventricular activation, and in most leads this is dominated by the upright R wave from the left ventricle. (As the depolarisation spreads towards the leads it produces a positive deflection.) In lateral leads such as leads I and V_6 the R wave is preceded by a small negative deflection (a Q wave) caused by activation from left to right of the interventricular septum. Septal activation is not normally detected in leads V_3, V_4, II, III and AVF, as these are at right angles to septal depolarisation. In leads AVR and V_1 the main direction of left ventricular activation is away from the electrode, giving a dominant S wave. The QRS axis is the mean frontal plane vector of the QRS complex, and can be estimated roughly by seeing which limb lead has the biggest R wave (see Figs 3.6 and 3.8). Normally it lies between 0° (largest R, smallest S in lead I) and 90° (largest R, smallest S in AVF).

Exercise (stress) ECG

By performing an ECG during progressively increasing exercise (usually on a treadmill) it is possible to detect stress-provoked arrhythmias, or evidence of ischaemia. Blood pressure (BP) recording and assessment of symptoms should be performed regularly throughout the test. Horizontal or downsloping ST segment depression of > 1 mm suggests ischaemia. Failure to achieve an increase in blood pressure, or the occurrence of a fall in pressure during exertion, is evidence of ventricular decompensation and is usually indicative of extensive ischaemia. The inability to achieve the predicted heart rate target renders the test inconclusive, rather than negative. An exercise

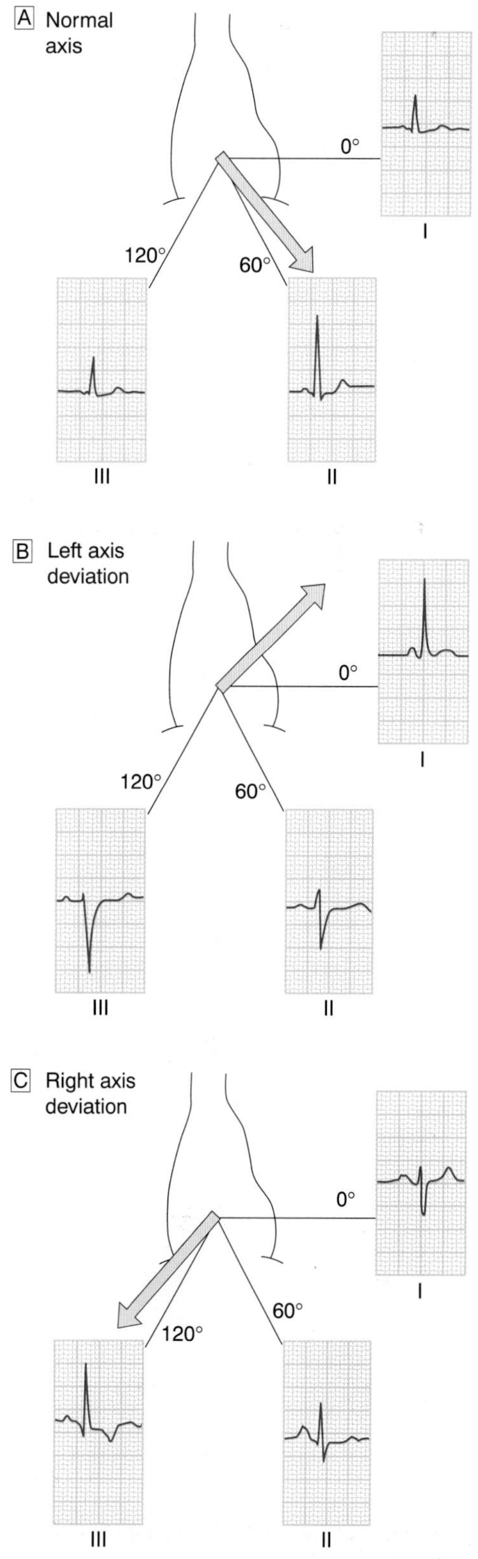

Fig. 3.8 The QRS axis. A Normal. B Left deviation. C Right deviation.

EXERCISE TEST: HIGH-RISK FINDINGS

- Low threshold for ischaemia (i.e. within stage 1 or 2 of the Bruce Protocol)
- Fall in BP on exercise
- Widespread, marked or prolonged ischaemic ECG changes
- Exercise-induced arrhythmia

ECG may be necessary to confirm the clinical diagnosis of ischaemic heart disease but is particularly useful for *risk stratification* in patients with coronary artery disease (see the information box).

Stress tests are *contraindicated* in the presence of unstable angina, decompensated heart failure, severe hypertension or severe outflow obstruction (e.g. aortic stenosis).

Ambulatory ECG (Holter monitoring)

Continuous recordings of one or more ECG leads may be obtained by attaching them to a small portable solid state or tape recorder. This technique is useful in detecting transient episodes of arrhythmia or ischaemia, which seldom occur fortuitously during the short time taken for routine 12-lead ECG recordings. Infrequent arrhythmias may be detected with a device which is placed over the chest during the symptomatic episode. This records the ECG for subsequent trans-telephonic transmission to a cardiac centre.

RADIOLOGY

A chest radiograph is useful for determining the size and shape of the heart, and the state of the pulmonary blood vessels and lung fields. Most information is given by a postero-anterior (PA) projection taken in full inspiration. Antero-posterior (AP) projections are convenient when the patient is confined to bed (e.g. in intensive care units) but result in magnification of the cardiac shadow because of the divergence of the radiograph beam.

An estimate of overall heart size can be made by comparing the maximum width of the cardiac outline with

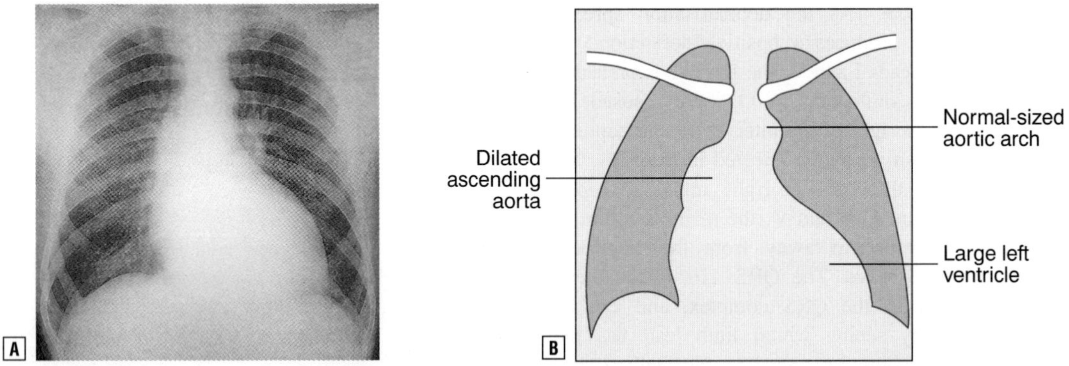

Fig. 3.9 [A] Chest radiograph from a patient with aortic regurgitation, left ventricular enlargement and dilatation of the ascending aorta. [B] Diagram to illustrate the position of major structures.

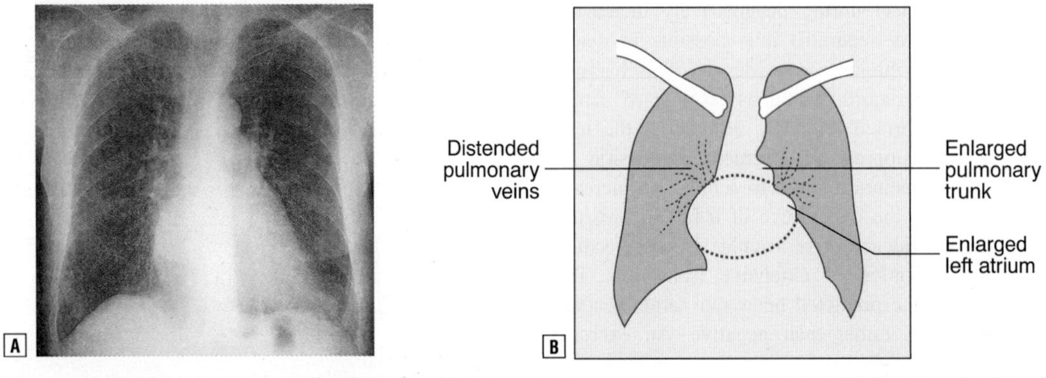

Fig. 3.10 [A] Chest radiograph of a patient with mitral stenosis and regurgitation indicating enlargement of the left atrium and prominence of the pulmonary artery trunk. **[B] Diagram to illustrate major structures.**

the maximum internal transverse diameter of the thoracic cavity. This 'cardiothoracic ratio' should be less than 0.5 cm and the transverse cardiac diameter less than 15.5 cm. Enlargement of the cardiac silhouette occurs with pericardial effusion, and apparent enlargement may be mimicked by mediastinal masses.

Dilatation of individual cardiac chambers can be recognised by the characteristic alterations they cause to the cardiac silhouette (see Figs 3.9 and 3.10, and also pp. 271–289).

- Left atrial dilatation results in prominence of the left atrial appendage, a double cardiac shadow to the right of the sternum and widening of the angle of the carina as the left main bronchus is pushed upwards.
- Right atrial enlargement projects from the right heart border towards the right lower lung field.
- Left ventricular dilatation causes prominence of the left lower heart border and enlargement of the cardiac silhouette. LV hypertrophy does not cause overall cardiac enlargement unless heart failure ensues.
- Right ventricular dilatation increases heart size and displaces the apex upwards. A lateral view may help to differentiate right and left ventricular enlargement.

Lateral or oblique projections may be useful in detecting aortic or mitral valve calcification, which may be obscured by the spine on the PA view. However, echocardiography is more sensitive.

ECHOCARDIOGRAPHY (ECHO)

This technique uses reflected ultrasound to study blood flow, the structure of the heart and the movement of valves and cardiac muscle. Ultrasound is reflected at interfaces, between blood and more solid tissues, so anatomic dimensions can be measured.

Two-dimensional (or cross-sectional) real-time echocardiography

Using a mechanical probe with rotating crystals, or an electronic equivalent, the ultrasound beam is swung rapidly back and forth over an arc or sector. The resulting information is synthesised into a two-dimensional map or picture of the position of the reflecting structures and presented on a television screen. The picture is the equivalent of a 'slice' through the heart, in a particular

INDICATIONS FOR ECHOCARDIOGRAPHY

- Diagnose and quantify severity of valve disease
- Evaluate congenital heart disease
- Assess ventricular function
- Detect pericardial effusion
- Identify vegetations in endocarditis
- Identify sources of embolism

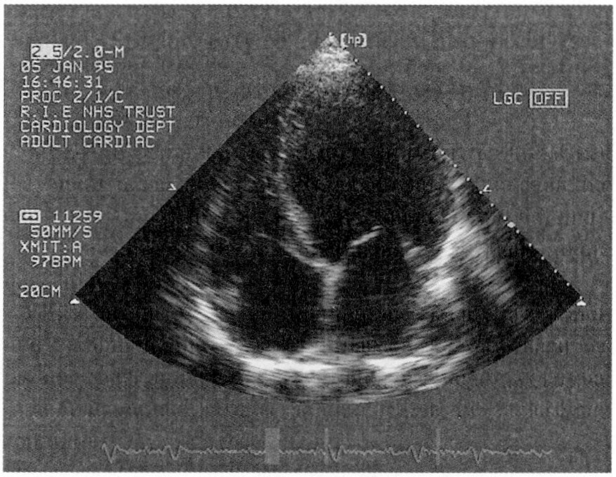

A

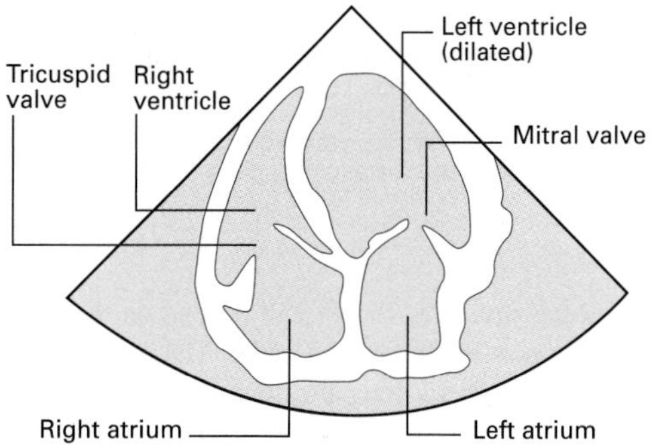

B

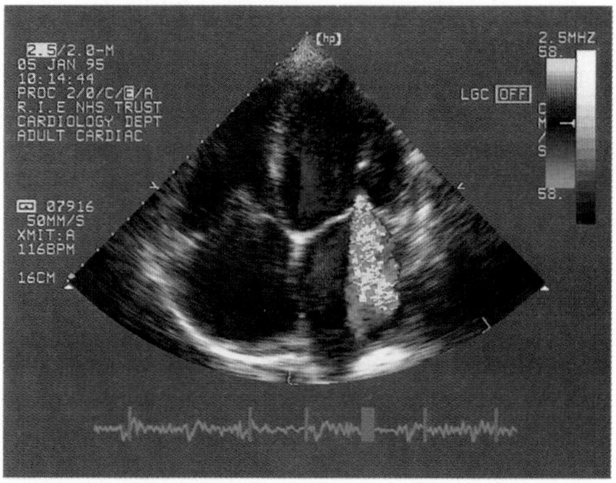

C

Fig. 3.11 Echocardiographic illustration of the principal cardiac structures in the 'four chamber' view. A Late diastole. B Diagram of major features. C Systole: colour-flow Doppler has been used to demonstrate mitral regurgitation which appears as a flame-shaped (yellow/blue) turbulent jet into the left atrium (see p. 202).

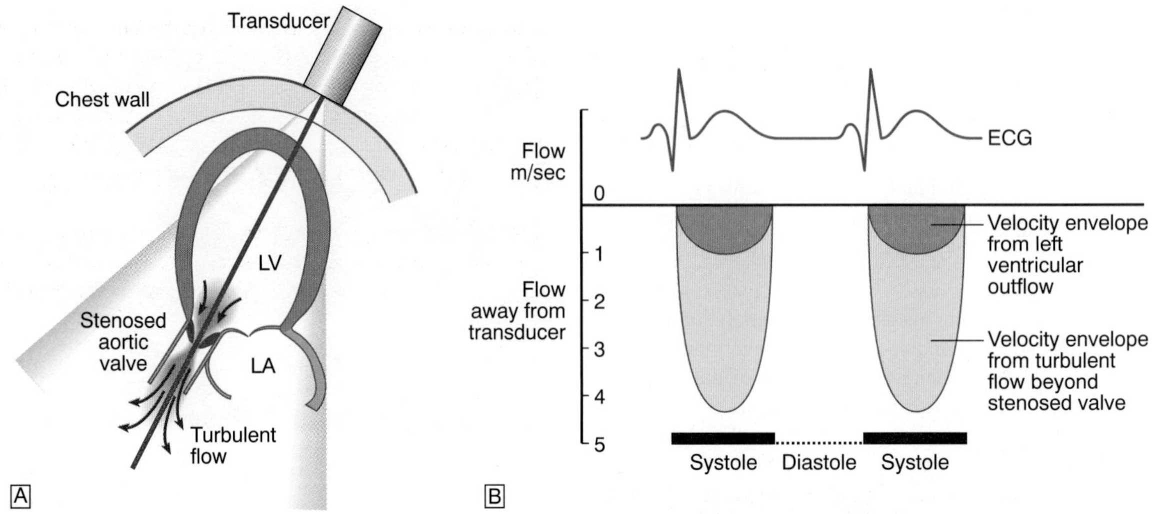

Fig. 3.12 Doppler echocardiography in aortic stenosis. A The aortic valve is imaged in a 'two chamber' view and a Doppler beam passed directly through the left ventricular outflow tract and the aorta into the turbulent flow beyond the stenosed valve. B The velocity of the blood cells is recorded to determine the maximum velocity and hence the pressure gradient across the valve: a velocity of > 4.0 m/sec, as in this example, usually indicates severe stenosis. The ratio of velocities from before the valve (left ventricular outflow) to beyond the valve (maximum velocity) indicates the degree of acceleration of blood and hence the severity of stenosis. A ratio of 4:1 indicates severe stenosis, as in this example.

plane, and the structures shown will depend on the position and orientation of the ultrasound probe. The beam oscillates very rapidly, and so the ultrasound image accurately reproduces the movement of structures in the living heart (hence 'real time') (see Fig. 3.11). This type of echocardiography is particularly valuable for detecting intracardiac masses, such as thrombi or tumours, or endocarditic vegetations. It is also very useful in defining complex structural abnormalities in congenital heart disease.

In M-mode echocardiography the ultrasound beam is focused into a narrow beam and structures are depicted graphically with respect to time and the ECG. This technique is particularly useful for accurate timing of cardiac events such as the opening and closing of valves.

Transoesophageal echocardiography

In this technique an ultrasound probe, in the shape of an endoscope, is passed into the oesophagus and positioned immediately behind the left atrium. This produces very clear images and in endocarditis, for example, it is often possible to see vegetations that are too small to be detected by ordinary echocardiography. The high-quality images that can be obtained make the technique particularly valuable for investigating patients with prosthetic (especially mitral) valve dysfunction, congenital abnormalities (e.g. atrial septal defect), and patients with systemic embolism in whom a cardiac defect is suspected but cannot be identified by transthoracic echocardiography.

Doppler echocardiography

This technique depends on the fundamental principle that sound waves reflected from moving objects, such as intracardiac red blood cells, undergo a frequency shift. The speed and direction of movement of the red cells, and thus of blood, can be detected in the heart chambers and great vessels. The greater the frequency shift, the faster the blood is moving. The derived information can be presented either as a plot of blood velocity against time for a particular point in the heart (see Fig. 3.12) or as a colour overlay on a two-dimensional real-time echo picture (colour flow Doppler, see Figs 3.11 and 3.13). Doppler echocardiography is valuable in detecting abnormal directions of blood flow, e.g. aortic or mitral reflux, and in estimating pressure gradients, e.g. the gradient across a stenosed aortic valve (see Fig. 3.12). Normal velocities are in the order of 1 m/sec, but in the presence of a stenosis flow velocity is increased. (For example, in severe aortic stenosis the peak (maximum) aortic velocity may be increased to 5 m/sec.) An estimate of the pressure gradient across a valve or lesion is given by the modified Bernoulli equation:

$$\text{Pressure gradient (mmHg)} = 4 \times (\text{peak velocity in m/sec})^2$$

Advanced echo techniques include intravascular ultrasound, which is used to define vessel wall abnormalities and guide interventional treatment, and Doppler myocardial imaging, which can be used to quantify systolic and diastolic myocardial function.

CARDIAC CATHETERISATION

In these techniques a specially designed catheter is inserted into a vein or artery and advanced into the heart under radiographic fluoroscopic guidance. This allows the operator to measure intracardiac pressures, take samples from individual cardiac chambers and obtain angiograms by injecting contrast media into an area of interest.

Coronary angiography is used to detect stenoses (see Fig. 3.14) and guide revascularisation procedures such as PTCA (percutaneous transluminal coronary angioplasty) in patients with coronary artery disease, and has become by far the most common indication for cardiac catheterisation in most countries. The procedure is usually accomplished by cannulating the right femoral or brachial artery, can often be completed without an overnight stay in hospital, and is safe, with serious complications occurring in less than 1 in 1000 cases.

Although cardiac catheterisation can be used to assess valve and congenital heart disease accurately, this is seldom necessary because the requisite information can usually

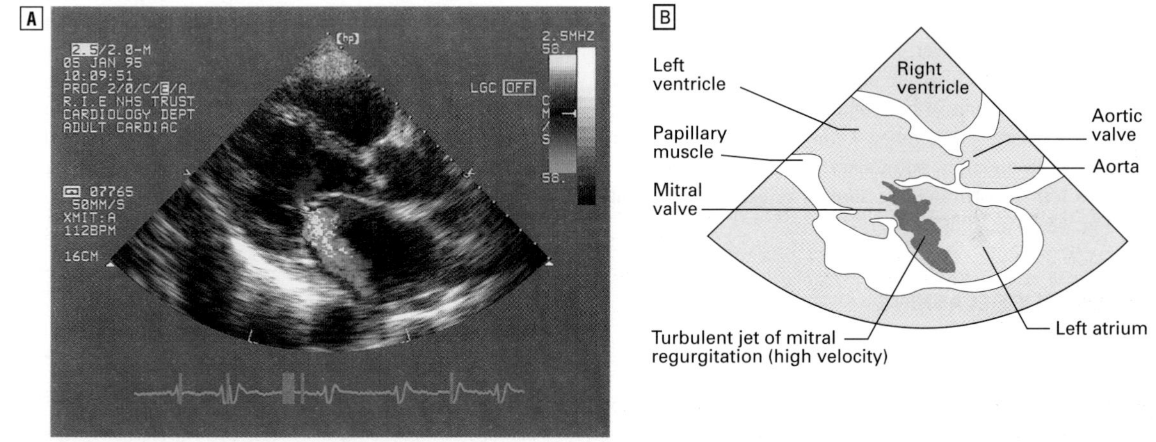

Fig. 3.13 A **Echocardiogram (systole)**. Real-time image of the heart (parasternal long axis view) showing turbulent jet (yellow/blue) of mitral regurgitation. B **Diagram to illustrate major features.**

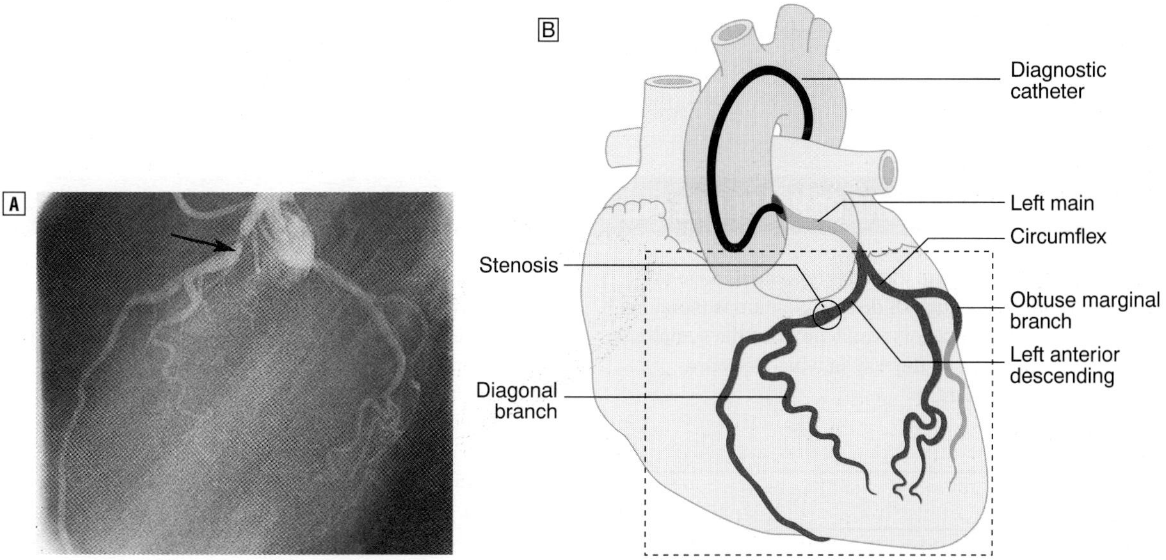

Fig. 3.14 A **Coronary artery angiogram** showing the left anterior descending and circumflex coronary arteries with a stenosis in the left anterior descending vessel. B **Diagram to illustrate vessels and branches.**

be obtained through non-invasive techniques such as Doppler echocardiography. Nevertheless, pressure measurements can be used to assess the severity of valvular stenoses, and measurement of oxygen saturation in samples withdrawn via the catheters at different sites in the heart can be used to detect and quantify intracardiac shunts. For example, a step up in oxygen saturation from 65% in the right atrium to 80% in the pulmonary artery is indicative of a large left to right shunt that might be due to a ventricular septal defect. Cardiac output can also be measured using dye dilution or thermodilution techniques.

Left atrial pressure can be measured directly by puncturing the interatrial septum, from the right atrium, with a special catheter. However, for most purposes a satisfactory approximation to left atrial pressure can be obtained by 'wedging' an end-hole or balloon catheter in a branch of the pulmonary artery. Thus, Swan–Ganz balloon catheters are often used to monitor pulmonary 'wedge' pressure as a guide to left heart filling pressure in critically ill patients (see Fig. 15.10, p. 1039).

RADIONUCLIDE SCANNING

The availability of gamma-emitting radionuclides with a short half-life has made it possible to use radionuclides for studying cardiac function non-invasively. The gamma rays are detected by means of a planar or tomographic camera and permit images of the heart to be reconstructed. Two techniques are available.

Blood pool scanning

The isotope is injected intravenously and mixes with the circulating blood. The gamma camera detects the amount of isotope-emitting blood in the heart at different phases of the cardiac cycle, and also the size and 'shape' of the cardiac chambers. By linking the gamma camera to the ECG it is possible to collect information over multiple cardiac cycles, allowing 'gating' to the systolic or diastolic phases of the cardiac cycle. Blood pool scanning provides an accurate and reproducible measure of left ventricular function, and is useful for detecting left ventricular aneurysms.

Myocardial scanning

This technique also uses gamma camera scintigraphy, but the object is usually to distinguish between ischaemic and non-ischaemic myocardium (using radioactive thallium or other tracers—see p. 249 and Fig. 3.54, p. 251) or between normal and infarcted myocardium (using radioactive pyrophosphate). More sophisticated quantitative information is available with positron emission tomography (PET), but this is largely a research tool and is only available in a few centres.

FURTHER INFORMATION ON FUNCTIONAL ANATOMY, PHYSIOLOGY AND INVESTIGATIONS

Chambers J 1995 Clinical echocardiography. BMJ Publishing Group, London
Feigenbaum H 1993 Echocardiography, 5th edn. Lea & Febiger, Philadelphia. *An authoritative reference source on echocardiography*
Hampton J R 1997 The ECG made easy, 5th edn. Churchill Livingstone, Edinburgh
Hampton J R 1997 The ECG in practice, 3rd edn. Churchill Livingstone, Edinburgh
Levick J R 1995 Introduction to cardiovascular physiology, 2nd edn. Butterworth, London. *The physiological basis of cardiac signs and investigations*
Munro J, Edwards C R W 1995 Macleod's clinical examination, 9th edn. Churchill Livingstone, Edinburgh

MAJOR MANIFESTATIONS OF HEART DISEASE

Heart disease gives rise to a relatively limited range of symptoms. Differentiation of disease conditions therefore requires emphasis on factors which provoke the symptoms and subtle differences in the way in which they are described by the patient.

CHEST PAIN

Chest pain is a common presentation of cardiac disease, but it can also signify disease of the lungs, the musculoskeletal system or, less commonly, the gastrointestinal system. It is useful to discriminate between central and peripheral or 'pleural type' pain (see the information box) and then to consider diagnostic approaches to patients presenting with these symptoms.

DIAGNOSTIC APPROACH TO THE PATIENT WITH CENTRAL CHEST PAIN

History

A number of key characteristics help to distinguish cardiac pain from that of other causes.

DIFFERENTIAL DIAGNOSIS OF CHEST PAIN
Central
Cardiac • Myocardial ischaemia (angina) • Myocardial infarction • Pericarditis • Mitral valve prolapse **Aortic** • Dissecting aneurysm • Dilating aneurysm • Aortitis (rare) **Pulmonary/mediastinum** • Massive embolus • Tracheitis • Mediastinal malignancy **Oesophageal** • Oesophagitis • Oesophageal spasm • Mallory–Weiss syndrome **Psychogenic** • Anxiety/cardiac neurosis **Neurological/skeletal** • Herniated intervertebral disc • Osteoarthritis • Trauma (impact injuries)
Peripheral
Lungs/pleura • Lobar pneumonia • Pneumothorax • Pulmonary infarction • Malignancy • Tuberculosis • Connective tissue disorders (rare) **Chest wall disorders** (simulating pleural pain) • Rib fracture/injury • Intercostal muscle injury • Epidemic myalgia (Bornholm disease) • Costochondritis (Tietze's syndrome) **Psychogenic** • Anxiety **Neurological/skeletal** • Herniated intervertebral disc • Herpes zoster • Thoracic outlet syndrome

Location

Cardiac pain is typically centrally located in the chest, on account of the derivation of the nerve supply to the heart and mediastinum. Pain only experienced at a peripheral site in the chest is rarely of cardiac origin (see the information box).

Radiation

Ischaemic pain, especially when severe, may radiate to the neck, jaw and upper or even lower arms. Pain situated over the left anterior chest, and radiating laterally, may have various other causes including pleural or lung pain, chest wall injury and anxiety.

Provocation

Anginal pain is precipitated by exertion (not after exertion) and is relieved by resting. With deteriorating or unstable angina, similar pain may be brought on by minimal exertion and may also occur at rest. In contrast, pain associated with a specific movement (bending, stretching, turning) is likely to be musculoskeletal in origin.

Character of the pain

Cardiac pain is typically described as dull, constricting or 'heavy'. It may not be appreciated as pain but as discomfort, and the constricting sensation can be described as breathlessness. Patients often use characteristic hand gestures (e.g. open hand or clenched fist) when describing ischaemic pain. Pleural pain is 'sharp' or 'catching' in quality and interrupts breathing, coughing or movement. It may originate from lung pleura or pericardium.

Pattern of onset

The pain of aortic dissection, massive pulmonary embolism or of pneumothorax is usually very sudden in onset (seconds). Myocardial infarction pain usually takes several minutes, or even longer, to develop; similarly, angina builds up gradually in proportion to the intensity of exertion.

Associated features

The severe pain of myocardial infarction, or massive pulmonary embolus, or aortic dissection is often accompanied by autonomic disturbance including sweating, nausea and vomiting. Breathlessness is associated with raised pulmonary capillary pressure or pulmonary oedema in myocardial infarction, and may accompany any of the respiratory causes of chest pain. Cough is characteristically associated with tracheitis, pneumonia or pulmonary oedema. Associated gastrointestinal symptoms may provide the clue to the source of non-cardiac chest pain (oesophageal reflux, oesophagitis, peptic ulceration or biliary disease).

Symptomatic features in the differential diagnosis of central chest pain

Angina

This is a choking or constricting chest pain which comes on with exertion, is relieved by rest, and is due to myocardial ischaemia. It is commonly felt retrosternally and may radiate to the left or more rarely the right arm, to the throat,

DIFFERENTIAL DIAGNOSIS OF CENTRAL CHEST PAIN AT REST FROM HISTORY

• Prolonged, continuous pain > 30 min • Tight or burning • Radiation to arms or jaw • Autonomic upset	→ Favours myocardial infarction
• Pain as above but not prolonged • No autonomic upset	→ Favours myocardial ischaemia
• Cataclysmic onset • Intrascapular • Tearing in nature	→ Consider aortic dissection
• Varies with position or respiration	→ Consider pericarditis
• Chest wall tenderness	→ Consider musculoskeletal cause

jaws and teeth, or through to the back. The pain may be described as squeezing, crushing, burning or aching, but seldom stabbing. Patients may describe a choking sensation simulating breathlessness.

The pain may be brought on or exacerbated by emotion, and is frequently made worse by large meals or a cold wind. It is relieved by nitrates (see p. 248). 'Unstable angina' describes a pattern of severe angina which may be precipitated by minimal exertion, or may occur spontaneously, and may culminate in infarction.

Myocardial infarction

The pain is similar in nature and distribution to angina but is more severe, persists at rest, and does not respond to nitrates. There are usually features of sympathetic nervous system activation, and vomiting is common. There may be anxiety and a frightening feeling of impending death (see p. 257). In some patients, and especially the elderly, the symptoms are atypical and may simulate other conditions.

Aortic dissection

The pain is severe, sharp and tearing, often felt in or penetrating through to the back, and is abrupt in onset (see p. 270).

Pericarditic pain

This is felt retrosternally, to the left of the sternum, or in the left or right shoulder. It characteristically varies in intensity with movement and the phase of respiration (see p. 299). It is described as 'sharp' and may catch the patient during inspiration or coughing.

Musculoskeletal chest pain

This is very variable in site and intensity but does not usually fall into the patterns described above. It may vary with posture or movement; can be brought on by exertion but often does not cease rapidly on resting; and is very commonly accompanied by local tenderness over a rib or costal cartilage.

Oesophageal pain

The pain can mimic that of angina very closely, is sometimes precipitated by exercise and may be relieved by nitrates. It is usually possible to elicit a history relating chest pain to eating, drinking or oesophageal reflux. It may coexist with angina.

Examination

In uncomplicated new-onset angina, physical examination is often normal. However, underlying risk factors may be evident, including hypertension and hyperlipidaemia (see p. 245). The physical features of myocardial infarction are those of the accompanying autonomic disturbance (sweating, pallor) or those of cardiac failure (fourth heart sound, pulmonary crepitations or florid oedema), or diminished output (cyanosis, peripherally poor perfusion). The patient usually looks 'ill'. *However, the absence of such signs does not exclude the diagnosis.*

Similar autonomic disturbance may accompany any cause of severe pain. Signs of pleural involvement (see below) provide important clues to the diagnosis, and it must be remembered that the inflammation may affect the pericardium and/or the lung pleura. Tachypnoea or dyspnoea and cyanosis may accompany pulmonary embolism, but more commonly there are no abnormal physical signs. *Thus, proceeding to examination without a careful history may be unhelpful.*

Investigations

Although cardiac investigations may reveal a specific abnormality, a lack of sensitivity means that a normal or non-specific result does not exclude the diagnosis of cardiac pain.

For example, the first ECG in patients presenting with infarction may not show characteristic changes in up to one-third of cases. On the other hand, where typical ECG signs of acute infarction are present, then the diagnosis is made and no other investigation should delay the start of treatment. The chest radiograph is not diagnostic in infarction, but may reveal pulmonary oedema. It should be performed in suspected aortic dissection or suspected pulmonary causes of chest pain. Although rapid-analysis cardiac enzymes are now available, insufficient enzyme (creatine kinase, troponin, myoglobin) is released in the first 1–2 hours of onset to be certain of the diagnosis. Thus the enzymes provide retrospective confirmation of infarction rather than a guide to immediate treatment (analgesia, aspirin, reperfusion).

Similarly, the resting ECG and chest radiograph are often normal in angina, even when caused by severe left main or three-vessel coronary disease. Exercise or stress-provoked tests are discussed later (see p. 249).

Arterial blood gases may help to guide therapy when the patient exhibits hypoxaemia or cyanosis (pulmonary embolus, extensive pneumonia) but should *not* be performed if the patient requires thrombolysis because of potential bleeding complications.

Echocardiography should be performed when cardiac failure is associated with valvular dysfunction or muscle impairment, but need not delay the start of treatment.

Patients with chest pain and acute cardiac failure require intensive monitoring (ECG, blood pressure, urinary output, oxygen saturation), and may even require haemodynamic monitoring (pulmonary artery, pulmonary capillary pressure, cardiac output and vascular resistance) in order to titrate inotropic drug support and monitor the need for further invasive treatment or ventilation.

Thus the sequence of investigations is guided by the history, the clinical signs and the suspected diagnosis.

DIAGNOSTIC APPROACH TO THE PATIENT WITH PERIPHERAL CHEST PAIN

History

Pleural pain is usually sharp, and worsens during the inspiratory phase of the ventilatory cycle (pleurisy). However, it can be dull and persistent, as exemplified by mesothelioma (see p. 387) and other malignant tumours involving the pleura. Sudden onset of pleural pain in the absence of preceding ill health should suggest pneumothorax or pulmonary infarction; a short history of ill health is suggestive of pneumonia, tuberculosis or viral myalgia, whereas a long history of ill health should arouse suspicion of malignant disease, tuberculosis or pneumonia in an immunocompromised patient. Similarly, significant weight loss is suggestive of malignancy or tuberculosis. There may be a history of conditions favouring development of a deep venous thrombosis (see p. 795) in pulmonary infarction, and arthralgia or rashes may suggest an underlying connective tissue disorder (see p. 855).

Examination

On general examination there may be pyrexia (in pneumonia, but also in established pulmonary infarction), cachexia suggestive of malignancy, signs of deep venous thrombosis, or stigmata of connective tissue diseases. On examination of the chest a pleural rub may be heard on auscultation, and it is important to determine whether a pleural effusion is present. Localised chest wall tenderness or pain on 'springing' the ribs is common in chest wall disorders but rare in pleural disease.

Investigations

The chest radiograph is nearly always abnormal in cases of pleural disease, and it may be diagnostic in pneumothorax (see p. 388). There may be pleural effusions which require further investigation (see below), and linear lower zone abnormalities are common in pulmonary infarction. Diffuse pulmonary shadowing is a common feature of infections in immunocompromised individuals, and bilateral upper zone abnormalities may be present in tuberculosis (but not in all cases).

Where pulmonary infarction is suspected, a ventilation/perfusion scan (see p. 309), CT scan with contrast or pulmonary angiography may be necessary to confirm the diagnosis, and ascending venography can be used to identify the site and extent of deep venous thrombosis. In bacterial pneumonia, sputum should be examined and cultured for pathogens and blood taken for white cell count and blood cultures. In cases of suspected tuberculosis, sputum should be stained and cultured for mycobacteria and a tuberculin test performed, but in the absence of sputum it is often necessary to obtain bronchial washings by bronchoscopy. The sputum can be examined for malignant cells, but in suspected pleural malignancy transthoracic needle biopsy or thoracoscopy is usually necessary to obtain a histological diagnosis.

If pleural effusion is present, in the case of a small or loculated effusion, ultrasonography may be necessary to identify the most favourable site where aspiration and biopsy can be performed. In large pleural effusions the investigation of choice is aspiration and pleural biopsy using an Abram's needle (see p. 310). The fluid should be examined for bacterial pathogens, tubercle bacilli, malignant cells and a differential white cell count. It is also useful to determine pleural fluid protein, glucose and lactate dehydrogenase (LDH) levels. High titres of rheumatoid factor, anti-DNA antibodies etc. may be found in pleural effusions complicating connective tissue diseases (see p. 386). Multiple pleural biopsies should be fixed and examined histologically. If a diagnosis is not established by pleural aspiration and biopsy, thoracoscopy may be necessary to permit direct visualisation and biopsy of abnormal tissue.

BREATHLESSNESS (DYSPNOEA)

See Chapter 4, p. 312.

ACUTE CIRCULATORY FAILURE

Shock is a loosely defined term used to describe the clinical syndrome that develops when there is critical impairment of tissue perfusion due to some form of acute circulatory failure.

There are numerous causes of shock and the condition is described on page 1031. However, the important features of the major causes of acute heart failure or cardiogenic shock are described below.

CAUSES OF CARDIOGENIC SHOCK

The common causes are illustrated in Figure 3.15. Echocardiography is very helpful when the diagnosis is in doubt.

Myocardial infarction

Although heart failure complicating myocardial infarction can be due to mechanical problems such as mitral regurgitation or a ventricular septal defect (see p. 264) it is usually due to left ventricular dysfunction.

Hypotension, oliguria, confusion and cold, clammy peripheries are the manifestations of a low cardiac output, whereas breathlessness, hypoxia, cyanosis and inspiratory crackles at the lung bases are features of pulmonary oedema. A chest radiograph (see Fig. 3.16) may reveal signs of pulmonary congestion when clinical examination is normal. If necessary, a Swan–Ganz catheter can be used to measure the pulmonary artery wedge (PAW) pressure (see Fig. 15.10, p. 1039).

These findings can be used to divide patients with acute myocardial infarction into four haemodynamic subsets (see the information box).

ACUTE MYOCARDIAL INFARCTION: PATIENT SUBSETS
Normal cardiac output. No pulmonary oedema
• The normal state of affairs; carries a good outlook and requires no treatment for heart failure
Normal cardiac output. Pulmonary oedema
• Usually due to moderate left ventricular dysfunction; should be treated with diuretics and vasodilators
Low cardiac output. No pulmonary oedema
• Often due to a combination of right ventricular infarction and hypovolaemia due to a reduced oral intake of fluids, vomiting and inappropriate diuretic therapy. Such patients have a poor prognosis and are difficult to manage, and it is usually advisable to insert a Swan–Ganz catheter and give i.v. fluids or plasma to raise the PAW pressure to between 14 and 16 mmHg
Low cardiac output. Pulmonary oedema
• Usually due to extensive left ventricular damage and carries a very poor prognosis. The patient may benefit from treatment with diuretics, vasodilators and inotropes (see p. 214)

The viable myocardium surrounding a fresh infarct may contract poorly for a few days. This phenomenon is known as *myocardial stunning* and means that, in this setting, it is often worth treating acute heart failure energetically in the

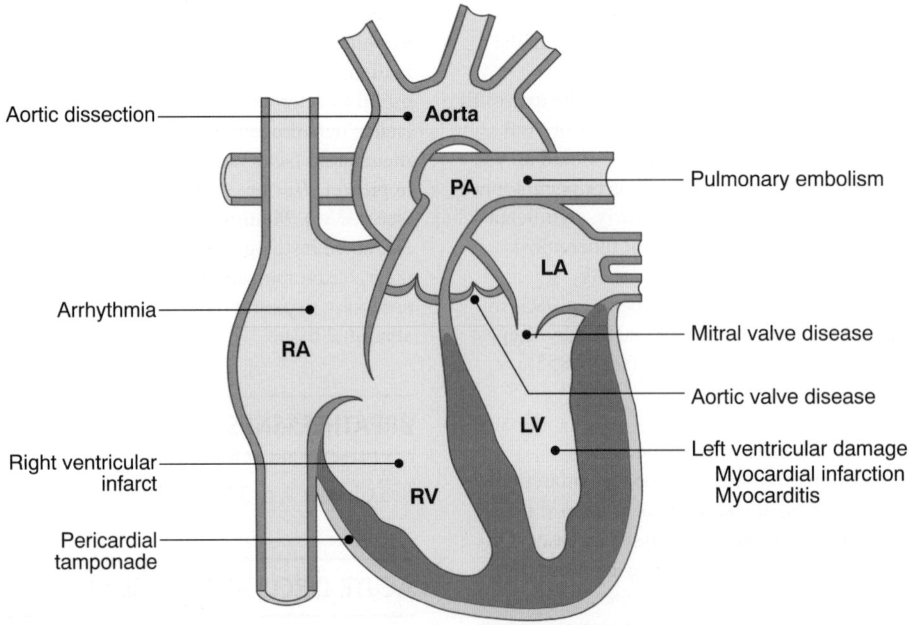

Fig. 3.15 Some common causes of cardiogenic shock.

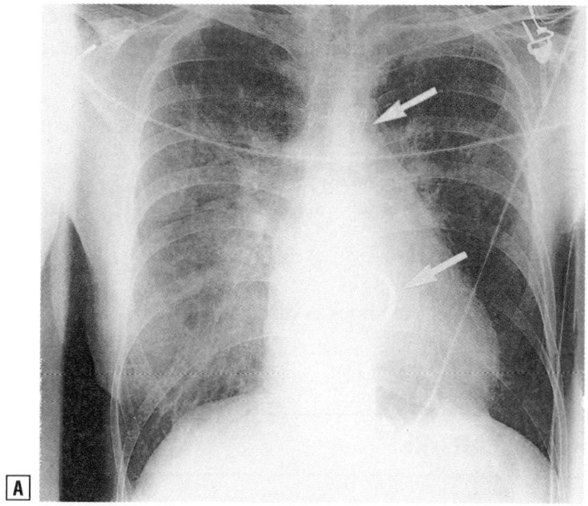

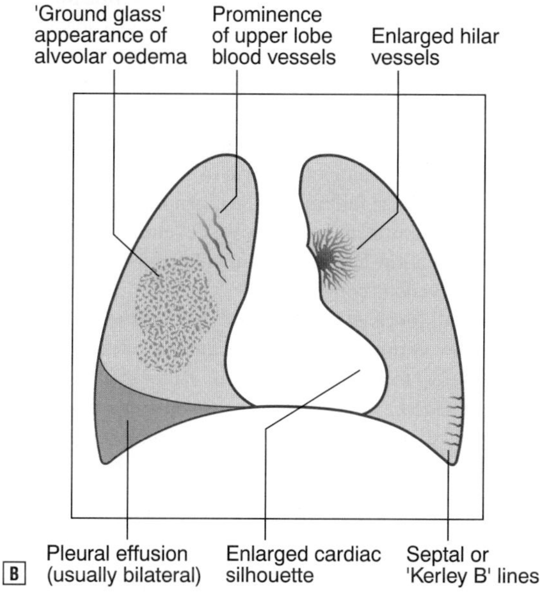

Fig. 3.16 A Chest radiograph demonstrating pulmonary oedema in a patient with a prosthetic mitral valve (bottom arrow). This was due to fracture of one of the valve struts; the disc had fallen out of the valve and lodged in the aortic arch (top arrow). **B The appearance of the chest radiograph in heart failure.**

hope and expectation that overall cardiac function will improve.

Acute massive pulmonary embolism

This may complicate leg or pelvic vein thrombosis and usually presents with sudden collapse. The clinical features are discussed on page 378.

Bedside echocardiography may be very helpful and usually demonstrates a small vigorous left ventricle with a dilated right ventricle; it is sometimes possible to see thrombus in the right ventricular outflow tract or main pulmonary artery. Spiral CT scanning of the chest with contrast will usually provide a definitive diagnosis and is preferable to pulmonary angiography, which may be hazardous.

Treatment (see p. 380) may utilise high-flow oxygen, anticoagulation, thrombolytic therapy and sometimes surgical embolectomy.

Pericardial tamponade

This condition is due to a collection of fluid or blood in the pericardial sac compressing the heart; the effusion may be small and is sometimes less than 100 ml. Sudden deterioration is frequently due to bleeding into the pericardial space.

Tamponade may complicate any form of pericarditis and is often due to malignant disease. Other causes include trauma and rupture of the free wall of the myocardium following myocardial infarction.

The important clinical features of the condition are listed in the information box.

CLINICAL FEATURES OF PERICARDIAL TAMPONADE

- Dyspnoea
- Collapse
- Tachycardia
- Hypotension
- Gross elevation of the venous pressure
- Soft heart sounds with an early third heart sound
- Pulsus paradoxus (a large fall in blood pressure during inspiration when the pulse may be impalpable)
- Kussmaul's sign (a paradoxical rise in the jugular venous pressure during inspiration)

An ECG may show features of the underlying disease, e.g. pericarditis or acute myocardial infarction. When there is a large pericardial effusion the ECG complexes are small and there may be electrical alternans (a changing axis with alternate beats caused by the heart moving in the bag of fluid). A chest radiograph may show an enlarged globular heart but can look normal. Echocardiography, which may be done at the bedside, is the best way of confirming the diagnosis, and helps to identify the optimum site for paracentesis.

Prompt recognition of tamponade is important because the patient usually responds dramatically to percutaneous pericardiocentesis (see p. 300) or surgical drainage.

Valvular heart disease

Acute left ventricular failure may be due to the sudden onset of aortic regurgitation, mitral regurgitation or prosthetic valve dysfunction (see Fig 3.16A). Some of the common causes of these problems are listed in the information box.

CAUSES OF ACUTE VALVE FAILURE
Aortic regurgitation
• Aortic dissection • Infective endocarditis • Ruptured sinus of Valsalva
Mitral regurgitation
• Papillary muscle rupture due to acute myocardial infarction • Infective endocarditis • Rupture of chordae due to myxomatous degeneration, or blunt chest wall trauma
Prosthetic valve failure
• Mechanical valves: fracture, jamming, thrombosis, dehiscence • Biological valves: degeneration with cusp tear

The clinical diagnosis of acute valvular dysfunction is sometimes difficult. Murmurs are often unimpressive because there is usually a tachycardia with a low cardiac output. Transthoracic echocardiography will establish the diagnosis in most cases; however, transoesophageal echocardiography is sometimes required to identify prosthetic mitral valve regurgitation.

Patients with acute valve failure usually require cardiac surgery and should be referred for urgent assessment in a cardiac centre.

The chest radiograph in left heart failure (see Fig. 3.16)

A rise in pulmonary venous pressure from left-sided cardiac failure first shows on the chest radiograph as an abnormal distension of the upper lobe pulmonary veins (with the patient in the erect position). The vascularity of the lung fields becomes more prominent and the pulmonary artery dilated (the right lower pulmonary artery should measure less than 16 mmHg). Subsequently, interstitial oedema causes thickened interlobular septa and dilated lymphatics (when pulmonary venous pressure is in the range 20–30 mmHg; normal is 5–14 mmHg). These are evident as horizontal lines in the costophrenic angles (septal or 'Kerley B' lines). More advanced changes due to alveolar oedema cause a hazy opacification spreading from the hilar regions, and pleural effusions (pulmonary venous pressure > 30 mmHg).

Management

Management of acute pulmonary oedema

This is a feature of acute left heart failure and needs urgent treatment:

- Sit the patient up in order to reduce pulmonary congestion.
- Give oxygen (high flow, high concentration).
- Use morphine (10 mg intravenous, intramuscular or subcutaneous) to alleviate breathlessness and reverse reflex peripheral vasoconstriction.
- Administer a powerful diuretic such as frusemide (40–80 mg intravenously); these drugs provide rapid relief because they are also vasodilators.

If these immediate measures prove inadequate, one may try to stimulate the heart using inotropic agents, or to reduce left ventricular load by using more powerful vasodilators.

Management of shock

The management of shock is discussed in detail in Chapter 15, page 1033.

HEART FAILURE

Heart failure is an imprecise term used to describe the state that develops when the heart cannot maintain an adequate cardiac output or can do so only at the expense of an elevated filling pressure. In the mildest forms of heart failure, cardiac output is adequate at rest and becomes inadequate only when the metabolic demand increases during exercise or some other form of stress.

In practice, heart failure may be diagnosed whenever a patient with significant heart disease develops the signs or symptoms of a low cardiac output, pulmonary congestion or systemic venous congestion.

Almost all forms of heart disease may lead to heart failure and it is important to appreciate that, like anaemia, the term refers to a clinical syndrome rather than a specific diagnosis. Good management depends on an accurate aetiological diagnosis, partly because in some situations a specific remedy may be available, but mainly because a clear understanding of the pathophysiology is essential to logical drug therapy.

Heart failure is frequently due to coronary artery disease, tends to affect elderly subjects and often leads to prolonged disability. In the United Kingdom most patients admitted to hospital with heart failure are more than 65 years old and remain inpatients for a week or more.

Although the outlook depends to some extent on the underlying cause of the problem, heart failure carries a very poor prognosis; approximately 50% of patients with severe heart failure will die within 2 years. Many patients die suddenly, often due to malignant ventricular arrhythmias or myocardial infarction.

Pathophysiology

The cardiac output is a function of the preload (the volume and pressure of blood in the ventricle at the end of diastole), the afterload (the arterial resistance) and myocardial contractility. The interaction of these variables is shown in Figure 3.17, which is based on Starling's Law of the heart.

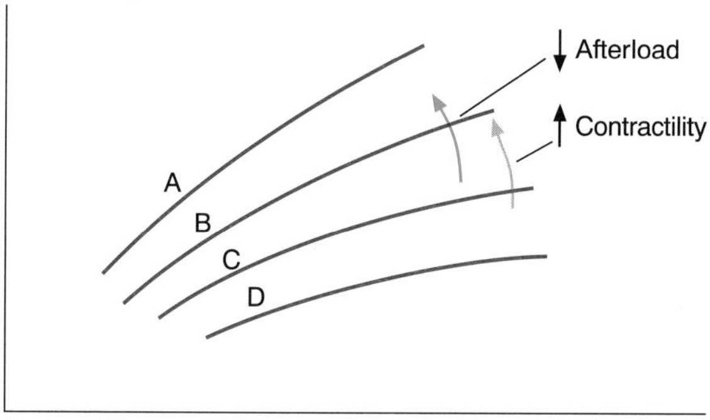

Fig. 3.17 Starling's Law. Normal (A), mild (B), moderate (C) and severe (D) heart failure. Ventricular performance is related to the degree of myocardial stretching. An increase in preload (end-diastolic volume, end-diastolic pressure, filling pressure or atrial pressure) will therefore enhance function; however, overstretching causes marked deterioration. In heart failure the curve moves to the right and becomes flatter. An increase in myocardial contractility or a reduction in afterload (arterial resistance/blood pressure) will shift the curve upwards and to the left.

Heart failure is associated with complex neurohormonal changes including activation of the renin-angiotensin-aldosterone axis and the sympathetic nervous system. At first these changes may help to optimise cardiac function by altering the afterload or preload and by increasing myocardial contractility (see Fig. 3.18). However, ultimately they become counterproductive and often reduce cardiac output by causing an inappropriate and excessive increase in peripheral vascular resistance. A vicious circle may be established because a fall in cardiac output will cause further neurohormonal activation and increasing peripheral vascular resistance.

The onset of pulmonary and/or peripheral oedema is due to high atrial pressures compounded by salt and water retention caused by impaired renal perfusion and secondary aldosteronism.

Types of heart failure

Heart failure can be described or classified in several ways.

Acute and chronic heart failure

Heart failure may develop suddenly, as in myocardial infarction, or gradually, as in progressive valvular heart disease. When there is gradual impairment of cardiac

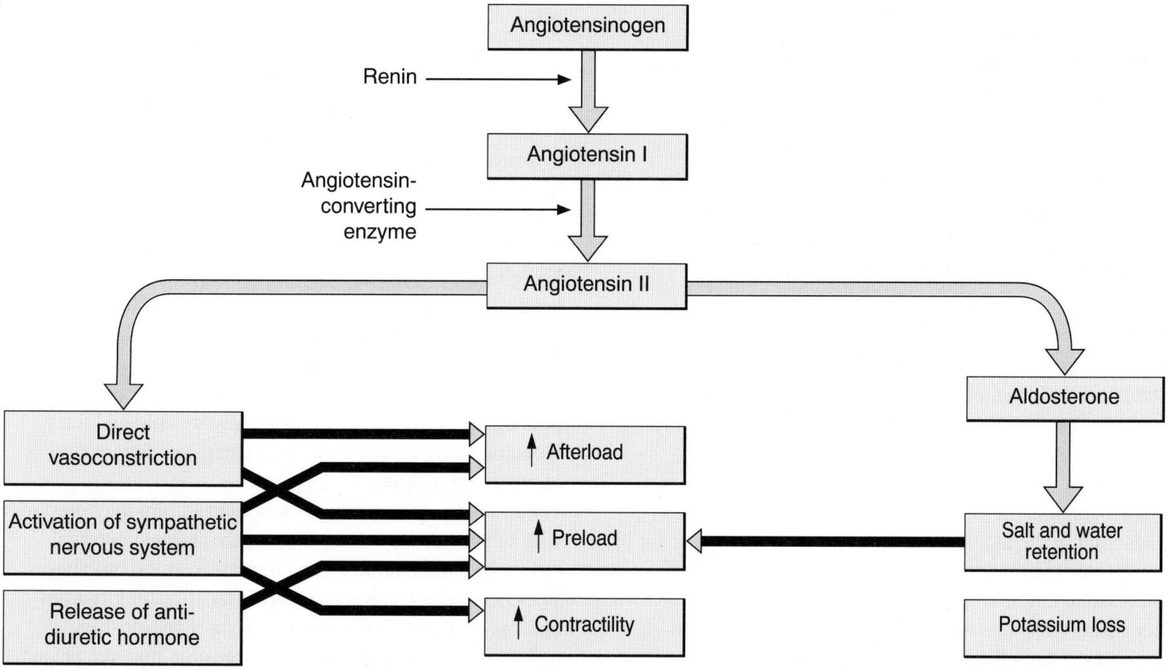

Fig. 3.18 The renin-angiotensin-aldosterone system in heart failure. Impaired renal perfusion and diuretic therapy lead to the release of renin with secondary changes in the afterload, preload and myocardial contractility.

function, a variety of compensatory changes (see the first information box) may take place. Although initially these changes may improve overall cardiac function, as the disease progresses they often become counterproductive.

The term *compensated* heart failure is sometimes used to describe a patient with impaired cardiac function in whom adaptive changes have prevented the development of overt heart failure. A minor event, such as an intercurrent infection, may precipitate overt heart failure in this type of patient (see the second information box).

COMPENSATORY CHANGES IN HEART FAILURE

Local changes

- Chamber enlargement
- Myocardial hypertrophy
- Increased heart rate

Systemic changes

- Activation of the sympathetic nervous system
- Activation of the renin-angiotensin-aldosterone system (see Fig. 3.18)
- Release of antidiuretic hormone
- Release of natriuretic peptides (atrial and brain natriuretic peptide—ANP and BNP)

FACTORS THAT MAY PRECIPITATE OR AGGRAVATE HEART FAILURE

- Myocardial ischaemia or infarction
- Intercurrent illness (e.g. infection)
- Arrhythmia
- Inappropriate reduction of therapy
- Administration of a drug with negative inotropic (e.g. β-adrenoceptor antagonist) or fluid-retaining properties (e.g. non-steroidal anti-inflammatory drugs, corticosteroids)
- Pulmonary embolism
- Conditions associated with increased metabolic demand (e.g. pregnancy, thyrotoxicosis, anaemia)
- Intravenous fluid overload (e.g. post-operative i.v. infusion)

Left, right and biventricular heart failure

The left side of the heart is a term for the functional unit of the left atrium and left ventricle, together with the mitral and aortic valves, whereas the right heart comprises the right atrium, right ventricle, tricuspid and pulmonary valves.

Left-sided heart failure. In this condition there is a reduction in the left ventricular output and/or an increase in the left atrial or pulmonary venous pressure. An acute increase in left atrial pressure may cause pulmonary congestion or pulmonary oedema; but a more gradual increase in the left atrial pressure may lead to reflex pulmonary vasoconstriction, which protects the patient from pulmonary oedema at the cost of increasing pulmonary hypertension.

Right-sided heart failure. In this condition there is a reduction in right ventricular output for any given right atrial pressure. Causes of isolated right heart failure include chronic lung disease (cor pulmonale), multiple pulmonary emboli, and pulmonary valvular stenosis.

Biventricular heart failure. Failure of the left and right heart may develop because the disease process (e.g. dilated cardiomyopathy or ischaemic heart disease) affects both ventricles, or because disease of the left heart leads to chronic elevation of the left atrial pressure, pulmonary hypertension and subsequent right heart failure.

Forward and backward heart failure

In some patients with heart failure the predominant problem is an inadequate cardiac output *(forward failure)* whilst other patients may have a normal or near-normal cardiac output with marked salt and water retention causing pulmonary and systemic venous congestion *(backward failure).*

Diastolic and systolic dysfunction

Heart failure may develop as a result of impaired myocardial contraction *(systolic dysfunction)* but can also be due to poor ventricular filling and high filling pressures caused by abnormal ventricular relaxation *(diastolic dysfunction).* The latter is commonly found in patients with left ventricular hypertrophy and occurs in many forms of heart disease, notably hypertension and ischaemic heart disease. Systolic and diastolic dysfunction often coexist, particularly in patients with coronary artery disease.

High output failure

Conditions that are associated with a very high cardiac output (e.g. a large AV shunt, beri-beri, severe anaemia or thyrotoxicosis) can occasionally cause heart failure. In such cases additional causes of heart failure are often present.

Clinical features

The clinical picture depends on the nature of the underlying heart disease, the type of heart failure that it has evoked and the neural and endocrine changes that have developed (see Table 3.1).

A low cardiac output causes fatigue, listlessness and a poor effort tolerance. The peripheries are cold and the blood pressure is low. Poor renal perfusion may lead to oliguria and uraemia.

Pulmonary oedema due to left heart failure may present with breathlessness, orthopnoea, paroxysmal nocturnal dyspnoea and inspiratory crepitations over the lung bases. The chest radiograph shows characteristic abnormalities (see pp. 209 and 210) and is usually a more sensitive indicator of pulmonary venous congestion than the physical signs.

In contrast, right heart failure produces a high jugular venous pressure, with hepatic congestion and dependent

Table 3.1 Causes of heart failure

Cause	Features	Examples
Reduced ventricular contractility	Progressive ventricular dilatation In coronary artery disease 'akinetic' or 'dyskinetic' segments contract poorly and may impede the function of the normal segments by distorting their contraction and relaxation patterns	Myocarditis/cardiomyopathy (global dysfunction) Myocardial infarction (segmental dysfunction)
Ventricular outflow obstruction (pressure overload)	Initially concentric ventricular hypertrophy allows the ventricle to maintain a normal output by generating a high systolic pressure. However, secondary changes in the myocardium and increasing obstruction eventually lead to failure with ventricular dilatation and rapid clinical deterioration	Hypertension, aortic stenosis (left heart failure) Pulmonary hypertension, pulmonary valve stenosis (right heart failure)
Ventricular inflow obstruction	Small vigorous ventricle Dilated hypertrophied atrium Atrial fibrillation is common and often causes marked deterioration because ventricular filling depends heavily on atrial contraction	Mitral stenosis Tricuspid stenosis Endomyocardial fibrosis and other disorders that cause a stiff myocardium, e.g. left ventricular hypertrophy Constrictive pericarditis
Ventricular volume overload	Dilatation and hypertrophy allow the ventricle to generate a high stroke volume and help to maintain a normal cardiac output. However, secondary changes in the myocardium eventually lead to impaired contractility and worsening heart failure	Mitral regurgitation (LV volume overload) Aortic regurgitation (LV volume overload) Atrial septal defect (RV volume overload) Ventricular septal defect Increased metabolic demand (high output)

peripheral oedema. In ambulant patients the oedema affects the ankles, whereas in bed-bound patients it collects around the thighs and sacrum. Massive accumulation of fluid may cause ascites or pleural effusion. Oedema may be due to other conditions (see the information box).

Chronic heart failure is sometimes associated with marked weight loss *(cardiac cachexia)* caused by a combination of anorexia and impaired absorption due to gastrointestinal congestion, poor tissue perfusion due to a low cardiac output, and skeletal muscle atrophy due to immobility.

DIFFERENTIAL DIAGNOSIS OF PERIPHERAL OEDEMA

- **Cardiac failure** (right or combined left and right heart failure, pericardial constriction, cardiomyopathy)
- **Chronic venous insufficiency**
- **Hypoalbuminaemia** (nephrotic syndrome, liver disease, protein-losing enteropathy)
  Often widespread, can affect arms and face
- **Drugs**
  Retaining sodium (fludrocortisone, non-steroidal anti-inflammatory agents)
  Increasing capillary permeability (nifedipine)
- **Idiopathic** (women > men)
- **Chronic lymphatic obstruction**

Complications

In advanced heart failure a number of non-specific complications may occur.

Uraemia. This reflects poor renal perfusion due to the effects of diuretic therapy and a low cardiac output. Treatment with vasodilators or dopamine may improve renal perfusion.

Hypokalaemia. This may be the result of treatment with potassium-losing diuretics or hyperaldosteronism caused by activation of the renin-angiotensin system and impaired aldosterone metabolism due to hepatic congestion. Most of the body's potassium is intracellular, and there may be substantial depletion of potassium stores even when the plasma potassium concentration is in the normal range.

Hyponatraemia. This is a feature of severe heart failure and may be caused by diuretic therapy, inappropriate water retention, or failure of the cell membrane ion pump.

Impaired liver function. Hepatic venous congestion and poor arterial perfusion frequently cause mild jaundice and abnormal liver function tests; reduced synthesis of clotting factors may make anticoagulant control difficult.

Thromboembolism. Deep vein thrombosis and pulmonary embolism may occur due to the effects of a low cardiac output and enforced immobility, whereas systemic emboli may be related to arrhythmias, particularly atrial fibrillation, or intracardiac thrombus complicating conditions such as mitral stenosis or LV aneurysm.

Arrhythmias. Atrial and ventricular arrhythmias are very common and may be related to electrolyte changes (e.g. hypokalaemia, hypomagnesaemia), the underlying structural heart disease, and the pro-arrhythmic effects of increased circulating catecholamines and some drugs (e.g. digoxin). Sudden death occurs in up to 50% of patients with heart failure and is often due to a ventricular arrhythmia. Frequent ventricular ectopic beats and runs of non-sustained ventricular tachycardia are common findings in patients with heart failure and are associated with an adverse prognosis; unfortunately, the outlook appears to be no better when anti-arrhythmic drugs are used to suppress these arrhythmias.

Investigations

Simple tests (e.g. urea, electrolytes, ECG, chest radiograph) may help to establish the nature and severity of the underlying heart disease and detect any complications (see below).

Echocardiography is a very useful investigation and should be considered in all patients with significant heart failure in order to:

- confirm the diagnosis
- detect hitherto unsuspected valvular heart disease (e.g. occult mitral stenosis) and other conditions that may be amenable to specific remedies
- identify patients who will benefit from long-term therapy with an angiotensin-converting enzyme inhibitor (see below).

Management of heart failure

General measures

Bed rest increases renal blood flow and may help to initiate a diuresis in a patient with severe heart failure. However, regular stamina-building exercise (e.g. brisk walking or swimming) has been shown to improve the outlook in patients with chronic heart failure.

Patients with heart failure should be advised to avoid a high dietary salt intake, excess alcohol, and salt- or fluid-retaining drugs (e.g. non-steroidal anti-inflammatory drugs—NSAIDs).

Drug therapy

Cardiac function can be improved by increasing contractility, optimising preload or decreasing afterload. The effects of these measures are illustrated in Figure 3.19. Drugs that reduce preload are most appropriate in patients with high end-diastolic filling pressures and evidence of pulmonary or systemic venous congestion (backward failure); drugs that reduce afterload or increase myocardial contractility are particularly valuable in patients with signs and symptoms of a low cardiac output (forward failure).

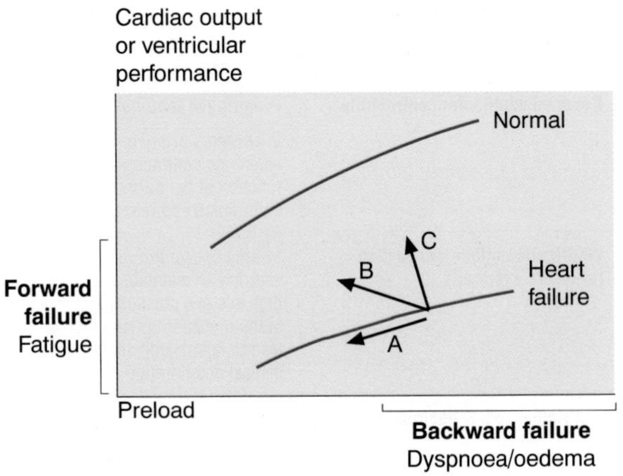

Fig. 3.19 The effect of treatment on ventricular performance curves in heart failure. Diuretics and venodilators (A), angiotensin-converting enzyme inhibitors and mixed vasodilators (B), and positive inotropic agents (C).

Diuretics. These are usually the first line of treatment. The main types, mode of action, and side-effects of these drugs are described on page 401. In heart failure, diuretics produce an increase in urinary sodium excretion, leading to a reduction in blood and plasma volume, and may also cause a small but significant degree of arterial and venous dilatation. Diuretic therapy will, therefore, reduce preload and improve pulmonary and systemic venous congestion; it may also cause a small reduction in afterload and ventricular volume leading to a fall in wall tension and increased cardiac efficiency.

Although a fall in preload (ventricular filling pressure) tends to reduce cardiac output, the 'Starling curve' in heart failure is flat so there may be a substantial and beneficial fall in filling pressure with little change in cardiac output (see Fig. 3.19). Nevertheless, excessive diuretic therapy may cause an undesirable fall in cardiac output with a rising blood urea, hypotension and increasing lethargy.

In severe heart failure treatment with combinations of diuretics from different classes (loop, thiazide and potassium-sparing) may increase the diuretic effect and may help to prevent hypokalaemia.

Vasodilators. The use of vasodilators in acute circulatory failure is described on page 1042. These drugs are also valuable in chronic heart failure; venodilators (e.g. organic nitrates) reduce preload, and arterial dilators (e.g. hydralazine) reduce afterload (see Fig. 3.19). However, their use is limited by pharmacological tolerance and hypotension, and treatment with angiotensin-converting enzyme inhibitors is usually preferable.

Angiotensin-converting enzyme (ACE) inhibitors. The advent of these drugs has been a major advance in the treatment of heart failure. They act to prevent the conversion of angiotensin I to angiotensin II, thereby counteracting salt and water retention, peripheral arterial and venous vasoconstriction, and activation of the sympathetic nervous system (see Fig. 3.18, p. 211). They will, therefore, interrupt the vicious circle of neurohumoral activation that is characteristic of moderate and severe heart failure and will also prevent the undesirable activation of the renin-angiotensin system caused by diuretic therapy.

The major benefit of ACE inhibitor therapy in heart failure is a reduction in afterload; however, there may also be an advantageous reduction in preload and a modest increase in the plasma potassium concentration. Treating heart failure with a combination of a potassium-losing diuretic and an ACE inhibitor therefore has many potential advantages.

Clinical trials have shown that in moderate and severe heart failure ACE inhibitors can produce a substantial improvement in effort tolerance and in mortality. Using data from the SOLVD (studies of left ventricular dysfunction) trial it has been calculated that treating 1000 heart failure patients with an ACE inhibitor for 3 years would prevent about 50 premature deaths and 350 hospital admissions. Recent trials have also established that ACE inhibitors can improve outcome and prevent the onset of overt heart failure in patients with poor residual left ventricular function following myocardial infarction (see p. 265).

Unfortunately these drugs can cause profound hypotension with postural symptoms and a deterioration in renal function (especially in patients with bilateral renal artery stenosis or pre-existing renal disease). Moreover, there may be a potentially catastrophic fall in blood pressure following the first dose of an ACE inhibitor, particularly if the drug is started in the presence of hypotension, hypovolaemia or hyponatraemia due to prior diuretic therapy. In stable patients, without hypotension (systolic BP > 100 mmHg), ACE inhibitors can usually be started in the community without problems. However, in other patients it is usually advisable to withhold diuretics for 24 hours before starting treatment with a low dose, while the patient is supine and under observation. If hypotension occurs, this can be counteracted by elevating the foot of the bed, intravenous saline or, in extreme circumstances, intravenous angiotensin II. Renal function must be monitored and should be checked a month after starting therapy.

- *Captopril* (average dose 25 mg 8-hourly) is a short-acting agent with an elimination half-life of 6–8 hours. Unwanted effects include hypotension, hyperkalaemia, deterioration in renal function, cough, skin rash, altered taste and neutropenia.
- *Enalapril* (average dose 20 mg daily) is a long-acting agent that is only active after conversion, in the liver, to the active metabolite enalaprilat. Unwanted effects are similar to those caused by captopril.
- *Lisinopril* (average dose 10 mg daily) has a long half-life and a similar range of side-effects.

Angiotensin II receptor antagonists (e.g. losartan—average dose 50 mg once daily). These drugs act by blocking the action of angiotensin II on the heart, peripheral vasculature and kidney and, in heart failure, produce beneficial haemodynamic changes that are similar to the effects of ACE inhibitors. However, their effect on mortality will not be clear until large-scale randomised controlled trials have been completed. In contrast to ACE inhibitors, they have no effect on the breakdown of bradykinin within the lungs and do not therefore cause cough; the two classes of drug may also have different effects on vascular regulation and cell growth.

Digoxin. This should be used as first-line therapy in patients with heart failure and atrial fibrillation, when it will usually provide adequate control of the ventricular rate together with a small positive inotropic effect. The dosage and side-effects are discussed on page 239.

The role of digoxin in the treatment of patients with heart failure and sinus rhythm is less certain. In a recent large randomised controlled trial among this patient population, treatment with digoxin had no effect on overall survival but did reduce the need for hospitalisation.

β-adrenoceptor antagonists ('β-blockers'). These drugs diminish the effects of sympathetic stimulation on the heart and, if given in standard doses, may precipitate acute on chronic heart failure. Nevertheless, recent trials have shown that, when given in very small incremental doses under carefully monitored conditions, they can increase ejection fraction, improve symptoms and reduce the frequency of hospitalisation in patients with chronic heart failure.

Amiodarone (see p. 239). This is a potent anti-arrhythmic drug which has little negative inotropic effect and is therefore valuable in patients with poor left ventricular function. Although not firmly established, there is growing interest in the prospect of using anti-arrhythmic drugs to prevent potentially fatal arrhythmias. However, clinical trials of amiodarone in heart failure have produced conflicting results and the drug is usually used to treat patients with symptomatic arrhythmias.

Other drugs. A variety of potentially useful oral positive inotropic agents have been developed but have been shown to *increase* mortality in clinical trials.

Anticoagulants are used to treat or prevent thromboembolism complicating atrial fibrillation.

Heart transplantation

Cardiac transplantation is an established and very successful form of treatment for patients with intractable heart failure. Coronary artery disease and dilated cardiomyopathy are the most common reasons for transplantation. The introduction of cyclosporin for immunosuppression has improved survival, which now exceeds 90% at 1 year. The use of transplantation is limited by the availability of donor hearts so it is generally reserved for young patients with severe symptoms.

Conventional heart transplantation is contraindicated in patients with pulmonary vascular disease due to long-standing left heart failure, complex congenital heart disease (e.g. Eisenmenger's syndrome) or primary pulmonary hypertension, because the right ventricle of the donor heart may fail in the face of increased pulmonary vascular resistance. However, heart-lung transplantation is an option for such patients and has also been used in the treatment of terminal respiratory disease such as cystic fibrosis.

Although cardiac transplantation usually produces a dramatic improvement in the recipient's quality of life, serious complications may occur:

- *Rejection.* In spite of routine therapy with cyclosporin A, azathioprine and corticosteroids, episodes of rejection are common and may present with heart failure, arrhythmias or subtle ECG changes; cardiac biopsy is often used to confirm the diagnosis before starting treatment with high-dose steroids.
- *Accelerated atherosclerosis.* Recurrent heart failure is often due to progressive atherosclerosis in the coronary arteries of the donor heart. This is not confined to patients who were transplanted for coronary artery disease and is probably a manifestation of chronic rejection. Angina is rare because the heart has been denervated.
- *Infection.* Opportunistic infection with organisms such as cytomegalovirus or aspergillus remains a major cause of death in transplant recipients.

HYPERTENSION

Definition

High blood pressure is a trait as opposed to a specific disease, and represents a quantitative rather than a qualitative deviation from the norm. Any definition of hypertension is therefore arbitrary.

Systemic blood pressure rises with age, and the incidence of cardiovascular disease (particularly stroke and coronary artery disease) is closely related to average blood pressure at all ages, even when BP readings are within the so-called 'normal range'.

The risks associated with a given blood pressure are dependent upon the combination of risk factors in the specific individual. These include age, gender (males > females), ethnic origin (blacks > whites), diet, smoking, family history, blood cholesterol, diabetes mellitus and pre-existing vascular disease.

During the last 30 years a series of randomised controlled trials have demonstrated that antihypertensive therapy (mostly with thiazide diuretics and/or β-adrenoceptor antagonists) reduces the incidence of stroke and, to a lesser extent, coronary artery disease. These benefits accrue even in groups with diastolic blood pressures as low as 90 mmHg and have been demonstrated in elderly subjects with blood pressure readings of less than 90 mmHg diastolic but more than 160 mmHg systolic. The relative benefit (approximately 30% reduction in risk of stroke) was similar in all patient groups, so the absolute benefit (total number of events prevented) of treatment is greatest in those at highest risk. For example, extrapolating from the Medical Research Council (MRC) Mild Hypertension Trial (1985), one would have to treat 566 young patients with bendrofluazide for 1 year to prevent 1 stroke (the equivalent figure for propranolol was 1423 patient years); whereas in the MRC trial of antihypertensive treatment in the elderly (1992), 1 stroke was prevented for every 286 patients treated for 1 year.

In the light of these observations a useful and practical definition of hypertension is *the level of blood pressure at which the benefits of treatment outweigh its costs and hazards.*

APPROACH TO NEWLY DIAGNOSED HYPERTENSION

Hypertension occasionally causes headache but, provided there are no complications, most patients remain asymptomatic. Accordingly, the diagnosis is usually made at routine examination or when a complication arises. A blood pressure check is advisable every 5 years in adults.

The objectives of the initial evaluation of a patient with high blood pressure readings are:

- to obtain accurate and representative measurements of blood pressure
- to identify any underlying cause (secondary hypertension)
- to recognise other risk factors for the development of cardiovascular disease
- to detect any complications (target organ damage) that are already present.

These goals can usually be attained by a careful history, clinical examination and some simple investigations.

History

The family history, lifestyle (exercise, diet, smoking habit) and other risk factors should be recorded. A careful history will also identify those patients with drug- or alcohol-induced hypertension and may elicit symptoms of other causes of secondary hypertension such as paroxysmal headache, palpitation and sweating in phaeochromocytoma. However, in most hypertensive patients symptoms are due to complications such as coronary artery disease (e.g. angina, breathlessness) or cerebrovascular disease.

Examination

Radio-femoral delay (coarctation of the aorta), enlarged kidneys (polycystic kidney disease), abdominal bruits (renal artery stenosis) and the characteristic facies and habitus of Cushing's syndrome are all examples of physical signs that may help to identify one of the causes of secondary hypertension (see below). Examination may also reveal features of important risk factors such as central obesity and hyperlipidaemia (tendon xanthomas etc.). Nevertheless, the majority of abnormal signs are due to the complications of hypertension.

Non-specific findings may include left ventricular hypertrophy (apical heave), accentuation of the aortic component of the second heart sound, and possibly a fourth heart sound. The optic fundi are often abnormal (see below) and there may be evidence of generalised atheroma or specific complications such as aortic aneurysm or peripheral vascular disease.

Investigations

Investigations are required to quantify risk, diagnose secondary hypertension and identify complications; some are advisable in all patients, while others are appropriate only in selected patients (see the information boxes).

Ambulatory blood pressure monitoring and echocardiography (to detect subtle degrees of left ventricular hypertrophy) are potentially useful investigations in patients with borderline hypertension when the need for antihypertensive treatment is in doubt.

Measurement of BP

A decision to embark upon antihypertensive therapy effectively commits the patient to life-long treatment, so it is vital that the BP readings on which this decision is based are as accurate as possible.

Measurements should be made, to the nearest 2 mmHg, in the sitting position with the arm supported, and repeated after 5 minutes' rest if the first recording is high. Remember that all modern guidelines on treatment are based on recordings of Korotkoff phase V diastolic BP (disappearance of sounds) not phase IV (muffling of sounds). To avoid spuriously high recordings in obese subjects, the cuff should contain a bladder that encompasses at least two-thirds of the circumference of the arm. Unless there is severe hypertension (readings of more than 200/120 mmHg), measurements should be repeated once a month for 3 months and treatment started only if the initial hypertension is sustained.

Exercise, anxiety, discomfort and unfamiliar surroundings can all lead to a transient rise in BP. Sphygmomanometry, particularly when performed by a doctor, can cause an unrepresentative surge in BP which has been termed '*white coat hypertension*', and as many as 20% of patients with apparent hypertension in the clinic may have a 'normal BP' when it is recorded by automated devices used in their own home. The risk of cardiovascular disease in these patients is less than that observed in patients with sustained hypertension but greater than that seen in normotensive subjects. Some studies suggest that home or ambulatory BP measurements can provide a better assessment of risk than casual clinic BP recordings, but these remain controversial and require confirmation.

HYPERTENSION: INVESTIGATION OF ALL PATIENTS

- Urinalysis for blood, protein and glucose
- Plasma urea and electrolytes
  N.B. Hypokalaemic alkalosis may indicate primary aldosteronism but is usually due to diuretic therapy
- Plasma creatinine
- Plasma cholesterol
- ECG: to detect left ventricular hypertrophy or evidence of coronary artery disease

HYPERTENSION: INVESTIGATION OF SELECTED PATIENTS

- Chest radiograph: to detect cardiomegaly, heart failure, coarctation of the aorta
- Ambulatory BP recording: to assess borderline or 'white coat' hypertension
- Echocardiogram: to detect or quantify left ventricular hypertrophy
- Renal ultrasound: to detect possible renal disease
- Renal angiography: to detect or confirm presence of renal artery stenosis
- Urinary catecholamines: to detect possible phaeochromocytoma
- Urinary cortisol and dexamethasone suppression test: to detect possible Cushing's syndrome
- Plasma renin activity and aldosterone: to detect possible primary aldosteronism

Secondary hypertension

In more than 95% of cases a specific underlying cause of hypertension cannot be found. Such patients are said to have *essential hypertension.*

The pathogenesis of essential hypertension is not clearly understood. Different investigators have proposed the kidney, the peripheral resistance vessels and the sympathetic nervous system as the seat of the primary abnormality. In reality the problem is probably multifactorial. Hypertension is more common in some ethnic groups, particularly American Blacks and Japanese, and approximately 40–60% is explained by genetic factors. Important environmental factors include a high salt intake, heavy consumption of alcohol, obesity and impaired intrauterine growth.

In about 5% of unselected cases, hypertension can be shown to be a consequence of a specific disease or abnormality leading to sodium retention and/or peripheral vasoconstriction *(secondary hypertension)*. The causes are listed in the information box.

CAUSES OF SECONDARY HYPERTENSION
Alcohol
Pregnancy (pre-eclampsia)
Renal disease (see Ch. 6)
• Renal vascular disease • Parenchymal renal disease, particularly glomerulonephritis • Polycystic kidney disease
Endocrine disease (see Ch. 8)
• Phaeochromocytoma • Cushing's syndrome • Primary hyperaldosteronism (Conn's syndrome) • Hyperparathyroidism • Acromegaly • Primary hypothyroidism • Thyrotoxicosis • Congenital adrenal hyperplasia due to 11-β-hydroxylase, or 17-hydroxylase deficiency • Liddle's syndrome • 11-β-hydroxysteroid dehydrogenase deficiency
Drugs
• e.g. Oral contraceptives containing oestrogens, anabolic steroids, corticosteroids, non-steroidal anti-inflammatory drugs, carbenoxolone, sympathomimetic agents
Coarctation of the aorta (see p. 292)

Secondary hypertension is more likely, and investigation therefore particularly appropriate, in:

- patients with clinical or biochemical features of a specific disorder
- young patients (< 30 years old)
- accelerated hypertension
- refractory hypertension.

Renal artery stenosis (see p. 439)

Fibromuscular dysplasia is a rare cause of renal artery stenosis in young people. In contrast, unilateral or bilateral atheroma of the renal arteries frequently causes or exacerbates hypertension in the elderly, particularly those who are heavy smokers. This form of renovascular disease may present with renal failure, refractory hypertension, flash pulmonary oedema or heart failure. A variety of tests, including renal ultrasound (discrepancy in kidney size) and captopril renography (unilateral renal dysfunction), may be indicative of renal artery disease but the diagnosis can only be definitively established or excluded by arteriography. Many patients, particularly those with renal failure or refractory hypertension, can be treated successfully by percutaneous balloon angioplasty with or without stent insertion; however, in complex cases surgery may be necessary.

Other risk factors

Careful assessment of all risk factors is particularly important in borderline hypertension, because the absolute benefit of antihypertensive treatment will be small and may not therefore justify the hazard and inconvenience in a patient with no other risk factors. The absolute benefit of treatment may be considerable, however, in a patient with multiple risk factors (diabetes, hyperlipidaemia, smoking etc.).

Complications (target organ damage)

The adverse effects of hypertension principally involve the blood vessels, the central nervous system, the retina, the heart and the kidneys and can usually be detected by simple clinical means.

Patients with hypertensive complications or target organ damage are at considerable risk and usually require specific antihypertensive treatment.

Blood vessels

In larger arteries (> 1 mm diameter) the internal elastic lamina is thickened, smooth muscle hypertrophied, and fibrous tissue deposited. The vessels dilate and become tortuous and their walls become less compliant. In smaller arteries (< 1 mm) hyaline arteriosclerosis occurs in the wall, the lumen narrows and aneurysms may develop. Widespread atheroma develops and may lead to coronary and/or cerebrovascular disease, particularly if other risk factors (e.g. smoking, hyperlipidaemia) are present.

These structural changes in the vasculature often perpetuate and aggravate hypertension by increasing peripheral vascular resistance, reducing renal function and inducing renal artery stenosis.

Hypertension is also implicated in the pathogenesis of aortic aneurysm and aortic dissection (see pp. 269–271).

Central nervous system

Stroke is a common complication of hypertension and may

be due to cerebral haemorrhage or cerebral infarction. Carotid atheroma and transient cerebral ischaemic attacks are more common in hypertensive patients. Subarachnoid haemorrhage is also associated with hypertension.

Hypertensive encephalopathy is a rare condition characterised by high blood pressure and neurological symptoms, including transient disturbances of speech or vision, paraesthesiae, disorientation, fits and loss of consciousness. Papilloedema is common. A CT scan of the brain often shows haemorrhage in and around the basal ganglia; however, the neurological deficit is usually reversible if the hypertension is properly controlled.

Retina

The optic fundi reveal a gradation of changes linked to the severity of hypertension; fundoscopy can, therefore, provide an indication of the arteriolar damage occurring elsewhere (see the information box).

HYPERTENSIVE RETINOPATHY	
• Grade 1	Arteriolar thickening, tortuosity and increased reflectiveness ('silver wiring')
• Grade 2	Grade 1 plus constriction of veins at arterial crossings ('arteriovenous nipping')
• Grade 3	Grade 2 plus evidence of retinal ischaemia (flame-shaped or blot haemorrhages and 'cotton wool' exudates)
• Grade 4	Grade 3 plus papilloedema

'Cotton wool' exudates are associated with retinal ischaemia or infarction, and fade in a few weeks (see Fig. 3.20A). 'Hard' exudates (small, white, dense deposits of lipid) and microaneurysms ('dot' haemorrhages) are more characteristic of diabetic retinopathy (see Fig. 7.18, p. 499).

Hypertension is also associated with central retinal vein thrombosis (see Fig. 3.20B).

Heart

The excess cardiac mortality and morbidity associated with hypertension is largely due to a higher incidence of coronary artery disease.

High blood pressure places a pressure load on the heart and may lead to left ventricular hypertrophy with a forceful apex beat and fourth heart sound. ECG or echocardiographic evidence of left ventricular hypertrophy is highly predictive of cardiovascular complications and these tests are therefore particularly useful in risk assessment.

Atrial fibrillation is common and may be due to diastolic dysfunction caused by left ventricular hypertrophy or the effects of coronary artery disease.

Severe hypertension can cause left ventricular failure, in the absence of coronary artery disease, particularly when renal function, and therefore sodium excretion, is impaired due to chronic renal failure or renal artery stenosis.

Kidneys

In addition to being a cause, renal disease may also be a result of hypertensive damage to the renal vessels. Long-standing hypertension may cause proteinuria and progressive renal failure (see p. 430).

'Malignant' or 'accelerated' phase hypertension

This rare condition may complicate hypertension of any aetiology and is characterised by accelerated microvascular damage with necrosis in the walls of small arteries and arterioles ('fibrinoid necrosis') and intravascular thrombosis.

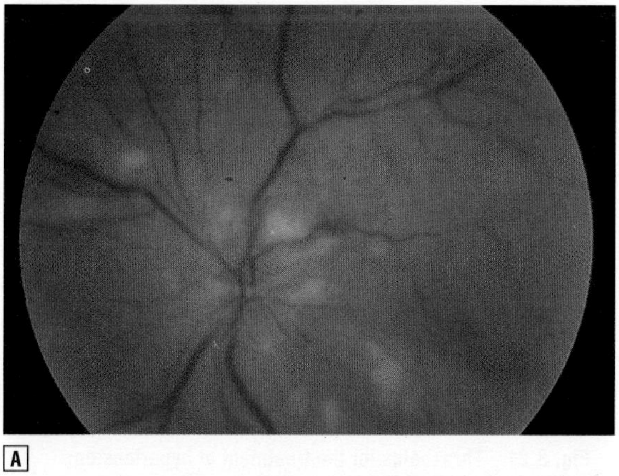
A

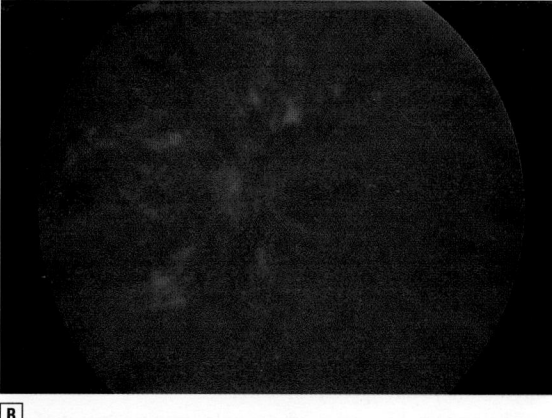
B

Fig. 3.20 **A** **Grade 4 hypertensive retinopathy** showing swollen optic disc, retinal haemorrhages and multiple cotton wool spots (infarcts). **B** **Central retinal vein thrombosis** showing swollen optic disc and widespread fundal haemorrhage, commonly associated with systemic hypertension.

The diagnosis is based on evidence of high blood pressure and rapidly progressive end-organ damage such as retinopathy (grade 3 or 4), renal failure and/or hypertensive encephalopathy (see above). Left ventricular failure may occur, and if this is untreated, death occurs within months.

Management

The object of treating systemic arterial hypertension is to reduce the risk of complications and improve survival. The benefits of treatment have to be weighed against side-effects and inconvenience, so it is important to treat the whole patient, not just the blood pressure. In view of these considerations it is not particularly helpful to set up arbitrary levels of blood pressure at which treatment should be commenced. However, the British Hypertension Society has published useful guidelines (see Fig. 3.21).

In most patients the aim of treatment is to reduce BP to less than 150/90 mmHg. However, this is often not achieved and in the UK the rule of halves has been observed: only half of all hypertensives are diagnosed, only half of these patients are on treatment, and blood pressure is well controlled in only half of those receiving therapy.

General measures

Diet. Reducing alcohol consumption and correcting obesity are both effective antihypertensive measures. Very low sodium diets (10–20 mmol/l) lower blood pressure but are unpalatable. Moderate sodium restriction (70–80 mmol/l) is helpful and can be accomplished by not adding salt to food and avoiding foods with a very high sodium content.

Risk factor modification. The effects of cigarette smoking and hypertension on cardiovascular morbidity are more than additive, and smoking should be strongly discouraged. Energetic treatment of hyperlipidaemia is also an effective means of risk reduction.

Exercise and relaxation. Regular exercise improves physical fitness and can lower blood pressure. Formal relaxation classes, meditation and biofeedback have all been shown to reduce blood pressure in small groups of patients; their efficacy is usually proportional to the enthusiasm of the teacher and the commitment of the participant. However, it is unusual for such treatment to replace the need for antihypertensive drug therapy.

Antihypertensive drug therapy

Many patients can be satisfactorily treated with a single antihypertensive drug, the choice of which will be determined by safety, convenience and freedom from side-effects. The remainder will require a combination of two, three or more antihypertensive agents.

The principal agents used in single-drug treatment of hypertension are thiazide diuretics, β-adrenoceptor antagonists and ACE inhibitors; calcium antagonists and some vasodilators are also effective.

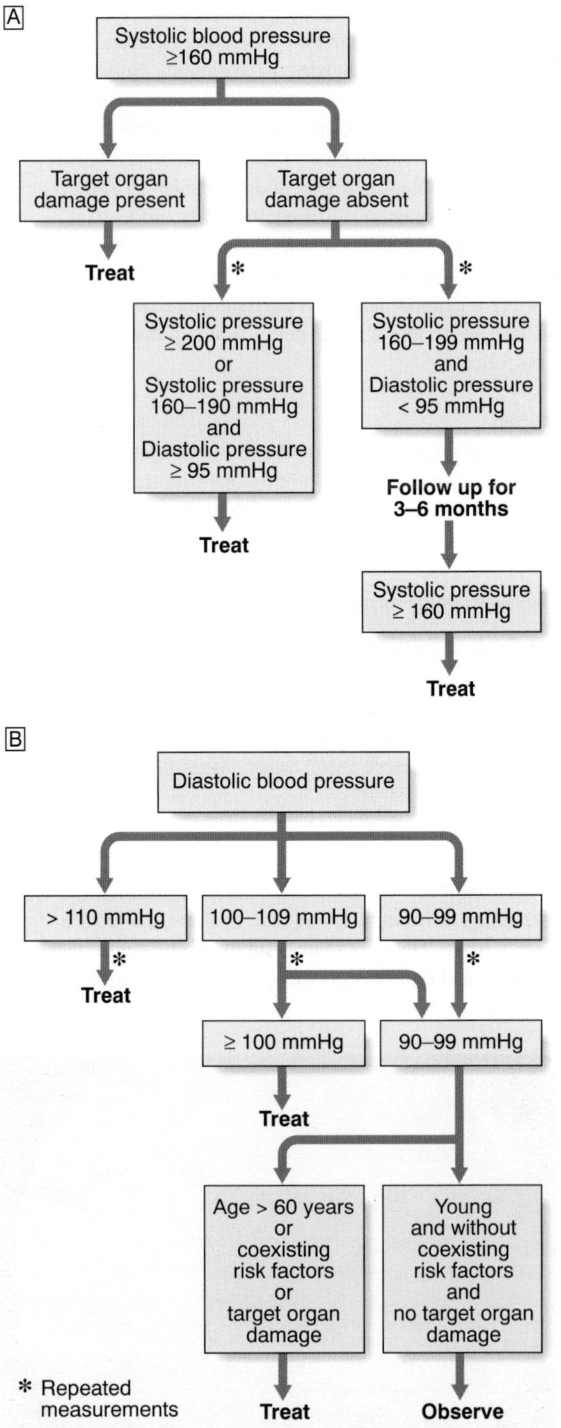

Fig. 3.21 Thresholds for the treatment of hypertension: British Hypertension Society guidelines. A Systolic. B Diastolic.

Drug therapy should be tailored to the specific needs of the individual patient, particularly if there are complicating medical conditions (e.g. asthma, vascular disease, diabetes). Many physicians start treatment with a β-adrenoceptor antagonist or a thiazide diuretic, depending on the likely side-effects and the presence of any relevant additional pathology. For example, β-adrenoceptor antagonists commonly cause cold extremities, and thiazide diuretics may cause impotence. On the other hand, a β-adrenoceptor antagonist is likely to benefit a patient with angina, whereas a diuretic or ACE inhibitor may be more appropriate if there is evidence of heart failure.

Thiazide and other diuretics. These diuretics and their adverse effects are discussed on page 401. The mechanism of their hypotensive action is incompletely understood, and it may take up to a month for the maximum effect to be observed. Thiazide diuretics may cause hyperuricaemia (precipitating gout) and glucose intolerance, but seldom cause postural hypotension.

A daily dose of 2.5 mg bendrofluazide or 0.5 mg cyclopenthiazide is appropriate. More potent loop-acting diuretics, such as frusemide (40 mg daily) or bumetanide (1 mg daily), have few advantages over thiazides in the treatment of hypertension unless there is substantial renal impairment or they are used in conjunction with an ACE inhibitor.

β-adrenoceptor antagonists. A large number of β-adrenoceptor antagonists ('β-blockers') are available and these differ in several important respects. Those with a short half-life are mostly available in slow-release, once-daily formulations. Metoprolol (100–200 mg daily), atenolol (50–100 mg daily) and bisoprolol (5–10 mg daily) are cardioselective and therefore preferentially block the cardiac β_1-adrenoceptors, as opposed to the β_2-adrenoceptors which mediate vasodilatation and bronchodilatation. Pindolol (15–30 mg daily) and oxprenolol (160–320 mg daily) have partial agonist (intrinsic sympathomimetic) activity and therefore tend to cause less bradycardia. Propranolol is subject to extensive first-pass metabolism, which means that a large and variable proportion of the drug is destroyed in its first passage through the liver. The dose of propranolol must, therefore, be carefully titrated according to the patient's individual needs. Propranolol is lipid-soluble and crosses the blood-brain barrier; this may explain why it commonly causes CNS side-effects such as nightmares, drowsiness and depression. In contrast, atenolol and bisoprolol are water-soluble and largely excreted unchanged through the kidneys; CNS side-effects are therefore less common. 'β-blockers' may aggravate asthma, heart failure and peripheral vascular disease, and may cause fatigue and muscle discomfort. The metabolic side-effects of β-blocking drugs include a tendency to increase plasma concentrations of cholesterol; they are, nevertheless, widely used and are especially useful in the presence of angina.

Labetalol (200 mg–2.4 g daily in divided doses) is a combined α- and β-adrenoceptor antagonist which is sometimes more effective than pure β-blockers and can be used as an infusion in malignant phase hypertension.

Angiotensin-converting enzyme (ACE) inhibitors (see p. 215). These drugs inhibit the conversion of angiotensin I to angiotensin II and have been a major advance in the treatment of moderate to severe hypertension. They have few side-effects and compliance tends to be good. They should be used with particular care in patients with impaired renal function or renal artery stenosis because they can reduce the filtration pressure in the glomeruli and precipitate renal failure. As in the treatment of cardiac failure, it is best to start with a small dose (e.g. captopril 6.25 mg daily) and build up to an effective maintenance dose (e.g. captopril 25–75 mg twice daily, enalapril 20 mg daily or lisinopril 10–20 mg daily). Side-effects include first-dose hypotension, cough, rash, proteinuria, hyperkalaemia, renal dysfunction and dysgeusia (an unpleasant metallic taste). *Electrolytes and creatinine should be checked before and 7–10 days after commencing therapy.*

Angiotensin II receptor antagonists (see p. 215). These drugs (e.g. losartan 50–100 mg daily, valsartan 40–160 mg daily) block the AT I angiotensin II receptor and have similar effects to ACE inhibitors; however, they do not influence bradykinin metabolism and do not therefore cause cough.

Calcium antagonists. Diltiazem (60–120 mg 8-hourly or 200–300 mg, slow-release, daily), amlodipine (5–10 mg daily) or nifedipine (30–90 mg daily) are effective and usually well-tolerated antihypertensive drugs. They are particularly useful when hypertension coexists with angina. Side-effects include flushing, palpitations, fluid retention and constipation. Diltiazem and verapamil may cause bradycardia.

Other drugs. A variety of vasodilators are used to treat hypertension. These include the α_1-adrenoceptor antagonists, such as prazosin (0.5–20 mg daily in divided doses), indoramin (25–100 mg twice daily) and doxazosin (1–4 mg daily), and drugs that act directly on vascular smooth muscle, such as hydralazine (25–100 mg 12-hourly) and minoxidil (10–50 mg daily). Side-effects include first-dose and postural hypotension, headache, tachycardia and fluid retention. Minoxidil also causes increased facial hair and is therefore unsuitable for female patients.

Centrally acting drugs, such as methyldopa (initial dose 250 mg 8-hourly) and clonidine (0.05–0.1 mg 8-hourly), are effective antihypertensive drugs but cause fatigue and are usually poorly tolerated.

Drug combinations. Some drugs have complementary actions (see the information box); for example, thiazides increase renin production while β-adrenoceptor antagonists depress it. A number of combination tablets have been marketed, but the proportion of the two drugs is not necessarily optimal for every patient.

LOGICAL ANTIHYPERTENSIVE DRUG COMBINATIONS		
• Diuretic	plus	β-adrenoceptor antagonist ACE inhibitor
• β-adrenoceptor antagonist	plus	Diuretic Calcium antagonist α-blocker
• ACE inhibitor	plus	Diuretic Calcium antagonist

The emergency treatment of accelerated phase or malignant hypertension

In accelerated phase hypertension it is unwise to lower blood pressure too quickly because this may compromise tissue perfusion (due to altered autoregulation) and can cause cerebral damage, including occipital blindness, and precipitate coronary or renal insufficiency. Even in the presence of cardiac failure or hypertensive encephalopathy a controlled reduction, to a level of about 150/90, over a period of 24–36 hours is ideal.

In most patients it is possible to avoid parenteral therapy and bring blood pressure under control with bed rest and oral drug therapy. Intravenous or intramuscular labetalol (2 mg/min to a maximum of 200 mg), intravenous nitroglycerin (0.6–1.2 mg/hr), intramuscular hydralazine (5 or 10 mg aliquots repeated at half-hourly intervals), and intravenous sodium nitroprusside (0.3–1.0 mg/kg body weight per minute) are all effective remedies but require careful supervision, preferably in an intensive care unit.

Refractory hypertension

The common causes of treatment failure in hypertension are non-compliance with drug therapy, inadequate therapy, and failure to recognise an underlying cause such as renal artery stenosis or phaeochromocytoma; of these, the first is by far the most prevalent. There is no easy solution to compliance problems, but simple treatment regimens, attempts to improve rapport with the patient, and careful supervision may all help.

ABNORMAL HEART SOUNDS AND MURMURS

The first clinical manifestation of heart disease may be the discovery of an abnormal sound on auscultation. Such a finding may be incidental—for example, during a routine childhood examination—or may be prompted by symptoms of heart disease.

Is the sound of cardiac origin?

Additional heart sounds and murmurs demonstrate a consistent relationship to a specific part of the cardiac cycle, whereas extra-cardiac sounds (e.g. pleural rub or venous

Table 3.2 Normal and abnormal heart sounds

Sound	Timing	Characteristics	Mechanisms	Variable features
First heart sound (S1)	Onset of systole	Usually single or narrowly split	Closure of mitral and tricuspid valves	Loud in hyperdynamic circulation (anaemia, pregnancy, thyrotoxicosis) or mitral stenosis Soft in heart failure or mitral regurgitation
Second heart sound (S2)	End of systole	Split on inspiration. Single on expiration	Closure of aortic and pulmonary valves. P2 delayed in inspiration	Fixed splitting with atrial septal defect. Wide but variable splitting with delayed right heart emptying (right bundle branch block or pulmonary stenosis) Reversed splitting due to delayed left heart emptying (e.g. left bundle branch block)
Third heart sound (S3)	Early in diastole	Low pitch, often heard as 'gallop'	From ventricular wall due to abrupt cessation of rapid filling	Common in young people, pregnancy or hyperdynamic states but pathological in other conditions
Fourth heart sound (S4)	End of diastole, just before S1	Low pitch Always a pathological finding	Ventricular origin (stiff ventricle and augmented atrial contraction) related to atrial filling	Absent in atrial fibrillation
Systolic clicks	Early or mid-systole	Brief, high-intensity sound	Valvular stenosis (aortic or pulmonary) Floppy mitral valve Prosthetic heart sounds from opening and closing of normally functioning mechanical valves	Click may be lost when stenotic valve becomes thickened or calcified Prosthetic clicks lost when valve obstructed by thrombus or vegetations
Opening snap (OS)	Early in diastole	High pitch, brief duration	Opening of stenosed leaflets of mitral valve	Moves closer to S2 as mitral stenosis becomes more severe. May be absent in calcified valve

hum) do not. Pericardial friction produces a characteristic scratching or crunching noise which often has two components corresponding to atrial and ventricular systole and may disappear or change with altered posture or respiration.

Is the sound pathological? (See Table 3.2)

Pathological sounds and murmurs are the product of accelerated or turbulent blood flow across structurally abnormal valves or congenital defects, or rapid ventricular filling due to abnormal loading conditions.

Some added sounds are physiological but may also occur in pathological conditions; for example, a third sound is common in young people and in pregnancy but is also a feature of heart failure. Similarly, a systolic murmur due to turbulence across the right ventricular outflow tract may occur in hyperdynamic states (e.g. anaemia, pregnancy) but may also be due to pulmonary stenosis or an intracardiac shunt (e.g. atrial septal defect) leading to volume overload of the right ventricle.

FEATURES OF A BENIGN OR INNOCENT HEART MURMUR

- Soft
- Mid-systolic
- Heard at left sternal edge
- No radiation
- No other cardiac abnormalities

AUSCULTATORY FEATURES OF HEART MURMURS

Systolic or diastolic? (timing)

- Time the murmur using heart sounds, carotid pulse and the apex beat

Duration?

- Does the murmur extend throughout systole or diastole or is it confined to a shorter part of the cardiac cycle?

How loud is it? (intensity)

- Grade 1 very soft (only audible in ideal conditions)
- Grade 2 soft
- Grade 3 moderate
- Grade 4 loud with associated thrill
- Grade 5 very loud
- Grade 6 heard without stethoscope

N.B. Diastolic murmurs are sometimes graded 1–4.

Where is it heard best? (location)

- Listen over the apex and base of the heart including the aortic and pulmonary areas

Where does it radiate?

- Evaluate radiation to the neck, axilla or back

What does it sound like? (pitch and quality)

- Pitch is determined by flow (high pitch indicates high-velocity flow)
- Is the intensity constant or variable?

Benign (physiological) murmurs (see the information box) do not occur in diastole, and systolic murmurs that radiate or are associated with a thrill are almost always pathological. An echocardiogram is often necessary to confirm the nature of an abnormal heart sound or murmur.

What are the important auscultatory characteristics of a heart murmur? (see the information box)

Whether a murmur is systolic or diastolic is best assessed by timing it with the apex beat or carotid pulse (see Figs 3.22 and 3.23). Changes in a murmur's intensity during the cardiac cycle are also an important clue to its origin. The duration, location, radiation and intensity of the murmur are all useful discriminants (see Table 3.3). Radiation of a murmur is determined by the direction of turbulent blood flow and is only detectable when there is a high-velocity jet—e.g. in mitral regurgitation (radiation from apex to axilla) or aortic stenosis (radiation from base to neck). Similarly, the pitch and quality of the sound can help to distinguish the murmur—e.g. the 'blowing' murmur of mitral regurgitation or the 'rasping' murmur of aortic stenosis.

Systolic murmurs associated with ventricular outflow tract obstruction occur in mid-systole and have a crescendo-

Table 3.3 Murmurs and their location

Type of murmur	Location
SYSTOLIC MURMURS	
Mid-systolic murmurs (crescendo-decrescendo)	
Aortic stenosis Pulmonary stenosis Hypertrophic cardiomyopathy Fallot's tetralogy Atrial septal defect (pulmonary flow)	Aortic area (radiating towards neck) and/or left sternal edge
Pansystolic murmurs	
Mitral regurgitation	Apex (radiating towards axilla)
Tricuspid regurgitation	Left sternal edge (low-pitched)
Ventricular septal defect	Left sternal edge (harsh, rasping)
Late-systolic murmurs	
Mitral valve prolapse Hypertrophic cardiomyopathy	Apex
DIASTOLIC MURMURS	
Early-diastolic murmurs	
Aortic regurgitation Pulmonary regurgitation, Graham Steell (pulmonary regurgitation due to pulmonary hypertension and mitral stenosis)	Left sternal edge
Mid-diastolic murmurs	
Mitral stenosis	Apex
Austin Flint (aortic regurgitation impairing mitral diastolic flow) Tricuspid stenosis	Left sternal edge
CONTINUOUS MURMURS	
Persistent ductus arteriosus	Upper left sternal edge
Venous hum (positional) Arteriovenous shunts	Anterior chest wall/elsewhere

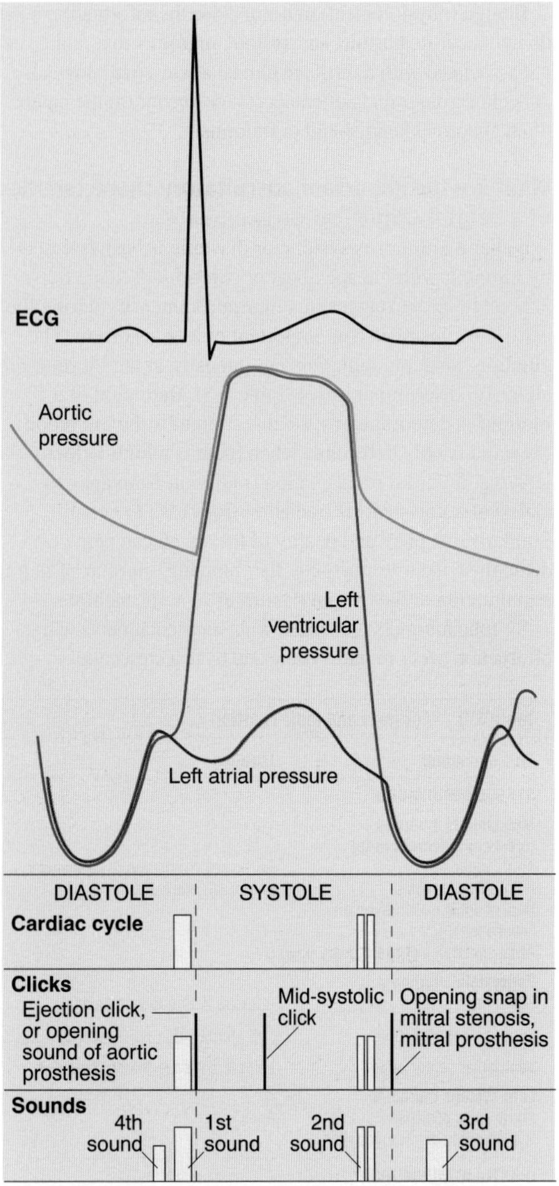

Fig. 3.22 The relationship of the cardiac cycle to the electrocardiogram, the left ventricular pressure wave and the position of heart sounds.

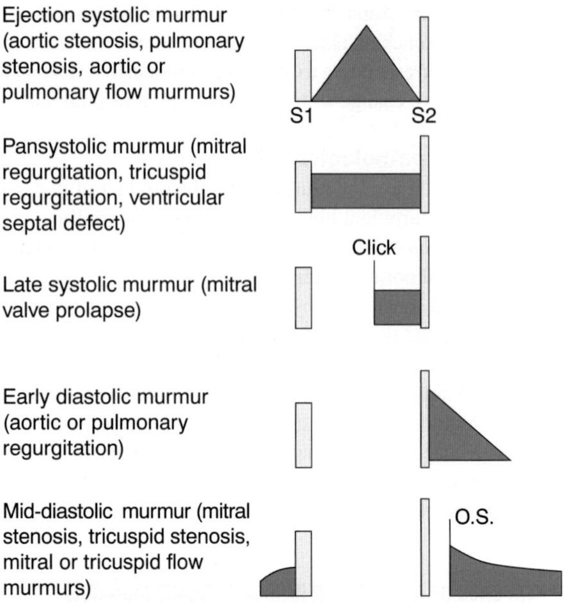

Fig. 3.23 The timing and pattern of cardiac murmurs.
(O.S. = opening snap)

decrescendo pattern, in keeping with the velocity of blood flow. Pansystolic murmurs maintain a constant intensity and extend from the first heart sound throughout systole (up to and beyond the second heart sound) and occur when blood leaks from a ventricle into a low-pressure chamber at an even or constant velocity (mitral regurgitation, tricuspid regurgitation, ventricular septal defect). Late-systolic murmurs also reflect the velocity of blood flow (e.g. dynamic obstruction of hypertrophic cardiomyopathy which occurs late in systole).

Mid-diastolic murmurs are due to accelerated or turbulent flow across the mitral or tricuspid valves. Early diastolic murmurs are due to regurgitation across the aortic or pulmonary valves and have a soft blowing quality with a decrescendo pattern.

Continuous murmurs result from a combination of systolic and diastolic flow (as in persistent ductus arteriosus). They should be distinguished from the sounds produced by flow in arterial shunts, a venous hum (high rates of venous flow in children) and extra-cardiac noises such as pericardial friction rub.

The characteristics of specific valve defects and congenital anomalies are described in the relevant sections later in the chapter.

PALPITATION

Palpitation is the term used to describe an abnormal subjective awareness of the heart beat. The symptom may be due to an abnormal rhythm, extrasystoles, a particularly forceful heart beat (e.g. increased stroke volume in aortic regurgitation) or anxiety. A provisional diagnosis can usually be made on the basis of a careful and thorough history (see Fig. 3.24). However, in order to make a

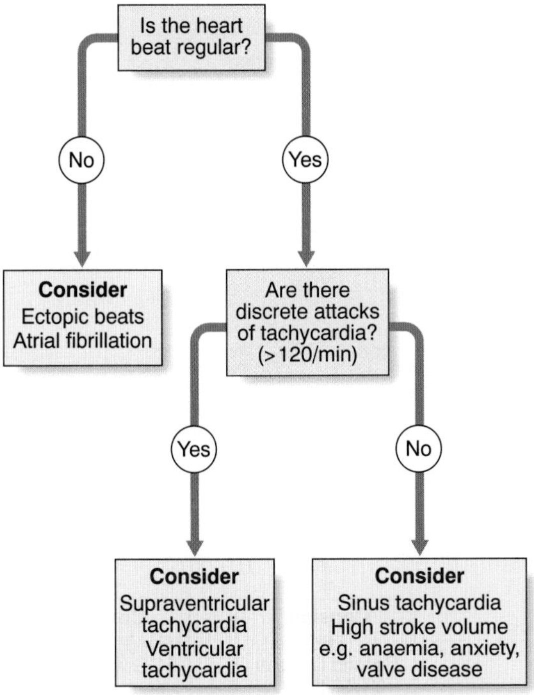

Fig. 3.24 A simple approach to the diagnosis of palpitation.

definitive diagnosis it may be necessary to obtain an ECG recording during an attack of typical palpitation by means of ambulatory ECG monitoring (see p. 200).

Accurate assessment of palpitation requires an exact description of the sensation (see the information box) and it is often helpful to ask patients to explain their symptoms by tapping out the heart beat on their chest or a table top.

THE EVALUATION OF PALPITATION: IMPORTANT QUESTIONS

• Is the palpitation continuous or intermittent?
• Is the heart beat regular or irregular?
• What is the approximate heart rate?
• Do symptoms occur in discrete attacks?
  Is the onset abrupt?
  How do attacks terminate?
• Are there any associated symptoms?
  e.g. Chest pain
  Lightheadedness
  Polyuria (a feature of supraventricular tachycardia—see p. 230)
• Are there any precipitating factors?
  e.g. Exercise
  Alcohol
• Is there clinical evidence of structural heart disease?
  e.g. Coronary artery disease
  Valvular heart disease

Extrasystoles (ectopic beats) are often perceived as a missed or a more forceful beat (see p. 232).

Palpitation is a very common and often frightening symptom. However, if there is no evidence of underlying structural heart disease the outlook is good, even if the patient's symptoms are due to an arrhythmia. Careful assessment and explanation will therefore often help to allay a patient's fears.

The diagnosis and management of individual arrhythmias are considered in detail on page 227.

SYNCOPE

The common causes of syncope, drop attacks or sudden loss of consciousness are listed in the information box. These conditions may also be responsible for recurrent episodes of dizziness, lightheadedness or presyncope.

Cardiac syncope is caused by a sudden drop in cardiac output and cerebral perfusion due to an arrhythmia or a mechanical problem. Inappropriate vasodilatation also causes symptoms by reducing cerebral perfusion.

Vasovagal syncope

This is mediated by the Bezold–Jarisch reflex and is usually triggered by a reduction in venous return due to prolonged standing, excessive heat or a large meal. Concomitant sympathetic activation then leads to vigorous contraction of the relatively underfilled ventricles and engages the reflex by stimulating ventricular

COMMON CAUSES OF SYNCOPE
Cardiac

• Arrhythmia
  Bradycardia (especially sinus node disease and atrioventricular block)
  Tachycardia (especially ventricular tachycardia)
• Mechanical (often effort-related)
  e.g. Ischaemic LV dysfunction
  Aortic stenosis
  Hypertrophic obstructive cardiomyopathy

Inappropriate vasodilatation
• Simple faint • Malignant vasovagal syndrome • Carotid sinus hypersensitivity • Micturition syncope • Postural (orthostatic) hypotension
Neurogenic
• Epilepsy • Transient ischaemic attacks
Metabolic
• Hypoglycaemia

mechanoreceptors. This produces parasympathetic (vagal) activation and sympathetic withdrawal causing bradycardia, vasodilatation or both. Head-up tilt testing can be used to confirm the diagnosis by inducing a typical attack. Treatment is often unnecessary but in severe cases, β-adrenoceptor antagonists, disopyramide and a dual-chamber pacemaker are all partially effective remedies.

Differential diagnosis

Whenever possible, an accurate description of the attack should be obtained from the patient and a witness. Particular attention should be paid to the recovery phase and possible precipitants or triggers such as medication, exercise and alcohol. In cardiac syncope, recovery is usually rapid, whereas patients with vasovagal syncope often feel nauseated and unwell for several minutes, and patients with neurogenic syncope usually take more than 5 minutes to recover. Table 3.4 lists some useful discriminants which can help to identify the likely mechanism of syncope.

A careful history and clinical examination will often reveal the cause of recurrent syncope without recourse to complex and expensive investigations. In the remaining cases the pattern and description of the patient's symptoms should indicate the probable mechanism of syncope and will therefore determine subsequent investigations (see Fig. 3.25). The discovery of common pathology (e.g. paroxysmal atrial fibrillation or cervical spondylosis in elderly subjects) does not necessarily explain the patient's complaint, and in many cases a definitive diagnosis can only be made if it is possible to provoke typical symptoms or demonstrate a close temporal relationship between the patient's symptoms and an arrhythmia.

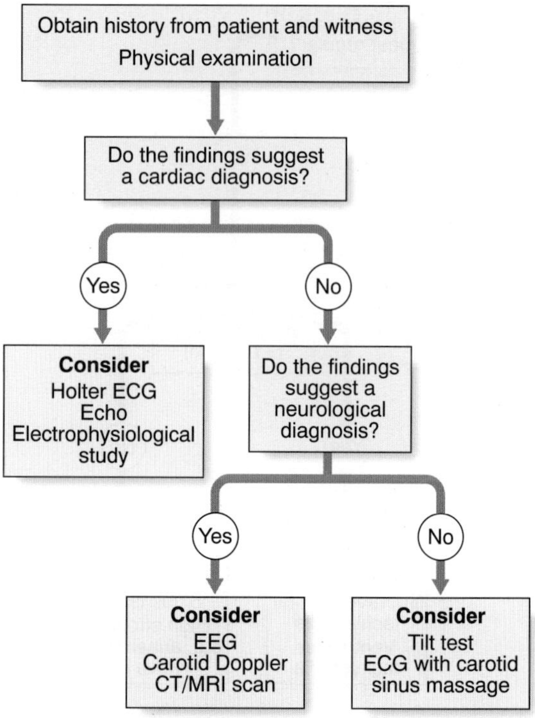

Fig. 3.25 A simple guide to the investigation and diagnosis of recurrent presyncope and syncope.

Table 3.4 Typical features of cardiac and neurogenic syncope

	Cardiac syncope	Neurogenic syncope
Premonitory symptoms	Lightheadedness Palpitation Chest pain Breathlessness	Headache Confusion Hyperexcitability Olfactory hallucinations 'Aura'
Unconscious period	Extreme 'death-like' pallor	Prolonged (> 1 min) unconsciousness Motor seizure activity* Tongue-biting Urinary incontinence
Recovery	Rapid recovery (< 1 min) Flushing	Prolonged confusion (> 5 min) Headache Focal neurological signs

* **N.B.** Cardiac syncope can also cause convulsions by inducing cerebral anoxia.

FURTHER INFORMATION ON MAJOR MANIFESTATIONS OF HEART DISEASE

Dargie H J, McMurray J J V 1994 Diagnosis and management of heart failure. British Medical Journal 308: 321–328
Management guidelines in essential hypertension: report of the second working party of the British Hypertension Society 1993 British Medical Journal 306: 983–987
O'Brien E T, Beevers D G, Marshall H J 1995 ABC of hypertension, 3rd edn. British Medical Journal Publishing Group, London
Task force of the European Society of Cardiology 1995 Guidelines on the diagnosis of heart failure. European Heart Journal 16: 741–751

DISORDERS OF HEART RATE, RHYTHM AND CONDUCTION

The heart beat is normally initiated by an electrical discharge from the sinoatrial (sinus) node. The atria and ventricles then depolarise sequentially as electricity passes through the specialised conducting tissue (see Fig. 3.26). The sinus node acts as a pacemaker and has its own intrinsic rate that is regulated by the autonomic nervous system; vagal activity slows the heart rate, and sympathetic activity accelerates it.

If the sinus rate becomes unduly slow, a lower centre may assume the role of pacemaker. This is known as an escape rhythm and may arise in the AV node (nodal rhythm) or the ventricles (idioventricular rhythm).

An arrhythmia is a disturbance in the electrical activity of the heart and may be paroxysmal or continuous. Bradycardia is defined as a rate of < 60/min, whereas tachycardia is the term used when the rate exceeds 100/min.

There are two underlying mechanisms for tachycardia:

- increased automaticity—when the tachycardia is sustained by repeated spontaneous depolarisation of an ectopic focus or single cell
- re-entry—when the tachycardia is initiated by an ectopic beat but sustained by a closed loop or re-entry circuit (see Fig. 3.27). Most tachyarrhythmias are due to re-entry.

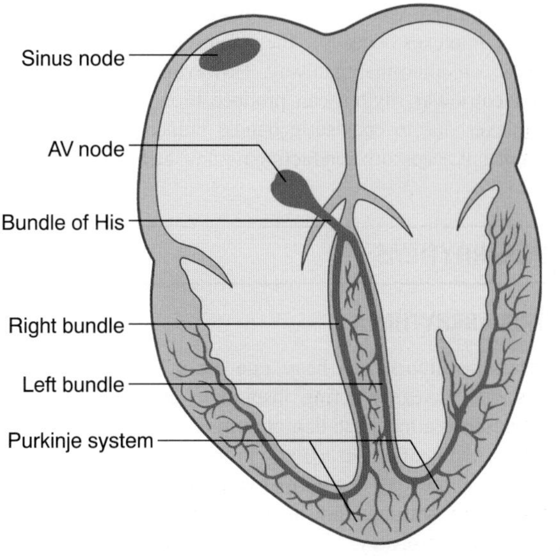

Fig. 3.26 The specialised conducting tissue of the heart.

An arrhythmia may be supraventricular (sinus, atrial or junctional) or ventricular. Supraventricular rhythms usually produce narrow QRS complexes because the ventricles are depolarised normally through the AV node and bundle of

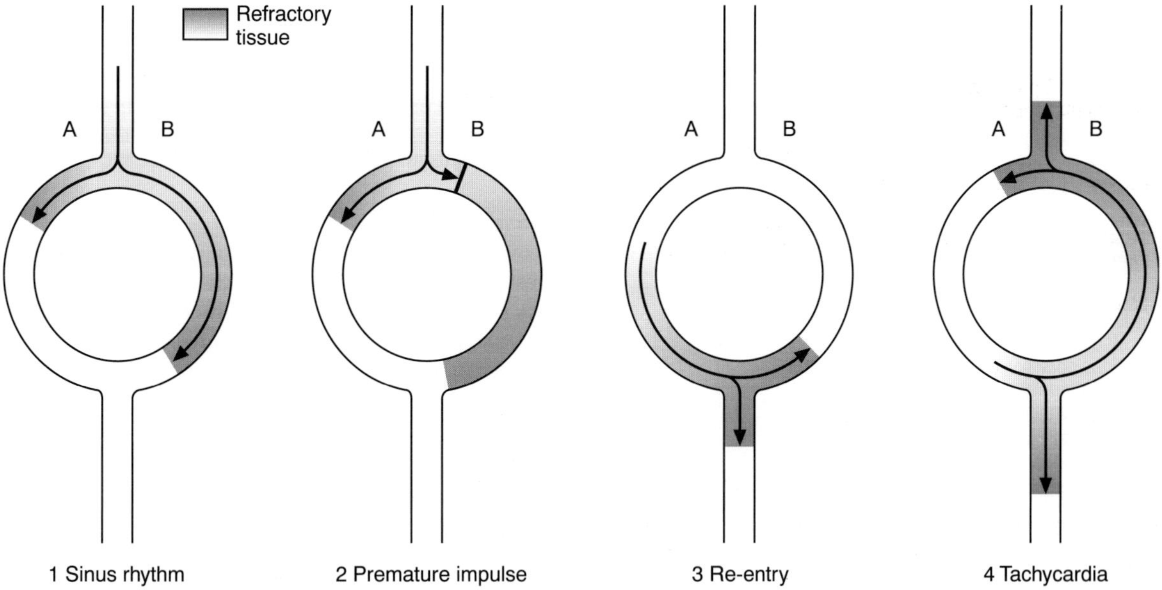

Fig. 3.27 The mechanism of re-entry. Re-entry can occur when there are two alternative pathways with different conducting properties (e.g. the AV node and an accessory pathway, or an area of normal tissue and an area of ischaemic tissue). In this example, pathway A conducts slowly and recovers quickly while pathway B conducts rapidly and recovers slowly. **(1)** In sinus rhythm each impulse passes down both pathways before entering a common distal pathway. **(2)** As the pathways recover at different rates a premature impulse may find pathway A open and B closed. **(3)** Pathway B may recover while the premature impulse travels selectively down pathway A. The impulse may then travel retrogradely up pathway B, setting up a closed loop or re-entry circuit. **(4)** This may initiate a tachycardia that will continue until the circuit is interrupted by a change in conduction rates or electrical depolarisation.

His. In contrast, ventricular rhythms produce broad bizarre QRS complexes because the ventricles are activated through an abnormal pathway. However, occasionally a supraventricular rhythm can produce broad or wide QRS complexes due to coexisting bundle branch block, or the presence of accessory conducting tissue (see below).

SINUS RHYTHMS

SINUS ARRHYTHMIA

Phasic alteration of the heart rate during respiration (the sinus rate increases during inspiration and slows during expiration) is a manifestation of normal autonomic nervous activity, and is often particularly pronounced in children. A complete absence of this normal variation in heart rate with breathing or with changes in posture may be a feature of autonomic neuropathy.

SINUS BRADYCARDIA

A sinus rate of less than 60/min may occur in normal people during sleep and is a common finding in athletes. Some pathological causes are listed in the information box. Acute symptomatic sinus bradycardia usually responds to intravenous atropine 0.6 mg.

SINUS TACHYCARDIA

This is defined as a sinus rate of more than 100/min, and is usually due to an increase in sympathetic activity associated with exercise, emotion or pathology (see the information box). The rate seldom exceeds 160/min, except in infants.

SOME PATHOLOGICAL CAUSES OF SINUS BRADYCARDIA AND TACHYCARDIA

Sinus bradycardia

- Myocardial infarction
- Sinus node disease (sick sinus syndrome)
- Hypothermia
- Hypothyroidism
- Cholestatic jaundice
- Raised intracranial pressure
- Drugs, e.g. β-adrenoceptor antagonist, digoxin, verapamil

Sinus tachycardia

- Anxiety
- Fever
- Pregnancy
- Anaemia
- Heart failure
- Thyrotoxicosis
- Phaeochromocytoma
- Drugs, e.g. β-adrenoceptor agonists (bronchodilators)

ATRIAL TACHYARRHYTHMIAS

ATRIAL ECTOPIC BEATS (EXTRASYSTOLES, PREMATURE BEATS)

These usually cause no symptoms but can give the sensation of a missed beat or an abnormally strong beat. The ECG (see Fig. 3.28) shows a premature but otherwise normal QRS complex; if visible, the preceding P wave has a different configuration because the impulse starts at an abnormal site.

ATRIAL TACHYCARDIA

An ectopic atrial tachycardia due to increased automaticity is rare but is sometimes a manifestation of digitalis toxicity. The ECG shows an atrial rate of 140–220/min with abnormal P waves often accompanied by atrioventricular block (e.g. 2:1, 3:1 or variable). Management is similar to that for atrial flutter (see below).

ATRIAL FLUTTER

In this condition a rapid atrial rate of around 300/min is associated with 2:1, 3:1, 4:1 or variable atrioventricular block. The ECG shows characteristic saw-toothed flutter waves (see Fig. 3.29). When there is regular 2:1 AV block it may be difficult to distinguish atrial flutter from supraventricular or sinus tachycardia because alternate flutter waves are buried in the QRS complexes. This should always be suspected when there is a narrow complex tachycardia of 150/min. Carotid sinus pressure or intravenous adenosine may help to establish the diagnosis by temporarily increasing the degree of AV block and revealing the flutter waves (see Fig. 3.30).

Management

Digoxin, β-adrenoceptor antagonists or verapamil can be used to control ventricular rate (see p. 236). However, in many cases it may be preferable to try and restore sinus rhythm by atrial overdrive pacing, DC (direct current) cardioversion or drug therapy. Amiodarone, propafenone or flecainide may be

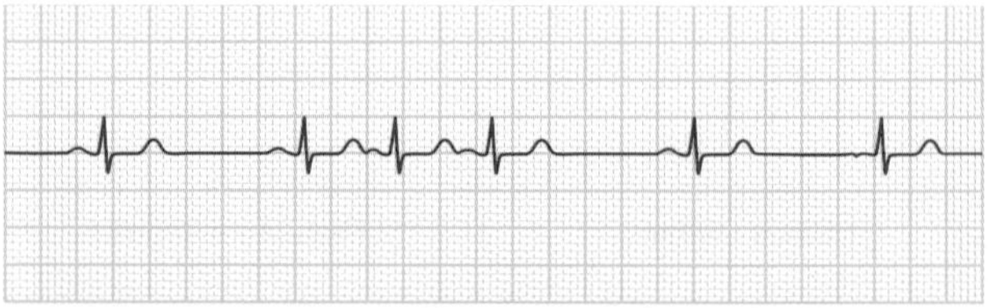

Fig. 3.28 Atrial ectopic beats. The first, second and fifth complexes are normal sinus beats. The third, fourth and sixth complexes are atrial ectopic beats with identical QRS complexes and abnormal (sometimes barely visible) P waves.

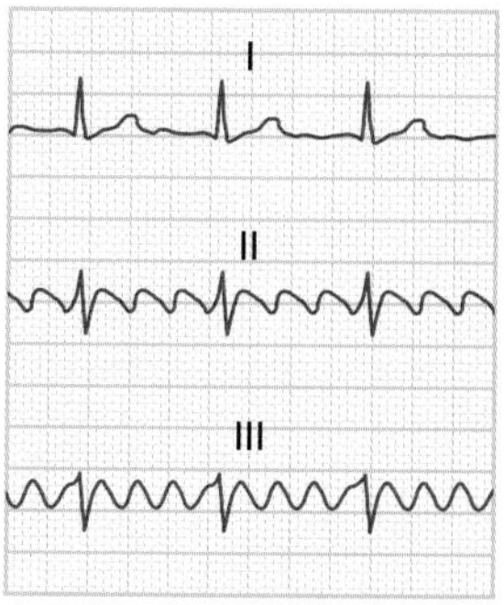

Fig. 3.29 Atrial flutter. Simultaneous recording showing atrial flutter with 3:1 block; flutter waves are only visible in leads II and III.

effective and can also be used to prevent recurrent episodes of atrial flutter (see p. 236). Disopyramide or quinidine can be used in conjunction with digoxin (see p. 236).

ATRIAL FIBRILLATION

In this arrhythmia the atria beat rapidly, chaotically and ineffectively; the ventricles respond at irregular intervals giving the characteristic 'irregularly irregular' pulse. The ECG (see Fig. 3.31) shows normal but irregular QRS complexes; there are no P waves but the baseline may show irregular fibrillation waves.

Atrial fibrillation (AF) is the most common sustained cardiac arrhythmia, with an overall prevalence of 0.5% in the adult population, rising to 10% or more in those over 75 years. Common causes are listed in the information box.

The onset of atrial fibrillation can cause palpitation and may precipitate or aggravate cardiac failure in patients with an abnormal heart, especially those with mitral stenosis or poor left ventricular function. Nevertheless, atrial fibrillation is often asymptomatic, particularly in the elderly.

Ineffective atrial contraction coupled with left atrial dilatation predisposes to stasis and may lead to thrombosis and systemic embolism. The risk of thromboembolism depends on the underlying cause (see below), and increases with the size of the left atrium and the age of the patient.

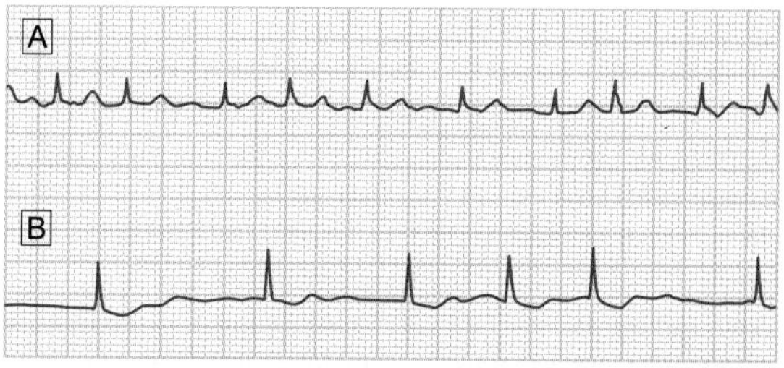

Fig. 3.31 Two examples of atrial fibrillation. The QRS complexes are irregular and there are no P waves. [A] There is usually a fast ventricular rate, often between 120 and 160/min, at the onset of atrial fibrillation. [B] However, in chronic atrial fibrillation the ventricular rate may be much slower due to the effects of medication and AV nodal fatigue.

COMMON CAUSES OF ATRIAL FIBRILLATION

- Coronary artery disease (including acute myocardial infarction)
- Valvular heart disease (especially rheumatic mitral valve disease)
- Idiopathic (lone atrial fibrillation)
- Hypertension
- Thyrotoxicosis
- Sinoatrial disease
- Alcohol
- Cardiomyopathy
- Congenital heart disease
- Pulmonary embolism
- Pericardial disease
- Pneumonia

Management

Digoxin, β-adrenoceptor antagonists ('β-blockers') or verapamil (see pp. 236–240) will reduce the ventricular rate by increasing the degree of AV block, and this alone may produce a striking improvement in overall cardiac function, particularly in patients with mitral stenosis. Treatment of the underlying cause (e.g. thyrotoxicosis, post-operative chest infection) may restore sinus rhythm; if not, elective DC cardioversion (see p. 243) should be considered. In

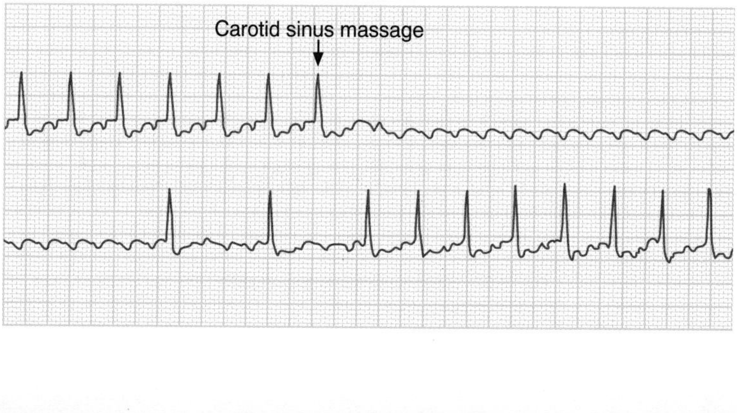

Fig. 3.30 Carotid sinus massage in atrial flutter: continuous trace. In this example, the diagnosis of atrial flutter with 2:1 block was established when carotid sinus massage produced temporary AV block revealing the flutter waves.

patients with paroxysmal atrial fibrillation and those who have undergone successful cardioversion, β-adrenoceptor antagonists (especially sotalol), flecainide, propafenone, disopyramide or amiodarone, but not digoxin, may help to preserve sinus rhythm (see pp. 236–240).

In exceptional cases, refractory atrial tachyarrhythmias can be treated by deliberately inducing complete heart block using surgery or transvenous catheter radiofrequency ablation; a permanent pacemaker must be implanted at the same time.

Atrial fibrillation is associated with a risk of systemic embolism or stroke, which may be reduced by anticoagulation treatment with warfarin. Before embarking on potentially hazardous treatment with warfarin, the patient's risk of embolism should be assessed (see the information box). This risk is so high in patients with mitral valve disease that anticoagulant treatment with warfarin is indicated, unless anticoagulation poses unacceptable risks. Patients who have already had a systemic or cerebral embolism are at high risk of a second event and, provided a CT scan has excluded cerebral haemorrhage, should also be anticoagulated with warfarin.

Older patients (> 65 years) with atrial fibrillation constitute the largest group and have an annual risk of stroke or systemic embolism of about 5%. Several large randomised trials have shown that this risk can be reduced by about two-thirds by treatment with warfarin, at the cost of an annual risk of bleeding of 1–1.5%. Aspirin reduces the risk of stroke by about one-fifth. Patients in these trials were often highly selected and may not represent patients encountered in routine clinical practice where also the risks of anticoagulant treatment may be higher than experienced in the setting of a tightly controlled clinical trial.

Certain clinical characteristics are associated with an increased risk of systemic embolism; echocardiography can also help to identify patients with atrial fibrillation who are at risk. The presence of one or more clinical or echocardiographic risk factors favours the prescription of warfarin (see the information box). Warfarin cannot be reliably administered to some patients and such patients should receive aspirin. The target international normalised ratio (INR) for warfarin should be 2.0–3.0.

RISK OF SYSTEMIC EMBOLISM OR STROKE WITH ATRIAL FIBRILLATION

High risk (> 10% per annum)
- Mitral valve disease
- Previous systemic embolism or stroke

Intermediate risk (approximately 5% per annum)
- > 65 years
- One or more clinical or echocardiographic risk factors

Low risk (< 1.5% per annum)
- < 65 years
- No evidence of clinical or structural heart disease

RISK FACTORS FOR EMBOLISM OR STROKE IN AF

Clinical	Echocardiographic
• Mitral valve disease • Previous embolism or stroke • Hypertension • Diabetes mellitus • Previous myocardial infarction • Previous congestive heart failure • Thyrotoxicosis	• Mitral valve disease • Valvular disease including mitral annular calcification • Large left atrium • Dilated left ventricle • Left ventricular aneurysm • Intracardiac thrombus

Young patients (< 65 years) with no evidence of structural or clinical heart disease have a very low risk of systemic embolism or stroke and do not require warfarin but may benefit from aspirin treatment.

JUNCTIONAL TACHYARRHYTHMIAS (SUPRAVENTRICULAR TACHYCARDIA)

AV NODAL RE-ENTRY TACHYCARDIA

This rhythm is due to re-entry within the AV node and produces a regular tachycardia with a rate of between 140 and 220; it tends to occur in hearts that are otherwise normal and may last from a few seconds to many hours. The patient is usually aware of a fast heart beat and may feel faint or breathless. Polyuria, due to the release of atrial natriuretic peptide, is sometimes a feature, and cardiac pain or heart failure may occur if there is coexisting structural heart disease. The ECG (see Fig. 3.32) usually shows a tachycardia with normal QRS complexes but occasionally there may be rate-dependent bundle branch block.

Management

Treatment is not always necessary. However, an attack may be terminated by carotid sinus massage or other measures that increase vagal tone (e.g. self-induced vomiting, Valsalva manoeuvre). Intravenous adenosine or verapamil will restore sinus rhythm in most cases. Suitable alternative drugs include β-adrenoceptor antagonists, disopyramide and digoxin. In an emergency the tachycardia should be terminated by DC cardioversion (see p. 243).

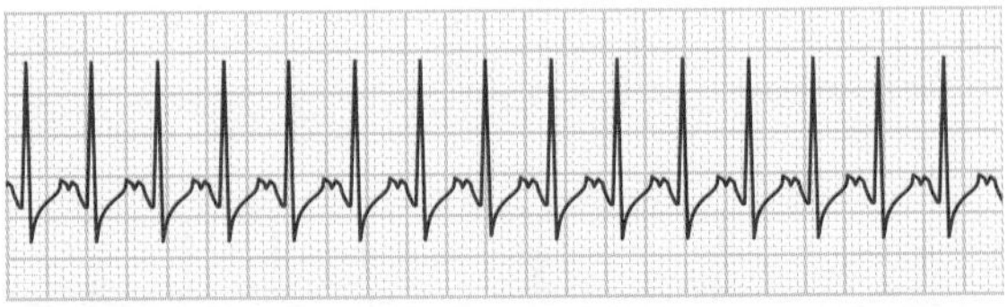

Fig. 3.32 Supraventricular tachycardia. The rate is 180/min and the QRS complexes are normal.

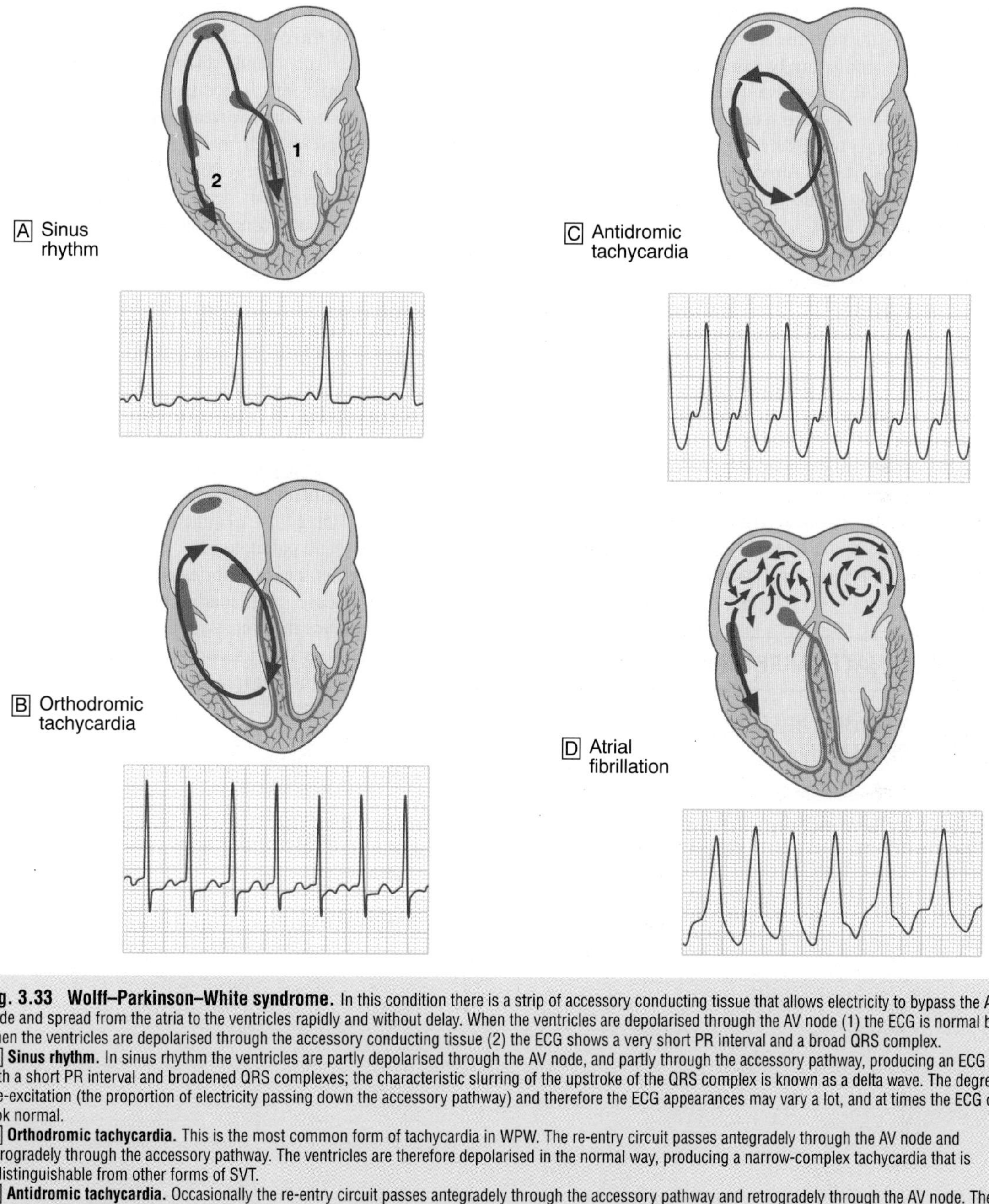

Fig. 3.33 Wolff–Parkinson–White syndrome. In this condition there is a strip of accessory conducting tissue that allows electricity to bypass the AV node and spread from the atria to the ventricles rapidly and without delay. When the ventricles are depolarised through the AV node (1) the ECG is normal but when the ventricles are depolarised through the accessory conducting tissue (2) the ECG shows a very short PR interval and a broad QRS complex.
A Sinus rhythm. In sinus rhythm the ventricles are partly depolarised through the AV node, and partly through the accessory pathway, producing an ECG with a short PR interval and broadened QRS complexes; the characteristic slurring of the upstroke of the QRS complex is known as a delta wave. The degree of pre-excitation (the proportion of electricity passing down the accessory pathway) and therefore the ECG appearances may vary a lot, and at times the ECG can look normal.
B Orthodromic tachycardia. This is the most common form of tachycardia in WPW. The re-entry circuit passes antegradely through the AV node and retrogradely through the accessory pathway. The ventricles are therefore depolarised in the normal way, producing a narrow-complex tachycardia that is indistinguishable from other forms of SVT.
C Antidromic tachycardia. Occasionally the re-entry circuit passes antegradely through the accessory pathway and retrogradely through the AV node. The ventricles are then depolarised through the accessory pathway, producing a broad-complex tachycardia.
D Atrial fibrillation. In this rhythm the ventricles are largely depolarised through the accessory pathway, producing an irregular broad-complex tachycardia which is often more rapid than the example shown.

If attacks are frequent or otherwise disabling, prophylactic oral therapy with any of the above drugs may be indicated. However, radiofrequency ablation may be curative and is often preferable to long-term drug treatment.

THE WOLFF–PARKINSON–WHITE (WPW) SYNDROME

In this condition there is an abnormal band of atrial tissue which connects the atria and ventricles and can electrically bypass the AV node. In normal sinus rhythm conduction takes place partly through the AV node and partly through the more rapidly conducting bypass tract. The ECG shows shortening of the PR interval and a 'slurring' of the QRS complex called a delta wave (see Fig. 3.33A). As the AV node and bypass tract have different conduction speeds and refractory periods, a re-entry circuit (see Fig. 3.27, p. 227) can develop, causing paroxysms of tachycardia (see Figs 3.33B and 3.33C). The onset of atrial fibrillation may produce very rapid ventricular rates because the bypass pathway lacks the rate-limiting properties of the normal AV node (see Fig. 3.33D). Atrial fibrillation is therefore a potentially dangerous arrhythmia in these patients and may cause collapse and syncope, and even lead to death.

Drug treatment is only indicated in symptomatic patients and is aimed at slowing the conduction rate and prolonging the refractory period of the bypass tract, using agents such as flecainide, disopyramide or amiodarone (see pp. 236–240); digoxin and verapamil increase conduction in the bypass tract and should be avoided. Transvenous catheter radiofrequency ablation of the bypass tract offers a cure and is the treatment of choice for most patients.

VENTRICULAR TACHYARRHYTHMIAS

VENTRICULAR ECTOPIC BEATS (EXTRASYSTOLES, PREMATURE BEATS)

The ECG shows premature broad bizarre QRS complexes which may be unifocal, when there is a single ectopic focus, or multifocal (varying morphology with multiple foci—see Fig. 3.34). 'Couplet' and 'triplet' are terms used to describe two or three successive ectopic beats, whereas a run of alternate sinus and ectopic beats is known as 'bigeminy'. Ectopic beats produce a low stroke volume because left ventricular contraction is premature and ineffective. The pulse is therefore irregular, with weak or missed beats. Patients are often asymptomatic but may complain of an irregular heart beat, missed beats or abnormally strong beats (due to the increased output of the post-ectopic sinus beat). The significance of ventricular ectopic beats (VEBs) depends on the nature of any underlying heart disease.

Ventricular ectopic beats in otherwise healthy subjects

VEBs are frequently found in normal people, and their prevalence increases with age. Ectopic beats in patients with otherwise normal hearts are often more prominent at rest, and tend to disappear with exercise. The outlook is excellent and treatment is unnecessary, although low-dose β-adrenoceptor antagonist treatment is sometimes used to suppress anxiety and palpitation.

VEBs are sometimes a manifestation of otherwise subclinical heart disease, particularly coronary artery disease. There is no evidence that anti-arrhythmic therapy is merited in such patients but the discovery of frequent ventricular ectopic beats might reasonably prompt some general cardiac investigations.

Ventricular ectopic beats associated with heart disease

Frequent VEBs are often observed during acute myocardial infarction but are of no prognostic significance and require no treatment. However, persistent frequent (> 10/hour)

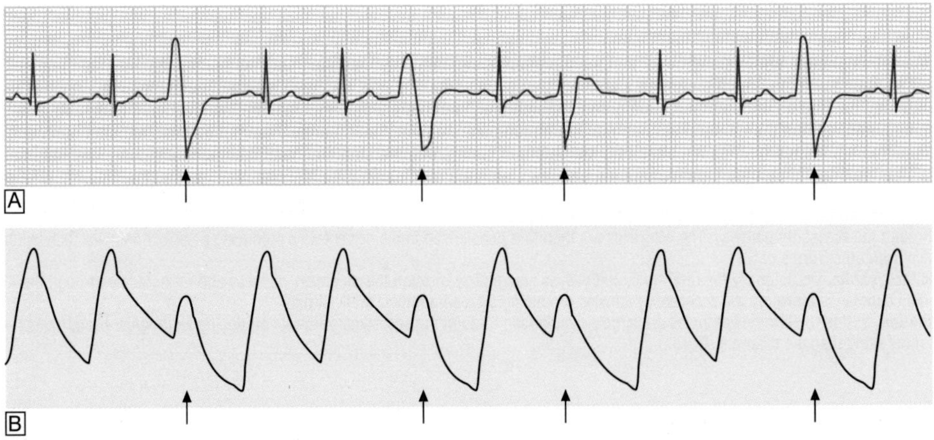

Fig. 3.34 Ventricular ectopic beats. [A] There are broad bizarre QRS complexes with no preceding P wave (arrows) in between normal sinus beats. Their configuration varies, so these are multifocal ectopics. [B] A simultaneous arterial pressure trace is shown. The ectopic beats result in a weaker pulse (arrows), which may be perceived as a 'dropped beat'.

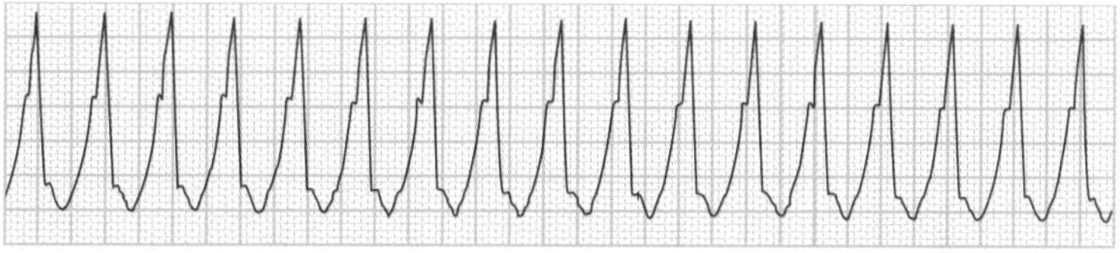

Fig. 3.35 Ventricular tachycardia: rhythm strip. Typical broad bizarre QRS complexes with a rate of 160/min.

ventricular ectopic activity in patients who have survived the acute phase of myocardial infarction is indicative of a poor long-term outcome. Unfortunately, anti-arrhythmic therapy does not improve, and may even worsen, the prognosis in these patients.

VEBs are common in patients with heart failure, when they are associated with an adverse prognosis; but again the outlook is no better if they are suppressed with anti-arrhythmic drugs. Effective treatment of the heart failure may suppress the ectopic beats.

VEBs are also a feature of digoxin toxicity, are sometimes found in mitral valve prolapse, and may occur as 'escape beats' in the presence of an underlying bradycardia. Treatment should always be directed at the underlying condition.

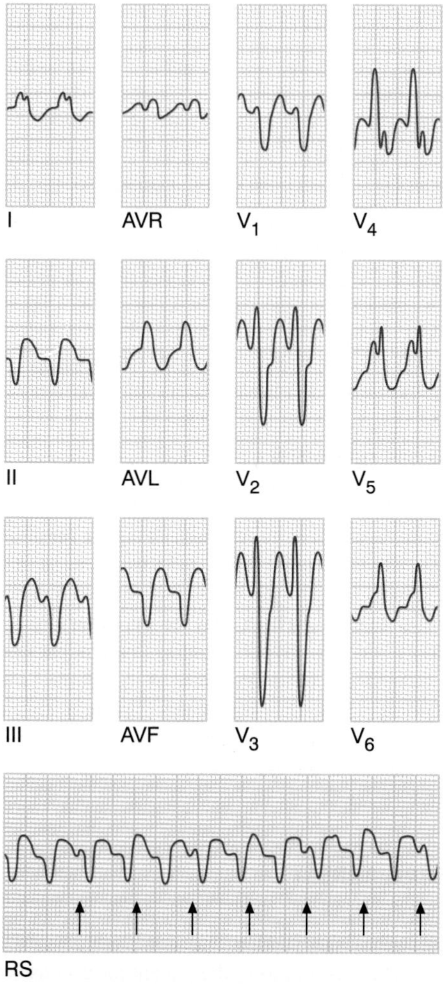

Fig. 3.36 Ventricular tachycardia: 12-lead ECG. The morphology of this tachycardia is typical of VT, with very broad QRS complexes and marked left axis deviation. In addition, there is AV dissociation; some P waves are visible and others are buried in the QRS complexes (arrows).

VENTRICULAR TACHYCARDIA

This is a grave arrhythmia because it is nearly always associated with serious heart disease and may degenerate into ventricular fibrillation. Patients may complain of palpitation or the symptoms of a low cardiac output such as dizziness, dyspnoea or even loss of consciousness (syncope). The ECG shows broad, abnormal QRS complexes with a rate of between 140 and 220 per minute (see Fig. 3.35) and may be difficult to distinguish from supraventricular tachycardia with bundle branch block or pre-excitation (Wolff–Parkinson–White syndrome). Features in favour of ventricular tachycardia are listed in the information box. A 12-lead (see Fig. 3.36), intracardiac (see Fig. 3.37) or oesophageal ECG may help to establish the diagnosis. When there is doubt it is safer to treat for ventricular tachycardia (VT), which is by far the most common cause of a broad-complex tachycardia.

The common causes of ventricular tachycardia include acute myocardial infarction, myocarditis, cardiomyopathy, and chronic ischaemic heart disease, particularly when it is associated with a ventricular aneurysm or poor left ventricular function.

Patients recovering from myocardial infarction sometimes have periods of idioventricular rhythm ('slow' ventricular tachycardia) at a rate only slightly above the preceding sinus rate. These episodes are usually self-limiting and asymptomatic, and do not require treatment. Other forms of ventricular tachycardia, if they last for more than a few beats, will require treatment, often as an emergency.

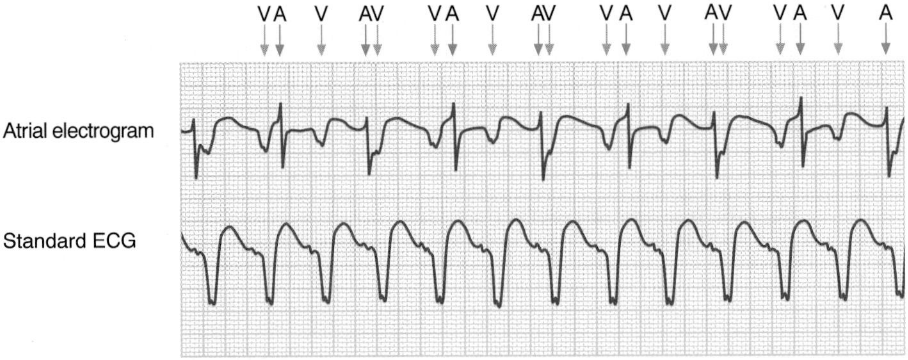

Fig. 3.37 Ventricular tachycardia: intracardiac ECG. A simultaneous recording of an atrial electrogram, obtained by placing a pacing lead in the right atrium, and an ordinary rhythm strip illustrating ventricular tachycardia with AV dissociation. Although the standard ECG shows a broad-complex tachycardia with no visible P waves, dissociated atrial activity is clearly visible in the atrial electrogram. (A = atrial depolarisation; V = ventricular depolarisation)

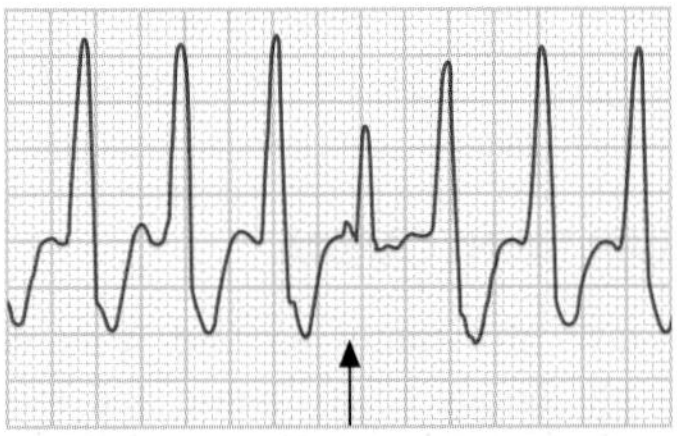

Fig. 3.38 Ventricular tachycardia: fusion beat (arrow). In ventricular tachycardia there is independent atrial and ventricular activity. Occasionally a P wave is conducted to the ventricles through the AV node. This may produce a normal sinus beat in the middle of the tachycardia (a capture beat); however, more commonly the conducted impulse fuses with an impulse from the tachycardia (a fusion beat). This phenomenon can only occur when there is AV dissociation and is therefore diagnostic of ventricular tachycardia.

FEATURES IN FAVOUR OF VENTRICULAR TACHYCARDIA IN THE DIFFERENTIAL DIAGNOSIS OF BROAD-COMPLEX TACHYCARDIA

- A history of myocardial infarction
- AV dissociation (pathognomonic)
- Capture/fusion beats (pathognomonic—see Fig. 3.38)
- Extreme left axis deviation
- Very broad QRS complexes (> 140 ms)
- No response to carotid sinus massage or i.v. adenosine

Management

Prompt action to restore sinus rhythm is required and in most cases should be followed by prophylactic therapy. Direct current cardioversion is often the initial treatment of choice but if this is not available or if the arrhythmia is well tolerated, intravenous lignocaine may be given as a bolus followed by an intravenous infusion (see Table 3.5, p. 237). Mexiletine, flecainide, disopyramide and amiodarone are suitable alternatives (see pp. 236–240). Hypokalaemia, hypomagnesaemia and acidosis must be corrected.

Oral prophylactic therapy with either mexiletine, disopyramide, propafenone or amiodarone (see pp. 236–240) is often necessary. The efficacy of such drug therapy should always be assessed by ambulatory ECG monitoring, by exercise testing or by invasive electrophysiological studies. If drug therapy fails, alternative treatments include the use of an automatic implantable cardioverter-defibrillator (see p. 244), or surgery to identify and resect the area of diseased myocardium which is responsible for the arrhythmia.

TORSADES DE POINTES

This is a type of ventricular tachycardia characterised by QRS complexes of continuously changing amplitude that appear to twist around the isoelectric line at a rate of 200–250/min. This arrhythmia is associated with prolongation of the QT interval, which may be hereditary but is more commonly due to hypokalaemia, hypomagnesaemia or toxic side-effects of drugs such as quinidine, sotalol or amiodarone. Specific treatments include intravenous magnesium and pacing, which increases the heart rate and therefore shortens the QT interval.

CARDIAC ARREST

This describes the sudden and complete loss of cardiac function. There is no pulse, the patient loses consciousness, and respiration ceases almost immediately; death is virtually inevitable unless effective treatment is given promptly. Cardiac arrest may be due to ventricular fibrillation, pulseless ventricular tachycardia, asystole or electromechanical dissociation.

Aetiology of cardiac arrest

Ventricular fibrillation

This is the most common and most easily treatable cause of sudden death. It may be due to myocardial infarction, ischaemia or electrocution. The presence of structural heart disease, electrolyte disturbance such as hypokalaemia, or inappropriate medication may increase susceptibility to ventricular fibrillation. The arrhythmia produces rapid ineffective uncoordinated movement of the ventricles, which therefore produce no pulse. The ECG (see Fig 3.39) shows chaotic, bizarre, irregular complexes.

Ventricular asystole

This occurs when there is no electrical activity of the ventricles and may be due to failure of the conducting tissue or massive ventricular damage complicating myocardial infarction. Cardiac massage or a blow to the chest can sometimes restore cardiac activity, although an artificial pacemaker may be needed to prevent further attacks.

Electromechanical dissociation

This occurs when there is no effective cardiac output despite the presence of normal or near-normal electrical activity; it may be caused by treatable conditions such as hypovolaemia or tension pneumothorax (see below) but is often due to cardiac rupture or massive pulmonary embolism and therefore carries a poor prognosis.

Management of cardiac arrest

Basic life support (BLS)

The management of the collapsed patient requires prompt assessment and restoration of the airway, breathing and circulation with basic life support (see Fig. 3.40), with the aim of maintaining the circulation until more definitive treatment with advanced life support can be administered.

Advanced life support (ALS)

Advanced life support (see Fig. 3.41) aims to restore normal cardiac rhythm by defibrillation where the cause of cardiac arrest is due to arrhythmia, and/or to restore cardiac output by correcting other reversible causes of cardiac

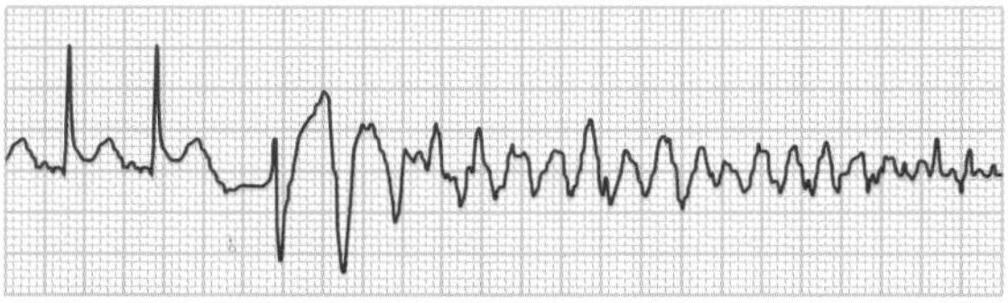

Fig. 3.39 Ventricular fibrillation. A bizarre chaotic rhythm initiated in this case by two ectopic beats in rapid succession.

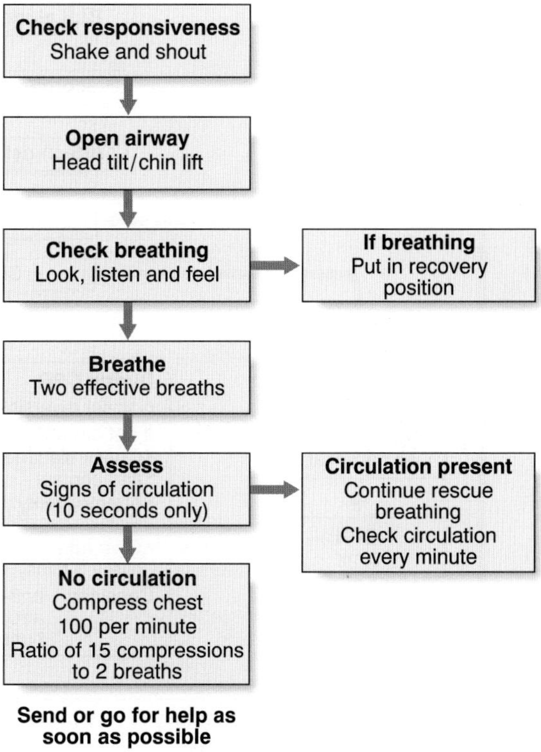

Fig. 3.40 Algorithm for adult basic life support.

arrest. ALS provides support to the circulation additional to BLS by administering intravenous drugs, and by passing an endotracheal tube (ETT) to administer positive pressure ventilation.

If cardiac arrest is witnessed, a precordial thump may sometimes convert ventricular fibrillation or tachycardia to normal rhythm, but this is futile if cardiac arrest has lasted longer than a few seconds.

The top priority in ALS is to assess the patient's cardiac rhythm by attaching a defibrillator/monitor. The most common arrhythmias causing cardiac arrest in adults are ventricular fibrillation (VF) or *pulseless* ventricular tachycardia (VT), and with prompt defibrillation these can usually be successfully treated. Defibrillation is firstly with 200 joules; if normal rhythm is not restored, a further shock of 200 joules is given; if unsuccessful, this is followed by a third shock of 360 joules. If these three shocks are unsuccessful, 1 mg of adrenaline (epinephrine) intravenously and a further 1 minute of cardiopulmonary resuscitation are given before trying a further sequence of up to three shocks each at 360 joules.

Cardiac arrest may be due to asystole which may occasionally be mimicked by ventricular fibrillation of low amplitude, or 'fine VF'. If asystole cannot be confidently

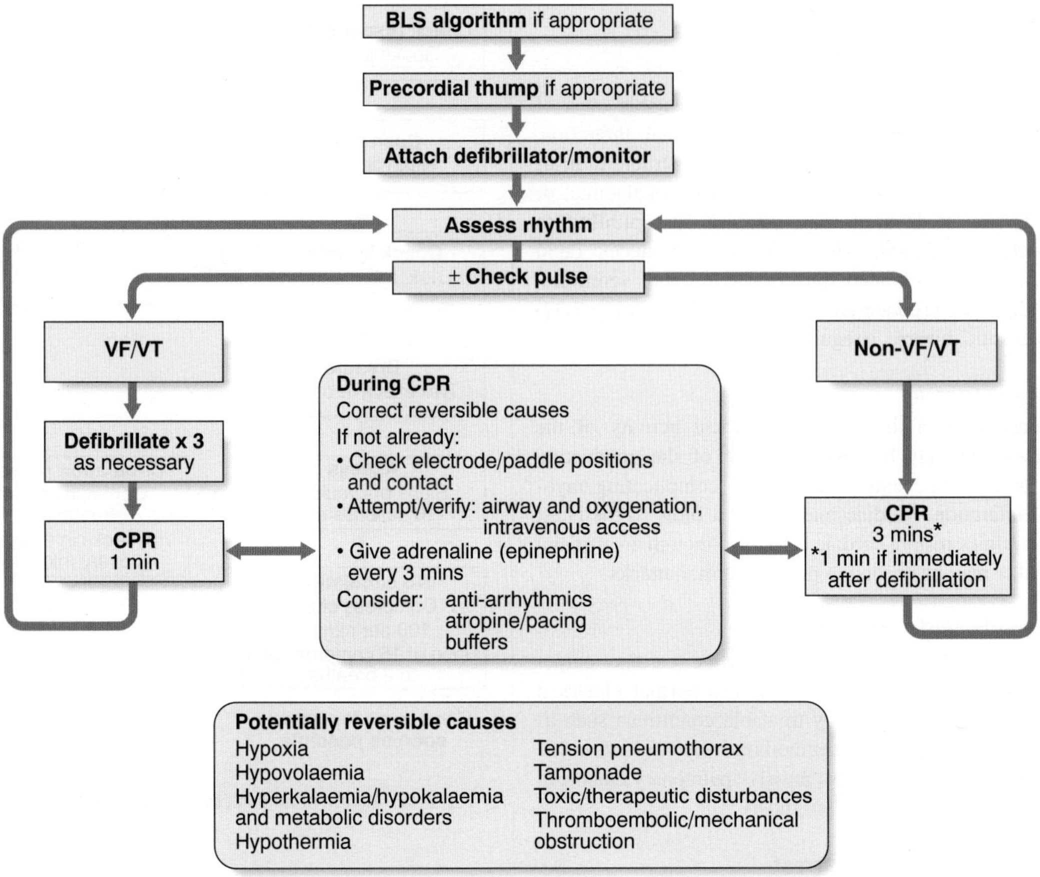

Fig. 3.41 Algorithm for adult advanced life support. (BLS = basic life support; VF = ventricular fibrillation; VT = pulseless ventricular tachycardia; CPR = cardiopulmonary resuscitation)

diagnosed, then the patient should be regarded as having 'fine VF' and defibrillated. If an electrical rhythm is present which would be expected to produce a cardiac output, 'electromechanical dissociation' is present. There are several potentially reversible causes which can be easily remembered by a list of four Hs and four Ts (see blue box, Fig. 3.41). In practical terms, electromechanical dissociation or definite asystole are treated without defibrillation by maintaining cardiopulmonary resuscitation (CPR) whilst seeking potentially reversible causes, i.e. following the 'non-VF/VT' limb of the ALS algorithm.

ANTI-ARRHYTHMIC DRUGS

The classification of anti-arrhythmic drugs

Some of the drugs used to treat individual arrhythmias have already been mentioned. These agents may be classified according to their mode of action or their main site of action (see the information boxes on p. 238). The main uses, dosages and side-effects of the most widely used drugs are summarised in Table 3.5.

Class I drugs

Class I drugs act principally by suppressing excitability and slowing conduction in atrial or ventricular muscle.

Quinidine. This is excreted in the urine and accumulates in renal failure. Gastrointestinal side-effects (abdominal discomfort, nausea and diarrhoea) are common; more serious side-effects include myocardial depression, ventricular tachycardia (often heralded by prolongation of the QT interval) and idiosyncratic autoimmune thrombocytopenia or haemolytic anaemia. Quinidine potentiates digoxin, by increasing plasma digoxin concentrations, and is subject to many other important drug interactions. In view of these problems it is usually used as a second- or third-line agent.

Table 3.5 The main uses, dosages and side-effects of the most widely used anti-arrhythmic drugs

Drug	Main uses	Route	Dose (adult)	Important side-effects
CLASS I				
Quinidine	Prevention of VEs and AF	Oral	Test dose: 250 mg Maintenance: 500 mg 12-hourly as quinidine bisulphate SR	GI upset, myocardial depression, torsades de pointes (see p. 234), haemolytic anaemia, potentiates digoxin and warfarin
Disopyramide	Prevention and treatment of all tachyarrhythmias	I.v. Oral	2 mg/kg at 30 mg/min then 0.4 mg/kg/hr (max 800 mg/day) 300–800 mg daily in divided dosage	Myocardial depression, hypotension, dry mouth, urinary retention
Lignocaine	Treatment and short-term prevention of VT and VF	I.v.	Bolus 50–100 mg 4 mg/min for 30 mins, then 2 mg/min for 2 hrs, then 1 mg/min for 24 hrs	Confusion, convulsions
Mexiletine	Prevention and treatment of ventricular tachyarrhythmias	I.v. Oral	Loading dose: 100–250 mg at 25 mg/min then 250 mg in 1 hr then 250 mg in 2 hrs Maintenance therapy: 0.5 mg/min 200–250 mg 8-hourly	GI irritation, confusion, dizziness, tremor, nystagmus, ataxia
Flecainide	Prevention and treatment of all tachyarrhythmias	I.v. Oral	2 mg/kg over 10 mins then 1.5 mg/kg/hr for 1 hr then 0.1 mg/kg/hr 50–100 mg 12-hourly	Myocardial depression, dizziness
Propafenone	Prevention and treatment of all tachyarrhythmias	Oral	150 mg 8-hourly for 1 week then 300 mg 12-hourly	Myocardial depression, dizziness
CLASS II				
Propranolol		I.v. Oral	1 mg over 1 min to a maximum of 10 mg 10–160 mg 6- or 8-hourly	
Metoprolol	Treatment and prevention of SVT and AF	I.v. Oral	5 mg over 2 mins to a maximum of 15 mg 50–100 mg 8- or 12-hourly	Myocardial depression, bradycardia, bronchospasm, fatigue, depression, nightmares, cold peripheries
Atenolol	Prevention of VEs and exercise-induced VT	I.v. Oral	2.5 mg at 1 mg/min repeated at 5-min intervals (max 10 mg) 50–100 mg daily	
Sotalol		I.v. Oral	10–20 mg slowly 40–160 mg 12-hourly	Sotalol can cause torsades de pointes (see p. 234)
CLASS III				
Amiodarone	Serious atrial and ventricular tachyarrhythmias, particularly in the WPW syndrome	I.v. Oral	5 mg/kg over 20–120 mins then up to 15 mg/kg/24 hr Initially 600–1200 mg/day then 1–200 mg daily	Photosensitivity, skin discoloration, corneal deposits, thyroid dysfunction, alveolitis, nausea and vomiting, hepatotoxicity, peripheral neuropathy, torsades de pointes (see p. 234), potentiates digoxin and warfarin
CLASS IV				
Verapamil	Treatment of SVT, control of AF	I.v. Oral	5–10 mg over 30 s 40–120 mg 8-hourly or 240 mg SR daily	Myocardial depression, hypotension, bradycardia, constipation
OTHER				
Adenosine	Treatment of SVT, aid to diagnosis in unidentified tachycardia	I.v.	3 mg over 2 s followed if necessary by 6 mg then 12 mg at intervals of 1–2 mins	Flushing, dyspnoea, chest pain
Digoxin	Treatment and prevention of SVT, control of AF	I.v. Oral	Loading dose: 0.5–1 mg (total). 0.5 mg over 30 mins then 0.25–0.5 mg 4- to 8-hourly to maximum total of 1 mg assessing response before each additional dose 0.5 mg 6-hourly then 0.125–0.25 mg daily	GI disturbance, xanthopsia, arrhythmias (see p. 239)

(SVT = supraventricular tachycardia; AF = atrial fibrillation; VE = ventricular ectopic; VT = ventricular tachycardia; VF = ventricular fibrillation; SR = sustained-release formulation; WPW = Wolff–Parkinson–White)

ANTI-ARRHYTHMIC DRUGS: PRINCIPLES OF USE
The drugs used to treat arrhythmias are potentially toxic and should be used carefully according to the following principles: • Many arrhythmias are benign and do not require specific treatment • Precipitating or causal factors should be corrected if possible. These may include excess alcohol or caffeine consumption, myocardial ischaemia, hyperthyroidism, acidosis, hypokalaemia and hypomagnesaemia • If drug therapy is required it is best to use as few drugs as possible • In difficult cases programmed electrical stimulation (electrophysiological study) may help to identify the optimum therapy • When dealing with life-threatening arrhythmias it is essential to ensure that prophylactic treatment is effective. Ambulatory monitoring, exercise testing and programmed electrical stimulation may be of value • Patients on long-term anti-arrhythmic drugs should be reviewed regularly and attempts made to withdraw therapy if the factors which precipitated the arrhythmias are no longer operative • Patients who do not respond to drug therapy may benefit from other forms of therapy such as antitachycardia pacing, radiofrequency ablation or arrhythmia surgery

Disopyramide. This has weak atropine-like effects and may cause urinary retention or precipitate glaucoma. It has a depressant effect on ventricular function and should be avoided in cardiac failure. The drug is cleared through the kidneys and liver. If it is used in patients with atrial flutter and AV block, there is a risk of a paradoxical increase in heart rate as the atria slow and 2:1 block changes to 1:1 conduction; this can be prevented by pre-treatment with digoxin.

Lignocaine. This must be given parenterally, and has a very short plasma half-life, so plasma concentration will depend on the rate of infusion. It is mainly used for the urgent treatment or prophylaxis of ventricular tachycardia or fibrillation.

CLASSIFICATION OF DRUGS WITH ANTI-ARRHYTHMIC PROPERTIES ACCORDING TO THEIR MAIN SITE OR SITES OF ACTION
Sinus node
• β-adrenoceptor antagonists, verapamil, diltiazem
AV node
• Adenosine, β-adrenoceptor antagonists, verapamil, diltiazem, digoxin
Ventricles
• Lignocaine, mexiletine
Atria, ventricles and accessory conducting tissue
• Quinidine, disopyramide, flecainide, propafenone, amiodarone

CLASSIFICATION OF ANTI-ARRHYTHMIC DRUGS ACCORDING TO THEIR EFFECT ON THE INTRACELLULAR ACTION POTENTIAL
Class I—membrane-stabilising agents (fast sodium channel blockers)
(a) Block Na^+ channel and prolong action potential • Quinidine, disopyramide **(b)** Block Na^+ channel and shorten action potential • Lignocaine, mexiletine **(c)** Block Na^+ channel with no effect on action potential • Flecainide, propafenone
Class II—β-adrenoceptor antagonists
• Propranolol, metoprolol, atenolol, l-sotalol
Class III—drugs whose main effect is to prolong the action potential
• Amiodarone, d-sotalol
Class IV—slow calcium channel blockers
• Verapamil, diltiazem
N.B. Some drugs (e.g. digoxin and adenosine) have no place in this classification, while others have properties in more than one class (e.g. amiodarone, which has actions in all four classes).

Mexiletine. This can be given intravenously or orally and is used for the treatment or prophylaxis of ventricular arrhythmias. Side-effects include nausea, vomiting, confusion, dizziness, tremor, nystagmus and ataxia. Metabolism is mainly hepatic and the drug may accumulate in liver disease.

Flecainide. This can be given intravenously or orally for the treatment or prophylaxis of supraventricular or ventricular arrhythmias and may be useful in the management of Wolff–Parkinson–White syndrome. Unfortunately, it is a potent myocardial depressant and cannot, therefore, be used safely in patients with poor left ventricular function. Like all anti-arrhythmic drugs it can in some circumstances be pro-arrhythmic and has been found to be hazardous in patients with a history of myocardial infarction. Flecainide is therefore contraindicated in ischaemic heart disease, except in patients with life-threatening ventricular arrhythmias who have been assessed by invasive electrophysiological studies.

Propafenone. This is indicated for the treatment or prophylaxis of all tachyarrhythmias and is particularly useful in paroxysmal atrial fibrillation, ventricular tachycardia and the Wolff–Parkinson–White syndrome. Propafenone is a class Ic drug but also has some β-adrenoceptor antagonist (class II) properties and may precipitate heart failure or heart block in susceptible patients. Important interactions with digoxin, warfarin and cimetidine have been described.

Class II drugs

This group comprises the β-adrenoceptor antagonists (β-blockers). The agents used most commonly are as follows.

Propranolol. This is not cardioselective and is subject to extensive first-pass metabolism in the liver. The effective oral dose is therefore unpredictable and must be titrated after starting treatment with a small dose. For the same reason intravenous propranolol is very potent. CNS side-effects (e.g. nightmares, sedation) are common because the drug readily crosses the blood–brain barrier.

Metoprolol. This is a cardioselective β-adrenoceptor antagonist and may therefore have fewer side-effects than propranolol. However, it is also lipid-soluble and therefore crosses the blood–brain barrier.

Atenolol. This is a cardioselective β-adrenoceptor antagonist with a long duration of action; it is largely excreted unchanged through the kidneys. CNS side-effects are rare because it is water-soluble.

Sotalol. This is a racemic mixture of two isomers with non-selective β-adrenoceptor antagonist (mainly l-sotalol) and class III (mainly d-sotalol) activity; it has a long half-life.

Class III drugs

Class III drugs act by prolonging the plateau phase of the action potential, thus lengthening the refractory period.

Amiodarone. This is the principal drug in this class although both disopyramide and sotalol have class III activity. Amiodarone has unusual pharmacokinetics and is effective against a wide variety of atrial and ventricular arrhythmias. It is probably the most effective drug currently available for controlling paroxysmal atrial fibrillation and the arrhythmias associated with the Wolff–Parkinson–White syndrome. Furthermore, it is very useful in preventing episodes of recurrent ventricular tachycardia, particularly in patients with poor left ventricular function. Amiodarone has an extraordinarily long tissue half-life (25–110 days). This means that the onset of action after oral and intravenous therapy is delayed; indeed it may take several months to reach steady state. For the same reason the drug's effects may last for weeks or months after treatment has been stopped. Side-effects are frequent (up to one-third of patients), numerous and potentially serious (see Table 3.5); they include photosensitisation, corneal deposits, gastrointestinal problems, thyroid dysfunction, liver disease and pulmonary fibrosis. Drug interactions are also common; for example, the effects of digoxin and warfarin are potentiated by amiodarone.

Class IV drugs

These block the 'slow calcium channel' which is particularly important for impulse generation and conduction in atrial and nodal tissue, although it is also present in ventricular muscle.

Verapamil. This is the most widely used anti-arrhythmic drug in this class; however, diltiazem has similar properties. Intravenous verapamil may cause profound bradycardia and/or hypotension and should not be used in conjunction with oral or intravenous β-adrenoceptor antagonists.

Table 3.6 Response to intravenous adenosine

Arrhythmia	Response
Supraventricular junctional tachycardia	Termination
Atrial fibrillation, atrial flutter	Transient AV block
Ventricular tachycardia	No effect

Other anti-arrhythmic drugs

Adenosine. Adenosine must be given intravenously and, like carotid sinus massage, produces transient AV block lasting a few seconds. Accordingly, it may be used to terminate junctional tachycardias when the AV node is part of the re-entry circuit or to help establish the diagnosis in difficult arrhythmias such as atrial flutter with 2:1 AV block or broad-complex tachycardia (see Tables 3.5 and 3.6).

Adenosine is given as an intravenous bolus according to an ascending dosage schedule. The initial dose is 3 mg given over 2 seconds. If there is no response after 1–2 minutes, 6 mg should be given and if necessary the physician should wait another 1–2 minutes before administering the maximum dose of 12 mg. Unwanted effects are short-lived and include flushing, breathlessness and chest pain. The effects of adenosine are greatly potentiated by dipyridamole and inhibited by theophylline and other xanthines.

Digoxin. This is a purified glycoside from the European foxglove, *Digitalis lanata*, which slows conduction and

DIGOXIN TOXICITY

Extra-cardiac manifestations

- Anorexia, nausea, vomiting
- Diarrhoea
- Altered colour vision (xanthopsia)

Cardiac manifestations

- Bradycardia
- Multiple ventricular ectopics
- Ventricular bigeminy (alternate ventricular ectopics)
- Paroxysmal atrial tachycardia
- Ventricular tachycardia
- Ventricular fibrillation

Management

- Stop digoxin
- Check urea, electrolytes and plasma digoxin level
- Correct hypokalaemia and/or dehydration
- Correct bradycardia using atropine (0.6 mg i.v.) and/or temporary pacing
- Treat atrial tachycardia with β-adrenoceptor antagonists
- Treat ventricular tachycardia with lignocaine
- In overdose, specific antidigoxin antibodies may be of value

N.B. Cardioversion carries an increased risk of provoking ventricular fibrillation.

prolongs the refractory period in the AV node. This effect helps to control the ventricular rate in atrial fibrillation and will often interrupt re-entry tachycardias involving the AV node. On the other hand, digoxin tends to shorten refractory periods and enhance excitability and conduction in other parts of the heart (including accessory conduction pathways); it may therefore increase atrial and ventricular ectopic activity and can lead to more complex atrial and ventricular tachyarrhythmias.

Digoxin is largely excreted by the kidneys, and the maintenance dose (see Table 3.5) should be reduced in children, the elderly and those with renal impairment. It is widely distributed and has a long tissue half-life so that effects may persist 24–36 hours after the last dose. Measurements of plasma digoxin concentration are useful in demonstrating that the dose being used is inadequate and in confirming a clinical impression of toxicity (see the information box).

SINOATRIAL DISEASE (SICK SINUS SYNDROME)

Sinoatrial disease can occur at any age, but is most common in the elderly. The underlying pathology is not understood but may involve fibrosis, degenerative changes and/or ischaemia of the sinus node. The condition is characterised by a variety of arrhythmias (see the information box) and may present with palpitation, dizzy spells, or syncope due to intermittent tachycardia, bradycardia, or pauses (sinoatrial block or sinus arrest) with no atrial or ventricular activity (see Fig. 3.42).

A permanent pacemaker may benefit patients with troublesome symptoms due to spontaneous bradycardias, or those with symptomatic bradycardias induced by drugs required to prevent tachyarrhythmias. Pacing the atrium may help to prevent episodes of atrial fibrillation; however, permanent pacing does not improve prognosis and is not indicated in patients who are asymptomatic.

COMMON FEATURES OF SINOATRIAL DISEASE

- Sinus bradycardia
- Sinoatrial block (sinus arrest)
- Paroxysmal supraventricular tachycardia
- Paroxysmal atrial fibrillation
- Atrioventricular block

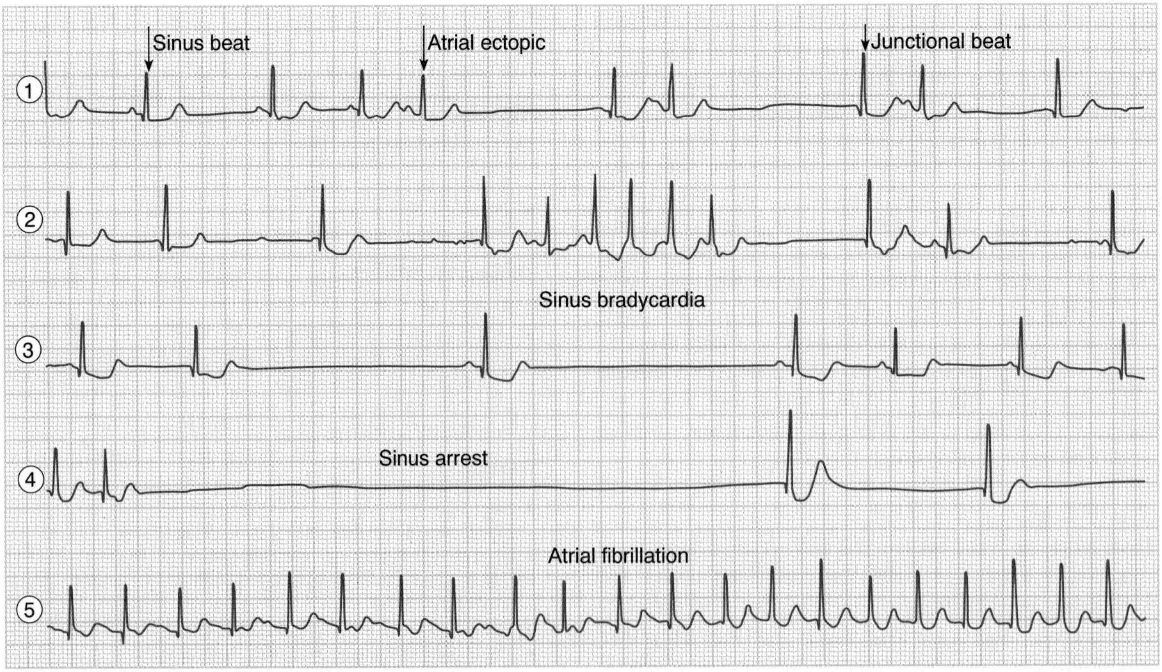

Fig. 3.42 Sinoatrial disease (sick sinus syndrome). A continuous rhythm strip from a 24-hour ECG tape recording illustrating periods of sinus rhythm, atrial ectopics, junctional beats, sinus bradycardia, sinus arrest and paroxysmal atrial fibrillation.

ATRIOVENTRICULAR AND BUNDLE BRANCH BLOCK

ATRIOVENTRICULAR (AV) BLOCK

Atrioventricular conduction is influenced by autonomic activity; AV block can therefore be intermittent and may only be evident when the conducting tissue is stressed by a rapid atrial rate. Accordingly, atrial tachyarrhythmias are often associated with AV block (see Fig. 3.29, p. 229).

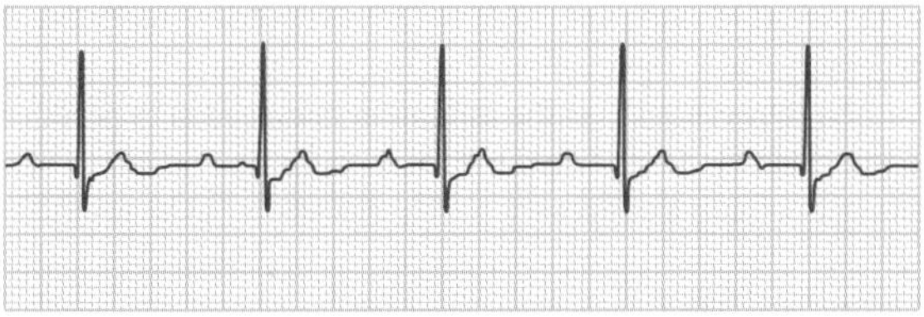

Fig. 3.43 First-degree heart block. The PR interval is prolonged and measures 0.26 seconds.

First-degree AV block

In this condition AV conduction is delayed so the PR interval is prolonged beyond the upper limit of normal (0.20 second). There are no symptoms and the diagnosis can only be made from the ECG (see Fig. 3.43).

Second-degree AV block

In this condition dropped beats occur because some impulses from the atria fail to get through to the ventricles.

In *Mobitz type I second-degree AV block* (see Fig. 3.44) there is progressive lengthening of successive PR intervals culminating in a dropped beat. The cycle then repeats itself. This is known as Wenckebach's phenomenon and is usually due to impaired conduction proximal to the bundle of His. The phenomenon may be physiological and is sometimes observed at rest or during sleep in athletic young adults with high vagal tone.

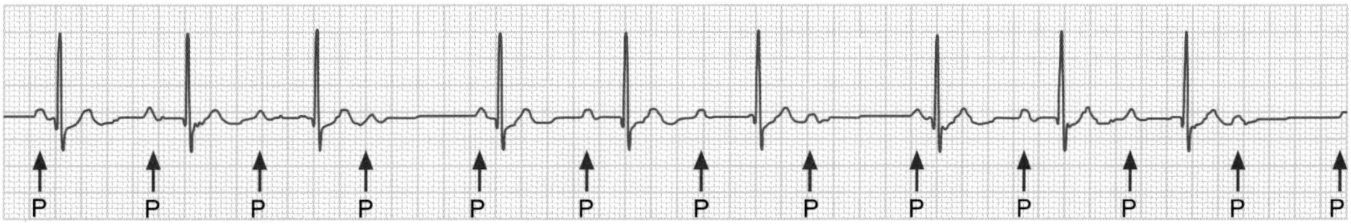

Fig. 3.44 Second-degree heart block (Mobitz type I—Wenckebach's phenomenon). The PR interval progressively increases until a P wave is not conducted. The cycle then repeats itself.

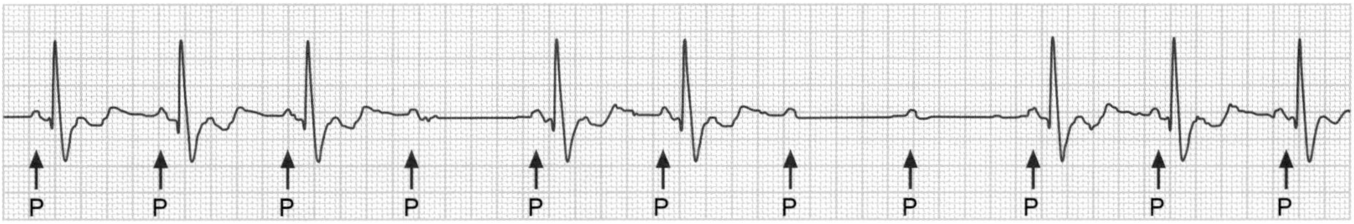

Fig. 3.45 Second-degree heart block (Mobitz type II). The PR interval of conducted beats is normal but some P waves are not conducted.

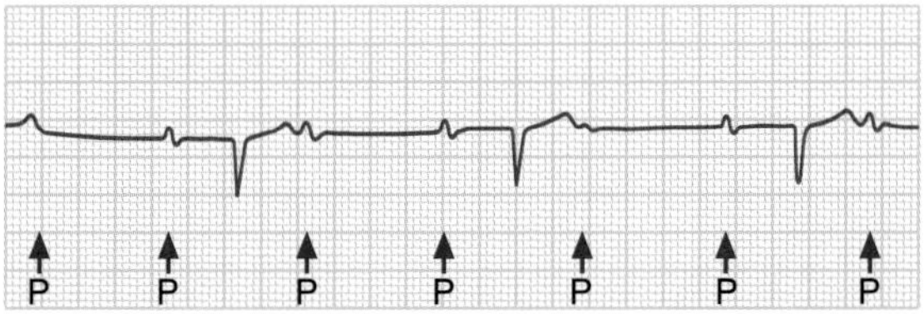

Fig. 3.46 Second-degree heart block with fixed 2:1 block. Alternate P waves are not conducted. This may be due to Mobitz type I or II block.

In *Mobitz type II second-degree AV block* (see Fig. 3.45) the PR interval of the conducted impulses remains constant but some P waves are not conducted. This is usually caused by disease below the bundle of His and is more serious than Mobitz type I.

In *2:1 AV block* (see Fig. 3.46) alternate P waves are conducted so it is impossible to distinguish between Mobitz type I and type II block.

Third-degree (complete) AV block (see Fig. 3.47)

When AV conduction fails completely, the atria and ventricles beat independently (AV dissociation). Ventricular

THE AETIOLOGY OF COMPLETE HEART BLOCK

Congenital

Acquired

- Idiopathic fibrosis
- Myocardial infarction/ischaemia
- Inflammation
  - Acute (e.g. aortic root abscess in infective endocarditis)
  - Chronic (e.g. sarcoidosis, Chagas disease)
- Trauma (e.g. cardiac surgery)
- Drugs (e.g. digoxin, β-adrenoceptor antagonist)

activity is maintained by an escape rhythm arising in the bundle of His (narrow QRS complexes) or the distal conducting tissues (broad QRS complexes). Distal escape rhythms tend to be slower and less reliable.

The aetiology is shown in the information box.

Complete heart block produces a slow (25–50/min) regular pulse that, except in the case of congenital complete heart block, does not vary with exercise. There is usually a compensatory increase in stroke volume with a large volume pulse and systolic flow murmurs. Cannon waves may be visible in the neck and the intensity of the first heart sound varies due to the loss of AV synchrony.

Adams–Stokes attacks

Episodes of ventricular asystole may complicate complete heart block or Mobitz type II second-degree AV block and can also occur in patients with sinoatrial disease (see Fig. 3.42). This may cause recurrent syncope or 'Adams–Stokes' attacks.

A typical episode is characterised by a sudden loss of consciousness, which frequently occurs without warning and may result in a fall. Convulsions (due to cerebral ischaemia) can occur if there is prolonged asystole. There is pallor and a death-like appearance during the attack, but when the heart starts beating again there is a characteristic flush. In contrast to epilepsy, recovery is rapid.

Management

AV block complicating acute myocardial infarction

Acute *inferior* myocardial infarction is often complicated by transient AV block because the right coronary artery supplies the junctional tissues and bundle of His. However, there is usually a reliable escape rhythm and if the patient remains well no treatment is required. Clinical deterioration due to second-degree or complete heart block may respond to atropine (0.6 mg intravenously, repeated as necessary) or, if this fails, a temporary pacemaker. In the vast majority of cases the AV block will resolve within 7–10 days.

Second-degree or complete heart block complicating acute *anterior* myocardial infarction is usually a sign of extensive myocardial damage and therefore carries a poor prognosis. Asystole may ensue and a temporary pacemaker should be inserted as soon as possible. If the patient presents with asystole, atropine (0.6 mg intravenously, repeated if necessary) and isoprenaline (1–5 mg in 500 ml 5% dextrose, infused intravenously at the minimum rate needed to produce a satisfactory heart rhythm) may help to maintain the circulation until a temporary pacing electrode can be inserted.

Chronic AV block

Patients with symptomatic bradyarrhythmias associated with AV block should receive a permanent pacemaker (see below).

Asymptomatic first-degree or Mobitz type I second-degree AV block does not require treatment but may be an indication of serious underlying heart disease.

A permanent pacemaker is usually indicated in patients with asymptomatic Mobitz type II second-degree or complete heart block because there is evidence that pacing can improve their prognosis. An exception may be made in young asymptomatic patients with congenital complete heart block who have a mean daytime heart rate of more than 50 per minute.

BUNDLE BRANCH BLOCK AND HEMIBLOCK

Interruption of the right or left branch of the bundle of His delays activation of the appropriate ventricle, broadens the

THE COMMON CAUSES OF BUNDLE BRANCH BLOCK

LBBB	RBBB
• Coronary artery disease • Hypertension • Aortic valve disease • Cardiomyopathy	• Normal variant • Right ventricular hypertrophy or strain, e.g. pulmonary embolism • Congenital heart disease, e.g. atrial septal defect • Coronary artery disease

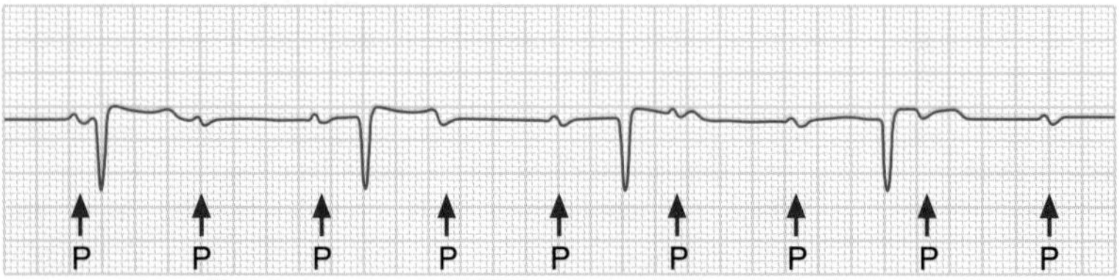

Fig. 3.47 Complete (third-degree) AV block. There is complete dissociation of atrial and ventricular complexes. The atrial rate is 80/min and the ventricular rate is 38/min.

QRS complex (0.12 seconds or more) and produces the characteristic alterations in QRS morphology shown in Figures 3.48 and 3.49.

Right bundle branch block (RBBB) is a common normal variant but left bundle branch block (LBBB) usually signifies important underlying heart disease. Both forms of bundle branch block may be due to conducting tissue disease but are also features of other types of heart disease (see the information box).

The left branch of the bundle of His divides into an anterior and posterior fascicle. Damage to the conducting tissue at this point (hemiblock) does not broaden the QRS complex, but alters the mean direction of ventricular depolarisation (mean QRS axis), causing left axis deviation in left anterior hemiblock and right axis deviation in left posterior hemiblock. The combination of right bundle branch and left anterior or posterior hemiblock is known as bifascicular block.

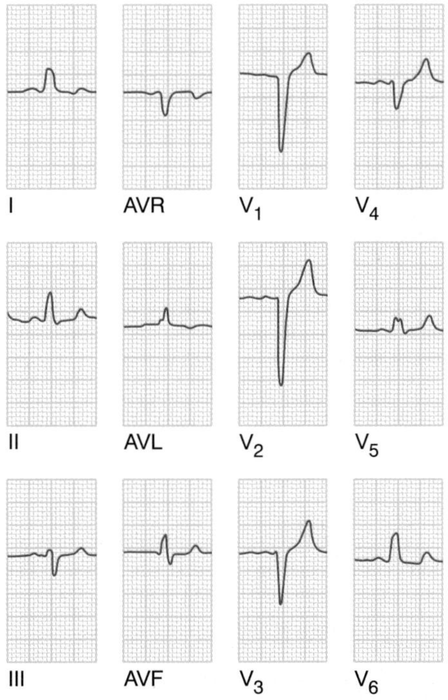

Fig. 3.49 Left bundle branch block. Note the wide QRS complexes with the loss of the Q wave or septal vector in lead I and 'M'-shaped QRS complexes in V_5 and V_6.

ELECTRICAL TREATMENT OF ARRHYTHMIAS

EXTERNAL DEFIBRILLATION AND CARDIOVERSION

The heart can be completely depolarised by passing a sufficiently large electrical current through it from an external source. This will interrupt any arrhythmia and produce a brief period of asystole which is usually followed by the resumption of normal sinus rhythm. Modern defibrillators deliver a direct current (DC), high-energy, short-duration shock via two electrodes coated with conducting jelly, positioned over the upper right sternal edge and the apex.

Energy applied during a critical period around the peak of the T wave may provoke ventricular fibrillation, so when this technique is used to treat organised rhythms such as atrial fibrillation or ventricular tachycardia the shock should be synchronised with the ECG, and is normally given 0.02 sec after the peak of the R wave. The precise timing of the discharge is not important in ventricular fibrillation.

In ventricular fibrillation and other emergencies the energy of the first shock should be 200 joules; there is no need for an anaesthetic if the patient is unconscious. Elective cardioversion requires a general anaesthetic. High-energy shocks may cause myocardial damage, so if there is no urgency it is appropriate to begin with a low-amplitude shock, going on to larger shocks if necessary. In atrial fibrillation a synchronised shock of 100 joules may restore sinus rhythm, and in more organised rhythms such as atrial flutter or supraventricular tachycardia, energies of 50 joules or less may suffice.

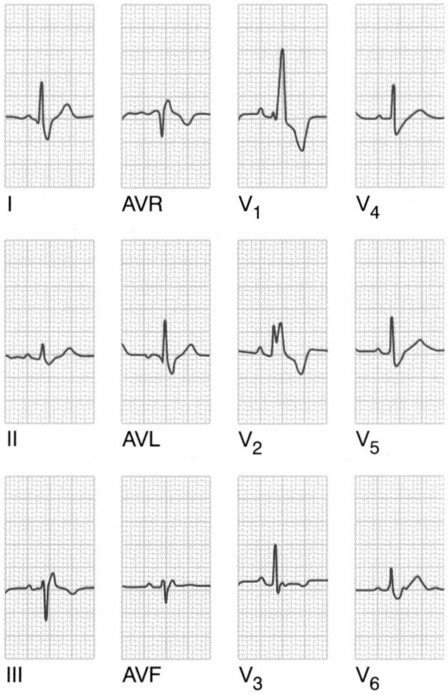

Fig. 3.48 Right bundle branch block. Note the wide QRS complexes with 'M'-shaped configuration in leads V_1 and V_2 and a wide S wave in lead I.

Digoxin toxicity increases the risk of untoward arrhythmias after cardioversion, and ideally digitalis therapy should be withdrawn 36 hours before elective cardioversion. Patients with long-standing atrial arrhythmias are at risk of systemic embolism before and after cardioversion, so it is wise to ensure that the patient is adequately anticoagulated for at least 4 weeks either side of the procedure.

Implantable cardioverter-defibrillator (ICD)

This sophisticated device is implanted transvenously like a permanent pacemaker and can deliver a tiered sequence of treatments for ventricular tachycardia, including competitive pacing, synchronised cardioversion with a low-energy shock, and defibrillation with a higher-energy shock (which can be painful). They can also pace the ventricles in the event of bradycardia. ICDs are more effective than anti-arrhythmic drugs in preventing sudden death in some high-risk patients, such as those who have been resuscitated from ventricular tachycardia or fibrillation that was not associated with acute myocardial infarction. They are extremely expensive and should only be implanted in carefully selected patients in specialist centres.

Radiofrequency catheter ablation

The aim of this technique is to interrupt a re-entry circuit by selectively damaging endocardial tissue with radiofrequency energy delivered through a transvenous catheter. Radiofrequency ablation has become the treatment of choice for symptomatic Wolff–Parkinson–White syndrome and is also used to treat other atrial and junctional tachycardias. The procedure is often time-consuming but does not require an anaesthetic and can produce a lifetime cure.

ARTIFICIAL PACEMAKERS

Temporary pacemakers

In an emergency it is sometimes possible to pace the heart by passing an electric current through electrodes placed on the chest wall, passed down the oesophagus, or inserted directly through the chest wall into the myocardium. None of these methods is satisfactory for more than a few minutes, if at all, and the most effective technique for temporary artificial pacemaking is to insert a bipolar pacing electrode via an antecubital, subclavian or femoral vein and position it under fluoroscopic control in the apex of the right ventricle. The electrode is then connected to an external pulse generator which can be adjusted to alter the energy output or pacing rate. The threshold is the lowest output that will reliably pace the heart and should be less than 1 volt at implantation. The generator should be set to deliver an output that is at least twice this figure, and may require daily adjustment because the threshold tends to rise, due to inflammation and oedema around the tip of the electrode.

Temporary pacing may be indicated in the management of transient heart block and other arrhythmias complicating acute myocardial infarction, as a safety measure in patients with heart block or sinoatrial disease (that does not require permanent pacing) undergoing a general anaesthetic, or as a prelude to permanent pacing. Complications include pneumothorax and other forms of trauma related to the insertion of the wire, local infection or septicaemia (usually *Staphylococcus aureus*), and pericarditis. Failure of the system may be due to lead displacement or a progressive increase in the threshold (exit block). The complication and failure rates increase with time and it is seldom wise to use a temporary pacing system for more than 10–14 days.

The ECG of a patient whose rhythm is controlled by an artificial ventricular pacemaker placed in the right ventricle shows regular broad QRS complexes with a left bundle branch block pattern. Each complex is immediately preceded by a 'pacing spike'. Nearly all pulse generators are used in the 'demand' mode so that a spontaneously generated QRS complex will inhibit the pacemaker.

Permanent pacemakers

Permanent artificial pacemakers utilise the same principles, but the pulse generator is implanted under the skin. Electrodes can be placed in the apex of the right ventricle, the right atrial appendage or both (see Fig. 3.50).

Most permanent pacemakers are programmable so the rate, output etc. can be altered by an external programmer using radiofrequency or magnetic signals. This facility allows the cardiologist to prolong the life of the pacemaker by choosing optimum settings and may provide the means to overcome a wide range of pacing problems. For example, programming can be used to increase output in the face of an unexpected increase in threshold, or to alter sensitivity if the pacemaker is inappropriately inhibited by electrical potentials generated in the pectoral muscles (myopotential inhibition).

Atrial pacing may be appropriate for patients with sinoatrial disease without AV block, and ventricular pacing is the only suitable mode for patients with continuous atrial fibrillation. In dual (atrial and ventricular) chamber pacing the atrial electrode can be used to detect spontaneous atrial activity and trigger ventricular pacing, thereby preserving atrioventricular synchrony and allowing the ventricular rate to increase together with the atrial rate during exercise and other forms of stress. Dual-chamber pacing is expensive but has many advantages when compared to simple ventricular pacing; these include superior haemodynamics leading to a better effort tolerance, a lower prevalence of atrial arrhythmias in patients with sinoatrial disease, and the ability to prevent or cure the 'pacemaker syndrome' (a fall in the blood pressure and dizziness precipitated by the start of ventricular pacing).

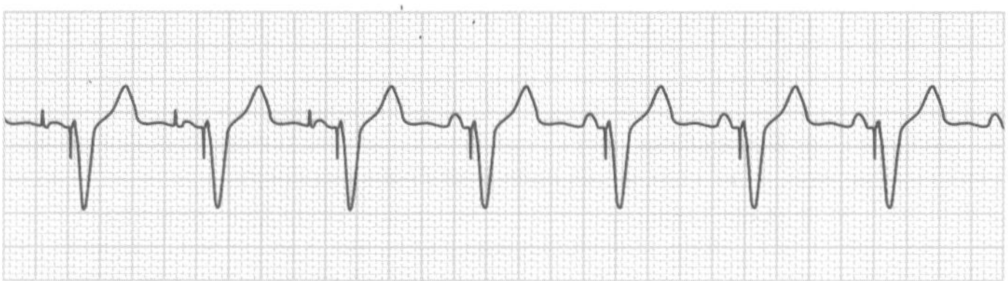

Fig. 3.50 Dual-chamber pacing. The first three beats show atrial and ventricular pacing with narrow pacing spikes in front of each P wave and QRS complex. The last four beats show spontaneous P waves with a different morphology and no pacing spike; the pacemaker senses or tracks these P waves and maintains AV synchrony by pacing the ventricle after an appropriate interval.

There are also 'rate-responsive' pacemakers which react (by changing the pacing rate) to parameters such as respiration or physical movement. This type of pacemaker helps to maintain an optimum heart rate and can be used in patients who are not suitable for atrial triggered pacing, e.g. patients with atrial fibrillation.

FURTHER INFORMATION ON DISORDERS OF HEART RATE, RHYTHM AND CONDUCTION

Bennett D H 1997 Cardiac arrhythmias, 5th edn. Butterworth–Heinemann, Oxford

Lip G Y H 1996 ABC of atrial fibrillation. British Medical Journal Publishing Group, London. *An excellent series of articles that were published in the BMJ during 1995 and 1996*

The 1998 European Resuscitation Council guidelines for adult advanced life support 1998 British Medical Journal 316: 1863–1869

ISCHAEMIC (CORONARY) HEART DISEASE

Coronary heart disease is the most common form of heart disease and the single most important cause of premature death in the developed world. In the UK one in four men and one in five women die from this disease; an estimated 300 000 people have a myocardial infarct each year and approximately 1.7 million people have angina. The death rates from coronary heart disease in the UK are among the highest in the world (more than 150 000 people died from coronary heart disease in the UK in 1995) but are falling. Unfortunately, the incidence of the condition is increasing rapidly in Eastern Europe and many developing countries.

PATHOPHYSIOLOGY, RISK FACTORS AND PREVENTION

Disease of the coronary arteries is almost always due to atheroma and its complications, particularly thrombosis. However, occasionally the coronary arteries are involved in other disorders such as congenital anomalies (e.g. anomalous origin, fistula or malformation of a major coronary artery), aortitis, polyarteritis and other connective tissue disorders.

ATHEROMA

Atheroma or atherosclerosis is a patchy focal disease of the arterial wall. Some arteries such as the radial artery and the internal mammary artery are largely spared, while others, notably the coronary arteries, are at high risk. Coronary artery, cerebral and peripheral vascular disease often co-exist but seldom develop at the same rate.

In Western countries atheromatous plaques begin to appear in the second and third decade of life. The nature and composition of these plaques change as they evolve (see Fig. 3.51).

Fatty streaks develop as circulating monocytes migrate into the intima, take up oxidised low-density lipoprotein (LDL) from the plasma, and become lipid-laden foam cells. As these foam cells die and release their contents, extracellular lipid pools appear. Local and systemic factors will determine whether a fatty streak resolves or progresses to an atheromatous lesion. In early atheroma, smooth muscle cells migrate into and proliferate within the plaque. As the lesion grows it encroaches into the lumen of the vessel and erodes the media.

A mature fibrolipid plaque has a core of extracellular lipid surrounded by smooth muscle cells and is separated from the lumen by a cap of collagen-rich fibrous tissue. Such plaques may rupture or fissure, allowing blood to enter and disrupt the arterial wall; this may compromise the lumen of the vessel and often precipitates thrombosis and local vasospasm. Plaque rupture may lead to rapid growth of the lesion or occlusion of the vessel and is thought to be the cause of most acute coronary syndromes.

The number and state of evolution of plaques both increase with age, but the rate of progression of individual plaques, even in the same patient, is very variable.

Clinical features

The clinical manifestations and pathological correlates of coronary artery disease are shown in Table 3.7.

Risk factors

Key factors influencing the development of coronary disease can be studied either in animal models or by looking for associations between clinical coronary disease and variables such as smoking and plasma cholesterol. Animal models do not accurately reproduce human pathology, and epidemio-

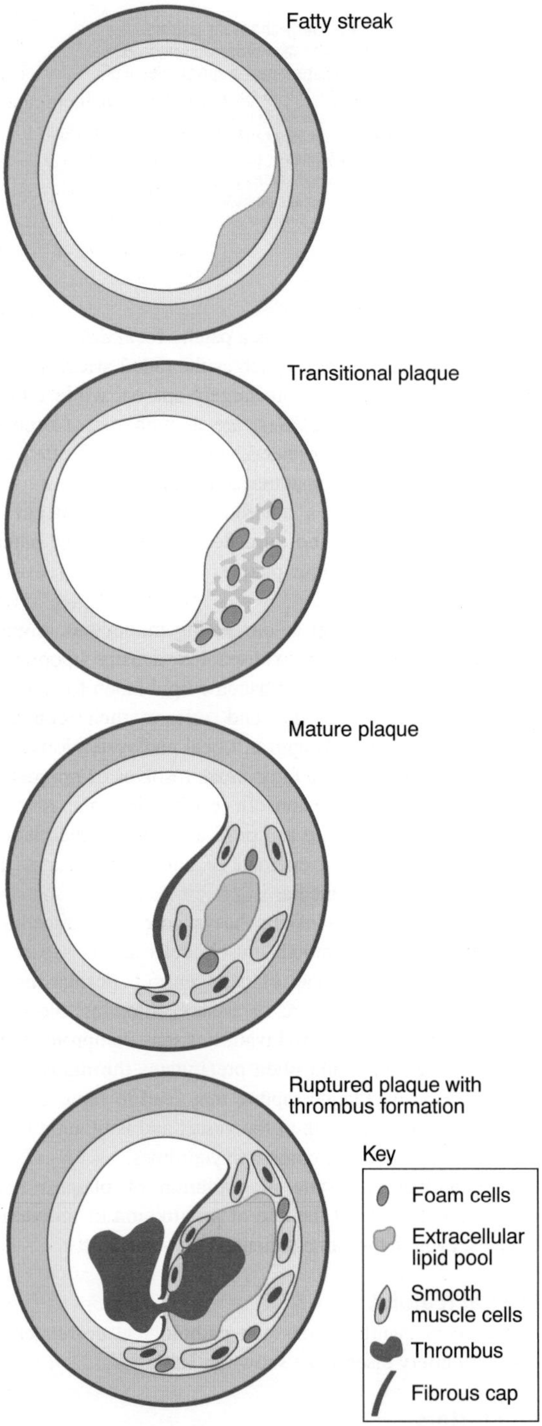

Fig. 3.51 The evolution of an atheromatous plaque.

Table 3.7 Coronary artery disease: clinical manifestations and pathology

Clinical problem	Pathology
Stable angina	Ischaemia due to fixed atheromatous stenosis of one or more coronary arteries
Unstable angina	Ischaemia caused by dynamic obstruction of a coronary artery due to plaque rupture with superimposed thrombosis and spasm
Myocardial infarction	Acute occlusion of a coronary artery due to plaque rupture and thrombosis and resulting in myocardial necrosis
Heart failure	Myocardial dysfunction due to infarction or ischaemia
Arrhythmia	Altered conduction due to ischaemia or infarction
Sudden death	Ventricular arrhythmia, asystole or massive myocardial infarction

SOME IMPORTANT RISK FACTORS FOR CORONARY ARTERY DISEASE

Fixed	Modifiable
• Age • Male sex • Family history	• Smoking • Hypertension • Lipid disorders • Diabetes mellitus • Haemostatic variables • Sedentary lifestyle • Obesity • Dietary deficiencies of antioxidant vitamins and polyunsaturated fatty acids

logical studies are often unable to distinguish between risk factors, which bear a causative relation to the disease, and risk markers, where the variable measured is not itself the cause but is linked to something which is.

Some risk factors for coronary disease are listed in the information box. Such factors amplify underlying genetic risk. For example, a monozygotic twin of an affected individual has an eight-fold, and a dizygotic twin a four-fold increased risk (compared to the general population) of dying from coronary heart disease.

The effect of risk factors is multiplicative rather than additive; thus people with a combination of risk factors (e.g. smoking, hypertension and diabetes) have the greatest risk of developing coronary heart disease. It is important to distinguish between *relative* risk (the proportional increase in risk) and *absolute* risk (the actual chance of an event). Thus a man of 35 with a plasma cholesterol of 10 mmol/litre who smokes 40 cigarettes a day is *relatively* much more likely to die from coronary disease within the next decade than a non-smoking woman of the same age with a normal cholesterol, but the *absolute* likelihood of his dying during this time is still small (high relative risk, low absolute risk).

The risk of suffering a coronary event is analogous to the risk of being involved in a road accident. An inexperienced driver in an old car with poor brakes, bald tyres and defective steering is much more likely to have an accident than an experienced driver in a new car. However, there is a random element which means that occasionally the good driver will have an accident a few minutes after leaving home.

- *Age and male sex.* Obviously these risk factors cannot be corrected; however, there is considerable evidence that hormone replacement therapy may reduce the risk of ischaemic heart disease in post-menopausal women.
- *Family history.* Coronary artery disease often runs in families. This may be due to genetic factors or the effects of a shared environment (similar diet, smoking habits etc.). At present it is estimated that about 40% of the risk of developing ischaemic heart disease is controlled by genetic factors, and 60% by environmental factors. Hyperlipidaemia, hyperfibrinogenaemia and abnormalities of other coagulation factors are often genetically determined.
- *Smoking.* Tobacco is probably the most important *avoidable* cause of coronary disease. There is a strong, consistent and dose-linked relationship between cigarette smoking and ischaemic heart disease. The relative risk is highest in young people and becomes significantly lower within 6 months of quitting.
- *Hypertension.* The incidence of coronary artery disease increases as blood pressure rises and the excess risk is related to both systolic and diastolic blood pressure. Antihypertensive drugs have been shown to reduce coronary mortality but by less than might have been anticipated (see p. 216).
- *Hypercholesterolaemia* (see pp. 532–537). Patients with familial hyperlipidaemia have a high incidence of premature coronary disease and many epidemiological studies have demonstrated a positive correlation between mean population plasma cholesterol concentration and morbidity and death from coronary disease. The excess risk is closely related to the plasma concentration of LDL cholesterol and is inversely related to the plasma high-density lipoprotein (HDL) cholesterol concentration. There is also a weak correlation between plasma triglyceride concentration and the incidence of coronary artery disease. Large-scale randomised clinical trials have shown that lowering high cholesterol concentrations mainly by drugs reduces the risk of cardiac events, including death, myocardial infarction and the need for subsequent revascularisation procedures. HMG CoA reductase inhibitors are the most effective form of lipid-lowering therapy and the largest absolute benefit is seen in those who have the highest absolute risk.
- *Diabetes mellitus.* This is associated with an increased incidence of ischaemic heart disease and with a tendency to diffuse coronary atheroma. Insulin resistance (normal glucose homeostasis with high levels of insulin) is associated with obesity and physical inactivity and is also a potent risk factor for coronary heart disease. These factors are thought to account for the high incidence of ischaemic heart disease in some Asian communities.
- *Haemostatic factors.* Platelet activation, and high levels of fibrinogen and factor VII are associated with an increased risk of myocardial infarction (coronary thrombosis). Nevertheless, these parameters are currently seldom measured in routine clinical practice.
- *Physical activity.* Regular exercise (brisk walking, cycling or swimming for 20 minutes two or three times a week) appears to have a protective effect which may be related to its ability to increase HDL cholesterol, lower blood pressure, reduce blood clotting, and promote collateral vessel development.
- *Obesity.* Obesity, particularly if central or truncal, is an independent risk factor, although it is often associated with other adverse factors such as hypertension, diabetes and physical inactivity.
- *Alcohol.* A moderate intake of alcohol (2–4 units a day) appears to offer some protection from coronary disease; however, heavy drinking is associated with hypertension and an excess of cardiac events.
- *Other dietary factors.* Diets deficient in fresh fruit, vegetables and polyunsaturated fatty acids are associated with an increased risk of coronary disease. This may be independent of the tendency of diets with a high polyunsaturated/saturated ratio to lower cholesterol. Low levels of vitamin C, vitamin E and other antioxidants may enhance the production of oxidised LDL (see Fig. 3.51) and are important independent risk factors for coronary disease.
- *Mental stress.* There is very little evidence to support the popular view that stress causes coronary heart disease; however, there is no doubt that stress can aggravate the symptoms of established heart disease.

Strategies for the prevention of coronary disease

Primary prevention

Two complementary strategies can be used to prevent coronary disease in apparently healthy but at-risk individuals. The *population strategy* aims to modify the risk factors of the whole population through diet and lifestyle advice on the basis that even a small reduction in smoking, average cholesterol etc. will produce substantial benefits. In contrast, the *targeted strategy* aims to identify and treat high-risk individuals, who usually have a combination of risk factors and can be identified by using composite scoring systems. However, these individuals are relatively few in number and constitute only a small proportion of those who will ultimately develop coronary disease.

Some reasonable public health advice is summarised in the information box.

POPULATION ADVICE TO PREVENT CORONARY DISEASE

- Do not smoke
- Take regular exercise
- Maintain 'ideal' body weight
- Eat a mixed diet rich in fresh fruit and vegetables
- Aim to get no more than 30% of energy intake from fat

Secondary prevention

There is strong and compelling evidence that the correction of risk factors, particularly smoking and hypercholesterolaemia, will improve the outlook for most patients with established coronary or vascular disease (secondary prevention). Individuals with documented coronary artery disease have a high absolute risk of subsequent cardiac events and therefore have most to gain from preventive measures (see Table 3.8).

Table 3.8 Examples of the benefits of long-term secondary prevention following myocardial infarction

Preventive measure	Events prevented per 1000 patient years of treatment
Smoking cessation	15 deaths 46 non-fatal myocardial infarctions (MIs)
Aspirin	7 deaths 9 non-fatal MIs 9 non-fatal strokes
β-adrenoceptor antagonist	21 deaths 21 non-fatal MIs
Statins (HMG CoA reductase inhibitors)	7 deaths 12 non-fatal MIs 3 non-fatal strokes 11 revascularisations 4 cases of heart failure

N.B. Even in a high-risk primary prevention population (the West of Scotland Study), four times as many people needed to be treated with a lipid-lowering agent to prevent a cardiac event compared to secondary prevention.

Many clinical events offer an unrivalled opportunity to introduce effective secondary preventive measures. For example, patients who have just survived a myocardial infarction or undergone a major procedure such as coronary artery bypass grafting are usually keen to help themselves and may be particularly receptive to appropriate lifestyle advice.

MYOCARDIAL ISCHAEMIA

ANGINA PECTORIS

Angina pectoris is the term used to describe discomfort due to transient myocardial ischaemia and constitutes a clinical syndrome rather than a disease; it may occur whenever there is an imbalance between myocardial oxygen supply and demand (see the information box).

FACTORS INFLUENCING MYOCARDIAL OXYGEN SUPPLY AND DEMAND

Oxygen demand	Oxygen supply
Cardiac work • Heart rate • Blood pressure • Myocardial contractility	Coronary blood flow* • Duration of diastole • Coronary perfusion pressure (aortic diastolic coronary sinus or right atrial diastolic pressure) • Coronary vasomotor tone Oxygenation • Haemoglobin • Oxygen saturation

* **N.B.** Coronary blood flow occurs mainly in diastole.

Coronary atheroma is by far the most common cause but angina is also a feature of aortic valve disease, hypertrophic cardiomyopathy and some other forms of heart disease.

Clinical features

The history is by far the most important factor in making the diagnosis. Stable angina is characterised typically by central chest pain that is precipitated by exertion and promptly relieved by rest.

Most patients describe a sense of oppression or tightness in the chest—'like a band round the chest'; 'pain' may be denied. When describing angina the victim often closes a hand around the throat, puts a hand or clenched fist on the sternum, or places both hands across the lower chest. The term 'angina' is derived from the Greek word for strangulation and many patients report a 'choking' sensation. Breathlessness is sometimes a prominent feature.

The pain may radiate to the neck or jaw and is often accompanied by discomfort in the arms, particularly the left, the wrists and sometimes the hands; the patient may also describe a feeling of heaviness or uselessness in the arms (referred pain). Occasionally the pain is epigastric or interscapular. Angina may occur at any of these places of reference without chest discomfort but a history of precipitation by effort, and relief by rest or sublingual nitrate, should still allow the condition to be recognised.

Symptoms tend to be worse after a meal, in the cold, and when walking uphill or into a strong wind (peripheral vasoconstriction, increased oxygen demand). Some patients find that the pain comes when they start walking and that later it does not return despite greater effort ('start-up angina'). Some experience the pain when lying flat (decubitus angina), and some are awakened by it (nocturnal angina).

Angina may also occur capriciously as a result of coronary arterial spasm; occasionally this is accompanied

CLINICAL SITUATIONS PRECIPITATING ANGINA
Common
• Physical exertion • Cold exposure • Heavy meals • Intense emotion
Rare
• Lying flat (decubitus angina) • Vivid dreams (nocturnal angina)

by transient ST elevation on the ECG (Prinzmetal's or variant angina).

Physical examination is frequently negative, but should include a careful search for evidence of:

- *important risk factors*—e.g. nicotine stains, hypertension, hyperlipidaemia (tendon xanthomas, thickening of the Achilles tendons, arcus lipidis etc.), diabetes, myxoedema
- *contributory disease*—e.g. obesity, anaemia, thyrotoxicosis, aortic valve disease
- *left ventricular dysfunction*—e.g. gallop rhythm, cardiomegaly, basal crackles, elevated venous pressure
- *generalised arterial disease*—e.g. carotid bruits, peripheral vascular disease.

Differential diagnosis

This includes musculoskeletal, pericardial and oesophageal pain. Musculoskeletal pains are provoked by specific movement rather than by walking, and background pain often persists at rest; there may be associated chest wall tenderness. The pain of pericarditis is provoked by changes in posture or deep inspiration. Angina occurring at rest may be confused with oesophagitis, with or without a hiatus hernia, but pain due to oesophagitis usually has a burning quality and is relieved by antacids. Oesophageal spasm, however, may cause a different type of pain which is difficult to distinguish from variant angina.

Investigations

Resting ECG

The ECG may show evidence of previous myocardial infarction but is normal in most patients. Occasionally there is T wave flattening or inversion in some leads, providing non-specific evidence of myocardial ischaemia or damage.

The most convincing ECG evidence of myocardial ischaemia is obtained by demonstrating reversible ST segment depression or elevation, with or without T wave inversion, at the time the patient is experiencing symptoms (whether spontaneous or induced by exercise testing).

Exercise ECG

A formal exercise tolerance test (ETT) is usually performed using a standard treadmill or bicycle ergometer protocol to ensure a progressive and reproducible increase in workload while monitoring the patient's ECG (preferably all 12 leads), blood pressure and general condition. Resuscitation facilities must be available and the test should be stopped if the patient develops significant chest pain or discomfort, a serious arrhythmia, a fall in blood pressure or marked ST segment changes. Planar or downsloping ST segment depression of 1 mm or more is indicative of ischaemia (see Fig. 3.52); upsloping ST depression is less specific and often occurs in normal individuals.

Exercise testing can be used to confirm or refute a diagnosis of angina and is also a useful means of assessing the severity of coronary disease and identifying high-risk individuals (see Table 3.9). For example, the amount of exercise which can be tolerated and the extent and degree of any ST segment change (see Fig. 3.53) provide a useful guide to the likely extent of coronary disease.

Exercise testing is not infallible and may produce false positive results in the presence of digoxin therapy, left ventricular hypertrophy, left bundle branch block or Wolff–Parkinson–White syndrome. The predictive accuracy of exercise testing is lower in women than men.

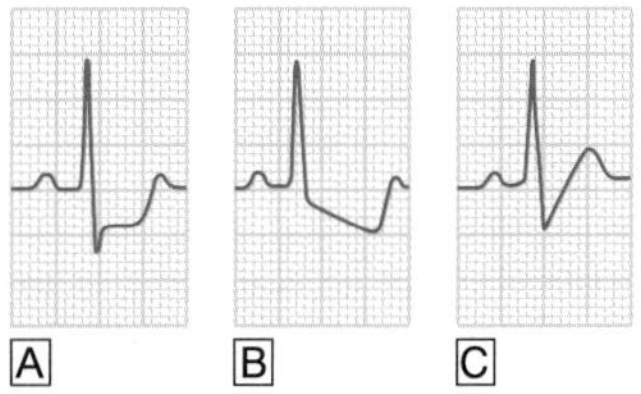

Fig. 3.52 Forms of exercise-induced ST depression. A Planar ST depression is usually indicative of myocardial ischaemia. B Downsloping depression also usually indicates myocardial ischaemia. C Upsloping depression, however, may be a normal finding.

Table 3.9 A guide to risk stratification in angina	
High risk	**Low risk**
Unstable angina Post-infarct angina	Predictable exertional angina
Poor effort tolerance	Good effort tolerance
Ischaemia at low workload (ETT)	Ischaemia only at high workload (ETT)
Left main or three-vessel disease	Single-vessel or minor two-vessel disease
Poor LV function	Good LV function
N.B. Patients may fall between these categories.	

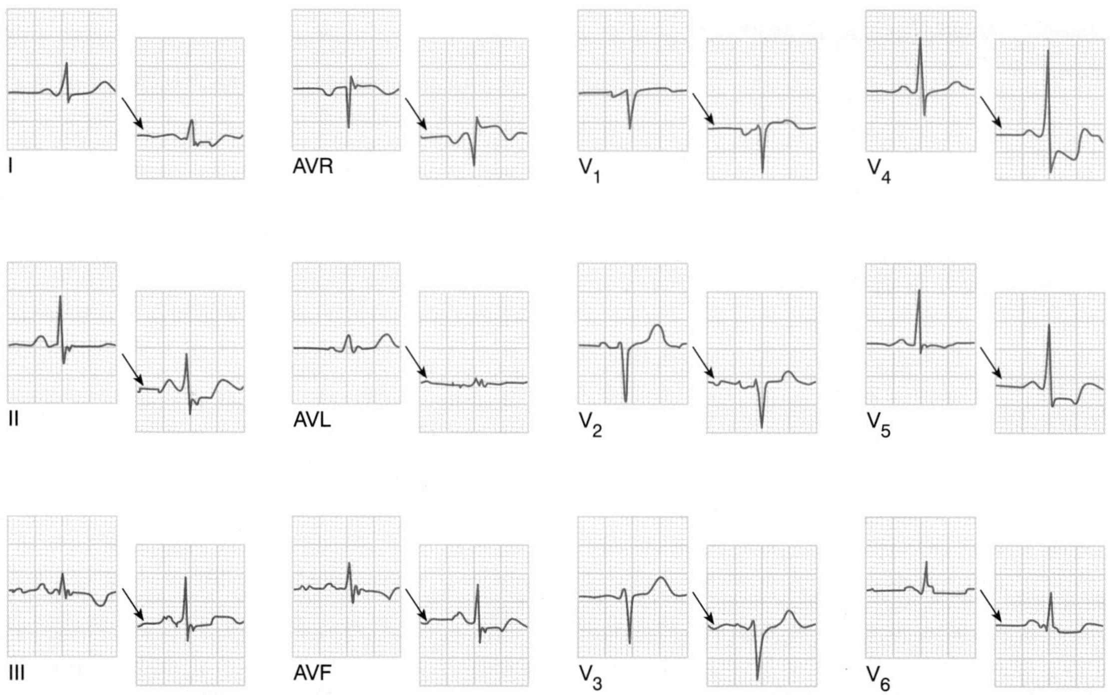

Fig. 3.53 A positive exercise test. The resting 12-lead ECG shows some minor T wave changes in the inferolateral leads but is otherwise normal. After 3 minutes' exercise on a treadmill there is marked planar ST depression in leads II, V_4 and V_5 (right offset). Subsequent coronary angiography revealed critical three-vessel coronary artery disease.

Isotope scanning

Myocardial perfusion scanning may be helpful in the evaluation of patients with an equivocal or uninterpretable exercise test and those who are unable to exercise; its predictive accuracy is higher than that of the exercise ECG. The technique involves obtaining scintiscans of the myocardium at rest and during stress after the administration of an intravenous radioactive isotope such as thallium 201 (^{201}Tl); it may be used in conjunction with conventional exercise testing or some form of pharmacological stress such as a controlled infusion of dobutamine. Thallium is an analogue of potassium and is taken up by viable perfused myocardium. A perfusion defect present during stress but not rest provides evidence of reversible myocardial ischaemia (see Fig. 3.54), whereas a persistent perfusion defect seen during both phases of the study is usually indicative of previous myocardial infarction.

Ventricular function can be measured by radionuclide blood pool scanning or echocardiography.

Coronary arteriography

This provides detailed information about the extent and nature of coronary artery disease (see Fig. 3.55) and is usually performed with a view to coronary bypass grafting or angioplasty (see p. 253). In some patients, diagnostic coronary angiography may be indicated when non-invasive tests have failed to elucidate the cause of atypical chest pain.

Management

The management of angina pectoris involves:

- a careful assessment of the likely extent and severity of arterial disease and any contributory factors
- the identification of high-risk patients
- the identification and control of significant risk factors (e.g. smoking, hypertension, hyperlipidaemia—see Secondary prevention above)
- the use of measures to control symptoms
- treatment to improve life expectancy.

Symptoms alone are a poor guide to the extent of coronary artery disease; exercise testing is therefore advisable in all patients who are potential candidates for revascularisation. A schema for the investigation and treatment of patients with angina is illustrated in the algorithm (see Fig. 3.56).

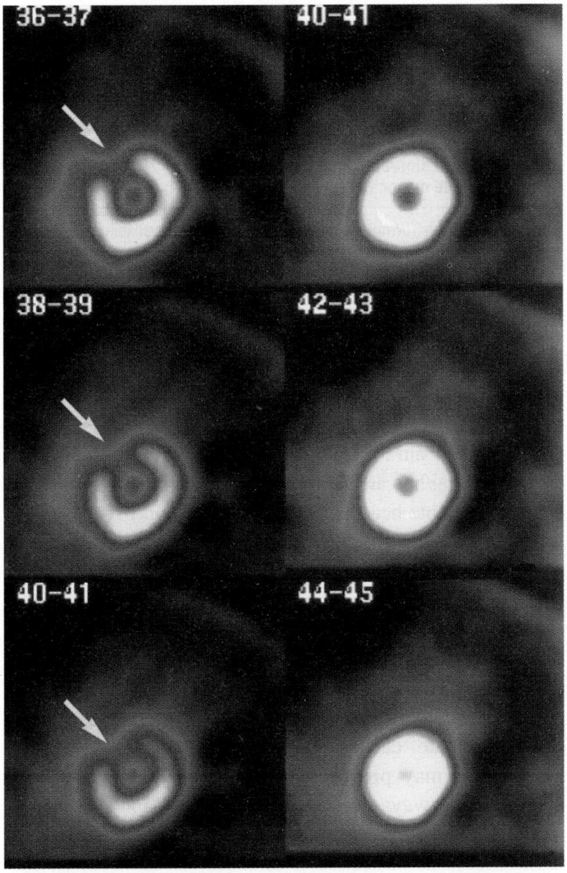

Fig. 3.54 A thallium scan showing reversible anterior myocardial ischaemia. The images are cross-sectional tomograms of the left ventricle. The resting scans (right) show even uptake of thallium and look like doughnuts; during stress (in this case a dobutamine infusion) there is reduced uptake of thallium, particularly along the anterior wall (arrows), and the scans look like crescents (left). Subsequent angiography showed a severe stenosis in the left anterior descending coronary artery (see Fig. 3.55).

ADVICE TO PATIENTS WITH ANGINA

- Do not smoke
- Aim at ideal body weight
- Take regular exercise (Exercise up to, but not beyond, the point of chest pain is beneficial and may promote collateral vessels.)
- Avoid severe unaccustomed exertion, and vigorous exercise after a heavy meal or in very cold weather
- Take sublingual nitrate before undertaking exertion that may induce angina

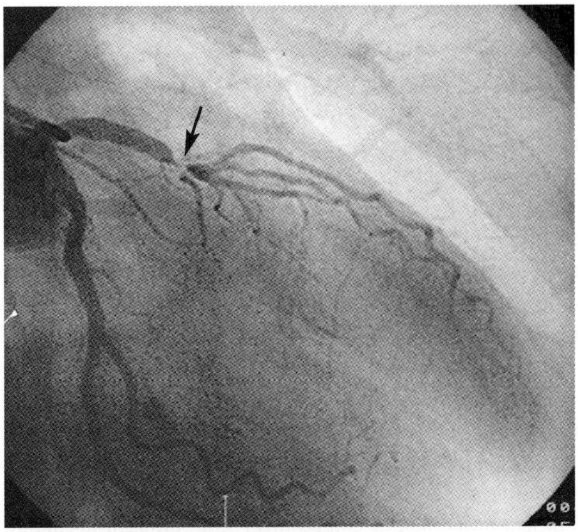

Fig. 3.55 Coronary angiogram from the patient with stable angina whose thallium scan is shown in Figure 3.54. There is a severe stenosis (arrow) of the left anterior descending coronary artery.

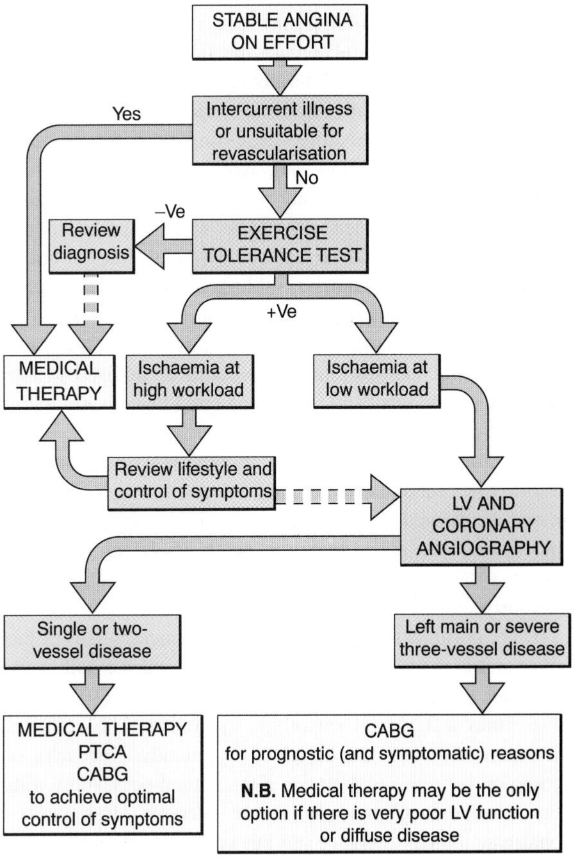

Fig. 3.56 A schema for the investigation and treatment of stable angina on effort. A myocardial perfusion scan can be used instead of an ETT in patients who cannot perform an exercise test. (PTCA = percutaneous transluminal coronary angioplasty; CABG = coronary artery bypass grafting)

The control of symptoms should start with an explanation of how they are caused. Most patients respond to a careful presentation of the problem emphasising the prospect of spontaneous improvement due to collateral development and can learn to help themselves by avoiding undue exertion and by using prophylactic sublingual nitrates.

Aspirin

Low-dose (75–300 mg) aspirin reduces the risk of adverse events such as myocardial infarction and should be prescribed for all patients with coronary artery disease indefinitely unless it causes troublesome dyspepsia or other side-effects.

Anti-anginal drug treatment

Four groups of drugs are used to help relieve or prevent the symptoms of angina: nitrates, β-adrenoceptor antagonists (β-blockers), calcium antagonists and potassium-channel activators.

Nitrates. These drugs act directly on vascular smooth muscle to produce venous and arteriolar dilatation; their beneficial effects in angina are due to a reduction in myocardial oxygen demand (lower preload and afterload) and an increase in myocardial oxygen supply (coronary vasodilatation).

Sublingual glyceryl trinitrate (GTN) administered from a metered-dose aerosol (400 μg per spray) or as a tablet (300 or 500 μg) allowed to dissolve under the tongue or crunched and retained in the mouth, will usually relieve an attack of angina in 2–3 minutes. Unwanted side-effects include headache (which may be more distressing than the angina), symptomatic hypotension and, rarely, syncope. To avoid these symptoms the tablet may be spat out as soon as angina is relieved. GTN tablets deteriorate when exposed to the atmosphere and should be replaced 8 weeks after the bottle has been opened; in contrast, sublingual nitrate sprays have a long shelf-life and can be used for many years.

Patients often need to be reassured that GTN is not dangerous or habit-forming and should be advised to use the drug prophylactically before engaging in exercise that is liable to provoke pain.

As sublingual GTN has a short duration of action (see Table 3.10), there has been much interest in ways of giving more prolonged nitrate therapy. GTN can be given percutaneously as a paste or patch (5–10 mg once or twice a day), or as a slow-release buccal tablet (1–5 mg 6-hourly).

GTN is subject to extensive first-pass metabolism in the liver and is therefore virtually ineffective when swallowed; however, other nitrates such as isosorbide dinitrate (10–20 mg, 3–6 times a day) and isosorbide mononitrate (20–60 mg, 1–3 times a day) can be given by mouth. Headache is common but tends to diminish if the patient perseveres with the treatment. Continuous nitrate therapy often causes pharmacological tolerance but this can be avoided by using a regimen that includes a nitrate-free period of 6–8 hours every day. A variety of once-daily proprietary preparations with a built-in nitrate-free period are available; it is usually best to schedule the medication so that drug levels are low during the night when the patient is inactive.

Table 3.10 Duration of action of some nitrate preparations

Preparation	Peak action	Duration of action
Sublingual GTN	4–8 mins	10–30 mins
Buccal GTN	4–10 mins	30–300 mins
Transdermal GTN	1–3 hrs	Up to 24 hrs
Oral isosorbide dinitrate	45–120 mins	2–6 hrs
Oral isosorbide mononitrate	45–120 mins	6–10 hrs

N.B. Slow-release formulations of all these drugs are available.

Intravenous nitrates (nitroglycerin 0.6 mg/hr or isosorbide dinitrate 1 mg/hr) are useful in the treatment of unstable angina and acute heart failure (see pp. 208 and 1040). These drugs can be adsorbed and degraded in the giving set and should be administered through polyethylene tubing. The infusion rate must be adjusted carefully according to the clinical response.

β-adrenoceptor antagonists. These drugs lower myocardial oxygen demand by reducing heart rate, blood pressure and myocardial contractility. Unfortunately, they can exacerbate cardiac failure and peripheral vascular disease and may provoke bronchospasm in patients with obstructive airways disease. The properties and side-effects of the 'β-blockers' are discussed on pages 221 and 238.

In theory, non-selective β-adrenoceptor antagonists may aggravate coronary vasospasm by blocking the coronary artery β_2-adrenoceptors and it is usually advisable to use a once-daily cardioselective preparation (e.g. atenolol 50–100 mg daily, SR metoprolol 200 mg daily, bisoprolol 5–10 mg daily).

A β-adrenoceptor antagonist drug should not be withdrawn abruptly because this may precipitate dangerous arrhythmias, worsening angina or myocardial infarction *(the β-blocker withdrawal syndrome).*

Calcium antagonists. These drugs inhibit the slow inward current caused by the entry of extracellular calcium through the cell membrane of excitable cells, particularly cardiac and arteriolar smooth muscle, and lower myocardial oxygen demand by reducing blood pressure and myocardial contractility.

Nifedipine, nicardipine and amlodipine often cause a reflex tachycardia; this may be counterproductive and it is often best to use these drugs in combination with a β-adrenoceptor antagonist. In contrast, verapamil and diltiazem are particularly suitable for patients who are not receiving a β-blocker because they inhibit conduction through the AV node and tend to cause a bradycardia. All the calcium antagonists reduce myocardial contractility and may aggravate or precipitate heart failure. Other unwanted effects include oedema, flushing, headache and dizziness.

Table 3.11 Calcium antagonists used for the treatment of angina

Drug	Dose	Feature
Nifedipine	5–20 mg 8-hourly*	May cause marked tachycardia
Nicardipine	20–40 mg 8-hourly	May cause less myocardial depression than the other drugs in this group
Amlodipine	2.5–10 mg daily	Ultra long-acting
Verapamil	120–240 mg 8-hourly*	Commonly causes constipation; useful anti-arrhythmic properties (see p. 239)
Diltiazem	60–120 mg 8-hourly*	Similar anti-arrhythmic properties to verapamil

* Once- or twice-daily slow-release preparations are available.

The dosage and some of the distinguishing features of these drugs are listed in Table 3.11.

Potassium-channel activators. These drugs (e.g. nicorandil 10–30 mg 12-hourly orally) have arterial and venous dilating properties but do not exhibit the tolerance seen with nitrates.

Although each of these groups of drug has been shown to be superior to placebo in relieving the symptoms of angina, there is little convincing evidence that one group is more effective than another. Moreover, many commonly used combinations of anti-anginal drugs have not been evaluated in well-controlled clinical trials. Nevertheless, it is conventional to start therapy with low-dose aspirin, sublingual GTN and a β-adrenoceptor antagonist, and then add a calcium channel antagonist or a long-acting nitrate later, if necessary. The goal of controlling angina with minimal side-effects and the simplest possible drug regimen is unlikely to be reached without a degree of trial and error.

Invasive treatment

Invasive options for the treatment of ischaemic heart disease include coronary angioplasty (sometimes called PTCA, for percutaneous transluminal coronary angioplasty), reversed saphenous vein bypass grafting and internal mammary artery grafting (sometimes called CABG, for coronary artery bypass grafting).

Coronary angioplasty (PTCA)

This is performed by passing a fine guidewire across a coronary stenosis under radiographic control and using it to position a balloon which is then inflated to dilate the stenosis (see Fig. 3.57). PTCA has many applications and can be used to provide complete or partial ('culprit lesion' angioplasty) revascularisation in patients with stable angina, unstable angina or myocardial infarction.

Coronary angioplasty is an effective symptomatic treatment for chronic stable angina and is mainly used in single or two-vessel disease; there is no evidence that it improves survival. Stenoses in bypass grafts can be dilated as well as those in the native coronary arteries, and the procedure is often used to provide palliative therapy for patients with recurrent angina after CABG.

The main complication of PTCA is occlusion of the vessel by thrombus or by a loose flap of intima (coronary artery dissection). This occurs in about 2–5% of procedures and may necessitate urgent coronary bypass grafting. The risk of complications and the likely success of the procedure are closely related to the morphology of the stenosis. Short, concentric, soft lesions on a straight segment of artery are ideal for this form of treatment. On the other hand, the outcome tends to be worse if the target lesion is complex, eccentric or calcified, lies on a bend or involves an important branch of the artery.

Recurrent angina is common (32% at 6 months in one study) and may require further angioplasty or bypass grafting. Re-stenosis is due to a combination of elastic recoil and smooth muscle proliferation which tends to occur within 3 months. Low-dose aspirin therapy is beneficial but does not prevent re-stenosis.

A coronary stent (see Fig. 3.57) is a piece of coated metallic 'scaffolding' that can be deployed on a balloon and used to maximise and maintain dilatation of a stenosed vessel after PTCA. Stenting reduces the risk of re-stenosis and can be used to treat complications of PTCA such as coronary artery dissection (bail-out stenting).

Coronary artery bypass grafting

This involves major surgery under cardiopulmonary bypass. The internal mammary arteries or reversed segments of the patient's own saphenous vein are used to bypass the major coronary artery stenoses (see Fig. 3.58). In general, the operative mortality is less than 1%; however, the risk is higher in elderly patients and those with poor left ventricular function.

Approximately 90% of patients are free of angina a year after surgery but less than 60% of patients are asymptomatic 5 or more years after CABG. Early post-operative angina is usually due to graft failure arising from technical problems during the operation or poor 'run off' due to disease in the distal native coronary vessels. Late recurrence of angina may be due to progressive disease in the native coronary arteries or graft degeneration. Less than 50% of vein grafts are patent 10 years after surgery, although internal mammary artery grafts last much longer.

Low-dose aspirin (75–150 mg daily) has been shown to improve graft patency and should be prescribed indefinitely

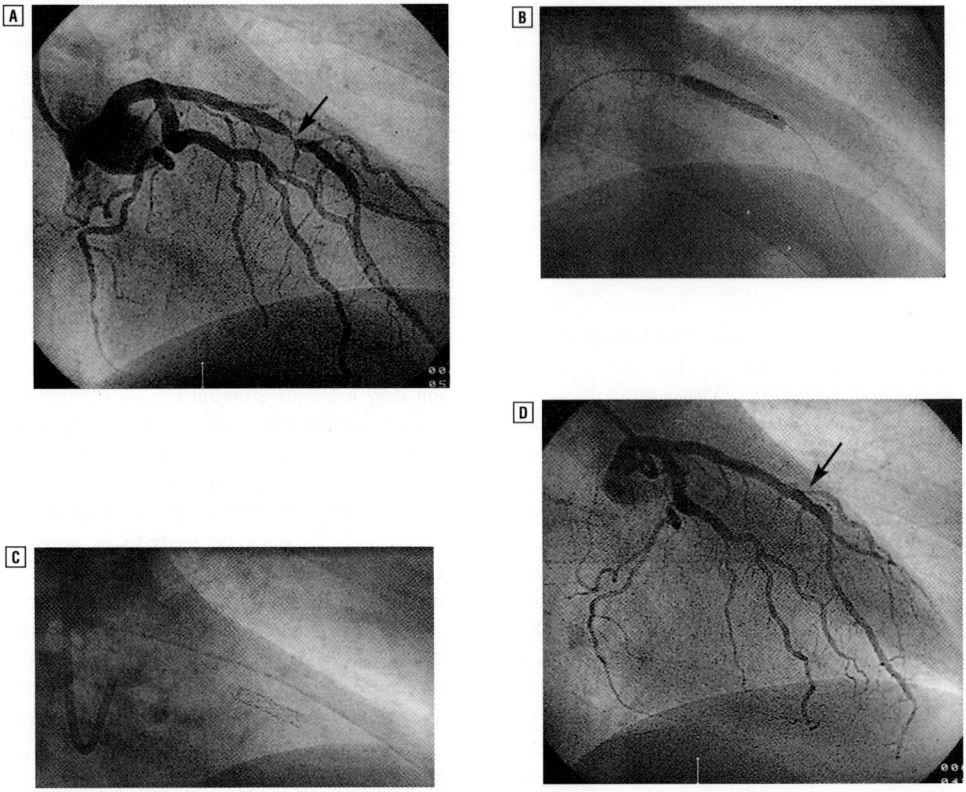

Fig. 3.57 Top: A sequence of coronary angiograms illustrating a successful angioplasty with stent insertion. A A stenosis in the left anterior descending coronary artery (arrow). B Inflation of balloon catheter with mounted stent passed into artery over a fine guidewire. C Balloon catheter has been removed showing inflated stent left in situ. D Final angiogram in focused projection showing elimination of stenosis (arrow).

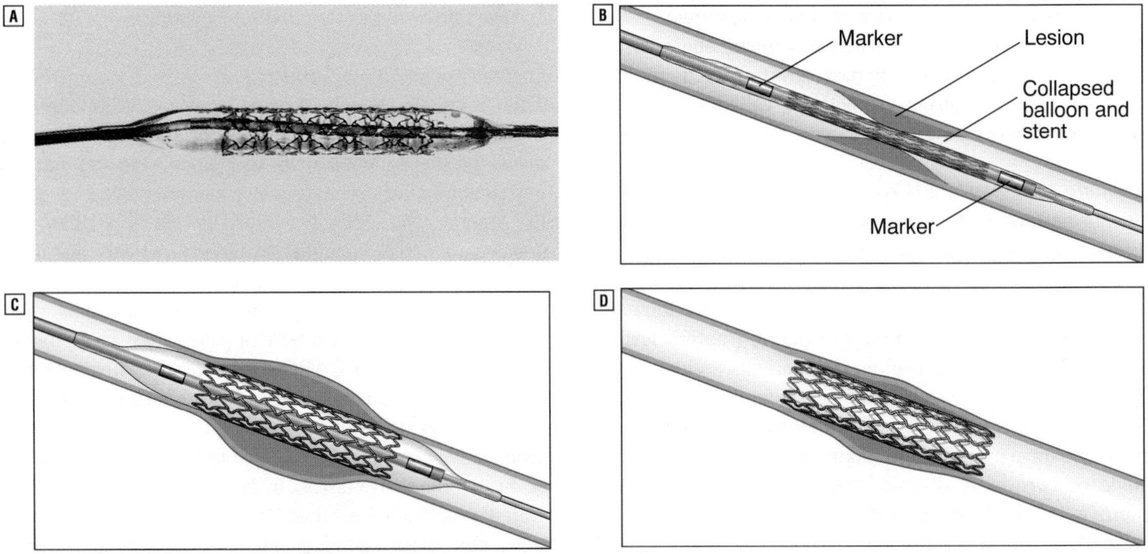

Fig. 3.57 Bottom: Photograph and schematic diagrams equivalent to sequence of angiograms above. A Photograph of stent mounted on balloon angioplasty catheter. B Balloon with mounted stent is placed across stenosis. C Balloon is inflated, stretching stent to normal size of arterial lumen. D Stent is left in place, holding open arterial lumen.

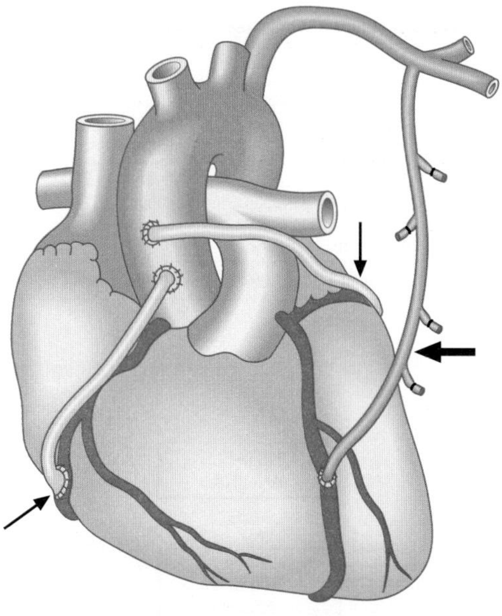

Fig. 3.58 A triple coronary artery bypass graft operation. Reversed saphenous vein grafts have been placed on the circumflex and right coronary arteries (small arrows) and the left internal mammary artery has been used to graft the left anterior descending coronary artery (arrow).

provided that it is well tolerated. Aggressive lipid-lowering therapy has also been shown to slow the progression of disease in the native coronary arteries and bypass grafts; total blood cholesterol should therefore be reduced to below 5.0 mmol/l whenever possible. There is a substantial excess cardiovascular morbidity and mortality in patients who continue to smoke after bypass grafting. Persistent smokers are twice as likely to die in the 10 years following surgery compared with those who quit at surgery.

Coronary artery bypass grafting has been shown to improve survival in patients with left main coronary stenosis, and symptomatic patients with three-vessel coronary disease (i.e. involving left anterior descending, circumflex and right coronary arteries) or two-vessel disease involving the proximal left anterior descending coronary artery. Improvement in survival is most marked in those who have undergone left internal mammary artery grafting and those with impaired left ventricular function before surgery.

Coronary angioplasty and coronary artery bypass grafting are compared in Table 3.12.

Prognosis

In general the prognosis of coronary artery disease is related to the number of diseased vessels (one-, two- or three-vessel coronary artery disease) and the degree of left ventricular dysfunction. A patient with single-vessel disease and good LV function has an excellent outlook (5-year survival > 90%), whereas a patient with severe LV dysfunction and extensive three-vessel disease has a poor prognosis (5-year survival < 30%) without revascularisation.

More than half of a group of patients with angina will live for 5 years, and a third for 10 years from the time of diagnosis. Spontaneous symptomatic improvement due to the development of collateral vessels is common.

UNSTABLE ANGINA

Unstable angina is the term used to describe patients who present with rapidly worsening angina (crescendo angina), severe angina at rest or prolonged and severe ischaemic chest pain without ECG or enzyme evidence of significant myocardial infarction. It may present as a new phenomenon or against a background of chronic stable angina.

The culprit lesion is usually a complex ulcerated or fissured atheromatous plaque with adherent platelet-rich thrombus and local coronary artery spasm (see Fig. 3.59). It is important to appreciate that coronary artery thrombosis is a dynamic process whereby the obstruction may grow by thrombosis and changes in plaque morphology, sometimes leading to complete occlusion of the vessel, or regress, sometimes only temporarily, due to the effects of platelet disaggregation endogenous thrombolysis. Episodes of myocardial ischaemia are due to an abrupt reduction in coronary blood flow caused by thrombosis or spasm

Table 3.12 Comparison between coronary angioplasty (PTCA) and coronary artery bypass grafting (CABG)

	PTCA	CABG
Principal use	Single-vessel disease; two-vessel disease; unstable angina	Left main stem stenosis; three-vessel disease
Mortality	< 1%	< 1%
Incidence of neurological complications	None	5% seldom permanent but stroke may occur
Hospital stay	24–36 hours	7–10 days
Return to work	2–5 days	2–3 months
Recurrence of angina	30% in 6 months; PTCA may be repeated	10% in 1 year, then 5% per year
Main complications	Myocardial infarction; emergency CABG; vascular damage related to the arterial puncture site	Diffuse left ventricular damage; perioperative MI; infection; wound pain

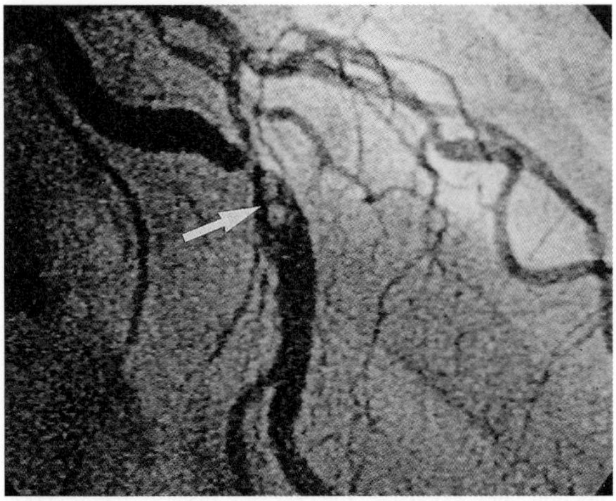

Fig. 3.59 Coronary angiogram from a patient with unstable angina. The angiogram demonstrates a complex stenosis of the circumflex coronary artery with a filling defect due to adherent thrombus (arrow).

(supply-led ischaemia). In contrast, stable angina is related to a fixed obstruction and usually precipitated by an increase in myocardial oxygen demand *(demand-led ischaemia).*

The ECG may show ST/T wave changes including ST depression, transient ST elevation and T wave inversion. The T wave changes are sometimes prolonged. Unstable angina may result in the release of specific intracellular cardiac enzymes (troponin T and I), and raised levels of such enzymes indicate an adverse prognosis.

Management

Patients should be admitted urgently to hospital because there is a 10–15% risk of death or acute myocardial infarction during the unstable phase and clinical trials have shown that appropriate medical therapy can reduce the incidence of adverse events by at least 50%.

The initial treatment should include bed rest, aspirin (75–300 mg daily), and a β-adrenoceptor antagonist (e.g. atenolol 50–100 mg daily or metoprolol 50–100 mg 12-hourly). Nifedipine can be added to the β-adrenoceptor antagonist but may cause an unwanted tachycardia if it is used alone; verapamil or diltiazem are therefore preferable if a β-adrenoceptor antagonist is contraindicated. In high-risk cases (see Table 3.13), heparin should be given either as an intravenous infusion of unfractionated heparin with dose adjusted according to the thrombin time, or as subcutaneous low molecular weight heparin (e.g. enoxaparin 1 mg/kg 12-hourly). If pain persists or recurs, infusions of intravenous nitrates (e.g. nitroglycerin 0.6–1.2 mg/hr or isosorbide dinitrate 1–2 mg/hr), or buccal nitrates may help.

Most patients respond rapidly to these measures and can be gradually mobilised. If there are no contraindications to

Table 3.13 Unstable angina: risk stratification

	High risk	Low risk
Clinical	Post-infarct angina Recurrent pain at rest Heart failure	No history of MI Rapid resolution of symptoms
ECG	ST depression Transient ST elevation Persistent deep T wave inversion	Minor or no ECG changes
Enzymes	Troponin T > 0.2 μg/ml	Troponin T < 0.2 μg/ml

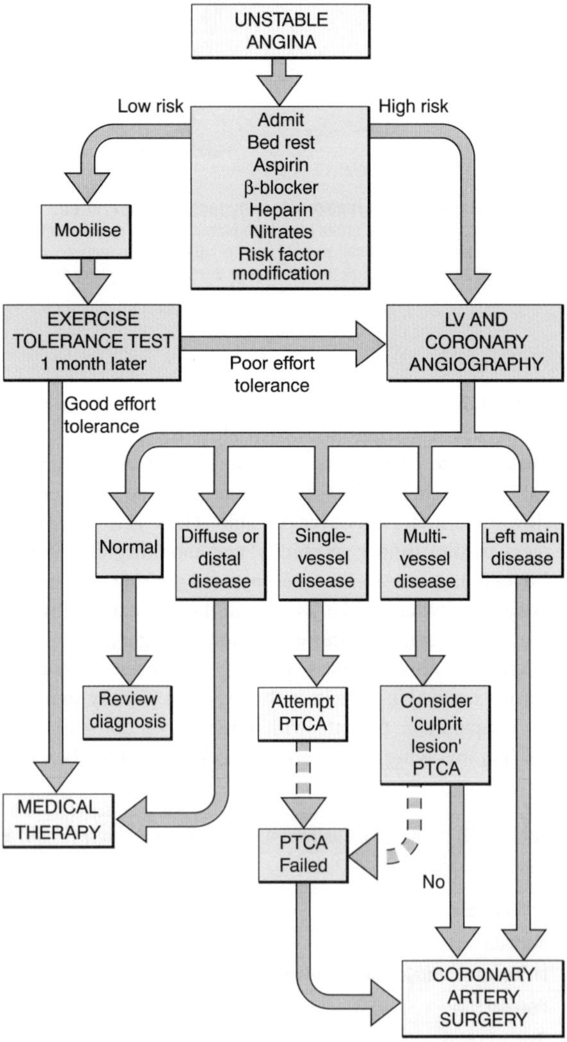

Fig. 3.60 A guide to the investigation and treatment of unstable angina. See Table 3.13 and text for identification of high- and low-risk patients.

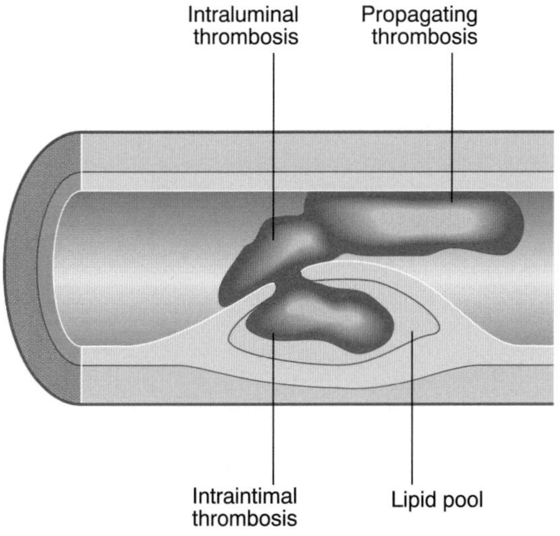

Fig. 3.61 Coronary artery thrombosis. Myocardial infarction is caused by occlusion of a coronary artery due to thrombus propagating from a ruptured atheromatous plaque.

surgery or angioplasty, exercise testing should be arranged 3–4 weeks later, when the plaque has stabilised, with a view to recommending coronary arteriography if the test is positive at a low workload.

Coronary arteriography should be considered in patients at high risk (see Table 3.13), including those who fail to settle on medical therapy, those with extensive ECG changes and those with severe pre-existing stable angina. This often shows single-vessel disease that is amenable to angioplasty. Balloon dilatation of the 'culprit lesion' may also be advisable in patients with multivessel disease. However, if the lesion is not suitable for angioplasty or there is a significant left main stem stenosis, the patient should be referred for urgent coronary artery bypass grafting.

A plan for the management of unstable angina is illustrated in Figure 3.60.

MYOCARDIAL INFARCTION

Myocardial infarction is almost always due to the formation of occlusive thrombus at the site of rupture of an atheromatous plaque in a coronary artery (see Fig. 3.61). The thrombus often undergoes spontaneous lysis over the course of the next few days, although by this time irreversible myocardial damage has occurred. Without treatment the infarct-related artery remains permanently occluded in 30% of patients. Many early deaths are due to ventricular fibrillation but in patients who survive the first few hours the outcome is largely determined by the extent of myocardial damage. The process of infarction takes at least 8 hours and therefore most patients present when it is still possible to salvage myocardium and improve outcome (see Fig. 3.62).

Clinical features

Pain is the cardinal symptom of myocardial infarction, but breathlessness, vomiting and collapse or syncope are common features. The pain occurs in the same sites as angina but is usually more severe and lasts longer; it is often described as a tightness, heaviness or constriction in the chest. At its worst the pain is one of the most severe which can be experienced and the patient's expression and pallor may vividly convey the seriousness of the situation.

Most patients are breathless and in some this is the only symptom. If syncope occurs it is usually due to an

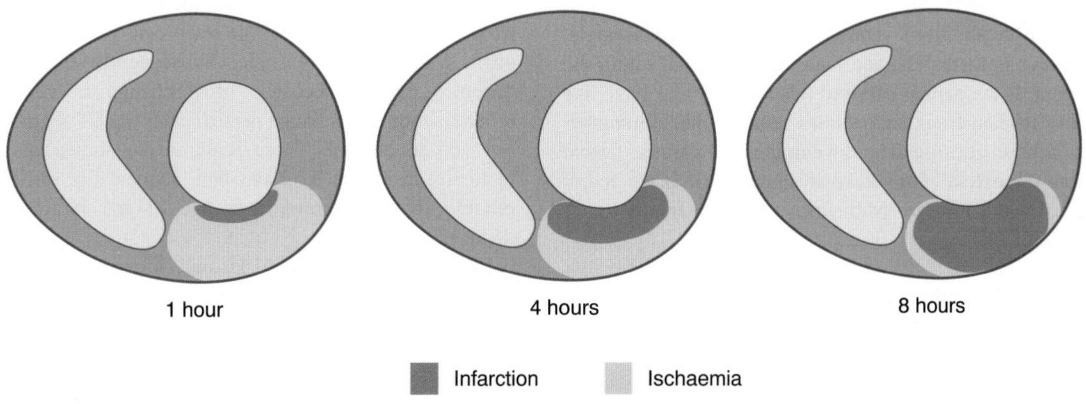

Fig. 3.62 The time course of myocardial infarction. The relative proportion of ischaemic, infarcting and infarcted tissue slowly changes over a period of 8–12 hours. In the early stages of myocardial infarction a significant proportion of the myocardium in jeopardy is potentially salvageable.

arrhythmia or profound hypotension. Vomiting and sinus bradycardia are often due to vagal stimulation and are particularly common in patients with inferior myocardial infarction. Nausea and vomiting may also be caused or aggravated by opiates given for pain relief.

Sometimes infarction occurs in the absence of physical signs.

Some myocardial infarcts pass unrecognised; these painless or 'silent' myocardial infarcts are particularly common in elderly and diabetic patients.

CLINICAL FEATURES OF MYOCARDIAL INFARCTION

Symptoms

- Prolonged cardiac pain
  Chest, throat, arms, epigastrium or back
- Anxiety
  Fear of impending death
- Nausea and vomiting
- Breathlessness
- Collapse/syncope

Physical signs

- Signs of sympathetic activation
  Pallor, sweating, tachycardia
- Signs of vagal activation
  Vomiting, bradycardia
- Signs of impaired myocardial function
  Hypotension, oliguria, cold peripheries
  Narrow pulse pressure
  Raised JVP
  Third heart sound
  Quiet first heart sound
  Diffuse apical impulse
  Lung crepitations
- Signs of tissue damage
  Fever
- Signs of complications
  e.g. Mitral regurgitation, pericarditis (see below)

Sudden death, from ventricular fibrillation or asystole, may occur immediately, and many deaths occur within the first hour. If the patient survives this most critical stage, the liability to dangerous arrhythmias remains, but diminishes as each hour goes by. The development of cardiac failure reflects the extent of myocardial damage and is the major cause of death in those who survive the first few hours of infarction.

Differential diagnosis

The differential diagnosis is wide and includes most causes of central chest pain or collapse (see p. 204).

Investigations

Electrocardiography

The ECG is usually a sensitive and specific way of confirming the diagnosis; however, it may be difficult to interpret if there is bundle branch block or evidence of previous myocardial infarction. Occasionally the initial ECG is normal and diagnostic changes appear a few hours later.

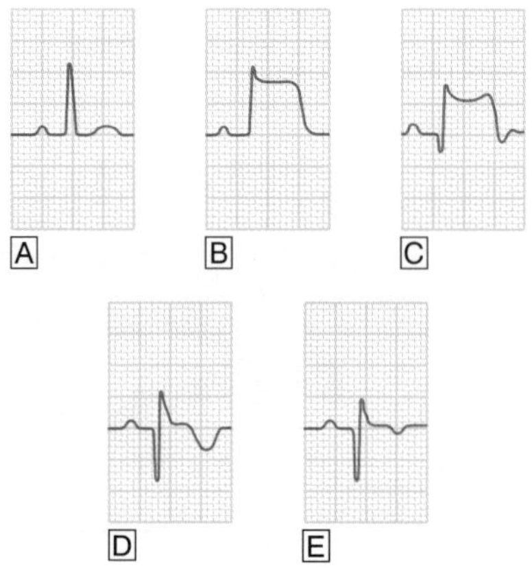

Fig. 3.63 The serial evolution of ECG changes in full thickness myocardial infarction. A Normal ECG complex. B Acute ST elevation ('the current of injury'). C Progressive loss of the R wave, developing Q wave, resolution of the ST elevation and terminal T wave inversion. D Deep Q wave and T wave inversion. E Old or established infarct pattern—the Q wave tends to persist but the T wave changes become less marked.

The rate of evolution is very variable. In general, stage B appears within minutes, stage C is within hours, stage D within days and stage E after several weeks or months. This diagrammatic representation should be compared with the actual ECGs in Figures 3.65, 3.66 and 3.67.

The earliest ECG change is usually ST elevation; later on there is diminution in the size of the R wave, and in transmural (full thickness) infarction a Q wave begins to develop. One explanation for the Q wave is that the myocardial infarct acts as an 'electrical window', transmitting the changes of potential from within the ventricular cavity, and allowing the ECG to 'see' the reciprocal R wave from the other wall of the ventricle. Subsequently the T wave becomes inverted because of a change in ventricular repolarisation; this change persists after the ST segment has returned to normal. These features are shown diagrammatically in Figure 3.63 and their sequence is sufficiently reliable for the approximate age of the infarct to be deduced.

In contrast to transmural lesions, subendocardial infarction causes ST/T wave changes (see Fig. 3.64) without Q waves or prominent ST elevation; this is often accompanied by some loss of the R waves in the leads facing the infarct.

The ECG changes are best seen in the leads which 'face' the infarcted area (see Fig. 3.6, p. 198). When there has been anteroseptal infarction, abnormalities are found in one or more leads from V_1 to V_4, while anterolateral infarction

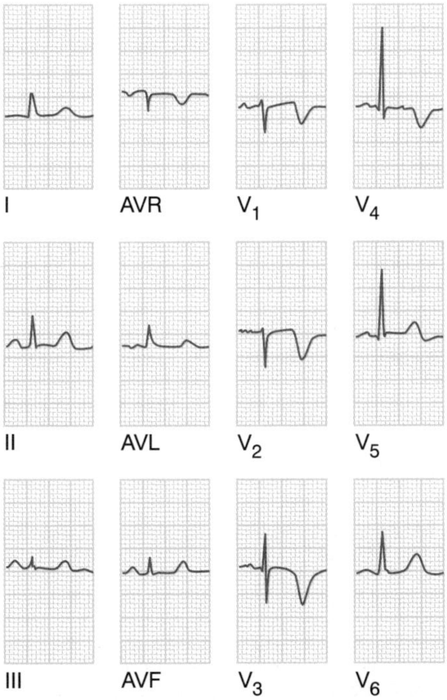

Fig. 3.64 Recent anterior subendocardial (partial thickness) infarction. There is deep symmetrical T wave inversion together with a reduction in the height of the R wave in leads V_1, V_2, V_3 and V_4.

produces changes from V_4 to V_6, in AVL and in lead I. Inferior infarction is best shown in leads II, III and AVF, while at the same time leads I, AVL and the anterior chest leads may show 'reciprocal' changes of ST depression (see Figs 3.65, 3.66 and 3.67). Infarction of the posterior wall of the left ventricle is not recorded in the standard leads by ST elevation or Q waves, but the reciprocal changes of ST depression and a tall R wave may be seen in leads V_1–V_4.

Plasma enzymes

Myocardial infarction causes a detectable rise in the plasma concentration of enzymes which are normally concentrated within cardiac cells. The enzyme most widely used in the detection of myocardial infarction is creatine kinase (CK). More sensitive and cardiospecific enzymes are CK-MB (mass assay) and troponin T and I. The troponins are

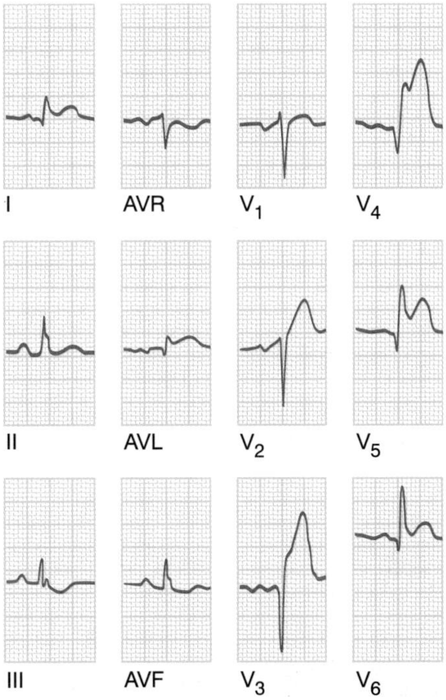

Fig. 3.65 Acute full thickness anterior myocardial infarction. This ECG was recorded from a 48-year-old man who had developed severe chest pain 6 hours earlier. There is ST elevation in leads I, AVL, V_2, V_3, V_4, V_5 and V_6, and there are Q waves in leads V_3, V_4 and V_5. Anterior infarcts with prominent changes in leads V_2, V_3 and V_4 are sometimes called 'anteroseptal' infarcts, as opposed to 'anterolateral' infarcts where the ECG changes are predominantly found in V_4, V_5 and V_6.

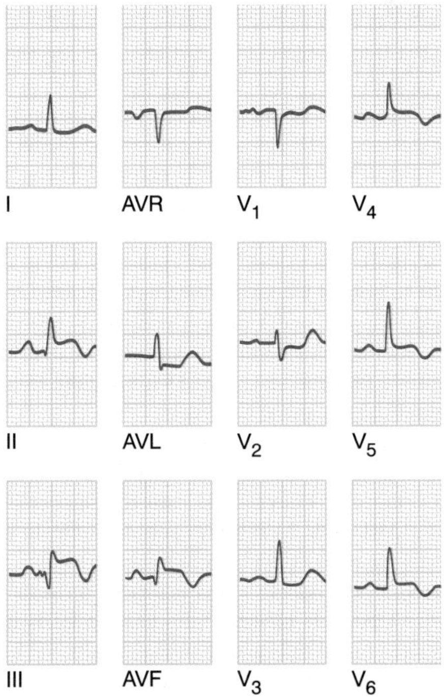

Fig. 3.66 Acute full thickness inferolateral myocardial infarction. This ECG was recorded from a 55-year-old woman who had developed severe chest pain 4 hours earlier. There is ST elevation in the inferior leads II, III and AVF and the lateral leads V_4, V_5 and V_6. There is also 'reciprocal' ST depression in leads AVL and V_2.

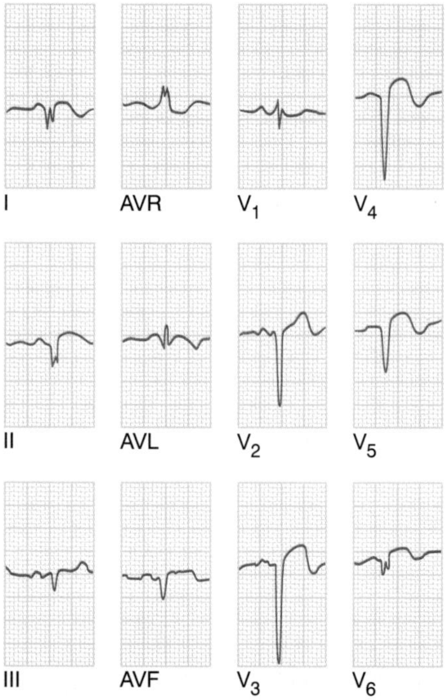

Fig. 3.67 Established anterior and inferior full thickness infarction. This ECG was recorded from a 70-year-old man who had presented with an acute anterior infarct 2 days earlier and had been treated for an inferior myocardial infarct 11 months before then. There are Q waves in the inferior leads (II, III and AVF) and Q waves with some residual ST elevation in the anterior leads (I and V_2–V_6).

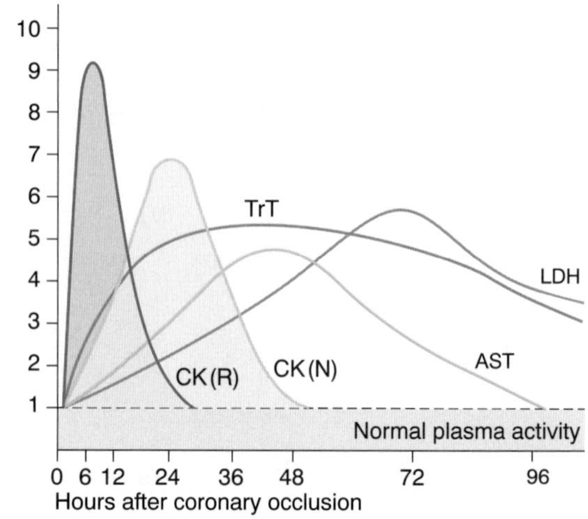

Fig. 3.68 Changes in plasma enzyme concentrations after myocardial infarction. Creatine kinase (CK) and troponin T (TrT) are the first to rise, followed by aspartate aminotransferase (AST) and then lactate (hydroxybutyrate) dehydrogenase (LDH). In patients treated with a thrombolytic agent reperfusion is usually accompanied by a rapid rise in plasma creatine kinase (curve CK (R)) due to a washout effect; if there is no reperfusion, the rise is less rapid but the area under the curve is often greater (curve CK (N)).

released within hours and remain elevated for at least 36 hours; they are also released, to a minor degree, in unstable angina. Aspartate aminotransferase (AST) and lactate dehydrogenase (LDH) can also be measured. Serial (usually daily) estimations are particularly helpful because it is the change in enzyme levels which is of diagnostic value (see Fig. 3.68).

CK starts to rise at 4–6 hours, peaks at about 12 hours and falls to normal within 48–72 hours. CK is also present in skeletal muscle, and a modest rise in CK (but not CK-MB) may sometimes be due to an intramuscular injection or vigorous physical exercise. Defibrillation causes significant release of cardiac enzymes.

AST starts to rise about 12 hours after infarction and reaches a peak on the first or second day, returning to normal within 3 or 4 days. LDH starts to rise after 12 hours, reaches a peak after 2 or 3 days and may remain elevated for a week or more (see Fig. 3.68); measurements of LDH are therefore appropriate when a patient presents several days after a possible infarct. Unfortunately, LDH is highly concentrated in red cells and abnormal results can be due to very mild haemolysis.

Other blood tests

A leucocytosis is usual, reaching a peak on the first day. The erythrocyte sedimentation rate becomes raised and may remain so for several days.

Chest radiography

This may demonstrate pulmonary oedema which is not evident on clinical examination (see Fig. 3.16, p. 209). The heart size is often normal but there may be cardiomegaly due to previous myocardial damage, coexisting cardiac disease or a pericardial effusion.

Cardiac ultrasound

Echocardiography can be performed at the bedside and is an invaluable technique for assessing left and right ventricular function and detecting important complications such as cardiac rupture, ventricular septal defect, mitral regurgitation and pericardial effusion.

Radionuclide scanning

A radionuclide ventriculogram (p. 204) can be used to assess left ventricular function and may provide useful prognostic information.

Early management

The earlier a patient with suspected acute myocardial infarction is brought within reach of a defibrillator, the better. In the UK most front-line ambulances are equipped with a semi-automatic advisory defibrillator. A patient with severe chest pain also requires urgent medical assessment and analgesia, so it is often appropriate to summon an ambulance and a general practitioner at the same time.

In general, all patients with suspected myocardial infarction should be admitted to hospital for further observation and monitoring. However, an exception may be made if the patient has a terminal illness or serious concomitant disease.

The essentials of the immediate management of acute myocardial infarction are listed in the information box.

EARLY MANAGEMENT OF ACUTE MYOCARDIAL INFARCTION

- Provide facilities for defibrillation
- Bed rest
- Oral aspirin
- High-flow oxygen
- I.v. access
- I.v. analgesia with opiates
- I.v. antiemetic
- Consider thrombolysis with i.v. streptokinase or alteplase
- Consider i.v. β-adrenoceptor antagonist
- Monitor ECG
- Detect and treat complications early

Patients are usually treated in a dedicated coronary care unit because this offers a convenient way of concentrating the necessary expertise, monitoring and resuscitation facilities. If there are no complications, the patient can be mobilised from the second day and discharged from hospital on the sixth or seventh day.

Analgesia

Intravenous opiates (initially morphine sulphate 10 mg or diamorphine 5 mg) and antiemetics (initially cyclizine 50 mg or prochlorperazine 12.5 mg) should be administered through an intravenous cannula and titrated against the response by giving repeated small aliquots until the patient is comfortable.

Intramuscular injections should be avoided because the clinical effect may be delayed by poor skeletal muscle perfusion and a painful haematoma may form following thrombolytic therapy.

Aspirin

Oral administration of 75–300 mg aspirin daily improves survival (30% reduction in short-term mortality) on its own, and enhances the effect of thrombolytic therapy. The first tablet (300 mg) should be given in a soluble or chewable form and the therapy should be continued indefinitely if there are no unwanted effects.

Thrombolytic drugs

Coronary thrombolysis helps restore coronary patency (see Fig. 3.69), preserves left ventricular function, and improves survival. Successful thrombolysis leads to reperfusion with relief of pain, resolution of acute ECG changes and sometimes transient arrhythmias. The sooner the patient is treated, the better the results will be; any delay will only increase the extent of myocardial damage—'minutes mean muscle'.

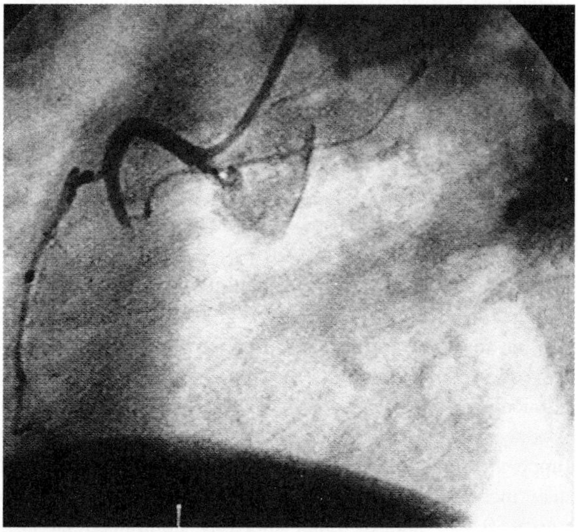

A

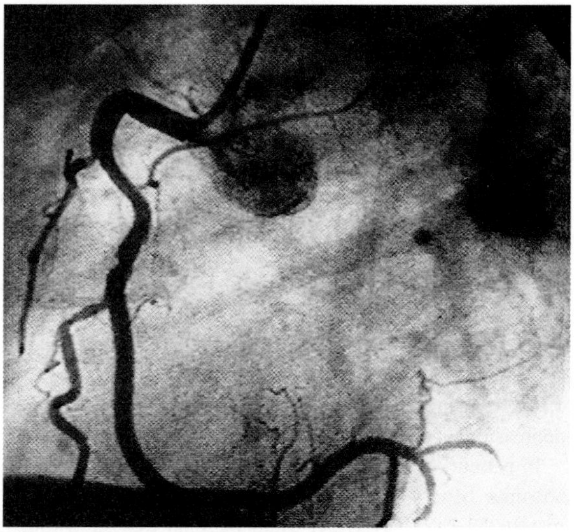

B

Fig. 3.69 Coronary angiograms from a patient with acute inferior myocardial infarction. A Complete occlusion of the proximal right coronary artery. B Appearance of the right coronary artery following successful thrombolytic therapy.

Clinical trials have shown that the appropriate use of these drugs can reduce the hospital mortality of myocardial infarction by between 25% and 50%. (Short-term mortality was reduced from 13% to 8% in the ISIS-2 trial.) Follow-up studies have demonstrated that this survival advantage is maintained for at least 8 years. The benefit is greatest in those patients who receive treatment within the first few hours, and the choice of agent is less important than the speed of treatment.

Streptokinase, 1.5 million units in 100 ml of saline given as an intravenous infusion over 1 hour, is a widely used regimen. Streptokinase is relatively cheap (approximately £60–£80 per dose in the UK) but is antigenic and occasionally causes serious allergic manifestations. The drug may also cause hypotension, which can often be managed by stopping and restarting the infusion at a slower rate. Circulating neutralising antibodies are formed following treatment with streptokinase and may persist for 5 years or more. These antibodies can render subsequent infusions of streptokinase ineffective so it is advisable to use another agent if the patient requires further thrombolysis in the next few years.

Alteplase (human tissue plasminogen activator or tPA) is a genetically engineered drug and is approximately 10 times more expensive than streptokinase; it is not antigenic and seldom causes hypotension. The standard regimen is given over 90 minutes (bolus dose of 15 mg, followed by 0.75 mg/kg of body weight, but not exceeding 50 mg, over 30 minutes and then 0.5 mg/kg body weight, but not exceeding 35 mg, over 60 minutes). As it is so expensive many units only use tPA if streptokinase is contraindicated by virtue of allergy, previous exposure, or profound hypotension. However, there is evidence that the drug may produce slightly better survival rates than streptokinase, particularly among high-risk patients.

An overview of all the large randomised trials confirms that thrombolytic therapy significantly reduces short-term mortality in patients with suspected myocardial infarction if it is given *within 12 hours* of the onset of symptoms and the ECG shows *bundle branch block* or *characteristic ST segment elevation* of greater than 1 mm in the limb leads or 2 mm in the chest leads. In contrast, thrombolysis appears to be of little net benefit in other patient groups, specifically those who present more than 12 hours after the onset of symptoms and those with a normal ECG or ST depression.

In patients with ST elevation or bundle branch block the absolute benefit of thrombolysis plus aspirin is approximately 50 lives saved per 1000 patients treated within 6 hours and 40 lives saved per 1000 patients treated between 7 and 12 hours after the onset of symptoms.

The major hazard of thrombolytic therapy is bleeding. Cerebral haemorrhage causes 4 extra strokes per 1000 patients treated and the incidence of other major bleeds is between 0.5% and 1%. Accordingly, it may be wise to withhold the treatment if there is a significant risk of serious bleeding. Some potential contraindications to thrombolytic therapy are outlined in the information box.

RELATIVE CONTRAINDICATIONS TO THROMBOLYTIC THERAPY (POTENTIAL CANDIDATES FOR PRIMARY ANGIOPLASTY)

- Active internal bleeding
- Previous subarachnoid or intracerebral haemorrhage
- Uncontrolled hypertension
- Recent surgery (within 1 month)
- Recent trauma (including traumatic resuscitation)
- High probability of active peptic ulcer
- Pregnancy

The potential benefits and risks of thrombolytic therapy must be assessed in every case. For example, it would be reasonable to give thrombolytic therapy to a patient who presents early with evidence of extensive anterior infarction despite a history of peptic ulceration; on the other hand, the risks of thrombolysis would probably exceed the benefits in a patient with a similar history of peptic ulceration who presents late with evidence of limited inferior myocardial infarction.

Angioplasty

Immediate or *primary* angioplasty (without thrombolysis) of the infarct-related coronary artery is a relatively safe and effective alternative to thrombolytic therapy. This form of treatment is particularly suitable for patients in whom the hazards of thrombolysis are high, but it is only available in centres where the appropriate facilities and expertise are available.

Although *rescue* angioplasty is sometimes undertaken in patients who do not respond to thrombolytic therapy, the benefits of this form of treatment are not well established at the present time.

Anticoagulants

Subcutaneous heparin (12 500 units twice daily for 7 days or until discharge from hospital), given in addition to oral aspirin, may prevent reinfarction after successful thrombolysis and reduce the risk of thromboembolic complications. Clinical trials have shown that this form of therapy produces a small reduction in short-term mortality (approximately 5 lives saved per 1000 patients treated) but also increases the risk of cerebral haemorrhage (0.56% versus 0.4%) and of other bleeding complications (1% versus 0.8%).

A period of treatment with warfarin should be considered if there is persistent atrial fibrillation, evidence of extensive anterior infarction, or if echocardiography shows mobile mural thrombus, because these patients are at increased risk of systemic thromboembolism.

β-adrenoceptor antagonists

Acute β-adrenoceptor antagonist use with intravenous atenolol (5–10 mg given over 5 minutes) or metoprolol (5–15 mg given over 5 minutes) relieves pain, reduces arrhythmias and improves short-term mortality in patients who present within 12 hours of the onset of symptoms, but should be avoided if there is heart failure, heart block or severe bradycardia. Chronic β-adrenoceptor antagonist therapy improves long-term survival, and should be given to all patients who can tolerate it.

Nitrates and other agents

Sublingual glyceryl trinitrate (300–500 μg) is a valuable first-aid measure in threatened infarction, and intravenous nitrates (nitroglycerin 0.6–1.2 mg/hour or isosorbide dinitrate 1–2 mg/hour) are useful for the treatment of left ventricular failure and the relief of recurrent or persistent ischaemic pain.

Large-scale trials have shown that there is no evidence of a survival advantage from the routine use of oral nitrate therapy, oral calcium antagonists or intravenous magnesium in patients with acute myocardial infarction.

Complications of infarction

Arrhythmias

Nearly all patients with acute myocardial infarction have some form of arrhythmia; in many cases this is mild and of no haemodynamic or prognostic significance. Various degrees of heart block (see pp. 241–243) are also common. Some common arrhythmias are listed in the information box; the diagnosis and management of these arrhythmias are discussed in detail on pages 227–245.

Pain relief, rest, reassurance and the correction of hypokalaemia can all play a major role in the prevention of arrhythmias.

Ventricular fibrillation. This occurs in about 5–10% of patients who reach hospital, and is thought to be the major cause of death in those who die before receiving medical attention. Prompt defibrillation will usually restore sinus rhythm. Moreover, the prognosis of patients who are successfully resuscitated in this way is identical to the prognosis of patients with acute myocardial infarction that is not complicated by ventricular fibrillation. The need to recognise and treat ventricular fibrillation quickly is one of the main foundations on which the policy of acute coronary care is built.

COMMON ARRHYTHMIAS IN ACUTE MYOCARDIAL INFARCTION

- Ventricular fibrillation
- Ventricular tachycardia
- Accelerated idioventricular rhythm
- Ventricular ectopics
- Atrial fibrillation
- Atrial tachycardia
- Sinus bradycardia (particularly after inferior MI)
- Heart block

Atrial fibrillation. This is common, frequently transient, and may not require treatment. However, if the arrhythmia causes a rapid ventricular rate with severe hypotension or circulatory collapse, cardioversion by means of an immediate synchronised DC shock should be considered. In other situations digoxin (see p. 239) is usually the treatment of choice. Atrial fibrillation (due to acute atrial stretch) is often a feature of impending or overt left ventricular failure and therapy may be ineffective if heart failure is not recognised and treated appropriately. Anticoagulation may be required.

Sinus bradycardia. This does not usually require treatment, but if there is hypotension or haemodynamic deterioration, atropine (0.6 mg intravenously) may be given.

Heart block (see section on AV block complicating acute myocardial infarction, p. 242). Heart block complicating *inferior* infarction is usually temporary and often resolves following thrombolytic therapy; it may also respond to atropine (0.6 mg intravenously repeated as necessary). However, if there is clinical deterioration due to second-degree or complete heart block, a temporary pacemaker should be considered. Heart block complicating *anterior* infarction is more serious, because asystole may suddenly supervene, and constitutes an indication for the insertion of a prophylactic temporary pacemaker (see p. 244).

Ischaemia

Post-infarct angina occurs in up to 50% of patients. Most patients have a residual stenosis in the infarct-related vessel despite successful thrombolysis, and this may cause angina if there is still viable myocardium downstream; nevertheless, there is no evidence that routine angioplasty improves outcome after thrombolysis. In some patients occlusion of a vessel may precipitate angina by disturbing a system of collateral flow that was compensating for disease in another vessel.

Patients who develop angina at rest or on minimal exertion following myocardial infarction should be managed in the same way as patients with unstable angina (see pp. 255–257). Intravenous nitrates (e.g. nitroglycerin 0.6–1.2 mg/hour or isosorbide dinitrate 1–2 mg/hour) and intravenous heparin (1000 units/hour, adjusted according to the thrombin time) may be helpful, and early coronary angiography with a view to angioplasty of the 'culprit' lesion should be considered.

Acute circulatory failure

Acute circulatory failure usually reflects extensive myocardial damage and indicates a bad prognosis. All the other complications of myocardial infarction are more likely to occur when acute heart failure is present.

The assessment and management of heart failure complicating acute myocardial infarction are discussed in detail on page 206.

Pericarditis

This may occur at any stage of the illness but is particularly common on the second and third day. The patient may recognise that a different pain has developed, even though it is at the same site, and often finds that the pain is positional and tends to be worse, or sometimes only appears, on inspiration. A pericardial rub may be audible.

The post-myocardial infarction syndrome *(Dressler's syndrome)* is characterised by persistent fever, pericarditis and pleurisy and is probably due to autoimmunity. The symptoms tend to occur a few weeks or even months after the infarct and often subside after a few days; prolonged or severe symptoms may require treatment with high-dose aspirin, a non-steroidal anti-inflammatory drug or even corticosteroids.

Mechanical complications

Part of the necrotic muscle in a fresh infarct may tear or rupture, with devastating consequences:

- Papillary muscle damage may cause acute pulmonary oedema and shock due to the sudden onset of severe mitral regurgitation with a loud pansystolic murmur and third heart sound. The diagnosis can be confirmed by Doppler echocardiography, and emergency mitral valve replacement may be necessary. Lesser degrees of mitral regurgitation are common, and may be transient.
- Rupture of the interventricular septum may cause left-to-right shunting through a ventricular septal defect. This usually presents with sudden haemodynamic deterioration accompanied by a new loud pansystolic murmur and may be difficult to distinguish from acute mitral regurgitation; however, patients with an acquired ventricular septal defect tend to develop right heart failure rather than pulmonary oedema. Doppler echocardiography and right heart catheterisation will confirm the diagnosis, and without prompt surgery the condition is usually fatal.
- Rupture of the ventricle may lead to cardiac tamponade and is usually fatal (see p. 209).

Embolism

Thrombus often forms on the endocardial surface of freshly infarcted myocardium; this may lead to systemic embolism and occasionally causes a stroke or ischaemic limb.

Venous thrombosis and pulmonary embolism may occur but have become less common due to the use of prophylactic anticoagulants and early mobilisation.

Impaired ventricular function, remodelling and ventricular aneurysm

Acute full thickness myocardial infarction is often followed by thinning and stretching of the infarcted segment *(infarct expansion)*; this leads to an increase in wall stress with progressive dilatation and hypertrophy of the remaining ventricle (*ventricular remodelling*—see Fig. 3.70). As the ventricle dilates, it becomes less efficient and heart failure may supervene. Infarct expansion occurs over a few weeks but ventricular remodelling may take years. Accordingly, heart failure often develops many years after acute myocardial infarction.

A left ventricular aneurysm develops in approximately 10% of patients and is particularly common when there is persistent occlusion of the infarct-related vessel. Heart failure, ventricular arrhythmias, mural thrombus and systemic embolism are all recognised complications of aneurysm formation. Other clinical features include a paradoxical

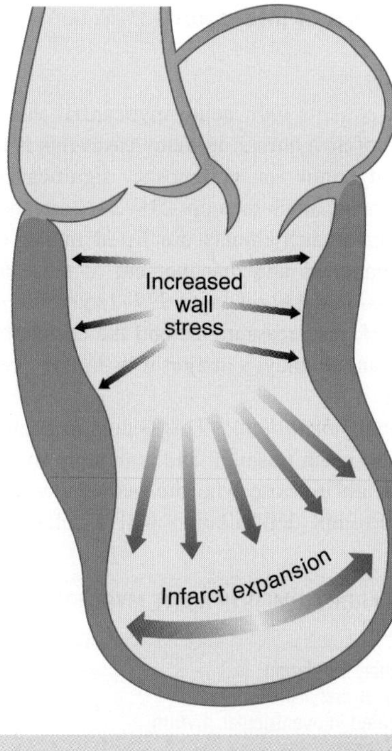

Fig. 3.70 Infarct expansion and ventricular remodelling. Full thickness myocardial infarction causes thinning and stretching of the infarcted segment (infarct expansion), which leads to increased wall stress with progressive dilatation and hypertrophy of the remaining ventricle (ventricular remodelling).

impulse on the chest wall, persistent ST elevation on the ECG, and sometimes an unusual bulge from the cardiac silhouette on the chest radiograph. Echocardiography is usually diagnostic. Surgical removal of a left ventricular aneurysm carries a high morbidity and mortality but is sometimes necessary.

Late management

Patients who have survived a myocardial infarction are at risk of further ischaemic events; any management strategy should therefore aim to identify those patients at high risk and introduce effective secondary prevention measures.

Risk stratification and further investigation

The prognosis of patients who have survived an acute myocardial infarction is related to the degree of myocardial damage, the extent of any residual myocardial ischaemia and the presence of significant ventricular arrhythmias.

Left ventricular function. The degree of left ventricular dysfunction can be crudely assessed from the physical findings (tachycardia, third heart sound, crackles at the lung bases, elevated venous pressure etc.), the ECG changes and the size of the heart on chest radiograph. However, formal measurements using echocardiography or radionuclide imaging are often valuable and may help to select patients for ACE inhibitor therapy among those without overt left ventricular failure (see below).

Ischaemia. Patients who are suitable candidates for revascularisation should undergo an exercise tolerance test approximately 4 weeks after the infarct; this will help to identify those individuals with significant residual myocardial ischaemia who require further investigation and may help to boost the confidence of the remainder.

If the exercise test is negative and the patient has a good effort tolerance the outlook is good, with a 1–4% chance of an adverse event in the next 12 months. In contrast, patients with residual ischaemia in the form of chest pain or ECG changes at low exercise levels are at high risk with a 15–25% chance of suffering a further ischaemic event in the next 12 months.

Coronary arteriography, with a view to angioplasty or bypass grafting, should therefore be considered in any patient with a strongly positive exercise tolerance test or significant angina on effort.

Arrhythmias. The presence of ventricular arrhythmias during the convalescent phase of myocardial infarction may herald sudden death and is associated with a poor prognosis. Although empirical anti-arrhythmic treatment appears to be of no value, and may even be hazardous, in this situation selected patients may benefit from sophisticated electrophysiological testing and specific anti-arrhythmic therapy.

Recurrent ventricular arrhythmias are sometimes manifestations of myocardial ischaemia or impaired LV function and may respond to appropriate treatment directed at the underlying problem.

Routine drug therapy

Aspirin. Low-dose aspirin therapy reduces the risk of further infarction and other vascular events by approximately 25% and should be continued indefinitely if there are no unwanted effects.

β-adrenoceptor antagonists. Continuous treatment with an oral β-adrenoceptor antagonist has been shown to reduce long-term mortality by approximately 25% among the survivors of acute myocardial infarction. Unfortunately, patients with bradycardia, heart block, hypotension, overt cardiac failure, asthma, chronic obstructive airways disease and significant peripheral vascular disease do not usually tolerate β-blockers.

Angiotensin-converting enzyme (ACE) inhibitors. Several clinical trials have shown that long-term treatment with an ACE inhibitor (e.g. captopril 50 mg 8-hourly, enalapril 10 mg 12-hourly, or ramipril 2.5–5 mg 12-hourly) can counteract ventricular remodelling, prevent the onset of heart failure, improve survival and reduce hospitalisation. The benefit of treatment is greatest in those with overt heart failure (clinical or radiological) but extends to patients with asymptomatic LV dysfunction. This form of therapy should therefore be considered in any patient who has sustained a myocardial infarct complicated by transient heart failure or poor residual left ventricular function (e.g. LV ejection fraction < 40%).

Risk factor modification

Smoking. The 5-year mortality of patients who continue to smoke cigarettes is double that of those who quit smoking at the time of their infarct. Giving up smoking is the single most effective contribution a patient can make to his or her own future.

Hyperlipidaemia. Convincing evidence from large-scale randomised clinical trials has demonstrated the importance of lowering plasma cholesterol following myocardial infarction. The aim is to reduce total cholesterol to less than 5.0 mmol/l, low-density lipoprotein (LDL) cholesterol to less than 3.4 mmol/l, and triglycerides to within the normal range. Lipids should be measured within 24 hours of presentation because there is often a transient (up to 3 months) and unrepresentative fall in blood cholesterol later on. Dietary advice should be given but is often ineffective. HMG CoA reductase enzyme inhibitors ('statins') can produce marked reductions in total (and LDL) cholesterol and have been shown to reduce the subsequent risk of death, reinfarction, stroke and the need for revascularisation (see Table 3.8, p. 248). These benefits extend to patients with relatively low or average blood cholesterol concentrations (e.g. > 5.0 mmol/l). Alternative treatments may be advisable in patients with mixed hyperlipidaemia or marked hypertriglyceridaemia (see p. 535).

Other risk factors. Maintaining an ideal body weight, taking regular exercise, and achieving good control of hypertension and diabetes may all improve the long-term outlook.

Mobilisation and rehabilitation

There is histological evidence that the necrotic muscle of an acute myocardial infarct takes 4–6 weeks to become replaced with fibrous tissue. Accordingly, it is conventional to restrict physical activities during this period. When there are no complications the patient can sit in a chair on the second day, walk to the toilet on the third day, return home in 5–7 days and gradually increase activity with the aim of returning to work in 4–6 weeks (unless this involves heavy physical activity). The majority of patients may resume driving after 4–6 weeks; however, in the UK vocational (e.g. heavy goods and public service vehicle) driving licence holders require special assessment.

Emotional problems such as denial, anxiety and depression are common, and must be recognised and dealt with accordingly. Many patients are severely and even permanently incapacitated as a result of the psychological rather than the physical effects of myocardial infarction, and all benefit from thoughtful explanation, counselling and reassurance at every stage of the illness. Many patients mistakenly believe that 'stress' was the cause of their heart attack and may restrict their activity inappropriately. The patient's spouse will also require emotional support, information and counselling.

Formal rehabilitation programmes based on graded exercise protocols with individual and group counselling are often very successful, and in some cases have been shown to improve the long-term outcome.

Prognosis

In almost a quarter of all cases of myocardial infarction death occurs within a few minutes without medical care. Half the deaths from myocardial infarction occur within 24 hours of the onset of symptoms and about 40% of all affected patients die within the first month.

Early death is usually due to an arrhythmia but later on the outcome is determined by the extent of myocardial damage. Unfavourable features include poor left ventricular function, heart block and persistent ventricular arrhythmias. The prognosis is worse for anterior than for inferior infarcts. Bundle branch block and high enzyme levels both indicate extensive myocardial damage. Old age, stress and social isolation are also associated with a higher mortality. In the absence of unfavourable features, the outlook is as good for those who survive ventricular fibrillation as for the others.

Of those who survive an acute attack, more than 80% live for a further year, about 75% for 5 years, 50% for 10 years and 25% for 20 years.

SUDDEN DEATH

This term can be applied when a person previously in apparent good health falls ill and dies within minutes or at most a few hours.

Approximately 30% of these patients have an identifiable non-cardiac cause of death, such as cerebral haemorrhage or a ruptured aortic aneurysm. However, in most cases death is attributable to coronary artery disease and is usually due to an arrhythmia related to acute myocardial infarction, ischaemia, heart failure or scarring from a previous myocardial infarct. An arrhythmia is probably also the cause of sudden death in patients with other cardiac abnormalities such as acute myocarditis, severe aortic stenosis, critical pulmonary stenosis and hypertrophic cardiomyopathy. A small group of patients who die suddenly have no obvious pathological cause of death on postmortem examination; a cardiac arrhythmia seems the most likely cause in this group as well.

Observations of patients who have died during ambulatory ECG monitoring suggest that ventricular fibrillation is the most common arrhythmia causing sudden death. In many cases of ventricular fibrillation prompt resuscitation can restore effective cardiac action (see pp. 235–236).

The survivors of an 'out-of-hospital' cardiac arrest require careful evaluation. If there is no evidence of acute myocardial infarction there is a high chance of recurrent cardiac arrest and the patient may benefit from specific anti-arrhythmic therapy. In patients with poor left ventricular function (ejection fraction < 20%) empirical therapy with amiodarone 200–300 mg daily may be used to reduce the risk of recurrence; others may benefit from drug treatment guided by electrophysiological studies or an implantable cardioverter-defibrillator (see p. 244).

Relatives of patients who have died suddenly often seek reassurance, and should be examined, if appropriate, for evidence of familial conditions such as hypertrophic cardiomyopathy, Marfan's syndrome and hyperlipidaemia. A family history of sudden death in childhood or young adult life is sometimes associated with prolongation of the QT interval on the ECG, and β-blockade may improve prognosis in this group.

FURTHER INFORMATION ON ISCHAEMIC (CORONARY) HEART DISEASE

Collins R, Peto R, Baigent C, Sleight P 1997 Aspirin, heparin and fibrinolytic therapy in suspected acute myocardial infarction. New England Journal of Medicine 336: 847–860. *An up-to-date review*
Davies M J (ed) 1993 Atherosclerosis. British Heart Journal 69: S1–S73. *This supplement to the British Heart Journal contains 10 excellent review articles on the pathophysiology and prevention of coronary artery disease*
Fox K A A 1997 Management of patients following myocardial infarction. Medicine 25 (11): 68–72
Task force of the European Society of Cardiology 1994 Prevention of coronary heart disease in clinical practice. European Heart Journal 15: 1300
Task force of the European Society of Cardiology 1996 Acute myocardial infarction: pre-hospital and in-hospital management. European Heart Journal 17: 43–63

VASCULAR DISEASE

PERIPHERAL ARTERIAL DISEASE

Disease of the peripheral arteries is most commonly due to atheroma. Less common causes are thromboembolism, vasculitis, Raynaud's disease and cold injury (frostbite). A variant of atheromatous peripheral vascular disease occurs in diabetics, with soft tissue ischaemia, infection, ulceration and peripheral neuropathy but preservation of the major pulses.

ATHEROMATOUS PERIPHERAL VASCULAR DISEASE

Clinical features

Atheromatous peripheral vascular disease is more common in men than women, is strongly associated with smoking, and affects the legs more than the arms. Patients are usually over 50 years old.

Symptoms

The most common presenting symptom is intermittent claudication—a discomfort or ache in the calves or buttocks precipitated by walking and relieved by rest. Pulses in the leg and foot are absent or diminished. Patients may also complain of cold feet or legs and discoloration due to peripheral cyanosis.

As the disease progresses rest pain may develop. This is characteristically worse at night, and the patient may get temporary relief by allowing the limb to hang over the side of the bed outside the bedclothes.

Signs

The peripheral pulses are diminished or absent and the feet may feel cold. Bruits may be audible over the abdominal aorta, iliac vessels or femoral arteries but are not a useful guide to the severity of the underlying disease. By the time the patient experiences rest pain in the limb, it is common for the skin to be pale or discoloured, and for hair growth to be absent. Small patches of skin necrosis (leg ulcers) may appear, often related to pressure points or minor injury. Finally, frank gangrene may occur, usually starting with one or more toes. This is characterised by dark discoloration, spreading proximally, severe pain and often infection, with a foul-smelling discharge.

Investigations

Although radiographs may show calcification in arteries, they are not sensitive indicators of the degree of arterial narrowing nor of its localisation. Measurement of the ratio of ankle to brachial cuff pressures has provided a useful marker of the extent of disease in epidemiological studies, but lacks sensitivity in an individual. Doppler ultrasound is often the initial investigation of choice and enables peripheral pulse pressure to be measured and sites of stenosis and occlusion to be identified; this then helps to select patients for angiography (see Fig. 3.71) and revascularisation. Ultrasound of the abdomen can detect vascular calcification and aneurysms in the abdominal aorta.

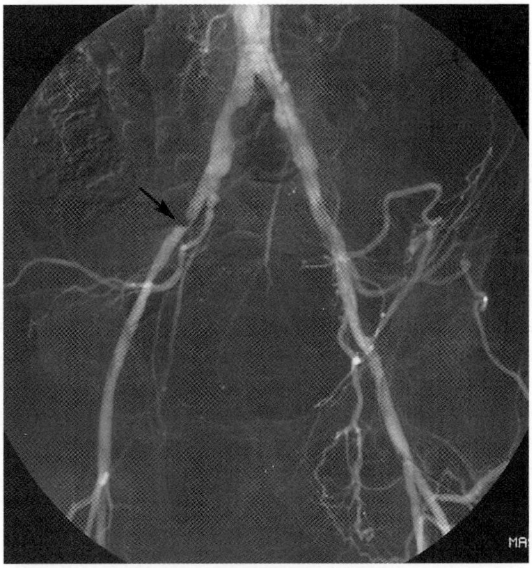

Fig. 3.71 Digital contrast angiogram of the distal aorta and iliac arteries in a patient with peripheral vascular disease. Multiple atheromatous plaques can be seen with a severe stenosis in the right iliac artery (arrow).

Angiography is used to define the anatomy and extent of disease with a view to revascularisation by balloon angioplasty or open surgery.

Management (see the information box)

Medical therapy with vasodilators is of little value. However, balloon angioplasty is useful for the relief of symptoms caused by iliac or femoral stenoses and aorto-iliac bypass surgery is an effective form of treatment when symptoms are due to disease of the proximal vessels.

MANAGEMENT OF PERIPHERAL ARTERIAL DISEASE
General measures
• Stop smoking • Low-dose aspirin • Correct risk factors • Lose weight if obese • Stop vasoconstrictor drugs • Optimise diabetic and hypertension control • Encourage exercise (increases collateral flow) • Avoid infection and trauma, arrange chiropody • Vasodilators/anticoagulants are unhelpful
Indications for revascularisation
• Acute ischaemia of the limb. The hallmarks are: acute pain, pallor, lack of pulse, paralysis. Embolectomy or surgical repair may be required and amputation may be necessary if intervention is delayed • Chronic ischaemia with impaired skin and tissue viability, non-healing ulcers • Disabling symptoms due to arterial stenoses or occlusions

Amputation may be necessary if the limb is painful, infected and not viable. Severe pain is sometimes due to ischaemic neuropathy and may respond to treatment with amitriptyline (25–50 mg at night).

The most common cause of death in peripheral vascular disease is myocardial infarction. Cerebrovascular disease and smoking-related lung disease are also common. A holistic approach is important because these associated diseases may require treatment in their own right and there is often much to be gained from secondary preventive measures; moreover, the presence of significant heart, lung or cerebrovascular disease may influence the potential risks and benefits of vascular surgery.

SUDDEN OCCLUSION OF A MAJOR ARTERY

This is commonly due to embolism from the heart as a result of mural thrombus after myocardial infarction, endocarditis, rheumatic heart disease or, rarely, an atrial myxoma. Emboli that precipitate acute clinical symptoms lodge most frequently at the aortic, iliac or popliteal bifurcations. The limb becomes painful, cold, numb and pale, and pulses distal to the occlusion disappear. Surgical embolectomy should be considered without delay, and is often performed under local anaesthesia.

VASCULITIS

Vasculitis is a generic term for inflammatory diseases affecting blood vessels. Vasculitides affecting medium-sized or large vessels may cause symptoms of peripheral artery disease. The most important are polyarteritis nodosa, giant cell arteritis and Takayasu's disease (pulseless disease or aortic arch syndrome) (see pp. 864–865). The clinical presentation and management of this group of diseases are detailed in Chapter 12.

RAYNAUD'S PHENOMENON AND RAYNAUD'S DISEASE

Clinical features

Raynaud's phenomenon is caused by intense vasospasm of peripheral arteries. On exposure to cold, the fingers (and less commonly the toes) become initially very pale from vasoconstriction. This is followed by cyanosis secondary to the poor blood flow. Eventually, when the blood flow returns, the digits become dusky, red and painful. Some causes are listed in the information box. When the condition occurs in isolation it is called *Raynaud's disease*. This occurs more frequently in women than in men, and is common, affecting about 5% of the population.

CAUSES OF RAYNAUD'S PHENOMENON

• Idiopathic (Raynaud's disease)
• Drugs
    β-adrenoceptor antagonists
    Ergotamine and derivatives
• Occupational exposure to vibrating tools
• Occupational exposure to cold
• Scleroderma/systemic sclerosis
• Cryoglobulinaemia
• CREST syndrome (Calcinosis, Raynaud's, oEsophageal hypomotility, Sclerodactyly, Telangiectasia)

Management

Patients should stop smoking, and vasoconstrictor drugs or β-adrenoceptor antagonists should be withdrawn. Cold exposure should be avoided. Nifedipine (5–10 mg 8-hourly) and other vasodilators are sometimes helpful.

DISEASES OF THE AORTA

Three types of condition may affect the aorta: aneurysm, dissection and aortitis (see Fig. 3.72, p. 270).

AORTIC ANEURYSM

An aortic aneurysm is an abnormal dilatation of the aortic wall. Aortic dissection has a different pathology and is considered separately.

Aetiology

Atheromatous disease

Atheroma may weaken the aortic wall and lead to local aneurysm formation. The most common site is the abdominal aorta between renal and iliac arteries. The descending thoracic aorta may be affected, but atheromatous aneurysms of the ascending aorta are rare.

POSSIBLE CAUSES OF ANEURYSM
• Atheromatous disease—affects ascending or descending aorta • Collagen vascular diseases—affect thoracic aorta: cystic medial necrosis, Marfan's syndrome, Ehlers–Danlos syndrome • Aortitis

Aneurysm formation involves destruction of elastin by proteolytic enzymes (decreased tissue metalloproteinase inhibition) in the aortic wall and increased pressure on the collagen matrix, especially in the presence of hypertension. Genetic abnormalities have been detected in type III collagen, predisposing to aneurysm formation.

Marfan's syndrome

Aneurysms associated with this disorder may rupture directly, or cause dissection. Patients usually present in the third to fifth decades; they may have the characteristic facial and skeletal features of the fully fledged syndrome, but 'formes frustes' occur. Marfan's syndrome is inherited as an autosomal dominant trait and may also cause mitral regurgitation. Chest radiography, ultrasound or CT scanning may detect aortic dilatation at an early stage. Elective replacement of the ascending aorta may be considered, but carries a mortality of 5–10%. Use of β-adrenoceptor antagonists may also reduce the risk of aortic dilatation and rupture. Pregnancy is particularly hazardous.

Aortitis causing aortic aneurysm

Syphilis is now a rare cause of aortitis. It can produce saccular aneurysms of the ascending aorta containing calcification.

Other conditions causing aortitis are: Takayasu's disease, Reiter's syndrome, giant cell arteritis and ankylosing spondylitis (see Ch. 12).

Thoracic aneurysms

Thoracic aortic aneurysms may produce chest pain similar to cardiac pain, associated with expansion of the aneurysm. If they extend proximally they may cause aortic valve regurgitation. They can also cause symptoms by compressing the trachea, main bronchus or superior vena cava. Occasionally, they may erode into the adjacent structures, causing haemorrhage, tamponade and death.

Abdominal aneurysms

Clinically, 'expansile' pulsation of an aneurysm must be distinguished from 'transmitted' pulsation from a normal aorta and the diagnosis is usually confirmed by ultrasound or CT scanning. The abdominal or chest radiograph may reveal calcification. The natural history of an aneurysm is expansion leading to eventual rupture.

Management

Elective surgical repair has a much lower mortality than emergency surgery for rupture. Suggested management for abdominal aneurysms is shown in the information box. The mortality for surgical repair of thoracic aneurysms is higher than that of abdominal aneurysms. Thoracic aortic aneurysms are therefore usually treated conservatively unless there are signs of progressive enlargement. In contrast, dissecting aneurysms of the ascending aorta usually require emergency surgical intervention (see below).

CLINICAL FEATURES OF ABDOMINAL ANEURYSMS
• More common in men than women, particularly those over 60 years of age
Symptoms
• Commonly asymptomatic (especially small aneurysms < 5 cm in diameter) • May present with backache, abdominal pain or limb claudication • May present acutely, with pain and hypotension from rupture
Signs
• Aneurysm may be palpable in abdominal aorta • Evidence of widespread vascular disease • Stigmata of distal embolisation • Haemodynamic collapse (hypotension, tachycardia, shock), with rupture of aneurysm

MANAGEMENT OF ABDOMINAL AORTIC ANEURYSMS
Symptoms of rupture
• Emergency surgery
Backache or abdominal pain
• Ultrasound, CT or angiography; consider surgery
Asymptomatic
• Ultrasound—if < 4 cm, serial ultrasound + follow up if > 4 cm, consider surgery

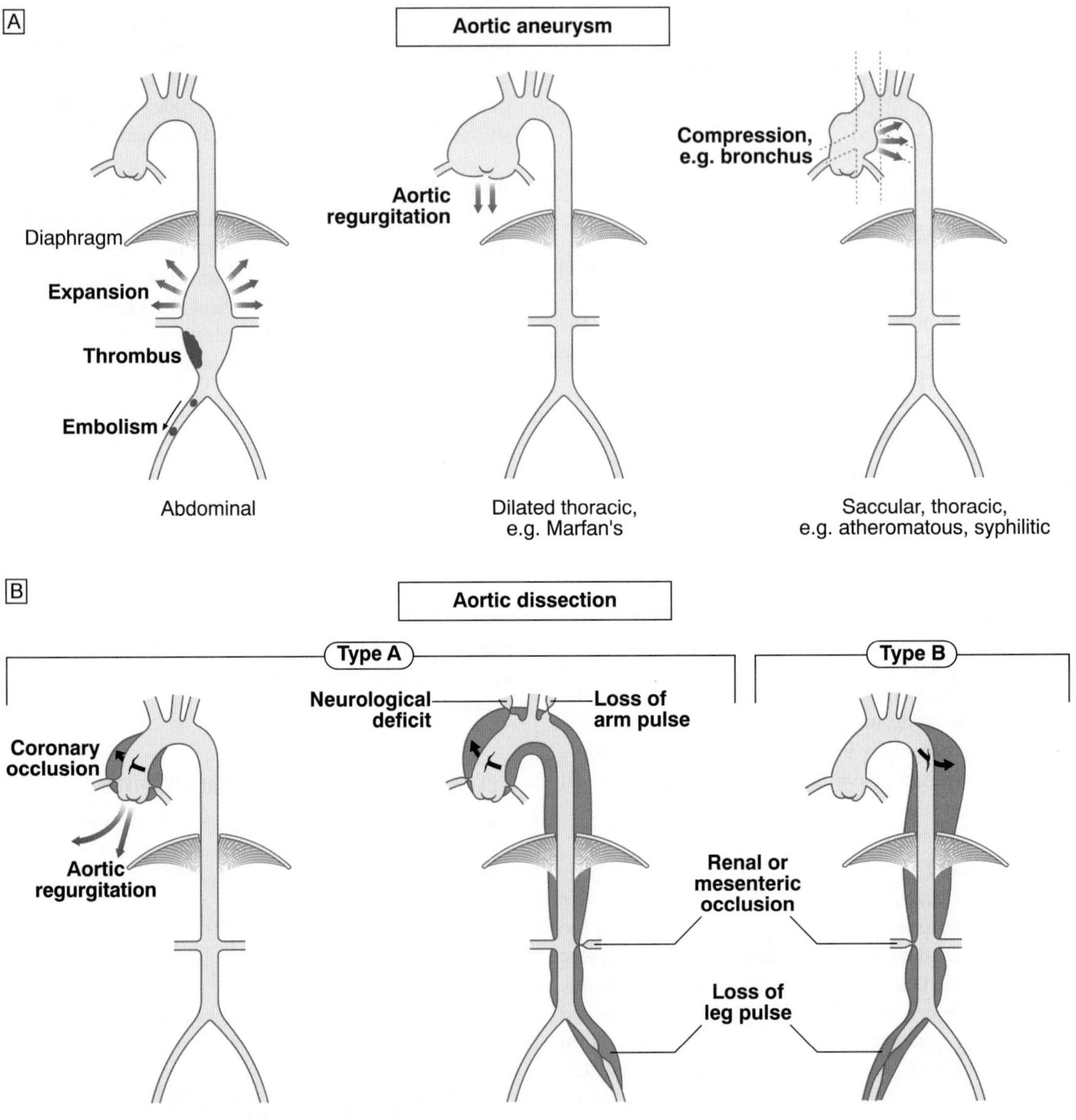

Fig. 3.72 Types of aortic disease and their complications. A Types of aortic aneurysm. B Types of aortic dissection.

AORTIC DISSECTION

Aortic dissection is caused by a tear in the intima of the aorta, exposing the diseased media to blood at intra-aortic pressure. The media is cleaved into two layers, creating a 'false lumen' in addition to the existing or 'true lumen'. The dissection may compromise branches of the aorta as it spreads along its length, causing, for example, cerebral, coronary or renal ischaemia. The false lumen may go on to rupture externally into the left pleural space or pericardium, or internally re-entering the true lumen.

Aortic dissection is classified anatomically and for clinical management into type A, which involves the ascending aorta, and type B, which involves only the descending aorta distal to the left subclavian artery. Type A dissections occur in two-thirds of cases and frequently extend into the descending aorta. The peak incidence is in the sixth and seventh decades of life, a history of hypertension is present in the large majority, and men are twice as frequently affected as women. Aortic dissection can occur in younger patients when there is an abnormality of the aortic media, although the causation in pregnancy is poorly understood (see the information box).

CONDITIONS ASSOCIATED WITH AORTIC DISSECTION
• Hypertension, in 80% of cases • Cystic medial degeneration of aortic wall, e.g. Marfan's syndrome, Ehlers–Danlos syndrome • Previous surgery to aorta, e.g. coronary bypass, aortic valve replacement • Pregnancy, usually third trimester

Clinical features

Symptoms

Clinical presentation is usually acute, with very sudden onset of extremely severe pain in the chest and back, often starting between the shoulder blades, migrating, and frequently described as 'tearing'.

Signs

On examination there may be hypertension and asymmetry of the brachial, carotid or femoral pulses. In type A dissection there may be signs of aortic reflux (e.g. early diastolic murmur).

Investigations

The chest radiograph characteristically shows broadening of the upper mediastinum and distortion of the aortic 'knuckle', but these appearances are not invariable. (They are absent in 40%.) A left-sided pleural effusion is common. The ECG may show left ventricular hypertrophy in patients with hypertension, or changes of myocardial infarction (usually inferior) if the dissection has extended into the coronary arteries. Doppler echocardiography may show aortic regurgitation, a dilated aortic root, and occasionally the flap of the dissection. Transoesophageal echocardiography is particularly helpful because transthoracic echocardiography can only image the first 3–4 cm of the ascending aorta. CT scanning and MRI are both highly specific, and angiography of the aortic arch is not usually needed unless these other imaging techniques are not available.

Management

Initial management involves control of hypertension (maintain systolic pressure < 100 mmHg) and definition of the site of origin and extent of the dissection. Type A dissecting aneurysms require emergency surgical repair under cardiopulmonary bypass. Type B aneurysms can often be treated medically, with bed rest and careful control of blood pressure. In Type B, surgical intervention may be needed if there is evidence of leakage or extension, or for renal or bowel ischaemia from the intimal flap.

FURTHER INFORMATION ON VASCULAR DISEASE

Iselbacher E M, Eagle K A, De Sauchs R W 1997 Diseases of the aorta. In: Braunwald E (ed) Heart disease. W B Saunders, Philadelphia

DISEASES OF THE HEART VALVES

A diseased valve may be narrowed (stenosed) or it may fail to close adequately, and thus permit regurgitation of blood. The term 'incompetence' may be used synonymously with regurgitation or reflux, but the latter descriptions are preferable. The principal causes of valve disease are summarised in the information box.

PRINCIPAL CAUSES OF VALVE DISEASE

Valve regurgitation	Valve stenosis
• Congenital • Acute rheumatic carditis • Chronic rheumatic carditis • Infective endocarditis • Syphilitic aortitis • Valve ring dilatation (e.g. dilated cardiomyopathy) • Traumatic valve rupture • Senile degeneration • Damage to chordae and papillary muscles (e.g. MI)	• Congenital • Rheumatic carditis • Senile degeneration

The aetiology of individual valve lesions is considered separately below.

RHEUMATIC HEART DISEASE

ACUTE RHEUMATIC FEVER

Aetiology and prevalence

Acute rheumatic fever is triggered by infection with specific strains of group A streptococci which possess antigens that cross-react with human connective tissue, particularly heart valve glycoprotein.

The condition usually affects children or young adults, and there is a familial variation in susceptibility. Its prevalence in Western Europe and North America has progressively declined to very low levels, but it remains common in parts of Asia, Africa and South America, where it is still the most common cause of acquired heart disease in childhood and adolescence.

Clinical features

Rheumatic fever is a systemic illness typically presenting with fever, anorexia, lethargy and joint pains. Arthritis occurs in approximately 75% of patients and other features

JONES CRITERIA FOR THE DIAGNOSIS OF RHEUMATIC FEVER

Major manifestations

- Carditis
- Polyarthritis
- Chorea
- Erythema marginatum
- Subcutaneous nodules

Minor manifestations

- Fever
- Arthralgia
- Previous rheumatic fever
- Raised ESR or C-reactive protein
- Leucocytosis
- First-degree or second-degree AV block

PLUS

- Supporting evidence of preceding streptococcal infection: recent scarlet fever, raised antistreptolysin O or other streptococcal antibody titre, positive throat culture

N.B. Evidence of recent streptococcal infection is particularly important if there is only one major manifestation.

include skin rashes, carditis and neurological features (see Fig. 3.73). The diagnosis according to the revised Jones criteria is based upon two or more major manifestations or one major and two or more minor manifestations. In both cases evidence of preceding streptococcal infection is required (antistreptococcal antibody; antistreptolysin antibody; positive culture for group A streptococcus; recent scarlet fever).

Carditis

This is the most important manifestation of rheumatic fever. Carditis presents as breathlessness (due to heart failure or pericardial effusion), palpitations or chest pain (usually due to peri- or pancarditis). Other features consist of tachycardia, cardiac enlargement and new or changed cardiac murmurs. A soft systolic murmur is common but non-specific. A soft mid-diastolic murmur (Carey Coombs murmur) is often due to valvulitis, with nodules forming

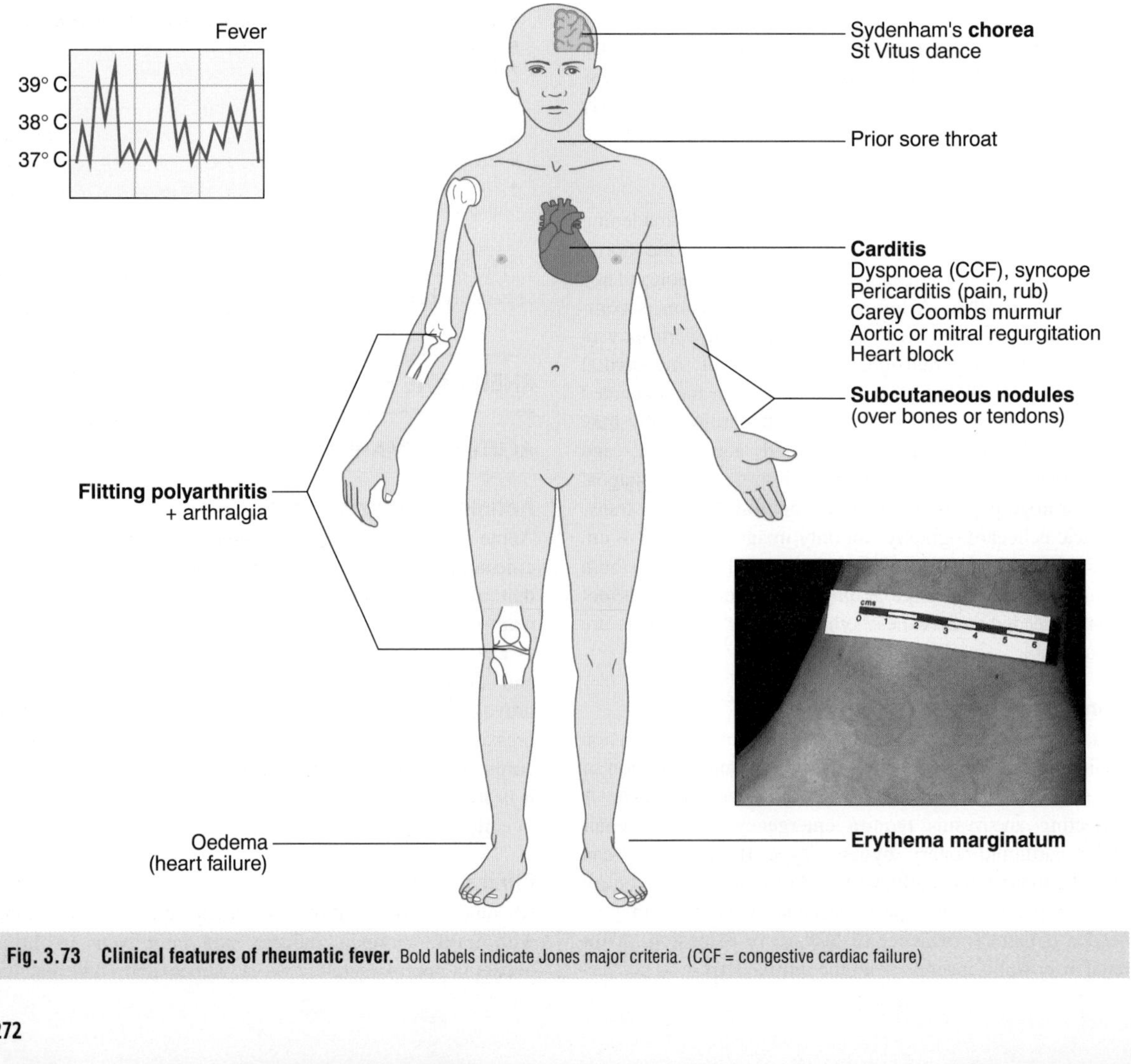

Fig. 3.73 Clinical features of rheumatic fever. Bold labels indicate Jones major criteria. (CCF = congestive cardiac failure)

on the mitral valve leaflets. There may be a pericardial friction rub which is often intermittent. Cardiac failure may result either from impaired function of ventricular muscle or from mitral or aortic incompetence and tends to occur in a 'fulminant' form of rheumatic fever that is more common in developing countries. Electrocardiographic changes include ST or T wave changes; conduction defects sometimes occur and may cause syncope.

Sydenham's chorea (St Vitus dance)

Central nervous system involvement may manifest late after the initial infection (6 months or more), with those affected exhibiting spasmodic unintentional movements and possibly altered speech. Spontaneous recovery is usual, though it may be followed by chronic cardiac disease.

Arthritis

The arthritis of rheumatic fever is often symmetrical, affecting large joints with acute painful inflammation which characteristically 'flits' from joint to joint (i.e. a migratory polyarthralgia). The joints affected include those of the limbs, spine, and sometimes the temporomandibular and costoclavicular joints. There is commonly, but not invariably, a history of sore throat 2–4 weeks before the onset of joint symptoms. In adults, joint symptoms tend to be more prominent than carditis; in children under 6 years old the converse may be true.

Skin lesions

The following may be present:

- *Erythema marginatum*, which occurs in 10–20% of children with rheumatic fever. It starts as red macules (blotches) which fade in the centre but remain red at the edges. The resulting red rings or 'margins' may coalesce or overlap (see Fig. 3.73).
- *Subcutaneous nodules*, which are uncommon, but associated with more severe carditis. They are small (< 0.5 cm), firm, painless, and best felt over bone or tendons. Typically the nodules are much smaller than those of rheumatoid arthritis.

Other systemic manifestations are rare, but include pleurisy, pleural effusion and pneumonia.

Investigations

These are listed in the information box.

It is important to note that while the systemic markers are non-specific, they may be useful in following progress of the disease. Furthermore, positive throat cultures are present only in a minority of patients at the time of clinical presentation and ASO titres are normal in about one-fifth of adult cases of rheumatic fever and most cases of chorea.

INVESTIGATIONS IN ACUTE RHEUMATIC FEVER
Evidence of a systemic illness (non-specific)
• Leucocytosis, raised ESR, raised C-reactive protein
Evidence of preceding streptococcal infection (specific)
• Throat swab culture: group A β-haemolytic streptococci (also from family members and contacts) • Antistreptolysin O antibodies (ASO titres): rising titres, or levels of > 200 units (adults), > 300 units (children)
Evidence of carditis
• Chest radiograph: cardiomegaly; pulmonary congestion • ECG: first- and second-degree heart block; features of pericarditis; T wave inversion; reduction in QRS voltages • Echocardiography: cardiac dilatation and valve abnormalities

Management

Treatment for acute rheumatic fever is directed towards limiting cardiac damage, relieving symptoms and eliminating the streptococcal infection.

Bed rest and supportive therapy

During the acute phase of rheumatic fever or during active carditis the patient should be rested in bed, as otherwise there is a risk of recurrence of signs and symptoms. Later, the patient may feel well, although temperature, leucocyte count and erythrocyte sedimentation rate (ESR) remain elevated. Bed rest must be continued until these indices of continuing disease activity have settled. In patients who have had carditis, it is conventional to continue bed rest for 2–6 weeks after the ESR and temperature have returned to normal. Prolonged bed rest, particularly in children or adolescents, produces problems of boredom and depression that need to be anticipated and managed.

Cardiac failure should be treated as necessary (see p. 214). Valve replacement may be required for severe mitral or aortic incompetence. Heart block is seldom progressive, and pacemaker therapy is rarely needed.

Aspirin

Aspirin will usually relieve the symptoms of arthritis rapidly and a prompt response (within 24 hours) helps to confirm the diagnosis. A reasonable starting dose is 60 mg/kg body weight per day, divided into six doses. In adults, 120 mg/kg per day may be needed up to the limits of tolerance or a maximum of 8 g per day. Mild toxic effects include nausea, tinnitus and deafness; more serious ones are vomiting, tachypnoea and acidosis. Aspirin should be continued until the ESR has fallen, and then gradually tailed off.

Corticosteroids

These produce more rapid symptomatic relief than aspirin, and are indicated in cases with carditis or severe arthritis. There is no evidence that long-term steroids are beneficial. Prednisolone or prednisone 1.0–2.0 mg/kg per day in divided doses should be continued until the ESR is normal, then gradually tailed off.

Antistreptococcal therapy

Eradication of streptococcal infections and prevention of recurrence are important. Benzathine penicillin 1.2 million units i.m. should be given on diagnosis, followed by oral phenoxymethyl-penicillin 500 mg 12-hourly for 10 days. Subsequent prophylaxis may be with oral phenoxymethyl-penicillin 500 mg continued for at least 5 years after the last attack and until the patient reaches at least 20 years of age. If compliance with an oral regimen is in doubt, then i.m. administration may be employed.

Recurrences are more common when cardiac disease is present and, if so, prophylaxis should continue until age 30. A sulphonamide, or erythromycin, may be used if the patient is allergic to penicillin.

Follow-up

Carditis most frequently occurs within 2 weeks of the onset of arthritis. Chronic rheumatic heart disease is much more common in patients who have carditis during the initial attack or during a recurrence. It is important to prevent recurrence by continuing antistreptococcal prophylaxis, and to recognise and follow up chronic valve lesions, but at the same time it is important not to induce a cardiac neurosis. Echocardiography is valuable in assessing valve problems. If it remains normal, follow-up can be discontinued 10 years after the initial attack.

CHRONIC RHEUMATIC HEART DISEASE

Chronic valvular heart disease develops subsequently in at least half of those affected by rheumatic fever with carditis. The predominantly affected valve is the mitral (in > 90%) and then less commonly the aortic, tricuspid and pulmonary. The lesions develop after 10–20 years in 'Western' countries but much earlier in developing countries.

Pathology

The main pathological process in chronic rheumatic heart disease is a progressive fibrosis particularly affecting the heart valves. This is in contrast to the destructive lytic process of acute rheumatic fever. The condition also affects the pericardium and myocardium and may contribute to heart failure and conduction disorders. For the mitral valve the result is shortening of the chordae tendineae, fusion of the commissures and a reduction in size of the valve orifice. The haemodynamic result is mitral stenosis with or without regurgitation. Similar disorders of the aortic and tricuspid valves produce distortion and rigidity of the cusps, and in consequence, stenosis and incompetence. Once damage has developed on a valve, the altered haemodynamic stresses on the valve perpetuate and extend the damage, even in the absence of a continuing rheumatic process.

MITRAL VALVE DISEASE

MITRAL STENOSIS

Aetiology and pathophysiology

Mitral stenosis is almost always rheumatic in origin. However, in the elderly, heavy calcification of the mitral valve apparatus can produce a syndrome similar to mitral stenosis. There is also a rare form of congenital mitral stenosis.

Some episodes of rheumatic fever may pass unrecognised and it is only possible to elicit a history of rheumatic fever or chorea in about half of the patients. Isolated mitral stenosis accounts for about 25% of all cases of rheumatic heart disease and an additional 40% have mixed mitral stenosis and regurgitation. Two-thirds of cases occur in women.

In rheumatic mitral stenosis the mitral valve orifice is slowly diminished by progressive fibrosis and calcification of the valve leaflets, fusion of the cusps and subvalvular apparatus. The flow of blood from the left atrium to the left ventricle is therefore restricted and left atrial pressure rises, leading to pulmonary venous congestion and breathlessness. There is dilatation and hypertrophy of the left atrium, and left ventricular filling becomes more dependent on left atrial contraction.

Any increase in heart rate shortens diastole (the time the mitral valve is open) and produces a further rise in left atrial pressure; situations that demand an increase in cardiac output will also increase left atrial pressure. Exercise and pregnancy are therefore poorly tolerated.

The mitral valve orifice is normally about 5 cm^2 in diastole and may be reduced to 1 cm^2 or less in severe mitral stenosis. Patients usually remain asymptomatic until the stenosis is at least moderately severe (approximately 2 cm^2 or less). At first, symptoms occur only on exercise; however, in severe stenosis left atrial pressure is permanently elevated and symptoms may occur at rest. Reduced lung compliance, due to chronic pulmonary venous congestion, contributes to breathlessness, and a low cardiac output may cause fatigue.

Atrial fibrillation due to progressive dilatation of the left atrium is very common. The onset of atrial fibrillation often precipitates pulmonary oedema because the accompanying tachycardia and loss of atrial contraction frequently lead to marked haemodynamic deterioration with a dramatic rise in left atrial pressure. In contrast, a more gradual rise in left atrial pressure tends to cause an increase in pulmonary vascular resistance, which leads to pulmonary artery hypertension and may protect the patient from pulmonary oedema.

A minority of patients (less than 20%) remain in sinus rhythm, which is often associated with a small fibrotic left atrium and severe pulmonary hypertension.

All patients with mitral stenosis are at risk from left atrial thrombosis and systemic thromboembolism, particularly those with atrial fibrillation. Prior to the advent of anticoagulant therapy, emboli caused a quarter of all deaths in this condition.

(Normal pressure values are shown in Fig. 3.74.)

Clinical features

The main features of mitral stenosis are shown in the information boxes.

Symptoms

The gradual reduction in the mitral valve orifice usually produces insidious onset of breathlessness, and pulmonary congestion may cause cough. Exercise tolerance may diminish very slowly over many years and patients often do not appreciate the extent of their disability. Eventually symptoms occur at rest. Acute pulmonary oedema or pulmonary hypertension can lead to haemoptysis. Systemic embolism is sometimes a presenting feature.

Asymptomatic mitral stenosis. The physical signs of mitral stenosis are often found before symptoms develop, and their recognition is of particular importance in pregnancy.

SYMPTOMS OF MITRAL STENOSIS

- Exertional dyspnoea, nocturnal dyspnoea, cough
- Ankle/leg oedema, abdominal swelling (right heart failure)
- Symptoms of acute pulmonary oedema (especially with pregnancy or AF)
- Symptoms secondary to arterial/venous emboli, e.g. stroke, haemoptysis, chest pain
- Symptoms of diminished cardiac output, e.g. fatigue

Signs

The stenotic valve prolongs atrial emptying, resulting in the leaflets remaining open at the onset of systole and closing with an unusually loud sound (S1) which may be palpable—the tapping apex beat. The turbulent flow, which is heralded

SIGNS OF MITRAL STENOSIS

- Atrial fibrillation
- Mitral facies
- Auscultation
  - Loud first heart sound, opening snap
  - Mid-diastolic murmur
- Signs of raised pulmonary capillary pressure
  - Crepitations, pulmonary oedema, effusions
- Signs of pulmonary hypertension
  - RV heave, loud P_2

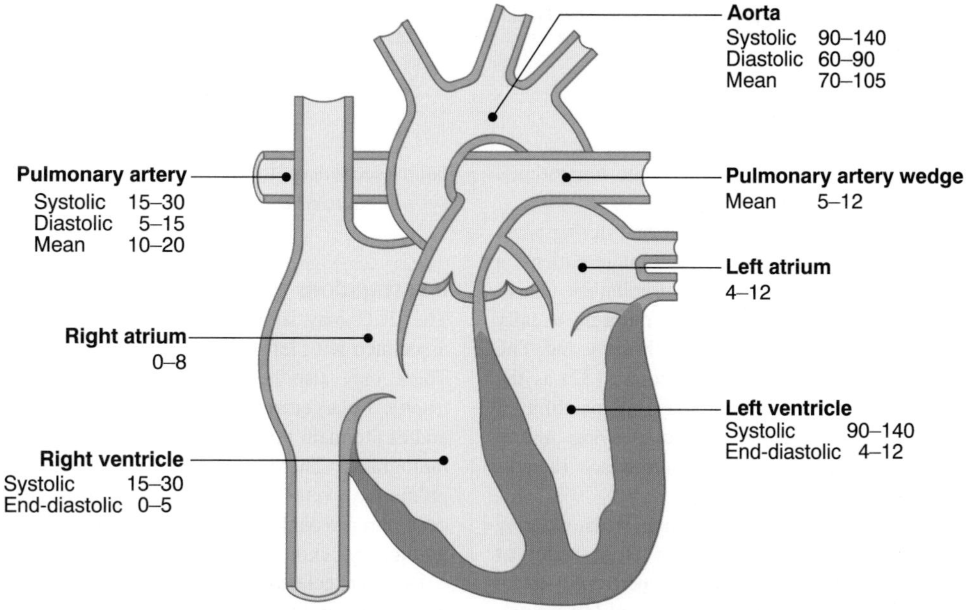

Fig. 3.74 Normal pressure values (mmHg) of the heart.

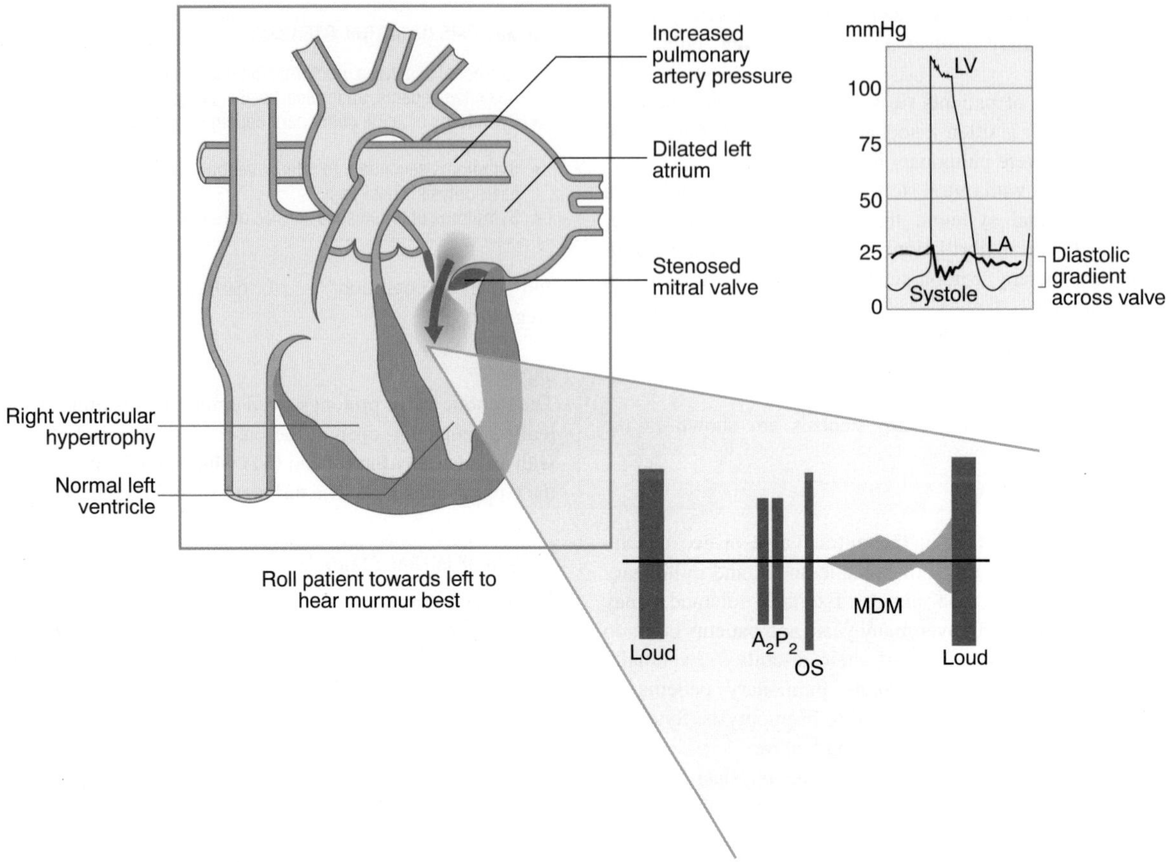

Fig. 3.75 Mitral stenosis: murmur and illustration of the diastolic pressure gradient between left atrium and left ventricle. (Mean gradient is reflected by the area between LA and LV in diastole.) The first heart sound is loud, there is an opening snap (OS) and mid-diastolic murmur (MDM) with presystolic accentuation.

by the opening snap, causes the characteristic low-pitched diastolic murmur, and often a thrill (see Fig. 3.75).

The murmur is accentuated by exercise and during atrial systole. Early in the disease or in asymptomatic patients a presystolic murmur may be the only auscultatory abnormality. In patients with symptoms the murmur usually extends from the opening snap to the first heart sound. The opening snap gets closer to the second sound (S2) as the stenosis becomes more severe, but may be inaudible if the valve is heavily calcified. Accompanying mitral regurgitation causes a pansystolic murmur which radiates towards the axilla.

The development of pulmonary hypertension may be demonstrated by an abnormal pulsation felt to the left of the sternum, due to right ventricular hypertrophy or to forward displacement of the heart by a dilated left atrium. Pulmonary hypertension may cause a loud pulmonary component of the second heart sound. Tricuspid regurgitation secondary to right ventricular dilatation causes a systolic murmur and systolic waves in the venous pulse.

Investigations

The ECG may show either the bifid P waves (P mitrale) associated with left atrial hypertrophy, or atrial fibrillation. There may also be evidence of right ventricular hypertrophy. Enlargement of the left atrium and its appendage and of the main pulmonary artery may be seen on the chest radiograph. There may be enlargement of the upper pulmonary veins and horizontal linear shadows in the costophrenic angles as indications of a high left atrial and pulmonary venous pressure.

Doppler echocardiography can provide the definitive evaluation of mitral stenosis; apart from confirming the diagnosis, it allows an assessment of its severity and it also provides information on the rigidity and state of calcifi-

INVESTIGATIONS IN MITRAL STENOSIS
ECG
• Left atrial hypertrophy (if not in AF) • Right ventricular hypertrophy
Chest radiograph
• Enlarged left atrium • Signs of pulmonary venous hypertension
Echo
• Thickened immobile cusps • Reduced valve area • Reduced rate of diastolic filling of LV
Doppler
• Pressure gradient across mitral valve • Pulmonary artery pressure
Cardiac catheterisation
• Pressure gradient between LA (or pulmonary wedge) and LV

cation of the valve cusps, the size of the left atrium, pulmonary artery pressure and the state of left ventricular function (see Fig. 3.76).

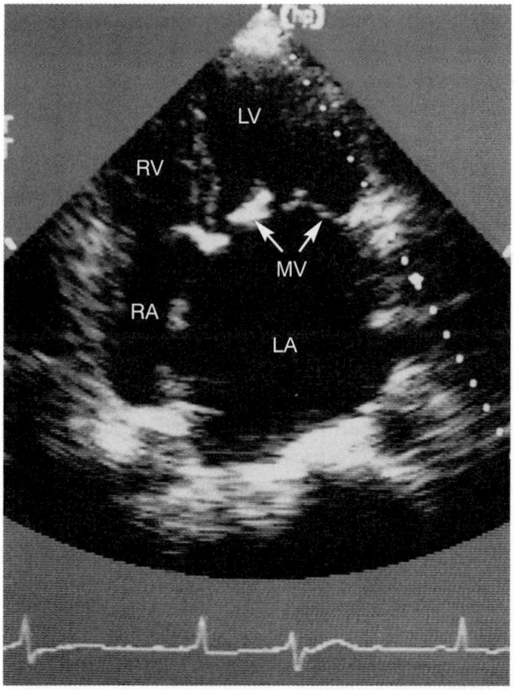

Fig. 3.76 Echocardiogram of a patient with mitral stenosis, apical view. Note that the left atrium is enlarged and bigger than the left ventricle. The left atrium also bulges towards the right atrium. The mitral valve (MV) is thickened and forms a dome shape in diastole as it fails to open fully (arrows).

Prior to the advent of echocardiography, cardiac catheterisation was used to confirm the severity of mitral stenosis by measurement of the gradient across the mitral valve from pressures recorded simultaneously in the left ventricle and left atrium (or pulmonary capillary wedge position). Cardiac catheterisation still has a role in assessing co-existing mitral regurgitation and coronary disease.

Management

Patients with minor symptoms should be treated medically, but the definitive treatment of mitral stenosis is by mitral valvotomy, balloon valvuloplasty or mitral valve replacement. If the patient remains symptomatic despite medical treatment, if pulmonary congestion persists, or if pulmonary hypertension develops, valvuloplasty or surgery is indicated.

Medical management

This consists of anticoagulants (see p. 796) to reduce the risk of systemic embolism, digoxin (0.125–0.25 mg/day) to control the ventricular rate in atrial fibrillation (or to prevent a rapid ventricular rate if atrial fibrillation should develop), diuretics to control pulmonary congestion (see p. 401) and antibiotic prophylaxis against infective endocarditis (see p. 289).

Mitral balloon valvuloplasty

This is the treatment of choice if the appropriate criteria are fulfilled (see the information box). Closed or open mitral valvotomy may be used if the facilities or expertise for valvuloplasty are not available.

CRITERIA FOR MITRAL VALVULOPLASTY
• Significant symptoms • Isolated mitral stenosis • No (or trivial) mitral regurgitation • Mobile, non-calcified valve/subvalve apparatus on echo • Left atrium free of thrombus

Mitral valve replacement

If there is substantial mitral reflux, or if the valve is rigid and calcified, then surgery rather than balloon valvuloplasty is indicated.

Monitoring and after-care

Clinical symptoms are a guide to the severity of mitral re-stenosis, but Doppler echocardiography provides a more accurate assessment. The ECG gives evidence of increasing pulmonary hypertension and the heart size on chest radiography is a useful but not infallible guide to severity. Patients who have had a mitral valvuloplasty or valvotomy should practise antibiotic prophylaxis against infective endocarditis (see p. 289) and should be followed up at 1–2-yearly intervals because re-stenosis may occur.

MITRAL REGURGITATION

Aetiology and pathophysiology

Rheumatic disease is the principal cause of mitral regurgitation in countries where rheumatic fever is common but elsewhere, including in the United Kingdom, other causes (see the information box) are more important.

CAUSES OF MITRAL REGURGITATION

- Mitral valve prolapse
- Dilatation of the mitral valve ring (e.g. Rheumatic fever, coronary artery disease, cardiomyopathy)
- Damage to valve cusps and chordae (e.g. Rheumatic heart disease, endocarditis)
- Damage to papillary muscle
- Myocardial infarction

Chronic mitral regurgitation causes gradual dilatation of the left atrium with little increase in pressure and therefore relatively few symptoms. However, breathlessness and pulmonary oedema will supervene if the left ventricle dilates and the left ventricular diastolic and left atrial pressures increase as a result of chronic volume overload. In contrast, acute mitral regurgitation tends to cause a rapid rise in left atrial pressure (because left atrial compliance is normal) and marked symptomatic deterioration.

Mitral valve prolapse

This is also known as 'floppy' mitral valve and is one of the more common causes of mild mitral regurgitation. It is caused by congenital anomalies or degenerative myxomatous changes and is sometimes a feature of connective tissue disorders such as Marfan's syndrome.

In the mildest forms of mitral prolapse the valve remains competent but bulges back into the atrium during systole, causing a mid-systolic click but no murmur. In the presence of a regurgitant valve the click is followed by a late systolic murmur. The murmur lengthens as regurgitation becomes more severe, and the combination of a click and late systolic murmur provides the clinical hallmark of mitral prolapse. Occasionally, multiple clicks are heard, or the click is obscured by the first heart sound; the pansystolic murmur may be indistinguishable from other causes of mitral regurgitation. The physical signs may vary with posture or respiration.

Progressive elongation of the chordae tendineae may lead to increasing mitral regurgitation, while if chordal rupture occurs, regurgitation may suddenly become severe. These complications are rare before the fifth or sixth decade.

Mitral prolapse is associated with an increased incidence of arrhythmias—these are usually benign but a small minority of patients have frequent and bizarre arrhythmias. Some patients with atypical chest pain are found to have mitral prolapse but this association is not specific. Telling patients that they have an abnormal valve sometimes exacerbates or perpetuates a cardiac neurosis. Mitral prolapse is more common than would be expected in young people with embolic stroke or transient cerebral ischaemic attacks, but the overall risk of this complication is exceedingly small. Haemodynamically significant mitral prolapse can predispose to infective endocarditis, and hence requires antibiotic prophylaxis, but overall the long-term prognosis is good.

Other causes of mitral regurgitation

Regurgitation can result from dilatation of the mitral valve ring in association with diseases involving the myocardium, such as rheumatic fever, extensive infarction, diphtheria, myocarditis or cardiomyopathy. Papillary muscle dysfunction commonly follows myocardial infarction. Rupture of the papillary muscles or chordae may also occur with infarction, resulting in acute severe pulmonary oedema. The valve cusps may also be damaged gradually from chronic rheumatic heart disease, in which case there is often coexisting mitral stenosis and/or aortic valve disease. Mitral regurgitation can develop rapidly with infective endocarditis.

Clinical features

These are summarised in the information box.

The symptoms depend on how suddenly the regurgitation develops. When the valve damage is a slow process the symptoms are similar to those in mitral stenosis. After acute myocardial infarction, the mitral regurgitation may be severe, and should be differentiated from ventricular septal rupture.

CLINICAL FEATURES OF MITRAL REGURGITATION

Symptoms

Acute mitral regurgitation
- Symptoms of acute pulmonary oedema and reduced cardiac output

Chronic progressive mitral regurgitation
- Exertional dyspnoea, nocturnal dyspnoea, palpitations (AF, atrial flutter, increased stroke volume)
- Symptoms of pulmonary oedema (esp. with pregnancy or AF)
- Symptoms of diminished cardiac output, e.g. fatigue
- Ankle/leg oedema, abdominal swelling (right heart failure)

Signs

- Atrial fibrillation/flutter
- Cardiomegaly—displaced hyperdynamic apex beat
- Apical pansystolic murmur ± thrill
- Soft S1, apical S3
- Signs of raised pulmonary capillary pressure crepitations, pulmonary oedema, effusions
- Signs of pulmonary hypertension may be present

The physical signs arise from the regurgitant jet which causes an apical systolic murmur (see Fig. 3.77). This often radiates into the axilla, and may be accompanied by a thrill. The apex beat is usually displaced to the left as a result of dilatation of the left ventricle. The abnormal valve closure is often associated with a quiet first heart sound; increased forward flow through the mitral valve may give rise to a loud third heart sound and even a short mid-diastolic murmur.

Investigations

The radiograph and ECG often give evidence of left atrial and/or left ventricular hypertrophy. Atrial fibrillation is common, as a consequence of atrial dilatation. Echocardiography provides information about the state of the mitral valve, but Doppler (or colour Doppler) echocardiography gives a better estimate of the extent of regurgitation (see Fig. 3.13, p. 203). At cardiac catheterisation the severity of mitral regurgitation may be indicated by the size of the *v* (systolic) waves in the left atrial or PAW trace, or by left

INVESTIGATIONS IN MITRAL REGURGITATION (MR)
ECG
• Left atrial hypertrophy (if not in AF) • Left ventricular hypertrophy
Chest radiograph
• Enlarged left atrium • Enlarged left ventricle • Signs of pulmonary venous hypertension • Signs of pulmonary oedema (if acute)
Echo
• Dilated LA, LV • Dynamic LV (unless LVF predominates)
Doppler
• Detects and quantifies regurgitation (see Fig. 3.13, p. 203)
Cardiac catheterisation
• Dilated LA, LV, mitral regurgitation • Pulmonary hypertension may be present (chronic MR) • Coexisting coronary artery disease

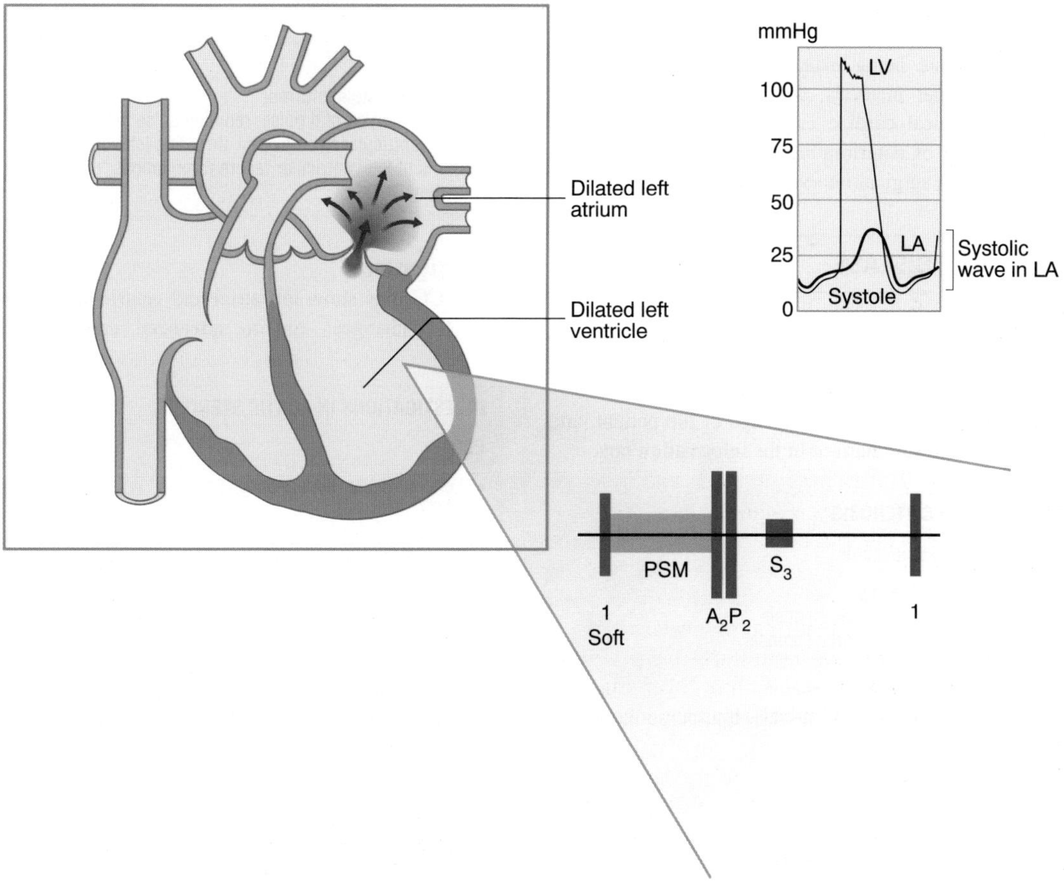

Fig. 3.77 Mitral regurgitation: radiation of the murmur to the axilla and illustration of systolic wave in left atrial pressure. The first sound is normal or soft and merges with a pansystolic murmur (PSM) extending to the second heart sound. A third heart sound occurs with severe regurgitation. The left atrium and ventricle become dilated.

ventricular angiography. However, this is not always reliable, as left atrial compliance may vary. In practice, a common problem lies in deciding the extent to which cardiac failure is due to mitral regurgitation and the extent to which it reflects impaired left ventricular function.

Management

If mitral regurgitation is due to myocardial disease, treatment when available is directed to the latter. When the valve disease is predominant and symptoms severe, mitral valve replacement or repair is indicated. Mitral regurgitation of moderate severity can be treated medically, as shown in the information box. Vasodilators can reduce the regurgitant fraction and are therefore particularly helpful.

MEDICAL MANAGEMENT OF MITRAL REGURGITATION
• Diuretics • Vasodilators, e.g. ACE inhibitors (see p. 215) • Digoxin if atrial fibrillation is present • Anticoagulants if atrial fibrillation is present • Antibiotic prophylaxis

Patients who are being managed medically should be reviewed at regular intervals; worsening symptoms, progressive radiological cardiac enlargement or echocardiographic evidence of deteriorating left ventricular function are indications for surgical intervention.

AORTIC VALVE DISEASE

AORTIC STENOSIS

Aetiology and pathophysiology

The likely aetiology varies with the age of the patient, and possible causes are summarised in the information box.

CAUSES OF AORTIC STENOSIS
Infants, children, adolescents
• Congenital aortic stenosis • Congenital subvalvular aortic stenosis • Congenital supravalvular aortic stenosis
Young adults to middle-aged
• Calcification and fibrosis of congenitally bicuspid aortic valve • Rheumatic aortic stenosis
Middle-aged to elderly
• Calcification of bicuspid valve • Senile degenerative aortic stenosis • Rheumatic aortic stenosis

Except in the congenital forms, aortic stenosis develops slowly; the cardiac output is maintained at the cost of a steadily increasing gradient across the aortic valve. The left ventricle becomes increasingly hypertrophied, and coronary blood flow may become inadequate. The fixed outflow obstruction limits the increase in cardiac output required on exercise. Patients may develop angina, left ventricular failure and arrhythmias, even in the absence of concomitant coronary disease. However, in elderly patients aortic stenosis and coronary atheroma frequently coexist.

Clinical features

Mild or moderate aortic stenosis is asymptomatic. The features are summarised in the information box. The characteristic murmur is illustrated in Figure 3.78.

CLINICAL FEATURES OF AORTIC STENOSIS
Symptoms
• Exertional dyspnoea • Angina • Pulmonary oedema • Exertional syncope • Sudden death
Signs
• Ejection systolic murmur • Slow-rising carotid pulse, reduced pulse pressure • Left ventricular hypertrophy, thrusting left ventricle • Signs of left ventricular failure (crepitations, pulmonary oedema)

Investigations

The ECG may show left atrial and ventricular hypertrophy and ST changes, and in advanced cases features of

INVESTIGATIONS IN AORTIC STENOSIS
ECG
• Left ventricular hypertrophy (usually) • LBBB
Chest radiograph
• May be normal. Sometimes enlarged left ventricle and dilated ascending aorta on PA view, calcified valve on lateral view
Echo
• Calcified valve, hypertrophied LV
Doppler
• Estimate of gradient
Cardiac catheterisation
• Systolic gradient between LV and aorta • Post-stenotic dilatation of aorta • Regurgitation of aortic valve may be present **N.B.** Cardiac catheter may only be required to determine if coronary disease is present.

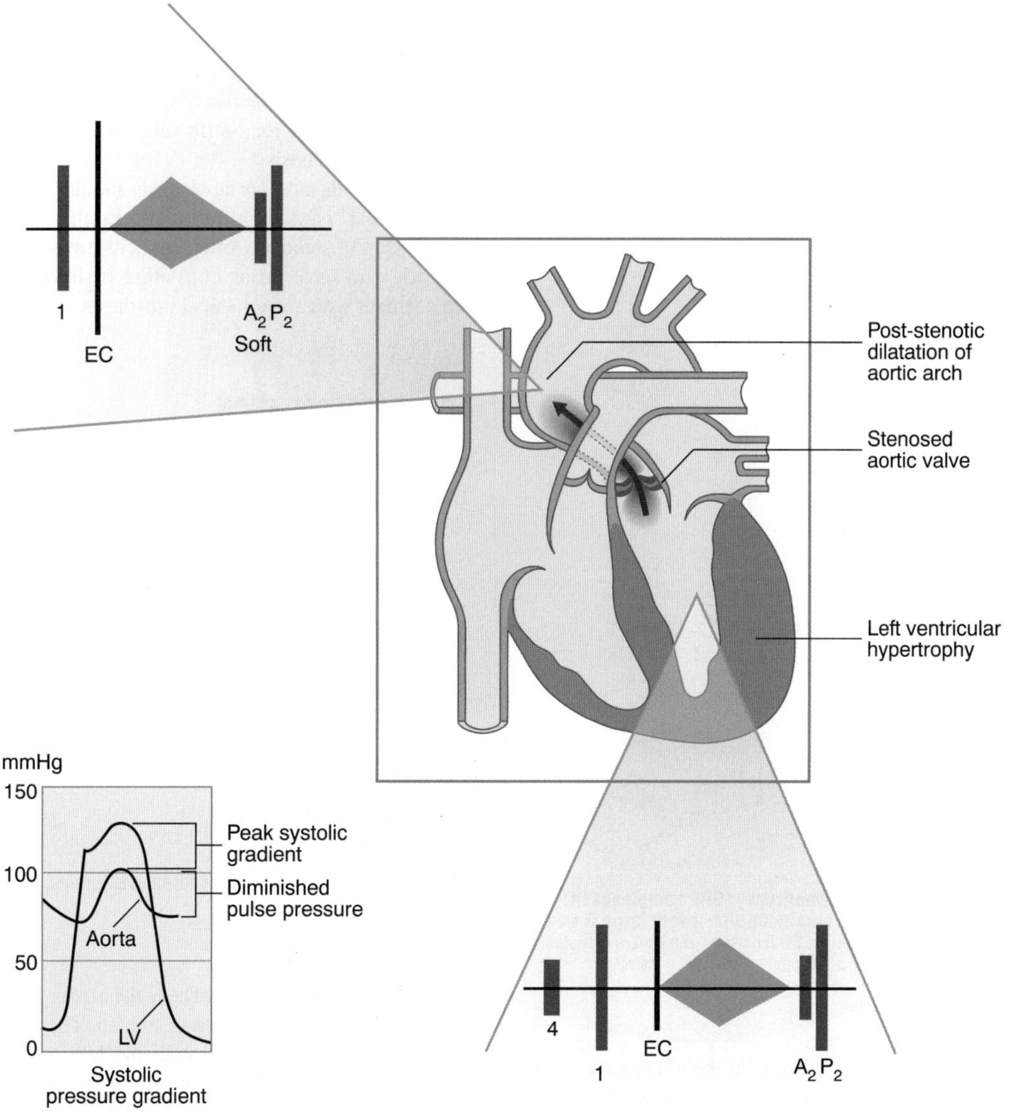

Fig. 3.78 Aortic stenosis: radiation of the murmur in aortic stenosis with left ventricular hypertrophy and enlargement of the ventricle. Pressure traces show the systolic gradient between left ventricle and aorta. The 'diamond shape' murmur may be heard in the aortic outflow and also at the apex. The aortic component of the second heart sound (A_2) is quiet or inaudible. An ejection click (EC) may be present with valvular aortic stenosis. Aortic stenosis may lead to left ventricular hypertrophy with a fourth sound at the apex and post-stenotic dilatation of the aortic arch.

hypertrophy are gross (see Fig. 3.79). LBBB is common. Downsloping ST segments and T inversion ('strain pattern') may be seen in leads reflecting the left ventricle. However, especially in the elderly, the ECG may be normal despite severe stenosis. The postero-anterior chest radiograph is frequently normal, but may show left ventricular enlargement and post-stenotic dilatation of the ascending aorta. A lateral radiograph, or magnetic resonance image, may show valve calcification, but the diagnosis is more readily made on echocardiography.

Echocardiography will show an abnormal aortic valve, which may be heavily calcified and disorganised, and a hypertrophied left ventricle. Doppler echocardiography permits calculation of the systolic gradient across the aortic valve from the velocity of the ejected jet of blood, and detects the presence or absence of aortic regurgitation.

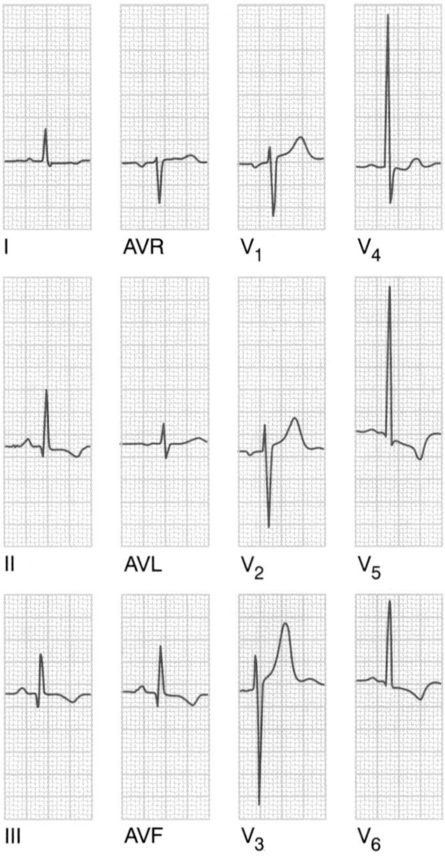

Fig. 3.79 Left ventricular hypertrophy: QRS complexes in limb leads have increased amplitude with a very large R wave in V_5 and S wave in V_2. There is ST depression and T wave inversion in leads II, III, AVF, V_5 and V_6: a 'left ventricular strain' pattern.

Cardiac catheterisation is indicated if the ultrasound studies are unsatisfactory or if it is necessary to assess the state of the coronary arteries.

Management

Patients with symptomatic aortic stenosis and a valve gradient indicative of moderate or severe stenosis (i.e. > 50 mmHg in the presence of a normal cardiac output at rest) should have aortic valve replacement. To wait too long exposes the patient to the risk of sudden death, or irreversible deterioration in ventricular function. However, prospective reviews of *asymptomatic* aortic stenosis in the elderly have revealed a relatively benign prognosis without surgery, and in such patients conservative management may be appropriate. Patients should be kept under review, as the development of angina, symptoms of low cardiac output, or heart failure are indications for surgery. Old age, per se, is not a contraindication to valve replacement, and results remain very good in experienced centres even into the ninth decade.

Aortic balloon valvuloplasty is useful in congenital aortic stenosis but is of no long-term value in elderly patients with calcific aortic stenosis.

Patients with mild aortic stenosis should be followed up with regular cardiac ultrasound examination to detect progression of stenosis. Anticoagulants are only required in patients who have atrial fibrillation or have had a valve replacement with a mechanical prosthesis.

AORTIC REGURGITATION

Aetiology and pathophysiology

The condition results from congenitally abnormal aortic cusps (e.g. bicuspid valves), or from valve damage due to rheumatic heart disease or infective endocarditis, or other rarer causes (see the information box).

CAUSES OF AORTIC REGURGITATION
Congenital
• Bicuspid valve, or disproportionate cusps
Acquired
• Rheumatic disease • Infective endocarditis • Trauma • Aortic dilatation: Marfan's syndrome, atheroma, syphilis, ankylosing spondylitis

When regurgitation is marked, the stroke output of the left ventricle may be doubled or trebled. The major arteries are then conspicuously pulsatile; the left ventricle dilates and hypertrophies and initially compensates for the regurgitation. The left ventricular diastolic pressure rises, at first only with exercise, and breathlessness develops. In contrast to chronic gradual onset regurgitation, acute regurgitation may result from damage to the aortic leaflets (endocarditis, trauma), and auscultatory signs may be masked by tachycardia and the abrupt rise in LV end-diastolic pressure (shortening or even abolishing the typical murmur).

Clinical features

These are listed in the information box. Until the onset of breathlessness, the only symptom may be an awareness of the heart beat, particularly when lying on the left side. This results from the increased stroke volume. Paroxysmal nocturnal dyspnoea may be the first symptom and peripheral oedema, or angina, may occur. The charac-

CLINICAL FEATURES OF AORTIC REGURGITATION (AR)
Symptoms
Mild to moderate AR • Often asymptomatic • Awareness of heart beat, 'palpitations' **Severe AR** • Symptoms of heart failure • Angina
Signs
Pulses • Large-volume or 'collapsing' pulse • Bounding peripheral pulses • Capillary pulsation in nail beds—Quincke's sign • Femoral bruit ('pistol shot')—Duroziez's sign • Head nodding with pulse—de Musset's sign **Murmurs** • Early diastolic murmur • Systolic murmur of increased stroke volume • Austin Flint murmur (soft mid-diastolic) **Other signs** • Thrusting apex, fourth heart sound, enlarged LV • Signs of heart failure

teristic murmur is illustrated in Figure 3.80. Although it is usually best heard to the left of the sternum, it is sometimes louder to the right. A thrill is uncommon. When the leak is small the murmur will be heard only if the steps shown in Figure 3.80 are followed; this is of crucial importance in the early detection of infective endocarditis affecting the aortic valve. A systolic murmur due to the increased stroke volume is common, and does not necessarily indicate stenosis. When the leak is large the diagnosis is usually easy, with gross pulsation in the large arteries, a collapsing pulse, a low diastolic and an increased pulse pressure. There is usually a thrusting apical impulse and often a presystolic impulse and a fourth heart sound. The regurgitant jet produces fluttering of the mitral leaflets and a soft mid-diastolic murmur; the latter is called an Austin Flint murmur.

In acute severe regurgitation the features of heart failure may predominate, the murmur may be short (or even absent), and there may be insufficient time for the ventricle to dilate. This possibility must be considered, especially in the context of endocarditis.

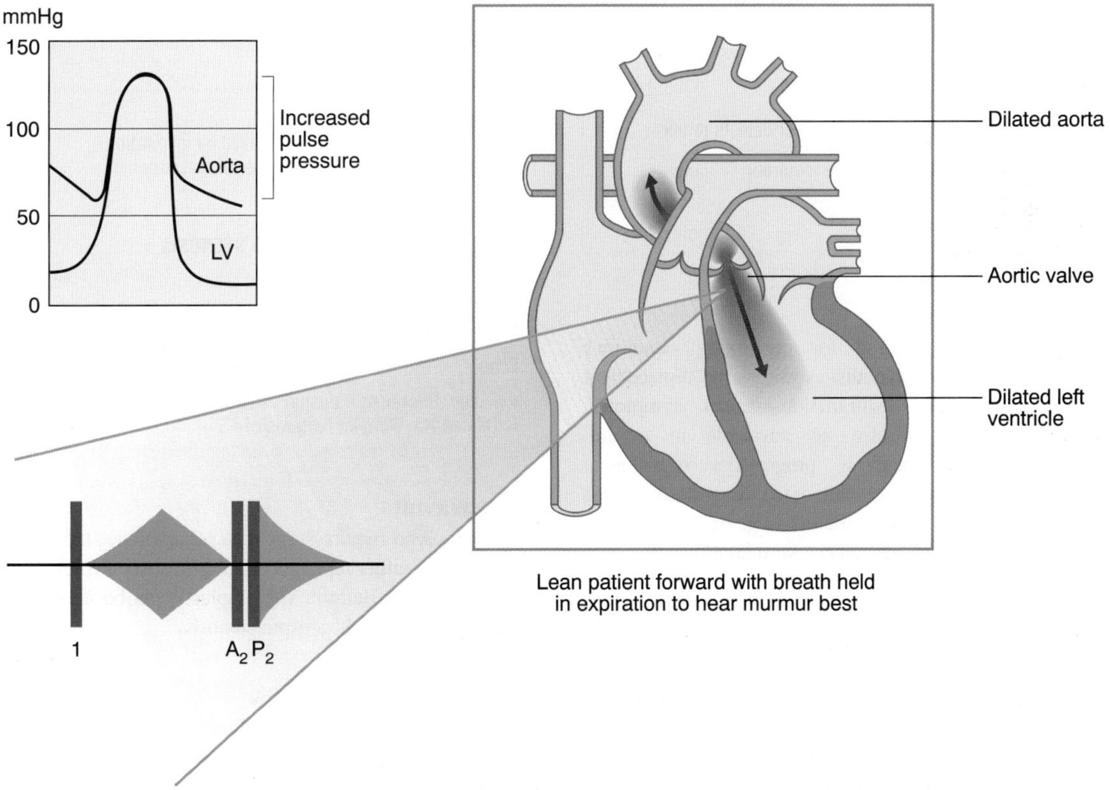

Fig. 3.80 Aortic regurgitation. The early diastolic murmur is best heard at the left sternal edge and may be accompanied by an ejection systolic murmur due to the enlarged stroke volume ('to and fro' murmur). Aortic regurgitation may lead to dilatation of the aortic arch and left ventricle.

Investigations

The chest radiograph characteristically shows cardiac and aortic dilatation, together with signs of left heart failure. When regurgitation is marked, the ECG may show left ventricular hypertrophy and ST changes. Echocardiography in aortic regurgitation shows a ventricle with vigorous contraction (until heart failure ensues). There may be fluttering of the anterior mitral leaflet in the regurgitant jet. The echocardiogram may reveal vegetations in infective endocarditis, and gives information about left ventricular function. Regurgitation is readily detected by Doppler or colour Doppler echocardiography. In severe acute aortic regurgitation the rapid rise in LV diastolic pressure may cause premature mitral valve closure. Cardiac catheterisation and aortography can be helpful in assessing severity, and dilatation of the aorta.

INVESTIGATIONS IN AORTIC REGURGITATION
ECG
• Initially normal, later LV hypertrophy and T wave inversion
Chest radiograph
• Cardiac dilatation, may be aortic dilatation • Features of left heart failure
Echo
• Dilated left ventricle • Hyperdynamic ventricle • Fluttering anterior mitral leaflet, Doppler detects reflux
Cardiac catheterisation (may not be required)
• Dilated LV, aortic regurgitation • Dilated aortic root

Management

Treatment may be required for underlying conditions such as endocarditis or syphilis. Aortic valve replacement is indicated if aortic regurgitation causes symptoms. However, surgery may also be advisable in asymptomatic patients if there is progressive radiological cardiomegaly or echocardiographic evidence of deteriorating left ventricular function. Vasodilators (e.g. ACE inhibitors) may prevent progressive left ventricular dilatation.

TRICUSPID VALVE DISEASE

TRICUSPID STENOSIS

Aetiology

Tricuspid stenosis is usually rheumatic in origin, and nearly always occurs in association with mitral and aortic valve disease. It is uncommon, with clinically evident tricuspid disease occurring in $<5\%$ of rheumatic heart disease. Isolated rheumatic tricuspid stenosis is very rare. Tricuspid stenosis and regurgitation are also associated with the carcinoid syndrome (see p. 652).

Clinical features

Usually the symptoms of the associated mitral and aortic valve disease predominate, but tricuspid stenosis causes symptoms of right heart failure including hepatic discomfort and ascites, and peripheral oedema.

The main clinical feature is a raised jugular venous pressure with a prominent *a* wave, and a slow *y* descent on account of the loss of the normal rapid RV filling (see p. 197). There may be presystolic hepatic pulsation, which represents a palpable *a* wave. There is a mid-diastolic murmur usually best heard at the lower left or right sternal edge; this is usually higher-pitched than the murmur of mitral stenosis and increased by inspiration.

CLINICAL FEATURES OF TRICUSPID STENOSIS (TS)
Symptoms
• Symptoms of associated mitral or aortic disease • Symptoms of right heart failure Abdominal swelling Hepatic discomfort Peripheral oedema Fatigue
Signs
• Raised JVP, prominent *a* wave • Mid-diastolic murmur—increased by inspiration • Right heart failure—ascites, peripheral oedema

INVESTIGATIONS IN TRICUSPID STENOSIS
Chest radiograph
• Enlarged RA (not specific for TS)
Echo
• Fused, thickened tricuspid valve • Dilated RA, Doppler features of TS

Management

In patients who require surgery to other valves, the tricuspid valve (TV) is either replaced or subjected to valvotomy at the time of surgery. Balloon valvuloplasty can be used to treat rare cases of isolated tricuspid stenosis.

TRICUSPID REGURGITATION

Aetiology and pathophysiology

Tricuspid regurgitation is common. The most frequent cause is described as 'functional', because the valve is not structurally abnormal but is stretched as a result of right ventricular dilatation (e.g. cor pulmonale).

CAUSES OF TRICUSPID REGURGITATION (TR)
Primary
• Rheumatic heart disease • Endocarditis, particularly in intravenous drug abusers • Ebstein's congenital anomaly
Secondary
• Right ventricular dilatation due to chronic left heart failure ('functional TR') • Right ventricular infarction • Pulmonary hypertension

SIGNS OF TRICUSPID REGURGITATION
• Raised JVP • Large systolic wave in JVP (*cv* wave) • Systolic hepatic pulsation • Pansystolic murmur (left sternal edge)—louder on inspiration

INVESTIGATIONS IN TRICUSPID REGURGITATION
Chest radiograph
• Dilated RA, RV
Echo
• RV dilatation • TV may be structurally abnormal (rheumatic disease, endocarditis, Ebstein's congenital anomaly) • Estimate PA pressure from Doppler

Symptoms are usually non-specific, and relate to reduced forward flow and venous congestion (tiredness, oedema, hepatic enlargement). The most prominent clinical feature is a large systolic wave in the jugular venous pulse (a *cv* wave replaces the normal *x* descent).

Management

Tricuspid regurgitation, which is due to right ventricular dilatation, gets better when the cause of right ventricular overload is corrected, e.g. by mitral valve replacement or by diuretic and vasodilator treatment of left ventricular failure.

Patients with a normal pulmonary artery pressure tolerate isolated tricuspid reflux without ill effects, and valves damaged by endocarditis do not always need to be replaced. A few patients with organic tricuspid valve damage and elevated pulmonary artery pressure may need tricuspid valve repair (annuloplasty) or replacement.

PULMONARY VALVE DISEASE

PULMONARY STENOSIS

Aetiology

The condition can occur in the carcinoid syndrome but is virtually always congenital, when it may be isolated or associated with other abnormalities such as Fallot's tetralogy (see p. 295).

Clinical features and management

The principal finding on examination is the ejection systolic murmur, loudest to the left of the upper sternum, and radiating towards the left shoulder. There may be a thrill, best felt when the patient leans forward and breathes out. The murmur is often preceded by an ejection sound. Delay in right ventricular ejection may cause wide splitting of the second heart sound. Severe pulmonary stenosis is characterised clinically by: a loud harsh murmur; an inaudible pulmonary closure sound (P_2); an increased right ventricular thrust; prominent *a* waves in the jugular pulse; ECG evidence of right ventricular hypertrophy; and post-stenotic dilatation in the pulmonary artery on the chest radiograph.

Mild to moderate isolated pulmonary stenosis is relatively common, does not usually progress, and does not require treatment. It is a low-risk lesion for infective endocarditis.

Severe pulmonary stenosis (resting gradient > 50 mmHg with a normal cardiac output) is treated by percutaneous pulmonary balloon valvuloplasty or, if unavailable, by surgical valvotomy. Long-term results are very good. Post-operative pulmonary regurgitation is common but benign.

CLINICAL FEATURES OF PULMONARY STENOSIS (PS)
Symptoms
• Symptoms of right heart failure • Symptoms of the carcinoid syndrome (see p. 652)
Signs
• Giant *a* wave in the JVP • RV hypertrophy and dilatation • Systolic murmur (upper left sternum)—increases on inspiration with increased pulmonary flow • Systolic thrill over pulmonary outflow • P2 soft and delayed • Valvular PS may have an ejection click

INVESTIGATIONS IN PULMONARY STENOSIS
Chest radiograph
• Prominent pulmonary artery (post-stenotic dilatation)
ECG
• Right atrial and RV hypertrophy
Echo
• Abnormal PV • Outflow gradient on Doppler

PULMONARY REGURGITATION

Pulmonary regurgitation is rarely an isolated phenomenon and is usually associated with pulmonary artery dilatation due to pulmonary hypertension. It may, for example, complicate mitral stenosis, producing an early diastolic decrescendo murmur at the left sternal edge that is difficult to distinguish from aortic regurgitation (Graham Steell murmur). The pulmonary hypertension may also be secondary to other disease of the left side of the heart, to primary pulmonary vascular disease, or to Eisenmenger's syndrome. Trivial pulmonary regurgitation is a frequent echocardiographic Doppler finding in normal individuals and is not of clinical significance.

INFECTIVE ENDOCARDITIS

Aetiology

Infective endocarditis is due to microbial infection of a heart valve (native or prosthetic), the lining of a cardiac chamber or blood vessel, or a congenital anomaly (e.g. septal defect). The causative organism is usually a bacterium, but may be a rickettsia (*Coxiella burnetii*—Q fever endocarditis), chlamydia or fungus.

INFECTIVE ENDOCARDITIS ON NATIVE VALVES: PREVALENCE OF ORGANISMS IN EUROPE AND NORTH AMERICA

Bacteria	
• Streptococci	
viridans	30–40%
Enterococci	10–15%
Other streptococci	20–25%
• Staphylococci	
aureus	9–27%
Coagulase negative	1–3%
• Gram-negative bacilli • Haemophilus • Anaerobes	Total 3–8%
Other organisms	
• Rickettsiae, fungi	Less than 2%

Streptococcus viridans (*S. mitis* and *S. sanguis*, α-haemolytic streptococci) are commensals in the upper respiratory tract and a common cause of periodontal infection. They may enter the blood stream on chewing, teeth-brushing or at the time of dental treatment. Other streptococci, including *S. faecalis*, *S. milleri* and *S. bovis*, may enter the blood from the bowel or urinary tract. *S. milleri* and *S. bovis* are sometimes associated with large bowel neoplasms.

Staphylococcus aureus is a common cause of acute endocarditis, originating from skin infections, abscesses or vascular access sites (e.g. intravenous and central lines), or intravenous drug abuse. It is a highly virulent and invasive organism, usually producing florid vegetations, valve destruction greater than in subacute endocarditis, and abscess formation. Other causes of acute endocarditis include *Streptococcus pneumoniae* and *Neisseria gonorrhoeae*.

Post-operative endocarditis follows cardiac surgery and affects native or prosthetic heart valves or other prosthetic materials. The most common organism is a coagulase-negative staphylococcus *(Staphylococcus albus)*. There is frequently a history of post-operative wound infection with the same organism.

In Q fever endocarditis (rickettsia) the patient often has a history of contact with farm animals. It commonly affects the aortic valve and may cause hepatic complications and purpura. Prolonged (life-long) antibiotic therapy may be required.

Gram-negative bacteria of the so-called HACEK group are slow-growing fastidious organisms that may only be revealed after prolonged culture and may be resistant to penicillin.

Brucella is associated with a history of contact with goats or cattle and often affects the aortic valve.

Fungi *(Candida, Aspergillus)* may attack previously normal or prosthetic valves. Abscesses and emboli are common, therapy is difficult (surgery is often required) and the mortality is high. Concomitant bacterial infection may be present.

Incidence

A community study of South-east Scotland revealed that the incidence of infective endocarditis was 16 cases per million per annum. In a large British study, the underlying heart disease was rheumatic heart disease in 24% of patients, congenital heart disease in 19%, and some other cardiac abnormality (e.g. calcified AV, floppy MV) in 25%. The remainder (32%) were not thought to have a pre-existing cardiac abnormality.

Pathophysiology

Endocarditis occurs at sites where the endothelium is damaged by a high-pressure jet of blood (ventricular septal defect, persistent ductus arteriosus, or regurgitant mitral or aortic valves) or on damaged valves. In intravenous drug addicts right heart valves are affected (especially tricuspid). Endothelial damage leads to the deposition of platelets and fibrin, which are colonised by blood-borne organisms, creating vegetations. The avascular valve tissue and presence of fibrin aggregates help to protect the proliferating organisms from host defence mechanisms. Affected valves develop vegetations composed of organisms, fibrin and platelets, and the vegetations may become large enough to cause obstruction or may break away as emboli. Regurgitation may develop or increase, owing to the perforation

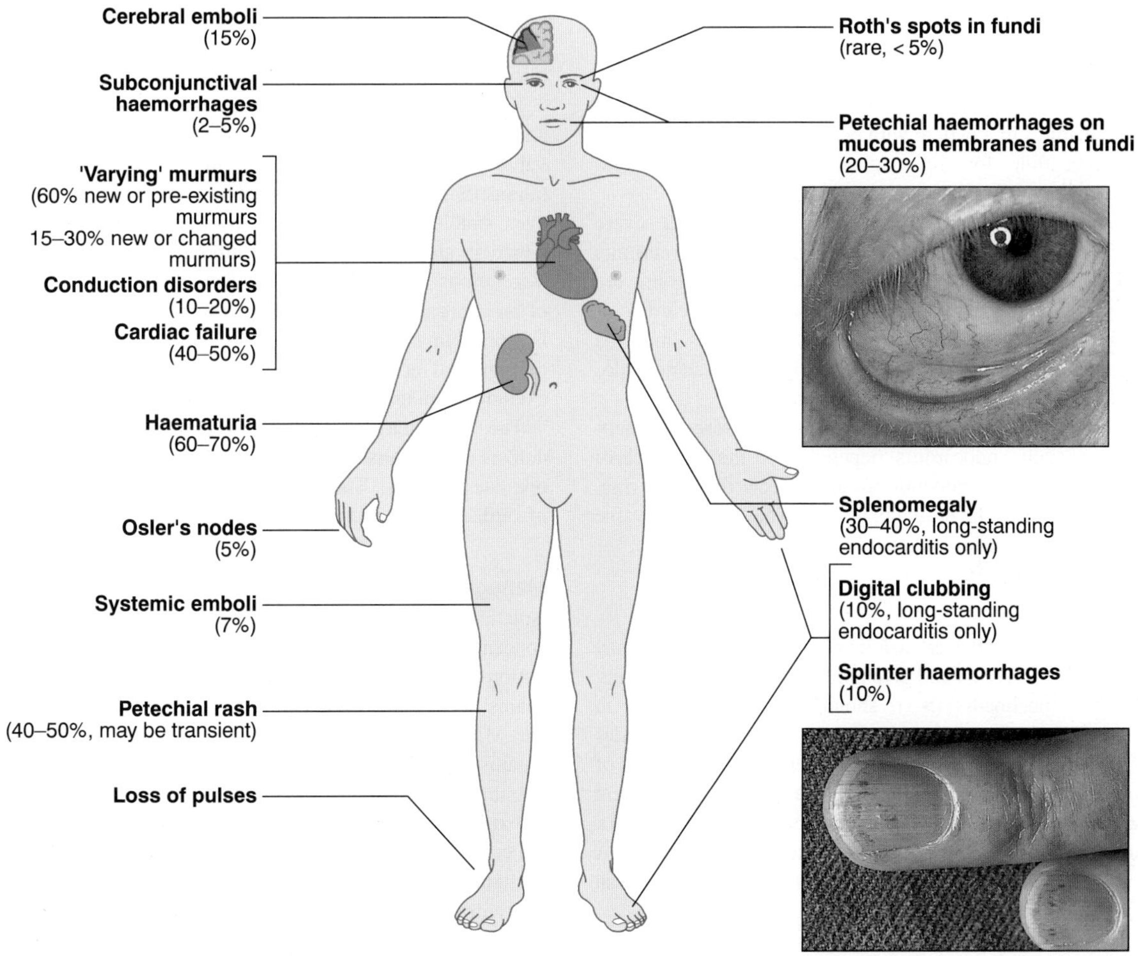

Fig. 3.81 Clinical features which may be present in endocarditis.

of a cusp or the disruption of chordae. Extra-cardiac manifestations result from emboli or from immune complexes, which may be responsible for vasculitis and skin lesions. Mycotic aneurysms may develop in arteries at the site of infected emboli. At postmortem it is common to find infarction of the spleen and kidneys, and sometimes an immune glomerulonephritis.

Clinical features

Possible clinical features in endocarditis, and their frequency, are given in Figure 3.81.

The clinical course of endocarditis

Prior to the advent of effective therapy, the illness often ran a stuttering course over several months, accompanied by the striking clinical stigmata. This pattern is now rare. Clinically, endocarditis has been divided into an acute and a more insidious 'subacute' form. The designation of acute and subacute forms has been questioned, as the clinical pattern is influenced not only by the organism, but also by the site of infection, prior antibiotic therapy and the presence of a valve or shunt prosthesis. Furthermore, the subacute form may abruptly develop acute life-threatening complications including valve disruption or emboli.

Subacute endocarditis. This should be suspected when a patient known to have congenital or valvular heart disease develops a persistent fever, complains of unusual tiredness, night sweats or weight loss, or develops new signs of valve dysfunction or heart failure. Less often, it presents as an embolic stroke or peripheral arterial embolism. Other features include purpura and petechial haemorrhages in the skin and mucous membranes, and splinter haemorrhages under the finger or toe nails. Osler's nodes are painful tender swellings at the fingertips, probably the result of vasculitis. They are rare. Digital clubbing is a late sign. The spleen is frequently palpable; in *Coxiella* infections the spleen and the liver may be considerably enlarged. Microscopic haematuria is common. The finding of any of these features in a patient with persistent fever or malaise is an indication for re-examination to detect hitherto unrecognised heart disease.

Acute endocarditis. This usually presents as a severe febrile illness with prominent and changing heart murmurs and petechiae. Clinical stigmata of chronic endocarditis are usually absent. Embolic events are common, and cardiac or renal failure may develop rapidly. Abscesses may be detected on echocardiography. Partially treated acute endocarditis behaves like subacute endocarditis.

Post-operative endocarditis. This may resemble subacute or acute endocarditis, depending on the virulence of the organism. The infection usually affects the valve ring. Any unexplained fever in a patient who has had heart valve surgery should be investigated for possible endocarditis.

Investigations

Blood culture is the crucial investigation because it may identify the infection and give guidance about management. Several specimens (> 3) should be taken prior to commencing therapy, and these need not wait for episodes of pyrexia. Aseptic technique is essential and the risk of contaminants must be minimised by sampling from different venepuncture sites. An indwelling line should not be used for cultures. Aerobic and anaerobic cultures are required. A knowledge of prior antibiotic treatment may allow an inactivating enzyme to be added and facilitate growth.

Elevation of the ESR, a normocytic, normochromic anaemia and leucocytosis are common but not invariable, and thrombocytopenia may be present. Measurement of plasma C-reactive protein (CRP) is more reliable than the ESR in assessing progress. Proteinuria may occur and microscopic haematuria is usually present.

Echocardiography is the key investigation for detecting and following the progress of vegetations, for assessing valve damage, and for detecting abscess formation. Vegetations (3–5 mm) can be detected by transthoracic echo, and even smaller ones (1–1.5 mm) by transoesophageal echo, which is also valuable for identifying abscess formation. Vegetations may be difficult to distinguish in the presence of an abnormal valve; the sensitivity of transthoracic echo is approximately 65% but more than 90% for transoesophageal echo. Failure to detect vegetations does not exclude the diagnosis and should not delay treatment.

The ECG may show the development of conduction defects (due to abscess formation) and occasionally infarction due to emboli. The chest radiograph may show evidence of cardiac failure and cardiomegaly.

Management

Isolation of the organism allows minimum inhibitory concentrations (MIC) and minimum bactericidal concentrations (MBC) of the antimicrobial drug to be measured against the specific organism. Plasma drug levels 4–8 times the MIC/MBC are usually effective in eradicating the organism. Any source of infection should be removed if possible; for example, a tooth with an apical abscess should be extracted.

Persisting infection is indicated by continuing fever, changing murmurs, and a persistently elevated ESR or CRP concentration. Antimicrobial therapy must be started before surgery.

A list of some common antimicrobial treatment regimens for common causative organisms is shown in Table 3.14.

Table 3.14 Antimicrobial treatment of common causative organisms in infective endocarditis

Organism	Antimicrobial	Dose	
Strep. viridans	Benzylpenicillin i.v. + gentamicin i.v.	1.2 g 4-hourly 80 mg 12-hourly	2 weeks for sensitive organisms (MIC ≤ 0.1 ml) 4 weeks for others
Strep. faecalis	Ampicillin or amoxycillin i.v. + gentamicin i.v.	2 g 4-hourly 80 mg 12-hourly	4 weeks 4 weeks
N.B. For gentamicin-resistant organisms give ampicillin/amoxycillin alone for 6 weeks and add streptomycin if sensitive			
Staphylococci			
Penicillin-sensitive	Benzylpenicillin i.v. + gentamicin i.v.	1.2 g 4-hourly 80–120 mg 8-hourly	4 weeks 1 week
Penicillin-resistant Methicillin-sensitive	Flucloxacillin i.v. + gentamicin i.v.	2 g 4-hourly 80–120 mg 8-hourly	4 weeks 1 week
Penicillin- and methicillin-resistant	Vancomycin i.v. + gentamicin i.v.	1 g 12-hourly 80–120 mg 8-hourly	4 weeks 1 week
N.B. The dose of gentamicin and vancomycin should be adjusted according to plasma drug concentrations. Renal function should be monitored during treatment with these drugs.			

INDICATIONS FOR CARDIAC SURGERY IN INFECTIVE ENDOCARDITIS

- Heart failure due to valve damage
- Failure of antibiotic therapy (persistent or uncontrolled infection)
- Large vegetations on left-sided heart valves with evidence or 'high risk' of systemic emboli
- Abscess formation

N.B. Patients with prosthetic valve endocarditis or fungal endocarditis often require cardiac surgery.

Prevention

Patients with valvular or congenital heart disease may be susceptible to infective endocarditis. Patients should be aware of the risk of endocarditis, the need to avoid bacteraemia, and the importance of maintaining good dental health. Potential sources of infection should be treated promptly. Antibiotic prophylaxis requires that the drug and dose chosen should be sufficient to kill the offending organism, but should only be given shortly before bacteraemia in order to reduce resistance (see Table 3.15).

Table 3.15 Antibiotic prophylaxis against endocarditis

Procedure	Antibiotic	Dose
Local anaesthetic		
Dental or upper respiratory tract procedures	Amoxycillin orally	3 g 1 hr before
If allergic to or received penicillin in last month	Clindamycin orally	600 mg 1 hr before
N.B. Previous endocarditis: treat as special-risk (see below).		
General anaesthetic		
Dental or upper respiratory tract procedures	Amoxycillin i.v. **plus** amoxycillin orally	1 g at induction 0.5 g 6 hrs later
If allergic to penicillin	Vancomycin i.v. infusion **plus** gentamicin i.v.	1 g over 1 hr before 120 mg
Genitourinary procedures or special-risk patients, i.e. prosthetic valve or previous endocarditis	Amoxycillin i.v. **plus** gentamicin i.v. **plus** amoxycillin orally	1 g 120 mg 0.5 g 6 hrs later
If allergic to penicillin	Vancomycin i.v. infusion **plus** gentamicin i.v.	1 g over 1 hr before 120 mg
N.B. Obstetric and gynaecological procedures or gastrointestinal surgery/instrumentation—treat only prosthetic valve patients (as for special-risk patients, above).		

FURTHER INFORMATION ON DISEASES OF THE HEART VALVES

American Heart Association Special Writing Committee on Rheumatic Fever, Endocarditis and Kawasaki Disease of the Council of Cardiovascular Disease in the Young 1992 (update) Guidelines for the diagnosis of rheumatic fever: Jones criteria. Journal of the American Heart Association 268: 2069–2073

British Cardiac Society and Research Unit of the Royal College of Physicians Working Group 1996 Valvular heart disease: investigation and management. Recommendations. Journal of the Royal College of Physicians of London 30: 309–315

British Society for Antimicrobial Chemotherapy Endocarditis Working Party 1992 Antibiotic prophylaxis of infective endocarditis. Lancet 339: 1292–1293

Dajani A S, Bisno A L, Chung K J et al 1990 Prevention of bacterial endocarditis. Recommendations of the American Heart Association. Journal of the American Medical Association 264: 2919–2922

CONGENITAL HEART DISEASE

Congenital heart disease usually presents during the first year of life but can present at any stage of life. Defects which are well tolerated, e.g. atrial septal defect, may cause no symptoms until adult life or may first be detected incidentally on routine examination or chest radiograph. There are growing numbers of patients who have had surgical correction of congenital defects in infancy or childhood who remain well for many years and subsequently re-present in later life (see the information box).

PRESENTATION OF CONGENITAL HEART DISEASE THROUGHOUT LIFE

Birth and neonatal period

- Cyanosis
- Heart failure

Infancy and childhood

- Cyanosis
- Heart failure
- Arrhythmia
- Murmur
- Failure to thrive

Childhood and adolescence

- Cyanosis due to shunt reversal (Eisenmenger's syndrome)

Adult

- Heart failure
- Murmur
- Arrhythmia
- Hypertension (coarctation)
- Late consequences of previous cardiac surgery, e.g. arrhythmia, heart failure

In utero the ductus arteriosus shunts blood from the pulmonary artery to the aorta, bypassing the lungs. The ductus arteriosus normally closes within a few days of birth and this may reveal underlying congenital heart disease (e.g. severe pulmonary stenosis), when pulmonary blood flow is dependent upon flow coming through the ductus arteriosus from the aorta. Cyanosis is caused by unoxygenated venous blood passing directly into the systemic circulation without passing through the lungs. This can be intermittent as, for example, in tetralogy of Fallot, where the degree of dynamic obstruction between the right ventricle and the pulmonary artery affects the degree of right-to-left shunting across the ventricular septal defect. Cyanosis may develop in adult life if a patient with a left-to-right shunt develops pulmonary hypertension and consequent reversal of the shunt from right to left, i.e. Eisenmenger's syndrome (see below).

Aetiology and incidence

The incidence of haemodynamically significant congenital cardiac abnormalities is about 0.8% of live births (see Table 3.16). Maternal infection or exposure to drugs or toxins may cause congenital heart disease. Maternal rubella infection is associated with persistent ductus arteriosus, pulmonary valvular and/or artery stenosis, and atrial septal defect. Maternal alcohol abuse is associated with septal defects and maternal lupus erythematosus is associated with congenital complete heart block. Genetic or chromosomal abnormalities such as Down's syndrome may cause septal defects, and gene defects have also been identified as causing specific abnormalities, e.g. Marfan's and DiGeorge's syndromes.

Clinical features

Symptoms may be absent, or the child may be noticed to be breathless, or may fail to attain normal growth and development. All degrees of severity occur. Some defects are not compatible with extrauterine life, or only for a short time. Clinical signs vary with the anatomical lesion. Cerebrovascular accidents and cerebral abscesses are complications of severe cyanotic congenital disease.

Table 3.16 Incidence and relative frequency of congenital cardiac malformations

Lesion	% of all CHD defects
Ventricular septal defect	30
Atrial septal defect	10
Patent ductus arteriosus	10
Pulmonary stenosis	7
Coarctation of aorta	7
Aortic stenosis	6
Tetralogy of Fallot	6
Complete transposition of great arteries	4
Others	20

Early diagnosis is important because many types of congenital heart disease are amenable to surgical treatment, but this opportunity may be lost if secondary changes—for example, pulmonary vascular damage—occur.

Principal features are illustrated in Figure 3.82.

Central cyanosis and digital clubbing

Central cyanosis of cardiac origin occurs when desaturated blood enters the systemic circulation without passing through the lungs (i.e. there is a right-to-left shunt). In the neonate, the most common cause of this is transposition of the great arteries, in which the aorta arises from the right ventricle and the pulmonary artery from the left. In older children, cyanosis is usually the consequence of a ventricular septal defect combined with severe pulmonary stenosis (tetralogy of Fallot) or with pulmonary vascular disease (Eisenmenger's syndrome). Prolonged cyanosis is associated with finger and toe clubbing.

Pulmonary hypertension

Persistently raised pulmonary flow (e.g. with left-to-right shunt) leads to increased pulmonary resistance followed by pulmonary hypertension. When the shunt is reversed cyanosis is evident (Eisenmenger's syndrome).

Growth retardation and learning difficulties

This may be a feature with large left-to-right shunts at ventricular or great arterial level but can also occur with other defects, especially if they form part of a genetic syndrome. Major intellectual impairment is uncommon in children with isolated congenital heart disease, but minor learning difficulties can occur both with and without cardiac surgery.

Syncope

In the presence of increased pulmonary vascular resistance or severe left or right outflow obstruction, exercise may provoke syncope. Systemic vascular resistance falls on exercise but pulmonary vascular resistance may rise, worsening right-to-left shunting and cerebral oxygenation.

Eisenmenger's syndrome

This occurs when increased pulmonary flow due to an initial left-to-right shunt produces severe pulmonary hypertension and *reversal* of the shunt (i.e. right-to-left shunting). Progressive changes (including obliteration of distal vessels) take place in the pulmonary vasculature, and once established, the increased pulmonary resistance is irreversible. Central cyanosis appears, and digital clubbing develops. The chest radiograph shows enlarged central pulmonary arteries and peripheral 'pruning' of the pulmo-

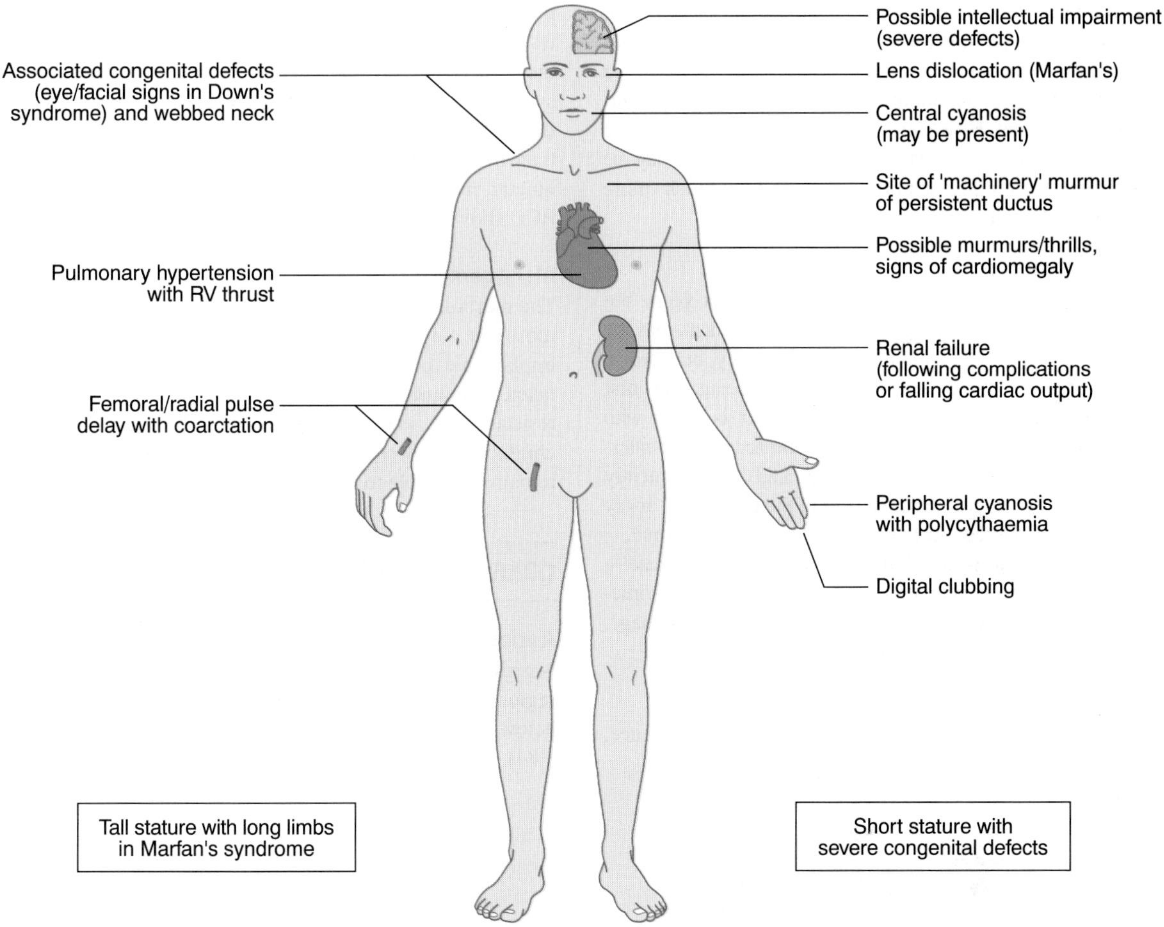

Fig. 3.82 Clinical features which may be present in various forms of congenital heart disease.

nary vessels. The ECG shows right ventricular hypertrophy. Eisenmenger's syndrome is more common with large ventricular septal defects or persistent ductus arteriosus than with atrial septal defects. Patients with the syndrome are at particular risk from abrupt changes in afterload which exacerbate right-to-left shunting (vasodilatation, anaesthesia, pregnancy).

Pregnancy

Most patients with surgically corrected congenital heart disease and many with palliated or untreated disease will tolerate pregnancy well. However, pregnancy is hazardous in the presence of conditions associated with cyanosis or severe pulmonary hypertension. For example, maternal mortality in patients with Eisenmenger's syndrome is more than 50% and sterilisation is usually recommended in such patients.

PERSISTENT DUCTUS ARTERIOSUS

Aetiology

During fetal life, before the lungs begin to function, most of the blood from the pulmonary artery passes through the ductus arteriosus into the aorta just below the origin of the left subclavian artery. Normally the ductus closes soon after birth but sometimes it fails to do so. Since the pressure in the aorta is higher than that in the pulmonary artery (PA), there will be a continuous arteriovenous shunt, the volume of which depends on the size of the ductus. As much as 50% of the left ventricular output may be recirculated through the lungs, with a consequent increase in the work of the heart. When the ductus is structurally intact, a prostaglandin synthetase inhibitor (indomethacin) may be used in the first week of life to induce closure. However, in the presence of a congenital defect with impaired lung perfusion (e.g. pulmonary stenosis and left-to-right shunt through the ductus), it may be advisable to improve oxygenation by maintaining the ductus open with prostaglandin treatment. However, such treatments are ineffective in an abnormal ductus. Persistence of the ductus may be associated with other abnormalities, and is much more common in females.

Clinical features

With small shunts there may be no symptoms for years, but when the ductus is large, growth and development may be retarded. Usually there is no disability in infancy, but cardiac failure may eventually ensue, dyspnoea being the first symptom. A continuous 'machinery' murmur is heard with late systolic accentuation, maximal in the second left intercostal space below the clavicle (see Fig. 3.83). It is frequently accompanied by a thrill. Enlargement of the pulmonary artery may be detected radiologically. The ECG is usually normal.

A large left-to-right shunt in infancy may cause a considerable rise in pulmonary artery pressure, and sometimes this leads to progressive pulmonary vascular damage. Pulses are increased in volume.

Persistent ductus with reversed shunting

With the resulting rise in pulmonary vascular resistance, pulmonary artery pressure rises further until it equals or exceeds aortic pressure. The shunt through the defect may then reverse, causing central cyanosis (Eisenmenger's syndrome, see p. 290). With a persistent ductus arteriosus this cyanosis may be more apparent in the feet and toes than in the upper part of the body. The murmur becomes quieter, may be confined to systole, or may disappear. The ECG shows evidence of right ventricular hypertrophy.

Management

The morbidity and mortality of surgical division is low, but most can now be closed at cardiac catheterisation with an implantable occlusive device. Closure should be undertaken in infancy if the shunt is significant and pulmonary resistance not elevated, but this may be delayed till later childhood in those with smaller shunts for whom closure remains advisable to reduce the risk of endocarditis.

COARCTATION OF THE AORTA

Aetiology

Narrowing of the aorta most commonly occurs in the region where the ductus arteriosus joins the aorta, i.e. just below the origin of the left subclavian artery (see Fig. 3.84). The condition is twice as common in males as

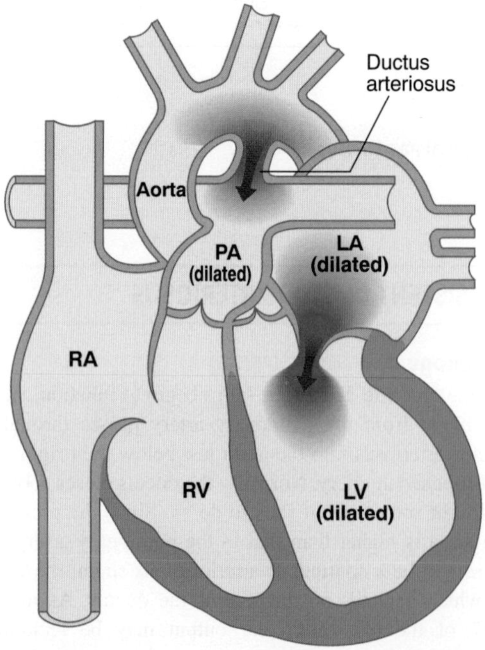

Fig. 3.83 Persistent ductus arteriosus. There is a connection between the aorta and the pulmonary artery with left-to-right shunting and dilatation of the pulmonary artery, left atrium and left ventricle.

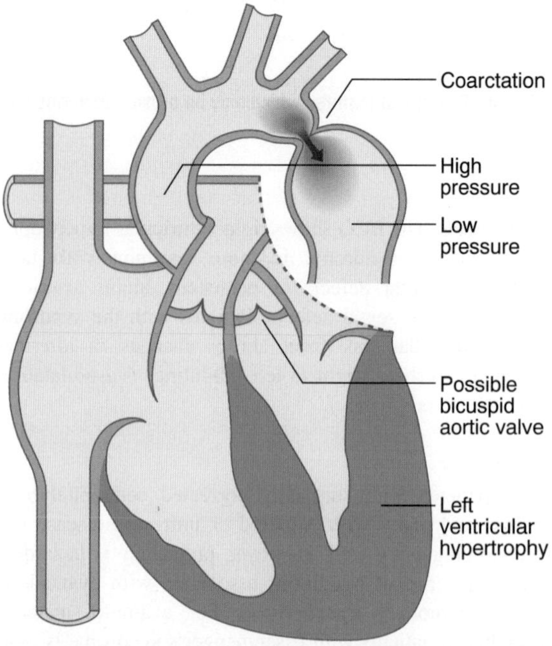

Fig. 3.84 Coarctation of the aorta.

females and occurs in 1:4000 children. It is associated with other abnormalities, of which the most frequent are bicuspid aortic valve and 'berry' aneurysms of the cerebral circulation. Acquired coarctation of the aorta is rare but may follow trauma, or be a complication of a progressive arteritis (Takayasu's disease, see p. 864).

Clinical features

Aortic coarctation is an important cause of cardiac failure in the newborn, but symptoms are often absent when it is detected in older children or adults. Headaches may occur from hypertension proximal to the coarctation, and occasionally weakness or cramps in the legs may result from decreased circulation in the lower part of the body. The blood pressure is raised in the upper body but normal or low in the legs. The femoral pulses are weak, and delayed in comparison with the radial. A systolic murmur is usually heard posteriorly, over the coarctation. There may also be an ejection systolic murmur in the aortic area due to the bicuspid valve. As a result of the aortic narrowing, collaterals form, mainly involving the peri-scapular and intercostal arteries. These may result in localised bruits.

Radiological examination in early childhood is often normal but at a later age may show changes in the contour of the aorta (indentation of the descending aorta, '3 sign'), and notching of the under-surfaces of the ribs from collaterals. Magnetic resonance imaging is ideal for demonstrating the lesion. The ECG may show left ventricular hypertrophy.

Management

In untreated severe cases, death may occur from left ventricular failure, dissection of the aorta or cerebral haemorrhage. Surgical correction is advisable in all but the mildest cases. If this is done sufficiently early in childhood persistent hypertension may be avoided. Patients repaired in late childhood or adult life often remain hypertensive or become hypertensive again. Recurrence of stenosis may occur as the child grows, and this may be managed by balloon dilatation, which is also under investigation as initial treatment. Coexistent aortic valve disease also requires long-term follow-up.

ATRIAL SEPTAL DEFECT

Aetiology

Atrial septal defect is one of the most common congenital heart defects, and occurs twice as frequently in females. Most are 'ostium secundum' defects, involving the fossa ovalis. 'Ostium primum' defects result from a defect in the atrioventricular septum and are associated with a 'cleft mitral valve' (split anterior leaflet).

Since the normal right ventricle is much more compliant than the left, a large volume of blood shunts through the defect from the left to the right atrium and then to the right ventricle and pulmonary arteries (see Fig. 3.85). As a result there is gradual enlargement of the right side of the heart and of the pulmonary arteries. Pulmonary hypertension and shunt reversal sometimes complicate atrial septal defect, but are less common and tend to occur later in life than with other types of left-to-right shunt.

Clinical features

Most children are free of symptoms for many years and the condition is often detected at routine clinical examination or following a chest radiograph. Dyspnoea, chest infections, cardiac failure and arrhythmias (e.g. atrial fibrillation) are other possible modes of presentation. The characteristic physical signs are the result of the volume overload of the right ventricle:

- wide fixed splitting of the second heart sound:
  —wide because of delay in right ventricular ejection, increased stroke volume and RBBB
  —fixed because the septal defect equalises left and right atrial pressures throughout the respiratory cycle
- a systolic flow murmur over the pulmonary valve.

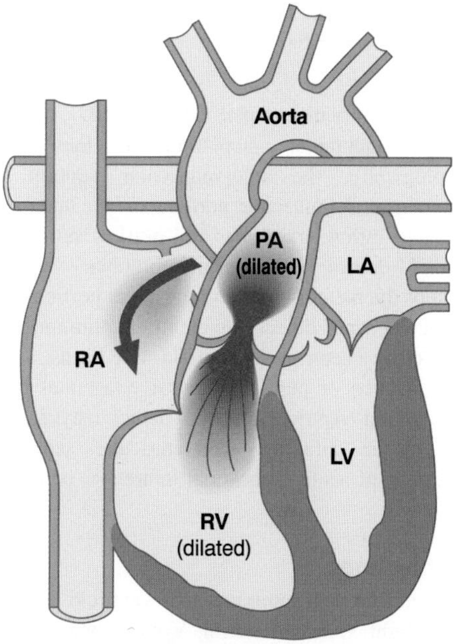

Fig. 3.85 Atrial septal defect. Blood flows across the atrial septum (arrow) from left to right. The murmur is produced by increased flow velocity across the pulmonary valve, as a result of left-to-right shunting and large stroke volume. The density of shading is proportional to velocity of blood flow.

In children with a large shunt there may be a diastolic flow murmur over the tricuspid valve. Unlike a mitral flow murmur, this diastolic murmur is usually high-pitched.

The chest radiograph shows enlargement of the heart, the pulmonary artery and pulmonary plethora. The ECG usually shows incomplete right bundle branch block because right ventricular depolarisation is delayed as a result of ventricular dilatation (with a 'primum' defect there is left axis deviation). Echocardiography demonstrates RV dilatation and hypertrophy and pulmonary artery dilatation, and can directly demonstrate the defect. The precise size and location of the defect can be shown by transoesophageal echocardiography.

Management

Atrial septal defects in which pulmonary flow is increased 50% above systemic flow (i.e. flow ratio of 1.5:1) are often large enough to be clinically recognisable and should be closed surgically. Closure can also be accomplished at cardiac catheterisation using implantable closure devices. The long-term prognosis thereafter is excellent unless pulmonary hypertension has developed. Pulmonary hypertension and shunt reversal are both contraindications to surgery.

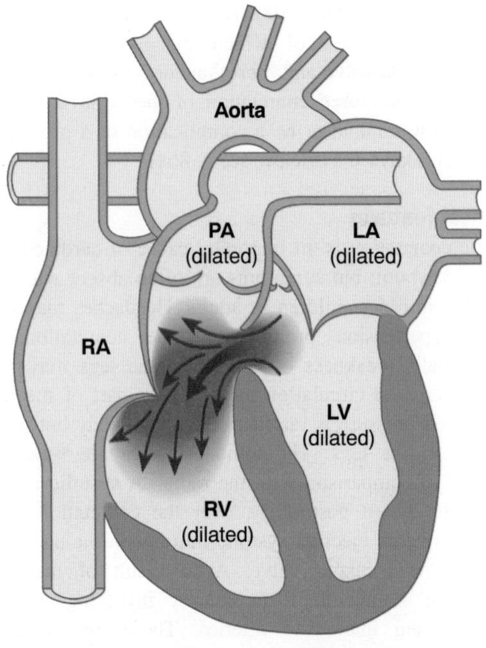

Fig. 3.86 Ventricular septal defect. In this example a large left-to-right shunt (arrow) has resulted in chamber enlargement.

VENTRICULAR SEPTAL DEFECT

Aetiology

Congenital ventricular septal defect (VSD) occurs as a result of incomplete septation of the ventricles. Embryologically, the interventricular septum has a membranous and a muscular portion, and the latter is further divided into inflow, trabecular and outflow portions. Most congenital defects are 'perimembranous', i.e. at the junction of the membranous and muscular portions.

Ventricular septal defects are the most common congenital cardiac defect, occurring once in 500 live births. The defect may be isolated or part of complex congenital heart disease. Acquired ventricular septal defect may result from rupture of an infarcted interventricular septum as a complication of acute myocardial infarction, or rarely from trauma.

Clinical features

Flow from the high-pressure left ventricle to the low-pressure right ventricle during systole produces a pansystolic murmur usually heard best at the left sternal edge but radiating all over the precordium (see Fig. 3.86). A small defect often produces a loud murmur (maladie de Roger) in the absence of other haemodynamic disturbance. Conversely, a large defect may produce a softer murmur, particularly if pressure in the right ventricle is elevated. This may be found to be the case immediately after birth, while pulmonary vascular resistance remains high, or when the shunt is reversed—Eisenmenger's syndrome (described above).

Congenital ventricular septal defect may present as cardiac failure in infants, as a murmur with only minor haemodynamic disturbance in older children or adults, or rarely as Eisenmenger's syndrome. In a proportion of infants, the murmur gets quieter or disappears. This may be due to *spontaneous closure* of the defect or to the development of Eisenmenger's syndrome.

Cardiac failure is usually absent in the immediate postnatal period but becomes apparent in the first 4–6 weeks of life (large defect). In addition to the murmur, there is prominent parasternal pulsation, tachypnoea and indrawing of the lower ribs on inspiration. The chest radiograph shows pulmonary plethora and the ECG shows right and left ventricular enlargement.

Management

Small ventricular septal defects require no specific treatment apart from endocarditis prophylaxis. Cardiac failure caused by a ventricular septal defect in infancy is initially treated medically with digoxin (10–20 μg/kg per day) and frusemide (1–3 mg/kg per day). Persisting failure is an indication for surgical repair of the defect. Closure devices to be delivered at cardiac catheterisation are being developed.

Doppler echocardiography helps to predict the small septal defects that are likely to close spontaneously. Eisenmenger's syndrome is avoided by monitoring (repeated ECG and echocardiography) for signs of rising pulmonary resistance and carrying out surgical repair when appropriate. Surgical closure is contraindicated in fully developed Eisenmenger's syndrome when heart-lung transplantation may be the only effective method of treatment.

Prognosis

Except in the case of Eisenmenger's syndrome, long-term prognosis is very good in congenital ventricular septal defect. Most patients with Eisenmenger's syndrome die in the second or third decade of life, but a few survive to the fifth decade without transplantation.

TETRALOGY OF FALLOT

The four components of the tetralogy are shown in Figure 3.87.

The RV outflow obstruction is most often subvalvular (infundibular), but may be valvular, supravalvular or a

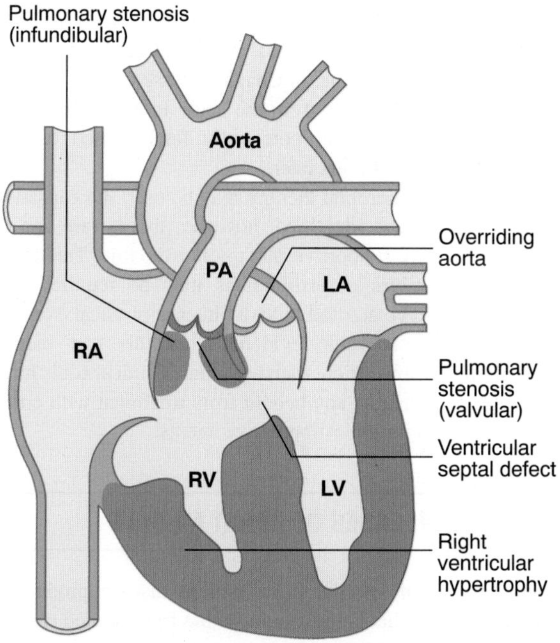

Fig. 3.87 Tetralogy of Fallot. The tetralogy comprises (1) pulmonary stenosis, (2) a ventricular septal defect, (3) overriding of the ventricular septal defect by the aorta, and (4) right ventricular hypertrophy.

combination of these. The VSD is usually large and similar in aperture to the aortic orifice. The combination results in elevated RV pressure and right-to-left shunting of cyanotic blood across the VSD.

Aetiology

The embryological cause is abnormal development of the bulbar septum which separates the ascending aorta from the pulmonary artery, and which normally aligns and fuses with the outflow part of the interventricular septum. The defect occurs in about 1 in 2000 births and is the most common cause of cyanosis in infancy (> 1 year).

Clinical features

Children are usually cyanosed but cyanosis may not be present in the neonate because it is only when right ventricular pressure rises to equal or exceed left ventricular pressure that a large right-to-left shunt develops. The subvalvular component of the RV outflow obstruction is dynamic, and may increase suddenly under adrenergic stimulation. The affected child suddenly becomes increasingly cyanosed, often after feeding or a crying attack, and may become apnoeic and unconscious. These attacks are called 'Fallot's spells'. In older children Fallot's spells are uncommon, but cyanosis becomes increasingly apparent, with stunting of growth, digital clubbing and polycythaemia. Some children characteristically obtain relief by squatting after exertion (this increases the afterload of the left heart and reduces the right-to-left shunting). The natural history before the development of surgical correction was variable, but most patients died in infancy or childhood.

On examination the most characteristic feature is usually the combination of cyanosis with a loud ejection systolic murmur in the pulmonary area (as for pulmonary stenosis). Cyanosis may be absent in the newborn, or in patients where right ventricular outflow obstruction is mild ('acyanotic tetralogy of Fallot'). Growth may be impaired.

Investigations

ECG shows right ventricular hypertrophy, and the chest radiograph shows an abnormally small pulmonary artery and a 'boot-shaped' heart. Echocardiography is diagnostic and demonstrates that the aorta is not continuous with the anterior ventricular septum.

Management

The definitive management is total correction of the defect by surgical relief of the pulmonary stenosis and closure of the ventricular septal defect. Primary surgical correction may be undertaken prior to age 5, except if the pulmonary arteries are too hypoplastic, when a palliative shunt may be performed (for example, an anastomosis between the pulmonary artery and subclavian artery). The shunt improves pulmonary blood flow and pulmonary artery development and may facilitate definitive correction at a later stage.

The prognosis after total correction is good, especially if the operation is performed in childhood. Follow-up is needed to identify residual pulmonary stenosis, recurrence of the septal defect, and rhythm disorders.

OTHER CAUSES OF CYANOTIC CONGENITAL HEART DISEASE

Other causes of cyanotic congenital heart disease are summarised in Table 3.17. Echocardiography is usually the definitive diagnostic procedure, supplemented if necessary by cardiac catheterisation.

Table 3.17 Other causes of cyanotic congenital heart diseases

Defect	Features
Tricuspid atresia	Absent tricuspid orifice, hypoplastic RV RA to LA shunt, VSD shunt, other anomalies Surgical correction *may* be possible
Transposition of the great vessels	Aorta arises from the morphological RV, pulmonary artery from LV Shunt via atria, ductus and possibly VSD Palliation by balloon atrial septostomy/ enlargement Surgical correction possible
Pulmonary atresia	PV atretic and pulmonary artery hypoplastic RA to LA shunt, pulmonary flow via ductus Palliation by balloon atrial septostomy Surgical correction may be possible
Ebstein's anomaly	TV is dysplastic and displaced into RV, right ventricle 'atrialised' Tricuspid regurgitation and RA to LA shunt Spectrum of severity Arrhythmias Surgical repair possible, but significant risks

FURTHER INFORMATION ON CONGENITAL HEART DISEASE

Perloff J K 1994 Clinical recognition of congenital heart disease, 4th edn. W B Saunders, Philadelphia. *A definitive text*

Perloff J K, Child J S 1997 Congenital heart disease in adults, 2nd edn. W B Saunders, Philadelphia

Redington A 1994 Practical guide to congenital heart disease in adults. W B Saunders, Philadelphia. *A brief text that is easy to read*

DISEASES OF THE MYOCARDIUM

Although the myocardium is involved in most types of heart disease, the terms 'myocarditis' and 'cardiomyopathy' are usually reserved for conditions that primarily affect the heart muscle. An international commission has recommended using specific terminology, e.g. 'sarcoid heart muscle disease', when the cause of heart muscle disease is known, and using the term 'cardiomyopathy' only if a cause cannot be identified.

ACUTE MYOCARDITIS

This is an acute inflammatory and potentially reversible condition that may complicate a wide variety of infections; inflammation may be due to infection of the myocardium or circulating toxins. Viral infection is the most common cause of myocarditis in the UK.

The clinical picture ranges from a symptomless disorder, sometimes recognised by the presence of an inappropriate tachycardia, to fulminant heart failure. ECG changes are common but non-specific. If necessary, the diagnosis can be confirmed by endomyocardial biopsy.

Although death may occur, due to a ventricular arrhythmia or rapidly progressive heart failure, in most patients the immediate prognosis is excellent. However, there is strong evidence that some forms of myocarditis may lead to chronic low-grade myocarditis or dilated cardiomyopathy (see below); for example, in Chagas disease (see p. 162) the patient usually recovers from the acute infection but often develops a chronic and potentially fatal dilated cardiomyopathy 10 or 20 years later.

Specific antimicrobial therapy may be used if a causative organism has been identified; however, this is rare and in most cases only supportive therapy is available. Treatment for cardiac failure or arrhythmias may be required and patients should be advised to avoid intense physical exertion because there is some evidence that this can induce potentially fatal ventricular arrhythmias. Clinical trials have failed to demonstrate any benefit from treatment with corticosteroids and immunosuppressive agents.

SPECIFIC DISEASES OF HEART MUSCLE

Many forms of specific heart muscle disease produce a clinical picture that is indistinguishable from dilated cardiomyopathy (e.g. connective tissue disorders, sarcoidosis, haemochromatosis, alcoholic heart muscle disease). In contrast, amyloidosis and eosinophilic heart disease produce symptoms and signs similar to those found in restrictive cardiomyopathy (see below), whereas the heart

SPECIFIC DISEASES OF HEART MUSCLE
Infections
• Viral, e.g. Coxsackie A and B, influenza, HIV • Bacterial, e.g. diphtheria • Protozoal, e.g. trypanosomiasis
Endocrine and metabolic disorders
• e.g. Diabetes, hypo- and hyperthyroidism, acromegaly, carcinoid syndrome, inherited storage diseases
Connective tissue diseases
• e.g. Systemic sclerosis, systemic lupus erythematosus, polyarteritis nodosa
Infiltrative disorders
• e.g. Haemochromatosis, haemosiderosis, sarcoidosis, amyloidosis
Endomyocardial fibrosis and eosinophilic heart disease
Toxins
• e.g. Drugs, alcohol, irradiation
Neuromuscular disorders
• e.g. Dystrophia myotonica, Friedreich's ataxia

disease associated with Friedreich's ataxia (see pp. 991–992) can mimic hypertrophic cardiomyopathy (see below).

Treatment and prognosis are determined by the underlying disorder. Abstention from alcohol may lead to a dramatic improvement in patients with alcoholic heart muscle disease.

CARDIOMYOPATHY

There are three types of cardiomyopathy (see Fig. 3.88).

Dilated cardiomyopathy

In this condition there is impaired ventricular contraction (often affecting both ventricles) leading to progressive left-sided and, later, right-sided heart failure. Men are affected more than twice as often as women. The condition is inherited as an autosomal dominant trait in approximately 20% of cases and usually presents as unexplained heart failure. Arrhythmia, thromboembolism and sudden death are common and may occur at any stage; sporadic chest pain is a surprisingly frequent symptom. The ECG usually shows non-specific changes but echocardiography is useful in establishing the

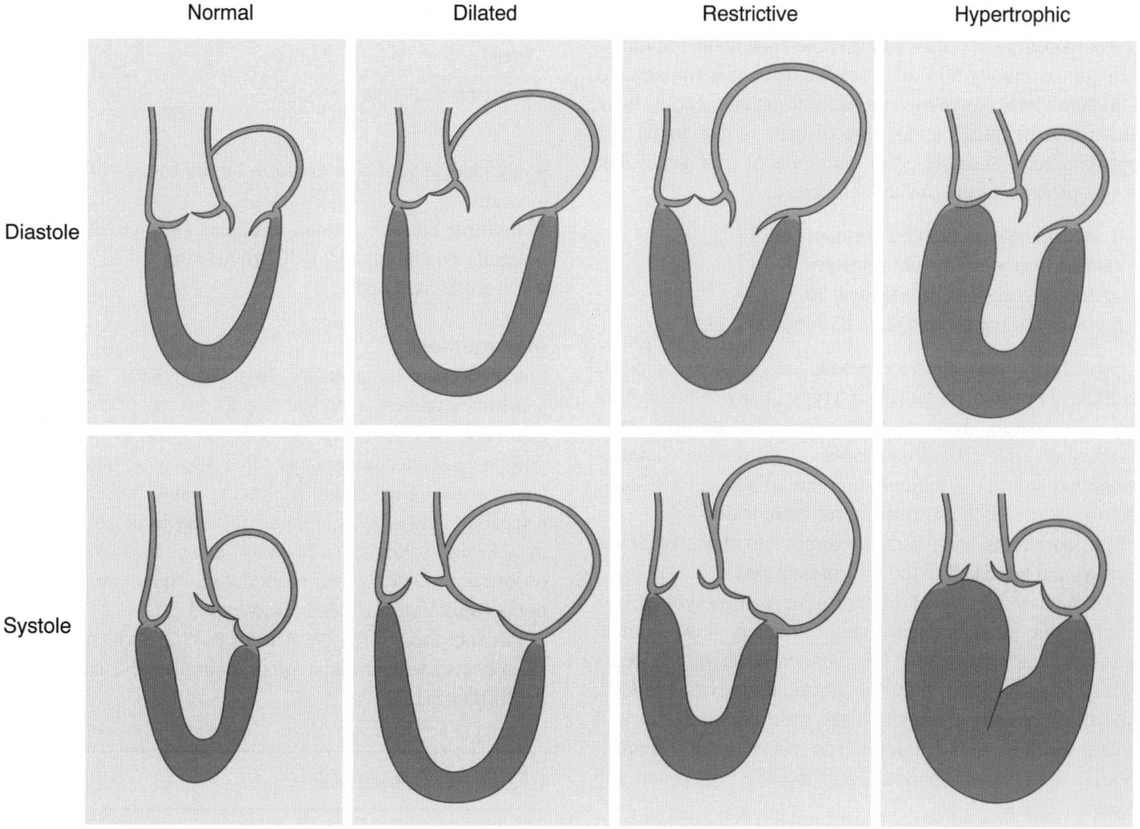

Fig. 3.88 The three types of cardiomyopathy.

diagnosis. The differential diagnosis includes most forms of specific heart muscle disease (e.g. alcoholic heart disease) and ischaemic heart disease. Treatment is aimed at controlling the resulting heart failure. Although some patients remain well for many years, the prognosis is generally poor and cardiac transplantation may be indicated.

Restrictive or obliterative cardiomyopathy

In this condition ventricular filling is impaired because the ventricles are 'stiff'. This leads to high atrial pressures with atrial hypertrophy, dilatation and later atrial fibrillation. The differential diagnosis includes endomyocardial fibrosis, eosinophilic heart muscle disease and amyloidosis. Diagnosis can be very difficult and may require complex Doppler echocardiography, CT or MRI scanning and endomyocardial biopsy. Treatment is usually symptomatic, but excision of fibrotic endocardium may benefit some patients. The prognosis is usually poor and transplantation may be indicated.

Hypertrophic cardiomyopathy

This is a familial condition characterised by inappropriate and elaborate ventricular hypertrophy with malalignment of the myocardial fibres. The hypertrophy may be generalised or largely confined to the interventricular septum (asymmetric septal hypertrophy) or the apex (apical hypertrophic cardiomyopathy—a variant which is common in the Far East).

In approximately 50% of cases the disease is transmitted as an autosomal dominant trait. Recent genetic studies have shown that in most patients the disease is due to one of approximately 70 single-point mutations of four genes that encode proteins of the cardiac sarcomere:

- β-myosin heavy chain on chromosome 14
- cardiac troponin T on chromosome 1
- α-tropomyosin on chromosome 15
- myosin-binding protein C on chromosome 11.

Heart failure may develop because the stiff non-compliant ventricles impede diastolic filling. Hypertrophy of the septum may also cause dynamic left ventricular outflow tract obstruction *(HOCM—hypertrophic obstructive cardiomyopathy)* and mitral regurgitation due to abnormal systolic anterior motion of the anterior mitral valve leaflet.

The symptoms and signs are similar to those of aortic stenosis and are listed in the information box.

The natural history of hypertrophic cardiomyopathy is variable but clinical deterioration is often slow. Annual mortality is approximately 1%. Sudden death often occurs during or just after vigorous physical activity; indeed, hypertrophic cardiomyopathy is the most common cause of sudden death in young athletes. The risk of sudden death is greatest in those who present early in life (< 30 years) and those who have:

- a history of a previous cardiac arrest or sustained ventricular tachycardia
- an adverse genotype and/or a family history of sudden death
- multiple episodes of non-sustained ventricular tachycardia on ambulatory ECG monitoring
- recurrent syncope.

CLINICAL FEATURES OF HYPERTROPHIC CARDIOMYOPATHY
Symptoms
• Angina on effort • Dyspnoea on effort • Syncope on effort • Sudden death
Signs
• Jerky pulse* • Palpable left ventricular hypertrophy • Double impulse at the apex (palpable fourth heart sound due to left atrial hypertrophy) • Mid-systolic murmur at the base* • Pansystolic murmur (due to mitral regurgitation) at the apex * Signs of left ventricular outflow tract obstruction which may be augmented by standing up (reduced venous return), inotropes and vasodilators (e.g. sublingual nitrate)

INVESTIGATIONS IN HYPERTROPHIC CARDIOMYOPATHY
Chest radiograph
• Non-specific changes only
ECG
• Left ventricular hypertrophy ± a wide variety of often bizarre abnormalities
Echo
• Usually diagnostic

Management

β-adrenoceptor antagonists help to relieve angina and sometimes prevent syncopal attacks but no pharmacological treatment is definitely known to improve prognosis. Arrhythmias are common and often respond to treatment with amiodarone. Dual-chamber pacing and surgery (partial resection of the septum or mitral valve replacement) are useful in selected patients, particularly those with outflow tract obstruction. Digoxin and vasodilators may increase outflow tract obstruction and should be avoided.

Patients thought to be at high risk of sudden death are often treated with amiodarone or an implantable cardioverter-defibrillator (ICD).

CARDIAC TUMOURS

Primary cardiac tumours are rare (< 0.2% of autopsies), but the heart and mediastinum may be the site of metastases.

Most primary tumours are benign (75%), and of these the majority are myxomas. The remainder are fibromas, lipomas, fibroelastomas and haemangiomas.

ATRIAL MYXOMA

Myxomas most commonly arise in the left atrium, as single or multiple polypoid tumours, attached by a pedicle to the interatrial septum. They are usually gelatinous but may be solid and even calcified, with superimposed thrombus.

The tumour may be detected incidentally (on echocardiography), or following investigation of pyrexia, syncope, arrhythmias or emboli. Occasionally the condition presents with malaise and features suggestive of a connective tissue disorder, including a raised ESR.

On examination the first heart sound is usually loud and there may be a murmur of mitral regurgitation with a variable diastolic sound (tumour 'plop') due to prolapse of the mass through the mitral valve.

The diagnosis is made on echocardiography and treatment is by surgical excision. If the pedicle is removed, less than 5% of tumours recur.

FURTHER INFORMATION ON DISEASES OF THE MYOCARDIUM

Maron B J 1997 Hypertrophic cardiomyopathy. Lancet 350: 127–133. *An up-to-date review*

Pisani B, Taylor D O, Mason J W 1997 Inflammatory myocardial disease and cardiomyopathies. American Journal of Medicine 102: 459–469

Richardson P, McKenna W, Bristow M 1996 Report of the 1995 World Health Organization/International Society and Federation of Cardiology Task Force on the definition and classification of cardiomyopathies. Circulation 93: 841–842

The cardiomyopathies. Supplement 1994 British Heart Journal 72: S1–S56. *A supplement devoted entirely to cardiomyopathy*

DISEASES OF THE PERICARDIUM

The normal pericardial sac contains about 50 ml of fluid, similar to lymph, which lubricates the surface of the heart. The pericardium limits distension of the heart, contributes to the haemodynamic interdependence of the ventricles, and acts as a barrier to infection. Nevertheless, congenital absence of the pericardium does not appear to result in significant clinical or functional limitations.

ACUTE PERICARDITIS

Aetiology

Pericardial inflammation may be due to infection, immunological reaction, trauma or neoplasm and sometimes remains unexplained. Pericarditis and myocarditis often coexist, and all forms of pericarditis may produce a pericardial effusion (see below), which, depending on the aetiology, may be fibrinous, serous, haemorrhagic or purulent.

AETIOLOGY OF ACUTE PERICARDITIS
Common
• Acute myocardial infarction • Viral (e.g. Coxsackie B, but often not identified)
Less common
• Uraemia • Malignant disease • Trauma (e.g. blunt chest injury) • Connective tissue disease (e.g. SLE)
Rare (in UK)
• Bacterial infection • Rheumatic fever • Tuberculosis

A fibrinous exudate may eventually lead to varying degrees of adhesion formation, whereas serous pericarditis often produces a large effusion of turbid, straw-coloured fluid with a high protein content.

A haemorrhagic effusion is often due to malignant disease, particularly carcinoma of the breast, carcinoma of the bronchus and lymphoma.

Purulent pericarditis is rare and may occur as a complication of septicaemia, by direct spread from an intrathoracic infection, or from a penetrating injury.

Clinical features

The characteristic pain of pericarditis is retrosternal, radiates to the shoulders and neck and is often aggravated by deep breathing, movement, a change of position, exercise and swallowing. A low-grade fever is common.

A pericardial friction rub is a high-pitched superficial scratching or crunching noise produced by movement of the inflamed pericardium, and is diagnostic of pericarditis; it is usually heard in systole but may also be audible in diastole and frequently has a 'to-and-fro' quality.

Investigations

The ECG shows ST elevation with upward concavity (see Fig. 3.89) over the affected area, which may be widespread. Later, there may be T wave inversion, particularly if there is a degree of myocarditis.

Management

The pain can usually be relieved by aspirin (600 mg 4-hourly), but a more potent anti-inflammatory agent such as indomethacin (25 mg 8-hourly) may be required. Corticosteroids may suppress symptoms but there is no evidence that they accelerate cure.

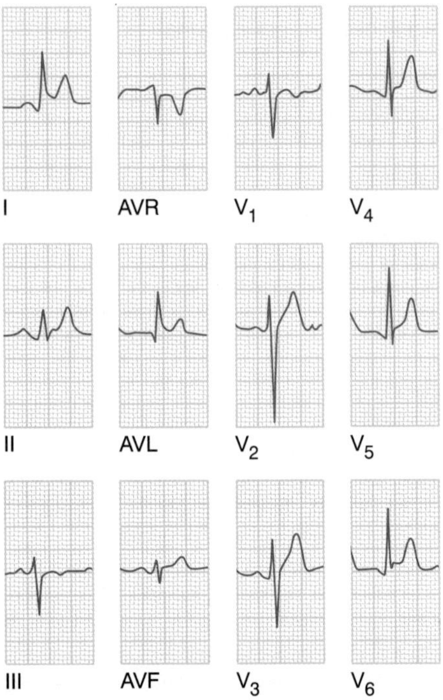

Fig. 3.89 ECG from a young man with acute pericarditis complicating acute myeloblastic leukaemia. Widespread ST elevation (leads I, II, AVL, V_3–V_6) is shown. The upward concave shape of the ST segments (see lead I) and the unusual distribution of ECG changes (involving anterior and inferior leads) may help to distinguish pericarditis from acute myocardial infarction.

In viral pericarditis recovery usually occurs within a few days or weeks, but there may be recurrences *(chronic relapsing pericarditis)*. Purulent pericarditis requires treatment with antimicrobial therapy, paracentesis and, if necessary, surgical drainage.

PERICARDIAL EFFUSION

If a pericardial effusion develops there is sometimes a sensation of retrosternal oppression. An effusion is difficult to detect clinically; although the heart sounds may become quieter, pericardial friction is not always abolished.

The QRS voltages on the ECG are often reduced in the presence of a large effusion. Serial chest radiographs may show a rapid increase in the size of the cardiac shadow over days or even hours, and when there is a large effusion the heart often has a globular or pear-shaped appearance. Echocardiography is the definitive investigation for pericardial effusion (see Fig. 3.90).

Cardiac tamponade

This term is used to describe acute heart failure due to compression of the heart by a large or rapidly developing effusion. Atypical presentations may occur when the effusion is loculated as a result of previous pericarditis or cardiac surgery. See also page 209.

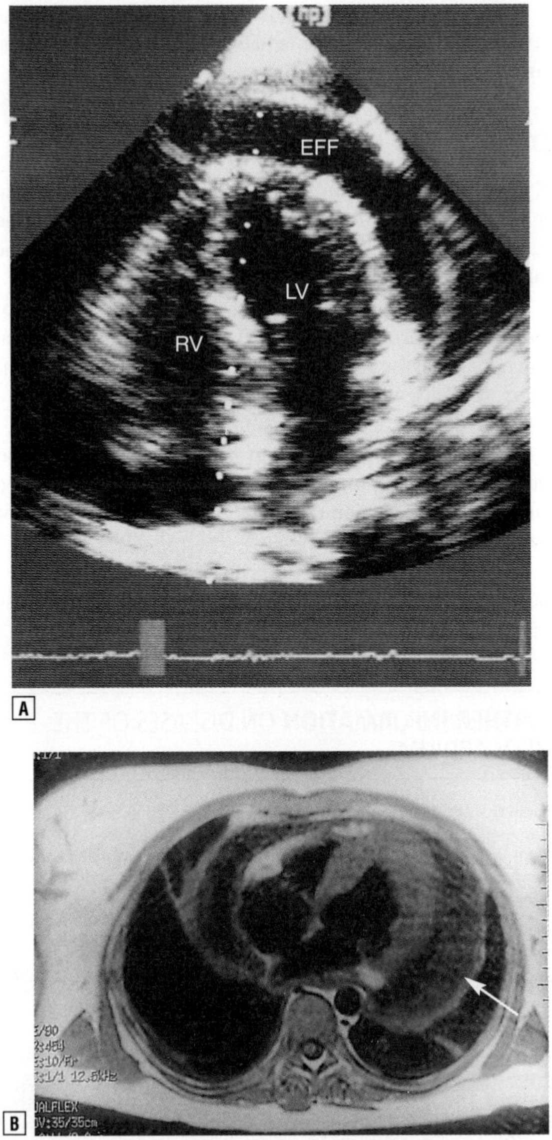

Fig. 3.90 A Echocardiogram (apical view) showing pericardial effusion (EFF). B MRI scan showing pericardial effusion (arrow).

Pericardial aspiration

Paracentesis of a pericardial effusion may be indicated for diagnostic purposes or for the treatment of cardiac tamponade.

The fluid may be aspirated by introducing a needle just medial to the cardiac apex or by inserting a needle below the xiphoid process and directing it towards the left shoulder. The route of choice will depend on the experience of the operator, the configuration of the patient and the position of the effusion. Simultaneous echocardiography is very helpful.

Complications of paracentesis include arrhythmias, damage to a coronary artery, and bleeding with exacerbation of tamponade as a result of injury to the right ventricle.

A few millilitres of fluid may be sufficient for diagnostic purposes; however, if therapeutic drainage is required, it is unwise to attempt aspiration of the whole effusion through a rigid needle and it may be safer to use a plastic cannula inserted over a needle or guidewire.

A viscous, loculated or recurrent effusion may require formal surgical drainage.

TUBERCULOUS PERICARDITIS

Tuberculous pericarditis may complicate pulmonary tuberculosis but may also be the first manifestation of the infection. In Africa a tuberculous pericardial effusion is a common feature of the acquired immunodeficiency syndrome (AIDS).

The condition typically presents with chronic malaise, weight loss and a low-grade fever. An effusion usually develops and the pericardium may become thick and unyielding, leading to pericardial constriction or tamponade. An associated pleural effusion is often present.

The diagnosis may be confirmed by aspiration of the fluid and direct examination or culture for tubercle bacilli. Treatment requires specific antituberculous chemotherapy (see p. 352). Corticosteroids may help to prevent the development of constrictive pericarditis.

CHRONIC CONSTRICTIVE PERICARDITIS

Constrictive pericarditis is due to progressive thickening, fibrosis and calcification of the pericardium. In effect, the heart is encased in a solid shell and cannot fill properly; the calcification may extend into the myocardium, so there may also be impaired myocardial contraction.

The condition often follows an attack of tuberculous pericarditis but can also complicate haemopericardium, viral pericarditis, rheumatoid arthritis and purulent pericarditis; it is often impossible to identify the original insult.

Clinical features

The symptoms and signs of systemic venous congestion are the hallmarks of constrictive pericarditis; atrial fibrillation is common and there is often dramatic ascites and hepato-

CLINICAL FEATURES OF CONSTRICTIVE PERICARDITIS

- Fatigue
- Rapid, low-volume pulse
- Pulsus paradoxus (an excessive fall in blood pressure during inspiration)
- Elevated JVP with a rapid *y* descent
- Kussmaul's sign (a paradoxical rise in the JVP during inspiration)
- Loud early third heart sound or 'pericardial knock'
- Hepatomegaly
- Ascites
- Peripheral oedema

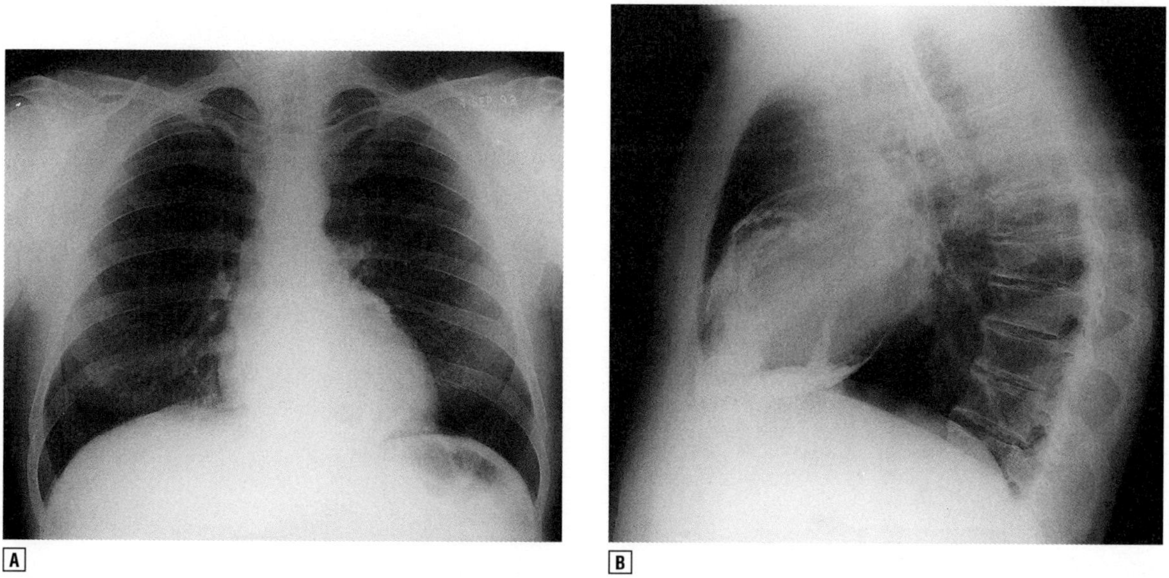

Fig. 3.91 Chest radiographs from a patient with severe heart failure due to chronic constrictive pericarditis. The heart is not enlarged and there is heavy calcification of the pericardium that is most visible on the lateral film. A PA radiograph. B Lateral radiograph.

megaly. Breathlessness is not a prominent symptom because the lungs are seldom congested.

The condition is sometimes overlooked and should be suspected in any patient with unexplained right heart failure and a small heart. A chest radiograph, which may show pericardial calcification (see Fig. 3.91), and echocardiography often help to establish the diagnosis. CT scanning and magnetic resonance imaging are also useful techniques for imaging the pericardium.

Constrictive pericarditis is often difficult to distinguish from restrictive cardiomyopathy and the final diagnosis may depend on complex echo-Doppler studies and cardiac catheterisation.

Management

Surgical resection of the diseased pericardium can lead to a dramatic improvement but carries a high morbidity and produces disappointing results in up to 50% of patients.

FURTHER INFORMATION ON GENERAL CARDIOLOGY

Braunwald E 1997 Heart disease: a textbook of cardiovascular medicine, 5th edn. W B Saunders, Philadelphia. *2000 pages—the definitive textbook of cardiology*

Julian D G, Cowan J C, McClenachan J 1998 Cardiology, 7th edn. W B Saunders, London. *A 400-page paperback textbook of general cardiology that is easy to read*

Opie L H 1997 Drugs for the heart, 4th edn. W B Saunders, Philadelphia. *A useful paperback that describes the drug treatment of all forms of heart disease*

Diseases of the respiratory system

4

G.K. CROMPTON • C. HASLETT • E.R. CHILVERS

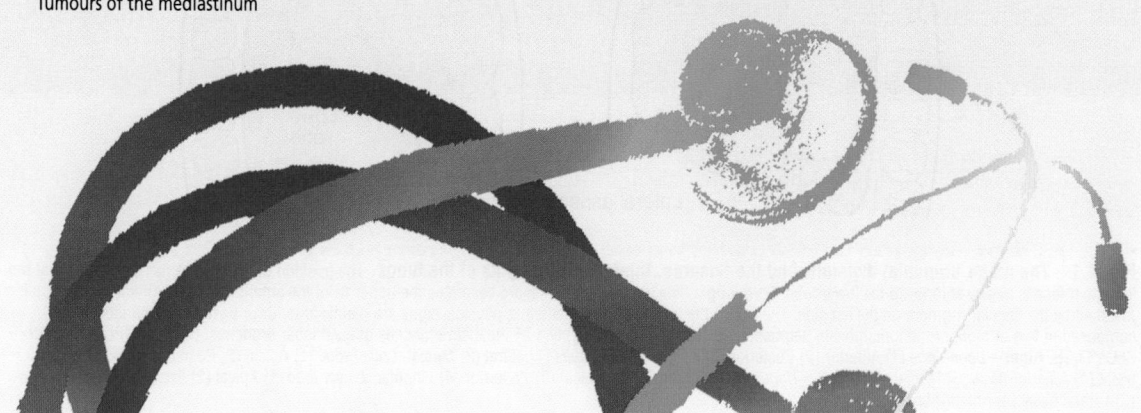

The lungs, with their combined surface area of greater than 500 m^2, are directly open to the external environment. Thus structural, functional or microbiological changes within the lungs can be closely related to epidemiological, environmental, occupational, personal and social factors. Primary respiratory diseases are responsible for a major burden of morbidity and untimely deaths, and the lungs are often affected in multisystem diseases.

Respiratory symptoms are the most common cause of presentation to the family practitioner. Asthma occurs in more than 10% of British children; bronchial carcinoma is the most common fatal malignancy in the developed world; the lung is the major site of opportunistic infection in those immunocompromised by the acquired immune deficiency syndrome (AIDS) or by anti-allograft and anticancer chemotherapeutic regimens; and the spectre of tuberculosis, particularly the emergence of multiple drug-resistant strains, is back with us.

A number of important research advances have occurred in recent years. The discovery of the genetic mechanism of cystic fibrosis provides a novel opportunity to develop gene therapy strategies to replace the defective gene. The lung is especially favoured for gene therapy since its airway epithelial cells are accessible to nebulised particles and the extensive microvascular pulmonary capillary endothelium is available to intravenously delivered agents. Finally, recent advances in our understanding of the cellular and molecular mechanisms underlying diseases such as asthma and the acute (formerly adult) respiratory distress syndrome (ARDS) are likely to lead to rational, mechanism-based therapy within the foreseeable future.

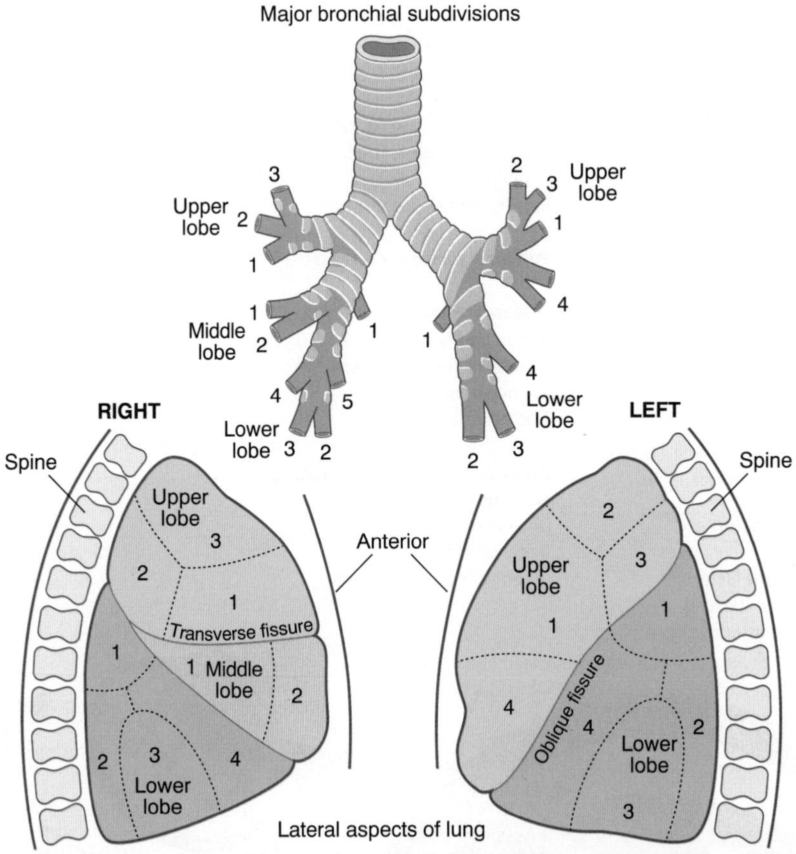

Fig. 4.1 The major bronchial divisions and the fissures, lobes and segments of the lungs. The position of the oblique fissure is such that the left upper lobe is largely anterior to the lower lobe. On the right side the transverse fissure separates the upper from the anteriorly placed middle lobe which is matched by the lingular segment on the left side. The site of the lobe determines whether physical signs are mainly anterior or posterior. Each lobe is composed of two or more bronchopulmonary segments, i.e. the lung tissue supplied by the main branches of each lobar bronchus. BRONCHOPULMONARY SEGMENTS: **Right**—*Upper lobe* (1) Anterior (2) Posterior (3) Apical. *Middle lobe* (1) Lateral (2) Medial. *Lower lobe* (1) Apical (2) Posterior basal (3) Lateral basal (4) Anterior basal (5) Medial basal. **Left**—*Upper lobe* (1) Anterior (2) Apical (3) Posterior (4) Lingular. *Lower lobe* (1) Apical (2) Posterior basal (3) Lateral basal (4) Anterior basal.

FUNCTIONAL ANATOMY, PHYSIOLOGY AND INVESTIGATIONS

APPLIED ANATOMY AND PHYSIOLOGY

The upper respiratory tract includes the nose, nasopharynx and larynx. It is lined by vascular mucous membranes with ciliated epithelium on their surfaces. The lower respiratory tract includes the trachea and bronchi. These form an interconnecting tree of conducting airways eventually joining, via around 64 000 terminal bronchioles, with the alveoli to form the acini. The lower respiratory tract is lined with ciliated epithelium as far as the terminal bronchioles. The larynx and large bronchi are supplied with sensory nerve receptors involved in the cough reflex.

Some knowledge of the patterns of branching of the lobar and segmental bronchi is necessary for interpreting investigations, including chest radiographs and CT scans. Major bronchial and pulmonary divisions are shown in Figure 4.1. (See also bronchoscopic appearances in Fig. 4.8, p. 310.)

The acinus is the gas exchange unit of the lung (see Fig. 4.2) and comprises branching respiratory bronchioles leading to clusters of alveoli. The alveoli are lined mostly with flattened epithelial cells (type I pneumocytes), but there are some, more cuboidal, type II pneumocytes. The latter produce surfactant, a mixture of phospholipids, which acts to reduce surface tension and counteract the tendency of alveoli to collapse. Type II pneumocytes also display a remarkable capacity to divide and reconstitute the type I pneumocytes after lung injury.

The right ventricle pumps blood against the relatively low pulmonary vascular resistance. Blood flows through a remarkably rich capillary network, intimately adjacent to alveoli (see Fig. 4.2), facilitating gas exchange. Increased pulmonary vascular resistance, due for example to thromboembolism (see p. 377) or to destructive changes caused by chronic obstructive pulmonary disease (COPD) (see p. 322), results in right ventricular hypertrophy, and eventually right heart failure (cor pulmonale) ensues.

GAS EXCHANGE, VENTILATION, BLOOD FLOW AND DIFFUSION

Gas exchange in the lungs is suboptimal unless there is sufficient ventilation, distributed uniformly to different parts of the lungs and matched by uniform distribution of blood flow. Furthermore, abnormal diffusion of oxygen or carbon dioxide across the alveolar-capillary membrane impairs gas exchange.

In clinical practice the important consequences of impaired gas exchange are hypoxaemia and hypercapnia.

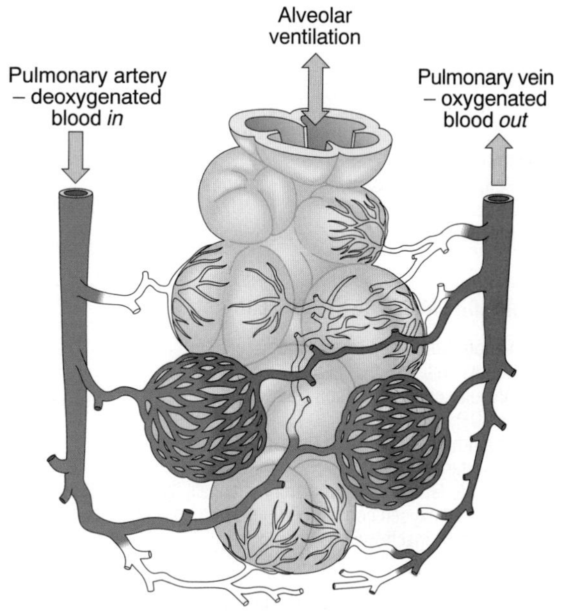

Fig. 4.2 The acinus—the basic gas exchange unit of the lung.

Hypercapnia ($PaCO_2$ > 6 kPa (45 mmHg)) is generally caused by conditions resulting in alveolar hypoventilation or ventilation-perfusion mismatch (see the information box on p. 306). Hypoventilation may be caused by depression of the respiratory centre in the medulla; in contrast, stimulation of the respiratory centre causes hypocapnia and respiratory alkalosis (see Table 4.1). Ventilation-perfusion mismatch is thought to be largely responsible for the hypercapnia of chronic obstructive pulmonary disease (COPD) and severe asthma.

Table 4.1 Some influences on the respiratory centre

Mechanism	Example
Stimulant	
Voluntary	Overbreathing
Upper brain-stem lesions	Central neurogenic hyperventilation
Input from receptors	Pain; muscles and joints; pulmonary afferents
Increased $PaCO_2$	Via central and peripheral chemoreceptors
Increased arterial hydrogen ion concentration	Via peripheral chemoreceptors
Decreased PaO_2 (< 8 kPa at rest)	Via peripheral chemoreceptors
Pyrexia	
Depressant	
Voluntary	Breath-holding
Brain-stem lesions	
Sedative drugs	Opiates, benzodiazepines
Hypothermia	

COMMON CAUSES OF HYPERCAPNIA (RAISED $PaCO_2$)

Central
- Brain-stem lesion
- Central sleep apnoea

Neuromuscular
- Peripheral neuropathy
- Myasthenia gravis
- Myopathies

Chest wall
- Kyphoscoliosis
- Ankylosing spondylitis
- Trauma

Pulmonary
- COPD (and emphysema)

COMMON CAUSES OF HYPOXAEMIA

Corrected by oxygen:
- Venous admixture effect (poorly ventilated lung)
- Alveolar underventilation (raised $PaCO_2$)
- Impairment of diffusion (less important at rest)

Not corrected:
- Right to left shunts (circulatory channels bypassing lungs)
- Reduced oxygen content (PaO_2 may be normal) (anaemia; inactivated haemoglobin)

Causes of hypoxaemia are shown in the information box. Blood flow wasted on perfusing poorly ventilated lung is probably the most important of these and contributes to the hypoxaemia found, for example, in bronchial obstruction (due to secretions, mucosal oedema, bronchoconstriction or tumours), destruction of elastic tissue (e.g. emphysema), pulmonary collapse, consolidation, fibrosis or oedema, and chest wall deformities. In conditions where the area of alveolar-capillary interface available for gas exchange is reduced (e.g. emphysema), impaired diffusion may contribute to hypoxaemia. This effect may not be significant at rest, but may limit the amount of oxygen which can be taken up during exercise.

Hypoxaemia due to ventilation-perfusion mismatch, hypoventilation or diffusion impairment is reversed by giving oxygen. In right to left shunts—as, for example, in congenital heart diseases and pulmonary vascular anomalies—blood does not pass through alveolar capillaries and therefore oxygen does not fully correct the hypoxaemia. Hypoxaemia also occurs if the oxygen-carrying capacity of the blood is reduced as, for example, in anaemia or carbon monoxide poisoning.

The normal arterial PaO_2 is over 12 kPa (90 mmHg) at the age of 20 and falls to around 11 kPa (82 mmHg) at 60. Above this age a further fall in PaO_2 of up to 1.3 kPa (10 mmHg) may occur on lying down because of closure of small airways in the dependent regions of the lungs.

Under physiological conditions hypoxaemia and hypercapnia both stimulate ventilation. In some patients with COPD, tolerance of chronic hypercapnia ensues, and in such patients administration of high concentrations of oxygen removes the remaining hypoxaemic stimulus for ventilation, resulting in worsening hypercapnia. Patients with COPD who have chronic hypercapnia should therefore receive, if required, low concentrations of oxygen (e.g. 24–28%), adjusted according to arterial blood gas analysis (see p. 312). Patients with pure asthma do not have chronic hypercapnia and it is therefore safe, and indeed important, to give high concentrations of oxygen during exacerbations of asthma (see p. 333).

LUNG DEFENCES

Each day our lungs are directly exposed to more than 7000 litres of air which contain varying amounts of inorganic and organic particles as well as potentially lethal bacteria and viruses. In general terms, physical mechanisms including cough are particularly important in defence of the upper airways, whereas the lower airways are protected by complex mucociliary mechanisms, by the antimicrobial properties of surfactant and the lung-lining fluids, and by resident alveolar macrophages.

Physical defences

Most large particles are removed from inspired air by the nose, which is composed of a 'stack' of fine aerodynamic filters comprising fine hairs and columnar ciliated epithelium which cover the turbinate bones. The larynx acts as a sphincter during cough and expectoration and is an essential mechanism protecting the lower airways during swallowing and vomiting.

Mucociliary clearance

Particles with a diameter greater than 0.5 μm which survive passage through the nose will be trapped by the lining fluid of the trachea and bronchi to be cleared by the 'mucociliary escalator' (see Fig. 4.3). This highly effective small particle clearance mechanism works by a complex interaction

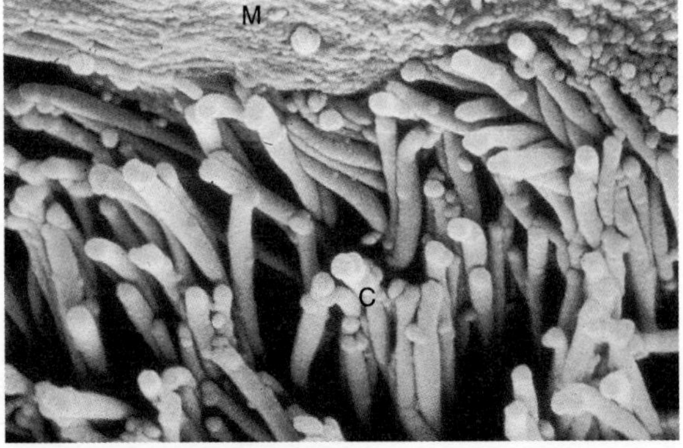

Fig. 4.3 The mucociliary escalator. Scanning electron micrograph of the respiratory epithelium showing large numbers of cilia (C) overlaid by the mucus 'raft' (M).

PROTECTIVE AGENTS IN THE LUNG-LINING FLUID

- Surfactant proteins—bacterial opsonisation
- Immunoglobulins (IgA, IgG, IgM)—bacterial opsonisation, generation of the immune response
- Complement—bacterial opsonisation, generation of the inflammatory response
- Bactericidal proteins—bacterial killing
- Proteinase inhibitors—protection of host tissues during the inflammatory response

between cilia, which are a series of small projections on the surface of respiratory epithelial cells, and mucus, which forms a 'raft' on top of the cilia. Particles are trapped by the mucus which is then swept by the cilia in a cephalic direction. Other important functions of mucus include: dilution of noxious substances; lubrication of the airways; and humidification of inspired air. Mucus, which is mostly secreted by goblet cells of the respiratory epithelium, is composed of 95% water, the mucus glycoproteins and a variety of other proteins (see the information box) which, although present in low concentrations, are likely to play an important role in the defence of the bronchial tree. A number of factors may reduce mucociliary clearance by interfering with ciliary function or by causing actual ciliary damage. These include: pollutants, cigarette smoke, local and general anaesthetic agents, bacterial products and viral infection. There is also a rare autosomal recessive condition (1 in 30 000 live births) called primary ciliary dyskinesia, which is characterised by repeated sinusitis and respiratory tract infections which progress to persistent lung suppuration and bronchiectasis, thus reinforcing the importance of ciliary clearance in antibacterial lung defences.

Surfactant and other defensive proteins

In addition to surface active properties which are so important in lung mechanics (see p. 311), surfactant contains a number of proteins, including surfactant protein A, which can opsonise bacteria and other particles, rendering them susceptible to phagocytosis by macrophages. Lung-lining fluids also contain other defensive proteins (see the information box) including immunoglobulins, complement, defensins (powerful antibacterial peptides) and a variety of antiproteinases which play an important role in protecting healthy tissues from damage which would be incurred by the release of proteinases from inflammatory cells during the inflammatory response (see p. 24).

Alveolar macrophages

These multipotent cells normally patrol the interior of the alveoli (see Fig. 4.4) where they display a formidable array of mechanisms by which they recognise and destroy bacteria and other foreign organic particles. The remarkably versatile resident macrophage can also 'call in reinforcements' by generating mediators which cause an inflammatory response

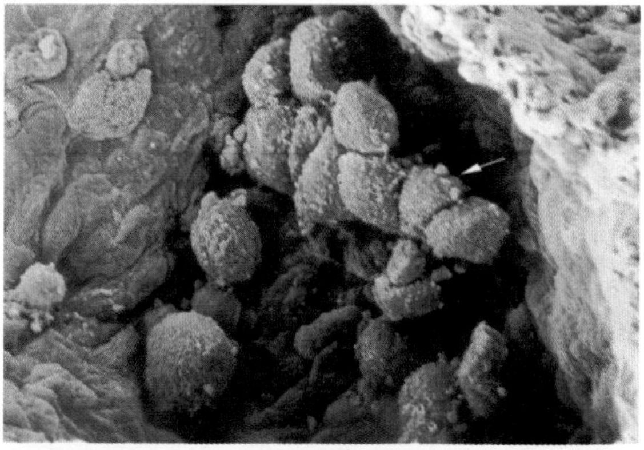

Fig. 4.4 Alveolar macrophages. Scanning electron micrograph showing alveolar macrophages (arrow) patrolling the alveolar spaces of the lung.

and attract granulocytes and monocytes (see p. 23). It may also generate an immune response by presenting antigens and by releasing specific lymphokines. Finally, the alveolar macrophage exerts important scavenging functions in the clearance of dead bacteria and other cells during the aftermath of infection and inflammation. Nevertheless, it is important to appreciate that the excessive or uncontrolled release of some of these powerful macrophage products may cause disordered inflammation or scarring responses which are likely to be important in the pathogenesis of a variety of inflammatory diseases including asthma, chronic bronchitis and emphysema, and other inflammatory/scarring conditions of the lung, e.g. fibrosing alveolitis.

INVESTIGATION OF RESPIRATORY DISEASE

It is essential to take a detailed history from the patient, and much can be learned from a careful physical examination (see Table 4.2 on p. 308). Routine haematological and biochemical investigations can provide indices of infection, immunosuppression and evidence of metastasis of lung tumours, but a number of special investigations are often required in the diagnosis and monitoring of lung disease.

IMAGING

The 'plain' chest radiograph

Many diseases, including bronchial carcinoma and pulmonary tuberculosis, cannot be detected at an early stage without a radiograph of the chest. A lateral film provides additional information about the likely nature and situation of a pulmonary, pleural or mediastinal abnormality.

Table 4.2 Summary of typical physical signs in the more common respiratory diseases

Pathological process	Movement of chest wall	Mediastinal displacement	Percussion note	Breath sounds	Vocal resonance	Added sounds
Consolidation as in lobar pneumonia	Reduced on side affected	None	Dull	High-pitched bronchial	Increased; whispering pectoriloquy	Fine crepitations[1] early; coarse crepitations later
Collapse due to obstruction of a major bronchus	Reduced on side affected	Towards lesion	Dull	Diminished or absent	Reduced or absent	None
Collapse due to peripheral bronchial obstruction	Reduced on side affected	Towards lesion	Dull	High-pitched bronchial	Increased; whispering pectoriloquy	None early; coarse crepitations later
Localised fibrosis and/or bronchiectasis	Slightly reduced on side affected	Towards lesion	Impaired	Low-pitched bronchial	Increased	Coarse crepitations
Cavitation (usually associated with consolidation or fibrosis)	Slightly reduced on side affected	None, or towards lesion	Impaired	Bronchial	Increased; whispering pectoriloquy	Coarse crepitations
Pleural effusion Empyema	Reduced or absent (depending on size) on side affected	Towards opposite side	Stony dull	Diminished or absent (occasionally bronchial)	Reduced or absent (occasionally increased)	Pleural rub in some cases (above effusion)
Pneumothorax	Reduced or absent (depending on size) on side affected	Towards opposite side	Normal or hyper-resonant	Diminished or absent (occasionally faint bronchial)	Reduced or absent	Tinkling crepitations when fluid present
Bronchitis: acute or chronic	Normal or symmetrically diminished	None	Normal	Vesicular with prolonged expiration	Normal	Rhonchi[2], usually with some coarse crepitations
Bronchial asthma	Symmetrically diminished	None	Normal	Vesicular with prolonged expiration	Normal or reduced	Rhonchi, mainly expiratory and high-pitched
Bronchopneumonia	Symmetrically diminished	None	May be impaired	Usually harsh vesicular with prolonged expiration	Normal	Rhonchi and coarse crepitations
Diffuse pulmonary emphysema	Symmetrically diminished	None`	Normal or hyper-resonant	Diminished vesicular with prolonged expiration	Normal or reduced	Expiratory rhonchi
Interstitial lung disease	Symmetrically diminished	None	Normal	Harsh vesicular with prolonged expiration	Usually increased	End-inspiratory crepitations not influenced by coughing

[1] Crepitations = crackles.
[2] Rhonchi = wheeze.

Comparison with previous radiographs may help to distinguish between a 'new' or progressive change which is thus potentially serious, and 'old' or static abnormalities which may be of no importance. In some diseases, such as chronic bronchitis and asthma, there is often no radiographic abnormality. In these diseases functional assessment (see p. 311) is of much more value in detecting abnormality.

Computed tomography (CT)

This has virtually taken over from conventional tomography in centres where it is available. Conventional tomography was valuable in determining the position and size of a pulmonary nodule or mass and whether calcification or cavitation was present. It was also useful in localising lesions for percutaneous needle biopsy and in assessing the mediastinum and thoracic cage. In all of these examples, however, except possibly for assessing the ribs, computed tomography is more sensitive and accurate. CT is now widely used in the pre-operative assessment of patients with lung cancer, particularly for assessing mediastinal spread, and the presence of metastases in the liver or adrenals. Its value in imaging the mediastinum can be greatly enhanced by using an intravenous contrast which outlines the mediastinal vessels. High-resolution CT is particularly useful in diagnosing interstitial fibrosis, and in identifying bronchiectasis (see Fig. 4.5).

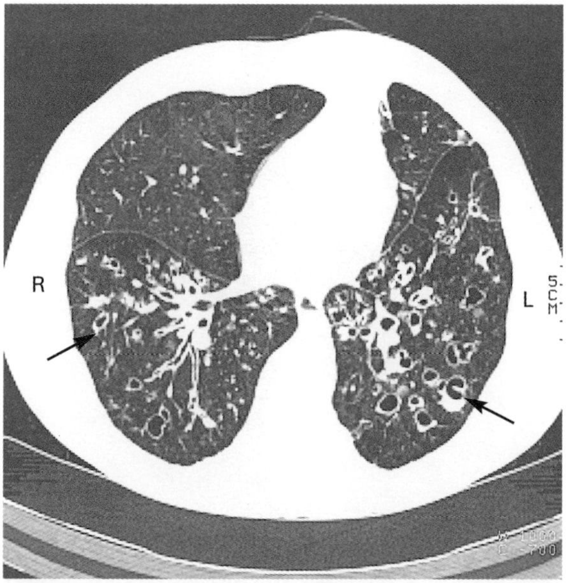

Fig. 4.5 Computed tomography of the thorax. This scan shows extensive dilatation of the bronchi (bronchiectasis) with thickened walls (arrows) in both lower lobes.

Ventilation-perfusion imaging

The main value of this technique is in the detection of pulmonary thromboemboli. ^{133}Xe gas is inhaled (the ventilation scan) and ^{99m}Tc-labelled macroaggregates of albumin, or albumin microspheres, are injected intravenously, the particles becoming transiently trapped in pulmonary microvessels and providing the 'perfusion' scan. Pulmonary emboli can be detected as a 'filling defect' in the perfusion scan (see Fig. 4.6), but patients with asthma, chronic bronchitis or other forms of obstructive airways disease may also have disordered pulmonary vascular distribution. However, in these patients the ventilation scan shows defects which match the areas of reduced perfusion on the perfusion scan, whereas the perfusion defects in pulmonary embolism are not matched to defects on the ventilation scan. Ventilation-perfusion scanning may also be useful in pre-operative assessment of the functional effects of lung cancer and bullae.

Pulmonary angiography

This is the definitive method of diagnosing pulmonary emboli, particularly in the acutely ill and shocked patient or when ventilation-perfusion scans are equivocal. Contrast medium is passed down a catheter inserted via the femoral vein into the main pulmonary artery. This catheter can also be used to measure pulmonary artery pressure and instil thrombolytic agents such as streptokinase. Digital subtraction angiography (DSA) is a technique whereby images obtained before contrast injection are digitised and subtracted from post-contrast images, thus removing bones and other background structures from the final digital images. This technique is more sensitive and requires much less contrast to obtain high-quality images (see Fig. 4.7).

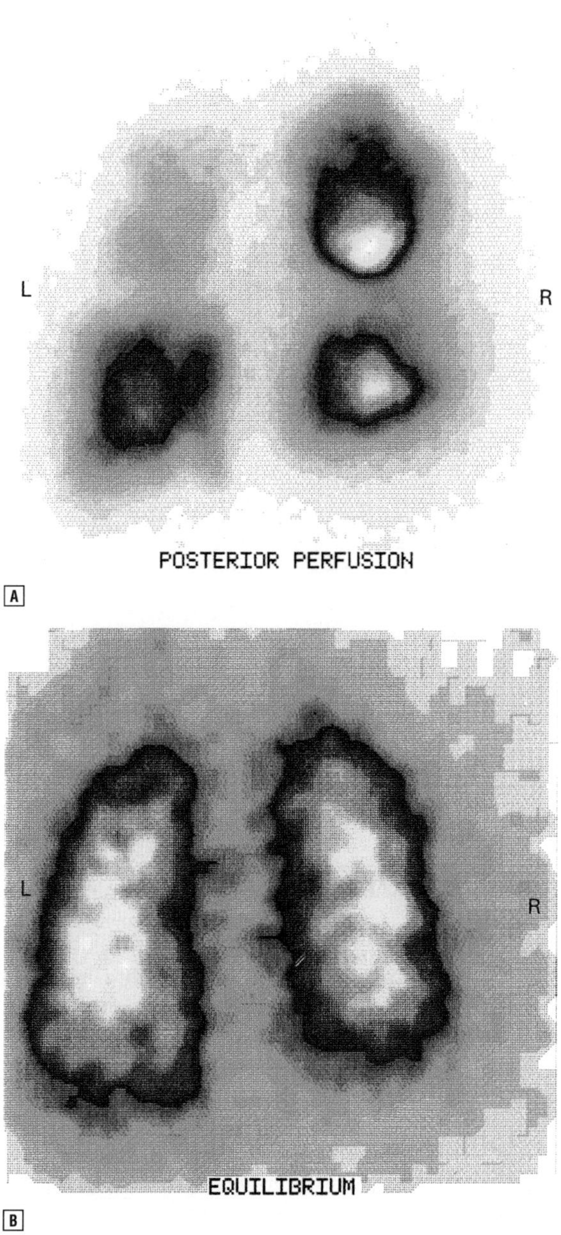

Fig. 4.6 Lung ventilation and perfusion scintigraphy. [A] Multiple perfusion defects present in left upper zone and right mid-zone of perfusion scan. [B] Normal ventilation scan. These appearances indicate a high probability of recent pulmonary embolism.

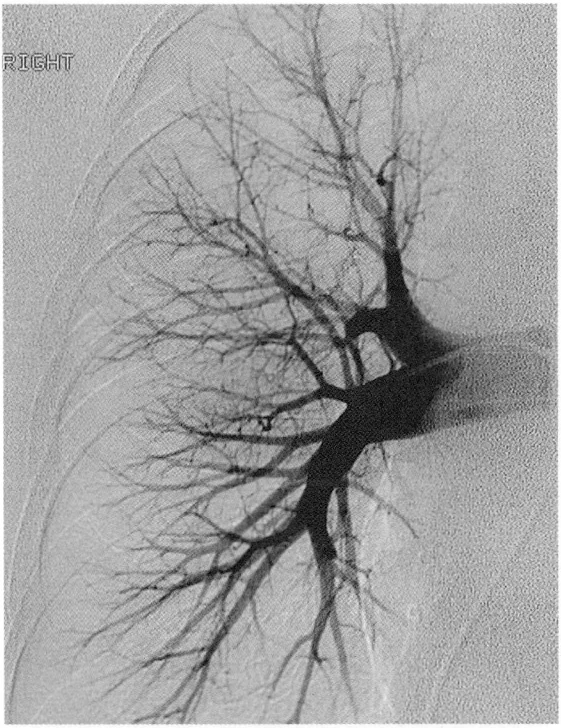

Fig. 4.7 Normal digital subtraction pulmonary angiogram of the right lung.

ENDOSCOPIC EXAMINATION

Laryngoscopy
The larynx may be inspected indirectly with a mirror or directly with a laryngoscope. Fibreoptic instruments allow a magnified view to be obtained.

Bronchoscopy
The trachea and larger bronchi (see Fig. 4.8) are inspected by a bronchoscope of either flexible fibreoptic or rigid type. Rigid bronchoscopy usually requires general anaesthesia. Structural changes, such as distortion or obstruction, can be seen. Abnormal tissue in the bronchial lumen or wall can be biopsied, and bronchial brushings, washings or aspirates can be taken for cytological or bacteriological examination. The range of direct vision is limited by the calibre of the subsegmental bronchi, but peripheral lesions can sometimes be reached by flexible biopsy forceps directed under fluoroscopic control. Small biopsy specimens of lung tissue taken by forceps passed through the bronchial wall (transbronchial biopsy) may reveal sarcoid granulomata or malignant diseases, but are generally too small to be of diagnostic value in diffuse interstitial lung disease (see pp. 365 and 370).

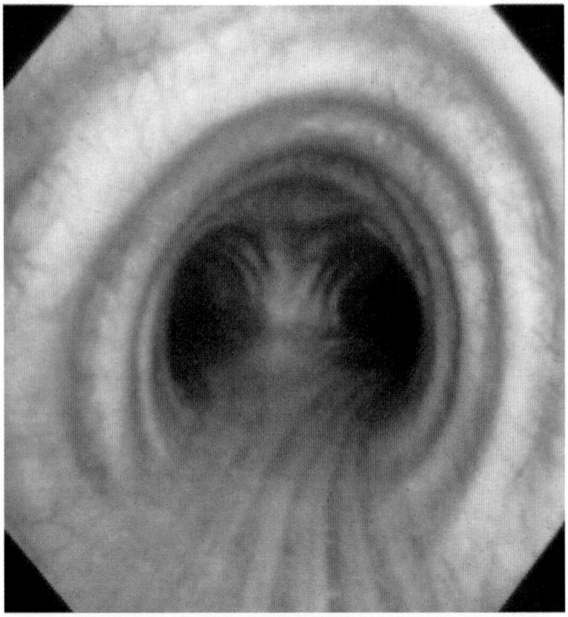

Fig. 4.8 Bronchoscopic appearances of the lower trachea, carina and the right and left main bronchi.

Mediastinoscopy
The mediastinoscope is introduced through a small incision at the suprasternal notch to give a view of the upper mediastinum. Biopsy of some mediastinal nodes is possible, which may be of value in obtaining a diagnosis and in determining whether a bronchial carcinoma has spread to the mediastinum and is, therefore, inoperable.

Pleural aspiration and biopsy
Pleural aspiration and biopsy using an Abram's needle is a 'blind' procedure but often provides histological evidence of the cause of pleural effusion. Transthoracic needle biopsy (often with radiological guidance) may be useful in obtaining a cytological diagnosis from a peripheral lung lesion. In difficult cases, thoracoscopy may be necessary to obtain diseased tissue, and the recent introduction of video-assisted thoracoscopic lung biopsy is likely to obviate the need for surgical thoracotomy in cases of interstitial lung disease when lung biopsy is required (see p. 370).

SKIN TESTS

The tuberculin test (see p. 352) may be of value in the diagnosis of tuberculosis. Skin hypersensitivity tests are useful in the investigation of allergic disease (see p. 328).

IMMUNOLOGICAL AND SEROLOGICAL TESTS

The presence of pneumococcal antigen (revealed by

counterimmunoelectrophoresis) in sputum, blood or urine may be of diagnostic importance. Exfoliated cells colonised by influenza A virus (see p. 340) can be detected by fluorescent antibody techniques. In blood, high or rising antibody titres to specific organisms (such as *Legionella, Mycoplasma, Chlamydia* or viruses) may eventually clinch a diagnosis suspected on clinical grounds. Precipitating antibodies may be found as a reaction to fungi such as *Aspergillus* (see p. 355) or to antigens involved in allergic alveolitis (see p. 371).

MICROBIOLOGICAL INVESTIGATIONS

Sputum, pleural fluid, throat swabs, blood and bronchial washings and aspirates can be examined for bacteria, fungi and viruses. In some cases, as when *M. tuberculosis* is isolated, the information is diagnostically conclusive but in other circumstances the findings must be interpreted in conjunction with the results of clinical and radiological examination.

HISTOPATHOLOGICAL AND CYTOLOGICAL EXAMINATION

Histopathological examination of biopsy material (obtained from pleura, lymph node or lung) often allows a 'tissue diagnosis' to be made. This is of particular importance in suspected malignancy or in elucidating the pathological changes in interstitial lung disease (see p. 365). Important causative organisms, such as *Mycobacterium tuberculosis*, *Pneumocystis carinii* or fungi may be identified in bronchial washings, brushings or transbronchial biopsies.

Cytological examination of exfoliated cells in sputum, pleural fluid or bronchial brushings and washings or of fine-needle aspirates from lymph nodes or pulmonary lesions can provide rapid evidence of malignancy. Cellular patterns in bronchial lavage fluid may help to distinguish pulmonary changes due to sarcoidosis (see p. 367) from those caused by fibrosing alveolitis (see p. 369) or allergic alveolitis (see p. 371).

LUNG FUNCTION TESTING

Most pulmonary function tests detect impairment and assess the effects of treatment or progress of the disease. (Some abbreviations used in pulmonary function testing are shown in Table 4.3.)

Fewer tests, such as measurements of exercise tolerance, assess disability or handicap. Some tests require a high degree of skill and elaborate apparatus, but others, e.g. FEV_1 and FVC, are simple routine procedures which can be undertaken by any doctor without special training.

Measurements of ventilatory capacity

The forced expiratory volume in one second (FEV_1), forced vital capacity (FVC) and vital capacity (VC) are obtained from maximal forced and relaxed expirations into a recording spirometer and compared with predicted values based on age, sex, height and ethnic group. Typical patterns of abnormality known as *obstructive* and *restrictive* ventilatory defects are shown in Table 4.4.

Table 4.3 Abbreviations used in pulmonary function testing

Abbreviation	Stands for
FEV_1	Forced expiratory volume in 1 second
FVC	Forced vital capacity
VC	Vital capacity (forced or relaxed)
PEF	Peak (maximum) expiratory flow
TLC	Total lung capacity
FRC	Functional residual capacity
RV	Residual volume
TLCO	Gas transfer factor for carbon monoxide
DLCO	Diffusing capacity for carbon monoxide
KCO	Transfer coefficient for carbon monoxide

Table 4.4 Patterns of abnormal ventilatory capacity

Test	Obstructive	Restrictive
FEV_1	↓↓	↓
VC	↓ or normal	↓↓
FEV_1/VC	↓	Normal or ↑

If an obstructive ventilatory defect is found, the response to bronchodilators in standard doses (salbutamol 200 μg from pressurised aerosol) or larger doses (salbutamol 2.5 mg by nebuliser) can be measured. Reversibility of airflow obstruction is found in asthma (see p. 326) and in some patients with COPD.

Peak expiratory flow (PEF) can be measured during forced expiration by a gauge or meter, which is simpler and cheaper than a spirometer. Reduced values indicate airflow obstruction, and serial measurements are of use in following circadian changes (see p. 330) and responses to therapy or to occupational exposure to allergens or sensitising agents. PEF is of little value in restrictive ventilatory defects.

Measurements of lung volumes

Normal landmarks and patterns of abnormality of lung volumes in obstructive and restrictive ventilatory defects are shown in Figure 4.9 on page 312. The values are obtained either by diluting helium (a non-toxic, non-absorbed gas) into the gas in the lungs, or in a whole body plethysmograph.

Measurements of gas transfer factor

The gas transfer factor (diffusing capacity) may be thought of as the conductance of the lungs for the gas being studied. It forms a useful overall estimate of the ability of the lungs to exchange gases, and is of particular value in interstitial lung disease (see p. 365), sarcoidosis (see p. 367) and

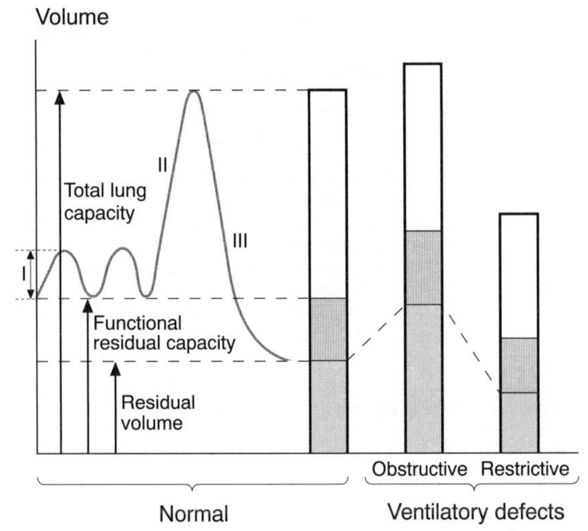

Fig. 4.9 Normal lung volumes and the changes which occur in obstructive and restrictive ventilatory defects. (I = 'tidal' volume; II = forced inspiration; III = forced expiration)

emphysema (see p. 322). It is normally estimated by measuring the uptake of carbon monoxide from a single breath of a 0.3% mixture in air.

Arterial blood gas analysis

Modern automatic analysers give a rapid direct readout of PaO_2, $PaCO_2$ and hydrogen ion concentration in arterial blood, often supplemented by derived variables (such as oxygen saturation and bicarbonate concentration) which may be of value in assessment of hypoxaemia or acid-base balance (see p. 398 and 410). Such measurements are of particular value in the management of respiratory failure (see p. 317), asthma (see p. 326) and acute respiratory distress syndrome (ARDS) (see p. 1035).

Ear or pulse oximeters allow continuous non-invasive measurement of arterial oxygen saturation, of value in assessing hypoxaemia and the effects of oxygen therapy.

Exercise tests

Exercise challenge is a self-evident test for detecting exercise-induced asthma (see p. 330). Formal exercise tests, in which cardiac and respiratory responses to bicycle or treadmill exercise are measured in the laboratory, are of value in detecting exercise hypoxaemia and in assessing disability due to respiratory disease.

'Everyday' exercise tests, such as measurement of the distance the patient can walk in 6 minutes, require no complex apparatus and assist in the assessment of disability, handicap and the response to treatment.

FURTHER INFORMATION ON FUNCTIONAL ANATOMY, PHYSIOLOGY AND INVESTIGATIONS

Gibson G J 1995 Respiratory function tests. In: Brewis R A L et al (eds) Respiratory Medicine. Baillière Tindall, London
Haslett C 1995 Non-immune defence mechanisms of the lung. In: Ledingham J et al (eds) Oxford Textbook of Medicine. Oxford University Press, Oxford
Leach R M, Treacher D F 1992 Oxygen transport: the relationship between oxygen delivery and consumption. Thorax 47: 971–978
Wagner P D, Rodriguez-Roisin R 1991 Clinical advances in pulmonary gas exchange. American Review of Respiratory Disease 143: 883–889

MAJOR MANIFESTATIONS OF LUNG DISEASE

DYSPNOEA

Breathlessness or dyspnoea can be defined as an unpleasant subjective awareness of the sensation of breathing. It is a common symptom of cardiac and respiratory disease, but it may occur as a result of disorders of other systems, e.g. diabetic ketoacidosis or severe anaemia. The term 'dyspnoea' is derived from the Greek roots *dys* (difficult, painful) and *pnoia* (breathing). Breathless patients with asthma or COPD often also describe a 'tight chest'. Pleural pain (see p. 384) of any cause is associated with limitation of breathing.

In broad physiological terms, patients usually perceive discomfort either from an increased ventilatory rate or drive, which can be provoked by a variety of factors, or from any disease which causes sufficient reduction of ventilatory capacity (see the information box). Other factors, however, including the stimulation of intra-

PHYSIOLOGICAL BASIS OF DYSPNOEA

Increased ventilatory rate	Reduced ventilatory capacity
• ↑ $PaCO_2$—e.g. COPD • ↓ PaO_2—e.g. cyanotic congenital heart disease, asthma, COPD • Acidaemia—e.g. diabetic ketoacidosis, lactic acidosis • Exercise • Fever	• ↓ Lung volume, e.g. restrictive lung diseases—pneumonia, pulmonary oedema, interstitial lung diseases • ↑ Resistance to airflow, e.g. asthma, COPD, upper airway or laryngeal obstruction • Pleural pain

Table 4.5 Some causes of dyspnoea

System	Acute dyspnoea at rest	Chronic exertional dyspnoea
Cardiovascular system	*Acute pulmonary oedema Pulmonary embolus Major neonatal congenital heart disease	*Chronic cardiac failure Chronic pulmonary thromboembolism Congenital heart disease
Respiratory system	*Acute severe asthma *Acute exacerbation of COPD *Pneumothorax *Pneumonia Acute respiratory distress syndrome Inhaled foreign body (especially in the child) Lobar collapse Laryngeal oedema (e.g. anaphylaxis)	*COPD *Chronic asthma Bronchial carcinoma Interstitial lung diseases: sarcoidosis, fibrosing alveolitis, extrinsic allergic alveolitis, pneumoconiosis Lymphatic carcinomatosis (may cause intolerable dyspnoea) Large pleural effusion(s)
Others	Metabolic acidosis (e.g. diabetic ketoacidosis, lactic acidosis, uraemia, overdose of salicylates, ethylene glycol poisoning) Hysterical hyperventilation	Severe anaemia

* Denotes a common cause.

pulmonary receptors (e.g. J receptors), augment the ventilatory response in many bronchopulmonary disorders.

It follows that diseases presenting with dyspnoea often have a multifactorial aetiology, e.g. acute respiratory infections may stimulate the respiratory rate as a consequence of fever, hypoxaemia and, in severe cases, by acidaemia or hypercapnia. They may also reduce ventilatory capacity by increasing bronchial resistance and by restricting ventilation because of pleural pain.

While it is useful to understand the physiological basis of dyspnoea, patients often present either as an emergency with acute breathlessness (with prominent symptoms even at rest) or with chronic dyspnoea on exertion, and it is useful therefore to describe the causes of dyspnoea in this fashion (see Table 4.5).

AN APPROACH TO THE DIFFERENTIAL DIAGNOSIS IN PATIENTS WITH CHRONIC EXERTIONAL DYSPNOEA

Chronic obstructive pulmonary disease (COPD)

There is usually a history of exertional dyspnoea, often associated with wheeze, over many months or years, with a steady chronic decline in exercise capacity (e.g. initially breathlessness on hills and stairs, but eventually after walking a few paces on the flat). Chronic cough productive of sputum, usually most troublesome in the mornings, is the rule and there is often a history of recurrent acute exacerbations. In late disease orthopnoea, nocturnal breathlessness and ankle swelling may supervene as a result of the development of cor pulmonale.

Central cyanosis at rest or after minimal exertion, wheeze and pursing of the lips during expiration, and intercostal indrawing during inspiration, are common examination findings. The antero-posterior diameter of the chest may be increased (barrel chest) and there may be a reduced crico-sternal distance with a 'tracheal tug' on inspiration.

The chest radiograph may show signs of hyperinflation and/or bullae; arterial blood gases may reveal hypoxaemia, hypercapnia and a raised plasma bicarbonate, indicating compensated type II respiratory failure. It is important to note that patients presenting with type II respiratory failure (see p. 318) may not be distressed by breathlessness. There will often be a severe obstructive defect on spirometry, with a low FEV_1 which may or may not improve after inhaled bronchodilators.

Heart disease

It is often difficult to differentiate breathlessness due to heart disease from that caused by lung disease. A history of cough, wheezing and nocturnal breathlessness may occur in cardiac failure as well as COPD. A history of angina or hypertension may be useful in implicating a cardiac cause.

On examination, an increase in heart size as judged by a displaced apex beat, a raised jugular venous pressure (JVP) and cardiac murmurs may implicate cardiac disease (although these signs can occur also in severe cor pulmonale). The chest radiograph may show cardiomegaly and an electrocardiogram (ECG) may provide evidence of left ventricular disease. Arterial blood gases may be of value, since in the absence of intracardiac shunts or severe, obvious pulmonary oedema, the PaO_2 in cardiac disease is not usually reduced significantly and the $PaCO_2$ is low or normal.

Interstitial or alveolar disease of the lung

A large number of conditions can cause interstitial lung disease (see p. 365), which may be difficult to distinguish from other conditions including infiltrating malignancy and chronic opportunistic lung infections (see the information box, p. 366). It is imperative to elicit a detailed history, including occupation and exposure to birds and other sources of organic agents which may provoke lung disease. The chest radiograph is nearly always abnormal, but early changes may be very subtle. Pulmonary function tests usually show a restrictive defect (reduced vital capacity) and reduced gas transfer (see p. 311). Arterial blood gases may show hypoxaemia, or haemoglobin desaturation may be detected by oximetry, particularly during formal exercise testing, which may be valuable in early disease, but $PaCO_2$ is seldom elevated, even in advanced disease.

Diseases of the chest wall or respiratory muscles

These are usually obvious on history, examination and chest radiography. Other rarer causes of alveolar hypoventilation, e.g. brain-stem defects, primary alveolar hypoventilation and alveolar hypoventilation in gross obesity, may cause disordered breathing and cyanosis, but these conditions are not usually associated with breathlessness.

Pulmonary thromboembolism

As will be considered below (see p. 377), pulmonary thromboembolism often presents with acute breathlessness with or without chest pain. However, this condition should also be suspected in patients at risk of venous thromboembolism (see p. 795) who present with more gradual onset of breathlessness. Leg swelling and an elevated JVP may make one suspicious but clearly can also occur in cardiac failure.

Psychogenic breathlessness

Breathlessness which is not caused by organic disease of the heart or lungs is common. It creates a particularly difficult clinical problem when it occurs in patients with pre-existing disease associated with dyspnoea, such as asthma or heart disease. It is possible in most patients to ascertain by careful questioning whether the sensation of breathlessness is different from that caused by exertion in the past, or dyspnoea associated with any pre-existing lung or heart disease. Psychogenic breathlessness is usually described as an 'inability to get enough air' into the lungs and this leads to extra deep breaths having to be taken. This form of breathlessness rarely disturbs sleep, but may be present after waking for another reason, and sometimes it is not made worse by exertion and may even be relieved by exercise. Specialist centres use a number of features to develop a 'points' score in the assessment of this problem, often called hyperventilation—see the information box. Occasionally, formal metabolic exercise testing may be required to be confident that patients have breathlessness which does not have an organic cause.

Overt 'hysterical hyperventilation', which usually is dramatic and is associated with pins and needles in the hands and feet, cramps and carpopedal spasm due to acute respiratory alkalosis, presents as a respiratory emergency but rarely creates a diagnostic problem. It must always, however, be included in the differential diagnosis of acute-onset breathlessness (see Table 4.5).

SOME FACTORS POINTING TO PSYCHOGENIC HYPERVENTILATION

- 'Inability to take a deep breath'
- Frequent sighing/erratic ventilation at rest
- Short breath-holding time in the absence of severe respiratory disease
- Difficulty in performing/inconsistent spirometry manoeuvres
- High score on Nijmegen questionnaire
- Induction of symptoms during submaximal hyperventilation
- Resting end-tidal $CO_2 < 4.5\%$

AN APPROACH TO THE PATIENT WITH ACUTE SEVERE DYSPNOEA

Acute severe breathlessness is one of the most common medical emergencies. The presentation is often dramatic and it is easy for the inexperienced clinician to be disconcerted. Although there are usually a number of possible causes, attention to the history and a rapid but careful examination will usually suggest a diagnosis which can often be confirmed by routine investigations, including chest radiograph, ECG, arterial blood gases and echocardiography. Some specific features aiding in the diagnosis of important causes of acute severe breathlessness are considered in detail in Table 4.6.

History

It is important to ascertain the rate of onset and severity of breathlessness and whether associated cardiovascular (chest pain, palpitations, sweating and nausea) or respiratory (cough, wheeze, haemoptysis, stridor) symptoms are present. A previous history of repeated episodes of left ventricular failure, asthma or exacerbations of COPD is valuable. Recent intake of drugs or a history of other diseases (renal, diabetes or anaemia) should be established. In the severely ill patient it may be necessary to obtain a brief history from friends, relatives or ambulance personnel. In children, particularly pre-school toddlers, the possibility of inhalation of a foreign body should always be considered.

Examination

The severity of the condition should be assessed immediately by the level of consciousness, degree of central cyanosis, evidence of anaphylaxis (urticaria or angio-oedema), patency of the upper airway, ability to speak (in phrases or sentences), and the cardiovascular status assessed by heart rate and rhythm, blood pressure

Table 4.6 Differential diagnosis of acute severe dyspnoea

Condition	History	Signs	Chest radiography	Arterial blood gases	ECG	Other tests
Left ventricular failure	Chest pain, orthopnoea, palpitations, *a previous cardiac history	Central cyanosis, JVP (→ or ↑), *sweating, cool extremities, *dullness and crepitations at bases	Cardiomegaly, *upper zone vessel enlargement, *overt oedema/pleural effusions	↓ PaO_2 ↓ $PaCO_2$	Sinus tachycardia, *signs of myocardial infarction, arrhythmia	*Echocardiography (↓ left ventricular function)
Massive pulmonary embolus	Recent surgery or other risk factors Chest pain, previous pleurisy, *syncope, *dizziness	Severe central cyanosis, *elevated JVP, *absence of signs in the lung (unless previous pulmonary infarction), shock (tachycardia, reduced blood pressure)	May be subtle changes only, prominent hilar vessels, *oligaemic lung fields	⇓ PaO_2 ↓ $PaCO_2$	Sinus tachycardia $S_1Q_3T_3$ pattern ↓ T (V_1–V_4) Right bundle branch block	*Echocardiography *V/Q scan *Pulmonary angiography
Acute severe asthma	*History of previous episodes, asthma medications, wheeze	Tachycardia and pulsus paradoxus Cyanosis (late) *JVP → *⇓ peak flow, rhonchi	*Hyperinflation only (unless complicated by pneumothorax)	↓ PaO_2 ↓ $PaCO_2$ (until late)	Sinus tachycardia (bradycardia with severe hypoxaemia—late)	
Acute exacerbation of COPD	*Previous episodes (admissions) If in type II respiratory failure, may not be distressed	Cyanosis *Signs of COPD (barrel chest, intercostal indrawing, pursed lips, tracheal tug) *Signs of CO_2 retention (warm periphery, flapping tremor, bounding pulses)	*Hyperinflation, minor signs of emphysema, signs of events precipitating exacerbation	↓ or ⇓ PaO_2 In type II failure $PaCO_2$ ↑, with ↑ [H^+] and ↑ bicarbonate	Nil, or signs of right ventricular failure (in cor pulmonale)	
Pneumonia	*Prodromal illness *Fever *Rigors *Pleurisy	Fever *Pleural rub *Consolidation Cyanosis (only if widespread)	*Pneumonic consolidation	↓ $PaCO_2$ ↓ PaO_2	Tachycardia	
Metabolic acidosis	*Evidence of diabetes/renal disease *Overdose of aspirin or ethylene glycol	Fetor (ketones) *Hyperventilation without physical signs in heart or lungs *Dehydration Air hunger (Kussmaul's respiration)	Normal	*PaO_2 normal ⇓ $PaCO_2$ ⇓ pH (↑ H^+)		
Psychogenic (a diagnosis of *exclusion*)	Previous episodes	**Not* cyanosed **No* heart signs **No* lung signs Carpopedal spasm	Normal	*PaO_2 normal ⇓ $PaCO_2$ *pH normal or ↑ (H^+ ↓)		End-tidal $PaCO_2$ *Low exercise tolerance test

* Denotes a valuable discriminatory feature.

and degree of peripheral perfusion. Then examination should be targeted on digital clubbing, clinical evidence of anaemia or polycythaemia, and any clinical features of diabetes, renal failure or any other chronic disease. A detailed examination of the respiratory system should include respiratory rate, pattern of breathing, position of the trachea and whether there are areas of hyper-resonance or dullness on percussion. Breath sounds should be compared on each side of the chest and at the bases, and the presence of abnormal sounds noted. The peak expiratory flow should be measured whenever possible. Leg swelling may suggest cardiac failure or venous thrombosis.

CHEST PAIN

See Chapter 3, page 204.

HAEMOPTYSIS

Coughing up blood, irrespective of the amount, is an alarming symptom and nearly always brings the patient to the doctor. A clear history should be taken to establish that it is true haemoptysis, and not haematemesis or epistaxis (nosebleed). Haemoptysis must always be assumed to have a serious cause until appropriate investigations have excluded bronchial carcinoma, thromboembolic disease, tuberculosis etc. (see the information box).

CAUSES OF HAEMOPTYSIS

Bronchial disease
- Carcinoma*
- Bronchiectasis*
- Acute bronchitis*
- Bronchial adenoma
- Foreign body

Parenchymal disease
- Tuberculosis*
- Suppurative pneumonia*
- Lung abscess
- Parasites (e.g. hydatid disease, flukes)
- Trauma
- Actinomycosis
- Aspergilloma

Lung vascular disease
- Pulmonary infarction*
- Polyarteritis nodosa
- Goodpasture's syndrome
- Idiopathic pulmonary haemosiderosis

Cardiovascular disease
- Acute left ventricular failure*
- Mitral stenosis*
- Aortic aneurysm

Blood disorders
- Leukaemia
- Haemophilia
- Anticoagulants

* More common causes.

Many episodes of haemoptysis are unexplained, even after full investigation, and are likely to be caused by simple bronchial infection. A history of repeated small haemoptyses, or blood-streaking of sputum, is highly suggestive of bronchial carcinoma. Chronic fever and weight loss may suggest tuberculosis. Pneumococcal pneumonia is often the cause of 'rusty'-coloured sputum but can cause frank haemoptysis, as can all the pneumonic infections which lead to suppuration or abscess formation (see p. 344). Bronchiectasis can cause catastrophic bronchial haemorrhage and in these patients there may be a history of previous tuberculosis or whooping cough in early life. In hospital practice pulmonary thromboembolism is the most common cause of haemoptysis. Major risk factors include immobilisation, malignant disease of any organ, cardiac failure and pregnancy.

Physical examination may reveal clues as to the underlying diagnosis, e.g. finger clubbing in bronchial carcinoma or bronchiectasis; other signs of malignancy such as cachexia, hepatomegaly, lymphadenopathy etc.; fever or chest signs of consolidation and pleurisy in pneumonia or pulmonary infarction; leg signs of deep venous thrombosis in a minority of patients with pulmonary infarction; and signs of systemic diseases including rash purpura, haematuria, splinter haemorrhages, lymphadenopathy or splenomegaly in the uncommon systemic diseases which may be associated with haemoptysis.

Management

In catastrophic acute haemoptysis, the patient should be nursed on the side of the suspected source of bleeding, haemodynamically resuscitated and then bronchoscoped, ideally under general anaesthesia using a rigid bronchoscope which allows optimal bronchial suction and which can be used to maintain ventilation during anaesthesia. Angiography and arterial embolisation, or even emergency pulmonary surgery, can be life-saving in the acute situation in the patient not known to have malignant disease.

In the vast majority of cases, however, the haemoptysis itself is not life-threatening and it is possible to follow a logical sequence of investigations which include:

- chest radiograph, which may give clear evidence of a localised lesion including pulmonary infarction, a tumour (malignant or benign), pneumonia or tuberculosis
- full blood count and other haematological tests including clotting screen
- bronchoscopy, which will often be necessary to exclude a central bronchial carcinoma (not visible on the chest radiograph) and to provide a tissue diagnosis in other cases of suspected bronchial neoplasia
- ventilation-perfusion lung scan, which is helpful in establishing a diagnosis of suspected pulmonary thromboembolic disease. Pulmonary angiography may be necessary in a minority of patients (see p. 309)
- CT. This is particularly useful in investigating peripheral chest radiograph lesions which may not be accessible to bronchoscopy; recent developments in spiral CT scanning, however, indicate that this investigation is also of value in the diagnosis of massive pulmonary embolism.

THE SOLITARY RADIOGRAPHIC PULMONARY LESION

Frequently patients present because they have been found to have an abnormal chest radiograph. A common clinical problem is often created by the adult with few or no symptoms, who has been found to have a single peripheral

THE SOLITARY PULMONARY NODULE	
Common causes	**Uncommon causes**
• Bronchial carcinoma • Single metastasis • Localised pneumonia • Lung abscess • Tuberculoma • Pulmonary infarct	• Benign tumours • Lymphoma • Arteriovenous malformation • Hydatid cyst • Bronchogenic cyst • Rheumatoid nodule • Pulmonary sequestration • Pulmonary haematoma • Wegener's granuloma • 'Pseudotumour'—fluid in a fissure • Aspergilloma (usually see air 'halo')

lesion (nodule) detected by chest radiography. There are many causes of the 'peripheral radiograph shadow', some of which are shown in the information box. Primary bronchial carcinoma is the most likely cause in a middle-aged or elderly adult, particularly if a smoker.

Investigations

Radiography

The single most important investigation is examination of previous radiographs, if they exist, since if a lesion has been present for more than 2 years and it has not changed, it can be assumed to be non-malignant. If there are no previous radiographs or if previous films are normal, CT can be of great value in defining the lesion more precisely, demonstrating the presence of calcification and cavitation within it and detecting multiple smaller lesions which may not be apparent on the conventional radiograph. CT will also show hilar and mediastinal lymphadenopathy, which is important in the staging of a primary bronchial carcinoma (see p. 361).

Sputum examination

Sputum (fresh specimen) should be examined for malignant cells (see Fig. 4.36, p. 362), and also for pathogenic organisms, if infection is suspected.

Invasive procedures

Bronchoscopy is unlikely to allow visualisation of a peripheral lesion, but a diagnosis of malignant disease or infection can be achieved by examination of bronchial washings and brushings obtained from the segment of lung in which the lesion is seen to be radiographically or on CT. Biopsy of the lesion via the bronchoscope may be possible with the aid of radiograph screening in some patients. Percutaneous fine-needle aspiration under radiographic or CT guidance has proved to be an effective procedure with few complications (pneumothorax and haemorrhage), and is increasingly being used in the investigation of the peripheral radiographic opacity. On occasion, a definitive diagnosis can only be made by surgical resection.

Whenever bacterial infection is included in the list of differential diagnoses an antibiotic such as amoxycillin should be given during the period in which the investigations are being performed; the patient should then undergo a repeat radiograph to see whether there has been a reduction in size of the opacity. In elderly patients in whom a primary malignant lesion is suspected, but who are considered unfit for any form of curative treatment, observation by repeat radiograph at intervals of a few weeks may be the most appropriate management decision. However, it is important to be confident that the lesion being observed is not active tuberculosis. If there is any doubt, and the patient cannot produce sputum for mycobacterial examination, bronchoscopy should be performed, in all but the very frail, in order to obtain bronchial washings for tuberculosis culture.

RESPIRATORY FAILURE AND SLEEP APNOEA

RESPIRATORY FAILURE

Respiratory failure results from a disorder in which lung function is inadequate for the metabolic requirements of the individual. Its classification into type I and type II relates to the absence or presence of hypercapnia (raised $PaCO_2$). A summary of respiratory failure and its characteristic blood gas abnormalities is shown in Table 4.7 on page 318.

Management of acute type I respiratory failure

The most common causes of acute type I respiratory failure are listed in the information box.

All patients should be treated with high-concentration ($\geq 35\%$) oxygen by oronasal mask. Young children may require to be treated in oxygen tents, since few of them tolerate masks. Very ill patients may require immediate tracheal intubation and mechanical ventilation (see p. 321). Effective management requires prompt diagnosis and treatment of the underlying disorder. Close monitoring is essential and arterial blood gases taken on presentation

COMMON CAUSES OF ACUTE TYPE I RESPIRATORY FAILURE
• Severe acute asthma (causes type II failure when life-threatening) • Acute exacerbation of COPD (also causes type II failure) • Left ventricular failure and other causes of pulmonary oedema • Pulmonary embolism • Pneumonia

Table 4.7 Respiratory failure

	Type I (PaO_2 < 8.0 kPa) ($PaCO_2$ < 6.6 kPa)		Type II (PaO_2 < 8.0 kPa) ($PaCO_2$ > 6.6 kPa)	
	Acute	**Chronic**	**Acute**	**Chronic**
Typical blood gases	PaO_2↓↓ $PaCO_2$↔or ↓ pH↔or ⇓ HCO_3↔	PaO_2↓ $PaCO_2$↔ pH↔ HCO_3↔	PaO_2↓ $PaCO_2$↑ pH↓ HCO_3↔	PaO_2↓ $PaCO_2$↑ pH↓ or ↔ HCO_3↑
Causes	Asthma Pulmonary embolus Pulmonary oedema Acute respiratory distress syndrome Pneumothorax Pneumonia	Emphysema Lung fibrosis Lymphangitis carcinomatosa R → L shunts Anaemia	Severe acute asthma Acute epiglottitis Inhaled foreign body Respiratory muscle paralysis Flail chest injury Sleep apnoea Brain-stem lesion Narcotic drugs	COPD Primary alveolar hypoventilation Kyphoscoliosis Ankylosing spondylitis
Therapy	Treat underlying cause High-concentration O_2 Mechanical ventilation if necessary	Treat underlying disorder Long-term O_2	Treat underlying disorder Controlled low-concentration O_2 Mechanical ventilation or tracheostomy if necessary	Treat underlying disorder Controlled long-term O_2 delivery Mechanical ventilatory support if necessary

should be checked within 20 minutes to establish that treatment has achieved acceptable PaO_2 levels. If there is no improvement despite treating the underlying condition, an early decision about mechanical ventilation is necessary, particularly in severe acute asthma. In acute left ventricular failure, massive pulmonary embolism and when pulmonary infarction or pneumonia is the cause of pleural pain, treatment with opiates is entirely appropriate, but these drugs should *never* be used in asthma or COPD, except immediately prior to and during assisted mechanical ventilation.

Management of type II respiratory failure

Acute

In acute type II respiratory failure, also known as asphyxia, CO_2 retention occurs and causes severe acute respiratory acidosis (see Table 4.7). Treatment is aimed at immediate or very rapid reversal of the precipitating event—e.g. dislodgement of a laryngeal foreign body or tracheostomy, fixation of ribs in a flail chest injury, reversal of narcotic poisons, treatment of acute severe asthma etc. In some cases it will be necessary to support ventilation temporarily by intubation and mechanical ventilation if the condition causing respiratory failure cannot immediately be reversed.

Chronic

The most common cause of chronic type II respiratory failure is COPD. Here CO_2 retention may occur on a chronic basis, the potential for acidaemia being corrected by renal conservation of bicarbonate, which results in the plasma pH remaining within the normal range. The status quo is often maintained until there is a further pulmonary insult (see the information box), such as an exacerbation of COPD which precipitates an episode of 'acute on chronic' respiratory failure.

SOME CAUSES OF 'ACUTE ON CHRONIC' TYPE II RESPIRATORY FAILURE

- Retention of secretions
- Bronchospasm
- Pulmonary embolus
- Cardiac failure
- Rib fractures/intercostal muscle tears
- Pneumothorax
- CNS depression (narcotic drugs)

The further acute increase in $PaCO_2$ results in acidaemia, and worsening hypercapnia may also lead to drowsiness and eventually coma. The principal aim of treatment in type II respiratory failure is to keep the patient alive and achieve a safe PaO_2 without inducing extremes of $PaCO_2$ or pH, while identifying and treating the precipitating condition (see the information box). It is important to note that in the patient who already has severe lung disease, only a small insult may be required to tip the balance towards catastrophic respiratory failure. Moreover, in contrast to acute severe asthma, in type II respiratory failure the patient with COPD, despite being critically ill with severe hypoxaemia, hypercapnia and acidaemia, may not be overtly distressed.

In the initial assessment it is important to evaluate the patient's conscious level and his or her ability to respond to commands, particularly the ability to cough effectively. This may give a preliminary indication of whether intubation and tracheal suction may be necessary to clear secretions or whether physiotherapy will be helpful. The decision regarding mechanical ventilation can be complex and difficult. Ideally, an early decision should be made, based mainly on whether there is a potentially remediable precipitating condition (see the information box) and whether the patient is likely to regain an acceptable quality of life. It is important to remember that while physical signs of CO_2 retention (confusion, flapping tremor, bounding pulses etc.) can be helpful if present, they are often unreliable; there is no substitute for arterial blood gases in the assessment of initial severity and response to treatment.

Prompt intervention may occasionally be necessary for some precipitating conditions, e.g. intercostal tube drainage of pneumothoraces, injection with local anaesthetic for fractured ribs and torn muscles, which can result in dramatic improvement of respiratory function (see the information box). Generally, however, treatment is empirical and includes low-concentration controlled oxygen therapy, physiotherapy, bronchodilators, broad-spectrum antibiotics and diuretics. While the dangers of hypercapnia have not been exaggerated, it is important to recognise that severe hypoxaemia *must* be reversed if the patient is not to suffer potentially fatal arrhythmias or severe cerebral complications. The aim of oxygen therapy is not necessarily to achieve a normal PaO_2; even a small increment of increase in the PaO_2 will often have a greatly beneficial effect on oxygen delivery to tissues since the arterial values of these patients are often on the very steep part of the oxygen saturation curve. If controlled oxygen treatment causes an increase in the $PaCO_2$ associated with a reduction in pH, mechanical ventilation may be required. Alternatively, treatment with respiratory stimulants such as doxapram can in some circumstances be used to stimulate ventilation over a 24–48-hour period while the precipitating condition is treated. Nasal positive pressure assisted ventilation (NPPV, see p. 321) may also be of value.

ASSESSMENT AND MANAGEMENT OF 'ACUTE ON CHRONIC' TYPE II RESPIRATORY FAILURE

Initial assessment

N.B. Patient may not appear distressed despite being critically ill.

- Conscious level (response to commands, ability to cough)
- CO_2 retention (warm periphery, bounding pulses, flapping tremor)
- Airways obstruction (wheeze, intercostal indrawing, pursed lips, tracheal 'tug')
- Right heart failure (oedema, raised JVP, hepatomegaly, ascites)
- Background functional status and quality of life
- Signs of precipitating event (see the information box on p. 318)

Investigations

- Arterial blood gases (severity of hypoxaemia, hypercapnia and acidaemia)
- Chest radiograph

Management

- Maintenance of airway
- Treatment of specific precipitating event (see the information box on p. 318)
- Frequent physiotherapy ± pharyngeal suction
- Nebulised bronchodilators
- Controlled oxygen therapy
  - Start with 24% controlled-flow mask
  - Aim for a $PaO_2 \geq 7$ kPa (a $PaO_2 < 5$ is very dangerous)
- Antibiotics
- Diuretics

Progress

- If $PaCO_2$ continues to rise or patient cannot achieve a safe PaO_2 without severe hypercapnia and acidaemia, respiratory stimulants (e.g. doxapram) or mechanical ventilation may be required

THE SLEEP APNOEA/HYPOPNOEA SYNDROME

In the past decade, it has been realised that 2–4% of the middle-aged population suffer the consequences of recurrent upper airway obstruction during sleep. They experience day-time sleepiness, especially in monotonous situations, and this results in a three-fold risk of road traffic accidents and a nine-fold risk of single-vehicle accidents. Difficulty with concentration, impaired work performance and impaired cognitive function, along with depression and irritability, are other features. The patient usually feels that he or she has been asleep all night but wakes feeling unrefreshed. Bed-partners will report loud snoring in all body postures and often will have noticed multiple breathing pauses.

The problem results from recurrent occlusion of the back of the throat during sleep, most often starting at the level of the soft palate. On inspiration the pressure in the throat is subatmospheric. During wakefulness upper airway dilating muscles—including palatoglossus and genioglossus—actively contract during each inspiration to preserve airway patency. During sleep, muscle tone generally declines, including that in the upper airway dilating muscles, and their ability to maintain patency falls. In most people sufficient tone persists to result in uncompromised breathing during sleep. However, in those who for some reason have a narrow throat when awake, upper airway opening muscle action is more important and when it falls during sleep the airway narrows. If the narrowing is slight, turbulent flow and the vibration and noise of snoring occur—around 40% of middle-aged men and 20% of middle-aged women snore. If the upper airway narrowing during sleep progresses to the point of occlusion or near-occlusion, sleeping subjects increase respiratory effort to try to breathe until the increased effort transiently awakens them, so briefly that they have no recollection, but long enough for the upper airway dilating muscles to open the airway again. Then a series of deep breaths are taken before the subject rapidly returns to sleep, snores and becomes apnoeic once more. This recurrent cycle of apnoea, awakening, apnoea, awakening ... may repeat itself many hundreds of times per night and the sleep fragmentation results in day-time sleepiness and impaired day-time performance. The awakenings are associated with surges in blood pressure which may lead to an increased frequency of hypertension, ischaemic heart disease and stroke.

Predisposing factors to the sleep apnoea/hypopnoea syndrome include being male, which doubles the risk probably due to a testosterone effect on the upper airway, and obesity, found in about half the patients and having the effect of narrowing the throat by parapharyngeal fat deposits. Acromegaly and hypothyroidism also predispose by submucosal infiltration narrowing the upper airway. The condition is often familial, and in these families the maxilla and mandible are back-set, thus narrowing the upper airway. Alcohol and sedatives predispose to snoring and apnoeas by relaxing the upper airway dilating muscles.

Investigations

Any person who falls asleep once per day when not in bed, who complains that his or her work is impaired by sleepiness or who is a habitual snorer with multiple witnessed apnoeas should be referred to a sleep or respiratory specialist, provided that the sleepiness does not result from inadequate time in bed or from shift work etc. Overnight studies of breathing, oxygenation and sleep quality are diagnostic (see Fig. 4.10) but the level of complexity of investigation will vary depending on probability of diagnosis, differential diagnosis and resources. The current threshold for abnormality is 15 apnoeas/hypopnoeas per hour of sleep, where an apnoea is a 10-second or longer breathing pause and a hypopnoea a 10-second or longer 50% reduction in breathing.

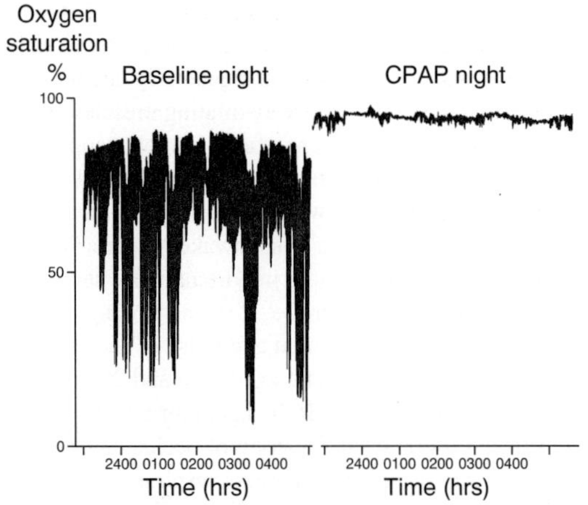

Fig. 4.10 Sleep apnoea/hypopnoea syndrome: overnight oxygen saturation trace. Trace for 46-year-old patient showing on left panel a night when he slept without continuous positive airway pressure (CPAP) and had 53 apnoeas plus hypopnoeas/hour, with 55 brief awakenings/hour and marked oxygen desaturation. Right panel shows the next night when he slept with a CPAP pressure of 10 cm H_2O which abolished his breathing irregularity and awakenings and improved his oxygenation.

Differential diagnosis

Narcolepsy is a much rarer cause of sleepiness, occurring in 0.05% of the population and associated sometimes with cataplexy (when muscle tone is lost in fully conscious people in response to emotional triggers and they may flop over), hypnagogic hallucinations (hallucinations at sleep onset) and sleep paralysis. Idiopathic hypersomnolence occurs in younger individuals and is characterised by long nocturnal sleeps.

Management

In a few patients advice to avoid evening alcohol and lose weight suffices, but most need to use continuous positive airway pressure (CPAP) delivered by nasal mask every night at home. CPAP keeps the throat open by making the upper airway pressure above atmospheric. The pressure for CPAP is set in the laboratory to the lowest that will prevent apnoeas, hypopnoeas and awakenings. The effect is dramatic (see Fig. 4.10) and CPAP results in marked improvements in symptoms, day-time performance, quality of life and survival. There is no evidence that upper airway surgery has any role in the management of the syndrome but mandibular advancement devices may be effective in some patients.

OXYGEN THERAPY

The delivery of oxygen to tissue mitochondria is controlled by factors exerting influences at various levels, including: inspired oxygen concentration (F_IO_2); alveolar ventilation; ventilation-perfusion distribution within the lung; haemoglobin and concentrations of agents such as carbon monoxide which may bind to haemoglobin; influences on the oxygen haemoglobin dissociation curve; cardiac output; and distribution of capillary blood flow within the tissues.

Many of the causes of hypoxaemia (see the information box on p. 317) are corrected by increasing the F_IO_2, but right to left shunting, either through circulatory channels bypassing the lung or through parts of the lung in which the alveoli are inaccessible to inspired oxygen, is less susceptible to such therapeutic approaches. The increased amount of dissolved oxygen carried by the blood which has perfused alveoli with a high PaO_2 can saturate the haemoglobin in small quantities of shunted blood, but persistence of cyanosis when 100% oxygen is breathed indicates that the shunt is larger than 20% of the cardiac output.

The consequences of severe hypoxaemia include: systemic hypotension, pulmonary hypertension, polycythaemia, tachycardia, and undesirable cerebral consequences ranging from confusion to coma.

The objectives of oxygen therapy are:

- to overcome the reduced partial pressure and quantity of oxygen in the blood
- to increase the quantity of oxygen carried in solution in the plasma, even when the haemoglobin is fully saturated.

Adverse effects

100% oxygen is both irritant and toxic if inhaled for more than a few hours. Premature infants develop retrolental fibroplasia and blindness if exposed to excessive concentrations. In adults, pulmonary oxygen toxicity (as manifested by pulmonary oedema) would not be expected to occur unless the patient had been treated with a concentration of greater than 40% oxygen for more than 24 hours.

Administration

Oxygen should always be prescribed in writing with clearly specified flow rates or concentrations.

- *High concentrations for short periods*, such as 60% oxygen via a high-flow mask, are particularly useful in acute type I respiratory failure such as commonly occurs in left ventricular failure or asthma.
- *Low concentrations*, via a 24% or 28% controlled-flow mask, are the most accurate method of delivering controlled oxygen therapy, particularly in type II respiratory failure. However, when a low concentration of oxygen is required continuously for more than a few hours, 1–2 litres per minute via nasal double cannulae allows patients to eat and to undergo physiotherapy etc. while continuing to receive oxygen. When high-flow masks are used, the oxygen should be humidified by passing it over warm water (as in the East–Radcliffe humidifier). This is not necessary with low-flow masks or nasal cannulae, as a high proportion of atmospheric air is mixed with oxygen.
- *Chronic oxygen delivery* from cylinders delivered to the home, or more conveniently from an oxygen concentrator, is often given via a low-concentration mask or nasal cannulae. Assessment for long-term oxygen therapy usually requires that the patients should have a PaO_2 of less than 7.3 kPa breathing air and an FEV_1 of less than 1.5 litres in the steady state (i.e. at least 1 month since the previous exacerbation) (see p. 325). Long-term chronic oxygen delivery has also been achieved by transtracheal microcatheters which have proved to be both oxygen-saving and of cosmetic benefit.

MECHANICAL VENTILATION

Patients with initially severe respiratory failure (type I or type II) or those who fail to improve despite optimal medical therapy may require mechanical ventilation. The various types of invasive (via an endotracheal tube) or non-invasive (via a face or nasal mask) ventilation are detailed on page 1044. In the majority of patients with respiratory failure intermittent positive pressure ventilation (IPPV) with full sedation is indicated. Nasal positive pressure ventilation (NPPV), delivered by a nasal mask, has proved to be of great value in the treatment of acute on chronic and chronic respiratory failure. Patients who benefit most from NPPV are those with skeletal deformity, especially kyphoscoliosis, and neuromuscular disease. However, NPPV can also be of value in some patients with central alveolar hypoventilation. It is now also being used in the acute situation in patients with COPD and type II respiratory failure, usually to try to avoid tracheal intubation and IPPV, but also in weaning such patients from mechanical ventilation.

LUNG TRANSPLANTATION

Lung transplantation is now widely used in the treatment of a number of selected patients with 'end-stage' cardiopulmonary disease. Transplantation of both heart and lungs was the first transplantation approach for many disorders (see the information box), but because of shortage of donor organs and improved surgical techniques, many double-lung and single-lung transplants are now being performed.

SOME INDICATIONS FOR HEART-LUNG TRANSPLANTATION

Parenchymatous lung disease	Pulmonary vascular disease
• Cystic fibrosis • Emphysema • Pulmonary fibrosis • Alveolar cell carcinoma • Lymphangioleiomyomatosis • Obliterative bronchiolitis	• Primary pulmonary hypertension • Thromboembolic pulmonary hypertension • Veno-occlusive disease • Eisenmenger's syndrome

Single-lung transplantation is being used, often with great initial success, in the treatment of restrictive lung diseases (e.g. fibrosing alveolitis), and also in granulomatous diseases such as sarcoidosis, pulmonary hypertension and emphysema. Single-lung transplantation is contraindicated in patients with chronic bilateral pulmonary infection (cystic fibrosis and bronchiectasis) and in patients with coexisting congenital or left heart disease.

Heart and lung transplantation is necessary for congenital cardiopulmonary problems such as Eisenmenger's syndrome, and is preferred by some surgeons for the treatment of primary pulmonary hypertension.

FURTHER INFORMATION ON MAJOR MANIFESTATIONS OF LUNG DISEASE

Antonelli M, Conti G, Rocco M et al 1998 A comparison of non-invasive positive pressure ventilation and conventional mechanical ventilation in patients with acute respiratory failure. New England Journal of Medicine 339: 429–435

Douglas N J, Polo O 1994 Pathogenesis of obstructive sleep apnoea hypopnoea syndrome. Lancet 344: 653–655

Ingbar D H (ed) 1994 Respiratory emergencies. Clinics in Chest Medicine: 383–551

Polo O, Berthon-Jones M, Douglas N J et al 1994 Management of obstructive sleep apnoea/hypopnoea syndrome. Lancet 344: 656–660

OBSTRUCTIVE PULMONARY DISEASES

CHRONIC OBSTRUCTIVE PULMONARY DISEASE (COPD)

Chronic obstructive pulmonary disease is the internationally preferred term encompassing chronic bronchitis, emphysema and some cases of chronic asthma. By definition COPD is a chronic, slowly progressive disorder characterised by airflow obstruction (FEV_1 < 80% predicted and FEV_1/VC ratio < 70%) which does not change markedly over several months. The impairment of lung function is largely fixed but may be partially reversible by bronchodilator therapy. Historically, the term 'chronic bronchitis' was used to define any patient who coughed up sputum on most days of at least 3 consecutive months for more than 2 successive years (provided other causes of cough had been excluded) and 'emphysema' referred to the pathological process of a permanent destructive enlargement of the airspaces distal to the terminal bronchioles. Although 'pure' forms of these two conditions do exist there is considerable overlap in the vast majority of patients.

The death rate from COPD currently exceeds 25 000/year (> 10-fold higher than asthma) in England and Wales and this condition accounts for over 10% of all hospital medical admissions in the United Kingdom.

Aetiology and natural history

The single most important cause of COPD is cigarette smoking and a direct correlation exists between the number of cigarettes smoked in pack years (1 pack year = 20 cigarettes smoked daily for 1 year) and the likelihood of developing the disease. Smoking is thought to have its effect by inducing persisting airway inflammation and causing a direct imbalance in oxidant/antioxidant capacity and proteinase/antiproteinase load in the lungs. Individual susceptibility to smoking is, however, very wide, with only 15% of smokers likely to develop clinically significant COPD. A small additional contribution to the severity of COPD has been reported in patients exposed to dusty or air-polluted environments. An association also exists between low birth weight, bronchial hyper-responsiveness (see p. 326) and the development of COPD. Alpha$_1$-antitrypsin deficiency can cause emphysema in non-smokers but this risk is increased dramatically in enzyme-deficient patients who smoke. Stopping smoking slows the average rate of decline in FEV_1 from 50–70 ml/year to 30 ml/year (i.e. equal to non-smokers) (see Fig. 4.11). Interestingly, there is no evidence that acute exacerbations or drug therapy affect the rate of decline of the FEV_1.

Pathology

Most patients develop airway wall inflammation, hypertrophy of the mucus-secreting glands and an increase in the number of goblet cells in the bronchi and bronchioles with a consequent decrease in ciliated cells. There is, therefore, less efficient transport of the increased mucus in the airways. Airflow limitation reflects both mechanical obstruction in the small airways and loss of pulmonary elastic recoil. Loss of alveolar attachments around such airways makes them more liable to collapse during expiration.

Emphysema is usually centriacinar, involving respiratory bronchioles, alveolar ducts and centrally located alveoli (see Fig. 4.12). More rarely, panacinar emphysema or paraseptal emphysema develops, with the latter responsible for blebs on the lung surface and/or giant bullae. Pulmonary vascular remodelling caused by persistent hypoxaemia results in pulmonary hypertension and right ventricular hypertrophy and dilatation.

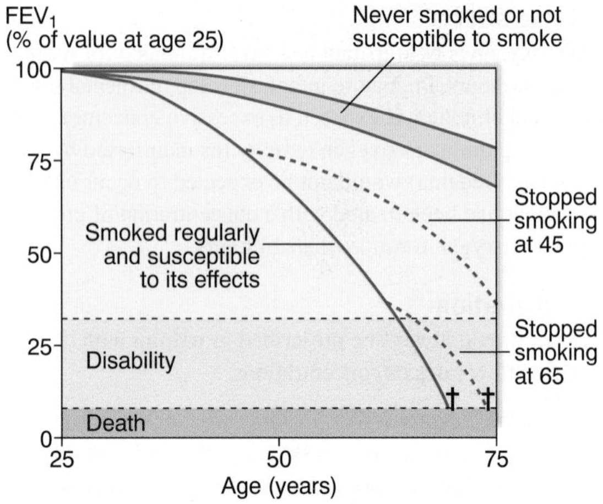

Fig. 4.11 Model of annual decline in FEV_1 with accelerated decline in susceptible smokers. On stopping smoking, subsequent loss is similar to that in healthy non-smokers.

Clinical features

The clinical state is dictated largely by the severity of disease (see Table 4.8). The disease generally starts with repeated attacks of productive cough, usually after colds

Table 4.8 Classification and diagnosis of COPD

Severity	Spirometry	Symptoms
Mild	FEV_1 60–79% predicted	Smoker's cough ± exertional breathlessness
Moderate	FEV_1 40–59% predicted	Exertional breathlessness ± wheeze; cough ± sputum
Severe	FEV_1 < 40% predicted	Breathlessness, wheeze and cough prominent; swollen legs

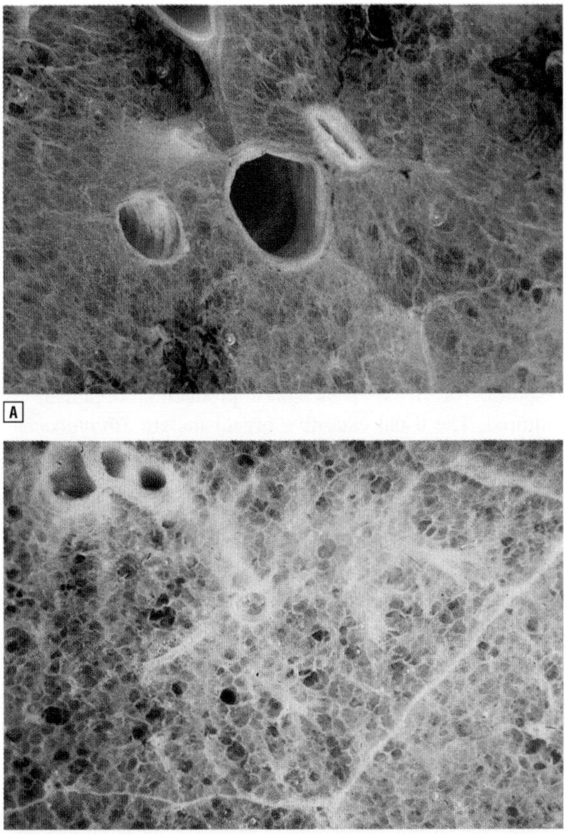

Fig. 4.12 The pathology of emphysema. A Normal lung. B Emphysematous lung showing gross loss of the normal surface area available for gas exchange.

during the winter months, which show a steady increase in severity and duration with successive years until cough is present all the year round. Thereafter, patients suffer recurrent respiratory infections, exertional breathlessness, regular morning cough, wheeze and occasionally chest tightness. Sputum may be scanty, mucoid, tenacious and occasionally streaked with blood during infective exacerbations. Frankly purulent sputum is indicative of bacterial infection which often occurs in these patients. Breathlessness is aggravated by infection, excessive cigarette smoking and adverse atmospheric conditions.

In patients with mild to moderate disease the respiratory examination may be normal. However, variable numbers of inspiratory and expiratory rhonchi, mainly low- and medium-pitched, are audible in most patients. Crepitations (crackles) which usually, but not always, disappear after coughing may be audible over the lower zones.

Physical signs associated with severe disease are outlined in the information box. These reflect pulmonary

CLINICAL ABNORMALITIES IN PATIENTS WITH ADVANCED AIRFLOW OBSTRUCTION

- Rhonchi, especially on forced expiration
- A reduction in the length of the trachea palpable above the sternal notch
- Tracheal descent during inspiration (tracheal 'tug')
- Contraction of the sternomastoid and scalene muscles on inspiration
- Excavation of the suprasternal and supraclavicular fossae during inspiration, together with indrawing of the costal margins and intercostal spaces
- Increased antero-posterior diameter of the chest relative to the lateral diameter; loss of cardiac dullness
- Loss of weight common (often stimulates unnecessary investigation)
- Pursed-lip breathing—physiological response to decrease air trapping
- Central cyanosis
- Flapping tremor and bounding pulse (due to hypercapnia)
- Peripheral oedema which may indicate cor pulmonale
- Raised JVP, right ventricular heave, loud pulmonary second sound, tricuspid regurgitation

hyperinflation, hypoxaemia, the development of cor pulmonale (pulmonary hypertension and right heart failure) and polycythaemia.

Investigations

Pulmonary function tests

The diagnosis and classification of COPD rests on objective demonstration of airways obstruction by spirometric testing (see Table 4.8). An abnormal FEV_1 (< 80% predicted), with an FEV_1/VC ratio of < 70% and little variation in serial PEF, strongly suggests COPD. A normal FEV_1 excludes the diagnosis. The relationship between FEV_1 and PEF is poor in COPD, and PEF in particular may underestimate the degree of airflow obstruction in these patients.

Reversibility testing to salbutamol and ipratropium bromide is necessary to detect patients with substantial increases in FEV_1 who are really asthmatic, and to establish the post-bronchodilator FEV_1 which is the best predictor of long-term prognosis. Significant reversibility is defined as a 15% and at least 200 ml increase in FEV_1. A similar objective response to a course of oral prednisolone (30 mg daily for 2 weeks) justifies prescription of regular inhaled steroids and should be performed in all patients with COPD.

Lung volumes show an increase in TLC and RV; the carbon monoxide transfer factor and coefficient are markedly reduced in patients with a severe emphysema component. Alveolar underventilation causes a fall in PaO_2 and often a permanent increase in $PaCO_2$, especially in severe cases. Measurement of arterial blood gases should be performed in all patients with severe COPD (FEV_1 < 40% predicted).

Exercise tests are of little diagnostic value but can provide an objective assessment of exertional dyspnoea.

Imaging

COPD cannot be diagnosed on a chest radiograph but this investigation is useful in excluding other pathology. In moderate and severe COPD the chest radiograph typically shows hypertranslucent lung fields with disorganisation of the vasculature, a low flat diaphragm or 'terracing' of the hemidiaphragms and prominent pulmonary artery shadows at both hila. Bullae may also be observed. CT can be used to quantify the extent and distribution of emphysema (see Fig. 4.13) but its clinical value is currently restricted to the assessment of bullous emphysema and the potential for lung volume reduction surgery or lung transplantation (see p. 325). Patients with α_1-antitrypsin deficiency typically display basal disease, compared with the predominantly apical disease seen in smokers with normal α_1-antitrypsin levels.

Haematology

Polycythaemia may develop but should not be assumed to be secondary without measurement of PaO_2. Venesection may be considered if the packed cell volume is > 50%.

Management

The treatment of patients with stable COPD is outlined in Figure 4.14.

Reduction of bronchial irritation

It is of extreme importance that the patient who smokes should stop completely and permanently. Participation in an active smoking cessation programme leads to a higher quit rate. Dusty and smoke-laden atmospheres should be avoided, which may involve a change of occupation.

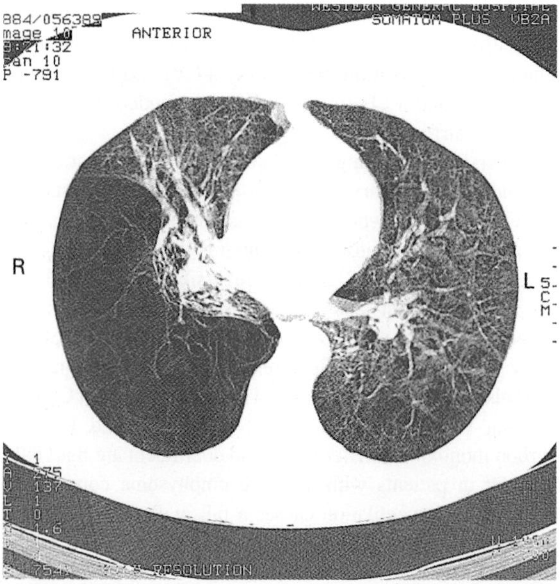

Fig. 4.13 Gross emphysema in the right lower lobe. High-resolution CT showing emphysema most evident in the right lower lobe.

Treatment of respiratory infection

Respiratory infection should be treated promptly because it aggravates breathlessness and may precipitate type II respiratory failure in patients with severe airflow obstruction. Purulent sputum is treated with amoxycillin 250 mg 8-hourly (clarithromycin 250–500 mg 12-hourly if penicillin-sensitive) pending sputum culture results. Co-amoxiclav 375 mg 8-hourly should be used if there is no response or if a β-lactamase-producing organism is cultured. The usual causative organisms are *Streptococcus pneumoniae* or *Haemophilus influenzae*. A 5–10-day course of treatment is usually effective. Well-informed, reliable patients can be given a supply of one of these drugs and start a course of treatment on their own initiative when the need arises.

Continuous suppressive antibiotic treatment is not advised as it is apt to promote the emergence of drug-resistant organisms within the respiratory tract. Influenza immunisation should be offered to all patients each year.

Bronchodilator and anti-inflammatory therapy

Short-acting β_2-adrenoceptor agonists or inhaled anticholinergics should be used as required and prior to exercise depending on the symptomatic response. In moderate and severe COPD these agents should be used regularly and in combination, and inhaled steroids added if a trial of oral corticosteroids produces objective improvement in the FEV_1 (see above). Theophyllines and long-acting β_2-adrenoceptor agonists are of limited value in COPD but may be of value in patients with demonstrated reversibility. There is no role for other anti-inflammatory drugs. It is vital to check inhaler use as many patients with COPD struggle to use metered-dose inhalers (MDIs) effectively; dry powder inhalers or large-volume spacer devices are hence often preferable. The use of home nebulisers to deliver high doses of bronchodilator drugs is controversial; treatment is expensive and may have important side-effects; however, a few patients may show significant objective or subjective improvements with such treatment.

Other measures

Exercise should be encouraged and outpatient-based pulmonary rehabilitation programmes, while not affecting the FEV_1, can improve exercise performance and reduce breathlessness. Obesity, poor nutrition, depression and social isolation should be identified and, if possible, improved. Expectorants, cough suppressants and mucolytic agents are of no proven benefit. Sedatives and opiate-based analgesic preparations are contraindicated.

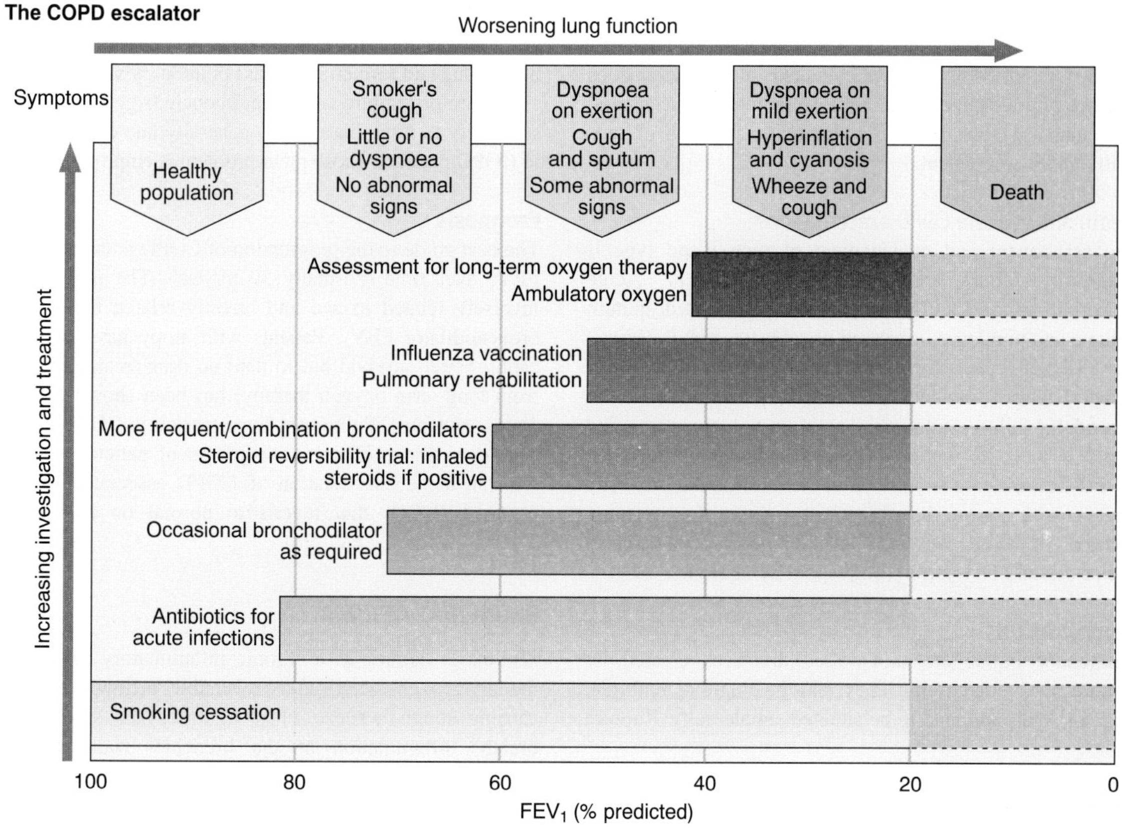

Fig. 4.14 Summary of management of COPD.

Long-term domiciliary oxygen therapy

Long-term low-concentration oxygen therapy (2 litres/min by nasal cannulae) decreases pulmonary hypertension, reduces secondary polycythaemia, improves neuro-psychological health and, most importantly, prolongs life in hypoxaemic COPD patients. The most efficient method of providing oxygen in this way is by an oxygen concentrator. Low-concentration oxygen should be administered for 15 hours or more per 24 hours. The criteria for the prescription of long-term oxygen therapy are given in the information box.

PRESCRIPTION OF LONG-TERM OXYGEN THERAPY (LTOT) IN COPD

- Arterial blood gases measured in clinically stable patient on optimal medical therapy on at least two occasions 3 weeks apart
- PaO_2 < 7.3 kPa irrespective of $PaCO_2$ and FEV_1 < 1.5 litres
- PaO_2 7.3–8 kPa plus pulmonary hypertension, peripheral oedema or nocturnal hypoxaemia
- Patient stopped smoking
- Use at least 15 hours/day at 2–4 litres/min to achieve PaO_2 > 8 kPa without an unacceptable rise in $PaCO_2$

Air travel

Medical assessment and clearance are required in all patients who are dyspnoeic on walking 50 m. In practice, all patients with a resting PaO_2 on air of < 9.0 kPa will require supplemental oxygen since at usual in-flight cabin pressures equivalent to 5–8000 feet the PaO_2 of such patients will fall below 7 kPa. Hypercarbia or gross hypoxaemia while breathing air (PaO_2 < 6.7 kPa) is a relative contraindication to air travel. Additional hazards include expansion of non-functioning emphysematous bullae and abdominal gases and drying of bronchial secretions.

Surgical intervention

A very small group of patients are suitable for surgical intervention. Young patients, particularly those with α_1-antitrypsin deficiency and severe disease, should be considered for lung transplantation (usually single-lung), and surgical removal of expanding or very large bullae may be indicated in some patients. Lung volume reduction surgery, in which the most severely affected areas of emphysematous lung are removed in order to improve pulmonary mechanics, particularly by enhancing diaphragmatic function, is currently under assessment.

Treatment of acute COPD exacerbations

The assessment and management of type I and type II respiratory failure are detailed on page 317. Acute exacerbations of COPD can present as increased sputum volume and purulence, increased breathlessness and wheeze, chest tightness and sometimes fluid retention. The differential diagnosis includes pneumonia, pneumothorax, left ventricular failure, pulmonary embolism, lung cancer and upper airway obstruction. The management of an acute COPD exacerbation is outlined in the information box. Any patient with severe breathlessness, cyanosis, worsening oedema, impaired conscious level or poor social circumstances should be referred for hospital admission.

Complications

Pulmonary bullae are thin-walled airspaces created by rupture of alveolar walls. They may be single or multiple, large or small and tend to be situated subpleurally. Rupture of subpleural bullae may cause pneumothorax (see p. 388) and occasionally bullae increase in size, compress functioning lung tissue and further embarrass pulmonary ventilation.

Respiratory failure and cor pulmonale (right heart failure secondary to lung disease) are generally late complications in COPD patients whose main problem is emphysema.

MANAGEMENT OF ACUTE COPD EXACERBATIONS

In the community

- Add or increase bronchodilator therapy
- Antibiotics (see p. 324)
- Oral corticosteroids *if* patient already on oral corticosteroids, *if* previous response to such treatment, *if* airflow obstruction fails to respond to bronchodilator therapy or *if* first presentation of disease (prednisolone 30 mg daily for 1 week)

In hospital

- Check arterial blood gases (ABGs), chest radiograph, ECG, full blood count, urea and electrolytes; measure FEV_1 +/– peak flow; send sputum for culture
- Oxygen: 24%–28% via mask, 2 litres/min by nasal prongs; check ABGs within 60 min and adjust according to PaO_2 (try to keep ≥ 7.5 kPa) and $PaCO_2$/pH
- Bronchodilators: nebulised β_2-adrenoceptor agonist (+ ipratropium bromide if severe) 4–6-hourly. If no response consider i.v. aminophylline infusion
- Oral corticosteroids: indicated as above
- Diuretics: indicated if JVP elevated and oedema present
- If pH < 7.26 and $PaCO_2$ is rising, consider ventilatory support (invasive or non-invasive IPPV, see p. 321). If not indicated (e.g. previous poor quality of life, significant co-morbidity) doxapram can be considered
- Prophylactic subcutaneous heparin

N.B. All patients should be reviewed 4–6 weeks after hospital discharge to assess ability to cope at home, FEV_1, inhaler technique and understanding of treatment, and the potential need for LTOT or a home nebuliser

Prognosis

The best guide to the progression of COPD is the decline in FEV_1 over time (normally 30 ml/year). The prognosis is inversely related to age and directly related to the post-bronchodilator FEV_1. Patients with atopy have a significantly better survival but to date no drug treatment (aside from long-term oxygen therapy) has been shown to affect disease outcome. Pulmonary hypertension in COPD implies a poor prognosis. The mean survival of patients admitted with an acute exacerbation of COPD associated with an elevated $PaCO_2$ that reverts to normal on recovery is 3 years.

BRONCHIAL ASTHMA

Asthma is defined as a chronic inflammatory disorder of the airways, characterised by reversible airflow obstruction causing cough, wheeze, chest tightness and shortness of breath. Inflammation of the bronchial wall involving eosinophils, mast cells and lymphocytes, together with the cytokine and inflammatory products of these cells, induces hyper-responsiveness of the bronchi so that they narrow more readily in response to a wide range of stimuli. Narrowing of the airway is usually reversible, but in some patients with chronic asthma the bronchial wall inflammation may lead to irreversible obstruction of airflow (see the information box).

The airflow obstruction, which characteristically fluctuates markedly, causes mismatch of alveolar ventilation and perfusion and increases the work of breathing. Being more marked during expiration it also causes air to be 'trapped' in the lungs. A narrowed bronchus can no longer

CARDINAL PATHOPHYSIOLOGICAL FEATURES OF ASTHMA

Airflow limitation

- Usually reverses spontaneously or with treatment

Airway hyper-responsiveness

- Exaggerated bronchoconstriction to a wide range of non-specific stimuli, e.g. exercise, cold air

Airway inflammation

- Eosinophils, lymphocytes, mast cells, neutrophils; associated oedema, smooth muscle hypertrophy and hyperplasia, thickening of basement membrane, mucous plugging, epithelial damage (see Fig. 4.15) be effectively cleared by coughing up the mucus formed by the disease process, and many of the bronchi become obstructed by mucus plugs (see Fig. 4.15). This is usually a conspicuous finding at autopsy. Respiratory arrest may occur within a few minutes after the onset of a severe episode. Death from asthma may also occur from alveolar hypoventilation and severe arterial hypoxaemia in the patient exhausted by a prolonged attack.

Bronchial asthma is a common disease; 15% of children report an episode of wheezing characteristic of asthma within the previous year, 5% have a diagnosis of asthma, and 1% have severe disabling asthma. In adults, 2–5% have a clinical diagnosis of asthma. Asthma prevalence has increased over the past few decades and until recently this trend was matched by a slow increase in asthma deaths (currently 1800/year in England and Wales). Of note, there appear to be major geographical variations in asthma, prevalence being highest in New Zealand, Australia and Britain and lowest in China and Malaysia. While air pollution is not causally linked to asthma, there is little doubt that it can contribute to asthma morbidity and mortality.

Pathophysiology

In the majority of patients who do not have a relevant occupational history, the cause of asthma is unknown. Current theories include early exposure to aero-allergens, early viral infections, diet or, paradoxically, fewer childhood infections resulting from improved public health standards. It remains useful, however, to classify asthma as early-onset or extrinsic asthma which usually occurs in

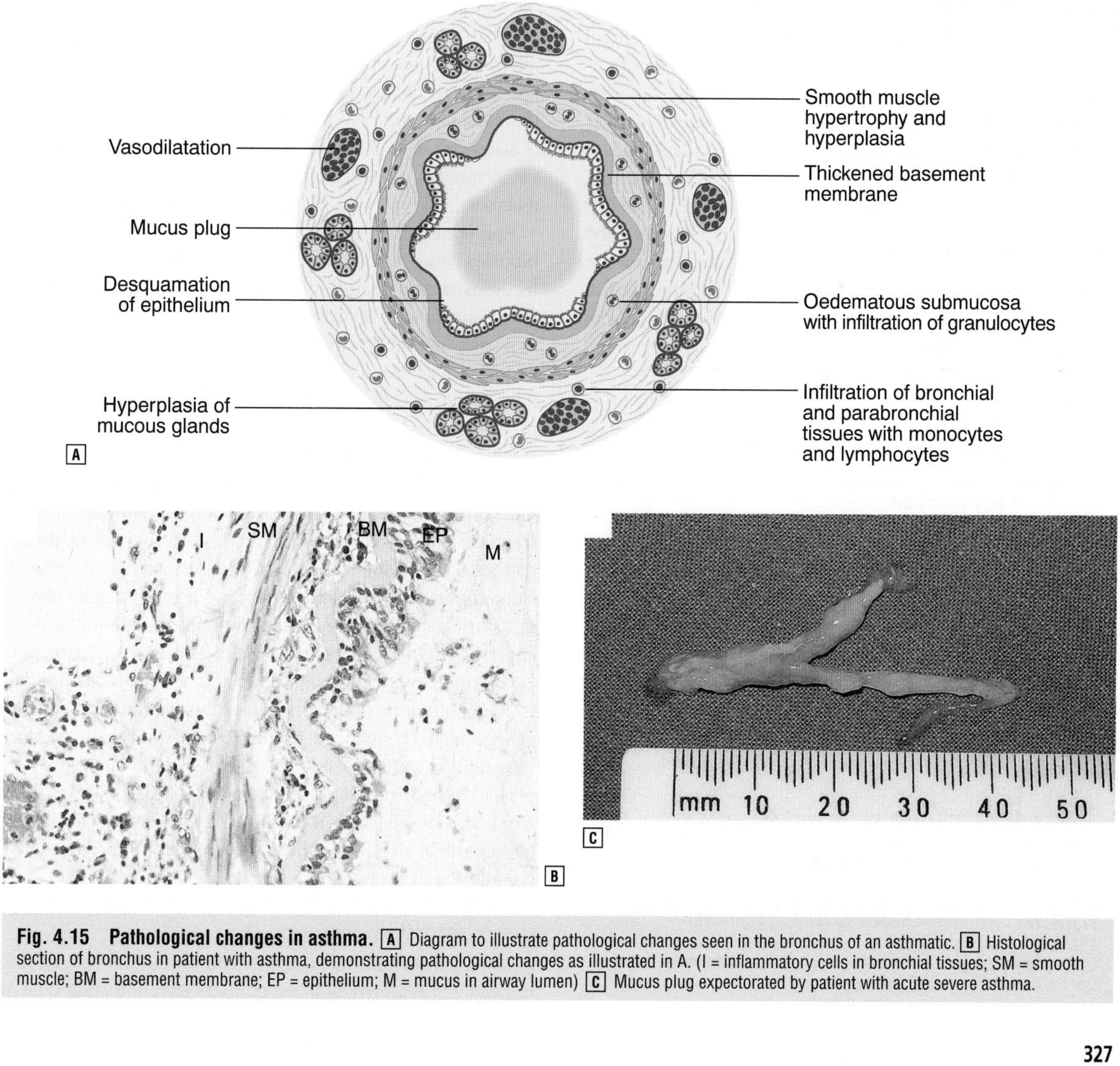

Fig. 4.15 Pathological changes in asthma. [A] Diagram to illustrate pathological changes seen in the bronchus of an asthmatic. [B] Histological section of bronchus in patient with asthma, demonstrating pathological changes as illustrated in A. (I = inflammatory cells in bronchial tissues; SM = smooth muscle; BM = basement membrane; EP = epithelium; M = mucus in airway lumen) [C] Mucus plug expectorated by patient with acute severe asthma.

atopic children and resolves in 80%, and late-onset or idiopathic non-atopic adult asthma which is chronic in the majority of cases.

Early-onset asthma (atopic)

It is common for asthma to begin in childhood, and generally it occurs in atopic individuals who readily form IgE antibodies to commonly encountered allergens. Asthma in these individuals is often referred to as 'atopic' asthma. These individuals can be identified by skin hypersensitivity tests which produce positive reactions to a wide range of common allergens. It is unusual for a single allergen to be the sole cause of asthma. Other allergic disorders such as allergic rhinitis and eczema are often present, and a family history of these disorders and of 'early-onset' asthma is common.

The allergens responsible for asthma in atopic individuals generally enter the bronchi with the inspired air and are derived from organic material such as pollen, mite-containing house dust, feathers, animal dander and fungal spores. Previous exposures to these agents will have stimulated the formation of IgE, and an 'anaphylactic antigen-antibody reaction' in the bronchi may follow further exposure to specific allergen (see Fig. 4.16). This causes the release, from cells such as the mast cell in the bronchial wall, of pharmacologically active substances which provoke an immediate asthmatic bronchoconstrictor response and often a secondary late reaction of allergic type in the bronchial wall (see Fig. 4.16). Much less frequently, similar effects may be produced by ingested allergens derived from certain foods such as fish, eggs, milk, yeast and wheat, which presumably reach the bronchi via the blood stream.

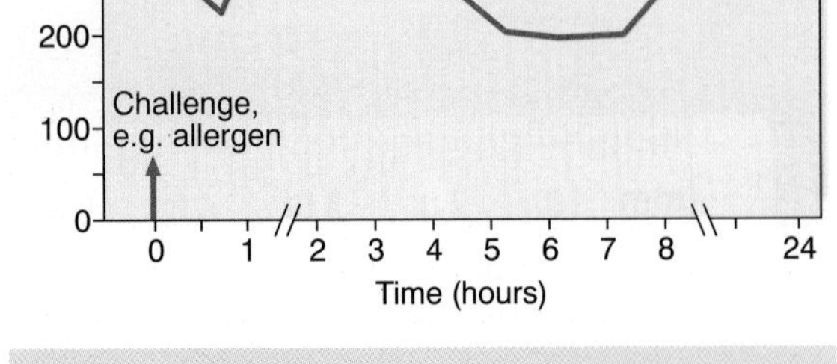

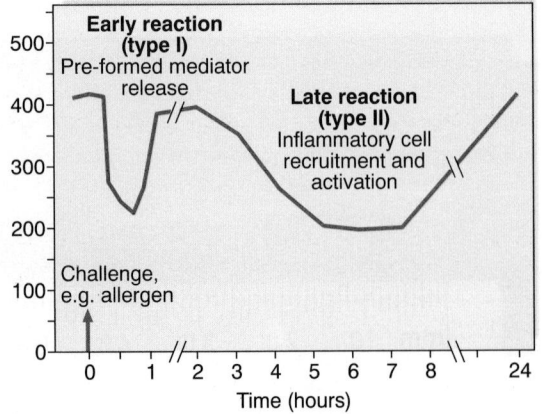

Fig. 4.16 Changes in peak flow following allergen challenge. A similar biphasic response is observed following a variety of different challenges. Occasionally an individual will develop an isolated late response with no early reaction.

The traditional view was that inhaled allergen interacted with surface mast cells through IgE-dependent mechanisms, causing these cells to release mediators such as histamine, which then act on receptors on smooth muscle cells and lead to bronchoconstriction. This is probably a mechanism of the early asthmatic reaction, but several different cells are involved in the perpetuation of the chronic inflammatory reaction in the bronchial wall that characterises asthma. Eosinophils play an important role, the asthmatic inflammatory reaction being characterised by a cellular infiltration rich in activated eosinophils. These cells release bioactive lipid mediators and oxygen radicals, and their granules contain toxic basic proteins including major basic protein, eosinophil cationic protein, eosinophil-derived neurotoxin and eosinophil peroxidase. T lymphocytes are present in increased numbers in asthmatic airways and immunological markers suggest that they are activated. They play an important role in orchestrating and perpetuating the chronic asthmatic response. To do this they must be programmed to release appropriate cytokines, such as interleukin-5 which, among other effects, delays eosinophil apoptosis and hence increases the longevity of these cells in the asthmatic airway. The number of airway macrophages is also increased in asthma and these cells may be activated via a number of mechanisms including a low-affinity IgE receptor.

Epithelial shedding is commonly observed in airway biopsies from asthmatic patients, and this has long been recognised as a feature of fatal asthma. Epithelial damage may contribute to airway hyper-responsiveness in a number of ways including the exposure of subepithelial nerve endings and additional access of inhaled allergen to inflammatory cells. Microvascular leakage is also a feature of asthma and may be triggered by many inflammatory mediators; it causes plasma exudation into the lumen of the airways that contributes to mucous plugging, decreased mucociliary clearance, release of kinins and complement fragments, and oedema of the airway wall which facilitates epithelial stripping. Although the sensitivity of airways smooth muscle to bronchoconstricting agents remains normal in asthma, the increase in muscle bulk around the airways appears to be a contributory factor in airflow obstruction. Likewise, airway inflammation induces an imbalance between cholinergic and peptidergic neuronal control, causing exaggerated bronchoconstrictor responses. Finally, airway remodelling with subendothelial fibrosis, goblet cell hyperplasia, smooth muscle and vascular changes may result in fixed airway obstruction. Asthma can, therefore, no longer be regarded as simple bronchoconstriction produced by contraction of bronchial muscle.

Late-onset asthma (non-atopic)

Asthma can begin at any age in non-atopic individuals and because the majority of these patients are adults this type of

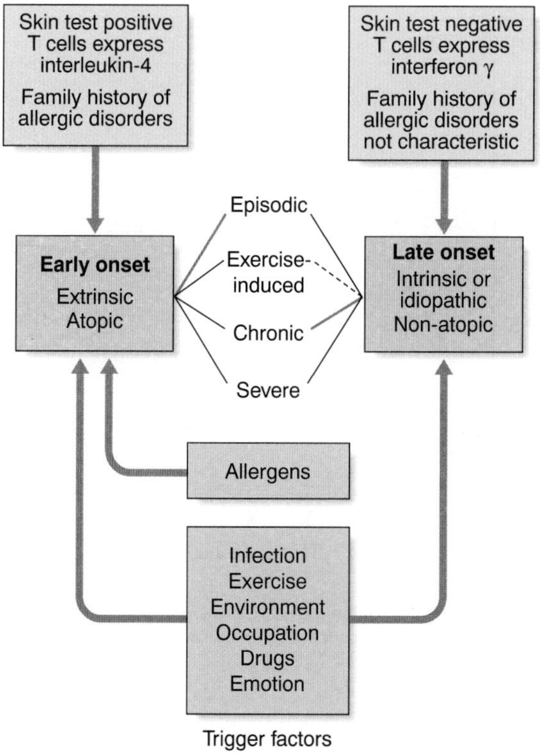

Fig. 4.17 Aetiology and types of asthma.

asthma is often called late-onset asthma. There is no clinical evidence that external allergens play a part in the production of the disease, to which the term 'intrinsic asthma' is sometimes applied (see Fig. 4.17).

Triggers of the asthmatic response

Allergens can trigger episodes of asthma in atopic patients but asthma is more often aggravated by non-specific factors such as cold air, tobacco smoke, dust and acrid fumes, respiratory viral infection and emotional stress. In children and young adults asthma almost invariably follows strenuous exertion (exercise-induced asthma) or exposure to cold air. Acute attacks of asthma may be caused by the inadvertent prescription or use of β-adrenoceptor antagonists, aspirin and non-steroidal anti-inflammatory drugs. Asthma also may develop because of exposure to dusts, organic materials, fumes and chemical substances in the working environment.

Clinical features

Bronchial asthma may be either episodic or chronic, and although there is a good deal of overlap between these two syndromes the distinction is clinically useful, particularly in terms of prognosis and management. There is a tendency for atopic individuals to develop episodic asthma, and non-atopic individuals chronic asthma (see Fig. 4.17).

Episodic asthma

In this form of the disease the patient has no respiratory symptoms or signs between episodes of asthma. Paroxysms of wheeze and dyspnoea may occur at any time and can be of sudden onset. Episodes of asthma can be triggered by allergens, exercise or viral infections such as the common cold, or may be apparently spontaneous. Attacks may be mild or severe and may last for hours, days or even weeks.

Severe acute asthma

This term has replaced 'status asthmaticus' as the description of life-threatening attacks of asthma. The patient usually adopts an upright position, fixing the shoulder girdle to assist the accessory muscles of respiration. During an attack the chest is held near the position of full inspiration and the percussion note may be hyper-resonant. Breath sounds, when not obscured by numerous high-pitched polyphonic expiratory and inspiratory rhonchi, are vesicular in character with prolonged expiration. There is often a cough which aggravates the respiratory distress. The respiratory symptoms are accompanied by tachycardia, pulsus paradoxus and sweating. In very severe asthma central cyanosis and bradycardia may occur and airflow may become so restricted that rhonchi are no longer produced; a 'silent chest' in such patients is an ominous sign.

Chronic asthma

Symptoms of chest tightness, wheeze and breathlessness on exertion, together with spontaneous cough and wheeze during the night and early morning, may be chronic unless controlled by appropriate therapy. Episodes of severe acute asthma can occur, and cough productive of mucoid sputum with recurrent episodes of frank respiratory infection is common in this type of asthma, which in adults may be difficult to distinguish from chronic bronchitis. Patients with untreated chronic asthma are seldom without expiratory rhonchi. Severe asthma persisting from childhood may cause a 'pigeon chest' deformity.

Investigations

A diagnosis of asthma is made on the basis of a compatible clinical history plus a demonstration of variable airflow obstruction (see the information box on p. 330) which may classically be seen as 'morning dipping' of the peak expiratory flow (see Fig. 4.18).

In more difficult situations where the above tests are negative, an exercise test, histamine or methacholine bronchial provocation test (see p. 331), occupational exposure test or trial of oral corticosteroids (e.g. prednisolone 30 mg daily for 2 weeks) may be required. An elevated sputum or peripheral blood eosinophil count or increased serum level

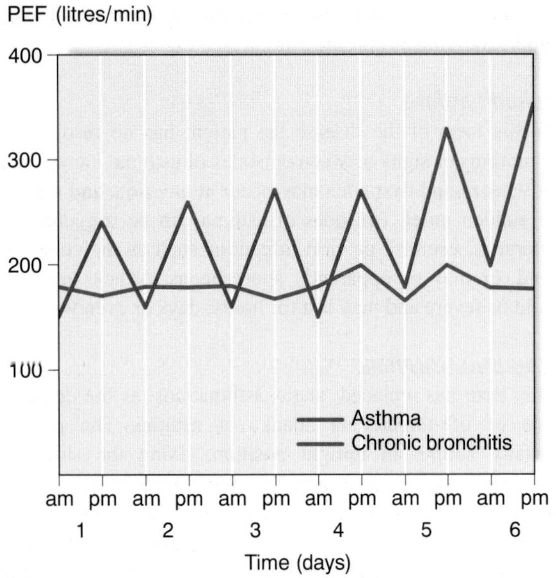

Fig. 4.18 'Morning dipping'. Serial recordings of peak expiratory flow (PEF) in patients with chronic bronchitis and asthma. Note sharp overnight fall (morning dip) and subsequent rise during the day in patients, with asthma, which does not occur in patients with chronic bronchitis.

MAKING A DIAGNOSIS OF ASTHMA
Compatible clinical history *plus either/or* • ≥ 15% improvement in FEV_1 or PEF following administration of a bronchodilator (see Fig. 4.19) *or* • ≥ 15% spontaneous change in PEF during 1 week of home monitoring (see Fig. 4.18)

of total or allergen-specific IgE (radioallergosorbent test—RAST) may also be helpful. It is particularly important, however, to be aware that wheeze is audible in many conditions other than asthma.

Pulmonary function tests

Measurement of the FEV_1 and VC or PEF provides a fairly reliable indication of the degree of airflow obstruction, and can also be used to determine whether and to what extent it can be relieved by bronchodilator drugs (see Fig. 4.19). These parameters are also used to examine whether asthma is provoked by exercise (see Fig. 4.20), hyperventilation or occupational exposure. Serial recordings of PEF are useful in distinguishing patients with chronic asthma from those with fixed or irreversible airflow obstruction associated with COPD. In asthma there is usually a marked diurnal variation in PEF, the lowest values being recorded in the mornings ('morning dipping') (see Fig. 4.18). Serial PEF recordings are also invaluable in the assessment of a patient's response to corticosteroid therapy and in the long-

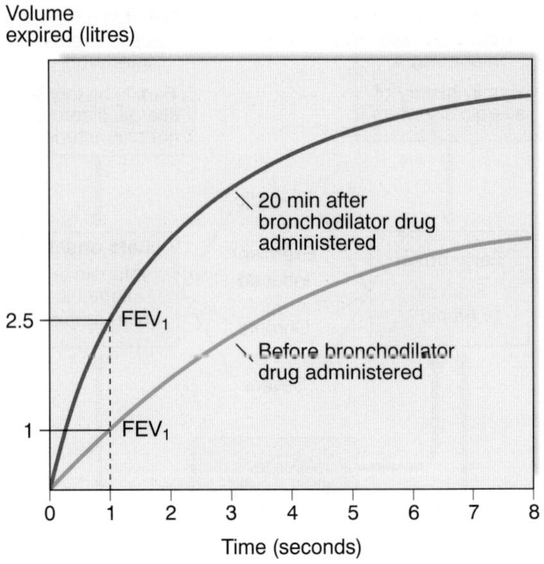

Fig. 4.19 Reversibility test. Forced expiratory manoeuvres before and 20 min after inhalation of a β_2-adrenoceptor agonist. Note the increase in FEV_1 from 1.0 to 2.5 litres.

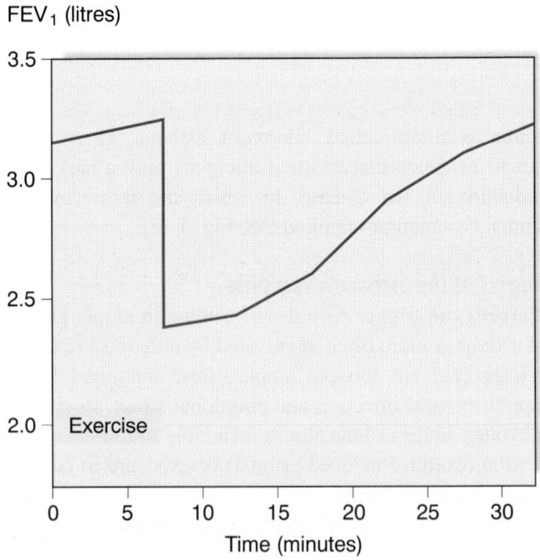

Fig. 4.20 Exercise-induced asthma. Serial recordings of forced expiratory volume in one second (FEV_1) in patient with bronchial asthma before and after 6 minutes of strenuous exercise. Note initial slight rise on completion of exercise, followed by sudden fall and gradual recovery. Adequate warm-up exercise or pretreatment with a β_2-adrenoceptor agonist, nedocromil sodium or a leucotriene antagonist (e.g. montelukast sodium) often protects against exercise-induced symptoms.

term monitoring of patients with poorly controlled disease. Also they are essential in monitoring response to treatment of severe acute asthma.

Measurement of bronchial reactivity can be of value in diagnosing asthma and in assessing the effects of treatment. This can be achieved by administering increasing concentrations of substances such as histamine and methacholine by inhalation until there is a 20% fall in FEV_1 or PEF. This concentration is called the PC_{20}. Patients with asthma show evidence of bronchoconstriction at much lower concentrations than normal subjects.

Radiological examination

In an acute attack of asthma the lungs appear hyperinflated. Between episodes the chest radiograph is usually normal. In long-standing chronic cases the appearances may be indistinguishable from hyperinflation caused by emphysema and a lateral view may demonstrate a 'pigeon chest' deformity. Occasionally, when a large bronchus is obstructed by tenacious mucus, there is an opacity caused by lobar or segmental collapse.

A chest radiograph should be performed in all patients with severe acute asthma. This is especially important if there is poor response to treatment and assisted ventilation is being contemplated, since pneumothorax is a rare but potentially fatal complication. The chest radiograph may rarely show mediastinal and subcutaneous emphysema in attacks of acute asthma.

Allergic bronchopulmonary aspergillosis may complicate chronic persisting asthma (see p. 354) and produce areas of segmental/subsegmental collapse.

Arterial blood gas analysis

Measurements of arterial blood gas pressures (PaO_2 and $PaCO_2$) are indispensable in the management of patients with severe acute asthma.

Management

The following principles for the management of patients with asthma are based closely on the guidelines for the management of asthma produced by the British Thoracic Society and the International Consensus Report on the diagnosis and management of asthma.

Avoidance

There are a few instances in which a single agent can be identified as the cause of attacks of asthma. The measures which can be taken to prevent or reduce exposure to these agents, and the degree of success likely to be achieved, are summarised in Table 4.9. However, the vast majority of asthmatic patients are hypersensitive to a wide range of allergens and attempts to avoid them all are impracticable.

Avoidance of day-to-day triggers such as exercise and cold air generally imposes inappropriate restrictions on lifestyle, and it is preferable to adjust treatment to cover exposure to these. Smoking should be discouraged.

Hyposensitisation

This involves the subcutaneous injection of initially very small but gradually increasing concentrations of extracts of allergens believed to be responsible for the patient's asthma. Hyposensitisation may be of some value when only a single allergen is implicated but it is not without risk of producing an acute anaphylactic reaction. This form of therapy has largely been abandoned in Britain because of the attendant risks. Hyposensitisation with a mixture of allergens is irrational and cannot be recommended.

Table 4.9 Allergens and other substances liable to provoke attacks of asthma

Causative agent	Preventive measures	Efficacy
Pollens	Try to avoid exposure to flowering vegetation Keep bedroom windows closed	Low
Mites in house dust	Use sealed mattress Hot-wash all bedding regularly Damp-dust and ventilate bedroom thoroughly	Uncertain
Animal dander	Avoid contact with dogs, cats, horses or other animals	High
Feathers in pillows or quilts	Substitute latex foam pillows and synthetic fibre quilts	High
Drugs (e.g. β-adrenoceptor antagonists, aspirin, NSAIDs)	Avoid all preparations of relevant drugs	High
Foods (including prepared foods or wine containing sodium metabisulphite)	Identify and eliminate from diet	Low*
Industrial chemicals (e.g. isocyanates, epoxy resins)	Avoid exposure to chemical, or change occupation	High

* More effective in control of eczema.

Management of chronic persistent asthma

Patient education plays a vital role in the management of patients with asthma. Treatment should be stepped up or down as required, with PEF monitoring being key to such decisions. The patient should be allowed to select the best inhaler device for himself or herself, and compliance and inhaler technique must be checked at every opportunity. All metered dose inhalers (MDIs) widely used in the UK will be reformulated over the next few years to replace conventional chlorofluorocarbons (CFCs) with new propellants hydrofluoroalkane (HFAs). These products will be equally effective and as safe as current CFC-containing MDIs but the aerosol characteristics are different and this may be noticed by patients. In patients with mild to moderate asthma (on step 1–3 medication—see below and Fig. 4.21) the aim of treatment should be to minimise all symptoms, permit unrestricted exercise and prevent exacerbations. In patients with more severe disease (on step 4–5 medication) the aim should be to achieve the best possible and most stable PEF, to improve symptoms and exercise capacity, and to reduce bronchodilator drug use as far as possible with the least adverse effects from the drugs used.

Step 1 Occasional use of inhaled short-acting β_2-adrenoceptor agonist bronchodilators. Short-acting bronchodilators, such as salbutamol or terbutaline, are used by inhalation as required for the relief of minor symptoms. If the patient is using β_2-adrenoceptor agonists more than once daily move to step 2. Beta$_2$-adrenoceptor agonist therapy alone is only recommended if it is used occasionally and when this allows the patient to lead an active normal life free from nocturnal and exercise-induced asthmatic symptoms.

Step 2 Regular inhaled anti-inflammatory agents. Inhaled short-acting β_2-adrenoceptor agonists are used as required *plus* an inhaled steroid (beclomethasone dipropionate or budesonide) up to 800 μg daily or fluticasone up to 400 μg daily. Alternatively, sodium cromoglycate or nedocromil sodium can be used instead of an inhaled corticosteroid, but these drugs are rarely effective outside childhood.

Step 3 High-dose inhaled corticosteroids, or low-dose inhaled corticosteroids plus a long-acting inhaled β_2-adrenoceptor agonist. Inhaled short-acting β_2-adrenoceptor agonists are used as required *plus* an inhaled corticosteroid in the dose range 800–2000 μg daily. Alternatively, a long-acting β_2-adrenoceptor agonist (e.g. salmeterol 50 μg 12-hourly) or a sustained-release theophylline may be added. When corticosteroids in high dose are inhaled via a conventional pressurised MDI the routine use of a large-volume spacer (holding chamber) is recommended. When dry powder inhalers are used, mouth rinsing and gargling with spitting out of the rinsing liquid after each treatment should be encouraged. Spacers and rinsing are recommended to decrease gastrointestinal absorption of swallowed drug, and to lower the risk of developing the local side-effect of oropharyngeal candidiasis.

Step 4 High-dose inhaled corticosteroids and regular bronchodilators. Inhaled short-acting β_2-adrenoceptor agonists are used as required with an inhaled corticosteroid (800–2000 μg daily) *plus* a sequential therapeutic trial of one or more of:

- inhaled long-acting β_2-adrenoceptor agonist (e.g. salmeterol, eformoterol fumarate)
- sustained-release oral theophylline
- leucotriene receptor antagonist (e.g. montelukast sodium)
- inhaled ipratropium bromide or oxitropium bromide

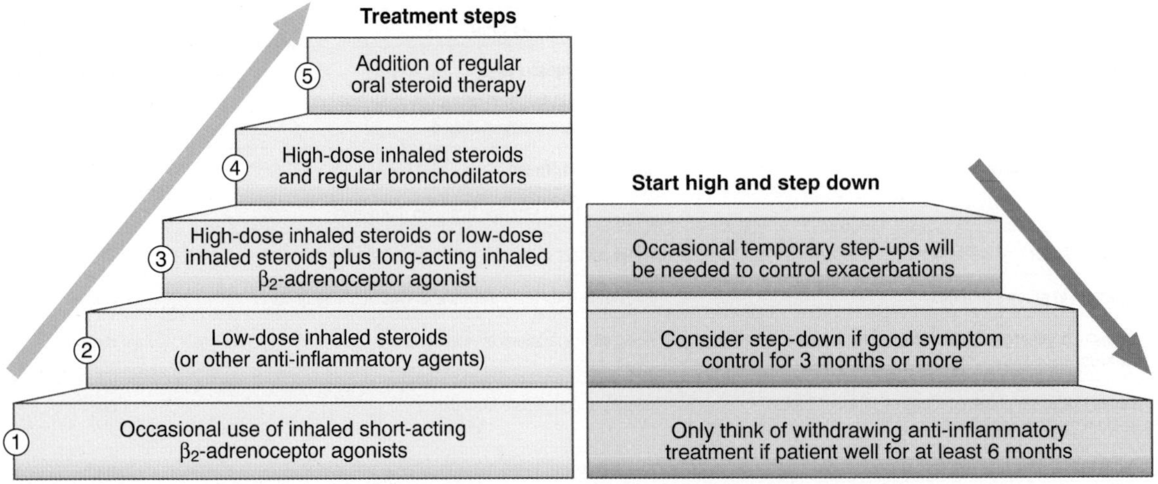
Treatment steps
5 Addition of regular oral steroid therapy
4 High-dose inhaled steroids and regular bronchodilators
3 High-dose inhaled steroids or low-dose inhaled steroids plus long-acting inhaled β2-adrenoceptor agonist
2 Low-dose inhaled steroids (or other anti-inflammatory agents)
1 Occasional use of inhaled short-acting β2-adrenoceptor agonists
Start high and step down
Occasional temporary step-ups will be needed to control exacerbations
Consider step-down if good symptom control for 3 months or more
Only think of withdrawing anti-inflammatory treatment if patient well for at least 6 months

Fig. 4.21 Concept of step-up and step-down drug treatment in asthma.

- long-acting oral β_2-adrenoceptor agonist (sustained-release salbutamol or terbutaline preparations)
- high-dose inhaled β_2-adrenoceptor antagonists
- sodium cromoglycate or nedocromil sodium.

Step 5 Addition of regular oral corticosteroid therapy. Step 4 treatment is given *plus* regular prednisolone tablets prescribed in the lowest amount necessary to control symptoms as a single daily dose in the mornings.

Using this 'stepwise' approach to asthma management (see Fig. 4.21), the initial treatment for each patient should be chosen individually depending upon severity of disease. In general it is better to start with a treatment regimen which is likely to achieve disease control rapidly and then 'step down' rather than to start with inadequate treatment and then have to 'step up'. Patient compliance is also likely to be better when symptom control is achieved rapidly. Regular review is important and if there has been good symptomatic control for 3–6 months a step down should be made. This is of particular importance in those taking oral and high-dose inhaled corticosteroids (steps 3–5).

Short-course oral corticosteroid treatments

Short courses of 'rescue' oral corticosteroids are often required to regain control of symptoms. For adults, 30–60 mg of prednisolone can be given initially and the same dose continued in a single daily dose each morning until 2 days after control is re-established. In children, a dose of 1–2 mg/kg body weight can be used. Tapering of the dose to withdraw treatment is not necessary unless given for more than 3 weeks. Indications for 'rescue' courses include:

- symptoms and PEF progressively worsening day by day
- fall of PEF below 60% of the patient's personal best recording
- onset or worsening of sleep disturbance by asthma
- persistence of morning symptoms until midday
- progressively diminishing response to an inhaled bronchodilator
- symptoms severe enough to require treatment with nebulised or injected bronchodilators.

Increase in dose of inhaled corticosteroid

Doubling the dose of inhaled corticosteroid is often advised to control minor exacerbations of asthma not severe enough to warrant treatment with oral prednisolone. This appears to be effective in many cases.

Management of acute severe asthma

The aims of management are to prevent death, to restore pulmonary function to the patient's best as quickly as possible, to maintain optimal pulmonary function and to prevent early relapse. The features of acute severe asthma are shown in the information box.

PEF should be recorded immediately in all patients unless they are too ill to cooperate. PEF measurements are most easily interpreted when expressed as a percentage of the predicted normal value or of the previous best obtained value on optimal treatment. When neither of these is known, decisions have to be made on the absolute value recorded, remembering that normal values vary with age, sex and height. In previously fit asthmatics, recordings of < 200 l/min are indicative of severe disease, and values of < 100 l/min must be taken as evidence of life-threatening asthma.

IMMEDIATE ASSESSMENT OF ACUTE SEVERE ASTHMA
Features of severity
• Pulse rate > 110 per min • Pulsus paradoxus • Unable to speak in sentences • PEF < 50% of expected
N.B. *Apparent* distress and respiratory rate may be misleading
Life-threatening features
• Cannot speak • Central cyanosis • Exhaustion, confusion, reduced conscious level • Bradycardia • 'Silent chest' • Unrecordable PEF
Arterial blood gases in life-threatening asthma
• A normal (5–6 kPa) or high CO_2 tension • Severe hypoxaemia (< 8 kPa) especially if being treated with oxygen • A low pH or high $[H^+]$

Immediate treatment

See Figure 4.22.

Oxygen

Oxygen should be given at the highest concentration available (usually 60%). High-concentration oxygen therapy does not cause or aggravate carbon dioxide retention in asthma, and the presence of carbon dioxide retention must not be interpreted as a contraindication for the use of high-concentration oxygen treatment. Thereafter, the concentration of oxygen used can be adjusted according to the arterial blood gas measurements. A PaO_2 of > 8.5–9 kPa should be maintained if possible.

High doses of inhaled β_2-adrenoceptor agonists

When possible, β_2-adrenoceptor agonists should be nebulised using oxygen. Salbutamol 2.5–5 mg or terbutaline 5–10 mg should be given initially and repeated within 30 minutes if necessary. When treatment is given outside hospital and oxygen is not available an air compressor can be used to drive the nebuliser. An alternative method of giving high doses of β_2-adrenoceptor agonists in general practice is multiple actuations of an MDI into a large-volume spacer device.

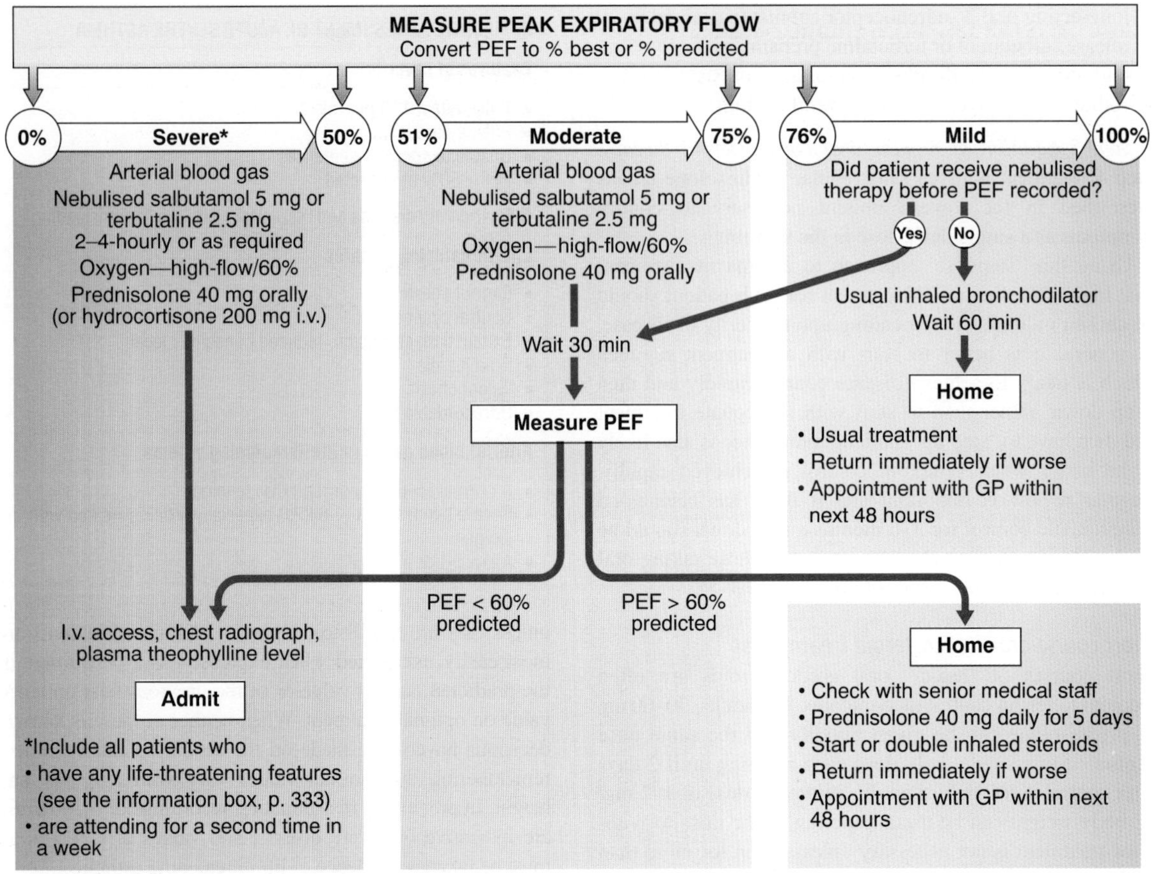

Fig. 4.22 Immediate treatment of patients with acute severe asthma.

Systemic corticosteroids

Systemic corticosteroids are necessary for the treatment of all cases of acute severe asthma. Intravenous hydrocortisone 200 mg (if the patient is unable to swallow or vomiting) or oral prednisolone 30–60 mg should be given initially.

Subsequent management

All patients must be closely supervised and oxygen therapy continued. If features of severity persist, additional measures may be required (see the first information box). Systemic corticosteroid treatment with oral prednisolone 30–60 mg daily is recommended for patients responding to treatment, but intravenous hydrocortisone 200 mg 6-hourly should be continued in the seriously ill. Mechanical ventilation is necessary as a life-saving procedure in a few patients. Indications for endotracheal intubation and intermittent positive ventilation are shown in the second information box.

Monitoring of treatment

PEF recordings should be made every 15–30 minutes to assess early response and as necessary thereafter. In hospital PEF values should be charted 4–6-hourly before and after inhaled bronchodilator treatments throughout the period of hospital stay.

Repeat measurement of arterial blood gas tensions and pH or H^+ within 1–2 hours is necessary in all patients if the first

CONTINUED MANAGEMENT OF ACUTE SEVERE ASTHMA

If features of severity persist:
- Ipratropium bromide 0.5 mg should be added to the nebulised β_2-adrenoceptor agonist
- An aminophylline infusion (500 µg/kg/hour) should be commenced with an initial slow i.v. injection (5 mg/kg over 20 minutes) in patients *not* on oral theophyllines. Infusion rates should be adjusted thereafter according to plasma theophylline levels. Alternatively, salbutamol or terbutaline (250 µg i.v. over 10 minutes) can be given
- Continue nebulised β_2-adrenoceptor agonist treatment every 15–30 minutes as necessary. Reduce to 4-hourly once clear clinical response
- Mechanical ventilation

INDICATIONS FOR ASSISTED VENTILATION IN ACUTE SEVERE ASTHMA

- Coma
- Respiratory arrest
- Exhaustion, confusion, drowsiness
- Deterioration of arterial blood gas tensions despite optimal therapy
  - PaO_2 < 8 kPa and falling
  - $PaCO_2$ > 6 kPa and rising
  - pH < 7.3 and falling

arterial sample showed features of life-threatening disease (see the information box, p. 333). Continuous monitoring of oxygen saturation by pulse oximetry is valuable in all patients to help assess response, especially in the very ill. Oximetry may also prevent the need to repeat an arterial puncture in most patients. When an aminophylline infusion is used in the treatment regimen, continuous therapy should be monitored by theophylline serum levels with the aim of achieving and maintaining a concentration of 55–110 μmol/1.

Prognosis

The prognosis of individual asthma attacks is generally good. There is occasionally a fatal outcome, especially if treatment is inadequate or delayed. Spontaneous remission is fairly common in episodic asthma, particularly in children, but rare in chronic asthma. Seasonal fluctuations can occur in both types of asthma. Atopic subjects with episodic asthma are usually worse in the summer when they are more heavily exposed to antigens, while chronic asthmatics are usually worse in winter months because of the increased frequency of viral infections.

Prior to discharge from hospital, patients should have been taking discharge medication (i.e. changed from nebulised drugs) for 24 hours and have a PEF of ≥75% predicted or personal best over that period. They should also have their own PEF meter, a written self-management plan, an adequate supply of medication and an appointment to be reviewed by their GP within 7 days.

BRONCHIECTASIS

Aetiology and pathogenesis

Bronchiectasis, the term used to describe abnormal dilatation of the bronchi, may be produced in different ways. It may be acquired or, less commonly, congenital. The causes are listed in the information box.

Bronchiectasis is usually secondary to severe bacterial infection in childhood, often as a complication of whooping cough or measles.

Bronchiectasis may be due to bronchial distension resulting from the accumulation of pus beyond a lesion obstructing a major bronchus, such as compression by tuberculous hilar lymph nodes, an inhaled foreign body or a bronchial tumour. Recurrent infection and chronic obstruction by viscid mucus are both factors in causing bronchiectasis in cystic fibrosis (see p. 337). Rarely, it may be the result of congenital dysfunction of the cilia, which is a feature of, for example, Kartagener's syndrome (bronchiectasis, sinusitis and transposition of the viscera).

CAUSES OF BRONCHIECTASIS

Congenital

- Ciliary dysfunction syndromes
  - Primary ciliary dyskinesia (immotile cilia syndrome)
  - Kartagener's syndrome
  - Young's syndrome
- Cystic fibrosis
- Primary hypogammaglobulinaemia

Acquired—children

- Pneumonia (complicating whooping cough or measles)
- Primary tuberculosis
- Foreign body

Acquired—adults

- Suppurative pneumonia
- Pulmonary tuberculosis
- Allergic bronchopulmonary aspergillosis
- Bronchial tumours

Pathology

The bronchiectatic cavities may be lined by granulation tissue, squamous epithelium or normal ciliated epithelium. There may also be inflammatory changes in the deeper layers of the bronchial wall and hypertrophy of the bronchial arteries. Chronic inflammatory and fibrotic changes are usually found in the surrounding lung tissue.

Clinical features

Bronchiectasis may involve any part of the lungs but the more efficient drainage by gravity of the upper lobes usually produces less serious symptoms and complications than when bronchiectasis involves the lower lobes.

The groups of clinical features that occur in more severe cases are shown in the information box.

Physical signs in the chest may be unilateral or bilateral. If the bronchiectatic airways do not contain secretions and there is no associated lobar collapse there are no abnormal physical signs. When there are large amounts of sputum in the bronchiectatic spaces numerous coarse crepitations can be heard over the affected areas. When collapse is present the character of the physical signs depends on whether or not the proximal bronchus supplying the collapsed lobe is patent (see Table 4.2, p. 308).

Investigations

Bacteriological and mycological examination of sputum

This is necessary in all patients but is especially important

SYMPTOMS OF BRONCHIECTASIS
Due to accumulation of pus in dilated bronchi
• Chronic productive cough usually worse in mornings and often brought on by changes of posture. Sputum often copious and persistently purulent in advanced disease
Due to inflammatory changes in lung and pleura surrounding dilated bronchi
• Fever, malaise and increased cough and sputum volume when spread of infection causes pneumonia, which is frequently associated with pleurisy. Recurrent pleurisy in the same site often occurs in bronchiectasis
Haemoptysis
• Can be slight or massive and is often recurrent. Usually associated with purulent sputum or an increase in sputum purulence. Can, however, be the only symptom in so-called 'dry bronchiectasis'
General health
• When disease is extensive and sputum persistently purulent a decline in general health occurs with weight loss, anorexia, lassitude, sleep sweating, and failure to thrive in children. In these patients digital clubbing is common

in bronchiectasis associated with cystic fibrosis and in any patient who has had numerous courses of antibiotic treatments.

Radiological examination

Bronchiectasis, unless very gross, is not usually apparent on the conventional chest radiograph. In advanced disease the cystic bronchiectatic spaces may be visible. Abnormalities produced by associated pulmonary infection and/or collapse are evident. A diagnosis of bronchiectasis can only be made with certainty by CT (see Fig. 4.5, p. 309).

Assessment of ciliary function

A screening test can be performed in patients suspected of having a ciliary dysfunction syndrome by assessing the time taken for a small pellet of saccharin placed in the anterior chamber of the nose to reach the pharynx, when the patient can taste it. This time should not exceed 20 minutes and is greatly prolonged in patients with ciliary dysfunction. It is possible to assess ciliary function by measuring ciliary beat frequency using biopsies taken from the nose. Whenever possible the ciliary ultrastructure should also be determined by electron microscopy.

Management

Postural drainage

The aim of this measure is to keep the dilated bronchi emptied of secretions. Efficiently performed, it is of great value both in reducing the amount of cough and sputum and in preventing recurrent episodes of bronchopulmonary infection. In its simplest form, postural drainage consists of adopting a position in which the lobe to be drained is uppermost, thereby allowing secretions in the dilated bronchi to gravitate towards the trachea, from which they can readily be cleared by vigorous coughing. 'Percussion' of the chest wall with cupped hands aids dislodgement of sputum, and a number of mechanical devices are available which cause the chest wall to oscillate, thus achieving the same effect as postural percussion and chest wall compression. The optimum duration and frequency of postural drainage depend on the amount of sputum but 5–10 minutes once or twice daily is a minimum for most patients. Forced expiratory manoeuvres ('huffing and puffing') are of help in augmenting the expectoration of sputum.

Antibiotic therapy

The policy governing the use of antibiotics in most patients with bronchiectasis is the same as that in chronic bronchitis (see p. 324). Some, especially those with cystic fibrosis, present difficult therapeutic problems because of secondary infection with bacteria such as staphylococci and Gram-negative bacilli, in particular *Pseudomonas* species. In these circumstances it may prove necessary to use oral ciprofloxacin (250–750 mg twice daily) or ceftazidime by intravenous injection or infusion (100–150 mg/kg daily in three divided doses). The bronchi of some patients with cystic fibrosis also become colonised by *Aspergillus fumigatus*.

Surgical treatment

It is essential to demonstrate exactly the extent of bronchiectasis by CT. Pulmonary function must also be carefully assessed. The most suitable cases for pulmonary resection are young patients in whom bronchiectasis is unilateral and confined to a single lobe or segment. Unfortunately, many of the patients in whom medical treatment proves unsuccessful are also unsuitable for pulmonary resection either because of extensive bronchiectasis or coexisting chronic lung disease. Resection of areas of bronchiectatic lung has no role in the management of the progressive forms of bronchiectasis—for example, those associated with ciliary dysfunction and cystic fibrosis.

Prognosis

The disease is progressive when associated with ciliary dysfunction and cystic fibrosis, and inevitably causes respiratory failure and right ventricular failure. In other patients the prognosis can be relatively good if postural drainage is performed regularly and antibiotics are used judiciously.

Prevention

As bronchiectasis commonly starts in childhood following

measles, whooping cough or a primary tuberculous infection, it is essential that these conditions receive adequate prophylaxis and treatment. The early recognition and treatment of bronchial obstruction are particularly important.

CYSTIC FIBROSIS

Epidemiology and pathogenesis

Cystic fibrosis (CF) is the most common severe autosomal recessive disease in Caucasians, occurring with a carrier rate of 1 in 25 and an incidence of about 1 in 2500 live births. CF is the result of mutations affecting a gene (located on the long arm of chromosome 7) which encodes for a chloride channel known as cystic fibrosis transmembrane conductance regulator (CFTR), which is essential for the regulation of salt and water movement across cell membranes. The most common CFTR mutation in Northern European and American populations is Δ 508, but numerous mutations have now been identified in this region. The genetic defect causes an increased sodium chloride content in sweat and increased electrical potential difference across the respiratory epithelium which can be detected in the nose (see Fig. 4.23) This results in much increased viscosity of secretions in the lung and other organs, which causes ciliary dysfunction and chronic bronchial infection. Recurrent exacerbations of bronchial infection predispose to bronchial wall damage, eventually causing bronchiectasis, often predominantly in the upper lobes initially but subsequently in all areas of both lungs, with the end result of death from respiratory failure. There are also disorders in the gut epithelium, and in the pancreas and liver (causing intestinal malabsorption, diabetes and hepatic cirrhosis). Most men with CF are infertile due to failure of development of the vas deferens. Population carrier screening is feasible, but unlikely to affect overall patient numbers significantly. However, early diagnosis can be achieved by neonatal screening, and in some cases by amniocentesis.

Clinical features

Lung function is normal at birth, which leads to the hope that if the basic defect can be corrected by gene therapy many of the sequelae (see the information box on p. 338) might be avoided. Bronchiectasis, however, usually develops at a young age. Initially the bacteria associated with CF are those expected in bronchiectasis of other causes (see p. 335), but infection with *Staphylococcus aureus* tends to be early in CF and the majority have *Pseudomonas* infection at an early age. Repeated lung infection, inflammation and scarring almost inevitably lead to respiratory failure and death.

Management

The management of established cystic fibrosis is that of

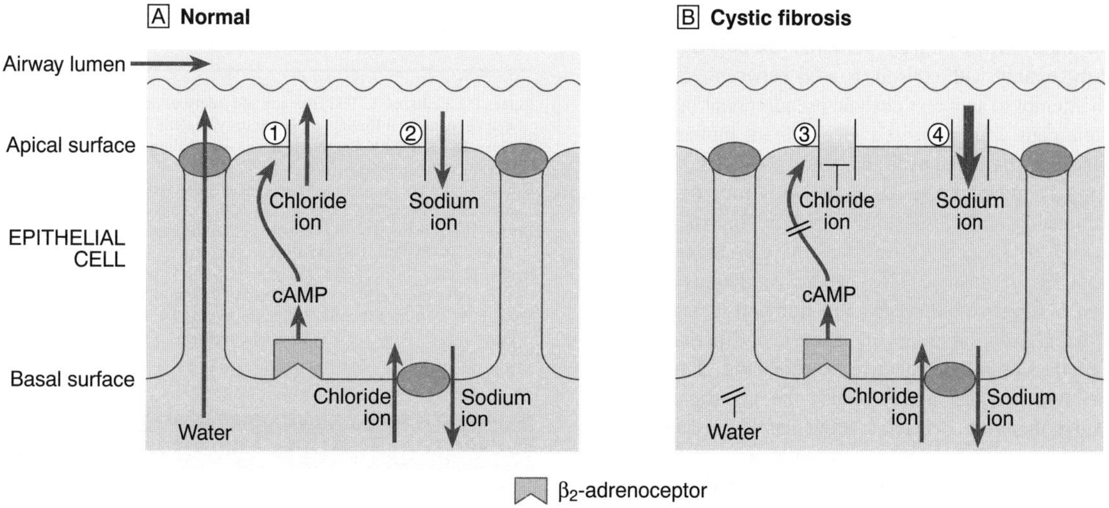

Fig. 4.23 Cystic fibrosis (CF): basic defect in the pulmonary epithelium. A The CF gene codes for a chloride channel (1) in the apical (lumenal) membrane of epithelial cells in the conducting airways. This channel is normally controlled by cyclic adenosine monophosphate (cAMP) and indirectly by β-adrenoceptor stimulation. It is one of several apical ion channels which together control the quantity and solute content of airway-lining fluid. Normal channels appear to inhibit the adjacent epithelial sodium channels (2). B In CF, one of many CF gene defects causes absence or defective function of this chloride channel (3). This leads to reduced chloride secretion and loss of inhibition of sodium channels with excessive sodium resorption (4) and dehydration of the airway lining. The resulting abnormal airway-lining fluid is believed to predispose to infection by mechanisms which are not fully understood.

COMPLICATIONS OF CYSTIC FIBROSIS

Respiratory
- Spontaneous pneumothorax
- Haemoptysis
- Nasal polyps
- Respiratory failure
- Cor pulmonale

Others
- Diabetes (11% of adults)
- Delayed puberty
- Male infertility
- Psycho-social problems
- Amyloidosis
- Arthropathy

Gastrointestinal
- Malabsorption
- Distal intestinal obstruction syndrome
- Biliary cirrhosis
- Increased frequency of gallstones

severe bronchiectasis (see p. 336). All patients with cystic fibrosis who produce sputum should have regular chest physiotherapy, which should be performed more frequently during exacerbations. Lung infections are usually predominantly caused by *Pseudomonas* species and *Staphylococcus aureus*. Unfortunately the bronchi of many CF patients eventually become colonised with pathogens which are resistant to most antibiotics; *Pseudomonas aeruginosa* and *Burkholderia cepacia* (previously known as *Pseudomonas cepacia*) are the main culprits. Infections with *Haemophilus influenzae* can be treated with a number of antibiotics and *Staphylococcus aureus* should be treated with flucloxacillin or erythromycin. Patients requiring frequent courses of intravenous antibiotics for the control of *Pseudomonas* infections can, with benefit, be taught self-administration via an indwelling central venous port and cannula, implanted subcutaneously in the chest wall to allow intravenous therapy at home. Nebulised antibiotic therapy, mainly with colistin, is used between exacerbations in an attempt to suppress chronic pseudomonal infection.

Treatment with nebulised recombinant human DNAase (rhDNAase) has been available since 1994. The aim of this therapy is to solubilise DNA derived from disintegrated inflammatory cells, which is a major contributor to the viscosity of bronchial secretions in CF, in which it is present in abundance. This expensive therapy has been shown to improve pulmonary function and increase patient well-being in a subgroup of patients, and perhaps also to reduce the number of infective exacerbations. There is also some evidence that it can reduce the neutrophil elastase load and, therefore, decelerate bronchial wall tissue damage. It has to be emphasised that this treatment is very expensive and is not of benefit to all patients, which makes clinical selection of patients for such treatment difficult. Aerosol α_1-antitrypsin treatment has been used to reduce the neutrophil elastase load, but this form of therapy is even less established than rhDNAase.

A number of patients with cystic fibrosis develop symptoms of bronchospasm, which can be treated effectively with bronchodilators following appropriate reversibility tests. Allergic bronchopulmonary aspergillosis (see p. 354) is also a well-recognised complication of CF. It is also common for 'atypical mycobacteria' to be cultured from the sputum of CF patients, but it is frequently difficult to determine whether these organisms are causing disease, or are benign 'colonisers' of the bronchiectatic airways which do not require specific therapy.

The prognosis of CF has greatly improved in the last decade, mainly because of better control of bronchial sepsis and maintenance of nutrition. The median survival of patients with CF is now predicted to be at least 40 years for children born in the 1990s. Organ transplantation remains last-resort therapy for patients with end-stage disease.

The potential for somatic gene therapy

The discovery of the CF gene and the fact that the lung defect is located in the respiratory epithelium (which is accessible by inhaled therapy) presents an exciting opportunity for gene therapy. The CF gene could be 'packaged' within a liposome or incorporated by genetic engineering into a modified viral vector and delivered to the respiratory epithelium with the aim of correcting the genetic defect. The feasibility of this approach is currently under investigation and initially promising results have been obtained in preliminary studies of the CF gene delivered to the nasal mucosa of CF patients. Studies of the delivery of the gene to the bronchi are in progress.

FURTHER INFORMATION ON OBSTRUCTIVE PULMONARY DISEASES

Barnes P J, Pedersen S 1993 Efficacy and safety of inhaled corticosteroids in asthma. American Review of Respiratory Disease 148: S1–S26

Bochner B S et al 1994 Immunological basis of allergic asthma. Annual Review of Immunology: 707–735

British Guidelines on Asthma Management 1997 1995 review and position statement. Thorax 52 (Suppl. 1): S1–S20

British Thoracic Society 1993 Guidelines on the management of asthma. Thorax 48 (Suppl. 2): S1–S24

British Thoracic Society 1997 Guidelines for the management of chronic obstructive pulmonary disease. Thorax 52 (Suppl. 5): S1–S28

Porteous D J, Dorin J R 1991 Cystic fibrosis 3: Cloning the cystic fibrosis gene—implications for diagnosis and treatment. Thorax 46: 46–55

INFECTIONS OF THE RESPIRATORY SYSTEM

Infections of the upper and lower respiratory tract continue to be a major cause of morbidity and mortality throughout the world, with patients at the extremes of age or with pre-existing lung disease or immune suppression being at particular risk. Viruses are the most frequent cause of upper respiratory illnesses, with bacteria being responsible for the majority of community- and hospital-acquired pneumonia in adults. Organisms such as *Mycoplasma*, *Coxiella* and *Chlamydia* are less common causes of severe pneumonia. Pulmonary infection by *Mycobacterium tuberculosis*, atypical mycobacteria and fungi results in diseases of a more chronic type. These are described separately.

UPPER RESPIRATORY TRACT INFECTIONS

The clinical features, complications and management of the common and most important upper respiratory tract infec-

Table 4.10 Common and most important upper respiratory tract infections: clinical features, complications and management

Infection	Clinical features	Complications	Management
Acute coryza (common cold)	Rapid onset. Burning and tickling sensation in nose. Sneezing. Sore throat. Blocked nose with watery discharge. Discharge usually green/yellow after 24–48 hrs (secondary infection). Nasal allergy can give rise to similar clinical features	Sinusitis. Lower respiratory tract infection (bronchitis/pneumonia). Hearing impairment, otitis media (due to blockage of Eustachian tubes)	Most do not require treatment. Paracetamol 0.5–1 g 4–6-hourly for relief of systemic symptoms. Nasal decongestant in some cases. Antibiotics not necessary in uncomplicated coryza
Acute laryngitis	Often a complication of acute coryza. Dry sore throat. Hoarse voice or loss of voice. Attempts to speak cause pain. Initially, painful and unproductive cough. Stridor in children (croup) because of inflammatory oedema leading to partial obstruction of a small larynx	Complications rare. Chronic laryngitis. Downward spread of infection may cause tracheitis, bronchitis or pneumonia	Rest voice. Paracetamol 0.5–1 g 4–6-hourly for relief of discomfort and pyrexia. Steam inhalations may be of value. Antibiotics not necessary in simple acute laryngitis
Acute laryngotracheo-bronchitis (croup)	Initial symptoms like common cold. Sudden paroxysms of cough accompanied by stridor and breathlessness. Contraction of accessory muscles and indrawing of intercostal spaces. Cyanosis and asphyxia in small children, if appropriate treatment not given	Asphyxia. Death. Superinfection with bacteria, especially *Strep. pneumoniae* and *Staph. aureus*. Viscid secretions may occlude bronchi	Inhalations of steam and humidified air/high concentrations of oxygen. Endotracheal intubation or tracheostomy to relieve laryngeal obstruction and allow clearing of bronchial secretions. Intravenous antibiotic therapy for seriously ill (co-amoxiclav or erythromycin). Maintain adequate hydration
Acute epiglottitis	Fever and sore throat, rapidly leading to stridor because of swelling of epiglottis and surrounding structures (infection with *H. influenzae*). Stridor and cough in absence of much hoarseness may distinguish acute epiglottitis from other causes of stridor	Death from asphyxia which may be precipitated by attempts to examine the throat—*avoid using a tongue depressor or any instrument* unless facilities for endotracheal intubation or tracheostomy are immediately available	Intravenous antibiotic therapy essential. Co-amoxiclav or chloramphenicol. Other measures as for acute laryngo-tracheobronchitis
Acute bronchitis and tracheitis	Often follows acute coryza. Irritating unproductive cough accompanied by retrosternal discomfort of tracheitis. Chest tightness, wheeze and breathlessness when bronchi become involved. Tracheitis causes pain on coughing. Sputum is initially scanty, mucoid, viscid and may be streaked with blood. After a day or so sputum becomes mucopurulent, more copious and, in tracheitis, often blood-stained. Acute bronchial infection may be associated with a pyrexia of 38–39°C and a neutrophil leucocytosis. Spontaneous recovery occurs over a few days in the majority of patients	Bronchopneumonia. Exacerbation of chronic bronchitis which often results in type II respiratory failure in patients with severe chronic obstructive airways disease. Acute exacerbation of bronchial asthma	Specific treatment rarely necessary in previously healthy individuals. Cough may be eased by pholcodine 5–10 mg 6–8-hourly. In patients with COPD (see p. 322) and asthma (see p. 333) aggressive treatment of exacerbations may be required. Amoxycillin 250 mg 8-hourly should be given to previously healthy patients who are thought to be developing bronchopneumonia (see also p. 343)
Influenza (a specific acute illness caused by a group of myxoviruses—two common types, A and B)	Sudden onset of pyrexia associated with generalised aches and pains, anorexia, nausea and vomiting. Degree of ill health ranges from mild to rapidly fatal. Usually harsh unproductive cough. Most patients do not develop complications and acute symptoms subside within 3–5 days, but may be followed by 'post-influenzal asthenia' which can persist for several weeks During epidemics the diagnosis is usually easy. Sporadic cases may have to be diagnosed by virus isolation, fluorescent antibody techniques or serological tests for specific antibodies	Tracheitis, bronchitis, bronchiolitis and bronchopneumonia. Secondary bacterial invasion by *Strep. pneumoniae*, *H. influenzae* and *Staph. aureus* may occur. Toxic cardiomyopathy may cause sudden death (rare). Encephalitis, demyelinating encephalopathy and peripheral neuropathy are also rare complications	Bed rest is advisable until fever has subsided. Paracetamol 0.5–1 g 4–6-hourly can be used to relieve headache and generalised pains. Pholcodine 5–10 mg 6–8-hourly may be given to suppress cough. Specific treatment for pneumonia (see p. 343) may be necessary

Table 4.11 Respiratory infections caused by viruses

Clinical syndrome	Usual cause (other causes in parentheses)
Epidemic influenza	Influenza A and B
'Influenza-like' illness	Adenoviruses, rhinoviruses (Enteroviruses)
Sore throat	Adenoviruses (Enteroviruses, parainfluenza viruses, influenza A and B in partially immune)
Common cold (coryza)	Rhinoviruses (Coronaviruses, enteroviruses, adenoviruses, respiratory syncytial virus)
'Feverish' cold	Rhinoviruses, enteroviruses (Influenza A and B, parainfluenza viruses, respiratory syncytial virus)
Croup	Parainfluenza 1, 2, 3 (Rhinoviruses, enteroviruses)
Bronchitis	Rhinoviruses, adenoviruses (Influenza A and B)
Bronchiolitis	Respiratory syncytial virus (Parainfluenza 3)
Pneumonia	Influenza A and B, chickenpox (Respiratory syncytial virus, parainfluenza, measles and adenoviruses in children and elderly)

tions are summarised in Table 4.10. The vast majority of these illnesses, of which acute coryza (common cold) is by far the most common, are caused by viruses (see Table 4.11). Immunity is short-lived and virus-specific. Other viral infections include acute laryngitis and acute laryngotracheobronchitis. Bacterial infection is the usual cause of acute tonsillitis, otitis media and epiglottitis.

Most patients with upper respiratory tract infections recover rapidly and specific investigation is indicated only in more severe illness. The possibility of acute epiglottitis, which represents a medical emergency, must be considered at all times (see Table 4.10). Viruses can be isolated from exfoliated cells collected on throat swabs, and may be identified retrospectively by serological tests. Certain viruses can be identified in exfoliated cells by the fluorescent antibody technique, allowing the pathogen to be identified more rapidly. Throat swabs may also be helpful if streptococcal pharyngitis is suspected, and examination of the blood will identify infectious mononucleosis (see p. 110). Radiographic examination may be required if an underlying chronic infection involving the sinuses is suspected.

PNEUMONIA

Pneumonia is defined as an acute respiratory illness associated with recently developed radiological pulmonary shadowing which is either segmental or affecting more than one lobe. As the setting in which a pneumonia develops has such major implications for the likely organisms involved and hence dictates the immediate choice of antibiotics, pneumonias are now classified as community-acquired, hospital-acquired, or those occurring in the immunocompromised host, or damaged lung (including suppurative and aspirational pneumonia).

COMMUNITY-ACQUIRED PNEUMONIA

This form of pneumonia is responsible for over 1 000 000 admissions per year in the UK. Infection is usually spread by droplet inhalation and while most patients affected are previously well, cigarette smoke, alcohol and corticosteroid therapy all impair ciliary and immune function. Other risk factors include old age, recent influenza infection, pre-existing lung disease and for certain forms of pneumonia contact with sick birds *(Chlamydia psittaci)* or farm environments *(Coxiella burnetii)*. Knowledge of the patient's recent travel history and local epidemics is also valuable. Appropriate investigation allows a microbiological diagnosis to be made in approximately 60% of patients with pneumonia. The term 'lobar pneumonia' is a radiological and pathological term referring to homogeneous consolidation (red hepatisation) of one or more lung lobes, often with associated pleural inflammation; bronchopneumonia refers to more patchy alveolar consolidation associated with bronchial and bronchiolar inflammation often affecting both lower lobes.

Clinical features

Patients present with a short illness of cough, fever and malaise, often associated with pleuritic chest pain which is occasionally referred to the shoulder or anterior abdominal wall. The cough is characteristically short, painful and at first dry, but later becomes productive and may become rust-coloured or even frankly blood-stained. The sudden onset of a high fever can result in rigors or, in children, vomiting or a febrile convulsion. Appetite is usually lost and headache is a frequent accompanying symptom. In patients with severe pneumonia confusion can be an early and dominant problem. Certain features may suggest a particular microbiological diagnosis (see Table 4.12).

Physical signs include a significant pyrexia, tachycardia, tachypnoea, evidence of hypoxaemia and not infrequently hypotension and confusion. Pleurisy often results in diminution of respiratory movement and a pleural rub on the affected side. At a variable time after onset, generally within 2 days, signs of consolidation appear (see p. 308), with impairment of the percussion note and high-pitched bronchial breath sounds. When resolution begins, numerous coarse crepitations are heard, indicating liquefaction of the alveolar exudate. If a pleural effusion develops, physical signs of fluid in the pleural space are usually found, but bronchial breath sounds can persist and the presence of an empyema (see p. 387) may be suspected only from the

Table 4.12 Clinical and radiological characteristics of community-acquired pneumonias caused by specific organisms

Organism	Frequency*	Clinical features	Radiological features
COMMON ORGANISMS			
Streptococcus pneumoniae	30%	Young to middle-aged, rapid onset, high fever, rigors, pleuritic chest pain, herpes simplex labialis, 'rusty' sputum	Lobar consolidation, one or more lobes
Chlamydia pneumoniae	10%	Young to middle-aged, large-scale epidemics or sporadic, often mild, self-limiting disease Associated sinusitis, pharyngitis, laryngitis White cell count often normal, liver transaminases elevated Usually diagnosed on serology	Small segmental infiltrates
Mycoplasma pneumoniae	9%	Children and young adults, autumn and 3–4-yearly cycles Insidious onset, headaches, systemic features, often few signs in chest Erythema nodosum, myocarditis, pericarditis, meningoencephalitis, rash, haemolytic anaemia	Patchy or lobar consolidation, hilar lymphadenopathy may be seen
Legionella pneumoniae	5%	Middle to old age, recent travel, local epidemics around point source, e.g. cooling tower Headache, malaise, myalgia, high fever, dry cough, gastrointestinal symptoms Confusion, hepatitis, hyponatraemia, hypoalbuminaemia	Shadowing may spread despite antibiotics and often slow to resolve
UNCOMMON ORGANISMS			
Haemophilus influenzae	3%	Often underlying lung disease, purulent sputum	Bronchopneumonia
Staphylococcus aureus	< 1%	Coexistent debilitating illness Often complicates viral pneumonia Can arise from, or cause, abscesses in other organs, e.g. osteomyelitis	Lobal or segmental. Abscess formation, residual cysts
Chlamydia psittaci	< 1%	Contact with sick birds Malaise, low-grade fever, protracted illness Hepatosplenomegaly	Patchy lower lobe consolidation
Coxiella burnetii		Farm or abattoir contact Chronic course, influenza-like illness, dry cough, conjunctivitis, hepatomegaly, endocarditis	Multiple segmental opacities
Klebsiella pneumoniae	< 1%	Systemic disturbance marked, widespread consolidation, often in upper lobes, purulent dark sputum, high mortality	Expansion of affected lobes
Actinomyces israelii	< 1%	Mouth commensal Cervicofacial, abdominal or pulmonary infection, empyema, chest wall sinuses, pus with 'sulphur grains'	Abscesses, pleural effusions and bone involvement
Primary viral pneumonias		Influenza, parainfluenza and measles can cause pneumonia commonly complicated by bacterial infection Respiratory syncytial virus seen mainly in infancy Varicella (chickenpox) can cause severe pneumonia	Chickenpox produces multiple miliary nodular shadows which may calcify

* No microbiological diagnosis established in approximately 40% of patients with community-acquired pneumonia admitted to hospital.

recurrence or persistence of pyrexia. Upper abdominal tenderness is sometimes apparent in patients with lower lobe pneumonia or if there is associated hepatitis.

Investigations

The main objectives of investigating patients with a clinically based diagnosis of pneumonia are:

- to obtain a radiological confirmation of the diagnosis
- to exclude other conditions that may mimic pneumonia (see the information box on p. 342)
- to obtain a microbiological diagnosis
- to help assess the severity of the pneumonia
- to identify the development of complications.

Radiological examination

In lobar pneumonia, the chest radiograph shows a homogeneous opacity localised to the affected lobe or segment; this usually appears within 12–18 hours of the onset of the illness (see Fig. 4.24 on p. 342). Radiological examination is also particularly helpful if a complication such as pleural effusion, intrapulmonary abscess formation or empyema is suspected. Hilar lymphadenopathy is occasionally seen in mycoplasma pneumonia, and lung cavities are more frequently observed in patients with staphylococcal or pneumococcal serotype 3 pneumonia. Follow-up radiological examination is essential as failure of a pneumonia to resolve may indicate underlying bronchial obstruction (e.g. a foreign body or carcinoma).

DIFFERENTIAL DIAGNOSIS OF PNEUMONIA
Pulmonary infarction
• Often presents like bacterial pneumonia, but pyrexia usually less, cough not as troublesome, haemoptysis much more common and the source of embolism may be apparent
Pulmonary/pleural tuberculosis
• Acute pulmonary tuberculosis can simulate pneumonia, but patients seldom as acutely ill. Tuberculous pleurisy may also present like a bacterial pleural infection
Pulmonary oedema
• Pulmonary oedema, especially if unilateral and localised, may be difficult to distinguish from pneumonia on the chest radiograph. Absence of fever and presence of heart disease favour a diagnosis of oedema
Inflammatory conditions below the diaphragm
• Conditions such as cholecystitis, perforated peptic ulcer, subphrenic abscess, acute pancreatitis and hepatic amoebiasis may be mistaken for lower lobe pneumonia associated with diaphragmatic pleurisy
Rare disorders
• Pulmonary eosinophilia (see p. 375), intrathoracic manifestations of connective tissue disorders (see p. 374), acute allergic alveolitis (see p. 371), Wegener's granulomatosis

Microbiological investigations

Every effort should be made to establish a microbiological diagnosis, as such information is invaluable in tailoring antibiotic therapy and in managing any complications. The identification of organisms such as *Legionella pneumophila* also has important public health implications. In patients who are severely ill, a microbiological diagnosis becomes essential and if sputum cannot be obtained, an attempt should be made to aspirate secretions or washings from the

MICROBIOLOGICAL INVESTIGATIONS IN PATIENTS WITH COMMUNITY-ACQUIRED PNEUMONIA
All patients
• Sputum—direct smear by Gram (see Fig. 4.25) and Ziehl–Neelsen stains. Culture and antimicrobial sensitivity testing • Blood culture—frequently positive in pneumococcal pneumonia • Serology—acute and convalescent titres to diagnose *Mycoplasma*, *Chlamydia*, *Legionella* and viral infections. Pneumococcal antigen detection in serum
Severe community-acquired pneumonia (see p. 344)
The above tests *plus* consider: • Tracheal aspirate, induced sputum, bronchoalveolar lavage, protected brush specimen or percutaneous needle aspiration. Direct fluorescent antibody stain for *Legionella* and viruses • Serology—*Legionella* antigen in urine. Pneumococcal antigen in sputum and blood. Immediate IgM for *Mycoplasma* • Cold agglutinins—positive in 50% of patients with *Mycoplasma*
Selected patients
• Throat/nasopharyngeal swabs—helpful in children or during influenza epidemic • Pleural fluid—should always be sampled when present in more than trivial amounts, preferably with ultrasound guidance

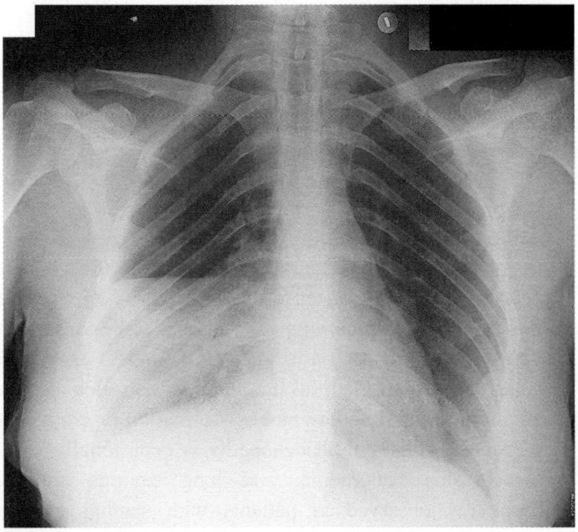

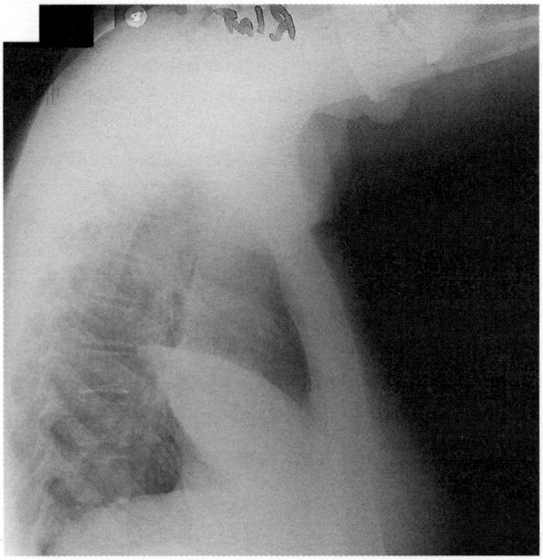

Fig. 4.24 Pneumonia of the right middle lobe. [A] Postero-anterior (PA) view: consolidation in right middle lobe with characteristic opacification beneath the horizontal fissure and loss of normal contrast between the right heart border and lung. [B] Lateral view: consolidation confined to the anteriorly situated middle lobe.

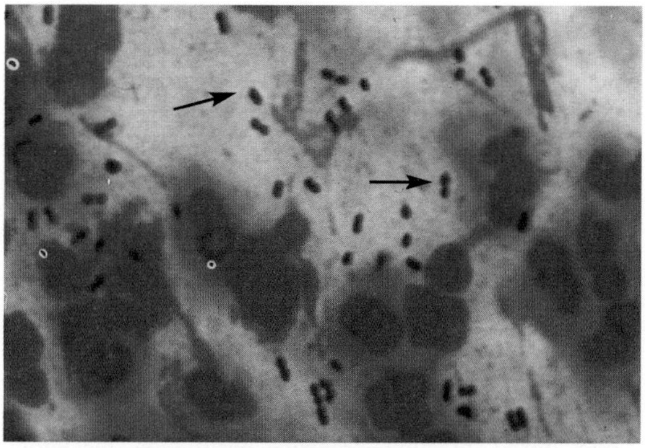

Fig. 4.25 Gram stain of sputum showing Gram-positive diplococci characteristic of *Strep. pneumoniae* (arrows).

FEATURES ASSOCIATED WITH A HIGH MORTALITY IN PNEUMONIA
Clinical
• Age 60 years or older • Respiratory rate > 30/min • Diastolic blood pressure 60 mmHg or less • Confusion • More than one lobe involved on chest radiograph • Presence of underlying disease
Laboratory
• Hypoxaemia (PaO_2 < 8 kPa) • Leucopenia (white blood cells < 4000 × 10^9/litre) • Leucocytosis (white blood cells > 20 000 × 10^9/litre) • Raised serum urea (> 7 mmol/l) • Positive blood culture • Hypoalbuminaemia

trachea or lower respiratory tract either by bronchoscopy or inserting a needle through the cricothyroid membrane. Some patients can be induced to produce sputum by the administration of nebulised hypertonic saline. A summary of the microbiological investigations required in patients with community-acquired pneumonia is provided in the information box.

Arterial blood gas measurements

These should be measured in all patients admitted to hospital with a diagnosis of pneumonia.

General blood tests

A high neutrophil leucocytosis favours a diagnosis of bacterial (particularly pneumococcal) pneumonia; patients with pneumonia caused by atypical agents tend to have a marginally raised or normal white cell count. A marked leucopenia indicates either a viral aetiology or overwhelming bacterial infection.

Assessment of disease severity

It is essential that in every patient with a clinical diagnosis of pneumonia an assessment is made to determine the severity of the disease. The use of simple clinical and laboratory parameters can determine very accurately those at high risk of death (see the information box) and forms an important guide to the level of patient monitoring required. This assessment also has an important bearing on antibiotic choice. As a simple guide, patients with two or more of the four cardinal markers of severity, namely a respiratory rate ≥ 30, a diastolic blood pressure ≤ 60 mmHg, a serum urea ≥ 7 mmol/l or the presence of confusion, have a 36-fold higher risk of dying compared with those patients without such features. Likewise, it is important to appreciate that a higher proportion of patients with mycoplasma pneumonia die compared to those with pneumococcal pneumonia and that in the latter condition coexistent septicaemia increases the mortality rate significantly.

Management

With appropriate intervention most patients respond promptly to antibiotic treatment. Delayed recovery suggests either that some complication such as empyema has developed or that the diagnosis is incorrect. Alternatively, the pneumonia may be secondary to a proximal bronchial obstruction or recurrent aspiration which delays recovery.

Oxygen

Oxygen should be administered to all hypoxaemic patients, and high concentrations (≥ 35%) should be used in all patients who do not have hypercapnia or advanced obstructive airways disease. Assisted ventilation should be considered at an early stage in all patients who remain significantly hypoxaemic despite adequate oxygen therapy. Most patients with moderate to severe pneumonia also require intravenous fluids and occasionally inotrope support (see p. 1042).

Antibiotic treatment

Antibiotics should be given as soon as a clinical diagnosis of pneumonia is made. If possible, culture specimens should be sent prior to starting antibiotics but such treatment should not be delayed if, for example, a sputum sample is not readily available. The antibiotic regimens currently recommended in uncomplicated and severe community-acquired pneumonia are detailed in the information box on p. 344. If *Strep. pneumoniae* is identified as the causative organism benzylpenicillin 1–2 g 6-hourly (i.v.) can be used in place of amoxycillin. Oral cephalosporins should not be used in the management of community-acquired pneumonia as they do not penetrate well into sputum or bronchial fluids and do not cover likely organisms. Patients with proven *Klebsiella* pneumonia should be treated

ANTIBIOTIC TREATMENT FOR COMMUNITY-ACQUIRED PNEUMONIA (CAP)
Uncomplicated CAP
• Amoxycillin 500 mg 8-hourly orally • *If patient allergic to penicillin* Clarithromycin 500 mg 12-hourly orally *or* Erythromycin 500 mg 6-hourly orally • *If staphylococcus is cultured or suspected* Flucloxacillin 1–2 g 6-hourly i.v. *plus* Clarithromycin 500 mg 12-hourly i.v. • *If Mycoplasma or Legionella is suspected* Clarithromycin 500 mg 12-hourly orally or i.v. *or* Erythromycin 500 mg 6-hourly orally or i.v. *plus* Rifampicin 600 mg 12-hourly i.v. in severe cases
Severe CAP
• Clarithromycin 500 mg 12-hourly i.v. *or* Erythromycin 500 mg 6-hourly i.v. *plus* • Co-amoxiclav 1.2 g 8-hourly i.v. *or* Ceftriaxone 1–2 g daily i.v. *or* Cefuroxime 1.5 g 8-hourly i.v. *or* Amoxycillin 1 g 6-hourly i.v. *plus* flucloxacillin 2 g 6-hourly i.v.

with gentamicin (dose according to patient age, weight, creatinine clearance and intended frequency of use) plus either ceftazidime 1 g 8-hourly (i.v.) or ciprofloxacin 200 mg 12-hourly (i.v. infusion). *Chlamydia pneumoniae* is a somewhat difficult organism to culture and hence most cases are diagnosed late or retrospectively on serological grounds. In proven or suspected (epidemic) cases, erythromycin or tetracycline is recommended. Psittacosis is treated with tetracycline 500 mg 6-hourly orally or 500 mg 12-hourly i.v., or erythromycin at an equivalent dose. Actinomycosis, which is now regarded as an anaerobic bacterial infection, responds best to benzylpenicillin 2–4 g 6-hourly (i.v.). Chickenpox pneumonia is usually treated with oral aciclovir 200 mg 5 times daily for 5 days.

In most cases of uncomplicated pneumococcal pneumonia a 7–10-day course of treatment is usually adequate, although treatment is usually required for 14 days or longer in patients with *Legionella*, staphylococcal or *Klebsiella* pneumonia.

Treatment of pleural pain

It is important to relieve pleural pain in order to allow the patient to breathe normally and cough efficiently. Mild analgesics such as paracetamol are rarely adequate and most patients require pethidine 50–100 mg or morphine 10–15 mg by intramuscular or intravenous injection. Opiates, however, must be used with extreme caution in patients with poor respiratory function.

Physiotherapy

Formal physiotherapy is not indicated in patients with community-acquired pneumonia; however, assisted coughing is important in patients who suppress cough because of pleural pain. The administration of analgesic drugs should be coordinated with this form of physiotherapy to optimise patient cooperation.

Complications

Assessing progress can be difficult in patients with pneumonia. Although the response to antibiotics may be rapid and dramatic, fever may persist for several days and the chest radiograph often takes several weeks or even months to resolve, especially in the elderly. Failure to respond to therapy may indicate use of the wrong antibiotic, mixed infection, bronchial obstruction, the wrong diagnosis (e.g. pulmonary thromboembolism) or the development of a complication (see the information box).

COMPLICATIONS OF PNEUMONIA
• Parapneumonic effusion—common • Empyema—see page 387 • Retention of sputum causing lobar collapse • Development of thromboembolic disease • Pneumothorax—particularly with *Staph. aureus* • Suppurative pneumonia/lung abscess—see below • ARDS, renal failure, multi-organ failure • Ectopic abscess formation *(Staph. aureus)* • Hepatitis, pericarditis, myocarditis, meningoencephalitis • Pyrexia due to drug hypersensitivity

SUPPURATIVE AND ASPIRATIONAL PNEUMONIA (INCLUDING PULMONARY ABSCESS)

Suppurative pneumonia is the term used to describe a form of pneumonic consolidation in which there is destruction of the lung parenchyma by the inflammatory process. Although microabscess formation is a characteristic histological feature of suppurative pneumonia, it is usual to restrict the term 'pulmonary abscess' to lesions in which there is a fairly large localised collection of pus, or a cavity lined by chronic inflammatory tissue, from which pus has escaped by rupture into a bronchus.

Suppurative pneumonia and pulmonary abscess may be produced by infection of previously healthy lung tissue with *Staph. aureus* or *Klebsiella pneumoniae*. These are, in effect, primary bacterial pneumonias associated with pulmonary suppuration. More frequently, suppurative pneumonia and pulmonary abscess develop after the inhalation of septic material during operations on the nose, mouth or throat under general anaesthesia, or of vomitus during anaesthesia or coma. In such circumstances gross oral sepsis may be a predisposing factor. Additional risk factors for aspiration pneumonia include bulbar or vocal cord palsy, achalasia or oesophageal reflux and alcoholism.

CLINICAL FEATURES OF SUPPURATIVE PNEUMONIA
Onset
• Acute or insidious
Symptoms
• Cough productive of large amounts of sputum which is sometimes fetid and blood-stained • Pleural pain common • Sudden expectoration of copious amount of foul sputum occurs if abscess ruptures into a bronchus
Clinical signs
• High remittent pyrexia • Profound systemic upset • Digital clubbing may develop quickly (10–14 days) • Chest examination usually reveals signs of consolidation; signs of cavitation rarely found • Pleural rub common • Rapid deterioration in general health with marked weight loss can occur if disease not adequately treated

Intravenous drug users are at particular risk of developing lung abscess, often in association with endocarditis affecting the pulmonary and tricuspid valves. Aspiration into the lungs of acid gastric contents can give rise to a severe haemorrhagic pneumonia often complicated by ARDS (see p. 1035). The clinical features of a suppurative pneumonia are summarised in the information box.

Bacterial infection of a pulmonary infarct or of a collapsed lobe may also produce a suppurative pneumonia or a lung abscess. The organism(s) isolated from the sputum include *Strep. pneumoniae*, *Staph. aureus*, *Strep. pyogenes*, *H. influenzae*, and in some cases anaerobic bacteria. In many cases, however, no pathogens can be isolated, particularly when antibiotics have been given.

Chest radiograph features

There is a homogeneous lobar or segmental opacity consistent with consolidation or collapse. A large, dense opacity, which may later cavitate and show a fluid level, is the characteristic finding when a frank lung abscess is present. Occasionally, a pre-existing emphysematous bulla becomes infected and appears as a cavity containing an air-fluid level.

Management

In many patients oral treatment with amoxycillin 500 mg 6-hourly is effective. If an anaerobic bacterial infection is suspected (e.g. from fetor of the sputum) oral metronidazole 400 mg 8-hourly should be added. Antibacterial therapy should be modified according to the results of microbiological examination of the sputum. Prolonged treatment for 4–6 weeks may be required in some patients with lung abscess. Removal or treatment of any obstructing endobronchial lesion is essential.

In contrast to uncomplicated community-acquired pneumonia, physiotherapy is of great value, especially when large abscess cavities have formed. It may not be possible to drain lower lobe cavities without postural coughing.

In most patients there is a good response to treatment and although residual fibrosis and bronchiectasis are common sequelae, these seldom give rise to serious morbidity. Abscesses that fail to resolve despite optimal medical therapy require surgical intervention.

HOSPITAL-ACQUIRED PNEUMONIA

Hospital-acquired or nosocomial pneumonia refers to a new episode of pneumonia occurring at least 2 days after admission to hospital. The term includes post-operative and certain forms of aspiration pneumonia, and pneumonia or bronchopneumonia developing in patients with chronic lung disease, general debility or those receiving assisted ventilation.

Aetiology

The factors predisposing to the development of pneumonia in a hospitalised patient are listed in the information box. The elderly are particularly at risk and this condition now occurs in 2–5% of all hospital admissions.

FACTORS PREDISPOSING TO NOSOCOMIAL PNEUMONIA
Reduced host defences against bacteria
• Reduced immune defences (e.g. corticosteroid treatment, diabetes, malignancy) • Reduced cough reflex (e.g. post-operative) • Disordered mucociliary clearance (e.g. anaesthetic agents) • Bulbar or vocal cord palsy
Aspiration of nasopharyngeal or gastric secretions
• Immobility or reduced conscious level • Vomiting, dysphagia, achalasia or severe reflux • Nasogastric intubation
Bacteria introduced into lower respiratory tract
• Endotracheal intubation/tracheostomy • Infected ventilators/nebulisers/bronchoscopes • Dental or sinus infection
Bacteraemia
• Abdominal sepsis • Intravenous cannula infection • Infected emboli

The most important distinction between hospital- and community-acquired pneumonia is the difference in the spectrum of pathogenic organisms, with the majority of hospital-acquired infections caused by Gram-negative bacteria. These include *Escherichia*, *Pseudomonas* and *Klebsiella* species. Infections caused by *Staph. aureus* (including multidrug-resistant—MRSA—forms) are also common in hospital, and anaerobic organisms are much more likely than in pneumonia acquired in the community. This profile of organisms in part reflects the high rate of colonisation of the nasopharynx of hospital patients with Gram-negative bacteria, together with the poor host defences and general inability of the severely ill or semiconscious patient to clear upper airway and respiratory tract secretions.

Clinical features

The clinical features and investigation of patients with hospital-acquired pneumonia are very similar to community-acquired pneumonia (see p. 340). In the elderly or debilitated patient who develops acute bronchopneumonia (or 'hypostatic pneumonia') symptoms of acute bronchitis are followed after 2 or 3 days by increased cough and sputum purulence associated with a rise in temperature. Breathlessness and central cyanosis may then appear, but pleural pain is uncommon. In the early stages the physical signs are those of acute bronchitis followed by the development of crepitations. There is a neutrophil leucocytosis and the chest radiograph shows mottled opacities in both lung fields, chiefly in the lower zones.

Management

Adequate Gram-negative coverage is usually obtained with:

- a third-generation cephalosporin (e.g. cefotaxime) *plus* an aminoglycoside (e.g. gentamicin)
- imipenem *or*
- a monocyclic β-lactam (e.g. aztreonam) *plus* flucloxacillin.

Aspiration pneumonia can be treated with co-amoxiclav 1.2 g 8-hourly plus metronidazole 500 mg 8-hourly. The nature and severity of most hospital-acquired pneumonias dictate that these antibiotics are all given i.v. at least initially.

Physiotherapy is of particular importance in the immobile and elderly, and adequate oxygen therapy, fluid support and monitoring are essential. The mortality from hospital-acquired pneumonia is high (approximately 30%).

PNEUMONIA IN THE IMMUNOCOMPROMISED PATIENT

Pulmonary infection is common in patients receiving immunosuppressive drugs and in those with diseases causing defects of cellular or humoral immune mechanisms. For example, patients with the acquired immune deficiency syndrome (AIDS) are susceptible to many types of pneumonia, in particular *Pneumocystis carinii* (see p. 103). It is important to recognise, however, that the common pathogenic bacteria are responsible for the majority of lung infections in immunocompromised patients (see Table 4.13). Despite this the Gram-negative bacteria, especially *Pseudomonas aeruginosa*, are more of a problem than Gram-positive organisms, and unusual organisms or those normally considered to be of low virulence or non-pathogenic may become 'opportunistic' pathogens. Likewise, infection is often due to more than one organism. *Pneumocystis carinii* and other fungi such as *Aspergillus fumigatus*, viral infections, cytomegalovirus and herpes-viruses, and infections with *M. tuberculosis* and other types of mycobacteria are all common causes of infection in patients who are immunocompromised.

Table 4.13 Common causes of immune suppression: associated lung infection

	Cause	Lung infection
Neutropenia	Cytotoxic drugs Agranulocytosis Acute leukaemia	*Staph. aureus* Gram-negative bacteria *Candida albicans* *Aspergillus fumigatus*
T cell defect (+/– B cell defect)	Lymphoma Chronic lymphocytic leukaemia (CLL) Immunosuppressive drugs Bone marrow transplants Splenectomy	*C. albicans* *Mycobacterium tuberculosis* *Pneumocystis carinii* Cytomegalovirus Gram-negative bacteria *Staph. aureus* *Strep. pneumoniae* *H. influenzae*
Antibody production	CLL Myeloma	*Strep. pneumoniae* *H. influenzae*

Clinical features

The patient usually presents with fever, cough, breathlessness and infiltrates on the chest radiograph. Patients may develop non-specific symptoms, and a high index of suspicion is required to determine the site and nature of the infection. In general, the onset of symptoms tends to be less rapid in patients with opportunistic organisms such as *Pneumocystis carinii* and mycobacterial infections. In *Pneumocystis carinii* pneumonia symptoms of cough and breathlessness can be present several days or weeks before the onset of systemic symptoms or even a chest radiograph abnormality.

Diagnosis

Lung biopsy offers the greatest chance of establishing a diagnosis if examination of sputum or bronchoalveolar lavage fluid has not revealed a pathogen. This, however, is a relatively high-risk and invasive procedure and should be reserved for patients in whom less invasive procedures fail to establish a diagnosis and in whom there has been no response to broad-spectrum antibiotic treatment. Some patients who cannot produce sputum can be induced to do so by the inhalation of nebulised hypertonic saline. Fibreoptic bronchoscopy should be performed early since a diagnosis can often be established by examination of lavage fluid, bronchial brushings or transbronchial biopsies.

Management

Whenever possible, treatment should be based on an established aetiological diagnosis. In practice, however, the cause of the pneumonia is frequently not known when treatment has to be started. Hence, broad-spectrum antibiotic therapy is required (e.g. a third-generation cephalosporin, or a quinolone, plus an antistaphylococcal antibiotic, or an antipseudomonal penicillin plus an aminoglycoside) and this treatment is thereafter tailored according to the results of investigations and the clinical response. The management of *P. carinii* infection is detailed on page 103.

TUBERCULOSIS

This disease, which a few years ago was considered to be almost under control in Western Europe and North America, has once again become a serious world-wide problem because of AIDS and the predicted spread of this specific communicable disease to the normal population. However, in developed countries there is still a tendency for tuberculosis to be overlooked, the diagnosis being made late or only at autopsy.

THOSE AT GREATEST RISK OF ACQUIRING TUBERCULOSIS

- Children, adolescents and young adults
- Contacts of patients with smear-positive pulmonary disease
- Immunocompromised individuals (e.g. AIDS patients and those on immunosuppressive therapy and corticosteroids)
- Those in close contact with many potential patients (e.g. health workers)
- Underprivileged people living in overcrowded conditions
- Pre-existing conditions—diabetes mellitus, gastric surgery, silicosis, alcoholism
- Asian and West Indian immigrants

Aetiology

Several types of mycobacteria are responsible for disease in humans, as shown in the information box.

Entry of the tubercle bacillus into the body or the alimentary or respiratory tract is not necessarily followed by a clinical illness, the development of which is dependent upon several other factors.

Pathology

The initial *'primary'* tuberculosis infection usually occurs in the lung (see Fig. 4.26) but occasionally in the tonsil or alimentary tract, especially the ileocaecal region. The primary infection differs from subsequent infections in that the primary focus in lung, tonsil or bowel is almost invariably accompanied by caseous lesions in the regional lymph nodes, such as the mediastinal, cervical or mesenteric groups respectively.

In most people, the primary infection and the associated lymph node lesions heal and calcify. In a few, healing, particularly in lymph nodes, is incomplete and viable tubercle bacilli may enter the blood stream. In consequence, tuberculous lesions may develop elsewhere. *'Haematogenous'*

TYPES OF MYCOBACTERIA CAUSING DISEASE IN HUMANS

Mycobacterium tuberculosis complex

- *Mycobacterium tuberculosis*—cause of most infections
- *Mycobacterium bovis*—endemic in cattle, spread to humans by milk. Now rare in UK

Opportunistic mycobacterial infections

- *Mycobacterium kansasii*
- *Mycobacterium xenopi*
- *Mycobacterium malmoense*
- MAIS complex*—*Mycobacterium avium, Mycobacterium intracellulare, Mycobacterium scrofulaceum*

Can be isolated from tap water and food animal tissues. Used to be a rare cause of disease but incidence is increasing in AIDS and other immunosuppressed patients

* In Cleveland, USA, in 1985 isolates of the MAIS complex outnumbered those of *Mycobacterium tuberculosis*. This was attributed to mycobacterial disease in AIDS patients

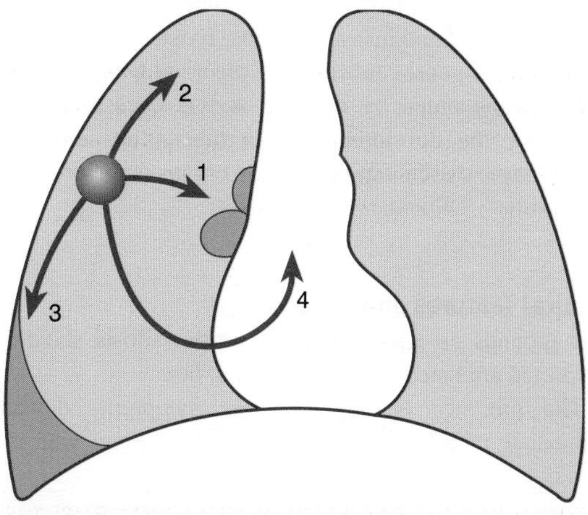

Fig. 4.26 Primary pulmonary tuberculosis. (1) Spread from primary focus to hilar and mediastinal lymph glands to form the 'primary complex', which in most cases heals spontaneously. (2) Direct extension of the primary focus—'progressive pulmonary tuberculosis'. (3) Spread to the pleura—tuberculous pleurisy and pleural effusion. (4) Blood-borne spread: *few bacilli*—pulmonary, skeletal, renal, genitourinary infection often months or years later; *massive spread*—miliary tuberculosis and meningitis.

lesions of this kind are more common in the lungs, bones, joints and kidneys, and lesions may develop months or even years after the primary infection.

Sometimes the primary infection does not heal. A pulmonary lesion, particularly when it occurs during adolescence or early adult life, may lead to progressive pulmonary tuberculosis. A tuberculous mediastinal lymph node, in children especially, may compress a lobar or segmental bronchus (rarely a main bronchus) and produce pulmonary collapse. Occasionally, the node may ulcerate through the bronchial wall and discharge caseous material into the lumen, with the production of acute tuberculous lesions in the related lobe or segment. Infection may also be carried by lymphatics from tuberculous mediastinal lymph nodes to the pleura or pericardium, with the production of tuberculous pleurisy or pericarditis. Comparable complications may occur when the primary lesion is in the tonsil or gut—for example, 'cold abscess' of the neck or tuberculous peritonitis.

Rarely a caseous tuberculous focus ruptures into a vein and produces acute dissemination throughout the body, a condition known as *acute miliary tuberculosis*. Meningitis often complicates this condition.

Progressive pulmonary tuberculosis may develop directly from a primary lesion or it may occur later following reactivation of an incompletely healed primary focus. Alternatively progressive pulmonary tuberculosis may be the result of reinfection.

Post-primary pulmonary tuberculosis is the term used to describe lung disease, the characteristic pathological feature of which is the tuberculous cavity, formed when the caseated and liquefied centre of a tuberculous pulmonary lesion is discharged into a bronchus. Extension of infection to the pleura causes tuberculous pleurisy, which is sometimes accompanied by effusion and is occasionally followed by the development of a tuberculous empyema. Blood-borne dissemination to other organs is uncommon in post-primary pulmonary tuberculosis.

Clinical features and diagnosis

The grounds on which pulmonary tuberculosis should be suspected are listed in the information box.

The presence of any of these symptoms demands immediate radiological examination of the lungs and, if an abnormality is found, the examination of at least three specimens of sputum for tubercle bacilli. The diagnosis can readily be made by microscopic examination of sputum smears stained by the Ziehl–Neelsen method when bacilli are numerous, whereas the auramine-phenol fluorescent test is of value in the detection of small numbers of tubercle bacilli. Culture of sputum, or of broncho-alveolar lavage fluid, fasting gastric washings or laryngeal swabs if no sputum can be obtained, is necessary when smears are negative and is essential for the detection of drug resistance (see p. 354). Drug-sensitivity tests can now be conducted rapidly by use of the Bactec radiometric method.

SYMPTOMS AND SIGNS WHICH SHOULD ALWAYS RAISE THE SUSPICION OF TUBERCULOSIS

- Persistent cough
- Haemoptysis
- Pleural pain not associated with an acute illness
- Spontaneous pneumothorax
- Lethargy
- Weight loss

In the vast majority of patients the diagnosis of pulmonary tuberculosis can be made with confidence by radiological examination of the chest and examination of the sputum. In some patients it is necessary to perform further radiological examination after a course of treatment with an antibiotic, such as amoxycillin, in order to exclude an acute inflammatory cause for an abnormal radiograph shadow.

The complications are shown in the information box.

Primary pulmonary tuberculosis

The primary infection usually occurs in childhood. A history of contact with a case of active pulmonary tuberculosis is obtained in many instances. In the vast majority of patients the primary infection produces no symptoms or signs and passes unnoticed unless routine radiological examination of the chest happens to be performed at the

COMPLICATIONS OF TUBERCULOSIS

- Pleurisy—with or without pleural effusion
- Pneumothorax—may follow rupture of cavity into pleural space
- Empyema or pyopneumothorax—serious complications of rupture of a tuberculous lesion into the pleural space
- Tuberculous laryngitis—usually only occurs in advanced pulmonary disease
- Tuberculous enteritis—follows the swallowing of heavily infected sputum in some patients with extensive pulmonary disease
- Ischiorectal abscess—consider tuberculosis in all cases. Tubercle bacilli can pass through rectal mucosa
- Blood-borne dissemination—uncommon complication of post-primary pulmonary disease except in the immunosuppressed
- Respiratory failure and right ventricular failure—late complications when disease has caused extensive pulmonary destruction and fibrosis
- Fungal colonisation of cavities—cavities which persist after antituberculosis treatment may become colonised with *Aspergillus fumigatus* and a ball of fungus (aspergilloma) may develop (see p. 355)

appropriate time or serial tuberculin tests show conversion from negative to positive.

In a few patients the primary infection produces a febrile illness which is generally mild and lasts for no more than 7–14 days. It is unusual for gross symptoms or focal signs to develop but a slight dry cough is occasionally present. The leucocyte count is normal but the erythrocyte sedimentation rate (ESR) is raised.

The primary infection may be accompanied by erythema nodosum, which is characterised by bluish-red, raised, tender, cutaneous lesions on the shins and less commonly on the thighs, and is associated in some patients with pyrexia and polyarthralgia. Erythema nodosum may be the first clinical indication of a tuberculous infection. The tuberculin reaction is always strongly positive in these patients and evidence of primary tuberculosis can usually be detected on the chest radiograph. Erythema nodosum is, however, seen in conditions other than primary tuberculosis—for example, sarcoidosis, streptococcal infections and drug reactions.

Occasionally, the primary pulmonary infection pursues a progressive course (see p. 347). Symptoms and signs due to its complications (see Fig. 4.26) may appear either during the course of the initial illness or after a latent interval of weeks or months. Such complications include pleurisy or pleural effusion (see p. 384), lobar or segmental collapse, acute miliary tuberculosis, tuberculous meningitis (see p. 350) and post-primary pulmonary tuberculosis (see below).

As primary pulmonary tuberculosis and its complications respond satisfactorily to antituberculous chemotherapy, which should be given in every case, the prognosis is excellent.

Miliary tuberculosis

Hitherto, miliary tuberculosis has occurred chiefly in children and young adults but with the changing demography of tuberculosis in many countries miliary tuberculosis is affecting persons in older age groups in whom it tends to take the form of an insidious illness—the 'cryptic' type—which is often difficult to diagnose.

The disease may start suddenly or may be preceded by a few weeks of vague ill health. In children and young adults systemic disturbance rapidly becomes profound. In particular there is a high pyrexia with drenching sweats during sleep, marked tachycardia, loss of weight and usually progressive anaemia. Cough and breathlessness are only occasionally present. There may be no abnormal physical signs in the lungs, although widespread crepitations may be heard late in the disease. The liver is often enlarged and the spleen may be palpable. Choroidal tubercles may be visible on ophthalmoscopy but are rarely present in the elderly. Leucocytosis is usually absent or slight. If chemotherapy is not given, death takes place within days or weeks.

'Cryptic' miliary tuberculosis

Diagnosis of this form of disseminated disease is shown in the information box.

'CRYPTIC' MILIARY TUBERCULOSIS

Diagnosis frequently made at autopsy—often not suspected during life

- Age group—adults and elderly, particularly females
- Symptoms—chest symptoms *rare*. Lassitude, weight loss and general debility
- Clinical signs—choroidal tubercles *rare*. Chest usually normal. Liver and occasionally spleen may be enlarged. Low-grade pyrexia common
- Chest radiograph—often normal
- Blood—neutropenia, pancytopenia and leukaemoid reaction quite common

The diagnosis of acute miliary tuberculosis can be made with confidence only when radiological examination of the chest shows the characteristic 'miliary' mottling symmetrically distributed throughout both lung fields or when choroidal tubercles are seen. The diagnosis can often be suspected at an earlier stage by the symptoms, progressive clinical deterioration, persistent pyrexia and splenomegaly.

Bacteriological confirmation should be sought by culture of sputum, urine or bone marrow. A liver biopsy may be diagnostic in difficult cases. Although the tuberculin reaction is usually positive in young patients a negative result does not exclude acute miliary tuberculosis, as tuberculin sensitivity is occasionally depressed in the later stages of the illness.

A therapeutic trial of chemotherapy with ethambutol or pyrazinamide and isoniazid in conventional doses (see p. 353) is indicated in patients suspected of having the cryptic form of miliary tuberculosis. Clinical improvement is usually evident within 10 days if the diagnosis is correct.

Post-primary pulmonary tuberculosis

Most of the morbidity and mortality from tuberculosis is caused by this form of the disease. In Western Europe and North America the majority of cases occur in middle-aged and elderly subjects, but AIDS has caused an increase among young adults. In developing countries it is most prevalent in adolescence and early adult life.

The lesions are most frequently situated in the upper lobes. The disease is often bilateral and occasionally a whole lobe may be consolidated in acute pneumonic tuberculosis.

The onset of post-primary pulmonary tuberculosis is usually insidious, with the gradual development of general symptoms or cough and sputum. Sometimes a dramatic event such as haemoptysis, pleural pain or a spontaneous pneumothorax marks the onset but the diagnosis is now frequently made by radiography before any dramatic symptoms have appeared.

At first no abnormal physical signs may be present but despite this an extensive lesion may be visible radiologically. The earliest physical signs consist of a few crepitations, usually situated over one or other lung apex posteriorly. Ultimately, physical signs of consolidation, cavitation and fibrosis may develop, and occasionally those of pleurisy with or without effusion, or spontaneous pneumothorax (see Table 4.2, p. 308).

Investigations. Radiological examination is of paramount importance for diagnosis in the early stages before physical signs appear and for assessment of the extent and progress of the disease.

The earliest radiological change is usually an ill-defined opacity or opacities usually situated in one of the upper lobes (see Fig. 4.27). In more advanced cases opacities are larger and more widespread and may be bilateral. Occasionally there is a dense homogeneous shadow involving the whole lobe ('pneumonic tuberculosis'). An area or areas of translucency within the opacities indicates cavitation; very large cavities may be visible in some cases. The presence of cavitation in an untreated patient usually indicates that the disease is active. When fibrosis is marked the trachea and mediastinal structures are displaced towards the side of the lesion.

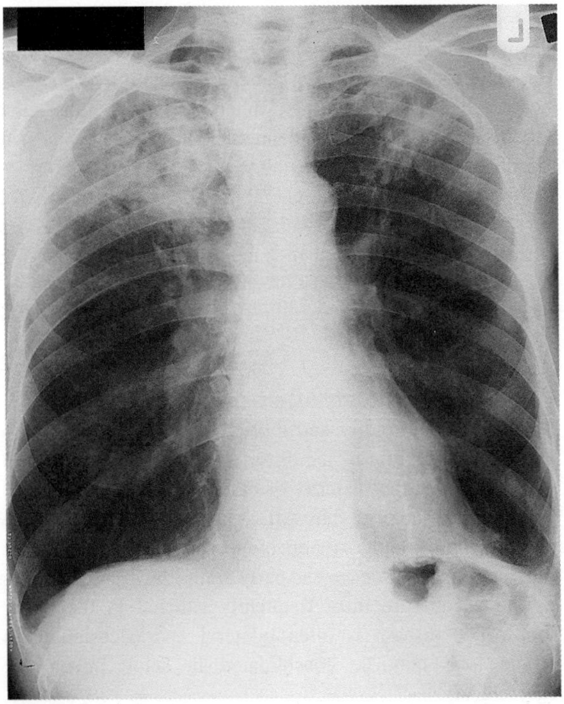

Fig. 4.27 Bilateral pulmonary tuberculosis. Upper lobe shadowing more obvious on the right.

The radiological appearances of pleural effusion and pneumothorax, which may accompany those of pulmonary tuberculosis, are described on pages 385 and 389.

Extra-pulmonary tuberculosis

Tuberculosis can affect any organ and tissue of the body (see Fig. 4.28).

Gastrointestinal tuberculosis. Tuberculous ulceration of the tongue can occur but is rare. Diarrhoea, malabsorption, intestinal obstruction and ascites can result from tuberculosis of the intestines and peritoneum. Peritoneal involvement is a common autopsy finding in patients who have died from undiagnosed disseminated disease.

Pericardium. Infection of the pericardial sac is uncommon but can give rise to pericardial effusion and tamponade (see p. 300). Constrictive pericarditis can be a late result of infection and is the consequence of fibrosis and calcification.

Genitourinary tuberculosis. Renal tuberculosis is a fairly common form of non-pulmonary tuberculosis but rarely gives rise to symptoms until the renal lesions are extensive. Haematuria and increased frequency of micturition can be caused by renal tuberculosis. Patients with 'sterile pyuria' should always be suspected of having tuberculosis, and at least three early morning urine specimens should be examined.

Infection of the fallopian tubes was a common cause of infertility; it can also give rise to salpingitis and tubal abscess. Epididymal tuberculosis presents as a painless craggy swelling which subsequently can form a sinus.

Central nervous system tuberculosis. Tuberculous meningitis is an extremely serious form of infection which can be associated with miliary tuberculosis but can also present in the absence of generalised disease. Headache, neck stiffness, vomiting and disordered consciousness are features of the disease, which can be fatal or result in permanent neurological deficit if not diagnosed and treated at an early stage. Cerebral tuberculomata are uncommon and may or may not present with focal neurological signs.

Lymph node tuberculosis. This is a very common manifestation of tuberculous disease, especially in Asians. Lymph node enlargement in any site can occur but cervical node involvement is most common. The enlargement of lymph nodes is usually painless. When caseation and liquefaction of the nodes occur, the swellings become fluctuant and sinus formation is common.

Bone and joint tuberculosis. Skeletal infection is relatively common and can lead to vertebral collapse, pyarthrosis, osteomyelitis and 'cold abscess' formation.

Tuberculous infection in other sites. Destruction by infection of the adrenal glands can give rise to Addison's

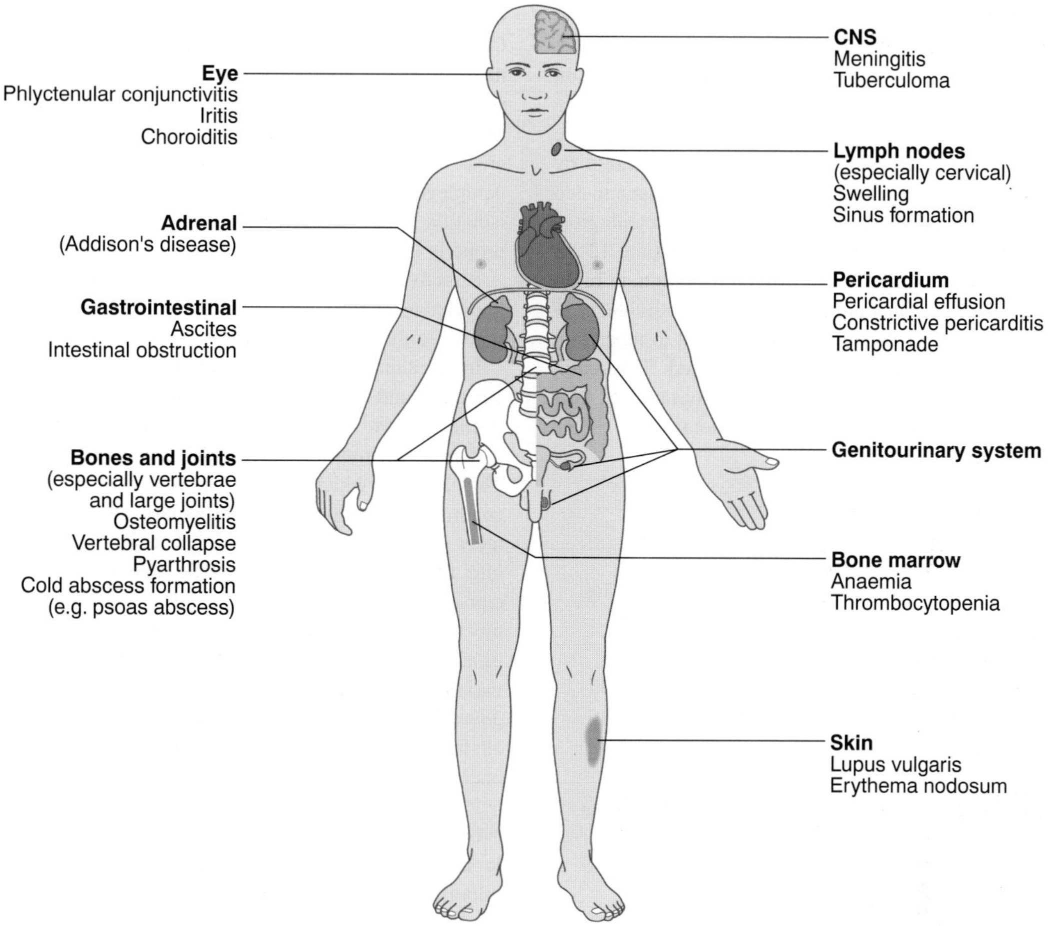

Fig. 4.28 Some of the extra-pulmonary tissues which can be affected by tuberculosis.

disease (see p. 589). Tuberculous infection of the skin is referred to as lupus vulgaris and erythema nodosum can be a manifestation of primary tuberculosis. Phlyctenular keratoconjunctivitis, iritis and choroiditis can occur in patients who have a tuberculous infection.

Non-Mycobacterium tuberculosis complex mycobacteria (atypical mycobacteria)

Mycobacteria of the non-*M. tuberculosis* complex are ubiquitous in the environment and have in the past been called atypical or opportunistic mycobacteria. Clinically important disease caused by these organisms was uncommon compared with tuberculosis, but there has been a recent increase in pulmonary and non-pulmonary infections, which is only in part explained by the susceptibility of immunocompromised individuals to infection with these organisms. Disseminated mycobacteriosis is a problem in AIDS. In general these mycobacteria show in vitro resistance to many of the antituberculosis drugs, and treatment is often difficult. The organisms which most often cause disease in humans are: *M. malmoense*, *M. kansasii*, *M. xenopi* and members of the *M. avium/intracellulare* group of mycobacteria.

MANAGEMENT OF TUBERCULOSIS

General principles of control and prevention

Case-finding

Mass radiography is no longer used in case-finding; the highest yield by far is by referral from general practitioners, and open-access chest radiography greatly assists. Contact examination also achieves a high case yield where it is focused on household contacts of sputum-smear positive patients, especially contacts under 25 years of age.

BCG vaccination

BCG (bacille Calmette–Guérin) is a strain of bovine TB of low virulence which is used for intradermal vaccination (0.1 ml of reconstituted freeze-dried vaccine), conferring protection for up to 7 years. Vaccination reduces the incidence of pulmonary tuberculosis in young adults by 80% and minimises the risk of serious disseminated disease—miliary tuberculosis and tuberculous meningitis. In the UK it is currently offered to schoolchildren at 12–13 years of age. Vaccination is also offered to infants in high-risk groups (e.g. Asian immigrants) and to individuals in endemic areas. Only those who do not respond to tuberculin tests (see the information box) are vaccinated. Tuberculin test responders are screened with chest radiography as they may require chemoprophylaxis or chemotherapy.

TUBERCULIN TESTS
Mantoux test
10 tuberculin units of purified protein derivative in 0.1 ml normal saline intradermally in flexor aspect of the forearm. Test is positive if 2–4 days later there is at least 5 mm induration with surrounding erythema. False negatives: • HIV—decreased cellular immunity • Miliary tuberculosis + late stages of tuberculous meningitis • Elderly patients • Immunosuppressive drugs
Heaf test (or tine test)
Multiple puncture technique, of value in population studies and contact tracing. Test read at 3 days: grades 0–2 (negative or weakly positive), 3–4 (strongly positive)

Chemoprophylaxis

Healed tuberculous scars may still contain viable bacteria and if cellular immunity is suppressed for any reason (e.g. corticosteroid treatment, cytotoxic chemotherapy) there may be recrudescence of disease. These patients and those identified from contact tracing and tuberculin testing as being at high risk will be given chemoprophylaxis (see the information box).

CHEMOPROPHYLAXIS OF TUBERCULOSIS
Isoniazid (5 mg/kg by mouth) daily for 1 year should be considered in: • Non-BCG vaccinated tuberculin-positive children under age 3 years—vulnerable in respect of miliary tuberculosis and tuberculous meningitis • Unvaccinated contacts who have recently become tuberculin-positive • Immunosuppressed patients • Adolescents with high degree of tuberculin sensitivity
Isoniazid (5 mg/kg by mouth) daily for 6 weeks should be considered in: • Infants of highly infectious patients—isoniazid-resistant BCG vaccine can be used with isoniazid chemoprophylaxis

Chemotherapy

Chemotherapy is the mainstay of modern treatment of tuberculosis, although the occasional patient still requires surgery for drainage of an empyema, caseating tuberculous lymph nodes or, more rarely, resection of bronchiectatic areas of the lung, or emergency surgery to prevent spinal paraplegia. Except where young children are at risk, isolation is not necessary, provided the patient is being properly treated by chemotherapy.

Effective treatment of tuberculosis is based on detailed knowledge of the drugs available so that the most appropriate regimen for the individual patient can be devised.

In Britain four drugs—rifampicin, isoniazid, pyrazinamide and ethambutol—are used as first-line treatment in most cases. Streptomycin is now rarely used except in patients with multiple drug resistance or hypersensitivity. Thiacetazone, which is cheap, is widely used in developing countries. Pyrazinamide is particularly useful in the treatment of tuberculous meningitis because it diffuses well into the cerebrospinal fluid. The role of drugs such as ciprofloxacin, which have in vitro activity against the tubercle bacillus but which have not been formally assessed in clinical trials, is uncertain. Apart from a few minor variations in dose and duration of treatment, the policy governing the use of antituberculosis drugs is the same for all forms of the disease. These drugs should be used in once-daily doses as shown in Table 4.14.

Adverse effects

In choosing a suitable drug regimen for individuals it is important to bear in mind those side-effects which are particularly liable to cause serious chronic disability, such as vestibular disturbance due to streptomycin, which must be prescribed with caution. Even with the relatively low dose recommended for ethambutol, a few patients develop optic neuritis and some are left with a permanent visual defect. This must be taken into consideration whenever ethambutol is prescribed, particularly in children.

Streptomycin, and occasionally isoniazid, ethambutol and rifampicin, may produce a hypersensitivity reaction, comprising pyrexia and an erythematous skin eruption which usually but not invariably develops 2–4 weeks after treatment is started. Rifampicin, which colours the urine orange-pink, is a potent liver enzyme inducer and should be used with appropriate caution when prescribed with other drugs such as oestrogens (e.g. oral contraceptives), warfarin, corticosteroids, oral hypoglycaemic drugs, phenytoin or digoxin. It should, if possible, be avoided in patients with liver disease. The principal adverse effects of the most commonly prescribed drugs are shown in Table 4.14.

Drug regimens

The 'short-course' regimens shown in the information box are virtually 100% effective in the treatment of tuberculosis.

Table 4.14 Daily doses and side-effects of commonly used antituberculosis drugs

Drug	Clinical setting	Daily dose	Side-effects
Rifampicin[1]	Children Adults weighing less than 50 kg and in the elderly Adults weighing more than 50 kg	10–20 mg/kg 450 mg 600 mg	Drug interactions, hypersensitivity hepatitis, vasculitis, fever, skin-flushing, nausea and abdominal pain, breathlessness and wheeze (intermittent regimens only) Rifampicin should not be given again to any patient in whom it has caused vasculitis
Isoniazid	Children Adults Intermittent regimen Miliary tuberculosis/meningitis Chemoprophylaxis	10 mg/kg 200–300 mg 15 mg/kg[2] 10–12 mg/kg[2] 5 mg/kg	Hypersensitivity, polyneuropathy, lack of mental concentration
Ethambutol	Children and adults: initial 8 weeks Subsequently In renal failure	25 mg/kg 15 mg/kg According to serum levels	Optic neuritis, hypersensitivity
Pyrazinamide	Children and adults	20–35 mg/kg (max. 2.5 g)	Hepatitis, gout, hypersensitivity
Streptomycin sulphate	Children Adults under 40 years and weighing more than 45 kg Adults 40–60 years or weighing less than 45 kg Adults over 60 years or in patients with renal failure Intermittent regimens	30 mg/kg 1 g 0.75 g According to serum levels 0.75–1 g	Vestibular disturbance, hypersensitivity Deafness (rare)

[1] Taken at least 30 minutes before breakfast. [2] Plus pyridoxine 10 mg to prevent peripheral neuropathy.

If primary drug resistance is suspected, quadruple therapy should be given as initial treatment.

Any patient who cannot be trusted to take antituberculosis drugs regularly should be kept in hospital for the initial (2-month) phase of treatment or be given supervised outpatient therapy. Thereafter for 10 months, the following should be given at home twice weekly (at 3- and 4-day intervals): streptomycin sulphate 1 g i.m., and isoniazid 15 mg/kg orally in a single dose, plus pyridoxine 10 mg. Pyridoxine is given to prevent peripheral neuropathy. This type of chemotherapy should be wholly supervised, the tablets being administered at the same time as the injection.

STANDARD DRUG REGIMENS

Total duration 6 months

Initial phase 2 months
- Pyrazinamide (plus ethambutol) in combination with isoniazid and rifampicin

Continuation phase 4 months
- Isoniazid and rifampicin

A four-drug combination should be chosen whenever there is a possibility of primary drug resistance. Three drugs—isoniazid, rifampicin in combination with pyrazinamide during the initial 2 months—are adequate for the majority of patients in the UK

Total duration 9 months

Initial phase 2 months
- Isoniazid plus rifampicin and ethambutol

Continuation phase 7 months
- Isoniazid plus rifampicin

Inexpensive treatment regimens

In developing countries it is sometimes impossible for economic reasons to adhere to ideal chemotherapeutic regimens.

12-MONTH REGIMENS, INEXPENSIVE AND REASONABLY EFFECTIVE

Twice-weekly

- Streptomycin 1 g i.m.
- Isoniazid 15 mg/kg plus pyridoxine 10 mg orally

The effectiveness of this regimen is nearly 100% in the absence of primary drug resistance if daily treatment with standard doses of streptomycin and isoniazid can be afforded for the first 2–3 months

Daily

- Isoniazid 300 mg
- Thiacetazone 150 mg

} single doses by mouth

Very cheap regimen which is 80–95% effective

Response to treatment

It is most unusual, even in advanced cases, for sputum cultures to remain positive for longer than 6 months if bacilli at the start of treatment are fully sensitive to the drugs used. Reliance must be placed on smear examination where facilities for sensitivity testing do not exist.

Drug-resistant tubercle bacilli

The treatment of patients infected with drug-resistant tubercle bacilli presents a problem requiring specialised knowledge. Additional drugs available for the treatment of such cases are: sodium aminosalicylate (commonly referred to as PAS—*p*-aminosalicylic acid, 5 g 12-hourly by mouth), ethionamide or prothionamide (0.75–1 g daily by mouth), capreomycin (0.7–1 g i.m. daily), cycloserine (0.75–1 g daily by mouth), ciprofloxacin and clarithromycin.

Corticosteroids

The evidence for the beneficial effects of corticosteroids in tuberculosis treatment is not great, except perhaps in tuberculosis of the meninges and ureters where, in combination with antituberculous drugs, it is thought to reduce the chance of secondary complications from excessive scarring. Prednisolone is also sometimes used in combination with antituberculosis drugs to treat fulminant disease.

Prognosis

There has been a remarkable decline in the mortality from pulmonary tuberculosis with the advent of effective chemotherapy. Provided the tubercle bacilli are not initially drug-resistant and chemotherapy is used correctly, a fatal outcome is uncommon even if the disease has reached an advanced stage when it is first recognised. Antituberculous chemotherapy has reduced the mortality of miliary tuberculosis to virtually zero, provided the diagnosis is made at an early stage. Late complications of respiratory failure and secondary infection with pyogenic bacteria or fungi can be prevented if pulmonary tuberculosis is diagnosed at a reasonably early stage and is efficiently treated.

RESPIRATORY DISEASES CAUSED BY FUNGI

Most fungi encountered by humans are harmless saprophytes but some species may, in certain circumstances, infect human tissue or promote damaging allergic reactions.

The term *mycosis* is applied to disease caused by fungal infection. Predisposing factors include metabolic disorders such as diabetes mellitus, toxic states (for example, chronic alcoholism), diseases in which immunological responses are disturbed such as AIDS, treatment with corticosteroids and immunosuppressive drugs, and radiotherapy. Local factors such as tissue damage by suppuration or necrosis and the elimination of the competitive influence of a normal bacterial flora by antibiotics may also facilitate fungal infection.

Diagnosis

The diagnosis of fungal disease of the respiratory system is usually made by mycological examination of sputum—microscopic examination of stained films for fungal hyphae being extremely important—supported by serological tests and in some cases by skin sensitivity tests.

ASPERGILLOSIS

Most cases of bronchopulmonary aspergillosis are caused by *Aspergillus fumigatus*, but other members of the genus (*A. clavatus*, *A. flavus*, *A. niger* and *A. terreus*) occasionally cause disease. The conditions associated with *Aspergillus* species are listed in the information box.

CLASSIFICATION OF BRONCHOPULMONARY ASPERGILLOSIS

- Atopic (allergic) asthma (see p. 328)
- Allergic bronchopulmonary aspergillosis (asthmatic pulmonary eosinophilia)
- Extrinsic allergic alveolitis *(Aspergillus clavatus)*
- Intracavitary aspergilloma
- Invasive pulmonary aspergillosis

ALLERGIC BRONCHOPULMONARY ASPERGILLOSIS (ABPA)

This is caused by hypersensitivity reactions to *A. fumigatus* involving the bronchial wall and peripheral parts of the lung. In the vast majority of patients it is associated with bronchial asthma, but it can occur in non-asthmatic patients and is a recognised complication of cystic fibrosis. It is one of the causes of pulmonary eosinophilia (see p. 375), since it is characterised by fleeting radiographic abnormalities associated with peripheral blood eosinophilia.

Clinical features

Fever, breathlessness, cough productive of bronchial casts and worsening of asthmatic symptoms can all be manifestations of ABPA, but frequently the diagnosis is suggested by abnormalities on routine chest radiographs of patients whose asthmatic symptoms are no worse than usual. When repeated episodes of ABPA have caused bronchiectasis, the symptoms and complications of that disease often overshadow those of asthma.

Investigations

The disease is characterised by recurrent transient radiograph abnormalities of two main types: diffuse pulmonary infiltrates and lobar or segmental pulmonary collapse. Permanent radiographic changes of bronchiectasis ('tram-line', ring and 'gloved-finger' shadows) are seen predominantly in the upper lobes in patients with advanced disease.

The diagnostic features are shown in the information box. Not all are required to make a confident diagnosis.

DIAGNOSTIC FEATURES OF ALLERGIC BRONCHOPULMONARY ASPERGILLOSIS

- Asthma (in the majority of cases)
- Peripheral blood eosinophilia > 0.5×10^9/litre
- Presence or history of chest radiograph abnormalities
- Positive skin test to an extract of *A. fumigatus*
- Serum precipitating antibodies to *A. fumigatus*
- Elevated total serum IgE
- Fungal hyphae of *A. fumigatus* on microscopic examination of sputum

Management

In the absence of safe and effective antifungal agents which can be given long-term, the main aims of therapy are:

- suppression of the immunopathological responses to *A. fumigatus* with low-dose oral corticosteroid therapy (prednisolone 7.5–10 mg daily)
- optimal, control of associated asthma
- prompt, effective management of exacerbations associated with new chest radiograph changes—prednisolone 40–60 mg daily and physiotherapy. If lobar collapse persists for more than 7–10 days bronchoscopy to remove impacted mucus should be performed to prevent the development of bronchiectasis.

INTRACAVITARY ASPERGILLOMA

Inhaled air-borne spores of *A. fumigatus* may lodge and germinate in damaged pulmonary tissue, and an 'aspergilloma' (a ball of aspergillus fungus) can form in any area of damaged lung in which there is a persistent abnormal space. The most common cause of such pulmonary damage is tuberculosis (see Fig. 4.29), but an aspergilloma can develop in an abscess cavity, a bronchiectatic space or even a cavitated tumour. Most, but not all, are caused by *A. fumigatus*.

Clinical features

An aspergilloma often produces no specific symptoms but may be responsible for recurrent haemoptysis, which is often severe. The presence of a fungus ball in the lung can also give rise to non-specific systemic features such as lethargy and weight loss.

Investigations

The development of a fungal ball within a cavity produces a tumour-like opacity on radiograph. An aspergilloma can usually be distinguished from a peripheral bronchial carcinoma by the presence of a crescent of air between the fungal ball and the upper wall of the cavity. Aspergillomata may be multiple.

Diagnosis

The diagnosis is usually suspected because of the chest radiograph findings. Serum precipitins to *A. fumigatus* can be demonstrated in virtually all patients. Sputum contains hyphal fragments on microscopy which are often only scanty, and is usually positive on culture. Less than 50% of patients exhibit skin hypersensitivity to extracts of *A. fumigatus*.

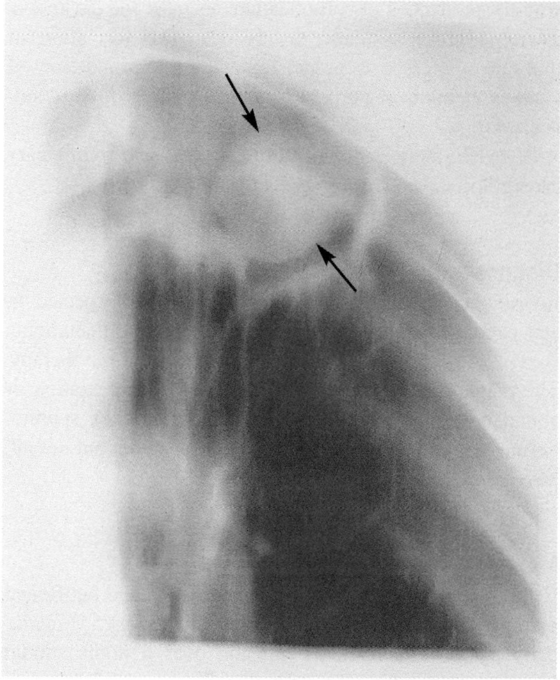

Fig. 4.29 Aspergilloma in left upper lobe cavity. Aspergilloma demonstrated using conventional tomography. Rounded fungal ball (arrows) separated from the wall of the cavity by a 'halo' of air.

Management

Specific antifungal therapy is of no value. Surgical removal of the aspergilloma is indicated in patients who have massive haemoptysis and in whom thoracotomy is not contraindicated because of poor respiratory reserve. Bronchial artery embolisation is an alternative approach to the management of recurrent haemoptysis.

INVASIVE PULMONARY ASPERGILLOSIS

Invasion of previously healthy lung tissue by *A. fumigatus* is uncommon but can produce a serious and often fatal condition which usually occurs in patients who are immunocompromised either by drugs or disease. The source of the infection can be an aspergilloma but this is by no means always so.

Clinical features

Spread of the disease throughout the lungs is usually rapid, with the production of consolidation, necrosis and cavitation. There is grave systemic disturbance. The formation of multiple abscesses is associated with the production of copious amounts of purulent sputum which is often blood-stained.

A much more indolent form of invasive pulmonary aspergillosis is now recognised.

Diagnosis

Invasive pulmonary aspergillosis should be suspected in any patient thought to have severe suppurative pneumonia (see p. 344) which has not responded to antibiotic therapy. The diagnosis can be established by the demonstration of abundant fungal elements in stained smears of sputum. Serum precipitins can be demonstrated in some, but not all, patients.

Management

If the diagnosis is established at an early stage antifungal therapy can be successful. Amphotericin 0.25–1 mg/kg daily by slow intravenous infusion over 6 hours should be given in combination with flucytosine 150–200 mg/kg daily by mouth or by intravenous infusion, in four divided doses. The combination of flucytosine and amphotericin prevents resistance to flucytosine developing and allows a smaller daily dose of amphotericin to be used than would be possible if this drug was used on its own. Liposomal amphotericin is recommended when toxicity precludes the use of conventional amphotericin. Itraconazole has been used successfully in the treatment of invasive aspergillosis.

Histoplasmosis, coccidioidomycosis, blastomycosis and cryptococcosis

See pages 146–148.

FURTHER INFORMATION ON INFECTIONS OF THE RESPIRATORY SYSTEM

British Thoracic Society 1993 Guidelines for the management of community-acquired pneumonia in adults admitted to hospital. British Journal of Hospital Medicine 49: 346–350

Court C A, Garrard C S 1992 Nosocomial pneumonia in the intensive care unit—mechanisms and significance. Thorax 47: 465–473

Crompton G K 1995 Bronchopulmonary aspergillosis. In: Brewis R A L, Corrin B, Geddes D et al (eds) Respiratory medicine, 2nd edn. W B Saunders, London

Moore-Gillon J 1997 Tuberculosis. In: Farthing M J G Horizons in Medicine no. 8. Royal College of Physicians, London, pp. 211–220

Neville K, Bromberg A, Bromberg R et al 1994 The third epidemic—multidrug-resistant tuberculosis. Chest 105: 45–48

TUMOURS OF THE BRONCHUS AND LUNG

Between 1995 and 1996 there were more than 35,800 lung cancer deaths in the UK. Bronchial carcinoma is by far the most common (> 90%) lung tumour; by comparison, benign tumours of the lung are rare. Primary carcinomas of other organs, in particular the breast, kidney, uterus, ovary, testes and thyroid, may give rise to metastatic pulmonary deposits, as may an osteogenic or other sarcoma. Bronchial tumours also represent the most common cause of obstruction to a major bronchus (see the information box).

CAUSES OF LARGE BRONCHUS OBSTRUCTION

Common

- Bronchial carcinoma or adenoma (see Table 4.16, p. 363)
- Enlarged tracheobronchial lymph nodes (malignant or tuberculous)
- Inhaled foreign bodies (especially right lung and in children)
- Bronchial casts or plugs consisting of inspissated mucus or blood clot (especially asthma, haemoptysis, debility)
- Collections of mucus or mucopus retained in the bronchi as a result of ineffective expectoration (especially post-operative following abdominal surgery)

Rare

- Aortic aneurysm
- Giant left atrium
- Pericardial effusion
- Congenital bronchial atresia
- Fibrous bronchial stricture (e.g. following tuberculosis)

The clinical and radiological manifestations of bronchial obstruction (see Figs 4.30 and 4.31) depend on the site of the obstruction, whether the obstruction is complete or partial, the presence or absence of secondary infection, and the extent of pre-existing lung disease. Signs of displacement of the mediastinum or elevation of the diaphragm only occur if a major portion of the lung becomes collapsed. Bacterial infection affecting the distal lung is almost inevitable whenever a major bronchus is significantly obstructed. Hence pneumonia is often the first clinical manifestation of a bronchial carcinoma, even when the degree of obstruction is insufficient to cause collapse.

The cause of bronchial obstruction should be determined at bronchoscopy; this procedure also enables biopsy of abnormal tissue and the removal of foreign bodies, mucus plugs or tenacious secretions.

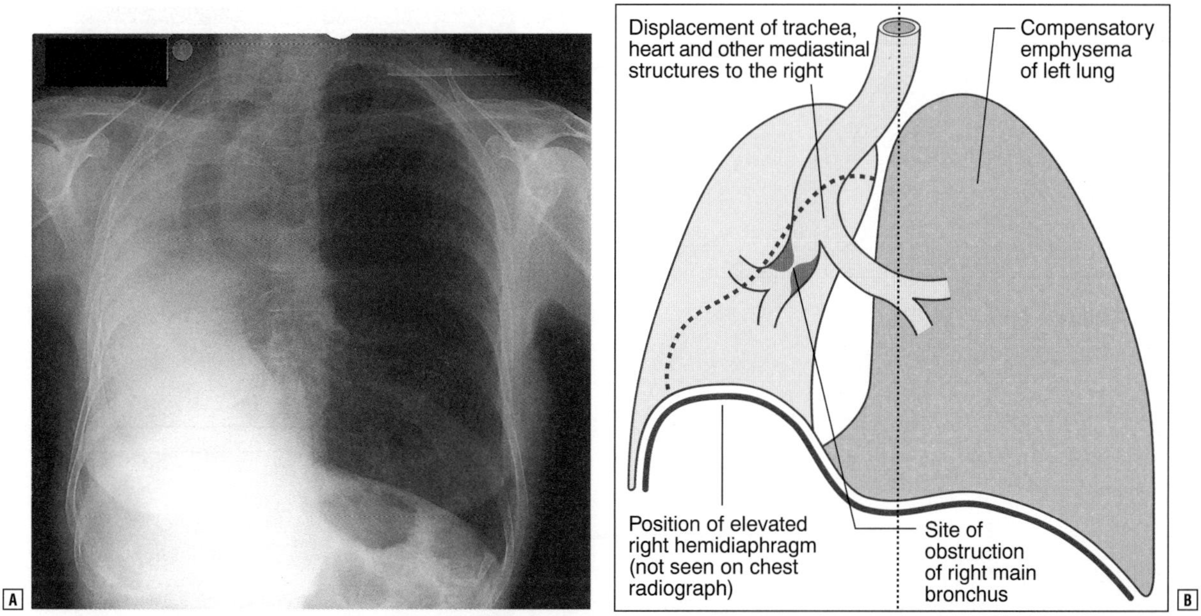

Fig. 4.30 Collapse of the right lung. Effects on neighbouring structures. [A] Chest radiograph. [B] Artist's impression.

PRIMARY TUMOURS OF THE LUNG

Aetiology

Cigarette smoking is by far the most important single factor in the causation of lung cancer. It is thought to be directly responsible for at least 90% of lung carcinomas, the risk being directly proportional to the amount smoked and to the tar content of cigarettes. For example, the death rate from the disease in heavy cigarette smokers is 40 times that in non-smokers. The effect of 'passive' smoking is more difficult to quantify but is currently believed to be a factor in 5% of all lung cancer deaths. Exposure to naturally occurring radon has been estimated to cause 5% of lung cancers. The incidence of lung cancer is also slightly higher in urban than in rural dwellers; this may reflect differences in atmospheric pollution (including tobacco smoke) or occupation since a number of industrial products (e.g. asbestos, beryllium, cadmium and chromium) are associated with lung cancer.

BRONCHIAL CARCINOMA

The incidence of bronchial carcinoma has increased dramatically during the 20th century (see Fig. 4.32, p. 359) and it is now the most common fatal malignancy in the developed world. It accounts for more than 50% of all male deaths from malignant disease and the incidence of lung cancer deaths is expected to climb over the next 20 years, with an increasing number unrelated to smoking (see the information box).

Pathology

Bronchial carcinomas arise from the bronchial epithelium or mucous glands. The common cell types are listed in Table 4.15.

When the tumour arises in a large bronchus symptoms arise early, but tumours originating in a peripheral bronchus

LUNG CANCER IN GREAT BRITAIN

- 36 000 deaths/year
- 25% of all cancer deaths
- 8% of all male deaths and 4% of all female deaths
- More than three-fold increase in deaths since 1950
- Most rapidly increasing cause of cancer death in women
- Most common cause of cancer death in men
- After breast cancer, the second most common cause of cancer death in women in England and Wales

Table 4.15 Common cell types of bronchial carcinoma

Cell type	%
Squamous	35%
Adenocarcinoma	30%
Small-cell	20%
Large-cell	15%

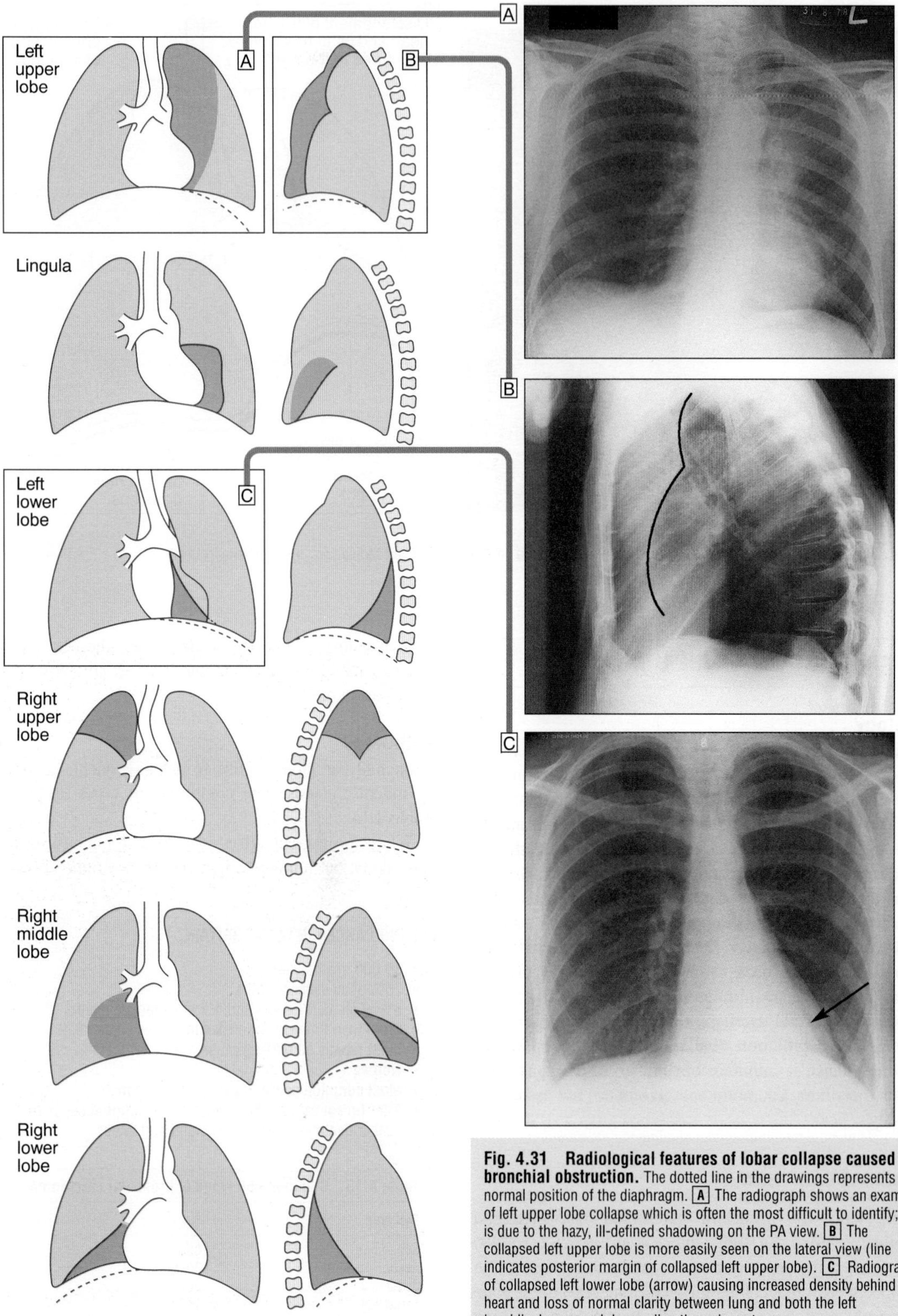

Fig. 4.31 Radiological features of lobar collapse caused by bronchial obstruction. The dotted line in the drawings represents the normal position of the diaphragm. **A** The radiograph shows an example of left upper lobe collapse which is often the most difficult to identify; this is due to the hazy, ill-defined shadowing on the PA view. **B** The collapsed left upper lobe is more easily seen on the lateral view (line indicates posterior margin of collapsed left upper lobe). **C** Radiograph of collapsed left lower lobe (arrow) causing increased density behind heart and loss of normal clarity between lung and both the left hemidiaphragm and descending thoracic aorta.

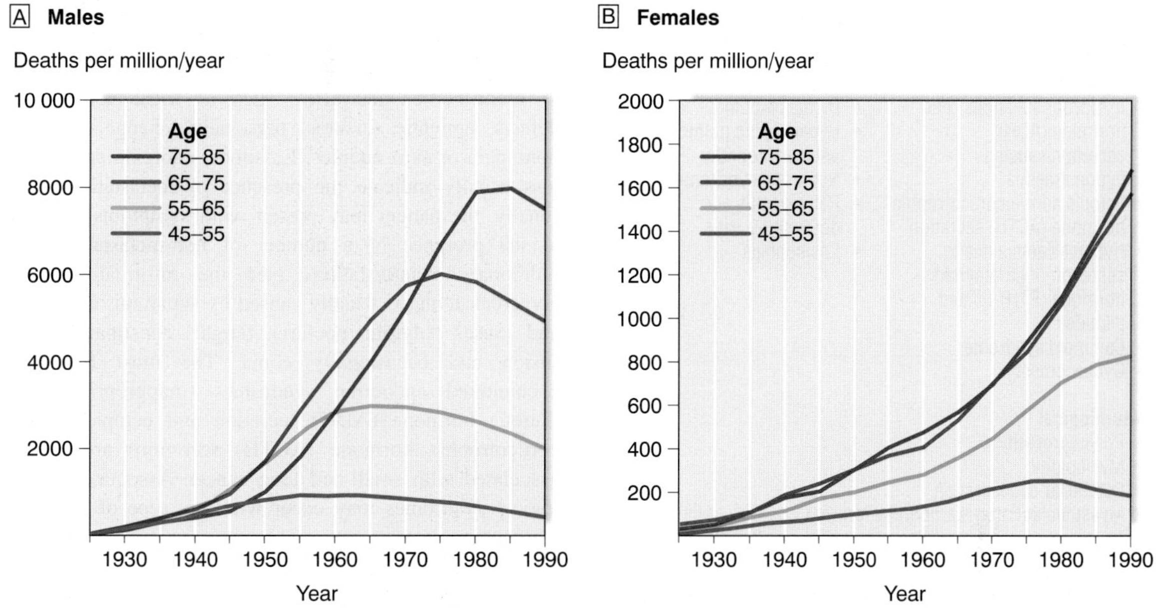

Fig. 4.32 Mortality trends from lung cancer in England and Wales, 1921–90 by age and year of death. A Males. B Females.
Note the recent decline in mortality from lung cancer in men, reflecting a change in smoking habit.

can attain a very large size without producing symptoms. Such a tumour, which is usually of the squamous type, may undergo central necrosis and cavitation, when it may have similar radiographic features to a lung abscess (see Fig. 4.33).

Bronchial carcinoma may involve the pleura either directly or by lymphatic spread and extend into the chest wall, invading the intercostal nerves or the brachial plexus and causing severe pain. The primary tumour, or tumour within lymph node metastases, may spread into the mediastinum and invade or compress the pericardium, oesophagus, superior vena cava, trachea, phrenic or left recurrent laryngeal nerves. Lymphatic spread to supraclavicular and mediastinal lymph nodes is also frequently observed. Blood-borne metastases occur most commonly in liver, bone, brain, adrenals and skin. Even a small primary tumour may cause widespread metastatic deposits and this is a particular characteristic of small cell-type lung cancers.

Clinical features

Lung cancer may present in a number of different ways. Most commonly, symptoms reflect local involvement of the bronchus, but may also arise from spread to the chest wall or mediastinum, from distant blood-borne spread, or less commonly as a result of a variety of non-metastatic paraneoplastic syndromes (see the information box).

Cough is the most common early symptom; sputum is purulent if there is secondary infection. Bronchial obstruction may lead to pneumonia, and a recurrent pneumonia at

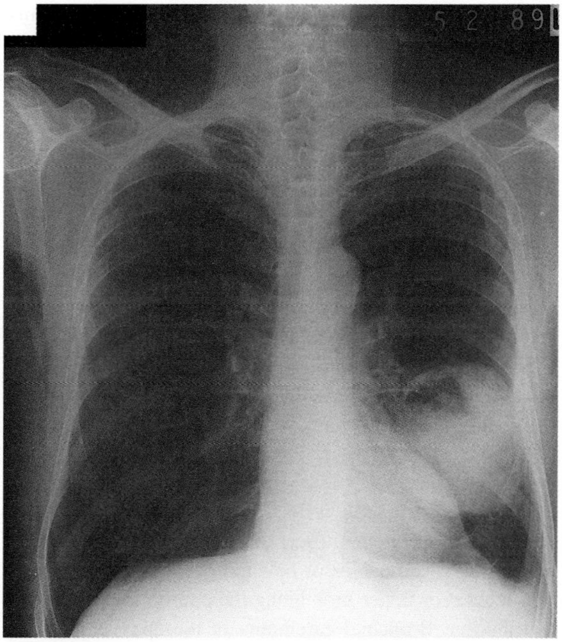

Fig. 4.33 Large cavitated bronchial carcinoma in left lower lobe.

NON-METASTATIC EXTRA-PULMONARY MANIFESTATIONS OF BRONCHIAL CARCINOMA

Endocrine
- Inappropriate antidiuretic hormone (ADH) secretion causing hyponatraemia
- Ectopic adrenocorticotrophic hormone (ACTH) secretion
- Hypercalcaemia due to secretion of parathyroid hormone (PTH)-related peptides
- Carcinoid syndrome
- Gynaecomastia

Neurological
- Polyneuropathy
- Myelopathy
- Cerebellar degeneration
- Myasthenia (Eaton–Lambert syndrome)

Other
- Digital clubbing
- Hypertrophic pulmonary osteoarthropathy
- Nephrotic syndrome
- Polymyositis and dermatomyositis
- Eosinophilia

the same site or one which is slow to respond to treatment, particularly in a cigarette smoker, should immediately suggest the possibility of bronchial carcinoma. A lung abscess may sometimes develop, leading to cough productive of large volumes of purulent sputum. A change in the character of the 'regular' cough of a smoker, particularly if it is associated with other new respiratory symptoms, should always alert the clinician to the possibility of bronchial carcinoma.

Haemoptysis is a common symptom, especially in tumours arising in large bronchi. Occasionally, central tumours invade large vessels, causing massive haemoptysis which may be fatal. Repeated episodes of scanty haemoptysis or blood-streaking of sputum in a smoker are highly suggestive of bronchial carcinoma and should always be investigated.

Breathlessness may reflect occlusion of a large bronchus, resulting in collapse of a lobe or lung or the development of a large pleural effusion. Stridor may occur where spread of the tumour to the subcarinal and paratracheal glands causes compression of the main bronchi or lower end of the trachea or, rarely, where the trachea is the site of the primary tumour.

Pleural pain usually reflects malignant invasion of the pleura, although it can reflect distal infection. Involvement of the intercostal nerves or brachial plexus may cause pain in the chest or upper limb along the appropriate nerve root distribution. Bronchial carcinoma in the apex of the lung ('superior sulcus tumour') may cause Horner's syndrome (ipsilateral partial ptosis, enophthalmos, a small pupil and hypohidrosis of the face—see Fig. 14.22, p. 971) due to involvement of the sympathetic chain at or above the stellate ganglion and/or Pancoast's syndrome (pain in the shoulder and inner aspect of the arm) caused by involvement of the lower part of the brachial plexus. Mediastinal spread may result in dysphagia.

The patient may also present with symptoms due to blood-borne metastases, such as focal neurological defects, epileptic seizures, personality change, jaundice, bone pain or skin nodules. Lassitude, anorexia and weight loss usually indicate the presence of metastatic spread. Finally, the patient may present with symptoms referable to the presence of a number of non-metastatic extra-pulmonary manifestations (see the information box). Hypercalcaemia is usually caused by squamous carcinoma and causes polyuria, nocturia, fatigue, constipation, confusion and occasionally coma. The most frequently encountered endocrine syndromes (inappropriate antidiuretic hormone (ADH) secretion and ectopic adrenocorticotrophic hormone (ACTH) secretion) are usually associated with small-cell lung cancer. Associated neurological syndromes may occur with any type of bronchial carcinoma.

Physical signs

Examination is usually normal unless there is significant bronchial obstruction, or the tumour has spread to the pleura or mediastinum. A tumour obstructing a large bronchus produces the physical signs of collapse (or occasionally obstructive emphysema) and may give rise to pneumonia that is characterised by a relative absence of physical signs and a slow response to treatment. A monophonic or unilateral rhonchus (wheeze) suggests the presence of a fixed bronchial obstruction, and the presence of stridor indicates obstruction at or above the level of the main carina. A hoarse voice associated with an ineffectual or 'bovine' cough usually indicates left recurrent laryngeal nerve palsy. Phrenic nerve paralysis causes unilateral diaphragmatic palsy and hence dullness to percussion and absent breath sounds at a lung base. Involvement of the pleura produces the physical signs of pleurisy or of pleural effusion (see p. 384). Bronchial carcinoma is also the most common cause of the superior vena cava syndrome, which presents initially as bilateral engorgement of the jugular veins and later as oedema affecting the face, neck and arms. Digital clubbing is often seen and may be a component part of a syndrome called hypertrophic pulmonary osteoarthropathy (HPOA), which is characterised by periostitis of the long bones, most commonly the distal tibia, fibula, radius and ulna. This gives rise to pain and tenderness in the affected joints and often pitting oedema over the anterior aspect of the shin. Radiographs of the painful bone show subperiosteal new bone formation. HPOA, while most frequently associated with bronchial carcinoma, can occur with other tumours and has been described in association with cystic fibrosis.

Investigations

The main aim of investigation is to confirm the diagnosis, establish the histological cell type and define the extent of the disease.

The common radiological features of bronchial carcinoma are illustrated in Figure 4.34. Further investigation to obtain

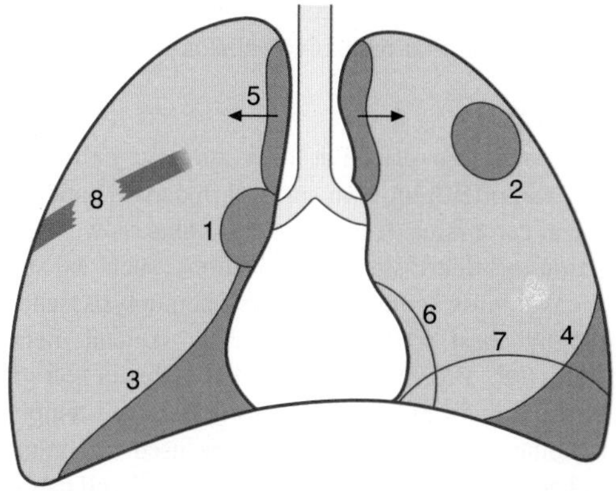

Fig. 4.34 Common radiological presentations of bronchial carcinoma. (See the information box below for details)

COMMON RADIOLOGICAL PRESENTATIONS OF BRONCHIAL CARCINOMA
1 Unilateral hilar enlargement
Central tumour. Hilar glandular involvement. Beware—peripheral tumour in apical segment of a lower lobe can look like an enlarged hilar shadow on the PA radiograph
2 Peripheral pulmonary opacity (see p. 316)
Usually irregular but well circumscribed. May have irregular cavitation within it. Can be very large
3 Lung, lobe or segmental collapse
Usually caused by tumour within the bronchus causing occlusion. Lung collapse can be produced by compression of the main bronchus by enlarged lymph glands
4 Pleural effusion
Usually indicates tumour invasion of pleural space; very rarely a manifestation of infection in collapsed lung tissue distal to a bronchial carcinoma
5–7 Broadening of mediastinum, enlarged cardiac shadow, elevation of a hemidiaphragm
Paratracheal lymphadenopathy may cause widening of the upper mediastinum. A malignant pericardial effusion will cause enlargement of the cardiac shadow. If a raised hemidiaphragm is caused by phrenic nerve palsy, screening will show it to move paradoxically upwards when patient sniffs
8 Rib destruction
Direct invasion of the chest wall or blood-borne metastatic spread can cause osteolytic lesions of the ribs

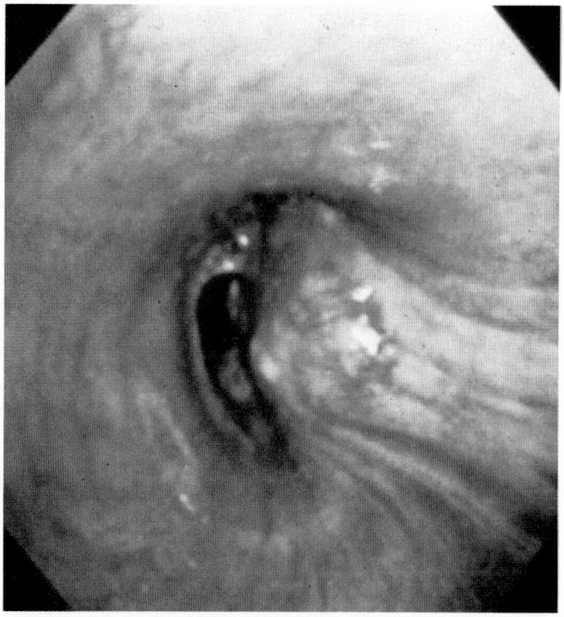

Fig. 4.35 Bronchoscopic view of a bronchogenic carcinoma. There is distortion of mucosal folds, partial occlusion of the airway lumen and abnormal tumour tissue.

a histological diagnosis and determine operability is nearly always indicated.

Bronchoscopy is usually the most useful investigation as it can provide tissue (biopsies and bronchial brush samples) for pathological examination and allow direct assessment of the proximity of central tumours to the main carina (see Fig. 4.35). If abnormal tissue is not visible at bronchoscopy, bronchial washings and directed biopsies can be taken from the lung segment in which the tumour is shown to be located on radiological examination. In patients who are not fit enough for a bronchoscopy, examination of sputum cytology can be a valuable diagnostic aid (see Fig. 4.36 on p. 362). Pleural biopsy is indicated in all patients with pleural effusions. If bronchoscopy fails to obtain a cytological diagnosis, percutaneous needle biopsy under CT guidance is appropriate for peripheral tumours or mediastinoscopy for patients with suspected mediastinal involvement. Not infrequently, thoracoscopy or thoracotomy is required to obtain a definitive histological diagnosis. In patients with metastatic disease the diagnosis can often be confirmed by needle aspiration or biopsy of enlarged lymph nodes, skin lesions, where indicated, liver or bone marrow.

After establishing a histological diagnosis, investigations should focus on determining whether the tumour is operable. This requires excluding involvement of central mediastinal structures or spread of tumour to distant sites and ensuring that the patient's respiratory and cardiac function

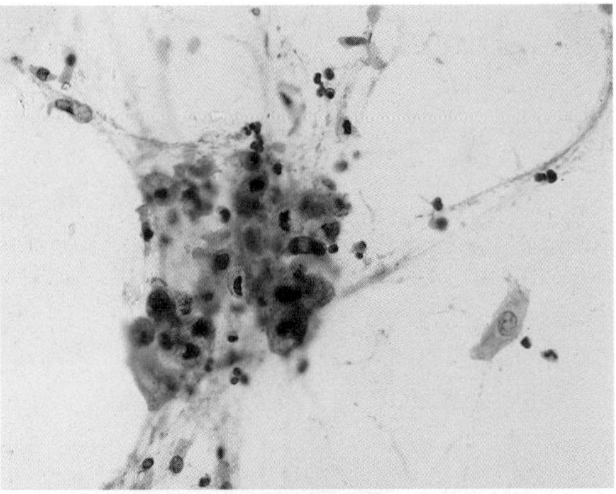

Fig. 4.36 Sputum sample showing a cluster of carcinoma cells. There is keratinlsation, showing orangeophillia of the cytoplasm, and non-keratinised forms are also seen. The nuclei are large and 'coal-black' in density. These are the features of squamous cell bronchogenic carcinoma.

is sufficient to allow surgical treatment (see the information box). The propensity of small-cell lung cancer to metastasise early dictates that very few patients with this tumour type are suitable for surgical intervention and that more detailed pre-operative staging is advisable before resection is contemplated. Head CT, radionuclide bone scanning, liver ultrasound and bone marrow biopsy can be reserved for patients with clinical, haematological or biochemical evidence of tumour spread to such sites.

Management

Cure can only be achieved by surgical resection. Unfortunately, in the majority of cases (approximately 85%) surgery is not possible or appropriate, and such patients can only be offered palliative therapy. Radiotherapy, and in some cases chemotherapy, can relieve distressing symptoms.

CONTRAINDICATIONS TO SURGICAL RESECTION IN BRONCHIAL CARCINOMA

- Distant metastasis (M1)
- Invasion of central mediastinal structures including heart, great vessels, trachea and oesophagus (T4)
- Malignant pleural effusion (T4)
- Contralateral mediastinal nodes (N3)
- FEV_1 < 0.8 litres
- Severe or unstable cardiac or other medical condition

N.B. In otherwise fit individuals, direct extension of tumour into the chest wall, diaphragm, mediastinal pleura, pericardium or to within 2 cm of the main carina does not exclude surgery. Though surgically resectable, patients with N2 (ipsilateral mediastinal) nodes may require neoadjuvant or adjuvant therapy.

Surgical treatment

As discussed, careful staging is essential prior to surgical resection and equal attention must be given to the patient's respiratory reserve and cardiac status. This, coupled with improvements in surgical and post-operative care, now offers 5-year survival rates of > 75% in stage I disease (N0, tumour confined within visceral pleura) and 55% in stage II disease, which includes resection in patients with ipsilateral peribronchial or hilar node involvement.

Radiotherapy

While much less effective than surgery, radical radiotherapy can offer long-term survival in certain patients with bronchial carcinoma. It is of greatest value, however, in the palliation of distressing complications such as superior vena caval obstruction, recurrent haemoptysis, and pain caused by chest wall invasion or by skeletal metastatic deposits (see Fig. 12.11A, p. 812). Obstruction of the trachea and main bronchi can also be relieved temporarily by radiotherapy. Radiotherapy can be used in conjunction with chemotherapy in the treatment of small-cell carcinoma and is particularly efficient at preventing the development of brain metastasis in patients who have had a 'complete' response to chemotherapy. Continuous hyperfractionated accelerated radiotherapy (CHART), in which a similar total dose is given in smaller but more frequent fractions, offers better survival prospects than conventional schedules.

Chemotherapy

The treatment of small-cell carcinoma with combinations of cytotoxic drugs, sometimes in combination with radiotherapy, can increase the median survival of patients with this highly malignant type of bronchial carcinoma from 3 months to well over a year. Combination chemotherapy leads to better outcomes than single-agent treatment. In particular, oral etoposide leads to more toxicity and worse survival than standard combination chemotherapy. Current recommendations include i.v. cyclophosphamide, doxorubicin and vincristine or i.v. cisplatin and etoposide. The above regimens are given every 3 weeks for 3–6 cycles. Nausea and vomiting peak for 3 days after each cycle of chemotherapy and are best treated with $5\text{-}HT_3$ receptor antagonists.

The use of combinations of chemotherapeutic drugs requires considerable medical skill and expertise and it is recommended that such treatment should only be given under the supervision of clinicians experienced in such treatment. In general, chemotherapy is far less effective in non-small-cell bronchial cancers. However, recent studies in such patients using platinum-based chemotherapy regimens have shown a 30% response rate associated with a small increase in survival.

Laser therapy

Laser treatment via a fibreoptic bronchoscope is essentially palliative, the aim being to destroy tumour tissue occluding major airways to allow re-aeration of collapsed lung. The best results are achieved in tumours of the main bronchi.

General aspects of management

As in other forms of carcinoma, effective communication, pain relief and attention to diet are important (see Ch. 16). Hypercalcaemia is an uncommon but important complication of lung cancer, particularly squamous cell carcinoma. Treatment in the acute situation involves intravenous rehydration, maintenance of a good urine output and administration of bisphosphonates. Thereafter, steroids may be effective and mithramycin may be necessary to maintain a normal blood calcium (see p. 576). Demeclocycline can be useful for controlling inappropriate ADH secretion in patients with small-cell lung cancer. The management of malignant pleural effusions is outlined on page 386.

Prognosis

The overall prognosis in bronchial carcinoma is very poor, with around 80% of patients dying within a year of diagnosis and less than 6% of patients surviving 5 years after diagnosis. The best prognosis is with well-differentiated squamous-cell tumours which have not metastasised and are amenable to surgical treatment. The clinical features and prognosis of other less common benign and malignant tumours of the lung are given in Table 4.16.

SECONDARY TUMOURS OF THE LUNG

Blood-borne metastatic deposits in the lungs may be derived from many primary tumours (see p. 356). The secondary deposits are usually multiple and bilateral. Often there are no respiratory symptoms and the diagnosis is made by radiological examination. Breathlessness may be the only symptom if a considerable amount of lung tissue has been replaced by metastatic tumour. Endobronchial deposits are uncommon but can cause haemoptysis and lobar collapse.

PULMONARY LYMPHATIC CARCINOMATOSIS

Lymphatic infiltration may develop in patients with carcinoma of the breast, stomach, bowel, pancreas or bronchus. This grave condition causes severe and rapidly progressive breathlessness associated with marked hypoxaemia. The diagnosis is often suggested by the chest radiograph, which shows diffuse pulmonary shadowing radiating from the hilar regions, often associated with septal lines.

TUMOURS OF THE MEDIASTINUM

The mediastinum can be divided into four major compartments with reference to the lateral chest radiograph (see Fig. 4.37, p. 364).

- superior mediastinum—above a line drawn between the lower border of the 4th thoracic vertebra and the upper end of the body of the sternum
- anterior mediastinum—in front of the heart
- middle mediastinum—between the anterior and posterior compartments
- posterior mediastinum—behind the heart.

A variety of conditions can present radiologically as a mediastinal mass (see the information box, p. 364).

Benign tumours and cysts arising within the mediastinum are frequently diagnosed when radiological examination of the chest is undertaken for some other reason. In general, they do not invade vital structures but may cause symptoms by compressing the trachea or occasionally the superior vena cava. A dermoid cyst may very occasionally rupture into a bronchus.

Table 4.16 Rarer types of lung tumour

Tumour	Status	Histology	Typical presentation	Prognosis
Adenosquamous carcinoma	Malignant	Tumours with areas of unequivocal squamous and adeno differentiation	Peripheral or central lung mass	Stage-dependent
Carcinoid tumour	Low-grade malignant	Neuro-endocrine differentiation	Bronchial obstruction, cough	95% 5-year survival with resection
Bronchial gland adenoma	Benign	Salivary gland differentiation	Tracheobronchial irritation/obstruction	Local resection curative
Bronchial gland carcinoma	Low-grade malignant	Salivary gland differentiation	Tracheobronchial irritation/obstruction	Local recurrence occurs
Hamartoma	Benign	Mesenchymal cells, cartilage	Peripheral lung nodule	Local resection curative
Bronchoalveolar carcinoma	Malignant	Tumour cells line alveolar spaces	Alveolar shadowing, productive cough	Variable, worse if multifocal

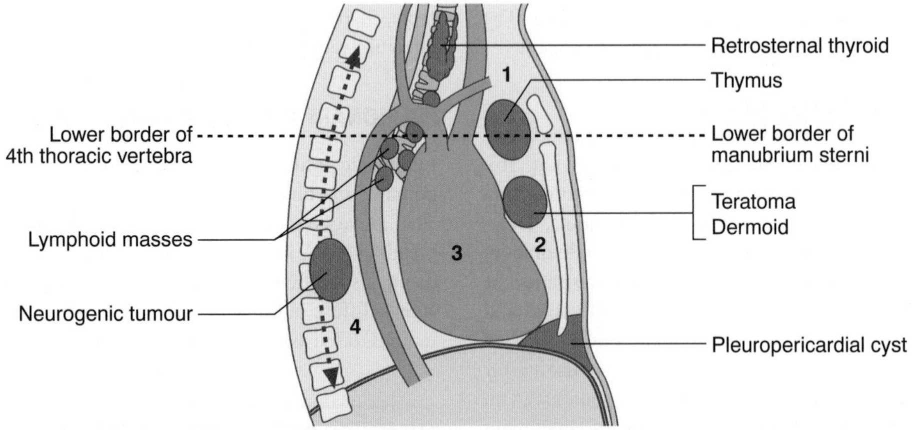

Fig. 4.37 The divisions of the mediastinum described in the diagnosis of mediastinal masses. (1) Superior mediastinum. (2) Anterior mediastinum. (3) Middle mediastinum. (4) Posterior mediastinum. Sites of the more common mediastinal tumours are also illustrated.

SOME CAUSES OF A MEDIASTINAL MASS

Superior mediastinum
- Retrosternal goitre
- Vascular lesion
  - Persistent left superior vena cava
  - Prominent left subclavian artery
- Thymic tumour
- Dermoid cyst
- Lymphoma
- Aortic aneurysm

Anterior mediastinum
- Retrosternal goitre
- Dermoid cyst
- Thymic tumour
- Lymphoma
- Aortic aneurysm
- Germ cell tumour
- Pericardial cyst
- Hernia through the diaphragmatic foramen of Morgagni

Posterior mediastinum
- Neurogenic tumour
- Paravertebral abscess
- Oesophageal lesion
- Aortic aneurysm
- Foregut duplication

Middle mediastinum
- Bronchial carcinoma
- Lymphoma
- Sarcoidosis
- Bronchogenic cyst
- Hiatus hernia

Malignant mediastinal tumours are distinguished by their power to invade as well as compress structures such as bronchi and lungs (see the information box on p. 365). As a result, even a small malignant tumour can produce symptoms, although as a rule the tumour has attained a considerable size before this happens. Included in this category are mediastinal lymph node metastases, lymphomas, leukaemia, malignant thymic tumours and germ cell tumours. Aortic and innominate aneurysms have destructive features resembling those of malignant mediastinal tumours.

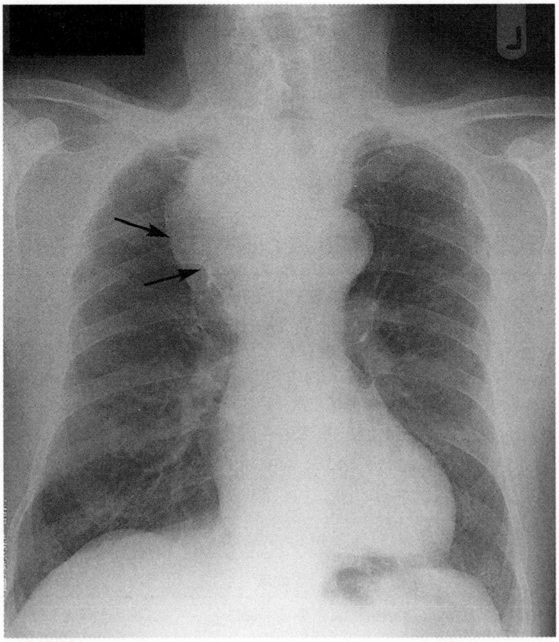

Fig. 4.38 Large mass (intrathoracic goitre—arrows) extending from right upper mediastinum.

Investigations

Radiological examination

A benign mediastinal tumour generally appears as a sharply circumscribed opacity situated mainly in the mediastinum but often encroaching on one or both lung fields (see Fig. 4.38). A malignant mediastinal tumour seldom has a clearly

SYMPTOMS AND SIGNS PRODUCED BY MALIGNANT INVASION OF THE STRUCTURES OF THE MEDIASTINUM

- Trachea and main bronchi
  Stridor, breathlessness, cough, pulmonary collapse
- Oesophagus
  Dysphagia, oesophageal displacement or obstruction on barium swallow examination
- Phrenic nerve
  Diaphragmatic paralysis
- Left recurrent laryngeal nerve
  Paralysis of left vocal cord giving rise to hoarseness and 'bovine' cough
- Sympathetic trunk
  Horner's syndrome
- Superior vena cava
  SVC obstruction results in non-pulsatile distension of neck veins, oedema and cyanosis of head, neck, hands and arms. Dilated anastomotic veins on chest wall
- Pericardium
  Pericarditis and/or pericardial effusion

defined margin and often presents as a general broadening of the mediastinal shadow. CT together with MRI are the investigations of choice for mediastinal tumours.

Bronchoscopy
Bronchoscopy should be carried out in most patients because bronchial carcinoma is a common cause of mediastinal tumour by secondary lymphatic spread.

Surgical exploration
If enlarged lymph nodes are suspected in the anterior mediastinum, tissue from these nodes can be removed for histological examination by mediastinoscopy. However, surgical exploration of the chest with removal of part or all of the tumour is often required to obtain a histological diagnosis.

Management
Benign mediastinal tumours should be removed surgically because most produce symptoms sooner or later. Some of them, particularly cysts, may become infected while others, especially neural tumours, have the potential to undergo malignant transformation. The operative mortality is low providing there is not a relative contraindication to surgical treatment such as coexisting cardiovascular disease, COPD or extreme age.

The treatment of lymphoma and leukaemia is described on pages 782 and 772, respectively. The management of malignant thymomas is surgical. Lymph node metastases from bronchial carcinoma often respond well, though temporarily, to radiotherapy or, in the case of small-cell carcinoma, to chemotherapy. Complications such as superior vena caval and tracheal obstruction can also be treated with radiotherapy or a combination of radiotherapy and chemotherapy, and the placement of internal stents is now possible for localised obstruction of both these structures.

FURTHER INFORMATION ON TUMOURS OF THE BRONCHUS AND LUNG

Management of lung cancer 1998 Effective Health Care Bulletin 4: 1–11
Spiro S G 1997 New approaches to lung cancer. In: Farthing M J E (ed) Horizons in Medicine no. 8. Royal College of Physicians, London, pp. 249–258
Woll P J 1991 Growth factors and lung cancer. Thorax 46: 924–929

INTERSTITIAL AND INFILTRATIVE PULMONARY DISEASES

INTERSTITIAL PULMONARY DISEASES

Interstitial lung diseases are a heterologous group of conditions caused by diffuse thickening of the alveolar walls with inflammatory cells and exudate (e.g. the acute respiratory distress syndrome—ARDS), granulomas (e.g. sarcoidosis), haemorrhage (e.g. Goodpasture's syndrome, see p. 444) and/or fibrosis (e.g. fibrosing alveolitis). Some are the result of exposure to known agents (e.g. asbestos), whereas in others, such as sarcoidosis, the cause is unknown. Lung disease may occur in isolation, or as part of a systemic connective tissue disorder—for example, in rheumatoid arthritis and systemic lupus erythematosus. Interstitial lung diseases may present acutely, as in acute drug reactions and ARDS, but more often the natural history is one of slowly progressive loss of alveolar-capillary gas exchange units over months or even years. This relentless progression of increased lung stiffness, disordered matching of ventilation and perfusion, and gas transfer defects results in worsening exertional dyspnoea which in many cases eventually progresses to respiratory failure, pulmonary hypertension, cor pulmonale and death.

Aetiology
There is a very wide range of causes of interstitial lung disease (see the information box). Some, like sarcoidosis,

SOME CAUSES OF INTERSTITIAL LUNG DISEASE

- Sarcoidosis
- Cryptogenic fibrosing alveolitis
- Exposure to organic dusts, e.g. farmer's lung, bird fancier's lung
- Exposure to inorganic dusts, e.g. asbestosis, silicosis
- As part of systemic inflammatory disease, e.g. acute respiratory distress syndrome, fibrosing alveolitis in connective tissue disorders
- Some forms of pulmonary eosinophilia
- Exposure to irradiation and drugs
- Rare disorders, e.g. alveolar proteinosis, histiocytosis

are quite common whereas others are rare. Despite the different causes and pathological processes involved, many interstitial lung diseases give rise to similar symptoms, physical signs, radiological changes and disturbances of pulmonary function and are therefore worthy of collective consideration. Nevertheless, the various underlying aetiologies present very different implications for prognosis and therapy. Moreover, interstitial lung diseases may be confused with other conditions (see the information box) with similar clinical and radiological features. Therefore a general approach to interstitial lung disease will be considered before a more detailed description of some specific disorders.

CONDITIONS WHICH MIMIC INTERSTITIAL LUNG DISEASES

Infection
- Viral pneumonia
- *Pneumocystis carinii*
- *Mycoplasma pneumoniae*
- Tuberculosis
- Parasites, e.g. filariasis
- Fungal infiltration

Malignancy
- Leukaemia and lymphoma
- Lymphatic carcinomatosis
- Multiple metastases
- Alveolar cell carcinoma

Pulmonary oedema

Pulmonary haemorrhage

Aspiration

Diagnosis of interstitial lung disease: a general approach

The first task is to differentiate the disorder from other conditions which can mimic interstitial lung diseases (ILDs) (see the information box), and then to determine which of the many causes of ILD is implicated. Establishing a diagnosis is important for a number of reasons. Firstly, there are prognostic implications; for example, sarcoidosis is usually self-limiting, whereas cryptogenic fibrosing alveolitis (see p. 369) is often fatal. Secondly, establishing a specific diagnosis will avoid inappropriate treatment; for example, the powerful immunosuppressive regimens used for some cases of cryptogenic fibrosing alveolitis would be undesirable if the underlying condition was extrinsic allergic alveolitis (see p. 371). Thirdly, some ILDs can be expected to respond better than others to treatment, e.g. a good response to corticosteroids could be predicted in sarcoidosis (see p. 367), whereas the prognosis would need to be more guarded in cryptogenic fibrosing alveolitis (see p. 370). Finally, a lung biopsy taken when the patient is already established on empirical immunosuppressive therapy is not only associated with a higher morbidity and mortality, but the tissue obtained is more difficult to interpret histologically, and therefore it is desirable to be confident about the diagnosis before starting any therapy.

Establishing a diagnosis often presents a considerable clinical challenge, necessitating meticulous attention to the history and physical signs together with the judicious and selective use of investigations.

History

The duration of disease may sometimes be difficult to ascertain. In the early stages particularly, gradually progressive shortness of breath on exertion may be the only symptom, and hence the patient may not present clinically until there is quite extensive lung pathology. It is clearly important to elicit a detailed history of exposure to organic dusts, inorganic dusts and drugs, including the degree and duration of such exposure. Contact with birds at home or in the working environment is the cause of the most common form of extrinsic allergic alveolitis, but enquiry about birds at home is often overlooked. A history of rashes or joint pains may suggest an underlying connective tissue disorder.

Physical signs

In many cases, especially in early disease, there may be few, if any, physical signs. In advanced disease tachypnoea and cyanosis may be obvious at rest, and there may be signs of pulmonary hypertension and right heart failure. Digital clubbing may be prominent, particularly in cryptogenic fibrosing alveolitis or asbestosis. There may be restriction of lung expansion and showers of end-inspiratory crepitations on auscultation over the lower zones posteriorly and laterally. Extra-pulmonary signs, including lymphadenopathy or uveitis, may be present in sarcoidosis (see the information box, p. 368) and arthropathies or rashes may suggest an ILD occurring as a manifestation of a connective tissue disorder (see p. 374).

Investigations

Laboratory investigations

No single blood test is diagnostic for a particular interstitial lung disease. Some laboratory tests may be useful in indicating systemic disease or providing crude indices of disease activity. The ESR and C-reactive protein may be non-specifically elevated. Serological tests may be of some value: antinuclear antibodies, rheumatoid factor etc. in connective tissue diseases, and anti-glomerular basement membrane antibodies in Goodpasture's syndrome (see p. 444). Serum levels of angiotensin-converting enzyme (ACE) may be elevated in sarcoidosis, but this test is not specific for sarcoidosis.

Radiology

The chest radiograph may show a fine reticular shadowing, a reticulo-nodular or even a nodular pattern of infiltration at the bases and peripherally (see Fig. 4.39A). In advanced disease there may be cystic areas and honeycombing.

High-resolution CT is extremely valuable in detecting early interstitial lung disease and assessing the extent and type of involvement (see Fig. 4.39B), and is also helpful in identifying hilar and paratracheal lymphadenopathy, particularly in sarcoidosis.

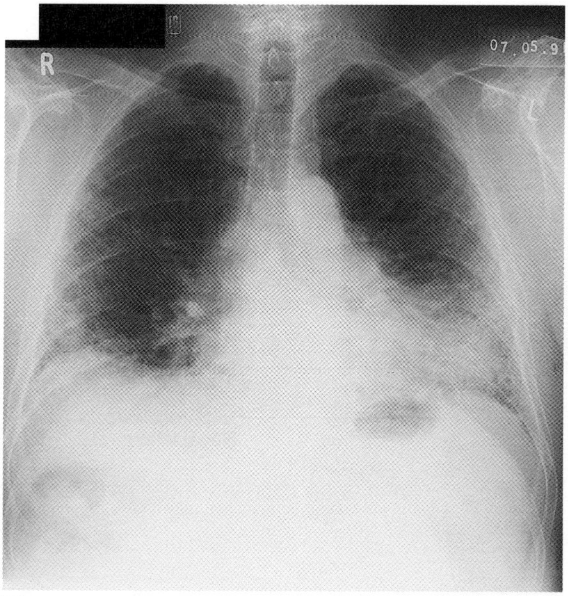

A

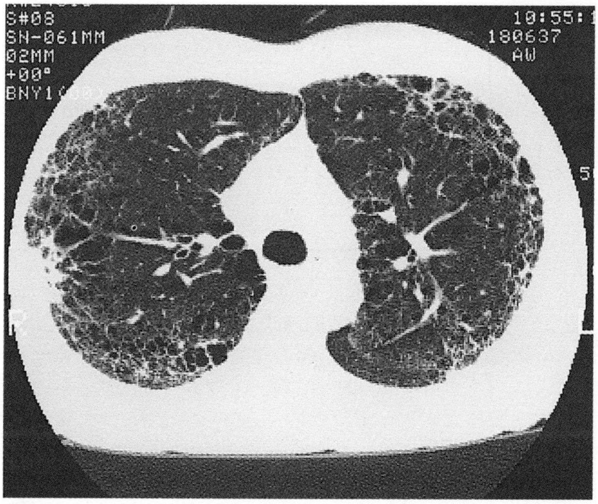

B

Fig. 4.39 Cryptogenic fibrosing alveolitis. A Chest radiograph showing bilateral, predominantly lower zone and peripheral coarse reticular-nodular shadowing and small lungs. B The CT shows honeycombing and scarring which is most marked peripherally.

Bronchoscopy and bronchoalveolar lavage

Bronchoalveolar lavage is not often of diagnostic value, but there are some important exceptions. Increased numbers of lymphocytes in bronchoalveolar lavage fluid occur in sarcoidosis and extrinsic allergic alveolitis, whereas a neutrophilia is suggestive of cryptogenic fibrosing alveolitis or pneumoconiosis. In the rare disease, alveolar proteinosis, copious lipoproteinaceous material is recovered in the lavage fluid, and large numbers of iron-laden macrophages are seen in pulmonary haemosiderosis (see Table 4.21, p. 376).

Histology. Examination of biopsy material is an important diagnostic procedure in most cases. Bronchial and transbronchial biopsies obtained via the fibreoptic bronchoscope will often establish the diagnosis in sarcoidosis and in some conditions which mimic interstitial lung disorders such as lymphatic carcinomatosis and certain infections. However, this approach provides only a small sample of tissue, and in less specific disorders such as cryptogenic fibrosing alveolitis a larger biopsy sample is usually necessary to yield a confident diagnosis. This used to necessitate a thoracotomy and open lung biopsy. However, the advent of video-assisted thoracoscopic (VAT) lung biopsy has considerably refined this procedure, with a reduction in morbidity.

SARCOIDOSIS

Sarcoidosis is a multisystem granulomatous disease. It is associated with imbalance between subsets of T lymphocytes and other disturbances of cell-mediated immunity, but the relationship between these phenomena and sarcoidosis has not yet been explained. The lesions are histologically similar to tuberculous follicles, apart from the absence of caseation and tubercle bacilli, but there is no convincing evidence that the disease is caused by any of the mycobacteria. Chronic beryllium poisoning produces a disease which mimics sarcoidosis both pathologically and clinically but exposure to beryllium is now extremely uncommon. Histological changes resembling those of sarcoidosis are occasionally seen in individual organs, such as lymph nodes, in conditions such as carcinoma and fungal infections, but these localised 'sarcoid reactions' are not associated with systemic sarcoidosis.

Pathology

The mediastinal and superficial lymph nodes, lungs, liver, spleen, skin, eyes, parotid glands and phalangeal bones are most frequently affected, but all tissues may be involved (see Figs 4.40 and 4.41 on pp. 368 and 369). The characteristic histological feature consists of non-caseating epithelioid follicles which usually resolve spontaneously, but fibrosis occurs in up to 20% of cases of pulmonary sarcoidosis and it is presently impossible to identify this group of patients prospectively. Sarcoidosis is seldom fatal unless it affects vital organs such as the heart or the central nervous system. Calcium metabolism may be disturbed, causing hypercalcaemia and, rarely, nephrocalcinosis and renal failure.

Clinical features

Since sarcoid lesions can develop in almost any tissue, there may be a number of unusual presentations, such as cardiac arrhythmias or cranial nerve palsies (see the information box). However, in most tissues the granulomas are usually 'silent' and the disease is most commonly detected

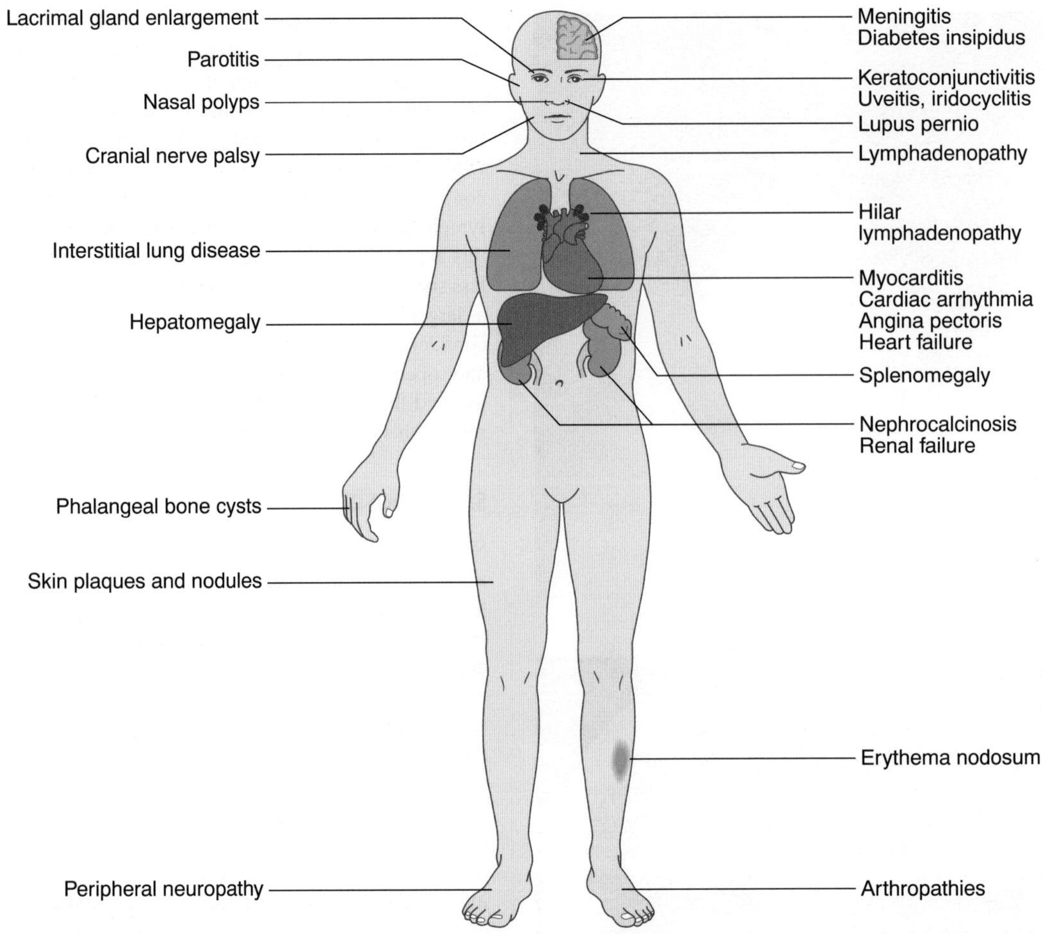

Fig. 4.40 The range of possible systemic involvement in sarcoidosis.

by an abnormal chest radiograph revealing bilateral hilar lymphadenopathy in an asymptomatic patient. With more extensive lung involvement there may be exertional dyspnoea or cough. Patients may also present with an 'acute' form of sarcoidosis, with erythema nodosum, arthropathy, uveitis and bilateral hilar lymphadenopathy. At the other extreme, patients with chronic and extensive sarcoidosis may complain of lassitude, fatigue, breathlessness and cough.

PRESENTATION OF SARCOIDOSIS

- Asymptomatic—abnormal routine chest radiograph (*c.*30%)
- Respiratory and constitutional symptoms (20–30%)
- Erythema nodosum and arthralgia (20–30%)
- Ocular symptoms (5–10%)
- Skin sarcoids (5%)
- Superficial lymphadenopathy (5%)
- Other (1%), e.g. hypercalcaemia, diabetes insipidus

Investigations

Skin sensitivity to tuberculin is depressed or absent in most patients, and the Mantoux reaction is, therefore, a useful 'screening' test; a strongly positive reaction to one tuberculin unit virtually excludes sarcoidosis. Although the diagnosis can often be made with a fair measure of confidence from the clinical and radiological features (see the information box) and the tuberculin test, it should, if possible, be confirmed histologically by biopsy of a superficial lymph node or of a skin lesion when these are present. Transbronchial lung biopsy frequently (in 70–85% of cases, even in those with apparently normal radiology) confirms the diagnosis. Bronchoalveolar lavage usually yields fluid with an increased proportion of lymphocytes.

The plasma level of angiotensin-converting enzyme (ACE) is often elevated. While not specific for sarcoidosis, this test may be valuable in the assessment of disease activity and response to treatment. The chest radiographical

CHEST RADIOGRAPH CHANGES IN SARCOIDOSIS
Stage I
• Radiograph shows bilateral hilar enlargement, usually symmetrical; paratracheal nodes often enlarged • Spontaneous resolution usually within 1 year in majority of cases. Often asymptomatic, but may be associated with erythema nodosum and arthralgia
Stage II
• Radiograph shows a combination of hilar glandular enlargement and pulmonary opacities which are often diffuse, but not always • Patients usually asymptomatic. Spontaneous improvement occurs in majority
Stage III
• Radiograph shows diffuse pulmonary shadows without evidence of hilar adenopathy. Evidence of pulmonary fibrosis may be present or develop • Disease less likely to resolve spontaneously. Pulmonary fibrosis can cause breathlessness, pulmonary hypertension and cor pulmonale

features have been used to stage sarcoidosis (see the information box).

When parenchymal lung disease is significant there may be disordered pulmonary function tests with a reduction in gas transfer and typical restrictive abnormalities occurring in more advanced disease, particularly if fibrosis has occurred.

In stage III sarcoidosis assessment of disease progression is by repeated measurement of lung volumes, carbon monoxide transfer factor and serial chest radiographs.

Hypercalcaemia may occur but seldom causes symptoms. Corticosteroid treatment may be necessary to avert renal complications of hypercalcaemia.

Management

Stage I and stage II disease usually resolves spontaneously and treatment is seldom required but occasionally patients with persistent erythema nodosum, pyrexia and arthralgia, or iridocyclitis require oral corticosteroid therapy for a short period.

Symptomatic stage III pulmonary sarcoidosis and sarcoidosis involving the eyes or other vital organs usually need to be treated with corticosteroids which may have to be continued for several years. Sarcoidosis usually responds rapidly to prednisolone 20–40 mg daily for 4 weeks; thereafter the disease is usually suppressed by a maintenance dose of 7.5–10 mg daily, or 20 mg daily on alternate days.

CRYPTOGENIC FIBROSING ALVEOLITIS

Cryptogenic fibrosing alveolitis (CFA) exemplifies many of the typical features of interstitial lung disease. By definition this form of fibrosing alveolitis is not associated with an overt systemic or connective tissue disorder, although the Epstein–Barr virus, exposure to metal and wood dusts, and certain drugs such as antidepressants have been reported to be associated with the disease. CFA is about twice as common among cigarette smokers than in non-smokers.

CFA is probably not a single disease entity but a group of diseases with similar pathological changes. It is characterised histologically by cellular infiltration and thickening of alveolar walls, together with large mononuclear cells in alveolar spaces. There is a variable degree of fibrosis and in

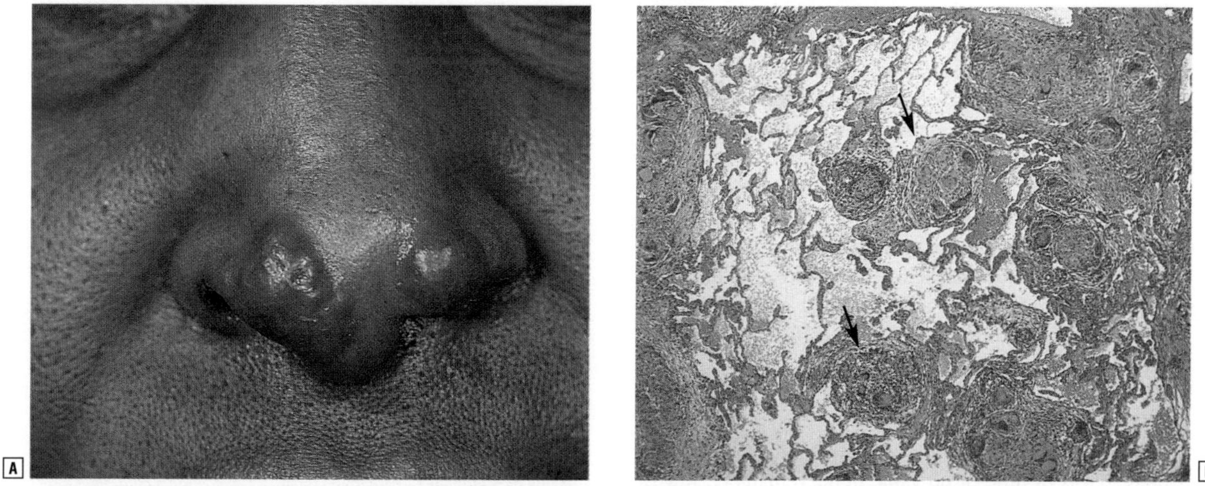

Fig. 4.41 Pathological lesions in sarcoidosis. A Nasal cutaneous sarcoid lesions. B Histology of sarcoidosis in the lung, showing non-caseating granulomas (arrows).

most cases progressive fibrosis occurs. Whatever the cause of fibrosing alveolitis, lung macrophages appear to become 'activated' and produce chemotactic and activating factors for neutrophils which injure tissues by the release of proteinases and oxidants. Lung macrophages are probably also involved in fibrosis by their release of fibronectin and a range of pro-fibrotic cytokines and growth factors which stimulate fibroblasts to proliferate and secrete scar tissue matrix proteins.

Clinical features

Progressive exertional breathlessness is usually the presenting symptom, often accompanied by persistent dry cough. In most patients there is gross clubbing of the fingers and toes. Chest expansion may be poor and numerous bilateral end-inspiratory crepitations are audible on auscultation, particularly over the lower zones posteriorly.

Investigations

Blood tests are of no value in confirming a diagnosis of CFA. However, rheumatoid factor and antinuclear factor can be detected in 30–50% of patients. Lactate dehydrogenase is elevated in most cases.

The chest radiograph shows diffuse pulmonary opacities which are usually most obvious in the lower zones and peripherally (see Fig. 4.39, p. 367). The hemidiaphragms are high and the lungs appear small. In advanced disease the chest radiographs may show 'honeycomb lung', in which diffuse pulmonary shadowing is interspersed with small cystic translucencies. 'Honeycomb lung' is also a characteristic feature of rare diseases such as histiocytosis X and tuberous sclerosis (see Table 4.21, p. 376). High-resolution CT can reveal a dramatic picture in late disease (see p. 367). It may be particularly useful in early disease when chest radiograph changes may be slight or absent.

Pulmonary function tests show a restrictive ventilatory defect with proportionate reduction in VC and FEV_1. The carbon monoxide transfer factor is low and there is an overall reduction in lung volume. In early disease there is arterial hypoxaemia on exercise; later, arterial hypoxaemia and hypocapnia are present at rest.

Bronchoalveolar lavage fluid usually contains increased numbers of neutrophils and eosinophils. Transbronchial biopsy is often of no help because the small size of the biopsy specimens does not allow the pathologist to differentiate between fibrosing alveolitis and other forms of pulmonary fibrosis. Lung biopsy is therefore necessary to establish a diagnosis in most patients.

Management

Treatment with corticosteroids is beneficial in about 30% of patients but is of little or no value in the remainder, few of whom survive for more than 5 years. A trial of prednisolone is indicated in most patients with progressive disease and should be given in a daily dose of 40–60 mg for 6–8 weeks. Assessment of response to this treatment is by repeat measurement of lung volumes, transfer factor and chest radiograph. Prednisolone should be withdrawn rapidly over a few weeks if there is no response. Should objective evidence of improvement be demonstrated the dose can be reduced gradually to a maintenance dose of 10 or 12.5 mg daily. In patients in whom it is not possible to reduce the dose of prednisolone below 15 or 20 mg daily without evidence of relapse, azathioprine in a dose of 1.5–2 mg/kg daily should be added in an attempt to reduce the dose of prednisolone to levels which are less likely to give side-effects. Alternative regimens include azathioprine 100 mg daily plus prednisolone 20 mg in a single oral morning dose on alternate days, or cyclophosphamide 2–3 mg/kg daily plus 20 mg prednisolone on alternate days.

Prognosis

The median survival time of untreated cases is about 4 years. Most deaths occur in patients over the age of 55, with males predominating. The rate of progression of pulmonary changes varies considerably from death within a few months to survival with minimal symptoms for many years. Occasionally the disease process may 'burn out', but in the majority of patients the disease is progressive, even in those who have responded to treatment. Single-lung transplantation should be considered in young patients with advanced disease.

LUNG DISEASES DUE TO EXPOSURE TO ORGANIC DUSTS

A wide range of organic agents may cause respiratory

Table 4.17 Some examples of lung diseases caused by organic dusts

Disorder	Source	Antigen/agent
Farmer's lung*	Mouldy hay, straw, grain	*Micropolyspora faenae* *Aspergillus fumigatus*
Bird fancier's lung*	Avian excreta, proteins and feathers	Avian serum proteins
Malt worker's lung*	Mouldy maltings	*Aspergillus clavatus*
Byssinosis	Textile industries	Cotton, flax, hemp dust
Air conditioner/ humidifier lung	Contamination of air conditioning	Thermophilic actinomycetes
Cheese worker's lung*	Mouldy cheese	*Aspergillus clavatus* *Penicillium casei*
Maple bark stripper's lung*	Bark from stored maple	*Cryptostroma corticale*

* Denotes lung disease presenting as extrinsic allergic alveolitis.

disorders (see Table 4.17). Disease results from a local immune response to animal proteins (e.g. bird fancier's lung) or fungal antigens in mouldy vegetable matter. The most common presentation has been termed extrinsic allergic alveolitis.

EXTRINSIC ALLERGIC ALVEOLITIS

In this condition the inhalation of certain types of organic dust produces a diffuse immune complex reaction in the walls of the alveoli and bronchioles.

The pathogenic mechanisms concerned in the production of extrinsic allergic alveolitis are not fully understood. It is thought that the disease develops in sensitised individuals mainly through a type III Arthus reaction, although type IV mechanisms are probably also important (see p. 34). When the antigen is inhaled, the immune complexes formed in antibody excess are precipitated very rapidly. Deposition of these immune complexes results in complement activation, causing a localised inflammatory reaction in the alveolar walls. Immunofluorescence has shown IgG, IgA and complement to be fixed in the pulmonary tissues when biopsy specimens are examined in the acute stages. The presence of granulomata in the alveolar walls provides some evidence for a type IV response also being involved. Bronchoalveolar lavage fluid from patients with extrinsic allergic alveolitis usually shows an increase in the number of lymphocytes.

Some of the agents which produce extrinsic allergic alveolitis, their source, and the names given to the resulting diseases are shown in Table 4.17. If patients with this disorder continue to be exposed to the relevant antigen they develop progressive lung fibrosis, leading to severe respiratory disability, pulmonary hypertension and cor pulmonale.

Clinical features

Extrinsic allergic alveolitis should be suspected when anyone regularly or intermittently exposed to organic dust complains, within a few hours of re-exposure to the same dust, of influenza-like symptoms including headache, muscle pains, malaise, pyrexia, dry cough and breathlessness without wheeze. When exposure is continuous, as is the case with the indoor pet bird at home, the presentation can be with breathlessness without systemic symptoms, and if the cause is not recognised this may result in the formation of irreversible pulmonary fibrosis.

Investigations

In the acute stage of the disease there may be end-inspiratory crepitations audible over both lungs. The chest radiograph shows diffuse micronodular shadowing, often more pronounced in the upper zones. Pulmonary function studies reveal a restrictive ventilatory defect with preservation or increase of the FEV_1/VC ratio. The PaO_2 is reduced and the $PaCO_2$ is often below normal because of over-ventilation. Diffusion capacity is impaired.

The diagnosis of extrinsic allergic alveolitis is usually based on the characteristic clinical and radiological features, together with the identification of a potential source of antigen at the patient's home or place of work. Reduction in the carbon monoxide transfer factor is the most sensitive functional abnormality. The diagnosis may be supported by a positive precipitin test or by more sensitive serological tests based on the enzyme-linked immunosorbent assay (ELISA) technique. However, it is also important to recognise that the great majority of farmers with positive precipitins do not have farmer's lung, and up to 15% of pigeon breeders may have positive serum precipitins and yet remain healthy. Where the diagnosis is suspected but the cause is not readily apparent it may be helpful to visit the patient's home or workplace. Occasionally, such as when a new agent is suspected, it may be necessary to prove the diagnosis by a provocation test; if positive, the inhalation of the relevant antigen is followed after 3–6 hours by pyrexia and a reduction in VC and gas transfer factor. Open lung biopsy may be necessary to establish a diagnosis.

Management

Mild forms of extrinsic allergic alveolitis rapidly subside when exposure to the antigen ceases. In acute cases prednisolone should be given for 3–4 weeks, starting with an oral dose of 30–40 mg per day. Severely hypoxaemic patients may require high-concentration oxygen therapy initially. Most patients recover completely, but the development of interstitial fibrosis causes permanent disability when there has been prolonged exposure to antigen.

BYSSINOSIS

Not all inhaled organic dusts cause interstitial infiltration. In byssinosis the initial lesion caused by cotton dust inhalation is acute bronchiolitis associated with symptoms and signs of generalised airflow obstruction, more in keeping with asthma. Initially, symptoms tend to recur after the weekend break ('Monday fever') but eventually become continuous. There is usually no radiological abnormality. Recovery usually follows removal from the dust hazard. Smokers have a greater incidence of byssinosis than non-smokers.

HUMIDIFIER FEVER

This is a disease with a similar pattern of symptoms to byssinosis. Fever and breathlessness may be a problem at the beginning of the week but often subside at the weekend. It is thought to be caused by water-borne micro-organisms from contaminated humidifiers in air-conditioning systems.

LUNG DISEASES DUE TO EXPOSURE TO INORGANIC DUSTS

In certain occupations, the inhalation of dusts, fumes or other noxious substances may give rise to specific pathological changes in the lungs. Generally, prolonged exposure to inorganic dusts (see Table 4.18) leads to diffuse pulmonary fibrosis (the pneumoconioses), although berylliosis causes an interstitial granulomatous disease similar to sarcoidosis. The dusts themselves cause little direct damage to the lung parenchyma and the pathological result depends largely on the inflammatory and fibrotic responses to the particular dust. The fibrogenic properties of mineral dusts vary, silica being markedly fibrogenic whereas iron and tin are almost inert. The most important types of pneumoconiosis are coal worker's pneumoconiosis, silicosis and asbestosis.

Industrial inorganic gases and fumes can cause other respiratory diseases including acute pulmonary oedema and asthma (see Table 4.19). Industrial lung diseases may also arise from exposure to organic dusts, e.g. farmer's lung and other extrinsic allergic alveolitides.

Clearly, it is essential to elicit a detailed occupational history, both present and past, since a diagnosis of occupational lung disease can easily be overlooked and the patient may be eligible for compensation. It must also be emphasised that in many types of pneumoconiosis a long period of dust exposure is required before radiological changes appear, and these may precede clinical symptoms.

Notes on diagnosis and claims for benefits in pneumoconiosis, occupational asthma and other related occupational diseases in Britain are contained in government pamphlets. New industrial processes are constantly being introduced and it is necessary to remain alert to the possibility that they may be associated with occupational lung disease.

COAL WORKER'S PNEUMOCONIOSIS

This disease follows prolonged inhalation of coal dust. The condition is subdivided into simple pneumoconiosis and progressive massive fibrosis for clinical purposes and for certification. It must be emphasised that for certification purposes in Britain the diagnosis rests at present on radiological and not clinical features.

Table 4.19 Some lung diseases due to inorganic gases and fumes

Cause	Occupation	Disease
Irritant gases (chlorine, ammonia, phosgene, nitrogen dioxide)	Various (industrial accidents)	Acute lung injury ARDS
Cadmium	Welding and electroplating	COPD
Isocyanates (e.g. epoxy resins, paints)	Plastic, paints; manufacture of epoxy resins and adhesives	Bronchial asthma Eosinophilic pneumonia

Simple coal worker's pneumoconiosis

This is categorised radiologically into three grades, depending on the size and extent of the nodulation present. It does not progress if the miner leaves the industry.

Progressive massive fibrosis

In this form of the disease, large dense masses, single or multiple, occur mainly in the upper lobes. These may be irregular in shape and may cavitate. Tuberculosis may be a complication. The disease can be disabling, may shorten life expectancy and may progress even after the miner leaves the industry.

Cough and sputum from associated chronic bronchitis are frequently present. The sputum may be black (melanoptysis). Progressive breathlessness on exertion occurs in the later stages, and respiratory and right ventricular failure supervene as terminal events. There may be no abnormal physical signs in the chest but where present they are those of chronic obstructive airways disease.

Antinuclear factor is present in the serum of about 15% of patients with coal worker's pneumoconiosis. Rheumatoid

Table 4.18 Some lung diseases caused by exposure to inorganic dusts

Cause	Occupation	Description	Characteristic pathological features
Coal dust **Silica**	Coal mining Mining, quarrying, stone dressing, metal grinding, pottery, boiler scaling	Coal worker's pneumoconiosis Silicosis	Focal and interstitial fibrosis, centrilobular emphysema, progressive massive fibrosis
Asbestos	Demolition, ship breaking, manufacture of fireproof insulating materials and brake-pads, pipe and boiler lagging	Asbestos-related disease	Interstitial fibrosis, pleural disease, carcinoma of larynx and bronchus
Iron oxide	Arc welding	Siderosis	Mineral deposition only
Tin oxide	Tin mining	Stannosis	
Beryllium	Aircraft, atomic energy and electronics industries	Berylliosis	Granulomata, interstitial fibrosis

factor is present in some patients in whom rheumatoid arthritis coexists, with rounded fibrotic nodules 0.5–5 cm in diameter. These are mainly in the periphery of the lung fields and the association is known as Caplan's syndrome. This syndrome may also occur in other types of pneumoconiosis.

SILICOSIS

This disease is becoming rare as the standards of industrial hygiene improve. It is caused by the inhalation of fine free crystalline silicone dioxide (silica) dust or quartz particles.

Silica is a most fibrogenic dust and causes the development of hard nodules which coalesce as the disease progresses. Tuberculosis may modify the silicotic process with ensuing caseation and calcification. The radiological features are similar to those seen in coal worker's pneumoconiosis, though the changes tend to be more marked in the upper zones. The hilar shadows may be enlarged, and 'egg-shell' calcification in the hilar lymph nodes is a distinctive feature but does not occur in all patients. The disease progresses even when exposure to dust ceases. The patient should, therefore, be removed from the offending environment as soon as possible. Clinical features are similar to those of coal worker's pneumoconiosis.

ASBESTOSIS

The main types of the fibrous mineral, asbestos, are chrysotile (white asbestos), which accounts for 90% of the world's production, crocidolite (blue asbestos) and amosite (brown asbestos). Exposure occurs in the mining and milling of the mineral and in a variety of occupations (see Table 4.18).

Asbestos may cause laryngeal carcinoma and a variety of pleural and lung pathologies (see Fig. 4.42). Of these, only asbestosis, diffuse pleural fibrosis and mesothelioma automatically qualify for industrial injury benefit in Britain. Asbestosis was defined by the Advisory Committee on Asbestos (1979) as 'fibrosis of the lungs caused by asbestos dusts which may or may not be associated with fibrosis of the parietal or pulmonary layer of the pleura'.

Pulmonary fibrosis caused by the inhalation of asbestos fibres is characterised by increasing exertion breathlessness. Digital clubbing is usually present and end-inspiratory crepitations are audible over the lower zones of both lungs.

The radiological changes are usually confined to the lower two-thirds of the lung fields and comprise mottled shadows with some streaky opacities and sometimes 'honeycombing' (see Fig. 4.42). As a result, the cardiac silhouette often appears 'shaggy'.

The most important physiological abnormalities are a reduced carbon monoxide transfer factor, decreased lung volumes and a restrictive ventilatory defect.

Respiratory and right ventricular failure eventually supervene. The incidence of bronchial carcinoma is much increased, and is at least 10-fold in persons suffering from asbestosis who also smoke.

The diagnosis is usually easy to establish from the history of exposure to asbestos, the clinical features of end-inspiratory crepitations and digital clubbing, the pulmonary function test abnormalities and the chest radiograph which also often shows pleural plaques (see Fig. 4.42). Lung biopsy may be required to confirm the diagnosis but is not without risk and should not be undertaken solely for the purpose of allowing patients to claim benefit.

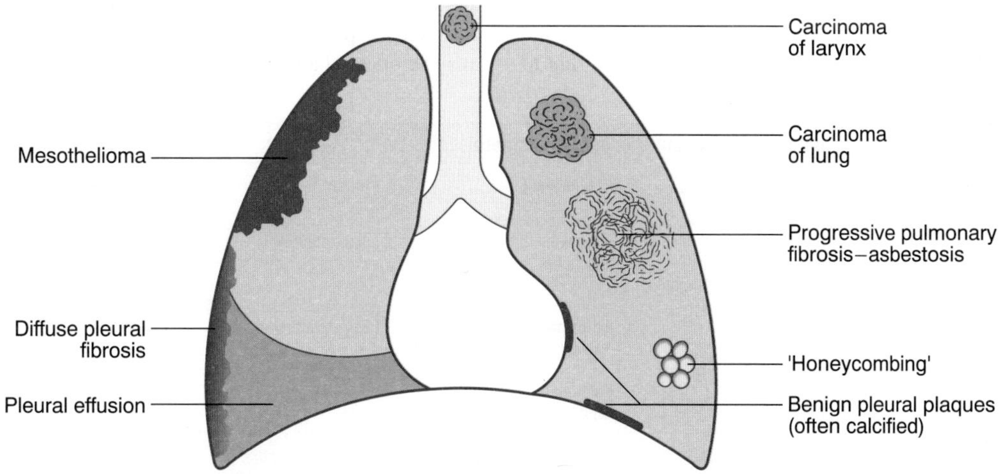

Fig. 4.42 Asbestos: the range of possible effects on the respiratory tract.

Management

No specific treatment is available. Corticosteroids are of no value in the management of asbestosis.

Prevention

Improvements in standards of industrial hygiene are now enforced by law in many countries; such measures as wearing respirators, damping dust and efficient ventilation systems are already proving effective in a number of industries.

LUNG DISEASES DUE TO SYSTEMIC INFLAMMATORY DISEASE

THE ACUTE (ADULT) RESPIRATORY DISTRESS SYNDROME

See page 1031.

RESPIRATORY INVOLVEMENT IN CONNECTIVE TISSUE DISORDERS

Fibrosing alveolitis is a recognised complication of most connective tissue diseases. The clinical features are usually indistinguishable from cryptogenic fibrosing alveolitis (see p. 369) and the response to immunosuppressive drugs is similarly unpredictable. Connective tissue disorders may also cause disease of the pleura, diaphragm and chest wall muscles (see Table 4.20). Pulmonary hypertension and cor pulmonale may result from advanced fibrosing alveolitis associated with connective tissue disorders.

Indirect associations between connective tissue disorders and respiratory complications include: those due to disease in other organs, e.g. thrombocytopenia causing haemoptysis; pulmonary toxic effects of drugs used to treat the connective tissue disorder; and secondary infection due to the disease itself, neutropenia or immunosuppressive drug regimens.

Rheumatoid disease

Fibrosing alveolitis is the most common pulmonary manifestation (rheumatoid lung). The clinical features, investigations, treatment and prognosis are similar to those of cryptogenic fibrosing alveolitis, although a rare variant of localised upper lobe fibrosis and cavitation has been described.

Pleural effusion is common, especially in men with seropositive disease. Effusions are usually small and unilateral but can be large and bilateral. Most resolve spontaneously. Biochemical testing shows an exudate (pleural protein > 30 g/l) with markedly reduced glucose levels and raised lactate dehydrogenase (LDH). Effusions that fail to resolve spontaneously may respond to a short course of oral prednisolone (30–40 mg daily), but some become chronic.

Pulmonary rheumatoid nodules do not usually cause symptoms and are detected on chest radiographs performed for other reasons. They are usually multiple and subpleural in site. Solitary nodules can look like primary bronchial carcinoma and when multiple the differential diagnosis includes pulmonary metastatic disease. Cavitation of nodules can raise the possibility of tuberculosis and cause pneumothorax. The combination of rheumatoid nodules and pneumoconiosis is known as Caplan's syndrome (see p. 373).

Bronchitis and bronchiectasis are both more common in rheumatoid patients. Rarely, the potentially fatal condition, obliterative bronchiolitis, may develop.

Systemic lupus erythematosus

Fibrosing alveolitis is a relatively uncommon manifestation of systemic lupus erythematosus. Pleuropulmonary involvement is more common in lupus than any other connective tissue disorder. Up to two-thirds of patients have repeated episodes of pleurisy, with or without effusions. Effusions may be bilateral and involve the pericardium.

Table 4.20 Respiratory complications of connective tissue disorders

Disorder	Airways	Parenchyma	Pleura	Diaphragm and chest wall
Rheumatoid arthritis	Bronchitis, obliterative bronchiolitis, bronchiectasis, crico-arytenoid arthritis, stridor	Fibrosing alveolitis, nodules, upper lobe fibrosis, infections	Pleurisy, effusion, pneumothorax	Poor healing of intercostal drain sites
Systemic lupus erythematosus	—	Fibrosing alveolitis, 'vasculitic' infarcts	Pleurisy, effusion	'Shrinking lungs'
Systemic sclerosis	Bronchiectasis	Pulmonary fibrosis, aspiration pneumonia	—	'Hidebound chest'
Dermatomyositis/ polymyositis	Bronchial carcinoma	Fibrosing alveolitis	—	Intercostal and diaphragmatic myopathy
Rheumatic fever	—	Pneumonia	Pleurisy, effusion	

Some patients with systemic lupus erythematosus present with exertional dyspnoea and orthopnoea but without overt signs of fibrosing alveolitis. The chest radiograph reveals elevated diaphragms, and pulmonary function testing shows reduced lung volumes. This condition has been described as 'shrinking lungs' and is thought to be caused by diaphragmatic myopathy.

Systemic sclerosis

Most patients with systemic sclerosis eventually develop diffuse pulmonary fibrosis; at necropsy more than 90% have evidence of lung fibrosis. In some patients it is indolent, but when progressive, like cryptogenic fibrosing alveolitis, the median survival time is around 4 years. Pulmonary fibrosis is rare in the CREST variant (see p. 859) of progressive systemic sclerosis.

Other pulmonary complications include recurrent aspiration pneumonias secondary to oesophageal disease. Rarely, sclerosis of the skin of the chest wall may be so extensive and cicatrising as to seriously restrict chest wall movement—the so-called 'hidebound chest'.

PULMONARY EOSINOPHILIA AND VASCULITIDES

This term is applied to a group of disorders of different aetiology in which lesions in the lungs produce a chest radiograph abnormality associated with an increase in the number of the eosinophil leucocytes in the peripheral blood. There is no satisfactory classification of this disparate group of disorders, but they can be divided into two main categories (see the information box).

Some causes of extrinsic pulmonary eosinophilia are also given in the information box. The most common disorder of this type in developed countries is allergic broncho-pulmonary aspergillosis (see p. 354) and in tropical countries the presence of microfilariae in the pulmonary capillaries (see p. 176) has to be considered.

PULMONARY EOSINOPHILIA

Extrinsic (cause known)

- Helminths
  e.g. *Ascaris, Toxocara, Filaria*
- Drugs
  Nitrofurantoin, para-aminosalicylic acid, sulphasalazine, imipramine, chlorpropamide, phenylbutazone
- Fungi
  e.g. *Aspergillus fumigatus*

Intrinsic (cause unknown)

- Cryptogenic eosinophilic pneumonia
- Churg–Strauss syndrome
- Hypereosinophilic syndrome
- Polyarteritis nodosa (rare)

CRYPTOGENIC EOSINOPHILIC PNEUMONIA

Cryptogenic eosinophilic pneumonia is more common in middle-aged females, and usually presents with malaise, fever, breathlessness and unproductive cough. The chest radiograph can show a variety of abnormal shadows, but they tend to be peripheral, often involve the upper zones and may be difficult to distinguish from the radiological features of pulmonary tuberculosis. Unless corticosteroids have been given, the peripheral blood eosinophil count is almost always very high, and the ESR and total serum IgE are elevated. Bronchoalveolar lavage reveals a very high proportion of eosinophils in the lavage fluid. Response to prednisolone (20–40 mg daily) is usually dramatic. Prednisolone treatment can usually be withdrawn after a few weeks without relapse, but long-term low-dose therapy is occasionally necessary to control the disease.

LUNG DISEASES DUE TO IRRADIATION AND DRUGS

RADIOTHERAPY

The lungs are exposed during radiotherapy treatment of lung tumours and also tumours of the breast, spine and oesophagus. The pulmonary effects of radiation are exacerbated by treatment with cytotoxic drugs, oxygen delivery and previous radiotherapy. Radiotherapy may cause acute damage to the lung, and also a chronic insidious scarring disease.

After pulmonary irradiation, acute radiation pneumonitis may present with cough and dyspnoea within 6–12 weeks. This acute form of lung damage may resolve spontaneously or respond to corticosteroid treatment. Chronic interstitial fibrosis presents later, usually with symptoms of exertional dyspnoea and cough. Established post-irradiation fibrosis does not usually respond to corticosteroid treatment.

DRUGS

Drugs may cause a number of parenchymal reactions including ARDS (see the information box on p. 376), eosinophilic reactions, and diffuse interstitial inflammation/scarring. Drugs can also cause other lung disorders including asthma (see p. 331), haemorrhage (e.g. anticoagulants, penicillamine) and occasionally pleural effusions and pleural thickening (e.g. hydralazine, isoniazid, methysergide). An ARDS-like syndrome of acute non-cardiogenic pulmonary oedema may present with dramatic onset of breathlessness, severe hypoxaemia and signs of alveolar oedema on the chest radiograph. This syndrome has been reported most frequently in cases of opiate overdose in drug addicts, but also after salicylate overdose, and there are occasional reports of its occurrence after therapeutic doses of drugs

DRUG-INDUCED RESPIRATORY DISEASE

Non-cardiogenic pulmonary oedema (ARDS)

- Hydrochlorothiazide
- Thrombolytics (streptokinase)
- I.v. β-adrenoceptor agonists (e.g. treatment of premature labour)
- Aspirin and opiates (in overdose)

Non-eosinophilic alveolitis

- Amiodarone, tocainide, flecainide, gold, nitrofurantoin, cytotoxic agents—especially bleomycin, busulphan, mitomycin C, methotrexate

Pulmonary eosinophilia

- Antimicrobials (nitrofurantoin, penicillin, tetracyclines, sulphonamides, nalidixic acid)
- Antirheumatic agents (gold, aspirin, penicillamine, naproxen)
- Cytotoxic drugs (bleomycin, methotrexate, procarbazine)
- Psychiatric drugs (chlorpromazine, dothiepin, imipramine)
- Anticonvulsants (carbamazepine, phenytoin)
- Others (sulphasalazine, nadolol)

Pleural disease

- Bromocriptine, amiodarone, methotrexate, methysergide
- Via induction of SLE—phenytoin, hydralazine, isoniazid

Asthma

- Via pharmacological mechanism (—β-adrenoceptor antagonists, cholinergic agonists, aspirin and NSAIDs)
- Idiosyncratic reaction (tamoxifen, dipyridamole)

including hydrochlorothiazides and some cytotoxic drugs.

Pulmonary fibrosis may occur in response to a variety of drugs, such as bleomycin and methotrexate, amiodarone and nitrofurantoin. Eosinophilic pulmonary reactions can also be caused by drugs. The pathogenesis may be an immune reaction similar to that in extrinsic allergic alveolitis, which specifically attracts large numbers of eosinophils into the lungs. This type of reaction is well described as a rare reaction to a variety of antineoplastic agents (e.g. bleomycin), antibiotics (e.g. sulphonamides), sulphasalazine and the anticonvulsants phenytoin and carbamazepine. Patients usually present with breathlessness, cough and fever. The chest radiograph characteristically shows patchy shadowing. Most cases resolve completely on withdrawal of the drug, but if the reaction is severe, rapid resolution can be obtained with corticosteroids.

RARE INTERSTITIAL LUNG DISEASES

See Table 4.21.

FURTHER INFORMATION ON INTERSTITIAL AND INFILTRATIVE PULMONARY DISEASES

Katzenstein A-L A, Myers J L 1998 Idiopathic pulmonary fibrosis: clinical relevance of pathologic classification. American Journal of Respiratory

Table 4.21 Rare interstitial lung diseases

Disease	Presentation	Chest radiograph	Course
Idiopathic pulmonary haemosiderosis	Haemoptysis, breathlessness, anaemia	Bilateral infiltrates often perihilar Diffuse pulmonary fibrosis	Rapidly progressive in children Slow progression or remission in adults Death from massive pulmonary haemorrhage, or cor pulmonale and respiratory failure
Alveolar proteinosis	Breathlessness and cough Occasionally fever, chest pain and haemoptysis	Diffuse bilateral shadowing, often more pronounced in the hilar regions Air bronchogram	Spontaneous remission in one-third Whole lung lavage effective therapy 50% remission after lavage Repeat lavage may be necessary
Histiocytosis X	Breathlessness, cough, pneumothorax	Diffuse interstitial shadowing progressing to honeycombing	Progressive leading to respiratory failure Poor response to immunosuppressive therapy in some
Neurofibromatosis	Breathlessness and cough in a patient with multiple organ involvement with neurofibromas including skin	Bilateral reticular nodular shadowing of diffuse interstitial fibrosis	Slow progression to death from respiratory failure Poor response to corticosteroid in some
Alveolar microlithiasis	No symptoms Breathlessness and cough	Diffuse calcified micronodular shadowing more pronounced in the lower zones	Slowly progressive to cor pulmonale and respiratory failure May stabilise in some Disodium etidronate may be effective
Lymphangioleiomyomatosis	Haemoptysis, breathlessness, pneumothorax and chylous effusion in females	Diffuse bilateral shadowing CT shows characteristic thin-walled cysts with well-defined walls throughout both lungs	Progressive to death within 10 years Oestrogen ablation and progesterone therapy of doubtful value Lung transplantation
Pulmonary tuberous sclerosis	Very similar to lymphangioleiomyomatosis except occasionally occurs in men		

Table 4.22 Categorisation of pulmonary thromboemboli

	Acute massive	Acute small/medium	Chronic microembolism
Pathophysiology	Major haemodynamic effects: ↓ cardiac output; acute right heart failure; disordered ventilation-perfusion ratio	Occlusion of segmental pulmonary artery → infarction ± effusion	Chronic occlusion of pulmonary microvasculature; pulmonary hypertension, right heart failure
Symptoms	Sudden syncope, faintness, central chest pain, apprehension, severe dyspnoea	Pleurisy, restricted breathing, haemoptysis	Exertional dyspnoea Late—exertional syncope, symptoms of right ventricular (RV) failure
Signs			
Cardiovascular	Major circulatory collapse; tachycardia; hypotension; ↑ jugular venous pressure; gallop rhythm; P_2 widely split (late)		May be nil early Late—RV heave, loud, split P_2 Terminal—signs of RV failure
Respiratory	Severe cyanosis, otherwise no local signs	Pleural rub, raised hemidiaphragm, crepitations, effusion (usually blood-stained)	
Other	↓ Urine output	Low-grade fever	
Investigations			
Chest radiograph	Often subtle; oligaemic lung fields, slight ↑ hilar shadows	Pleuropulmonary opacities; pleural effusion; linear shadows; raised hemidiaphragm	Enlarged pulmonary trunk; enlarged heart, prominent RV
ECG	$S_1Q_3T_3$ (see Fig. 4.43) T wave ↓ V_1–V_4 Right bundle branch block		Signs of RV hypertrophy and 'strain'
Blood gases	↓ $Pa\text{O}_2$; ↓ $Pa\text{CO}_2$	(↓ $Pa\text{CO}_2$)	Exertional ↓ $Pa\text{O}_2$ or desaturation (on formal exercise testing)
V/Q scan	Major areas of ↓ perfusion	Perfusion defect(s) not matched on the ventilation scan	May be no abnormality
Pulmonary angiography	Definitive diagnosis	Definitive diagnosis	May be no abnormality; may need lung biopsy to confirm diagnosis

and Critical Care Medicine 157: 1301–1315
Rom W N, Travis W D, Brody A R 1991 Cellular and molecular mechanism of asbestos-mediated disease. American Review of Respiratory Disease 143: 408–422
Rose C, King T E 1992 Controversies in hypersensitivity pneumonitis. American Review of Respiratory Disease 145: 1–2
Seaton A 1994 Management of the patient with occupational lung disease. Thorax 49: 627–629

PULMONARY VASCULAR DISEASE

PULMONARY THROMBOEMBOLISM

Aetiology and incidence

Pulmonary embolism most commonly results from detachment of vascular thrombus from the leg (70–80%) or pelvis (10–15%). Other rare causes of pulmonary embolism include amniotic fluid, placenta, air, fat, tumour (e.g. choriocarcinoma), parasites such as schistosomes, and septic emboli from endocarditis affecting the pulmonary or tricuspid valves. Effectively, the prophylaxis of pulmonary embolism is that of the prophylaxis and treatment of deep venous thrombosis (see pp. 796–797). Pulmonary thromboembolism is one of the most common acute severe pulmonary illnesses and accounts for at least 30 000 deaths per annum in the UK. Symptomatic pulmonary emboli occur in up to 1% of all post-operative patients. However, the autopsy incidence is 10–25% and in one-third of these, pulmonary embolism is a major contributor to death. A significant proportion are not suspected in life. Thus continued awareness of the possibility of pulmonary embolism in high-risk groups and willingness to pursue the diagnosis on the grounds of clinical suspicion are likely to reduce morbidity and save lives.

Pathophysiology

The pathophysiological consequences, clinical presentations, physical signs and results of investigations can be most easily understood if pulmonary emboli are classified on a basis of size—massive; small or medium-sized; and multiple microemboli (see Table 4.22).

Massive emboli become lodged in the proximal pulmonary arteries and chambers of the right heart, causing an acute and catastrophic reduction in cardiac output and right heart failure with major disruption in pulmonary ventilation-perfusion relationships due to very large areas of the lung being ventilated but not perfused.

Small and medium-sized emboli occlude segmental arteries, causing pulmonary infarction, pleural pain, haemoptysis and reduction in surfactant production. This is often associated with localised loss of lung volume. Fever, which is usually low-grade, is common in patients with established infarction.

In the rare condition of multiple microemboli, showers of tiny emboli occlude the capillary beds of the lung. Due to collateral vascular supply from bronchial vessels there is no infarction but insidious loss of the microvascular bed supplying the gas exchange units of the lung. Patients with this condition may present with atypical exertional dyspnoea but often the condition is not suspected until there are late complications, including severe pulmonary hypertension and right ventricular failure.

Clinical features

Massive pulmonary thromboembolism

Patients classically present several days after a major operation or other predisposing event with central chest pain, acute dyspnoea and apprehension. Symptoms due to sudden loss of cerebral and coronary blood flow occur, secondary to obstruction of the right ventricular outflow, and are often prominent. These include faintness, syncope and circulatory arrest. Pleurisy and haemoptysis are uncommon, although they may have occurred as a result of a previous 'sentinel' smaller embolus causing infarction. (Up to one-third of massive embolic events are preceded by a sentinel embolus.) Unlike other causes of acute severe dyspnoea (see p. 313), which are frequently associated with orthopnoea, the patient with massive embolisation may be more comfortable lying flat. On examination, there is a sinus tachycardia and other signs of low cardiac output including hypotension, impaired cerebration and peripheral vasoconstriction. Tachypnoea and central cyanosis will be obvious and the JVP elevated. A right ventricular gallop rhythm is an important physical sign in the first 24 hours, and a widely split P_2 may be detected.

Despite the major disorder of gas exchange there may be few, if any, signs on percussion and auscultation of the chest. If a patient (particularly one with a predisposing condition) is tachypnoeic, cyanosed, and lacks major chest signs but does have signs of reduced cardiac output and raised JVP, the diagnosis is massive pulmonary embolism until proven otherwise.

Small or medium-sized emboli

Pleuritic chest pain and breathlessness are the most frequent presenting symptoms. In pulmonary infarction, haemoptysis occurs in about 50% of patients. Clinically there may be a pleural rub and crepitations audible on auscultation, and since many patients also have pyrexia and non-specific chest radiographic abnormalities it is often difficult to differentiate pulmonary infarction from pneumonia. There may be clinical evidence of pleural effusion; this may be genuine, or be simulated by elevation of a hemidiaphragm which is common in pulmonary infarction, especially in those patients with pleural pain. Central cyanosis and signs of right heart failure are uncommon unless there has been extensive bilateral infarction.

Multiple microemboli

Thromboembolic pulmonary hypertension is a rare condition and may in certain patients reflect the development of thrombus formation within the pulmonary vascular tree or organisation of previous large thrombi rather than true microembolic events. It usually presents with exertional breathlessness, followed by angina and dizziness or syncope after minimal exertion. It is often difficult to differentiate thromboembolic pulmonary hypertension from primary pulmonary hypertension (see p. 381) in which in situ thrombus formation occurs.

Investigations

Massive pulmonary embolism

The chest radiograph is of little help, but may show signs of

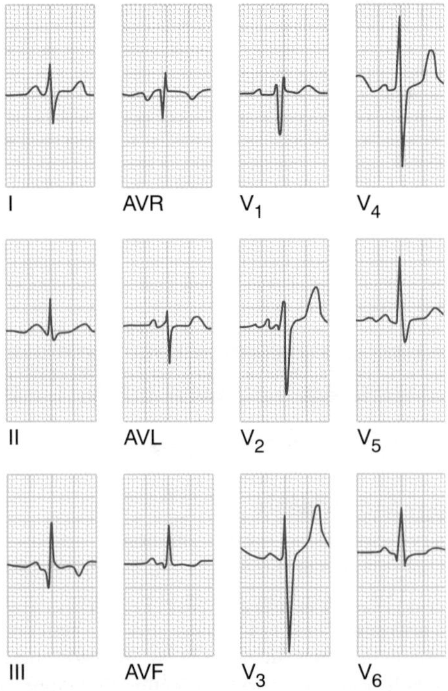

Fig. 4.43 ECG from patient with pulmonary embolism showing '$S_1Q_3T_3$' pattern.

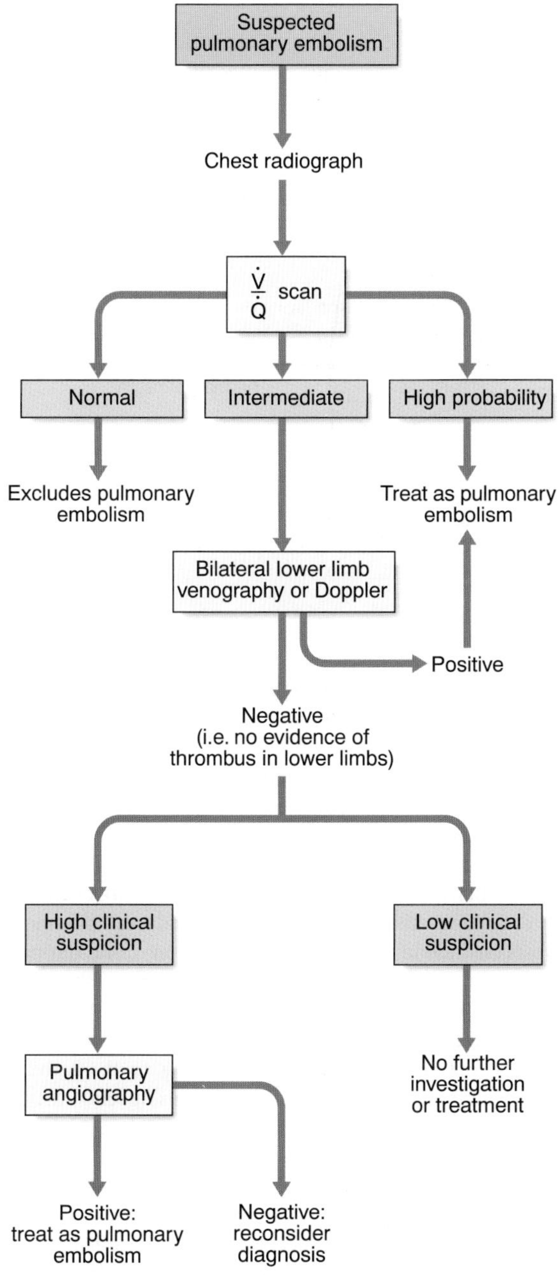

Fig. 4.44 Algorithm for the investigation of pulmonary thromboembolism.

pulmonary oligaemia which has to be predominantly unilateral to be detected. Bedside echocardiography is of particular value if the embolus is visualised in the right atrium, ventricular outflow tract or main pulmonary artery. It may also demonstrate right ventricular dilatation and hypokinaesia, and may exclude conditions such as pericardial tamponade and aortic dissection that may mimic massive pulmonary embolism. A number of suggestive ECG patterns have been described (see Ch. 3 and Fig. 4.43), the $S_1Q_3T_3$ pattern being the most characteristic, but no ECG changes are diagnostic. Arterial blood gas analysis typically shows hypoxaemia which is often associated with hypocapnia.

A high-probability diagnosis of massive pulmonary embolism can be made by a perfusion or ventilation-perfusion lung scan (see p. 309), but a definitive diagnosis can only be achieved by pulmonary angiography and/or spiral CT.

Pulmonary infarction

The investigation of patients with a suspected pulmonary embolism without cardiovascular compromise is shown in Figure 4.44. The chest radiograph, although never diagnostic, often shows abnormalities which should always alert the clinician to the possibility of pulmonary thromboembolism (see Fig. 4.45 on p. 380). Bilateral lower zone pleuropulmonary shadows, especially if linear and horizontal, are rarely seen in any condition other than pulmonary thromboembolism. Pleural effusion and elevation of a hemidiaphragm are other radiographic features of this disease. The wedge-shaped peripheral pulmonary shadow is uncommon. The chest radiograph abnormalities can change rapidly and the conversion of a non-specific lower zone shadow into a linear shadow, in 24–48 hours, is common and should raise the possibility of pulmonary infarction if this diagnosis has not previously been considered. Ventilation-perfusion lung scanning shows perfusion abnormalities which are not matched on the ventilation scan (see Fig. 4.6, p. 309). Radioisotope lung scanning may be misleading if not performed early. In some cases, a search for the source of emboli by lower limb venography and/or Doppler studies of the leg veins can support the diagnosis. Pulmonary angiography is rarely necessary; spiral CT scanning will not demonstrate thrombus in subsegmental arteries.

Electrocardiography is usually unhelpful, but may show right ventricular hypertrophy in patients who have chronic pulmonary thromboembolism. Arterial blood gas analysis may show hypoxaemia and hypocapnia in the early stages of extensive infarction. There is often a peripheral blood leucocytosis, and the patient may have a pyrexia.

Chronic microembolic disease (thromboembolic pulmonary hypertension)

As stated above, in the past this disease may have been diagnosed in patients with primary pulmonary hypertension since in situ thrombosis occurs in severe pulmonary hypertension and this makes diagnosis difficult even at autopsy.

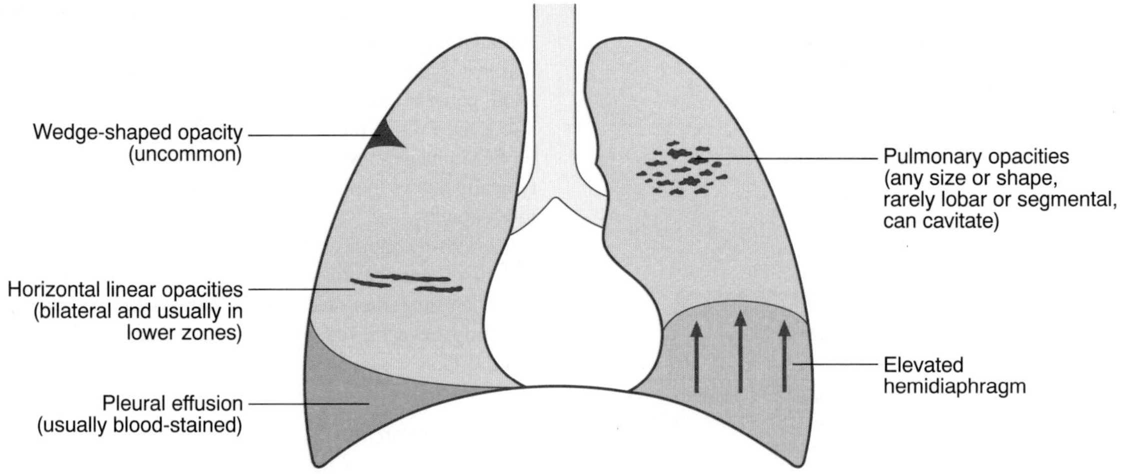

Fig. 4.45 Features of pulmonary thromboembolism/infarction on chest radiograph.

Pulmonary hypertension is difficult to diagnose unless it is severe. The chest radiograph shows enlargement of central pulmonary arteries and paucity of vascular markings in the peripheral parts of the lungs. Radioisotope scans are invariably abnormal but pulmonary angiography may not be able to differentiate thromboembolic from primary pulmonary hypertension. Pulmonary artery pressures should be measured prior to or during angiography, and right heart catheter studies are necessary if the effects of vasodilators are to be assessed.

Electrocardiography and echocardiography show hypertrophy and dilatation of the right heart. Echocardiography can be used to estimate the degree of pulmonary hypertension. Arterial blood gas analysis reveals hypoxaemia at rest or during exercise.

Management

General measures

Opiates may be necessary to relieve pain and distress, but should be used with great caution in the hypotensive patient. Resuscitation by external cardiac massage may be successful in the moribund patient by dislodging and breaking up a large central embolus. Transcatheter suction embolectomy can achieve similar results. The use of inotropic agents is of limited value since in massive pulmonary embolism the hypoxic, dilated right ventricle is near-maximally stimulated by endogenous catecholamines. Diuretics and vasodilators should be avoided at all times. Oxygen should be given to all hypoxaemic patients in a concentration necessary to restore arterial oxygen tension to as near normal as possible.

Anticoagulation

Anticoagulation remains the mainstay of treatment in pulmonary thromboembolic disease. Heparin (see p. 796) is necessary in all patients with massive pulmonary embolism and most patients with pulmonary infarction. Heparin should be given to all patients suspected of having pulmonary embolism, unless there is a contraindication, and then withdrawn if the diagnosis is disproved; this intervention substantially reduces mortality by preventing further embolic events, and also reduces mediator-induced pulmonary vasoconstriction and bronchoconstriction from thrombin activation and platelet aggregation. Therapy should be initiated with a bolus intravenous injection of 5000–10 000 units and thereafter i.v. therapy continued with a daily dose of 400–600 units/kg adjusted according to the activated partial thromboplastin time (aPTT). Bolus injection therapy can be used but is more difficult to monitor, and wide swings of anticoagulation are more likely with this route of administration. The optimal duration of therapy is not known, but for major thromboembolic episodes should be at least a week. Low molecular weight heparin has been shown to be as effective as standard dose unfractionated heparin, and is as effective when given subcutaneously. This form of heparin, which is more expensive than the unfractionated drug, may become the treatment of choice for pulmonary thromboembolic disease since subcutaneous administration simplifies therapy.

Oral anticoagulant treatment has no place in the immediate treatment of life-threatening thromboembolic disease, but should be used in the majority of patients who have been treated initially with heparin in whom the diagnosis is secure and there are no contraindications. Oral anticoagulants do not act immediately and, therefore, there should be an overlap with heparin therapy, usually of 3–4 days. (For oral anticoagulant control, see p. 796.)

The duration of anticoagulant therapy should be a few weeks in patients in whom the cause of the thromboembolism has been established and no longer exists (e.g. immobility and the contraceptive pill), a few months in those patients in whom the disease is apparently spontaneous, and long-term if thromboembolism is recurrent.

Thrombolytic therapy

The aim of thrombolytic therapy (see p. 261, as for myocardial infarction) is to actively dissolve the embolus, but unlike the treatment of coronary artery thrombosis, it has not yet been convincingly shown to be better than well-controlled heparin treatment. However, this form of treatment must be seriously considered in patients with massive pulmonary embolism in whom the diagnosis has been proven by angiography or spiral CT.

Embolectomy

Surgical removal of the embolus is rarely indicated but should be considered if possible in the moribund patient who fails to respond to thrombolytic therapy over the first hour.

Venous interruption

Venous interruption procedures are designed to prevent further emboli reaching the lungs. This form of treatment should only be considered in patients who have recurrent emboli in spite of well-controlled anticoagulant therapy, or in patients in whom long-term anticoagulant therapy is not possible.

PRIMARY PULMONARY HYPERTENSION

This is a rare condition, occurring more frequently in females, particularly children and young adults. Some cases are probably caused by multiple small pulmonary emboli or a poorly understood thrombotic process occurring locally in the pulmonary arteries, but in many others the aetiology is obscure. Pulmonary hypertension can be drug-induced (e.g. amphetamine-derived appetite suppressants). The pathological features, which include medial hypertrophy and fibrinoid necrosis, occur in all branches of the pulmonary arterial tree and result in pulmonary vascular obstruction, severe pulmonary hypertension and right heart failure. Patients usually present with dyspnoea on exertion, but physical signs may be unimpressive until right heart failure sets in. The diagnosis may be suspected after exercise-induced desaturation, and is confirmed by unexplained severe pulmonary hypertension with right heart pressures which may exceed systemic levels. Most patients die within 2–3 years of the onset of symptoms and anticoagulation or treatment with vasodilators appears to have little efficacy. Heart-lung transplantation should be considered early.

FURTHER INFORMATION ON PULMONARY VASCULAR DISEASE

Becker D M, Philbrick J T, Selby J B 1992 Inferior vena cava filters: indications, safety, effectiveness. Archives of Internal Medicine 152: 1985–1994

British Thoracic Society guidelines 1997 Suspected acute pulmonary embolism: a practical approach. Thorax 52 (Suppl. 4): S1–S24

Editorial 1998 Low molecular weight heparin for venous thromboembolism. Drugs and Therapeutics Bulletin 36: 25–29

DISEASES OF THE NASOPHARYNX, LARYNX AND TRACHEA

DISEASES OF THE NASOPHARYNX

ALLERGIC RHINITIS

This is a disorder in which there are episodes of nasal congestion, watery nasal discharge and sneezing. It may be seasonal or perennial.

Aetiology

Allergic rhinitis is due to an immediate hypersensitivity reaction in the nasal mucosa. The antigens concerned in the seasonal form of the disorder are pollens from grasses, flowers, weeds or trees. Grass pollen is responsible for hay fever (pollenosis), the most common type of seasonal allergic rhinitis in northern Europe; in the UK this disorder is at its peak between May and July.

Perennial allergic rhinitis may be a specific reaction to antigens derived from house dust, fungal spores or animal dander but similar symptoms can be caused by physical or chemical irritants—for example, pungent odours or fumes, including strong perfumes, cold air and dry atmospheres. The term vasomotor rhinitis is often used for this type of nasal problem because in this context the term 'allergic' is a misnomer.

Clinical features

In the seasonal type there are frequent sudden attacks of sneezing, with profuse watery nasal discharge and nasal obstruction. These attacks last for a few hours and are often accompanied by smarting and watering of the eyes and conjunctival infection. In the perennial variety the symptoms are similar but more continuous and generally less severe. Skin hypersensitivity tests with the relevant antigen are usually positive in seasonal allergic rhinitis and are thus of diagnostic value, but these tests are less useful in perennial rhinitis.

Management

The following symptomatic measures, singly or in combination, are usually effective in both seasonal and perennial allergic rhinitis:

- an antihistamine drug such as loratadine 10 mg daily by mouth
- sodium cromoglycate nasal spray, one metered dose of a 2% solution into each nostril 4–6 times daily
- beclomethasone dipropionate or budesonide aqueous nasal spray, one or two doses of 50 µg into each nostril twice daily.

Patients failing to respond to these measures may obtain symptomatic relief from intramuscular injection of a long-acting corticosteroid preparation but this form of treatment should be reserved for occasional use in patients whose symptoms are very severe and seriously interfere with school, business or social activities. Vasomotor rhinitis is often difficult to treat, but may respond to ipratropium bromide, administered into each nostril three or four times daily.

Prevention

In the seasonal type an attempt should be made to reduce exposure to pollen—for example, by avoiding country districts and keeping indoors as much as possible with windows closed during the pollen season, especially when pollen counts are reported to be high. The prevention of perennial rhinitis consists of avoiding, as far as possible, exposure to any identifiable aetiological factors but this is often difficult or impossible.

LARYNGEAL DISORDERS

Acute infections have already been described (see Table 4.10, p. 339). Other disorders of the larynx include chronic laryngitis, laryngeal tuberculosis (see p. 339), laryngeal paralysis and laryngeal obstruction. Tumours of the larynx are relatively common. For detailed information on these conditions the reader should refer to a textbook of diseases of the ear, nose and throat.

CHRONIC LARYNGITIS

The common causes of this condition are listed in the information box.

SOME CAUSES OF CHRONIC LARYNGITIS

- Repeated attacks of acute laryngitis
- Excessive use of the voice, especially in dusty atmospheres
- Heavy tobacco smoking
- Mouth-breathing from nasal obstruction
- Chronic infection of nasal sinuses

Clinical features

The chief symptom is hoarseness and the voice may be lost completely (aphonia). There is irritation of the throat and a spasmodic cough. The disease pursues a chronic course frequently uninfluenced by treatment, and in long-standing cases the voice is often permanently impaired.

Differential diagnosis

The causes of chronic hoarseness are listed in the information box.

CAUSES OF CHRONIC HOARSENESS

Consider if hoarseness persists for more than a few days:
- Tumour of the larynx
- Tuberculosis
- Laryngeal paralysis
- Inhaled corticosteroid treatment

These conditions must be considered in the differential diagnosis if hoarseness does not improve within a few weeks. In some patients a chest radiograph may bring to light an unsuspected bronchial carcinoma or pulmonary tuberculosis. If no such abnormality is found, laryngoscopy should be performed, usually by a specialist in otolaryngology.

Management

The voice must be rested completely. This is particularly important in public speakers. Smoking should be prohibited. Some benefit may be obtained from frequent inhalations of medicated steam.

LARYNGEAL PARALYSIS

Aetiology

Paralysis is due to interference with the motor nerve supply of the larynx. It is nearly always unilateral and, by reason of the intrathoracic course of the left recurrent laryngeal nerve, usually left-sided. One or both recurrent laryngeal nerves may be damaged at thyroidectomy or by carcinoma of the thyroid. Rarely, the vagal trunk itself is involved by tumour, aneurysm or trauma.

Clinical features

Hoarseness

This always accompanies laryngeal paralysis, whatever its cause. Paralysis of organic origin is seldom reversible, but when only one vocal cord is affected hoarseness may improve or even disappear after a few weeks, following a compensatory adjustment whereby the unparalysed cord crosses the midline and approximates with the paralysed cord on phonation.

'Bovine cough'

A characteristic feature of organic laryngeal paralysis is a cow-like cough which results from the loss of the explosive phase of normal coughing consequent upon the failure of the cords to close the glottis. Difficulty in bringing up sputum, which some patients experience, is also explained on the same basis. A normal cough in patients with partial loss of voice or aphonia virtually excludes laryngeal paralysis.

Stridor

Stridor is occasionally present but is seldom severe, except when laryngeal paralysis is bilateral.

Diagnosis

Laryngoscopy is necessary to establish the diagnosis of laryngeal paralysis with certainty. The paralysed cord lies in the so-called 'cadaveric' position, midway between abduction and adduction.

Management

The cause of laryngeal paralysis should be treated if that is possible. In unilateral paralysis the voice may be improved by the injection of Teflon into the affected vocal cord. In bilateral organic paralysis, tracheal intubation, tracheostomy or a plastic operation on the larynx may be necessary.

HYSTERICAL HOARSENESS AND APHONIA

Hoarseness or complete loss of voice may occur as a manifestation of hysteria. There are often clues in the history to suggest a diagnosis of hysteria but laryngoscopy may be necessary to exclude a pathological cause of the voice abnormality. In hysteria only the voluntary movement of adduction of the vocal cords is seen to be impaired.

LARYNGEAL OBSTRUCTION

Laryngeal obstruction is more liable to occur in children than in adults because of the smaller size of the glottis. Some important causes are given in the information box.

CAUSES OF LARYNGEAL OBSTRUCTION

- Inflammatory or allergic oedema, or exudate
- Spasm of laryngeal muscles
- Inhaled foreign body
- Inhaled blood clot or vomitus in an unconscious patient
- Tumours of the larynx
- Bilateral vocal cord paralysis
- Fixation of both cords in rheumatoid disease

Clinical features

Sudden complete laryngeal obstruction by a foreign body produces the clinical picture of acute asphyxia—violent but ineffective inspiratory efforts with indrawing of the intercostal spaces and the unsupported lower ribs, accompanied by cyanosis. Unrelieved, the condition progresses rapidly to coma and death within a few minutes. When, as in most cases, the obstruction is incomplete at first, the main clinical features are progressive breathlessness accompanied by stridor and cyanosis. There is indrawing of the intercostal spaces and lower ribs on both sides with each inspiratory effort. In such cases the great danger is that complete laryngeal obstruction may occur at any time and result in sudden death.

Management

Transient attacks of laryngeal obstruction due to exudate and spasm, which may occur with acute laryngitis in children (see p. 339) and with whooping cough, are potentially dangerous but can usually be relieved by the inhalation of steam.

Laryngeal obstruction from all other causes carries a high mortality and demands prompt treatment. The following measures may have to be employed.

Relief of obstruction by mechanical measures

When a foreign body is known to be the cause of the obstruction in children it can often be dislodged by turning the patient head downwards and squeezing the chest vigorously. In adults this is often impossible, but a sudden forceful compression of the upper abdomen (Heimlich manoeuvre) may be effective. In other circumstances the cause of the obstruction should be investigated by direct laryngoscopy which may also permit the removal of an unsuspected foreign body, or the insertion of a tube past the obstruction into the trachea. Tracheostomy must be performed without delay if these procedures fail to relieve laryngeal obstruction, but except in dire emergencies this operation should be performed in an operating theatre by a surgeon.

Treatment of the cause

In cases of diphtheria, antitoxin should be administered, and for other infections the appropriate antibiotic should be given. In angio-oedema complete laryngeal occlusion can usually be prevented by treatment with adrenaline 0.5–1 mg (0.5–1 ml of 1:1000) intramuscularly, chlorpheniramine maleate 10–20 mg by slow intravenous injection and intravenous hydrocortisone sodium succinate 200 mg.

TRACHEAL DISORDERS

ACUTE TRACHEITIS

See Table 4.10, page 339.

TRACHEAL OBSTRUCTION

External compression by enlarged mediastinal lymph nodes containing metastatic deposits, usually from a bronchial carcinoma, is a more frequent cause of tracheal obstruction than the uncommon primary benign or malignant tumours. Rarely, the trachea may be compressed by an aneurysm of the aortic arch, or in children by tuberculous mediastinal lymph nodes. Tracheal stenosis is an occasional complication of tracheostomy, prolonged intubation, Wegener's granulomatosis or trauma.

Clinical features

Stridor can be detected in every patient with severe tracheal narrowing. Endoscopic examination of the trachea should be undertaken without delay to determine the site, degree and nature of the obstruction.

Management

Localised tumours of the trachea can be resected, but reconstruction after resection may present complex technical problems. Endobronchial laser therapy, tracheal stents and radiotherapy are alternatives to surgery. The choice of treatment depends upon the nature of the tumour and the general health of the patient. Radiotherapy or chemotherapy may temporarily relieve compression by malignant lymph nodes and tracheal stents introduced bronchoscopically may be of temporary value. Benign tracheal strictures can sometimes be dilated but may have to be resected.

TRACHEO-OESOPHAGEAL FISTULA

This may be present in new-born infants as a congenital abnormality. In adults it is usually due to malignant lesions in the mediastinum, such as carcinoma or lymphoma, eroding both the trachea and oesophagus to produce a communication between them. Swallowed liquids enter the trachea and bronchi through the fistula and provoke coughing.

Management

Surgical closure of a congenital fistula, if undertaken promptly, is usually successful. There is usually no curative treatment for malignant fistulae and death from overwhelming pulmonary infection rapidly supervenes.

DISEASES OF THE PLEURA, DIAPHRAGM AND CHEST WALL

DISEASES OF THE PLEURA

PLEURISY

Pleurisy is not a diagnosis but simply the term used to describe the result of any disease process involving the pleura and giving rise to pleuritic pain or evidence of pleural friction. Pleurisy is a common feature of pulmonary infarction and may be an early manifestation of pleural invasion in pulmonary tuberculosis or by a pulmonary tumour.

Clinical features

Pleural pain is the characteristic symptom. On examination rib movement is restricted and a pleural rub is present in many cases, particularly when the patient takes a deep breath. It is not heard when the breath is held except near the pericardium, where a so-called pleuropericardial rub may be present. The other clinical features depend upon the nature of the disease causing the pleurisy. There may be complete clinical recovery or an effusion may develop, depending upon the underlying cause.

Every patient must have a chest radiograph but a normal radiograph does not exclude a pulmonary cause for the pleurisy. A preceding history of cough, purulent sputum and pyrexia is presumptive evidence of a pulmonary infection which may not have been severe enough to produce a radiographic abnormality or which may have resolved before the chest radiograph was taken.

Management

The primary cause of pleurisy must be treated. The symptomatic treatment of pleural pain is described on page 344.

PLEURAL EFFUSION

This term is used when serous fluid accumulates in the pleural space. The condition of purulent effusion or empyema is described on page 387. The passive transudation of fluid into the pleural cavity (hydrothorax) occurs in cardiac failure and in conditions causing hypoproteinaemia, such as nephrotic syndrome, liver failure and severe malnutrition. Some causes of pleural effusion are shown in the information box, and Table 4.23 on page 386.

Pleural effusion may be unilateral or bilateral. Bilateral effusions often occur in cardiac failure, but are also seen in much less common disorders such as the connective tissue diseases and hypoproteinaemia. The cause of the majority of pleural effusions can be identified if a careful history is taken and a comprehensive clinical examination performed.

CAUSES OF PLEURAL EFFUSION

Common	Uncommon
• Pneumonia • Tuberculosis • Pulmonary infarction • Malignant disease • Subdiaphragmatic disorders (subphrenic abscess, pancreatitis etc.) • Cardiac failure	• Hypoproteinaemia (nephrotic syndrome, liver failure, malnutrition) • Connective tissue diseases • Acute rheumatic fever • Post-myocardial infarction syndrome • Meigs' syndrome (ovarian tumour plus effusion) • Myxoedema • Uraemia • Asbestos-related benign pleural effusion • Yellow nail syndrome

Where the cause is obscure, a lead may be given by enquiry regarding travel abroad, occupation—for example, exposure to asbestos, contact with tuberculosis, risk factors for thromboembolism such as oral contraception, recent immobilisation or operation. Detailed investigations as described below may, however, be necessary.

Clinical features

The symptoms and signs of pleurisy often precede the development of effusion but the onset in some patients may be insidious. Breathlessness is the only symptom related to the effusion and the severity depends on the size and rate of accumulation of the fluid. The physical signs in the chest are those of fluid in the pleural space (see p. 308).

Investigations

Radiological examination

The chest radiograph shows a dense uniform opacity in the lower and lateral parts of the hemithorax, shading off above and medially into translucent lung (see Fig. 4.46). Occasionally the fluid is localised below the lower lobe ('subpulmonary effusion'), the appearances simulating an elevated hemidiaphragm. A localised opacity may be seen when the effusion is loculated—for example, in an interlobar fissure.

Ultrasonography

This investigation is valuable to differentiate between a loculated pleural effusion and pleural tumour and also helps to localise an effusion prior to aspiration and pleural biopsy.

Pleural aspiration and pleural biopsy

Absolute proof that an effusion is present can be obtained only by the aspiration of fluid. Pleural biopsy is always indicated whenever a diagnostic aspiration of pleural fluid is performed because the chances of obtaining a diagnosis from pleural biopsy material are much greater than by examination of the pleural liquid alone. A pleural biopsy needle should be

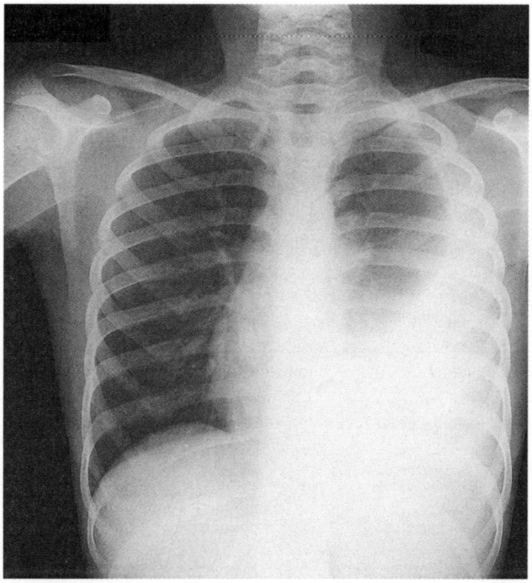

Fig. 4.46 Pleural effusion. Chest radiograph showing the characteristic opacification of a large left-sided effusion.

inserted through an intercostal space at the area of maximum dullness on percussion and at the site of maximum radiological opacity as shown by postero-anterior and lateral films, or at a site determined by ultrasound. At least 50 ml of fluid should be withdrawn, aliquots being placed in separate containers for microbiological examination including culture for tuberculosis, and cytological and biochemical examination. Whenever there is a strong suspicion of tuberculosis a large volume of pleural liquid should be submitted to the laboratory. Pleural biopsies should be taken after pleural liquid has been aspirated for diagnostic purposes.

The appearance of the fluid is straw-coloured, blood-stained, purulent or chylous. The protein content gives an indication as to whether the effusion is an exudate (> 30 g/l) or a transudate (< 30 g/l). The predominant cell type (neutrophil, eosinophil, lymphocyte, red blood cell) provides useful information, and fluid should always be examined for malignant cells.

There is a high amylase level in effusions secondary to acute pancreatitis. Pleural effusions secondary to rheumatoid disease contain a low glucose, high LDH and, if chronic, a high concentration of cholesterol.

Other investigations

Estimation of the total and differential peripheral blood leucocyte count, a tuberculin test, and examination of the sputum for tubercle bacilli and malignant cells should be routine in most situations. A chest radiograph may disclose an underlying pulmonary lesion and indicate its nature. If

Table 4.23 Pleural effusion: main causes and features

Cause	Appearance of fluid	Type of fluid	Predominant cells in fluid	Other diagnostic features
Tuberculous	Serous, usually amber-coloured	Exudate	Lymphocytes (occasionally polymorphs)	Positive tuberculin test Isolation of *M. tuberculosis* Positive pleural biopsy (80%)
Malignant disease	Serous, often blood-stained	Exudate	Serosal cells and lymphocytes Often clumps of malignant cells	Positive pleural biopsy (40%) Evidence of malignant disease elsewhere
Cardiac failure*	Serous, straw-coloured	Transudate	Few serosal cells	Other evidence of left heart failure Response to diuretics
Pulmonary infarction*	Serous or blood-stained	Exudate	Red blood cells Eosinophils	Contralateral evidence of infarction Source of embolism Factors predisposing to venous thrombosis
Rheumatoid disease*	Serous Turbid if chronic	Exudate	Lymphocytes (occasionally polymorphs)	Rheumatoid arthritis Rheumatoid factor in serum Cholesterol in chronic effusion; low glucose
Systemic lupus erythematosus*	Serous	Exudate	Lymphocytes and serosal cells	Other manifestations of SLE Antinuclear factor or anti-DNA in serum
Acute pancreatitis	Serous or blood-stained	Exudate	No cells predominate	High amylase (greater than in serum)
Obstruction of thoracic duct	Milky	Chyle	None	Chylomicrons

* Effusion often bilateral.

the lung is obscured by a massive effusion the radiograph should be repeated after a large volume of fluid has been aspirated. Other investigations which may be of help include bronchoscopy, biopsy or aspiration of the scalene lymph node, thoracoscopy and serological tests for antinuclear and rheumatoid factors.

The main diagnostic features and more important causes of pleural effusion are shown in Table 4.23.

Management

Aspiration of pleural fluid may be necessary to relieve breathlessness. It is inadvisable to remove more than 1 litre on the first occasion because 're-expansion' pulmonary oedema occasionally follows the aspiration of larger amounts. A pneumothorax may be produced even by a careful operator, and a chest radiograph must always be taken after the procedure.

Treatment of the underlying cause—for example, heart failure, pneumonia, pulmonary embolism or subphrenic abscess—will often be followed by resolution of the effusion. However, certain conditions require special measures as detailed below.

Post-pneumonic pleural effusion

Pleural effusions complicating pneumonia require aspiration to ensure that an empyema has not developed, and to prevent pleural thickening.

Tuberculous pleural effusion

Patients with tuberculous effusions should always receive antituberculosis chemotherapy (see p. 352). Aspiration is required initially if the effusion is large and causing breathlessness. The addition of prednisolone 20 mg daily by mouth for 4–6 weeks will promote rapid absorption of the fluid, obviate the need for further aspiration and may prevent fibrosis, but it is rarely necessary if a rifampicin-containing regimen is used.

Malignant effusions

Effusions caused by malignant infiltration of the pleural surfaces re-accumulate rapidly. To avoid the distress of repeated aspirations, an attempt should be made to drain all fluid via an intercostal tube then obliterate the pleural space (pleurodesis) by the injection of substances which produce an inflammatory reaction and extensive pleural adhesions. The agents most frequently used are tetracycline, kaolin and bleomycin.

ASBESTOS-RELATED PLEURAL DISEASE

Benign pleural plaques

These areas of pleural thickening do not produce clinical symptoms and are usually identified on routine chest radiograph. They are often calcified and in the early stage are best seen on oblique films. They are most commonly observed on the diaphragm and anterolateral pleural surfaces (see Fig. 4.47).

Benign pleural effusion

This is considered to be a specific asbestos-related entity

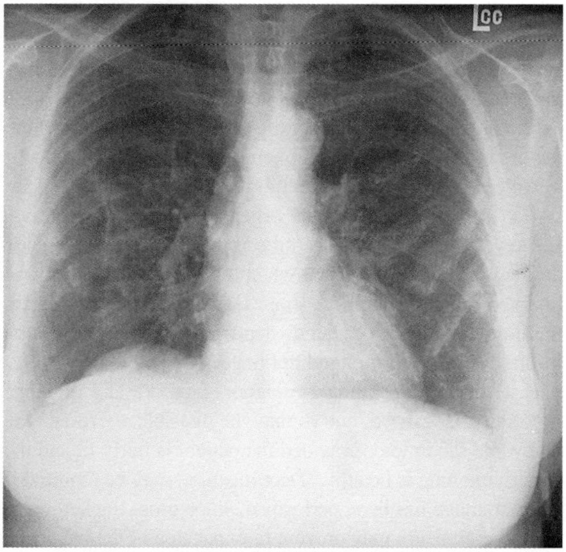

Fig. 4.47 Asbestos-related benign pleural plaques. Chest radiograph showing extensive calcified pleural plaques ('candle wax' appearance), particularly marked on the diaphragm and lateral pleural surfaces.

and may be associated with pleural pain, fever and leucocytosis. The pleural liquid may be blood-stained, and differentiation of this benign condition from a malignant effusion caused by mesothelioma can be difficult. The disease is self-limiting but may cause considerable pleural fibrosis which sometimes leads to breathlessness.

Mesothelioma of the pleura

This malignant tumour of the pleura is usually caused by exposure to asbestos which may be trivial. Blue asbestos is thought to be the most potent cause of mesothelioma. Clinical presentation is frequently with chest pain. A pleural effusion, often blood-stained, may develop and cause breathlessness. A diagnosis can be confirmed histologically by pleural biopsy in some patients, but tumour masses may later develop in the chest wall at the site of the biopsy. Thoracotomy is seldom justified as a diagnostic procedure in patients with suspected mesothelioma. There is no curative treatment and chest wall pain is often difficult to control.

Diffuse pleural fibrosis

Diffuse pleural fibrosis is a much more important pleural manifestation of asbestos fibre inhalation than pleural plaque formation, since it can restrict chest expansion and cause breathlessness. The restrictive defect caused by diffuse pleural fibrosis tends to progress.

EMPYEMA

This term describes the presence of pus in the pleural space. The pus may be as thin as serous fluid or so thick that it is difficult or impossible to aspirate even through a wide-bore needle. Microscopically, neutrophil leucocytes are present in large numbers. The causative organism may or may not be isolated from the pus. An empyema may involve the whole pleural space or only part of it ('loculated' or 'encysted' empyema) and is almost invariably unilateral.

Aetiology

Empyema is always secondary to infection in a neighbouring structure, usually the lung. The principal infections liable to produce empyema are the bacterial pneumonias and tuberculosis. Hence, over 40% of patients with community-acquired pneumonia develop an associated pleural effusion and about 15% of these become secondarily infected. Other causes are infection of a haemothorax and rupture of a subphrenic abscess through the diaphragm. Empyema has become relatively unusual because pulmonary infection can now be so readily controlled by antibacterial therapy.

Pathology

Both layers of pleura are covered with a thick, shaggy inflammatory exudate. The pus in the pleural space is often under considerable pressure and if the condition is not adequately treated there may be rupture into a bronchus from which pus is expectorated, or through an intercostal space with the formation of a subcutaneous abscess or sinus. A bronchopleural fistula is produced and a pyopneumothorax is formed when an empyema ruptures into a bronchus.

The only way in which an empyema can heal is by irradication of the infection and apposition of the visceral and parietal pleural layers with obliteration of the empyema space by organisation of the intervening exudate. This cannot occur unless re-expansion of the compressed lung is secured at an early stage by removal of all the pus from the pleural space. Re-expansion of the lung cannot take place if:

- there is delay in treatment or inadequate drainage and the visceral pleura becomes grossly thickened and rigid
- the pleural layers are kept apart by air entering the pleura through a bronchopleural fistula
- disease in the lung, such as bronchiectasis, bronchial carcinoma or pulmonary tuberculosis, renders it incapable of re-expansion.

In all these circumstances an empyema tends to become chronic, and healing may not take place without recourse to thoracic surgery.

Clinical features

An empyema should be suspected in patients with pul-

CLINICAL FEATURES OF EMPYEMA
Systemic features
• Pyrexia; usually high and remittent • Rigors, sweating, malaise and weight loss • Polymorphonuclear leucocytosis
Local features
• Pleural pain; breathlessness; cough and sputum usually because of underlying lung disease; copious purulent sputum if empyema ruptures into a bronchus (bronchopleural fistula) • Clinical signs of fluid in the pleural space

monary infection if there is persistence or recurrence of pyrexia despite the continued administration of a suitable antibiotic. In other cases the illness produced by the primary infective lesion may be so slight that it passes unrecognised and the first definite clinical features are due to the empyema itself.

Once an empyema has developed, two separate groups of clinical features are found. These are shown in the information box.

Investigations

Radiological examination

The appearances are indistinguishable from those of pleural effusion. When air is present in addition to pus (pyopneumothorax), a horizontal 'fluid level' marks the interface of liquid and air if the film is taken in the erect position.

Aspiration of pus

This confirms the presence of an empyema. Ultrasonography is recommended to identify the optimal place to undertake pleuracentesis, which is best performed with a wide-bore needle.

Bacteriological examination of pus

This may help to determine the cause of the empyema. The pus is frequently sterile when antibiotics have been given. The distinction between tuberculous and non-tuberculous disease can be difficult and often requires pleural histology and culture.

Management

Treatment of non-tuberculous empyema

When the patient is acutely ill and the pus is thin in consistency an intercostal tube should be inserted under ultrasound guidance into the most dependent part of the empyema space and connected to a water-seal drain system. If the initial aspirate reveals turbid fluid or frank pus, or if loculations are seen on ultrasound, the tube should be put on suction (5–10 cm water), flushed with 20 ml normal saline 6-hourly and streptokinase (250 000 U in 100 ml normal saline) inserted daily for 3 days. Urokinase should be used if streptokinase has been given within the preceding year or the patient is known to have streptokinase antibodies. Finally, an antibiotic should be given to which the organism causing the empyema is sensitive.

An empyema can often be aborted if these measures are started early enough and the organisms are drug-sensitive. If, however, the intercostal tube is not providing adequate drainage, which can happen when the pus thickens, surgical intervention is required. A short segment of rib is resected, the empyema cavity cleared of pus, and a wide-bore tube inserted to allow prolonged drainage.

If a chronic empyema is diagnosed before any drainage procedure is carried out it may be feasible to resect the empyema sac in toto, provided the patient is fairly fit and the underlying lung is healthy. 'Decortication' may be required if open drainage has been performed, since gross thickening of the visceral pleura may prevent re-expansion of the lung.

Treatment of tuberculous empyema

Antituberculosis chemotherapy must be started immediately and the pus in the pleural space should be aspirated through a wide-bore needle until it ceases to re-accumulate. In many patients no other treatment is necessary but surgery is occasionally required to ablate a residual empyema space.

SPONTANEOUS PNEUMOTHORAX

The two chief causes of spontaneous pneumothorax are:

- rupture of a subpleural emphysematous bulla or pleural bleb, or the pulmonary end of a pleural adhesion
- rupture of a subpleural tuberculous focus.

The first cause is very much more common in Britain. Other conditions which rarely give rise to pneumothorax include staphylococcal lung abscess, pulmonary infarction, bronchial carcinoma and most forms of chronic obstructive and fibrotic lung disease.

Pathology

There are three types of spontaneous pneumothorax (see Fig. 4.48). In a 'closed' pneumothorax communication between the pleura and lung seals off as the lung deflates and does not reopen (see Fig. 4.48A). With an 'open' pneumothorax the communication is generally with a bronchus (bronchopleural fistula) and does not seal off when the lung collapses. The air pressure in the pleural space approximates to atmospheric pressure both on inspiration and expiration and the lung cannot re-expand. Moreover, the large bronchial communication facilitates the transmission of infection from the air passages into the pleural space and empyema is a common complication. The term 'open' is also applied to a pneumothorax resulting

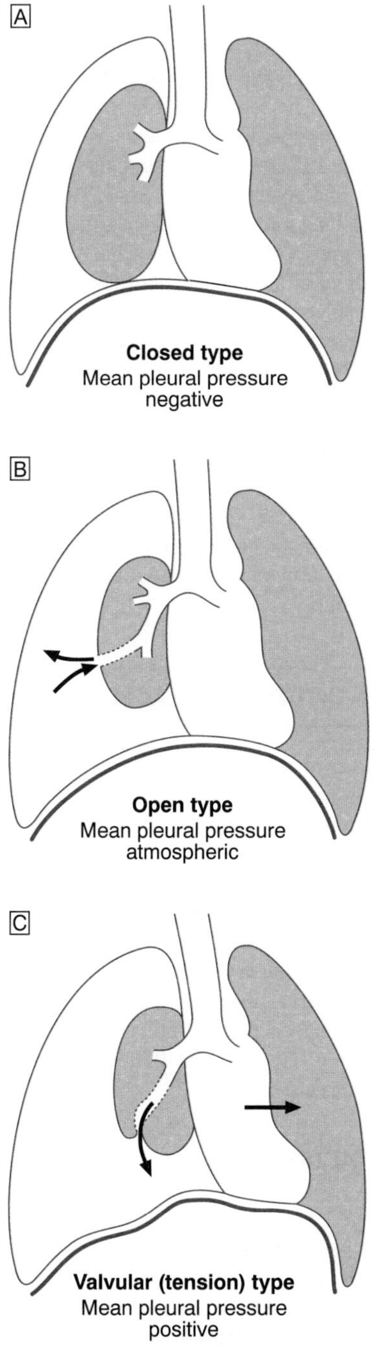

Fig. 4.48 Types of spontaneous pneumothorax. A Closed type. B Open type. C Valvular (tension) type.

from a penetrating wound of the chest wall (see Fig. 4.48B). Finally, a tension pneumothorax may develop if the communication between the pleura and lung persists but is small and acts as a one-way valve which allows air to enter the pleural space during inspiration and coughing but prevents it from escaping. Very large amounts of air may be trapped in the pleural space and the intrapleural pressure may rise to well above atmospheric levels. This causes not only compression of the underlying deflated lung but also mediastinal displacement towards the opposite side, with consequent compression of the opposite lung and cardiovascular compromise (see Fig. 4.48C).

Clinical features

The onset is usually sudden, with pain or a feeling of tightness on the affected side of the chest that may be aggravated by deep breathing. The patient becomes increasingly breathless and in severe cases cyanosed. Physical signs in the chest are of air in the pleural space (see p. 308) but when the pneumothorax is small and localised there may be no abnormal signs and it may be revealed only by a radiograph.

Closed spontaneous pneumothorax

Breathlessness, which is seldom severe unless there is underlying bronchopulmonary disease, gradually abates over the course of a few days. Progressive spontaneous absorption of air takes place and re-expansion of the lung is usually complete within a few weeks, depending upon the initial size of the pneumothorax. Pleural infection is uncommon in this type of pneumothorax.

Open spontaneous pneumothorax

This usually follows rupture of an emphysematous bulla, a small pleural bleb, a tuberculous cavity or a lung abscess into the pleural space. The onset is similar to that of the closed type but breathlessness does not improve and, when the cause is tuberculosis or lung abscess, pyrexia and systemic disturbance soon ensue. There are the physical and radiological signs of air, or air and fluid, in the pleural space. Acid-fast bacilli can be isolated from the pleural fluid in tuberculosis.

Tension pneumothorax

A tension or valvular pneumothorax produces the most dramatic clinical picture. Breathlessness is rapidly progressive and is accompanied by central cyanosis. Death may occur from asphyxia within a few minutes, but usually the course of events is less rapid and medical attention can be obtained in time to avert a fatal outcome.

Investigations

The chest radiograph usually shows a sharply defined edge of the deflated lung which may be more easily seen when the film is taken in expiration. There is complete translucency between this and the chest wall, with no lung markings. The degree of pulmonary deflation varies. Care

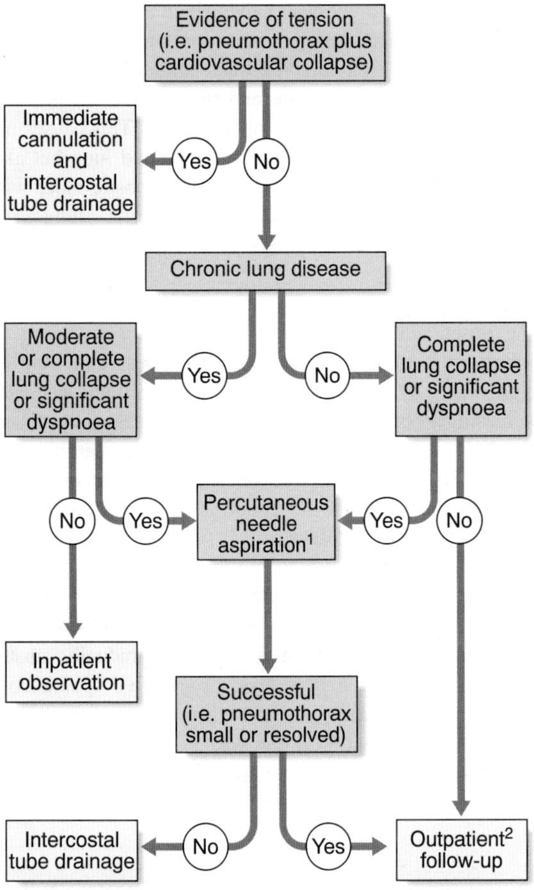

Fig. 4.49 Management of spontaneous pneumothorax. (1) Aspirate in the 2nd intercostal space anteriorly in mid-clavicular line using a 16 F cannula; discontinue if resistance felt, patient coughs excessively, or 2–5 litres of air removed. (2) Beware: the post-aspiration chest radiograph is not a reliable indicator of whether a pleural leak remains and hence all patients should be told to attend again immediately in the event of noticeable deterioration.

must be taken to differentiate between large emphysematous bullae and a pneumothorax. Radiographs also show the degree of mediastinal displacement and give information regarding the presence or absence of pleural fluid and underlying pulmonary disease.

Management

It is now recognised that percutaneous aspiration is a simple, effective and well-tolerated alternative to intercostal tube drainage in patients presenting with a spontaneous pneumothorax (see Fig. 4.49). However, even a small pneumothorax may cause severe respiratory failure in patients with COPD and hence such patients are more likely to require intercostal tube drainage and inpatient observation. If required, an intercostal drain should be inserted in the 4th, 5th or 6th intercostal space in the mid-axillary line following blunt dissection through to the parietal pleura. The tube should be advanced in an apical direction, connected to an underwater seal and secured firmly to the chest wall. Clamping of the drain is unnecessary and potentially dangerous. The drain should be removed 24 hours after the lung has fully re-inflated and bubbling stopped. If bubbling in the underwater bottle stops prior to full re-inflation, then the tube is either blocked, kinked or displaced.

Patients presenting with a spontaneous pneumothorax should not fly for 3 months and should be advised to stop smoking and about the risks of a further attack.

Recurrent spontaneous pneumothorax

Recurrent pneumothorax, particularly if bilateral, should be treated by obliteration of at least one pleural space. This can be achieved by introduction of an irritant substance such as kaolin, or by pleural abrasion or parietal pleurectomy at thoracotomy.

DISEASES OF THE DIAPHRAGM

Abnormalities of the diaphragm are common and may be congenital or acquired. Both hemidiaphragms are displaced downwards and functionally impaired by diseases which cause pulmonary hyperinflation, notably emphysema. Diaphragmatic function can also be impaired in neuromuscular disorders, connective tissue diseases and skeletal deformities such as thoracic scoliosis. Paralysis of the diaphragm is usually unilateral and caused by lesions of one phrenic nerve. Bilateral hemidiaphragm weakness or paralysis can occur in polyneuropathies, the most common being the Guillain–Barré syndrome (infective polyneuropathy).

CONGENITAL DISORDERS

Diaphragmatic hernias

Congenital defects of the diaphragm can allow herniation of abdominal viscera. Posteriorly situated hernias through the foramen of Bochdalek are more common than anterior hernias through the foramen of Morgagni.

Eventration of the diaphragm

Abnormal elevation of one hemidiaphragm, more often the left, results from total or partial absence of muscular development of the septum transversum. Most eventrations are asymptomatic and are detected by chance on radiograph in adult life, but severe respiratory distress can be caused in infancy if the diaphragmatic muscular defect is extensive.

CAUSES OF ELEVATION OF A HEMIDIAPHRAGM

- Phrenic nerve paralysis
- Eventration of the diaphragm
- Decrease in volume of one lung, e.g. lobectomy, unilateral pulmonary fibrosis
- Severe pleuritic pain
- Pulmonary infarction
- Subphrenic abscess
- Large volume of gas in the stomach or colon
- Large tumours or cysts of the liver

Other oesophageal abnormalities
These include defects of the oesophageal hiatus, congenital absence and duplication of the diaphragm. The diaphragm may be involved in most primary muscle disorders.

ACQUIRED DISORDERS

Diaphragmatic paralysis
Phrenic nerve damage leading to paralysis of a hemidiaphragm is most often produced by bronchial carcinoma but can also be the result of a number of neurological disorders, injury or disease of cervical vertebrae and tumours of the cervical cord. Trauma to the neck, including birth injuries, surgery and stretching of the phrenic nerve by mediastinal masses and aortic aneurysms may also lead to diaphragmatic paralysis. Sometimes no cause can be found.

Paralysis of one hemidiaphragm results in loss of approximately 20% of ventilatory capacity, but this is not usually noticed by otherwise healthy individuals.

Diagnosis is suggested by elevation of the hemidiaphragm on chest radiograph and is confirmed by screening or ultrasonography, which show paradoxical movement of the paralysed hemidiaphragm on sniffing.

Other acquired diaphragmatic disorders
Hiatus hernia is common (see p. 624) and diaphragmatic rupture usually caused by a crush injury may not be detected until years after the injury. Peripheral neuropathies of any type can involve the diaphragm, as can disorders affecting the anterior horn cells, e.g. poliomyelitis. Connective tissue disorders such as systemic lupus erythematosus, and hypothyroidism and hyperthyroidism, may cause diaphragmatic weakness. Respiratory disorders which cause pulmonary hyperinflation, e.g. emphysema, and those which result in small stiff lungs, e.g. diffuse pulmonary fibrosis, decrease diaphragmatic efficiency and predispose to fatigue. Severe skeletal deformity, such as kyphosis, causes gross distortion of diaphragmatic muscle configuration and gross mechanical disadvantage.

DEFORMITIES OF THE CHEST WALL

THORACIC KYPHOSCOLIOSIS

Abnormalities of alignment of the dorsal spine and their consequent effects on thoracic shape may be caused by:

- congenital abnormality
- vertebral disease including tuberculosis, osteoporosis and ankylosing spondylitis
- trauma
- neuromuscular disease such as poliomyelitis.

Simple kyphosis causes less pulmonary embarrassment than kyphoscoliosis.

Kyphoscoliosis, if severe, restricts and distorts expansion of the chest wall, causing maldistribution of the ventilation and blood flow in the lungs. Patients with severe deformity may develop type II respiratory failure, pulmonary hypertension and right ventricular failure; survival beyond middle age is uncommon. The tempo of deterioration is often accelerated by bacterial infection in the bronchi and lungs.

PECTUS CARINATUM

Pectus carinatum (pigeon chest) is almost always caused by severe asthma during childhood. Very occasionally this deformity can be produced by rickets or occurs without any obvious explanation.

PECTUS EXCAVATUM

In pectus excavatum (funnel chest) the body of the sternum, usually only the lower end, is curved backwards. The heart is displaced to the left and may be compressed between the sternum and the vertebral column, but only rarely is there associated disturbance of cardiac function. The deformity may restrict chest expansion and reduce vital capacity. The impairment of cardiac or pulmonary function is seldom sufficient to warrant surgical correction but an operation may be indicated for cosmetic reasons.

FURTHER INFORMATION ON DISEASES OF THE PLEURA, DIAPHRAGM AND CHEST WALL

Miller A C, Harvey J E 1993 Guidelines for the management of spontaneous pneumothorax. British Medical Journal 307: 114–116

Disturbances in water, electrolyte and acid-base balance

5

C.P. SWAINSON • A.D. CUMMING

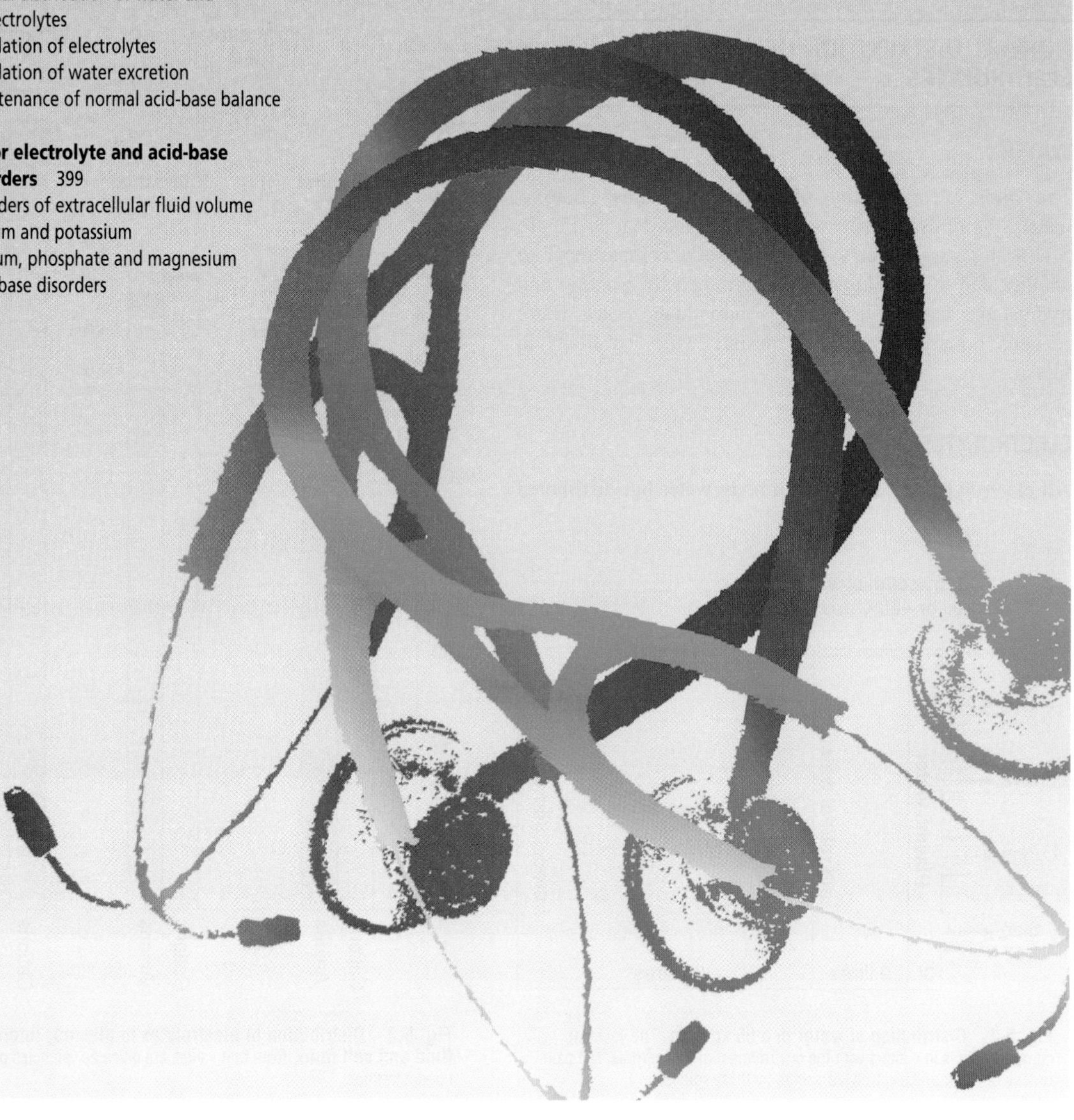

Disturbances in water, electrolyte and acid-base balance are common problems encountered in general medical and surgical practice. Some are trivial, but others are associated with a high mortality and require urgent assessment and treatment. The kidneys play an important part in maintaining normal water, electrolyte and acid-base balance. Many of these disturbances occur in older patients with moderate, often undiagnosed, chronic renal failure whose homeostatic abilities are compromised.

The anatomy of the kidney and the physiology of glomerular function are described in Chapter 6.

PHYSIOLOGY OF ELECTROLYTES, WATER AND ACID-BASE

NORMAL DISTRIBUTION OF WATER AND ELECTROLYTES

WATER

The body of a healthy 65 kg man contains approximately 40 litres of water, distributed as shown in Figure 5.1. Water passes freely from one body compartment to another and its distribution is determined by osmotic and hydrostatic forces. In healthy individuals body water remains remarkably constant despite wide variations in intake.

ELECTROLYTES

All electrolytes are dissolved in body water but distributed differently in the various compartments (see Fig. 5.2). The effective osmolality (tonicity) of plasma and interstitial fluid is determined by the concentrations of sodium (Na^+) and chloride (Cl^-), while that of the intracellular fluid is determined by the concentrations of potassium (K^+), magnesium (Mg^{++}), phosphate PO_4^{--} and sulphate SO_4^{--}. The amount of hydrogen ion [H^+] in the extracellular fluid (ECF) is tiny (40 nmol/l) and much can be buffered by cationic proteins such as albumin and haemoglobin. The differences in ionic composition of cells and the interstitial fluid are essential to normal cell function. They are maintained by a number of active bidirectional pumps in both the apical and basolateral membranes, such as Na^+/K^+ ATPase (see Fig. 5.3).

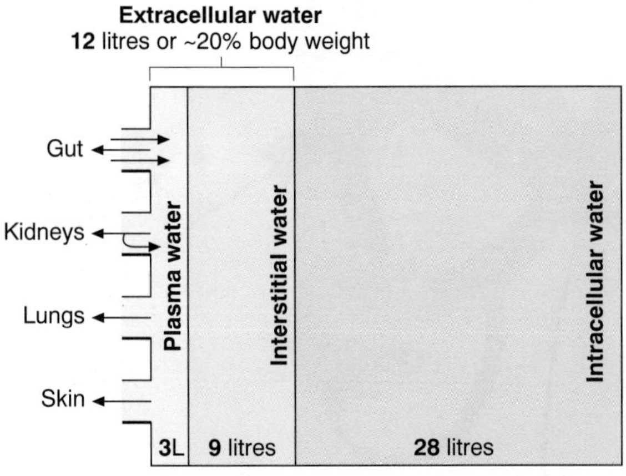

Fig. 5.1 Distribution of water in a 65 kg man. The vascular compartment is in contact with the environment at four portals. Net gain or loss of water and electrolytes occurs by these routes.

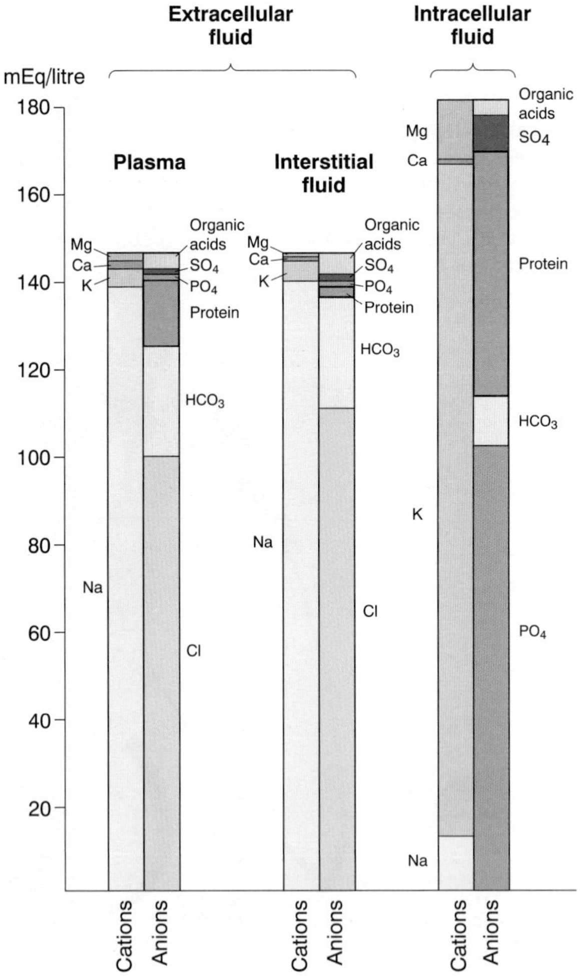

Fig. 5.2 Distribution of electrolytes in plasma, interstitial fluid and cell fluid. Note that values are given as valencies not concentrations.

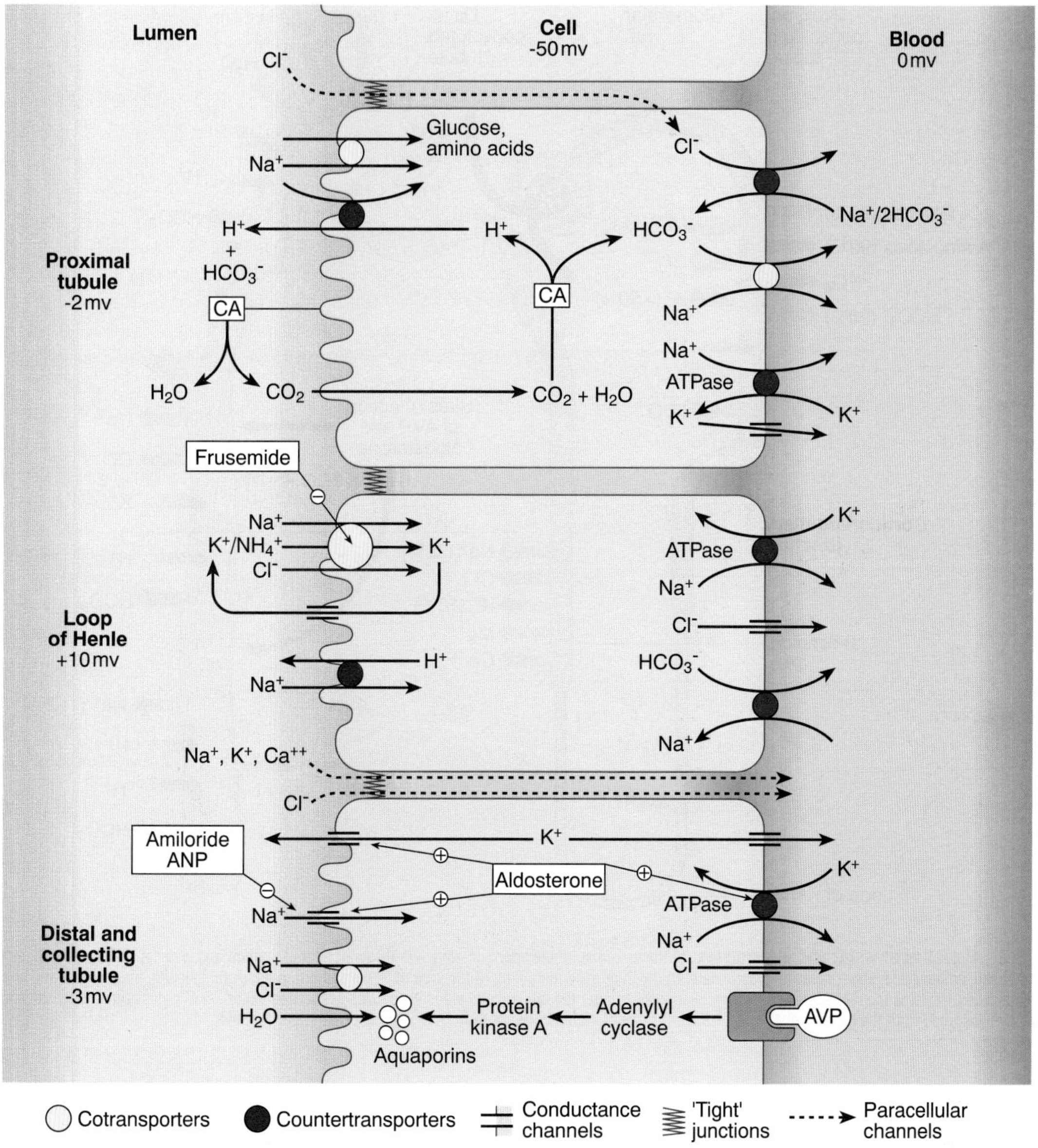

Fig. 5.3 Electrolyte transport in kidney. Kidney cells regulate electrolyte reabsorption and secretion by a mixture of cotransporters (e.g. sodium with glucose and amino acids), countertransporters (another ion, e.g. K^+ or HCO_3^-) and ion-specific conductance channels. The figure shows these major transport systems for each of the three main segments of the nephron. Their activity contributes to the changing potential difference (in mv) between the lumen and blood. The basolateral Na^+/K^+ ATPase is a major driving force for electroneutral cotransport by maintaining a low intracellular Na^+ and lumen-negative cell interior. Na^+/H^+ exchange occurs in most nephron segments. Potassium leaves the cell through conductance channels driven by a concentration gradient. Chloride either moves through a paracellular route or through conductance channels in the basolateral membrane. In the loop of Henle, an $Na^+/K^+/Cl^-$ cotransporter uses K^+ recycled from the cell interior and is the major component of sodium transport that is inhibited by loop diuretics. The distal tubule and collecting duct sodium conductance channels are inhibited by thiazide diuretics, amiloride and atrial natriuretic peptide (ANP), and stimulated by aldosterone. Aldosterone also stimulates potassium conductance channels and the Na^+/K^+ ATPase. At the bottom of the figure, arginine vasopressin (AVP) is shown binding to the V2 receptor in the basolateral membrane; this triggers a series of steps that result in the exocytosis of aquaporins (water channels) at the luminal membrane, thus allowing increased water transport through the cell.

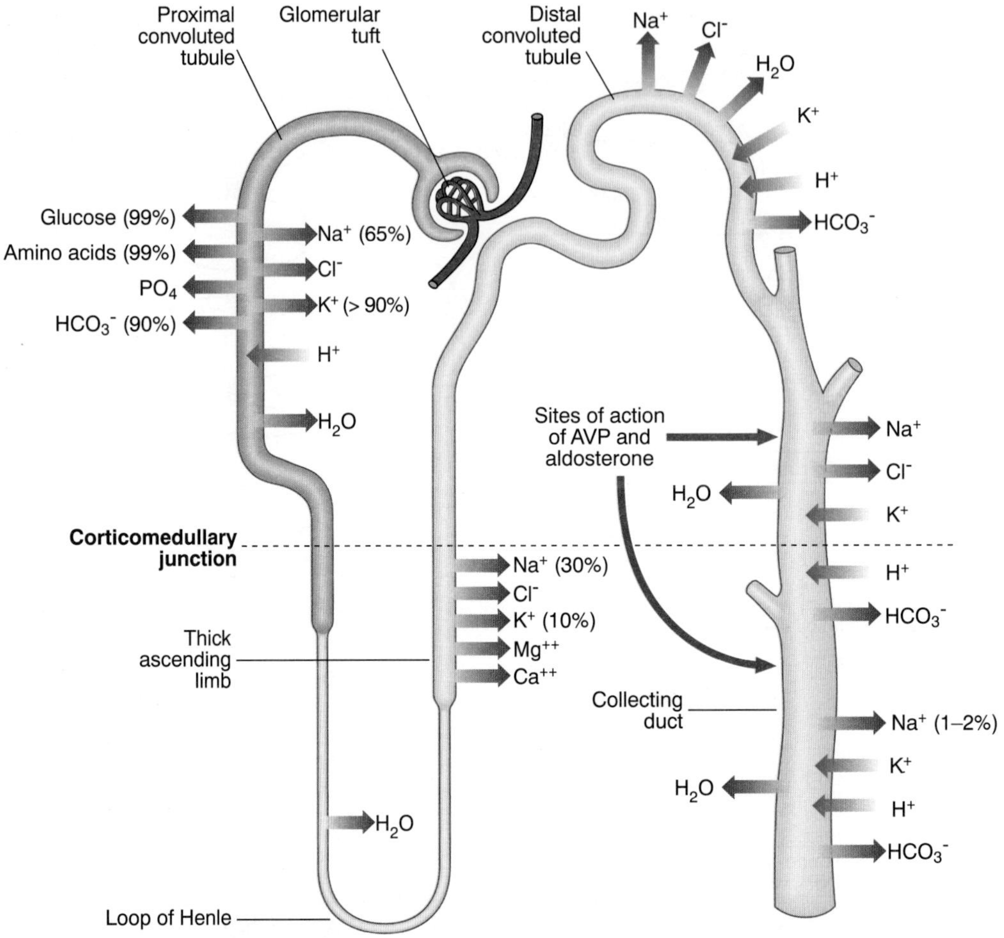

Fig. 5.4 Excretion of water and electrolytes. In the proximal tubule approximately two-thirds of filtered sodium and water is reabsorbed, together with glucose, amino acids, phosphate and bicarbonate. In the thick ascending limb of the loop of Henle sodium, potassium, calcium, magnesium and chloride are reabsorbed, whilst in the distal tubule sodium is reabsorbed under the influence of aldosterone with associated excretion of potassium and hydrogen ions. Water is reabsorbed from the distal nephron under the influence of arginine vasopressin (AVP) and the hypertonic medulla.

REGULATION OF ELECTROLYTES

SODIUM AND POTASSIUM

This depends upon selective reabsorption and secretion of electrolytes by the renal tubules. Figure 5.3 shows the major transport mechanisms present in renal tubular cells. Figure 5.4 shows the sites of reabsorption and secretion of the major electrolytes. Sodium is absorbed actively with glucose and amino acids in the proximal tubule, and in exchange with H^+ in all nephron segments.

Control of proximal tubular reabsorption of sodium and water is poorly understood. It is linked to the glomerular filtration rate (GFR) so that the fraction reabsorbed is normally constant. An increase in ECF volume is associated with reduced reabsorption of sodium and water at this site. Among the mechanisms proposed are angiotensins, atrial natriuretic peptide, changes in physical forces operating across peritubular capillary walls, increased local release of dopamine, and other unidentified natriuretic factors.

Most of the remaining sodium and chloride is reabsorbed without water in the thick ascending limb of the loop of Henle (see Fig. 5.3 middle). This is the single effect which is multiplied by the countercurrent loops of the tubule and peritubular capillaries. The result serves to establish an osmotic gradient in the interstitium from ~ 300 mosm in the outer medulla to > 1000 mosm around the terminal collecting duct. As in the proximal tubule, reabsorption of sodium in the ascending limb is flow-dependent; the amount reabsorbed varies directly with the proportion of filtrate delivered to the site. The diuretic drug frusemide competes with chloride for the luminal cotransport exchanger, thus inhibiting absorption of sodium, potassium and chloride.

Unabsorbed sodium passes into the distal tubule, collecting tubule and collecting duct. Here the cell membrane is relatively impermeable to chloride. Much of the sodium is reabsorbed 'in exchange' for potassium and hydrogen ions, which diffuse from cell to lumen down a lumen-negative electrochemical gradient created by active sodium transport (see Fig. 5.3 lower). The cells lining this part of the nephron can sustain a large concentration gradient for sodium between tubular and peritubular fluids. Thus in a sodium-depleted individual the concentration of sodium in the urine can be reduced to almost zero. At this site sodium transport is stimulated by aldosterone and prostaglandins, and inhibited by atrial natriuretic peptide and kinins.

More than 90% of filtered potassium (K^+) is reabsorbed actively in the proximal tubule and ascending limb. Urinary K^+ is largely derived from cells in the distal nephron (see Fig. 5.4), where active absorption of sodium creates a lumen-negative potential difference. An electrochemical gradient is created by active transport of potassium from the peritubular fluid into the cells (see Fig. 5.3), a process stimulated by aldosterone, while the intraluminal potential, negative with respect to the peritubular fluid, favours diffusion of potassium from cells to lumen (hence the hypokalaemia of Conn's syndrome). Drugs which lower aldosterone concentrations (e.g. ACE inhibitors) and block its action (e.g. spironolactone, amiloride) cause hyperkalaemia more easily when GFR is low. Factors influencing the rate of potassium excretion are shown in the information box.

FACTORS INCREASING K^+ EXCRETION

- Rise in tubular cell K^+, e.g. hyperaldosteronism, alkalosis
- High urine flow rate
- Avid Na^+ reabsorption
- Excess poorly reabsorbed anions, e.g. phosphate, ketones

The dual actions of the adrenocortical and antidiuretic hormones on the renal tubules play an important role in determining the total sodium, potassium and water content of the body. The rate of secretion of vasopressin is determined mainly by changes in osmolality of the blood but increases also in response to pain, stress and a reduction in ECF volume. Aldosterone secretion is increased by reduction in renal perfusion pressure and the sodium chloride concentration of the fluid reaching the macula densa. These stimuli increase secretion of renin by the juxtaglomerular apparatus (JGA); this in turn acts on its substrate angiotensinogen to produce the decapeptide angiotensin I. This is cleaved by angiotensin-converting enzyme (ACE), which converts angiotensin I to angiotensin II, and this stimulates synthesis of aldosterone by the adrenal cortex, thus tending to restore ECF volume.

CALCIUM, PHOSPHATE AND MAGNESIUM

Filtered calcium (that fraction not bound to plasma proteins) is reabsorbed throughout the nephron in a fashion similar to sodium; thus the rate of excretion of calcium usually varies with that of sodium. Parathyroid hormone (PTH) enhances tubular reabsorption of sodium and calcium, which contributes to the development of hypercalcaemia in primary hyperparathyroidism. Vitamin D_3 may stimulate proximal tubular calcium reabsorption.

Phosphate is filtered from plasma and reabsorbed principally by the proximal tubule, normally at close to its maximum capacity, so that in most circumstances the GFR is the major determinant of urinary phosphate excretion. Tubular phosphate reabsorption is reduced by PTH, contributing to the low plasma phosphate in primary and secondary hyperparathyroidism.

Most filtered magnesium is reabsorbed, partly under the influence of PTH, in the thick ascending limb of the loop of Henle. Tubular handling of calcium, phosphate and magnesium is influenced by various drugs, including diuretics, leading to low plasma concentrations and clinical symptoms in some cases.

REGULATION OF WATER EXCRETION

About two-thirds of the filtered water is reabsorbed with an equivalent amount of sodium in the proximal tubules. The remainder passes through the distal nephron where its reabsorption (see Fig. 5.4) is regulated by the antidiuretic hormone, arginine vasopressin (AVP). Figure 5.3 (bottom) illustrates how AVP acts to open specific water channels (aquaporins) in vesicles close to the luminal membrane. AVP binds to a specific V2 receptor for which analogue drugs are in development. *In the presence of AVP* the collecting duct becomes permeable to water, which is then passively reabsorbed in response to the high concentrations of sodium, chloride and urea in the medullary interstitium. The urine thus becomes concentrated. *In the absence of AVP* the distal nephron is almost impermeable to water. The active tubular reabsorption of sodium and chloride without water in the thick ascending limb of the loop of Henle results in the formation of a dilute urine.

MAINTENANCE OF NORMAL ACID-BASE BALANCE

Oxidative metabolism of proteins, fats and carbohydrate generates acid products which must be excreted to maintain body fluids within an optimal hydrogen ion concentration. Acid-base control involves *body buffers, lung function* and *kidney function* (in order of speed of response).

THE CO_2-BICARBONATE BUFFER SYSTEM

The most important buffer system is the CO_2-bicarbonate system. Arterial blood H^+ concentration ($[H^+]$) depends on the concentrations of carbonic acid (H_2CO_3 1.2 mmol/l in health), CO_2 (at a partial pressure of 5.2 kPa) and bicarbonate (24 mmol/l).

This is an 'open' buffer system because the bicarbonate and CO_2 components are under physiological control, reacting to changes in hydrogen ion concentration:

$$H^+ + HCO_3^- \leftrightarrow H_2CO_3 \leftrightarrow H_2O + CO_2$$

(regulated by kidneys) *(regulated by lungs)*

$[H^+]$ = dissociation constant (K) × $[CO_2]/[HCO_3^-]$
i.e. $[H^+]$ depends on the ratio of $[CO_2]$ to $[HCO_3^-]$

If H^+ ions are added to the blood (metabolic acidosis, e.g. poisoning by an acid) the equation is *pushed* to the right, and ventilation increases, via stimulation of chemoreceptors, to blow off CO_2. If the $[CO_2]$ rises, as in type II respiratory failure, the equilibrium is *pushed* to the left, increasing $[H^+]$ (respiratory acidosis). To compensate, the kidney must excrete more H^+ and regenerate more bicarbonate to set up a new equilibrium. In contrast, if H^+ ions are lost (e.g. as a result of vomiting in pyloric stenosis), the equation is *pulled* to the left (metabolic alkalosis). To bring the $[H^+]$ back to normal, more CO_2 is needed, and $[CO_2]$ rises through reduced ventilation by the lungs. Voluntary or involuntary hyperventilation leads to a fall in $[CO_2]$, and the equation is *pulled* to the right, with a fall in $[H^+]$ (respiratory alkalosis).

The process of compensation takes time, particularly renal compensation. Therefore acute disorders are less likely to be compensated than chronic ones. Compensation may be complete (H^+ concentration restored to normal) or partial (H^+ concentration still abnormal).

OTHER BUFFER SYSTEMS

Apart from the CO_2-bicarbonate system, other buffers include haemoglobin in red cells and hydroxyapatite in bone. These are 'closed' buffer systems which can be saturated. Haemoglobin in red cells is the major buffer that transfers H^+ and CO_2 from tissues to the lungs. Some CO_2 is transported reversibly bound to haemoglobin as a carbamino compound, but most is converted to H_2CO_3 since red cells are rich in carbonic anhydrase, which catalyses this reaction in either direction. Hydrogen ions from H_2CO_3 are taken up by Hb after it has given up oxygen to the tissues, while the HCO_3^- moves from red cells to plasma in exchange for chloride (chloride shift, see Fig. 5.5). Most of the carbonic acid added to the blood therefore appears as HCO_3^- rather than as acid. As blood passes through the lungs the process is reversed, and the CO_2 formed is exhaled. Not all acids can be oxidised completely to CO_2 and water. Such compounds as phosphoric acid and sulphuric acid from the diet are excreted by the kidneys as 'fixed acids'. A number of organic acids are important in disease. For example, excess lactate builds up in tissues starved of oxygen and results in a 'lactic acidosis' because of excess H^+ from reduced phosphorylated nucleotides (NADPH) in mitochondria.

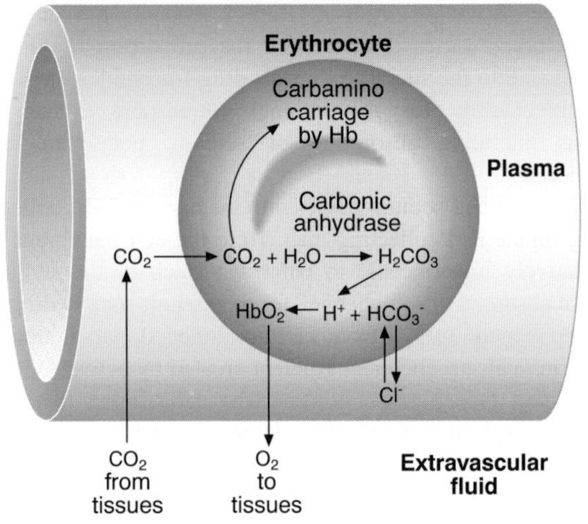

Fig. 5.5 Transport of CO_2.

The kidney is crucial in the response to changes in H^+ concentration (see Fig. 5.6). In proximal tubular cells, CO_2 derived from cellular metabolism or diffusion from the tubular lumen combines with water to form carbonic acid, which dissociates to H^+ and a bicarbonate ion. The H^+ ion is actively pumped into the tubular lumen, where it 'traps' filtered bicarbonate to form carbonic acid. Catalysed by luminal carbonic anhydrase, carbonic acid in the lumen dissociates to water and CO_2, which (unlike bicarbonate) is able to back-diffuse into the tubular cell, to continue the cycle. The original intracellular bicarbonate ion is actively cotransported with sodium into the interstitium, and hence the circulation. The net effect is that for each proton excreted, one bicarbonate ion is returned to the blood, so that bicarbonate reserves are regenerated. Filtered bicarbonate ions are reabsorbed mainly by this mechanism up to a threshold plasma concentration of 25 mmol/l. Above

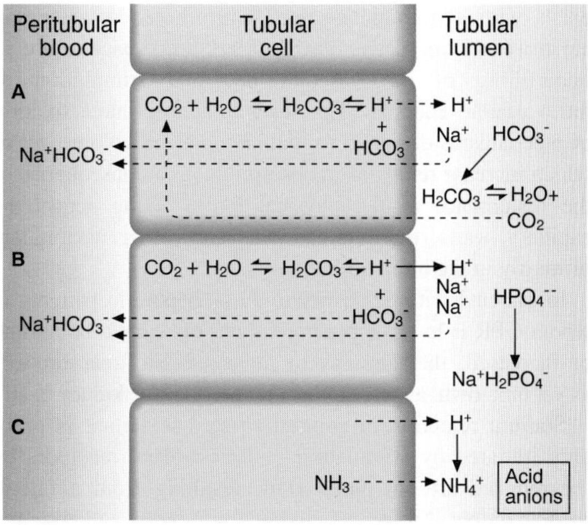

Fig 5.6 Hydrogen ion excretion. [A] Carbonic acid is generated from CO_2 and H_2O in tubular cells. Hydrogen ions (H^+) from this acid are secreted into the tubular lumen in exchange for sodium, which is reabsorbed into the blood along with bicarbonate ions liberated from the carbonic acid. Secreted H^+ combines with filtered bicarbonate to form carbonic acid; this 'traps' filtered bicarbonate and carbonic anhydrase catalyses the conversion of carbonic acid to CO_2 and water. [B] Some hydrogen ions are buffered by filtered disodium hydrogen phosphate in the tubular fluid forming dihydrogen sodium phosphate. [C] Other hydrogen ions are buffered by ammonia (NH_3) to form the weak acid NH_4^+. Anions of inorganic and organic acids are excreted largely as ammonium salts.

this level, reabsorption is incomplete and the excess is eliminated in the urine.

Active H^+ secretion continues all along the nephron. When most of the filtered bicarbonate has been reabsorbed, secreted hydrogen ions are taken up by other bases in the tubular fluid. The corresponding conjugate acids are excreted in the urine. Filtered bases, of which disodium hydrogen phosphate is the most important, accept about one-third of the hydrogen ions destined for excretion (see Fig. 5.6). This allows secretion of H^+ ions to continue without too high an opposing concentration gradient. The amount excreted in this way is limited by the magnitude of the hydrogen ion gradient between blood and tubular fluid which can be sustained by cells in the distal nephron. The urine pH cannot be reduced much below 4.5. Two-thirds of secreted protons are therefore accepted by the base ammonia (NH_3) formed within the tubular cell from glutamine. NH_3 enters the acid urine by non-ionic diffusion and accepts a proton to form the weak acid, NH_4^+. The luminal cell membrane is relatively impermeable to this charged particle, and it is excreted in the urine (see Fig. 5.6).

A healthy person eating a mixed diet excretes 40–80 mmol of hydrogen ion in the urine daily. When the rate of production of protons is increased (e.g. in diabetic ketoacidosis) the healthy kidney produces larger quantities of ammonia and up to 500 mmol/day of hydrogen ions may be excreted in the urine, mainly as NH_4^+. By contrast, when a diet consisting mainly of fruit and vegetables is taken, sodium di- and trihydrogen phosphate and bicarbonate are excreted and tubular secretion of ammonium ions is suppressed.

In the distal tubule and collecting duct, sodium is reabsorbed in exchange for either potassium or hydrogen ions, under the influence of aldosterone. When intracellular potassium is low, H^+ is preferentially exchanged, and vice versa. Hence the observed clinical associations between hypokalaemia and alkalosis, and hyperkalaemia and acidosis (although acidosis also inhibits the Na^+/K^+ ATPase which pumps potassium into cells). Diuretics which block sodium reabsorption in the loop of Henle, by increasing the delivery of sodium to the distal tubular exchange site, cause increased loss of both H^+ ions and potassium (hypokalaemic alkalosis).

FURTHER INFORMATION ON PHYSIOLOGY OF ELECTROLYTES, WATER AND ACID-BASE

Burckhardt G, Greger R 1992 Principles of electrolyte transport across plasma membranes of renal tubular cells. In: Windhager E E (ed) Handbook of physiology, section 8: 639–658. Oxford University Press, New York

Cohen R M, Feldman G M, Fernandez P C 1997 The balance of acid, base and charge in health and disease. Kidney International 52: 287–293

López-Nieto C E, Brenner B 1997 Molecular basis of inherited disorders of renal solute transport. Current Opinion in Nephrology and Hypertension 6: 411–421

Rossier B C, Alpern R J (eds) 1997 Molecular cell biology and physiology of solute transport. Current Opinion in Nephrology and Hypertension 6: 423–459

Zeidel M L, Strange K, Emma F, Harris H W 1993 Mechanisms and regulation of water transport in the kidney. Seminars in Nephrology 13: 155–167

MAJOR ELECTROLYTE AND ACID-BASE DISORDERS

Clinical assessment

Most patients exhibit few and subtle signs. Gross physical signs are usually associated with severe abnormalities and a correspondingly high mortality. Major electrolyte disturbances are most commonly associated with abnormalities of neurological or muscular function. A history of recent acute illness or surgery, drug ingestion or poisoning is always important. Careful review of fluid and weight charts may show discrepancies in intake and output.

DISORDERS OF EXTRACELLULAR FLUID VOLUME

SODIUM AND WATER EXCESS

In health the total body Na^+ is kept within narrow limits despite considerable day-to-day variation in intake. Western dietary sodium is variable but is commonly 150–200 mmol/day. A common presentation of salt and water excess is oedema, breathlessness and signs of congestive cardiac failure.

Aetiology

Accumulation of Na^+ occurs when renal excretion fails to keep pace with the amount ingested. Since Na^+ retention is accompanied by retention of an approximately iso-osmotic amount of water, the volume of the ECF is increased but ECF Na^+ concentration is not materially altered. Generalised oedema due to accumulation of fluid in the interstitial spaces is the clinical consequence of expansion of the ECF, and becomes evident when the ECF volume is increased by about 15%.

The appearance of generalised oedema requires:

1. a change in the forces acting upon the microcirculation which determine distribution of water and electrolytes between intravascular and interstitial fluid
2. renal retention of Na^+ and water in the face of increased body Na^+ and expansion of the ECF.

The sequence of events depends on the underlying disease and its stage of development (see Fig. 5.7). The simplest pattern is seen in patients with minimal change nephropathy (see p. 443), in which heavy proteinuria coexists with a normal or raised GFR. Loss of water and electrolytes from plasma into the interstitial space results in underfilling of the vascular bed and stimulation of intravascular receptors. This leads to appropriate activation of mechanisms designed to maintain plasma volume, all of which increase renal Na^+ reabsorption. As a consequence of the disturbance of the physical forces acting across the capillary walls, the retained Na^+ and water accumulate primarily in the interstitium.

In patients with acute nephritis, or nephrotic patients in whom GFR is low, the plasma volume appears to be normal or increased; the stimulus to increased Na^+ reabsorption, as yet unknown, appears to be a property of the kidney itself.

Sodium retention in congestive cardiac failure is probably initiated by stimulation of intra-arterial receptors by the reduced arterial blood flow, resulting from a fall in cardiac output. An increase in both pulmonary and systemic venous pressure leads to sequestration of retained Na^+ and water in the interstitial spaces of both circuits; this further reduces effective arterial flow. The problem is compounded by loss of the normal natriuretic response to atrial dilatation. Atrial natriuretic peptide concentrations in plasma are raised, but the kidney apparently fails to respond.

In hepatic cirrhosis, gross distortion of intrahepatic architecture gives rise to obstruction to hepatic venous outflow, to portal hypertension and to the development of

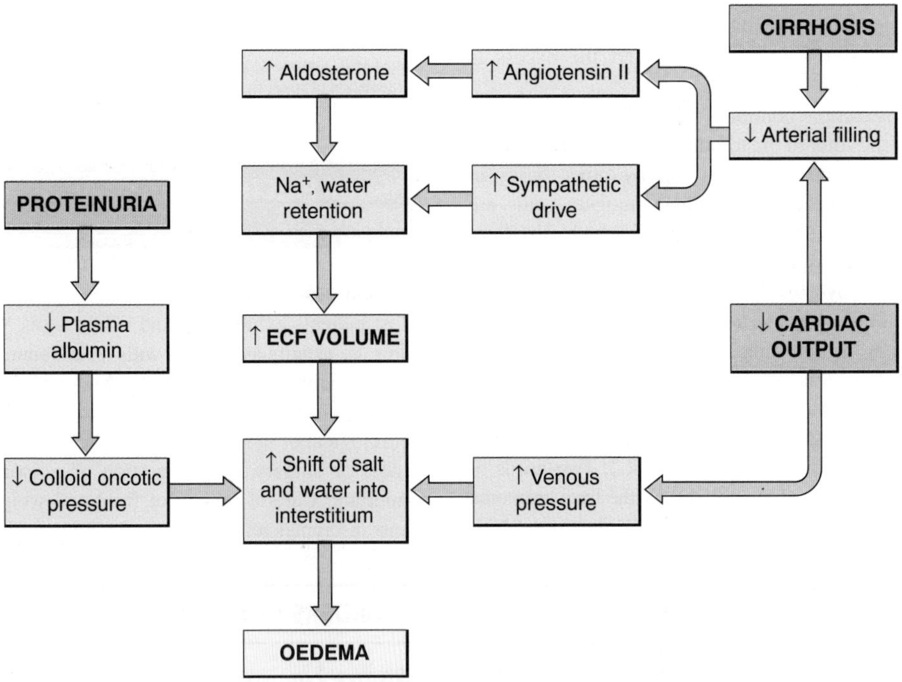

Fig. 5.7 The main forces acting to increase renal sodium and water reabsorption are shown for proteinuria, heart failure and cirrhosis.

portasystemic shunts (see p. 707). Receptors within the hepatic circulation are thought to respond to increased hepatic venous pressure, and to initiate Na^+ retention via sympathetic hepatorenal reflexes. There may also be relative underfilling of the vascular system, due to dilatation of the systemic circulation and to sequestration of fluid in the peritoneal cavity; this may further stimulate renal sodium retention through neuro-endocrine mechanisms, such as renin-angiotensin-aldosterone activation.

Knowledge of this subject is incomplete and changing rapidly, but clearly in all these disorders, stimuli arising from an underperfused section of the vascular tree are important in initiating and maintaining renal Na^+ retention despite increased total body Na^+. Conditions associated with generalised oedema are shown in the information box.

CONDITIONS ASSOCIATED WITH GENERALISED OEDEMA

- Cardiac failure
- Nephrotic syndrome, acute nephritic syndrome
- Acute oliguric renal failure; advanced chronic renal failure (GFR < 15 ml/min)
- Hepatic cirrhosis, acute liver failure, hepatic vein thrombosis
- Protein-losing enteropathy
- Starvation, thiamine deficiency
- Premenstrual fluid retention, pregnancy
- Acute anaphylaxis
- Drugs which cause sodium retention
  - Antihypertensives (calcium channel blockers, vasodilators)
  - Corticosteroids
  - Non-steroidal anti-inflammatory drugs (NSAIDs)
  - Oestrogens
  - Liquorice, carbenoxolone

Clinical features

These depend to some extent on the distribution of retained fluid and are described under the various diseases.

Management

The principles of management are simple and are shown in the information box.

MANAGEMENT OF OEDEMA

- Restrict dietary sodium to 100 mmol/day ('no added salt') or 50 mmol in severe cases
- Diuretics
- Specific treatment directed at the cause, e.g. ACE inhibitor in heart failure, corticosteroids in minimal change nephropathy

Diuretic therapy

Drugs which block Na^+ reabsorption also increase urinary volume, because reabsorption of water in the nephron is passive and depends on Na^+ reabsorption.

Table 5.1 provides information about commonly used diuretics. The choice of drug depends upon the severity of the oedema and whether or not the patient is resistant to the

Table 5.1 Commonly used diuretic drugs

Class	Drugs	Principal sites of action in nephron	Extrarenal actions	Principal side-effects of the group
High-potency diuretics	Frusemide	1 Inhibition of reabsorption of NaCl in thick ascending limb of loop of Henle 2 Minor inhibition of reabsorption of NaCl in proximal tubule 3 Increase renal blood flow	Increase venous capacitance	Postural hypotension, K^+ depletion, Mg^{++} depletion, alkalosis, hyperuricaemia, hyperglycaemia, hypersensitivity (rash, myelosuppression, hepatic dysfunction, interstitial nephritis)
	Bumetanide	As above		Ototoxicity
	Ethacrynic acid	As above		
Medium-potency diuretics	Benzothiadiazines (thiazides)	1 Inhibition of reabsorption of NaCl in early distal tubule (diluting site) 2 Inhibition of reabsorption of NaCl in proximal tubule 3 Some inhibit reabsorption of $NaHCO_3$ in proximal and distal tubules (minor)	Antihypertensive	K^+ depletion, alkalosis, hyponatraemia, hyperuricaemia, hyperglycaemia, hyperlipidaemia, hypersensitivity (rash, myelosuppression, acute pancreatitis, hepatic dysfunction, interstitial nephritis)
	Metolazone	As above 1 and 2		
Low-potency diuretics	Acetazolamide	Inhibits reabsorption of $NaHCO_3$ in proximal and distal tubule	Decreased rate of formation of aqueous humour in the eye	K^+ depletion, acidosis, drowsiness, hypersensitivity (rash, myelosuppression, interstitial nephritis), renal stones
K^+-sparing low-potency diuretics	Spironolactone	Aldosterone antagonist inhibits aldosterone-sensitive Na^+/K^+ exchange in collecting tubule	Gynaecomastia	Hyperkalaemia, acidosis
	Triamterene	Inhibits reabsorption of Na^+ in collecting tubule, thus indirectly inhibits K^+ secretion at that site		Renal stones containing triamterene, acute renal failure when given with indomethacin
	Amiloride	As triamterene		Hyperkalaemia

effects of diuretics. Mild cases, e.g. ankle oedema in an elderly person with cardiac failure, usually respond to a combination of moderate salt restriction and benzothiadiazine diuretic. Hydrochlorothiazide 50–100 mg/day or bendrofluazide 5–10 mg/day may be given or, if a slower and more prolonged diuresis is desired, chlorthalidone 50 mg/day can be used. More severe cases should receive a high-potency diuretic—oral frusemide 40–120 mg/day or bumetanide 1–3 mg/day—with a diet containing about 100 mmol/day Na^+. Intravenous frusemide, 20–40 mg, is valuable in treating acute pulmonary oedema. Intravenous ethacrynic acid should be avoided because of ototoxicity. Causes of resistance to the effects of diuretics are given in the information box.

CAUSES OF DIURETIC RESISTANCE

- Reduced renal function
- Volume depletion and secondary hyperaldosteronism
- Profound hypoproteinaemia

Patients with chronic renal failure often respond to large doses of oral frusemide (250 mg–1 g) or bumetanide (5–10 mg). If this fails, a combination of one of these diuretics with metolazone (5–10 mg) or bendrofluazide (10 mg) may succeed, since these drugs act synergistically. In patients with resistant oedema due to cirrhosis or severe cardiac failure whose renal function is not compromised, a combination of spironolactone (100–200 mg) or amiloride (20 mg) with frusemide or bumetanide may induce diuresis. These lower-potency drugs are poor diuretics alone, but are of value when combined with a loop diuretic, as they inhibit Na^+ reabsorption in exchange for K^+ or H^+ in the distal nephron. Since they reduce K^+ excretion they must not be given along with K^+ supplements, nor used when renal function is impaired, lest dangerous hyperkalaemia results.

Adverse effects of diuretic therapy on water and electrolyte balance

Potassium depletion. High- and medium-potency diuretics, which deliver an increased amount of Na^+ to the distal nephron, induce K^+ depletion (see p. 407), especially when given repeatedly over long periods and when combined with a low Na^+ diet. Symptoms of K^+ deficiency may arise before satisfactory loss of oedema has been achieved and are then superimposed upon clinical features of Na^+ and water accumulation. This is liable to occur during the treatment of severe heart failure (see p. 213) and may be responsible for the development of digoxin toxicity before the heart failure has been controlled. In hepatic disease with ascites and oedema, K^+ depletion may aggravate or precipitate hepatic encephalopathy.

Prophylactic administration of K^+ is essential when diuretics are given frequently. Potassium chloride 3–4 g/day in divided doses is given, usually as slow-release or effervescent tablets.

Metabolic alkalosis. See page 413.

Sodium depletion and reduced blood volume. Overtreatment with diuretics results in Na^+ and water depletion. This may occur when high-potency drugs are given over prolonged periods without adequate supervision. The clinical features of Na^+ and water depletion are described below.

Patients with severe oedema resistant to therapy sometimes develop clinical features of reduced blood volume while still oedematous. In these cases hypotension, tachycardia and a raised blood urea are often associated with a low plasma [Na^+]. Such patients usually suffer from advanced cardiac, hepatic or renal disease associated with hypoproteinaemia. Persistent attempts to reduce the oedema usually lead to further deterioration. Diuretics should be withheld temporarily and a more liberal salt intake permitted. Cautious infusion of 25–100 g plasma protein solution or 20–40 g salt-poor albumin over a period of 3 or 4 hours to increase the blood volume may help. Signs of circulatory overload are an indication to stop the infusion.

Hyponatraemia. Patients with severe oedema may develop hyponatraemia because they are unable to excrete water normally (see p. 405). This is exacerbated by the use of thiazides or metolazone which interfere with urinary dilution. The clinical features associated with hyponatraemia and its management are discussed on pages 405–406.

SODIUM AND WATER DEPLETION

Volume depletion is a more accurate term than dehydration, which refers to hypernatraemia secondary to water loss.

Aetiology and assessment

Loss of salt and water occurs with any of the conditions in Table 5.2. There will usually be a good clinical history or a chart review will demonstrate excessive loss of fluids via urine or elsewhere.

It is important to assess *volume status* to facilitate diagnosis and rational treatment. Postural hypotension, the jugular venous pressure (JVP) and the presence or absence of oedema are the main clinical signs which point to whether a patient has a normal plasma volume, is volume-depleted or is overloaded. The severity of volume depletion can be judged using the criteria described in the information box.

Management

Principles are given in the information box. These patients require restoration of plasma volume, which can be achieved with NaCl 0.9% solution supplemented by plasma expanders (e.g. plasma protein solutions, colloidal starch etc.) or sodium bicarbonate 1.26% solution when severe

Table 5.2 Causes of sodium and water depletion

Underlying mechanism	Clinical condition
Loss from alimentary tract	**External loss** Vomiting Aspiration of GI contents Fistulae Diarrhoea Villous adenoma of large bowel **Sequestration of fluid in bowel** Ileus Intestinal obstruction
Loss in urine	**Extrarenal factors acting on kidney** Osmotic diuresis Diabetes mellitus Mannitol Diuretics Metabolic acidosis Adrenocortical insufficiency **Renal disease** Diuretic phase acute tubular necrosis Post-obstructive diuresis Chronic renal insufficiency Proximal renal tubular acidosis Medullary cystic disease Congenital polycystic disease Chronic interstitial nephritis
Loss in sweat	Fever Hot environment
Loss in exudates and transudates, 'third' space losses	**Loss from body surfaces** Burns Extensive dermatitis **Loss into body cavities or soft tissues** Ascites Peritonitis Acute pancreatitis Rhabdomyolysis Inferior vena cava thrombosis

CLINICAL EVALUATION OF SALT AND WATER DEPLETION

Mild (< 2 litres in adult)

- Thirst
- Concentrated urine

Moderate (2–3 litres in adult)

As above, plus:
- Dizziness, weakness
- Oliguria (< 400 ml/day)
- Postural hypotension > 20 mmHg systolic
- Low JVP

Severe (> 3 litres in adult)

As above, plus:
- Confusion, stupor
- Systolic BP < 100 mmHg
- Tachycardia (not in elderly), low pulse volume
- Cold extremities, poor capillary return
- Reduced skin turgor ('doughy')

metabolic acidosis is also present. The JVP and blood pressure should be monitored. Acutely ill patients or those with heart disease will require a central venous pressure (CVP) line and monitoring. Intake of water should be restricted in patients who are also hyponatraemic and dextrose 5% solution should not be administered until the plasma sodium is within the normal range.

GUIDELINES FOR REPLACEMENT OF VOLUME DEFICIT

Mild

- 0.9% saline 1 litre i.v. 6–12-hourly

Moderate

- 0.9% saline 1 litre i.v. over 2–4 hours
- 0.9% saline 1–2 litres i.v. 6–8-hourly

Severe

- Gelatin/starch/plasma protein solution 0.5–1 litre over 1–3 hours
- 0.9% saline 2 litres i.v. over 4–6 hours
- 0.9% saline 1 litre 6-hourly until replaced

N.B. Initial treatment must be reviewed frequently to ensure satisfactory improvement and to avoid precipitating cardiac failure. CVP monitoring is often indicated in patients with a history of heart disease or in the elderly. Maintenance treatment depends on the nature and amount of continuing losses which should be measured—potassium, calcium and magnesium may be needed.

SODIUM AND POTASSIUM

HYPERNATRAEMIA

The plasma sodium concentration is an indication of the water added to or leaving body fluids. Hypernatraemia usually indicates a lack of water. The water content of the body is reduced both absolutely and relative to the Na^+ content, so that the osmolar concentration of all body fluids rises.

Aetiology

Water intake is usually about 2 litres/day but is variable and tends to be less in females. An adult in a temperate climate loses between 0.5 and 1 litre of water/day in expired air and by evaporation from the skin. This loss can be increased considerably by a rise in temperature and sweating. Water can be conserved by the kidneys up to a limit determined by renal concentrating ability (up to 1200 mosm/kg) and the amount of solutes that need to be excreted; a high solute load requires an obligatory high urine output.

The causes of water depletion (see Table 5.3) are most commonly a reduced intake, and an increase in insensible loss in elderly patients with infection. Excessive loss of water in the urine (diabetes insipidus) due to impaired concentrating ability is much less common but can be seen after serious head injury.

Table 5.3 Causes of pure or predominant water depletion

Underlying mechanism	Clinical condition
Reduced intake	Water unavailable Voluntary water intake reduced, e.g. in infants, the aged, people who are depressed or apathetic Coma Inability to swallow Nausea Primary hypodipsia
Increased loss from skin	Fever, hyperthyroidism Hot environment
Increased loss from respiratory tract	Hyperventilation, fever High altitudes
Increased loss in urine due to marked impairment of urinary concentrating mechanism	**Deficiency of vasopressin (AVP)** Diabetes insipidus **Renal tubular unresponsiveness to AVP** (nephrogenic diabetes insipidus) Hypercalcaemia, K^+ depletion Chronic interstitial nephritis Amyloidosis, obstructive uropathy Medullary cystic disease Drugs, e.g. lithium Congenital **Solute diuresis** Diabetes mellitus Enteral or parenteral feeds with high solute concentration

Hypernatraemia is also encountered in children forced to ingest salt (in order to induce vomiting after self-poisoning) and in adults on high protein/calorie nasogastric feeding who are given insufficient water to excrete the high solute load.

Clinical features

These are shown in the information box.

CLINICAL FEATURES OF PREDOMINANT WATER DEPLETION
Mild (1–2 litres in adult)
• Thirst • Concentrated urine
Moderate (2–4 litres in adult)
• Marked thirst, difficulty swallowing • Dizziness, mild confusion/aggression and weakness • Oliguria, concentrated urine • Rising plasma urea and Na^+
Severe (4–10 litres in adult)
• Severe thirst • Confusion, coma, muscle weakness • 'Doughy' skin and tissues • Tachycardia, low BP • Oliguria, concentrated urine • Raised plasma urea, Na^+ and Hb

Consequences of water depletion

As water is lost from the body the ECF becomes hypertonic and the plasma [Na^+] rises. Water migrates from cells to re-establish osmotic equilibrium, and intracellular dehydration develops when more than 8% of body water is lost. Renal reabsorption of Na^+ and Cl^- and excretion of K^+ increase secondary to secretion of aldosterone. Retained Na^+ and Cl^- increase ECF tonicity and facilitate transfer of water from cells. The overall loss of water is thus shared by the intracellular and extracellular compartments, so that the circulatory disturbance in water depletion is much less marked than in salt and water depletion of comparable magnitude.

Diagnosis

Diagnosis is made from the history, clinical findings and the presence of hypernatraemia. A measurement of urine osmolality will be helpful; if this is > 600 mosm/kg a renal cause is most unlikely. The urine should be tested for glucose, and renal function checked by measurement of plasma urea and creatinine concentrations. Marked polyuria of more than 3 litres/day and urine osmolality of < 200 mosm/kg suggest AVP-deficient diabetes insipidus or one of the renal lesions in Table 5.3.

Management

Management of water depletion in adults is given in the information box. It can often be prevented by ensuring an adequate intake in ill patients and this is especially important in patients receiving enteral feeds. Fluid charts and daily weights are useful to monitor progress. It is essential that large water deficits are replaced gradually over several days to avoid rapid shift of water into cells, which can cause severe disturbance of neurological function. Where there is a specific cause (e.g. diabetes insipidus, diabetes mellitus, hypercalcaemia) then this requires rigorous specific therapy in addition to water replacement.

GUIDELINES FOR REPLACEMENT OF WATER DEFICIT	
Mild	
• Water 2 litres by mouth or 5% dextrose i.v.	6–12 hours
Moderate	
• 5% dextrose 2–4 litres i.v.	24 hours
Severe	
• 0.9% saline 1 litre i.v. • 5% dextrose 4 litres i.v. • 5% dextrose 2–4 litres i.v. + oral water	1 hour 24 hours 24–48 hours
Maintenance treatment	
• 5% dextrose + oral water to balance urine + insensible loss until plasma Na^+ and urea normal	

HYPONATRAEMIA

Hyponatraemia reflects a change in the proportion of sodium and water in plasma, rather than a change in sodium content. Hyponatraemia is common in patients with volume depletion because of excessive AVP stimulating water retention.

Pseudohyponatraemia is seen with gross hyperlipidaemia. Older autoanalysers measure the sodium in the whole sample and report a low value when the true concentration in the plasma water is normal; the plasma appears obviously lipaemic.

Aetiology

Healthy adults can drink up to 20 litres/day and the kidneys will respond with a vigorous water diuresis. However, patients with restricted renal function, including older persons, cannot respond in this way and may become hyponatraemic with much smaller volumes. Most patients regulate their intake of water through the thirst mechanism, but some mentally disturbed patients may voluntarily drink excessive fluids and develop hyponatraemia. Patients cannot regulate their own fluid intake when on intravenous fluids or a tube feed.

The more common causes of hyponatraemia are shown in the information box in relation to the assessment of volume status. A number of disease processes and drugs interfere with normal water excretion and Table 5.4 shows the causes of hyponatraemia grouped according to pathogenesis. Hyponatraemia can be caused where water is transferred out from cells because of a sudden rise in plasma osmolality. This may occur in uncontrolled diabetes mellitus with hyperglycaemia or following the administration of an osmotic diuretic, e.g. mannitol.

The most common pathogenesis of hyponatraemia is *sodium and water depletion*, where the loss of salt from the body exceeds the reduction in total body water, often because patients continue to drink water in the early stages of the illness. Major causes are given in Table 5.2. Hyponatraemia in these patients is maintained by excessive AVP secretion which has been stimulated by volume depletion, or pain and stress. The stimulus to AVP secretion, which occurs when the plasma volume is reduced by about 5%, overrides osmoreceptor-mediated signals to switch off AVP production as plasma osmolality falls. The urine thus shows paradoxical concentration in the face of dilute body fluids.

The last group of conditions associated with hyponatraemia are those in which the increase in total body water exceeds a simultaneous increase in body sodium. In these conditions the retention of sodium is associated with a simultaneous inability to excrete water. This is often mediated at the kidney level by both excessive sodium retention at proximal sites and excessive inappropriate AVP secretion because of 'effective volume' depletion.

AETIOLOGY OF HYPONATRAEMIA

Low ECF

- Volume depletion (e.g. diabetic ketoacidosis, vomiting and/or diarrhoea, bowel obstruction, burns)
- Cirrhosis
- Adrenal failure
- Salt-losing renal disease

Normal ECF

- Nephrotic syndrome
- Hypothyroidism
- Diuretics
- NSAIDs
- Post-operative pain and analgesia

High ECF

- Cardiac failure
- Renal failure
- Syndrome of inappropriate secretion of ADH (SIADH)

Table 5.4 Causes of hyponatraemia

Pathogenesis	Clinical condition	Extracellular fluid volume
Increased total body water	SIADH Adrenocortical failure Hypothyroidism Hypopituitarism Psychogenic polydipsia	Slightly increased; no oedema
Relative increase in extracellular water	Uncontrolled diabetes mellitus Administration of mannitol	Normal or slightly reduced
Reduction in total body sodium exceeds reduction in total body water	Any cause of mixed Na^+ and water depletion (Table 5.2)	Reduced
Increase in total body water exceeds increase in total body sodium	Cardiac failure Liver failure Nephrotic syndrome Cirrhosis Renal failure Diuretics	Increased Oedema common

Diagnosis

Clinical assessment of plasma volume is crucial in assessing the contribution of sodium depletion or excess to the overall picture. The *history*, including recent drug ingestion, review of fluid balance charts and weight, followed by careful clinical examination, paying attention to the conditions listed in Table 5.4, will generally identify a cause. Hyponatraemia may be associated with a mild confusional state, lassitude and sleepiness, progressing to gross confusion, myoclonic jerks and generalised seizures. Serious clinical signs occur in patients in whom the plasma sodium has changed abruptly or is very low (< 110 mmol/l).

This is a medical emergency, as the mortality is about 40% and the risk of neurological damage (central pontine myelinolysis) is high.

Additional laboratory tests

The plasma urea and creatinine will be required to assess renal function. The urinary sodium and osmolality are helpful in judging the contributions of renal sodium loss and of AVP. Hyponatraemia with a high urine osmolality (AVP effect) and a low urinary sodium (sodium and water loss) is an *appropriate* response to volume depletion. If plasma volume is thought to be normal or is increased, then a high urine osmolality indicates an *inappropriate* excess of AVP—the syndrome of inappropriate secretion of ADH (SIADH). Causes of SIADH are shown in the information box.

CONDITIONS ASSOCIATED WITH THE SYNDROME OF INAPPROPRIATE SECRETION OF ADH (SIADH)
Neoplasm
• Carcinoma of bronchus (small cell), pancreas, duodenum, ureter, bladder, prostate, lymphoma, thymoma, mesothelioma
Disorders of CNS
• Meningitis, encephalitis, brain abscess, head injury, cerebral tumour, cerebral vascular accident, hydrocephalus, cerebral or cerebellar atrophy, delirium tremens, psychosis, Guillain–Barré syndrome
Non-malignant pulmonary lesions
• Tuberculosis, pneumonia (bacterial, viral)
Drugs
• Narcotics, phenothiazines, carbamazepine, tricyclic antidepressants, monoamine oxidase inhibitors, clofibrate, vincristine, vinblastine, cyclophosphamide*, chlorpropamide, non-steroidal anti-inflammatory drugs*
Miscellaneous
• Pain, post-operative period, nausea
* Potentiate effect of ADH (AVP) on collecting duct.

Management

Management will often need to be started before the results of all investigations are available. In some cases it will be necessary to await the results of endocrine investigations before coming to a definite diagnosis, but these will be uncommon.

All patients are best managed by restriction of water intake and further details are given in the information box. In patients with severe neurological symptoms the plasma sodium should be raised more rapidly by giving hypertonic NaCl solution intravenously. A loop diuretic may be required in these patients to prevent volume overload.

GUIDELINES FOR TREATMENT OF HYPONATRAEMIA
Plasma Na > 120 mmol/l
• Water restriction to 0.5 litre • 0.9% saline if volume deplete • Stop drugs/treat specific cause
Plasma Na > 110–120 mmol/l
• Water restriction < 0.5 litre • 0.9% saline i.v. (if not in ECF excess) 1 litre 12-hourly • Add frusemide 20–40 mg oral if overloaded
Plasma Na < 110 mmol/l or with neurological signs
• 1.8% or 3% saline *slowly* i.v. to raise plasma Na 0.5 mmol/l/hour • Add frusemide 20 mg i.v. if overloaded or CVP rises rapidly

Frequent monitoring of the plasma sodium and overall fluid balance is essential.

Transfer of water from cells

Patients with uncontrolled diabetes mellitus and hyponatraemia are treated with isotonic fluids and insulin. Where mannitol is the underlying cause, no active treatment should be necessary, as it is excreted over 6–8 hours.

Sodium and water depletion

See page 402.

Sodium and water excess

See page 399. These patients require sodium restriction (50–80 mmol/day) as well as water restriction and careful use of a loop diuretic. Where the hyponatraemia is caused by a drug, then withdrawal of the drug and water restriction are usually sufficient. Hyponatraemia caused by diuretics may require volume expansion with NaCl 0.9% solution.

HYPERKALAEMIA

The principal causes of hyperkalaemia are given in Table 5.5. Most K^+ is inside cells, so changes in the *distribution* of K^+ between plasma and intracellular fluid can have a marked effect on the plasma K^+ concentration. The Na^+/K^+ ATPase which transports potassium into cells in exchange for sodium is pH-sensitive. In diabetic ketoacidosis, hyperkalaemia is relatively common because of metabolic acidosis (shift of potassium out of cells) and hypovolaemia (impaired K^+ excretion), despite an overall K^+ deficit accumulated during the period of osmotic diuresis. During treatment with insulin, hyperkalaemia rapidly resolves and may be followed by a significant hypokalaemia.

Pseudohyperkalaemia is caused by the release of K^+ in vitro from abnormal or damaged cells, such as the abnormal white blood cells in acute leukaemia. It is also common in

Table 5.5 Causes of hyperkalaemia

Underlying mechanism	Clinical condition
Increased intake	I.v. fluid containing K^+, high K^+ foods Drugs containing K^+
Tissue breakdown	Bleeding into soft tissues, GI tract or body cavities Haemolysis, rhabdomyolysis Catabolic states
Shift of K^+ out of cells	Tissue damage (e.g. following ischaemia, shock) Acidosis Insulin deficiency Aldosterone deficiency β-adrenoceptor antagonists ECF hypertonicity
Impaired excretion	**Renal disease** Acute renal failure Severe chronic renal failure (GFR < 15 ml/min) Impaired tubular secretion of K^+ (systemic lupus erythematosus, transplanted kidney, amyloidosis, sickle-cell disease) **Acute circulatory failure** **Drugs which inhibit renal K^+ secretion** Aldosterone antagonists, amiloride **Abnormalities of renin-angiotensin-aldosterone axis** Addison's disease, adrenal enzyme deficiencies Primary hypoaldosteronism, hyporeninaemic hypoaldosteronism, β-adrenoceptor antagonists, NSAIDs, ACE inhibitors
Pseudohyperkalaemia	Release of K^+ in vitro from abnormal blood cells or incorrectly handled specimens

poorly handled blood specimens which have been left for too long at room temperature before separation and analysis.

Diagnosis

Hyperkalaemia must be suspected in the circumstances outlined in the information box and confirmed by urgent analysis. Clinical signs of hyperkalaemia are rare. Patients may complain of tingling around the lips or in the fingers but are more likely to present with collapse due to a dangerous bradyarrhythmia. This may be the first and only sign of hyperkalaemia and an irregular pulse should be checked with an electrocardiogram (ECG). Typical ECG changes are shown in Figure 5.8. Patients may also develop severe muscular weakness resulting in a flaccid paralysis, loss of tendon jerks, abdominal distension and ileus. These patients require emergency treatment, and clinical suspicion should be confirmed by an emergency plasma K^+ estimation.

SUSPECT HYPERKALAEMIA

- Release of K^+ from dead/injured cells, e.g. tissue damage, rhabdomyolysis, haemolysis, GI bleeding
- Rapid administration of K^+ by mouth or intravenously
- Impaired renal excretion of K^+, including severe renal failure, use of K^+-sparing diuretics (spironolactone, amiloride, triamterene)
- Acidosis

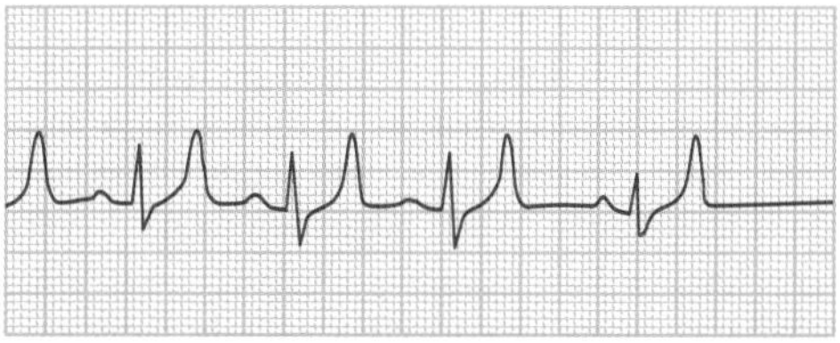

Fig. 5.8 Changes in the ECG associated with hyperkalaemia. The T waves are tall, peaked and tent-like, and the PR interval and QRS complexes are lengthened. In severe cases, the P wave disappears and the QRS complex widens further, with loss of the T wave.

Hyperkalaemia is dangerous because cardiac arrest can occur when the plasma K^+ exceeds 7 mmol/l, and this may be the earliest and only manifestation. The blood results must be acted on immediately.

Management

Hyperkalaemia should be prevented in conditions associated with oliguria. The established case can be dealt with by the measures shown in the information box. Recurrence of hyperkalaemia should then be prevented by dietary restriction of foods rich in K^+ and further use of Calcium Resonium 15–30 g 2–3 times daily. Patients with renal failure may require dialysis.

MANAGEMENT OF ACUTE HYPERKALAEMIA

- Identify and treat cause
- Inject 10–20 ml 10% calcium gluconate i.v. over 10 min (reduces risk of cardiac arrest)
- Inject 50 ml 50% glucose i.v. Monitor plasma glucose; give insulin if hyperglycaemia occurs. Monitor plasma K^+ after 20–30 min and repeat if necessary
- Start infusion of 10–20% dextrose 500 ml 4–6-hourly (to minimise rebound ↑ K^+)
  Alternative Salbutamol 0.5 mg i.v. in 5% dextrose over 15 min
- Calcium Resonium (exchange resin, binds K^+ in exchange for calcium) may be given, 15–30 g orally
- If metabolic acidosis present—infuse sodium bicarbonate 1.26% 500 ml 6–8-hourly until plasma $[HCO_3^+]$ in normal range. **N.B.** Watch for circulatory overload
- Correct volume depletion and/or respiratory acidosis if present
- Use haemodialysis/haemofiltration or peritoneal dialysis if the above fail

HYPOKALAEMIA

Dietary intake of K^+ is 60–80 mmol/day; over 85% is excreted in the urine and the remainder in stools. The maintenance of K^+ balance depends on regulation of urinary K^+ excretion. Potassium excretion is increased when cell K^+ rises (in alkalosis), when urine flow is high and when there is active reabsorption of sodium mediated by increased aldosterone. When potassium intake is very low, urinary excretion falls gradually to about 5 mmol/day, but this small continuing loss, together with the daily stool loss of 8–10 mmol, results in moderate K^+ depletion. Most of body potassium is in cells and uptake is stimulated by insulin, β-adrenoceptor agonists, aldosterone and alkalosis.

The causes of potassium depletion are given in Table 5.6. Most of the gastrointestinal disorders listed are associated with loss of Na^+ and water as well as K^+, and result in volume depletion. The increase in circulating aldosterone leads to additional loss of K^+ in urine. A number of drugs, including most diuretics, promote potassium loss.

Diagnosis

Hypokalaemia may be suggested by tiredness and muscular weakness, which in extreme cases can result in the patient being unable to walk or climb stairs. Neurological functions are usually normal, but tingling in the fingers, apathy, paralysis and coma may be present in extreme cases. Long-standing hypokalaemia damages renal tubular structures and results in a failure of the antidiuretic response to vasopressin (nephrogenic diabetes insipidus). Patients with hypokalaemia may therefore present with nocturia or marked polyuria and polydipsia. The ECG may be helpful (see Fig. 5.9) and the development of arrhythmias on a combination of digoxin and diuretics should raise clinical suspicion.

Plasma K^+ is low in most cases of K^+ depletion. However, in the presence of severe ECF depletion, metabolic acidosis or deficiency of insulin or aldosterone, clinically significant K^+ depletion may develop without a change in plasma K^+—for example, in untreated diabetic ketoacidosis. Conversely, patients suffering from metabolic alkalosis, or who have been taking excessive insulin or β-adrenergic agonists, may have a low plasma K^+ despite a normal total body K^+ because of movement of K^+ into cells. The diagnosis depends on careful assessment of the clinical history, including drugs, and examination for gastrointestinal or renal disease. The urinary K^+ may be helpful, as a value of < 20 mmol/day excludes renal K^+ loss, while a urinary K^+ of > 30 mmol/day is strongly suggestive of a renal cause.

Table 5.6 Causes of potassium depletion

Underlying mechanism	Clinical condition
Reduced intake	Diet containing adequate calories and insufficient potassium Potassium-free intravenous fluid
Loss from alimentary tract	**External loss** Vomiting Aspiration of GI contents Fistulae Diarrhoea[1] Acute Chronic (laxative addicts, malabsorption syndrome) Villous adenoma large bowel Ureterosigmoidostomy **Sequestration of fluid in bowel** Ileus Intestinal obstruction
Loss in urine	**Extrarenal factors acting on kidney** Primary aldosteronism[2] Bartter's syndrome Gitelman's syndrome Secondary aldosteronism (e.g. renovascular disease, accelerated hypertension,[2] cirrhosis, cardiac failure, nephrotic syndrome) Cushing's syndrome[2] Diabetic ketoacidosis Metabolic alkalosis Chronic metabolic acidosis Drugs, e.g. diuretics, amphotericin B, corticosteroids,[2] liquorice,[2] carbenoxolone[2] **Renal disease** Recovery phase of acute tubular necrosis Following relief of urinary tract obstruction Renal tubular acidosis

[1] Considerable amounts of potassium may be lost in diarrhoea.
[2] Associated with hypertension.

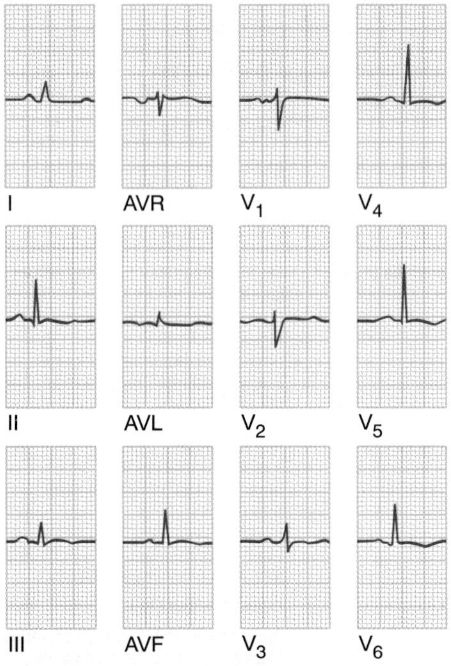

Fig. 5.9 Changes in the ECG associated with hypokalaemia. Sinus rhythm with normal QRS complexes. The T waves are flattened and U waves are present in most leads.

Bartter's and Gitelman's syndromes are rare, sometimes familial and often asymptomatic, potassium-losing conditions. Gitelman's syndrome is distinguished by hypomagnesaemia and urinary magnesium loss. Bartter's syndrome is caused by a mutation in the gene encoding the $Na^+/K^+/NH_4^+/Cl^-$ cotransporter in the loop of Henle (see Fig. 5.3), or in genes encoding calcium or potassium channels. Blood pressure is normal and most patients require life-long treatment with oral potassium supplements. Neither ACE inhibitors nor NSAIDs have been shown to have therapeutic effects.

Management

Potassium depletion can be treated by giving a K^+ salt orally or intravenously. The former route is preferable as it is less potentially hazardous. Oral KCl (1 g = 13.4 mmol K^+) is satisfactory unless a metabolic acidosis is present. These preparations may cause gastrointestinal irritation; oesophageal and small bowel erosions and strictures are uncommon complications. A diet rich in K^+, i.e. containing fruit and fruit juices, coffee, milk and animal protein, is helpful.

In ill patients and those with marked clinical features, intravenous KCl is needed. Associated salt and water deficiency should be treated first and intravenous administration of potassium avoided until urine output is established. Between 80 and 100 mmol K^+/day is usually sufficient. No more than 20 mmol of K^+ should be given in any 3-hour period.

Prevention is better than cure, and strategies for prevention are shown in the information box.

PREVENTION OF POTASSIUM DEPLETION
Diuretics
• Additional KCl 20–60 mmol/day. (N.B. Not with potassium-sparing diuretics or patients on ACE inhibitors.) Plasma K^+ should be monitored
Corticosteroids
• Some patients on high doses need potassium supplements
I.v. fluids
• Most patients will need 60 mmol/day K^+ distributed over 24 hours. The plasma K^+ should be monitored daily

CALCIUM, PHOSPHATE AND MAGNESIUM

Calcium metabolism in health and disease is discussed on pages 517 and 575.

HYPOPHOSPHATAEMIA

Most body phosphate (80%) is in the bony skeleton, and around 20% in cells, predominantly muscle. Phosphate molecules are critical to many biochemical processes, including cell energetics (ATP), intracellular signalling (cAMP) and nucleic acid synthesis. A body deficit of phosphate therefore has widespread effects. In the presence of a plasma phosphate less than 0.4 mmol/l (normal range 0.8–1.4 mmol/l), widespread cell dysfunction and death may occur. Rapid changes in plasma phosphate usually reflect redistribution from plasma to cells. In this respect, phosphate behaves similarly to potassium, and enters cells in association with insulin-stimulated carbohydrate metabolism. In clinical situations where carbohydrate is administered acutely, with a background of impaired nutrition and a total body phosphate deficit, severe hypophosphataemia may ensue, with the consequences shown in the information box above. This is referred to as the nutritional recovery syndrome. Alkalosis also stimulates a shift into cells. Causes of hypophosphataemia are shown in the information box.

CONSEQUENCES OF HYPOPHOSPHATAEMIA AND PHOSPHATE DEPLETION
• Muscle pain and weakness, increased plasma creatine kinase • Respiratory muscle weakness • Cardiac arrhythmias • Neuroencephalopathy—confusion, convulsions, coma • Haemolysis • Hypercalciuria, hypermagnesuria

CAUSES OF REDUCED PLASMA PHOSPHATE CONCENTRATION
Hyperparathyroidism (by increased urinary excretion)
• Primary • Secondary e.g. Vitamin D deficiency/osteomalacia Malabsorption Familial hypophosphataemic rickets
Increased carbohydrate metabolism and insulin action (by shift into cells)
• Intravenous glucose infusions • Insulin infusion • Treatment of diabetic ketoacidosis • Parenteral nutrition • Nutritional recovery syndrome
Alkalosis (by shift into cells)
• Metabolic, e.g. bicarbonate infusion • Respiratory, e.g. artificial hyperventilation
Reduced oral absorption of phosphate
• Oral phosphate-binding agents, e.g. aluminium hydroxide • Starvation (only minor reduction because of ↓ carbohydrate metabolism) • Chronic alcoholism, alcohol withdrawal
Phosphate removal
• Haemodialysis • Peritoneal dialysis
Extracellular fluid volume expansion
N.B. Hypophosphataemia is often multifactorial in origin.

Management

In many cases, and particularly if there is no prior body phosphate depletion, hypophosphataemia is transient and of no clinical significance. The duration and severity should be taken into account when deciding on treatment. Sustained values of < 0.4 mmol/l require therapy. Oral treatment is preferred. Milk is a good source (up to 2 litres/day) or oral supplements such as Phosphate-Sandoz (16 mmol phosphate, 20 mmol sodium, 3 mmol potassium per tablet), one 3–6 times daily. Intravenous therapy should be given with care, and in general should not exceed 18 mmol/24 hours of a mixed phosphate solution. Plasma concentrations of calcium, phosphate, potassium and magnesium must be closely monitored during treatment.

HYPERPHOSPHATAEMIA

This is most commonly seen in acute or chronic renal failure, or in states of massive cell necrosis, such as acute rhabdomyolysis, acute haemolysis, or in neoplastic disease treated by chemotherapy (tumour lysis syndrome). Sustained hyperphosphataemia is associated with a risk of metastatic calcification, secondary stimulation of the parathyroid glands, and symptoms such as pruritus. Treatment with oral phosphate binders and/or dialysis may be required (see Ch. 6).

MAGNESIUM DEFICIENCY AND EXCESS

Disorders of magnesium metabolism are occasionally responsible for otherwise puzzling clinical features.

Aetiology of magnesium depletion

The important causes of magnesium depletion are shown in Table 5.7.

Clinical features of magnesium depletion

These are predominantly neuromuscular, with tremor and choreiform movements. Depression, confusion, agitation, epileptic fits and hallucinations also occur. The diagnosis can be confirmed by finding a plasma magnesium concentration of less than 0.7 mmol/l. Since most magnesium is intracellular, a body deficit can be present with a normal plasma concentration.

Gitelman's syndrome is characterised by hypokalaemia and hypomagnesaemia and is caused by a mutation in the thiazide-sensitive NaCl cotransporter in the distal tubule (see Fig. 5.3). The hypokalaemia can be treated successfully with amiloride. Blood pressure is normal.

Management of magnesium depletion

Magnesium is very poorly absorbed orally, and oral supplements are of little value. The condition is best treated by giving 30–50 mmol magnesium chloride intravenously in a litre of isotonic saline or 5% dextrose over 12–24 hours.

Table 5.7 Causes of magnesium depletion

Underlying mechanism	Clinical condition
Reduced intake	Protein-energy malnutrition (PEM) Prolonged administration of Mg^{++}-free intravenous fluids
Loss from GI tract	Vomiting Chronic diarrhoea (malabsorption, laxative abuse) Fistulae; aspiration of GI contents
Losses in urine	**Extrarenal factors acting on the kidney** Drugs, e.g. loop diuretics, gentamicin, cisplatin Ketoacidosis Chronic alcoholism Hyperparathyroidism Primary or secondary aldosteronism **Renal disease** Gitelman's syndrome Post-obstructive diuresis Diuretic phase of acute tubular necrosis Renal tubular acidosis
Miscellaneous	Acute pancreatitis Excessive lactation

Thereafter 15–20 mmol magnesium should be infused daily until plasma Mg^+ is normal. When renal function is impaired the amount of magnesium should be halved.

Magnesium excess

This mainly occurs in acute or chronic renal failure, and may contribute to the central nervous system disturbance associated with severe uraemia. Treatment is that of the underlying condition.

ACID-BASE DISORDERS

There are four main types of disturbance of hydrogen ion concentration (see Table 5.8); *acidosis* and *alkalosis* may be either *respiratory* or *metabolic* in origin. These may be *pure* or *mixed* disorders, and their effects are eventually modified by compensatory changes. Changes in arterial blood [H^+], $PaCO_2$ and plasma [HCO_3^-] in acid-base disturbances are shown in Table 5.8.

Clinical assessment

Disturbances in acid-base balance may be accompanied by mild central nervous system dysfunction and abnormalities of respiration. The history, particularly of chronic diseases such as diabetes or obstructive airways disease, and of recent acute illness or drug ingestion, is important. Often the cause is obvious because acid-base disturbances accompany a variety of serious acute disorders. Assessment of volume status is also important in these patients as it will help to guide therapy.

Table 5.8 Changes in arterial blood [H⁺], *Pa*CO_2 and plasma [HCO_3^-] in acid-base disturbances

Disorder	[H⁺]	*Pa*CO_2	HCO_3^-
Metabolic acidosis			
Acute	↑	→	↓
Compensated (by ↑ ventilation)	↗ or →	↓	↓
Metabolic alkalosis			
Acute	↓	→	↑
Compensated (by ↓ ventilation)	↘ or →	↑	↑
Respiratory acidosis			
Acute (duration—hours)	↑	↑	→
Compensated (duration—days) (by renal retention of HCO_3^-)	↗ or →	↑	↑
Respiratory alkalosis			
Acute	↓	↓	→
Compensated (by ↑ renal excretion of HCO_3^-)	↘ or →	↓	↓

METABOLIC ACIDOSIS

Metabolic acidosis is characterised by a reduction in plasma bicarbonate and a consequent rise in [H⁺]. The *Pa*CO_2 is reduced secondarily by hyperventilation, which mitigates the rise in [H⁺] (see Table 5.8). The relationship between [H⁺] and *Pa*CO_2 in stable acid-base disorders is well defined; diagrams such as Figure 5.10 are sometimes helpful in defining the nature and extent of the disturbance.

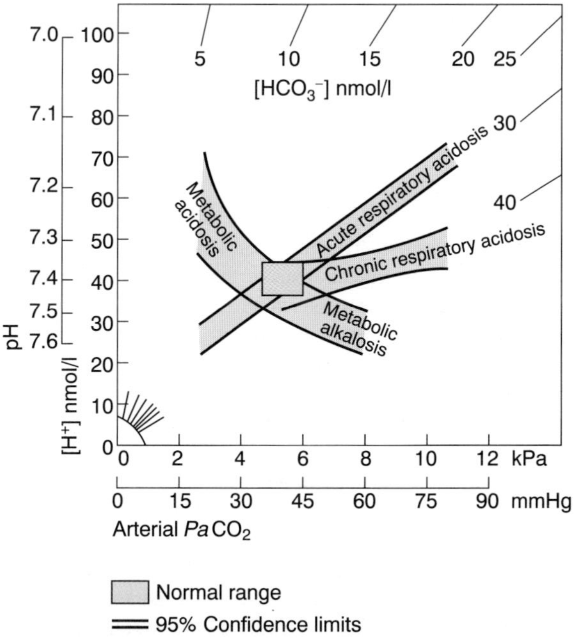

Fig. 5.10 Diagram showing changes in blood [H⁺]. The rectangle indicates limits of normal reference ranges for [H⁺] and *Pa*CO_2. The bands represent 95% confidence limits of single disturbances in human blood in vivo. When the point obtained by plotting [H⁺] against *P* does not fall within one of the labelled bands, compensation is incomplete or a mixed disorder is present (Flenley D 1971 Lancet 1: 1921).

The *anion gap* represents those negative ions not normally measured in clinical practice. These include phosphate and sulphate, lactate, ketoacids and albumin. A convenient formula is:

$$\text{Anion gap} = \text{plasma } Na^+ - (\text{plasma } Cl^- + \text{plasma } HCO_3^-)$$

Values in health range from 8 to 14 mmol/l. In some types of metabolic acidosis, reduced bicarbonate in plasma is accompanied by an increase in plasma chloride, leading to a normal anion gap. Where excessive acid is added to the plasma, either by disordered metabolism or by addition of exogenous acid, or there is failure of acid excretion, the anion gap is increased. This should prompt attempts to identify the abnormal anion(s) and correct the underlying problem (see Table 5.9). A low anion gap is occasionally seen in multiple myeloma, in lithium poisoning and in severe hypercalcaemia or hypermagnesaemia.

Aetiology

The physiological disturbances which give rise to metabolic acidosis are shown in the information box, and conditions in which these develop are listed in Table 5.9. In most situations, metabolic acidosis is accompanied by sodium and water depletion, and the aetiology of this is also indicated in Table 5.9.

DISTURBANCES WHICH GIVE RISE TO METABOLIC ACIDOSIS

- Overproduction of acids other than H_2CO_3
- Ingestion of acids or potential acids
- Failure to excrete acids other than H_2CO_3 at a rate equal to their generation
- Loss of the base bicarbonate in urine or from the GI tract

Lactic acidosis occurs when the rate of production of lactic acid from pyruvate in muscle, skin, brain and erythrocytes exceeds the rate of removal by liver and kidney. As indicated by the equation

$$[\text{lactate}] = K[\text{NADH}]/[\text{NAD}] \times [\text{pyruvate}] \times [H^+]$$

lactate production increases when oxidative metabolism is reduced, glycolysis is increased, and [pyruvate] and [NADH] rise. Causes of lactic acidosis are shown in the information box. Those in Group A are associated with hypotension and/or severe tissue hypoxia. Disorders in Group B are not, but are associated with impaired mitochondrial respiration and increased lactate production.

Diabetic ketoacidosis is discussed on page 493. In chronic renal failure, the most important factor limiting H⁺ excretion is reduced production of NH_4^+ by the diminished mass of tubules (see p. 435). Distal (type 1) renal tubular acidosis (RTA) is a failure of hydrogen ion secretion, whereas proximal (type II) RTA is a failure to reabsorb filtered bicarbonate.

Table 5.9 Causes of metabolic acidosis

Mechanism	Clinical disorders	Accumulating acid	Anion gap[1]	Cause of associated Na^+ depletion
Addition of excessive acid to plasma				
1 Disorders of intermediary metabolism	Ketoacidosis	Aceto-acetic β-hydroxybutyric	Increased	Loss in urine with anion of abnormal acid
	Lactic acidosis	Lactic	Increased	Loss in urine with anion of abnormal acid
2 Addition of exogenous substances	Methanol poisoning	Formic	Increased	Loss in urine with anion of abnormal acid
	Ethylene glycol poisoning	Glycolic, oxalic	Increased	Loss in urine with anion of abnormal acid
	Salicylate poisoning[2]	Various organic	Increased	Loss in urine with anion of abnormal acid
Failure to excrete acid at a normal rate				
1 Inadequate renal NH_4^+ production	Chronic renal failure	Sulphuric, phosphoric etc. produced by metabolism	Increased	Impaired renal Na^+ conservation
2 Inability to maintain $[H^+]$ gradient between blood and urine	Distal renal tubular acidosis	Hydrochloric	Normal	Reduced Na^+/H^+ exchange in distal tubule
3 Oliguria	Acute renal failure	Sulphuric, phosphoric etc. produced by metabolism	Increased	Usually absent
Loss of bicarbonate				
1 In urine	Proximal renal tubular acidosis	Hydrochloric	Normal	Reduced Na^+/H^+ exchange in proximal tubule
	Carbonic anhydrase inhibitors, e.g. acetazolamide	Hydrochloric	Normal	Reduced Na^+/H^+ exchange throughout nephron
2 From GI tract	Diarrhoea, fistulae	Hydrochloric	Normal	Loss of Na^+ in GI secretions
	Ureterosigmoidostomy	Hydrochloric	Normal	Loss of Na^+ in GI secretions

[1] Anion gap = plasma Na^+ – (plasma Cl^- + plasma HCO_3^-); normal 8–14 mmol/l.
[2] Especially in children; in adults respiratory alkalosis usually predominates.

CAUSES OF LACTIC ACIDOSIS

Group A

- Shock from any cause (septic shock most common)
- Respiratory failure
- Poisoning with cyanide or carbon monoxide
- Severe anaemia

Group B

- Diabetes mellitus
- Hepatic failure
- Severe infection
- Drugs (biguanides such as metformin, salicylates, isoniazid, sorbitol)
- Toxins (ethanol, methanol)
- Congenital enzyme defects

Clinical features

The most obvious clinical consequence is stimulation of respiration by the raised $[H^+]$. In severe cases, respirations become deep and sighing (Kussmaul's respiration). When the $[H^+]$ exceeds 70 nmol/l, myocardial function is compromised, cardiac output falls, and this, in conjunction with peripheral vasodilatation, results in a fall in blood pressure. Such patients are frequently confused or drowsy.

In many cases the clinical picture is determined by the underlying disorder and the presence of concomitant Na^+ and water depletion.

Management

The cause of acidosis should be identified and treated whenever possible. Treatment of ketoacidosis and lactic acidosis results in metabolism of the accumulated acids to CO_2 and water, a process which regenerates bicarbonate. Any associated sodium and water depletion should be corrected using intravenous isotonic sodium chloride solution. This neutral solution might be expected to have relatively little influence on the acidity of body fluids. However, provided kidney function is normal, it will usually correct a metabolic acidosis of moderate severity. Adequately perfused kidneys will generate HCO_3^- and retain this along with the infused sodium, rejecting the chloride in the urine.

In the presence of renal disease, or of markedly reduced renal function due to the sodium and water depletion, renal generation of bicarbonate is impaired. Approximately 30% of the total requirement for sodium and water should then be given as isotonic (1.26%) sodium bicarbonate. Blood $[H^+]$ and $[HCO_3^-]$ should be monitored, and infusion of sodium bicarbonate stopped when $[H^+]$ is normal.

In cardiogenic shock or after cardiac arrest, acidosis develops without sodium depletion. Treatment with i.v. sodium bicarbonate is usually unnecessary. Treatment of diabetic ketoacidosis and of lactic acidosis in diabetes is described on pages 495–496. In chronic renal failure, oral sodium bicarbonate supplements may be required on a long-term basis.

METABOLIC ALKALOSIS

Metabolic alkalosis, which is less common than metabolic acidosis, is characterised by an increase in plasma bicarbonate, a fall in blood [H^+], and a small compensatory rise in $PaCO_2$ (see Fig. 5.11 and Table 5.8). In health, when plasma HCO_3^- rises above normal, the filtered load of HCO_3^- exceeds the tubular reabsorptive capacity, so that urinary excretion of HCO_3^- increases rapidly. It is therefore very difficult to produce metabolic alkalosis in the presence of normal renal function.

Aetiology

Commonly several factors contribute to the development of metabolic alkalosis. It is convenient to consider an initiation phase, in which plasma [HCO_3^-] increases, and a maintenance phase during which the raised plasma [HCO_3^-] is sustained because of altered renal function (see the information box).

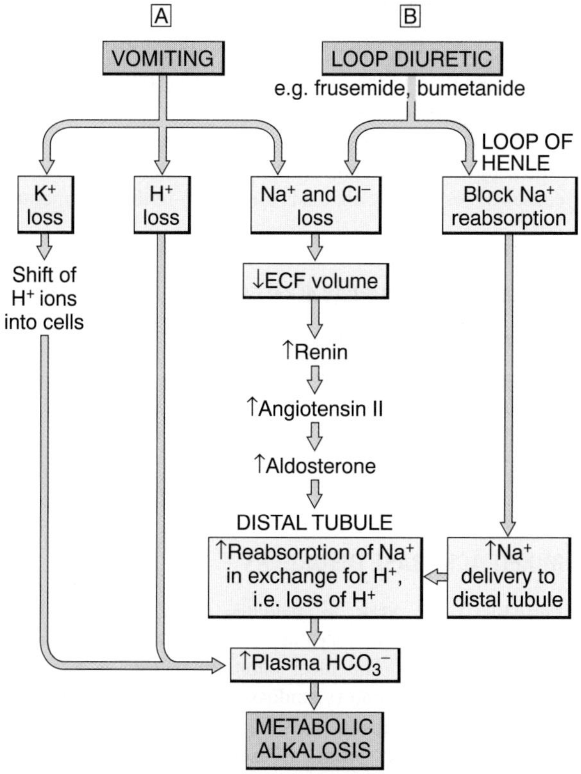

Fig. 5.11 Simplified scheme showing pathogenesis of metabolic alkalosis. A Metabolic alkalosis due to loss of gastric contents. B Metabolic alkalosis due to use of loop diuretics.

CONDITIONS IN WHICH METABOLIC ALKALOSIS CAN BE SUSTAINED (increased proportion of filtered sodium reabsorbed with bicarbonate)

- Strong stimulus to reabsorb sodium (i.e. hypovolaemia), particularly in the presence of a low plasma chloride, and thus reduced filtered chloride
- Increased secretion of H^+ by renal tubular cells:
  - Increased delivery of sodium to the distal nephron (e.g. by loop diuretics)
  - High $PaCO_2$ (e.g. chronic respiratory failure)
  - Tubular cell K^+ depletion
  - Increased mineralocorticoid activity

Important causes are shown in Table 5.10. When H^+ ions are secreted into the gastric lumen, bicarbonate from parietal cells is added to the blood; this is subsequently neutralised by reabsorption of the secreted H^+ in the small bowel. Loss of H^+ in vomitus or because of gastric aspiration therefore initiates metabolic alkalosis. The disturbance is sustained because loss of sodium, chloride, water and potassium in the gastric secretions gives rise to extracellular fluid depletion, hypochloraemia and a potassium deficit. All of these enhance the renal reabsorption of sodium in exchange for H^+ (see Fig. 5.11).

In potassium deficiency, the alkalosis is initiated by shift of H^+ from ECF into cells, and maintained by enhanced secretion of protons by the K^+-depleted distal tubular cells. In conditions where there is an excess of mineralocorticoid,

Table 5.10 Most common causes of metabolic alkalosis

Underlying mechanism	Clinical condition
Loss of Na^+, Cl^-, H^+ and water (ECF depletion)	Vomiting or aspiration of gastric contents Congenital chloridorrhoea[1] Administration of diuretics (benzothiadiazines, frusemide, bumetanide)
Potassium depletion	See Table 5.6[2]
Excessive mineralocorticoid activity	Primary aldosteronism Cushing's syndrome Bartter's syndrome Adrenal enzyme defects Secondary aldosteronism Administration of liquorice, e.g. carbenoxolone
Administration of exogenous alkali	Oral or i.v. HCO_3^-, citrate[3] Administration of gluconate, acetate, lactate

[1] A rare disorder associated with loss of H^+ and Cl^- in diarrhoeal stools.
[2] Alkalosis is uncommon in K^+ depletion due to primary renal disease.
[3] Present in transfused blood.

such as primary aldosteronism, alkalosis is initiated and sustained by corticosteroid-stimulated reabsorption of sodium in exchange for H^+ in the distal nephron. Potassium is also lost, which further stimulates renal Na^+/H^+ exchange.

In the presence of a reduced GFR, or any factor which enhances bicarbonate reabsorption (see the information box), administration of exogenous base (e.g. some antacid preparations) will cause alkalosis.

Consequences of metabolic alkalosis

The alkalosis causes reduced ventilation and a compensatory increase in $PaCO_2$ which shifts H^+ towards normal. This stimulates renal H^+ secretion so that bicarbonate regeneration is enhanced and the urine remains acidic.

Clinical features

Alkalosis rarely causes specific clinical symptoms. Acute alkalosis may cause tetany, either spontaneous or induced by Trousseau's manoeuvre (see p. 579). This is due primarily to the acute fall in plasma ionised calcium, although enhanced release of acetylcholine is another cause of increased neuromuscular excitability. Apathy, confusion and drowsiness may occur in severe cases, although this is often multifactorial. Severe long-standing alkalosis may be associated with reduced renal function and uraemia.

Management

In patients without renal disease, restoration of the ECF volume and the plasma chloride and potassium concentrations will remove the stimulus to renal H^+ secretion, and allow renal excretion of the excess bicarbonate. In patients who have lost gastric contents, e.g. in pyloric outlet obstruction, this should be done with isotonic (0.9%) sodium chloride solution (3–6 litres per 24 hours) and sufficient KCl to restore the K^+ deficit (40–60 mmol/day). Patients who require continuous aspiration of gastric contents in preparation for surgery should have the volume of aspirate replaced by intravenous infusion of an equal amount of isotonic (0.9%) sodium chloride solution containing KCl (20 mmol/l).

Alkalosis associated with K^+ deficiency is corrected by sufficient KCl to restore body K^+ to normal (see p. 409). Diuretic-induced alkalosis can be difficult to correct. If possible, the diuretic should be stopped for a few days and the intake of sodium chloride increased. If this is not possible (e.g. in severe cardiac failure) or ineffective, the carbonic anhydrase inhibitor acetazolamide (500–1000 mg daily) should be substituted for the diuretic for a few days to induce excretion of bicarbonate. Any K^+ deficit must be corrected. When alkalosis is due to mineralocorticoid excess, the underlying disorder must be treated. Restriction of dietary sodium and correction of K^+ deficiency with KCl mitigates the alkalosis.

RESPIRATORY ACIDOSIS

This arises when the effective alveolar ventilation fails to keep pace with the rate of CO_2 production. As a result, $PaCO_2$, blood $[HCO_3^-]$ and $[H^+]$ all rise.

The kidney responds by increased H^+ secretion, so that the urine becomes acid, bicarbonate is added to the blood, and the blood $[H_2CO_3]$ is partially restored. The distinction between respiratory acidosis and metabolic alkalosis can usually be made from knowledge of the cause of the disturbance, and the fact that characteristically the $[H^+]$ is raised in respiratory acidosis and reduced in metabolic alkalosis (see Table 5.8).

Aetiology and clinical features of respiratory acidosis are described on page 398.

RESPIRATORY ALKALOSIS

This occurs when there is excessive loss of CO_2 due to over-ventilation of the lungs. $PaCO_2$ and $[H^+]$ fall. The low $PaCO_2$ results in reduced renal Na^+/H^+ exchange, loss of bicarbonate in the urine, and a fall in plasma bicarbonate which mitigates the fall in blood $[H^+]$. The more common causes of respiratory alkalosis are shown in the information box.

CAUSES OF RESPIRATORY ALKALOSIS

- Hysterical overbreathing
- Assisted ventilation, if excessive
- Lobar pneumonia
- Pulmonary embolism
- Meningitis, encephalitis
- Salicylate poisoning
- Hepatic failure

MIXED ACID-BASE DISORDERS

Particularly in very ill patients, there may be both metabolic and respiratory factors contributing to an acid-base disturbance. The most common pattern is a mixed metabolic and respiratory acidosis (see the case example on p. 415). Nomograms such as Figure 5.10 are often useful for clarifying such complex cases. Management involves the treatments outlined above for each element of the disturbance.

FURTHER INFORMATION ON MAJOR ELECTROLYTE AND ACID-BASE DISORDERS

Abraham W T, Schrier R W 1994 Body fluid volume regulation and health in disease. Advances in Internal Medicine 39: 23–47
Arieff A I 1993 Management of hypernatraemia. British Medical Journal 307: 305–308
Brater D C 1998 Diuretic therapy. New England Journal of Medicine 339: 387–395
Gennari F J 1998 Hypokalaemia. New England Journal of Medicine 339: 451–458
Latta K, Hisano S, Chan J C 1993 Perturbations in potassium balance. Clinics in Laboratory Medicine 13: 149–156
Narins R G (ed) 1994 Clinical disorders of fluid and electrolyte metabolism, 5th edn. McGraw-Hill, New York
Pearce S H 1998 Straightening out the renal tubule: advances in the molecular basis of the inherited tubulopathies. Quarterly Journal of Medicine 91: 5–12
Preuss H G 1993 Fundamentals of clinical acid-base evaluation. Clinics in Laboratory Medicine 13: 103–116

CASE EXAMPLES *(Answers are on page 416)*

Question 5.1
A 60-year-old female is admitted with a short history of abdominal pain and vomiting. On examination, BP is 120/60, she is cold and confused and there is a tender swelling in the groin.

Electrolytes (mmol/l): Urea 12, Na^+ 122, K^+ 3.0, HCO_3^- 18
a. What is a likely explanation?
b. What treatment would you give?

Question 5.2
A 24-year-old man is admitted with a fractured tibia after a road traffic accident. He gives a history of intermittent lethargy and difficulty climbing stairs. He has not been taking any medication and there is no history of diarrhoea or vomiting. BP is 112/64.

Electrolytes (mmol/l): Urea 4.0, Na^+ 141, K^+ 2.2, HCO_3^- 28
a. What is the likely diagnosis?
b. What treatment would you give?

Question 5.3
A 32-year-old man is admitted in a very ill state. He had been drinking with friends, but had not been seen for some hours. On admission he is barely conscious and is breathing heavily.

Arterial blood gases: $[H^+]$ 98 nmol/l, $PaCO_2$ 2.7 kPa, HCO_3^- 6 mmol/l, PaO_2 13 kPa
a. What is the likely diagnosis?
b. How would you confirm it?
c. What treatment would you give?

Question 5.4
A 44-year-old lady with a long history of indigestion begins to vomit at home. She becomes unwell after 4 days and is admitted to hospital because of marked muscle weakness.

Arterial blood gases: $[H^+]$ 28 nmol/l, $PaCO_2$ 6.5 kPa, HCO_3^- 40 mmol/l, PaO_2 10.3 kPa, plasma potassium 2.1 mmol/l
a. What is the likely diagnosis?
b. What treatment would you give?

Question 5.5
A 56-year-old man, who has smoked heavily for many years, develops a worsening cough with purulent sputum, and is admitted to hospital because of difficulty in breathing. He is drowsy and cyanosed.

Arterial blood gases: $[H^+]$ 65 nmol/l, $PaCO_2$ 9.5 kPa, HCO_3^- 28 mmol/l, PaO_2 6.2 kPa
a. What is the likely diagnosis?
b. What treatment would you give?

Question 5.6
A 13-year-old schoolboy is brought to the casualty department having become acutely unwell in the headmaster's office. He is alert and agitated, the respiratory rate is 35/min, and he complains of tingling in his hands.

Arterial blood gases: $[H^+]$ 29 nmol/l, $PaCO_2$ 2.8 kPa, HCO_3^- 22 mmol/l, PaO_2 16 kPa
a. What is the likely diagnosis?
b. What treatment would you give?

Question 5.7
A 64-year-old man develops a chest infection and goes to bed. He is given antibiotics by his GP, but fails to improve; 48 hours later he is admitted to hospital. He is semiconscious, has a blood pressure of 80/40 mmHg and feels cold to the touch.

Arterial blood gases: $[H^+]$ 75 nmol/l, $PaCO_2$ 5.8 kPa, HCO_3^- 14 mmol/l, PaO_2 8 kPa
a. What is the acid-base disturbance?
b. Other than chest infection/pneumonia, what else could he be suffering from?
c. What other tests would you perform?
d. What treatment would you give?

Question 5.8
A 76-year-old woman is admitted, having been found on the floor at home. She has signs of a right hemiplegia, and is thought to have been lying for up to 48 hours.

Electrolytes (mmol/l): Urea 12, Na^+ 168, K^+ 4.8, HCO_3^- 23
a. What is the likely diagnosis?
b. What treatment would you give?

Question 5.9
An 18-year-old woman is transferred from a psychiatric unit to a medical ward. She is confused and has marked muscle weakness. Her pulse is irregular. She had been admitted 5 days previously for inpatient management of severe anorexia nervosa.

Electrolytes (mmol/l): Urea 3, Na^+ 138, K^+ 3.2, HCO_3^- 23
a. What other biochemical test would you perform?
b. What is the likely diagnosis?
c. What treatment would you give?

Question 5.10
A 54-year-old man is admitted suffering from confusion and drowsiness. He is a smoker and has finger clubbing.

Electrolytes (mmol/l): Urea 2.4, Na^+ 108, K^+ 3.5, HCO_3^- 26
a. What other biochemical test would you perform?
b. What is the likely diagnosis?
c. What treatment would you give?

ANSWERS TO CASE EXAMPLES

Question 5.1

a. Obstructed bowel (femoral hernia) and vomiting lead to volume depletion with hyponatraemia, hypokalaemia and metabolic acidosis. Small-bowel fluids are alkaline and rich in potassium.
b. 0.9% saline i.v. 1 litre over 2 hours followed by 0.9% saline + 20 mmol KCl/litre 6-hourly until volume is restored and she is fit for surgery.

Question 5.2

a. **Bartter's syndrome**, a rare tubular disorder in which sodium escapes from reabsorption in the loop of Henle, and is delivered in excess to the distal tubule, where it is reabsorbed in exchange for secretion of potassium. Normal blood pressure distinguishes it from primary aldosteronism (Conn's syndrome).
b. Urine K^+ was 60 mmol/l, confirming a renal cause; it should be less than 20 mmol/l in the presence of hypokalaemia. Oral KCl 8 tablets/day restored plasma K^+ to 3.3 mmol/l and relieved symptoms.

Question 5.3

a. Severe acute **metabolic acidosis**, due to poisoning—his drink had probably been 'spiked' with methanol, which is metabolised to formic acid. Low $PaCO_2$ reflects partial respiratory compensation.
b. Blood and urine to laboratory for toxicology analysis—measurement of lactate, methanol, ethylene glycol.
c. Give intravenous 1.26% sodium bicarbonate to restore safe $[H^+]$ (≈ 70 nmol/l) over 12–24 hours. Give intravenous fluids to establish a diuresis, and to facilitate renal excretion of methanol and formic acid. If blood methanol level is high, give oral ethanol to slow competitively metabolism of methanol. Consider haemodialysis if any evidence of renal failure.

Question 5.4

a. **Metabolic alkalosis**, due to pyloric stenosis, due in turn to chronic duodenal ulcer. Vomiting has caused loss of potassium, H^+, sodium and chloride. There is a total body deficit of sodium, which stimulates tubular sodium reabsorption in the distal tubule (which can only be in exchange for either H^+ or K^+). The kidney therefore cannot conserve H^+ or K^+. Also, because of chloride deficit, more bicarbonate is reabsorbed than normal.
b. Isotonic (0.9%) sodium chloride solution, 3–6 litres per day, to correct associated sodium chloride deficit. This removes the stimulus to sodium reabsorption and allows the kidney to conserve H^+ and K^+. Some intravenous K^+ will also be necessary (40–60 mmol/day). Surgery will be required to correct pyloric stenosis.

Question 5.5

a. Acute **respiratory acidosis**, due to an infective exacerbation of obstructive pulmonary disease. If his respiratory failure became **chronic**, with a persistent rise in $PaCO_2$, the kidney would compensate by retaining bicarbonate, e.g.

   H^+ 43 nmol/l, $PaCO_2$ 8.5 kPa, HCO_3^- 38 mmol/l, PaO_2 8.1 kPa

b. Try to improve respiratory function—nebulised bronchodilators, physiotherapy, antibiotics, controlled low-flow oxygen (e.g. 28%).

Question 5.6

a. Acute **respiratory alkalosis**, due to hyperventilation induced by anxiety. The tingling is due to a fall in plasma ionised calcium caused by the alkalosis.
b. Calm him down by reassurance and discussion, and persuade him to breathe slowly.

Question 5.7

a. **Mixed metabolic and respiratory acidosis**—although the $PaCO_2$ is within normal limits, it should be much lower for this degree of acidosis if it were purely metabolic.
b. **Septicaemia**, leading to lactic acidosis and renal failure, or respiratory failure due to pneumonia; he could also have diabetes mellitus with ketoacidosis. If he is on metformin for type II diabetes, lactic acidosis becomes even more likely.
c. **Plasma urea, electrolytes:**
   - urea 25.4 mmol/l (renal failure)
   - K^+ 6.5 mmol/l (↓ excretion due to renal failure; shift out of cells due to acidosis)
   - glucose 33 mmol/l (indicates uncontrolled diabetes)
   - blood lactate 11 mmol/l (high—indicates lactic acidosis).
d. Intravenous insulin to control diabetic ketoacidosis; i.v. fluids .(0.9% NaCl, 5% dextrose) to correct hypovolaemia and restore renal function; i.v. bicarbonate only if acidosis does not respond to these measures; antibiotics and chest physiotherapy.

Question 5.8

a. **Hypernatraemia**, caused by lack of access to water, in face of continued losses through the kidneys and insensible losses through the skin.
b. Water replacement, in the form of 5% dextrose. A reasonable choice would be 3 litres i.v. over 24 hours, with regular monitoring of the plasma sodium, aiming to reach a normal plasma sodium within 48 hours.

Question 5.9

a. Estimation of plasma phosphate—0.07 mmol/l (normal 0.8–1.2 mmol/l).
b. The **'nutritional recovery syndrome'**, also known as re-feeding hypophosphataemia. There is an underlying total body deficit of phosphate due to previous starvation. After feeding, there is a sudden increase in incorporation of phosphate into adenosine triphosphate (ATP) when glucose metabolism increases. A plasma phosphate of < 0.4 mmol/l can be associated with widespread cellular dysfunction.
c. Phosphate replacement. This is best done orally. If the patient cannot take tablets, i.v. phosphate solution should be given, not more than 30 mmol/day to avoid causing hypocalcaemia. Calcium, phosphate and magnesium must be monitored during therapy.

Question 5.10

a. Plasma and urine osmolality—plasma 243 mosm/kg, urine 632 mosm/kg.
b. **Dilutional hyponatraemia**, due to the syndrome of inappropriate ADH secretion (SIADH). The normal response to a low plasma osmolality is to pass a very dilute urine. Any degree of urinary concentration, as shown here, is abnormal and suggests an excess of vasopressin. He is likely to have underlying carcinoma of the bronchus.
c. Water restriction (500 ml/day). Careful administration of hypertonic (e.g. 1.8%) sodium chloride i.v., aiming to raise plasma sodium by not more than 0.5 mmol/l/hour. Occasionally, demeclocycline, which is toxic to the collecting duct and therefore inhibits the action of vasopressin, may be used in persistent cases.

Diseases of the kidney and urinary system

6

A.M. DAVISON • A.D. CUMMING • C.P. SWAINSON • N. TURNER

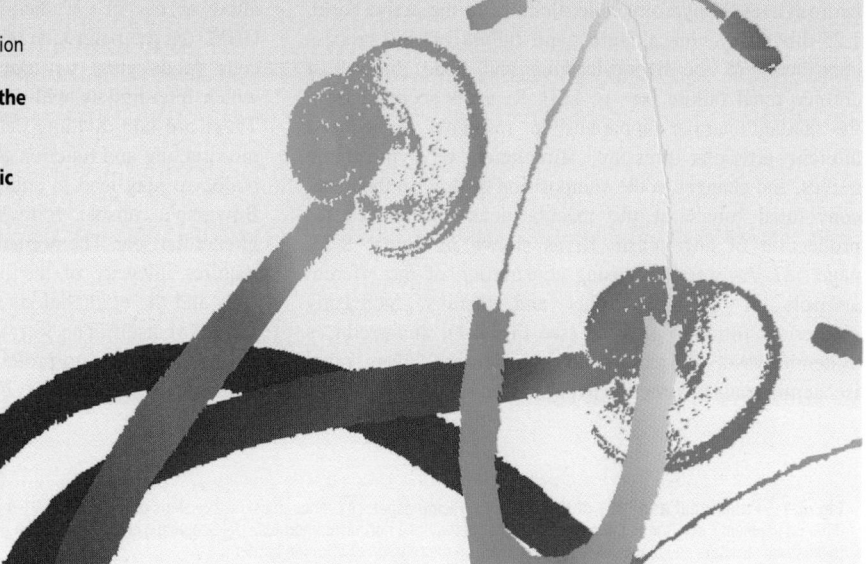

Renal medicine ranges from the management of common conditions to the use of complex technology to replace renal function. Since it is possible to do this, the practice of nephrology extends to involvement in the management of multisystem diseases where renal function is threatened or lost, and to transplantation, by which loss of renal function is most effectively replaced.

FUNCTIONAL ANATOMY, PHYSIOLOGY AND INVESTIGATIONS

MAJOR RENAL FUNCTIONS

In health, the volume and composition of body fluids are tightly regulated. The kidneys are largely responsible for maintaining this state, although for some components there are also controls of intake (e.g. water) or absorption (e.g. calcium). This is achieved by making large volumes of an ultrafiltrate of plasma (120 ml/min, 170 litres/day) at the glomerulus, and selectively reabsorbing components of the ultrafiltrate at points along the nephron, as shown in Figure 5.4, page 396). Many of these processes are tightly controlled and some are the targets of drug action.

In addition, the kidney has hormonal functions. Three of these are particularly important. The kidney is the main source of erythropoietin, which is produced by interstitial peritubular cells in response to hypoxia. Replacement of erythropoietin reverses the anaemia of chronic renal failure. The kidney is essential for vitamin D metabolism. It hydroxylates 25-hydroxycholecalciferol to the active form, 1,25-dihydroxycholecalciferol, and failure of this process contributes to the hypocalcaemia and bone disease of chronic renal failure (see p. 433). Renin is secreted from the juxtaglomerular apparatus in response to reduced afferent arteriolar pressure, stimulation of sympathetic nerves, and changes in the composition of fluid in the distal convoluted tubule at the macula densa. Renin causes production of angiotensin II, as shown in Figure 8.22, page 587. As well as causing constriction of the efferent arteriole of the glomerulus and thereby increasing glomerular filtration pressure (see Fig. 6.1), this produces systemic vasoconstriction and hypertension. Thus renal ischaemia leads to systemic hypertension.

FUNCTIONAL ANATOMY

Adult kidneys are 11–14 cm (three vertebral bodies) in length, and are located retroperitoneally on either side of the aorta and inferior vena cava. The right kidney is usually a few centimetres lower because the liver lies above it. Both kidneys rise and descend several centimetres with respiration.

Each kidney contains approximately 1 million nephrons. There is a rich blood supply, 20–25% of cardiac output, although there is considerable physiological variation in this. Intralobular branches of the renal artery give rise to the glomerular afferent arterioles. The basement membrane around the glomerular capillaries and the cells lying on either side of it form the filtration barrier (see Fig. 6.1). This allows free passage of water and small solutes; cells and large molecules are retained in the glomerular capillaries. Variations in the calibre of the afferent and efferent arterioles control the filtration pressure at the glomerular basement membrane (GBM). This is normally tightly regulated in order to maintain a constant glomerular filtration rate (GFR) despite varying systemic blood pressure and renal perfusion pressure. In response to a reduction in perfusion pressure, constriction of the efferent arteriole restores filtration pressure. This response of the efferent arteriole is dependent on angiotensin II production. The efferent arteriole goes on to supply the distal nephron and medulla.

The glomerulus contains three main cell types (see Fig. 6.1). The GBM is produced by fusion of the basement membranes of epithelial and endothelial cells. Both of these cells are specialised in structure and function. The glomerular endothelial cells contain pores (fenestrae) which allow access of circulating molecules to the underlying GBM. On the outer side of the GBM, glomerular epithelial cells (podocytes) put out multiple long foot processes which interdigitate with those of adjacent epithelial cells. These are non-dividing cells whose integrity is critical to the structure and function of the glomerulus. The death of a podocyte may lead to adhesion of the underlying GBM to Bowman's capsule, followed by the formation of a focal glomerular scar. The normal filtration barrier (see Fig. 6.1E) requires integrity of the junctions between the epithelial cells and the epithelial slit diaphragm apparatus as well as the GBM itself. The filtration barrier at the glomerulus is normally absolute to proteins the size of albumin (67 kDa) or larger, with those of 20 kDa or less able filter freely.

Fig. 6.1 Functional anatomy of the kidney. *(Facing page)* [A] Anatomical relationships of the kidney. [B] A single nephron. For the functions of different segments, see Figure 5.4, page 396. [C] Histology of a normal glomerulus. [D] Schematic cross-section of a glomerulus showing five capillary loops, to illustrate structure and show cell types. [E] Electron micrograph of filtration barrier.

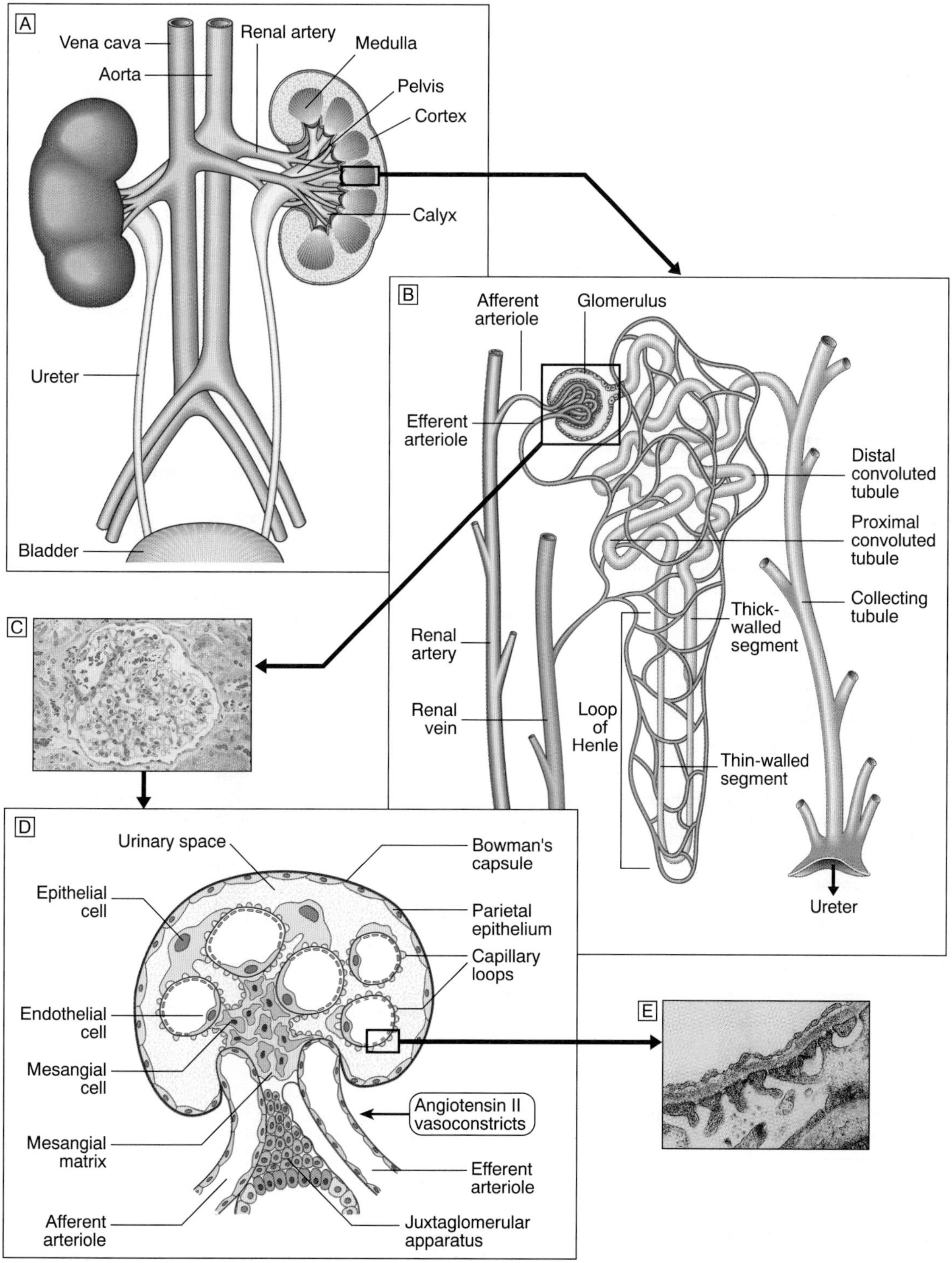
A
Vena cava
Aorta
Renal artery
Medulla
Pelvis
Cortex
Calyx
Ureter
Bladder
B
Afferent arteriole
Glomerulus
Efferent arteriole
Distal convoluted tubule
Proximal convoluted tubule
Collecting tubule
Thick-walled segment
Renal artery
Renal vein
Loop of Henle
Thin-walled segment
Ureter
C
D
Urinary space
Bowman's capsule
Epithelial cell
Parietal epithelium
Capillary loops
Endothelial cell
Mesangial cell
Angiotensin II vasoconstricts
Mesangial matrix
Efferent arteriole
Afferent arteriole
Juxtaglomerular apparatus
E

Between these sizes there is a gradient of clearance, the behaviour of individual molecules being influenced by their shape and charge. Anionic (negatively charged) proteins are relatively less freely filtered than cationic proteins. Little lipid is filtered. Mesangial cells lie in the central region of the glomerulus. They have similarities to vascular smooth muscle cells (e.g. contractility), but also some macrophage-like properties. In health, bone marrow-derived macrophages are occasionally found in glomeruli and in the interstitium.

Tubular cells are polarised, with a brush border (proximal tubular cells) and other specialised functions at their apex, lying on their own basement membrane at their base. Interstitial cells between tubules are less well understood. Fibroblast-like cells in the cortex are capable of producing erythropoietin in response to hypoxia. In the medulla, lipid-laden interstitial cells are believed to be important in prostaglandin production.

INVESTIGATION OF RENAL DISEASE

TESTS OF FUNCTION

Blood urea is a poor guide to renal function as it varies with protein intake, liver metabolic capacity and renal perfusion (see Fig. 6.2). Creatinine is a more reliable guide as it is produced from muscle at a constant rate and almost completely filtered at the glomerulus. As very little creatinine is secreted by tubular cells the creatinine clearance provides a reasonable approximation of the glomerular filtration rate. If muscle mass remains constant, changes in creatinine concentration reflect change in GFR. However, an increase outwith the normal range is not seen until GFR is reduced by about 50%, and isolated measurements of creatinine give a misleading impression of renal function in those with unusually small amounts (and occasionally in those with very large amounts) of muscle. More accurate measurement of GFR is now most easily undertaken by ascertaining the clearance of ^{51}Cr-labelled ethylenediaminetetraacetic acid (EDTA). This has largely replaced estimation of inulin clearance in clinical practice.

Urine volume gives a poor guide to renal function unless it is inappropriate to the circumstances. Between 300 and

CAUSES OF POLYURIA

- Excess fluid intake
- Osmotic, e.g. hyperglycaemia
- Cranial diabetes insipidus (loss of antidiuretic hormone—ADH)—see page 557
- Nephrogenic diabetes insipidus (tubular dysfunction)
  Genetic tubular cell defects: ADH receptor, aquaporin mutations
  Drugs/toxins: lithium, diuretics, hypercalcaemia
  Interstitial renal disease (see text)

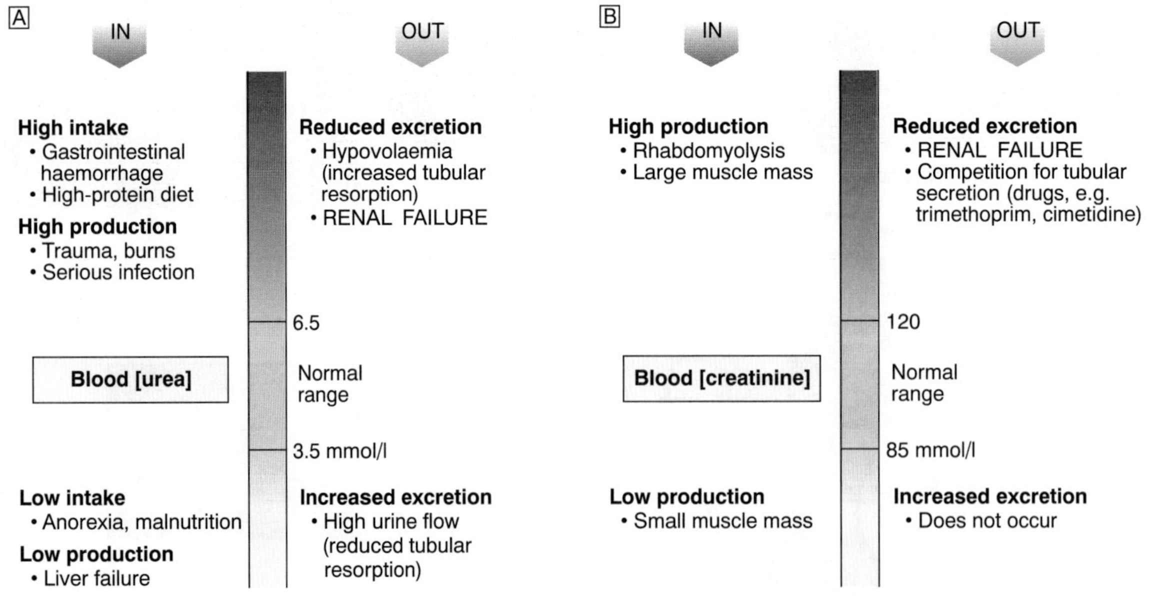

Fig. 6.2 Factors affecting blood levels of urea and creatinine. Factors affecting intake and production are shown to the left ('in'); those affecting excretion are shown to the right ('out'). A Urea. B Creatinine. Intake is omitted here as dietary creatinine (from meat) only rarely has a substantial influence on blood levels.

500 ml/day are needed to excrete solutes at maximum concentration on a normal diet. Complete anuria suggests either an acute vascular event or total urinary obstruction; even in the most severe intrinsic renal disorders some urine is usually still produced. Polyuria, which refers to the production of an excess volume of urine, may have a number of causes (see the information box).

Tests of tubular function, including concentrating ability, ability to excrete a water load and ability to excrete acid, are valuable in some circumstances.

IMAGING TECHNIQUES

Plain radiographs may show renal outlines if perinephric fat and bowel gas shadows permit. Opaque calculi and calcification within the renal tract may also be shown.

Renal ultrasound

This quick, non-invasive technique is the first and often the only required method of renal imaging. It can show renal size and position, dilatation of the collecting system (suggesting obstruction, see Fig. 6.3), distinguish tumours and cysts, and show other abdominal, pelvic and retroperitoneal pathology. In addition, it can image the bladder and estimate completeness of emptying in suspected bladder outflow obstruction. Images are often less clear in obese individuals. Ultrasonographic density of the renal cortex is increased and corticomedullary differentiation lost in chronic renal disease.

Doppler techniques are used to show blood flow and its characteristics in extrarenal and larger intrarenal vessels. The resistivity index is the ratio of peak systolic and diastolic velocities, and is influenced by the resistance to flow through small intrarenal arteries. It may be elevated in various diseases, including acute glomerulonephritis and rejection of a renal transplant. Severe renal artery stenosis causes damping of flow in intrarenal vessels, with slowed systolic upstroke, but ultrasound is incompletely evaluated for detecting renal artery stenosis. Thrombus in the renal vein may be identified, and will cause secondary abnormalities of the arterial waveform and swelling of the kidney.

The disadvantages of renal ultrasound are that it is operator-dependent and that the printed images convey only a fraction of the information gained by performing (or observing) the investigation in real time.

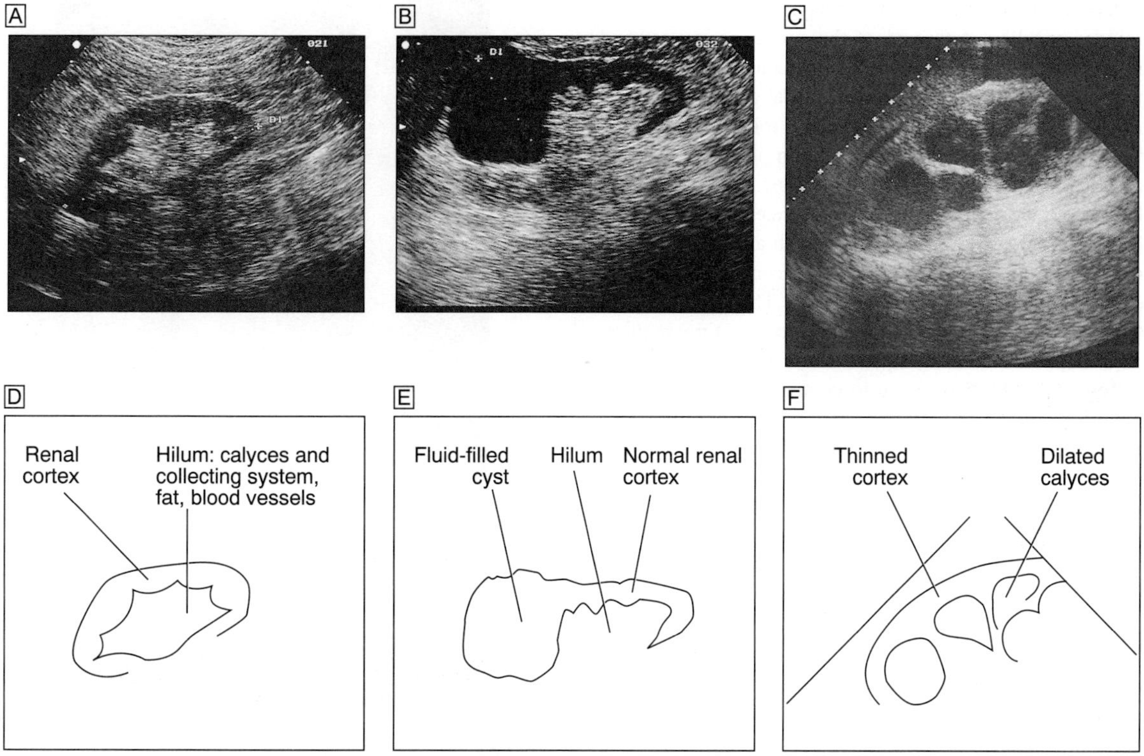

Fig. 6.3 Renal ultrasound. A Normal kidney. B A simple cyst occupies the upper pole of an otherwise normal kidney. C The renal pelvis and calyces are dilated by a chronic obstruction to urinary outflow. The thinness of the remaining renal cortex indicates chronicity. D, E and F The diagrams beneath show the anatomical features.

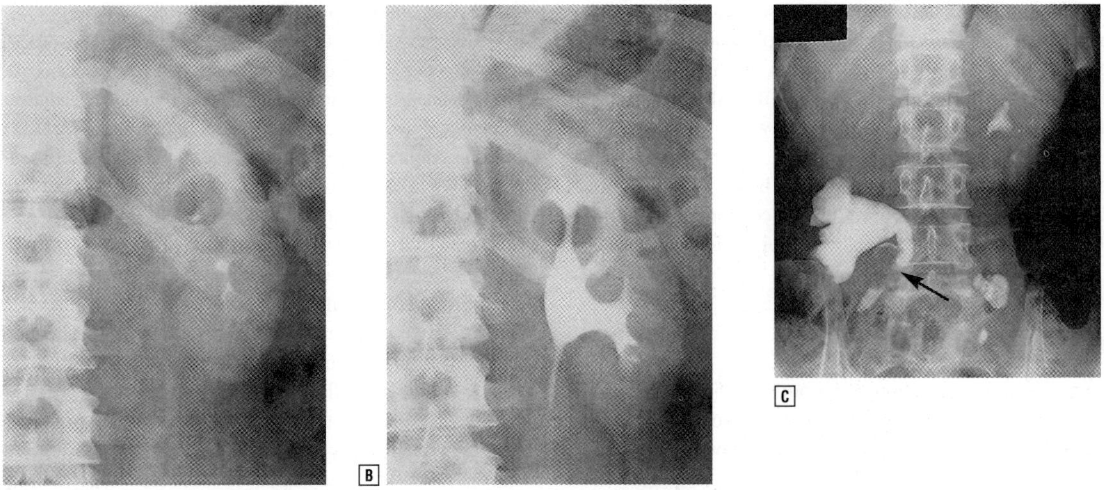

Fig. 6.4 Intravenous urograms. [A] Nephrogram phase at 1 minute. [B] Collecting system at 5 minutes. [C] Intravenous urogram showing a later view of a normal collecting system on the patient's left, with obstruction of the right system by a transitional cell carcinoma of the upper ureter, shown as a filling defect (arrow).

Intravenous urography (IVU)

While intravenous urography has been largely replaced by ultrasound for routine renal imaging, this technique provides excellent definition of the collecting system and ureters, and remains better than ultrasound for examining renal papillae, stones and urothelial malignancy (see Fig. 6.4). Radiographs are taken at intervals following administration of an intravenous bolus of an iodine-containing compound that is excreted by the kidney. An early image (1 minute after injection) will demonstrate the nephrogram phase of renal perfusion in patients with an adequate renal arterial supply. This is followed by contrast filling the collecting system, ureters and bladder. The disadvantages of this technique are the need for an injection, time requirement, dependence on adequate renal function for good images, and risk of exposure to contrast medium (allergy, nephrotoxicity). This last risk also applies to other techniques using contrast media, notably arteriography and computed tomography. Contrast nephrotoxicity is more likely in patients with diabetes mellitus or myeloma, and in those with pre-existing renal impairment. It can be reduced by avoiding dehydration and diuretics and by using less hyperosmotic (and more expensive) contrast media.

Pyelography

Antegrade pyelography requires the insertion of a fine needle into the pelvicalyceal system under ultrasound or radiographic control. Contrast is injected to outline the collecting system, and particularly to localise obstruction. This approach is much more difficult and hazardous in a non-obstructed kidney. In the presence of obstruction, percutaneous nephrostomy drainage can be established, and

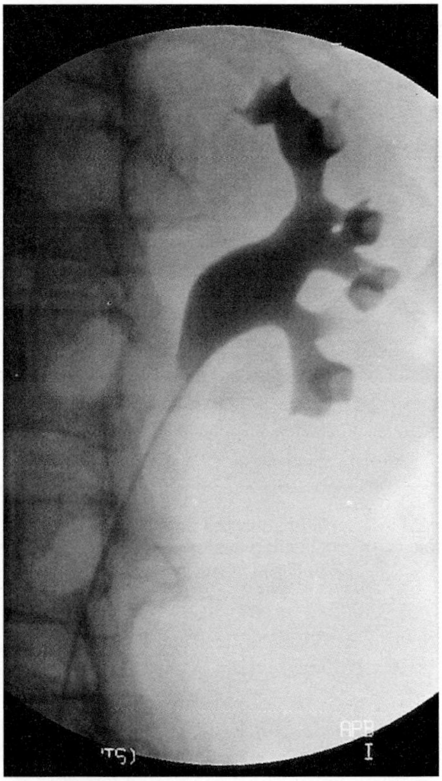

Fig. 6.5 Retrograde pyelography. The best views of the normal collecting system are shown by pyelography. A catheter has been passed into the left renal pelvis at cystoscopy. The anemone-like calyces are sharp-edged and normal. (Compare with the obstructed system shown in Figure 6.4C above.)

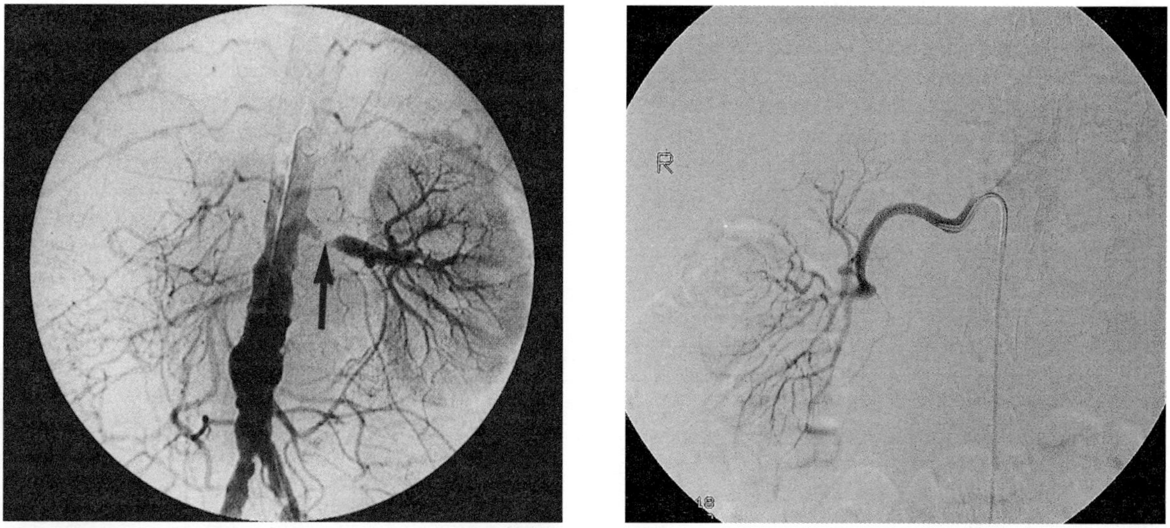

A B

Fig. 6.6 Renal arteriograms. A Digital subtraction arteriogram following injection of contrast material into the aorta showing renal artery stenosis. The right renal artery is absent. The left renal artery is stenosed (arrow), but contrast medium has passed the stenosis and the developing nephrogram can be seen. The abdominal aorta is severely irregular and atheromatous. B In another patient, a catheter has been passed beyond a stenosis at the ostium of the right renal artery in preparation for balloon dilatation/stenting.

often stents passed beyond any obstruction. Retrograde pyelography can be performed by inserting catheters into the ureteric orifices at cystoscopy (see Fig. 6.5).

Micturating cystourethrography

This is used to diagnose vesico-ureteric reflux and to assess its severity. The bladder is filled with contrast medium through a urinary catheter and films are taken while the patient voids (see Fig. 6.24, p. 451). It is used in combination with urodynamic studies in the assessment of disordered bladder emptying and urethral abnormalities, or sometimes for investigating patients with recurrent urinary infections, renal scars or renal failure of unknown cause.

Renal arteriography and venography

The main indication for renal arteriography is to investigate suspected renal artery stenosis or haemorrhage (see Fig. 6.6). In the absence of computed tomography it is also valuable for defining renal tumours. Balloon dilatation and stenting of the renal artery may be undertaken therapeutically, and bleeding vessels or arteriovenous fistulae occluded.

Venography is performed by placing a catheter into the inferior vena cava via the femoral vein, and is used to diagnose renal vein thrombosis (a complication of nephrotic syndrome) or extension of renal tumour (see Fig. 6.7).

Both techniques entail exposure to contrast medium and, in the presence of atherosclerotic disease, cholesterol emboli

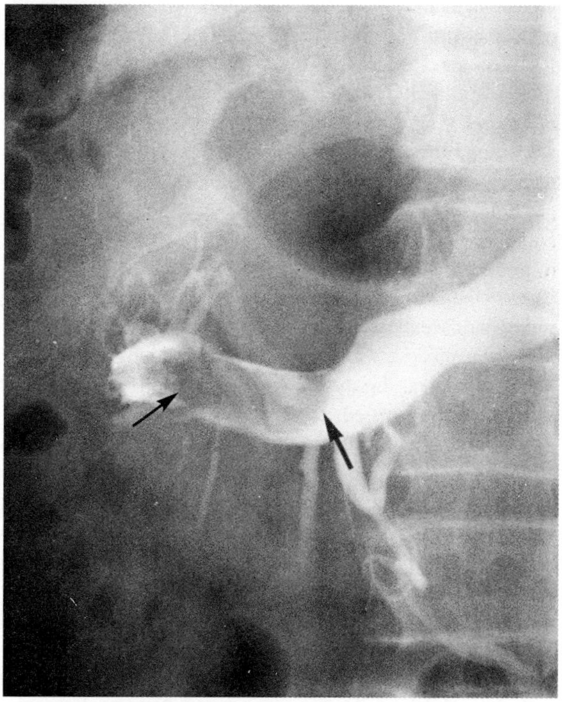

Fig. 6.7 Renal venography. Contrast has been injected into the renal vein and demonstrates renal vein thrombosis (arrows).

are a potentially serious consequence of intra-arterial manipulations.

Computed tomography (CT)

While not routinely of greater value than ultrasound, CT is particularly useful for characterising mass lesions within the kidney (see Fig. 6.8), or combinations of cysts with masses. It gives clearer definition of the retroperitoneal anatomy and, unlike ultrasound, is aided by increased amounts of fat, as this outlines organs and structures.

Spiral CT is a rapid-sequence technique, with images obtained immediately following a bolus injection of intravenous contrast media to outline vascular structures. It produces high-quality images of the main renal vessels and, when used to screen for possible renal artery stenosis in secondary hypertension, has the advantage of providing renal and adrenal (phaeochromocytoma, hyperaldosteronism) images at the same time.

Magnetic resonance imaging (MRI)

This technique is undergoing rapid development; however, the latest modifications are still not widely available. Despite this, MRI offers excellent resolution and distinction between different tissues, and a variety of methods for non-invasive arterial imaging (magnetic resonance angiography) are being developed. Gadolinium-based contrast media appear not to be nephrotoxic, but are expensive; they can produce good images of main renal vessels. These techniques are likely to develop further, and the relative places of spiral CT and MR angiography in non-invasive screening for renal artery stenosis have yet to be defined.

SPECIAL TESTS

Radionuclide studies

These studies require the injection of gamma ray-emitting radiopharmaceuticals which are taken up and excreted by the kidney, a process which can be monitored by an external gamma camera. In this way, the function of individual kidneys can be assessed.

Diethylenetriaminepentaacetic acid labelled with technetium (^{99m}Tc-DTPA) is excreted by glomerular filtration. Following injection of DTPA, computer analysis of uptake and excretion can be used to provide information regarding the arterial perfusion of each kidney. In renal artery stenosis, transit time is prolonged, peak activity delayed and excretion reduced. In less severe but still significant stenosis, a single dose of an angiotensin-converting enzyme (ACE) inhibitor ('captopril renography') can, by inhibiting the compensatory efferent glomerular arteriolar constriction induced by angiotensin II, induce these changes in a kidney that previously perfused normally. In patients with obstruction of the outflow tract, persistence of the nuclide in the renal pelvis is seen, and a loop diuretic fails to accelerate its disappearance.

Dimercaptosuccinic acid labelled with technetium (^{99m}Tc-DMSA) is filtered by glomeruli and partially bound to proximal tubular cells. Following intravenous injection, images of the renal cortex show the shape, size and function of each kidney (see Fig. 6.9). This is a sensitive method of demonstrating early cortical scarring that is of particular value in children. It is possible to assess the relative contribution of each kidney to total function.

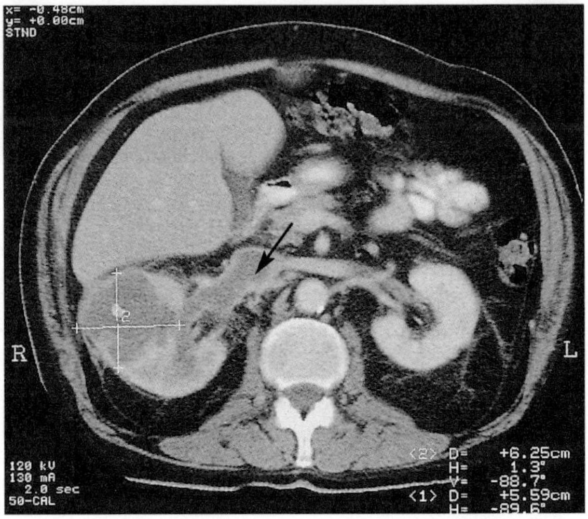

Fig. 6.8 Computed tomography. The right kidney is expanded by a low-density tumour which fails to take up contrast material. Tumour is shown extending into the renal vein and inferior vena cava (arrow).

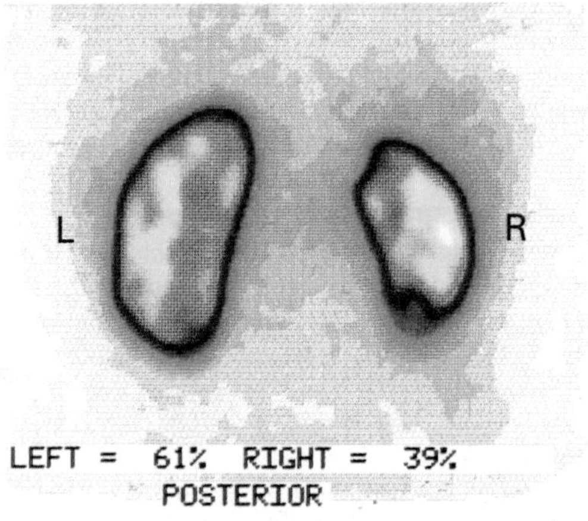

Fig. 6.9 DMSA isotope renogram. A posterior view is shown of a normal left kidney and a small right kidney (with evidence of cortical scarring at upper and lower poles) which contributes only 39% of total renal function.

Renal biopsy

Renal biopsy is used to establish the nature and extent of renal disease in order to judge the prognosis and need for treatment. The indications, contraindications and complications are given in the information box. The procedure is performed with ultrasound guidance to ensure accurate needle placement into a renal pole. Radiographic screening after contrast administration or other methods may also be used. Light microscopy, electron microscopy and immunohistological assessment of the specimen may all be required.

RENAL BIOPSY

Indications
- Acute renal failure that is not adequately explained
- Chronic renal failure with normal-sized kidneys
- Nephrotic syndrome or glomerular proteinuria in adults
- Nephrotic syndrome in children that has atypical features or is not responding to treatment
- Isolated haematuria with 'renal' characteristics or associated abnormalities

Contraindications
- Disordered coagulation or thrombocytopenia
- Uncontrolled hypertension
- Kidneys < 60% predicted size
- Solitary kidney (except transplants) (relative contraindication)

Complications
- Pain, usually mild
- Bleeding into urine, usually minor but may produce clot colic and obstruction
- Bleeding around the kidney, occasionally massive and requiring angiography with intervention, or surgery
- Arteriovenous fistula, rarely clinically significant

MAJOR MANIFESTATIONS OF RENAL DISEASE

URINARY ABNORMALITIES

HAEMATURIA

Haematuria may indicate bleeding from anywhere in the renal tract (see Fig. 6.10). Dipstick tests are very sensitive and can identify all significant bleeding, less than the amounts that are visible. Microscopy shows that normal individuals have occasional red cells in the urine, and positive tests are normal during menstruation, but persistent haematuria requires explanation, particularly in older age groups or others at risk of carcinoma of the bladder or other malignancy. Urine microscopy (see Fig. 6.11) is valuable in establishing the cause of bleeding. The presence of white blood cells and organisms may suggest infection; the presence of red cell casts indicates glomerular bleeding; a high proportion of dysmorphic erythrocytes (best seen by phase-contrast microscopy) likewise supports glomerular bleeding. In the absence of firm evidence of intrinsic renal disease, renal ultrasound and cystoscopy should be the first investigations in older patients.

Glomerular bleeding implies that the GBM is fractured. It may be seen physiologically following very strenuous exertion. Other causes of red or dark urine may sometimes be confused with haematuria (see the information box). If haematuria occurs with pointers to renal disease, further investigations should be directed towards looking for inflammatory renal disease, usually including renal biopsy. Isolated microscopic haematuria without evidence of malignancy or features of significant renal disease (no hypertension, normal renal function, insignificant amounts of protein in the urine) may be managed by observation alone. Although it occasionally gives warning of significant renal disease (e.g. Alport's syndrome, IgA nephropathy), it is commonly caused by the usually benign condition of thin GBM disease (see p. 442), insignificant vascular malformations, renal cysts or renal stones. In 'loin pain-haematuria' syndrome, benign glomerular bleeding is associated with episodic loin pain. Recurrent episodes of gross haematuria in association with respiratory infections are characteristic of IgA nephropathy (see p. 446).

CAUSES OF RED OR DARK URINE

- Haematuria
- Haemoglobinuria: red urine, stick test for blood positive, but no red cells on microscopy
- Myoglobinuria: in rhabdomyolysis. Very dark or black urine. Stick test for blood positive, but no red cells on microscopy
- Food dyes: beetroot (anthocyanins)
- Drugs: phenolphthalein (pink when alkaline), senna and other anthroquinones (orange), rifampicin (orange), L-dopa (darkens on standing)
- Porphyria (urine turns dark on standing; see p. 540)
- Alkaptonuria (see p. 826)

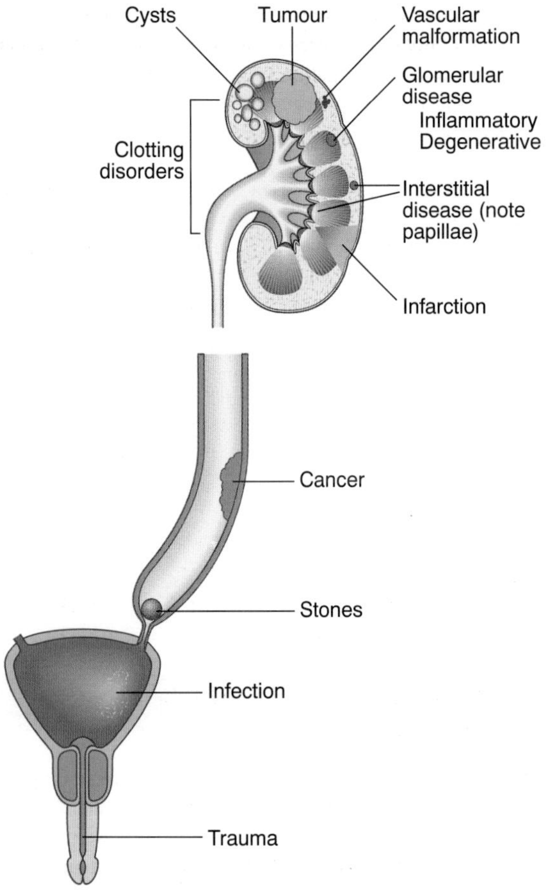

Fig. 6.10 Causes of haematuria. See the information box on page 425 for other causes of red or dark urine.

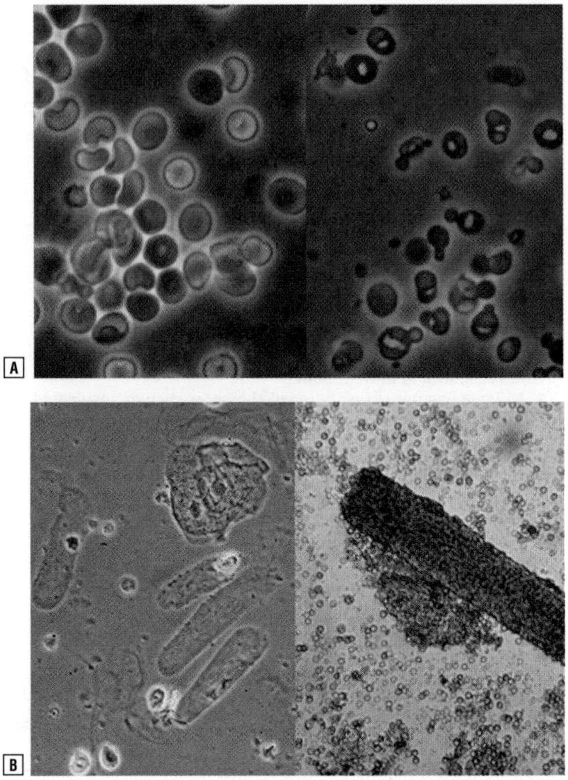

Fig. 6.11 Urine microscopy. A Phase contrast images of red blood cells (x 400) showing on the right glomerular bleeding with many dysmorphic forms including acanthocytes (tear-drop forms), and on the left bleeding from lower in the urinary tract. B On the left, phase contrast images show hyaline casts, a normal feature of urine (x 160). On the right, numerous red cells and a large red cell cast in acute glomerular inflammation (x 100, not phase contrast).

PROTEINURIA

Patients are usually unaware of proteinuria, although it may make urine froth easily. Moderate amounts of low molecular weight protein are normally filtered at the glomerulus. Usually these proteins are reabsorbed by tubular cells so that less than 150 mg/day should appear in the urine. Low molecular weight proteins appearing in the urine in larger quantities than this point to failure of reabsorption by damaged tubular cells, i.e. tubular proteinuria. This can be demonstrated by analysis of the size of excreted proteins, or by specific assays for such proteins (e.g. β_2-microglobulin, molecular weight 12 kDa). The amounts of such protein rarely exceed 1.5–2 g/24 hrs, and proteinuria greater than this almost always indicates significant glomerular disease.

Glomerular lesions allow filtration of larger serum proteins. The presence of albumin in the urine is a sure sign of glomerular abnormality. Albumin is the dominant serum protein, with a molecular weight of 67 kDa. Assays for this specific protein can identify the very early stages of glomerular disease in disorders with a predictably progressive course, such as diabetic nephropathy. Persistent microalbuminuria has also been associated with an increased risk of atherosclerosis and other diseases; neither the mechanism of proteinuria, nor an explanation of these associations has yet been found. Relatively minor leakage of albumin into the urine may also occur transiently after vigorous exercise, during fever, in heart failure, and in some other disease states, accounting for some positive stick tests in these circumstances. Such proteinuria should not reach nephrotic levels, and tests should be repeated after the stimulus is no longer present. Occasionally, proteinuria occurs only during the day, and the first morning sample is negative. In the absence of other signs of renal disease, such 'orthostatic proteinuria' is usually regarded as benign.

Patients with a clone of B lymphocytes secreting free immunoglobulin light chains (molecular weight 25 kDa) filter these freely into the urine, and Bence Jones protein can then be identified in fresh urine samples. This may occur in amyloidosis (see p. 541) and other plasma cell dyscrasias, but is particularly important as a marker for myeloma. Some light chains are toxic to tubular cells, and cause myeloma kidney. Bence Jones protein is poorly identified by stick tests for urinary protein; specific tests must be performed.

Twenty-four hour collections of urine are arduous and often inaccurate. Use of the protein/creatinine ratio in single samples makes allowance for the variable dilution. For an individual with an average muscle mass and normal rate of creatinine generation, a ratio of 120 (derived from [urine protein] in mg/l divided by the [urine creatinine] in mmol/l) corresponds to a protein excretion rate of approximately 1 g/24 hrs, and a ratio of 400 to 3.5 g/24 hrs. Regardless of absolute muscle mass, changes in this ratio can give valuable information about the progression of renal disease (see Tables 6.1 and 6.2).

Low levels of proteinuria without other evidence of renal disease may be managed by observation alone, but are a marker for later development of hypertension and overt renal disease. Nephrotic levels of proteinuria, or lesser levels in the presence of haematuria, hypertension or renal impairment, are usually an indication for renal biopsy.

In many types of renal disease, the severity of proteinuria is a marker for an increased risk of progressive loss of renal function, and direct toxicity has been suggested. The evidence for this is mostly circumstantial, but treatments that are effective at lowering the risk of progression (e.g. ACE inhibitors in diabetic nephropathy) also reduce proteinuria.

Table 6.1 Proteinuria

Excretion rate	Protein/creatinine (mg/mmol)*	Significance
< 0.15 g/24 hrs		Normal
0.3–0.5 g/24 hrs		Stick tests positive
0.5–2 g/24 hrs	50–200	Source equivocal
> 2.5 g/24 hrs	> 300	Glomerular disease likely
> 3.5 g/24 hrs	> 400	'Nephrotic range': always glomerular

* See text.

Table 6.2 Albumin excretion: alternative ways of expressing the normal range

Sample	Normal value
24-hr urine collection	< 30 mg/24 hrs
Timed sample from ambulant patient	< 20 μg/min
Timed overnight sample or from recumbent patient	< 10 μg/min
Albumin/creatinine ratio on a random urine sample	< 2.5 mg/mmol (male) < 3.5 mg/mmol (female)

Note > 300 mg/24 hrs (200 μg/min) is frank proteinuria.

NEPHROTIC SYNDROME

When substantial amounts of protein are lost in the urine, a series of secondary phenomena occur. It is these that constitute the nephrotic syndrome, although they begin to occur at levels of proteinuria lower than 'nephrotic range' (3.5 g/24 hrs). One formal definition of the nephrotic syndrome requires serum albumin < 30 g/litre, evidence of fluid retention or oedema, and more than 3.5 g of proteinuria/day. The diseases that cause nephrotic syndrome always affect the glomerulus (see the information box) and tend to be non-inflammatory, or subacute examples of inflammatory glomerulonephritis.

The consequences and complications of the nephrotic syndrome are listed in the second information box. Oedema accumulates predominantly in the lower limbs in adults, extending to the genitalia and lower abdomen as it gets

COMMON CAUSES OF NEPHROTIC SYNDROME

Non-inflammatory glomerulonephritis

- Minimal change nephropathy
- Focal and segmental glomerulosclerosis (FSGS)
- Membranous nephropathy

Proliferative/inflammatory glomerulonephritis

- Mesangiocapillary glomerulonephritis (MCGN)
- Other 'subacute' proliferative nephritis
- Systemic lupus erythematosus (SLE) (with a variety of histopathological types)

Systemic diseases

- Diabetic nephropathy
- Amyloidosis

CONSEQUENCES AND COMPLICATIONS OF NEPHROTIC SYNDROME

Oedema

- Caused by avid sodium retention and hypoalbuminaemia

Hypercoagulability

- Presumed relative loss of inhibitors of coagulation
- Venous thromboembolism is common and sometimes fatal

Hypercholesterolaemia

- High rate of arterial occlusions and disease

Infection

- Especially by pneumococci
- Associated with hypogammaglobulinaemia

more severe. In the morning, the upper limbs and face may be more affected. In children, ascites occurs early and oedema is often seen only in the face. Blood volume may be normal, reduced or increased. Avid renal sodium retention is an early and universal feature.

Management of nephrotic syndrome has four elements:

- Establish cause.
- Treat cause if possible.
- Treat symptoms.
- Prevent complications.

There are important age-related differences in the incidence of different causes. In neonates, congenital aetiologies are most common, with minimal change nephropathy the dominant diagnosis in older children. In later life there is a progressive increase in the incidence of membranous nephropathy and focal segmental glomerulosclerosis (FSGS). Diabetes mellitus and amyloidosis rarely cause nephrotic syndrome in childhood.

In children with minimal change nephropathy, initial management includes administration of high-dose corticosteroids. In older patients, and in children where this therapy is unsuccessful, a renal biopsy is essential unless there is strong evidence for a specific aetiology (e.g. a long history of diabetes, with other microvascular complications and a demonstrated progression from microalbuminuria, and with hypertension but no haematuria).

Symptomatic oedema is controlled by diuretics and a low-sodium diet (no added salt). In severe nephrotic syndrome very large doses of combinations of diuretic acting on different parts of the nephron (e.g. loop diuretic plus thiazide plus amiloride) may be required. In occasional patients with evidence of hypovolaemia, intravenous salt-poor albumin infusions may help to establish a diuresis. Over-diuresis risks secondary impairment of renal function through hypovolaemia. Venous thromboembolism is guarded against by anticoagulation. There is a case for routine anticoagulation in all patients with chronic or severe nephrotic syndrome. Hypercholesterolaemia is now commonly treated with lipid-lowering drugs (e.g. HMG CoA reductase inhibitors, see p. 537) because of the very high levels encountered and the high incidence of atherosclerotic disease. However, controlled trials have not been reported for this patient group. The risk of infection with pneumococci is especially high in children, who should be offered immunisation.

SYSTEMIC MANIFESTATIONS OF RENAL DISEASE

The broad categories of renal and urinary tract disease, and the typical manifestations that they may cause, are indicated in Figure 6.12. Symptoms related directly to the kidneys are uncommon in intrinsic or pre-renal disorders, and identification of such diseases is further complicated by

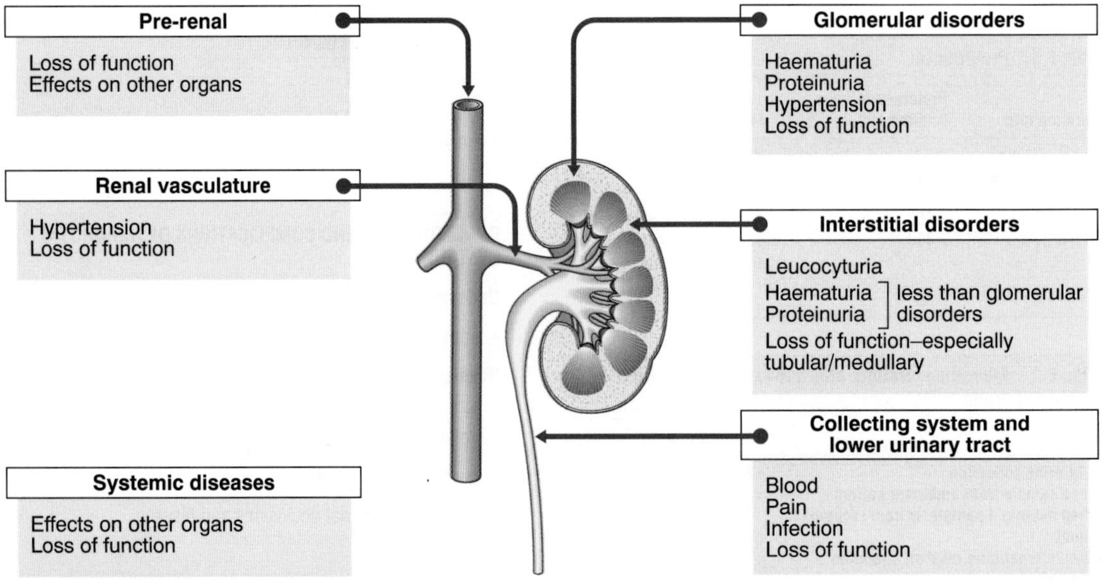

Fig. 6.12 Manifestations of renal and urinary tract disease.

the fact that loss of renal function is, with some exceptions, only recognised clinically at a late stage. Exceptions include the polyuria or sodium-wasting of some tubular disorders. More commonly, sodium retention and fluid imbalance lead to hypertension and oedema.

While non-inflammatory and subacute inflammatory/proliferative glomerular disorders may present with nephrotic syndrome, inflammatory glomerular disorders more typically cause haematuria in association with early signs of disturbed renal function, such as hypertension. If progressive, obvious signs of impaired excretion of water and solutes develop. The onset of these features in close succession has been described as the nephritic syndrome, but in pure form this condition is seen rarely, except in countries where post-infectious glomerulonephritis is common. Mixed inflammatory and nephrotic features are more common. It is important to recognise such disease, especially if renal impairment is progressing, as the inflammatory group includes some of the most treatable renal disorders.

RENAL FAILURE

This term is used primarily to denote failure of the excretory function of the kidneys, leading to retention of nitrogenous waste products of metabolism. Various other aspects of renal function may fail at the same time, including the regulation of fluid and electrolyte status and the endocrine function of the kidney. A wide range of clinical manifestations may therefore occur. The most fundamental categorisation of renal failure is into acute or chronic renal failure.

ACUTE RENAL FAILURE

Acute renal failure (ARF) refers to a sudden and usually reversible loss of renal function, which develops over a period of days or weeks. An increase in plasma creatinine concentration to greater than 200 μmol/l is often used as the biochemical definition. A reduction in urine volume occurs usually, but not always. There are many possible causes (see Fig. 6.13), and it is frequently multifactorial. The clinical picture is often dominated by the underlying condition. If the cause cannot be rapidly corrected and renal function restored, temporary renal replacement therapy may be required (see p. 438). Many of the underlying disorders giving rise to ARF are complex and carry a high mortality, but if the patient survives, normal or nearly normal renal function usually returns.

REVERSIBLE PRE-RENAL ACUTE RENAL FAILURE

Pathogenesis

The kidney can regulate its own blood flow and glomerular filtration rate over a wide range of perfusion pressures. When the perfusion pressure falls, as in hypovolaemia,

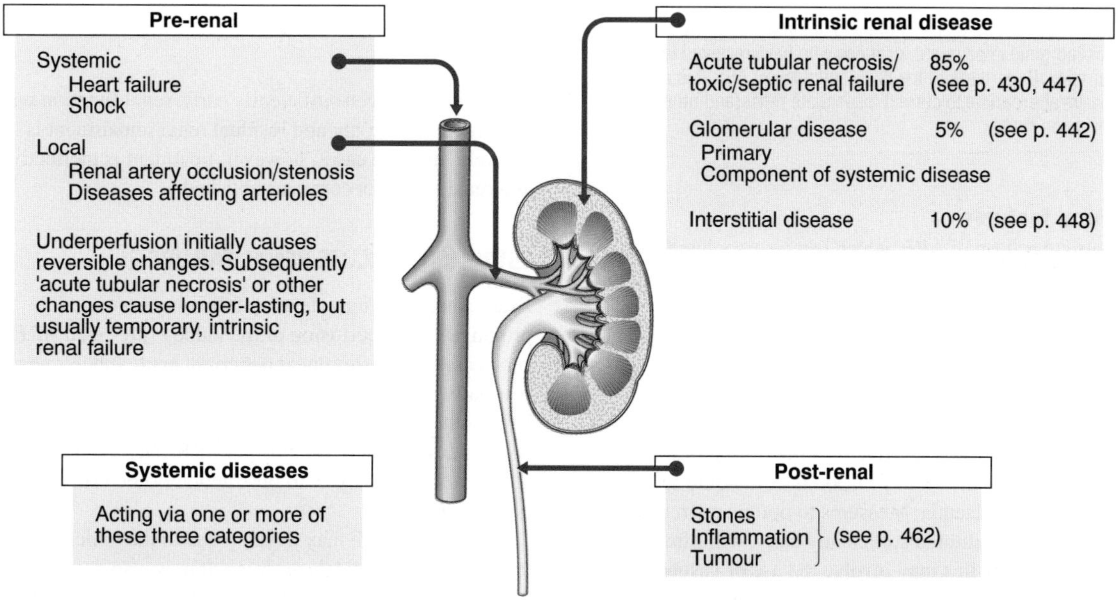

Fig. 6.13 Causes of acute renal failure.

shock, heart failure or narrowing of the renal arteries, the resistance vessels in the kidney dilate to facilitate flow. This is partly mechanical, due to decreased stretch of the vessel walls, and partly neurohumoral. Vasodilator prostaglandins are important, and this mechanism is markedly impaired by non-steroidal anti-inflammatory drugs (see p. 466).

If autoregulation of blood flow fails, the glomerular filtration rate can still be maintained by means of selective constriction of the post-glomerular (efferent) arteriole. This is mediated through release of renin and generation of angiotensin II, which preferentially constricts this vessel. ACE inhibitors interfere with this response.

More severe or prolonged underperfusion of the kidney may lead to failure of these compensatory mechanisms. Blood flow and filtration rate decline. The renal tubules are intact, and become hyperfunctional—i.e. tubular reabsorption of sodium and water is increased, partly through physical factors and partly through the influence of angiotensins, aldosterone and vasopressin. This leads to the formation of a low volume of urine which is concentrated (high osmolality) but low in sodium (see the information box).

DIAGNOSIS OF PRE-RENAL ACUTE RENAL FAILURE

- A compatible history
- The clinical findings
- A progressive increase in blood urea and plasma creatinine
- Urine osmolality > 600 mOsm/kg; urine sodium < 20 mmol/l; urine/plasma urea ratio of >10:1

The urinary findings depend on the kidneys' ability to respond to inadequate perfusion by intense conservation of sodium and water. They may therefore not be found in patients with pre-existing renal impairment, or those who have received loop diuretics. Regardless of the likely aetiology of ARF, it is almost always appropriate to correct inadequate renal (and other organ) perfusion swiftly.

Clinical features

A particular form of ARF, which can be associated with a decreased urinary sodium concentration, is seen in septic patients. The causation is multifactorial. In part it may reflect the action on the kidney of bacterial endotoxin and other mediator substances which are activated in the sepsis syndrome. Most septic patients, if they are volume resuscitated, show vasodilatation of the systemic circulation; this leads to a relative underfilling of the arterial tree, and the kidney responds as it would to absolute hypovolaemia. Measures to optimise circulatory parameters, if instituted sufficiently early, will often restore kidney function; this may involve the use of vasoconstrictor agents such as noradrenaline. When it is severe or prolonged, sepsis is also an important cause of established ARF with acute tubular necrosis.

There may be a marked reduction of blood pressure and signs of poor peripheral perfusion, such as delayed capillary return. However, pre-renal ARF may occur without systemic hypotension. Postural hypotension (a fall in blood pressure of ≥ 20/10 mmHg from lying to standing) is a valuable sign of hypovolaemia. The cause of the reduced renal perfusion may be obvious, but concealed blood loss can occur into the gastrointestinal tract following trauma (particularly where there are fractures of the pelvis or femur) and into the pregnant uterus. Large volumes of intravascular fluid are lost into tissues after crush injuries or burns, or in severe inflammatory skin diseases or sepsis. Metabolic acidosis and hyperkalaemia are often present.

Management

The underlying cause of the ARF must be established and corrected. When hypovolaemia is present, the blood volume must be restored as rapidly as possible, by replacing with blood, plasma or isotonic saline (0.9%), depending on what has been lost. If metabolic acidosis is severe, isotonic sodium bicarbonate (e.g. 500 ml of 1.26%) may be included as part of the replacement fluid. In most cases, however, restoration of blood volume will restore kidney function and allow correction of acidosis. It is often helpful to monitor the central venous pressure or pulmonary wedge pressure as an adjunct to clinical examination in determining the rate of administration of fluid.

Patients with cardiogenic or septic shock (see p. 1027), in addition to optimisation of their volume status, may require invasive haemodynamic monitoring to assess cardiac output and systemic vascular resistance, and the use of inotropic drugs to restore an effective blood pressure.

Prognosis

If treatment is given sufficiently early, renal function will usually return rapidly and residual renal impairment is unlikely. In some cases, however, treatment is ineffective and renal failure becomes established.

ESTABLISHED ACUTE RENAL FAILURE

Established ARF may develop following severe or prolonged underperfusion of the kidney (pre-renal ARF). In such cases, the histological pattern of acute tubular necrosis is usually seen. The features of this condition are described later in the chapter (see p. 447). Alternatively, patients may present de novo with established ARF, due to intrinsic disease of the kidney or to obstruction of the urinary tract (see Fig. 6.13).

Established ARF may develop due to the toxic effects on the kidney of chemicals or drugs. It may also develop in conditions affecting the intrarenal arteries and arterioles, such as vasculitis, accelerated hypertension and disseminated intravascular coagulation. Glomerular diseases can produce acute deterioration in renal function, particularly those which run a rapid course, such as crescentic glomerulonephritis. Acute allergic interstitial nephritis (see p. 448), which is often due to drugs, may cause ARF.

ARF can result from obstruction at any point in the urinary tract (see p. 462). If there are two functioning kidneys, ureteric obstruction only causes uraemia if it is bilateral. A history of loin pain, haematuria, renal colic, nocturia or difficulty in micturition suggests the diagnosis. Often the onset is clinically silent, and the obstruction is only discovered on investigation. An ultrasound examination of kidneys and ureters should, therefore, be carried out in any patient with unexplained renal failure.

Clinical features

These reflect the causal condition, such as trauma, septicaemia or systemic disease, together with features associated with renal failure. Patients are usually oliguric (urine volume < 500 ml daily). Anuria (complete absence of urine) is rare and usually indicates acute urinary tract obstruction or vascular occlusion. In about 20% of cases, the urine volume is normal or increased, but with a low GFR and a reduction of tubular reabsorption (non-oliguric acute renal failure). Excretion is inadequate despite good urine output, and the plasma urea and creatinine increase. In ARF, the rate of rise in plasma urea and creatinine is determined by the rate of catabolism (tissue breakdown). In ARF associated with severe infections, major surgery or trauma, the daily rise in plasma urea often exceeds 5 mmol/l.

Disturbances of water, electrolyte and acid-base balance arise; hyperkalaemia is common, particularly with massive tissue breakdown, haemolysis or metabolic acidosis. Since it causes ventricular arrhythmias, it must be controlled (see p. 406). Patients may have dilutional hyponatraemia, having received inappropriate amounts of intravenous water, e.g. as 5% dextrose or having continued to drink freely despite oliguria. Metabolic acidosis develops, unless it is prevented by loss of hydrogen ions through vomiting or aspiration of gastric contents. Hypocalcaemia, due to reduced renal production of 1,25-dihydroxycholecalciferol, is common.

At first the patient may feel well but, unless dialysis is instituted, clinical features linked to retention of metabolic waste products eventually appear. Initially these are anorexia, nausea and vomiting. Later, drowsiness, apathy and confusion, muscle twitching, hiccoughs, fits and coma occur. The respiratory rate is increased due to acidosis, pulmonary oedema or respiratory infection. Pulmonary oedema may result from the administration of excessive amounts of fluids and because of increased pulmonary capillary permeability (acute respiratory distress syndrome, see p. 1031). Anaemia is common due to excessive blood loss, haemolysis or decreased erythropoiesis. There is a bleeding tendency due to disordered platelet function and disturbances of the coagulation cascade. Gastrointestinal haemorrhage may occur, often late in the illness, although this is less common with effective dialysis and the use of agents that reduce gastric acid production. Severe infections may complicate ARF because humoral and cellular immune mechanisms are depressed in renal failure.

Management

Emergency resuscitation

Hyperkalaemia (a plasma K^+ concentration > 6 mmol/l) must be treated to prevent the development of life-threatening cardiac arrhythmias. This is detailed on page 406.

The circulating blood volume, if it is low, must be corrected by transfusion with appropriate fluids. This may require monitoring of central venous or pulmonary wedge pressure. Patients with pulmonary oedema usually require dialysis to remove sodium and water.

Determination of the cause of ARF and specific treatment of the underlying cause

The cause may be obvious or revealed by initial simple investigations (e.g. ultrasound showing obstruction). If not, a range of investigations, including renal biopsy, may be necessary. In many cases, more than one factor contributes to the renal dysfunction.

There is no specific treatment for acute tubular necrosis. Some other causes of ARF may require specific therapy. Obstruction should be relieved urgently. Corticosteroids and immunosuppressive drugs are of value in ARF due to systemic vasculitis and some other causes of rapidly progressive glomerulonephritis (see p. 443). Corticosteroids may also be indicated in acute tubulo-interstitial nephritis (see p. 448). Control of blood pressure is critical in acute renal failure due to accelerated hypertension (see p. 441). Plasma infusion and plasma exchange may be indicated in microangiopathic diseases (see p. 441).

If pelvic or ureteric dilatation is found, percutaneous nephrostomy is undertaken to decompress the urinary system (see p. 422). Dialysis can usually be avoided. Injection of dye through the nephrostomy tube (antegrade pyelography) reveals the site of the obstruction.

Once obstruction has been relieved and blood chemistry has returned towards normal, the underlying cause is identified and treated wherever possible (see p. 462). Sometimes obstruction is caused by pelvic malignancies, such as carcinoma of the cervix, uterus or colon, which are so advanced that intervention is inadvisable.

General management of established ARF

In established ARF, the aims are to control fluid and

electrolyte balance, maintain nutrition, control the biochemical abnormalities and protect the patient from infection. Drugs must be used with particular care. Renal replacement therapy may be required (see p. 438).

Fluid and electrolyte balance. After initial resuscitation, daily fluid intake should equal urine output, plus an additional 500 ml to cover insensible losses; febrile patients require more. Since sodium and potassium are retained, intake of these substances should be restricted. If abnormal losses occur, as in diarrhoea, additional fluid and electrolytes are required. The patient should be weighed daily. Large changes in body weight, or the development of oedema or signs of fluid depletion indicate that fluid intake should be reassessed.

Protein and energy intake. In patients in whom it is hoped to avoid dialysis, dietary protein is restricted to about 40 g/day. Attempts are made to suppress endogenous protein catabolism by giving as much energy as possible in the form of fat and carbohydrate. Patients treated by dialysis may have more protein (70 g protein daily, 10–12 g nitrogen). In some patients, feeding via a nasogastric tube may be helpful. Parenteral nutrition may be required because of vomiting or diarrhoea, or if the bowel is not intact, or to give adequate energy and nitrogen to hypercatabolic patients.

Recovery from acute renal failure

This is usually indicated by a gradual return of urine output, and subsequently a steady improvement in plasma biochemistry towards normal. Some patients, primarily those with acute tubular necrosis or after relief of chronic urinary obstruction, develop a 'diuretic phase' (see p. 463). Fluid should be given to replace the urine output as appropriate, and supplements of sodium chloride, sodium bicarbonate and potassium chloride may be needed to compensate for increased urinary losses. After a few days, urine volume falls to normal as the concentrating mechanism is restored.

Prognosis

In uncomplicated ARF, such as that due to simple haemorrhage or drugs, mortality is low even when renal replacement therapy is required. In ARF complicated by serious infection and failure of multiple organs, mortality is 50–70%. Outcome is determined by the severity of the underlying disorder and by complications rather than by renal failure itself.

Table 6.3 Important causes of chronic renal failure

Disease	Proportion of ESRF in Scotland[1]	Proportion of ESRF in USA[2]	Comments
Congenital and inherited			
Polycystic kidney disease	7%	3%	
Congenital hypoplasia/dysplasia	1%	1%	
Other inherited	1%	1%	Alport's syndrome (see p. 442) is the most frequent cause within this group
Vascular disease			
Renal artery stenosis	6%	2%	
Hypertension	4%	27%	Variation by nation/racial group—partly due to variation in diagnostic labels, but also to true variations in disease incidence (e.g. common in black races, rare in white)
Glomerular disease	19%	11%	Many varieties contribute, but IgA disease is the most common
Interstitial disease	14%	5%	Includes chronic pyelonephritis, reflux nephropathy and analgesic nephropathy
Systemic diseases			
Diabetes mellitus	17%	37%	Varies by race and region (see p. 504)
SLE	1%	1%	
Other	7%	3%	
Malignancy			
Myeloma	2%	1%	
Aetiology uncertain	18%	4%	
Other causes	3%	4%	

(ESRF = end-stage renal failure, renal failure requiring regular dialysis or transplantation for survival)

[1] Scottish data: 1993–7, from the Scottish Renal Registry.
[2] US data: 1991–5, from the United States Renal Data System 1997 Annual Data Report.

CHRONIC RENAL FAILURE

Chronic renal failure (CRF) is an irreversible deterioration in renal function which classically develops over a period of years. Initially, it is manifest only as a biochemical abnormality. Eventually, loss of the excretory, metabolic and endocrine functions of the kidney leads to the development of the clinical symptoms and signs of renal failure, which are sometimes referred to as uraemia.

The social and economic consequences of CRF are considerable. In Britain 70–80 new patients per million of the adult population are accepted for long-term dialysis treatment each year; the availability of dialysis and transplantation has transformed the outlook for such patients. Figures are much higher in some other countries because of differences in regional and racial incidences of disease as well as because of differences in medical practice.

Aetiology

CRF may be caused by any condition which destroys the normal structure and function of the kidney. Important causes are shown in Table 6.3. A presumptive diagnosis of a chronic form of glomerulonephritis may be made if there is proteinuria, haematuria and hypertension in the absence of any other cause of renal failure, but a precise diagnosis is not always established. Patients often have bilateral small kidneys, and in that situation renal biopsy is usually inadvisable because of the difficulty in making a histological diagnosis in severely damaged kidneys and the fact that treatment is unlikely to improve renal function significantly.

Pathogenesis

Disturbances in water, electrolyte and acid-base balance contribute to the clinical picture in patients with chronic renal failure, but the exact pathogenesis of the clinical syndrome of uraemia is unknown. Many substances present in abnormal concentration in the plasma have been suspected of being 'uraemic toxins', and uraemia is probably caused by accumulation of various intermediary products of metabolism.

Clinical features

In early CRF, the patient is often asymptomatic. Renal failure may present as a raised blood urea and creatinine found during routine examination, often accompanied by hypertension, proteinuria or anaemia. When renal function deteriorates slowly, patients may remain asymptomatic until the GFR is 20 ml/min or less (normal 80–120 ml/min). Nocturia, due to the loss of concentrating ability and osmotic load per nephron, is often an early symptom. Then, because of the widespread effects of renal failure, symptoms and signs may develop related to almost every body system (see Fig. 6.14). Patients may present with complaints which are not obviously renal in origin, such as tiredness or breathlessness.

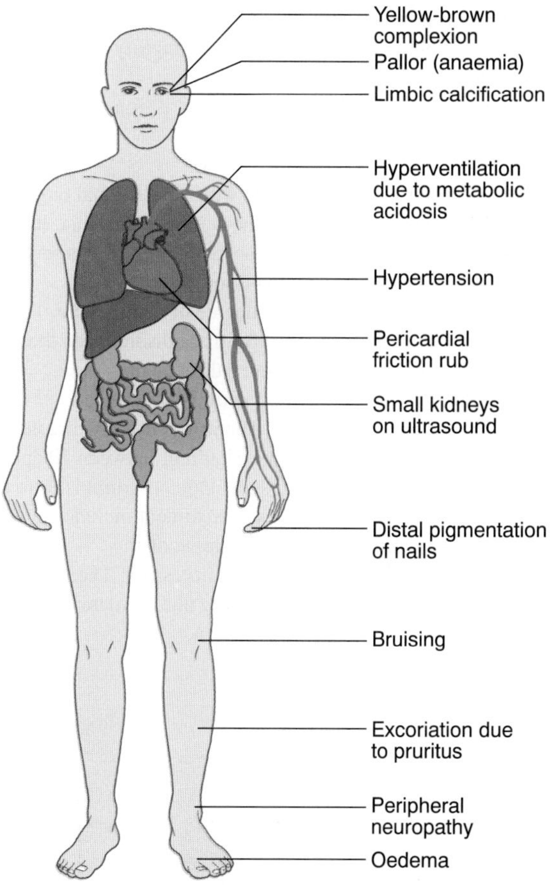

Fig. 6.14 Clinical features of advanced chronic renal failure.

In end-stage renal failure, patients appear ill and anaemic. They do not necessarily retain fluid, and may show signs of sodium and water depletion. There may be unusually deep respiration related to metabolic acidosis (Kussmaul's respiration), anorexia and nausea. Later, hiccoughs, pruritus, vomiting, muscular twitching, fits, drowsiness and coma ensue.

Anaemia

Anaemia is common, usually correlates with the severity of renal failure and contributes to many of the non-specific symptoms of CRF. Several mechanisms are implicated, including:

- relative deficiency of erythropoietin
- diminished erythropoiesis due to the toxic effects of uraemia on marrow precursor cells

- reduced red cell survival
- increased blood loss due to capillary fragility and poor platelet function
- reduced dietary intake and absorption of iron and other haematinics.

Plasma erythropoietin is usually within the normal range and thus inappropriately low for the degree of anaemia. In patients with polycystic kidneys, anaemia is often less severe or absent, and in some interstitial disorders it appears disproportionately severe for the degree of renal failure. This is probably because of the effects of these disorders on the interstitial fibroblasts that secrete erythropoietin.

Recombinant human erythropoietin is effective in correcting the anaemia of CRF. Therapy is usually directed towards achieving a target haemoglobin of between 10 and 12 g/l. It must be injected, and subcutaneous administration is most effective. Complications of treatment include increased blood pressure, and adjustment of antihypertensive medication is often necessary. There is also an increase in blood coagulability and an increased incidence of thrombosis of the arteriovenous fistulae used for haemodialysis. If anaemia is corrected slowly, these effects are less common. Erythropoietin is less effective in the presence of iron deficiency, active inflammation or malignancy, or in patients with aluminium overload which may occur in dialysis. These factors should be sought and, if possible, corrected before treatment.

Renal osteodystrophy

This metabolic bone disease which accompanies CRF consists of a mixture of osteomalacia, hyperparathyroid bone disease (osteitis fibrosa), osteoporosis and osteosclerosis (see Fig. 6.15). Osteomalacia results from diminished activity of the renal 1-α-hydroxylase enzyme, with failure to convert cholecalciferol to its active metabolite 1,25-dihydroxycholecalciferol. A deficiency of the latter leads to diminished intestinal absorption of calcium, hypocalcaemia and reduction in the calcification of osteoid. Osteitis fibrosa results from secondary hyperparathyroidism. The parathyroid glands are stimulated by the low plasma calcium, and also by

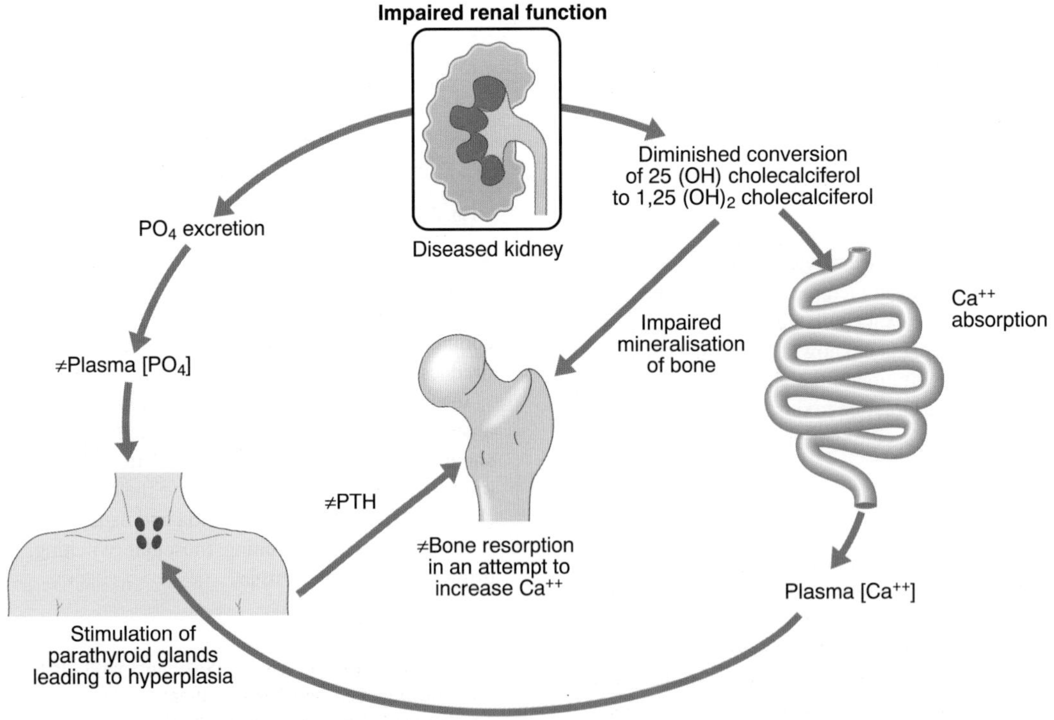

Fig. 6.15 Pathogenesis of renal osteodystrophy. Decreased hydroxylation of cholecalciferol by the diseased kidney results in a diminution in plasma 1,25-dihydroxycholecalciferol. The effect of this is to reduce intestinal absorption of calcium, resulting in a reduction in the plasma calcium with a consequent stimulation of the parathyroid glands to increase parathyroid hormone (PTH) secretion. The increased PTH has an effect on bone by causing increased osteoclastic activity with consequent bone resorption. In addition, the diminished 1,25-dihydroxycholecalciferol results in impaired mineralisation of bone. The net result is bone which exhibits increased osteoclastic activity and increased osteoid as a consequence of decreased mineralisation.

hyperphosphataemia. In some patients tertiary or autonomous hyperparathyroidism with hypercalcaemia develops. Osteoporosis occurs in many patients, possibly related to mild malnutrition. Osteosclerosis is seen mainly in the sacral area, at the base of the skull, and in the vertebrae; the cause of this unusual reaction is not known.

Myopathy

Generalised myopathy is due to a combination of poor nutrition, hyperparathyroidism, vitamin D deficiency and disorders of electrolyte metabolism. Muscle cramps are common, and quinine sulphate may be helpful. The 'restless leg syndrome', where the patient's legs are jumpy during the night, may be troublesome and is often improved by clonazepam.

Neuropathy

There is demyelination of medullated fibres, the longer fibres being involved earlier. Sensory neuropathy may cause paraesthesiae. Motor neuropathy may present as foot drop. Uraemic autonomic neuropathy may explain delayed gastric emptying, diarrhoea and postural hypotension. Clinical manifestations of neuropathy appear late in the course of chronic renal failure. They improve and may resolve once dialysis is established.

Endocrine function

A number of hormonal abnormalities may be present, of which the most important are hyperprolactinaemia and hyperparathyroidism. In women, amenorrhoea is common. In both sexes there is loss of libido and sexual function, at least in part related to hyperprolactinaemia (see p. 551). Treatment with bromocriptine is sometimes useful.

The half-life of insulin is prolonged in CRF due to reduced tubular metabolism of insulin, and insulin requirements may decline in diabetic patients in end-stage CRF. However, there is also a post-receptor defect in insulin action, leading to relative insulin resistance. This latter abnormality is improved by dialysis treatment. Changes in carbohydrate metabolism depend on which factors predominate.

Cardiovascular disorders

Hypertension develops in approximately 80% of patients with CRF. In part, this is caused by sodium retention. Chronically diseased kidneys also tend to hypersecrete renin, leading to high circulating concentrations of renin, angiotensin II and aldosterone. This is exaggerated if there is renal underperfusion related to renal vascular disease. Hypertension must be controlled, as it causes further vascular and glomerular damage and worsening of renal failure. Atherosclerosis is common and may be accelerated by hypertension. Vascular calcification may develop and be sufficiently severe to cause inadequate perfusion of the limbs. Pericarditis is common in untreated or inadequately treated end-stage renal failure. It may lead to pericardial tamponade and, later, constrictive pericarditis.

Acidosis

Declining renal function is associated with metabolic acidosis (see p. 411), which is often asymptomatic. Sustained acidosis results in protons being buffered in bone in place of calcium, thus aggravating metabolic bone disease. Acidosis may also contribute to reduced renal function and increased tissue catabolism. The plasma bicarbonate should be maintained above 18 mmol/l by giving sodium bicarbonate supplements. The dose is determined by clinical trial, commencing with 1 g 8-hourly and increasing as required. The increased sodium intake may induce hypertension or oedema; calcium carbonate (up to 3 g daily) is an alternative agent that is also used as a binder of dietary phosphate.

Infection

Cellular and humoral immunity are impaired, with increased susceptibility to infection. Infections are the second most common cause of death in dialysis patients, after cardiovascular disease.

Management

There are several aspects to the management of CRF:

- identify the underlying renal disease
- attempt to prevent further renal damage
- look for reversible factors which are making renal function worse
- attempt to limit the adverse effects of the loss of renal function
- institute renal replacement therapy (dialysis, transplantation) when appropriate.

At presentation the nature of the underlying disease should be determined if possible, by history, examination, testing of biochemistry, immunology, radiology and biopsy. The degree of renal failure is assessed and complications are documented. In some cases, the cause may be amenable to

REVERSIBLE FACTORS IN CHRONIC RENAL FAILURE

- Hypertension
- Reduced renal perfusion
  - Renal artery stenosis
  - Hypotension due to drug treatment
  - Sodium and water depletion
  - Poor cardiac function
- Urinary tract obstruction
- Urinary tract infection
- Other infections: increased catabolism and urea production
- Nephrotoxic medications

specific therapy, e.g. immunosuppression in some types of glomerulonephritis. A search is made for reversible factors, correction of which results in improved renal function (see the information box).

In patients with irreversible renal failure, various measures can reduce symptoms and may slow progression to end-stage renal failure.

Retarding the progression of CRF

Unless dialysis or transplantation is provided, CRF is eventually fatal. Once the plasma creatinine exceeds about 300 μmol/l there is usually progressive deterioration in renal function irrespective of aetiology. The rate of deterioration is very variable between patients, but is relatively constant for an individual patient. A plot of the reciprocal of the plasma creatinine concentration against time allows the physician to predict when dialysis will be required, and to detect any unexpected worsening of renal failure (see Fig. 6.16). Changes in the slope may reflect changes in treatment (e.g. blood pressure control).

Control of blood pressure

In many types of renal disease, but particularly in diseases affecting glomeruli, control of blood pressure may retard the rate of deterioration of GFR. This has been proven for diabetic nephropathy, but is probably true for other diseases as well, particularly those associated with heavy proteinuria. No threshold for this effect has been found; reduction of any level of blood pressure is beneficial.

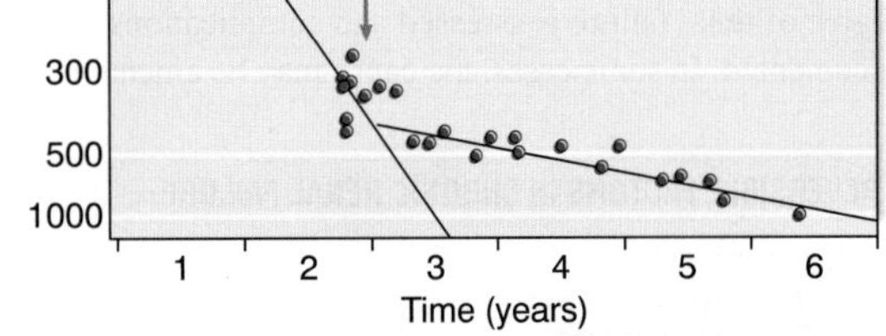

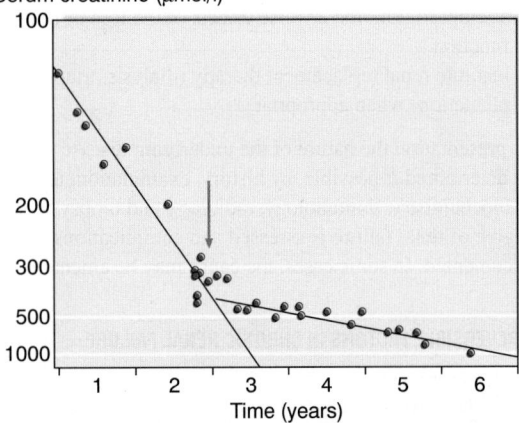

Fig. 6.16 Plot of the reciprocal of serum creatinine concentration against time over a 6-year period in a patient with progressive renal failure caused by membranous nephropathy. Serial plasma creatinine estimations permit prediction of the time to end-stage renal disease. The 'break point' (arrow) at which the gradient of the line is dramatically reduced was associated with a 6-month course of treatment with chlorambucil and prednisolone.

Various target blood pressures have been suggested—for example, 130/85 for CRF alone, lowered to 125/75 for those with proteinuria greater than 1 g/day. For older patients, a more practical target might be a maximum blood pressure equal to the 75th centile for their age. The very high incidence of left ventricular hypertrophy, heart failure and occlusive vascular disease in patients with long-standing renal disease also justifies vigorous efforts to control blood pressure.

ACE inhibitors have been shown to be more effective at retarding progression of renal failure than other therapies giving an equal lowering of systemic blood pressure in diabetes and in other types of glomerular disease. This may be because they reduce glomerular perfusion pressure by dilating the efferent arteriole, an effect which causes an immediate reduction in GFR when therapy is initiated. Reduction in proteinuria is a good prognostic sign, but it is not clear if this is causally related to prognosis. Apart from ACE inhibitors, angiotensin II receptor antagonists also reduce glomerular perfusion pressure, and the same effect may be achieved by some non-dihydropyridine calcium antagonists and possibly by other agents in the future.

Diet

In experimental studies, progressive renal disease can be retarded by various manipulations of diet, most notably by restriction of dietary protein. In human studies results have been less clear-cut; low-protein diets are difficult to adhere to and carry a risk of inducing malnutrition. This remains a controversial area but, for most patients living in areas where renal replacement therapy is available, severe protein restriction is not generally recommended. Moderate restriction (to 60 g protein per day) should be accompanied by adequate intake of calories to prevent malnutrition. Anorexia and muscle loss may indicate a need to commence dialysis treatment.

Lipids

Hypercholesterolaemia is almost universal in patients with significant proteinuria, and increased triglyceride levels are also common in patients with CRF. As well as influencing the development of vascular disease, it has been suggested that this may accelerate the progression of chronic renal disease. It is only the introduction of HMG CoA reductase inhibitors (see p. 537) that has made it possible to achieve substantial reductions in lipids in chronic renal disease, but there have been no long-term studies in this group of patients. However, many believe that the high incidence of vascular disease in CRF justifies the treatment of these abnormalities in advance of proof from controlled trials.

Electrolytes and fluid

Due to the reduced ability of the failing kidney to concentrate the urine, a relatively high urine volume is needed to excrete products of metabolism, and a fluid intake of around 3 litres/day is desirable. Some patients with so-called 'salt-wasting' disease may require a high sodium and water intake, including supplements of sodium chloride and sodium bicarbonate, to prevent fluid depletion and worsening of renal function. This is most often seen in patients with renal cystic disease, obstructive uropathy, reflux nephropathy or other tubulo-interstitial diseases and is not seen in patients with glomerular disease. These patients benefit from taking 5–10 g/day (85–170 mmol/day) of sodium chloride by mouth. It is usual to start with 2–3 g/day and increase the dose as required. The limit for additional salt is set by the development of systemic or pulmonary oedema, or aggravation of hypertension. Sodium bicarbonate may be substituted in part for sodium chloride when acidosis requires correction.

Limitation of potassium intake (e.g. 70 mmol/day) and sodium intake (e.g. 100 mmol/day) may be required in late CRF if there is evidence of accumulation. Disproportionate fluid retention in milder renal failure, sometimes leading to episodic pulmonary oedema, is particularly associated with renal artery stenosis.

Osteodystrophy

Plasma calcium and phosphate should be kept as near to normal as possible. Hypocalcaemia is corrected by giving 1-α-hydroxylated synthetic analogues of vitamin D. The dose is adjusted to avoid hypercalcaemia. This will usually prevent or control osteomalacia, although it is sometimes resistant, presumably because of other factors inhibiting bone mineralisation. Hyperphosphataemia is controlled by dietary restriction of foods with high phosphate content (milk, cheese, eggs) and the use of phosphate-binding drugs. These agents form insoluble complexes with dietary phosphate and prevent its absorption (e.g. calcium carbonate 500 mg with each meal). Aluminium hydroxide also has a phosphate-binding effect (aluminium hydroxide capsules 300–600 mg before each meal). To prevent aluminium toxicity, the dose of aluminium hydroxide should be kept to a minimum and should be administered immediately before meals. Secondary hyperparathyroidism is usually prevented or controlled by these measures, but in severe bone disease with autonomous parathyroid function, parathyroidectomy may become necessary.

Prognosis

The tendency of renal impairment to progress was described above (see Fig. 6.16), along with ways of influencing that progression.

Information about the long-term prognosis for patients on dialysis or following transplantation is limited because these techniques have been available only for the past 30 years and technology is changing rapidly. Nevertheless, dialysis and transplantation can be considered as highly effective forms of treatment, with a 5-year survival of approximately 80% for home haemodialysis, 80% following renal transplantation, 60% for hospital haemodialysis and 50% for continuous ambulatory peritoneal dialysis (CAPD). These figures are not directly comparable because of patient selection—many older patients and those with systemic diseases such as diabetes mellitus are treated by CAPD. They also conceal a very large increase in death rates from certain causes, but particularly vascular disease, in comparison with an age-matched population. However, they indicate how the prognosis of end-stage renal disease is now much better than that of many other potentially fatal diseases.

REPLACEMENT OF RENAL FUNCTION

The ability to replace the function of the kidney by artificial means has been available to physicians for 40 years. The excretory function of the kidney can be partially replaced by dialysis or haemofiltration techniques. These treatment methods can be used in the management of acute or chronic renal failure. They do not replace endocrine and metabolic functions, which can only be achieved by renal transplantation. Best results in patients with CRF are obtained by an integrated management programme, using the most appropriate form of therapy—haemodialysis, continuous ambulatory peritoneal dialysis or transplantation— depending on the clinical circumstances (see Fig. 6.17).

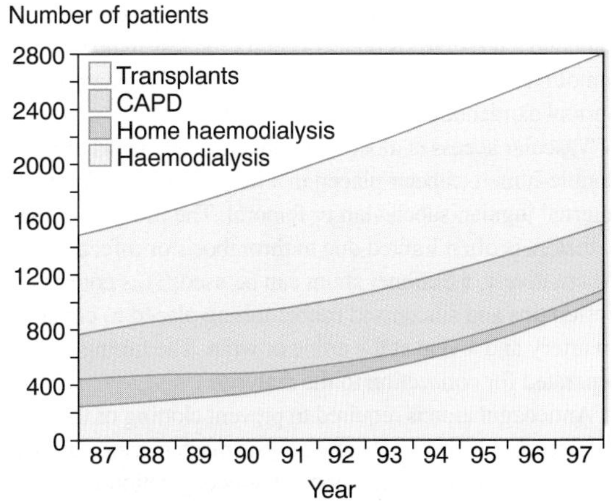

Fig. 6.17 Growth of renal replacement therapy. The figure shows the number of patients in Scotland with functioning renal transplants, on continuous ambulatory peritoneal dialysis (CAPD), and on home and hospital haemodialysis. Other countries show similar trends. The most expensive modality, hospital haemodialysis, shows the fastest rise, a trend that is likely to continue. (Figures from the Scottish Renal Registry.)

RENAL REPLACEMENT IN ACUTE RENAL FAILURE

The indications for renal replacement therapy in ARF are as follows:

- Increased plasma urea or creatinine concentration: in general, a plasma urea greater than 30 mmol/l and creatinine greater than 600 μmol/l are undesirable, but much depends on factors such as the rate of biochemical deterioration (i.e. increase in urea and creatinine concentration) and the risks of dialysis for the patient involved.
- Hyperkalaemia: while this can usually be controlled by medical measures in the short term (see p. 406), dialysis is often required for definitive control.
- Fluid overload: if not controlled by fluid restriction and diuretics.
- Uraemic pericarditis (uncommon in ARF).

The principal options for renal replacement in ARF are haemodialysis, acute high-volume haemofiltration, continuous (arteriovenous or venovenous) haemofiltration or haemodiafiltration, and peritoneal dialysis.

Intermittent techniques

Haemodialysis

Although continuous techniques are being used increasingly in the management of ARF, intermittent haemodialysis is still an important treatment modality in most renal units. The principles of therapy are similar to its use in chronic renal failure (see below). In ARF, most patients can be treated by 3–4 hours of haemodialysis, either daily in catabolic patients or on alternate days. Dialysis regimens are adjusted to maintain a pre-dialysis urea concentration less than 30 mmol/l, adequate control of potassium and phosphate, and normal extracellular fluid volume status.

Vascular access is most often obtained by means of a double-lumen catheter placed in a major vein, commonly the internal jugular, subclavian or femoral. The lifespan of these catheters is often limited due to thrombosis or infection. Alternatively, a Scribner shunt can be used. This consists of Teflon tips and siliconised rubber tubing placed to connect an artery and a vein at the ankle or wrist. The tubing is then separated for connection to the dialyser.

Anticoagulation is required to prevent clotting of the extracorporeal circuit. Haemodialysis machines are equipped to infuse heparin; the efficiency of anticoagulation is monitored by the activated clotting time (ACT). It has been claimed that the use of prostacyclin for anticoagulation is associated with a lower risk of bleeding on dialysis, and many units use this in selected patients.

Acute high-volume haemofiltration

This technique involves the rapid removal and replacement of 12–20 litres of plasma ultrafiltrate over 3–4 hours, using an artificial membrane with a very high ultrafiltration capacity, on a daily or alternate-day basis. The fluid removed is replaced by haemofiltration fluid. It is claimed that this technique induces less circulatory instability than haemodialysis.

Continuous techniques

These include continuous arteriovenous haemofiltration (CAVH) and continuous venovenous haemofiltration (CVVH). These systems cause less haemodynamic disturbance than conventional haemodialysis, and are widely used in patients with ARF who are unstable and require intensive care. In CAVH the extracorporeal blood circuit is driven by the arteriovenous pressure difference. Poor filtration rates and clotting of the filter may result from low arterial pressure and/or elevated central venous pressure. CVVH is pump-driven, allowing a reliable extracorporeal circulation. Most patients are managed by removal and replacement of 1 litre of filtrate per hour (equivalent to a GFR of 15 ml/min).

Peritoneal dialysis

This has been supplanted in most centres by the techniques outlined above. It is less efficient than haemodialysis, and seldom achieves good biochemical control in catabolic patients. It is not feasible after recent abdominal surgery, but can be useful in patients with cardiovascular instability, e.g. after cardiac surgery. A trocar and cannula system is used for acute peritoneal access, and 500 ml volumes of peritoneal dialysis fluid are infused and drained cyclically. Flow can be regulated manually or by an automatic cycler. Cloudy effluent indicates the development of peritonitis, in which case the catheter should be removed immediately and appropriate antibiotics given (e.g. vancomycin and gentamicin to cover the most common organisms).

RENAL REPLACEMENT IN CHRONIC RENAL FAILURE

Haemodialysis

In CRF, haemodialysis should be started when, despite adequate medical treatment, the patient has advanced renal failure, and before he or she develops serious complications. This often occurs with a plasma creatinine of 800–1000 μmol/l. Vascular access is required; an arteriovenous fistula should be formed, usually in the forearm, when the serum creatinine is around 600 μmol/l, so that it has time to become established; increased pressure in the veins leading from the fistula causes distension and thickening of the vessel wall (arterialisation). Large-bore needles can then be inserted into the vein to provide access for each haemodialysis treatment. If this is not possible, plastic cannulae in central veins can be used for short-term access. Haemodialysis is usually carried out for 3–5 hours three times weekly. Most patients notice a gradual improvement in symptoms during the first 6 weeks of treatment. Plasma urea and creatinine are lowered by each treatment but do not return to normal. Accepted standards of dialysis adequacy, which relate the clearance of urea to total body water, are adhered to in most units. Some patients are able to carry out their treatment at home. Many patients lead normal and active lives, and patient survival for more than 20 years is commonplace.

Continuous ambulatory peritoneal dialysis (CAPD)

CAPD is a form of long-term dialysis involving insertion of a permanent Silastic catheter into the peritoneal cavity. Two litres of sterile, isotonic dialysis fluid are introduced and left in place for a period of approximately 6 hours. During this time, metabolic waste products diffuse from peritoneal capillaries into the dialysis fluid down a concentration gradient. The fluid is then drained and fresh dialysis fluid introduced. This cycle is repeated four times daily, during which time the patient is mobile and able to undertake normal daily activities. It is particularly useful in young children, in elderly patients with cardiovascular instability and in patients with diabetes mellitus. Its long-term use may be limited by episodes of bacterial peritonitis, but some patients have been treated successfully for more than 10 years.

Recently, automated peritoneal dialysis (APD) has come into use. This system uses a mechanical device to perform the fluid exchanges during the night, leaving the patient free during the day.

Renal transplantation

This offers the possibility of restoring normal kidney function and correcting all the metabolic abnormalities of CRF. The kidney graft is taken from a cadaver donor or from a relative. ABO (blood group) compatibility between donor and recipient is essential, and it is usual to select donor kidneys on the basis of human leucocyte antigen (HLA) matching as this improves graft survival. Results of kidney transplantation have improved significantly in recent years. Three-year graft survival is in the region of 80%, while 3-year patient survival is approximately 90%.

Long-term immunosuppressive therapy is required. Many therapeutic regimens have been used, but the most common involves a combination of prednisolone, cyclosporin A and azathioprine. There is concern about the long-term nephrotoxicity of cyclosporin, and some centres routinely withdraw this if renal function is satisfactory 6–12 months post-transplant. The role of newer immunosuppressive agents such as tacrolimus (FK506) and mycophenolate mofetil is currently being established by clinical trials.

Immunosuppression is associated with an increased incidence of infection, particularly opportunistic infections, and an increased incidence of malignant neoplasms, especially of the skin. Approximately 50% of patients will have some skin malignancy by 15 years post-transplant. None the less, transplantation does offer the best hope of complete rehabilitation and is the most cost-effective of the treatment options for chronic renal failure. Lymphomas are rare but occur early and are often related to infection with herpesvirus, especially Epstein–Barr virus (see p. 110).

FURTHER INFORMATION ON MAJOR MANIFESTATIONS OF RENAL DISEASE

Edelstein C L, Ling H, Schrier R W 1997 The nature of renal cell injury. Kidney International 51: 1341–1351

Edelstein C L, Ling H, Wangsiripaison A, Schrier R W 1997 Emerging therapies for acute renal failure. American Journal of Kidney Diseases 30 (suppl 4): S89–S95

Klahr S, Levey A S, Beck G J et al 1994 The effects of dietary protein restriction and blood-pressure control on the progression of chronic renal disease. New England Journal of Medicine 330: 877–884

Lewis E J, Hunsicker L G, Bain R P et al 1993 The effect of angiotensin-converting enzyme inhibition on diabetic nephropathy. New England Journal of Medicine 329: 1456

Quarello F, Iadarola G M (eds) Analysis of urinary sediment. From the website of the Italian Society of Nephrology, http://www.sin-italia.org/imago/sediment/sed.htm

Scottish Intercollegiate clinical guidelines on asymptomatic haematuria, asymptomatic proteinuria and diabetic renal disease are available at http://pc47.cee.hw.ac.uk/sign/

Thadhani R, Pascual M, Bonventre J V 1996 Acute renal failure. New England Journal of Medicine 334: 1448–1460

United States Renal Data System (USRDS) Report 1997 http://www.med.umich.edu/usrds/

Walker R 1997 General management of end-stage renal disease. British Medical Journal 315: 1429–1432

RENAL VASCULAR DISEASES

Adequate blood supply is critical for all aspects of renal function. Hence, diseases which affect the renal blood vessels can cause any and all of the clinical manifestations of renal disease. They are particularly likely to cause acute or chronic renal failure and secondary hypertension.

RENAL ARTERY STENOSIS

While disease of the renal arteries is a well-known cause of secondary hypertension, it is also an increasingly recognised cause of renal failure, particularly in the elderly—a condition known as ischaemic nephropathy.

Pathology

Overall, the most common cause is atheromatous narrowing of the renal artery. This is more common in older patients, and rare below the age of 50. It is frequently, but not always, associated with degenerative vascular disease elsewhere in the body. In younger patients, fibromuscular dysplasia is a more likely cause. This is a congenital band of fibrous tissue around the artery, which, as the patient grows, causes progressive narrowing of the vessel. It most commonly presents with hypertension in patients aged 15–30 years. In both types, if the stenosis is haemodynamically significant, an area of post-stenotic dilatation develops distal to the narrowed area. Stenosis is classed as ostial, proximal or distal according to the part of the vessel affected, and is quantified in terms of the degree of narrowing. Stenosis of less than 50% is not usually considered to be haemodynamically significant. In unilateral disease, the unaffected kidney will show changes of hypertensive nephrosclerosis; the renal parenchyma on the stenosed side may be relatively protected from the effects of hypertension, but will have a reduced GFR due to underperfusion.

Investigations

If the stenosis is long-standing, a reduction in kidney size occurs, which can be detected by ultrasound examination. Since renovascular disease is often asymmetrical or unilateral, a discrepancy in size between the two kidneys on ultrasound is a useful pointer to the diagnosis, along with hypertension, renal impairment or vascular disease elsewhere. Renal isotope scanning may show delayed uptake of isotope and reduced excretion by an affected kidney. The definitive investigation is renal arteriography, and this is required before treatment is undertaken.

RENAL ARTERY STENOSIS

Renal artery stenosis is more likely if:
- Hypertension is severe, *or* of recent onset, *or* difficult to control
- Kidneys are asymmetrical in size
- There is evidence of vascular disease elsewhere (especially in lower limbs)

Management and prognosis

Untreated, atheromatous renal artery stenosis will progress to complete arterial occlusion and loss of kidney function in about 15% of cases; this figure is increased with more severe degrees of stenosis. If the progression is gradual, collateral vessels may develop and some function may be preserved. Even if the main arterial supply is lost, the kidney receives some blood supply from capsular blood vessels. These will not support kidney function, but may be sufficient to prevent infarction and loss of kidney structure. Fibromuscular dysplasia does not usually cause renal artery occlusion, and will usually stabilise once the patient stops growing.

Treatment options are as follows:

- medical treatment (antihypertensive therapy, low-dose aspirin and lipid-lowering drugs if appropriate)
- angioplasty, with or without mechanical stenting after balloon dilatation
- surgical resection of the stenosed segment and re-anastomosis.

At present there is no conclusive data to indicate the overall superiority of one approach over another. Angioplasty is widely used, and recent studies suggest that stenting of the vessel improves the success rate. Surgery is usually reserved for technically difficult cases, particularly those with ostial stenosis or multiple stenotic areas. Conservative medical treatment may be appropriate if there is widespread atheromatous disease of the aorta and elsewhere, leading to an increased risk of cholesterol embolisation after intervention.

DISEASES OF SMALL INTRARENAL VESSELS

A number of conditions are associated with acute damage and occlusion of small blood vessels (arterioles and capillaries) in the kidney. They are associated to varying degrees with similar changes elsewhere in the body. A common feature of these syndromes is microangiopathic haemolytic anaemia, in which haemolysis occurs as a consequence of damage incurred during passage through the abnormal vessels. Fragmented red cells can be seen on a blood film and are a hallmark of small-vessel disease. The main conditions associated with damage and occlusion of small intrarenal vessels are:

- thrombotic microangiopathy (haemolytic uraemic syndrome and thrombotic thrombocytopenic purpura)
  —associated with verotoxin-producing *Escherichia coli*
  —other (familial, drugs, cancer etc.)
- disseminated intravascular coagulation
- malignant hypertension (see Fig. 6.18)
- small-vessel vasculitis (see p. 866)
- systemic sclerosis (scleroderma)
- atheroemboli ('cholesterol' emboli).

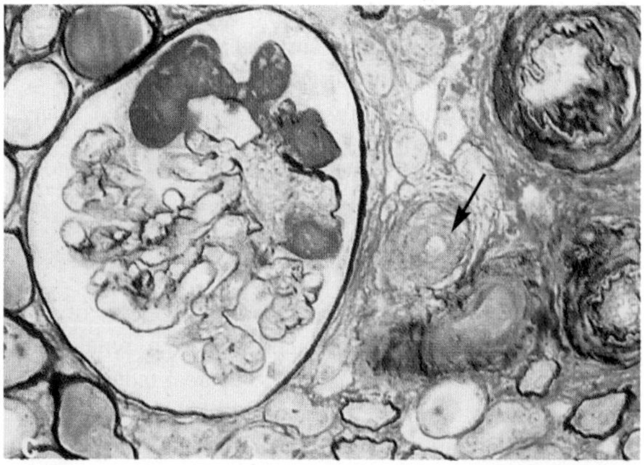

Fig. 6.18 Glomerular capillary thrombosis in malignant hypertension. Similar changes occur in thrombotic microangiopathy. The adjacent arteriole (arrow) shows gross intimal thickening.

Thrombotic microangiopathy

Haemolytic uraemic syndrome (HUS) and thrombotic thrombocytopenic purpura (TTP) are best regarded as on a spectrum of manifestations of thrombotic microangiopathy. The common feature of these disorders is damage to endothelial cells of the microcirculation, which is followed by cell swelling, platelet adherence and thrombosis. The manifestations are determined by the vascular beds most affected: kidneys in HUS, brain in TTP. Both disorders are characterised by a severe microangiopathy and a marked reduction in the platelet count and haemoglobin concentration. Other features of intravascular haemolysis—raised bilirubin and lactate dehydrogenase, decreased haptoglobins—are also present.

Thrombotic microangiopathy associated with *E. coli* infection (especially O157 serotypes) is a relatively new condition that is associated with the spread of verotoxin-producing organisms. Although the bacteria live as commensals in the gut of cattle and other domestic livestock, they can cause haemorrhagic diarrhoea in humans when the infection is contracted from contaminated food products, water or other infected individuals. In a proportion of cases, verotoxin produced by the organisms enters the circulation and binds to specific glycolipid receptors that are expressed particularly on the surface of microvascular endothelial cells. In children, this causes diarrhoea-associated (D+) HUS, although in more severe cases the brain and other organs are also affected. D+HUS is now the most common cause of acute renal failure in children in developed countries. In adults, the disease may more closely resemble TTP, but both adults and children usually recover, often after 5–15 days of dialysis. No specific treatments have been shown to help.

Other causes of thrombotic microangiopathy have a less certain outlook and are more likely to recur (sometimes after renal transplantation). Familial examples may reflect an abnormality of endothelial cell defence against damage or thrombosis. The disease may occur post-partum, in response to certain drugs (especially chemotherapy), after bone marrow transplantation, in malignancy and apparently spontaneously. Plasma exchange using fresh frozen plasma appears able to replace a deficient substance and enable recovery to occur in many of these examples.

Disseminated intravascular coagulation

In this condition, the most prominent abnormality is consumption of clotting factors due to uncontrolled thrombosis in the microvasculature, leading to severe deficiency of these proteins in the plasma and a tendency to haemorrhage from larger vessels. There may also be thrombocytopenia. Associated conditions include septic shock, in which bacterial endotoxin directly activates the coagulation cascade; obstetric complications; disseminated cancer; and other causes of massive internal bleeding or coagulation activation or depletion. Treatment consists of maintaining haemostasis with replacement of clotting factors as required and correcting the underlying condition, if possible.

Malignant hypertension

Malignant or accelerated hypertension (see p. 218) is of such severity as to cause acute damage to arterioles. It is often symptomatic, with headache, impaired vision and, finally, manifestations of renal failure (see Fig. 6.18). It is usually associated with the features of microangiopathy described above. In the absence of a previous history, it may be difficult to distinguish these patients from HUS with marked hypertension. They will usually respond to effective control of blood pressure, although renal function is permanently lost in 20% of cases.

Small-vessel vasculitis

This condition is described on page 866; there is immunological injury to arterioles and capillaries which may lead to a thrombotic microangiopathy, as above.

Systemic sclerosis (scleroderma)

This generalised disorder of connective tissue is described on page 858. Renal involvement is the most serious feature of the disease, and is characterised by intimal cell proliferation and luminal narrowing of intrarenal arteries and arterioles. Clinically, it usually presents as 'scleroderma renal crisis', with severe hypertension, microangiopathic features and progressive oliguric renal failure. There is intense intrarenal vasospasm, and plasma renin activity is markedly elevated. Use of ACE inhibitors to control the hypertension has improved the 1-year survival from 20% to 75%; about 50% of patients continue to require renal replacement therapy, however.

Atheroembolic renal disease ('cholesterol' emboli)

This is caused by showers of cholesterol-containing micro-emboli, arising in atheromatous plaques in major arteries. It occurs in patients with widespread atheromatous disease, usually after interventions such as surgery or arteriography. Clinical features are loss of kidney function, haematuria and proteinuria, and sometimes eosinophilia and inflammatory features which may mimic small-vessel vasculitis. Accompanying signs of microvascular occlusion in the lower limbs (ischaemic toes, livedo reticularis) are common but not invariable. There is no specific treatment.

FURTHER INFORMATION ON RENAL VASCULAR DISEASES

Kaplan B S, Meyers K E, Schulman S L 1998 The pathogenesis and treatment of hemolytic uremic syndrome. Journal of the American Society of Nephrology 8: 1126–1133

Kumar A, Asim M, Davison A M 1998 Taking precautions with ACE inhibitors. British Medical Journal 316: 1921–1930

GLOMERULAR DISEASES

Glomerular diseases may cause any of a characteristic range of abnormalities (see Fig. 6.12, p. 428). Here, glomerular diseases are divided into inherited and acquired groups, with the acquired group further divided into inflammatory/immune and non-inflammatory groups.

INHERITED GLOMERULAR DISEASES

ALPORT'S SYNDROME

A number of uncommon diseases may affect the glomerulus in childhood, but the most important disease affecting adults is Alport's syndrome. It may be caused by mutations or deletions of any of three genes, but most cases arise from the COL4A5 gene on the X chromosome. The underlying problem is a progressive degeneration of the GBM (see Fig. 6.19). Some other basement membranes containing the same collagen isoforms are similarly affected, notably in the cochlea.

No treatment has been devised to slow this process, but patients with Alport's syndrome are good candidates for renal replacement therapy as they are young and usually otherwise healthy. Some of these patients develop an immune response to the normal collagen antigens present in the GBM of a transplanted kidney, and in a small minority anti-GBM disease develops and destroys the allograft.

ALPORT'S SYNDROME
• The second most common inherited cause of renal failure (polycystic kidney disease being the most common) • Hallmark is progressive degeneration of GBM (see Fig. 6.19) • Caused by abnormalities of tissue-specific isoforms of type IV (basement membrane) collagen • Associated with sensorineural deafness (to high tone first) and some ocular abnormalities • Most cases associated with mutations of COL4A5, encoding α5 (IV) collagen, located at Xq22
X-linked disease
• Affected males usually develop end-stage renal failure in late teens or twenties • Female carriers usually have haematuria, but rarely develop significant renal disease
Autosomal recessive disease
• Females and males equally affected • Carriers may have microscopic haematuria

THIN GBM DISEASE

In thin GBM disease there is glomerular bleeding, usually only at the microscopic or stick-test level, without associated hypertension, proteinuria or reduction of GFR. The glomeruli appear normal by light microscopy, but on electron microscopy the GBM is abnormally thin. The prognosis is good. This syndrome accounts for a large proportion of 'benign familial haematuria', and is an autosomal dominant condition with an excellent prognosis. Some families may be carriers of autosomal recessive Alport's syndrome, but this cannot account for all cases.

GLOMERULONEPHRITIS

Although glomerulonephritis literally means 'inflammation of glomeruli', the term is used to include other types of glomerular disease with a presumed immunological causation, even though there is no histological evidence of inflammation.

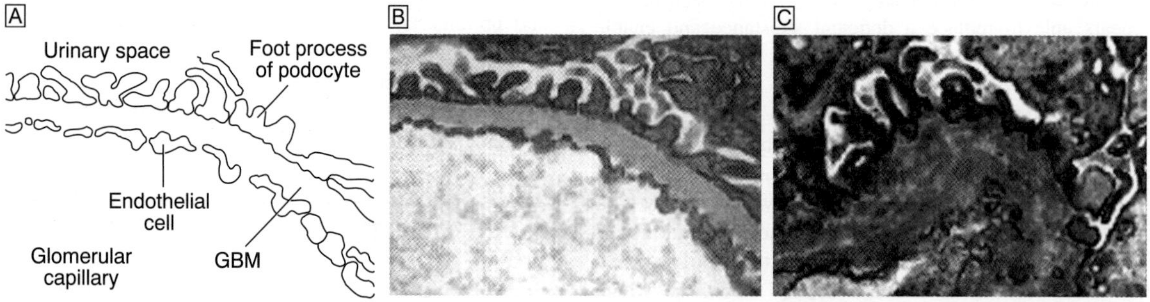

Fig. 6.19 Alport's syndrome. [A] Diagrammatic structure of the normal GBM. [B] The normal GBM (electron micrograph) contains mostly the tissue-specific α3, α4 and α5 chains of type IV collagen. [C] In Alport's syndrome this network is disrupted and replaced by α1 and α2 chains. Although the GBM appears structurally normal in early life, in time thinning appears, progressing to thickening, splitting and degeneration.

Classifications of glomerulonephritis are confusing. The original clinical classification (nephrotic, nephritic) has largely given way to histopathological categorisation, but this is being supplemented by division according to pathogenesis—where this process is understood. Here the mechanisms of glomerulonephritis are discussed and related to the major histopathological types (see Table 6.4). Examples of some important types are then discussed.

Mechanisms of glomerulonephritis

Most glomerulonephritis is presumed to be immunologically mediated. For some diseases there is direct evidence of this—e.g. the anti-GBM antibodies seen in Goodpasture's disease. Deposition of antibody is seen in many types of glomerulonephritis (see Table 6.4). In many, the presumed mechanisms involve cellular immunity, which is more difficult to investigate and prove. Associations with particular major histocompatibility complex types suggest involvement of the immune system, as the function of these molecules is to present antigens to lymphocytes. The response of several types of glomerulonephritis to immunosuppressive drugs provides further indirect evidence. In most cases the targets of immunity are likely to be glomerular antigens (see Fig. 6.20).

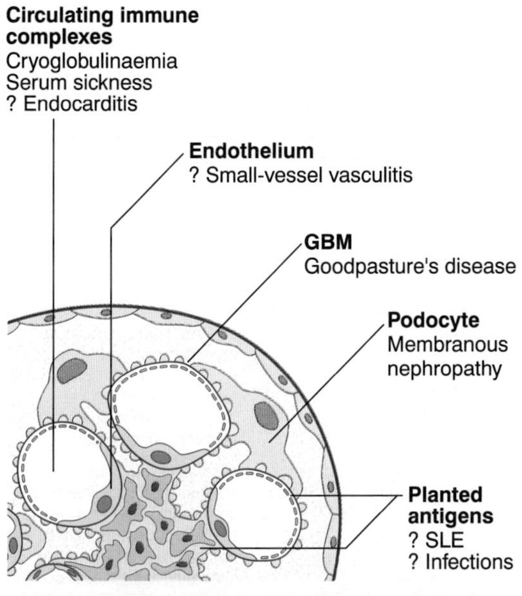

Fig. 6.20 Targets of immunity and autoimmunity in glomerulonephritis. The diagram also shows where antibodies and antigen-antibody (immune) complexes may be seen: subepithelial, between podocyte and GBM; intramembranous, within the GBM; subendothelial, between endothelial cell and GBM; and mesangial, within the mesangial matrix (compare with Fig. 6.21).

Although deposition of circulating immune complexes was previously thought to be a common mechanism of glomerulonephritis, it now seems likely that most granular deposits of immunoglobulin within glomeruli are caused by 'in situ' formation of immune complexes about glomerular antigens, or about other antigens ('planted' antigens, e.g. viral or bacterial antigens) that have localised in glomeruli. Where known, the pathogenesis of a particular form of glomerulonephritis is indicated in Table 6.4. Bacterial infections, usually subacute (typically subacute bacterial endocarditis), may cause a variety of histological patterns of glomerulonephritis, but usually with plentiful immunoglobulin deposition, and often with evidence of complement consumption (low C3).

LOW SERUM COMPLEMENT AND GLOMERULONEPHRITIS

- Post-infection glomerulonephritis
- Subacute bacterial infection—especially endocarditis
- SLE
- Cryoglobulinaemia
- Mesangiocapillary glomerulonephritis—usually type II

Crescent formation occurs when the GBM is disrupted and fibrin is deposited in the urinary space. Proliferation of surrounding epithelial cells, and of invading macrophages, causes the characteristic appearance (see Fig. 6.21, p. 445). Crescent formation may therefore occur in any of the 'inflammatory' types of nephritis if they enter an aggressive phase (e.g. IgA nephropathy); however, severe rapidly progressive glomerulonephritis (RPGN) with crescent formation is commonly associated with only a relatively small number of conditions (see the information box). As most of these require specific treatment to prevent renal failure, early recognition of RPGN is important.

COMMON CAUSES OF RAPIDLY PROGRESSIVE GLOMERULONEPHRITIS (RPGN)

- Systemic vasculitis (focal necrotising glomerulonephritis)
- SLE
- Goodpasture's (anti-GBM) disease
- Aggressive phase of other inflammatory nephritis (e.g. IgA nephropathy, post-infections (post-streptococcal) glomerulonephritis)

Crescent formation is usually seen in these circumstances and the term 'crescentic nephritis' is often used interchangeably with RPGN.

MINIMAL CHANGE NEPHROPATHY AND PRIMARY FOCAL SEGMENTAL GLOMERULOSCLEROSIS (FSGS)

Patients with minimal change nephropathy and a subgroup

Table 6.4 Glomerulonephritis: types, associations and causes

	Histology	Immune deposits	Pathogenesis	Association	Clinical features
Minimal change	Normal, except on electron microscopy, where fusion of podocyte foot processes is seen (occurs in many types of proteinuria)	None	Unknown	Atopy, HLA-DR7 Drugs	Acute and often severe nephrotic syndrome. Good response to corticosteroids. Dominant cause of idiopathic nephrotic syndrome in childhood
Focal segmental glomerulosclerosis (FSGS)	Segmental scars in some glomeruli No acute inflammation Foot process fusion seen in primary FSGS with nephrotic syndrome	Non-specific trapping in focal scars	Unknown; in some, circulating factors increase glomerular permeability	Healing of previous focal glomerular injury HIV infection, heroin abuse, other nephropathy	*Primary FSGS* presents as idiopathic nephrotic syndrome but less responsive to treatment than minimal change. May progress to renal impairment, can recur after transplantation *Secondary FSGS* presents with variable proteinuria and outcome
Focal segmental (necrotising) glomerulonephritis	Segmental inflammation and/or necrosis in some glomeruli May be crescent formation	Variable according to cause, but typically negative (or 'pauci-immune')	Small-vessel vasculitis	Primary or secondary small-vessel vasculitis	Usually implies presence of systemic disease, and responds to treatment with corticosteroids and cytotoxic agents. Check antineutrophil cytoplasm antibodies (ANCA), antinuclear antibodies (ANA)
Membranous nephropathy	Thickening of GBM Progressing to increased matrix deposition and glomerulosclerosis	Granular subepithelial IgG	Antibodies to a podocyte surface antigen, with complement-dependent podocyte injury	HLA-DR3 (for idiopathic) Drugs Heavy metals Hepatitis B virus Malignancy	Usually idiopathic; common cause of adult idiopathic nephrotic syndrome. One-third progress; may respond to chlorambucil/prednisolone Associated HLA class II allele varies in different populations
IgA nephropathy	Increased mesangial matrix and cells Focal segmental nephritis in acute disease	Mesangial IgA	Unknown	Usually idiopathic Liver disease	Very common disease with range of presentations, but usually including haematuria and hypertension (see text)
Mesangiocapillary glomerulonephritis (MCGN) (= membranoproliferative glomerulonephritis, MPGN)					
Type I	Mesangial cells interpose between endothelium and GBM	Subendothelial	Deposition of circulating immune complexes or 'planted' antigens	Bacterial infection Hepatitis B virus Cryoglobulinaemia (± hepatitis C virus infection)	Usually proteinuria, may be haematuria. Most common pattern found in association with subacute bacterial infection No proven treatments except where cause can be treated
Type II	Mesangial cells interpose between endothelium and GBM	Intramembranous dense deposits	Associated with complement con-sumption caused by autoantibodies	C3 nephritic factor and partial lipodystrophy	Also known as dense deposit disease
Post-infectious	Diffuse (uniformly in all glomeruli) proliferation of endothelial and mesangial cells Infiltration by neutrophils and macrophages May be crescent formation	Subendothelial	Immune response to streptococcal infection Cross-reactive epitopes or other explanation	Streptococcal and other infections	Now rare in developed countries except in some racial/socio-economic groups. Presents with severe sodium and fluid retention, hypertension, haematuria, oliguria. Usually resolves spontaneously
Goodpasture's disease (anti-GBM)	Usually crescentic nephritis	Linear IgG along GBM	Autoimmunity to $\alpha3$ chain of type IV collagen	HLA-DR15 (previously known as DR2)	Associated with lung haemorrhage, but either may occur alone. Treat with cortico-steroids, cyclophosphamide and plasma exchange to remove circulating autoantibodies
Lupus nephritis	Almost any histological type	Always positive and often profuse Pattern varies according to type	Some anti-DNA antibodies also bind to glomerular targets	Complement deficiencies Complement consumption	Very variable presentation; sometimes as renal disease alone without systemic features Responds to cytotoxic therapy in addition to prednisolone

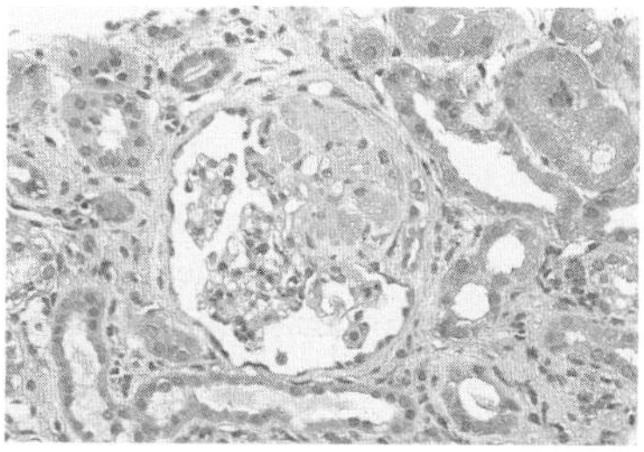

B Focal segmental glomerulosclerosis

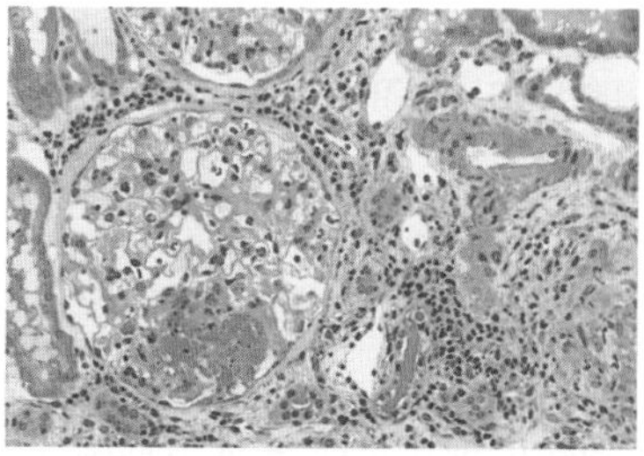

C Focal necrotising glomerulonephritis

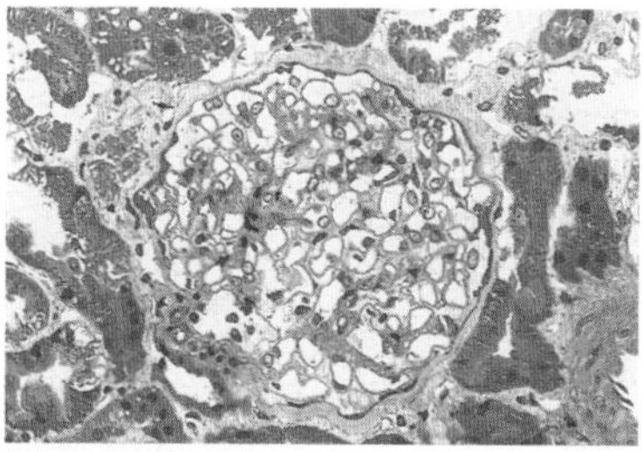

A Normal glomerulus

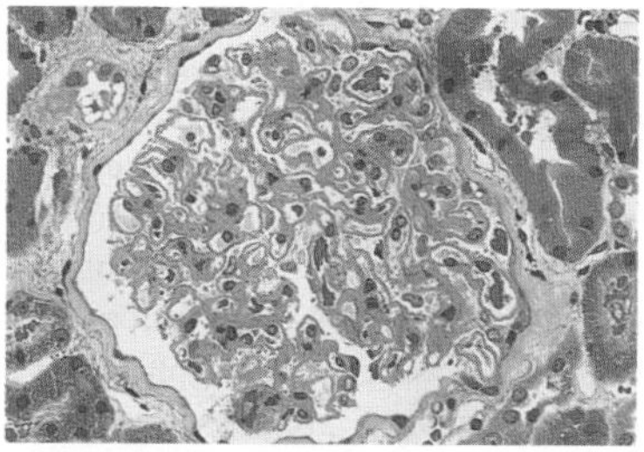

D Membranous nephropathy

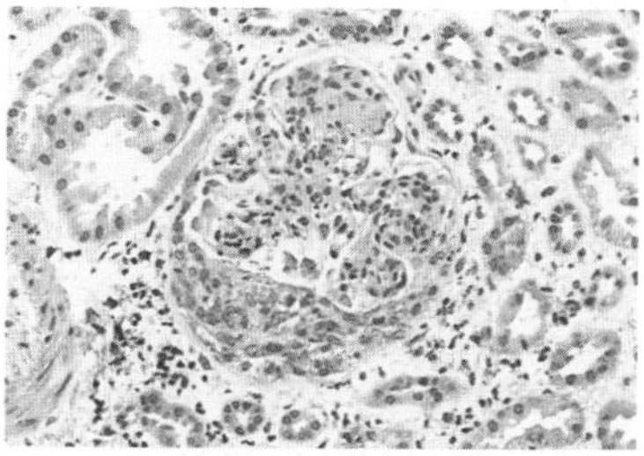

E Crescentic glomerulonephritis

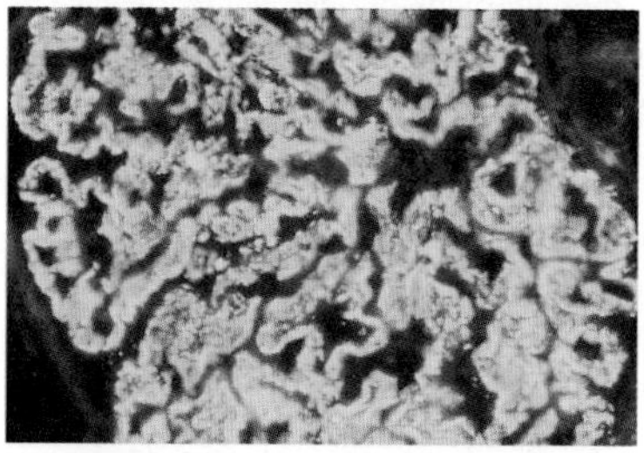

F Granular IgG deposits in membranous nephropathy

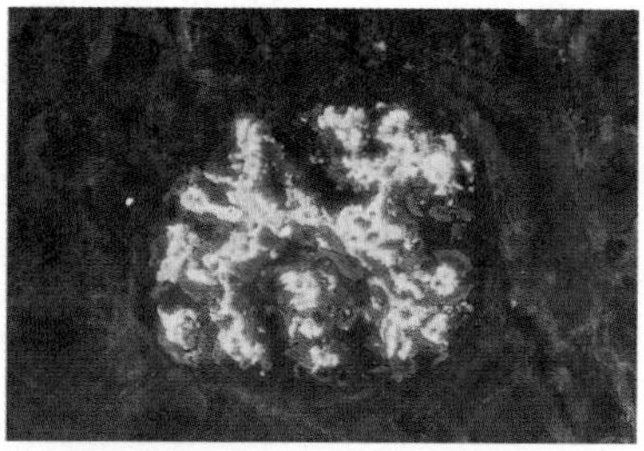

G Mesangial IgA deposits in IgA nephropathy

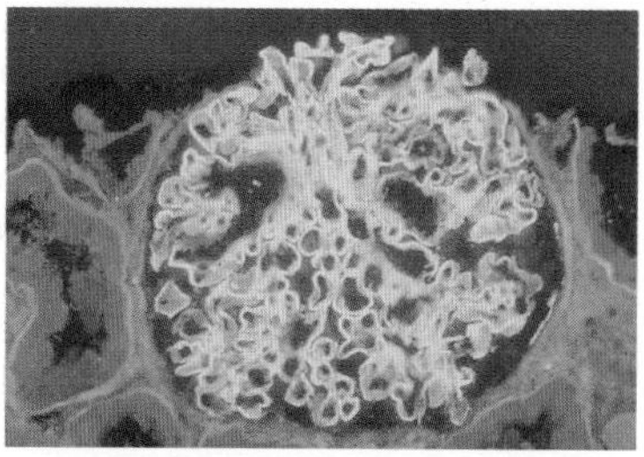

H Linear IgG deposits in Goodpasture's disease

Fig. 6.21 Histopathology of glomerular disease. Patterns of disease seen by light microscopy are shown in the upper images. The lower three images show patterns of immunoglobulin deposition in different conditions.
A A normal glomerulus. Note the open capillary loops and the thinness of their walls—'should look as if you could cut yourself on them'. B Focal segmental glomerulosclerosis. The portion of the glomerulus at 2 o'clock shows loss of capillary loops and cells, which are replaced by matrix. C Focal necrotising glomerulonephritis. The portion of the glomerulus at 6 o'clock is replaced by bright pink material with some 'nuclear dust'. Neutrophils may be seen elsewhere in the glomerulus. There is surrounding interstitial inflammation. Disease of this type is most commonly associated with small-vessel vasculitis (see text) and may progress to crescentic nephritis (see E). D Membranous nephropathy. The capillary loops are thickened (compare with the normal glomerulus) and there is expansion of the mesangial regions by matrix deposition. However, there is no gross cellular proliferation or excess of inflammatory cells. E Crescentic glomerulonephritis. The lower part of Bowman's space is occupied by a semicircular formation ('crescent') of large pale cells, compressing the glomerular tuft. This is usually seen in aggressive inflammatory types of glomerulonephritis.

Antibody deposition in the glomerulus shown by direct immunofluorescence.
F Granular deposits of IgG along the basement membrane in a subepithelial pattern, typical of membranous nephropathy. G IgA deposits in the mesangium, as seen in IgA nephropathy. H Ribbon-like linear deposits of anti-GBM antibodies along the GBM in Goodpasture's disease. Glomerular structure is well preserved in all of these examples.

of patients with FSGS can be seen as opposite ends of a spectrum of conditions causing the idiopathic nephrotic syndrome. Minimal change disease occurs at all ages but accounts for most cases of nephrotic syndrome in childhood and is the underlying diagnosis in about one-quarter of adult patients with nephrotic syndrome. Proteinuria usually remits on high-dose corticosteroids (1 mg/kg prednisolone for 6 weeks), although some patients who respond incompletely or relapse frequently need maintenance corticosteroids, cytotoxic therapy or other agents. Minimal change disease does not progress to renal impairment; the main problems are those of nephrotic syndrome and complications of treatment.

FSGS is a histological description, and similar appearances are found in patients with a number of different causes for renal disease. The primary FSGS group that present with idiopathic nephrotic syndrome and no other cause for renal disease typically show no or a poor response to corticosteroid treatment and often progress to renal failure; the disease frequently recurs after renal transplantation—when sometimes proteinuria recurs almost immediately. Cases between these extremes are common, however. A proportion of patients do show a response to steroids and other treatments used in minimal change disease. As FSGS is a focal process, abnormal glomeruli may not be seen if only a few are sampled, leading to an initial diagnosis of minimal change nephropathy. Juxtamedullary glomeruli are more likely to be affected in early disease.

In other patients with the histological appearances of FSGS, focal scarring reflects healing of previous focal glomerular injury, such as haemolytic uraemic syndrome, cholesterol embolism or vasculitis. In others, it seems to represent particular types of nephropathy—for instance, those associated with heroin abuse, human immunodeficiency virus (HIV) infection and massive obesity. Associations with numerous other forms of injury and renal disorders are reported. There is no specific treatment for most of these. HIV nephropathy may improve with corticosteroid treatment.

MEMBRANOUS NEPHROPATHY

This is the most common cause of nephrotic syndrome in adults. A proportion of cases are associated with known causes (see Table 6.4), but most are idiopathic. Of this group, approximately one-third remit spontaneously, one-third remain in a nephrotic state, and one-third show progressive loss of renal function. Short-term treatment with high doses of corticosteroids and alkylating agents may improve both the nephrotic syndrome and the long-term prognosis. However, because of the toxicity of these regimens, most nephrologists reserve such treatment for those with severe nephrotic syndrome or deteriorating renal function.

IgA NEPHROPATHY AND HENOCH–SCHÖNLEIN PURPURA

IgA nephropathy is the most commonly recognised type of glomerulonephritis and can present in many ways. Haematuria is almost universal, proteinuria usual, and hypertension very common. There may be severe proteinuria and nephrotic syndrome, or in some cases progressive loss of renal function. The disease is a common cause of end-stage renal failure. A particular hallmark of the disease in some individuals is acute exacerbations, often with gross haematuria, in association with minor respiratory infections. This may be so acute as to resemble acute post-infectious glomerulonephritis, with fluid retention, hypertension and oliguria with dark or red urine. Characteristically, the latency from clinical infection to nephritis is short—a few days or less. These episodes usually subside spontaneously.

In children, and occasionally in adults, a systemic vasculitis occurring in response to similar infections is called Henoch–Schönlein purpura. A characteristic petechial rash (cutaneous vasculitis) and abdominal pain (gastrointestinal vasculitis) usually dominate the clinical picture, with mild glomerulonephritis being indicated by haematuria. When the disease occurs in older children or adults the glomerulonephritis is usually more prominent. Renal biopsy shows mesangial IgA deposition and appearances indistinguishable from acute IgA nephropathy.

Occasionally, IgA nephropathy progresses rapidly. Crescent formation may be seen. The response to treatment usually seems poor; controlled trials of immunosuppression are in progress. The management of less acute disease is largely directed towards the control of blood pressure in an attempt to prevent or retard progressive renal disease.

ACUTE POST-INFECTION GLOMERULONEPHRITIS

This is most commonly seen after streptococcal infections, but can occur in response to other infections. It is much more common in children than adults and is now rarely seen in many parts of the developed world. The latency is usually about 10 days after a throat infection, suggesting an immune mechanism rather than direct infection. The latency after skin infection is longer. As for rheumatic fever, only certain streptococcal strains are associated with this complication.

An acute nephritis of varying severity occurs with avid sodium retention and oedema, hypertension, reduction of GFR, proteinuria, haematuria and reduced urine volumes. Characteristically, this gives the urine a red or smoky appearance. There are low serum concentrations of C3 and C4 and evidence of streptococcal infection (ASO titre, culture of throat swab, and other tests if skin infection is suspected).

Renal function begins to improve spontaneously within 10–14 days, and management by fluid and sodium restriction and use of diuretic and hypotensive agents are usually adequate. The renal lesion in almost all children and most adults seems to resolve completely despite the apparent severity of the glomerular inflammation and proliferation seen histologically.

GLOMERULONEPHRITIS ASSOCIATED WITH CHRONIC INFECTION

The association of subacute bacterial infection with an inflammatory glomerulonephritis was mentioned above. World-wide, glomerulonephritis associated with malaria, hepatitis B, leishmaniasis and other chronic infections is very common, although these are much less common in developed countries. The most common histological patterns are membranous and membranoproliferative lesions, although many other types may be seen; FSGS associated with HIV infection is increasingly prevalent. Proving a causative relationship between renal disease and infection in individual cases is extremely difficult. Acute and chronic infections may also cause interstitial renal disease (see below).

NON-INFLAMMATORY GLOMERULAR DISEASES

A number of diseases distort glomerular architecture and function by altering the structure or production of normal glomerular components, or by deposition of extraneous materials, without provoking inflammation. Some types of primary glomerulonephritis that do this have been discussed above. Almost all the other diseases in which this occurs are haematological or systemic disorders, in which the glomerulus is only one of the structures involved. Major examples are shown in Table 6.5 and discussed in more detail below, along with systemic diseases that affect other parts of the kidney.

Table 6.5 Non-inflammatory glomerular diseases

Disease	Initial changes	Refer to
Minimal change nephropathy	Loss of glomerular epithelial cell architecture	p. 443
Membranous nephropathy	Thickening of GBM	p. 446
Diabetes mellitus	Thickening of GBM Mesangial matrix expansion	p. 504
Amyloidosis	Deposition of fibrils throughout glomerulus	p. 541
Light chain disease	Immunoglobulin light chain deposition in GBM (rare)	
Fibrillary glomerulonephritis	Fibril deposition in GBM (rare)	

FURTHER INFORMATION ON GLOMERULAR DISEASES

Barsoum R S 1998 Malarial nephropathies. British Medical Journal 13: 1588–1597

Mason P D, Pusey C D 1994 Glomerulonephritis: diagnosis and treatment. British Medical Journal 309: 1557–1563 (published erratum 1995 310: 116)

TUBULO-INTERSTITIAL DISEASES

Tubulo-interstitial disease refers to a heterogeneous group of conditions characterised by structural change and dysfunction of renal tubular structures and the surrounding interstitium. The clinical presentation is often renal failure, either acute and reversible, or chronic, and commonly with electrolyte abnormalities, e.g. hyperkalaemia and acidosis. Proteinuria (and albuminuria) is rarely > 1g/24 hrs but low molecular weight proteinuria is common (e.g. retinol binding protein, β_2-microglobulin, lysozyme). Haematuria and pyuria are frequent in acute and chronic disease.

ACUTE TUBULAR NECROSIS

This is the most common cause of the clinical syndrome of acute renal failure, described on pages 429–432. Two categories of acute tubular necrosis (ATN) are recognised—cases due to ischaemia, which are more common, and the nephrotoxic type, caused by chemical or bacterial toxins. In practice, multiple factors are common.

Pathogenesis

Ischaemic tubular necrosis usually follows a period of shock, during which renal blood flow is greatly reduced. Measurements during the oliguric phase of ATN indicate that even when the systemic circulation has been restored, renal blood flow remains about 20% of normal. This is due to swelling of the endothelial cells of glomeruli and peritubular capillaries, and oedema of the interstitium. Blood flow is further reduced by vasoconstrictors such as thromboxane, vasopressin, noradrenaline and angiotensin II, partly counterbalanced by the release of intrarenal vasodilator prostaglandins. Thus, in ischaemic ATN, there is reduced delivery of oxygen to the tubular cells, which are very metabolically active, particularly in the thick ascending limb of the loop of Henle. Their high oxygen requirement is largely driven by the active reabsorption of sodium, and even in health the renal medulla is critically balanced in terms of oxygen delivery and consumption.

The ischaemic insult causes peroxidation of cell membrane lipids, influx of calcium and cell swelling.

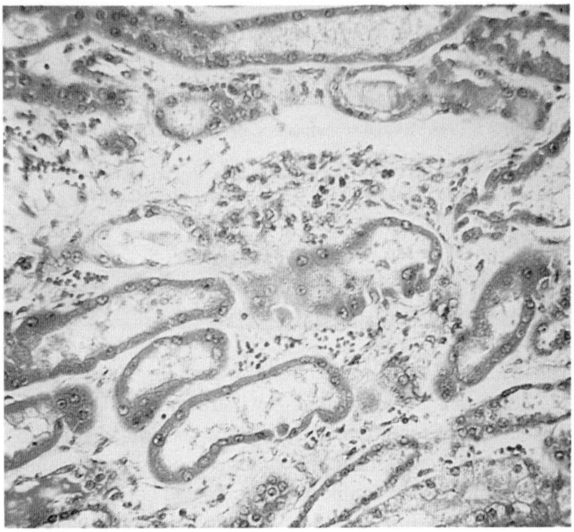

Fig. 6.22 Acute tubular necrosis.

Mitochondrial function is impaired, leading to anaerobic glycolysis and intracellular acidosis, and ultimately to lysosomal disruption, denaturation of proteins and DNA, and apoptosis of tubular cells (see Fig. 6.22). There is loss of adhesion between tubular cells and the basement membrane, leading to shedding of cells into the tubular lumen, where they may contribute to tubular obstruction. Focal breaks in the tubular basement membrane develop; these allow tubular contents to leak into the interstitial tissue.

In nephrotoxic ATN, a similar sequence occurs, but it is initiated by direct toxicity of the causative agent to tubular cells. Mechanisms of cell damage include the production of reactive oxygen species and peroxidation of membrane lipids, binding of toxins or drugs to target intracellular proteins to interfere with cellular respiration, or inhibition of cell protein synthesis. Examples include the aminoglycoside antibiotics, such as gentamicin; the cytotoxic agent cisplatin; and the antifungal drug amphotericin B.

Fortunately, tubular cells can regenerate and re-form the basement membrane. If the patient is supported during the regeneration phase, kidney function returns. There is often a diuretic phase—urine output increases rapidly and remains excessive for several days before returning to normal. This is due in part to loss of the medullary concentration gradient, which normally allows concentration of the urine in the collecting duct, and which depends on active tubular transport and continued delivery of filtrate to the ascending limb of the loop of Henle. Both factors are disturbed during ATN. The medullary concentration gradient is gradually 'washed out', and is not re-established until glomerular filtration and tubular function are restored. Not all patients have a diuretic phase, depending on the severity of the renal damage and the rate of recovery.

Pathology

In ATN the glomeruli are relatively normal, although there may be endothelial cell swelling and fibrin deposition. There are scattered breaks in tubular basement membranes, swelling and vacuolation of tubular cells, and in places apoptosis and necrosis of tubular cells with shedding of cells into the lumen (see Fig. 6.22). During the regenerative phase there is increased tubular mitotic activity. The interstitium is oedematous and infiltrated by inflammatory cells. Where the condition is caused by drugs, the interstitial inflammatory infiltrate may be more marked and constitute acute interstitial nephritis (see below).

INTERSTITIAL NEPHRITIS

ACUTE INTERSTITIAL NEPHRITIS

Acute interstitial nephritis (AIN) refers to acute inflammation within the tubulo-interstitium. Precipitating causes include drugs and toxins, and a variety of systemic diseases and infections (see the information box).

AETIOLOGY OF ACUTE INTERSTITIAL NEPHRITIS

Drugs
- Penicillins
- NSAIDs
- Allopurinol
- Frusemide

Systemic disease
- Sarcoidosis
- Sjögren's syndrome
- Myeloma

Infections
- Leptospirosis
- Tuberculosis
- Pyelonephritis
- Cytomegalovirus, hantavirus

Renal biopsies (see Fig. 6.23) show intense inflammation, with polymorphonuclear leucocytes and lymphocytes surrounding tubules and blood vessels, and occasional eosinophils (especially in drug-induced disease).

Diagnosis

Less than 30% of patients with drug-induced AIN have a generalised drug hypersensitivity reaction (fever, rash, eosinophilia). However, eosinophils may be found in the urine of up to 70%. Careful history, examination and specific tests may point to the diagnosis but a renal biopsy is usually required to be definitive. The degree of chronic inflammation in a biopsy is also a useful predictor of the eventual outcome for renal function. Many patients are not oliguric despite moderately severe ARF and patients with non-oliguric ARF should always be investigated for AIN.

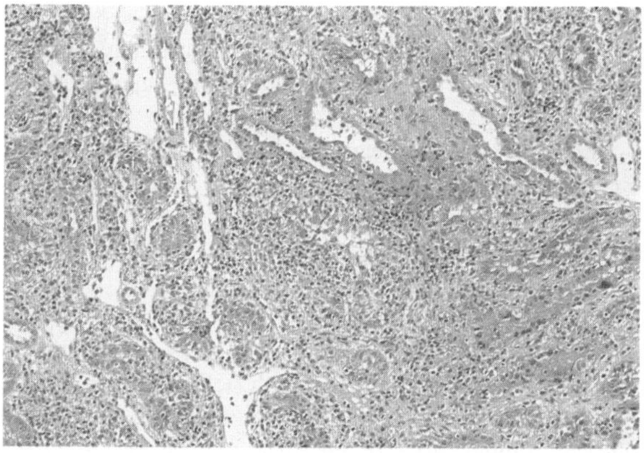

Fig. 6.23 Acute interstitial nephritis. Widespread interstitial infiltrate of inflammatory cells producing considerable destruction of normal architecture.

Management

ARF can be managed conservatively (see p. 430) and dialysis is only required for symptomatic or ill patients with a blood urea > 30 mmol/l. Many patients with drug-induced AIN will recover following withdrawal of the drug. Corticosteroids are frequently used but there is only anecdotal evidence of their effectiveness and some patients recover fully without them. Other specific causes should be treated (see relevant chapters).

CHRONIC INTERSTITIAL NEPHRITIS

Aetiology

Chronic interstitial nephritis (CIN) is a heterogeneous group of diseases causing chronic inflammation within the tubulo-interstitium. Causes are summarised in Table 6.6.

Any chronic glomerular disease can precipitate CIN although the mechanisms are not clear. In experimental animals, tubular cells may express class II HLA antigens and adhesion molecules and interact with T cells and macrophages. In vasculitis and SLE, there is clearly inflammation of the blood vessels as well as the tubules. Granulomas are characteristic of sarcoidosis and Wegener's granulomatosis while multinucleate giant cells are commonly associated with tubular casts in myeloma kidney. NSAIDs and phenacetin-containing compound analgesics have been associated with analgesic nephropathy (see below), which affects the inner medulla most severely, leading to papillary necrosis.

Clinical features

Most patients present in adult life with CRF, hypertension and small kidneys. CRF is often moderate (urea < 25 mmol/l) but, because of tubular dysfunction, electrolyte abnormalities are typical of more severe CRF (e.g. hyperkalaemia, acidosis). Urinalysis is non-specific. A minority of patients present with hypotension, polyuria and features of sodium and water depletion (low blood pressure, low jugular venous pressure) suggesting severe damage to collecting ducts ('salt-losing nephropathy'). Impairment of urine-concentrating ability and sodium conservation places patients with CIN at risk of superimposed ARF with even moderate salt and water depletion during an acute illness.

Table 6.6 Classification of chronic interstitial nephritis

Type of disease	Examples
Chronic glomerular disease	Varying degrees of interstitial nephritis may be found in association with almost any type of glomerulonephritis
Immune/inflammatory disease	Sarcoidosis, Sjögren's syndrome, SLE, primary autoimmune tubulo-interstitial nephritis, chronic transplant rejection, amyloidosis
Tumours	Myeloma
Drugs	All drugs causing AIN, especially NSAIDs, and compound analgesics (analgesic nephropathy)
Metabolic/congenital	Wilson's disease, hypokalaemia, medullary sponge kidney Hypercalciuria, hyperoxaluria, sickle-cell nephropathy
Toxins	Mushrooms, lead, Chinese herbs, Balkan nephropathy

The combination of interstitial nephritis and tumours of the collecting system is seen in Balkan nephropathy, so called because of where cases are found, and has been attributed to ingestion of fungal toxins, particularly ochratoxin A, present in food made from stored grain. A plant toxin, aristolochic acid, has been blamed for a rapidly progressive syndrome caused by Chinese herbs. Hyperkalaemia may be disproportionate in CIN or in diabetic nephropathy because of hyporeninaemic hypoaldosteronism (see p. 457). Renal tubular acidosis is seen most often in myeloma, sarcoidosis and amyloidosis (see p. 541).

Management

CRF will require conservative management (see p. 435). A full diagnostic workup for the conditions in Table 6.6 may help to identify a specific drug or toxin which can be withdrawn or suggest a specific diagnosis for treatment.

Acidosis can be corrected with oral sodium bicarbonate. Hyperkalaemia will require further measures (see p. 406).

ANALGESIC NEPHROPATHY

Renal papillary necrosis and CIN due to long continued

ingestion of analgesic drugs account for between 5% and 17% of end-stage renal disease in European countries. In animals, lesions can be induced with almost any NSAID. In humans, mixtures containing aspirin and phenacetin were historically important, but probably all NSAIDs can induce the lesion if taken regularly, even in small doses. Dehydration, which reduces medullary blood flow and results in concentration of the drugs in the renal medulla, is an important contributory factor.

Pathology

Diffuse interstitial fibrosis and tubular atrophy develop. Acute papillary necrosis is common, and is probably the initial lesion in most cases. A recognised complication is the development of carcinoma of the uroepithelium (renal pelvis, ureter or bladder).

Clinical features

Patients have usually taken prescribed or over-the-counter analgesic preparations for many years for headaches, backache, rheumatoid arthritis or osteoarthrosis. Asymptomatic disease may be disclosed when abnormalities of blood or urine are found during medical examination. Patients with moderate renal impairment present with malaise, thirst and polyuria due to impaired urinary concentration. Recurrent urinary infection is common. Approximately 60% of patients are hypertensive but 10% may be 'salt-losing'. Renal damage is predominantly tubular; failure to conserve sodium and renal tubular acidosis are common. Renal colic, ureteric obstruction and acute renal failure may be caused by the passage of fragments of necrotic papillae, which can be recognised by microscopic examination of the urine. ARF may also follow urinary infection or a sudden increase in the intake of analgesics. Many cases present with established CRF. Analgesic nephropathy may be part of a widespread syndrome associated with analgesic abuse, which includes peptic ulceration, anaemia, skin pigmentation and premature ageing.

Investigations

Apart from the history of drug ingestion, the diagnosis can sometimes be made on the basis of radiological findings and biochemical evidence of tubular dysfunction. The appearance of the papillae on IVU or retrograde pyelography is often characteristic. The contrast medium appears as a small tract within the papillary substance; later, the papillae may separate, giving a ring shadow. Urine usually contains red cells, and sterile pyuria is common. Proteinuria rarely exceeds 1 g/24 hrs at presentation, but tends to increase as renal failure develops.

Management

Analgesic preparations must be discontinued and 25% of patients will show some recovery of function; otherwise irreversible renal failure develops. Treatment also consists of maintaining a fluid intake of 2–3 litres/day, treating hypertension and infections, and providing supplements of sodium chloride and sodium bicarbonate to restore ECF volume and correct metabolic acidosis where necessary. Regular follow-up is essential. When renal function is severely impaired, the regimen for management of CRF should be instituted (see p. 435).

SICKLE-CELL NEPHROPATHY

The longer survival of patients with sickle-cell disease (see p. 764) means that a larger proportion live to develop chronic complications of microvascular occlusion. In the kidney these changes are most pronounced in the medulla, where the vasa recta are the site of sickling because of hypoxia and hypertonicity. Loss of urinary concentrating ability and polyuria are the earliest changes; distal renal tubular acidosis and impaired potassium excretion are typical. Papillary necrosis (as seen in analgesic nephropathy) is very common. A minority of patients develop end-stage renal failure. This is managed according to the usual principles, but response to recombinant erythropoietin is understandably poor. Patients with sickle trait have an increased incidence of unexplained microscopic haematuria, and occasionally overt papillary necrosis.

REFLUX NEPHROPATHY (CHRONIC PYELONEPHRITIS)

This is a chronic interstitial nephritis resulting from urinary tract infection associated with vesico-ureteric reflux (VUR) in early life. The incidence of reflux nephropathy is not known. About 12% of patients in Europe requiring treatment for end-stage renal disease are said to have renal scarring, but the precise diagnostic criteria are variable.

Pathogenesis

In the absence of urinary tract abnormalities, acute pyelonephritis in patients over the age of 5 years rarely leads to serious chronic renal disease. The most important predisposing factor is the presence of severe VUR in children. Reflux of urine from the bladder into the ureter during voiding is normally prevented because the ureter passes through the vesical wall obliquely and is occluded during contraction of the bladder. Abnormality of the intramural ureter allows reflux to occur and bacteria from the bladder may then reach the kidney. VUR may be unilateral or bilateral, and its severity varies. In mild cases (grades I, II) small amounts of urine pass a short distance up the ureter during voiding, returning to the bladder after cessation of micturition to form residual urine. In severe cases (grades III, IV) reflux occurs up the entire length of the ureter (see Fig. 6.24); this results in an increase in intrapelvic pressure, and the collecting ducts of the compound renal papillae are forced open and urine refluxes into the renal parenchyma as far as the cortex.

VUR is most often congenital, but can be due to obstructive lesions at the bladder neck (e.g. urethral valves). VUR in utero causes renal scars at birth and during the first year of life. In young children with recurrent urinary tract infection (UTI), scars are found in 8–13%, and VUR is usually demonstrable on the side of the scarred kidney. Reflux diminishes as the child grows, and usually disappears. It is rarely demonstrable in an adult with a scarred kidney due to infection in childhood. Severe reflux in young children interferes with renal growth. When UTI occurs in the presence of obstruction or stasis, whatever the cause, permanent damage may result in any age group.

In pregnant women scarring may result from UTI. The hormonal changes of pregnancy cause reduced ureteric motility and ureteric dilatation and may also facilitate the establishment of infection in the renal parenchyma.

Once CIN is established, destruction of renal tissue continues despite the absence of recurrent infections. Possible explanations include damage to the remaining functioning glomeruli by progressive ischaemia resulting from lesions of blood vessels sustained during acute infections, or survival of bacterial variants in the hypertonic medullary tissue.

Pathology

The changes, which are not diagnostic, may be unilateral or bilateral and of any grade of severity. Gross scarring of the kidneys, commonly at the poles, is seen with reduced size and narrowing of the cortex and medulla. Renal scars are juxtaposed to dilated calyces. Histologically, there is patchy fibrosis with chronic inflammatory cell infiltration, tubular atrophy, periglomerular fibrosis and eventual disappearance of nephrons. The arteries and arterioles may show sclerosis and narrowing. In patients who develop heavy proteinuria and hypertension, renal biopsies show glomerulomegaly and focal glomerulosclerosis (see p. 443), and this may develop in the unscarred kidney of patients with severe unilateral scarring.

Clinical features

In many cases no symptoms arise directly from the renal lesions, and the patient consults the doctor because of lassitude, vague ill health or symptoms of uraemia. Discovery of hypertension or proteinuria on routine examination may be the first indication of the disease. Symptoms arising from the urinary tract may also be present and include frequency of micturition, dysuria and aching lumbar pain. Occasionally, weakness and fainting result from salt loss in

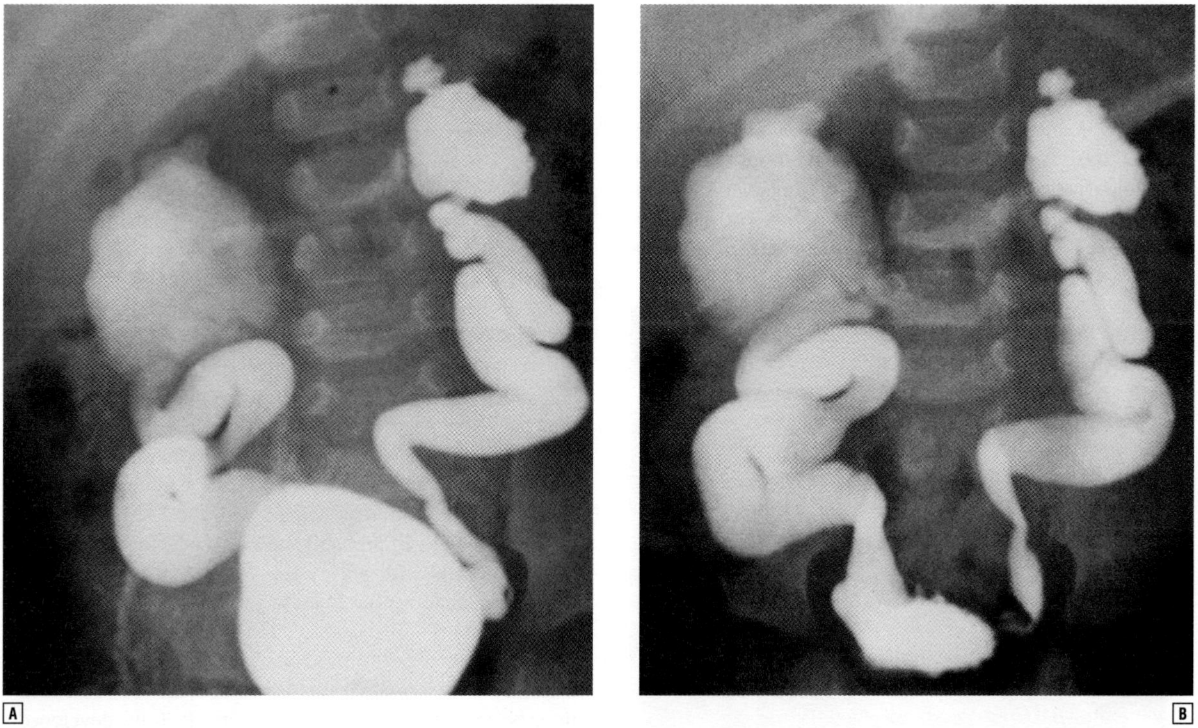

A B

Fig. 6.24 Micturating cystograms. A The bladder has been filled by contrast medium through a urinary catheter. Even before micturition there was gross vesico-ureteric reflux into widely distended ureters and pelvicalyceal systems. B The bladder is now empty except for a small residual pool, but contrast medium is retained in both collecting systems.

the urine. Pyuria and proteinuria < 1 g/24 hrs are common but not invariable. Renal calculi are more common.

A number of women present with hypertension and/or proteinuria in pregnancy. In some patients a positive family history is obtained with an autosomal dominant pattern of inheritance.

Investigations

The IVU shows the diagnostic features. The kidneys are reduced in size and there is localised contraction of the renal substance associated with clubbing of the adjacent calyces (see Fig. 6.25). Culture of the urine is mandatory. When infection is present, *E. coli* is the most common organism. Other agents include *Proteus*, *Pseudomonas aeruginosa* and staphylococci. Investigations such as rectal and vaginal examination, cystoscopy and renal ultrasound are performed to identify any abnormality causing obstruction to the flow of urine. A radionuclide renogram with post-micturition scanning or cysto-urethrogram will demonstrate VUR. Renal function should be assessed by estimation of the blood urea and creatinine, plasma electrolytes and creatinine clearance.

Management

Chronic infection may be difficult to eradicate. Attempts should be made to correct abnormalities of the urinary tract, including congenital malformations, and to remove calculi. An antibiotic to which the organism is sensitive should be given for 7 days. If the infection is not eradicated, suppressive therapy may be required for months (see Table 6.9, p. 460), the antibiotic being changed in response to the changing pattern and sensitivity of the organisms. Simple measures outlined in the information box on page 460 should be adopted. If pyonephrosis develops or persistent renal infection or pain is unilateral, nephrectomy may be indicated.

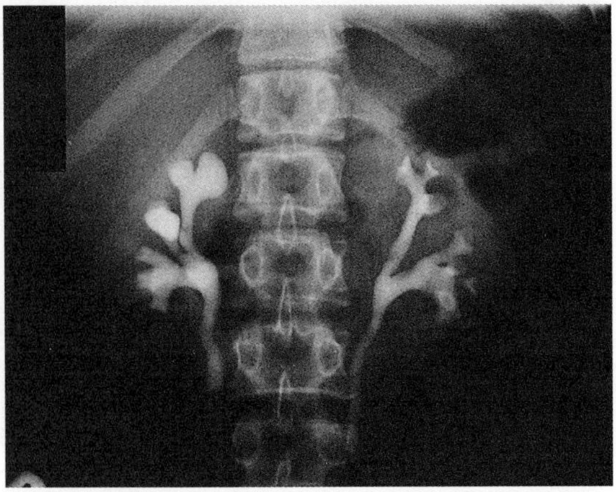

Fig. 6.25 Chronic pyelonephritis. Intravenous urogram revealing clubbing of the calyces which is particularly marked in the upper right pole. The appearances on the left are virtually normal.

The usual principles applying to the management of chronic renal failure apply (see p. 435). Rarely, hypertension is cured by the removal of the diseased kidney. The role of surgery in correction of VUR is limited because most childhood reflux tends to disappear spontaneously. Local treatments, e.g. the injection of Teflon paste, are currently under investigation.

A salt-losing state may develop in reflux nephropathy and other tubulo-interstitial disorders, and these features should be managed as described on page 437.

Prognosis

Many children with small or unilateral scars have a good prognosis, provided renal growth is normal. A small proportion with severely scarred kidneys will develop hypertension and CRF as teenagers; reflux nephropathy is a common cause of malignant hypertension in this age group. A number of adults present with hypertension, proteinuria and CRF in their fourth decade, while others present with either infection or hypertension alone, some in pregnancy. Many adults give no clear history of childhood infection. However, the prognosis for most patients with scarred kidneys is very good.

CYSTIC KIDNEY DISEASES

POLYCYSTIC KIDNEY DISEASE

Infantile polycystic kidney disease is rare; inherited as an autosomal recessive trait, it is associated with hepatic fibrosis, and is often fatal in the first year of life due to renal or hepatic failure. Adult polycystic kidney disease (APKD) (see Fig. 6.26) is common, affecting approximately 80/100 000 of the general population. It is inherited as an autosomal dominant trait, males and females being equally affected. The common PKD 1 gene on chromosome 16 encodes a very large transmembrane protein, polycystin, the function of which is still obscure. A milder and rarer form of the disease is associated with the PKD 2 gene on chromosome 4. It probably encodes a calcium channel which interacts with polycystin. Occasional families have disease linked to neither of these genes.

Pathology

Small cysts of proximal tubular epithelium are present in infancy and enlarge at a variable rate. In fully developed APKD the kidneys are asymmetrically enlarged and contain numerous cysts. These differ in size and are surrounded by a variable amount of parenchyma which often shows extensive fibrosis and arteriolosclerosis.

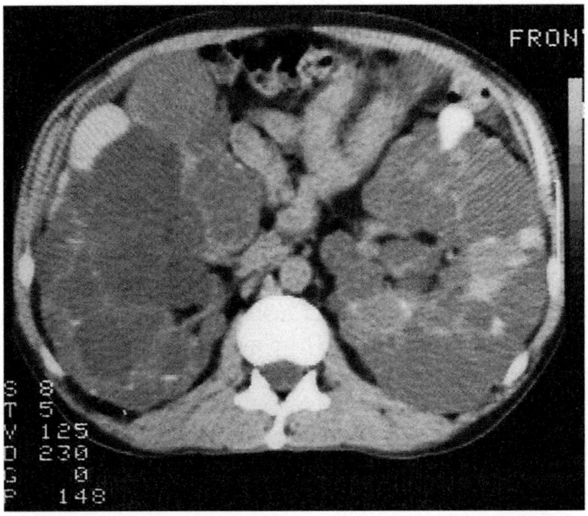

Fig. 6.26 Polycystic kidney disease. Two very large polycystic kidneys shown by CT.

Clinical features

Affected subjects are usually asymptomatic until late in life. After the age of 20 there is often an insidious onset of hypertension, which may or may not be associated with deterioration of renal function. Common clinical features are shown in the information box.

Often one or both kidneys can be palpated, and the surface may be nodular. Other diseases in which the kidneys may be palpably enlarged are hydronephrosis/pyonephrosis, solitary cyst, renal tumours and renal amyloid. The right kidney, and occasionally the lower pole of the left kidney, may be felt on clinical examination in normal slim adults.

About 30% of patients with APKD have hepatic cysts, but disturbance of liver function is rare. Berry aneurysms of cerebral vessels are an associated feature, especially in patients with a family history of this condition, and about 10% of patients have a subarachnoid haemorrhage. Mitral and aortic regurgitation are frequent but rarely severe, and colonic diverticula and abdominal wall hernias are recognised associations. There is a gradual reduction in renal function. However, the mean age of starting dialysis treatment in patients heterozygous for the PKD1 mutation is 57 years; 50% of patients never require chronic dialysis.

ADULT POLYCYSTIC KIDNEY DISEASE: COMMON CLINICAL FEATURES

- Vague discomfort in loin or abdomen due to increasing mass of renal tissue
- Acute loin pain or renal colic due to haemorrhage into a cyst
- Hypertension
- Haematuria
- Urinary tract infection
- Renal failure

Investigations

The diagnosis is made on the basis of clinical findings, family history and ultrasound, which is a sensitive method for demonstrating cysts. Now that the gene defects responsible for APKD have been identified, it is possible to make a specific genetic diagnosis.

Management

Good control of blood pressure is sensible, since uncontrolled hypertension accelerates the development of renal failure. Urinary infections must be treated promptly. Patients with impaired ability to conserve sodium ('salt-losing') require supplements of sodium chloride and sodium bicarbonate. The regimen for management of CRF will be needed as renal function deteriorates (see p. 435).

Screening and counselling

Screening by ultrasound can be used to detect asymptomatic cases of APKD amongst the relatives of patients. Screening and counselling should be offered to those over 18 years, although a negative result cannot exclude the disease entirely. Ultrasound is even less reliable in the 10–18-year group, and CT may be required to exclude or confirm cysts. A diagnosis made in early adult life allows regular monitoring of blood pressure and renal function, and permits genetic counselling to be given before most patients start their family. It does, however, have implications for life insurance, mortgages and employment, and not everyone offered screening will accept it. Specific genetic testing may be used both for screening and for antenatal diagnosis.

CYSTIC DISEASES OF THE RENAL MEDULLA

Cysts predominantly in the renal medulla are found in two different conditions. In medullary sponge kidney (see Fig. 6.27) the cysts are confined to the papillary collecting ducts. The condition is not usually genetic; its aetiology is unknown. Affected patients, usually adults, present with pain, haematuria, stone formation or urinary infection. The diagnosis is made by ultrasound or IVU. Contrast medium is seen to fill dilated or cystic tubules, which are sometimes calcified. The prognosis is generally good.

In medullary cystic disease small cortical cysts are also present, and these lead to progressive destruction of the nephron. This condition, characterised by thirst and polyuria (due to nephrogenic diabetes insipidus), occurs in younger patients, and there is often a family history. Sometimes affected patients are 'salt-losing', which aggravates the degree of renal failure. Even when treated appropriately, serious renal failure is usual.

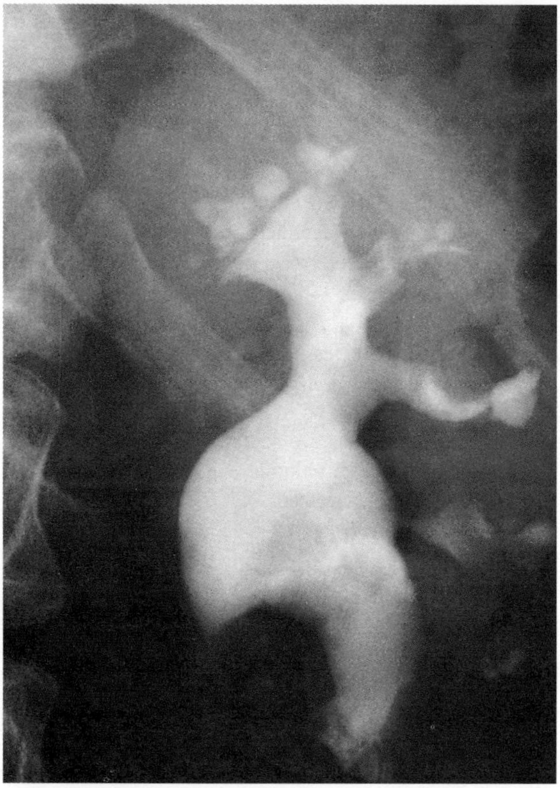

Fig. 6.27 Medullary sponge kidney. Intravenous pyelogram showing contrast medium filling both the collecting system and cavities arising from collecting ducts, especially within papillae of the upper pole. The cavities have been likened to bunches of grapes. Plain radiography may show calcification in the same regions.

ISOLATED DEFECTS OF TUBULAR FUNCTION

Renal glycosuria is a benign defect of tubular reabsorption of glucose, usually inherited as an autosomal recessive trait. Glucose appears in the urine in the presence of a normal blood glucose concentration (see p. 480).

Cystinuria is a rare condition in which reabsorption of filtered cystine, ornithine, arginine and lysine is defective. The high concentration of cystine in urine leads to cystine stone formation (see p. 463). Other uncommon tubular disorders include vitamin D-resistant rickets, in which reabsorption of filtered phosphate is reduced; nephrogenic diabetes insipidus, in which the tubules are resistant to the effects of vasopressin; and Bartter's and Gitelman's syndromes, in which there is sodium-wasting and hypokalaemia (see p. 407).

The term 'Fanconi's syndrome' is used to describe generalised proximal (especially) tubular dysfunction. Notable abnormalities include low blood phosphate and uric acid, the finding of glucose and amino acids in urine, and proximal renal tubular acidosis (see below). In addition to the causes of interstitial nephritis described above, some congenital metabolic disorders are associated with Fanconi's syndrome, notably Wilson's disease, cystinosis and hereditary fructose intolerance.

RENAL TUBULAR ACIDOSIS (RTA)

RTA results from a failure of either reabsorption of bicarbonate in the proximal tubule or acidification of the urine in the distal tubule. There may be little or no overall reduction in renal function. In both types, gene defects are described; otherwise the causes are those of diseases affecting the renal interstitium (see Table 6.6, p. 449), or the specific effects of toxins or drugs. Some disorders predominantly affect the distal tubule and are associated with distal RTA. These include hypercalciuria (see below), hyperoxaluria, amphotericin, solvents, medullary sponge kidney, sickle-cell disease and chronic urinary obstruction.

Distal renal tubular acidosis (classical or type 1)

In this condition the ability to form a very acid urine is lost, and the urine pH cannot be reduced to less than 5.3 even in the presence of severe systemic acidosis. This defect is due to failure of the collecting ducts to secrete hydrogen ions or to sustain the gradient for hydrogen ions between the luminal fluid and the tubular cell. Two types have been described. In complete distal RTA there is persistent hyperchloraemic acidosis. In the incomplete form, the plasma bicarbonate is normal, but the urine pH does not fall to less than 5.3 after ammonium chloride administration. Anorexia and fatigue are common, and there is hypercalciuria, hyperphosphaturia, and consequent stone formation and nephrocalcinosis. Loss of Na^+/H^+ exchange in collecting ducts leads to loss of sodium in urine and fluid depletion. Osteomalacia develops because of calcium loss and buffering of retained H^+ in bone. Children present with failure to thrive, polyuria and thirst.

Management consists of determining and dealing with the underlying cause where possible. Bicarbonate supplements should be given in a dose sufficient to keep the plasma bicarbonate in excess of 18 mmol/l. Large doses may be required, starting with a dose of 1g of sodium bicarbonate 8-hourly and increasing the dose until the desired plasma bicarbonate is achieved and there are no signs of sodium depletion (see p. 437). When hypokalaemia is present, a mixture of sodium and potassium bicarbonate should be given. Initially, about half of the total bicarbonate supplement is given as the potassium salt. The proportion of potassium bicarbonate is determined by regular monitoring of plasma potassium. Patients with osteomalacia may require 1α-hydroxycholecalciferol (alfacalcidol) or calcitriol.

Proximal renal tubular acidosis (type 2)

This may occur as an isolated defect (primary proximal RTA). More commonly, this occurs as part of Fanconi's syndrome. Proximal tubular Na^+/H^+ exchange is impaired, resulting in decreased bicarbonate reabsorption, large losses of bicarbonate in the urine, and a marked reduction in plasma bicarbonate. Once the plasma bicarbonate has fallen to about 12 mmol/l, the reduced filtered load can be reabsorbed by the proximal tubular cells, and the amount of bicarbonate reaching the distal tubule is negligible. In these circumstances, it is possible to show that the collecting duct cells can secrete hydrogen ions against a gradient, so that the urine pH falls to less than 5.3. There is frequently associated hyperchloraemia, potassium depletion and hypocalcaemia. Distinction of proximal and distal RTA requires special tests not considered here.

Any underlying cause should be treated if possible. The plasma bicarbonate should be maintained at a level greater than 18 mmol/l with appropriate supplements of sodium bicarbonate. Very large amounts of bicarbonate are needed, and it is recommended that the starting dose should be 1 mmol/kg daily. A 500 mg sodium bicarbonate capsule provides 6 mmol of bicarbonate. In those patients with hypokalaemia, a proportion of the dose, determined by monitoring plasma potassium, is given as potassium bicarbonate. Where necessary, calcium supplements and 1α-hydroxycholecalciferol are given.

FURTHER INFORMATION ON TUBULO-INTERSTITIAL DISEASES

Blantz R C 1998 Pathophysiology of pre-renal azotemia. Kidney International 53: 512–523

De Broe M E, Elseviers M M 1998 Current concepts: analgesic nephropathy. New England Journal of Medicine 338: 446–452

Watson M L 1997 Complications of polycystic kidney disease. Kidney International 51: 353–365

CONGENITAL ABNORMALITIES OF THE KIDNEYS

Congenital anomalies of the urinary tract affect more than 10% of infants and, if not immediately lethal, may lead to complications in later life. About 1 in 500 infants is born with only one kidney. Although usually compatible with normal life, this is often associated with other abnormalities. Polycystic kidney disease (see p. 452) is the most common inherited cause of severe renal disease. The next most common, Alport's syndrome, is considered on page 442. Other cystic diseases are considered above. Other inherited disorders affecting the kidney include tumour syndromes (see p. 468), conditions caused by mutations in transporter or exchanger molecules (see above) and a variety of rare conditions not discussed here.

RENAL INVOLVEMENT IN SYSTEMIC DISEASES

The kidneys may be directly involved in a number of multisystem diseases or secondarily affected by diseases of other organs. Involvement may be at a pre-renal, glomerular, interstitial or post-renal level. Many of the diseases are described in other sections of this chapter or in other chapters of the book. Table 6.7 lists some diseases in which renal involvement may be a prominent feature. Cancer, systemic vasculitis, SLE, diabetes mellitus and pregnancy are considered in further detail here.

Table 6.7 Systemic conditions affecting the kidney*

Disease	Mechanism
Vascular/cardiovascular	
Heart failure	Pre
Hypertension	Vasc
Atherosclerosis	Pre
Atheroemboli	Vasc
Thrombotic microangiopathy (HUS, TTP)	Vasc
Haematological	
Sickle-cell disease	Int
Plasma cell dyscrasias	
Myeloma	Int, other
Amyloidosis	Glom
Cryoglobulinaemia	Glom
Inflammatory/immunological	
Systemic vasculitis (SVV)	Glom
SLE	Glom
Systemic sclerosis	Vasc
Sjögren's syndrome	Int
Rheumatoid disease	Glom, other
Sarcoidosis	Int
Metabolic	
Diabetes	Glom
Hypercalcaemia	Tub
Hypokalaemia	Tub
Hepatorenal syndrome	Vasc
Infections (direct/remote/immune)	
Viral	Int
Bacterial	Glom, int
Other	Glom, int
Toxic states (direct/immune	
Drugs	Int, glom, obstr
Toxins	Int, glom, obstr
Diseases of pregnancy	
Pre-eclampsia	Glom

* The most common or major way in which the kidney is affected is shown as follows: pre = pre-renal; vasc = vascular (affecting arteries, arterioles or glomerular capillaries); glom = glomerular; int = interstitial; tub = tubular; obstr = intrarenal precipitation and obstruction.

MALIGNANT DISEASES

Cancer is not shown as a separate cause in Table 6.7, but may affect the kidney in many ways (see the information box).

RENAL EFFECTS OF MALIGNANCIES
Direct involvement
• Kidney: hypernephroma, lymphoma • Urinary tract: e.g. urothelial tumours, cervical carcinoma
Immune reaction
• Glomerulonephritis: especially membranous nephropathy • Systemic vasculitis (rarely): usually ANCA-negative
Metabolic consequences
• Hypercalcaemia • Uric acid crystal formation in tubules: usually in tumour lysis syndromes
Remote effects of tumour products
• Light chains in myeloma, amyloidosis • Antibodies in cryoglobulinaemia

SYSTEMIC VASCULITIS

The varieties and classification of systemic vasculitis are considered on page 862. Renal involvement is most commonly associated with small-vessel vasculitis (SVV), in which capillaritis may profoundly affect glomerular function. This causes an inflammatory glomerulonephritis that is focal in nature; focal necrosis is characteristic (see Table 6.4 and Fig. 6.21, pp. 444 and 445). The most important causes of this syndrome, microscopic polyangiitis and Wegener's granulomatosis, are usually associated with antibodies to neutrophil granule enzymes (ANCA, see p. 866). Vasculitis in other organs may give clues to the underlying systemic disorder and its subtype—e.g. ENT involvement and granulomatous lung disease in Wegener's granulomatosis. The similarity of alveolar and glomerular capillaries means that pulmonary haemorrhage, the consequence of capillaritis affecting alveoli, frequently occurs together with rapidly progressive glomerulonephritis (see p. 443). In some patients a focal glomerulonephritis with or without crescent formation may occur alone, with ANCA, as a kidney-limited form of systemic vasculitis. ANCA alone are not diagnostic of SVV. Importantly, ANCA have been described in chronic infections with associated renal disease, including endocarditis, HIV and tuberculosis. Inappropriate immunosuppression in these circumstances may be disastrous.

Treatment of the primary types of SVV with cyclophosphamide and corticosteroids is life-saving. Death from extrarenal manifestations of the disease is prevented, and renal function can be salvaged in acute disease, even if the glomerulonephritis is so severe as to cause oliguria.

Henoch–Schönlein purpura was discussed above, with IgA nephropathy. It is another SVV, in which similar focal nephritis is seen by light microscopy. However, instead of being pauci-immune (minimal or no immunoglobulin deposition in the glomeruli), mesangial deposits of IgA are seen, as in IgA nephropathy. ANCA are not usually detected. The disease is usually episodic and self-limiting, but severe progressive renal (or other) disease sometimes justifies the use of immunosuppressive treatment.

In addition to these common disorders, SVV sometimes occurs in the setting of other systemic inflammatory disorders, and the kidneys may be affected in these. Common examples include SLE and rheumatoid arthritis.

Medium- to large-vessel vasculitis, in the absence of involvement of small vessels, only causes renal disease when arterial involvement leads to hypertension or renal infarction.

SYSTEMIC LUPUS ERYTHEMATOSUS (SLE)

Renal involvement in SLE occurs in approximately 30% of patients within 1 year of diagnosis and a further 20% of patients by 5 years, although it is clinically silent in many. It usually manifests as glomerulonephritis although serologically, and sometimes clinically, overlapping syndromes (e.g. mixed connective tissue disorder, Sjögren's syndrome) may be associated with interstitial nephritis. As indicated in Table 6.4 (see p. 444), SLE can produce almost any histological pattern and an accordingly wide range of clinical features from florid rapidly progressive glomerulonephritis (RPGN, see p. 443) to chronic nephrotic syndrome. Most typically, patients present with subacute disease, with inflammatory features (haematuria, hypertension, variable renal impairment) accompanied by heavy proteinuria that often reaches nephrotic levels. The most common histological pattern is an inflammatory, diffusely proliferative glomerulonephritis with distinct features to suggest lupus. Controlled trials have shown that the risk of end-stage renal failure (ESRF) in this type of disease is significantly reduced by cyclophosphamide treatment, often given as regular intravenous pulses.

Significant renal involvement has traditionally been described as a poor prognostic factor in SLE. It usually signifies a need for more powerful (and therefore more hazardous) treatment, but in most, renal failure can be prevented. Drug side-effects are important; over-reliance on high doses of corticosteroids to control disease leads to substantial toxicity over many years. Cytotoxic agents carry the predictable risks of bone marrow suppression, infection, infertility and secondary malignancy. The risks of teratogenic effects and loss of fertility are particularly important, as many patients are young women.

Many patients go into relative remission from SLE once ESRF has developed. This may be because ESRF itself is an immunosuppressed state, as indicated by the incidence of bacterial infections in ESRF of all causes. Patients with ESRF caused by SLE are usually good candidates for dialysis and transplantation. Although it is one of the diseases that may recur in renal allografts, the immunosuppression required to prevent allograft rejection usually keeps SLE suppressed at the same time.

DIABETES MELLITUS

In patients with diabetes, the steady advance from microalbuminuria to dipstick-positive proteinuria, the development of hypertension and the progression to frank nephrotic syndrome are described on page 504. Not all patients require renal biopsy to establish the diagnosis, but non-diabetic renal disease causes proteinuria in up to 8% of diabetic patients and hence other treatable causes of renal disease should be excluded.

Once overt diabetic nephropathy has developed, hypotensive agents reduce the rate of loss of renal function. ACE inhibitors have an effect over and above that caused by reduction of blood pressure by reducing intraglomerular pressure. Some non-dihydropyridine calcium antagonists have similar effects on proteinuria, and may therefore be useful if ACE inhibitors or angiotensin receptor antagonists cannot be used. Blood pressure lowering should be aggressive. Beneficial effects have been shown at all levels of blood pressure and multiple agents may be required.

Management of nephrotic syndrome is according to usual principles (see p. 427). However, the presence of other diabetic complications often makes the management of nephrotic syndrome and renal impairment more difficult, and fluid retention is often particularly severe. Cardiovascular and peripheral vascular disease and autonomic neuropathy make changes in fluid balance associated with hypoproteinaemia, oedema and renal impairment more difficult to tolerate, and drug side-effects often compound this. Hyperkalaemia may be a difficult feature because of hyporeninaemic hypoaldosteronism, in which reduced renin production from prorenin and reduced release of aldosterone occur. Volume expansion and atrial natriuretic peptide may contribute to this. Gastroparesis and disordered bowel motility are frequently exacerbated, and irregular intake and absorption of food, plus alterations in the bioavailability of insulin due to reduced elimination of insulin and other changes in metabolism that occur as renal function deteriorates, usually lead to a deterioration of blood glucose control. Hypoglycaemic episodes are common in diabetic patients with renal failure. For these reasons, patients with diabetes commonly benefit from commencing renal replacement therapy at an earlier stage than other patients with ESRF, as this permits control of fluid balance and blood pressure with fewer drugs and enables some stabilisation to be achieved. Although the mortality of diabetic patients on dialysis and with renal transplants remains higher than that of other patients and management is often more difficult (see Fig. 6.28), survival rates are improving and their quality of life, especially following renal transplantation, may be good.

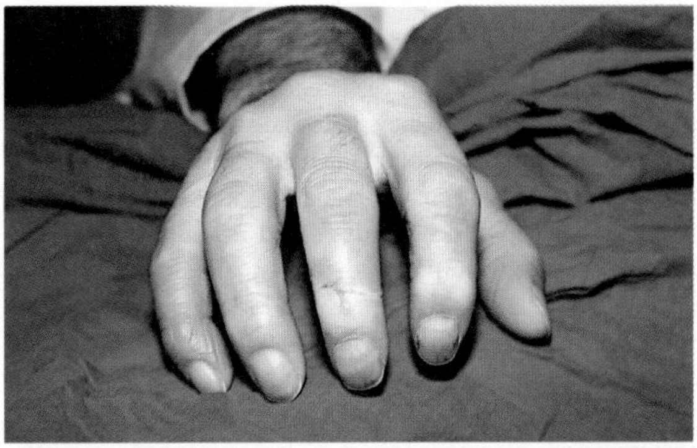

Fig. 6.28 The ischaemic hand of a diabetic patient with end-stage renal disease (ESRD). Symptoms and signs were precipitated by formation of an arteriovenous fistula for haemodialysis. The photograph illustrates the difficulties of managing ESRD in diabetes.

PREGNANCY

Pregnancy is a systemic condition, but not a disease. Physiological adaptations begin in the first few weeks. Peripheral vascular resistance declines, blood volume, cardiac output and GFR increase, and there is usually a reduction in blood pressure and plasma creatinine and urea values in the first trimester. Recordings of blood pressure and urine testing from the first clinic visit are valuable if problems arise later.

Some conditions are more common in pregnancy, the manifestations of others are modified by the physiological changes of pregnancy, and a few diseases are unique to pregnancy (see the information box). Pyelonephritis is more common, perhaps because of the reduced tone in the urinary collecting system and ureters, which causes a 'baggy' appearance on IVU and a somewhat dilated appearance on ultrasound. Proteinuria caused by glomerular disease is always exacerbated, and nephrotic syndrome may develop without any alteration in the underlying disease in individuals who had only slight proteinuria before pregnancy. This gives a particular risk of venous thrombo-

DISEASES UNIQUE TO PREGNANCY

- Hyperemesis gravidarum
- Septicaemia related to abortion and normal delivery
- Pre-eclampsia and related syndromes
- Post-partum haemolytic-uraemic syndrome (HUS)
- Placental abruption (may cause disseminated intravascular coagulation)
- Amniotic fluid embolism

embolism, which is now the leading cause of maternal deaths in developed countries.

Systemic autoimmune diseases are typically relatively quiescent during pregnancy, but tend to relapse in the first few weeks and months following delivery. Patients with such diseases who may become pregnant should be aware of the extra associated risks. Drugs used should be safe in pregnancy wherever possible. During pregnancy, therapy should not usually be stopped, but blood pressure targets may be modified (after discussion with the patient) and agents altered to those of proven safety.

Pre-existing renal disease increases the fetal and maternal risk of pregnancy, to a degree dependent on the level of renal function, proteinuria and hypertension. Similar consideration should be given to counselling and therapy.

Pre-eclampsia and related disorders

Pre-eclampsia is a systemic disorder that occurs in or near the third trimester of pregnancy. Its aetiology is unknown, although a number of risk factors are described (see the information box).

RISK FACTORS FOR PRE-ECLAMPSIA

- First pregnancy
- First pregnancy with a new partner
- Pre-eclampsia in previous pregnancies
- Age < 20 years or > 35 years
- Multiple pregnancy (singleton < twin < triplets etc.)
- Pre-existing hypertension
- Pre-existing renal disease

Pre-eclampsia is traditionally defined by the triad of oedema, proteinuria and hypertension. However, oedema is common in late pregnancy, proteinuria is a late sign, and while hypertension is usually present, it may be relative, mild, or even absent in certain variants of pre-eclampsia. Furthermore, all these features occur in renal disease, and may be exacerbated by pregnancy. Differentiating the two may be important, as pre-eclampsia is a progressive disease presenting increasing risk to the fetus and the mother, whereas in renal disease continuing the pregnancy may permit delivery of a healthier, more mature baby.

The only effective management for pre-eclampsia is delivery. Hypertension is a consequence, not the cause, of the disorder, and treatment is only justified to lower it from severe and immediately dangerous levels (e.g. higher than 180/110). Treating lower levels has been shown to confer no benefit, and exposes the fetus to additional drugs. If life-threatening complications are not present and the baby is immature, corticosteroids may be given to induce maturation of fetal lungs, and delivery postponed while mother and baby are closely observed. Magnesium sulphate has been shown to reduce the incidence of eclamptic convulsions.

FEATURES AND COMPLICATIONS OF PRE-ECLAMPSIA AND RELATED DISEASES

Clinical signs

- Hypertension
- Proteinuria
- Oedema
- Other evidence of the clinical syndromes listed below

Investigations

- Uric acid levels increased (before renal impairment apparent)
- Platelets decreased
- Reduced GFR (late)
- Increased pressor response to angiotensin II (only of research value)
- Fetus small for dates and growing slowly
- Fetal distress (late)

Clinical syndromes

- Eclampsia: severe hypertension, encephalopathy and fits
- Disseminated intravascular coagulation
- Thrombotic microangiopathy: may also occur post-partum (post-partum HUS)
- Acute fatty liver of pregnancy
- 'HELLP': haemolysis, elevated liver enzymes, low platelets (thrombotic microangiopathy with abnormal liver function)

Acute renal failure may occur in the setting of most of these syndromes. Cortical necrosis (irreversible infarction of the renal cortex) is more likely to occur in pregnancy as a complication of some of these disorders.

FURTHER INFORMATION ON RENAL INVOLVEMENT IN SYSTEMIC DISEASES

Davison J M 1997 Management of pre-existing disorders in pregnancy: renal disease. Prescribers' Journal 37: 46–53

Scottish Intercollegiate clinical guidelines on diabetic renal disease are available at http://pc47.cee.hw.ac.uk/sign/

INFECTIONS OF THE KIDNEY AND URINARY TRACT

INFECTIONS OF THE LOWER URINARY TRACT

When the urinary tract is anatomically and physiologically normal, and local and systemic defence mechanisms are intact, bacteria are confined to the lower end of the urethra. Urinary tract infection (UTI) implies multiplication of organisms in the urinary tract, and is defined by the presence of more than 100 000 organisms per ml in a midstream sample of urine (MSU).

CLINICAL PRESENTATION OF URINARY TRACT INFECTION
• Asymptomatic bacteriuria • Symptomatic acute urethritis and cystitis • Acute prostatitis • Acute pyelonephritis • Septicaemia (usually Gram-negative bacteria)

Such infections are much more common in women, about one-third of whom have a UTI at some time. The prevalence of UTI in women is about 3% at the age of 20, increasing by about 1% in each subsequent decade. In males UTI is uncommon except in the first year of life and in men over 60, in whom a degree of urinary tract obstruction due to prostatic hypertrophy is common. UTI causes considerable morbidity, and in a small minority of cases, renal damage and chronic renal failure.

Pathogenesis

Urinary tract infections may be uncomplicated or complicated; the latter may result in permanent renal damage, the former rarely (if ever) do so. Uncomplicated infections are almost invariably due to a single strain of organism.

UNCOMPLICATED AND COMPLICATED URINARY TRACT INFECTION
Uncomplicated
• Anatomically and physiologically normal urinary tract • Normal renal function • No associated disorder which impairs defence mechanisms
Complicated
• Abnormal urinary tract, e.g. obstruction, calculi, vesico-ureteric reflux, neurological abnormality, in-dwelling catheter, chronic prostatitis, cystic kidney, analgesic nephropathy, renal scarring • Impaired renal function • Associated disorder which impairs defence mechanisms (e.g. diabetes mellitus, immunosuppressive therapy)

Outside hospitals, *E. coli* derived from the faecal reservoir accounts for about 75% of infections, the remainder being due to *Proteus*, *Pseudomonas* species, streptococci or *Staphylococcus epidermidis*. In hospital a greater proportion of infections are due to organisms such as *Klebsiella* or streptococci, but faecal *E. coli* still predominates. Certain strains of *E. coli* have a particular propensity to invade the urinary tract. They possess surface fimbriae, at the tips of which are lectin molecules which bind to glycolipid or glycoprotein surface receptors on the urothelium.

The first stage in the development of UTI is colonisation of the periurethral zone with pathogenic faecal organisms. The urothelium of susceptible persons may have more receptors to which virulent strains of *E. coli* become adherent. In women, the ascent of organisms into the bladder is facilitated by the short urethra and absence of bactericidal prostatic secretions. Sexual intercourse causes minor urethral trauma and may transfer bacteria from the perineum into the bladder. Instrumentation of the bladder may also introduce organisms. Multiplication of organisms then depends on a number of factors, including the size of the inoculum and virulence of the bacteria (see the information box).

FACTORS WHICH LIMIT MULTIPLICATION OF ORGANISMS IN THE URINARY TRACT
• A high rate of urine flow • Regular complete bladder emptying • Urinary glycosaminoglycans (Tamm–Horsfall mucoprotein) which may bind to *E. coli*, thus preventing their attachment to urothelium • Mucosal defences: thin surface layer of glycosaminoglycans, secretions of IgA and IgG, mucosal phagocytosis

Table 6.8 Investigation of patients with acute urinary tract infection

Investigation	Indications
Culture of MSU or urine obtained by suprapubic aspiration	All patients
Microscopic examination of urine for white cells, red cells and casts	All patients
Dipstick examination of urine for blood, protein and glucose	All patients
Full blood count	Infants; children; adults with acute pyelonephritis or prostatitis
Plasma urea, electrolytes, creatinine	Infants; children; acute pyelonephritis; recurrent UTI
Blood culture	Fever, rigors or evidence of septic shock
Pelvic examination	Women with recurrent UTI
Rectal examination	Men (to examine prostate)
Intravenous urography (IVU) including film of bladder after voiding, to identify physiological and anatomical abnormalities	Infants; children Men after single UTI Women who (1) have acute pyelonephritis; (2) have recurrent UTI after urinary tract treatment; (3) have had UTI or covert bacteriuria in pregnancy (IVU 6 weeks after delivery)
Renal ultrasonography	Alternative to IVU to identify obstruction, cysts, calculi
Micturating cysto-urethrography (MCU) to identify and quantitate vesico-ureteric reflux and disturbed bladder emptying	Infants; children with abnormal IVU; any patient thought to have a disturbance of bladder emptying
Cystoscopy	Patients with chronic haematuria; patients with a suspected bladder lesion

Residual urine left after voiding interferes with mucosal defence mechanisms; thus patients with bladder outflow obstruction, gynaecological abnormalities, pelvic floor weakness or neurological problems are susceptible to infection. In those with vesico-ureteric reflux (see p. 450) urine expelled into the ureters during voiding returns to the bladder when it relaxes. Injury to the mucosa and the presence of a foreign body in the bladder also depress vesical defence mechanisms.

Clinical features

There is often an abrupt onset of frequency of micturition and dysuria. Scalding pain is felt in the urethra during micturition. Cystitis may give rise to suprapubic pain during and after voiding. After the bladder has been emptied, there may be an intense desire to pass more urine due to spasm of the inflamed bladder wall. Systemic symptoms are usually slight or absent. Suprapubic tenderness is often present. Urine may have an unpleasant odour and appear cloudy. Gross haematuria may occur. The diagnosis depends on:

- the characteristic clinical features
- demonstration of more than 10^6/ml organisms in a midstream specimen of urine, or any organisms in urine from a suprapubic aspiration.

The presence of pus cells in the urine (pyuria) is common but not invariable. Children, men and women with recurrent infection or signs of pyelonephritis must be more fully investigated, as shown in Table 6.8.

Management

Table 6.9 shows antibiotic regimens for treatment of UTI in adults. Ideally, results of urine culture and sensitivities should be available before treatment, but if the patient is in discomfort treatment may be started while awaiting the result. Since infection is usually due to *E. coli*, initial use of trimethoprim or amoxycillin is rational. The antibiotic can be changed if a resistant organism is identified or the response is unsatisfactory. Symptomatic relief usually occurs within 48 hours. A 3-day course is adequate and is superior to single-dose treatment. A fluid intake of at least 2 litres/day is helpful.

Failure to eradicate an organism suggests that one of the complicating factors listed on page 459 is present. Investigations should be performed to diagnose the underlying

PROPHYLACTIC MEASURES TO BE ADOPTED BY WOMEN WITH RECURRENT URINARY INFECTIONS

- Fluid intake of at least 2 litres/day
- Regular emptying of bladder (3-hour intervals by day and before retiring)
- Ensure complete emptying of bladder
- Double micturition if reflux present. (The patient should be advised, particularly before retiring for the night, to empty the bladder and then attempt to empty the bladder a second time approximately 10–15 minutes later)
- Emptying bladder before and after intercourse
- Application of 0.5% cetrimide cream to periurethral area before intercourse

This regimen is started after completion of a curative course of treatment and continued for several months.

Table 6.9 Antibiotic regimens for treatment of urinary tract infections in adults[1]

	Treatment of presumed urinary tract infection		Treatment of presumed pyelonephritis		Treatment of acute prostatitis		Prophylactic or suppressive therapy
Drug	Dose	Duration of course	Dose	Duration of course	Dose	Duration of course	Dose
Trimethoprim	300 mg daily	3 days	300 mg daily	7 days	200 mg 12-hourly	4–6 weeks	100 mg/night
Ampicillin or amoxycillin	250 mg 8-hourly	3 days	250–500 mg 8-hourly	7 days			250 mg/night
Gentamicin[2]			3–5 mg/kg i.v. daily[2]	7 days			
Cefuroxime[1]			250 mg 12-hourly oral or 750 mg 6–8-hourly i.v.	7 days Start treatment i.v. in seriously ill patient			
Ciprofloxacin[1]	250–500 mg 12-hourly	3 days	250–500 mg 12-hourly oral or 100 mg 12-hourly i.v.	7 days	250 mg 12-hourly	4–6 weeks	
Cephalexin							250 mg/night
Erythromycin					250 mg 6-hourly	4–6 weeks	

[1] Modification of dosage is necessary when renal function is severely impaired.
[2] Dose determined by plasma [creatinine] and [gentamicin]. Given in divided doses.

problem, which should be treated appropriately. Failing this, after a further course of antibiotics, suppressive antibiotic therapy can be used to prevent recurrent symptoms, septicaemia and renal damage, as outlined in Table 6.9. Urine is cultured regularly and the antibiotic changed as required.

Reinfection with another organism, or with the same organism after an interval, is not uncommon, particularly in sexually active women. Simple measures may prevent recurrence (see the information box). If these fail, freedom from attacks may be achieved by taking a single nightly dose of a suitable antibiotic after voiding and before going to bed (see Table 6.9).

COVERT OR ASYMPTOMATIC BACTERIURIA

This is defined as more than 10^6/ml organisms in the MSU of apparently healthy asymptomatic patients. Approximately 1% of children under the age of 1, 1% of schoolgirls, 0.03% of schoolboys and men, 3% of non-pregnant adult women and 5% of pregnant women have covert bacteriuria. There is no evidence that this condition causes chronic renal scarring in non-pregnant adults with normal urinary tracts. When it occurs in infants, pregnant women or in an abnormal urinary tract, investigation and treatment (see Tables 6.8 and 6.9) are required.

URETHRAL SYNDROME

Some patients, usually female, have symptoms suggestive of urethritis and cystitis but no bacteria are cultured from the urine. Possible explanations include infection with organisms not readily cultured by ordinary methods (e.g. chlamydia, certain anaerobes), allergy to toilet preparations or disinfectants, urethral congestion related to sexual intercourse, and post-menopausal atrophic vaginitis. Antibiotics are not indicated.

ACUTE PROSTATITIS

This is often accompanied by perineal pain and considerable systemic disturbance. The prostate is usually very tender. The diagnosis is confirmed by a positive culture from urine or from urethral discharge obtained after prostatic massage. The treatment of choice is trimethoprim or erythromycin, which penetrate prostatic secretions. A 4–6-week course is required (see Table 6.9).

INFECTIONS OF THE UPPER URINARY TRACT AND KIDNEY

The proportion of patients with cystitis or bacteriuria in whom the kidney is involved is unknown, but a figure of 50% has been suggested. Clinically, it is often impossible to know if renal infection is present.

Pathogenesis

Bacterial infection of the renal parenchyma is usually due to ascent of organisms via the ureter, although it can be blood-borne. About 75% of infections are due to *E. coli*, the remainder to *Proteus* species, *Klebsiella*, staphylococci or streptococci. Commonly, one or more complicating factors are present (see the information box, p. 459) but in infants and women infection can occur in the absence of such factors. Stasis within the urinary tract compromises its defences. Renal cysts or scars facilitate infection. The renal medulla is susceptible to infection because of the low oxygen tension, high osmolality and high concentrations of H^+ and ammonia that interfere with the function of leucocytes. The high osmolality probably favours conversion of bacteria to antibiotic-resistant L-forms.

ACUTE PYELONEPHRITIS

Pathology

The renal pelvis is inflamed and small abscesses in the renal parenchyma are often evident. Histological examination shows focal infiltration by polymorphonuclear leucocytes and the presence of these cells within the tubules.

Clinical features

There is sudden onset of pain in one or both loins, radiating to the iliac fossae and suprapubic area. About 30% of patients have dysuria due to associated cystitis. Fever is present, and rigors and vomiting may occur. Septicaemia with hypotension may supervene. Tenderness and guarding are usually present in the lumbar region. There is a leucocytosis. Microscopic examination of urine reveals pus cells, organisms, red cells and epithelial cells.

Acute pyelonephritis in infants and children may present as fever without localising symptoms. The initial feature may be a convulsion; apathy, abdominal distension and diarrhoea may occur. In a febrile child, urine should always be examined for pus cells and organisms.

Rarely, acute papillary necrosis follows an attack of acute pyelonephritis. Fragments of renal papillae are excreted in the urine and can be identified histologically. This complication, which may lead to acute renal failure, is particularly liable to occur in patients with diabetes mellitus or chronic urinary obstruction. It is also seen (without infection) in analgesic nephropathy and sickle-cell disease.

Differential diagnosis

Acute pyelonephritis should be distinguished from acute appendicitis, diverticulitis, cholecystitis and salpingitis, and also from perinephric abscess due to infection by *Staph. aureus*. In this condition there is marked pain and tenderness in the renal region, and often bulging of the loin on the affected side. Patients are extremely ill, with fever, leucocytosis and a positive blood culture. Urinary symptoms are absent, and urine contains neither pus cells nor organisms.

Management

Table 6.8 on page 459 shows the necessary investigations. Diagnosis depends on the clinical features and results of urine culture. Renal tract ultrasound examination should be performed without delay. Antibiotic regimens for adults are shown in Table 6.9. In less severe cases oral trimethoprim, amoxycillin or ciprofloxacin can be used. Severe cases require intravenous therapy. Urine culture should be repeated during the course, and 7 and 21 days after treatment.

RENAL TUBERCULOSIS

Tuberculosis of the kidney is invariably secondary to tuberculosis elsewhere (see p. 347) and occurs as a result of blood-borne infection. The initial lesion develops in the renal cortex and, if untreated, may ulcerate into the pelvis, with consequent involvement of the bladder, epididymis, seminal vesicles and prostate. The disease tends to occur in young people, and may present with recurrent haematuria and dysuria due to secondary involvement of the bladder. In addition, the general features of tuberculosis, i.e. malaise, fever, lassitude and weight loss, may be present. Chronic renal failure may result from destruction of kidney tissue, or be due to obstruction of the urinary tract when lesions heal by fibrosis. Culture of the urine by ordinary methods may be sterile in spite of pyuria, and indeed sterile pyuria is an indication to perform special cultures for tubercle bacilli. The extent of the infection with regard to the lower urinary tract should be ascertained by cystoscopic examination.

FURTHER INFORMATION ON INFECTIONS OF THE KIDNEY AND URINARY TRACT

Cattell W R (ed) 1996 Infections of the kidney and urinary tract. Oxford Clinical Nephrology series, Oxford University Press, Oxford

Kunin C M 1997 Urinary tract infections: detection, prevention and management, 5th edn. Williams & Wilkins, Baltimore

Stamm W E, Hooton T M 1993 Management of urinary tract infections in adults. New England Journal of Medicine 329: 1328–1334

OBSTRUCTION OF THE URINARY TRACT

Obstruction to the flow of urine from the kidney is a common disorder. It causes urinary stasis and an increase in

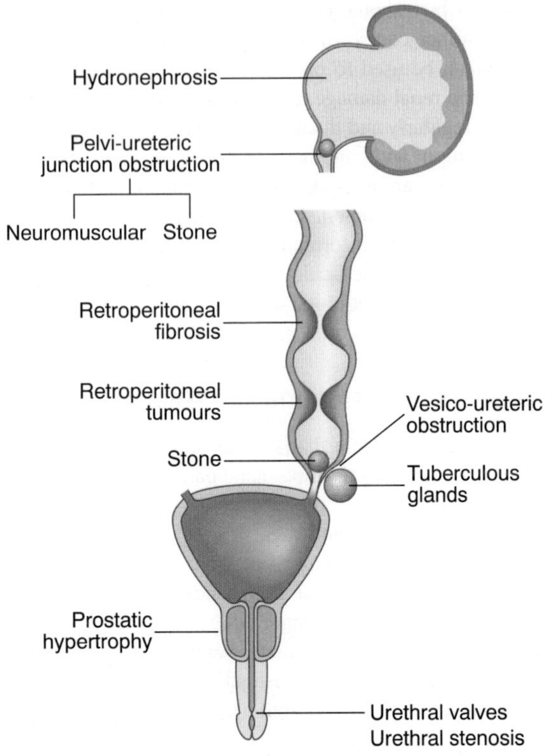

Fig. 6.29 Obstruction of the urinary tract. Obstruction to the urinary tract can arise at the pelvi-ureteric junction, in the ureter, at the vesico-ureteric junction, at the bladder and also in the urethra.

pressure above the obstruction, which in turn predispose to infection, stone formation and renal failure. Obstruction may occur at any level, but is most common at the pelvi-ureteric junction, at the bladder neck or in the urethra (see Fig. 6.29). Obstruction at the pelvi-ureteric junction causes hydronephrosis. Obstruction of the ureter causes hydroureter and subsequently hydronephrosis. Obstruction of the bladder neck or urethra distends the bladder, causes hypertrophy of its muscle (seen on cystoscopic examination as trabeculation), and subsequently leads to hydroureter and hydronephrosis. If obstruction is unrelieved, slowly progressive destruction of renal tissue occurs. Superimposed infection often results in a rapid deterioration of renal function.

Aetiology

Obstruction may be due to a structural lesion, or to a congenital neuromuscular defect which prevents the contraction wave and thus the flow of urine.

Clinical features

These vary with the cause and site of the lesion. When the obstruction is above the bladder, renal colic may occur, especially if the onset is sudden. More commonly, the obstruction is gradual, and aching pain in the loins, sometimes aggravated by drinking, develops. Superimposed infection causes malaise, fever, dysuria and sometimes septicaemia. Haematuria is common. In partial obstruction, transmission of the increased hydrostatic pressure to the kidney interferes with the counter-current concentrating mechanism and, paradoxically, may result in polyuria. Occasionally, a hydronephrotic kidney is palpable. Sometimes the patient presents with anuria and acute renal failure (see p. 429). Intermittent anuria suggests a diagnosis of a renal stone or retroperitoneal fibrosis. Outflow obstruction below the bladder causes difficulty in micturition. The urinary stream is thin in calibre and poor in force. Complete urinary retention may occur with consequent distension of the bladder, which may be visible and palpable as a swelling of the lower abdomen. Anuria or overflow incontinence may ensue. In the latter event, catheterisation reveals the presence of residual urine in the bladder after the patient has voided. Infection is extremely common.

Investigations

Rectal or vaginal examination should be carried out to detect prostatic enlargement or pelvic tumour.

Ultrasound examination will detect dilatation of the renal pelvis and upper ureter (see Fig. 6.3, p. 421). It is particularly valuable in acute renal failure, when it can be combined with percutaneous nephrostomy to relieve the obstruction, followed by antegrade pyelography to identify the site of the lesion (see p. 422).

Intravenous urography can also be used to diagnose obstruction; when obstruction is present, the nephrogram and pyelogram are both delayed, dilatation of the outflow system is seen, and the site of obstruction can often be identified. A post-voiding film should be performed to detect bladder abnormalities.

Neither ultrasound nor IVU can distinguish a distended urinary tract in which there is no resistance to flow (e.g. after pregnancy) from genuine urinary tract obstruction. However, this distinction can often be made by a diuretic renogram (see p. 424). Cystoscopy, pyelography, urethrography and cystometry may be required to define lesions in the bladder, urethra or lower ureter, and for removal of stones or debris from the ureter or bladder. Culture of urine and, if the patient is systemically unwell, of blood should be carried out. Assessment of renal function is essential.

Management

The ultimate objective is to remove the source of obstruction, but temporary drainage of the urinary tract may be required in order to preserve renal function, relieve symptoms and treat infection. Obstruction of the bladder neck or urethra should be relieved using a urethral or, rarely, a suprapubic catheter. Obstruction of the upper urinary tract can be treated by insertion of a catheter into the renal pelvis under ultrasound guidance (percutaneous nephrostomy).

Relief of obstruction may be followed by a massive diuresis (post-obstructive diuresis) due to impaired tubular function, loss of the medullary concentration gradient, and the diuretic effect of retained solute and water. In this situation, electrolyte losses must be replaced intravenously. When obstruction is incomplete, or is due to stones or debris which are likely to be passed spontaneously, temporary drainage is rarely necessary unless infection supervenes. Antibiotics are required to treat severe infection or to cover surgical procedures. Dialysis may be necessary before surgery.

Once the underlying lesion has been identified and renal function assessed, definitive treatment is often possible, e.g. removal of stones or transurethral resection of the prostate. When obstruction is irremediable, the ureters may be anastomosed to an isolated loop of ileum opening on to the abdominal wall (ileal conduit). Alternatively, in-dwelling stents may be left in one or both ureters and changed at regular intervals to prevent infection.

Patients who have undergone treatment for urinary tract obstruction should thereafter have periodic assessment of renal function. Unilateral nephrectomy may be indicated because of persistent infection and, occasionally, hypertension due to renin production in the damaged kidney.

URINARY TRACT CALCULI AND NEPHROCALCINOSIS

Aetiology

Urinary calculi consist of aggregates of crystals and small amounts of proteins and glycoprotein, but their genesis is poorly understood. Different types of stone occur in different parts of the world, and dietary factors probably play a part in determining the varying patterns. In Britain, stones in which the crystalline component consists of calcium oxalate are the most common (39% of calculi in one survey). In the same study, 14% of stones contained both calcium oxalate and calcium phosphate, 13% calcium phosphate alone, and 15% contained magnesium ammonium phosphate (struvite). Small numbers of cystine stones and uric acid stones were found.

In developing countries, bladder stones are common, particularly in children. In developed countries the incidence of childhood bladder stones is low, and renal stones in adults are more common. One survey found that 4% of the population has stones in the urinary tract, but the prevalence varies in different areas. It is surprising that stones and nephrocalcinosis are not more common, since some of the constituents are present in urine in concentrations which exceed their maximum solubility in water. However, urine contains proteins, glycosaminoglycans, pyrophosphate and citrate which, by forming complexes, may keep otherwise insoluble salts in solution.

Table 6.10 Risk factors for renal stone formation

Risk factor	Type of stone
Obstruction of urinary tract	Phosphate
Infection of urinary tract	Phosphate
Repeated dehydration (occupation, climate)	All types
Hypercalciuria	Calcium oxalate
Hyperoxaluria	Calcium oxalate
Hypocitraturia	Calcium
Inherited disorders	
Cystinuria	Cystine
Xanthinuria	Xanthine
Gout, myeloproliferative disorders	Urate
Medullary sponge kidney	Calcium

Certain conditions are frequently associated with stone formation (see Table 6.10).

The pH of urine influences the formation of stones. An alkaline urine tends to increase precipitation of calcium phosphate, and may be responsible for calcium phosphate stones in patients with renal tubular acidosis. The solubility of uric acid and cystine is reduced in acid urine. In developed countries most calculi occur in healthy young men in whom investigations reveal no clear cause for stone formation. Multiple aetiological factors are probably present in such cases, and it is likely that an alteration in the relative proportions of crystalloids and glycosaminoglycans in the urine is of particular importance.

Pathology

Urinary concretions vary greatly in size. There may be particles like sand anywhere in the urinary tract, or large round stones in the bladder. Staghorn calculi fill the whole renal pelvis and branch into the calyces (see Fig. 6.30); they are usually associated with previous pyelonephritis. Deposits of calcium may be present throughout the renal parenchyma, giving rise to nephrocalcinosis. This is especially liable to occur in patients with chronic pyelonephritis, renal tubular acidosis, hyperparathyroidism, vitamin D intoxication and healed renal tuberculosis.

Clinical features

These vary according to the size, shape and position of the stone, and the nature of any underlying condition. Renal calculi or nephrocalcinosis may be present for years without giving rise to symptoms, and may be discovered during radiological examination for another disorder. More commonly, patients present with pain, recurrent urinary infection or clinical features of urinary tract obstruction. The most common complaint arising from renal calculi is intermittent dull pain in the loin or back, increased by movement. Protein, red cells or leucocytes may appear in the urine.

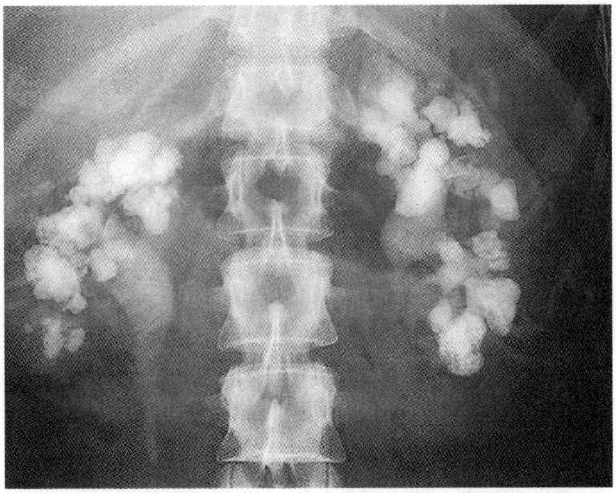

Fig. 6.30 Bilateral staghorn calculi shown on an intravenous pyelogram. Some dye is being excreted by the right kidney, with little function on the left.

When a stone becomes impacted in the ureter, an attack of renal colic develops. The patient is suddenly aware of pain in the loin, which radiates round the flank to the groin and often into the testis or labium, in the sensory distribution of the first lumbar nerve. The pain steadily increases in intensity to reach a maximum in a few minutes. The patient is restless, and generally tries unsuccessfully to obtain relief by changing position and by pacing the room. There is pallor, sweating and often vomiting, and the patient may groan in agony. Frequency, dysuria and haematuria may occur. The intense pain usually subsides within 2 hours, but may continue unabated for hours or days. The pain is usually constant during attacks, though slight fluctuations in severity may occur. Contrary to general belief, attacks rarely consist of intermittent severe pains coming and going every few minutes.

Investigations

The diagnosis of renal colic is usually easily made from the history and by finding red cells in the urine. Any patient suspected of having stones should have radiographs of the urinary tract. If there is doubt about the cause of pain an IVU during an attack may help. When the pain is due to a stone in the ureter, the radiograph shows a dense renal shadow and the appearance of dye in the renal pelvis is delayed (see Fig. 6.31). Subsequently, the site of obstruction may be visible. CT (without contrast) is more sensitive but less readily available. It may show 'non-radio-opaque' stones.

Appropriate investigations should be undertaken to discover any underlying disorder (see Table 6.11).

Management

The immediate treatment of loin pain or renal colic is bed

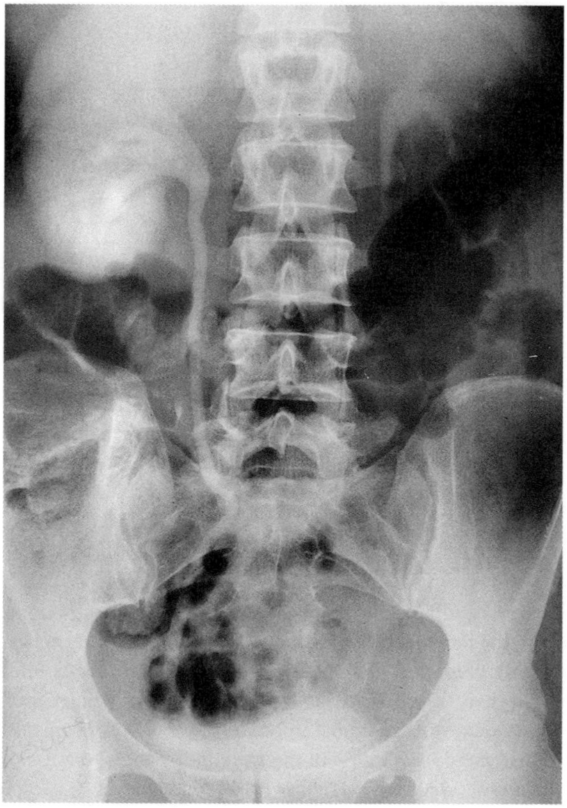

Fig. 6.31 Unilateral obstruction. Intravenous urogram of a patient with a stone (not visible) at the lower end of the right ureter. This film, taken 2 hours post-injection, demonstrates persistence of contrast medium in the right kidney, pelvicalyceal system and ureter, whereas only a small amount remains visible in the normal left pelvicalyceal system.

CONDITIONS ASSOCIATED WITH HYPERCALCIURIA AND HYPEROXALURIA

Hypercalciuria

Causes of hypercalcaemia
- Hyperparathyroidism, vitamin D excess, myeloma, sarcoidosis etc.

Hypercalciuria without hypercalcaemia
- High intake (dairy produce)
- Renal tubular acidosis
- Cushing's syndrome
- Prolonged immobilisation
- 'Idiopathic'
  Increased absorption from gut
  Reduced renal tubular readsorption

Hyperoxaluria
- High intake (fruit and vegetables)
- Increased absorption
  Ileal disease
  Low calcium diet

rest, application of warmth to the site of pain and administration of analgesia, e.g. a diclofenac suppository (100 mg). In severe cases, pethidine (100 mg), morphine (10–20 mg) and antispasmodic drugs, e.g. atropine sulphate (0.8 or 1.2 mg), may be given intramuscularly. If possible, the patient should drink 2 litres of fluid daily. Small stones, less than 5 mm in diameter, are usually passed spontaneously, but larger stones may require active intervention. Immediate action is required if anuria, bilateral hydronephrosis or significant infection, such as pyonephrosis, develops.

Attempts to dissolve calculi have failed, but lithotriptors may be used to fragment stones. Using this apparatus, shock waves are focused on the stone and fragments are passed in the urine. The technique requires free drainage of the tract below the stones.

Table 6.11 Investigation of patients with renal calculi

Investigation	Interpretation
Investigation of urinary tract	
Examination of urine for protein and red and white blood cells	Indicates abnormality of urinary tract
Quantitative urine culture (MSU)	Urinary infection
Plain radiograph of abdomen	Shows opaque calculi, nephrocalcinosis
IVU	Shows calculi, obstruction, abnormalities of urinary tract, e.g. medullary sponge kidney
Investigation of renal function	
Blood urea, plasma creatinine Creatinine clearance	Indicates renal function
Investigation to determine underlying cause	
Chemical analysis of the calculus	Provides information as to what investigations to pursue
Plasma calcium, phosphate	Hypercalcaemia
Plasma PTH	If hypercalcaemia present, to investigate possible hyperparathyroidism
24-hr urine calcium (× 2)	Hypercalciuria
Plasma urate and 24-hr urine urate (× 2)	In patients with urate or calcium stones
24-hr urine cystine (× 2)	In patients with cystine stones
24-hr urine oxalate (× 2)	Hyperoxaluria
Acidification of urine	Distal renal tubular acidosis (see p. 454)

Stones in the renal pelvis can be removed by open operation, endoscopically via a percutaneous nephrostomy or fragmented using the lithotriptor. Ureteric stones can be removed endoscopically via the bladder or a percutaneous nephrostomy, or can be pushed up into the renal pelvis and then removed through a nephrostomy or disintegrated by lithotripsy. Bladder stones are removed or fragmented during cystoscopy. Rarely, cystotomy is needed to remove large stones. Antibiotic cover should be given for stone removal.

INDICATIONS FOR INTERVENTION IN RENAL CALCULI

- The patient is anuric
- The ureter or pelvi-ureteric junction is obstructed, totally or partially, by a stone unlikely to pass spontaneously or one which has not moved for several weeks
- Infection is present
- The patient has intolerable or recurrent pain

In the longer term, a daily urine output of at least 2 litres is advisable in all patients with stone disease. Fluid intake should therefore be about 3 litres per day—more if the climate or the patient's occupation causes much sweating. Suitable measures should be instituted to correct any known cause of stone formation. Preparations containing vitamin D must be avoided.

Idiopathic hypercalciuria can be helped by reduction of sodium intake, and by the use of a thiazide diuretic. Reduction of calcium intake is not recommended unless it is very high, as it may lead to a negative overall calcium balance and reduction of bone mass, and causes increased oxalate absorption and excretion.

Citrate excretion can be increased by daily administration of potassium citrate or potassium bicarbonate. Alternatively, lemon juice may be a good dietary source. Hypokalaemia should be prevented as it leads to a reduction in citrate excretion.

In patients with recurrent oxalate stones, foods rich in this salt, such as rhubarb and spinach, should be avoided. Persons who have passed several uric acid or urate stones benefit from allopurinol, 100–300 mg daily, depending on renal function. Allopurinol also has a place in treating calcium oxalate stone disease, since urates may contribute by acting as a nidus for stone formation.

Phosphate-containing calculi are formed only in alkaline urine; hence acidifying the urine by giving ammonium chloride may be effective. In contrast, cystine and urate stones may be prevented, or sometimes dissolved, by giving sufficient sodium bicarbonate to make the urine persistently alkaline, and ensuring a high urine output of 2–4 litres/day. When these measures fail or are unacceptable to the patient, treatment with penicillamine, a chelating agent, in a dose of 1–1.5 g daily may be tried, although it is frequently associated with significant side-effects.

FURTHER INFORMATION ON URINARY TRACT CALCULI AND NEPHROCALCINOSIS

Bushinsky D A 1998 Nephrolithiasis. American Journal of Kidney Diseases 9: 917–924

Wickham J E 1993 Treatment of urinary tract stones. British Medical Journal 307: 1414–1417

DRUGS AND THE KIDNEY

PRESCRIBING IN RENAL DISEASE

Many drugs and drug metabolites are excreted by the kidney. The presence of renal impairment alters the required dose and frequency of those which are affected. This is discussed in Chapter 19 (see p. 1104).

DRUG-INDUCED RENAL DISEASE

The susceptibility of the kidney to damage by drugs stems from the fact that it is the route of excretion of many water-soluble compounds, including drugs and their metabolites. Some may reach high concentrations in the renal cortex as a result of proximal tubular transport mechanisms. Others are concentrated in the medulla by the operation of the counter-current system. The same applies to some toxins.

Toxic renal damage may occur at all levels (see Table 6.12), and sometimes by more than one mechanism. Very commonly, drugs contribute as one of multiple insults to the development of acute tubular necrosis. Haemodynamic renal impairment, acute tubular necrosis, and allergic reactions if recognised early enough, are usually reversible. However, other types, especially those associated with extensive fibrosis, are less likely to be reversible. Table 6.12 indicates some important mechanisms and examples. Numerically, reactions to NSAIDs and ACE inhibitors are the most important.

Non-steroidal anti-inflammatory drugs (NSAIDs)

NSAIDs have the predictable effect of impairing renal function in individuals where compensatory mechanisms are maintaining renal function (e.g. heart failure, cirrhosis, sepsis and renal impairment of almost any type), and may precipitate acute tubular necrosis in susceptible patients. This is a class effect that is related to alteration of essential prostaglandin-mediated vasodilatation. In addition, idiosyncratic immune reactions may occur: minimal change nephrotic syndrome and acute interstitial nephritis (see p. 448)—and frequently these may occur together. Analgesic nephropathy (see p. 449) is an occasional complication of long-term use.

Table 6.12 Mechanisms and examples of drug- and toxin-induced renal disease

Mechanisms	Drug or toxin*	Comments
Haemodynamic	NSAIDs	Especially as a cofactor. Via inhibition of prostaglandin synthesis
	ACE inhibitors	Reduce efferent glomerular arteriolar tone. Toxic in the presence of renal artery stenosis and other conditions of renal hypoperfusion
	Radiographic contrast media	Effect mediated via intense vasoconstriction, but this may not be the primary effect of these drugs
Acute tubular necrosis	Aminoglycosides, amphotericin	In most examples there is evidence of direct tubular toxicity, but haemodynamic and other factors probably contribute
	Paracetamol	May occur with or without serious hepatotoxicity
	Others	Drugs often act as one of several cofactors
	Radiographic contrast media	May be secondary to precipitation in tubules. Frusemide is a cofactor
Loss of tubular/collecting duct function	Lithium	Dose-related, partially reversible loss of concentrating ability
	Cisplatin	
	Aminoglycosides, amphotericin	At lower exposures than cause ATN
Immune (glomerular)	Penicillamine, gold	Membranous nephropathy
	Mercury and heavy metals	Membranous nephropathy
	Penicillamine	Crescentic or focal necrotising glomerulonephritis in association with ANCA and systemic small-vessel vasculitis
	NSAIDs	Minimal change nephropathy
Immune (interstitial)	NSAIDs, penicillins, many others	Acute interstitial nephritis
Chronic interstitial nephritis (alone)	Lithium	As a consequence of acute toxicity. Otherwise, controversial
	Cyclosporin, tacrolimus	The major problem with these drugs
	Lead, cadmium	Consequence of chronic toxicity
	Bence Jones protein	Only some light chains are nephrotoxic
	Ochratoxin and other fungal toxins	Produced by *Aspergillus* species. Putative cause of Balkan nephropathy
	Aristolochic acid and other plant toxins	Found in Aristolochia clematis. Putative cause of 'Chinese herb' nephropathy
Chronic interstitial nephritis (with papillary necrosis)	Various analgesics	See text (p. 449)
Obstruction (crystal formation)	Aciclovir	Crystals of the drug form in tubules. Aciclovir is now more common than the original example of sulphonamides
	Chemotherapy	Uric acid crystals forming as a consequence of tumour lysis (typically a first-dose effect in haematological malignancy)
Retroperitoneal fibrosis	Methysergide*, practolol*	Idiopathic is more common

*These drugs are no longer in use in the UK.

Angiotensin-converting enzyme (ACE) inhibitors

ACE inhibitors abolish the compensatory angiotensin II-mediated vasoconstriction of the glomerular efferent arteriole that occurs to maintain glomerular perfusion pressure distal to a renal artery stenosis (see Fig. 6.1, p. 419). If the stenosis is bilateral, or occurs in a single functioning kidney, an acute deterioration in renal function occurs. These drugs are increasingly used in patient groups at high risk of atherosclerotic renal artery stenosis, so the reaction is common, and monitoring of renal function before and after initiation of therapy is essential.

TUMOURS OF THE KIDNEY AND GENITO-URINARY TRACT

TUMOURS OF THE KIDNEY

RENAL CARCINOMA

Between 1% and 2% of malignant tumours arise in the kidney. Renal adenocarcinoma, the most common form, occurs most frequently in adult men. Occasionally, the affected kidney contains multiple tumours, or both kidneys are involved.

Pathology

The tumour, which is composed of large cells with clear cytoplasm, arises from the proximal tubular epithelium. The cut surface appears yellow, and large tumours contain haemorrhagic or cystic areas. Local spread is by penetration of the renal capsule and invasion of renal veins. Spread to the opposite kidney occurs via the veins. The tumour is vascular, and metastasises to regional lymph nodes, bone, lung and liver.

Clinical features

Haematuria is the most common presenting symptom. About 20% of patients present late with haematuria, pain in the loin or renal colic, and a palpable mass in the flank. In 30%, changes due to systemic effects of tumour metabolites are the first indication of disease (see Table 6.13). These effects resolve after nephrectomy and must not be attributed to

Table 6.13 Syndromes associated with renal carcinoma

Findings	% of patients with renal tumour with this finding	Comments
Raised ESR	55	Changes in serum proteins associated with many tumours
Hypertension	37	Secretion of renin by tumour
Anaemia	36	Depression of erythropoiesis +/– haematuria
Weight loss	34	Tumour products depress appetite
Pyrexia	17	Circulating pyrogens
Abnormal liver function	14	This may disappear after nephrectomy
Raised alkaline phosphatase	9	Secreted by tumour?
Hypercalcaemia	5	Parathyroid hormone-like peptide secretion by tumour
Polycythaemia	4	Erythropoietin secretion
Neuromyopathy	3	Tumour-associated antibodies to nerve tissue
Amyloidosis	2	Possibly associated with immunological reactions to the tumour

metastases. Approximately 30% of patients present with established metastases.

Investigations

Investigations are designed to demonstrate the presence of a solid tumour, to make a specific histological or cytological diagnosis, and to determine the extent of local, lymph node and haematogenous spread of the tumour.

Ultrasound examination reveals the mass and differentiates it from simple cysts and most other pathologies. It can also demonstrate invasion of the renal vein and local lymph nodes. IVU is less sensitive but usually shows splaying and distortion of the collecting system, or a cyst. Cyst fluid or tumour cells can be aspirated under ultrasound control and the cytology examined. The size of the tumour can be assessed from the IVU and ultrasound. CT is of value in determining spread through the renal capsule (see Fig. 6.8, p. 424). Invasion of the renal vein and vena cava can usually be shown by ultrasound, although occasionally pre-operative venography is required (see Fig. 6.7, p. 423). Spread to lymph nodes can be assessed by CT, and haematogenous metastases detected by chest radiograph, CT and radionuclide bone scanning.

Management

Early surgery affords the only real prospect of cure. The treatment of choice is removal of the affected kidney, en bloc, within the perinephric fascia. Simultaneous removal of the adrenal gland and regional lymph nodes is performed. The 5-year survival for tumours confined to the kidney is 60–75%. For all grades of tumour it is approximately 30%.

Partial nephrectomy may be performed for carcinoma of a solitary kidney or tumour involving both kidneys. If all renal tissue must be removed, chronic dialysis is instituted. Treatment of advanced disease is unsatisfactory. Nephrectomy or arterial embolisation of the kidney may be necessary for loin pain or haematuria. Radiotherapy often relieves pain due to metastases, and progesterone-like hormones may slow the advance of metastatic disease. However, neither radiotherapy, chemotherapy, hormonal therapy nor immunotherapy has had a substantial impact on the prognosis.

NEPHROBLASTOMA (WILMS TUMOUR)

This is the second most common malignant tumour of the kidney. It presents in the first decade, and often in the first year of life, most commonly as an abdominal mass. Haematuria tends to occur late in the disease. The tumour is radiosensitive, and responds to chemotherapy (see p. 1056). The best hope of cure is early diagnosis.

TUMOUR SYNDROMES

Two uncommon inherited conditions are associated with the formation of multiple renal tumours in adult life. In tuberous sclerosis (see p. 916) replacement of renal tissue by multiple angiomyolipomas (tubers) may occasionally cause renal failure in adult life. Other organs affected include the skin (adenoma sebaceum on the face) and brain (seizures and mental retardation). Von Hippel–Lindau syndrome is associated with the formation of multiple renal cysts and tumours, including multiple renal adenomas and carcinomas. Other problems include CNS haemangioblastomas and hypertension caused by phaeochromocytoma. Bilateral nephrectomy may need to be undertaken. Both of these conditions are transmitted as autosomal dominant traits.

Patients with a very long history of renal impairment (usually on long-term dialysis) often develop multiple renal cysts. These are associated with increased erythropoietin production, and sometimes with the development of renal cell carcinoma.

TUMOURS OF THE RENAL PELVIS, URETER AND BLADDER

These are histologically similar to each other, usually being transitional cell carcinomas. They spread locally by direct invasion, and also by implantation to other parts of the urinary tract. While some are benign, e.g. papillomas, all urinary tract tumours are liable to recur, even after apparently adequate treatment. The bladder is by far the most common site. Epidemiological studies have shown that males are more often affected, and that this tumour is particularly likely to develop in patients who work in industries such as dyeing and printing, where there may be exposure to aniline, in areas endemic for urinary schistosomiasis, in heavy smokers and as a complication of analgesic nephropathy and Balkan nephropathy.

Clinical features

Painless haematuria is commonly the sole presenting symptom. Unexplained frequency, dysuria or symptoms due to urinary tract obstruction also occur. The features of urinary infection may be superimposed.

Investigations

Patients with haematuria but normal ultrasound examination should have an IVU. Carcinoma in the renal pelvis appears as an abnormality on the urogram (see Fig. 6.4C, p. 422). If the IVU is normal, cystoscopy is performed, unless the patient is young and the haematuria obviously associated with urinary infection. In such a case the patient should be followed up, and cystoscopy carried out if haematuria persists. Biopsy of suspicious lesions can be performed at cystoscopy. Urinary cytology may indicate the need for cystoscopy or an initial investigation. Local spread from tumours of the renal pelvis is apparent on CT. Local spread of bladder tumours is assessed by bimanual examination under anaesthesia, from appearances at cystoscopy and from the histology. Spread to lymph nodes is assessed by CT, and metastasis elsewhere by chest radiograph, bone scan and liver function tests.

Management

Renal pelvic and ureteric tumours are treated by nephroureterectomy. Radiotherapy and chemotherapy are of little value. These patients may develop bladder tumours later, and therefore require regular follow-up by cystoscopy. Localised, well-differentiated bladder tumours (approximately 60% of such tumours) are treated by diathermy. Cystoscopy should be performed at yearly intervals thereafter to detect recurrence. Treatment of histologically malignant tumours or those which have spread beyond the bladder mucosa is unsatisfactory. Extensive superficial tumour can be treated by intravesical chemotherapy, and locally invasive lesions with radiotherapy. If this fails or the patient has severe bladder symptoms, total cystectomy and transplantation of the ureters into an ileal conduit may be required. Systemic methotrexate and cisplatin have been used to treat metastases but results are poor. Analgesics and palliative radiotherapy are used to relieve pain. The 5-year survival of patients with superficial well-differentiated lesions is 90%, whilst in those with invasive, poorly differentiated tumours it is 30%.

PROSTATIC DISEASE

BENIGN PROSTATIC HYPERTROPHY

This is most commonly found in men over 60, and may be associated with diminished androgen secretion. Histologically, the inner zone of the gland undergoes hyperplasia and hypertrophy, and there is an increase in fibromuscular stroma. The enlarged prostate obstructs the outflow of urine by compressing, displacing, distorting and elongating the prostatic urethra, with the effects on bladder and renal function referred to on page 462. Clinical features are those of progressive obstruction to urinary flow. Acute urinary retention may arise if the gland suddenly increases in size because of superimposed infection or congestion, or if cardiac failure develops in the elderly. In this situation, the patient has a sudden desire to micturate but is unable to do so, and the bladder becomes tense and tender. Chronic retention may pass unnoticed for some time, but there is a gradual increase in the volume of urine which remains in the bladder after micturition. Haematuria due to urethral bleeding may also occur and may be the presenting symptom. On rectal examination the prostate may feel large, elastic and uniform in consistency. When the median lobe alone is affected, the prostate feels normal and the condition can be recognised only by cystoscopy. Alpha-adrenoceptor antagonists may provide symptomatic relief. Transurethral resection of prostatic tissue is the treatment of choice to relieve the outflow obstruction.

PROSTATIC CARCINOMA

Adenocarcinoma of the prostate accounts for 70% of all cancers in men and causes 19 deaths/100 000 males annually in the UK, mostly in men over 50. Autopsy reports indicate that many men over 80 have latent foci of prostatic cancer.

Clinical features

Prostatic carcinoma may be found incidentally on examination of tissue removed during transurethral resection for supposedly benign prostatic hypertrophy. It may also present with symptoms of urethral obstruction similar to those of the benign condition. Local spread can cause pain, incontinence and sometimes acute renal failure due to involvement of the lower ends of both ureters. Patients may present with bone pain due to metastases. On examination per rectum, the prostate is hard and the median furrow often obliterated. Spread of tumour is often associated with increased serum prostate-specific antigen (PSA) which acts as a tumour marker.

Investigations

The diagnosis depends on the clinical findings and examination of biopsy material. Local invasion is assessed by bimanual examination under anaesthesia and by ultrasound. Screening for metastasis includes measurement of serum PSA, isotope bone scan, radiographs of bones and chest, and liver function tests.

Management

When asymptomatic disease is discovered incidentally, it may be best to defer treatment until symptoms develop, particularly in older men. Nevertheless, radical prostatectomy, pelvic radiotherapy and hormonal treatment designed to deprive the tumour of androgens have been advocated for these cases. When symptoms or evidence of local spread are present, radiotherapy or androgen deprivation is indicated. The latter can be achieved by administration of oestrogens or gonadotrophin-releasing hormone analogues, or by orchidectomy. Stilboestrol has a useful palliative action. The dose should be restricted to 1–3 mg daily by mouth, as larger doses, in addition to their feminising effects, are associated with an increased risk of cardiovascular complications. Alternatively, a gonadotrophin-releasing hormone analogue such as buserelin can be given by subcutaneous injection as 500 mg 8-hourly for 7 days. Thereafter, 100 mg doses delivered by a metered-dose nasal spray are instilled into the nostrils 4-hourly. During the early days of therapy, tumour growth may increase. Cyproterone acetate, which blocks the effect of androgens on target tissue, can be used as a second-line drug, 100 mg orally 8-hourly. Transurethral resection may be required to relieve obstruction. Metastatic disease can be treated by androgen deprivation or palliative radiotherapy or, if these measures fail, hypophysectomy. Trials of chemotherapy are in progress.

TESTICULAR TUMOURS

These are the most common form of malignant disease in men aged 25–34 years. The lesion may be a seminoma arising from spermatogonia, a teratoma from totipotential germ cells, or a combined tumour. These tumours occur in otherwise fit young men and should nowadays be regarded as curable. Early diagnosis and appropriate specialist treatment are essential.

Clinical features

A seminoma presents as a painless, often uniform, rapid enlargement of the testis. A teratoma causes more nodular changes and may secrete chorionic gonadotrophin, producing gynaecomastia. The tumour may be overlooked if obscured by a hydrocele or if the examination is inadequate. Some cases present with metastases.

Investigations

Spread to regional lymph nodes can be demonstrated by CT. Screening for metastases should include chest radiograph and liver function tests.

Management

The tumour should be removed using the inguinal approach. Histology gives some idea of prognosis. A seminoma confined to the testicle or with metastasis below the diaphragm is treated by radiotherapy, to which it is very sensitive. More widespread seminoma requires chemotherapy; this is the treatment of choice for teratoma. The usual agents are cisplatin and bleomycin. Circulating tumour markers (alphafetoprotein, human chorionic gonadotrophin and lactic dehydrogenase) are of help in assessing response to treatment and for monitoring patients in remission.

FURTHER INFORMATION ON TUMOURS OF THE KIDNEY AND GENITOURINARY TRACT

Farmer A, Noble J 1997 Drug treatment for benign prostatic hyperplasia. British Medical Journal 314: 1215–1216

Mulley A G Jnr, Barry M J 1998 Controversy in managing patients with prostate cancer. British Medical Journal 316: 1919–1920

Diabetes mellitus, and nutritional and metabolic disorders

7

B.M. FRIER • A.S. TRUSWELL • J. SHEPHERD • A. DE LOOY • R. JUNG

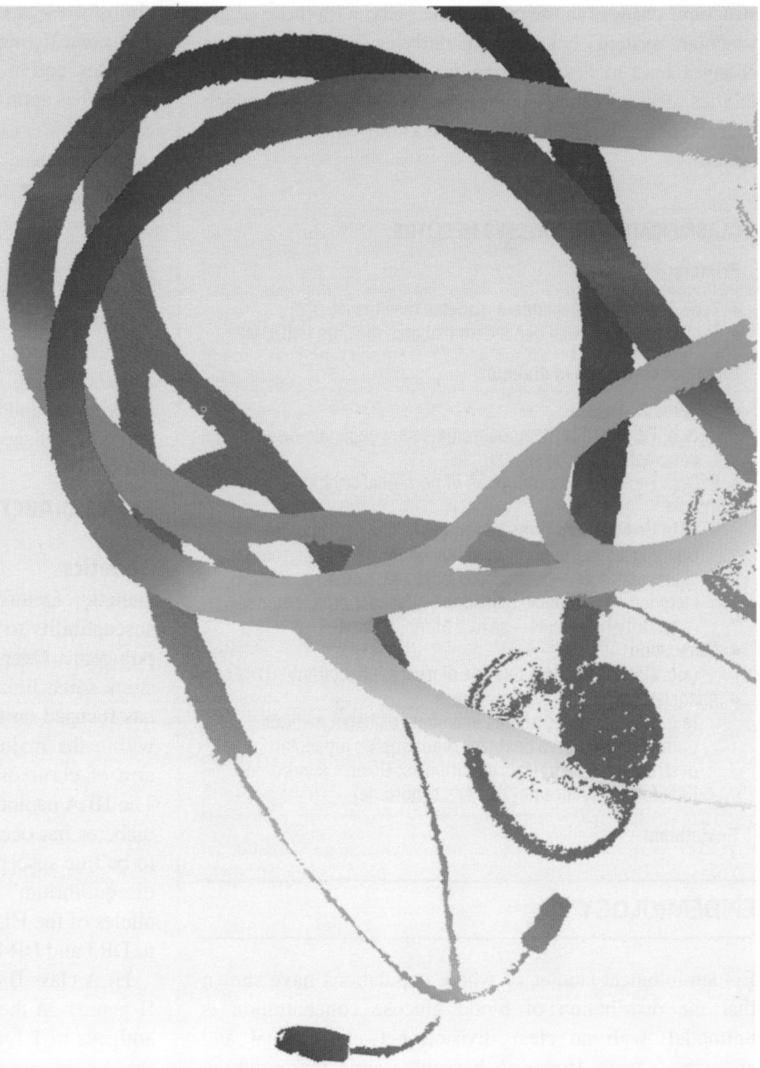

DIABETES MELLITUS

Diabetes mellitus is a clinical syndrome characterised by hyperglycaemia due to absolute or relative deficiency of insulin. This can arise in many different ways (see the information box). Lack of insulin affects the metabolism of carbohydrate, protein and fat, and causes a significant disturbance of water and electrolyte homeostasis. Death may result from acute metabolic decompensation while long-standing metabolic derangement is frequently associated with permanent and irreversible functional and structural changes in the cells of the body, with those of the vascular system being particularly susceptible. These changes lead to the development of well-defined clinical entities, the so-called 'complications of diabetes' which characteristically affect the eye, the kidney and the nervous system.

CLASSIFICATION OF DIABETES MELLITUS
Primary
• Type 1 or insulin dependent diabetes mellitus (IDDM) • Type 2 or non-insulin dependent diabetes mellitus (NIDDM)
Other specific types of diabetes
• Pancreatic disease (e.g. Pancreatitis, haemochromatosis, neoplastic disease, pancreatectomy, cystic fibrosis) • Excess endogenous production of hormonal antagonists to insulin (e.g. Growth hormone—acromegaly, glucocorticoids—Cushing's syndrome, thyroid hormones—hyperthyroidism, catecholamines—phaeochromocytoma, human placental lactogen—pregnancy, glucagon—glucagonoma, counter-regulatory hormones—severe burns, trauma) • Medication (e.g. Corticosteroids, thiazide diuretics, phenytoin) • Associated with genetic syndromes (e.g. DIDMOAD—diabetes insipidus, diabetes mellitus, optic atrophy, nerve deafness; lipoatrophy; muscular dystrophies; Friedreich's dystrophies; Down's syndrome; Klinefelter's syndrome; Turner's syndrome)
Gestational

EPIDEMIOLOGY

Epidemiological studies of whole populations have shown that the distribution of blood glucose concentration is unimodal, with no clear division between normal and abnormal values. However, hyperglycaemia represents an independent risk factor for the development of disease of both small and large blood vessels. Diagnostic criteria for diabetes (see Table 7.5, p. 481) have therefore been selected on the basis of identifying those who have a degree of hyperglycaemia which, if untreated, is associated with a significantly increased risk of developing (principally micro-)vascular disease. The implication of these criteria is that there is no such thing as 'mild' diabetes not requiring effective treatment.

Diabetes is world-wide in distribution and the incidence of both types of primary diabetes, i.e. type 1 or insulin dependent diabetes mellitus (IDDM) and type 2 or non-insulin dependent diabetes mellitus (NIDDM), is rising. However, the prevalence of both varies considerably in different parts of the world and this is probably due to differences in genetic and environmental factors. The prevalence of both types in Britain is between 1 and 2% but almost 50% of cases of type 2 diabetes remain undetected. The great majority of cases seen world-wide have primary diabetes, and in Europe and North America the ratio of type 2:type 1 is approximately 7:3.

AETIOLOGY

Although the precise aetiology of both main types of primary diabetes is uncertain, environmental factors interact with a genetic susceptibility to determine which of those with the genetic predisposition develop the clinical syndrome, and the timing of its onset. However, both the pattern of inheritance and the environmental factors differ in type 1 and type 2 diabetes.

TYPE 1 DIABETES (IDDM)

Genetics

Genetic factors account for about one-third of the susceptibility to type 1 diabetes, the inheritance of which is polygenic. Over 20 different regions of the human genome show some linkage with type 1 diabetes but most interest has focused on the human leucocyte antigen (HLA) region within the major histocompatibility complex on the short arm of chromosome 6; this locus is designated *IDDM 1*. The HLA haplotypes DR3 and/or DR4 predispose to type 1 diabetes but occur too frequently in Caucasian populations to be true susceptibility genes. These alleles are in 'linkage disequilibrium' with true susceptibility loci (probably alleles of the HLA-DQA1 and DQB1 genes which lie close to DR3 and DR4), i.e. they tend to be transmitted together.

HLA class II antigens (which are coded by the LA class II genes) on the surface of cells present foreign and self-antigens to T lymphocytes and play a key role in initiating the autoimmune response. Some polymorphisms of the HLA-DQB1 gene that result in specific amino-acid substitutions in the β chains of class II antigens may affect the ability of the class II molecule to accept and present autoantigens derived from pancreatic islet beta cells, and will so determine whether or not autoimmune damage will take place. Variants of the DQ β chain which carry an uncharged amino-acid residue (e.g. alanine, serine or valine) at position 57 appear to be diabetogenic, whereas the presence of aspartate is protective against type 1 diabetes.

The region of the insulin gene on chromosome 11p (now designated *IDDM 2*) is also linked with type 1 diabetes. Insulin or its precursors may act as a beta-cell autoantigen or alternatively the level of insulin production could determine the activity of the beta cell and its expression of other autoantigens. Other weaker diabetes susceptibility loci include *IDDM 3*, *IDDM 4* and *IDDM 5* which lie on chromosomes 15q, 11q and 6q respectively, but their gene products and modes of action are unknown.

Environmental factors

Although genetic susceptibility appears to be a prerequisite for the development of type 1 diabetes, the concordance rate between monozygotic twins is less than 40%, and environmental factors have an important role in promoting clinical expression of the disease.

Viruses

The evidence that viral infection might cause some forms of type 1 diabetes is derived from studies where virus particles known to cause cytopathic or autoimmune damage to β cells have been isolated from the pancreas. Several viruses have been implicated, including infection with mumps, Coxsackie B4, retroviruses, rubella (in utero), cytomegalovirus and Epstein–Barr virus, although the putative mechanisms by which they may induce type 1 diabetes differ.

Diet

Circumstantial evidence supports the proposition that dietary factors may, at least in certain circumstances, influence the development of type 1 diabetes. Bovine serum albumin (BSA), a major constituent of cow's milk, has been implicated in triggering type 1 diabetes. It has been shown that children who are given cow's milk early in infancy are more likely to develop type 1 diabetes than those who are breastfed. BSA may cross the neonatal gut and raise antibodies which, because of the close homology between BSA, the β chain of HLA class II antigens and a heat-shock protein expressed by beta cells, could cross-react with, and cause damage to, beta cell components.

Various nitrosamines (found in smoked and cured meats) and coffee have been proposed as potentially diabetogenic factors. In susceptible animals such as the diabetes-prone BB rat, various dietary proteins (e.g. gluten) may be essential for the expression of clinical type 1 diabetes.

Stress

Stress may progress the development of type 1 diabetes by stimulating the secretion of counter-regulatory hormones and possibly by modulating immune activity.

EVIDENCE THAT TYPE 1 DIABETES IS A T CELL-MEDIATED AUTOIMMUNE DISEASE

- HLA-linked genetic predisposition
- Association with other autoimmune disorders
- Circulating islet cell cytoplasmic and surface and insulin-autoantibodies in new cases
- Presence of circulating T-cell abnormalities
- Mononuclear cell infiltration of pancreatic islets resulting in selective destruction of insulin-secreting cells
- Recurrence of insulitis and selective destruction of insulin-secreting cells in pancreatic grafts
- Induction of remission by immunosuppressive drugs such as cyclosporin

Immunological factors

The information box summarises the evidence that type 1 diabetes is a slow T cell-mediated autoimmune disease. Family studies have produced evidence that destruction of the insulin-secreting cells in the pancreatic islets takes place over many years. Hyperglycaemia accompanied by the classical symptoms of diabetes occurs only when 90% of beta cells have been destroyed. In humans and animals with spontaneous type 1 diabetes the immune system retains the capacity to recognise and destroy transplanted pancreatic beta cells indefinitely.

Pancreatic pathology

The pathological picture in the pre-diabetic pancreas in type 1 diabetes is characterised by:

- 'insulitis' (see Fig. 7.1, p. 474)—that is, infiltration of the islets with mononuclear cells containing activated macrophages, helper cytotoxic and suppressor T lymphocytes, natural killer cells and B lymphocytes
- the initial patchiness of this lesion, with, until a very late stage, lobules containing heavily infiltrated islets seen adjacent to unaffected lobules
- the striking beta cell specificity of the destructive process, with the glucagon and other hormone-secreting cells in the islet invariably remaining intact.

Islet cell antibodies can be detected before the clinical development of type 1 diabetes and have a variable predictive value as a marker of disease (see Table 7.1, p. 474). However, at present they are not suitable for screening programmes, and disappear with increasing duration of diabetes.

TYPE 2 DIABETES (NIDDM)

Type 2 diabetes commonly occurs in subjects who are obese and insulin-resistant but these two factors alone are insufficient to cause diabetes unless accompanied by impaired beta cell function.

Genetics

Genetic factors are more important in the aetiology of type

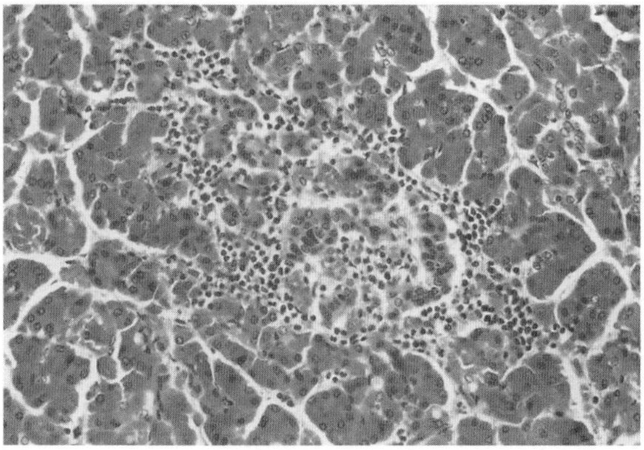

A

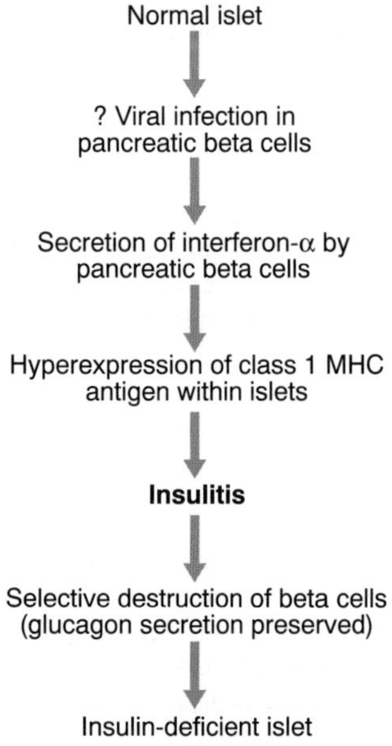

B

Fig. 7.1 Proposed pathogenesis of type 1 diabetes.
A Insulitis, showing chronic inflammatory cell infiltrate in a pancreatic islet. B Proposed sequence of events in the development of type 1 diabetes. (MHC = major histocompatibility complex)

Table 7.1 Islet cell antibodies in type 1 diabetes

	Predictive value* First-degree relatives	General population
Islet cell antibodies	20–50%	20–30%
Islet cell surface antibodies	ND	ND
Cytotoxic islet cell antibodies	ND	ND
Insulin autoantibodies	< 50%	ND
Glutamate decarboxylase (GAD65)	< 50%	ND

(ND = not determined)
* Predictive value estimated during long-term follow-up until development of type 1 diabetes in marker-positive healthy individuals.

2 than type 1 diabetes, as shown by studies in monozygotic twins where concordance rates for type 2 diabetes approach 100%. Molecular genetics has allowed the identification of certain specific, and clinically identifiable, forms of type 2 diabetes, which are the result of single gene defects (see Table 7.2). However, these subtypes, such as the syndrome of maturity onset diabetes of the young (MODY), are uncommon and constitute less than 5% of all cases of type 2 diabetes.

The majority of cases of type 2 diabetes are multifactorial in nature, with interaction of environmental and genetic factors. The nature of the genetic contribution is largely unknown, but it is evident that several genes are involved. In this polygenic model, inheritance of abnormalities in individual genes would not be sufficient to cause type 2 diabetes directly, but would confer an increased (or decreased) susceptibility. A variety of candidate susceptibility genes have been investigated, such as those for insulin, the insulin receptor, glucose transporters and glycogen synthase, but to date little or no association has been shown with multifactorial type 2 diabetes.

Environmental factors

Lifestyle

Epidemiological studies of type 2 diabetes provide evidence that overeating, especially when combined with obesity and underactivity, is associated with the development of type 2 diabetes. Other more direct studies have shown that middle-aged diabetic patients eat significantly more and are fatter and less active than their non-diabetic siblings. Although the majority of middle-aged diabetic patients are obese, only a few obese people develop diabetes. Obesity probably acts as a diabetogenic factor (through increasing resistance to the action of insulin) in those genetically predisposed to develop type 2 diabetes.

Malnutrition in utero

Retrospective analysis of the birth weight of males born in England in the 1930s has demonstrated an inverse relationship between weight at birth and at 1 year, and the development of type 2 diabetes in late adulthood. It is proposed (but not yet proven) that malnutrition in utero and in infancy may damage beta cell development at a critical period, predisposing to type 2 diabetes later in life.

Age

Age is an important risk factor for type 2 diabetes. In Britain over 70% of all cases of diabetes occur after the age of 50 years. Type 2 diabetes is principally a disease of the middle-aged and elderly, affecting 10% of the population over the age of 65.

Table 7.2 Single gene disorders associated with subtypes of type 2 diabetes

Gene	Inheritance	Metabolic abnormality	Clinical features
Hepatocyte nuclear factor 4α (HNF 4α)	Autosomal dominant	Impaired insulin secretion	Rare, progressive form of early onset disease (MODY 1)
Glucokinase	Autosomal dominant	Impaired insulin secretion	Mild and relatively stable early onset disease (MODY 2)
Hepatocyte nuclear factor 1α (HNF 1α)	Autosomal dominant	Impaired insulin secretion	Progressive early onset disease (MODY 3)
Mitochondrial DNA	Maternal	Impaired insulin secretion	Diabetes may be associated with deafness or MELAS syndrome
Insulin	Autosomal dominant	Defective insulin produced	Very rare
Insulin receptor	Autosomal dominant or recessive	Impaired insulin signalling	Severe insulin resistance
(MODY = maturity onset diabetes of the young; MELAS = syndrome of mitochondrial encephalopathy, lactic acidosis and stroke)			

Pregnancy

During normal pregnancy, insulin sensitivity is reduced through the action of placental hormones and this affects glucose tolerance. The insulin-secreting cells of the pancreatic islets may be unable to meet this increased demand in women genetically predisposed to develop either of the primary types of diabetes. The term 'gestational diabetes' refers to hyperglycaemia occurring for the first time during pregnancy (see p. 506). Repeated pregnancy may increase the likelihood of developing permanent diabetes, particularly in obese women; 80% of women with gestational diabetes ultimately develop permanent clinical diabetes requiring treatment.

Pathogenesis of type 2 diabetes

Insulin resistance

Increased hepatic production of glucose and resistance to the action of insulin in muscle are invariable in both obese and non-obese patients with type 2 diabetes. Insulin resistance may be due to any one of three general causes: an abnormal insulin molecule, an excessive amount of circulating antagonists, or target tissue defects. The last is the most common cause of insulin resistance in type 2 diabetes and seems to be the predominant abnormality in those with more severe hyperglycaemia.

A characteristic feature of type 2 diabetes is that it is often associated with other medical disorders including obesity, hypertension and hyperlipidaemia. It has been suggested that this cluster of conditions, all of which predispose to cardiovascular disease, is a specific entity (the 'metabolic syndrome' or 'syndrome X'), with insulin resistance being the primary defect (see Fig. 7.2).

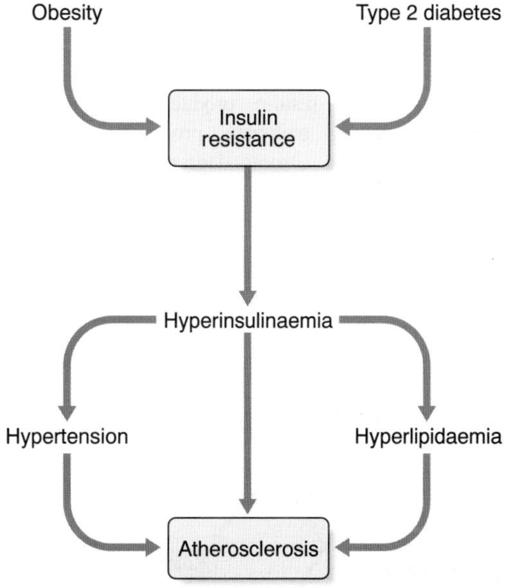

Fig. 7.2 Associations between insulin resistance, hyperinsulinaemia and promotion of atherosclerosis. Hypertension, hyperlipidaemia and central (abdominal) obesity are commonly associated with type 2 diabetes and this cluster of medical conditions is known as the 'metabolic syndrome'. Affected individuals have premature or accelerated macrovascular disease (coronary, cerebral and peripheral vascular disease).

Pancreatic beta cell failure

In type 2 diabetes there is only moderate reduction in the total mass of pancreatic islet tissue consistent with a measurable though, when related to the blood glucose level, reduced concentration of insulin in plasma. However, some pathological changes are typical of type 2 diabetes, the most consistent of which is deposition of amyloid. This is accompanied by atrophy of the normal tissue, particularly islet epithelial cells. Islet amyloid is composed of insoluble fibrils formed from islet amyloid polypeptide (also known as amylin). Small quantities of islet amyloid are very common in elderly non-diabetic patients, and the role of islet amyloid in the pathogenesis of type 2 diabetes is uncertain. Deposition of amyloid is probably not a cause of diabetes but rather reflects a pathological process which is increased in type 2 diabetes. More extensive amyloidosis is, however, found in patients who have progressed to insulin replacement therapy, suggesting that islet function may become compromised by amyloid deposition.

While beta cell numbers are reduced by 20–30% in type 2 diabetes, alpha cell mass is unchanged and glucagon secretion is increased, and this may contribute to the hyperglycaemia. Insulin resistance tends to raise blood glucose and stimulate insulin secretion to prevent hyperglycaemia. When the maximal insulin secretory capacity has been exceeded, any further increase in fasting blood glucose levels causes a decline in insulin generation (see Fig. 7.3). Possible mechanisms for beta cell decompensation include glucotoxicity, an intrinsic failure of insulin production, a switch to abnormal processing pathways producing biologically inactive products and chronic degranulation of the beta cell.

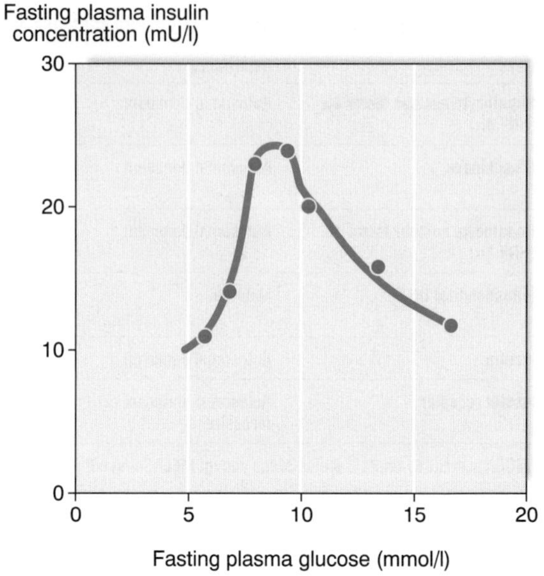

Fig. 7.3 Insulin secretory capacity in type 2 diabetes. In the natural history of pancreatic beta cell function in type 2 diabetes, insulin secretion initially increases to compensate for insulin resistance, but eventually fails, leading to type 2 diabetes. The fasting plasma insulin concentrations associated with the fasting plasma glucose are shown. This profile has been termed the 'Starling curve of the pancreas'.

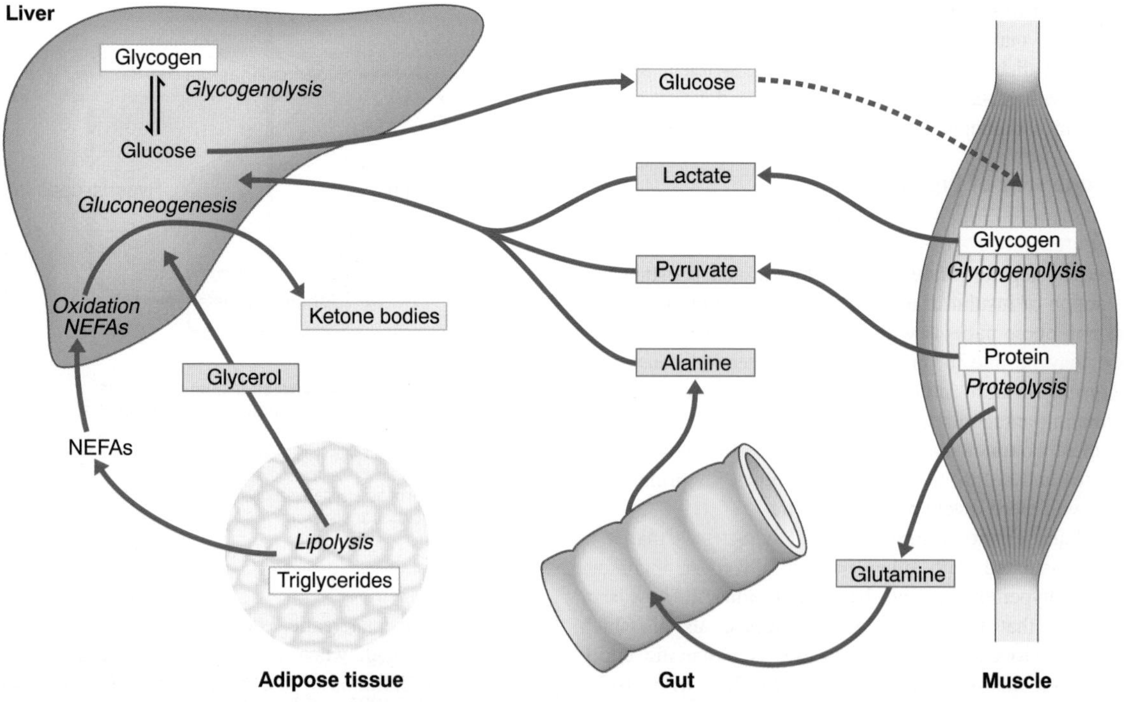

Fig. 7.4 Major gluconeogenic substrates and their tissues of origin. Insulin suppresses gluconeogenesis and promotes glycogenolysis. It promotes the peripheral uptake of glucose, particularly in skeletal muscle, and encourages storage (as muscle glycogen) and protein synthesis. Insulin promotes lipogenesis and suppresses lipolysis. These processes are reversed in the absence of insulin.

PATHOPHYSIOLOGY

Normal glucose metabolism and homeostasis

In humans, blood glucose is tightly regulated by homeostatic mechanisms and maintained within a narrow range of 3.5–6.5 mmol/l. A balance is preserved between the entry of glucose into the circulation from the liver, supplemented by intestinal absorption after meals, and glucose uptake by peripheral tissues, particularly skeletal muscle. A steady supply of glucose is essential for the brain, which uses glucose as its principal metabolic fuel.

When intestinal glucose absorption declines between meals, hepatic glucose output is increased in response to the counter-regulatory hormones, glucagon and adrenaline, and it falls during prolonged starvation as other metabolic fuels derived from fat become more important. The liver produces glucose by gluconeogenesis and glycogen breakdown. The main substrates for gluconeogenesis are shown in Figure 7.4.

Insulin is the only anabolic hormone and it has profound effects on the metabolism of carbohydrate, fat and protein (see Table 7.3, p. 478). Insulin is secreted from pancreatic beta cells into the portal circulation, with a brisk increase in response to a rise in blood glucose (e.g. after meals). Some characteristics of normal insulin secretion are shown in Figure 7.5. Insulin lowers blood glucose by suppressing hepatic glucose production and stimulating peripheral glucose uptake, mainly in skeletal muscle and fat, mediated by the glucose transporter, GLUT 4.

Adipocytes (and the liver) synthesise triglyceride from non-esterified fatty acids (NEFAs) and glycerol. Insulin stimulates lipogenesis and inhibits lipolysis, so preventing fat catabolism. Lipolysis, mediated by triglyceride lipase, is stimulated by catecholamines, and liberates NEFAs which can be oxidised by many tissues. Their partial oxidation in the liver provides energy to drive gluconeogenesis and also produces ketone bodies (acetoacetate, which can be oxidised to 3-hydroxybutyrate or condensed to acetone) which are generated in hepatocyte mitochondria. Ketone bodies are organic acids which, when formed in small amounts, are oxidised and utilised as metabolic fuel. However, the rate of utilisation of ketone bodies by peripheral tissues is limited, and when the rate of production by the liver exceeds their removal, hyperketonaemia results. Ketogenesis is regulated by the supply of NEFAs reaching the liver and is therefore enhanced by insulin deficiency and release of the counter-regulatory hormones that stimulate lipolysis.

Metabolic disturbances in diabetes

The hyperglycaemia of diabetes develops because of an absolute (type 1 diabetes) or a relative (type 2 diabetes)

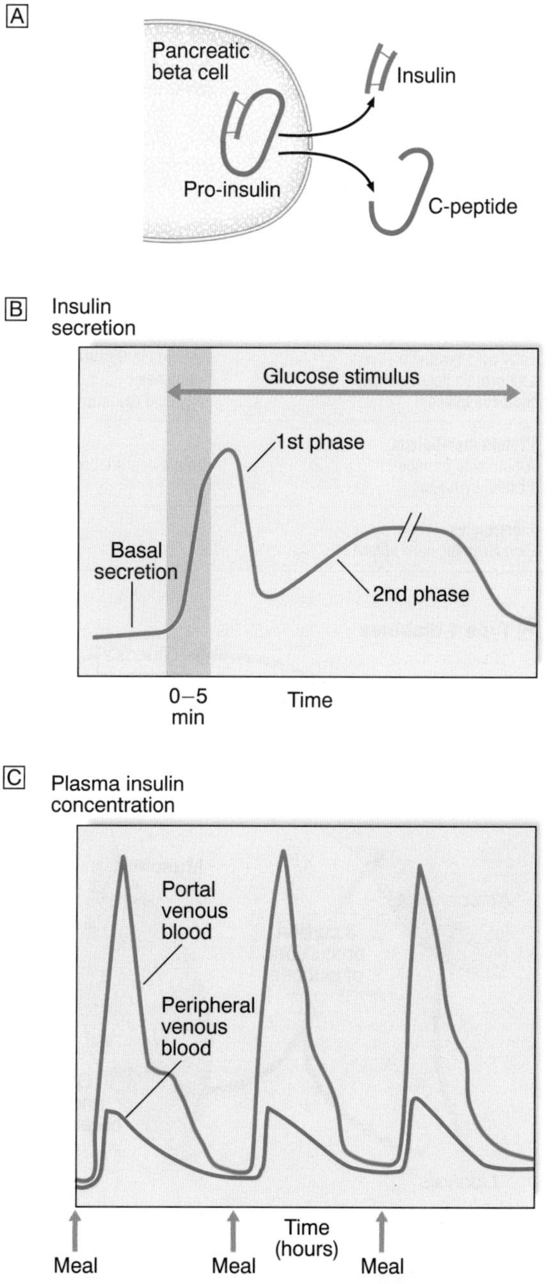

Fig. 7.5 Normal physiology of insulin secretion. A Pro-insulin in the pancreatic beta cell is cleaved to release insulin and equimolar amounts of inert C-peptide (connecting peptide). Measurement of C-peptide can be used to assess endogenous insulin secretory capacity. B An acute first phase of insulin secretion occurs in response to an elevated blood glucose, followed by a sustained second phase. C Plasma insulin concentrations are much higher in the portal vein than in peripheral venous blood.

Table 7.3 Actions of insulin

Increase (anabolic effects)	Decrease (anticatabolic effects)
Carbohydrate metabolism	
Glucose transport (muscle, adipose tissue)	Gluconeogenesis
Glucose phosphorylation	Glycogenolysis
Glycogenesis	
Glycolysis	
Pyruvate dehydrogenase activity	
Pentose phosphate shunt	
Lipid metabolism	
Triglyceride synthesis	Lipolysis
Fatty acid synthesis (liver)	Lipoprotein lipase (muscle)
Lipoprotein lipase activity (adipose tissue)	Ketogenesis
	Fatty acid oxidation (liver)
Protein metabolism	
Amino acid transport	Protein degradation
Protein synthesis	
Electrolytes	
Cellular potassium uptake	

deficiency of insulin, resulting in decreased anabolic and increased catabolic effects. In both type 1 and type 2 diabetes, insulin's actions are also impaired by insensitivity of target tissues. While this is a fundamental defect in type 2 diabetes, hyperglycaemia can also induce insulin resistance through glucose toxicity. The pathophysiological processes in type 1 and type 2 diabetes are shown in Figure 7.6.

Figure 7.7 relates the metabolic consequences of lack of insulin to its symptoms. Glycosuria occurs when the plasma glucose concentration exceeds the renal threshold (the capacity of renal tubules to reabsorb glucose from the glomerular filtrate) at approximately 10 mmol/l. The severity of the classical osmotic symptoms of polyuria and polydipsia is related to the degree of glycosuria. If hyperglycaemia develops slowly over months or years, as in type 2 diabetes, the renal threshold for glucose rises, and the symptoms of diabetes are mild. This is one reason for the large number of undetected cases of type 2 diabetes, many of whom are discovered coincidentally.

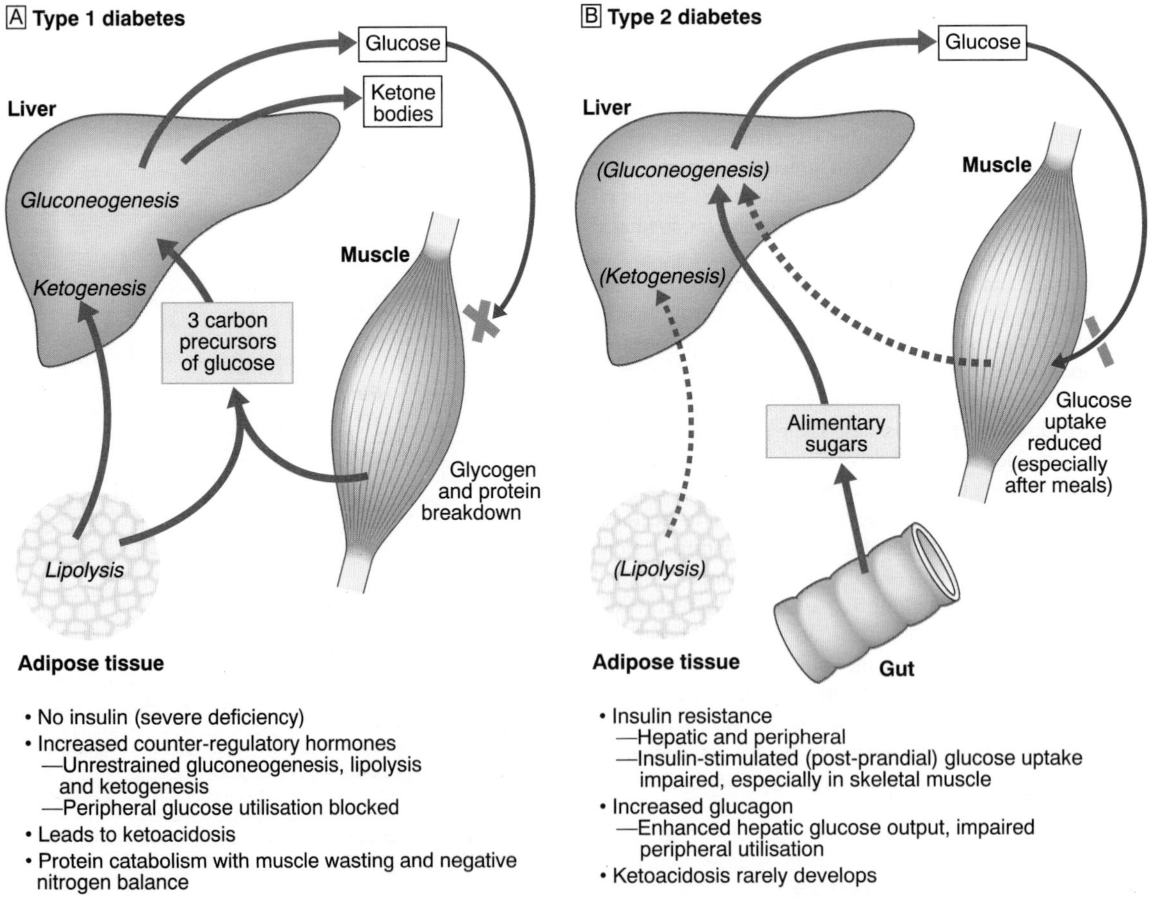

Fig. 7.6 Pathophysiological processes in diabetes mellitus. A Type 1 diabetes. B Type 2 diabetes.

Table 7.4 Comparative clinical features of type 1 and type 2 diabetes

	Type 1	Type 2
Age at onset	< 40 years	> 50 years
Duration of symptoms	Weeks	Months to years
Body weight	Normal or low	Obese
Ketonuria	Yes	No
Rapid death without treatment with insulin	Yes	No
Autoantibodies	Yes	No
Diabetic complications at diagnosis	No	20%
Family history of diabetes	No	Yes
Other autoimmune disease	Yes	No

CLINICAL FEATURES

The clinical features of the two main types of diabetes are compared in Table 7.4. While the distinction between type 1 and type 2 diabetes is broadly true in relation to the features listed, overlap occurs, particularly in age at onset of diabetes, duration of symptoms and family history. A few young people have a form of type 2 diabetes designated maturity onset diabetes of the young (MODY; see Table 7.2, p. 475) while some middle-aged and elderly patients present with typical autoimmune type 1 diabetes. Some patients with apparent type 2 diabetes have evidence of autoimmune activity against pancreatic beta cells, and may have a slowly evolving variant of type 1 diabetes. Insulin-deficient forms of type 2 diabetes in middle-aged patients may be difficult to identify at diagnosis, and classification of the type of diabetes can be difficult.

The classical symptoms of thirst, polyuria, nocturia and rapid weight loss are prominent in type 1 diabetes, but are often absent in patients with type 2 diabetes, many of whom are asymptomatic or have non-specific complaints such as chronic fatigue and malaise. Uncontrolled diabetes is associated with an increased susceptibility to infection and patients may present with skin sepsis (boils) and genital candidiasis, and complain of pruritus vulvae or balanitis.

Patients with type 1 diabetes often have no physical signs attributable to diabetes, but weight loss is common. In the fulminating case with ketoacidosis, the striking features are those of salt and water depletion, with loss of skin turgor, furred tongue and cracked lips, tachycardia, hypotension and reduced intra-ocular pressure. Breathing may be deep and sighing, the breath is usually fetid and the sickly-sweet

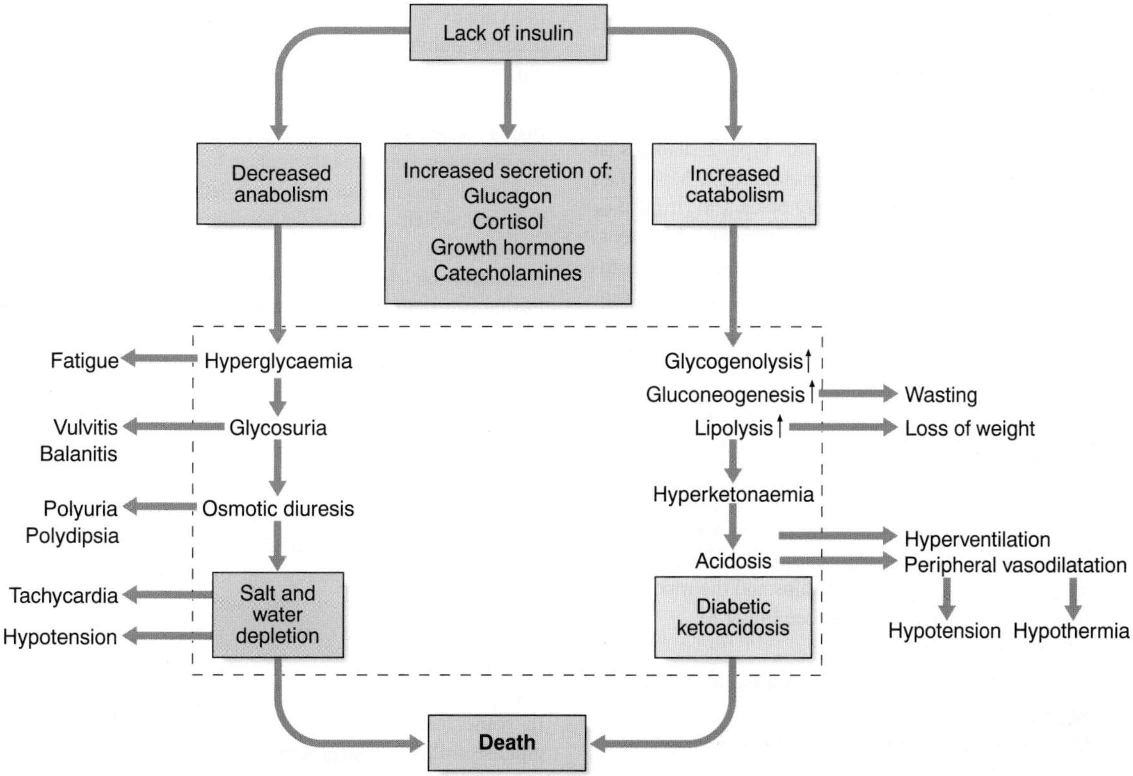

Fig. 7.7 Pathophysiological basis of the symptoms and signs of untreated or uncontrolled diabetes mellitus.

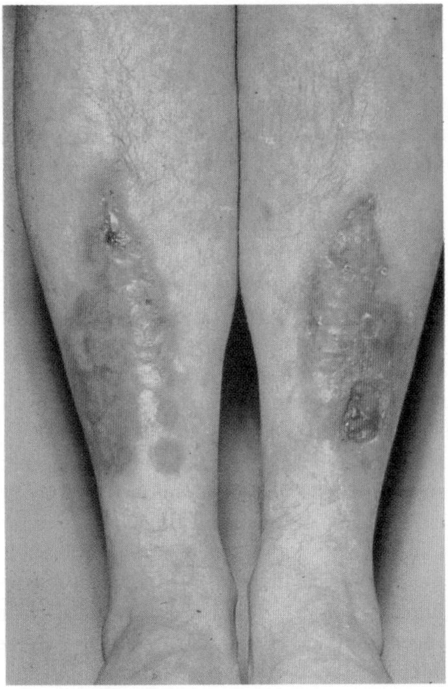

Fig. 7.8 Necrobiosis lipoidica diabeticorum. The usual site is the pre-tibial surface of the lower limbs.

smell of acetone may be apparent. Mental apathy, confusion or a reduced conscious level may be present.

The physical signs in patients with type 2 diabetes at diagnosis depend on the mode of presentation. More than 70% are overweight, and obesity may be central (truncal or abdominal). Hypertension is present in 50% of patients with type 2 diabetes. Although hyperlipidaemia is also common, skin lesions such as xanthelasma and eruptive xanthomata are relatively rare. Sometimes patients present with one or more of the long-term complications of diabetes. They may complain of paraesthesiae, pain and muscle weakness in the legs with signs of peripheral neuropathy or foot ulceration, or deterioration of vision from cataracts or retinopathy. Signs of macrovascular disease are common and may include diminished or impalpable pulses in the feet, bruits over the carotid or femoral arteries and ischaemic toes. Cutaneous features of diabetes include a dermopathy with trophic brownish scars on the shins and the much rarer necrobiosis lipoidica diabeticorum (see Fig. 7.8).

DIAGNOSIS

When the symptoms suggest diabetes the diagnosis may be confirmed by a random blood glucose concentration greater than 11 mmol/l, usually with concurrent glycosuria.

DIAGNOSIS OF DIABETES

Patient complains of symptoms suggesting diabetes

- Test urine for glucose and ketones
- Measure random or fasting blood glucose. Diagnosis confirmed by:
  Fasting plasma glucose > 7 mmol/l
  Random plasma glucose > 11 mmol/l

Indications for oral glucose tolerance test

- Random plasma glucose 7–11 mmol/l

N.B. HbA_{1c} is not used for diagnosis.

Urine testing

Testing the urine for glucose is the usual procedure for detecting diabetes, using sensitive glucose-specific dipstick methods. If possible, the test for urinary glucose should be performed on urine passed 1–2 hours after a meal since this will detect more cases of diabetes than a fasting urine specimen. Glycosuria always warrants full assessment.

The greatest disadvantage of using urinary glucose as a diagnostic or screening procedure is the individual variation in renal threshold. Thus some undoubtedly diabetic individuals will have a negative urine test while other non-diabetic individuals with a low renal threshold for glucose will give a positive result. Estimation of the blood glucose concentration, using an accurate laboratory method rather than a side-room technique, is therefore essential in making the diagnosis (see the information box).

Ketone bodies can be identified by the nitroprusside reaction, which is primarily specific for acetoacetate and is conveniently carried out using tablets or test papers. Ketonuria may be found in normal people who have been fasting or exercising strenuously for long periods, who have been vomiting repeatedly, or who have been eating a diet high in fat and low in carbohydrate. Ketonuria is therefore not pathognomonic of diabetes but, if associated with glycosuria, the diagnosis of diabetes is practically certain.

Renal glycosuria

Apart from diabetes, the most common cause of glycosuria is a low renal threshold for glucose (see Fig. 7.9), which is common during pregnancy and in young people and is a more frequent cause of glycosuria than diabetes. Renal glycosuria is a benign condition unrelated to diabetes.

Alimentary (lag storage) glycosuria

In some individuals a rapid but transitory rise of blood glucose follows a meal and the concentration exceeds the normal renal threshold; during this time glucose will be present in the urine. This response to a meal or to an oral glucose load is benign and is described as a 'lag storage'

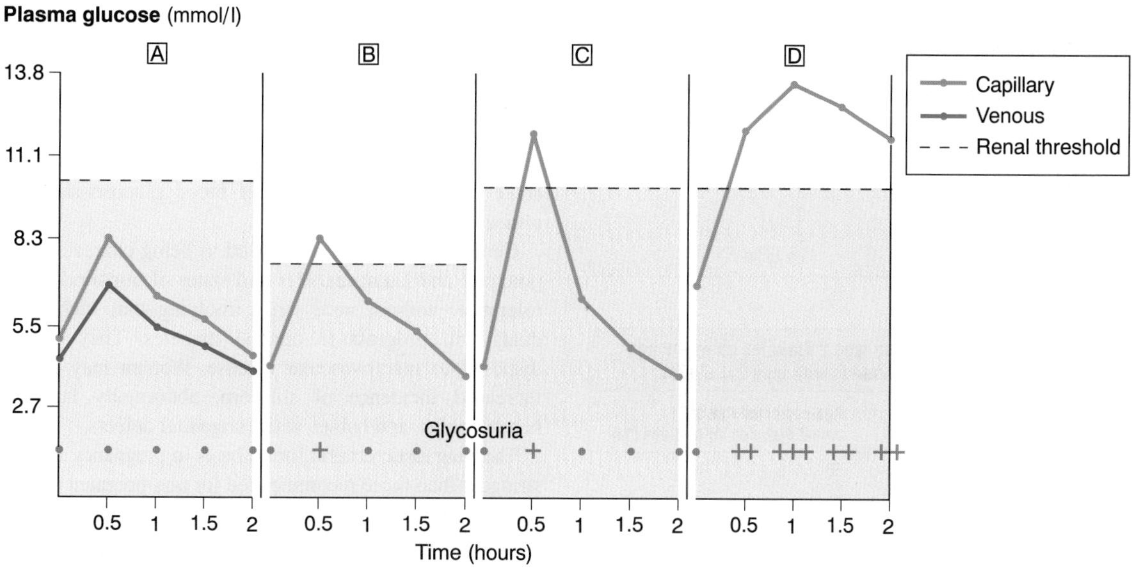

Fig. 7.9 The glucose tolerance test: blood glucose curves after 75 g glucose by mouth. A Normal curve. B Normal curve but with a low renal threshold leading to renal glycosuria. C Alimentary (lag storage) glycosuria. D Diabetes mellitus of moderate severity.

blood glucose curve, although alimentary glycosuria is a better term (see Fig. 7.9). It may occur in normal people or after gastric surgery, when it is caused by rapid gastric emptying leading to more rapid absorption of glucose into the circulation, and is sometimes observed in patients with hyperthyroidism, peptic ulceration or hepatic disease.

Glycosuria during pregnancy

Glycosuria is common in normal pregnancy (because the renal threshold for glucose falls secondary to an increase in the glomerular filtration rate) and in late pregnancy lactose appears in the urine. However, the finding of reducing substances in the urine of a pregnant woman should never be ignored and in all cases blood glucose should be measured to identify gestational diabetes. Since even minimal hyperglycaemia in pregnancy is associated with increased perinatal mortality and morbidity it is important to detect and treat these cases effectively.

The oral glucose tolerance test (OGTT)

When random blood glucose values are elevated but are not diagnostic of diabetes, glucose tolerance is usually assessed by the glycaemic response to oral ingestion of a glucose load (see the information box).

The diagnostic criteria for diabetes mellitus and normality recommended by the World Health Organization (WHO) in 1980 are shown in Table 7.5. The values are based on the threshold for risk of developing vascular disease. Intermediate readings are classified as 'impaired glucose tolerance' (IGT) and indicate the need for further evaluation. Many patients with IGT progress to frank diabetes with time, and it may be necessary, therefore, to keep such patients under review and to repeat the OGTT at a later date.

The diagnostic criteria are currently under review and the American Diabetes Association has proposed to define

ORAL GLUCOSE TOLERANCE TEST (OGTT)

- Unrestricted carbohydrate diet for 3 days before tests
- Fasted overnight
- Rest before test (30 min); no smoking; seated
- Plasma glucose measured before 75 g glucose load and at 30-min intervals for 2 hrs

Table 7.5 Oral glucose tolerance test: diagnostic criteria

	Plasma glucose	Whole blood glucose
	Venous (capillary) (mmol/l)	**Venous (capillary) (mmol/l)**
Diabetes		
Fasting	> 7.8 (> 7.8)*	> 6.7 (> 6.7)
2 hrs after glucose load	> 11.1 (> 12.2)	> 10.0 (> 11.1)
Impaired glucose tolerance		
Fasting	7.8 (7.8)	< 6.7 (< 6.7)
2 hrs after glucose load	7.8–11.0 (8.9–12.1)	6.7–9.9 (7.8–11.0)

* This value is under review and is likely to be lowered to 7.0 mmol/l.

N.B. Venous blood glucose concentration is lower than capillary blood. Whole blood glucose is lower than plasma because red blood cells contain relatively little glucose.

Table 7.6 Overall risk of developing type 1 diabetes in an individual who has a first-degree relative with type 1 diabetes

Relative with type 1 diabetes	% risk
Identical twin	35
Non-identical twin	20
HLA-identical sibling	16
Non-HLA-identical sibling	3
Father	9
Mother	3
Both parents	Up to 30

Table 7.7 Risk of developing type 2 diabetes up to the age of 80 years for siblings of probands with type 2 diabetes

Age at onset of type 2 diabetes in proband	Age-corrected risk of type 2 diabetes for siblings (%)
25–44	53
45–54	37
55–64	38
65–80	31

diabetes by a fasting plasma glucose of 7.0 mmol/l or above, and to introduce a classification of 'fasting hyperglycaemia' or 'impaired fasting glucose', when the fasting plasma glucose is between 5.8 and 6.9 mmol/l. This would exclude some cases of diabetes shown by the OGTT, and hence the WHO is currently recommending retention of this test.

In addition to patients with established clinical diabetes, two other categories are recognised. *Potential* diabetics are persons with a normal OGTT who have an increased risk of developing diabetes for genetic reasons, e.g. an individual who has a first-degree relative with diabetes (see Tables 7.6 and 7.7). *Latent* diabetics are persons in whom the OGTT is normal but who are known to have given an abnormal result under conditions imposing a burden on the pancreatic beta cells, e.g. during pregnancy, infection, myocardial infarction or other severe stress, or during treatment with corticosteroids, thiazide diuretics or other diabetogenic drugs. 'Stress hyperglycaemia' usually disappears after the acute illness has resolved, but blood glucose should be remeasured.

Certain features are recognised as being characteristic of potential and latent diabetes and states of impaired glucose tolerance, without necessarily implying that such individuals will progress to clinical diabetes. They are predisposed to macrovascular disease. Women may have an increased incidence of stillborn, abnormally large and heavy babies, and babies with congenital defects.

The diagnostic criteria for diabetes in pregnancy are more stringent than those recommended for non-pregnant subjects. Pregnant women with impaired glucose tolerance should be referred urgently to a specialist unit for full evaluation.

MANAGEMENT

Three methods of treatment are available for diabetic patients: diet alone, diet and an oral hypoglycaemic drug, and diet and insulin. Approximately 50% of new cases of diabetes can be controlled adequately by diet alone, 20–30% will need an oral hypoglycaemic drug and 20–30% will require insulin. Regardless of aetiology, the type of treatment required is determined by the circulating plasma insulin concentration. In clinical practice the age and weight of the patient at diagnosis are closely related to the

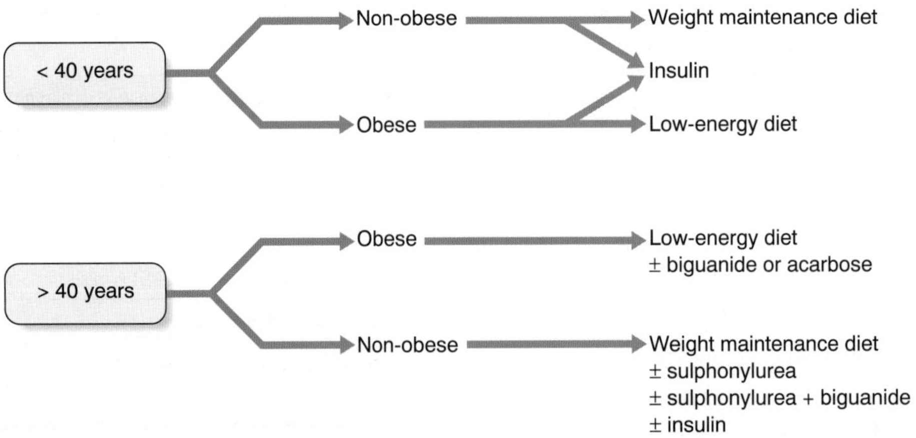

Fig. 7.10 The long-term treatment of diabetes. The treatment required by any individual can be determined by considering age and weight at diagnosis.

plasma insulin and usually indicate the type of treatment required (see Fig. 7.10). However, in each individual case the regimen adopted is effectively chosen by therapeutic trial.

The importance of lifestyle changes such as taking regular exercise, observing a healthy diet, reducing alcohol consumption and stopping smoking should not be underestimated in improving glycaemic control, but many people, particularly the middle-aged and elderly, find them difficult to sustain.

DIETARY MANAGEMENT

General principles

Dietary measures are required in the treatment of all diabetic patients to achieve the overall therapeutic goal: normal metabolism. The purposes of dietary treatment are set out in the information box.

AIMS OF DIETARY MANAGEMENT

- Abolish symptoms of hyperglycaemia
- Avoid hypoglycaemia associated with therapeutic agents (insulin, sulphonylureas)
- Reduce overall blood glucose and minimise fluctuations
- Avoid 'atherogenic' diets or those which may aggravate diabetic complications (e.g. high protein intake in nephropathy)
- Achieve weight reduction in obese patients to reduce insulin resistance, hyperglycaemia and dyslipidaemia

Daily energy intake

It is important that all diabetic patients consume a diet containing an appropriate energy content as this greatly influences glycaemic control. An individual patient's daily energy requirement involves consideration of factors such as age, sex, actual weight in relation to desirable weight, activity and occupation. However, although a dietary history is useful to establish an individual's habitual eating pattern and to assess what types of food are consumed regularly, it is not essential that all patients have their dietary energy content quantified formally. Formulae are available for estimating total energy expenditure and this information may be of value when prescribing a realistic diet for the obese patient. One successful approach is to agree appropriate dietary changes with the patient which will induce a daily 500 kcal deficit; such a weight-reducing diet may be less restrictive than the patient has anticipated.

Table 7.8 shows the approximate proportion of energy derived from carbohydrate, protein and fat in the British national diet. The intake of fat is therefore normally high, with a large proportion consisting of saturated fat, and is considered to be atherogenic; in the diabetic patient it is recommended that the percentage of calories derived from carbohydrate should be increased and that from fat reduced. It is important to explain to the individual patient that the 'diabetic diet' is simply a 'healthy diet' that is recommended for the population in general.

Table 7.8 Proportion of energy derived from carbohydrate, protein and fat

	UK national diet	Recommended diabetic diet
Energy	Maintains BMI of 25 kg/m^2	To approach BMI of 22 kg/m^2
Carbohydrate	45%	50–55%
Fat	40%	30–35%
Saturated fatty acids	17%	< 10%
Monounsaturated	11%	10–15%
Polyunsaturated	6%	< 10%
Protein	12–15%	10–15%

BMI = body mass index (weight [kg]/height^2 [m^2])

Carbohydrate and non-starch polysaccharide (dietary fibre)

A suitable diet for diabetic persons should have 50% of the daily caloric intake derived from carbohydrate, of which significant amounts should be in the form of non-starch polysaccharide (NSP), as dietary fibre. This can be subdivided into soluble and insoluble types. The consumption of 15 g soluble fibre (present in beans, peas, pulses, oats, fruit and vegetables) can produce a 10% reduction in fasting blood glucose, glycated haemoglobin and low-density lipoprotein (LDL) cholesterol. However, sustaining this indefinitely requires a high level of motivation, and is difficult to achieve if the daily intake is less than 1500 kcal. The inclusion of insoluble NSP (in wholemeal bread and breakfast cereals) aids satiety and may benefit weight control but the effect on lowering blood glucose is minimal. The most useful effect of a high-carbohydrate diet is to facilitate the maintenance of a much less atherogenic low-fat diet.

Restricted consumption of mono- and disaccharides (fructose, sucrose and glucose) is advised as part of healthy eating guidelines. Foods which contain a lot of sucrose are often high in fat and their intake should be limited. Sugar-free drinks should be used and unsweetened fruit juices restricted. Confectionery, puddings, biscuits and cakes should be limited, as should quenching thirst with milk when appetite is normal.

Classification of foods according to their acute effect on the blood glucose concentration ('glycaemic index') has been suggested as a means of determining the optimal carbohydrate foods for diabetic patients, but is not widely used.

Fat

As diabetes is a risk factor for macrovascular disease, the

intake of fat should be restricted to 30–35% of energy with less than 10% as saturated fat, less than 10% as polyunsaturated fat, and 10–15% as monounsaturated fat. The latter is associated with an improved plasma lipid profile (reduction in total and LDL cholesterol without lowering high-density lipoprotein (HDL) cholesterol) in type 2 diabetes. The use of monounsaturated oils in the diet (e.g. olive oil, rapeseed oil, peanut oil, some types of spreads, avocados and some types of nuts) is also beneficial. Weight loss in obese patients with type 2 diabetes greatly assists in lowering plasma lipids, but many patients find the reduction of dietary fat intake very difficult to achieve.

Alcohol

In general, diabetic individuals should take the same precautions regarding alcohol intake as the general population. However, account must be taken of:

- the energy and carbohydrate content of alcoholic drinks
- the inhibition of gluconeogenesis by alcohol which may potentiate the hypoglycaemic action of sulphonylureas and insulin
- the similarity of the features of inebriation and hypoglycaemia which may be confused by observers
- the tendency of alcohol to predispose towards the development of lactic acidosis in patients taking a biguanide (see p. 486)
- the fact that alcohol can induce a 'disulfiram type' of reaction in some patients taking chlorpropamide.

Abstinence should be encouraged if obesity, hypertension or hypertriglyceridaemia is present.

Salt

Diabetic patients should follow the advice given to the general population, namely to reduce sodium intake to no more than 6 g daily. Further restriction of sodium intake (to less than 3 g daily) is important in the management of hypertensive diabetic patients.

Diabetic foods and sweeteners

Low-calorie and sugar-free drinks are useful for patients with diabetes. These drinks usually contain non-nutritive sweeteners. Many 'diabetic foods' contain sorbitol or fructose which are relatively high in energy, may be expensive and may have gastrointestinal side-effects. They are not recommended as part of the diabetic diet.

The non-nutritive sweeteners saccharin, aspartame, sucramate and acesulphame K are the most widely used and provide means for reducing energy intake without loss of palatability.

Types of diabetic diet

Two basic types of diet are used in the treatment of diabetes: low-energy, weight-reducing diets and weight maintenance diets. The beneficial effect of weight reduction on the mortality rate of obese non-diabetic persons is well known and applies even more strikingly to the obese diabetic patient. Management of obese people (both diabetic and non-diabetic) with a diet low in refined and high in unrefined carbohydrate and restricted in total energy content results in increased insulin sensitivity. This promotes a decline in blood glucose in the obese diabetic patient. The precise mechanism of this effect is uncertain. Reduction in body weight increases this effect, encouraging a rise in the plasma insulin concentration in many patients so that additional therapy can often be avoided.

Low-energy, weight-reducing diets

Dietary prescriptions which cause a daily deficit of 500 kcal provide a realistic diet and induce a weekly weight loss of around 0.5 kg. Rapid weight reduction may provoke loss of lean body tissue, and in the elderly care must be taken to avoid the omission of essential nutrients, vitamins and minerals. Caloric restriction is essential for the obese diabetic patient treated with insulin to try to minimise the weight gain which insulin can promote. In such individuals, the omission of snacks between meals is often necessary.

Weight maintenance diets

These are necessary for individuals with a normal body mass index (BMI, see p. 526) and ideally should be high in carbohydrate and low in fat, with particular attention being paid to the type of fat ingested. While total energy intake remains constant, the percentage of energy from macronutrients should be altered as described above.

Diets for insulin-treated diabetes

A regular pattern of meals (and snacks) is important to maintain a constant daily intake of carbohydrate, and protects against hypoglycaemia. Simple information on the relative carbohydrate content of foods can be provided where appropriate. Carbohydrate exchanges are now seldom used as a method of controlling carbohydrate intake as the exchange system is inaccurate and makes no allowance for the glycaemic effect or for the fat content of foods.

A useful meal-planning tool is the plate model (see Fig. 7.11) which encourages the inclusion of carbohydrate as the main part of the meal in conjunction with vegetables, and limits the consumption of protein-containing foods. The daily inclusion of five portions of fruit and vegetables is recommended. Children and pregnant women with diabetes require specialised dietetic advice.

ORAL HYPOGLYCAEMIC DRUGS

Various drugs are effective in reducing hyperglycaemia in patients with type 2 diabetes. Although their mechanisms of action are different, most depend upon a supply of endo-

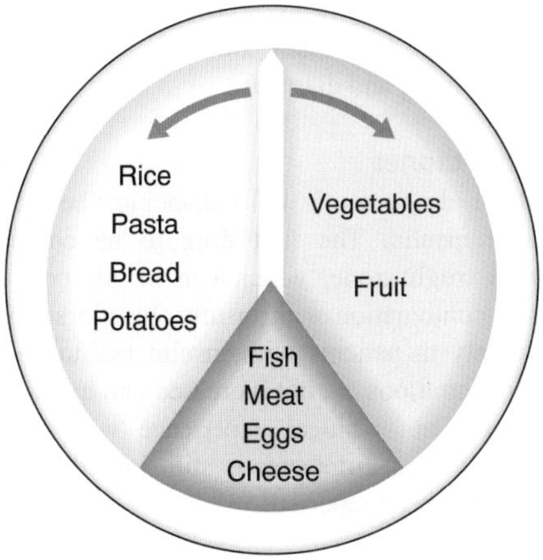

Fig. 7.11 A 'plate model' for meal planning. The plate is divided into three sections. The smallest section (one-fifth of total area) is for the meat, fish, eggs or cheese, and the remainder divided in roughly equal proportions between the staple food (rice, pasta, potatoes, bread etc.) and vegetables or fruit.

genous insulin and they therefore have no hypoglycaemic effect in patients with type 1 diabetes. The sulphonylureas and the biguanides have been the mainstay of treatment for many years but novel agents are now available, such as the insulin-enhancing agents, the thiazolidinediones, and the alpha-glucosidase inhibitors, which delay carbohydrate digestion and absorption of glucose. The effects of these drugs are compared in Table 7.9.

Sulphonylureas

Mechanism of action

The principal effect of sulphonylureas is mediated through stimulation of the release of insulin from the pancreatic beta cell, but they may also exert extrapancreatic effects, particularly in reducing the hepatic release of glucose and diminishing insulin resistance.

Indications for use

Sulphonylureas are valuable in the treatment of non-obese patients with type 2 diabetes who fail to respond to dietary measures alone. Although sulphonylureas will lower the blood glucose concentration of obese patients with type 2 diabetes, such patients should be treated energetically in the first instance by dietary measures alone since treatment with sulphonylureas is often associated with an increase in weight, which will increase insulin resistance and eventually aggravate the total disability. This leads to secondary failure to respond to the drugs, and progression to treatment with insulin. The main differences between the individual compounds lie in their potency, length of action and cost.

First-generation sulphonylureas (chlorpropamide, tolazamide and tolbutamide) are not commonly prescribed in modern practice although tolbutamide, the mildest of the sulphonylureas, is very well tolerated and rarely causes toxic reactions. Its duration of action is relatively short so the usual maintenance dose is 250–500 mg administered 8- or 12-hourly. Tolbutamide is a useful drug in the elderly in whom the risk and the consequences of inducing hypoglycaemia are increased. Chlorpropamide has a biological half-life of about 36 hours and is taken once daily, the usual maintenance dose being between 100 and 350 mg daily. Chlorpropamide may cause severe and prolonged hypoglycaemia. Larger doses are associated with an increased risk of toxic effects such as cholestatic jaundice, skin rash and blood dyscrasia, and can occasionally induce the syndrome of inappropriate antidiuretic hormone secretion (SIADH).

Of the second-generation sulphonylureas, glipizide and gliclazide are widely used and cause few side-effects, but glibenclamide is prone to induce severe hypoglycaemia and should also be avoided in the elderly. The dose-response of these drugs is most effective at low dosage; little additional hypoglycaemic benefit is obtained when the dose is increased to maximal levels. Several drugs can potentiate the hypoglycaemic effect of sulphonylureas by displacing them from their plasma protein-binding sites, e.g. salicylates, phenylbutazone, and antifungal agents.

Patients with type 2 diabetes who fail to respond to initial treatment with sulphonylureas are considered 'primary treatment failures'. The incidence of primary treatment

Table 7.9 Effects of oral hypoglycaemic drugs used in addition to dietary measures in the treatment of type 2 diabetes

	Insulin	Sulphonylureas	Metformin	Acarbose	Troglitazone
Reduce basal glycaemia	Yes	Yes	Yes	Slight	Yes
Reduce post-prandial glycaemia	Yes	Yes	Yes	Yes	Yes
Raise plasma insulin	Yes	Yes	No	No	No
Increase body weight	Yes	Yes	No	No	No
Improve lipid profile	Yes	No	Slight	Slight	Partial
Risk of hypoglycaemia	Yes	Yes	No	No	No
Tolerability	Good	Good	Moderate	Moderate	Good

failure depends mainly on the criteria for initial selection and patient compliance with diet. Patients with 'secondary failure' are not a homogeneous group; they include some with type 1 diabetes who have an absolute deficiency of insulin, some with insulin-deficient diabetes who present as type 2 diabetes and others with significant circulating plasma insulin levels who are usually obese and have failed to lose weight while supposedly taking a low-energy diet. Failure to comply with the diet is the most common precipitant of secondary treatment failure. With continuing follow-up, 'secondary failure' affects 3–10% of patients each year.

Biguanides

The biguanides are less widely used than the sulphonylureas because of a higher incidence of side-effects, particularly gastrointestinal symptoms.

Mechanism of action

The mechanism of action of these compounds has not been precisely defined. They have no hypoglycaemic effect in non-diabetic individuals but, in diabetes, insulin sensitivity and peripheral glucose uptake are increased. There is some evidence that they also impair glucose absorption by the gut and inhibit hepatic gluconeogenesis. Although secretion of some endogenous insulin is mandatory for their hypoglycaemic action, these compounds do not increase insulin secretion and hypoglycaemia does not occur.

Indications for use

Metformin is the only biguanide available. Its administration is not associated with a rise in body weight and it may therefore be preferred for the obese patient. In addition, as the hypoglycaemic effect of metformin is synergistic with that of the sulphonylurea drugs, there is a case for combining the two when either alone has proved inadequate. Metformin is given with food 8- or 12-hourly. The usual starting dose is 500 mg 12-hourly with a gradual increase as required to a maximum of 1 g 8-hourly. Its use is contraindicated in patients with impaired renal or hepatic function and in those who take alcohol in excess because the risk of lactic acidosis is significantly increased in such patients. It should be discontinued, at least temporarily, if any other serious medical condition develops, especially those causing severe shock or hypoxaemia. In such circumstances, treatment with insulin should be substituted.

Alpha-glucosidase inhibitors

The alpha-glucosidase inhibitors delay carbohydrate absorption in the gut by selectively inhibiting disaccharidases. Acarbose is currently available and is taken in a dose of 50–100 mg with each meal. It principally lowers post-prandial blood glucose, modestly improves overall glycaemic control and reduces HbA_{1c}. Acarbose can be combined with a sulphonylurea. The main side-effects are flatulence, abdominal bloating and diarrhoea.

Thiazolidinediones

These novel drugs work by enhancing the actions of endogenous insulin. The first drug to be commercially available is troglitazone, which can be prescribed either alone or in combination with insulin. Insulin sensitivity is improved only in patients with insulin resistance, plasma insulin concentrations are not increased and hypoglycaemia is not a problem. Clinical experience with the use of troglitazone in type 2 diabetes is still limited, and hepatic dysfunction has been reported.

Combined oral hypoglycaemic therapy and insulin

In diabetic patients who are requiring increasing doses of a sulphonylurea or biguanide, either alone or in combination, the introduction of a single dose of an intermediate-acting insulin (usually isophane), administered at bedtime, may improve glycaemic control and delay the development of overt pancreatic beta cell failure. The exogenous insulin suppresses the hepatic glucose output during the night and lowers fasting blood glucose. This treatment is ineffective in diabetic patients who have no evidence of endogenous insulin secretion, i.e. those who are C-peptide-negative. The combination of bedtime isophane insulin with metformin has been shown to be the regimen least likely to promote weight gain. For patients who are approaching secondary failure to oral medication, this provides a simple and effective introduction to self-treatment with insulin with very little risk of hypoglycaemia.

INSULIN

Manufacture and formulation

Insulin was discovered in 1921 and its clinical application transformed the management of type 1 diabetes, until then a fatal disorder. Until the 1980s insulin was obtained by extraction and purification from pancreata of cows and pigs (bovine and porcine insulins) and many patients continue to use animal insulins. The use of recombinant DNA technology has enabled large-scale production of human insulin. Recently, rDNA and protein engineering techniques that alter the amino acid sequence of insulin have been used to produce 'monomeric' analogues of insulin, which are more rapidly absorbed from the site of injection.

The duration of action of short-acting, unmodified insulin ('soluble' or 'regular' insulin), which is a clear solution, can be extended by the addition of protamine and zinc at neutral pH (isophane or NPH insulin) or excess zinc ions (lente insulins). These modified 'depot' insulins are cloudy preparations. Pre-mixed formulations containing short-acting

Table 7.10 Duration of action (in hours) of insulin preparations

Insulin	Onset	Peak	Duration
Monomeric (insulin analogues)	< 0.5	0.5–2.5	3–4.5
Short-acting (soluble, regular)	0.25–1	1–4	4–8
Intermediate-acting (isophane, lente)	1–3	3–8	7–14
Long-acting (bovine ultralente)	2–4	6–12	12–30

and isophane insulins in various proportions are available. The time characteristics of insulins are shown in Table 7.10.

In many countries, the insulin concentrations in available formulations have been standardised at 100 units/ml.

Insulin delivery

Insulin is injected subcutaneously into recommended sites, namely the anterior abdominal wall, upper arms, outer thighs and buttocks. Accidental intramuscular injection often occurs in children and thin adults. The rate of absorption of insulin may be influenced by many factors other than the insulin formulation, including the site, depth and volume of injection, skin temperature (warming), local massage and exercise. Absorption is also delayed from areas of lipohypertrophy at injection sites (see Fig. 7.12). This results from the local trophic action of insulin, so repeated injection at the same site should be avoided. Other routes of administration (intravenous and intraperitoneal) are reserved for specific circumstances.

Insulin is administered using a disposable plastic syringe with a fine needle (which can be reused several times) in preference to the traditional glass syringe and metal needle which require repeated sterilisation. Pen injectors with insulin in cartridge form are popular and convenient and are also available as pre-loaded disposable pens. They do not necessarily improve glycaemic control.

'Open-loop' systems are battery-powered portable pumps providing continuous subcutaneous or intravenous infusion of insulin, delivered at variable rates without reference to the blood glucose concentration. In practice, the 'loop' is closed by the patient performing blood glucose estimations and the use of these devices requires a high degree of patient motivation; they are prone to pump failure and rapid onset of ketoacidosis. These systems will not be suitable for general therapeutic use until they are less expensive and incorporate an automatic failure alarm in the form of a miniaturised glucose sensor.

Short-acting insulin has to be injected at least 30 minutes before a meal to allow adequate time for absorption. Many patients find this inconvenient and ignore this requirement. However, the rapidly absorbed insulin analogues can be administered 5–10 minutes before food and their peak action coincides more closely with the post-prandial rise in blood glucose (see Table 7.10).

Once absorbed into the blood stream, insulin has a half-life of about 7 minutes. It is cleared mainly by the liver and also the kidneys; plasma insulin concentrations are elevated in patients with liver disease or renal failure. The rate of clearance is also affected by binding to insulin antibodies (associated with the use of animal insulins).

Complications of insulin therapy are listed in the information box.

SIDE-EFFECTS OF INSULIN THERAPY

- Hypoglycaemia
- Weight gain
- Peripheral oedema (insulin causes salt and water retention in the short term when started)
- Insulin antibodies (animal insulins)
- Local allergy (rare)
- Lipodystrophy at injection sites (see Fig. 7.12)

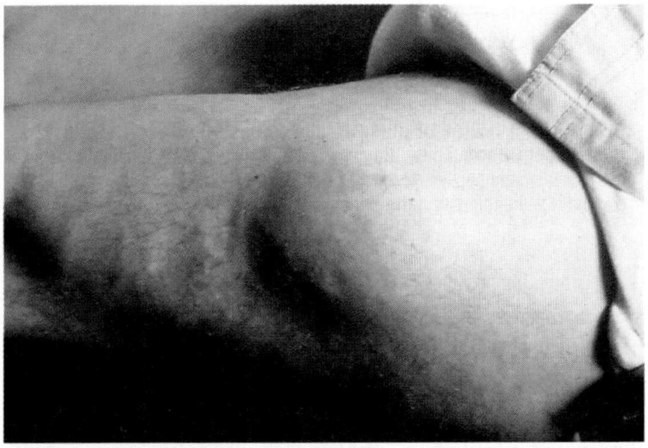

Fig. 7.12 Lipohypertrophy at insulin injection site.

Insulin regimens

Various insulin regimens are used in the treatment of diabetes. The choice of regimen depends on the desired degree of glycaemic control, the patient's lifestyle and his or her ability to adjust the insulin dose. Most patients require two or more injections of insulin daily. Once-daily injections rarely achieve satisfactory glycaemic control and are reserved either for some elderly patients or those who retain significant endogenous insulin secretion and have a low insulin requirement.

Twice-daily administration of a short-acting and intermediate-acting insulin (usually soluble and isophane insulins), given in combination before breakfast and the evening meal, is the simplest and most commonly used regimen. Individual requirements vary considerably but usually two-thirds of the total daily requirement of insulin is given in the morning in a ratio of 1:2, short:intermediate-acting insulins. The remaining one-third is given in the evening, and doses are adjusted according to blood glucose monitoring.

Several pre-mixed formulations are available containing different proportions of soluble and isophane insulins (e.g. 10:90; 20:80; 30:70; and 50:50). These are of value in patients who have difficulty mixing insulins, but are inflexible as the individual components cannot be adjusted independently.

Multiple injection regimens have been developed, with short-acting insulin being taken before each meal, and intermediate-acting insulin being injected at bedtime (basal-bolus regimen). This type of regimen allows greater freedom of timing of meals and is of value to individuals with variable day-to-day activities, but snacks may have to be taken between meals to prevent hypoglycaemia. The use of pen injectors has improved the acceptability of multiple injection regimens. The time action profile of different insulin regimens, compared to the secretory pattern of insulin in the non-diabetic state, is shown in Figure 7.13.

The management of children and teenagers presents particular problems which should be addressed in specialised clinics.

THERAPEUTIC GOALS

The aim of treatment is to achieve as near normal metabolism as is practicable. The nearer the body weight approaches the ideal level and the closer the blood glucose concentration is kept to normal, the more the total metabolic profile is improved and the lower the incidence of vascular disease and specific diabetic complications (see p. 489).

The ideal management for diabetes would allow the patient to lead a completely normal life, to remain not only

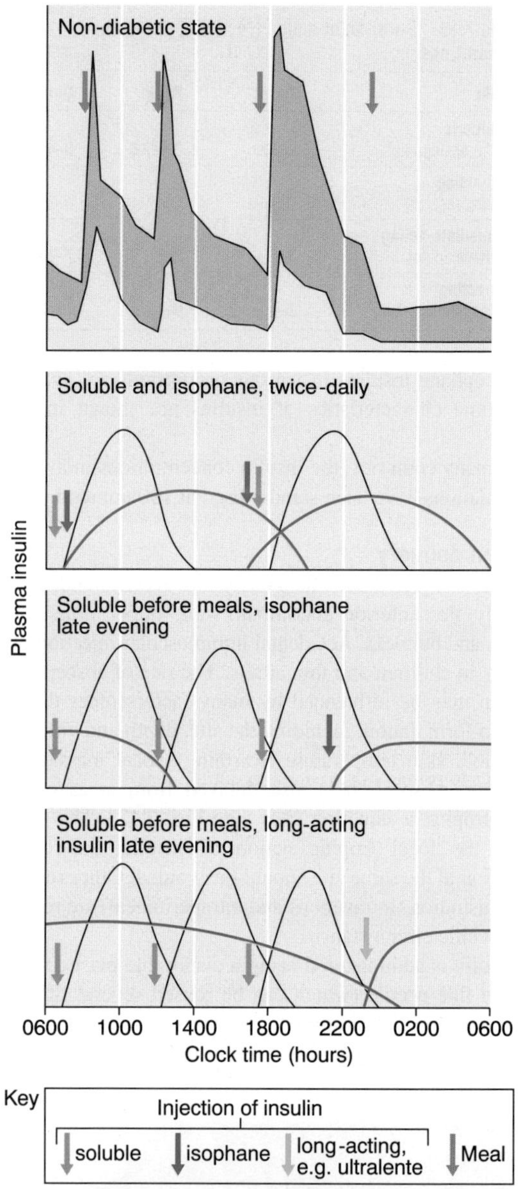

Fig. 7.13 Profiles of plasma insulin associated with different insulin regimens. These are compared to the normal secretory pattern in a non-diabetic person (top panel). These are theoretical patterns of plasma insulin and may differ considerably in individuals.

symptom-free but in good health, to achieve a normal metabolic state and to escape the long-term complications of diabetes. Although a few diabetic patients die from acute metabolic complications (ketoacidosis and hypoglycaemia), the major problem is the excess mortality and serious morbidity suffered as a result of the long-term complications of diabetes; the factors associated with these are

FACTORS ASSOCIATED WITH INCREASED MORTALITY AND MORBIDITY IN DIABETIC PATIENTS

- Duration of diabetes
- Early age at onset of disease
- High glycated Hb
- Raised blood pressure
- Proteinuria
- Obesity
- Hyperlipidaemia

THE CURRENT 'COST' OF DIABETES IN THE UK

- 30% reduction in life expectancy
- Most common cause of blindness in 20–65 age group
- 600 patients reach end-stage renal failure per annum
- Lower limb amputation rate increased 25-fold
- Use of hospital beds increased 6-fold
- 4.5% of total National Health Service budget

listed in the first information box on page 488. As indicated in the second information box, the cost to the community and to the individual patient is enormous.

Metabolic control and development of long-term complications of diabetes

Duration of diabetes and poor glycaemic control are most closely associated with vascular complications. A graded relationship has been demonstrated between the duration and degree of sustained hyperglycaemia, however caused and at whatever age it develops, and the risk of vascular disease. There is nothing 'mild' about type 2 diabetes as regards the development of complications.

The possibility of reversing early vascular disease by improving metabolic control has been examined in several prospective, randomised, controlled clinical trials involving patients with early background retinopathy and minimal proteinuria. None of these studies produced any evidence of reversal of either retinopathy or nephropathy, and in some cases retinopathy worsened abruptly soon after control was improved. Despite this, in the long term the rate of progression of both retinopathy and nephropathy was reduced by continuing better control. These studies stimulated a search for markers of early reversible retinal, renal and neural dysfunction, and shifted the emphasis in the management of diabetes to primary prevention of complications.

The Diabetes Control and Complications Trial (DCCT) was set up in type 1 diabetic patients to answer the question: are diabetic complications preventable? Recent analysis of the data generated during the 9 years of this large and very carefully designed study (see Further information, p. 509) demonstrated a 60% overall reduction in the risk of developing diabetic complications in those on intensive therapy with strict glycaemic control (mean HbA_{1c} around 7%), compared with those on conventional therapy (mean HbA_{1c} around 9%). In this study no single factor other than glycaemic control had a significant effect on outcome.

The conclusions which can be drawn from this landmark study are clear and incontrovertible:

- diabetic complications are preventable
- the aim of treatment should be 'near-normal' glycaemia, while at the same time avoiding serious hypoglycaemic episodes in insulin-treated patients.

In the DCCT, weight gain was common and severe hypoglycaemic episodes occurred three times more often in the patients with strict glycaemic control. Although there was no associated increase in deaths, major macrovascular events or neurological/cognitive defects, this increased risk of hypoglycaemia may alter the risk-benefit ratio of good control in certain patients. Thus less intensive treatment may be indicated:

- in those with impaired awareness of hypoglycaemia
- in those with severe macrovascular disease (particularly if they have a past history of myocardial infarction or cerebrovascular accident)
- for those who are very old and frail
- for very young (pre-school) children.

A large study of patients with type 2 diabetes, the UK Prospective Diabetes Study (UKPDS) has shown that diabetic complications are reduced by good glycaemic control and effective treatment of hypertension, irrespective of the type of therapy used.

ASSESSMENT OF GLYCAEMIC CONTROL

Urine testing

Semi-quantitative pre-prandial urine testing to assess blood glucose control has major limitations, particularly in patients with type 1 diabetes, but also in type 2 diabetes patients where a raised renal threshold for glucose may mask persistent hyperglycaemia. Negative urine tests fail to distinguish between normal and low blood glucose levels, which is a particular disadvantage since the aim of treatment is a normal blood glucose level while avoiding hypoglycaemia. However, urine glucose testing with visually read strips is still used by many patients with type 2 diabetes and is satisfactory in patients treated with diet alone or in those taking oral therapy who have stable glycaemic control.

Blood testing

Wherever possible, patients (particularly those treated with insulin) should be taught to perform capillary blood glucose measurements at home, using blood glucose test strips read either visually or with a glucose meter. The great advantage of self-monitoring of capillary blood glucose concentration is that information is available immediately and permits the well-informed and motivated patient to make appropriate adjustments in treatment (particularly in insulin dose) on a day-to-day basis. Thus ketoacidosis can be avoided, compliance with dietary measures encouraged and a normal or near-normal metabolism achieved while avoiding frequent and disabling hypoglycaemia. Single random blood glucose estimations obtained at routine clinic visits are of limited value and the main disadvantage of profiles obtained in hospital inpatients or day patients is that they are obtained in a highly artificial situation.

Glycated haemoglobin

Glycated haemoglobin (GHb) provides an accurate and objective measure of glycaemic control over a period of weeks to months. Several minor components of adult haemoglobin (HbA_1) can be separated from unmodified haemoglobin (HbA_0) by ion-exchange chromatography (see

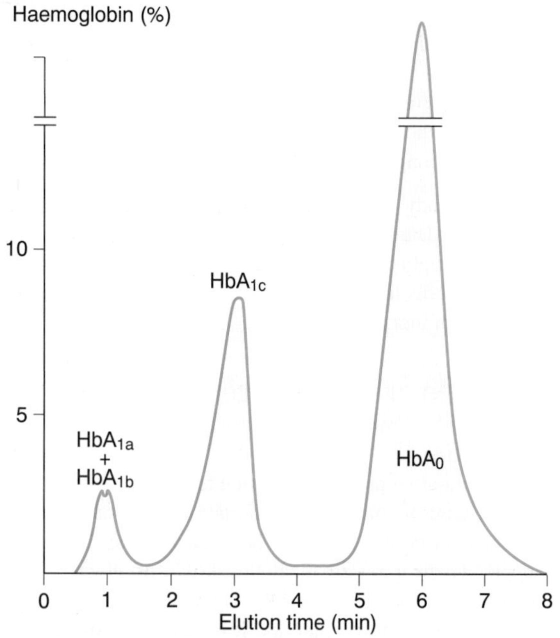

Fig. 7.14 Elution profile of human haemoglobin with ion exchange chromatography (HPLC). HbA_0 is unmodified haemoglobin, and minor components of HbA_{1a}, and HbA_{1b} and HbA_{1c} can be identified; they are reported collectively as total HbA_1.

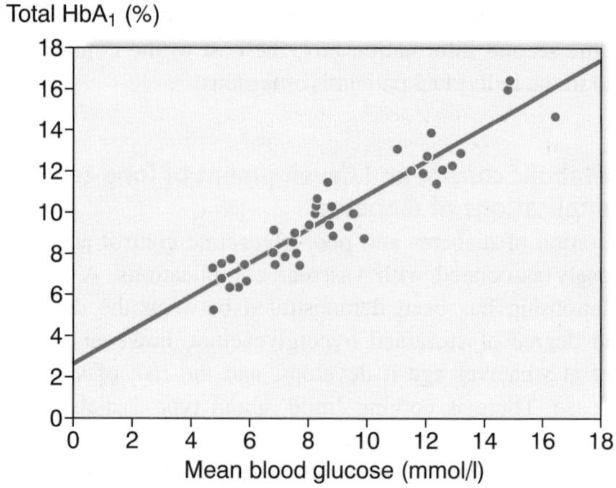

Fig. 7.15 The relationship between glycated haemoglobin (shown as total HbA_1) and mean blood glucose levels in the previous 3 months. Each dot represents the mean blood glucose concentration for a single patient. Each patient collected capillary blood samples before and 2 hours after each main meal for 24 hours every 2 weeks for 3 months. Glycated haemoglobin is expressed here as total HbA_1 but HbA_{1c} is often reported alone, and has a non-diabetic range that is lower than total HbA_1.

Fig. 7.14), and these haemoglobin moieties are increased in diabetes by the slow non-enzymatic covalent attachment of glucose and other sugars (glycation). The rate of formation of GHb is directly proportional to the ambient blood glucose concentration; a rise of 1% in GHb corresponds to an approximate increase of 2 mmol/l in average blood glucose. The close relationship between GHb and mean blood glucose is shown in Figure 7.15. Although GHb concentration reflects the integrated blood glucose control over the lifespan of the erythrocyte (120 days), the estimate is weighted by changes in glycaemic control occurring in the month before measurement (representing 50% of the GHb concentration). As GHb is affected more by recent than earlier events, a large shift in blood glucose control is rapidly accompanied by a change in GHb, detectable within 2–3 weeks.

Various assay methods can be used to measure GHb, but because of a current lack of consensus on a suitable reference method and the non-standardisation of methodology, a local non-diabetic reference range must be ascertained, and this precludes direct comparison of GHb values between laboratories. GHb estimates may be erroneously diminished in people with anaemia or during pregnancy, and with some assay methods may be difficult to interpret in patients who have uraemia or a haemoglobinopathy. In clinical practice, GHb is usually measured once or twice yearly to assess glycaemic control, permitting appropriate changes in treatment and identifying inconsistency with the patient's records of home blood glucose monitoring. GHb also provides an index of risk for developing diabetic complications. It is not used in the diagnosis of diabetes and is often normal in patients with impaired glucose tolerance.

Glycated serum proteins ('fructosamine') can be measured and, because of their shorter half-life, give an indication of glycaemic control over the preceding 2 weeks. Other than diabetic pregnancy, this is generally too short a time period to make clinical decisions on therapeutic management.

Blood lipids

The concentration of serum lipids, total cholesterol, HDL cholesterol and triglyceride is another important index of overall metabolic control in diabetic patients and should be monitored regularly. Ideally, the triglyceride concentrations should be measured in the fasting state.

EDUCATING PATIENTS

It is essential that diabetic patients learn to handle all aspects of their management as quickly as possible and this can be done on an outpatient basis. However, patients requiring insulin have to be seen daily at first and, if this is not practicable, admission to hospital will be necessary.

Every patient with type 1 diabetes who is capable of learning must be taught how to perform capillary blood glucose estimations and tests of urinary ketones, to keep a record of the results and to understand their significance.

Those requiring insulin need to learn how to measure their dose of insulin accurately with an insulin syringe or pen device, to give their own injections and to adjust the dose themselves on the basis of blood glucose estimations and other factors such as illness, exercise and hypoglycaemic episodes. They must be familiar with the symptoms associated with hypoglycaemia (see the information box, p. 492). They must therefore have a working knowledge of diabetes and also ready access to medical advice when the need arises. Information should be provided about driving (statutory regulations and practical advice). Provision of such education is time-consuming but only in this way can patients safely undertake normal activities while maintaining good control.

It is a wise precaution for diabetic patients who are taking insulin or an oral hypoglycaemic drug to carry a card stating their name and address, the fact that they have diabetes, the nature and dose of any insulin or other drugs they may be taking, and giving the name, address and telephone number of their family doctor and any specialist diabetic clinic they attend.

LONG-TERM SUPERVISION

Diabetes is a complex disorder which progresses in severity with time, so diabetic patients should be seen at regular intervals for the remainder of their lives, either at a specialist diabetic clinic or by their general practitioner provided he or she has a particular interest and training in diabetes. A checklist for follow-up visits is detailed in the information box below. The frequency of visits is very variable, ranging from weekly during pregnancy to annually in the case of patients with well-controlled type 2 diabetes.

CHECKLIST FOR FOLLOW-UP VISITS OF PATIENTS WITH DIABETES MELLITUS

- Body weight
- Urinalysis of fasting specimen for glucose, ketones, albumin (both macro- and microalbuminuria)
- Glycaemic control
  - GHb (HbA_{1c})
  - Inspection of home blood glucose monitoring record
- Hypoglycaemic episodes
  - Number of serious (requiring assistance in treatment) and mild episodes
  - Time when 'hypos' experienced
- Blood pressure (supine and erect)
- Visual acuity
  - Ophthalmoscopy (with pupils dilated)
- Lower limbs
  - Peripheral pulses
  - Tendon reflexes
  - Perception of vibration sensation
  - Feet: ulceration, callous skin indicating pressure areas, nails, need for chiropody

ACUTE COMPLICATIONS OF DIABETES

HYPOGLYCAEMIA

Hypoglycaemia occurs often in diabetic patients treated with insulin but relatively infrequently in those taking a sulphonylurea drug. The risk of hypoglycaemia is the most important single factor limiting the attainment of the therapeutic goal, namely near-normal glycaemia. In most instances the patient has no difficulty in recognising the symptoms of hypoglycaemia and can take appropriate remedial action. However, in certain circumstances (e.g. during sleep) and particularly in certain types of patient (e.g. patients with a long duration of type 1 diabetes), warning symptoms are not always perceived by the patient even when awake so that appropriate action is not taken and neuroglycopenia then unconsciousness ensue.

MORBIDITY OF SEVERE HYPOGLYCAEMIA IN DIABETIC PATIENTS

CNS
- Coma
- Convulsions
- Brain damage
- Impaired cognitive function
- Intellectual decline
- Vascular events: transient ischaemic attack, stroke

Heart
- Cardiac arrhythmias
- Myocardial ischaemia

Eye
- Vitreous haemorrhage
- ? Worsening of retinopathy

Other
- Hypothermia
- Accidents (including road traffic accidents)

Severe hypoglycaemia, defined as 'hypoglycaemia requiring the assistance of another person for recovery', can result in serious morbidity (see the information box above) and has a recognised mortality of 2–4% in insulin-treated patients. The unrecognised mortality is probably significantly higher than this. Sudden death during sleep in otherwise healthy young patients with type 1 diabetes has been described, and hypoglycaemia-induced cardiac arrhythmia has been implicated. Severe hypoglycaemia is very disruptive and impinges on many aspects of the patient's life including employment, driving and sport.

Symptoms of hypoglycaemia

Common symptoms of hypoglycaemia are listed in the information box on page 492. They comprise two main groups: those related to acute activation of the autonomic nervous system and those secondary to glucose deprivation of the brain (neuroglycopenia). Symptoms of hypoglycaemia are idiosyncratic and the ability to recognise their onset is an important aspect of the initial education of diabetic patients treated with insulin.

SYMPTOMS OF HYPOGLYCAEMIA

Autonomic
- Sweating
- Trembling
- Pounding heart
- Hunger
- Anxiety

Neuroglycopenic
- Confusion
- Drowsiness
- Speech difficulty
- Inability to concentrate
- Incoordination

Non-specific
- Nausea
- Tiredness
- Headache

Awareness of symptoms

If short-acting (soluble) insulin is administered to a normal person, symptoms of hypoglycaemia are usually experienced when the venous or capillary blood glucose is around 2.5–3.0 mmol/l. In diabetic patients who are chronically hyperglycaemic the same symptoms may develop at a higher blood glucose level; conversely, patients who have strict glycaemic control (GHb within the non-diabetic range) or who experience frequent hypoglycaemia may not experience any symptoms even when the blood glucose concentration is well below 2.5 mmol/l. This therapy-induced loss of awareness of hypoglycaemia is usually reversible if glycaemic control is relaxed.

The incidence of impaired perception of the onset of symptoms of hypoglycaemia and an altered symptom profile increases steadily with the duration of insulin treatment, and almost 50% of patients with type 1 diabetes are affected after 20 years of diabetes. This chronic form of hypoglycaemia unawareness may not be reversible; frequency of severe hypoglycaemia is increased six-fold, and intensive insulin therapy should be avoided. In affected patients the usual therapeutic goals need to be modified and frequent self-monitoring of blood glucose is mandatory.

Counter-regulatory responses

In response to a falling blood glucose, there is normally increased secretion of counter-regulatory hormones which counter the blood glucose-lowering effect of insulin. Glucagon and adrenaline are the most important of these. Hypoglycaemia-induced secretion of glucagon becomes impaired in most patients within 5 years of developing type 1 diabetes and after several years many patients also develop a defective adrenaline response to hypoglycaemia so that if hypoglycaemia develops, glucose recovery may be seriously compromised. Autonomic neuropathy may contribute to the deficient adrenaline response but those who develop deficient counter-regulatory responses may also have impaired central activation of neuro-endocrine secretion. Counter-regulatory deficiency cosegregates with impaired awareness of hypoglycaemia, suggesting a common pathogenetic mechanism within the brain. The glycaemic thresholds for the onset of hormonal secretion and symptoms are altered in affected patients, i.e. blood glucose has to fall to a much lower level to trigger these responses.

Causes and prevention

The main causes of hypoglycaemia in patients taking insulin or a sulphonylurea drug are listed in the information box.

CAUSES OF HYPOGLYCAEMIA

- Missed, delayed or inadequate meal
- Unexpected or unusual exercise
- Alcohol
- Poorly designed insulin regimen, particularly that predisposing to nocturnal hypoglycaemia
- Deficient glucose counter-regulation/impaired awareness of hypoglycaemia
- Gastroparesis due to autonomic neuropathy
- Unrecognised other endocrine disorder, e.g. Addison's disease
- Malabsorption
- Factitious (deliberately induced)
- Errors in oral hypoglycaemic agent or insulin dose/schedule/administration

The incidences of most common causes of hypoglycaemia can all be reduced by adequate patient education. Exercise-induced hypoglycaemia (see Fig. 7.16) occurs in treated, well-controlled, insulin-treated diabetic patients because a key factor in the normal adaptation to exercise, namely decreased secretion of endogenous insulin, does not occur. Patients should be taught that if strenuous or protracted exercise is anticipated the preceding dose of insulin should be reduced (the degree of reduction varying widely in individual patients but often being substantial) and extra carbohydrate ingested. All patients taking insulin should carry glucose tablets (e.g. Dextrosol 2.5 g glucose per tablet) at all times.

The incidence of nocturnal hypoglycaemia in patients with type 1 diabetes treated conventionally with a twice-daily injection regimen is difficult to establish but is certainly high. The common problem is that many insulin regimens in current use produce inappropriate nocturnal hyperinsulinaemia. When an intermediate-acting depot insulin such as isophane is taken before the main evening meal at 1700–1900 hrs, its peak action will coincide with the period of maximum sensitivity to insulin, namely 2300–0200 hrs. As nocturnal hypoglycaemia does not usually waken the sleeping patient, and the usual warning symptoms are not perceived, it is often undetected. However, on direct questioning, patients may admit to poor quality of sleep, morning headaches, 'hangover', chronic fatigue and vivid dreams or nightmares. Sometimes a

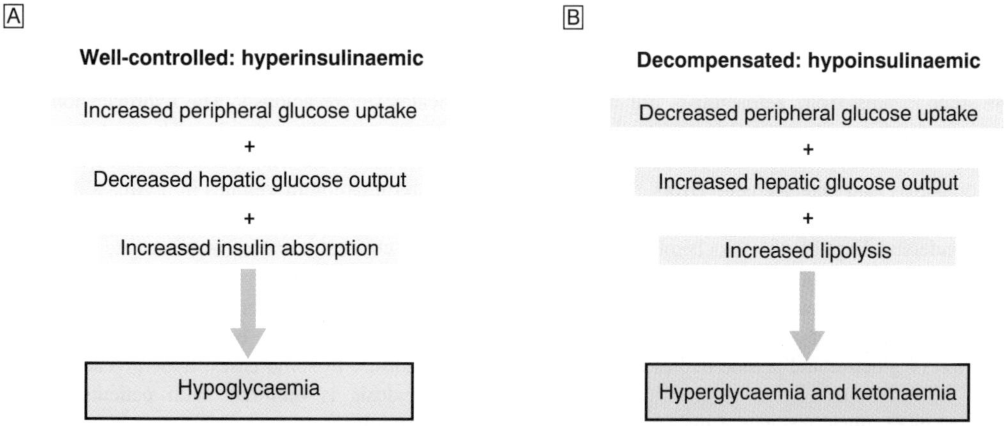

Fig. 7.16 The effect of exercise in diabetic patients being treated with insulin. A Well-controlled hyperinsulinaemic patients. B Decompensated hypoinsulinaemic patients.

relative may observe sweating (which may be profuse), restlessness, twitching or even convulsions. The only reliable way to make the diagnosis is to measure the blood glucose during the night. The times of maximum risk of biochemical hypoglycaemia are between 2300 and 0200 hrs and between 0500 and 0700 hrs. One approach to treatment is to defer administration of the evening dose of intermediate-acting insulin. In most cases this solves the problem provided that the depot insulin is not taken earlier than 2300 hrs. It is a sensible precaution for patients to measure the blood glucose before they go to bed and to take additional carbohydrate if the reading is less than 6.0 mmol/l.

Management

Treatment of acute hypoglycaemia depends on the severity of the hypoglycaemia and whether the patient is conscious and able to swallow. Treatment may simply require oral carbohydrate if hypoglycaemia is recognised early. If the patient is unable to swallow, parenteral glucose (30–50 ml of 50% dextrose) or glucagon (1 mg by intramuscular injection) should be administered. Glucagon, in addition to increasing hepatic breakdown of glycogen, stimulates the secretion of insulin and therefore should not be used to treat hypoglycaemia induced by an oral hypoglycaemic drug. The recommended dose of intravenous dextrose in children is 0.2 g/kg. A viscous gel solution (Hypostop) can be applied into the buccal cavity in children, although jam or honey may be just as effective.

As soon as the patient is able to swallow, glucose should be given orally. Full recovery may not occur immediately. Further, when hypoglycaemia has occurred in a patient using a long- or intermediate-acting insulin or a sulphonylurea, particularly chlorpropamide, the possibility of recurrence should be anticipated.

The development of cerebral oedema should be considered in patients who fail to regain consciousness after blood glucose is restored to normal. Other causes of impaired consciousness, such as alcoholic intoxication, a post-ictal state or cerebral haemorrhage, should be excluded. Cerebral oedema has a high mortality and morbidity and requires urgent treatment with mannitol and/or dexamethasone, and high-dose oxygen.

Following recovery it is important to try to identify a cause and make appropriate adjustments to the patient's therapy. Unless the reason for a hypoglycaemic episode is clear, the patient should reduce the next dose and subsequent doses of insulin by 20% and seek medical advice about further adjustments in dose. Patient education on the potential risks of inducing hypoglycaemia, regular blood glucose monitoring and treatment, including the need to have an accessible supply of glucose (and glucagon), are fundamental to prevention of this potentially dangerous side-effect of treatment. Relatives and friends also need to be familiar with the symptoms and signs of hypoglycaemia and should be instructed as to how this should be managed (including how to give an intramuscular injection of glucagon).

DIABETIC KETOACIDOSIS

Diabetic ketoacidosis is a major medical emergency and remains a serious cause of morbidity, principally in patients with type 1 diabetes. The average mortality in developed countries is 5–10% and is higher in the elderly. A significant number of new patients still present in diabetic ketoacidosis; in established diabetes a common course of events is that patients develop an intercurrent infection, lose their appetite, and either stop or drastically reduce their dose of insulin in the mistaken belief that under these circumstances less insulin is required. Any form of stress, particularly that produced by infection, may precipitate severe ketoacidosis, even in patients with type 2 diabetes. Although some deaths from ketoacidosis are associated with severe medical conditions such as acute myocardial infarction or septicaemia, others are the consequence of delays in diagnosis and management errors. No obvious precipitating cause can be found in many cases.

A clear understanding of the biochemical basis and pathophysiology of this problem is essential for its efficient treatment. Ketoacidosis is caused by insulin deficiency and an increase in catabolic hormones, leading to hepatic overproduction of glucose and ketone bodies (see Fig. 7.6, p. 478).

The cardinal biochemical features of diabetic ketoacidosis are:

- hyperglycaemia
- hyperketonaemia
- metabolic acidosis.

The hyperglycaemia causes a profound osmotic diuresis leading to dehydration and electrolyte loss, particularly of sodium and potassium. The metabolic acidosis forces hydrogen ions into cells, displacing potassium ions, which may be lost in urine or through vomiting.

The information box shows the average loss of fluid and electrolytes in moderately severe diabetic ketoacidosis in an adult. About half the deficit of total body water is derived from the intracellular compartment and occurs comparatively early in the development of acidosis with relatively few clinical features; the remainder represents loss of extracellular fluid sustained largely in the later stages. It is at this time that marked contraction of the size of the extracellular space occurs, with haemoconcentration, a decreased blood volume, and finally a fall in blood pressure with associated renal ischaemia and oliguria.

Every patient in diabetic ketoacidosis is potassium-depleted, but the plasma concentration of potassium gives very little indication of the total body deficit. Plasma potassium may even be raised initially due to disproportionate loss of water and catabolism of protein and glycogen. However, soon after insulin treatment is started there is likely to be a precipitous fall in the plasma potassium due to dilution of extracellular potassium by administration of intravenous fluids, the movement of potassium into cells as a result of treatment with insulin, and the continuing renal loss of potassium.

AVERAGE LOSS OF FLUID AND ELECTROLYTES IN AN ADULT WITH DIABETIC KETOACIDOSIS OF MODERATE SEVERITY

- Water: 6 litres
- Sodium: 500 mmol
- Chloride: 400 mmol
- Potassium: 350 mmol

The severity of ketoacidosis can be assessed rapidly by measuring the plasma bicarbonate; less than 12 mmol/l indicates severe acidosis. The hydrogen ion concentration gives an even more precise measure but requires arterial blood. There is no simple and accurate quantitative method for determination of ketones in plasma although a test strip (Ketostix) can be used as a semiquantitative guide to the plasma concentration of acetoacetate and acetone. The magnitude of the hyperglycaemia does not correlate with the severity of the metabolic acidosis; moderate elevation of blood glucose may be associated with life-threatening ketoacidosis. In some cases, hyperglycaemia predominates and acidosis is minimal, with patients presenting in a hyperosmolar state.

Clinical features

The clinical features of ketoacidosis are listed in the first information box below. The state of consciousness is very variable in patients with diabetic ketoacidosis; coma is uncommon. A patient with dangerous ketoacidosis requiring urgent treatment may walk into the consulting room. For this reason the term 'diabetic ketoacidosis' is to be preferred to 'diabetic coma', which implies that there is no urgency until unconsciousness supervenes. In fact, it is imperative that energetic treatment is started at the earliest possible stage.

Abdominal pain is sometimes a feature of diabetic ketoacidosis, particularly in children. Serum amylase may be elevated but rarely indicates coexisting pancreatitis. Although leucocytosis invariably occurs, this represents a stress response and does not necessarily indicate infection;

CLINICAL FEATURES OF DIABETIC KETOACIDOSIS

Symptoms	Signs
• Polyuria, thirst	• Dehydration
• Weight loss	• Hypotension
• Weakness	• Tachycardia
• Nausea, vomiting	• Air hunger (Kussmaul breathing)
• Leg cramps	• Smell of acetone
• Blurred vision	• Hypothermia
• Abdominal pain	• Confusion, drowsiness, coma (10%)

COMPLICATIONS OF DIABETIC KETOACIDOSIS

- Cerebral oedema
  May be caused by rapid reduction of blood glucose or use of hypotonic fluids
  High mortality; treat with mannitol, oxygen
- Acute respiratory distress syndrome
  Arterial hypoxaemia; pulmonary infiltrates
- Thromboembolism
- Disseminated intravascular coagulation (rare)
- Acute circulatory failure

pyrexia may not be present initially because of vasodilatation secondary to acidosis. Complications of diabetic ketoacidosis are described in the information box, bottom right, page 494.

Management

Diabetic ketoacidosis is a medical emergency which should be treated in hospital, preferably in a high-dependency area. Treatment must be monitored by laboratory measurement of plasma glucose, urea and electrolytes, and arterial pH (H^+ concentration) and bicarbonate, estimated initially at intervals of 1–2 hours.

The principal components of treatment are:

- the administration of short-acting (soluble) insulin
- fluid replacement
- potassium replacement
- the administration of antibiotics if infection is present.

Guidelines for the management of ketoacidosis are shown in Table 7.11, p. 496 and the information box.

MANAGEMENT OF DIABETIC KETOACIDOSIS
Average fluid deficit
• 6 litres 3 litres from extracellular compartment: replaced by saline 3 litres from intracellular compartment: replaced by dextrose
Capillary blood glucose measurement
• A capillary blood glucose measurement giving a reading of ≥ 17 mmol/l using visually read glucose strips can be very misleading since the actual blood glucose concentration is often considerably higher when measured accurately in the laboratory. Therefore an accurate measurement should be taken at an early stage
Additional procedures
The following may be required: • Catheterisation if after 3 hrs no urine passed • Nasogastric tube to keep stomach empty (in unconscious or semi-conscious patients) • Central venous line if cardiovascular system compromised so that volume of fluid given can be adjusted accurately • Plasma expander if BP does not rise with i.v. saline • Antibiotic if infection demonstrated or suspected
Monitor
• Blood glucose and electrolytes hourly for 3 hrs and every 2–4 hrs thereafter • Temperature, pulse, respiration, BP hourly • Urinary output and ketones • ECG, plasma osmolality, arterial pH in some cases

Insulin

If an intravenous infusion of insulin (see Table 7.11) is not possible, a loading dose of 10–20 units of soluble insulin can be given by intramuscular injection, immediately followed by 4–6 units hourly thereafter. The blood glucose concentration should fall by 3–6 mmol/l per hour. A more rapid fall in blood glucose should be avoided as hypoglycaemia can be precipitated and the serious complication of cerebral oedema may develop. If blood glucose does not fall within 2 hours after commencing treatment, the dose of insulin should be doubled until a satisfactory response is obtained. Ketosis, dehydration, acidaemia, infection and stress combine to produce severe insulin resistance in some cases but most will respond to a low-dose insulin regimen. When the blood glucose concentration has fallen to 10–15 mmol/l the dose of insulin should be reduced to 1–4 units hourly. Restoration of insulin by subcutaneous injection should not be instituted until the patient is able to eat and drink normally.

Fluid replacement

Intravenous fluid replacement is required since, even when the patient is able to swallow, fluids given by mouth may be poorly absorbed. The extracellular fluid deficit should be replenished by infusing isotonic saline (0.9% NaCl). Early and rapid rehydration is essential, otherwise the administered insulin will not reach the poorly perfused tissues. If the plasma sodium is greater than 155 mmol/l, 0.45% saline may be given initially instead of 0.9%.

The intracellular water deficit must be replaced by using 5% or 10% dextrose and not by more saline. It is best given when the blood glucose concentration approaches normal. An accurate record of fluid balance must be maintained.

Potassium

As the plasma potassium is often high at presentation, treatment with intravenous potassium chloride should be started cautiously (see Table 7.11) and carefully monitored. Sufficient should be given to maintain a normal plasma concentration and large amounts may be required (100–300 mmol in the first 24 hours). Cardiac rhythm should be monitored in severe cases because of the risk of electrolyte-induced cardiac arrhythmia.

Bicarbonate

In patients who are severely acidotic (pH < 7.0, $[H^+]$ > 100 nmol/l) the infusion of sodium bicarbonate (300 ml 1.26% over 30 minutes into a large vein) should be considered, with the simultaneous administration of potassium. Its use is controversial, however, and should only be considered in exceptional circumstances. Complete correction of the acidosis should not be attempted.

Antibiotics

Infections must be carefully sought and vigorously treated since it may not be possible to abolish ketosis until they are controlled.

Table 7.11 Guidelines for the management of diabetic ketoacidosis

Time (hrs)	Insulin (use only short-acting (soluble) insulin)	Fluid (i.v.)	Potassium (i.v.)	Other
0	Start i.v. insulin infusion 5 U/hr (Alternatively, 10–20 U i.m. followed by 5 U/hr i.m. thereafter)	Start i.v. 0.9% saline infusion, 1 litre in 30 min		Check capillary blood glucose. If ≥ 17 mmol/l obtain venous blood for urgent laboratory measurement of glucose, Na, K, Cl, CO_2, urea and pH or $[H^+]$. Test urine for ketones
0.5	Continue insulin 5 U/hr i.v.	0.5 litre of 0.9% saline in 30 min	If plasma K^+ > 5.5 mmol/l give no KCl; 3.5–5.5 mmol/l give 20 mmol KCl/l of infused fluid; < 3.5 mmol/l give 40 mmol KCl/l of infused fluid	If plasma Na^+ > 155 mmol/l give 0.45% rather than 0.9% saline until Na^+ falls to 140 mmol/l. If pH < 7.0 ($[H^+]$ > 100 nmol/l) give 300–500 ml 1.26% sodium bicarbonate over 30 min into large vein
1	Continue insulin 5 U/hr i.v.	0.5 litre of 0.9% saline in 1 hr	As above	Recheck biochemistry
2	Continue insulin 5 U/hr i.v. (higher rate if fall in blood glucose < 3 mmol/hr)	0.5 litre of 0.9% saline in 2 hrs	As above	Recheck biochemistry
	When blood glucose < 15 mmol/l Reduce rate of insulin infusion to 1–4 U/hr	Change to 5% glucose infusion 0.5 litre/2 hrs	Continue i.v. K^+ supplements	Continue to check biochemistry every 2–4 hrs
Continue with regimen until fluid deficit replaced, ketonuria abolished and adequate oral intake of carbohydrate feasible.				
N.B. These guidelines for a typical 'average' case should be modified appropriately in the individual patient after considering the blood biochemistry and clinical features, e.g. see below for information on treatment of non-ketotic hyperosmolar diabetic coma.				

NON-KETOTIC HYPEROSMOLAR DIABETIC COMA

This condition is characterised by severe hyperglycaemia (> 50 mmol/l) without significant hyperketonaemia or acidosis. Severe dehydration and pre-renal uraemia are common. This condition usually affects elderly patients, many with previously undiagnosed diabetes. Mortality is over 40%. Its treatment differs from that of ketoacidosis in two main respects. Firstly, these patients are usually relatively sensitive to insulin and approximately half the dose of insulin recommended for the treatment of ketoacidosis should usually be employed. Secondly, the plasma osmolality should be measured or, less accurately, calculated using the following formula based on plasma values in mmol/l:

$$\text{Plasma osmolality} = 2[Na^+] + 2([K^+] + [\text{glucose}] + [\text{urea}])$$

The normal value is 280–300 mmol/kg and the conscious level is depressed when it is high (> 340 mmol/kg). Saline (0.45%) should be given until the osmolality approaches normal, when 0.9% should be substituted. The rate of fluid replacement should be regulated on the basis of the central venous pressure, and plasma sodium concentration checked frequently. Thromboembolic complications are common, and prophylactic subcutaneous administration of heparin is recommended.

LACTIC ACIDOSIS

In coma due to lactic acidosis the patient is likely to be taking a biguanide for type 2 diabetes and is very ill and overbreathing but not so profoundly dehydrated as is usual in coma due to ketoacidosis. The patient's breath does not smell of acetone, ketonuria is mild or even absent yet the plasma bicarbonate and pH are markedly reduced (pH < 7.2). The diagnosis is confirmed by a high (usually > 5.0 mmol/l) concentration of lactic acid in the blood. Treatment is with intravenous sodium bicarbonate sufficient to raise the plasma pH to above 7.2, along with insulin and glucose. Despite energetic treatment, the mortality in this condition is > 50%. Sodium dichloroacetate may be given to lower blood lactate.

ACUTE CIRCULATORY FAILURE

Acute circulatory failure occurring in any of these types of acute metabolic decompensation should be treated as described on page 1033.

LONG-TERM COMPLICATIONS OF DIABETES

The long-term results of treatment of diabetes are disappointing in many patients (see p. 497). Table 7.12 and

Table 7.12 Mortality in diabetes

	Mortality ratio (diabetics vs matched controls)	
Overall	2.6	$p < 0.001$
Coronary heart disease **Cerebrovascular disease** **Peripheral vascular disease**	2.8	$p < 0.001$
All other causes including renal failure	2.7	$p < 0.05$

APPROXIMATE FIGURES FOR CAUSES OF DEATH IN TREATED DIABETIC PATIENTS

- Atherosclerosis 70%
- Renal failure 10%
- Cancer 10%
- Infections 6%
- Diabetic ketoacidosis 1%
- Other 3%

the information box show that the excess mortality incurred by diabetic patients is mainly caused by large blood vessel disease, which is common in treated diabetic patients and accounts for about 70% of all deaths, mostly from myocardial infarction and stroke. The pathological changes associated with atherosclerosis in diabetic patients are similar to those seen in the non-diabetic population but they occur earlier in life and are more extensive and severe. Diabetes enhances the effects of the other major cardiovascular risk factors, smoking, hypertension and hypercholesterolaemia (see Fig. 7.17). Hyperinsulinaemia may promote atherogenic changes in blood lipids and blood coagulability and raise arterial blood pressure. A metabolic (insulin resistance) syndrome has been described in which the cosegregation of various conditions is associated with premature and severe macrovascular disease (see the information box and Fig. 7.2, p. 475).

Disease of small blood vessels is a specific complication of diabetes and is termed diabetic microangiopathy. It

METABOLIC SYNDROME (SYNDROME X)

Features include:
- Type 2 diabetes or impaired glucose tolerance
- Low HDL cholesterol; elevated triglycerides
- Hypertension
- Central (android) obesity
- Increased plasminogen activator inhibitor-1
- Hyperuricaemia

This constellation of risk factors for atherosclerosis is sometimes called the 'insulin resistance syndrome' as hyperinsulinaemia is a central feature. It is associated with macrovascular disease (coronary, cerebral and peripheral arteries) and an excess mortality

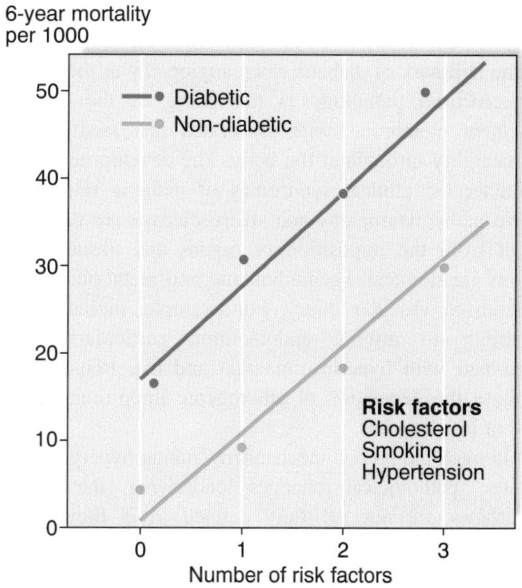

Fig. 7.17 Diabetes mellitus as a risk factor for coronary heart disease (CHD). Three major factors—smoking, hypertension and raised cholesterol—are associated with risk of CHD in the general population. The presence of diabetes mellitus produces an increment in risk in addition to these conventional factors.

contributes to mortality by causing renal failure due to diabetic nephropathy.

Both types of vascular disease also cause substantial morbidity and disability: e.g. blindness due to diabetic retinopathy; difficulty in walking, chronic ulceration of the feet, bowel and bladder dysfunction due to diabetic neuropathy; and angina, cardiac failure, intermittent claudication and gangrene due to atherosclerosis.

Pathophysiology

Some of the numerous biochemical and functional

PATHOGENESIS OF DIABETIC VASCULAR AND NEUROPATHIC COMPLICATIONS: POSSIBLE MECHANISMS

Biochemical consequences of hyperglycaemia

- Non-enzymatic glycation
- Oxidative-reductive stress
- Increased polyol pathway activity
- Intracellular *myo*-inositol depletion
- Increased diacylglycerol synthesis
- Increased protein kinase C activity

Functional abnormalities

- Haemodynamic disturbances
- Haemorrheological and coagulation abnormalities
- Microvascular hypertension
- Endothelial dysfunction
- Increased capillary permeability

abnormalities found in long-standing poorly controlled diabetic patients are listed in the information box.

The hallmark of diabetic microangiopathy at the level of ultrastructural pathology is thickening of the capillary basement membrane, with associated increased vascular permeability throughout the body. The development of the characteristic clinical syndromes of diabetic retinopathy, nephropathy, neuropathy and atherosclerosis are thought to result from the imposition of organ- and tissue-specific factors (anatomical, haemodynamic and metabolic) on the generalised vascular injury. For example, increased permeability of arterial endothelium, particularly when combined with hyperinsulinaemia and hypertension, will increase the deposition of atherogenic lipoproteins in the wall of large vessels.

Although the precise mechanisms linking hyperglycaemia to the pathological changes underlying the clinical syndromes are not yet fully defined, it is thought that increased metabolism of glucose to sorbitol via the polyol pathway is of central importance in pathogenesis, since haemodynamic, vascular permeability and structural changes in capillaries are prevented in diabetic animals by treatment with a variety of structurally different aldose-reductase inhibitors. Glycation of structural proteins and the production of advanced glycation end-products, with their deposition in various tissues, along with possible free radical-mediated damage, may underlie some of the structural and functional abnormalities of diabetic complications. Likewise, an increase in glycolytic metabolites within the cell contributes to enhanced synthesis of diacylglycerol which has been linked via the activation of protein kinase C to the various vascular abnormalities listed in the information box.

Whatever the mechanism of the noxious effect of long-standing hyperglycaemia, it has been shown (both in experimental animal models and in long-term clinical studies in human diabetes) that the nearer the overall blood glucose concentration is to normal, the fewer and less severe are the abnormalities listed in the information box, and the lower the incidence of the clinical syndromes arising from micro- and macroangiopathy.

DIABETIC RETINOPATHY

Diabetic retinopathy is the most common cause of blindness in adults between 30 and 65 years of age in developed countries. Although the precise mechanisms underlying its development are still not completely defined, retinal photocoagulation is an effective treatment provided it is given at an early stage when the patient is usually symptomless. This means that regular ophthalmoscopy, with the pupils fully dilated, is mandatory in all diabetic patients.

Clinical features

The clinical features characteristic of diabetic retinopathy are listed in the information box. These occur in varying combinations in different patients. Abnormalities of the capillary bed, which are not clinically visible, are the earliest lesions. They include capillary dilatation and closure.

CLINICAL FEATURES OF DIABETIC RETINOPATHY

- Microaneurysms
- Retinal haemorrhages
- Hard exudates
- Soft exudates
- Venous changes
- Neovascularisation
- Pre-retinal haemorrhage
- Vitreous haemorrhage
- Fibrosis

Microaneurysms

In most cases these are the earliest clinical abnormality detected. They appear as minute, discrete, circular, dark red spots near to, but apparently separate from, the retinal vessels (see Fig. 7.18A). They look like tiny haemorrhages but photographs of injected preparations of retina show that they are in fact minute aneurysms arising mainly from the venous end of capillaries near areas of capillary closure.

Haemorrhages

These most characteristically occur in the deeper layers of the retina and hence are round and regular in shape and described as 'blot' haemorrhages (see Fig. 7.18A). The smaller ones may be difficult to differentiate from microaneurysms and the two are often grouped together as 'dots and blots'. Superficial flame-shaped haemorrhages may also occur, particularly if the patient is hypertensive.

Hard exudates

These are characteristic of diabetic retinopathy. They vary in size from tiny specks to large confluent patches and tend to occur particularly in the perimacular area (see Fig. 7.18B). They result from leakage of plasma from abnormal retinal capillaries and overlie areas of neuronal degeneration.

Soft exudates

Sometimes referred to as 'cotton wool spots', these are similar to those seen in hypertension, and also occur particularly within five disc diameters of the optic disc. They represent arteriolar occlusions causing retinal ischaemia and are most often seen in rapidly advancing retinopathy or in association with uncontrolled hypertension.

Intraretinal microvascular abnormalities

Intraretinal microvascular abnormalities (IRMA) are dilated, tortuous capillaries which represent the remaining patent capillaries in an area where most have been occluded.

Neovascularisation

This may arise from mature vessels on the optic disc or the

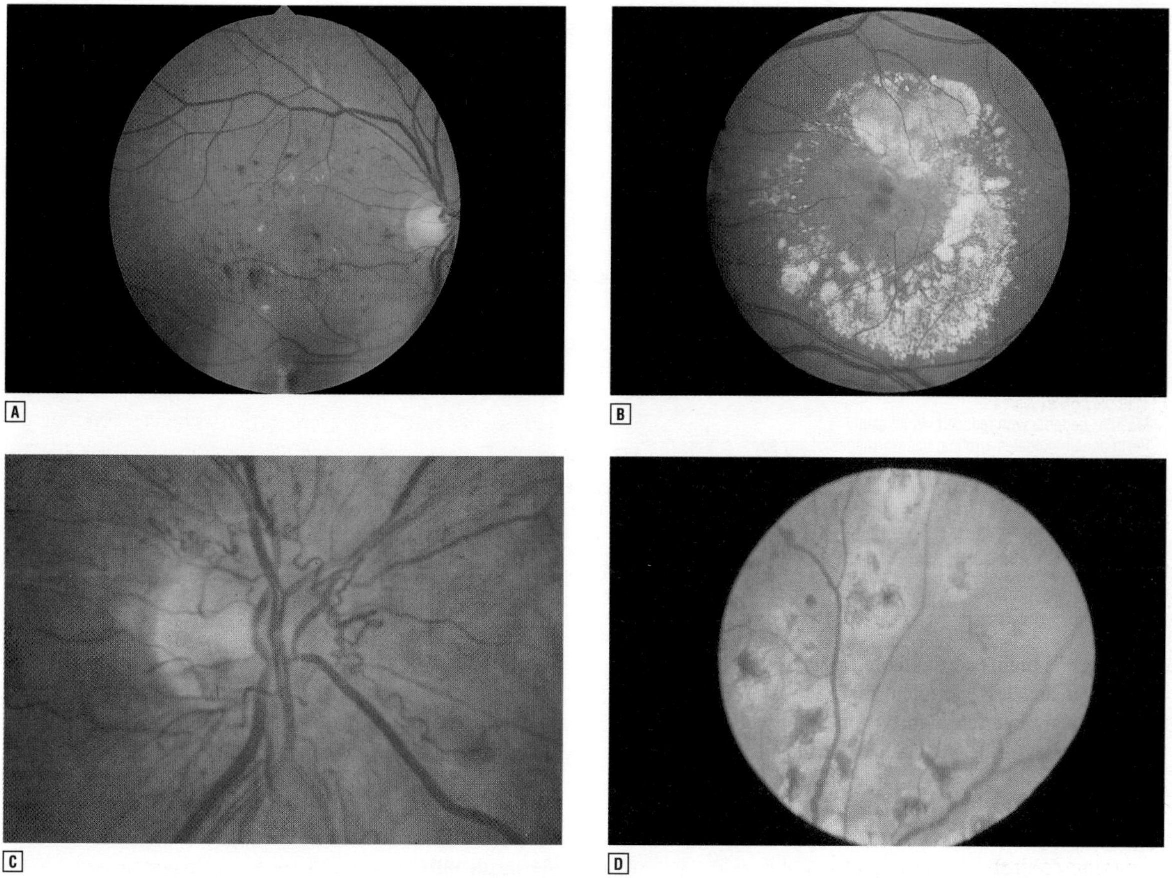

Fig. 7.18 Examples of diabetic eye disease. [A] Background diabetic retinopathy showing dot and blot haemorrhages and a few hard exudates. [B] Diabetic maculopathy with ring of exudates surrounding macula. [C] Proliferative diabetic retinopathy showing new vessels at upper and lower edges of optic discs. [D] Photocoagulation scars in retina treated with laser therapy.

retina in response to areas of ischaemic retina. The earliest appearance is that of fine tufts of delicate vessels forming arcades on the surface of the retina (see Fig. 7.18C). As they grow, they may extend forwards towards the vitreous. They are fragile and leaky and are liable to rupture, causing haemorrhage which may be intraretinal, pre-retinal ('sub-hyaloid') or into the vitreous. Serous products leaking from these new vessel systems stimulate a connective tissue reaction, retinitis proliferans. This first appears as a white, cloudy haze among the network of new vessels. As it extends, the new vessels may be obliterated and the surrounding retina covered by a dense white sheet. At this stage, bleeding is less common but retinal detachment can occur due to contraction of adhesions between the vitreous and the retina.

Venous changes

These include venous dilatation (an early feature probably representing increased blood flow), 'beading' (sausage-like changes in calibre) and increased tortuosity including 'oxbow lakes' or loops. These latter changes often indicate widespread capillary non-perfusion.

Classification

A classification of diabetic retinopathy, based on prognosis for vision and indications for specialist referral, is shown in Table 7.13, p. 500.

Microaneurysms, abnormalities of the veins, and small blot haemorrhages and hard exudates situated in the periphery will not interfere with vision unless they are associated with macular oedema in the perimacular or macular area. This is not easy to detect by ophthalmoscopy but should be suspected, particularly if there is marked impairment of visual acuity in association with mild peripheral non-proliferative retinopathy and no other obvious pathology.

New vessels may be completely symptomless until sudden visual loss occurs from a haemorrhage into the vitreous. Although these frequently resolve, the risk of

Table 7.13 Classification of diabetic retinopathy based on prognosis for vision

Type of retinopathy	Prognosis	Action required
Non-proliferative 'background' retinopathy without maculopathy Venous dilatation Peripheral Microaneurysms Small blot haemorrhages Small hard exudates	No immediate threat to vision	Maximise control of blood glucose, lipids and pressure Give advice to stop smoking and reduce intake of alcohol Observe carefully, i.e. fundoscopy *with dilated pupils* every 6–12 months Refer for specialist opinion if rate of progression increases significantly
Pre-proliferative retinopathy and/or maculopathy Venous loops and beading Clusters/sheets of microaneurysms and small blot haemorrhages and/or large retinal haemorrhages Intraretinal microvascular abnormalities Multiple soft exudates Macular oedema with reduced visual acuity Perimacular exudates ± retinal haemorrhages of any size	Sight-threatening; refer for specialist opinion	At this stage rapid lowering of the blood glucose may result in abrupt worsening of retinopathy with the appearance of soft exudates and an increased number of haemorrhages; it may be safer to lower the blood glucose gradually over a period of months
Proliferative retinopathy and/or exudative maculopathy Pre-retinal haemorrhage Neovascularisation Fibrosis Exudative maculopathy	Urgent review and treatment by specialist mandatory	

recurrence is high, and the more frequent the haemorrhage, the slower and less complete the recovery. Fibrous tissue may seriously interfere with vision by obscuring the retina and/or causing further retinal haemorrhage or detachment.

Prevention

Glycaemic control

Good glycaemic control, particularly in the early years following the development of diabetes, reduces the risk of developing retinopathy. Early diagnosis followed by effective treatment is particularly important for those with type 2 diabetes, 20% of whom present with established retinopathy, which in some is untreatable. In others, retinopathy is diagnosed only when the patient is referred for a specialist opinion after years of ineffective treatment of type 2 diabetes. Hyperglycaemia promotes retinal hyperperfusion, so a rapid reduction in blood glucose may cause an initial deterioration of retinopathy by causing relative ischaemia. Improvement in glycaemic control should therefore be effected gradually. The rate of progression of retinopathy is still significantly less in intensively treated patients than in matched control subjects.

Screening

Regular screening for retinopathy is essential in all diabetic patients but is particularly important in those with risk factors. These include early onset, long duration of diabetes, hypertension, poor glycaemic control, pregnancy, use of the oral contraceptive pill, smoking, excessive alcohol consumption, and evidence of microangiopathy elsewhere, particularly in patients with neuropathy and proteinuria. Screening can be undertaken in specialist diabetes centres, by the patient's GP if sufficiently experienced, or by trained optometrists. A non-mydriatic camera or a digital imaging system may be utilised in a retinal screening programme, but the problem remains that many diabetic patients receive no regular supervision.

Management

Severe non-proliferative and proliferative retinopathy can be treated with retinal photocoagulation and has been shown to reduce severe visual loss by 85%, and maculopathy by 50%. Photocoagulation is used:

- to destroy areas of retinal ischaemia (since it is thought that this plays a major role in the development of neovascularisation)
- to seal leaking microaneurysms and reduce macular oedema
- to obliterate new vessels directly on the retinal surface (but not on the optic disc).

Two types of photocoagulation are available: xenon-arc (white light) and laser beam (monochromatic green light). The latter is more comfortable for the patient and the smaller size of beam allows greater accuracy in delivering shots. This simple procedure can be done under local anaesthesia and in skilled hands carries little risk and can be very effective. Panretinal photocoagulation is frequently employed. New vessels can be eliminated, with vision being maintained in up to 90% of patients who have new vessels on the retina and/or disc; macular oedema can also be treated with laser therapy. Successfully treated patients must be reviewed regularly to check for further development of new vessels. Extensive photocoagulation scarring can cause significant visual field loss, which may interfere with driving ability.

Vitrectomy may be used in selected cases with advanced diabetic eye disease where visual loss is due to vitreous haemorrhage which has failed to clear, or retinal detachment resulting from retinitis proliferans.

The more severe types of retinopathy may be accompanied by the development of new vessels on the anterior surface of the iris: 'rubeosis iridis'. These vessels may obstruct the drainage angle of the eye and the outflow of aqueous fluid, causing secondary glaucoma. The main method of management is the prevention of extension of the rubeosis by early retinal photocoagulation.

Cataract

Very rarely a type of cataract specific to diabetes occurs in young patients with poorly controlled diabetes. Senile cataract occurs commonly in elderly diabetic patients but is probably no more frequent than in non-diabetic people. The indications for cataract extraction are similar to those for the non-diabetic population and depend on the degree of visual impairment caused by the cataract. An additional indication in diabetes is when adequate assessment of the fundus is precluded or laser treatment to the retina is prevented. The extracapsular method of extraction is preferable in diabetes with implantation of an intraocular lens.

DIABETIC NEUROPATHY

This is a relatively early and common complication affecting approximately 30% of diabetic patients. Although in a few patients it can cause severe disability, it is symptomless in the majority. Like retinopathy it occurs secondary to the metabolic disturbance and the prevalence is related to the duration of diabetes and the degree of metabolic control. Although there is evidence that the central nervous system is affected in long-term diabetes, the clinical impact of diabetes is mainly manifest on the peripheral nervous system.

Pathology

The main pathological features are listed in the information box. They can occur in motor, sensory and autonomic nerves.

DIABETIC NEUROPATHY—HISTOPATHOLOGY

- Axonal degeneration of both myelinated and unmyelinated fibres
  - Early: axon shrinkage
  - Later: axonal fragmentation; regeneration
- Thickening of Schwann cell basal lamina
- Patchy, segmental demyelination
- Abnormalities of intraneural capillaries: thickening of basement membrane and microthrombi

Classification

Various classifications of diabetic neuropathy have been proposed. One is shown in the information box. None of the proposed classifications is entirely satisfactory since motor, sensory and autonomic nerves may be involved in varying combinations so that clinically mixed syndromes usually occur.

CLASSIFICATION OF DIABETIC NEUROPATHY

Somatic	Visceral (autonomic)
• Polyneuropathy Symmetrical, mainly sensory and distal Asymmetrical, mainly motor and proximal • Mononeuropathy (including mononeuritis multiplex)	• Cardiovascular • Gastrointestinal • Genitourinary • Sudomotor • Vasomotor • Pupillary

Clinical features

Symmetrical sensory polyneuropathy

This is frequently asymptomatic. The most common signs found on physical examination are diminished perception of vibration sensation distally, 'glove-and-stocking' impairment of all other modalities of sensation and loss of tendon reflexes in the lower limbs. Sensory abnormalities dominate the clinical presentation. Symptoms include paraesthesiae in the feet and, rarely, in the hands, pain in the lower limbs (dull, aching and/or lancinating, worse at night, and mainly felt on the anterior aspect of the legs), burning sensations in the soles of the feet, cutaneous hyperaesthesia and an abnormal gait (commonly wide-based) often associated with a sense of numbness in the feet. Muscle weakness and wasting develop only in advanced cases, but subclinical motor nerve dysfunction is common. The toes may be clawed with wasting of the interosseous muscles, which results in increased pressure on the plantar aspects of the metatarsal heads with the development of callous skin at these and other pressure points. Electrophysiological tests demonstrate slowing of both motor and sensory conduction, and tests of vibration sensitivity and thermal thresholds are abnormal. A diffuse small-fibre neuropathy causes altered perception of pain and temperature and is associated with autonomic neuropathy; characteristic features include foot ulcers, Charcot arthropathy and symptomatic autonomic dysfunction.

Asymmetrical motor diabetic neuropathy

Sometimes called diabetic amyotrophy, this presents as severe and progressive weakness and wasting of the proximal muscles of the lower (and occasionally the upper) limbs. It is commonly accompanied by severe pain mainly felt on the anterior aspect of the leg, and hyperaesthesia and paraesthesiae are common. Sometimes there may also be marked loss of weight ('neuropathic cachexia'). The patient may look extremely ill and may be unable to get out of bed. Tendon reflexes may be absent on the affected side(s). Sometimes there are extensor plantar responses and the cerebrospinal fluid protein is often raised. This condition is thought to involve acute infarction of the lower motor neurons of the lumbosacral plexus. Other lesions involving this plexus, such as neoplasms and lumbar disc disease, must be excluded. Recovery usually occurs within 12 months and management is mainly supportive.

Mononeuropathy

Either motor or sensory function can be affected within a single peripheral or cranial nerve. Unlike the gradual progression of distal symmetrical and autonomic neuropathies, mononeuropathies are severe and of rapid onset; they eventually recover. The nerves most commonly affected are the 3rd and 6th cranial nerves, resulting in diplopia, and the femoral and sciatic nerves. Rarely, involvement of other single nerves results in paresis and paraesthesiae in the thorax and trunk (truncal radiculopathies). Nerve compression palsies commonly affect the median nerve, giving the clinical picture of carpal tunnel compression syndrome, and less commonly the ulnar nerve. Lateral popliteal nerve compression occasionally causes foot drop.

Autonomic neuropathy

This is not necessarily associated with peripheral somatic neuropathy. Either parasympathetic or sympathetic nerves may be predominantly affected in any one system or more. Although autonomic neuropathy can affect virtually all bodily systems in any one patient, involvement tends to be patchy. The information box lists the symptoms and signs arising from autonomic neuropathy affecting the various systems. The development of autonomic neuropathy is less clearly related to poor metabolic control than somatic neuropathy, and improved control rarely results in amelioration of symptoms. Within 10 years of developing overt symptoms of autonomic neuropathy, 30–50% of patients are dead—many from sudden cardiorespiratory arrest, the cause of which is unknown. Patients with postural hypotension have the highest subsequent mortality.

Management

Management of peripheral sensorimotor and autonomic neuropathies is outlined in Table 7.14.

Erectile failure (impotence) affects 30% of diabetic males and is often multifactorial. Although neuropathy and vascular causes are common, psychological factors, including depression, anxiety and reduced libido, may be partly responsible. Alcohol and antihypertensive drugs such as thiazide diuretics and β-adrenoceptor antagonists may cause sexual dysfunction and, rarely, patients may have an endocrine cause such as testosterone deficiency or hyperprolactinaemia.

CLINICAL FEATURES OF AUTONOMIC NEUROPATHY

Cardiovascular
- Postural hypotension
- Resting tachycardia
- Fixed heart rate
- Sudden cardiorespiratory arrest

Gastrointestinal
- Dysphagia, due to oesophageal atony
- Abdominal fullness, nausea and vomiting, unstable diabetes, due to delayed gastric emptying ('gastroparesis')
- Nocturnal diarrhoea ± faecal incontinence
- Constipation, due to colonic atony

Genitourinary
- Difficulty in micturition, urinary incontinence, recurrent infection, due to atonic bladder
- Impotence and retrograde ejaculation

Sudomotor
- Gustatory sweating
- Nocturnal sweats without hypoglycaemia
- Anhidrosis—fissures in the feet

Vasomotor
- Feet feel cold, due to loss of skin vasomotor responses
- Dependent oedema, due to loss of vasomotor tone and increased vascular permeability
- Bullous formation

Pupillary
- Decreased pupil size
- Resistance to mydriatrics
- Delayed or absent response to light

THE DIABETIC FOOT

The foot is a frequent site for complications in patients with diabetes and for this reason foot care is particularly important. The clinical features are listed in the information box on page 503.

Tissue necrosis in the feet is a common reason for hospital admission in diabetic patients. Such admissions tend to be prolonged and not unusually end with amputation at various levels.

Aetiology

Foot ulceration occurs as a result of trauma (often trivial) in the presence of neuropathy and/or peripheral vascular disease, with infection occurring as a secondary phenomenon following ulceration of the protective epidermis. In most cases all three components are involved but sometimes neuropathy or ischaemia may predominate. The

Table 7.14 Management of peripheral sensorimotor and autonomic neuropathies

Condition	Management
Pain and paraesthesiae from peripheral somatic neuropathies	Intensive insulin therapy (strict glycaemic control) Tricyclic antidepressants (amitriptyline, imipramine) Anticonvulsants (carbamazepine, phenytoin) Capsaicin (topical)
Postural hypotension	Support stockings Fludrocortisone α-adrenoceptor agonist (midodrine) Flurbiprofen
Gastroparesis	Dopamine agonists (metoclopramide, domperidone) Cisapride Erythromycin
Diarrhoea	Loperamide Broad-spectrum antibiotics
Constipation	Stimulant laxatives (senna)
Atonic bladder	Sympathomimetic drugs (carbachol) Anticholinesterase drugs (distigmine)
Excessive sweating	Anticholinergic drugs (propantheline, poldine) Clonidine Topical antimuscarinic agent (glycopyrrolate)
Erectile failure (impotence)	Papaverine or prostaglandin E_1 (alprostadil) (injected into corpus cavernosum) Phosphodiesterase inhibitor (sildenafil) Vacuum tumescence devices Implanted penile prostheses Psychological counselling

CLINICAL FEATURES OF DIABETIC FOOT

Neuropathy	Ischaemia
Symptoms • None • Paraesthesiae • Pain • Numbness	**Symptoms** • None • Claudication • Rest pain
Structural damage • Ulcer • Sepsis • Abscess • Osteomyelitis • Digital gangrene • Charcot joint	**Structural damage** • Ulcer • Sepsis • Gangrene

clinical features of these two types of foot are compared in the information box. Pure ischaemia accounts for a minority of foot ulcers in diabetic patients, with most being either neuropathic or neuro-ischaemic in type (see Fig. 7.19).

The main factors involved in the development of foot ulceration are shown in Figure 7.20. The most common cause of ulceration is a plaque of callous skin beneath which tissue necrosis occurs. This eventually breaks through to the surface.

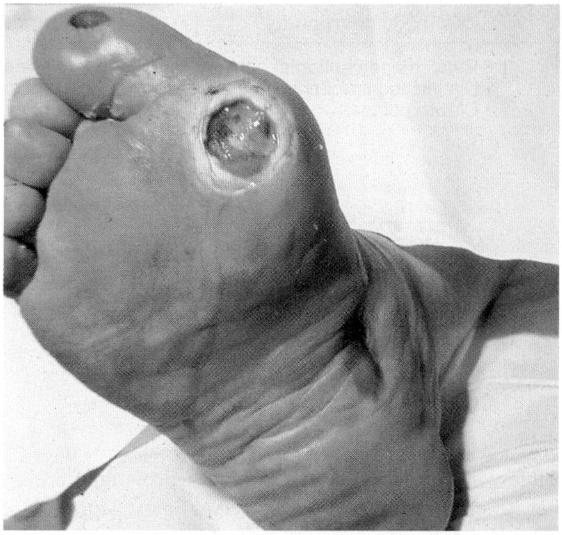

Fig. 7.19 Neuropathic foot ulcer in diabetic patient. Note the site of the ulcer on a weight-bearing area, the callus formation round the margins of the ulcer and the associated infection.

Management

The main components of medical management are listed in the information box. Removal of callous skin with a scalpel is usually best done by a podiatrist who has specialist training and experience in diabetic foot problems. Effective treatment of local infection with appropriate antibiotics is essential, and may have to be continued for protracted periods; osteomyelitis may be extremely difficult to eradicate. Charcot arthropathy with disorganisation of joints may cause serious deformity. Angiography may be necessary if the foot is ischaemic or ulcers are very slow to heal. Measures to improve glycaemic control may be

MANAGEMENT OF DIABETIC FOOT ULCERS

- Remove callous skin
- Treat infection
- Avoid weight-bearing
- Ensure good diabetic control
- Control oedema
- Undertake angiogram to assess feasibility of vascular reconstruction in some cases

Diabetic foot: practice points

- Prevention is the most effective way of dealing with the problem of tissue necrosis in the diabetic foot
- A specialist chiropodist (podiatrist) is an integral part of the diabetes team to ensure regular and effective chiropody and to educate patients in care of the feet

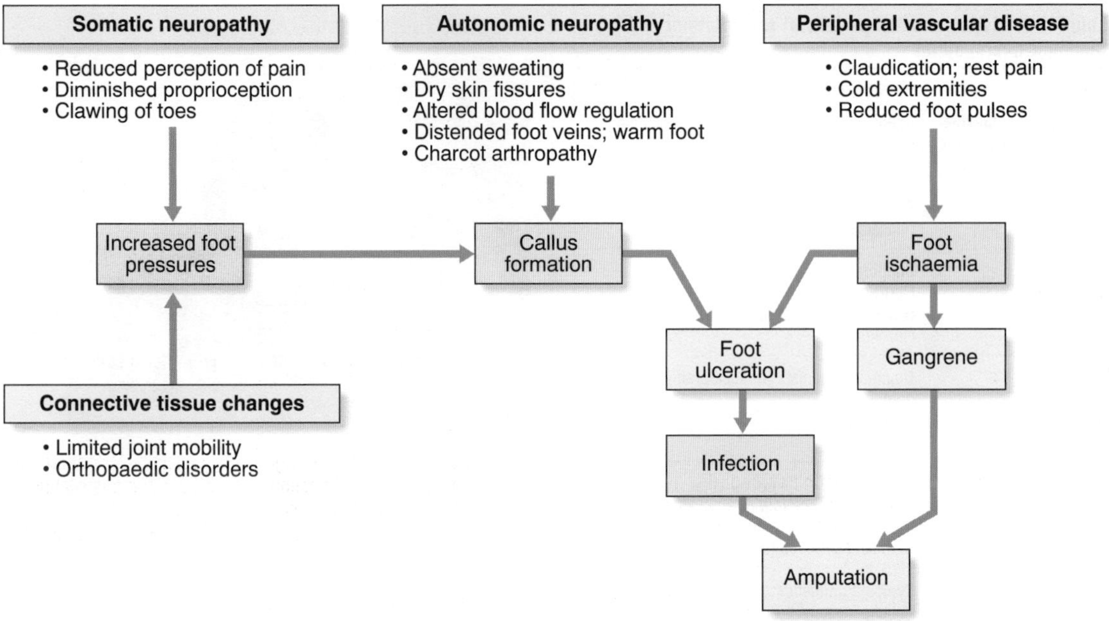

Fig. 7.20 Pathways leading to foot ulceration and amputation in diabetic foot disease. Inter-relationships of aetiological factors and principal clinical features are shown.

necessary to promote healing. Amputation may be unavoidable if there is extensive tissue and/or bony destruction or intractable ischaemic pain at rest in a limb in which vascular reconstruction has failed or is impossible due to extensive large blood vessel disease.

DIABETIC NEPHROPATHY

Diabetic nephropathy is an important cause of morbidity and mortality, and is now among the most common causes of end-stage renal failure (ESRF) in developed countries. As it occurs with other microvascular and macrovascular complications, management is frequently difficult and the benefits of prevention are very great.

About 30% of patients with type 1 diabetes have developed diabetic nephropathy after 20 years, but the risk after this time falls to less than 1% per year, and from the outset the risk is not equal in all patients (see the information box). There are hints that the overall incidence may be falling as standards of control have improved.

RISK FACTORS FOR DEVELOPING DIABETIC NEPHROPATHY

- Poor control of blood glucose
- Long duration of diabetes
- Presence of other microvascular complications
- Racial group (e.g. incidence high in Asian races, Pima Indians)
- Pre-existing hypertension
- Family history of diabetic nephropathy
- Family history of hypertension

The pattern of progression of renal abnormalities in diabetes is shown schematically in Figure 7.21. Pathologically, the first changes (seen at the time of microalbuminuria) are thickening of the glomerular basement membrane and accumulation of matrix material in the mesangium. Subsequently, nodular deposits (see Fig. 7.22) are characteristic, and glomerulosclerosis worsens (time of heavy proteinuria) until glomeruli are progressively lost and renal function deteriorates.

Microalbuminuria is an important indicator of risk of developing overt diabetic nephropathy, although it is also found in other conditions (see p. 505). It is therefore most reliable as an indicator of diabetic nephropathy within the first 10 years of type 1 diabetes (the majority will progress to overt nephropathy within a further 10 years), and less reliable in older patients with type 2 diabetes, in whom other diseases may account for it. Progressively increasing albuminuria, or albuminuria accompanied by hypertension, is much more likely to be due to early diabetic nephropathy.

If there is evidence for incipient nephropathy, vigorous efforts should be made to reduce the risk of progression by:

- improved control of blood glucose
- reduction of blood pressure

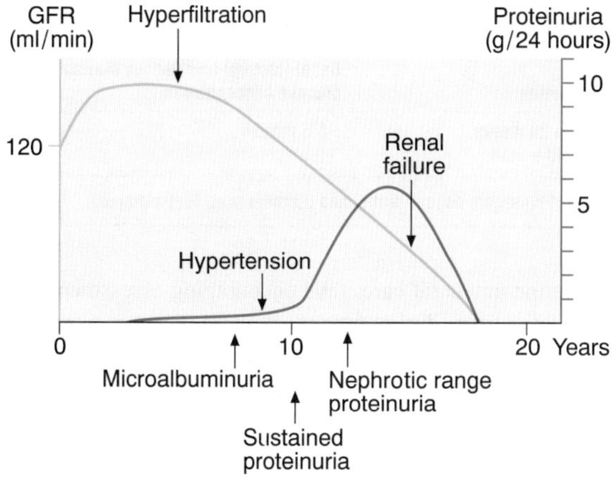

Fig. 7.21 Natural history of diabetic nephropathy. In the first few years of type 1 diabetes mellitus there is hyperfiltration which declines fairly steadily to return to a normal value at approximately 10 years. After about 10 years there is sustained proteinuria and by approximately 14 years it has reached the nephrotic range. Renal function continues to decline, with the end stage being reached at approximately 16 years.

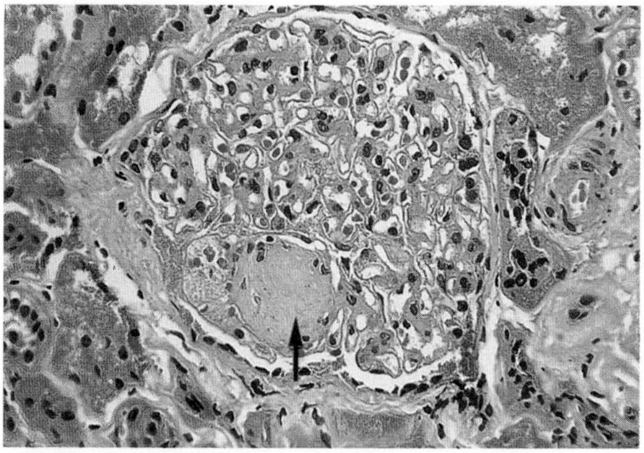

Fig. 7.22 Nodular diabetic glomerulosclerosis. There is thickening of basement membranes and mesangial expansion, and a Kimmelstiel–Wilson nodule (arrow).

- institution of angiotensin-converting enzyme (ACE) inhibitor therapy.

ACE inhibitors have been shown to provide greater benefit than equal blood pressure reduction achieved with other drugs (see p. 221). There may be particular problems with their use in diabetic nephropathy because of hyperkalaemia (see p. 406) and renal artery stenosis. Non-dihydropyridine calcium antagonists (diltiazem, verapamil) may be suitable alternatives in these circumstances.

Diabetic control becomes difficult as renal impairment progresses. Treatment with biguanides (metformin) should be abandoned when creatinine is higher than 150 μmol/l as the risk of lactic acidosis is increased. Long-acting sulphonylureas should be replaced by short-acting agents that are metabolised rather than excreted.

Renal replacement therapy (see p. 437) carries additional difficulties for diabetic patients. Renal transplantation can dramatically improve the life of many. However, large blood vessel disease causing cardiac failure and peripheral vascular disease, and microvascular disease causing neuropathy and retinopathy show continued progression. The progression of recurrent diabetic nephropathy in the allograft is usually too slow to be a serious problem. Coronary heart disease is the major cause of death. The place of pancreatic transplantation (generally carried out at the same time as renal transplantation), which can slow or reverse microvascular disease, is still uncertain and only available to a few.

SCREENING FOR MICROALBUMINURIA

- Identifies nephropathy in type 1 diabetes; independent predictor of macrovascular disease in type 2 diabetes
- Risk factors include increased blood pressure, poor glycaemic control, smoking
- Measured as albumin excretion rate (AER) of 20–200 μg/min (30–300 mg/24 hrs); requires timed collection of urine (overnight)
- Random urine sample can estimate urinary albumin:creatinine ratio (3–30 mg/mmol) (abnormal values: male > 2.5, female > 4.5)

Who to screen

- Type 1 diabetes annually from 5 years after diagnosis
- Type 2 diabetes annually from time of diagnosis

Abnormal tests

- Exclude recent (24 hrs) vigorous exercise, fever; ensure no heart failure, urine infection, prostatitis, not menstruating
- Confirm observation twice within 3–6 months
- Look for hypertension (or increased pressure within normal values)

SPECIAL PROBLEMS IN MANAGEMENT

PREGNANCY AND DIABETES

Problems in diabetic pregnancy

Pregnancy in diabetic women is associated with an increased perinatal mortality rate (that is, stillbirths and neonatal deaths within the first week of life). The main causes of this are intrauterine death in the third trimester of pregnancy, prematurity (due to a high incidence of spontaneous premature labour and of elective premature delivery in an attempt to avoid late intrauterine death), low birth weight and congenital malformation. Birth trauma is also more common due to a high incidence of excessively large, macrosomic babies.

Management of pregnancy in established diabetic women

All the above problems are directly related to poor metabolic control and largely disappear if near-normoglycaemia is maintained before and at conception and during pregnancy and delivery. The therapeutic goals and the components of a successful diabetic pregnancy are listed in the information box.

MANAGEMENT OF PREGNANCY IN WOMEN WITH ESTABLISHED DIABETES

Pre-pregnancy counselling

- Pregnancy planned

Before and at conception and during pregnancy

- Maintain good glycaemic control, i.e. HbA_{1c} within the range 6.5–8.0% by use of 3–4 injections of insulin daily
- Do not strive for normoglycaemia at the expense of hypoglycaemia. Check blood glucose during the night periodically
- Check overnight sample of urine for ketones regularly; increase intake of carbohydrate and dose of insulin to abolish ketonuria

Gestational diabetes

Gestational diabetes, defined as hyperglycaemia diagnosed for the first time in pregnancy, is a common problem. It occurs in individuals who have an inherited predisposition to develop diabetes and may take the form of either type 1 or type 2 diabetes. The hyperglycaemia may not disappear after delivery. It is associated not only with increased rates of perinatal mortality and neonatal morbidity but also with a high incidence (possibly as great as 80% at 25 years post-partum) of subsequent clinical diabetes (both type 1 and type 2) in the mother. Normalisation of metabolism, whether by treatment with dietary measures alone or, more commonly, with additional treatment usually in the form of insulin, undoubtedly reduces the fetal risk; its effect on diminishing the maternal risk of subsequent diabetes is less certain.

A screening procedure for gestational diabetes involving the measurement of true venous plasma glucose concentration 1 hour after a 50 g oral glucose load, followed by a formal 3-hour 100 g oral glucose tolerance test in suspicious cases, has been validated but is complicated. An accurate laboratory measurement of the basal (i.e. fasting or more than 3 hours after a meal) prevailing venous true plasma glucose concentration can be recommended for the following reasons:

- It is a simple test which avoids the need for special preparation and can be incorporated readily as part of routine antenatal care, thus encouraging assessment two or three times during pregnancy in all pregnant women.
- It is more physiological and relevant to the clinical problem, since the prevailing maternal blood glucose concentration is the important thing as far as the fetus is concerned.

Table 7.15 Screening for gestational diabetes

Gestation	Basal (fasting) true venous plasma glucose concentration
Up to 20 weeks	> 5.5 mmol/l
20–40 weeks	> 6.5 mmol/l

Note Investigate patient further and consider need for treatment.

Thus this measurement selects those in need of treatment. Table 7.15 gives the basal plasma glucose concentrations which indicate the need to consider instituting treatment.

Glycated haemoglobin is unreliable as a screening test for gestational diabetes and for assessing glycaemic control during pregnancy because:

- it is too insensitive
- it changes too slowly
- it is affected by things other than changes in the blood glucose concentration, such as the influx of new red cells into the circulation
- it reflects the overall integrated mean blood glucose concentration; it gives no information about fluctuations in the blood glucose level and may therefore be misleading.

Although measurements of glycated serum proteins ('fructosamine') may be more useful than glycated haemoglobin in pregnancy (since its rate of turnover is of the order of 2–4 weeks), it can only complement and not substitute for measurement of the blood glucose concentration which is the cornerstone of management in diabetic pregnancy.

Management of diabetes at delivery

Due to the risk of sudden intrauterine death in the third trimester, diabetic women traditionally were delivered at 36–38 weeks' gestation. Today, improved metabolic control makes later delivery possible and most are now delivered between 38 and 39 weeks' gestation after induction of labour, or if necessary by caesarian section; an increasing number also proceed to spontaneous vaginal delivery at term.

On the morning of delivery the usual breakfast and insulin should be replaced by an intravenous infusion of 10% dextrose with 10 units of short-acting (soluble) insulin added to each 500 ml. This should be given at a rate of 100 ml hourly. The blood glucose concentration should be monitored at intervals of 1–2 hours and the concentration of insulin adjusted to keep the blood glucose concentration within the range of 5–6 mmol/l. An alternative, easier and better method is to give the insulin separately from the glucose infusion by means of a constant rate infusion pump at a rate of 1–2 units hourly. Whatever method is used, administration of insulin should be stopped immediately on delivery and subcutaneous insulin resumed according to need, as determined by capillary blood glucose estimations. Little or no insulin may be required for 12 hours after delivery. Thereafter, the pre-pregnancy dose of subcutaneously administered insulin can be gradually resumed. Lactating diabetic mothers require additional dietary carbohydrate to avoid hypoglycaemia being precipitated.

SURGERY AND DIABETES

Surgery, whether performed electively or in an emergency, causes catabolic stress and invariably elicits secretion of cortisol, catecholamines, glucagon and growth hormone both in normal and diabetic subjects. This results in increased glycogenolysis, gluconeogenesis, lipolysis, proteolysis and insulin resistance, while the release of endogenous insulin is suppressed. In the non-diabetic person these metabolic effects lead to a secondary increase in the secretion of insulin which exerts a restraining and controlling influence. In diabetic patients there is either absolute deficiency of insulin (type 1 diabetes) or insulin secretion is delayed and impaired (type 2 diabetes) so that in untreated or poorly controlled diabetes the uptake of metabolic substrate is significantly reduced, catabolism is increased and ultimately metabolic decompensation in the form of diabetic ketoacidosis may develop in both types of diabetic patients. Starvation will exacerbate this process. In addition, hyperglycaemia impairs phagocytic function (leading to reduced resistance to infection) and wound healing. Thus surgery must be carefully planned and managed in the diabetic patient, with particular emphasis on good metabolic control, along with avoidance of hypoglycaemia which is particularly dangerous in the unconscious or semi-conscious patient.

Pre-operative assessment

Careful pre-operative assessment is mandatory and is summarised in the information box. Much of this can be done on an outpatient basis but, if cardiovascular or renal function is impaired, there are signs of neuropathy (particularly autonomic), diabetic control is poor, and alterations need to be made to the patient's usual treatment, then admission to hospital some days before operation will be required.

Perioperative management

The management of diabetic patients undergoing surgery requiring general anaesthesia is summarised in Figure 7.23.

PRE-OPERATIVE ASSESSMENT IN DIABETIC PATIENTS

- Assess cardiovascular and renal function
- Check for signs of neuropathy, particularly autonomic
- Assess glycaemic control
  Measure HbA_{1c}
  Monitor pre-prandial blood glucose four times daily
- Review treatment of diabetes
  Replace long-acting with intermediate and short-acting insulin
  Stop metformin and long-acting sulphonylureas; replace with insulin if necessary

Post-operatively, the glucose/insulin/potassium infusion should be continued until the patient's intake of food is adequate, when the normal insulin or tablet regimen can be resumed. If the intravenous infusion has to be continued for more than 24 hours, plasma electrolytes and urea should be measured and urinary ketones checked daily. If the infusion is prolonged, the concentration of potassium may require adjustment, and if dilutional hyponatraemia occurs a parallel saline infusion may be necessary. If fluids need to be restricted, e.g. in patients with cardiovascular or renal disease, the rate of infusion can be halved by using a 20% dextrose solution and doubling the concentration of insulin and potassium. The insulin requirement is likely to be higher than that indicated in Figure 7.23 in patients with hepatic disease, obesity or sepsis and in those being treated with corticosteroids or undergoing cardiopulmonary bypass surgery.

Surgical emergencies

If the patient is significantly hyperglycaemic and/or ketoacidotic, this should be corrected first with an intravenous infusion of saline and/or glucose plus insulin, 6 units per hour, and potassium as required. Subsequently, treatment is as described in Figure 7.23, page 508.

Emergency surgery in a patient with well-controlled insulin-dependent diabetes depends on when the last subcutaneous injection of insulin was given. If this was recent, an infusion of glucose alone may be sufficient, but frequent monitoring is essential.

MEDICAL EMERGENCIES

Hyperglycaemia is often found in patients who have sustained an acute myocardial infarction. In some, this represents stress hyperglycaemia, some have previously undiagnosed diabetes and many have established diabetes. Hyperglycaemia should be treated with insulin and, in patients with type 2 diabetes, oral hypoglycaemic agents should be stopped in the peri-infarct period. Recent studies have suggested that conversion to insulin therapy in type 2 patients with acute myocardial infarction may reduce their long-term mortality from coronary heart disease.

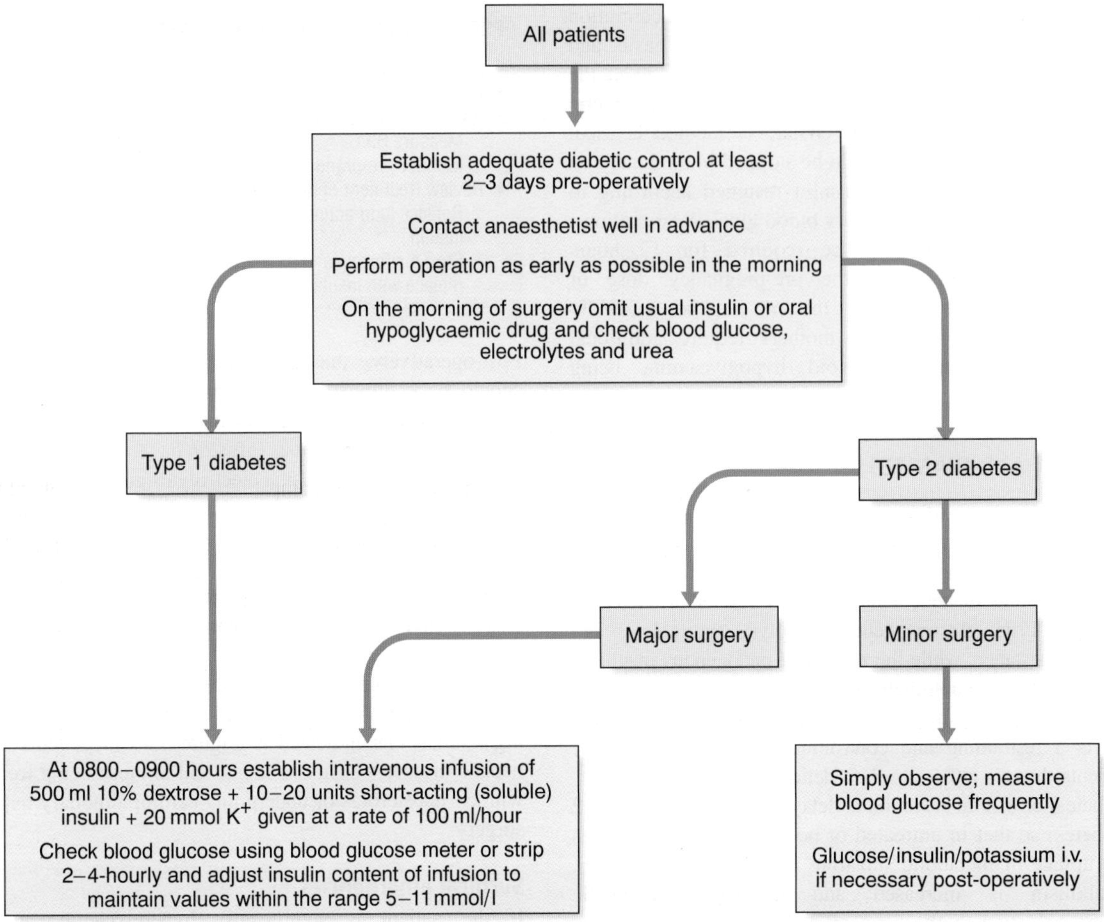

Fig. 7.23 Management of diabetic patients undergoing surgery and general anaesthesia.

PROSPECTS IN DIABETES MELLITUS

The prevalence of both primary types of diabetes is rising steadily, with increasing longevity particularly affecting the frequency of type 2 diabetes in an ageing population. Increasing obesity in Westernised cultures is exacerbating the problem and a global epidemic of diabetes is predicted within the next decade.

Management

The scale of the clinical problem presented by diabetic patients with severe vascular disease, the knowledge that diabetic complications are preventable with good glycaemic control, the introduction of better methods of assessing diabetic control, the realisation that at present good control is achieved in only a minority of diabetic patients, and increased understanding of the deficiencies and limitations of conventional treatment with insulin, have led to a search for better methods of treating type 1 diabetes.

Pancreatic transplantation presents particular problems relating to the exocrine pancreatic secretions, and long-term immunosuppression is necessary. While results are steadily improving, they remain significantly less good than for renal transplantation. Xenotransplantation with a porcine pancreas may be an alternative approach. However, it is questionable whether it will ever be considered justifiable to transplant young diabetic patients before vascular disease is clinically apparent.

Transplantation of isolated pancreatic islets (often into the liver in animal studies) is an attractive concept theoretically; it is safe and the problem of the exocrine secretions is avoided. Progress is being made towards meeting the needs of supply, encapsulation and storage but the problems of bioincompatibility, rejection and autoimmune destruction remain. Nevertheless, the development of methods of inducing tolerance to transplanted islets means that this may still prove the most promising approach in the long term.

Alternative methods and routes of insulin delivery are being sought other than subcutaneous injection which has the disadvantage of delivering insulin into the systemic and not the portal circulation. A wider range of insulin analogues is being developed, and nasal and oral routes and transcutaneous patch technology are being explored. Other therapeutic agents such as glucagon-like peptide (GLP-1) are being investigated, and novel oral hypoglycaemic drugs are being evaluated, including beta-cell stimulators called meglitinides (e.g. repaglinide).

Primary prevention of diabetes

From a public health standpoint the only cost-effective way of dealing with diabetes is to prevent it.

Type 2 diabetes is associated with an affluent lifestyle that is likely to arise in genetically predisposed individuals who eat too much and exercise too little. Effective health education could do much to reduce the incidence of clinically expressed disease, while screening for diabetes (particularly in high-risk groups such as the first-degree relatives of known cases) and more vigorous and early treatment of impaired glucose tolerance would reduce the incidence of serious vascular disease in these patients. The promotion of healthy diets with reduction in refined carbohydrate and saturated fats, and avoidance of being overweight, combined with regular exercise, has shown promising results in the primary prevention of type 2 diabetes.

In type 1 diabetes, the fact that the islet insulin-secreting cells are destroyed slowly over several years before clinical presentation offers the hope that, in the future, it may be possible to prevent type 1 diabetes. This depends on:

- the availability of accurate, predictive markers for the development of clinical diabetes in genetically predisposed individual subjects
- an understanding of the precise sequence of events leading to pancreatic beta cell destruction
- the development of methods of intervention based on specifically targeted immunomodulation which could be applied early in the pre-diabetic period before most of the insulin-secreting cells have been destroyed.

Treatment of diabetic complications

Treatment with aminoguanidine, an inhibitor of the formation of advanced glycation end-products, has been shown to prevent damage to the retina, kidney, nerve and artery in diabetic animals. It has low toxicity and is undergoing preliminary trials in humans with chronic diabetic complications.

FURTHER INFORMATION ON DIABETES MELLITUS

Diabetes Control and Complications Trial Research Group 1993 The effect of intensive treatment of diabetes on the development and progression of long-term complications in insulin-dependent diabetes mellitus. New England Journal of Medicine 329: 977–986

Frier B M and Fisher B M (eds) 1993 Hypoglycaemia and diabetes: clinical and physiological aspects. Edward Arnold, London

Pickup J C and Williams G (eds) 1997 Textbook of Diabetes, 2nd edn. Blackwell Science, Oxford

SIGN website for information on diabetic nephropathy

UK Prospective Diabetes Study (UKPDS) Group 1998 Intensive blood-glucose control with sulphonylureas or insulin compared with conventional treatment and risk of complications in patients with type 2 diabetes (UKPDS 33). Lancet 352: 837–853

NUTRITIONAL FACTORS IN HEALTH AND DISEASE

No medical history is complete without inquiring about the patient's food and drink intake; what people eat is one of the major environmental influences on health. The complexity of achieving good nutrition in individuals is recognised as a major challenge which can only be achieved by a team effort, including the patient and his or her family. This chapter will address primarily the medical aspects of nutrition and malnutrition.

Like immune reactions and infections, variations in nutrition can affect any organ of the body or several at once. Different areas of human nutrition are of interest to different specialists; for example, cardiologists are interested in dietary fats and plasma lipids, nephrologists in protein deficiency and in potassium excess, gastroenterologists in multiple deficiencies from malabsorption, in dietary fibre and in hypersensitivity to wheat and milk.

Diet is an important factor in the development of many chronic degenerative diseases, e.g. coronary heart disease, hypertension, diabetes mellitus, cirrhosis of the liver, gallstones, urinary tract stones, dental caries and diverticular disease, and in carcinomas such as those in the stomach, liver and large bowel. These diseases take a long time to develop and, for many, exactly which dietary components are involved, and how closely, remain uncertain. All medical specialties, and especially those in general practice, have an important role to play in prevention of disease and in health promotion. Modifications of a Western diet to reduce the risk of coronary heart disease are set out in the first information box on page 510.

Poor nutrition can lead to disease; however, disease may also precipitate malnutrition. Malnutrition in hospitalised patients is increasingly recognised and leads to many clinical complications.

NUTRITIONAL DISORDERS

Nutritional disorders can be classified as shown in the second information box on page 510.

MODIFICATIONS OF A WESTERN DIET THAT REDUCE THE RISK OF CORONARY HEART DISEASE

- Avoid or treat overweight by dietary restraint and appropriate regular exercise
- Restrict total fat intake to 30% of calories or less
- Restrict saturated plus trans-fatty acids to 10% of total calories or less
- ω-6 polyunsaturated fatty acid (mostly linoleic) intake should be between 6% and 10% of calories
- The remaining fat is from monounsaturated fatty acids (mostly oleic), i.e. 10–14% of calories
- Increase consumption of fish (providing very long chain ω-3 polyunsaturated fatty acids)
- Increase intake of whole-grain cereals, and green and orange vegetables and fruits (providing antioxidant vitamins and dietary fibre)
- Moderate intake of dietary cholesterol

CLASSIFICATION OF NUTRITIONAL DISORDERS
Undernutrition
• Insufficient food energy causing starvation (adults) or marasmus (children)
Malnutrition
• Deficiency of protein or other essential nutrients (see Table 7.16)
Obesity
• From prolonged positive energy balance
Nutrient excess
• Acute or chronic, e.g. iron, vitamin D, saturated fat
Effect of toxicants in foods
• e.g. In coeliac disease, urticaria, favism, migraine

Malnutrition

Deficiency diseases seldom present in pure form. More often than not they are secondary to some other illness or extreme change in living conditions, e.g. during hospitalisation. Not all the members of a community are equally affected; individuals with some physical or mental abnormality usually show clinical manifestations first. Young children, and the elderly and disabled are the most vulnerable.

When malnutrition occurs it is unlikely to involve only one nutrient. Even if the clinical features suggest a single deficiency, biochemical tests usually reveal depletion of other nutrients. Treatment should therefore not be confined to large intakes of the nutrient whose deficiency is indicated by the clinical signs. Furthermore, malnourished patients are particularly liable to infection, which may constitute the presenting illness or which may occur in modified form because malnutrition has suppressed some of the characteristic signs. Much of the skill in diagnosing patients with malnutrition is being aware of and disentangling predisposing illnesses, other associated malnutrition, and complicating diseases.

Undernutrition leading to secondary malnutrition

Starvation refers to severe undernutrition derived from a prolonged inadequacy of food intake and results in severe nutrient depletion or malnutrition. The effects of starvation will be more specifically discussed under protein-energy malnutrition (see p. 515).

Even in developed countries, seriously ill people or those in hospital for long periods are very likely to develop some degree of nutritional depletion including protein-energy malnutrition and/or particular deficiencies, e.g. of folate, potassium or iron. It has been estimated that up to 50% of hospitalised patients may demonstrate nutritional depletion at any one time. It is important to monitor patients' nutrition and provide appropriate support, both during hospitalisation and on discharge, not least because nutritionally depleted patients demonstrate functional consequences of nutritional depletion. These consequences depend on the degree and type of depletion, but sooner or later malnutrition will have some or even all of the following effects:

- reduced cellular and humoral responses to infections
- muscular weakness, reduced ability to cough, susceptibility to bronchopneumonia
- impaired healing of wounds (traumatic and surgical)
- atrophic surface epithelium with reduced protective secretions more easily penetrated by bacteria, especially in the gastrointestinal tract
- bed sores and ulcers
- reduced haemopoiesis
- reduced ability to metabolise drugs
- mental impairment
- dehydration
- specific types of malnutrition, e.g. Wernicke's encephalopathy.

Controlled prospective studies show that patients with features of malnutrition have more post-operative complications, more infections, longer hospital stays and a higher mortality. In some diseases nutritional support has been demonstrated to improve outcome, e.g. in inflammatory bowel disease, in burns and in patients with enterocutaneous fistulae. In many other conditions such data are not yet available; however, it is sensible to assess the nutritional status of each patient individually. If his/her status is subnormal, one should assess the range of support available, as it is possible to maintain or improve patients' nutrition even when the gastrointestinal tract is not functioning.

The causes of nutritional depletion are listed in the information box. A patient in any of these categories is at increased risk of malnutrition, though it may have not yet

CAUSES OF UNDERNUTRITION LEADING TO NUTRITIONAL DEPLETION

- Insufficient food
- Persistent regurgitation or vomiting
- Anorexia
- Malabsorption, e.g. small intestine disease
- Increased basal metabolic rate, e.g. thyrotoxicosis, prolonged infections, trauma, febrile illness
- Loss of calories in urine, e.g. glycosuria in diabetes mellitus
- Cachexia in some cases of cancer

developed. Before using technical methods to work out a detailed nutritional profile, the first step is to identify patients at high or increased nutritional risk. A systematic investigation of nutritional health should be undertaken and normally consists of four components:

- dietary history
- clinical examination
- anthropometry
- laboratory investigations.

Dietary history

In medical use this is usually qualitative: has the patient been eating too little food, or omitted any major foods? Is an unusual diet being taken? Quantitative nutrient intake is best assessed by a dietitian who is skilled in the area of dietary assessment. An estimate by one of four methods of weights of all foods eaten can be used: dietary history, 24-hour recall, food diary or food frequency questionnaire. By using food tables, usually in computer form, the daily intake of the major nutrients can be obtained. This can be compared with the recommended nutrient intake (dietary reference value), a simplified version of which is shown in Table 7.16. An intake below the dietary reference value indicates a risk of malnutrition but does not establish it because:

- the days on which food intake was estimated may have been unrepresentative
- the physiological requirements for different nutrients range by a factor of about 2 and the dietary reference values are set to cover the requirements of all healthy people
- for some nutrients, e.g. vitamins A and B_{12}, there are considerable reserves in the body.

Table 7.16 Size of adult requirements for essential nutrients

Adult daily requirement	Essential nutrients
Gram amounts	
1 kg (1 l)	Water
50–100 g	Available carbohydrate
50 g	Protein (8–10 essential amino acids)
1–5 g	Na, Cl, K, essential fatty acids
0.4–1 g	Ca, P
Milligram amounts	
300 mg	Mg
40 mg	Vit C
*c.*15 mg	Niacin, vit E, Fe, Zn
5–10 mg	Pantothenate, Mn
1–2 mg	Vit A, thiamin, riboflavin, vit B_6, F, Cu
Microgram amounts	
200 µg	Folate, Mo
*c.*100 µg	Biotin, I, Se
2–10 µg	Vit B_{12}, vit D, vit K, Cr

Figures are approximate, in places rounded to fit with others on a line. The range of requirements for different nutrients is about 10^9. In addition, sulphur is required in the form of the amino acids, methionine and cysteine; cobalt is required in the form of vitamin B_{12}.

Clinical examination

Thinness, oedema, pallor, weakness and other signs described in this chapter may be found, but one should not wait for the classic features of a deficiency disease before intervening with nutritional support. The primary illness may obscure or confuse signs of malnutrition.

Anthropometry

Changes of body weight reflect the water and/or energy (calorie) balance. If there is no unusual loss of water, each kilogram lost corresponds to 6–7000 kcal of energy (i.e. mostly adipose tissue), unless there is increased protein catabolism when the energy value of weight lost is less. Regular weighing of patients in hospital is valuable in management but it is difficult in paralysed and very sick patients, those nursed at strict bed rest, or those with splints, intravenous lines, catheters and drains. Weighing-beds are scarce in most hospitals. Wasting of both subcutaneous fat and muscle mass should be monitored. If weighing is impractical, these observations are more critical. Clinical estimation can be made more objective by measuring mid-arm circumference (see Table 7.17). The relative contributions of fat and muscle can be calculated (mid-arm muscle circumference = arm circumference − triceps skinfold), but accurate measurement of skinfold thickness requires special calipers. Harpenden or Holtain calipers are recommended.

Table 7.17 Reference standards for mid-arm circumference (mm)

	Men			Women		
	Centiles			Centiles		
Age	50th	10th	5th	50th	10th	5th
19–24	308	272	262	265	230	221
25–34	319	282	271	277	240	233
35–44	326	287	278	290	251	241
45–54	322	281	267	299	256	242
55–64	317	273	258	303	254	243
65–74	307	263	248	299	252	240

Laboratory investigations

Investigations consist of those that indicate the protein status, and biochemical tests for micronutrient deficiencies.

While the plasma albumin concentration can be used to assess visceral protein depletion, this value reflects synthetic rate, distribution in body pools, tissue catabolism or loss of protein from the body and hence it is important not to equate hypoproteinaemia with protein malnutrition. Injury, inflammation and the presence of liver disease all reduce the plasma albumin concentration. The ratio of C-reactive protein to albumin therefore provides a better estimate of protein depletion. Plasma transferrin and prealbumin are sometimes used as more sensitive indices of visceral and protein status but both can be influenced by other conditions. Urinary nitrogen (or urea nitrogen) reveals the degree of protein catabolism. A reduced total lymphocyte count indicates the possibility of impaired cell-mediated immunity, of which protein depletion is one cause. Biochemical tests for vitamins and some other essential nutrients are listed in Table 7.18. As with other tests in chemical pathology there can be both false positives and negatives. Each result needs to be evaluated with critical understanding; for example, serum vitamin B_{12} is increased in acute hepatitis, and alkaline phosphatase may not be elevated if rickets is accompanied by PEM.

In general, when the dietary intake of a nutrient is inadequate (less than obligatory losses) the individual goes through three stages:

- adaptation to the low intake (i.e. urine excretion falls)
- biochemical change indicating impaired function or cellular depletion
- overt clinical deficiency disease.

NUTRIENT AND ENERGY REQUIREMENTS

All foods provide both nutrients and energy. If energy requirements are not being met then it is highly unlikely that nutrient supply will be adequate, unless the diet has been carefully managed and computed, such as in a diet prescribed for weight loss. Meeting energy requirements is a fundamental and principal goal of nutrition.

Table 7.18 Biochemical methods used in diagnosing nutritional deficiencies

	Principal methods		
Nutrient	**Indicating reduced intake**	**Indicating impaired function (IF) or cell depletion (CD)**	**Supplementary methods**
Protein	Urinary nitrogen	Plasma albumin (IF)	Fasting plasma amino acid pattern
Vitamin A	Plasma carotene	Plasma retinol	Relative dose response
Thiamine	Urinary thiamine	Red blood cell transketolase and TPP effect (IF)	
Riboflavin	Urinary riboflavin	Red blood cell glutathione reductase and FAD effect (IF)	
Niacin	Urinary *N′* methyl-nicotinamide	Red cell NAD	Fasting plasma tryptophan
Vitamin B_6	Urinary 4-pyridoxic acid and/or plasma pyridoxal phosphate	Red blood glutamic oxalacetic transaminase and PP effect (IF)	Urinary xanthurenic acid after tryptophan load
Folate	Plasma folate	Red blood cell folate (CD)	Urinary FIGLU after histidine load
Vitamin B_{12}	Plasma holotranscobalamin II	Plasma vitamin B_{12}	Schilling test
Vitamin C	Plasma ascorbate	Leucocyte ascorbate (CD)	Urinary ascorbate
Vitamin D	Plasma 25-hydroxycholecalciferol	Raised plasma alkaline phosphatase (bone isoenzyme) (IF)	Plasma 1,25 OH vitamin D
Vitamin E	Plasma tocopherol/cholesterol ratio	Red cell haemolysis with H_2O_2 in vitro (IF)	
Vitamin K	Plasma phylloquinone	Plasma prothrombin	PIVKA II
Sodium	Urinary sodium	Plasma sodium	
Potassium	Urinary potassium	Plasma potassium	Total body potassium by counting ^{40}K
Iron	Plasma iron and transferrin	Plasma ferritin (CD)	Stainable iron in bone marrow
Magnesium	Plasma magnesium	Red cell magnesium	
Iodine	Urinary (stable) iodide	Plasma thyroxine (IF)	Plasma thyroid-stimulating hormone
Zinc	Plasma zinc	White blood cell zinc	Hair zinc
Selenium	Plasma selenium	Plasma glutathione peroxidase	
Calcium*			Total bone mineral

* There are no reliable simple methods for assessing calcium status.
(FAD = flavin adenine dinucleotide; NAD = nicotinamide adenine dinucleotide; TPP = thiamine pyrophosphate; FIGLU = formimino glutamic acid; PIVKA II = protein induced by vitamin K absence II)

ENERGY REQUIREMENTS

The largest component of energy expenditure is attributed to the lean body mass and is known as the basal metabolic rate (BMR). The lean body mass (related to weight and height) declines with age and is lower in women than men. Extra energy is required for growth, for pregnancy and lactation, for muscular activity and when febrile. There is considerable variation in energy expended between individuals of the same size, age, sex and activity. Adaptation occurs to an inadequate energy intake and to a lesser degree to superfluous energy intake. The largest variable in determining energy requirements is the energy attributed to exercise and movement. There are two units in use for energy: kilocalories and kilojoules (1 kcal = 4.184 kJ). Though both are metric, joules are SI units and are preferred in Europe for scientific usage. Approximate daily energy requirements are listed in Table 7.19. Adult requirements for essential nutrients are given in Table 7.16, page 511.

ENERGY-YIELDING NUTRIENTS

Three nutrients can act as energy substrates: carbohydrate, fat and protein. Protein has a profoundly negative effect on appetite and its use as an energy substrate should not be contemplated for this and other biochemical reasons. Carbohydrate and fat are the most important energy substrates and have an additional functional role.

Carbohydrates

The word 'carbohydrate' generically covers three substrates: simple sugars (e.g. sucrose), complex polysaccharides or starches (long-chain molecules), and dietary fibre or non-starch polysaccharides (not available for enzymic digestion by humans). The 'available' carbohydrate (starches and sugars) supplies a major part of the energy in a normal diet (4 kcal/g). No individual carbohydrate is an essential nutrient as the body can make it for itself from protein. However, if the available carbohydrate intake is less than 100 g per day, ketosis is likely to occur. Sugars are found in fruits, milk (lactose) and some vegetables. Starches are mostly found in cereals, root vegetables and legumes. The major carbohydrates in food are listed in the information box.

Table 7.19 Daily energy requirements

Circumstances	Requirements
Healthy females	
At rest	1600 kcal (6.7 MJ)
Light work	2000 kcal (8.4 MJ)
Heavy work	2250 kcal (9.4 MJ)
Healthy males	
At rest	2000 kcal (8.4 MJ)
Light work	2700 kcal (11.3 MJ)
Heavy work	3500 kcal (14.6 MJ)

SOURCES OF CARBOHYDRATES IN FOOD

Available sugars

- Monosaccharides—ribose, glucose, fructose
- Disaccharides—sucrose, lactose, maltose

Available polysaccharides

- Starch, glycogen, synthetic glucose polymers

Unavailable polysaccharides

- Most forms of dietary fibre

Sugars

Sugars are classified by the UK Department of Health as intrinsic (naturally incorporated in the cellular structure of fruits, milk etc.) or extrinsic (extracted, refined, concentrated, e.g. beet or cane sucrose). Intrinsic sugars and the foods that contain them are thought to be more acceptable nutritionally than extrinsic sugars because they are associated with other nutrients naturally present in the food. Extrinsic sugars are one of the factors that can contribute to the development of dental caries if eaten/sucked frequently.

Starches

Starches in cereal foods (wheat, rice), root foods (potatoes, cassava) and legumes are the nutrients which provide the largest proportion of calories in most diets around the world unless these diets are unusually high in fat or sugars. Although all starches are polymers of glucose, linked by the same 1–4 glycosidic linkages, they do not all behave in the same way when they are eaten.

Some starches are digested promptly by salivary and then pancreatic amylase and produce a steep rise in blood glucose. Other starches are more slowly digested, because they are protected in the structure of the food, because of the crystal structure or because the molecule is unbranched (amylose). After ingestion, the blood glucose rise is flatter and lower. The glycaemic index (see the information box) quantifies the effect of different carbohydrates on the blood glucose after a test meal. A small percentage of dietary starch may completely escape digestion in the small

GLYCAEMIC INDEX

- The glycaemic index is the incremental area under the 2-hour plasma glucose curve after eating the amount of a food containing 50 g carbohydrate ÷ the corresponding area after 50 g of glucose in water
- The glycaemic index is high for bread, potatoes and glucose, and lower for pasta, legumes and whole-grain cereals. The index may be useful in constructing therapeutic diets for diabetes (see p. 483)

intestine and pass unchanged into the large intestine, where it is fermented by the resident bacteria. This resistant starch thus behaves in much the same way as dietary fibre and is thought to confer a beneficial effect on the intestinal mucosa.

Dietary fibre

Dietary fibre, or non-starch polysaccharides, is the natural packing of plant foods. It can be defined as those parts of food which are not digested by human enzymes. The principal classes of dietary fibre are cellulose, hemicelluloses, lignins, pectins and gums. These are all polysaccharides (i.e. carbohydrates) except lignin, which occurs with cellulose in the structure of plants. Pectins and gums are viscous, not fibrous.

Some types of dietary fibre, notably the hemicellulose of wheat, increase the water-holding capacity of colonic contents and the bulk of faeces. They relieve simple constipation, appear to prevent diverticulosis and may reduce the risk of cancer of the colon. Other, viscous, indigestible polysaccharides like pectin and guar gum have greater effect in the upper gastrointestinal tract. They tend to slow gastric emptying, contribute to satiety, and may flatten the glucose tolerance curve and reduce plasma cholesterol concentration.

Dietary fibre (and resistant starch) is partly fermented in the large intestine by resident bacterial flora, yielding a small quantity of volatile fatty acids which are absorbed through the colonic mucosa. Flatus formation is common. There are as yet no official recommended intakes for dietary fibre, but the present average intakes of about 15–20 g/day in affluent countries are thought to be too low.

Fats

With their high calorie value (9 kcal/g), fats are useful to people with a large energy requirement due to expenditure. On the other hand, their high energy density makes them an insidious cause of obesity for sedentary people. Saturated fats, especially those containing myristic (14:0) and palmitic (16:0) acids, increase plasma low-density lipoproteins and total cholesterol. Monounsaturated fatty acids contain one double bond, e.g. oleic acid (18:1 ω9). Polyunsaturated fatty acids, with two or more double bonds, are in two main groups, depending on the distance of their first double bond, counting from the methyl (ω) end of the molecule. The principal polyunsaturated fatty acid in plant seed oils is linoleic acid (18:2 ω6). This and its elongated ω6 derivatives γ-linolenic acid (18:3 ω6) and arachidonic acid (20:4 ω6) are the essential fatty acids (EFAs), and are precursors of prostaglandins and eicosanoids and part of the structure of lipid membranes in all cells.

The ω3 series of polyunsaturated fatty acids, e.g. eicosapentaenoic (20:5 ω3) and docosahexaenoic (22:6 ω3), occur in fish oils and in the lipids of the human brain and retina. They are inhibitors of thrombosis and appear to act by competitively antagonising thromboxane A_2 formation. Purified fish body oils, e.g. omega-3 marine triglycerides, are one of the treatment options which may reduce the tendency to thrombosis—for instance, in people with coronary heart disease. They lower plasma triglyceride levels.

Essential fatty acid deficiency

This is rare in humans but has been reported in patients fed solely by total parenteral nutrition for long periods without fat emulsions. If only sufficient glucose and amino acids are given, they inhibit free fatty acid mobilisation from adipose tissue (where there is usually a moderate store of linoleic acid) and tissues in the rest of the body become depleted. There is a scaly dermatitis and the diagnosis can be confirmed biochemically by an increased ratio of eicosatrienoic acid (20:3 ω9) to arachidonic in plasma lipids.

Proteins

These are made up of some 20 different amino acids, of which nine are indispensable for normal synthesis of the different proteins in the body and for maintaining nitrogen balance in adults. These are listed in the information box. Arginine is also needed in infants. Methionine can substitute for cysteine and phenylalanine for tyrosine but not vice versa. The term 'indispensable' is preferred to the older term 'essential' because dispensable (non-essential) amino acids (glycine, alanine etc.) as well as indispensable amino acids are all essential at the cellular level. 'Indispensable' is used to mean 'required in the diet'. The dispensable amino acids can be synthesised in the body by transamination provided there is a sufficient supply of amino groups.

The nutritive value of different proteins depends on the relative proportions of indispensable amino acids they contain (sometimes called its biological value). Proteins of animal origin, particularly from eggs, milk and meat, are generally of higher biological value than the proteins of vegetable origin which are low in one or more of the indispensable amino acids. However, when two different vegetable proteins are eaten together (e.g. a cereal and a legume), their amino acid patterns can complement one another and produce a mix of indispensable amino acids with an adequate protein nutritive value. This is the principle of protein supply in a vegan or totally vegetarian diet.

ESSENTIAL OR INDISPENSABLE AMINO ACIDS

(In approximate ascending order of size requirement)

- Tryptophan
- Histidine
- Methionine + cysteine
- Threonine
- Isoleucine
- Valine
- Phenylalanine + tyrosine
- Lysine
- Leucine

The usual recommendation for an adequate protein intake is 10% of the total calories, i.e. about 65 g per day for the average adult. The minimum requirement is around 40 g of protein with a high proportion of indispensable amino acids or a high biological value.

PROTEIN-ENERGY MALNUTRITION (PEM)

PEM IN ADULTS

The predominant form of protein-energy malnutrition in adults is undernutrition, i.e. the result of a sustained negative energy (calorie) balance. This may be due to insufficient food supply or, where food is available, to anorexia, increased energy requirements or increased energy losses. Gross features of visceral protein deficiency (see kwashiorkor, p. 516) are rare in starvation; they are seen in some cases of hospital malnutrition (see p. 525) in whom there is excessive turnover or excessive loss (e.g. in burns) of body protein. Depletion of sodium, potassium and magnesium is common, often from diarrhoea, together with vitamins, especially thiamin, folate and vitamin C. The main causes of undernutrition and starvation are listed in the information box on page 511.

The features of severe undernutrition seen in adults and older children are detailed below; the effects of severe undernutrition in young children (marasmus) are described on page 516.

Clinical features

- Loss of weight in adults, cessation of growth in children.
- Thirst, weakness, feeling cold, nocturia, amenorrhoea and impotence, craving for food.
- Lax, pale, dry skin with loss of turgor and, occasionally, pigmented patches.
- Hair thinning or loss (except in adolescents).
- Cold and cyanosed extremities, pressure sores.
- Muscle wasting, loss of subcutaneous fat, subnormal arm circumference.
- Oedema, which may be present without hypoalbuminaemia ('famine oedema').
- Subnormal body temperature, slow pulse, low blood pressure and small heart.
- Distended abdomen, with diarrhoea.
- Diminished tendon jerks.
- Apathy, loss of initiative, depression, introversion, aggression if food is nearby.
- Susceptibility to infections (see the information box).

The high mortality rate in famine situations is often due to infections, e.g. typhus or cholera epidemics. The usual signs of infection may not appear. In advanced starvation, patients become completely inactive and may assume a flexed, fetal position. In the last stage of starvation, death comes quietly and often quite suddenly. The very old are most vulnerable. All organs are atrophied at necropsy, except the brain which tends to maintain its weight.

INFECTIONS ASSOCIATED WITH PEM

Patients with marasmus, kwashiorkor and starvation have increased susceptibility to:

- Gastroenteritis and Gram-negative septicaemia
- Respiratory infections, especially bronchopneumonia
- Certain viral diseases, especially measles and herpes simplex
- Tuberculosis
- Streptococcal and staphylococcal skin infections
- Helminthic infestations

Investigations

In a famine it is usually only possible to measure the body weight, estimate the patient's height and grade the severity of undernutrition by calculating the body mass index (weight [kg]/height^2 [m^2]). Where other investigations are possible, plasma free fatty acids are found to be increased; there is ketosis and a mild metabolic acidosis. Plasma glucose is low but albumin concentration is often maintained because the liver is still functioning normally. Insulin secretion is diminished, glucagon and cortisol tend to increase, reverse T3 replaces normal triiodothyronine. The resting metabolic rate falls, partly because of reduced lean body mass. The urine has a fixed specific gravity and creatinine excretion becomes low. There may be a mild anaemia, leucopenia and thrombocytopenia. The erythrocyte sedimentation rate is normal unless there is infection. Tests of delayed skin sensitivity, e.g. to tuberculin, are falsely negative. The electrocardiogram shows sinus brachycardia and low voltage.

Management

Whether in a famine or in wasting secondary to disease, people or patients need to be graded according to body mass index. People with mild starvation are in no danger; those with moderate starvation need extra feeding. People who are severely underweight need hospital-type care. Between 1500 and 2000 kcal/day will prevent the downward progress of undernutrition.

In severe starvation there is atrophy of the intestinal epithelium and of the exocrine pancreas, and the bile is dilute. When food becomes available, it should be given in small amounts at first. Food should be palatable and similar to the usual staple meal—for example, a cereal with some sugar, milk powder and oil. Salt should be restricted and a micronutrient supplement may be desirable (e.g. potassium, magnesium, multivitamins). During refeeding, a weight gain of 5% body weight per month indicates satisfactory progress.

Circumstances and resources are different in every famine but many problems are non-medical and concern organisation, infrastructure, liaison, politics, procurement, security and ensuring that food is distributed on the basis of need. Lastly, plans must be made for the future for prevention and/or intervention earlier if similar circumstances prevail. Management of undernutrition secondary to disease is discussed on page 525.

Prevention

Preventive measures for PEM are listed in the information box.

UNICEF'S INEXPENSIVE MEASURES TO PREVENT PEM
Mnemonic GOBI
G for growth monitoring
• The mother or father keeps a simple growth chart—the Road to Health card—in a cellophane envelope and brings the child to a clinic regularly for weighing and advice
O for oral rehydration
• The UNICEF formula (NaCl 3.5 g, $NaHCO_3$ 2.5 g, KCl 1.5 g, glucose 20 g or sucrose 40 g per litre of clean water) is saving many lives from gastroenteritis
B for breastfeeding
• This is a matter of life and death in a poor community with no facilities for hygiene. Additional food—which should be prepared from locally available foods—is not usually needed until 6 months of age
I for immunisation
• This provides protection against measles, diphtheria, pertussis, tetanus, tuberculosis and poliomyelitis

PROTEIN-ENERGY MALNUTRITION IN YOUNG CHILDREN

Whereas severe malnutrition in adults is usually the result of famine or secondary to major illness, malnutrition in young children is endemic in many developing countries where severe PEM affects around 2% and mild to moderate forms affect 20% or more.

Two types of severe malnutrition are described but many cases show features of both types ('marasmic kwashiorkor'). Marasmus is more common than kwashiorkor.

Marasmus

This refers to severe undernutrition in an infant or young child. The cause is a diet very low in energy, protein and other essential nutrients. Typically it is a disease of infants of poor parents living in the cities of developing countries; the child is weaned early, the parents have difficulty paying for the feeds, and there is no access to clean water or kitchen equipment to prepare food without bacterial contamination. The combination of malnutrition and poor hygiene predisposes to gastroenteritis, with diarrhoea and poor appetite, that further depletes the child's energy reserves.

The child is very thin, with no subcutaneous fat and wasted muscles. The abdomen shows gaseous distension, and diarrhoea is usual. Body weight is reduced below 60% of the WHO standard. In contrast to kwashiorkor, there is no oedema and skin and hair changes are mild or absent. The child is not usually anorexic.

Kwashiorkor

This type of malnutrition occurs most often in the second year of life in a child weaned from the breast on to a starchy diet very low in protein, such as cassava, yam, plantain, sweet potato or a cereal that has been refined and diluted. Such a child may appear in moderate health until its protein requirements are increased by an infection, e.g. gastroenteritis, measles or malaria.

Clinically, the child, although not thin, is miserable and apathetic (see Fig. 7.24). There are symmetrical skin changes maximal around the napkin area; these areas are at first pigmented and thickened, then cracks appear and lead to denuded areas of shallow pigmentation. The hair alters colour from black to blond, reddish or grey and becomes thin and sparse.

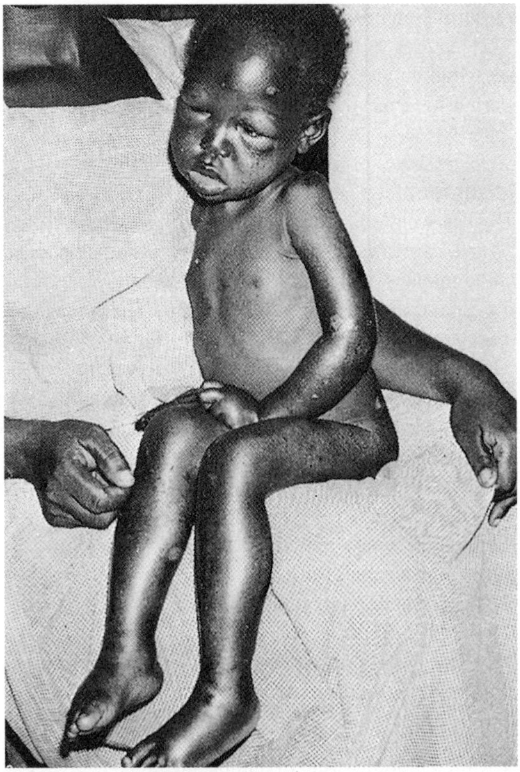

Fig. 7.24 A child with kwashiorkor. Note the oedema of the face, feet and hands, and skin lesions.

Table 7.20 Management of marasmus or kwashiorkor

	Features	Action
Resuscitation	Dehydration, electrolyte imbalance Acidosis, hypoglycaemia Hypothermia and infection	Refeed at 150 kcal/day building up volumes per day; use flour, dried skimmed milk, oil, sugar and multivitamin powder
Subclinical	Underweight (80% below medium standard) or stunted Increased susceptibility to gastroenteritis and respiratory infections	Diagnose as mild to moderate PEM; institute refeeding of protein and energy-rich foods, especially fat-containing ones

The essential pathological feature of kwashiorkor is acute protein depletion affecting mainly the liver, pancreas and gut. With depletion of amino acids, the liver cannot synthesise plasma albumin (hence the oedema) or very low density lipoprotein (hence the fatty liver). Why the viscera bear the brunt of protein depletion in these cases is still not entirely clear. Free radical damage may play a part.

Management of marasmus or kwashiorkor

The principles of management are given in Table 7.20.

The first phase is resuscitation. Dehydration, electrolyte disturbances, acidosis, hypoglycaemia and hypothermia should be corrected. A search must be made for infections and appropriate treatment given. Malnourished children are very susceptible to a number of infections and may not exhibit the usual responses of pyrexia and leucocytosis.

Refeeding consists of gradually working up energy to 150 kcal/kg and protein to 1.5 g/kg per day. The feeds given are essentially the same for both types of severe PEM but in kwashiorkor the child's anorexia requires more intensive hand feeding. Feeds vary in different centres but are usually based on dried skimmed milk mixed with flour, sugar and oil and given 5–6 times a day. Potassium, magnesium and a multivitamin mixture are also needed.

Severe PEM is associated with a mortality of around 20%, even in well-equipped hospitals. In children who recover the liver returns to normal. There is some evidence that children who have suffered chronic severe marasmus may have retarded brain growth with impaired IQ.

INORGANIC NUTRIENTS

Sixteen or more inorganic elements are essential for humans, as shown in the information box.

Deficiency disease is known for each of the elements listed, due to inadequate diet or from excessive losses. Toxic effects have also been observed from self-medication and disordered absorption/excretion, which occurs largely because of competition for protein-carriers between inorganic nutrients. Side-effects are most serious with selenium, iron and zinc.

ESSENTIAL INORGANIC NUTRIENTS

- Sodium (see p. 396)
- Potassium (see p. 396)
- Chloride, magnesium (see p. 397)
- Calcium
- Phosphorus
- Iron
- Zinc
- Copper
- Chromium
- Selenium
- Manganese
- Molybdenum
- Iodine
- Fluoride
- Cobalt[1]
- Sulphur[2]

[1] Physiologically active only in the form of vitamin B_{12}.
[2] Required in the form of the amino acids methionine and cysteine.

Calcium

Calcium is the most abundant cation in the body and powerful homeostatic mechanisms exist for maintaining circulating ionised calcium levels (see p. 397). If calcium intake is truly inadequate, bone mineralisation may be impaired in children and bone loss accelerated in adults. Small changes in total bone calcium can be measured as a research procedure using dual-energy X-ray absorptiometry (DEXA).

In adults, around 70% of the calcium ingested is excreted in faeces; during growth and lactation the efficiency of absorption increases. Calcium absorption may be impaired either by lack of vitamin D, by small intestinal disease and malabsorption, or by foods containing oxalate (e.g. spinach) or phytate (whole-grain cereals) which can form insoluble salts with calcium. The reference nutrient intake of calcium in the UK is 700 mg/day; dietary sources are listed in the information box. The potential benefits of a high calcium intake to ameliorate age-related bone loss are discussed on page 869.

DIETARY SOURCES OF CALCIUM

- Milks, cheeses, yoghurt, eggs
- Fish eaten with bone, e.g. sardines, pilchards
- Some shellfish
- Some nuts, e.g. almonds, peanuts
- Some vegetables, e.g. chick peas, beans
- Bread (if fortified)

Phosphorus

Dietary deficiency is rare. Usual dietary intakes are rather higher than for calcium, about 1.5 g/day. Total body phosphorus is about 700 g, mostly in the bones. Phosphate deficiency occurs:

- in premature infants fed on human milk
- in patients with renal tubular phosphate loss

- due to prolonged high dosage of aluminium hydroxide
- sometimes when alcoholics are refed with high-carbohydrate foods
- in patients on TPN if not enough phosphate is provided.

The features of deficiency are hypophosphataemia and muscle weakness secondary to ATP deficiency.

Iron

An account of iron metabolism and the measures for the prevention and treatment of iron deficiency anaemia is given on pages 757–759. This is one of the most important nutritional causes of ill health in Britain and other developed countries.

There is no physiological mechanism for the secretion of iron so maintenance of its homeostasis depends on iron absorption. Although dietary iron is poorly absorbed (5–15% of intake), the normal daily loss of iron, from desquamated surface cells, is 1 mg and requires a daily intake of 8 mg (at 15% absorption). As blood is the tissue richest in iron (1 ml contains 0.5 mg of iron), a regular loss of only 2 ml/day doubles the iron requirement. On average 30 mg of iron is lost during menstruation and hence premenopausal women require about twice as much iron as men, i.e. 15 mg/day.

A mixed diet with average amounts of meat and vegetables contains about 12–15 mg of iron. Cheap, monotonous, high-carbohydrate diets based on refined wheat flour contain much less. Foods rich in iron are listed in the information box.

Dietary iron overload is occasionally observed and results in iron accumulation in the liver and, rarely, cirrhosis. Haemochromatosis results from an inherited increase in iron absorption and is described on page 718.

DIETARY SOURCES OF IRON

Haem iron	Non-haem iron
• Muscle meat (red more than white) • Organ meat (e.g. liver) • Fish and shellfish	• Oatmeal • Legumes (peas, beans), nuts, dried fruit • Wholemeal bread • Iron-fortified cereal foods • Red wine • Chocolate

N.B. Foods or meals rich in vitamin C enhance iron absorption

Iodine

This is present in seafoods and in trace amounts in soil, water and most foods. Iodine is, however, lacking in the highest mountainous areas of the world, e.g. the Alps and the Himalayas. About 400 million people are estimated to have an inadequate iodine intake, half showing endemic goitre. Elimination of iodine deficiency disorders (IDD) is a public health priority for WHO.

When visible goitres are found in 10% or more of adolescents this indicates that the whole community has very low urinary iodine, e.g. < 30 mg per 1 g creatinine. Where most women have endemic goitre, 1% or more of the babies are born with cretinism (characterised by mental defect and dwarfism) and there is a higher prevalence than usual of deafness, slowed reflexes and poor learning in the remaining population. The adult requirement for iodine is about 100 μg/day.

The best way of preventing cretinism is by injecting all women of child-bearing age with 1–2 ml of iodised poppy seed oil (475–950 mg iodine) every 5 years.

Zinc

Zinc is an essential component of many enzymes including carbonic anhydrase, alcohol dehydrogenase and alkaline phosphatase. In PEM, associated zinc deficiency causes thymic atrophy, and zinc supplements may accelerate the healing of skin lesions, and promote general well-being and improved appetite. Low plasma zinc is not a reliable index of whole body zinc depletion.

CAUSES FOR NEGATIVE ZINC BALANCE AND LOW PLASMA ZINC IN ADULTS

• Intestinal disease • Nephrotic syndrome • Chronic alcoholism • Burns	• Anorexia nervosa • Haemodialysis • Diabetes mellitus • Chronic febrile illnesses

Acute zinc deficiency has been reported in patients receiving prolonged zinc-free i.v. alimentation and caused diarrhoea, mental apathy, a moist eczematoid dermatitis especially round the mouth, and loss of hair. The UK reference nutrient intake for zinc is 7 mg for women and 9.5 mg for men.

In the Middle East chronic deficiency has been described in association with dwarfism and hypogonadism. The best dietary sources are listed in the information box.

DIETARY SOURCES OF ZINC

- Oysters (very high)
- Liver, beef, lamb, other meats
- Wholemeal wheat flour and bread, oatmeal, wheat bran
- Sardines, crab
- Breakfast cereals
- Nuts, legumes

Selenium

Selenium deficiency has been reported to cause cardiomyopathy in children and a myopathy in adults, and is included as a supplement in patients receiving long-term TPN. Selenium is part of the enzyme glutathione peroxidase, which helps prevent hydroperoxides from accumulating in lipids of cell membranes. Some of the functions of selenium and vitamin E overlap. A second function is as part of the enzyme responsible for conversion of thyroxine to triiodothyronine in liver microsomes.

Other minerals

Copper metabolism is abnormal in Wilson's disease (see p. 718). Deficiency occasionally occurs in young children; the main features are anaemia, retarded growth and skeletal rarefaction.

Chromium facilitates the action of insulin. Deficiency has been reported in some children with PEM and as a rare complication of prolonged parenteral nutrition, presenting as hyperglycaemia.

Fluoride

Fluoride has an important influence on the prevention of dental caries. Most adults ingest between 1 and 3 mg of fluoride daily. If water contains 1 part per million (p.p.m.) of fluoride the incidence of dental caries is low. Soft waters usually contain no fluoride, whilst very hard waters may contain over 10 p.p.m. The fluoride in foodstuffs is of little importance; the exceptions are sea fish, which may contain 5–10 p.p.m., and tea; where consumption is frequent the adult intake from this source may be as much as 3 mg daily.

The benefit of fluoride is greatest when it is taken before the permanent teeth erupt, while their enamel is being laid down, as it increases its resistance to acid attack.

The deliberate addition of traces of fluoride (at 1 p.p.m.) to those public water supplies which are deficient is now a widespread practice in many countries.

Chronic fluoride poisoning is occasionally seen in localities where the water supply contains > 10 p.p.m. fluoride or in workers handling cryocite (sodium ammonium fluoride), used in smelting aluminium. This causes increases in bone density and calcification of ligaments and tendinous insertions of muscles.

Sodium, potassium and magnesium

The roles of sodium, potassium and magnesium are discussed in Chapter 5.

THE VITAMINS

Vitamins are organic substances in food which are required in very small amounts but which cannot be synthesised in the body. Twelve vitamins have been demonstrated to have clinical effects in humans (see Table 7.21).

Deficiencies of vitamins still occur in developed countries, e.g. of folate, thiamin and vitamins D and C. Some of these are induced by diseases or drugs. In developing countries deficiency diseases are more prevalent; for example, vitamin A deficiency is a major cause of blindness.

Table 7.21 Names of vitamins

Recommended name*	Alternative name(s)	Usual pharmaceutical preparation
Vitamin A	Retinol	Retinol ester
Vitamin B complex		
Thiamin	Vitamin B_1	Thiamin HCl
Riboflavin	Vitamin B_2	Riboflavin
Niacin	Nicotinic acid and nicotinamide vitamin B_3	Nicotinamide
Vitamin B_6	Pyridoxine	Pyridoxine HCl
Pantothenic acid		Calcium pantothenate
Biotin		Biotin
Folate	Folacin	Folic acid
Vitamin B_{12}	Cobalamin	Cyanocobalamin or hydroxocobalamin
Vitamin C	Ascorbic acid	Ascorbic acid
Vitamin D	Vitamin D_2 and D_3	(Ergo)calciferol
Vitamin E		α-tocopherol
Vitamin K		Vitamin K_1

* Where there is only one substance with vitamin activity (e.g. thiamin, riboflavin), the International Union of Nutritional Sciences recommends that the chemical name be used. Where there are several compounds with vitamin activity, names like vitamin A or vitamin E cover them all.

Some vitamins have pharmacological actions above the intake that prevents classic deficiency disease, e.g. vitamin A is used (with precautions) for acne.

Taking vitamin tablets is fashionable in affluent countries and a few practitioners recommend 'megavitamin therapy' of some vitamins. Doctors therefore need to know the features of both deficiency and overdosage of the major vitamins. Side-effects are most serious with high dosage of three vitamins: A, B_6 and D.

VITAMIN A (RETINOL)

Retinol is a fat-soluble substance and its functions include the following:

- In vision, 11-*cis* retinaldehyde is the initial part of the photoreceptor complex in rods and cones.
- Another form of the vitamin, retinoic acid, induces differentiation of epithelial cells by binding to specific nuclear receptors which turn on responsive genes. In vitamin A deficiency, mucus-secreting cells are replaced by keratin-producing cells.
- Vitamin A has been called the anti-infective vitamin. Deficient children suffer more severe respiratory infections and gastroenteritis, and increased mortality.

On the world scale, vitamin A deficiency is estimated to cause 500 000 new cases of blindness a year in young children, mostly in Asia, and WHO is giving high priority to the prevention of vitamin A deficiency.

DIETARY SOURCES OF RETINOL AND CAROTENE

- Liver (richest natural source of retinol)
- Milk, butter, cheese
- Egg yolk
- Fish liver oils and red palm oil
- Carrots (richest source of carotene) and dark green leafy vegetables
- Some yellow and red fruits (apricots, melon, pumpkin)

(Retinol or carotene is added to margarine in Britain and other countries)

Retinol is found only in foods of animal origin (see the information box); liver is the richest source. However, about two-thirds of vitamin A intake in Britain (and total intake in vegans) comes from carotenes (chiefly β-carotene).

All the carotenoids, including lycopene and lutein, with or without vitamin A activity, are antioxidants. Initial claims that vitamin A may give partial protection against some cancers have not been substantiated.

Night blindness

Night blindness is the earliest sign of vitamin A deficiency, and is particularly common in poor people living in underdeveloped countries; it can occur in patients with malabsorption. The diagnosis of vitamin A deficiency is supported by low plasma vitamin A concentration and is confirmed by marked improvement in dark adaptation following therapeutic doses of retinol.

Xerophthalmia

The earliest sign is xerosis conjunctivae—a dry, thickened and pigmented bulbar conjunctiva with a peculiar smoky appearance. Bitot's spots are glistening white plaques of desquamated thickened conjunctival epithelium, usually triangular in shape and firmly adherent to the underlying conjunctiva (see Fig. 7.25). When dryness spreads to the cornea it takes on a dull, hazy, lacklustre appearance due to keratinisation, and xerophthalmia is said to be present.

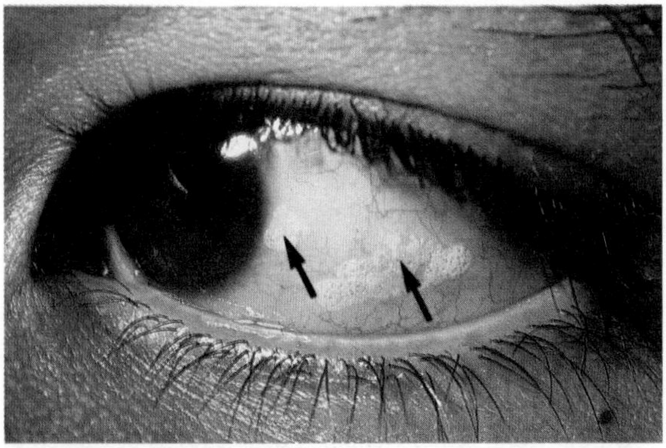

Fig. 7.25 Bitot's spots showing the white triangular plaques (arrows).

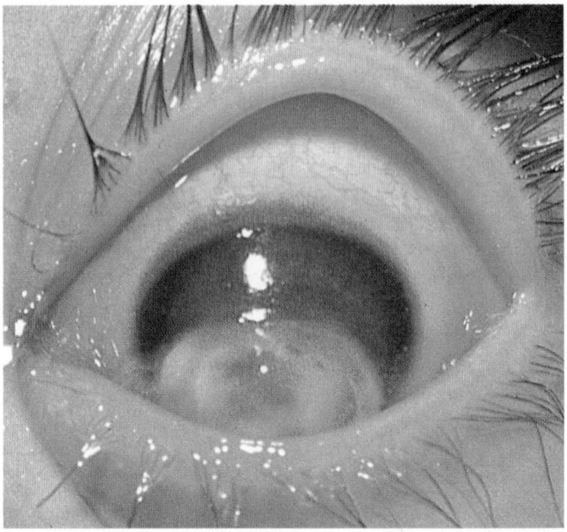

Fig. 7.26 Keratomalacia secondary to vitamin A deficiency in a 14-month-old child. There is colliquative necrosis affecting the greater part of the cornea. The relative sparing of the superior aspect of the cornea is typical.

In young children, xerophthalmia is almost always due to recent vitamin A deficiency and is usually associated with PEM. In older children and in adults, exposure to dust and glare may produce similar changes. Once the cornea is involved, the process can rapidly progress to keratomalacia.

Keratomalacia

This disease is a frequent cause of blindness among Indians, Indonesians and other rice-eating people of Asia; it also occurs in parts of Africa, the Middle East and Latin America and is frequently associated with PEM in young children. As the cornea undergoes ulceration and necrosis, the epithelia beyond the eye are involved (see Fig. 7.26). These children have a high mortality from infections.

Management

Immediately on diagnosis a single large dose of 60 mg retinol as palmitate or acetate (200 000 i.u.) should be given orally or, if there is vomiting or severe diarrhoea, by i.m. injection. The oral dose should be repeated the next day and again prior to discharge or at a follow-up visit. Underlying conditions such as PEM must be treated.

Prevention

In countries where vitamin A deficiency is endemic, pregnant women should be advised to eat dark green leafy vegetables and yellow fruits to build up stores of retinol in the fetal liver. Babies should also be given such vegetables or locally available carotene-rich fruits. In communities where xerophthalmia occurs, single prophylactic oral doses of 60 mg retinol (200 000 i.u.) as palmitate given to pre-school children significantly reduce the mortality from gastroenteritis and respiratory infections; a similar large dose is indicated in any child with measles.

Toxicity

Single large doses in children, as above, are well tolerated. The most serious side-effects of repeated moderate or high doses of retinol are liver damage, hyperostosis and teratogenicity. Women in developed countries who are pregnant are therefore advised not to take vitamin A supplements. Acute overdose leads to nausea and headache, increased intracranial pressure and skin desquamation.

THIAMIN (VITAMIN B_1)

Thiamin pyrophosphate (TPP) is an essential co-enzyme for the decarboxylation of pyruvate to acetylco-enzyme A. This is the bridge between anaerobic glycolysis and the tricarboxylic acid (Krebs) cycle. TPP is also the co-enzyme for transketolase in the hexose monophosphate shunt pathway and for decarboxylation of α-ketoglutarate to succinate in the Krebs cycle. Consequently, when thiamin is deficient:

- The cells cannot metabolise glucose aerobically; this is likely to affect the nervous system first, since it depends entirely on glucose for its energy requirements.
- There is accumulation of pyruvic and lactic acid, which produce vasodilatation and increase cardiac output.
- There is a risk of 'wet' beriberi, a high-output cardiac failure state associated with few ECG changes and a prompt response to thiamin.
- There is a risk of Wernicke's encephalopathy: 'quiet' confusion, ophthalmoplegia, nystagmus and ataxia. These respond to thiamin, but a memory disorder (Korsakoff's psychosis) may remain and is sometimes very persistent.
- There is a risk of 'dry' beriberi, a peripheral polyneuropathy presenting with paraesthesia, cramps and impaired sensation.

High-carbohydrate diets, heavy alcohol intake or intravenous glucose infusions predispose to or aggravate thiamin deficiency. The body contains only 30 mg of thiamin (30 times the adult daily requirement) and deficiency starts after about a month on a thiamin-free diet, sooner than for any other vitamin. Sources of thiamin are listed in the information box.

Management of severe thiamin deficiency

Wernicke's encephalopathy should be treated without delay with 50 mg thiamin hydrochloride by slow i.v. injection followed by 50 mg i.m. daily for a week. Response is within 2–3 days and this confirms the diagnosis. The memory disorder (Korsakoff's psychosis) takes longer to improve and some degree of memory impairment often persists.

In developed countries the prevention of beriberi and Wernicke's encephalopathy is related to the control of alcoholism. Bread and cereal foods are fortified with thiamin in most industrial countries. In the chronic alcoholic, vitamin B complex tablets can prevent the complications of thiamin deficiency.

DIETARY SOURCES OF THIAMIN

- Wheatgerm, wholemeal wheat flour and bread
- Yeast, legumes, nuts
- Pork, duck, Marmite, cod's roe
- Oatmeal, fortified breakfast cereals
- White bread if flour is enriched

RIBOFLAVIN

Riboflavin (vitamin B_2) is a constituent of the flavoproteins which are part of the oxidation chain in the mitochondria. It is a yellow-green fluorescent compound soluble in water. It is decomposed under alkaline conditions by heat and is also destroyed by exposure to ultraviolet (UV) light. The requirement is 1.2 mg per day. Clinical deficiency is rare but may lead to angular stomatitis, cheilosis and nasolabial dyssebacea.

DIETARY SOURCES OF RIBOFLAVIN

- Liver, kidney, meats
- Milk, yoghurt, cheese
- Marmite, wheatgerm
- Mushrooms, broccoli, avocado
- Fortified white flour and breakfast cereals

NIACIN (NICOTINIC ACID AND NICOTINAMIDE)

Nicotinamide is an essential part of the two important pyridine nucleotides, NAD and NADP—nicotinamide adenine dinucleotide (phosphate)—which play a key role in intermediate metabolism. NAD is also the co-enzyme for alcohol dehydrogenase. Nicotinic acid and nicotinamide have equal biological activity and are considered together in foods under the generic term 'niacin'. Both are water-soluble and resistant to heat.

A special feature of this vitamin is that it is normally synthesised in the body in limited amounts from tryptophan; 60 mg of tryptophan yields 1 mg of nicotinamide. For this reason niacin equivalents in a diet are calculated by adding together the niacin plus 1/60 of the tryptophan intake. Eggs and cheese are examples of foods that contain little preformed niacin but provide niacin equivalents from tryptophan.

DIETARY SOURCES OF NIACIN (PRE-FORMED)

- Liver, kidney, red meat, fish
- Peanuts, legumes
- Wholemeal wheat, bran
- Yeast (brewer's), Marmite
- Coffee

Pellagra

Pellagra is a nutritional disease due to deficiency of niacin, formerly endemic among the poor who subsisted chiefly on maize. Pellagra remains in parts of Africa. In developed countries it is occasionally seen in alcoholics and in patients with chronic small intestinal disease.

Clinical features

Pellagra can develop in only 8 weeks in individuals eating diets that are very deficient in niacin and tryptophan. It has been called the disease of the three Ds: dermatitis, diarrhoea and dementia. Characteristically, there is erythema resembling severe sunburn, appearing symmetrically over the parts of the body exposed to sunlight and especially on the neck. The skin lesions may progress to vesiculation, cracking, exudation and crusting with ulceration and sometimes secondary infection (see Fig. 7.27).

In the alimentary tract the diarrhoea is often associated with anorexia, nausea, glossitis and dysphagia. This reflects the presence of a non-infective inflammation that extends throughout the gastrointestinal tract.

In severe deficiency, delirium occurs acutely, with dementia developing in chronic cases.

Biochemical tests to confirm the diagnosis are urinary N methylnicotinamide or red cell NAD.

Management

Nicotinamide is given in a dose of 100 mg 8-hourly by mouth; it can be given parenterally. The response is usually rapid; within 24 hours the erythema of the skin diminishes, the diarrhoea ceases and a striking improvement occurs in the patient's behaviour and mental attitude.

PYRIDOXINE (VITAMIN B_6)

Pyridoxine, pyridoxal and pyridoxamine are three closely related compounds with similar physiological actions. The active form of the vitamin in humans is pyridoxal 5-phosphate, the co-enzyme for a large number of different enzyme systems involved in the metabolism of amino acids. Vitamin B_6 is available in most foods, and requirements are related to protein intake, 15 mg/g protein, or an average of 1.4 mg/day in the UK.

Certain drugs, such as isoniazid and penicillamine, act as chemical antagonists to pyridoxine and cause deficiency. Some cases of sideroblastic anaemia respond to treatment with pyridoxine.

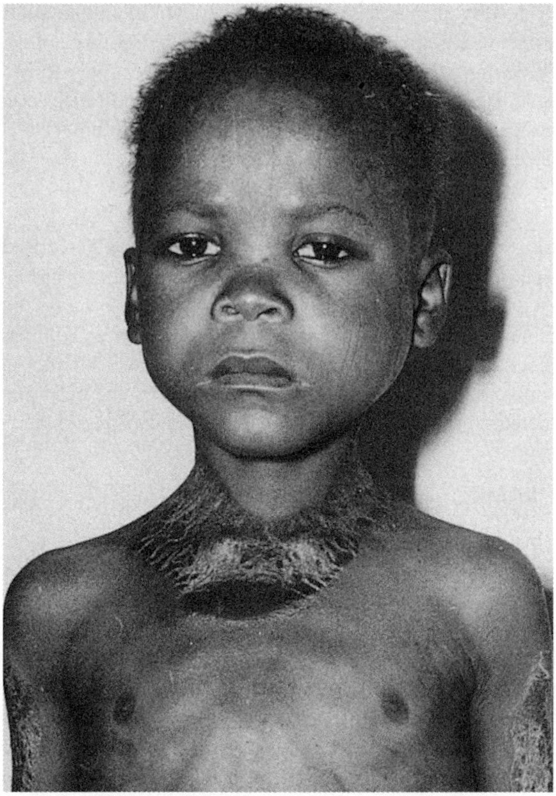

Fig. 7.27 Pellagra in a girl of 5 years. This skin lesion on the neck (Casal's collar) is pathognomonic of niacin deficiency.

Vitamin B_6 deficiency is rare but can occur in women taking oral contraceptives, and may be responsible for the mild depression which affects a small proportion of such women.

Megavitamin doses of vitamin B_6 (50 mg/day or more) taken for several months can cause a sensory polyneuropathy.

BIOTIN

Biotin functions as a co-enzyme for four carboxylases involved in carbohydrate, fatty acid and amino acid metabolism. The clinical features of deficiency include scaly dermatitis, alopecia, paraesthesia and urinary excretion of organic acids, e.g. propionic and 3-hydroxypropionic. A form of seborrhoeic dermatitis of infants responds to biotin.

VITAMIN B_{12} AND FOLATE

These vitamins and the haematological disorders due to their deficiency are discussed on pages 759 and 760. Although the requirements for vitamin B_{12} are very small

(1.5 μg/day), it is only found in animal products and hence vegans are at risk of deficiency. The normal liver contains enough stores to cover requirements for several years.

Vitamin B_{12} and the nervous system

Severe prolonged vitamin B_{12} deficiency (causes are listed on p. 759) may cause megaloblastic anaemia and/or neurological degeneration. In some cases the neurological disease predominates; this may be because a good intake of folate maintains erythropoiesis. Vitamin B_{12}, but not folate, is needed for the integrity of myelin. In severe deficiency there is insidious, diffuse and uneven demyelination. It may be clinically manifest as peripheral neuropathy or spinal cord degeneration affecting both posterior and lateral columns ('subacute combined degeneration of the spinal cord') or there may be cerebral manifestations (resembling dementia) or optic atrophy. Plasma vitamin B_{12} (before treatment) is very low; treatment with hydroxocobalamin should produce improvement but it may be slow.

Folic acid in the prevention of neural tube defects

Three major birth defects—spina bifida, anencephaly and encephalocele—all result from imperfect closure of the neural tube which takes place 3–4 weeks after conception. Prevention trials, including a large multicentre study by the Medical Research Council (UK) of recurrent neural tube defects, have shown that folic acid reduces recurrence or occurrence of these deformities by about 70%, but it must be taken prior to and following conception. In a prospective study in Dublin, red cell folate levels were lower in cases than in controls but did not fall within the deficient range. Folate is directly involved in DNA and RNA synthesis and it seems that a higher than normal level is required during embryonic development. The UK Department of Health (1991) advises that women who have experienced a pregnancy affected by neural tube defect should take 5 mg of folic acid daily from before conception and throughout the first trimester. In addition, all women planning a pregnancy are advised to include good sources of folate in their diet.

GOOD SOURCES OF FOLATE

- Brussels sprouts
- Fortified breakfast cereals
- Spinach, asparagus, beetroot
- Orange, avocado, melon
- Potatoes, cauliflower, peas, parsnips
- Marmite and Bovril
- Wholemeal bread
- Dried beans
- Kidney

Liver is the richest source of folate but an alternative source is advised in early pregnancy because of its high vitamin A content.

DIETARY SOURCES OF VITAMIN C

- Blackcurrants, guavas
- Green peppers, broccoli, cauliflower (raw)
- Oranges and other citrus fruits
- Brussels sprouts, cabbage
- Potatoes
- Liver (the only animal food that contains it)

VITAMIN C (ASCORBIC ACID)

Ascorbic acid is the most active reducing agent in the aqueous phase of living tissues and is easily and reversibly oxidised to dehydroascorbic acid.

Ascorbic acid is very easily destroyed by heat, increased pH and light, and is very soluble in water. Hence many traditional cooking methods reduce or eliminate it. The recommended adult intake is 30–75 mg/day in different countries.

It has been suggested that high-dose vitamin C improves immune function (including resistance to the common cold) and cholesterol turnover but such effects remain unproven. Daily intakes of more than 1 g/day have been reported to cause diarrhoea and the formation of renal oxalate stones.

Scurvy

Scurvy is the clinical manifestation of vitamin C deficiency. It occurs in people who have eaten no fruit or vegetables, or taken no vitamin supplements for 2–3 months. It is most likely to be seen in vagrants or in association with famines.

Ascorbic acid deficiency results in defective formation of collagen and there is in consequence impaired healing of wounds, capillary haemorrhage and subnormal platelet adhesiveness (normal platelets are rich in ascorbate).

Clinical features

The pathognomonic clinical sign is swollen and spongy gums, particularly the papillae between the teeth ('scurvy buds'). These bleed easily. There may be perifollicular, petechial or spontaneous bruising. Haemorrhage may occur into a joint or into the gastrointestinal tract. The patient is usually anaemic. Another characteristic is that fresh wounds fail to heal. Patients with scurvy are also at risk of sudden death, apparently from cardiac failure.

For treatment, a dose of 250 mg vitamin C 8-hourly by mouth should saturate the tissues quickly. The general deficiencies of the patient's former diet also need to be corrected. If the patient is anaemic, iron and sometimes folic acid are indicated.

Trauma, surgery and burns, infections, smoking and certain drugs—adrenocortical steroids, aspirin, indomethacin and tetracycline—all increase the requirement for vitamin C. Consequently, hospital patients often require more than the recommended intake.

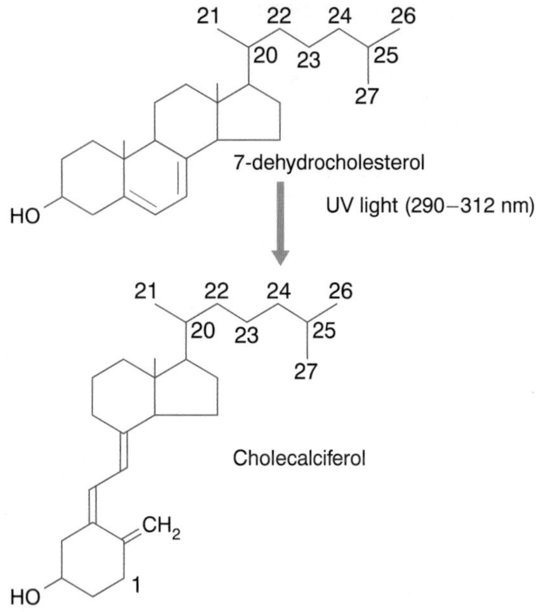

Fig. 7.28 Biosynthesis of vitamin D in the skin.

VITAMIN D

The natural form, cholecalciferol, is a modified steroid. It is formed in the skin by the action of UV light on 7-dehydrocholesterol, a minor companion of cholesterol (see Fig. 7.28). Cholecalciferol is formed in a few animal foods—fatty fish, eggs, liver and dairy foods—and it is concentrated in fish liver oils. The pharmaceutical form of pure vitamin D is (ergo)calciferol, made by the action of UV light on ergosterol (a sterol found in fungi). Ergocalciferol is added (in controlled amounts) to margarines and (in North America) to milk.

Cholecalciferol itself is not biologically active, and converted in the liver to 25-hydroxycholecalciferol 25 (OH) D_3 which is further hydroxylated in the kidneys mainly to 1,25-dihydroxycholecalciferol 1,25 (OH_2) D_3. This second product is the active form of vitamin D (see Fig. 8.16, p. 575).

The nutritional requirement is usually 2.5–5 µg/day. Older people and dark-skinned people make less vitamin D in their skin. In chronic intestinal diseases there can be malabsorption of vitamin D and in chronic kidney disease production of the active form is impaired. The clinical results of vitamin D deficiency are rickets (described on p. 871) in growing children, or osteomalacia and myopathy in adults.

DIETARY SOURCES OF VITAMIN D

- Fish liver oils, e.g. cod liver oil
- Fatty fish (herring, mackerel, salmon, sardines, tuna)
- Fortified margarine
- Infant milk formulas
- Eggs
- Liver

Vitamin D is toxic in large dosage; it causes hypercalcaemia. Hypervitaminosis D is mentioned on pages 576 and 465.

VITAMIN E

Alpha-tocopherol is the most potent of eight related fat-soluble substances with vitamin E activity. Vitamin E and carotenoids are the main fat-soluble antioxidants in the body. Vitamin E prevents oxidation of polyunsaturated fatty acids in cell membranes by free radicals. The first feature of human deficiency is a mild haemolytic anaemia which has been described only in premature infants and in malabsorption. Early oral administration reduces the severity of retrolental fibroplasia in premature infants given oxygen. In chronic fat malabsorption, e.g. in cystic fibrosis, ataxia and visual scotomas occur which respond to vitamin E.

More recently it has been suggested that, as a lipid-soluble antioxidant, vitamin E may reduce atherogenesis by protecting low-density lipoprotein from oxidation. The present recommended intake of vitamin E in the UK and USA is 7–10 mg/day in men, and 5–8 mg in women. If the intake of polyunsaturated fat is high, vitamin E intake should be increased. Rich sources include vegetable oils, whole-grain cereals and nuts.

VITAMIN K

Vitamin K is the coagulation vitamin and is required for the synthesis of an unusual amino acid, γ-carboxyglutamic (gla). Gla residues are part of the protein molecule of four of the coagulation factors, II, VII, IX and X. The gla residues confer on these proteins the capacity to bind to phospholipid surfaces in the presence of calcium.

Adequate amounts are normally supplied in the average diet (leafy vegetables and liver), or synthesised by bacteria in the colon. Vitamin K has important roles in three situations. In the newborn, primary deficiency can occur because placental transfer of vitamin K is inefficient, the neonatal bowel has not yet acquired bacteria and breast milk contains little of the vitamin. Vitamin K_1 is given routinely to newborn babies to prevent haemorrhagic disease of the newborn. In obstructive jaundice, dietary vitamin K is not absorbed and it is very important to administer the vitamin before biliary surgery. Thirdly, warfarin and related anticoagulants (see p. 797) act by antagonising vitamin K.

NUTRITIONAL DEPLETION AND SUPPORT IN HOSPITAL PATIENTS

NUTRITIONAL DEPLETION

PEM is the most important nutritional depletion in hospital patients but is not always obvious and tends to be overshadowed by the primary disease. Energy (calories) and protein cannot be given as capsules or an injection and providing enough of them parenterally is technically difficult and expensive.

At one end of the range semi-starvation is seen, for example, in anorexia nervosa or obstruction of the oesophagus; at the other end is hypoalbuminaemic malnutrition, which is sometimes called 'adult kwashiorkor'. This form is to be expected in a patient with increased protein catabolism and/or losses—for example, after burns or severe trauma—who has been receiving only intravenous glucose and water, and where plasma albumin is low. There can be oedema, and cell-mediated immunity is impaired. Types of micronutrient deficiency likely to occur in hospital are detailed in the second information box.

The intake of vitamins and other micronutrients can be boosted by giving these in a pharmaceutical preparation, by mouth or by injection. When a multivitamin preparation is given it is important to check that it contains all the major vitamins (including folic acid).

HOSPITAL PATIENTS AT INCREASED RISK OF MALNUTRITION

- Severely underweight: weight for height < 80% predicted
- Recent weight loss of 10% or more of usual body weight
- Alcoholism
- Malabsorption syndromes
- Increased metabolic rate: burns, trauma, severe infections, prolonged fever
- Increased losses, e.g. fistulae, draining wounds, renal dialysis, haemorrhage
- No food by mouth for over a week while receiving simple intravenous fluids (glucose/electrolytes/water)
- Antinutrients or catabolic drugs, e.g. immunosuppressants, cancer chemotherapy, adrenocorticol steroids
- Radiotherapy

MICRONUTRIENT DEFICIENCY IN HOSPITAL

- Thiamin—patient starving or vomiting 3 weeks if given i.v. glucose may develop Wernicke's encephalopathy
- Folate
- Vitamin B_{12} (prolonged nitrous oxide anaesthesia)
- Vitamin C—losses increased by stress; wound healing requires increased supply
- Vitamin K—from biliary obstruction, antibiotics
- Iron—from bleeding
- Zinc

NUTRITIONAL SUPPORT

The main aim of nutritional support is to get water, energy and protein into the patient. There are four principal routes and two or more can be used together.

Oral supplements

The ordinary diet can be reinforced with energy (calorie)-dense and/or protein-rich supplements.

Enteral feeding

This is usually given by a fine-bore plastic nasogastric tube but sometimes a gastrostomy or jejunostomy is used. Percutaneous gastrostomy (PEG) is useful for long-term enteral feeding. It is more convenient for the patient and reduces the risk of aspiration. The indications for and use of enteral feeding in critically ill patients are detailed on page 1047. There are a wide range of enteral preparations that can be administered either by a bolus, over a short time, or by continuous drip.

Parenteral feeding by a peripheral vein

This is easily established and is used for supplementary energy and/or fluid support. Glucose infusions can be given up to a concentration of 10% only, due to the risk of phlebitis. Since 2.5 litres of 10% glucose provides only 250 g of glucose and 1000 kcal, energy requirements cannot be achieved unless i.v. lipid emulsion is also given.

Parenteral feeding by central venous alimentation

This allows administration of more concentrated glucose infusions (25–35%). Although it is possible to provide all a patient's energy needs in this way, there are disadvantages in giving such a high carbohydrate intake: for instance, high insulin levels and essential fatty acid deficiency. It is probably best to give about 30% of energy as fat emulsion, along with glucose, amino acids and micronutrients. The day's prescription can be made up in a single sterile 3-litre bag container. A stable patient with intestinal failure usually requires 2500 kcal of energy, partly from glucose/electrolyte solutions, partly from an intravenous lipid preparation, e.g. Intralipid (which contains essential fatty acids), and partly from an intravenous preparation of mixed crystalline L-amino acids, e.g. Aminoplex, Synthamin or Vamin N. The amino acid infusion usually provides 10–12 g nitrogen/day. This is equivalent to 63–75 g of protein/day. In patients on total parenteral nutrition the minor nutrients, which are taken for granted in a normal diet, all have to be provided (see Table 7.16, p. 511). TPN costs considerably more than enteral feeding.

Indications

TPN is life-saving in patients with major disease of the small intestine in which the functioning gut mass is below the amount necessary for adequate digestion and absorption of nutrients. Intestinal failure can be acute (e.g. severe inflammatory bowel disease) or chronic (e.g. massive resection of small bowel, high gastrointestinal fistula).

DIETARY MODIFICATION AS TREATMENT: THE THERAPEUTIC DIET

Some diseases, notably coeliac disease, hepatic encephalopathy and phenylketonuria, are not caused by disturbed nutrition, but for each of them a specific modification of the usual diet, the therapeutic diet, is the principal treatment. The therapeutic diet may be life-saving. In other conditions, e.g. chronic renal failure, diabetes mellitus and mild hypertension, the appropriate therapeutic diet usually complements other modes of treatment. The prescription for a diet should state the nature of the modification(s), the degree of each modification, the planned duration of these, and any compensation for essential nutrients reduced as a result of the modifications. A dietitian is trained specifically to advise on the nature and degree of modification and then to construct and advise individuals on their therapeutic diet.

Changes to the patient's usual diet need to be carefully computed and explained. Unrealistic or unnecessary restrictions can reduce the nutritional adequacy of the diet; this is especially serious in children on modified diets where growth may be compromised.

OBESITY

'Overweight' and 'obesity' are terms commonly used to describe individuals with increased body fat. Measuring fat in humans requires special instruments and so excess weight is usually defined by measuring the body mass index (BMI).

Body mass index

BMI is calculated by measuring a person's weight in kilograms and then dividing by that person's height in metres squared (kg/m^2). For example, an adult weighing 70 kg with a height of 1.75 metres has a BMI of $70/1.75^2 = 22.9$. The advantage of this index rather than the use of weight alone is that it is height-independent, such that tall and short people of similar proportions have a similar BMI. The internationally accepted range of BMIs in adults is shown in the information box. Ideal body weight may also be defined as 100%, with overweight as 101% to 119% and obese as > 120% of normal.

For children weight excess can also be classified according to the BMI using standardised reference curves. A child whose BMI is above the 99.6% centile for age is usually considered overweight and requires remedial action. However, the child with a BMI of 98–99.6% may also have a weight problem, but in certain individuals, such as boys who are stocky and muscular, the BMI may appear in the 'high' range and yet not be indicative of excess fat. This makes the BMI in children far less reliable as an indicator of excess fat than in adults.

BMI RANGES IN ADULTS

• Acceptable range	18.5–24.9
• Overweight	25.0–29.9
• Obese	30.0–39.9
• Morbidly obese	≥ 40

Fat content

Body fat content may be measured using a number of techniques. The simplest method involves measuring skinfold thickness at four sites (biceps, triceps, subscapular and suprailiac) using a spring-loaded caliper and then applying the values to published equations. More exacting methods employ underwater weighing, isotopic measurement of whole body potassium content—an index of lean (non-fat) mass, or impedance analysis. The latter depends on the difference in electrical resistance between lean tissue and fat. Normal body fat content of an adult is 10–20% in men and 20–30% in women. While abdominal fat can be measured using CT or MRI, the ratio of waist circumference to height, or measuring the sagittal diameter of the abdomen at the level of L4/5, provides a useful index of intra-abdominal fat content.

Body fat distribution

There are two major types of fat distribution in adult obesity (see Fig. 7.29). Some adults store their fat mainly around the hips and thighs, which gives them a 'pear' shape known as gynoid distribution; this is characteristic of women. The second type found in both sexes is the storage of fat primarily in the abdomen, producing an 'apple' shape known as android distribution. This latter type can also be seen in mildly overweight people and is important to document as it is more closely related to disease risk than the BMI alone. To check for abdominal obesity one measures the waist-hip ratio. This is the waist circumference in centimetres divided by the hip circumference in centimetres. The waist circumference is usually measured half-way between the superior iliac crest and the rib cage in the mid-axillary line, whereas the hip circumference is measured one-third of the distance between the superior iliac spine and the patella. The diseases associated with abdominal obesity include hypertension, hyperlipidaemia, insulin resistance, diabetes mellitus and cardiovascular diseases. This is a risk if the waist-hip ratio is > 0.95 in males or

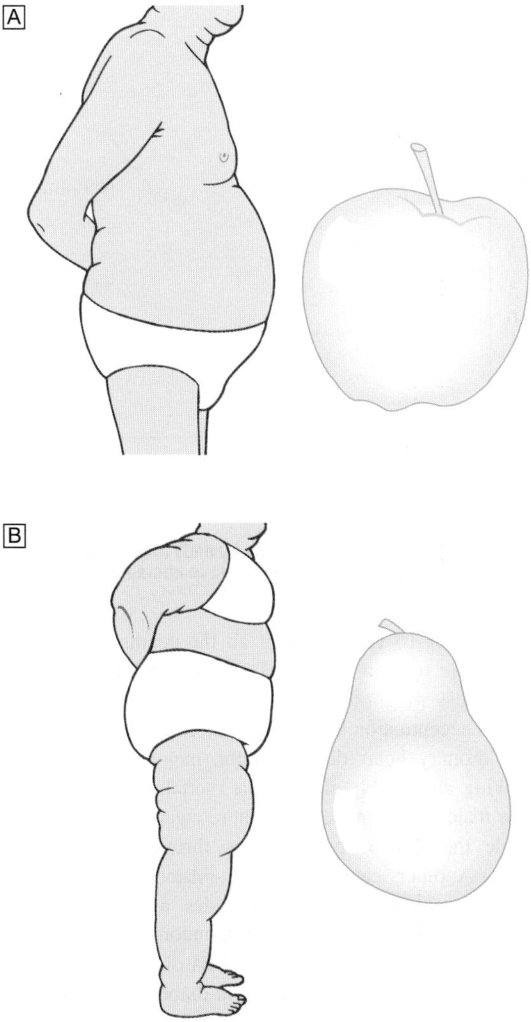

Fig. 7.29 Fat distribution. A Abdominal fat distribution (apple shape). B The gynoid distribution of where the fat is deposited, mainly on the hips and thighs (pear shape).

> 0.8 in females. Lately, research has indicated that measurement of waist circumference alone might suffice to define disease risk of intra-abdominal fat, as shown in Table 7.22.

Weight of the nation

The prevalence of excess weight in the UK adult population is shown in Table 7.23.

Table 7.22 Co-morbidity risk with waist circumference

	Increased risk	Substantial risk
Men	≥ 94 cm (= 37 inches)	≥ 102 cm (= 40 inches)
Women	≥ 80 cm (= 32 inches)	≥ 88 cm (= 35 inches)

Table 7.23 Prevalence of excess weight in UK adults (1996)

	Overweight	Obese	Total with excess weight
Men	44%	15%	59%
Women	32%	17%	49%

The proportion of the population in the UK with obesity has doubled over the last two decades. Other European countries have a greater problem, especially in women, with a prevalence of female obesity of 30% in Italy and 44% in Russia.

Aetiology of obesity

Weight gain is due to an imbalance between energy intake and energy expenditure. A modest but persistent excess intake of 50 kcal (0.2 MJ) per day will result over a 4-year period in a slow but progressive rise in weight of 10 kg. To carry this excess weight the body requires increased muscle mass, and the metabolism associated with this and the associated metabolic demands increase the body's metabolic rate to the extent that energy expenditure then matches the increased intake and weight stabilises out at a higher level. If intake rises progressively or expenditure is reduced by decreasing exercise, then weight rise will continue. An extra 10 kg indicates an extra 70 000 stored kcal. This storage potential explains why it takes so long to lose weight, for an energy reduction of 600 kcal per day (2.5 MJ) from the usual intake will require over 100 days of compliance to lose 10 kg. Once the person has lost weight, then a permanent change in intake and/or energy expenditure amounting to 300 kcal (1.25 MJ) per day of less intake or of extra exercise will be required to maintain this weight loss.

Behavioural changes

The behavioural changes conducive to weight gain are as follows:

- High-fat diets do not switch off appetite as well as carbohydrates and protein. Also fat induces very little energy expenditure when consumed as most is stored. Studies have shown that the prevalence of obesity is greatest in those eating the highest fat intake.
- Snacking and the loss of formalised meal patterns reduce the conscious recognition of foods eaten.
- Consumption of energy-dense foods (and drinks), often high in fat and sugar but low in bulk, increase energy intake substantially.
- Alcohol promotes weight gain as it provides substantial energy, and can stimulate appetite and loosen restraint.
- Decreasing physical activity with age accounts for the age-related weight gain. This difference can be as much as 700 kcal (2.9 MJ) per day when comparing a sports-keen young man and an inactive retired person of 65 years.

- Declining overall levels of physical activity in society occur with sedentary jobs, a change in social circumstance and sedentary pastimes; e.g. the television-watching 'couch potato'.
- Giving up smoking induces a fall in energy expenditure equivalent to 9 kcal per cigarette and an increase in food intake. The average weight gain is 2.8 kg in males and 3.8 kg in females. Nevertheless, the risk of smoking is so substantial that a rise in weight of 11 kg would be required to negate the benefit of giving up smoking 20 cigarettes per day.

Familial and genetic predisposition

Familial and genetic predisposition plays a role in weight gain. There are a number of known genetic conditions, such as Prader–Willi syndrome and mutations in the leptin gene, which produce a syndrome complex associated with obesity. However, such conditions are rare and are unlikely to have a bearing on the causation of obesity in the general population. Studies on families with obesity have implicated over 20 genes on at least 12 chromosomes, emphasising the polygenic influence on the development of obesity. Likewise, obese individuals have been found to have paradoxically elevated levels of leptin, a hormone normally produced by adipose tissue, that acts at the level of the hypothalamus to suppress appetite. This latter finding suggests that obesity may be analogous to type 2 diabetes, where patients have large amounts of insulin in their blood but are unable to respond to it. Overall, the genetic contribution to weight gain in susceptible families ranges from 25% to 40%, with the genetic determination of selective intra-abdominal fat deposition being greater at 30–50%.

Drugs

Certain drugs may contribute to weight gain; these include corticosteroids, tricyclic antidepressants, valproate, sulphonylureas for diabetes and some steroidal contraceptives.

Endocrine causes

Defined endocrine causes are rare, probably accounting for less than 1% of all weight gain in the population. Cushing's syndrome (see p. 581) causes substantial weight gain, especially in the abdominal region. Some hypothalamic tumours, such as craniopharyngioma, are associated with the development of obesity, whereas hypothyroidism causes weight gain possibly by reducing metabolic rate.

The risks of obesity

Excess weight increases mortality. In Framingham, USA, where the population has undergone long-term surveillance, the risk of death increased by 1% for each 0.5 kg weight rise between the ages of 30 and 42 years and by 2% between the ages of 50 and 62 years. In another study of women in the USA aged 30–55 years with a BMI of 29 or greater,

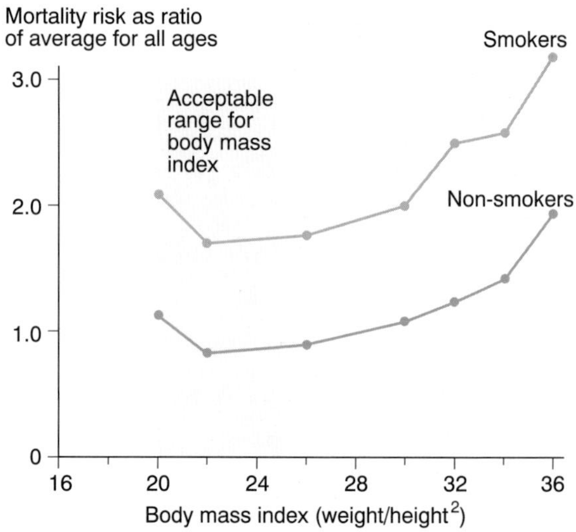

Fig. 7.30 Variations in mortality by body mass index in smokers (> 20 cigarettes per day) and in non-smokers.

followed for 16 years, half of all the deaths were directly attributable to their obesity. This relationship of mortality with excess weight (see Fig. 7.30) shows a J-shaped curve, with an accentuation in the rise in mortality above a BMI of 30. Coronary heart disease is the major cause of death. Smoking appreciably elevates the mortality curve, such that those males who smoke 20 or more cigarettes per day have double the risk of non-smokers throughout the weight range. Another cause of weight-related death is cancer, especially colorectal cancer in males and cancer of the gallbladder, biliary passages, breast, endometrium and cervix in females. A maintained weight loss of 9 kg in women is associated with a 25% reduction in diabetic, cardiovascular and cancer mortality.

Complications of weight gain are outlined in the first information box on page 529. The greatest risk is from diabetes mellitus. This occurs above a BMI of 22 with a five-fold rise in risk in females at a BMI of 25 (two-fold in males), a 28-fold risk at a BMI of 30 (seven-fold in males) and a 93-fold risk above a BMI of 35 (42-fold in males). A 10% increase in weight in men increases the risk of coronary heart disease by 38%, a 20% rise in weight by 86%. This is mainly related to associated alterations in lipid profile and hypertension. A 10% weight gain is associated with a rise in systolic pressure of about 6 mmHg and diastolic pressure by 4 mmHg; those who are genetically more susceptible exhibit the greater effect.

Management

The management of weight excess depends on the clinical assessment of the individual (see the second information box on p. 529) and includes the co-morbid risk factors such as

COMPLICATIONS OF OBESITY

- Type 2 diabetes mellitus
- Hypertension
- Stroke; also related to hypertension
- Hyperlipidaemias
- Coronary heart disease; related to hyperlipidaemia, hypertension and blood rheology
- Cancers: post-menopausal breast, endometrium, ovarian, gallbladder and colonic cancers
- Gallstones
- Lower limb: arthritis of the hip, knee and foot; varicose veins
- Breathlessness; sleep apnoea
- Infertility, hirsutism
- Pregnancy complications: neural tube defects, perinatal mortality, pre-eclampsia, gestational diabetes, pre-term labour, caesarian sections, deep vein thrombosis
- Stress incontinence, abdominal hernias
- Psychological: depression
- Social: disability on low income, reduced employment prospects

hypertension, hyperlipidaemia, diabetes mellitus and cardiovascular disease. The most appropriate treatment plan takes into account such risk factors but in addition the BMI (see Table 7.24). The aim at the outset is to achieve a modest weight loss of 10% since this is sufficient to achieve a significant improvement in health (see the information box on the right). It is also highly unlikely that an ideal weight will be achievable and to strive for this is likely to demoralise both patients and their advisers!

Management of weight can be considered in five modules, as follows.

ASSESSMENT OF THE OBESE PATIENT

History

- Smoking habit
- Current drug therapies that affect weight
- Alcohol intake
- Risk factors such as angina, myocardial infarction, stroke, intermittent claudication

Examination

- BMI; weight in indoor clothing without shoes; height without shoes
- Waist circumference
- Blood pressure

Tests

- Urinalysis
- Gamma-glutamyl transferase: for alcoholic liver disease
- Lipid profile
- Thyroid-stimulating hormone
- Blood glucose: random and fasting

Psychological

- Depression and eating disorders

Table 7.24 Management plan for obesity

BMI	Assessment	Advice
18.5–24.9	Weight steady in adult life	Healthy eating plan
	Gained > 5 kg in adult life	Weight maintenance with increased exercise
25–29.9	No other risk factors	Healthy eating plan
	Risk factors present	Weight reduction plan
	Waistline problem	Weight reduction plan
≥ 30		Weight reduction plan

THE BENEFITS OF A SUSTAINED 10% REDUCTION IN WEIGHT FOR THE OBESE

Mortality

- 20–25% fall in total mortality
- 30–40% fall in diabetes-related deaths
- 40–50% fall in obesity-related cancer deaths

Angina

- Reduces symptoms by 90%
- 33% increase in exercise tolerance

Blood pressure

- Fall of 10 mmHg systolic pressure
- Fall of 20 mmHg diastolic pressure

Lipids

- Fall by 10% in total cholesterol
- Fall by 15% in low-density lipoprotein (LDL) cholesterol
- Fall by 30% in triglycerides
- Increase by 8% in high-density lipoprotein (HDL) cholesterol

Diabetes

- Reduces risk of developing diabetes by > 50%
- Fall of 30–50% in fasting glucose
- Fall of 15% in HbA_{1c}

Rheology

- Decreases blood viscosity by 20–27%
- Decreases red cell aggregation by 20%

Module 1 Weight reduction

This aims to provide a 3-month structured management plan designed to meet the needs of each individual patient:

- Support from a trained health-care professional in a group setting since greater weight loss is achieved using groups than with individual consultations. This may reflect the interplay and mutual support of the individuals in the group.
- Diet consisting of a moderate reduction in energy intake of about 600 kcal (2.5 MJ) less than expenditure assessed on weight, sex and age (published formulae are used). This produces a greater weight loss than stricter diets (e.g. 1000 kcal) probably as compliance is better. Most diets aim to reduce fat intake. Starvation diets are

PRINCIPLES OF BEHAVIOURAL MODIFICATION

Issues to be discussed in group behavioural therapy are:
- Self-monitoring using a food diary
- Need for long-term lifestyle change
- Need to modify eating habits
- Need to assess present exercise level and ideas to increase this if necessary
- Importance of restricting occasions and situations when inappropriate types or amounts of food are eaten
- Separation of eating from other activities
- Planning of daily food intake
- Understanding of food labels and adapting recipes with regard to fat, salt, sugar and fibre
- Possibility of changes to individual eating style
- Identification of the causes of negative emotions and stress
- Recognition that eating may be related to stress
- Need to self-monitor feelings and emotions
- Dealing with situations that interfere with everyday food choices, e.g. eating out, holidays, family pressure and cost

potentially dangerous due to a risk of sudden death from heart disease exacerbated by profound loss in muscle and the development of arrhythmias secondary to elevated free fatty acids and deranged electrolytes. The dietary change should involve the patient's entire household.

- Behavioural modification therapy which is designed to support a process of change in the individual's attitude, perception and behaviour as regards food intake, lifestyle and physical activity. The information box provides some examples of the topics covered in a structured programme.
- Promotion of increased physical activity which can be maintained long-term. Such exercise need not be over-exertional because health gain is achieved at modest levels of exercise, as long as these are maintained. Walking briskly for 30 minutes each day can contribute 100–200 kcal (0.4–0.8 MJ) of energy expenditure daily, resulting in an additional weight loss of 1 kg per month.

Module 2 Weight maintenance plan

The weight reduction module is followed by a 3-month structured programme emphasising weight maintenance although continued weight loss may be an option for some. This again emphasises therapy in groups, with continued behavioural therapy, promotion of exercise and diet modification. Exercise in this module is designed to prevent weight regain once weight has been lost by dietary restriction.

Module 3 Drug therapy

Historically, two groups of appetite suppressant drugs were available, namely those affecting the hypothalamic catecholaminergic pathway (e.g. amphetamines, diethylpropion, phentermine and mazindol), and those affecting the hypothalamic serotinergic system (fenfluramine, dexfenfluramine). However, due to the cerebral stimulant properties of the first group and the high incidence of valvular heart disease and pulmonary hypertension seen in patients taking fenfluramine, dexfenfluramine and phentermine, these agents, even if available, are not recommended.

Two new drugs are to be licensed shortly in the UK. Orlistat inhibits pancreatic and gastric lipases decreasing ingested triglyceride hydrolysis. This produces a 30% reduction in dietary fat absorption which can contribute to a caloric deficit of about 0.8 MJ (200 kcal) per 24 hours. Adverse side-effects are mainly related to the effect of the fat malabsorption on the gut, namely loose stools, faecal urgency and flatus. The second drug is sibutramine which reduces food intake through β_1-adrenoceptor and 5-$HT_{2A/2C}$ receptor agonist activity. Metabolic rate may also be enhanced via stimulation of peripheral β_3-adrenoceptors. Weight loss achieved with this agent is 3–5 kg better than placebo with 6 months' therapy and is associated with an improvement in lipid profile. Side-effects include dry mouth, constipation and insomnia whereas the noradrenergic effects of the drug can increase heart rate and blood pressure in some.

Recent evidence suggests that such therapy should only be considered in those with a BMI > 30 who have failed to lose 10% weight after at least 3 months of a structured weight reduction programme consisting of dietary advice, behavioural modification and exercise. An obesity reduction drug could then be prescribed for 3 months in the first instance as long as there are no contraindications. If after 3 months' therapy the patient fails to lose 5% weight from the outset then the drug should cease. If, however, weight loss does exceed 5%, then the drug may be continued, with careful monitoring for adverse events.

Treatment of depression in obese patients with tricyclic antidepressants often produces weight gain, resulting in drug non-compliance. The new class of antidepressants which inhibit serotonergic uptake, such as fluoxetine, also reduce weight. Weight is lost for about 6 months on this class of drug but then is regained for reasons unknown and, therefore, these drugs are not recommended for the treatment of obesity without depression. Bulk-forming drugs and diuretics should not be used to enhance fat loss. Thyroid replacement therapy should only be used in the obese person when there is evidence of biochemical hypothyroidism.

Module 4 Very low calorie diets

Very low calorie diets (VLCDs) produce weight losses of 1.5–2.5 kg/week compared to 0.5 kg on conventional diets. VLCDs are mainly used for short-term rapid weight loss. In the UK, the recommendation is that VLCDs should only be considered by those with a BMI > 30 and under the supervision of an experienced physician/nutritionist. The composition of the diet should ensure a minimum of 50 g of protein each day for men and 40 g of protein for women to minimise muscle degradation. Energy content should be minimum 400 kcal (1.65 MJ) for women of height < 1.73 m and 500 kcal (2.1 MJ) for all men and women taller than 1.73 m. Side-effects tend to be a problem in the early stages of the diet, especially orthostatic hypotension, headache, diarrhoea and nausea.

Module 5 Bariatric surgery

Two procedures now dominate surgical practice, namely vertical banded gastroplasty and gastric bypass. Vertical banded gastroplasty involves the construction of a small stomach pouch fashioned by vertical stapling to restrict both gastric outlet and size (see Fig. 7.31). A newer technique involves a rubber ring placed around the stomach; the degree of constriction is varied by expanding the ring with saline via a tube connected to the abdominal wall. This latter technique allows adjustment at a later date as well as removal by minimal access surgery. Gastric bypass (Roux-en-Y) involves fashioning a pouch of low volume (less than 30 ml) by stapling across the stomach and then connecting a limb of small intestines as a conduit for food, hence bypassing the distal stomach, duodenum and upper jejunum (see Fig. 7.31B). The following recommendations apply:

- Most patients seeking such surgery should have a BMI > 40 but those with a BMI > 35 may be considered if there is a high-risk, life-threatening co-morbid condition or severe physical incapacity.
- All patients should be given the opportunity to lose weight on a supervised, expert-run programme.
- Multidisciplinary team evaluation is essential and surgery should only be contemplated in well-informed and motivated patients.
- Surgery should be undertaken by an experienced surgeon in a setting which incorporates expert medical surveillance and access to respiratory support.
- Life-long medical surveillance after surgery is a necessity.

Mortality is low in experienced centres but post-operative respiratory problems, wound infection, dehiscence, staple leaks, stomal stenosis, marginal ulcers and venous thrombosis are common. In the later post-operative period other problems may arise, such as pouch and distal oesophageal dilatation, persistent vomiting, dumping and micronutrient deficiencies, particularly of folate, vitamin B_{12} and iron which are of concern especially to women contemplating pregnancy.

Hypertension, hyperlipidaemia and diabetic glycaemic control are markedly improved in this group of patients where no other therapy is as effective.

Jaw wiring with the use of milk and other liquid diets can be most efficacious but rapid weight regain once the jaws are unwired is usual. This is why this technique is usually reserved for those requiring to lose significant weight rapidly for some operation or life event. Apronectomy is usually advocated to remove an overhang of abdominal fat, especially if infected, ulcerated or a nuisance. This operation is of no value for long-term weight reduction if appetite remains unrestricted. Jejunoileal bypass has an unacceptable mortality and morbidity (60%) and is now no longer recommended.

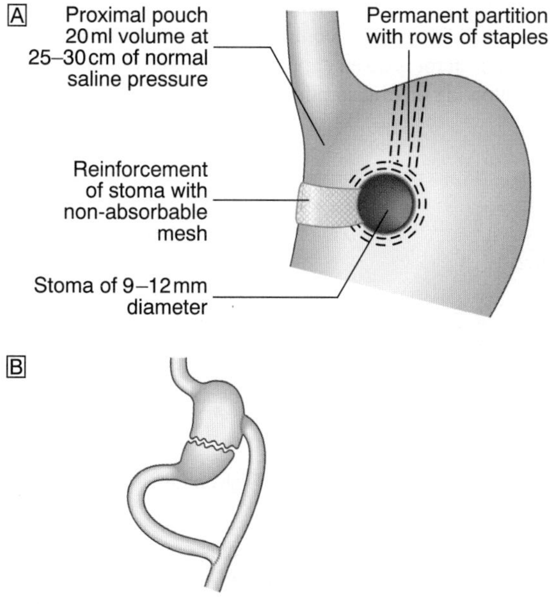

Fig. 7.31 Bariatric surgical procedures. A Vertical banded gastroplasty. B Roux-en-Y gastric bypass.

FURTHER INFORMATION ON NUTRITIONAL FACTORS IN HEALTH AND DISEASE

Department of Health 1991 Dietary reference values for food energy and nutrients for the United Kingdom: report of the panel on dietary reference values of the Committee on Medical Aspects of Food Policy. HMSO, London

Finer N (ed) 1997 Obesity. British Medical Bulletin 53: 2

Jones C M, Taylor G O, Whittle J G et al 1997 Water fluoridation, tooth decay in 5-year-olds and social deprivation measured by the Jarman score: analysis of data from British dental surveys. British Medical Journal 315: 514–517

Jung R T 1990 A colour atlas of obesity. Mosby–Wolfe, London

McWhirter J P, Pennington C R 1994 Incidence and recognition of malnutrition in hospital. British Medical Journal 308: 945–948

Mann J I, Truswell A S 1998 Essentials of human nutrition. Oxford University Press, Oxford

Medical Research Council Vitamins Study Research Group 1991 Prevention of neural tube defects: results of the Medical Research Council vitamins study. Lancet 338: 131–137

Scottish Intercollegiate Guidelines Network 1996 Obesity in Scotland: integrating prevention with weight management. A national clinical guideline for use in Scotland no. 8. Royal College of Physicians, Edinburgh

Souba W W 1997 Nutritional support. New England Journal of Medicine 336: 41–48

World Health Organization 1985 Report of a joint FAO/WHO/UNU expert consultation: energy and protein requirements. Technical Report Service 724. WHO, Geneva

OTHER METABOLIC DISORDERS

In medicine the term 'metabolic' is usually restricted to disorders which can best be described in biochemical terms.

Metabolic disorders may be classified in various ways: for example, by the specific enzyme deficiency responsible for the disorder, the body system principally affected or the predominant feature of the disorder (e.g. carbohydrate, amino acid, lipid or mineral metabolism).

Many relatively rare inborn errors of metabolism result from inactivity of a particular enzyme, usually by inheritance of a mutation in either or both alleles of the relevant gene. The mutated genes responsible for such diseases have frequently been identified by molecular methods described in Chapter 1. The chromosomal locations and nature of many of these genes are given in Chapter 20.

Common metabolic disorders are also influenced by genetic factors, usually requiring more than one predisposing gene and accentuated by environmental influences (see Fig. 1.30, p. 38). For example, numerous genes are implicated in diabetes mellitus and are reviewed in Table 1.11, page 56.

A few examples of other metabolic disorders are given below.

Carbohydrate. Aside from diabetes mellitus, rare genetic errors usually inherited as autosomal recessive traits can lead to abnormalities in the metabolism of galactose (galactosaemia), fructose (fructosuria) and glycogen (glycogen storage diseases such as von Gierke's disease). Further details are provided in Table 20.3, page 1130.

Amino acids. These are generally relatively rare diseases (e.g. cystinuria and the Fanconi syndrome). Phenylketonuria is rare but particularly important since the mental retardation which results can be avoided if the disease is detected in the neonatal period and treated with a special diet.

Purines. Gout is a classic example of a metabolic disorder and is described on page 831.

LIPOPROTEIN DISORDERS

Lipoprotein metabolism

Cholesterol and triglyceride are indispensable structural and metabolic components of all animal cells. Since they are hydrophobic they require to be transported through the aqueous environment of the plasma, encapsulated (see Fig. 7.32) in a shell of phospholipid and special proteins (called apolipoproteins), forming a family of lipid-protein particles or lipoproteins (see Table 7.25). The apolipoproteins play an essential role not only in maintaining the structure of the particles but also in directing their metabolism by acting as recognition proteins for a variety of plasma enzymes and cell membrane receptors (see Table 7.26).

Lipoprotein metabolism can be thought of in terms of three interconnected transport pathways focusing on the liver (see Fig. 7.33, p. 534). One, the exogenous pathway, is responsible for the digestion, absorption and tissue dissemination of dietary fat. About 100 g of triglyceride and 0.5 g of cholesterol flow through it each day. Digestive enzymes in the intestinal lumen hydrolyse these fats to free cholesterol, fatty acids and mono- and diglycerides, which combine with bile salts to form the water-soluble micelles responsible for carrying the lipids to absorptive sites in the small intestine. Under normal circumstances triglyceride absorption is virtually complete, while only about 50% of the cholesterol is taken up, the rest being lost in the faeces.

Following their absorption into the intestinal enterocytes,

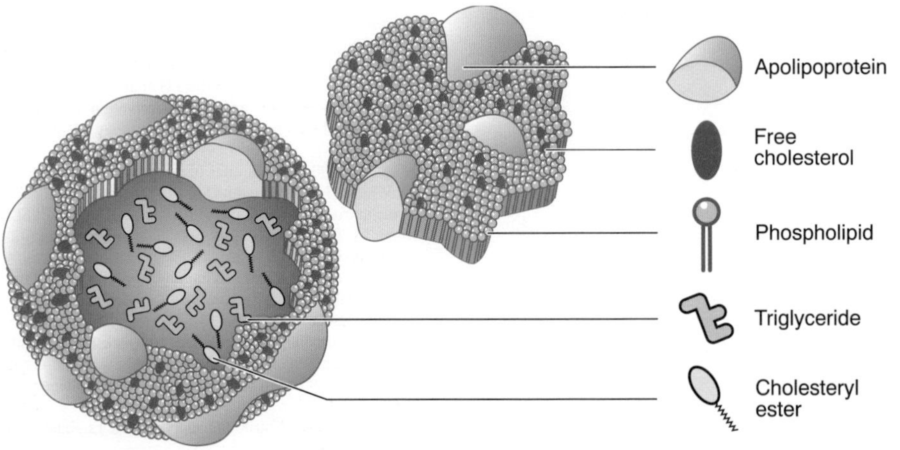

Fig. 7.32 Structural characteristics of a typical lipoprotein.

Table 7.25 Structure and functions of the four main lipoproteins

Lipoprotein	Main apolipoproteins	Functions
Chylomicron	B_{48}, AI, CII, E	Main transporter of dietary triglyceride; synthesised in the gut after a meal; not present in normal fasting plasma
Very low density lipoprotein (VLDL)	B_{100}, CII, E	Main carrier of endogenous triglyceride; synthesised in liver; precursor of LDL
Low-density lipoprotein (LDL)	B_{100}	Main cholesterol-carrier in blood; generated from VLDL in the blood stream
High-density lipoprotein (HDL)	AI, AII	Smallest but most abundant lipoprotein; transports cholesterol from peripheral tissues to liver for excretion; cardioprotective

Table 7.26 Properties of some human apolipoproteins

Apolipoprotein	Molecular weight	Site of synthesis	Functions
AI	28 000	Liver, intestine	Main HDL protein Activates lecithin:cholesterol acyltransferase (LCAT)
B_{100}	549 000	Liver	Main structural protein of VLDL and LDL Involved in triglyceride and cholesterol transport Binds to LDL receptor
B_{48}	254 000	Intestine	N-terminal 50% of B_{100} Lacks LDL receptor binding site Main structural protein of chylomicrons
CII	8850	Liver	Activates lipoprotein lipase (LPL) Directs chylomicron and VLDL triglyceride hydrolysis
E	34 000	Liver, intestine, macrophages, glial cells	Binds to LDL receptor and probably also to another specific liver receptor Important in brain lipid transport

the component parts of the dietary fat are reconstituted to re-form triglyceride and cholesteryl ester which are packaged in chylomicrons and secreted into the intestinal lymphatics, through which they reach the blood stream via the thoracic duct. In the circulation triglyceride is gradually removed by the action of the enzyme lipoprotein lipase (LPL), located on the endothelial surface of capillary beds in adipose tissue and cardiac and skeletal muscle. This process eviscerates the chylomicron, causes some of its surface phospholipid and protein to be shed into the plasma as a precursor of high-density lipoprotein (HDL), and leaves a remnant which is taken up rapidly by the liver; in the process, dietary cholesterol is deposited in that organ. There the sterol may be incorporated into hepatocyte membranes, oxidised to bile acids or repackaged into the endogenous triglyceride-rich counterpart of the chylomicron, the very low density lipoprotein (VLDL).

Among its many synthetic activities, the liver is responsible for the continuous production of VLDL which, in the fasting state, represents the body's primary source of circulating triglyceride energy. This particle is subject to the same lipase-mediated digestion process as the chylomicron, except that in this case the resulting particle (intermediate density lipoprotein—IDL) is not cleared rapidly by the liver. Instead, it undergoes additional remodelling to produce a cholesterol-enriched particle (low-density lipoprotein—LDL) with a plasma half-life of about 3 days. LDL is ultimately removed from the circulation by the high-affinity LDL receptor pathway, or by other less well-understood scavenger mechanisms thought to lead to the incorporation of LDL cholesterol into atheromatous plaques. Raised levels of LDL cholesterol therefore predispose to coronary heart disease (CHD).

In contrast to LDL, cholesterol-rich HDL particles protect against CHD. They are synthesised in the liver and intestine and also generated in part by lipolysis of chylomicra and VLDL. Defective triglyceride lipolysis in the blood stream, which results in hypertriglyceridaemia, is also associated with low circulating HDL levels. The actual function of HDL is to remove cholesterol from peripheral tissues through the action of the plasma enzyme, lecithin:cholesterol acyltransferase (LCAT), and transport it centripetally for hepatic excretion. This process is thought to be anti-atherogenic, consistent with the observation that raised levels of circulating HDL reduce the risk of CHD.

Disorders of lipoprotein metabolism

Lipoprotein disorders or dyslipidaemias are among the most common metabolic diseases seen in clinical practice. They are important because they may lead to a number of sequelae including CHD, dermatological manifestations (xanthelasmata and xanthomata), pancreatitis and (more rarely) neurological and ocular anomalies. Both hyper- and hypolipidaemias are recognised.

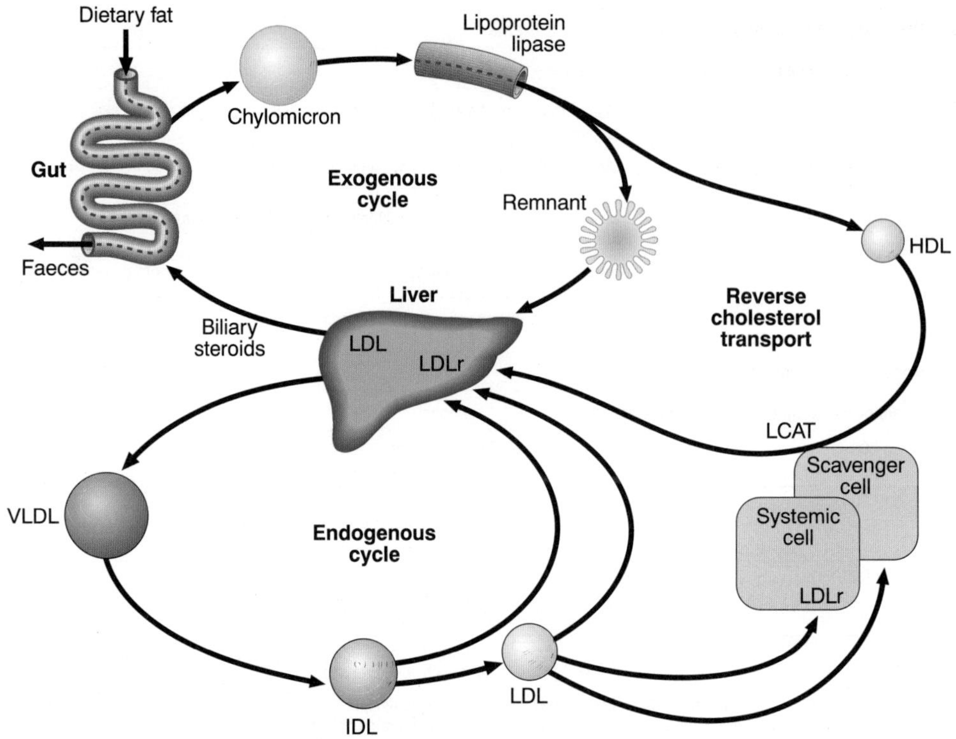

Fig. 7.33 Lipid transport through the plasma.

THE HYPERLIPIDAEMIAS

Hyperlipidaemia is common and can be divided into primary anomalies, which cannot be linked to an identifiable underlying disease, or secondary manifestations of some other condition (see Table 7.27). The latter usually disappear when the underlying condition is treated.

Table 7.27 Common causes of secondary hyperlipidaemia

Disease	Dominant lipid and lipoprotein abnormality
Diabetes mellitus **Chronic renal failure**	Raised triglyceride, VLDL, low HDL
Drugs e.g. Thiazides, β-adrenoceptor antagonists	Raised triglyceride, VLDL, low HDL
Oestrogen replacement therapy	Raised triglyceride, raised HDL
Alcohol excess	Raised triglycerides, VLDL, raised HDL
Hypothyroidism **Nephrotic syndrome**	Raised cholesterol, LDL

PRIMARY HYPERLIPIDAEMIA

Classification

There is at present no satisfactory comprehensive classification of lipoprotein disorders. Initially, attempts were made to define the abnormalities on the basis of their laboratory presentation. This classification, attributed to Fredrickson and colleagues, is still clinically valuable (see Table 7.28) but fails to identify the molecular or genetic defect(s) responsible for the conditions. Consequently, patients with a particular genetic defect may fall into two or more of the five Fredrickson categories, and progression of the condition or treatment may cause a patient to move from one category to another.

Recently, attempts have been made to introduce a genetic classification system (see Table 7.28) but, as different molecular defects are discovered, this approach has become increasingly complex and in the immediate future is unlikely to be of wide clinical use.

All hyperlipidaemias result from a complex interaction between genetic predisposition and dietary indiscretion. Two conditions in particular—familial hypercholesterolaemia and familial combined hyperlipidaemia—are frequently encountered in clinical practice and are primarily genetic in origin. A family history of hyperlipidaemia or early CHD

Table 7.28 Classification of the hyperlipoproteinaemias

Fredrickson type	Genetic classification	Defect	Clinical sequelae
I	Lipoprotein lipase deficiency Apo CII deficiency	Mutated or absent LPL Mutated LPL activator	Pancreatitis
II	Familial hypercholesterolaemia Apo B_{3500} defect Familial combined hyperlipidaemia	Deficient LDL receptor binding Reduced LDL catabolism Over-production of B_{100}-containing particles	CHD
III	Apo E_2 homozygosity	Mutated apo E plus precipitating environmental factor	CHD and PVD
IV	Familial combined hyperlipidaemia	Over-production of B_{100}-containing particles	CHD
V	Familial hypertriglyceridaemia	Unknown	Pancreatitis

(CHD = coronary heart disease; PVD = peripheral vascular disease)

should be sought in individuals with substantially raised plasma cholesterol or triglyceride.

Familial hypercholesterolaemia

Familial hypercholesterolaemia is a common autosomal dominant condition affecting about 1 in 500 of the population and results from a defect in the LDL receptor gene (more than 150 such defects have been identified so far). A mutation in apo B_{100} (called the B3500 defect since amino acid 3500 is mutated) produces the same clinical picture since the mutant protein fails to bind to the LDL receptor. Patients may develop excessive tissue deposits of cholesterol around the eye (xanthelasmata, see Fig. 7.34A, p. 536; corneal arcus, see Fig. 7.34B) or in tendons (xanthomata, see Fig. 7.34C), although in many instances the first evidence of the problem is a myocardial infarction occurring at an early age. Approximately 50% of affected individuals will have a myocardial infarction by the age of 50.

Familial combined (mixed) hyperlipidaemia

This common inherited condition, whose genetic origin is uncertain, is characterised by the familial concurrence of hypercholesterolaemia (raised LDL), hypertriglyceridaemia (raised VLDL), and sometimes both simultaneously, in different members of the same family (see Fig. 7.35, p. 536). Approximately 1 in 250 of the population suffers from the problem, which results from a combination of hepatic overproduction of the B_{100}-containing particles VLDL and/or LDL, and a partial defect in triglyceride lipolysis. Plasma HDL cholesterol levels are therefore usually low. CHD is common, but physical stigmata like xanthomata and premature corneal arcus do not feature.

Elevated plasma cholesterol and triglyceride concentrations are both linked to an increased risk of CHD, and this increases further when HDL is also low. High triglyceride and low HDL levels are often associated with insulin resistance and hypertension, producing a constellation of conditions of very high risk for macrovascular disease, the metabolic syndrome or 'syndrome X'. The latter reaches its full expression in patients with type 2 diabetes.

Management of hyperlipidaemia

The management of hyperlipidaemia aims to reduce the risk of CHD but ought to be seen as only one arm of a global strategy designed to achieve that objective. Smoking, hypertension, diabetes mellitus and other major risk factors, where present, also require attention.

Dietary management of hyperlipidaemia

Most patients who present with hyperlipidaemia suffer from a polygenic predisposition to raised blood lipids which is aggravated or unmasked by dietary or lifestyle indiscretions. Diets rich in cholesterol or saturated animal fats tend to raise blood (LDL) cholesterol while high carbohydrate intakes or excessive alcohol consumption may increase plasma (VLDL) triglyceride.

The first-line management of any primary hyperlipidaemia should always be dietary modification. This may be time-consuming and difficult but its importance should not be underestimated. Dietary management as a sole therapy should be pursued for 3–6 months before its effect is evaluated. The principal dietary guidelines for reducing both plasma cholesterol and triglyceride are shown in Figure 7.36. This diagram illustrates the standard lipid-lowering dietary guidelines which are currently recommended, but these obviously require some translation for patient use.

In essence, it is recommended that red meat and dairy consumption be reduced, while that of vegetables, fruit and pulses be increased, together with more fish being eaten (especially oily fish such as mackerel, salmon and tuna). In addition to modifying the composition of the diet, weight reduction to achieve ideal body weight coupled with exercise is important as both of these will help to improve glucose tolerance and lower blood pressure in addition to their effects on plasma lipids.

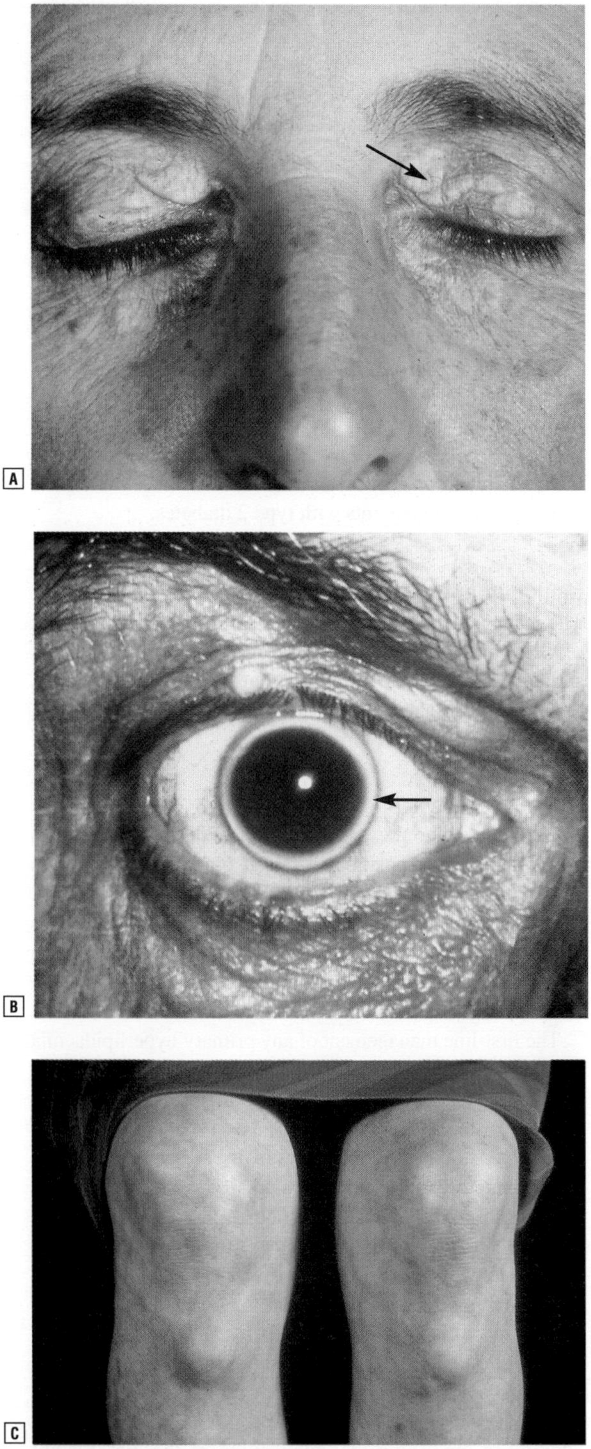

Fig. 7.34 Clinical manifestations of familial hypercholesterolaemia. A Xanthelasma (arrow). B Corneal arcus (arrow). C Xanthoma. These are commonly seen on Achilles or patellar tendons or on tendons on the dorsa of hands or feet.

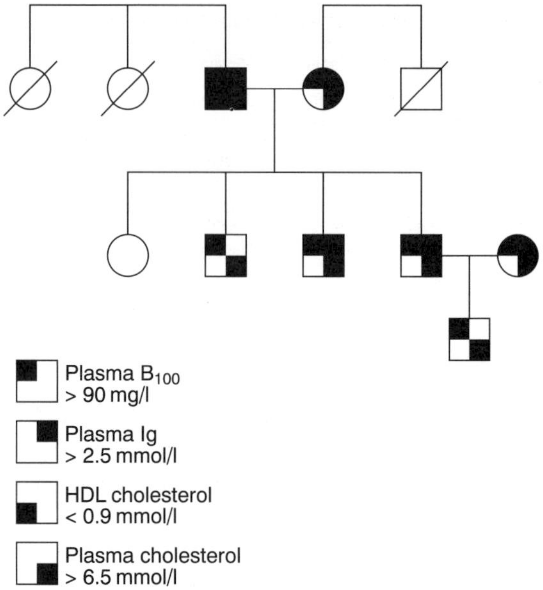

Fig. 7.35 Typical inheritance pattern of familial combined hyperlipidaemia.

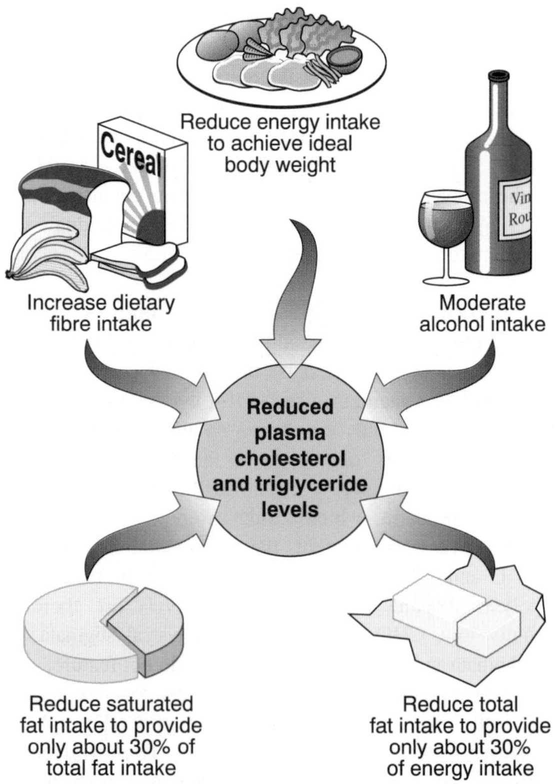

Fig. 7.36 Lipid-lowering dietary guidelines.

Table 7.29 Lipid-lowering drugs and their actions

Drug group	Principal actions
HMG CoA reductase inhibitors (e.g. simvastatin, pravastatin)	Inhibit cholesterol biosynthesis in the liver Activate hepatic LDL receptor Increase LDL catabolism Lower plasma and LDL cholesterol
Bile acid sequestrant resins (e.g. cholestyramine, colestipol)	Block intestinal reabsorption of bile acids Divert hepatic cholesterol into bile acid production Activate hepatic LDL receptors Lower plasma and LDL cholesterol
Fibrates (e.g. bezafibrate, fenofibrate)	Activate LPL Increase VLDL lipolysis Lower plasma triglyceride and raise HDL; reduce plasma LDL
Nicotinic acid and its derivatives	Inhibit lipolysis within adipocytes Reduce plasma free fatty acid levels Lower hepatic VLDL synthesis and secretion Lower triglyceride and increase HDL

Drug therapy for hyperlipidaemia

Drug therapy for hyperlipidaemia, if required, should be viewed as an adjunct to dietary management and other lifestyle changes. There is currently a range of lipid-lowering drugs available with a variety of actions (see Table 7.29). The most common drugs for the treatment of primary hypercholesterolaemia are HMG CoA reductase inhibitors (the 'statins') and the bile acid sequestrant resins. The most common drugs for the treatment of primary hypertriglyceridaemia or combined hyperlipidaemia are the fibrates or nicotinic acid and its derivatives.

THE HYPOLIPOPROTEINAEMIAS

The hypolipoproteinaemias are rare but, when they do occur, they often present with spectacular clinical features. They are of two main types. The first, abetalipoproteinaemia or hypobetalipoproteinaemia, results from defective secretion of apolipoprotein B-containing lipoproteins (chylomicra, VLDL, IDL and LDL). This results in fat malabsorption, ataxic neuropathy, retinitis pigmentosa and acanthocytosis. There is no definitive treatment, though administration of vitamin E may curb many of the morbid consequences of the condition.

The second deficiency state, Tangier disease, is associated with defective production of apolipoprotein A-containing HDL particles. As a result, transport of cholesterol to the liver for excretion is obstructed and sterol esters accumulate in unusual peripheral sites within the reticulo-endothelial system (e.g. tonsils, intestinal lymph nodes) and the cornea. Relapsing neuropathy is a feature of the condition, which has no specific treatment.

SPONTANEOUS HYPOGLYCAEMIA

Multiple causes of hypoglycaemia are recognised in humans. By far the most common is 'iatrogenic', which results from treatment with insulin or sulphonylurea drugs in patients with diabetes mellitus (see p. 485). Occasionally, hypoglycaemia is the presenting feature of an illness or occurs as an important epiphenomenon and is then considered to be 'spontaneous'. Hypoglycaemia is a biochemical abnormality, arbitrarily defined as a blood glucose concentration below 2.2 mmol/l. A blood glucose of this level is almost always pathological and requires active investigation to establish the cause.

Since the human brain is vitally dependent on a continuous supply of glucose as its principal source of energy, disruption of glucose availability will rapidly cause malfunction from neuroglycopenia. Multiple counter-regulatory mechanisms therefore exist to prevent a dangerous decline in blood glucose, including the secretion of hormones such as glucagon and adrenaline, suppression of endogenous insulin secretion, and neurally activated release of neurotransmitters.

The main factors affecting glucose homeostasis are: the intake of nutrients, gastric emptying and intestinal absorption, hepatic production of glucose and the secretion of insulin and counter-regulatory hormones. The prevailing blood glucose concentration reflects the rate of glucose influx into, and efflux from, the circulation. Blood glucose is normally maintained within a narrow range of 3.5–6.5 mmol/l with very limited excursions associated with starvation and the ingestion of food.

Classification

The most useful classification of hypoglycaemia is based upon aetiology (see the information box, p. 538). Subdivision of hypoglycaemia into 'fasting' and 'reactive' types is now outdated. The spectrum of causes of hypoglycaemia varies between hospital and community practice. In hospitalised patients, hypoglycaemia is associated with diabetic therapy, chronic renal failure, liver disease, infections, shock, pregnancy, neoplasia and burns. In the community, the majority of cases of hypoglycaemia are associated with the inadvertent misuse of insulin or excessive alcohol consumption. Other causes are rare.

Clinical features

Hypoglycaemia is usually episodic. Symptomatic features which are common with acute insulin-induced hypoglycaemia (e.g. sweating, tremor, hunger and anxiety, see p. 492) are

CAUSES OF HYPOGLYCAEMIA IN ADULTS

Pancreatic
- Insulinoma: benign, malignant, multiple and microadenomatosis
- Islet hyperplasia: nesidioblastosis or functional hyperinsulinism
- Pancreatitis
- Pluriglandular syndrome

Toxic hypoglycaemia
- Therapeutic hypoglycaemic agents: insulin*, sulphonylureas*
- Alcohol*
- Drugs, e.g. quinine, salicylates, propranolol, pentamidine
- Poisons, e.g. certain types of mushroom

Extrapancreatic neoplasms
- Mesenchymal tumours*
- Haemangiopericytoma
- Primary hepatic carcinoma
- Various other tumours

Autoimmune hypoglycaemia
- Autoimmune insulin syndrome
- Anti-insulin receptor antibodies

Essential reactive hypoglycaemia
- Post-gastrectomy: gastrointestinal motility disorders
- Alcohol-provoked

Liver and kidney disease
- Hepatocellular disease
- Advanced renal failure
- Congestive cardiac failure

Endocrine disease
- Pituitary insufficiency
- Adrenocortical insufficiency
- Hypothyroidism
- Selective hypothalamic insufficiency

Inborn errors of metabolism
- Adult glycogenolysis (liver glycogen disease)
- Hereditary fructose intolerance

Miscellaneous
- Sepsis
- Prolonged starvation: anorexia nervosa
- Dialysis
- Excessive exercise
- Diseases of the nervous system

* Indicates a common cause.

often absent in patients with spontaneous hypoglycaemia. A low blood glucose should be suspected in patients with altered consciousness, convulsions, abnormal neurological findings or odd behaviour. A high index of suspicion of hypoglycaemia should be maintained even when an obvious cause of cerebral abnormality is apparent, such as hemiplegic stroke, alcoholic intoxication or cerebral malaria. An accurate and reliable history may be difficult to obtain from the patient and an objective account from witnesses may be invaluable. Subacute or chronic neuroglycopenia often presents with deteriorating cognitive function over months or years, and psychiatric features may be prominent. In many instances, the only indication that hypoglycaemia is responsible is the finding of a low blood glucose on routine biochemical screening.

Investigations

A firm diagnosis of hypoglycaemia is usually based on 'Whipple's triad':

1. Symptoms are associated with fasting or exercise.
2. Symptoms are relieved by glucose.
3. A low blood glucose is demonstrated biochemically.

In addition, hypoglycaemia is often associated with inappropriately elevated plasma insulin concentrations.

Suspected hypoglycaemia (blood glucose < 2.5 mmol/l) should be confirmed by laboratory analysis of venous blood or capillary glucose. Test strips for capillary blood glucose, which are used for monitoring diabetes, are neither sufficiently sensitive nor accurate in the hypoglycaemic range and are often misread. Blood should be collected during the emergency presentation, both to confirm hypoglycaemia and for additional analyses, e.g. hormones (insulin, C-peptide), alcohol and drugs, which may identify a cause. This can prevent subsequent unnecessary and costly investigation, and is of forensic and medico-legal importance in cases such as attempted suicide or deliberate poisoning.

The nature and timing of the blood samples for glucose measurement are of importance. The possible development of a large arteriovenous difference after glucose absorption precludes the use of oral glucose load tests in the evaluation of causes of hypoglycaemia. It should also be noted that plasma glucose concentration is 15% higher than that estimated from whole venous blood.

Provocative tests for investigating suspected hypoglycaemia are summarised in the information box. Most patients with recurrent spontaneous hypoglycaemia will have a low blood glucose (< 2.5 mmol/l) after an overnight fast (18 hours), but this should be confirmed on three

INVESTIGATION OF SPONTANEOUS HYPOGLYCAEMIA

Provocation tests
- Fasting
  Blood glucose and insulin measured following overnight (18 hrs) fast (× 3); prolonged fast (72 hrs) rarely needed
- Exercise
  Blood glucose measured following 30 min vigorous exercise on treadmill or bicycle

Dynamic suppression tests
- C-peptide suppression test: i.v. infusion of 0.125 U/kg soluble insulin for 60 min with measurement of plasma glucose, insulin and C-peptide at 30-min intervals

separate occasions. In normal persons, blood glucose levels do not fall during exercise but in affected individuals hypoglycaemia may be precipitated by vigorous exercise for 30 minutes. A prolonged fast (72 hours) is rarely necessary, being a non-specific test which should be reserved for patients with demonstrated hyperinsulinism who have not developed symptomatic neuroglycopenia after overnight fasting or with exercise.

Plasma concentrations of insulin, C-peptide, pro-insulin and other hormones such as insulin-like growth factor-I and II may be estimated during confirmed hypoglycaemia. Characteristic patterns of plasma glucose and insulin are associated with different causes of hypoglycaemia. A diagnosis of endogenous hyperinsulinism depends upon evidence of inappropriate insulin and/or C-peptide secretion in the presence of hypoglycaemia.

Other provocative tests, such as the measurement of plasma C-peptide during insulin-induced hypoglycaemia (C-peptide suppression test) may be of value in the investigation of insulin-secreting tumours.

Tumour-induced hypoglycaemia

Insulinomas are pancreatic islet-cell tumours that secrete insulin and usually cause recurrent fasting hypoglycaemia.

These are rare tumours (about 1–2 cases/million population per year) but are one of the more common causes of fasting hypoglycaemia in non-diabetics. Often the patient has had symptoms for many years prior to presentation. These may include drowsiness on waking or a variety of other symptoms which may result in referral to a neurologist or psychiatrist (fits, 'funny turns', faintness, abnormal behaviour, paraesthesiae). These characteristically occur before meals and are relieved by food or a sweet drink. The tumours are often relatively small (0.5–5 mm in diameter) and may be found in any part of the pancreas. About 10% of them are malignant. The key to diagnosis is the demonstration of fasting hyperinsulinaemia (i.e. a plasma insulin which is inappropriately high for the blood glucose—see the information box) and a failure of suppression of insulin secretion, as judged by plasma C-peptide levels, during insulin-induced hypoglycaemia. The tumours can be localised by MRI or contrast-enhanced helical CT. Endoscopic or laparoscopic ultrasound are very successful techniques in skilled hands. Transhepatic portal venous sampling to measure plasma insulin concentrations and selective angiographic techniques are only used where other imaging tests have failed to locate the tumour. For non-malignant tumours surgery is the treatment of choice but if the tumour cannot be located or is malignant then medical therapy may be appropriate (see below).

Hypoglycaemia may also occur as a preterminal feature of advanced malignancy, particularly in patients with extensive hepatic metastases, and also with some very large tumours such as fibrosarcoma. Some tumours secrete substances with insulin-like activity, but this is uncommon. An alternative mechanism for tumours affecting the liver is the loss of hepatic gluconeogenesis.

Reactive hypoglycaemia and post-prandial syndrome

True reactive hypoglycaemia may occur in patients who have had previous gastric surgery or who have gastro-intestinal motility disorders and this may be a manifestation of the 'dumping' syndrome. However, some individuals describe symptoms suggestive of, but not actually due to, hypoglycaemia occurring 1–2 hours after food. This is often investigated inappropriately with an extended oral glucose tolerance test. An oral liquid glucose load often provokes a fall in blood glucose to below 3.0 mmol/l in normal individuals, and in view of the potential arterio-venous glucose difference, misinterpretation of these results may provoke an erroneous diagnosis of reactive hypoglycaemia. The suggested mechanisms for these symptoms include meal-induced hypotension, hyperventilation and altered glycaemic thresholds for neuroglycopenia.

These patients should be evaluated with ambulatory blood glucose measurements or with a standard mixed meal with serial measurements of plasma glucose and insulin and recording of symptoms. Occasionally, asynchronous plasma concentrations of glucose and insulin may be demonstrated but the meal provocation test rarely provokes symptomatic or biochemical hypoglycaemia, in contrast to the extended oral glucose tolerance test which may yield false-positive results and has to be interpreted with caution.

Management

Emergency treatment

The emergency treatment of acute hypoglycaemia should not be withheld to await the establishment of a biochemical diagnosis.

Reversal of hypoglycaemia is most effectively achieved with intravenous glucose given as 30–50 ml of 50% dextrose. Localised thrombophlebitis is a hazard. On regaining consciousness, the patient should be given oral carbohydrate, and a continuous intravenous infusion of dextrose (5% or 10%) may be necessary to prevent recurrence of hypoglycaemia. Intramuscular glucagon (1 mg) may be of value but may be ineffective if hepatic glycogen stores are depleted, as in prolonged starvation, severe inanition, and alcohol-induced or protracted hypoglycaemia.

Long-term treatment

Treatment of the underlying cause of hypoglycaemia will depend principally upon the specific diagnosis. Tumour-induced hypoglycaemia may require prolonged medical therapy if the tumour is not resectable surgically or cannot

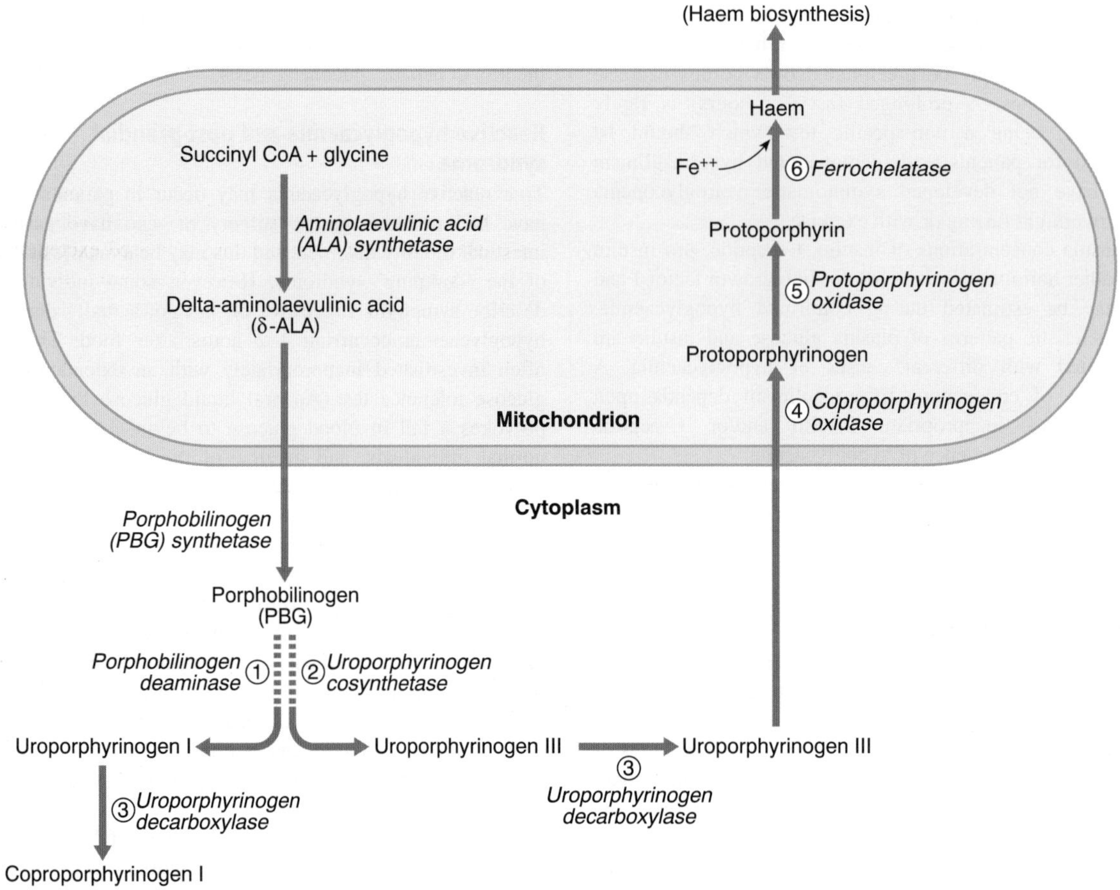

Fig. 7.37 Metabolic pathways for haem synthesis. A block in porphyria metabolism at the following sites results in a particular form of porphyria: (1) PBG deaminase—acute intermittent porphyria; (2) Uroporphyrinogen cosynthetase—congenital (erythropoietic) porphyria; (3) Uroporphyrinogen decarboxylase—porphyria cutanea tarda; (4) Coproporphyrinogen oxidase—hereditary coproporphyria; (5) Protoporphyrinogen oxidase—variegate porphyria; (6) Ferrochelatase—erythropoietic protoporphyria.

be located. Drugs such as diazoxide, combined with chlorothiazide, are beneficial and inhibit insulin secretion. Octreotide (a long-acting synthetic analogue of somatostatin) may be useful in some patients with malignant insulin-secreting tumours. The doses of these drugs have to be determined on the basis of the response. Patients with true reactive hypoglycaemia usually respond to dietary measures with the exclusion of highly refined sugars (such as sucrose) and the use of frequent, regular meals high in fibre content. Acarbose may also be beneficial.

THE PORPHYRIAS

Haem is the ferrous iron complex of protoporphyrin IX which functions as a prosthetic group for the haemoproteins; its biosynthesis occurs in all aerobic cells (see Fig. 7.37). The porphyrias are a heterogeneous group of rare disorders associated with inherited or acquired abnormalities of enzymes involved in the biosynthesis of haem, resulting in overproduction, accumulation and excretion of the intermediate compounds, the porphyrins, and/or the porphyrin precursors—delta-aminolaevulinic acid (ALA) and porphobilinogen (PBG). The enzyme delta-ALA synthase is a rate-limiting step in the rate of production of haem, and an increase in its activity results in overproduction of porphyrins and/or their precursors, ALA and PBG. Porphyrins are categorised as uro-, copro- or protoporphyrins depending on their structure, and both uro- and coproporphyrins can be excreted in the urine. If there is overproduction and excretion of PBG then the urine may turn reddish-brown on standing, and excess PBG can be demonstrated with the use of Ehrlich's aldehyde reagent.

The excess production of porphyrins and their precursors occurs either in the liver (hepatic porphyria) or in the bone

CLASSIFICATION AND PRINCIPAL FEATURES OF THE PORPHYRIAS

Hepatic	Erythropoietic
Acute intermittent porphyria (AIP) • Autosomal dominant • Porphobilinogen synthase abnormality • Precipitated by drugs and alcohol • Abdominal pain, polyneuropathy, hypertension, neuropsychiatric disorders	**Congenital porphyria** • Autosomal recessive • Uroporphyrinogen synthase abnormality • Extreme sensitivity to sunlight (severe scarring) • Dystrophy of nails and teeth, blindness
Variegate porphyria • Autosomal dominant • Protoporphyrinogen oxidase abnormality • Features of AIP and cutaneous porphyria • Bullous eruption with sunlight	**Erythropoietic protoporphyria** • Autosomal dominant • Ferrochelatase abnormality • Cutaneous photosensitivity, hepatic dysfunction
Hereditary coproporphyria • Autosomal dominant • Similar to variegate porphyria • Very rare	
Porphyria cutanea tarda • Autosomal dominant • Hepatic uroporphyrinogen decarboxylase abnormality • Association with alcohol; hepatic tumour	

marrow (erythropoietic porphyria). The classification of the porphyrias is shown in the information box. The hepatic porphyrias present clinically as acute disorders, with the exception of porphyria cutanea tarda. The clinical features of an acute episode, which is frequently precipitated by drugs, hormones or alcohol, are abdominal pain and vomiting, peripheral neuropathy, confusion or psychosis, and tachycardia and hypertension. The acute attacks are all associated with overproduction and increased excretion of the porphyrin precursors ALA and PBG. Overproduction of porphyrins results in cutaneous photosensitivity (see p. 889). Management of acute episodes is mainly supportive, but an adequate carbohydrate intake should be maintained and haematin infusion (haem arginate) should be given in severe attacks.

AMYLOIDOSIS

Amyloidosis is characterised by the extracellular aggregation under deposition of any of a number of proteins that characteristically associates into amyloid fibrils. These deposits have the ability to take up Congo red, a histological stain that is commonly used to demonstrate their nature. All known amyloid deposits also contain glycosaminoglycans and a glycoprotein, serum amyloid P component (SAP), in addition to the major fibril-forming protein.

Formation of amyloid fibrils is favoured by the production

Table 7.30 Types of amyloidosis and proteins causing them

Fibril-forming protein	Normal (N) or abnormal (A) sequence	Location of deposits	Syndrome
Amyloid A protein	N	Kidney, other	Reactive (AA) amyloidosis Amyloidosis of familial Mediterranean fever is identical
Immunoglobulin light chain	N	Kidney, heart, gut, nerves	AL amyloidosis (caused only by certain light chains, $\lambda > \kappa$)
β2-microglobulin (β2-m)	N	Bones, joints, other	Dialysis-associated amyloid β2-m accumulates in renal failure
Prion protein (PrP^{C})	N or A	Brain	Spongiform encephalopathies Although PrP^{Sc} formation is central, amyloid fibril formation is a variable component and may not be critical
Islet amyloid peptide	N	Islets of Langerhans	Type 2 diabetes mellitus (? causative)
Transthyretin	N	Variable	Senile amyloidosis Focal/systemic Rarely severe, usually a histological diagnosis
Transthyretin, apo A1, fibrinogen α, lysozyme, cystatin C	A	Various	Inherited syndromes usually affecting distinct organs according to type Rare
β-amyloid precursor	A	Brain	A-β amyloid: familial Alzheimer's disease
β-amyloid precursor	N	Brain	A-β amyloid: Alzheimer's disease

of some abnormal proteins, or by overproduction or accumulation of certain normal proteins. Abnormal proteins are the usual cause of the rare inherited amyloid syndromes. In prion diseases, the sequence of the protein is normal, but a pathological, alternatively folded protein conformation is 'infectious' in that it can trigger a similar structural change in other molecules. Sequence polymorphisms may increase susceptibility to switching to the abnormal (Pr^{c} to Pr^{sc}) conformation.

Although amyloid is relatively resistant to dissolution by proteases, there may be quite extensive turnover, at least in some types. This means that therapy that reduces the production of the fibril-forming protein may lead to resolution of the disease.

The list of diseases associated with amyloid deposition is now long. In systemic amyloidosis the deposition occurs at multiple locations, although with different favoured sites according to the protein being deposited. Local deposition accounts for other disorders, some of which are listed in Table 7.30. The two major acquired types of systemic amyloidosis are discussed in more detail below. Interestingly, they never involve the brain, although inherited and acquired localised forms of amyloid commonly do.

Primary (AL) amyloidosis

The protein deposited in primary amyloidosis is a normal immunoglobulin light chain (intact or N-terminal fragments of Igκ or Igλ) that is overproduced by an aberrant B-cell clone. Amyloidosis is one of many possible pathological consequences of monoclonal overproduction of an immunoglobulin or immunoglobulin fragment. Amyloidosis commonly occurs without other overt disease ('benign' gammopathy), but it may also occur in myeloma or B-cell lymphoma. Renal disease (nephrotic syndrome, renal impairment) is often the presenting feature. Involvement of the heart (restrictive cardiomyopathy, dysrhythmia), gut (malabsorption, motility disturbance) and tongue (macroglossia) are also common, and there may be peripheral neuropathy and autonomic neuropathy at presentation or later. Progression is usually rapid and relentless, with a median survival of only 1–2 years from the time of diagnosis. There is little to offer other than supportive management, although recently aggressive chemotherapeutic regimens have been advocated for younger patients who are able to tolerate such treatment.

Reactive (AA) amyloidosis

In reactive amyloidosis the protein deposited is a normal serum protein, amyloid A component (AA), an acute-phase reactant that is produced in the liver in response to inflammation. It is an apolipoprotein component of HDL, but its precise function, and why it behaves as an acute-phase protein, are not known. Reactive amyloidosis occurs only in association with long-standing inflammation (usually more than 10 years) in susceptible individuals. The most common causes are chronic arthritis—for example, rheumatoid arthritis and juvenile chronic arthritis—and chronic infections such as leprosy, tuberculosis, bronchiectasis and osteomyelitis. Renal disease (nephrotic syndrome, progressing to renal impairment) is often the first specific feature. Hepatosplenomegaly is usual. The disease is progressive unless the cause can be rectified—for instance, by eradication of the infection or suppression of arthritis. However, involvement of the heart and gut is less common and less severe than in AL amyloid, and the rate of progression and prognosis are dependent on the underlying disease but are generally slower.

Diagnosis of amyloidosis

Amyloidosis is best diagnosed by biopsy of an affected organ. Biopsies of rectal mucosa or abdominal fat may suggest the diagnosis, but can be negative and may be misleadingly positive (for example, many forms of renal disease occur in association with chronic arthritis or infection). The type of amyloidosis can be ascertained by special tests, for example by antibodies to show κ or λ light chains on tissue deposits or in B cells in the bone marrow. In AL amyloid, even if there is no circulating paraprotein, Bence Jones protein (Ig light chains) can usually be detected in the urine. Radioisotope scanning using labelled SAP is available in some centres as an aid to diagnosis and monitoring of treatment of both of the major types of systemic amyloidosis.

FURTHER INFORMATION ON OTHER METABOLIC DISORDERS

Endo A 1992 The discovery and development of HMG CoA reductase inhibitors. Journal of Lipid Research 33: 1569–1582

European Atherosclerosis Society 1994 Guidelines. Atherosclerosis 110: 121–161

Falk R H, Comenzo R L, Skinner M 1997 The systemic amyloidoses. New England Journal of Medicine 337: 898–909

Klag M J, Ford D E, Mead L A et al 1993 Serum cholesterol in young men and subsequent cardiovascular disease. New England Journal of Medicine 328: 313–318

Marks V, Teale J D 1993 Hypoglycaemia in the adult. Baillière's Clinical Endocrinology and Metabolism 7: 705–729

Pyorala K, de Backer G, Graham I et al 1994 Prevention of coronary heart disease in clinical practice. European Heart Journal 15: 1300–1331

Shepherd J 1994 Lipoprotein metabolism. Drugs 47: 1–10

Endocrine disease

8

C.R.W. EDWARDS • A.D. TOFT • B.R. WALKER

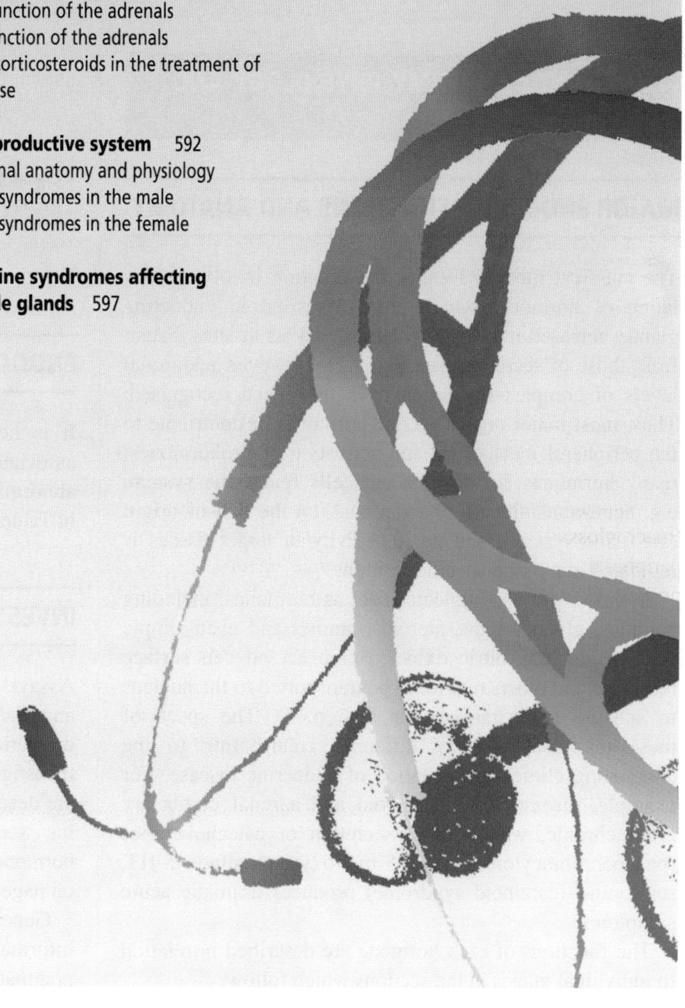

The body has two major control systems which allow specialised tissues to function in an integrated way: the nervous system and the endocrine system. Endocrinology concerns the synthesis, secretion and action of hormones. These are chemical messengers which coordinate the activities of different cells.

There are a large number of diseases of endocrine glands, but World Health Organization statistics indicate that they are a relatively rare cause of death (1–5%). Some endocrine diseases are common, particularly those of the thyroid gland, reproductive system and the β cells of the pancreas (see Ch. 7). For example, thyroid dysfunction occurs in > 10% of the population in areas with iodine deficiency, e.g. the Himalayas, and 4% of women aged 20–30 years in the United Kingdom. However, even rare endocrine syndromes cause important morbidity and present a particular diagnostic challenge to primary care clinicians who may see very few such patients during their working lives.

FUNCTIONAL ANATOMY, PHYSIOLOGY AND INVESTIGATIONS

MAJOR ENDOCRINE FUNCTIONS AND ANATOMY

The classical model of endocrine function involves regulation of hormones which are synthesised in endocrine glands, released into the circulation, and act at sites distant from those of secretion (see Fig. 8.1). However, additional levels of complex regulation have now been recognised. Thus, most major organs secrete hormones or contribute to the peripheral metabolism and activation of prohormones; many hormones act on adjacent cells (paracrine system, e.g. neurotransmitters), or even back on the cell of origin (autocrine system); and the sensitivity of target tissues is regulated in a tissue-specific fashion.

A wide variety of molecules act as hormones, including peptides, glycoproteins, steroids, amines and even simple compounds (e.g. nitric oxide). Some act on cell surface receptors and others require to be transported to the nucleus to activate gene transcription (see p. 5). The speed of these processes is very different, contributing to the contrasting clinical presentation of endocrine disease. For example, diseases of the thyroid and adrenal cortex are often chronic, while excess secretion of catecholamines (phaeochromocytoma) or 5-hydroxytryptamine—5-HT, serotonin—(carcinoid syndrome) produces dramatic acute symptoms.

The functions of each hormone are described in relation to individual glands in the sections which follow.

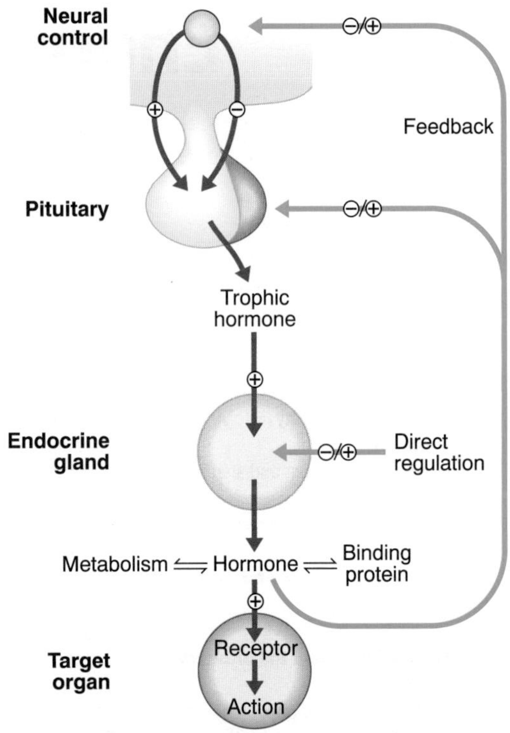

Fig. 8.1 An archetypal endocrine axis. Regulation by negative feedback and direct control is shown along with the equilibrium between active circulating free hormone and bound or metabolised hormone.

ENDOCRINE PATHOLOGY

It is not surprising that such a sophisticated system is associated with a large number of congenital and acquired abnormalities. Most endocrine diseases can be classified as in Table 8.1.

INVESTIGATION OF ENDOCRINE DISEASE

Assays are now available for most circulating hormones, and the resolution of imaging techniques has increased dramatically. As a result, a potentially bewildering array of investigations is available for endocrine disorders. Many are described in relation to individual glands in the following sections. Approximate adult reference values for hormone concentrations in plasma are given in Chapter 20, on page 1136.

General principles of endocrine testing are shown in the information box on page 546. The choice of test is often pragmatic; some tests are intellectually attractive, but

Table 8.1 Classification and examples of endocrine diseases

	Hormone excess	Hormone deficiency	Hormonal hypersensitivity	Hormonal resistance	Non-functioning endocrine tumours
Mechanism	Primary gland overproduction Secondary to excess trophic substance	Primary gland failure Secondary to deficient trophic hormone	Failure of inactivation of hormone Target organ overactivity/ hypersensitivity	Failure of activation of hormone Target organ resistance	
Hypothalamus and posterior pituitary	Syndrome of inappropriate antidiuretic hormone (SIADH)	Cranial diabetes insipidus Isolated releasing hormone deficiencies	Familial acromegaly	Nephrogenic diabetes insipidus	Craniopharyngioma
Anterior pituitary	Prolactinoma Acromegaly Cushing's disease	Hypopituitarism		Laron dwarfism Adrenocorticotrophic hormone (ACTH) receptor deficiency	Adenoma
Adrenal cortex	Conn's syndrome Cushing's syndrome Congenital adrenal hyperplasia Androgen-secreting tumour	Addison's disease Congenital adrenal hyperplasia	11β-hydroxysteroid dehydrogenase deficiency Liddle's syndrome	Glucocorticoid resistance Pseudohypoaldosteronism	Carcinoma (usually functioning)
Adrenal medulla	Phaeochromocytoma				
Ovary	Polycystic ovarian syndrome Granulosa cell tumours	Menopause Autoimmune gonadal failure Turner's syndrome			Cysts Carcinoma
Parathyroid	Hyperparathyroidism	Autoimmune or post-surgical hypo-parathyroidism		Pseudohypoparathyroidism	
Pancreas (endocrine)	Zollinger–Ellison syndrome Insulinoma Glucagonoma	Diabetes mellitus		Insulin resistance syndromes	
Testis	Leydig cell tumour	Klinefelter's syndrome Autoimmune gonadal failure Haemochromatosis		Androgen resistance syndromes 5α-reductase deficiency	
Thyroid	Graves' disease Multinodular goitre Adenoma Subacute thyroiditis	Hashimoto's thyroiditis Atrophic hypothyroidism		Thyroid hormone resistance 5'-monodeiodinase deficiency	Differentiated carcinoma Medullary carcinoma Lymphoma
Others		Osteomalacia		Vitamin D-resistant rickets	

research has shown them to have poor predictive value (e.g. the metyrapone test in Cushing's syndrome); local access to reliable sampling facilities and laboratory measurements is an important consideration.

EXAMPLES OF ENDOCRINE TESTING: PITUITARY FUNCTION

These principles are illustrated in the testing of anterior pituitary function, e.g. in a patient with a pituitary macro-adenoma (see the information box on p. 549). As described in detail in the section on pituitary disease, pituitary tumours are associated with local complications of the tumour, hypersecretion (most commonly of prolactin or growth hormone), and/or hyposecretion (of any pituitary hormone).

Prolactin is not secreted in pulsatile fashion, although it rises with significant mental stress. Assuming that the patient was not distressed by venepuncture, a random measurement of serum prolactin is sufficient to diagnose hyperprolactinaemia. In contrast, growth hormone is secreted in pulsatile fashion. A high random level cannot be interpreted as acromegaly unless the diagnosis is confirmed by failure of growth hormone to be suppressed (by the insulin-induced rise in insulin-like growth factor 1) during an oral glucose tolerance test.

PRINCIPLES OF ENDOCRINE INVESTIGATION
Functional considerations
• Release of many hormones is pulsatile, so random measurement may be invalid and sequential or dynamic tests may be required • Abnormalities are often characterised by loss of normal regulation of hormone secretion
Dynamic biochemical tests
• If hormone deficiency is suspected, choose a stimulation test • If hormone excess is suspected, choose a suppression test • The more tests there are to choose from, the less likely that any single test is infallible, so don't interpret one result in isolation
Imaging
• Secretory cells also take up substrates, which can be labelled • Most endocrine glands have a high prevalence of 'incidentalomas', so don't scan unless the biochemistry confirms endocrine dysfunction or the primary problem is a tumour
Biopsy (rarely indicated)
• Many endocrine tumours are difficult to classify histologically (e.g. adrenal carcinoma and adenoma)

The means of testing for hypopituitarism also depends on the hormone in question. A common test, which is still employed in some centres, involved the simultaneous administration of thyrotrophin-releasing hormone (TRH), gonadotrophin-releasing hormone (GnRH) and insulin (to induce hypoglycaemic stress and stimulate adrenocorticotrophic hormone (ACTH) and growth hormone). However, this is a hazardous procedure and research has shown that assessment of the target glands for most of these hormones provides equally reliable results. Details of each test are given in the sections on individual glands below.

Viewing the pituitary gland by magnetic resonance imaging reveals 'abnormalities' of the pituitary fossa in as many as 10% of middle-aged patients. It should therefore only be performed if there is a clear biochemical abnormality or in a patient who presents with clinical features of pituitary tumour (see p. 547). Functional imaging is rarely used, e.g. with radio-labelled octreotide, a somatostatin analogue.

Surgical biopsy is usually only performed as part of a therapeutic operation. Conventional staining identifies pituitary tumours as either chromophobe, acidophil or basophil. Classically, acidophil tumours are associated with growth hormone or prolactin excess, basophil tumours are associated with ACTH hypersecretion, and chromophobe tumours are non-functioning. However, many chromophobe tumours are associated with hormonal excess. Immunohistochemistry using specific antisera against the pituitary hormones is more valuable in identifying the hormone(s) secreted by specific pituitary cells. It is not possible for histology to predict whether a pituitary tumour will regrow rapidly and invade local structures.

FURTHER INFORMATION ON FUNCTIONAL ANATOMY, PHYSIOLOGY AND INVESTIGATIONS

Trainer P J, Besser G M 1995 The Bart's endocrine protocols. Churchill Livingstone, Edinburgh

MAJOR MANIFESTATIONS OF ENDOCRINE DISEASE

The large number of endocrine diseases present in many different ways. Classical syndromes are described in relation to individual glands in the following sections. In addition, endocrine diseases are often part of the differential diagnosis of common complaints discussed in other chapters of this book, including electrolyte abnormalities (see Ch. 5), hypertension (see Ch. 3), obesity (see Ch. 7) and osteoporosis (see Ch. 12).

THE HYPOTHALAMUS AND THE PITUITARY GLAND

FUNCTIONAL ANATOMY AND PHYSIOLOGY

The pituitary gland is enclosed in the sella turcica and bridged over by a fold of dura mater called the diaphragma sellae, with the sphenoidal air sinuses below and the optic chiasm above. The cavernous sinuses are lateral to the pituitary fossa and contain the 3rd, 4th and 6th cranial nerves and the internal carotid arteries. The gland is composed of two lobes, anterior and posterior, and is connected to the hypothalamus by the infundibular stalk, which has portal vessels carrying blood from the median eminence of the hypothalamus to the anterior lobe and nerve fibres to the posterior lobe (see Fig. 8.2).

The functions of the pituitary hormones are shown in Figure 8.3. Substances produced in the hypothalamus and released into the portal blood either stimulate or inhibit anterior pituitary hormone secretion. These are regulated by

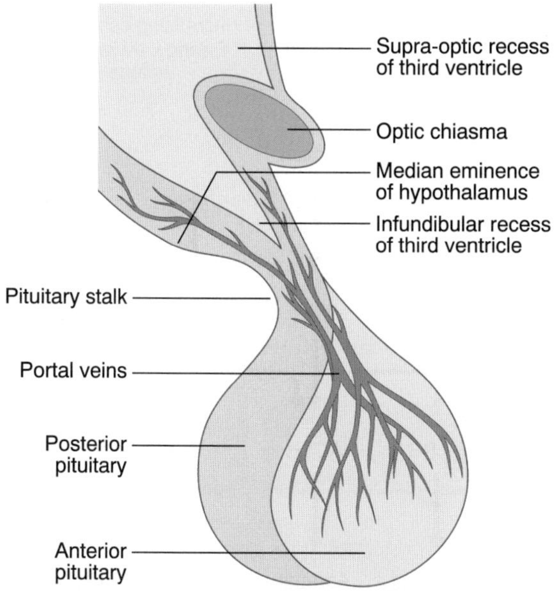

Fig. 8.2 Anatomical relationships of human pituitary.

a wide variety of stimuli of nervous, metabolic, physical or hormonal origin, in particular feedback control by hormones produced by the target glands (thyroid, adrenal cortex and gonads). Some pituitary peptides, especially the ACTH precursor, have several actions in peripheral tissues (see Fig. 8.4). Posterior pituitary hormones are synthesised in the hypothalamus and transported down nerve axons to be released from the posterior pituitary.

CLINICAL SYNDROMES ASSOCIATED WITH HYPOTHALAMIC AND PITUITARY DISEASE

Diseases of the hypothalamus and pituitary are rare and present with a wide variety of clinical features. However, they are treatable conditions, so it is important to consider these diagnoses when patients present by any of the routes listed in the information box.

PITUITARY AND HYPOTHALAMIC TUMOURS

NON-FUNCTIONING PITUITARY TUMOURS

Aetiology

Pituitary tumours are usually benign adenomas. Interpretation of their pathology is described on page 546.

ROUTES OF PRESENTATION OF HYPOTHALAMIC/PITUITARY DISEASE

Local complications from tumours

- Upwards extension
  - Chiasmal compression and visual field defect
  - Compression of pituitary stalk and disconnection hyperprolactinaemia
  - Rarely, hydrocephalus
- Lateral extension: dysfunction of cranial nerves 3, 4 and 6
- Downwards extension: rarely, 'nasal polyps'
- Stretch of dura mater: headache
- Acute infarction/haemorrhage: pituitary apoplexy

Increased hormone secretion

- Classical syndromes
  - Acromegaly
  - Hyperprolactinaemia
  - Cushing's syndrome
  - Rarely, luteinising hormone/follicle-stimulating hormone or thyroid-stimulating hormone secreting tumours

Decreased hormone secretion

- Panhypopituitarism
- Isolated hormone deficiency: short stature
- Hypothalamic syndrome

Incidental finding

- e.g. Skull radiograph or head CT scan performed for another reason

Primary carcinoma of the pituitary gland is rare, but a metastatic tumour from a primary in the breast, lung, kidney or elsewhere may occur in the hypothalamus and reduce pituitary function. Other tumours—for example, pinealoma, ependymoma or meningioma—may be associated with disturbance of the pituitary or hypothalamus. Conditions such as sarcoidosis or syphilis may mimic pituitary tumours.

Clinical features

These vary, depending on the type of lesion in the pituitary gland and the effect of that lesion on surrounding structures. Clinical features which result from secretion of excess hormones are described below. Tumours which do not secrete excess hormones—non-functioning adenomas—present with hypopituitarism or features resulting from local expansion of the tumour. Headache is the most common but least specific symptom. Pituitary tumours only cause features of hypothalamic or posterior pituitary dysfunction if they expand sufficiently to impinge on the hypothalamus, since pressure on the posterior pituitary does not interfere with its function.

Compression of the neural connections between the retina and occipital cortex leads to impaired visual fields. Although the classical visual field abnormalities associated with compression of the optic chiasm are bitemporal

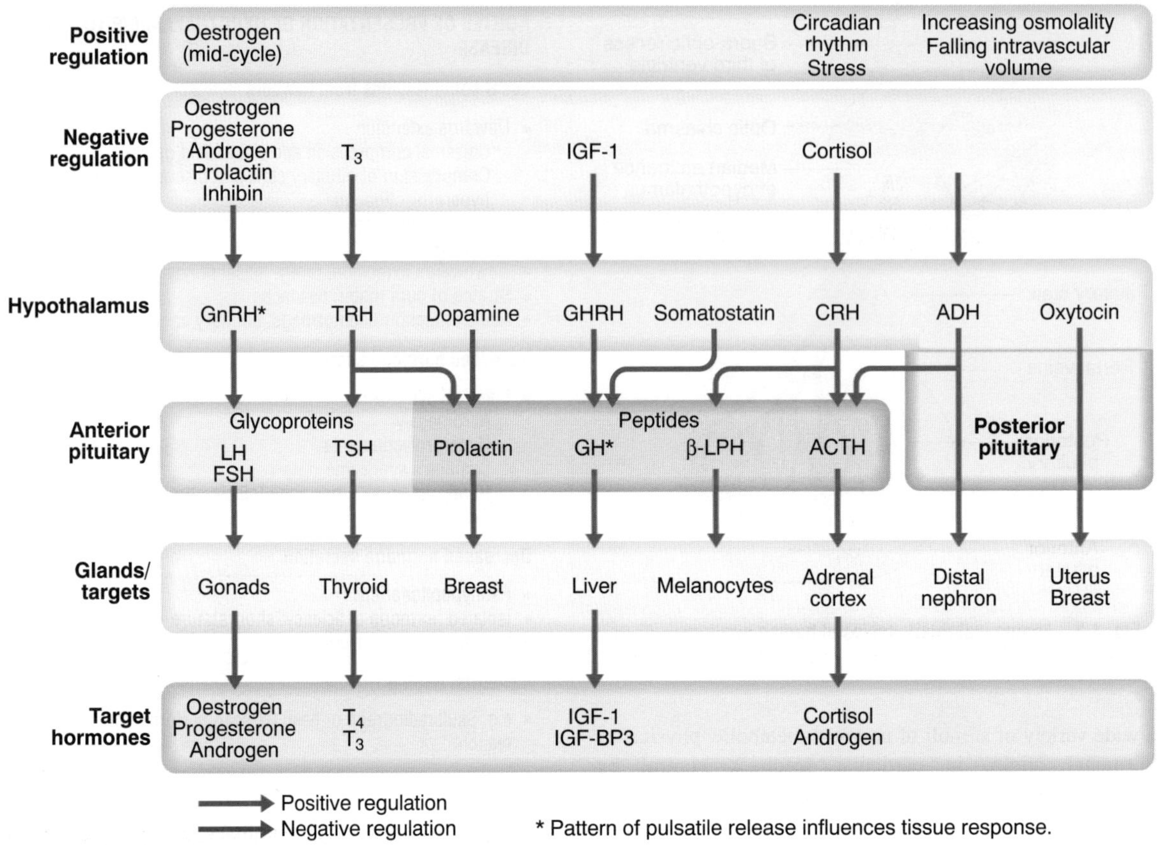

Fig. 8.3 Functional relationships of the pituitary. (CRH = corticotrophin-releasing hormone; ADH = antidiuretic hormone, arginine vasopressin; GnRH = gonadotrophin-releasing hormone; GHRH = growth hormone-releasing hormone; TRH = thyrotrophin-releasing hormone; TSH = thyroid-stimulating hormone; LH = luteinising hormone; FSH = follicle-stimulating hormone; GH = growth hormone; ACTH = adrenocorticotrophic hormone; IGF-1 = insulin-like growth factor 1; IGF-BP3 = IGF-binding protein 3; T_3 = triiodothyronine; T_4 = thyroxine; β-LPH = β-lipotrophic hormone)

hemianopia or upper quadrantanopia, any type of visual field defect may result from suprasellar extension of a pituitary tumour because it may compress the optic nerve (unilateral loss of acuity or scotoma), the optic chiasm, or the optic tract (homonymous hemianopia). Optic atrophy may be apparent on ophthalmoscopy. Diplopia and strabismus may follow pressure on the 3rd, 4th or 6th cranial nerves.

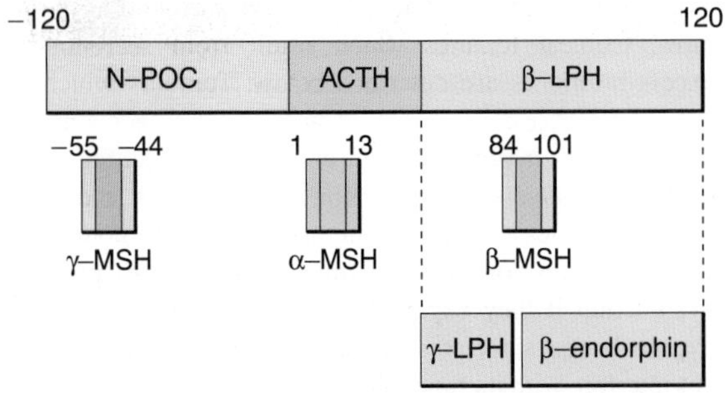

Fig. 8.4 ACTH/LPH precursor, pro-opiocortin (POC). The hatched areas represent the common core melanocyte-stimulating hormone (MSH) sequence within different molecules. β-LPH is further broken down to γ-LPH and β-endorphin.

Although hydrocephalus is described with pituitary tumours, it is important to recognise that they do not behave like 'brain tumours', in that they are usually slowly progressive, and do not cause neurological impairment or raised intracranial pressure. This is an important concept to get across to patients at an early stage.

Investigations

All patients with pituitary tumours should have the tests described in the information box. The imaging technique with the highest resolution is *magnetic resonance imaging* (MRI; see Figs 8.5 and 8.6), which will establish whether

STRATEGY OF INVESTIGATION OF PATIENTS WITH PITUITARY AND HYPOTHALAMIC DISEASE

Identify hypopituitarism

ACTH deficiency
- Short ACTH stimulation test (see p. 555)
- Only if uncertainty in interpretation of short ACTH stimulation test (e.g. acute presentation) then insulin tolerance test

Luteinising hormone (LH)/follicle-stimulating hormone (FSH) deficiency
- In the male, measure random serum testosterone
- In the pre-menopausal female, ask if she has regular menses
- In the post-menopausal female, measure random serum LH and FSH (which would normally be > 30 mU/l)

Thyroid-stimulating hormone (TSH) deficiency
- Measure random serum thyroxine
- Note that TSH is often detectable in pituitary disease, due to inactive isoforms in the blood

Growth hormone deficiency
(Only investigate if growth hormone replacement therapy being contemplated; see p. 556)
- Measure immediately after exercise
- Consider other stimulatory tests (see p. 555)

Cranial diabetes insipidus
(Only investigate if patient complains of polyuria/polydipsia, which may be masked by ACTH or TSH deficiency)
- Exclude other causes with blood glucose, potassium and calcium measurements
- Water deprivation test (see p. 558) or 5% saline infusion test

Identify hormone excess

- Measure random serum prolactin
- Investigate for acromegaly (glucose tolerance test) or Cushing's syndrome (see p. 583) if there are clinical features

Establish the anatomy and diagnosis

- Consider visual field testing
- Image the pituitary and hypothalamus by MRI or CT

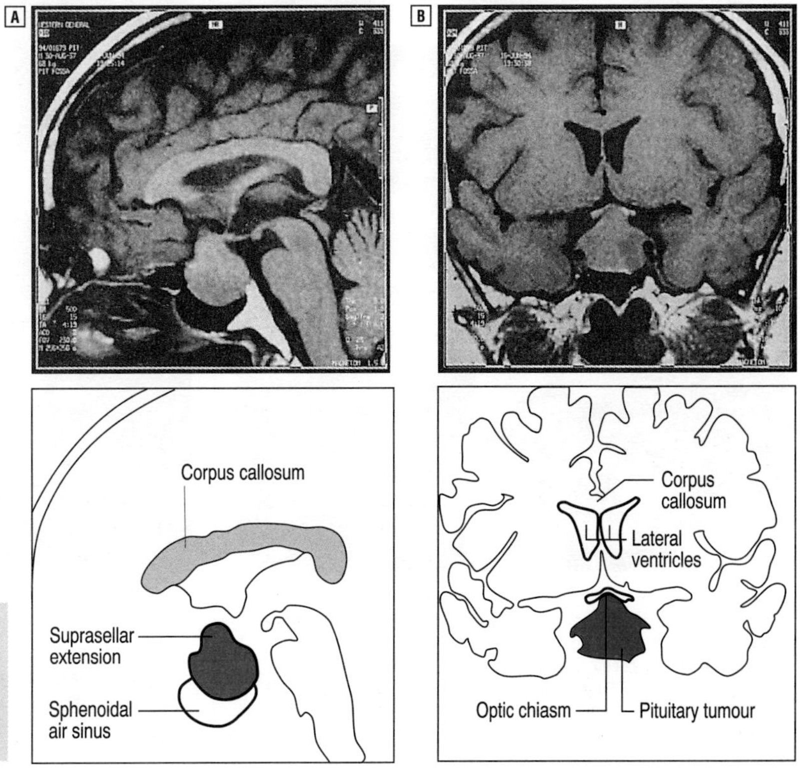

Fig. 8.5 Magnetic resonance image of a pituitary macroadenoma.
[A] Suprasellar extension of large pituitary tumour (lateral view). [B] Coronal view of pituitary tumour showing suprasellar extension and compression of the optic chiasm.

the tumour is a macroadenoma (> 10 mm diameter) or a microadenoma (< 10 mm diameter). If this is not available, computed tomography (CT) is reliable for identifying macroadenomas. The distinction of size of tumour is important mainly because microadenomas are not associated with hypopituitarism or compression of local structures and are only treated if they are secreting excess hormones. Some tumours are diagnosed from incidental abnormalities on a skull radiograph and an example is shown in Figure 8.7.

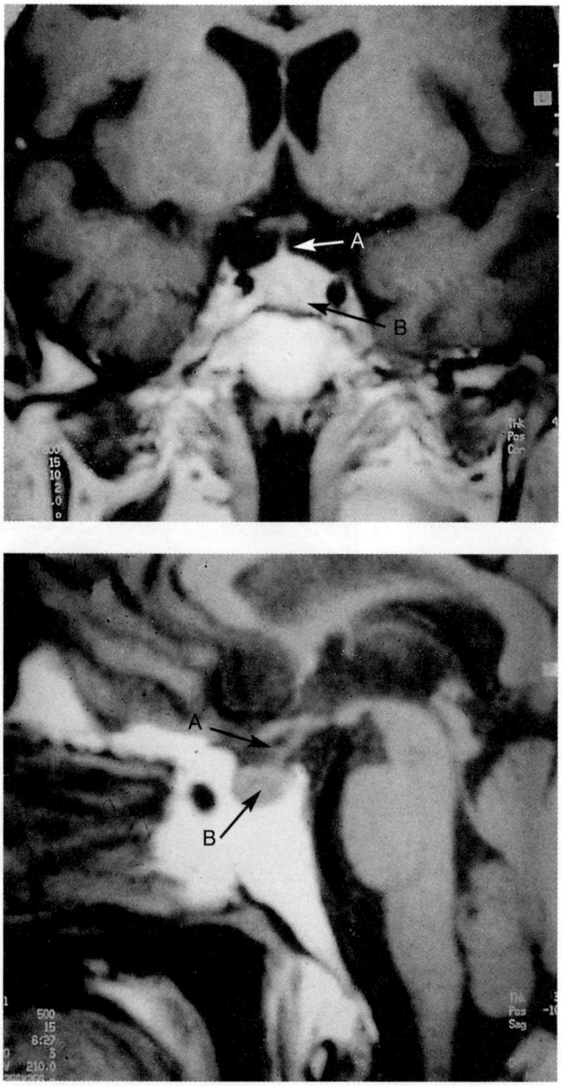

A B

Fig. 8.6 Magnetic resonance images of a left-sided pituitary microadenoma. A Coronal section. B Sagittal section. The left side of the pituitary is bulky and the infundibular stalk (arrow A in both figures) is deviated to the right but the lesion (arrow B in both figures) is poorly defined, < 10 mm in diameter, and does not extend outside the pituitary fossa.

However, a normal skull radiograph does not exclude a pituitary tumour and this investigation is no longer indicated when a tumour is suspected. If the clinical features suggest hormonal hypersecretion then this must be assessed as detailed below.

Management

Modalities of treatment for pituitary tumours are shown in Table 8.2.

If there is evidence of pressure on visual pathways then urgent treatment is required. The chances of recovery of a visual field defect are proportional to the duration of symptoms; recovery is very unlikely if the defect has been present for longer than 4 months. The only medical therapy which shrinks macroadenomas is dopamine agonists for macroprolactinomas (see below). It is crucial that serum

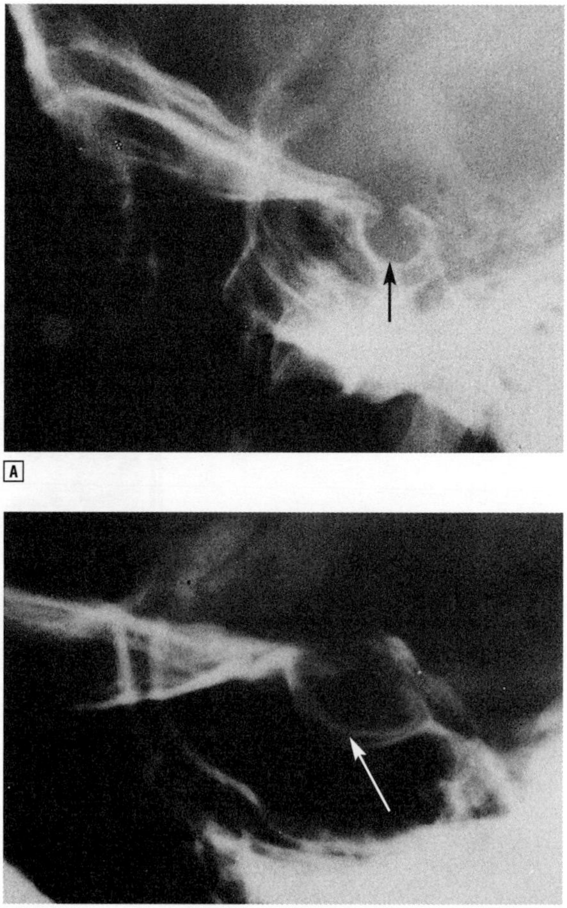

A B

Fig. 8.7 Lateral skull radiographs. A A normal pituitary fossa (arrow). B Expansion of the pituitary fossa causing a 'double-floor' appearance (arrow).

Table 8.2 Therapeutic modalities for hypothalamic and pituitary tumours

	Surgery	Radiotherapy	Medical	Comment
Non-functioning pituitary macroadenoma	++	+	–	
Prolactinoma	+	+	++ Dopamine agonists	Dopamine agonists cause macroadenomas to shrink
Acromegaly	++	+	+ Octreotide + Dopamine agonists	Octreotide does not cause macroadenomas to shrink
Cushing's disease	++	+	–	Radiotherapy is used in children and to prevent Nelson's syndrome
Craniopharyngioma	++	+	–	

++ First-line therapy; + second-line therapy.

prolactin is measured before emergency surgery is performed. If the prolactin is > 4000 mU/l then a therapeutic trial of bromocriptine for just a few days may successfully shrink the tumour and make surgery unnecessary.

Most operations on the pituitary are performed by the trans-sphenoidal approach pioneered by Harvey Cushing. The pituitary fossa is approached from an incision under the upper lip via the sphenoid sinus. Transfrontal surgery via a craniotomy is reserved for very large tumours and craniopharyngiomas because it has higher morbidity. It is uncommon to be able to resect a macroadenoma completely.

Following decompression imaging is repeated after a few months and, if there is any residual tumour, external radiotherapy is given to reduce the risk of recurrence. Radiation therapy is not useful in patients requiring urgent therapy because it takes many months or years to be effective and there is a risk of acute swelling of the tumour. The implantation of yttrium in the pituitary fossa is an alternative form of irradiation used only in certain specialist centres. The same is true for proton beam therapy.

All operations on the pituitary carry a risk of damaging normal endocrine function; this risk increases with the size of the primary tumour. Radiation therapy carries a life-long risk of hypopituitarism (50–70% in the first 10 years) and annual pituitary function tests are required. There is also concern that radiotherapy, which is delivered through the temporal lobes, might impair cognitive function and even induce primary brain tumours, but these side-effects have not been quantified and are likely to be rare.

Non-functioning tumours are followed up by repeated imaging at intervals which depend on the size of the tumour and whether or not radiotherapy has been administered.

CRANIOPHARYNGIOMA

Craniopharyngiomas are benign tumours which develop in cell rests of Rathke's pouch, and may be located within the sella turcica, or commonly in the suprasellar space. They are often cystic and/or calcified. They occur more commonly in young people than do pituitary adenomas. They may present with pressure on adjacent structures, hypopituitarism, or a hypothalamic syndrome, as described below. Craniopharyngiomas can rarely be reached by the trans-sphenoidal route, and surgery involves a craniotomy, with a relatively high risk of hypothalamic damage and other complications. Surgery is unlikely to be curative, and radiotherapy should probably be given, although there is uncertainty about its efficacy. Unfortunately, craniopharyngiomas often recur, requiring repeated surgery and inevitably causing considerable morbidity, usually from hypothalamic obesity and/or visual failure.

SYNDROMES OF PITUITARY HORMONE EXCESS

HYPERPROLACTINAEMIA

Aetiology

Elevation of plasma prolactin levels is a common finding and may arise from a variety of causes which are listed in the information box. Even though the list is long, it is usually possible to reach a presumptive diagnosis by taking a careful history, especially with regard to drug therapy.

Clinical features

Hippocrates was one of the first to observe that milk secretion was associated with decreased gonadal function. The cardinal features of hyperprolactinaemia are galactorrhoea and hypogonadism. In women this causes secondary amenorrhoea, oligomenorrhoea or menorrhagia, and anovulation with infertility. In men there is decreased libido, erectile impotence, reduced shaving frequency and lethargy. Men usually present with symptoms at a later stage than women and are more likely to have a macroadenoma.

CAUSES OF ELEVATED PLASMA PROLACTIN
Physiological
• Stress • Pregnancy • Lactation
Drugs
• Dopamine antagonists Antipsychotics (phenothiazines and butyrophenones) Antidepressants Antiemetics (e.g. metoclopramide, domperidone) • Dopamine-depleting drugs Reserpine Methyldopa • Oestrogens Oral contraceptive pill
Pathological
• Common Disconnection hyperprolactinaemia (e.g. non-functioning pituitary macroadenoma) Prolactinoma (usually microadenoma) Primary hypothyroidism • Uncommon Hypothalamic disease Pituitary tumour secreting prolactin and growth hormone Renal failure • Rare Chest wall reflex (e.g. nipple stimulation) Wet-nursing reflex (e.g. baby crying) Post-herpes zoster Ectopic source

Care should be taken to establish whether galactorrhoea is bilateral. Although unilateral galactorrhoea may be caused by prolactin excess, there should be a high index of suspicion of a breast carcinoma with nipple discharge.

Patients with macroadenomas may also have any of the clinical features of non-functioning pituitary tumours (see p. 547).

Investigations

The upper limit of normal for many assays of serum prolactin is 360 mU/l. During pregnancy and lactation physiological levels may reach 20 000 mU/l. In non-pregnant and non-lactating patients, levels of 360–1000 mU/l are likely to be induced by stress or drugs and a repeat measurement is indicated. Levels between 1000 and 4000 mU/l are likely to be due to drugs, a microprolactinoma, or disconnection hyperprolactinaemia (due to pressure on the infundibular stalk and loss of dopamine inhibition of prolactin secretion). Levels above 4000 mU/l are highly suggestive of a prolactinoma, and the higher the level, the bigger the tumour. Some macroprolactinomas cause levels as high as 100 000 mU/l. Dynamic tests of prolactin secretion, such as a TRH test or assessment of the response to bromocriptine, do not assist in the differential diagnosis.

Patients with prolactin excess should have tests of gonadal function (see p. 549), and thyroxine (T_4) and thyroid-stimulating hormone (TSH) measured to exclude primary hypothyroidism causing TRH-induced prolactin excess. Unless the prolactin falls after withdrawal of relevant drug therapy, a serum prolactin of > 1000 mU/l is an indication for an MRI scan (or a CT scan) of the hypothalamus and pituitary. Patients with macroadenomas also need tests for hypopituitarism (see p. 549). A glucose tolerance test to assess whether there is accompanying growth hormone excess is indicated if there are clinical features of acromegaly.

MRI will detect all macroadenomas and around 70% of microadenomas. In patients with a normal scan and no other cause of prolactin excess, the presumptive diagnosis is a small microadenoma.

Management

Medical

In almost all cases of hyperprolactinaemia dopamine agonist therapy will normalise prolactin levels with return of gonadal function. If gonadal function does not return despite effective lowering of prolactin then there may be associated gonadotrophin deficiency or, in the female, the onset of the menopause. Several dopamine agonists are now available, as shown in Table 8.3.

Dopamine agonist therapy is likely to be long-term in the majority of patients. However, it has been possible to withdraw bromocriptine without recurrence of hyperprolactinaemia after 10 years' treatment in some patients with microadenoma. Also, after the menopause suppression of prolactin is only required in microadenomas if galactorrhoea is troublesome. In patients with macroadenomas drugs can only be withdrawn after curative surgery or radiotherapy and under close supervision.

In general, patients with prolactin excess should avoid drugs which stimulate prolactin, including oestrogens.

Surgical

Dopamine agonists not only lower prolactin levels but shrink the majority of prolactin-secreting macroadenomas. Thus, surgical decompression is not usually necessary unless the macroadenoma is cystic. However, in patients who are intolerant of dopamine agonists, microadenomas can be removed selectively by trans-sphenoidal surgery with a cure rate of about 80%. The cure rate for surgery in macroadenomas is substantially lower.

Radiotherapy

External irradiation may be required for some macroadenomas to prevent regrowth if dopamine agonists are stopped.

Table 8.3 Dopamine agonist therapy: drugs used to treat prolactinomas

	Oral dose*	Advantages	Disadvantages
Bromocriptine	2.5–15 mg/day 8–12-hourly	Available for parenteral use Short half-life: useful in treating infertility Proven long-term efficacy	Ergotamine-like side-effects (nausea, headache, postural hypotension, constipation) Frequent dosing so poor compliance
Cabergoline	250–1000 μg/week 2 doses/week	Long-acting, so missed doses less important Reported to have fewer ergotamine-like side-effects	Unsuitable for treating infertility
Quinagolide	50–150 mg/day Once daily	A non-ergot with few side-effects in patients intolerant of the above	Untested in pregnancy
Pergolide			An older drug with bromocriptine-like side-effects; no longer used

* Tolerance develops for the side-effects. All of these agents, especially bromocriptine, must be introduced at low dose and increased over weeks. If several doses of bromocriptine are missed, the process must start again.

Pregnancy

Hyperprolactinaemia often presents with infertility so dopamine agonist therapy is often followed by pregnancy. Patients with microadenomas are advised to withdraw bromocriptine as soon as pregnancy is confirmed (e.g. by urinary human chorionic gonadotrophin (hCG) test on the third day after a missed period). In contrast, macroprolactinomas may enlarge rapidly under oestrogen stimulation and these patients continue dopamine agonist therapy and need measurement of prolactin levels and visual fields during pregnancy. All patients are advised to report headache or visual disturbance promptly.

ACROMEGALY AND GIGANTISM

Aetiology

Acromegaly is caused by growth hormone (GH) secretion from a pituitary tumour, usually a macroadenoma. Other causes, such as ectopic production of growth hormone-releasing hormone (GHRH; e.g. from a pancreatic tumour), are extremely rare.

GH acts directly on some tissues, but most of its biological effects are accounted for by stimulation of secretion of insulin-like growth factor 1 (IGF-1) and its binding proteins from the liver. IGF-1 circulates in a ternary complex, bound with a protein, IGF-BP3, and an acid-labile subunit. There is a whole family of IGF-binding proteins (numbering 10 at the time of writing) and some act as hormones themselves. They may be important not only in clinical disorders of GH secretion, but also in carcinogenesis and atheroma. This area is a major focus of research and a likely source of future therapeutic strategies.

Clinical features

If GH hypersecretion occurs before epiphyses have fused then gigantism will result. More commonly, GH excess occurs in adult life, after epiphyseal closure, and acromegaly ensues. If hypersecretion starts in adolescence and persists into adult life then the two conditions may be combined. The clinical features are listed in the information box. The most common complaints are headache and sweating.

Patients with macroadenomas may also have any of the clinical features of non-functioning pituitary tumours (see p. 547).

CLINICAL FEATURES OF ACROMEGALY

Soft tissue changes

- Skin thickening
- Increased sweating
- Headache
- Increased sebum production
- Enlargement of lips, nose and tongue
- Increased heel pad thickness
- Arthropathy
- Myopathy
- Carpal tunnel syndrome
- Visceromegaly (e.g. thyroid, heart, liver)

Acral enlargement

- Large hands (difficult to remove rings)
- Large feet (increasing shoe size)

Other bone changes

- Growth of lower jaw—prognathism
- Skull growth—prominent supraorbital ridges with large frontal sinuses
- Kyphosis
- Osteoarthritis

Metabolic effects

- Glucose intolerance (25%)
- Diabetes mellitus (10%)
- Hypertension (25% associated with increased body sodium)

Long-term complications

- Atheromatous disease (two- to three-fold relative risk)
- Colonic cancer (two- to three-fold relative risk)

Investigations

These patients should be investigated in the same way as patients with non-functioning pituitary tumours (see p. 549). In about 30% of patients prolactin levels are elevated. In addition, the clinical diagnosis must be confirmed by measuring GH levels during an oral glucose tolerance test (see Fig. 8.8). In normal subjects plasma GH suppresses to below 2 mU/l. In acromegaly it does not suppress and in about 50% of patients there is a paradoxical rise. IGF-1 levels are also high.

The diagnosis of acromegaly is more difficult in patients with insulin deficiency, either type I or long-standing type II diabetes mellitus. GH may fail to suppress following a glucose load in these patients because inadequate insulin secretion results in failure to stimulate IGF-1 from the liver. It is IGF-1 which in turn suppresses GH secretion. This is important because acromegaly can cause diabetes mellitus by exacerbating insulin resistance. However, in diabetics without acromegaly, IGF-1 levels are low but in acromegalics they are high.

Management

Surgical

Trans-sphenoidal surgery may result in cure of GH excess, especially in patients with microadenomas. More often, surgery serves to debulk the tumour and further therapy is required, according to post-operative imaging and glucose tolerance test results.

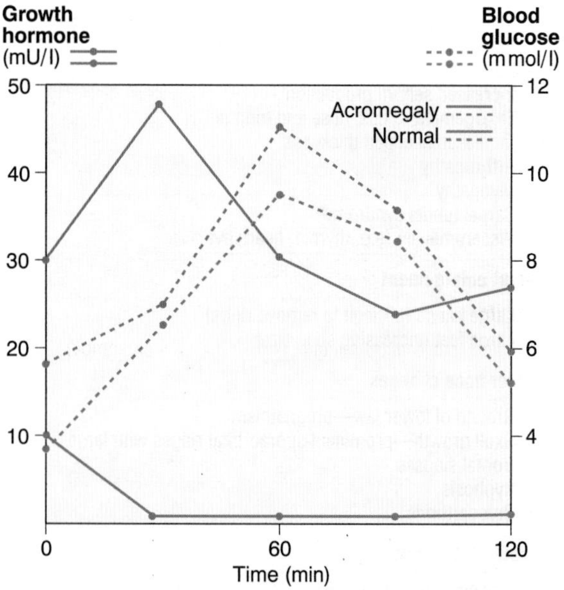

Fig. 8.8 Oral glucose tolerance tests in a normal subject and a patient with acromegaly with measurement of blood glucose and plasma growth hormone. Note the suppression of growth hormone secretion of < 2 mU/l in the normal subject, and failure to suppress (sometimes accompanied by paradoxical elevation) in acromegaly. Glucose tolerance may also be impaired in acromegaly.

Medical

There is debate about whether medical therapy should be employed for all patients with persisting acromegaly after surgery, or only for those with troublesome symptoms or demonstrable complications. Octreotide, a long-acting analogue of somatostatin, lowers GH, usually to < 10 mU/l. Importantly, octreotide does not shrink GH-secreting tumours. It is administered as a subcutaneous injection 2 or 3 times a day, but slow-release preparations for monthly injection have been produced recently. Octreotide inhibits gallbladder motility, so that ultrasound scans to detect gallstones and 'holidays' from the drug to allow emptying of biliary sludge may be important. Dopamine agonists are less potent in lowering GH, but may be helpful, especially in patients with associated prolactin excess.

Radiotherapy

External radiotherapy stops tumour growth and lowers GH levels. However, GH levels fall slowly and there is a risk of hypopituitarism.

CUSHING'S DISEASE

This rare pituitary tumour is dealt with in the section on Cushing's syndrome on page 581.

SYNDROMES OF PITUITARY AND HYPOTHALAMIC HORMONE DEFICIENCY

ANTERIOR PITUITARY HORMONE DEFICIENCY: ADULT HYPOPITUITARISM

Aetiology

The causes of hypopituitarism are shown in Table 8.4.

Clinical features

These depend on the underlying lesion. Congenital defects of the hypothalamus usually present with short stature (see p. 558). With progressive lesions of the pituitary there is a characteristic sequence of loss of pituitary hormone secretion. Growth hormone secretion is often the earliest to be lost. In adults, this produces lethargy, muscle weakness and increased fat mass but these features are not obvious in isolation. Next, luteinising hormone (LH) secretion becomes impaired with, in the male, loss of libido and impotence and, in the female, oligomenorrhoea or amenorrhoea. Later, in the male there may be gynaecomastia

Table 8.4 Causes of hypopituitarism

Site of lesion	Common deficiencies/ causes	Rare deficiencies/ causes
Hypothalamus		
Congenital	GnRH (Kallmann's syndrome) GHRH	TRH Corticotrophin-releasing factor (CRF)
Acquired	Craniopharyngioma Head injury Surgery Radiotherapy	Sarcoidosis Tuberculosis Histiocytosis X 1° or 2° tumour
Pituitary	Pituitary tumour Surgery Radiotherapy Head injury Local meningioma	2° tumour Post-partum necrosis (Sheehan's syndrome) Autoimmune Haemorrhage (apoplexy) Haemochromatosis

Table 8.5 Coma in a patient with hypopituitarism

Possible cause	Measure	Mechanism
Hypoglycaemia	Blood glucose and insulin	Lack of growth hormone and cortisol causing increased sensitivity to insulin
Water intoxication	Plasma Na^+, K^+ and urea—all low	Cortisol and thyroxine required for renal water excretion
Hypothermia	Rectal temperature	Hypothyroidism

and decreased frequency of shaving. In both sexes axillary and pubic hair eventually become sparse or even absent. The skin becomes characteristically finer and wrinkled. Follicle-stimulating hormone (FSH) secretion tends to be lost later than LH.

The next hormone to be lost is usually ACTH, resulting in symptoms of cortisol insufficiency. In contrast to primary adrenal insufficiency (see p. 589), zona glomerulosa function is not lost and hence angiotensin II-induced aldosterone secretion maintains normal plasma potassium. However, there may be postural hypotension and a dilutional hyponatraemia for three reasons:

- failure of vasoconstriction in the absence of cortisol results in pooling of blood in the legs on standing
- antidiuretic hormone (ADH) release is enhanced by hypotension and cortisol deficiency
- cortisol is required for normal water excretion by the kidney.

In contrast to the pigmentation of Addison's disease a striking degree of pallor is usually present, principally because of lack of stimulation of melanocytes by β-lipotrophic hormone (β-LPH) in the skin.

Finally, TSH secretion is lost with consequent secondary hypothyroidism. This contributes further to apathy and cold intolerance. In contrast to primary hypothyroidism frank myxoedema is not seen.

Untreated severe hypopituitarism eventually results in coma (see Table 8.5). This may be precipitated by some mild infection or injury.

Investigations

The strategy of investigation of pituitary disease is described on pages 545 and 549. Specific dynamic tests for diagnosing hormone deficiency are described in the information boxes. Other biochemical tests, such as the GnRH and TRH tests, are only useful in specific unusual circumstances, such as Kallmann's syndrome and in differentiating thyroid hormone resistance syndromes from TSH-secreting tumours, respectively.

Management

Further assessment and treatment of the causes of hypopituitarism are described above. In treating hormonal deficiencies, the aim should be to provide adequate substitution therapy according to the deficiencies demonstrated.

ACTH STIMULATION TEST

Use

- Diagnosis of primary or secondary adrenal insufficiency
- Relies on ACTH-dependent adrenal atrophy in secondary adrenal insufficiency, so may not detect acute ACTH deficiency

Dose

- 250 μg tetracosactrin (synacthen) by intramuscular injection at any time of day

Blood samples

- 0 and 30 minutes for plasma cortisol

Results

- Normal subjects 30-minute plasma cortisol > 550 nmol/l

TESTS OF GROWTH HORMONE SECRETION

GH levels are commonly undetectable, so a choice from the range of stimulation tests is required:

- 1 hour after going to sleep
- Frequent sampling during sleep
- Post-exercise
- Insulin-induced hypoglycaemia
- Clonidine
- Arginine
- Glucagon

Note that in pre-pubertal patients, priming with sex steroid is required before stimulation tests are performed.

INSULIN TOLERANCE TEST
Use
• Assessment of hypothalamic-pituitary-adrenal axis • Assessment of growth hormone deficiency • Indicated when there is doubt from other tests above
Contraindications
• Ischaemic heart disease • Epilepsy • Severe hypopituitarism (0800 hrs plasma cortisol < 180 nmol/l)
Dose
• 0.15 U/kg body weight soluble insulin intravenously
Aim
• To produce adequate hypoglycaemia (signs of neuroglycopenia—tachycardia and sweating—with blood glucose < 2.2 mmol/l)
Blood samples
• 0, 30, 45, 60, 90 and 120 minutes for blood glucose, plasma cortisol and growth hormone
Results
• Normal subjects GH > 20 mU/l • Normal subjects cortisol > 550 nmol/l

Cortisol replacement

Hydrocortisone (another name for cortisol) should be started if there is ACTH deficiency. Suitable doses are described in the section on adrenal disease (see p. 590). Mineralocorticoid replacement is not required.

Thyroid hormone replacement

Thyroxine 0.1–0.15 mg once daily should be given. Unlike primary hypothyroidism, measuring TSH is not helpful in adjusting the replacement dose, because patients with hypopituitarism often secrete glycoproteins which are measured in the TSH assays but are not bioactive. The aim is to maintain serum T_4 in the upper part of the reference range. This is required to ensure adequate levels of triiodothyronine (T_3), the active hormone, in target tissues, since all T_3 in these patients is derived from circulating T_4 and not secreted by the thyroid gland. It is dangerous to give thyroid replacement to patients with adrenal insufficiency without first giving glucocorticoid therapy, since this may precipitate adrenal crisis.

Sex hormone replacement

This is indicated if there is gonadotrophin deficiency to restore normal sexual function and to prevent osteoporosis. *Male* sex hormone replacement is shown in Table 8.6.

In *pre-menopausal females* the treatment is cyclical oestrogen therapy on days 1–21 and progestogen on days 14–21. This is administered most conveniently as an oral contraceptive pill. If oestrogenic side-effects (fluid retention, weight gain, hypertension, thrombosis and family history of breast cancer) are a concern, then a lower-dose oral or transdermal cyclical hormone replacement therapy is appropriate. In *post-menopausal females* the decision whether to give sex hormone replacement therapy is based on the same criteria as in patients without hypopituitarism (see p. 597).

Patients wishing fertility are usually given injections of gonadotrophins several times a week (hCG for LH action and human or equine extracted FSH). If there is a hypothalamic cause for the hypopituitarism then pulsatile GnRH therapy with a portable infusion pump is an alternative. Note that the pituitary GnRH receptors respond to pulsatile stimulation; continuous administration of GnRH or its analogues will suppress rather than stimulate LH/FSH secretion. The duration of gonadotrophin therapy depends on the duration and cause of hypogonadism. In both sexes the treatment requires specialist supervision, especially in females in whom there is a risk of multiple ovulation and the hyperstimulation syndrome, characterised by capillary leak with circulatory shock, pleural effusions and ascites.

Growth hormone replacement

Growth hormone is administered to young patients with growth hormone deficiency, renal failure or Turner's syndrome to assist them to attain their growth potential.

Table 8.6 Options for androgen replacement therapy

Preparation	Dose	Route of administration	Frequency	Comment
Depot testosterone esters	250–500 mg	Intramuscular injection	Every 2–4 weeks	Tends to 'wear off' before next dose is due
Transdermal patches	1–2 patches	To skin	Daily	Consistent circulating testosterone levels but 10% incidence of skin hypersensitivity
Testosterone undecanoate	40–120 mg	Oral	12-hourly	Variable blood levels and risk of liver dysfunction
Testosterone implant	600–800 mg	Subcutaneous	Every 3–6 months	Effective but causes scarring at site of implantation

Until recently, GH was discontinued once the epiphyses had fused and GH was not given to adults. However, although hypopituitary adults receiving 'full' replacement with hydrocortisone, thyroxine and sex steroids are usually much improved by these therapies, they often remain lethargic and unwell compared with a healthy population. Recent studies suggest that they feel better, and have objective improvements in their fat/muscle ratios and other metabolic parameters, if they are also given GH replacement. The principal side-effect is sodium retention, manifest as peripheral oedema or carpal tunnel syndrome. For this reason, GH replacement is started at a low dose (0.125 iu/kg body weight/week divided into daily subcutaneous injections) and increased over a period of 3 months, with monitoring of the response by measurement of serum IGF-1 levels.

HYPOTHALAMIC AND POSTERIOR PITUITARY DEFICIENCY SYNDROMES

Causes of hypothalamic disease are shown in Table 8.4, p. 555. Although commonly associated with anterior pituitary dysfunction, there are clinical features which are directly related to the hypothalamus and which occasionally present in isolation. These include hyperphagia and obesity, disturbance of temperature regulation leading most commonly to hypothermia in temperate climates and hyperthermia in the tropics, and disturbances of water balance.

DIABETES INSIPIDUS

This uncommon disease is characterised by the persistent excretion of excessive quantities of dilute urine, and thirst. Diabetes insipidus can be divided into *cranial diabetes insipidus*, in which there is deficient production of ADH, and *nephrogenic diabetes insipidus*, in which the renal tubules are unresponsive to ADH.

Aetiology

Causes of diabetes insipidus are listed in the information box.

Clinical features

The most marked symptoms are polyuria and polydipsia. The patient may pass 5–20 or more litres of urine in 24 hours. This is of very low specific gravity and osmolality (less than plasma usually). If the patient has an intact thirst mechanism, is conscious and has access to oral fluids, then he or she can maintain adequate fluid intake. However, in the unconscious patient or one with damage to the hypothalamic thirst centre diabetes insipidus is potentially lethal. If there is associated cortisol deficiency then diabetes insipidus may not be manifest until glucocorticoid replacement therapy is given. The differential diagnosis includes diabetes mellitus and primary polydipsia, a condition which is seen most often in patients with established psychiatric disease.

CAUSES OF DIABETES INSIPIDUS

Cranial

- Genetic defect
  - Dominant
  - Recessive (DIDMOAD syndrome—association of diabetes insipidus with diabetes mellitus, optic atrophy and deafness)
- Hypothalamic or high stalk lesion
  - e.g. Craniopharyngioma, head injury, surgery, histiocytosis X, sarcoidosis, pituitary tumour with suprasellar extension, basal meningitis, encephalitis
- Idiopathic

Nephrogenic

- Genetic defect
  - Sex-linked recessive
  - Cystinosis
- Metabolic abnormality
  - Hypokalaemia
  - Hypercalcaemia
- Drug therapy
  - Lithium
  - Demeclocycline
- Poisoning
  - Heavy metals

Investigations

Diabetes insipidus is confirmed if, in the face of elevated plasma osmolality (i.e. > 300 mOsm/kg), either ADH is not measurable in serum or the urine is not maximally concentrated (i.e. is < 660 mOsm/kg). Sometimes, random simultaneous samples of blood and urine will confirm the diagnosis, or refute the diagnosis by demonstrating a urine osmolality > 660 mOsm/kg. More often, a dynamic test is required. Most centres use a water deprivation test, described in the information box. An alternative is to infuse hypertonic saline (5% saline) and measure the threshold and gradient of ADH secretion in response to increasing plasma osmolality. Thirst can also be assessed during these tests on a visual analogue scale. In primary polydipsia the urine may be excessively dilute because of chronic diuresis which 'washes out' the solute gradient across the loop of Henle, but plasma osmolality is low rather than high.

DDAVP (see below) should not be administered to patients with primary polydipsia, since it will prevent excretion of water and risks severe water intoxication if the patient continues to drink fluid to excess.

In nephrogenic diabetes insipidus appropriate further tests include plasma electrolytes, calcium and investigation of the renal tract (see Chs 5 and 6). Anterior pituitary

WATER DEPRIVATION TEST
Use
To establish a diagnosis of diabetes insipidus, and differentiate cranial from nephrogenic causes
Protocol
• No coffee, tea or smoking on the test day • Free fluids until 0730 hrs on the morning of the test, but discourage patients from 'stocking up' with extra fluid in anticipation of fluid deprivation • No fluids from 0730 hrs • Attend at 0830 hrs for body weight, plasma and urine osmolality • Record body weight, urine volume, urine and plasma osmolality and thirst score on a visual analogue scale every 2 hours for up to 8 hours • Stop the test if the patient loses 3% of body weight • If plasma osmolality reaches > 300 mOsm/kg and urine osmolality < 660 mOsm/kg, then administer DDAVP (see text) 2 μg i.m.
Interpretation
• Diabetes insipidus is confirmed by a plasma osmolality > 300 mOsm/kg with a urine osmolality < 660 mOsm/kg • Cranial diabetes insipidus is confirmed if urine osmolality rises to > 660 mOsm/kg after DDAVP • Nephrogenic diabetes insipidus is confirmed if DDAVP does not concentrate the urine

function and suprasellar anatomy should be assessed in patients with cranial diabetes insipidus as indicated on page 549.

Management

Treatment of cranial diabetes insipidus is with des-amino-des-aspartate-arginine vasopressin (desmopressin, DDAVP), an analogue of ADH with a longer half-life. This is usually administered via the mucous membrane of the nose, either as a metered dose spray or using a manual aerosol device. DDAVP is also available as tablets, although bioavailability of peptides after oral administration is very low and rather unpredictable. In sick patients, DDAVP is given by intramuscular injection. The dose of DDAVP required to keep the patient in water balance must be determined by measuring plasma sodium concentrations and/or osmolality. The principal hazard is excessive treatment resulting in water intoxication and hyponatraemia. Inadequate treatment results in thirst and compensatory increase in fluid intake in the conscious patient. The ideal dose prevents nocturia but allows a degree of polyuria from time to time before the next dose (e.g. DDAVP nasal dose 5 μg in the morning and 10 μg at night).

Polyuria in nephrogenic diabetes insipidus is improved by thiazide diuretics (e.g. bendrofluazide 2.5–5 mg/day), amiloride (5–10 mg/day) and non-steroidal anti-inflammatory drugs (e.g. indomethacin 15 mg 8-hourly), although the last of these carries a risk of reducing glomerular filtration rate.

SHORT STATURE

Patients with short stature may present during teenage years, sometimes as a result of parental pressure. In most, failure to grow is associated with delayed puberty, although there are exceptions (see the information box). Although the mechanisms which initiate puberty are not fully understood, and are in part genetic, there is probably a threshold of body weight which acts as a trigger for normal puberty in boys (mean ± 2 SD for stage 1 is 12 ± 2.5 years; for stage 4 is 13.7 ± 2 years) and girls (stage 1 at 11.2 ± 2 years; menarche at 13 ± 1.9 years). Youngsters with delayed puberty are often underweight at presentation and have been small as children. Rarely, failure to progress into puberty is not investigated, so that the long bone epiphyses are not closed by sex steroids and final height is tall rather than short. These individuals have characteristic eunuchoid proportions, with long arms and legs relative to trunk height.

CAUSES OF SHORT STATURE
With delayed puberty
• Constitutional/familial • Systemic illness (e.g. asthma, malabsorption, coeliac disease, cystic fibrosis, renal failure) • Psychological stress • Anorexia nervosa • Excessive physical exercise • Hypogonadism (see the information box on p. 547; also Turner's syndrome in girls) • Other endocrine disease (e.g. Cushing's syndrome, primary hypothyroidism, pseudohypoparathyroidism)
Without delayed puberty
• Isolated growth hormone deficiency • Previous precocious puberty with closure of epiphyses (e.g. congenital adrenal hyperplasia, histiocytosis X, McCune–Albright syndrome) • Prior problem restricting growth now resolved (e.g. intra-uterine growth restriction, congenital heart disease) • Skeletal abnormality (e.g. achondroplasia, mucopolysaccharidoses)

Clinical assessment

Patients with short stature and delayed puberty require a general history and examination. The heights of the parents and older siblings and the age of their pubertal development may support a diagnosis of constitutional pubertal delay. In 95% of normal children final height is within 8.5 cm of the mean parental height. The presence of anosmia suggests possible Kallmann's syndrome due to isolated GnRH deficiency. Previous growth measurements in childhood, which can usually be obtained from the school health records, are useful since growth hormone-deficient children have usually always been small, whereas a change in growth velocity resulting in 'crossing the centiles' is more likely to reflect recent pathology. Patients with growth hormone deficiency are characteristically 'chubby', with increased subcutaneous fat, and so are short but not underweight. Some light axillary and pubic hair may develop because of adrenal androgen production, even though the patient is hypogonadal. Gynaecomastia should be interpreted as on page 593.

Current weight and height and assessment of pubertal development should be charted against centiles for normals (see the information box). The psychological impact of short stature and sexual immaturity on the young patient needs careful consideration since this is the principal determinant of whether specific treatment is appropriate.

ASSESSMENT OF PUBERTAL DEVELOPMENT (MARSHALL AND TANNER)	
Pubic hair	
PH1	No pubic hair
PH2	Sparse growth of straight light hair
PH3	Spreads over pubes; darker, coarser, curlier
PH4	Adult in character but smaller area
PH5	Extends on to thighs and towards umbilicus in men
Male genitalia	
G1	Infantile
G2	Testes < 4 ml
G3	Scrotal enlargement; testes 8–10 ml; lengthening of penis
G4	Testes > 12 ml; glans penis development
G5	Adult genitalia with testes > 15 ml
Breast	
B1	Pre-adolescent; elevation of papilla only
B2	Breast bud; elevation of breast and papilla; increased areolar diameter
B3	Further enlargement and elevation
B4	Projection of areola and papilla above contour of breast
B5	Mature; projection of papilla alone due to recession of areola

Investigations

Before blood sampling, ask the patient to exercise (e.g. by running up and down the stairs or round the car park until breathless) to stimulate growth hormone secretion (normal > 15 mU/l). Measure growth hormone, testosterone (in boys), oestradiol (in girls), LH and FSH, and perform screening tests for systemic illness, including haematology, renal function, liver function and thyroid function. Antigliadin and antimyosin antibodies are a useful screen for coeliac disease. A GnRH test may be helpful both to diagnose hypothalamic GnRH deficiency (usually Kallmann's syndrome) and to predict whether puberty is approaching (children have a predominant rise in FSH, but LH rises towards puberty). A plain radiograph of the wrist should be compared with a set of standard films to obtain a bone age. Bone age is delayed in pubertal delay and hypogonadism and is advanced in other conditions, e.g. following precocious puberty.

Further tests for growth hormone deficiency and primary and secondary hypogonadism are described above. Note that normal growth hormone responses to stimulation in peripubertal children require priming of the pituitary with sex steroids for a few days beforehand, and that growth hormone secretion is impaired by any other systemic illness. The demonstration of hypergonadotrophic hypogonadism should be followed by chromosomal analysis to establish Turner's (45, XO) or Klinefelter's (47, XXY) syndromes.

Management

Treatments of specific endocrine abnormalities are discussed elsewhere. Puberty can be induced in patients with constitutional delay using low doses of oral oestrogen in girls (e.g. ethinyloestradiol 2 μg daily) or testosterone in boys (e.g. depot testosterone ester injections 50 mg i.m. each month). Higher doses carry a risk of early fusion of epiphyses. This therapy should be given in a specialist clinic and progress monitored until endogenous puberty is established and priming therapy can be discontinued, usually in less than a year.

Isolated growth hormone deficiency is treated by daily subcutaneous injection of growth hormone. Growth hormone also has an established role in Turner's syndrome and in chronic renal failure. Its use in short children without a demonstrable endocrine abnormality is controversial; although it accelerates current growth, it does not result in an increase in final height.

Patients who have already gone through puberty and whose epiphyses have fused cannot be induced to grow further.

FURTHER INFORMATION ON THE HYPOTHALAMUS AND THE PITUITARY GLAND

De Boer H, Blok G J, Van Der Veen E A 1995 Clinical aspects of growth hormone deficiency in adults. Endocrine Reviews 16: 63–86

De Groot L J 1995 Endocrinology. W B Saunders, Philadelphia

Grinspoon S K, Biller B M K 1994 Laboratory assessment of adrenal insufficiency. Journal of Clinical Endocrinology and Metabolism 79: 923–931

THE THYROID GLAND

FUNCTIONAL ANATOMY AND PHYSIOLOGY

The thyroid secretes predominantly thyroxine (T_4), and only a small amount of triiodothyronine (T_3); approximately 85% of T_3 is produced by monodeiodination of T_4 in other tissues such as liver, muscle and kidney. T_4 is probably not metabolically active until converted to T_3, and may be regarded as a prohormone. T_3 and T_4 circulate in plasma almost entirely (> 99.9%) bound to transport proteins, mainly thyroxine-binding globulin (TBG). It is the minute fraction of unbound or free hormone which diffuses into tissues and exerts its metabolic action. It is possible to measure the concentration in plasma of total or free T_3 and T_4 but the advantage of the free hormone measurements is that they are not influenced by changes in concentration of binding proteins; in pregnancy, for example, TBG levels are increased and total T_3 and T_4 may be raised but free thyroid hormone levels are normal.

Production of T_3 and T_4 in the thyroid is stimulated by thyrotrophin (thyroid-stimulating hormone, TSH), a glycoprotein released from the thyrotroph cells of the anterior pituitary in response to the hypothalamic tripeptide, thyrotrophin-releasing hormone (TRH) (see p. 548). A circadian rhythm of TSH secretion can be demonstrated with a peak at 0100 hrs and trough at 1100 hrs, but the variation is small and does not influence the timing of blood sampling for assessment of thyroid function.

There is a negative feedback of thyroid hormones on the thyrotrophs such that in hyperthyroidism, when plasma concentrations of T_3 and T_4 are raised, TSH secretion is suppressed, and in hypothyroidism due to disease of the thyroid gland low T_3 and T_4 are associated with high circulating TSH levels. The anterior pituitary is very sensitive to minor changes in thyroid hormone levels within the normal range. Although the reference range for total T_4 is 60–150 nmol/l, a rise or fall of 20 nmol/l in an individual in whom the level is usually 100 nmol/l would on the one hand be associated with undetectable TSH and on the other hand with a raised TSH. The combination of 'normal' T_3 and T_4 and suppressed or raised TSH is known as subclinical hyperthyroidism and subclinical hypothyroidism respectively (see Table 8.7).

Non-thyroidal illness

In ill patients, e.g. in myocardial infarction or pneumonia, not only is there a decreased peripheral conversion of T_4 to T_3 but also alterations in the concentrations of binding proteins and in their affinity for thyroid hormones. In addition TSH levels may be subnormal, as a result of the illness itself or the use of drugs, such as dopamine or corticosteroids; or it may even rise into the hypothyroid range during convalescence. It follows that the biochemical assessment of thyroid function may be difficult in such patients, often dependent upon the type of assay used, and should not be undertaken unless there is strong clinical evidence of thyroid disease requiring urgent treatment.

HYPERTHYROIDISM

Hyperthyroidism is the clinical syndrome which results from exposure of the body tissues to excess circulating levels of free thyroid hormones. It is a common disorder with a prevalence of about 20/1000 females; males are affected five times less frequently.

Aetiology

It is important to identify the cause of hyperthyroidism (see Table 8.8) in order to prescribe appropriate treatment. In over 90% of patients hyperthyroidism is due to Graves' disease, multinodular goitre or an autonomously functioning solitary thyroid nodule (toxic adenoma). Excess pituitary secretion of TSH which may or may not originate from a

Table 8.7 Patterns of thyroid function test results in patients with thyroid disease

Type of disease	T_4	T_3	TSH
Conventional hyperthyroidism (95% of cases)	Raised	Raised	Undetectable
T_3-hyperthyroidism (5% of cases)	Normal[1]	Raised	Undetectable
Subclinical hyperthyroidism	Normal[1]	Normal[1]	Undetectable
Primary hypothyroidism	Low	Not indicated[2]	Raised (usually > 10 mU/l)
Subclinical hypothyroidism	Normal[3]	Not indicated[2]	Raised
Secondary hypothyroidism i.e. pituitary or hypothalamic disease	Low	Not indicated[2]	Undetectable[4]

[1] Usually upper part of reference range.
[2] Measurement of T_3 is not a sensitive indicator of hypothyroidism and should not be requested.
[3] Usually lower part of reference range.
[4] May be normal or even slightly raised due to the production of immunoreactive forms of TSH which have no biological activity.

Table 8.8 Causes of hyperthyroidism and their relative frequencies in a series of 2087 patients presenting to the Royal Infirmary, Edinburgh, in a 10-year period

Cause	Frequency (%)
Graves' disease	76
Multinodular goitre	14
Autonomously functioning solitary thyroid nodule	5
Thyroiditis	
Subacute (de Quervain's)*	3
Post-partum*	0.5
Iodide-induced	
Drugs (e.g. amiodarone)*	1
Radiographic contrast media*	–
Iodine prophylaxis programme*	–
Extra-thyroidal source of thyroid hormone excess	
Factitious hyperthyroidism*	0.2
Struma ovarii*	–
TSH-induced	
Inappropriate TSH secretion by pituitary	0.2
Choriocarcinoma and hydatidiform mole	–
Follicular carcinoma ± metastases	0.1

* These causes of hyperthyroidism are characterised by a negligible radio-iodine uptake test result.

tumour, intrinsic thyroid-stimulating activity of human chorionic gonadotrophin in hydatidiform mole and choriocarcinoma, ovarian teratoma containing thyroid tissue (struma ovarii), and metastatic differentiated carcinoma of the thyroid are extremely rare causes.

Clinical features

Hyperthyroidism usually develops insidiously and most patients have had symptoms for at least 6 months before presentation. Almost every system is affected and the clinical features are listed in the information box. There is great individual variation in the dominant features; for example, the initial presentation may be to a cardiologist on account of palpitations, to a dermatologist because of pruritus, or to a gastrointestinal clinic with diarrhoea. Weight loss in older patients may be associated with anorexia, raising the possibility of carcinoma. Atrial fibrillation, which is seldom seen in young patients unless there is severe long-standing disease, is common in the elderly. In children, medical attention may be sought because of behaviour disorders, deteriorating academic performance or a premature growth spurt.

GRAVES' DISEASE

Graves' disease is distinguished clinically from other forms of hyperthyroidism by the presence of diffuse thyroid enlargement, ophthalmopathy and rarely pretibial myxoedema. It can occur at any age but is unusual before puberty and most commonly affects the 30–50-year-old age group.

CLINICAL FEATURES OF HYPERTHYROIDISM

Goitre

- Diffuse ± bruit[1]
- Nodular

Gastrointestinal

- Weight loss despite normal or increased appetite[2]
- Hyperdefaecation[2]
- Diarrhoea and steatorrhoea
- Anorexia[2]
- Vomiting

Cardiorespiratory

- Palpitations[2], sinus tachycardia, atrial fibrillation[3]
- Increased pulse pressure
- Ankle oedema in absence of cardiac failure
- Angina, cardiomyopathy and cardiac failure[3]
- Dyspnoea on exertion[2]
- Exacerbation of asthma

Neuromuscular

- Nervousness, irritability, emotional lability[2], psychosis
- Tremor
- Hyper-reflexia, ill-sustained clonus
- Muscle weakness, proximal myopathy, bulbar myopathy[3]
- Periodic paralysis (predominantly Chinese)

Dermatological

- Increased sweating[2], pruritus
- Palmar erythema, spider naevi
- Onycholysis
- Alopecia
- Pigmentation, vitiligo[1]
- Digital clubbing[1]
- Pretibial myxoedema[1]

Reproductive

- Amenorrhoea/oligomenorrhoea
- Infertility, spontaneous abortion
- Loss of libido, impotence

Ocular

- Lid retraction, lid lag[1]
- Grittiness[1], excessive lacrimation[2]
- Chemosis[1]
- Exophthalmos[1], corneal ulceration[1]
- Ophthalmoplegia[1], diplopia[1]
- Papilloedema[1], loss of visual acuity[1]

Other

- Heat intolerance[2]
- Fatigue[2], apathy[3]
- Gynaecomastia
- Lymphadenopathy[1]
- Thirst
- Osteoporosis[3]

[1] Features of Graves' disease only.
[2] The most common symptoms of hyperthyroidism, irrespective of its cause.
[3] Features found particularly in elderly patients.

Pathogenesis

Graves' disease is the major immunologically mediated form of hyperthyroidism, the other being post-partum thyroiditis (see p. 566). The hyperthyroidism results from the production of IgG antibodies directed against the TSH-receptors on the thyroid follicular cell which stimulate thyroid hormone production and, in the majority, goitre formation. These antibodies are termed thyroid-stimulating immunoglobulins or TSH-receptor antibodies (TRAb) and can be detected in the serum of most patients with Graves' disease. Why these antibodies are produced is not clear but there are important genetic and environmental considerations.

In Caucasians there is an association of Graves' disease with HLA-B8, DR3 and DR2, and with inability to secrete the water-soluble glycoprotein form of the ABO blood group antigens coded for on chromosomes 6 and 19 respectively. Family studies show that 50% of monozygotic twins are concordant for hyperthyroidism as opposed to 5% of dizygotic twins. The trigger for the development of hyperthyroidism in genetically susceptible individuals may be infection with viruses or bacteria. Certain strains of the gut organisms *Escherichia coli* and *Yersinia enterocolitica* possess cell-membrane TSH-receptors. The production of antibodies to these microbial antigens which might cross-react with the TSH-receptor on the host thyroid follicular cell could result in the development of hyperthyroidism. Stress is usually dismissed as aetiologically unimportant but many experienced endocrinologists are impressed from time to time by the temporal relationship between the onset of hyperthyroidism and a major life event such as the death of a close relative.

The concentration of TRAb in the serum is presumed to fluctuate because of the natural history of Graves' disease (see Fig. 8.9). The ultimate thyroid failure in some patients is thought to result from the presence of yet another immunoglobulin, a blocking antibody against the TSH-receptor, and from tissue destruction by cytotoxic antibodies and cell-mediated immunity.

The pathogenesis of the ophthalmopathy and dermopathy is less well understood. Both are immunologically mediated but TRAb is not implicated. Within the orbit there is proliferation of fibroblasts which secrete hydrophilic glycosaminoglycans. The resulting increased interstitial fluid content, combined with a chronic inflammatory cell infiltrate, causes marked swelling of the extra-ocular muscles (see Fig. 8.10) and a rise in retrobulbar pressure. The eye is displaced forwards (proptosis, exophthalmos) and in more severe cases there is optic nerve compression.

Clinical features

Goitre

The diffusely enlarged gland is usually 2–3 times the normal volume and increased blood flow may be manifest by a thrill or bruit. In some patients, particularly the elderly, no thyroid enlargement is palpable or the gland may be nodular. The largest goitres tend to occur in young men.

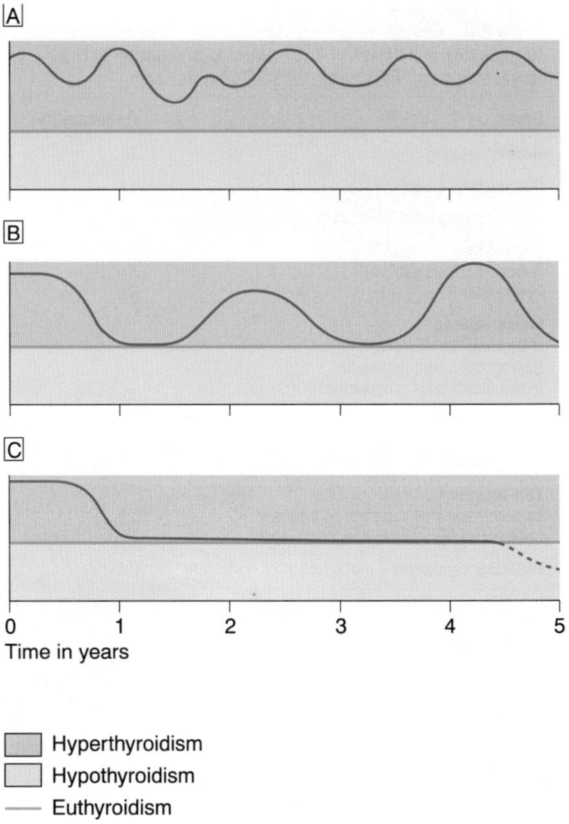

Fig. 8.9 Natural history of the hyperthyroidism of Graves' disease. A and B The majority (60%) of patients have either prolonged periods of hyperthyroidism of fluctuating severity, or periods of alternating relapse and remission. C It is the minority who experience a single short-lived episode followed by prolonged remission and, in some cases, by the eventual onset of hypothyroidism.

Ophthalmopathy

This is only present in 50% of patients when first seen but may also develop after successful treatment of the hyperthyroidism of Graves' disease, or precede its development by many years (exophthalmic Graves' disease). It is more common in cigarette smokers. The most frequent presenting symptoms are related to increased exposure of the cornea resulting from proptosis and lid retraction. There may be excessive lacrimation made worse by wind and bright light, and pain may be due to conjunctivitis or corneal ulceration. In addition there may be loss of visual acuity and/or visual field resulting from corneal oedema or optic nerve compression. If the extra-ocular

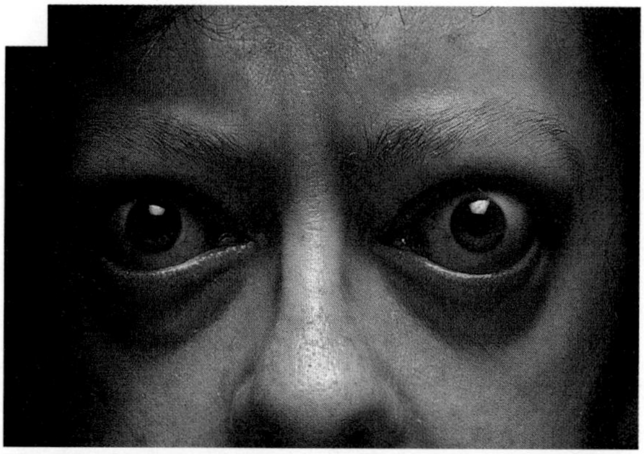

A

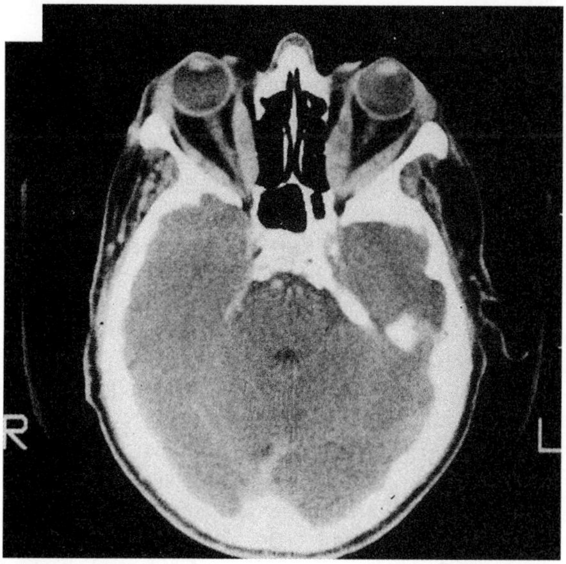

B

Fig. 8.10 Graves' disease. A Bilateral ophthalmopathy in a 42-year-old man, developing 2 years after successful treatment of hyperthyroidism with ^{131}I. The main symptoms were those of diplopia in all directions of gaze and reduced visual acuity in the left eye. The periorbital swelling is due to retrobulbar fat prolapsing into the eyelids, and increased interstitial fluid as a result of raised intra-orbital pressure. B Transverse CT scan of the orbits of the same patient, showing the extra-ocular muscles enlarged to three times their normal bulk. This is most obvious at the apex of the left orbit, causing compression of the optic nerve and reduced visual acuity.

muscles are involved and do not act in concert, diplopia will result.

Pretibial myxoedema

This infiltrative dermopathy takes the form of raised pink-coloured or purplish plaques on the anterior aspect of the leg, extending on to the dorsum of the foot. The lesions may be itchy and the skin may have a *peau d'orange* appearance with growth of coarse hair; less commonly, the face and arms may be affected.

Investigations

A clinical diagnosis can usually be made but, in view of the likely need for prolonged medical treatment or destructive therapy, it is essential to confirm the diagnosis biochemically by more than one test of thyroid function. Serum T_3 and T_4 concentrations are elevated in the majority, but T_4 is in the upper part of the normal range and T_3 is raised (T_3-thyrotoxicosis) in 5% of patients, particularly those with recurrent hyperthyroidism following surgery or a course of antithyroid drugs. TSH is less than 0.1 mU/l. Measurement of ^{131}I uptake by the thyroid and TRAb may be of value in diagnosing Graves' disease if exophthalmos, goitre and pretibial myxoedema are not present (see Fig. 8.11, p. 566). Other non-specific abnormalities are given in the information box.

NON-SPECIFIC BIOCHEMICAL ABNORMALITIES IN HYPERTHYROIDISM

Hepatic dysfunction
- Slightly raised concentrations of bilirubin, alanine aminotransferase and γ-glutamyl transferase; elevated alkaline phosphatase derived from bone and liver

Mild hypercalcaemia (5%)

Glycosuria
- Associated diabetes mellitus
- 'Lag storage' (see p. 480)

Management of hyperthyroidism of Graves' disease

Table 8.9 compares the different treatments. If it were possible to predict with confidence the natural history of the hyperthyroidism in an individual patient at presentation, it would be appropriate to give an antithyroid drug for 12–18 months to those in whom a single episode was anticipated and to advise destructive therapy with ^{131}I or surgery for those likely to experience recurrent disease. With the exception of young men with large goitres and those with severe hyperthyroidism, such a prediction is not possible. For patients under 40 years of age many centres adopt the empirical approach of prescribing a course of carbimazole and recommending surgery if relapse occurs. Although there is no evidence that thyroid carcinoma or leukaemia is induced by therapeutic ^{131}I, or that its use results in an increased frequency of congenital malformation among subsequent offspring, radioactive iodine treatment is usually reserved in the UK for patients over the age of 40.

Table 8.9 Comparison of the different treatments for the hyperthyroidism of Graves' disease

Management	Indications	Contraindications	Disadvantages/complications
Antithyroid drugs e.g. carbimazole	First episode in patients < 40 yrs	Hypersensitivity Breastfeeding (propylthiouracil suitable)	> 50% relapse rate usually within 2 years of stopping drug
Subtotal thyroidectomy	1. Recurrent hyperthyroidism after course of antithyroid drugs in patients < 40 yrs 2. Initial treatment in males with large goitres and in those with severe hyperthyroidism, i.e. total T_3 > 9.0 nmol/l 3. Poor drug compliance	Previous thyroid surgery Dependence upon voice, e.g. opera singer, lecturer[1]	Transient hypocalcaemia (10%) Hypoparathyroidism (1%) Recurrent laryngeal nerve palsy[1] (1%)
Radio-iodine	1. Patients > 40 yrs[2] 2. Recurrence following surgery irrespective of age 3. Other serious illness, e.g. multiple sclerosis irrespective of age	Pregnancy or planned pregnancy within 6 months of treatment	Hypothyroidism, approx. 40% in 1st year, 80% after 15 years Most likely treatment to result in exacerbation of exophthalmos

[1] It is not only vocal cord palsy which alters the voice following thyroid surgery; the superior laryngeal nerves are frequently transected and result in minor changes in voice quality.
[2] In certain parts of the world, ^{131}I is used more liberally and prescribed for young women in the 20–40 age group.

Antithyroid drugs

The most commonly used are carbimazole and its active metabolite, methimazole (not available in the UK). Propylthiouracil is equally effective but the dose is 10 times that of carbimazole. These drugs reduce the synthesis of new thyroid hormones by inhibiting the iodination of tyrosine. Carbimazole also has an immunosuppressive action, leading to a reduction in serum TRAb concentrations, but this is not enough to influence the natural history of the hyperthyroidism significantly.

CARBIMAZOLE

Dosage
- 0–3 weeks: 40–60 mg daily in divided doses
- 4–8 weeks: 20–40 mg daily in divided doses
- Maintenance: 5–20 mg daily

Duration of treatment
- 18–24 months

Adverse effects
- Rash (2%)
- Agranulocytosis (0.2%)

There is subjective improvement within 10–14 days of starting carbimazole and the patient is usually clinically and biochemically euthyroid at 3–4 weeks. The maintenance dose is determined by measurement of T_4 and TSH, attempting to keep both hormones within their respective reference ranges. In most patients it can be taken as a single daily dose and is continued for 18–24 months in the hope that during this period permanent remission will occur. Unfortunately, hyperthyroidism recurs in at least 50%, usually within 2 years of stopping treatment. Rarely, despite good drug compliance, T_4 and TSH levels fluctuate between those of hyperthyroidism and hypothyroidism at successive review appointments, presumably due to rapidly changing concentrations of TRAb. In such patients satisfactory control can be achieved by blocking thyroid hormone synthesis with carbimazole 10 mg 8-hourly and adding T_4 150 mg daily as replacement therapy.

The adverse effects of the antithyroid drugs develop within 7–28 days of starting treatment. Agranulocytosis cannot be predicted by routine measurement of white blood cell count, and is fortunately reversible. Patients should be warned to stop the drug and contact their medical attendant immediately should a severe sore throat develop. Cross-sensitivity between the antithyroid drugs is unusual and another member of the group can be substituted with good effect.

Subtotal thyroidectomy

Patients must be rendered euthyroid before operation. The antithyroid drug is stopped 2 weeks before surgery and replaced by potassium iodate 170 mg daily orally. This maintains euthyroidism in the short term by inhibiting thyroid hormone release and reduces the size and vascularity of the gland, making surgery technically easier. Complications of surgery are rare (see Table 8.9). One year after surgery 80% of patients are euthyroid, 15% permanently hypothyroid and 5% remain thyrotoxic. Thyroid failure within 6 months of operation may be temporary. Long-term follow-up of patients treated surgically is necessary, as the late development of hypothyroidism and recurrence of thyrotoxicosis are well recognised.

Radioactive iodine

^{131}I acts either by destroying functioning thyroid cells or by inhibiting their ability to replicate. The variable radiosensitivity of the gland means that the choice of dose is empirical. In most centres 185–370 MBq (5–10 mCi) is given orally, the dose depending upon clinical assessment of goitre size. This regimen is effective in 75% of patients within 4–12 weeks. During the lag period symptoms can be controlled by β-blocker or, in more severe cases, by carbimazole starting 48 hours after radio-iodine administration. If hyperthyroidism persists at 12 weeks a further dose of ^{131}I should be employed. The disadvantage of ^{131}I treatment is that the majority of patients eventually develop hypothyroidism and long-term follow-up is therefore necessary.

β-adrenoceptor antagonists

A non-selective β-adrenoceptor antagonist, such as propranolol (160 mg daily in divided doses) or nadolol (40–80 mg once daily), will alleviate but not abolish symptoms of hyperthyroidism within 24–48 hours. β-adrenoceptor antagonists cannot be recommended for long-term treatment, but they are extremely useful in the short term, e.g. patients awaiting hospital consultation or following ^{131}I therapy. Propranolol alone or in combination with iodine has been used in the preparation of patients for subtotal thyroidectomy, but this treatment cannot be recommended as standard practice.

Management of ophthalmopathy

The majority of patients require no treatment other than reassurance. Lid retraction will usually resolve when the patient becomes euthyroid, and exophthalmos usually lessens gradually over a period of 2–3 years. For those with symptomatic ophthalmopathy, methylcellulose eyedrops will counter the gritty discomfort of dry eyes, and tinted glasses or side shields attached to spectacle frames will reduce the excessive lacrimation triggered by sun or wind. Corneal ulceration is an indication for lateral tarsorrhaphy or a lid-lengthening procedure. Persistent diplopia can be corrected by extra-ocular muscle surgery but this should be delayed until the degree of diplopia is stable.

Papilloedema, loss of visual acuity or visual field defect requires urgent treatment with prednisolone 60 mg daily if blindness is to be prevented. Close cooperation between endocrinologist and ophthalmologist is necessary and, if significant improvement is not evident within 7–10 days, orbital decompression is indicated.

Management of dermopathy

The pretibial myxoedema of Graves' disease rarely requires to be treated. Local injections of triamcinolone or the application of betamethasone ointment under occlusive dressings may be effective.

TOXIC MULTINODULAR GOITRE

Like Graves' disease, this form of hyperthyroidism is more common in women. The mean age of presentation is 60 years. Thyroid hormone levels are usually only slightly elevated but, as an older age group is affected, cardiovascular features such as atrial fibrillation or cardiac failure tend to predominate. Treatment is usually with a large dose of ^{131}I (555–1850 MBq, 15–50 mCi), as the gland is relatively resistant to radiation. Hypothyroidism is less common than after treatment of Graves' disease. If there is significant tracheal compression or retrosternal extension of the goitre, partial thyroidectomy is indicated. Long-term treatment with antithyroid drugs is not appropriate as relapse is invariable after drug withdrawal.

TOXIC ADENOMA

The presence of a toxic solitary nodule is the cause of less than 5% of all cases of hyperthyroidism. The nodule is a follicular adenoma which autonomously secretes excess thyroid hormones and inhibits endogenous TSH secretion with subsequent atrophy of the rest of the thyroid gland. The adenoma is usually greater than 3 cm in diameter. In some cases spontaneous resolution of hyperthyroidism has occurred as a result of infarction of the adenoma.

Most patients are female and over 40 years of age. Although most nodules are palpable, the diagnosis can be made with certainty only by isotope scanning (see Fig. 8.11). The hyperthyroidism is usually mild and in almost 50% of patients the plasma T_3 alone is elevated (T_3-thyrotoxicosis). Treatment is by hemithyroidectomy or by ^{131}I (555–1110 MBq, 15–30 mCi). Permanent hypothyroidism does not occur following surgery and is unusual after treatment with ^{131}I, since the atrophic cells surrounding the nodule will have received little or no irradiation.

HYPERTHYROIDISM ASSOCIATED WITH A LOW IODINE UPTAKE

In patients with hyperthyroidism, the thyroid uptake of ^{131}I is usually high but a low or negligible uptake of iodine occurs in some rarer causes. If the radioactive iodine uptake test is not routinely performed in patients with thyrotoxicosis who do not have obvious Graves' disease or nodular goitre, the correct diagnosis may not be made and inappropriate treatment may be given.

Subacute (de Quervain's) thyroiditis

Subacute thyroiditis is a virus-induced (Coxsackie, mumps or adenovirus) inflammation of the thyroid gland which results in release of colloid and its constituents into the circulation.

This form of hyperthyroidism is characterised by pain in the region of the thyroid gland which may radiate to the angle of jaw and the ears and is made worse by swallowing, coughing and movement of the neck. The

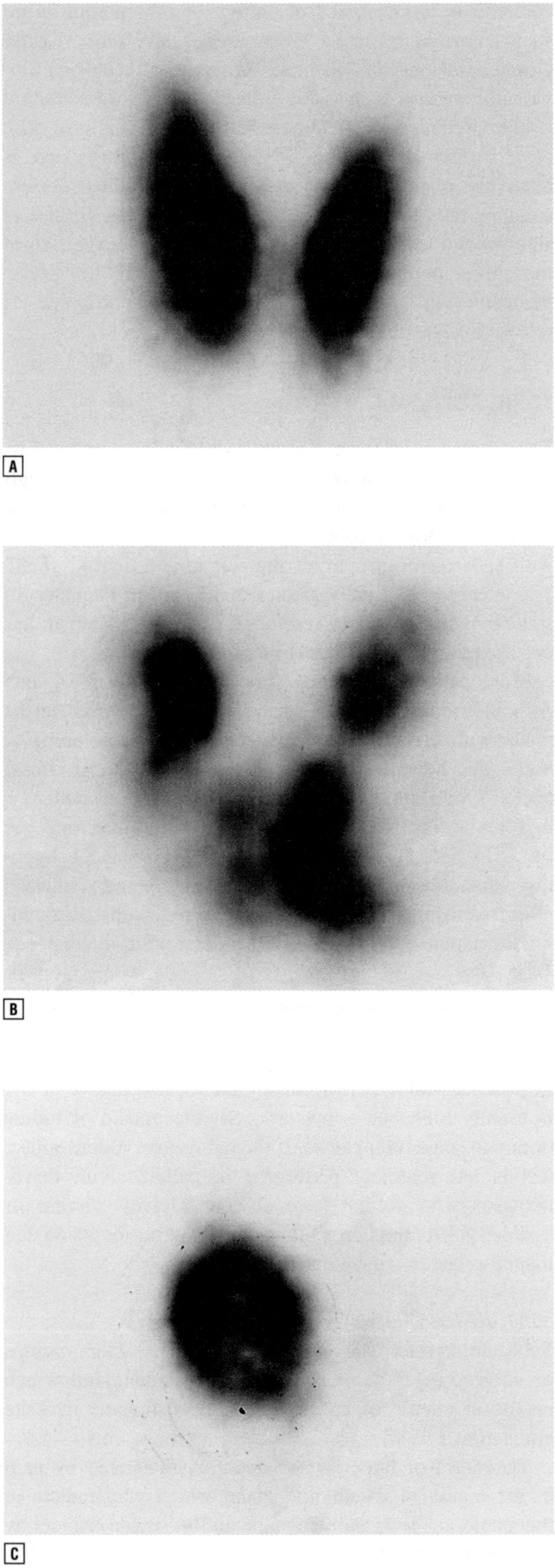

A

B

C

thyroid is usually palpably enlarged and tender. Systemic upset is common. Affected patients are usually females aged 20–40 years.

Thyroid hormone levels are raised for 4–6 weeks until the preformed colloid is depleted. The iodine uptake is low because the damaged follicular cells are unable to trap iodine and because endogenous TSH secretion is suppressed. Low-titre thyroid autoantibodies appear transiently in the serum, and the ESR is usually raised. The hyperthyroidism is followed by a period of hypothyroidism which is usually asymptomatic, and finally by full recovery of thyroid function within 4–6 months. The pain and systemic upset usually respond to simple measures such as aspirin or other non-steroidal anti-inflammatory drugs. Occasionally, however, it may be necessary to prescribe prednisolone 40 mg daily for 3–4 weeks. The hyperthyroidism is mild and treatment with propranolol 160 mg daily is usually adequate. Antithyroid drugs are of no benefit.

Post-partum thyroiditis

The maternal immune response which is modified during pregnancy to allow survival of the fetal homograft is enhanced after delivery and may unmask previously unrecognised subclinical autoimmune thyroid disease. Surveys have shown that transient biochemical disturbances of thyroid function, i.e. hyperthyroidism, hypothyroidism, and hyperthyroidism followed by hypothyroidism, lasting a few weeks occur in 5–10% of women within 6 months of delivery. Those affected are likely to possess antithyroid peroxidase (microsomal) antibodies in the serum in early pregnancy. Thyroid biopsy shows a lymphocytic thyroiditis. Symptoms of thyroid dysfunction are rare and there is no association between postnatal depression and abnormal thyroid function tests. However, symptomatic hyperthyroidism presenting for the first time within 6 months of childbirth is unlikely to be due to Graves' disease, and the diagnosis of post-partum thyroiditis can be confirmed by a negligible radio-iodine uptake.

If treatment of the hyperthyroid phase is necessary, a β-adrenoceptor antagonist should be prescribed and not an antithyroid drug. Post-partum thyroiditis tends to recur after subsequent pregnancies and eventually patients progress over a period of years to permanent hypothyroidism.

Fig. 8.11 ^{99m}-Technetium scans of patients with hyperthyroidism. A Graves' disease, showing diffuse uptake of isotope. B Multinodular goitre with maximum activity confined to individual nodules; such an appearance is not always associated with a palpable thyroid. C Right-sided toxic adenoma with lack of uptake of isotope by normal dormant gland due to suppression of serum TSH. Isotope thyroid scanning is no longer a routine investigation but may be of value in determining the cause of hyperthyroidism in patients with no palpable goitre or other indicators such as exophthalmos or pretibial myxoedema.

A similar painless form of thyroiditis, unrelated to pregnancy, has been increasingly recognised in North America and Japan, and accounts in these countries for up to 20% of all cases of hyperthyroidism.

Iodine-induced hyperthyroidism

The administration of iodine, either in prophylactic iodinisation programmes in iodine-deficient parts of the world or as a radiographic contrast medium, may result in the development of hyperthyroidism which is usually mild and self-limiting. Affected individuals are thought to have underlying thyroid autonomy, such as nodular goitre or Graves' disease in remission. This form of hyperthyroidism is now most often seen as a result of treatment with the anti-arrhythmic agent, amiodarone, which contains significant amounts of iodine. In some patients amiodarone causes a thyroiditis-like picture and mild transient hyperthyroidism, but in those with thyroid autonomy severe thyrotoxicosis may be precipitated and may even present for the first time up to 6 months after the drug has been stopped due to its slow release from adipose tissue. Treatment is with an antithyroid drug for as long as amiodarone is prescribed.

Assessment of thyroid function may be difficult in patients taking amiodarone, as the drug inhibits the peripheral conversion of T_4 to T_3. As a result, in euthyroid individuals it is not uncommon to record markedly elevated serum T_4 concentrations and even suppressed serum TSH, but serum T_3 is usually in the lower part of the normal range. In those developing hyperthyroidism, serum T_3 is clearly elevated but, if the value is equivocal, the decision to treat will depend upon the presence of other features of thyroid disease, such as goitre and ophthalmopathy.

Factitious hyperthyroidism

This uncommon condition occurs when someone takes excessive amounts of a thyroid hormone preparation, most often thyroxine. The exogenous T_4 suppresses pituitary TSH secretion and hence iodine uptake, serum thyroglobulin and release of endogenous thyroid hormones. As a result the T_4:T_3 ratio (approximately 30:1 in conventional hyperthyroidism) is increased to approximately 70:1 because circulating T_3 in factitious thyrotoxicosis is derived exclusively from the peripheral monodeiodination of T_4. The combination of negligible iodine uptake, high T_4:T_3 ratio and a low or undetectable thyroglobulin is diagnostic and has made what was often a difficult diagnosis much simpler.

SPECIAL PROBLEMS

Hyperthyroidism in pregnancy

The coexistence of pregnancy and hyperthyroidism is unusual as anovulatory cycles are common in thyrotoxic patients and autoimmune disease tends to remit during pregnancy. The hyperthyroidism is almost always caused by Graves' disease.

The hyperthyroidism is treated with carbimazole, which crosses the placenta and also treats the fetus, whose thyroid gland is exposed to the action of maternal TRAb. It is important to use the smallest dose of carbimazole (optimally less than 15 mg per day) which will maintain maternal (and presumably fetal) free hormones and TSH within their respective normal ranges in order to avoid fetal hypothyroidism and goitre.

The patient should therefore be reviewed every 4 weeks and it is a wise precaution to discontinue carbimazole 4 weeks before the expected date of delivery to avoid any possibility of fetal hypothyroidism at the time of maximum brain development. If the assay is available measurement of TRAb in the maternal serum at this stage is valuable; a high titre identifies those fetuses at particular risk of developing neonatal hyperthyroidism.

If maternal hyperthyroidism occurs after delivery and the patient wishes to continue breastfeeding, propylthiouracil (see p. 564) is the drug of choice as it is excreted in the milk to a much lesser extent than carbimazole.

If subtotal thyroidectomy is necessary because of poor drug compliance or hypersensitivity, it is most safely performed in the middle trimester. Radioactive iodine is absolutely contraindicated as it invariably induces fetal hypothyroidism.

Hyperthyroidism in childhood

Graves' disease is almost invariably the cause of thyrotoxicosis in childhood and usually presents in the second decade. Treatment should be with carbimazole until the patient is about 18 years of age in an attempt to guarantee the important stages in the physical and educational development of the child.

Atrial fibrillation

Hyperthyroidism is a major cause of atrial fibrillation. Characteristically, the ventricular rate is little influenced by digoxin but responds to the addition of a β-adrenoceptor antagonist. The dysrhythmia is present in about 10% of all patients with thyrotoxicosis but the incidence increases with age so that almost half of all males over the age of 60 are affected (see Fig. 8.12). It is increasingly recognised that subclinical hyperthyroidism may be a risk factor for atrial fibrillation. Cardioversion will establish stable sinus rhythm in up to 50% of patients but should not be contemplated until serum thyroid hormone and TSH concentrations have been restored to normal. Anticoagulation is indicated: aspirin in the elderly but warfarin in younger patients and in those with cardiomegaly or thrombus in the atria demonstrated by transoesophageal echocardiography.

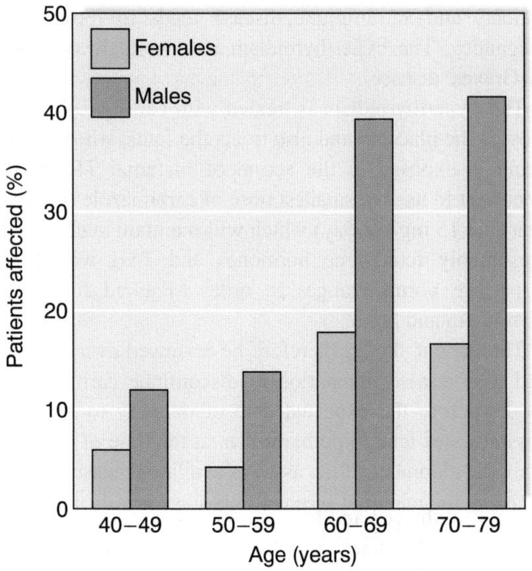

Fig. 8.12 Incidence of atrial fibrillation in different age groups of male and female patients with hyperthyroidism.

Hyperthyroid crisis

This is a rare and life-threatening increase in the severity of the clinical features of hyperthyroidism. The most prominent signs are fever, agitation, confusion, tachycardia or atrial fibrillation and, in the older patient, cardiac failure. It is a medical emergency and, despite early recognition and treatment, the mortality rate is 10%. Thyrotoxic crisis is most commonly precipitated by infection in a patient with previously unrecognised or inadequately treated hyperthyroidism. It may also develop shortly after subtotal thyroidectomy in an ill-prepared patient or within a few days of ^{131}I therapy when acute irradiation damage may lead to a transient rise in serum thyroid hormone levels.

Patients should be rehydrated and given a broad-spectrum antibiotic. Propranolol is rapidly effective orally (80 mg 6-hourly) or intravenously (1–5 mg 6-hourly). Sodium iopodate 500 mg per day orally will restore serum T_3 levels to normal in 48–72 hours. It is a radiographic contrast medium which not only inhibits the release of thyroid hormones, but also reduces the conversion of T_4 to T_3 and is therefore more effective than potassium iodate or Lugol's solution. Carbimazole 15 mg 8-hourly orally inhibits the synthesis of new thyroid hormone. If the patient is unconscious or uncooperative carbimazole can be administered rectally with good effect, but no preparation is available for parenteral use.

Sodium iopodate and propranolol can be withdrawn after 10–14 days and the patient maintained on carbimazole.

Subclinical hyperthyroidism

This term is used to describe clinically euthyroid patients in whom serum thyroid hormone concentrations are normal but usually in the upper part of the reference range, and TSH is undetectable in the absence of non-thyroidal illness. Subclinical hyperthyroidism occurs most often in patients with exophthalmic Graves' disease (50%), multinodular goitre (25%) and in a variable proportion following therapy of hyperthyroidism. Although there is evidence from studies of hepatic, renal and cardiac function that such patients are probably mildly hyperthyroid, treatment is not usually instituted. There is a significant risk of overt hyperthyroidism developing and follow-up is indicated.

HYPOTHYROIDISM

PRIMARY HYPOTHYROIDISM

In primary hypothyroidism there is an intrinsic disorder of the thyroid gland, e.g. following ^{131}I therapy for Graves' disease, in which low levels of thyroid hormones are associated with raised TSH. The classification is shown in the information box.

CLASSIFICATION OF PRIMARY HYPOTHYROIDISM	
Spontaneous atrophic	**Goitrous**
Post-ablative (post-^{131}I)	Hashimoto's thyroiditis
Subclinical	Drug-induced
Transient	Iodine deficiency
Congenital	Dyshormonogenesis

Spontaneous atrophic hypothyroidism, thyroid failure following ^{131}I or surgical treatment of hyperthyroidism and the hypothyroidism of Hashimoto's thyroiditis account for over 90% of cases in those parts of the world which are not iodine-deficient. The prevalence of primary hypothyroidism is 10/1000 but increases to 50/1000 if patients with subclinical hypothyroidism (normal T_4, raised TSH) are included. The female:male ratio is approximately 6:1.

SPONTANEOUS ATROPHIC HYPOTHYROIDISM

This form of primary hypothyroidism increases in incidence with age and, like Graves' disease and Hashimoto's thyroiditis, is an organ-specific autoimmune disorder. There is destructive lymphoid infiltration of the thyroid, ultimately leading to fibrosis and atrophy. There is also evidence for the presence of TSH-receptor antibodies which block the effects of endogenous TSH. In some patients there is a history of Graves' disease treated with antithyroid drugs

10–20 years earlier and, very occasionally, patients with this form of hypothyroidism develop Graves' disease. As with any of the immunologically mediated thyroid disorders, patients are at risk of developing other organ-specific autoimmune conditions such as type I diabetes mellitus, pernicious anaemia and Addison's disease, and autoimmune disease is not uncommon in their first- and second-degree relatives.

Clinical features

These depend on the duration and severity of the hypothyroidism. In the patient in whom complete thyroid failure has developed insidiously over months or even years many of the clinical features listed in the information box are likely to be present. A consequence of prolonged hypothyroidism is the infiltration of many body tissues by the mucopolysaccharides, hyaluronic acid and chondroitin sulphate, resulting in a low-pitched voice, poor hearing, slurred speech due to a large tongue, and compression of the median nerve at the wrist. Infiltration of the dermis gives rise to non-pitting oedema or myxoedema which is most marked in the skin of the hands, feet and eyelids. The resultant periorbital puffiness is often striking and, when combined with facial pallor due to vasoconstriction and anaemia, or a lemon-yellow tint to the skin due to carotenaemia, purplish lips and malar flush, the clinical diagnosis is simple. Most cases of hypothyroidism are not so obvious, however, and unless the diagnosis is positively entertained in a middle-aged woman complaining of symptoms such as tiredness, weight gain or depression, or with the carpal tunnel syndrome, an opportunity for early treatment will be missed. On the other hand, many patients are asymptomatic and thyroid failure is detected by screening during hospital admission or by routine testing of thyroid function in patients known to be at risk of developing hypothyroidism, e.g. following ^{131}I therapy of Graves' disease. It is in this group of patients that there is often little or no subjective benefit from thyroxine replacement therapy.

CLINICAL FEATURES OF HYPOTHYROIDISM

General
- Tiredness, somnolence
- Weight gain
- Cold intolerance
- Hoarseness
- Goitre

Cardiorespiratory
- Bradycardia, hypertension, angina, cardiac failure*
- Xanthelasma
- Pericardial and pleural effusion*

Neuromuscular
- Aches and pains, muscle stiffness
- Delayed relaxation of tendon reflexes
- Carpal tunnel syndrome, deafness
- Depression, psychosis*
- Cerebellar ataxia*
- Myotonia*

Haematological
- Macrocytosis
- Anaemia
  - Iron deficiency (pre-menopausal women)
  - Normochromic
  - Pernicious

Dermatological
- Dry, flaky skin and hair, alopecia
- Purplish lips and malar flush, carotenaemia
- Vitiligo
- Erythema ab igne (Granny's tartan)
- Myxoedema

Reproductive
- Menorrhagia
- Infertility
- Galactorrhoea*
- Impotence*

Gastrointestinal
- Constipation
- Ileus*
- Ascites*

* Rare but well-recognised features.

Investigations

Serum T_4 is low and TSH raised, usually in excess of 20 mU/l. T_3 concentrations do not discriminate reliably between euthyroid and hypothyroid patients and should not be measured. Other non-specific abnormalities include elevation of the enzymes lactate dehydrogenase and creatine kinase, raised cholesterol and triglyceride levels, and low serum sodium. In severe prolonged hypothyroidism the electrocardiogram (ECG) classically demonstrates sinus bradycardia with low voltage complexes and ST/T wave abnormalities.

Management

Hypothyroidism should be treated with thyroxine, which is available as 25, 50 and 100 μg tablets. It is customary to start slowly and a dose of 50 μg per day should be given for 3 weeks, increasing thereafter to 100 μg per day for a further 3 weeks and finally to 150 μg per day. In the elderly and in patients with ischaemic heart disease the initial dose should be 25 μg per day. Thyroxine should always be taken as a single daily dose as it has a plasma half-life of approximately 7 days. The correct dose of thyroxine is that which restores serum TSH to normal. There is some evidence that the finding of an undetectable TSH concentration indicates over-treatment even in the presence of a normal T_4, although in certain circumstances, e.g. Hashimoto's thyroiditis and differentiated thyroid carcinoma, the aim is to suppress TSH without inducing overt hyperthyroidism.

Patients feel better within 2–3 weeks. Reduction in weight and periorbital puffiness occurs quickly, but the restoration of skin and hair texture and resolution of any effusions may take 3–6 months (see Fig. 8.13).

SPECIAL PROBLEMS

Ischaemic heart disease

Around 5% of patients with long-standing hypothyroidism complain of angina at presentation or develop it during

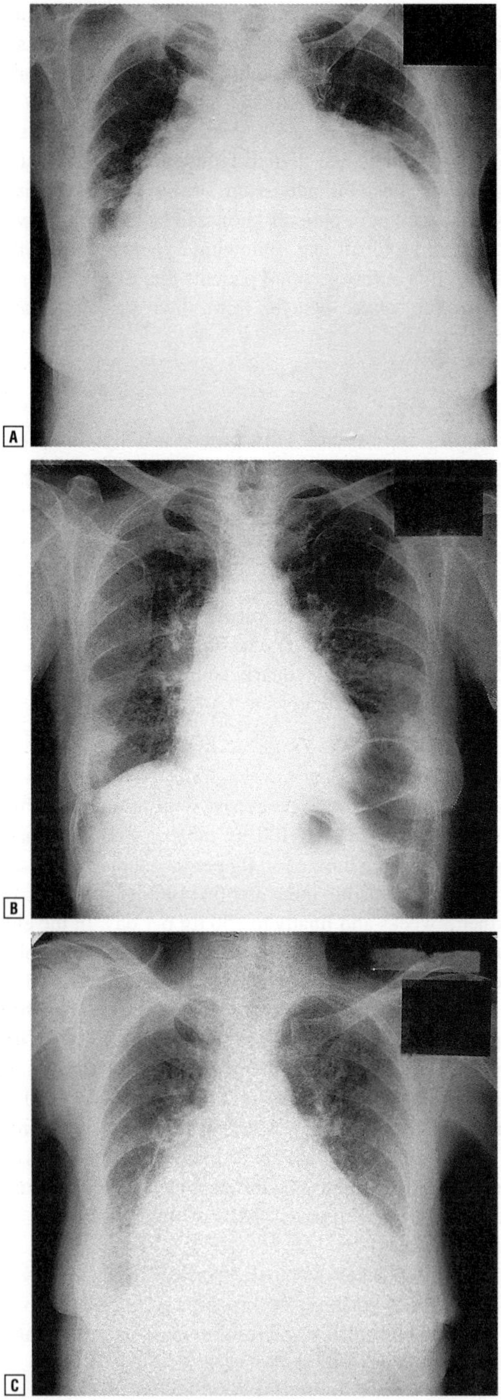

Fig. 8.13 Sequential chest radiographs in a patient with severe long-standing hypothyroidism. A Before treatment. Cardiomegaly is due to a combination of dilatation and pericardial effusion. B After treatment with thyroxine for 9 months. C Recurrence of cardiomegaly 2–3 years after patient stopped taking thyroxine.

treatment with thyroxine. Although angina may remain unchanged in severity or paradoxically disappear with restoration of metabolic rate, exacerbation of myocardial ischaemia, infarction and sudden death are well-recognised complications, even using doses of thyroxine as low as 25 μg per day. Approximately 40% of patients with angina cannot tolerate full replacement therapy despite the use of β-adrenoceptor antagonists and vasodilators. Although there is still reluctance to operate on patients with untreated or partially treated hypothyroidism, coronary artery surgery and balloon angioplasty can safely be performed in such patients and, if successful, allow full replacement dosage of thyroxine in the majority.

Hypothyroidism in pregnancy

Until recently it was thought that the dose of thyroxine did not need to be changed during pregnancy. However, on the basis of serum TSH measurements most pregnant women with primary hypothyroidism require an increase in the dose of thyroxine of some 50 μg daily. One explanation for this phenomenon is the well-recognised increase in serum thyroxine-binding globulin concentration during pregnancy, resulting in a decrease in serum free thyroid hormone concentrations which cannot be compensated for by thyroidal secretion. Serum TSH and free T_4 should be measured during each trimester and the dose of thyroxine adjusted to maintain a normal TSH.

Myxoedema coma

This is a rare presentation of hypothyroidism in which there is a depressed level of consciousness, usually in an elderly patient who appears myxoedematous. Body temperature may be as low as 25°C, convulsions are not uncommon and cerebrospinal fluid (CSF) pressure and protein content are raised. Mortality rate is 50% and survival depends upon early recognition and treatment of hypothyroidism and other factors contributing to the altered consciousness level, e.g. drugs such as phenothiazines, cardiac failure, chest infection, dilutional hyponatraemia, hypoxaemia and hypercapnia due to hypoventilation.

Myxoedema coma is a medical emergency and treatment must begin before biochemical confirmation of the diagnosis. Thyroxine is not usually available for parenteral use and triiodothyronine is given as an intravenous bolus of 20 μg followed by 20 μg 8-hourly until there is sustained clinical improvement. In survivors there is a rise in body temperature within 24 hours and, after 48–72 hours, it is usually possible to substitute oral thyroxine in a dose of 50 μg per day. Unless it is apparent that the patient has primary hypothyroidism, e.g. thyroidectomy scar or goitre, the thyroid failure should be assumed to be secondary to hypothalamic or pituitary disease and treatment given with hydrocortisone sodium succinate 100 mg intramuscularly 8-hourly, pending the results of T_4, TSH and cortisol concentrations (see Table 8.5, p. 555). Other measures include slow rewarming by wrapping the patient in a space blanket, cautious use of intravenous fluids, broad-spectrum antibiotics and high-flow oxygen. Occasionally, if hypoxaemia, hypercapnia and respiratory acidosis persist, assisted ventilation may be necessary.

Ensuring compliance

Patients often do not take long-term medication in the recommended dose and thyroxine is no exception (see Fig. 8.13). It is, therefore, important to measure thyroid function every 1–2 years once the dose of thyroxine is stabilised and at each visit to reinforce the need for regular medication. In some patients in whom tablet-taking is erratic, thyroxine is taken diligently or even in excess for the few days prior to a clinic visit, resulting in the seemingly anomalous combination of a high serum T_4 and high TSH.

Inappropriate thyroxine therapy

In some patients treatment with thyroxine may have been started in the past without biochemical confirmation of the diagnosis for a variety of complaints such as obesity, tiredness or alopecia and may have been given for many years to patients in whom thyroid failure could have been short-lived, e.g. post-partum thyroiditis. Thyroxine should be stopped and serum T_4 and TSH concentrations measured 4–6 weeks later. This period allows for any thyroxine-induced suppression of pituitary thyrotrophs to recover and a biochemical distinction to be made between primary and secondary hypothyroidism. If the patient is truly hypothyroid, lack of thyroxine for 4–6 weeks will be relatively easily tolerated.

GOITROUS HYPOTHYROIDISM

The following conditions are not always associated with hypothyroidism and should therefore be included in the differential diagnosis of a euthyroid patient with goitre.

Hashimoto's thyroiditis

This is the most common cause of goitrous hypothyroidism. It typically affects 20–60-year-old women who present with a small or moderately sized diffuse goitre which is characteristically firm or rubbery in consistency. The goitre may be soft, however, and impossible to differentiate from simple goitre by palpation alone. Thyroid status depends upon the relative degrees of lymphocytic infiltration, fibrosis and follicular cell hyperplasia within the gland but 25% of patients are hypothyroid at presentation. In the remainder, serum T_4 is normal and TSH normal or raised but these patients are at risk of developing overt hypothyroidism in future years. In 90% of patients with Hashimoto's thyroiditis thyroid peroxidase antibodies are present in the serum. In those under the age of 20 years the antinuclear factor (ANF) may be positive.

Thyroxine therapy is indicated not only for hypothyroidism but also for goitre shrinkage. In this context the dose of thyroxine should be sufficient to suppress serum TSH to undetectable levels without inducing hyperthyroidism (usually 150 μg daily but in some patients 200 μg daily).

Drug-induced hypothyroidism

Lithium carbonate. This is widely used for the treatment of manic-depressive illness. Like iodide, lithium inhibits the release of thyroid hormones. Although the most common evidence of thyroid dysfunction is a raised serum TSH, some patients, usually those with underlying autoimmune thyroiditis, develop goitre and hypothyroidism.

Iodine. When taken for prolonged periods iodine may cause goitrous hypothyroidism in patients with underlying autoimmune thyroiditis. This is usually seen in those with chronic respiratory diseases given expectorants containing potassium iodide, or in patients receiving the antidysrhythmic drug, amiodarone, which contains a significant amount of iodine.

Iodine deficiency

In certain parts of the world, such as the Andes, Himalayas and central Africa, where there is dietary iodine deficiency, thyroid enlargement is common (more than 10% of the population) and is known as endemic goitre. Most patients are euthyroid and have normal or raised TSH levels. In general the more severe the iodine deficiency, the greater the incidence of hypothyroidism.

Dyshormonogenesis

Dyshormonogenesis is an unusual genetically determined defect in thyroid hormone synthesis. The mode of inheritance is autosomal recessive. Although several forms have been described, the most common results from deficiency of the intrathyroidal peroxidase enzyme. Homozygous individuals present with congenital hypothyroidism; heterozygotes present in the first two decades of life with goitre, normal thyroid hormone levels and a raised TSH. The combination of dyshormonogenetic goitre and nerve deafness is known as Pendred's syndrome.

TRANSIENT HYPOTHYROIDISM

This is often observed during the first 6 months after subtotal thyroidectomy or ^{131}I treatment of Graves' disease, in the post-thyrotoxic phase of subacute thyroiditis and in post-partum thyroiditis (see Fig. 8.14). In these conditions thyroxine treatment should not be necessary as the patient is usually asymptomatic during the short period of thyroid failure. In some neonates transplacental passage of TSH-

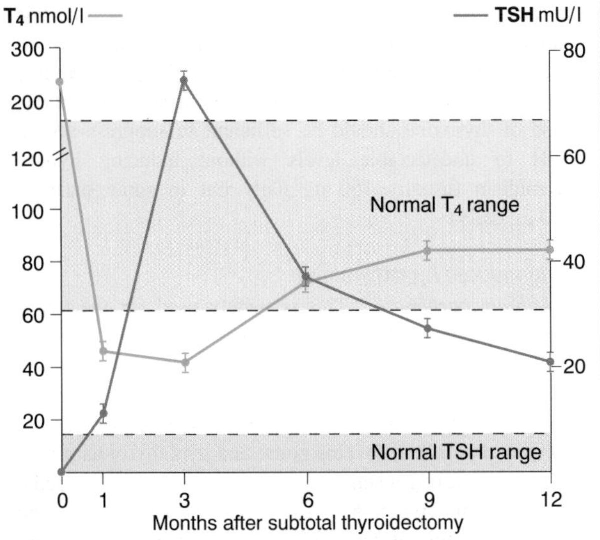

Fig. 8.14 Total T_4 and TSH levels before and after subtotal thyroidectomy in a series of patients with temporary hypothyroidism.

receptor-blocking antibodies from a mother with autoimmune thyroid disease is a cause of hypothyroidism which, like neonatal thyrotoxicosis, is temporary.

SUBCLINICAL HYPOTHYROIDISM

Subclinical hypothyroidism is a term used to describe asymptomatic patients who are clinically euthyroid, with thyroid hormone levels at the lower end of the reference range, but with raised serum TSH. It is most often encountered after ^{131}I or surgical treatment of hyperthyroidism and may persist for many years. The present consensus is that these patients are mildly hypothyroid and failure to recognise this is a reflection of the poor discrimination of clinical examination. Thyroxine should be given in a dose of 50–150 μg daily—sufficient to restore TSH concentrations to normal.

CONGENITAL HYPOTHYROIDISM

It has long been recognised that early treatment with thyroxine is essential to prevent irreversible brain damage in children with congenital hypothyroidism. Thyroid failure, however, is difficult to diagnose clinically in the first few weeks of life. Routine screening of TSH levels in blood spot samples obtained 5–7 days after birth has revealed an incidence of approximately 1 in 3000, resulting from either thyroid agenesis, ectopic or hypoplastic glands, or dyshormonogenesis. Congenital hypothyroidism is thus six times more common than phenylketonuria.

It is now possible to start thyroid replacement therapy within 2 weeks of birth. Developmental assessment of infants treated at this early stage has revealed no differences between cases and controls in most children.

SECONDARY HYPOTHYROIDISM

This form is much less common than primary hypothyroidism. There is atrophy of an inherently normal thyroid gland caused by failure of TSH secretion in patients with hypothalamic or anterior pituitary disease, e.g. pituitary macroadenoma (see p. 554). Note that TSH is not always low in secondary hypothyroidism.

SIMPLE GOITRE

This is the term used to describe diffuse or multinodular enlargement of the thyroid which occurs sporadically and is of unknown aetiology. It is likely, however, that suboptimal dietary iodine intake, minor degrees of dyshormonogenesis and stimuli such as epidermal growth factor and growth-stimulating immunoglobulins are important in the development of simple goitre. Affected patients are euthyroid, usually female and often have a family history of goitre.

SIMPLE DIFFUSE GOITRE

This form of goitre usually presents between the ages of 15 and 25 years, often during pregnancy, and tends to be noticed not by the patient but by friends and relatives. Occasionally, there is a tight sensation in the neck, particularly when swallowing. The goitre is soft and symmetrical and the thyroid is enlarged to 2–3 times normal size. There is no tenderness, lymphadenopathy or overlying bruit. Concentrations of T_3, T_4 and TSH are normal and no thyroid autoantibodies are detected in the serum. No treatment is necessary and in most cases the goitre regresses. In some, however, the unknown stimulus to thyroid enlargement persists and as a result of recurrent episodes of hyperplasia and involution during the following 10–20 years the gland becomes multinodular with areas of autonomous function (simple multinodular goitre, see Fig. 8.15).

SIMPLE MULTINODULAR GOITRE

Presentation is rare before middle age. The patient may have been aware of goitre for many years, perhaps slowly increasing in size. Rarely, medical advice may have been sought because of painful swelling lasting a few days caused by haemorrhage into a nodule or cyst. The goitre is nodular or lobulated on palpation and may extend

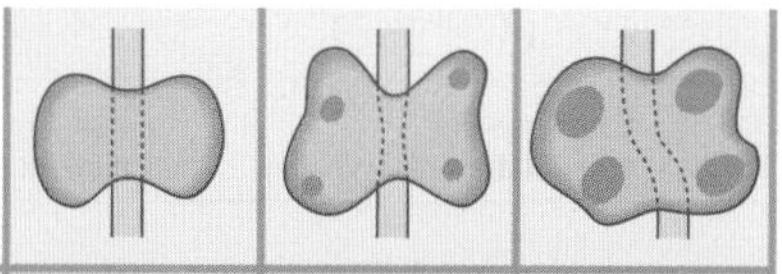

Age (in years)	15–25	35–55	> 55
Goitre	Diffuse	Nodular	Nodular
Tracheal compression/ deviation	No	Minimal	Yes
T_3, T_4	Normal	Normal	Raised
TSH	Normal	Normal or undetectable	Undetectable

Fig. 8.15 Natural history of simple goitre.

retrosternally. Very large goitres may cause mediastinal compression with stridor, dysphagia and obstruction of the superior vena cava. Hoarseness due to recurrent laryngeal nerve palsy can occur but is strongly suggestive of thyroid carcinoma. Serum T_3 and T_4 are normal and in the majority are associated with normal TSH. In approximately 25%, thyroid hormone levels are in the upper part of their respective normal ranges and TSH is undetectable (subclinical hyperthyroidism). Radiographs of the thoracic inlet may show tracheal displacement or compression, intrathyroidal calcification and the extent of retrosternal extension. A flow-volume loop (see Ch. 4) will detect cases with significant extra-thoracic tracheal compression which can be confirmed by CT scanning.

If the goitre is small no treatment is necessary other than annual review, as the natural history is progression to a toxic multinodular goitre. Partial thyroidectomy is indicated for large goitres which cause mediastinal compression or which are cosmetically unattractive. Unfortunately, recurrence 10–20 years later is not uncommon and cannot be prevented by the long-established custom of treatment with thyroxine, which may serve to aggravate any associated hyperthyroidism.

SOLITARY THYROID NODULE

Palpable thyroid nodules occur in approximately 5% of females and are even more commonly found at post-mortem examination. Whereas multinodular goitre is benign, solitary nodules may be malignant. In those who seek medical attention it is important, therefore, to determine whether the nodule is benign, e.g. cyst or colloid nodule, or malignant. With the exception of haemorrhage into a cyst when thyroid enlargement is of rapid onset and painful, or the presence of cervical lymphadenopathy which is highly suggestive of carcinoma, it is rarely possible to make this distinction on clinical grounds alone. However, a solitary nodule presenting in childhood or adolescence, particularly if there is a past history of head and neck irradiation, or presenting in the elderly, should raise the suspicion of malignancy. Very occasionally, a secondary deposit from a renal, breast or lung carcinoma presents as a painful, rapidly growing solitary thyroid nodule.

Investigations

The most useful is fine-needle aspiration of the nodule. This is performed in the outpatient clinic without local anaesthetic, using a standard 21 gauge venepuncture needle and a 20 ml syringe. Aspiration may be therapeutic in the small proportion of patients in whom the swelling is a pure cyst, although recurrence on more than one occasion is an indication for surgery. Usually 2–3 aspirates are taken from the nodule. Cytological examination will differentiate benign (80%) from suspicious or definitely malignant nodules (20%), of which half are confirmed as cancer at surgery. The advantage of fine-needle aspiration over long-established tests such as isotope and ultrasound scanning is that a much higher proportion of patients avoid surgery. The limitation of the method is that it cannot differentiate between follicular adenoma and carcinoma.

It is important to measure serum T_3, T_4 and TSH in all patients with a solitary thyroid nodule. The finding of undetectable TSH is very suggestive of an autonomously functioning thyroid adenoma which can only be confirmed by thyroid isotope scanning (see Fig. 8.11, p. 566), is for practical purposes always benign, and is treated with ^{131}I or surgery.

MALIGNANT TUMOURS

Primary thyroid malignancy is rare, accounting for less than 1% of all carcinomas, and has a prevalence of 25 per million. As shown in Table 8.10 it can be classified according to the cell type of origin. With the exception of medullary carcinoma, thyroid cancer is always more common in females.

DIFFERENTIATED CARCINOMA

In most patients, presentation is with a palpable solitary nodule.

Papillary carcinoma

This is the most common of the malignant thyroid tumours

Table 8.10 Malignant thyroid tumours

Origin of tumour	Type of tumour	Frequency (%)	Usual age of presentation (years)	Approximate 20-year survival (%)
Follicular cells	Differentiated carcinoma			
	Papillary	70	20–40	95
	Follicular	10	40–60	60
	Undifferentiated carcinoma			
	Anaplastic	5	> 60	< 1
Parafollicular C cells	Medullary carcinoma	5–10	> 40*	50
Lymphocytes	Lymphoma	5–10	> 60	10

* Patients with medullary carcinoma as part of multiple endocrine neoplasia type II may present in childhood.

and accounts for 90% of irradiation-induced thyroid cancer. It may be multifocal, and spread is to regional cervical lymph nodes. Some patients present with cervical lymphadenopathy and no apparent thyroid enlargement and the primary lesion may be less than 10 mm in diameter.

Follicular carcinoma

This is always a single encapsulated lesion. Spread to cervical lymph nodes is rare. Metastases are blood-borne and are most often found in bone, lungs and brain.

Management

This is usually by total thyroidectomy followed by a large dose of ^{131}I (3000 MBq, ~ 80 mCi) in order to ablate any remaining thyroid tissue, normal or malignant. Thereafter, long-term treatment with thyroxine in a dose sufficient to suppress TSH (usually 150–200 μg daily) is important as there is some evidence that differentiated thyroid carcinoma may be TSH-dependent. Follow-up is by measurement of serum thyroglobulin which should be low or undetectable in patients taking a suppressive dose of thyroxine. A level in excess of 15 μg/l is strongly suggestive of tumour recurrence or metastases which may be detected by whole-body scanning with ^{131}I and may respond to further radioiodine therapy.

Prognosis

Most patients have an excellent prognosis when treated appropriately. Patients under 50 years of age with papillary carcinoma can anticipate a near-normal life expectancy if the tumour is less than 2 cm in diameter, confined to the thyroid and cervical nodes and of low-grade malignancy histologically. Even for patients with distant metastases at presentation the 10-year survival is approximately 40%.

ANAPLASTIC CARCINOMA AND LYMPHOMA

These two conditions are difficult to distinguish clinically but this is easier with cytological examination of fine-needle aspiration biopsy. Patients are usually elderly women in whom there is rapid thyroid enlargement over 2–3 months. The goitre is hard and symmetrical. There is usually stridor due to tracheal compression and hoarseness due to recurrent laryngeal nerve palsy. There is no effective treatment of anaplastic carcinoma although radiotherapy may afford temporary relief of mediastinal compression. The prognosis for lymphoma which may arise from pre-existing Hashimoto's thyroiditis is better. External irradiation often produces dramatic goitre shrinkage and, when combined with chemotherapy, may result in survival for 5 years or more.

MEDULLARY CARCINOMA

This tumour arises from the parafollicular C cells of the thyroid. In addition to calcitonin, the tumour may secrete 5-HT, various peptides of the tachykinin family, ACTH and prostaglandins. As a consequence carcinoid syndrome and Cushing's syndrome have been described in association with medullary carcinoma.

Patients usually present in middle age with a firm thyroid mass. Cervical lymphadenopathy is common, but distant metastases are rare initially. Serum calcitonin levels are raised and are useful in monitoring response to treatment. Despite the very high levels of calcitonin found in some patients, hypocalcaemia is extremely rare.

Treatment is by total thyroidectomy with removal of affected cervical nodes. Since the C cells do not concentrate iodine there is no role for ^{131}I therapy. Prognosis is very variable, some patients surviving 20 years or more and others less than 1 year.

Medullary carcinoma of the thyroid is part of the multiple endocrine neoplasia type II syndrome (see p. 598).

RIEDEL'S THYROIDITIS

This is not a form of thyroid cancer but the presentation is similar and the differentiation can usually only be made by thyroid biopsy. It is an exceptionally rare condition of unknown aetiology in which there is extensive infiltration of the thyroid and surrounding structures with fibrous tissue. There may be associated mediastinal and retroperitoneal fibrosis. Presentation is with a slow-growing goitre which is irregular and stony-hard. There is usually tracheal and oesophageal compression necessitating partial thyroidectomy. Other recognised complications include recurrent laryngeal nerve palsy, hypoparathyroidism and eventually hypothyroidism.

FURTHER INFORMATION ON THE THYROID GLAND

Franklyn J A 1994 The management of hyperthyroidism. New England Journal of Medicine 330: 1731–1738
Lindsay R S, Toft A D 1997 Hypothyroidism. Lancet 349: 413–417
Sawin C T, Geller A, Wolf P A et al 1994 Low serum thyrotropin concentrations as a risk factor for atrial fibrillation in older patients. New England Journal of Medicine 331: 1249–1252

THE PARATHYROID GLANDS

FUNCTIONAL ANATOMY AND PHYSIOLOGY

The four parathyroid glands lie behind the lobes of the thyroid. The parathyroid glands are not regulated by the pituitary gland, but respond directly to changes in serum ionised calcium concentrations. Parathyroid hormone (PTH) is a single-chain polypeptide of 84 amino acids which is synthesised by the chief cells and released in response to a fall in serum ionised calcium concentration. This hormone interacts with vitamin D and its metabolites in regulating calcium absorption and excretion. Its actions are shown in Figure 8.16. In summary, PTH has direct effects which promote reabsorption of calcium from renal tubules and bone. PTH also has indirect effects, mediated by increasing conversion of 25-hydroxycholecalciferol (i.e. 25-hydroxy-vitamin D) to the more potent hormone 1,25-dihydroxycholecalciferol, which results in increased calcium absorption from food and enhanced mobilisation of calcium from bone.

PTH plays a central role in regulating calcium homeostasis because vitamin D and dietary calcium are rarely deficient. Moreover, 99% of total body calcium is in bone, but this pool is in dynamic equilibrium with the extracellular fluid by processes of bone resorption and deposition. The initial effect of PTH on bone is to stimulate osteolysis, returning calcium from bone to extracellular fluid. Prolonged exposure of bone to PTH is associated with increased osteoclastic activity, extensive bone remodelling and osteoblastic repair. Abnormalities of vitamin D are described in Chapter 12. Hypercalcaemia is one of the most common presentations of endocrine disease.

In some species calcitonin, a hormone secreted from the parafollicular C cells of the thyroid gland, also regulates calcium metabolism. However, although calcitonin is a useful tumour marker in medullary carcinoma of thyroid

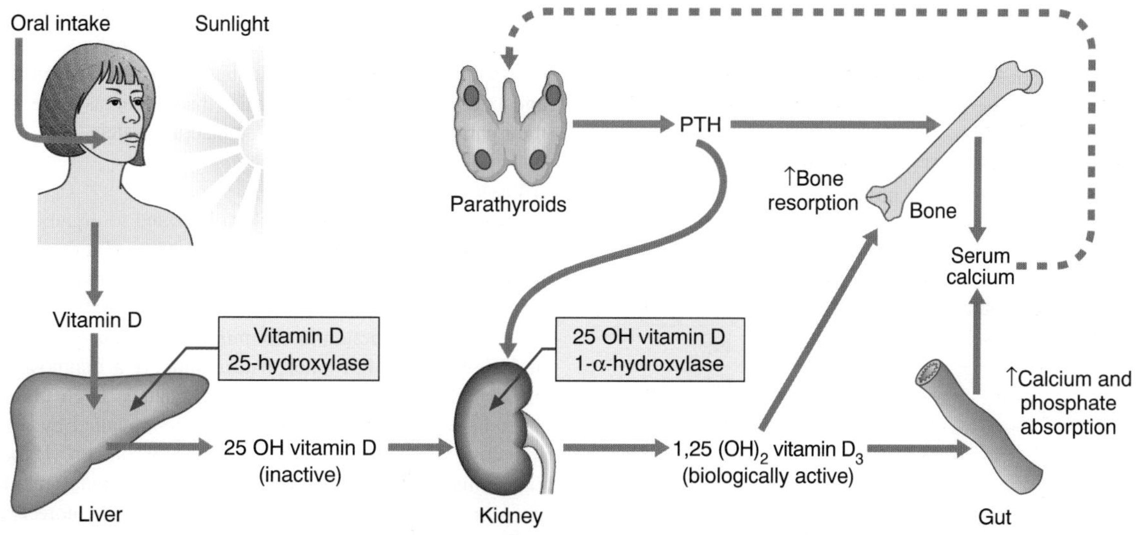

Fig. 8.16 Outline of calcium homeostasis showing interactions between parathyroid hormone (PTH) and vitamin D. Calcium in serum exists as 50% ionised (Ca^{++}), 10% non-ionised or complexed with organic ions such as citrate and phosphate, and 40% protein-bound, mainly to albumin. It is the ionised calcium concentration which regulates PTH production.

(see p. 574), it is of no clinical relevance to calcium homeostasis in humans.

HYPERPARATHYROIDISM AND HYPERCALCAEMIA

Aetiology

Hypercalcaemia has always presented with its diverse clinical manifestations described below but, more recently, a large number of patients with asymptomatic hypercalcaemia have been detected by increased use of automated biochemical screening. The causes of hypercalcaemia are listed in the information box.

CAUSES OF HYPERCALCAEMIA
With normal or elevated (i.e. inappropriate) PTH levels
• Primary or tertiary hyperparathyroidism • Lithium-induced hyperparathyroidism • Familial hypocalciuric hypercalcaemia
With low (i.e. suppressed) PTH levels
• Malignancy e.g. Lung, breast, renal, ovarian, colonic and thyroid carcinoma • Multiple myeloma • Elevated 1,25(OH)$_2$-vitamin D e.g. Intoxication or sarcoidosis • Thyrotoxicosis • Paget's disease with immobilisation • Milk-alkali syndrome • Thiazide diuretics

It is customary to distinguish three categories of hyperparathyroidism, as shown in Table 8.11. In primary hyperparathyroidism there is usually autonomous secretion of parathyroid hormone (PTH) by a single parathyroid adenoma varying in size from a few millimetres to several centimetres in diameter. Secondary hyperparathyroidism is present when there is hyperplasia with increased PTH secretion in an attempt to compensate for prolonged hypocalcaemia. Its effect is to restore serum calcium levels at the expense of the stores of calcium in bone. In a very small proportion of cases of secondary hyperparathyroidism continuous stimulation of the parathyroids may result in adenoma formation and autonomous PTH secretion. This is known as tertiary hyperparathyroidism.

Table 8.11 Hyperparathyroidism

Type	Serum calcium	PTH
Primary Single adenoma (90%) Multiple adenomata (4%) Nodular hyperplasia (5%) Carcinoma (1%)	Raised	Not suppressed
Secondary Chronic renal failure Malabsorption Osteomalacia and rickets	Low	Raised
Tertiary	Raised	Not suppressed

Primary hyperparathyroidism is the most common of the parathyroid disorders with a prevalence of about 1 in 800. It is 2–3 times more common in women than men and 90% of patients are over 50 years of age. It also occurs in all of the familial multiple endocrine neoplasia syndromes, as described on page 598.

Clinical features and diagnosis

Symptoms and signs of hypercalcaemia include polyuria and polydipsia, renal colic, lethargy, anorexia, nausea, dyspepsia and peptic ulceration, constipation, depression, drowsiness and impaired cognitive function. Some of these are brought to mind by the adage 'bones, stones and abdominal groans'. About 50% of patients with primary hyperparathyroidism are asymptomatic. In others, these symptoms may go unrecognised until patients present with renal calculi (5% of first stone formers and 15% of recurrent stone formers have primary hyperparathyroidism), with or without impaired renal function, or acute dehydration and profound hypercalcaemia. Hypertension is common in hyperparathyroidism. Parathyroid tumours are almost never palpable.

A family history of renal tract stones and/or neck surgery raises the possibility of multiple endocrine neoplasia (see p. 598). However, familial hypocalciuric hypercalcaemia is a rare but important catch for the unwary. This autosomal dominant disorder is associated with a defective calcium receptor in the parathyroid gland, but is always asymptomatic and uncomplicated. Occasionally, these patients have had their parathyroid glands removed inappropriately.

Investigations

About 50% of circulating calcium is bound to organic ions such as citrate or phosphate and to proteins. Total calcium measurements need to be corrected if serum albumin is low, by adjusting the value for calcium upwards by 0.1 mmol/l for each 6 g/l reduction in albumin. Low plasma phosphate and elevated alkaline phosphatase support a diagnosis of primary hyperparathyroidism or malignancy. High plasma phosphate and alkaline phosphatase accompanied by renal impairment suggest tertiary hyperparathyroidism. Hypercalcaemia may cause nephrocalcinosis and renal tubular impairment resulting in hyperuricaemia and hyperchloraemia.

The most discriminant investigation is the measurement of PTH using a specific immunoradiometric assay. Older assays were not able to distinguish PTH from PTH-related peptide. If PTH is normal or elevated and urinary calcium is elevated, then hyperparathyroidism is confirmed. If PTH is low, and no other cause is apparent, then malignancy with or without bony metastases is likely. PTH-related peptide can be measured in these patients, but this is not generally necessary. Unless the source is obvious the patient should be screened for malignancy with a chest radiograph, isotope bone scan, myeloma screen (erythrocyte sedimentation rate, serum protein electrophoresis, immunoglobulins and urinary Bence Jones protein), serum angiotensin-converting enzyme (elevated in sarcoidosis), and further imaging as appropriate.

Skeletal and radiological changes in primary hyperparathyroidism

Osteitis fibrosa, in which there is increased bone resorption by osteoclasts with fibrous replacement in the lacunae, is the characteristic skeletal disorder of primary hyperparathyroidism. These changes may present clinically as bone pain and tenderness, fracture and deformity. Rarely, primary hyperparathyroidism may present as a local swelling, usually of the mandible, due to an isolated cyst. Chondrocalcinosis is due to deposition of calcium pyrophosphate crystals within articular cartilage. This typically affects the menisci at the knees and can result in secondary degenerative arthritis or predispose to attacks of acute pseudogout, especially following parathyroidectomy.

There are characteristic changes on plain radiographs. In the early stages there may be demineralisation, and subperiosteal erosions may be noted in the phalanges (see Fig. 8.17). These are most marked on the radial side of the middle phalanx. There may also be resorption of the terminal phalanges. A 'pepper-pot' appearance may be seen on lateral radiographs of the skull. Cystic changes are rare. In nephrocalcinosis, scattered opacities may be visible within the renal outline. There may be soft tissue calcification in arterial walls, in soft tissues of hands, and in the cornea. However, changes on plain radiographs are features of long-standing hyperparathyroidism, and these investigations are not required either to confirm the diagnosis or as a criterion for surgery.

Localisation of parathyroid tumours

If primary hyperparathyroidism is confirmed biochemically, imaging to locate the adenoma or differentiate adenomas from hyperplasia is not necessary. In over 90% of patients an experienced surgeon will locate the adenoma without difficulty. If surgical exploration has been unsuccessful, however, ultrasonography, selective neck vein catheterisation with PTH measurements, CT scanning and subtraction imaging may prove useful. In this last technique the neck is imaged during the successive injections of two short-lived isotopes: ^{201}thallium (^{201}Tl) (taken up by thyroid and parathyroid), followed by ^{99m}-technetium (^{99m}Tc) (taken up by thyroid only). Computer subtraction of the two images leaves a parathyroid image if an adenoma is present.

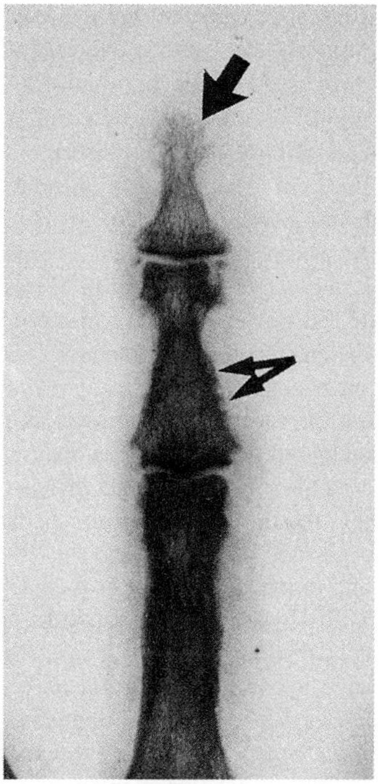

Fig. 8.17 Radiograph of subperiosteal erosions (lower arrows) in a phalanx with terminal resorption (top arrow) in a patient with primary hyperparathyroidism.

Management

Treatment of malignant hypercalcaemia is described in the information box.

TREATMENT OF MALIGNANT HYPERCALCAEMIA

- Rehydration with normal saline
  - To replace as much as a 4–6 litre deficit
  - May need monitoring with central venous pressure in old age or renal impairment
- Bisphosphonates, e.g. pamidronate 90 mg i.v. over 4 hours
  - Causes a fall in calcium which is maximal at 2–3 days and lasts a few weeks
  - Unless the cause is removed, follow up with an oral bisphosphonate
- Additional rapid therapy may be required in very ill patients
  - Forced diuresis with saline and frusemide
  - Glucocorticoids, e.g. prednisolone 40 mg daily
  - Calcitonin
  - Haemodialysis
- Treat the cause

Treatment of primary hyperparathyroidism

The only long-term treatment for primary hyperparathyroidism is surgery, with excision of the parathyroid adenoma or debulking of hyperplastic glands. The selection of patients who require surgery is difficult. They include those with clear-cut symptoms or documented complications such as peptic ulceration, renal stones, renal impairment or osteopenia. However, a large number of patients have only vague symptoms or are asymptomatic. These should be reviewed every 6–12 months, with assessment of symptoms, renal function, serum calcium and perhaps bone mineral density.

At operation the surgeon ideally attempts to locate and assess all parathyroid tissue. Problems may arise from the variability in number and site of the glands, especially if some lie within the thyroid or superior mediastinum. The current management of hyperplasia is to remove all four glands and to transplant some of the excised tissue to the forearm. If hypercalcaemia returns, part of the transplant can be removed under local anaesthetic.

Post-operative hypocalcaemia is not uncommon during the first 2 weeks while residual suppressed parathyroid tissue recovers. It is usually mild or asymptomatic and can be controlled with oral calcium supplements, e.g. 80 mmol daily. It is recognised that patients with particularly high pre-operative serum calcium levels and obvious bone or renal damage are especially likely to develop prolonged symptomatic hypocalcaemia after operation, as there is a major net shift of calcium into healing bone. This hypocalcaemia can be minimised by giving 1α-hydroxycholecalciferol 2 mg daily for 48 hours before surgery and continuing for 1–2 weeks after operation. Intravenous calcium gluconate (as 10 ml of 10% solution which can be given 3–4-hourly) and oral calcium supplements may also be necessary.

Treatment of severe hypercalcaemia is described in the information box on malignant hypercalcaemia. Note that hypercalcaemia in patients with primary hyperparathyroidism responds less well to glucocorticoids and bisphosphonates than in malignancy. Urgent neck surgery is sometimes required, but strenuous attempts should be made to replace fluid deficits and lower the serum calcium concentration before administering an anaesthetic.

HYPOPARATHYROIDISM AND HYPOCALCAEMIA

Aetiology

Hypocalcaemia is much less common than hypercalcaemia. Its *differential diagnosis* is shown in Table 8.12. Although almost all laboratories routinely report total serum calcium concentrations, it is the ionised concentration which is biologically important. The most common cause of hypocalcaemia is a low serum albumin with normal ionised calcium concentration. Correction of total serum calcium concentration for serum albumin is described on page 576. Conversely, ionised calcium may be low in the face of normal total serum calcium if the serum is alkalotic (see Ch. 5).

The most common cause of hypoparathyroidism is damage to the parathyroid glands or their blood supply during *thyroid surgery*, although this complication occurs in only 1% of thyroidectomies. Transient hypocalcaemia

Table 8.12 Differential diagnosis of hypocalcaemia

	Total serum calcium concentration	Ionised serum calcium concentration	Serum phosphate concentration	Serum PTH concentration	Comments
Hypoalbuminaemia	↓	→	→	→	See correction factor, page 576
Alkalosis Respiratory, e.g. hyperventilation Metabolic, e.g. Conn's syndrome	→	↓	→	→ or ↑	See Chapter 5
Vitamin D deficiency	↓	↓	↓	↑	See Chapter 12
Chronic renal failure	↓	↓	↑	↑	Due to impaired vitamin D hydroxylation Serum creatinine ↑
Hypoparathyroidism Post-surgical Idiopathic Infantile	↓	↓	↑	↓	
Pseudohypoparathyroidism	↓	↓	↑	↑	Characteristic phenotype
Acute pancreatitis	↓	↓	→ or ↓	↑	Usually clinically obvious Serum amylase ↑

develops in 10% of patients 12–36 hours following subtotal thyroidectomy for Graves' disease.

Idiopathic hypoparathyroidism may develop at any age, and is sometimes associated with autoimmune disease of the adrenal, thyroid or ovary, especially in young people.

Pseudohypoparathyroidism is usually an autosomal dominant syndrome in which there is tissue resistance to the effects of PTH. The PTH-receptor is normal but there is a defective post-receptor mechanism.

Clinical features

Tetany occurs in all syndromes in which ionised calcium concentrations are low. Additional features are specific to different aetiologies.

Tetany

Low ionised calcium concentrations cause increased excitability of peripheral nerves. Magnesium depletion should also be considered as a possible contributing factor, particularly in malabsorption, diuretic therapy or alcohol excess.

In *children*, a characteristic triad of carpopedal spasm, stridor and convulsions occurs, though one or more of these may be found independently of the others. The hands in carpal spasm adopt a characteristic position. The metacarpophalangeal joints are flexed, the interphalangeal joints of the fingers and thumb are extended and there is opposition of the thumb *(main d'accoucheur)*. Pedal spasm is much less frequent. Stridor is caused by spasm of the glottis. *Adults* complain of tingling in the hands, feet and around the mouth. Less often there is painful carpopedal spasm, while stridor and fits are rare.

Latent tetany may be present when signs of overt tetany are lacking. It is best recognised by eliciting *Trousseau's sign*. Inflation of the sphygmomanometer cuff on the upper arm to more than the systolic blood pressure is followed by carpal spasm within 3 minutes. A less specific sign of hypocalcaemia is that described by Chvostek, in which tapping over the branches of the facial nerve as they emerge from the parotid gland produces twitching of the facial muscles.

Other features

Prolonged hypocalcaemia in hypoparathyroidism may cause grand mal epilepsy, psychosis, cataracts, calcification of basal ganglia and papilloedema. In addition, there is an association with mucocutaneous candidiasis, particularly affecting finger nails, mouth and oesophagus. In pseudohypoparathyroidism there is no associated mucocutaneous candidiasis, but patients may have mental retardation and characteristically there are skeletal abnormalities such as short stature and short 4th and 5th metacarpals and metatarsals. The term 'pseudo-pseudohypoparathyroidism' is given to patients exhibiting the above skeletal abnormalities but in whom serum calcium concentration and other biochemistry are normal.

Management

Control of tetany

Alkalosis can be reversed acutely if arterial PCO_2 is increased by rebreathing expired air in a paper bag or administering 5% CO_2 in oxygen.

Injection of 20 ml of a 10% solution of calcium gluconate slowly into a vein will raise the serum calcium concentration immediately. An intramuscular injection of 10 ml may also be given to obtain a more prolonged effect. In severe cases of alkalotic tetany, intravenous calcium gluconate often relieves the spasm, while specific treatment of the alkalosis, which will vary with the cause, is being applied (see Ch. 5). If tetany is not relieved by giving calcium, the administration of magnesium may be required.

Chronic control of hypocalcaemia

Commercial preparations of parathyroid hormone are unsatisfactory for the treatment of parathyroid insufficiency because they have to be given by frequent injections, and soon become ineffective because of antibody formation. Substitution therapy for persistent hypoparathyroidism and for pseudohypoparathyroidism is provided by 1α-hydroxycholecalciferol (alfacalcidol) which is hydroxylated in the liver to 1,25-dihydroxycholecalciferol (calcitriol). The dose of these preparations is 0.5–3 μg daily. It is important to monitor the serum calcium level every 3–6 months once the dose has been stabilised. Serum PTH can also be monitored in pseudohypoparathyroidism.

FURTHER INFORMATION ON THE PARATHYROID GLANDS

Bilezikian J P 1993 Management of hypercalcemia. Journal of Clinical Endocrinology and Metabolism 77: 1445–1449

THE ADRENAL GLANDS

FUNCTIONAL ANATOMY AND PHYSIOLOGY

Adrenal anatomy is shown in Figure 8.18. Histologically, the cortex is divided into three zones, but these function as two units which produce corticosteroids in response to humoral stimuli. By contrast, the medulla is a component of the sympathetic nervous system which secretes catecholamines. Pathways for the biosynthesis of corticosteroids are shown in Figure 8.19 and the principal functions of adrenal hormones are shown in the information box on page 581.

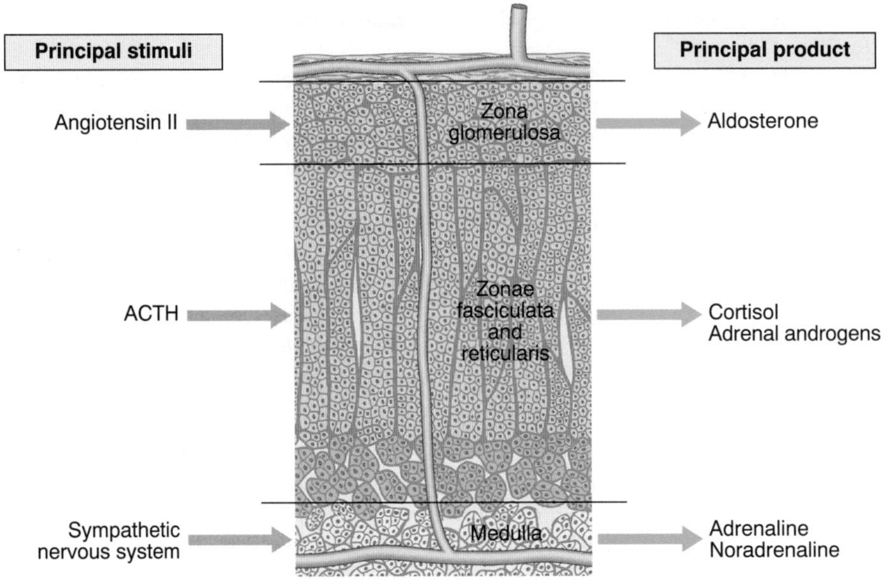

Fig. 8.18 Structure and function of the adrenal gland.

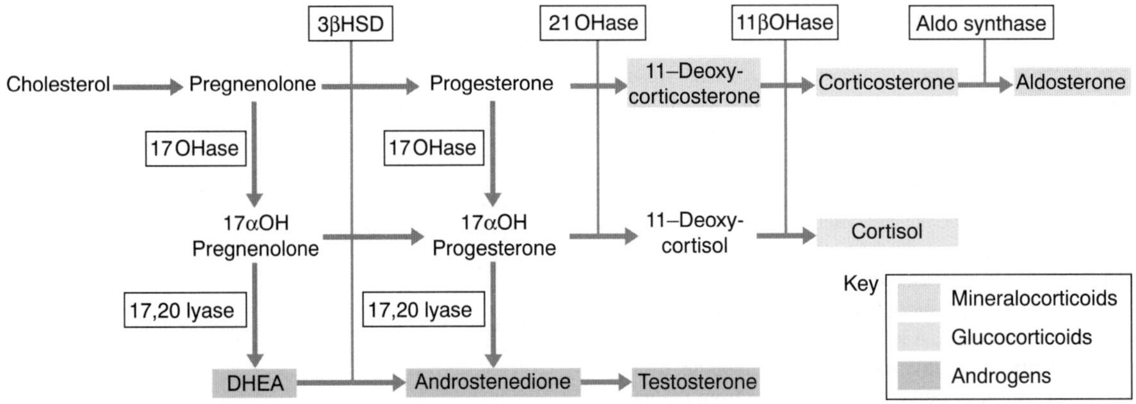

Fig. 8.19 The major pathways of synthesis of adrenal corticosteroids. (DHEA = dehydroepiandrosterone; OHase = hydroxylase; HSD = hydroxysteroid dehydrogenase)

Glucocorticoids

Cortisol is the major glucocorticoid in humans, although corticosterone also has glucocorticoid activity. ACTH has a diurnal pattern of secretion so that cortisol levels are highest in the morning on waking and lowest in the middle of the night. Cortisol rises dramatically during stress, including any illness. This elevation, and the resultant actions listed in the information box, protect key metabolic functions at the expense of others (e.g. maintaining cerebral glucose supply during starvation) and puts an important 'brake' on potentially damaging inflammatory responses to infection and injury. The clinical importance of cortisol deficiency is therefore most obvious at times of stress.

In the circulation more than 95% of cortisol is bound to protein, principally cortisol-binding globulin. It is the free fraction which is biologically active via glucocorticoid receptors (see Ch. 1) which regulate the transcription of many genes in many cells. Cortisol can also activate mineralocorticoid receptors, but it does not normally do so because cells containing mineralocorticoid receptors also express an enzyme, 11β-hydroxysteroid dehydrogenase

PRINCIPAL FUNCTIONS OF ADRENAL HORMONES
Glucocorticoids
• Carbohydrate metabolism regulation (e.g. ↑ gluconeogenesis) • ↑ Protein catabolism • Immunomodulation • Cardiovascular regulation (e.g. ↑ blood pressure)
Mineralocorticoids
• Sodium retention (in distal nephron, sweat duct, colon, salivary gland) • Potassium excretion
Catecholamines
• ↑ Heart rate • Modulate vascular tone (vasoconstriction by noradrenaline and vasodilatation by adrenaline) • Antagonise insulin action

type 2 (11β-HSD), which converts cortisol to its inactive metabolite, cortisone. Loss of this protection of mineralocorticoid receptors by inhibition of 11β-HSD (e.g. by liquorice) results in cortisol acting as a potent sodium-retaining steroid.

Mineralocorticoids

Aldosterone is the body's most important sodium-retaining hormone, which acts via mineralocorticoid receptors. 11-deoxycorticosterone also has mineralocorticoid activity. The principal stimulus to aldosterone secretion is angiotensin II, a peptide produced by activation of the renin-angiotensin system (see Fig. 8.22, p. 587). Renin secretion from the juxtaglomerular apparatus is stimulated by low perfusion pressure in the afferent arteriole, low sodium filtration leading to low sodium concentrations at the macula densa, and increased sympathetic nerve activity. As a result, renin is increased in hypovolaemia and renal artery stenosis, and standing levels of renin are about double those when lying down.

Catecholamines

In humans, only a small proportion of circulating noradrenaline is derived from the adrenal medulla; much more is released from other nerve endings. However, the methyltransferase enzyme responsible for the conversion of noradrenaline to adrenaline is induced by glucocorticoids. Blood flow in the adrenal is centripetal so that the medulla is bathed in high concentrations of cortisol and is the major source of circulating adrenaline. In the absence of functioning adrenal medullae, e.g. after bilateral adrenalectomy, there appear to be no clinical consequences attributable to deficiency of circulating catecholamines. The contribution of these compounds as circulating hormones to homeostasis in humans is therefore uncertain.

Adrenal androgens

The control of adrenal androgen production is unclear. Certainly ACTH plays a role. However, there may be a separate androgen-stimulating hormone (ASH) which is responsible for the adrenarche and results in initial pubic hair development before puberty.

HYPERFUNCTION OF THE ADRENALS

GLUCOCORTICOID EXCESS: CUSHING'S SYNDROME

Aetiology

Causes of Cushing's syndrome are shown in the information box. By convention, pituitary-dependent cortisol excess, as described by Harvey Cushing, is called Cushing's disease. By far the most common cause is iatrogenic, due to prolonged immunosuppression with synthetic glucocorticoids such as prednisolone. Amongst endogenous causes, Cushing's disease is the most common (~ 80%). Both Cushing's disease and adrenal tumour are four times more common in women than men. In contrast, ectopic ACTH syndrome (often due to a small-cell carcinoma of the bronchus) is more common in men.

CLASSIFICATION OF CUSHING'S SYNDROME
ACTH-dependent
• Pituitary-dependent bilateral adrenal hyperplasia (i.e. Cushing's disease) • Ectopic ACTH syndrome (e.g. bronchial carcinoid, small-cell lung carcinoma, pancreatic carcinoma) • Iatrogenic (ACTH therapy)
Non-ACTH-dependent
• Iatrogenic (chronic glucocorticoid therapy, e.g. for asthma) • Adrenal adenoma • Adrenal carcinoma
Pseudo-Cushing's syndrome, i.e. cortisol excess as part of another illness
• Alcohol excess (biochemical and clinical features) • Major depressive illness (biochemical features only, some clinical overlap) • Primary obesity (mild biochemical features, some clinical overlap)

Clinical features

In both the clinical assessment and investigation of a patient with possible Cushing's syndrome, it is helpful to divide the assessment into two stages:

1. Does the patient have Cushing's syndrome?
2. If the answer to 1. is yes, what is the cause?

Table 8.13 Clinical features of Cushing's syndrome

Symptoms	(%)	Signs	(%)
Weight gain	91	Obesity	97
Menstrual irregularity	84	Plethora	94
Hirsutism	81	Moon face	88
Psychiatric	62	Hypertension	74
Backache	43	Bruising	62
Muscle weakness	29	Striae	56
		Muscle weakness	56

Does the patient have Cushing's syndrome?

The features common to all causes of glucocorticoid excess are indicated in Table 8.13 and Figure 8.20. Weight gain is the most common symptom and obesity the most frequent sign. The distribution of fat is classically described as centripetal (like a lemon on toothpicks) but generalised obesity may be just as common. Of course, most patients with obesity do not have Cushing's syndrome. Features which have the best predictive value in favour of Cushing's syndrome in an obese patient are bruising, myopathy and hypertension. However, any clinical suspicion of cortisol excess is best resolved by screening investigations.

Psychiatric disturbance, usually depression, is also common in Cushing's syndrome, but much more common in patients who do not have glucocorticoid excess. Unfortunately, major depressive illness is itself associated with elevated cortisol secretion, which resolves when mood improves. Depression does not cause other clinical features of Cushing's syndrome. Any clinical suspicion of cortisol excess in a depressed patient requires careful investigation.

Alcohol excess is another reversible cause of elevated cortisol secretion which does cause clinical features of Cushing's syndrome, the 'alcoholic pseudo-Cushing's syndrome'. This diagnosis is strongly suggested by a recent history of alcohol excess but can only be proven if the biochemical abnormalities resolve during a period of abstinence.

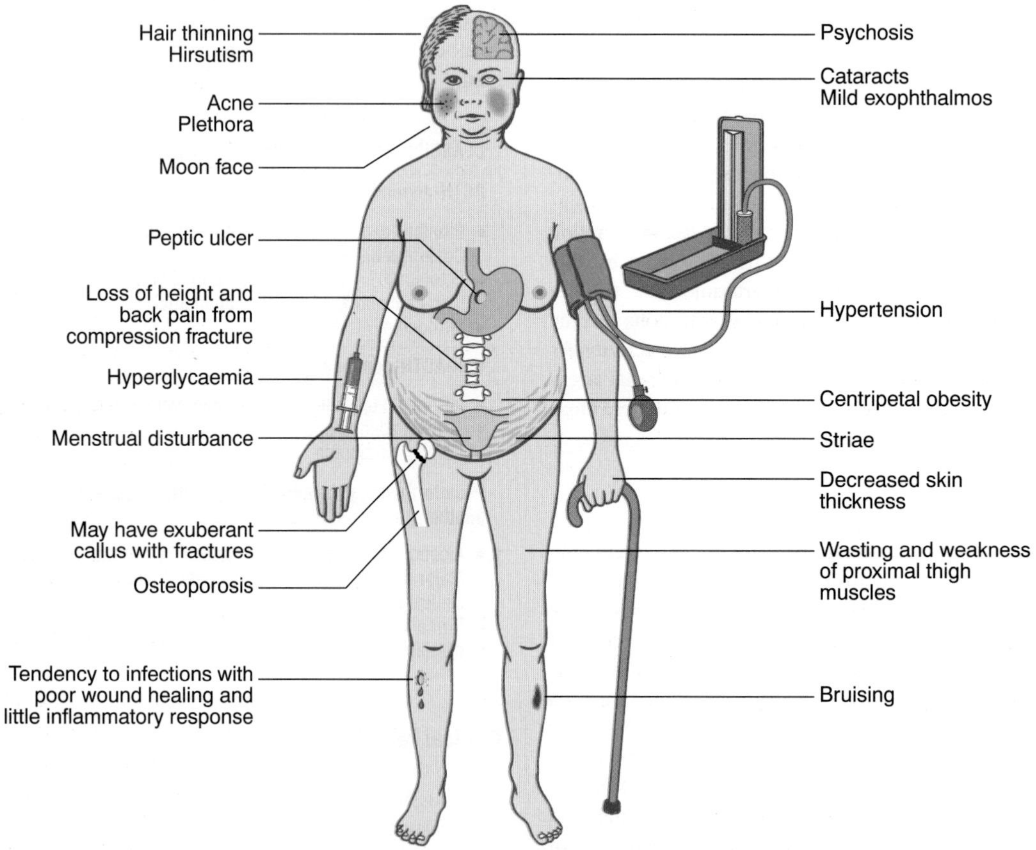

Fig. 8.20 Cushing's syndrome: clinical features common to all causes.

Table 8.14 Tests for Cushing's syndrome

Test	Protocol	Interpretation
Urine free cortisol	24-hr timed collection (some centres use overnight collections corrected for creatinine)	Normal range depends on assay
Overnight dexamethasone suppression test	1 mg orally at midnight; measure plasma cortisol at 0800–0900 hrs	Plasma cortisol < 60 nM excludes Cushing's
Diurnal rhythm of plasma cortisol	Sample for cortisol at 0900 hrs and at 2300 hrs (requires acclimatisation to ward for at least 48 hrs)	Evening level > 75% of morning level in Cushing's
Low-dose dexamethasone suppression test	0.5 mg 6-hourly for 48 hrs; sample 24-hr urine cortisol and 0900 hr plasma cortisol during second day	Urine cortisol < 100 nmol/day or plasma cortisol < 60 nM excludes Cushing's
Insulin tolerance test	See page 556	Peak plasma cortisol > 120% of baseline excludes Cushing's
High-dose dexamethasone suppression test	0.5 mg 6-hourly for 48 hrs; sample 24-hr urine cortisol at baseline and during second day	Urine cortisol < 50% of basal suggests pituitary-dependent disease; > 50% basal suggests ectopic ACTH syndrome
Corticotrophin-releasing hormone test	100 μg ovine CRH i.v. and monitor plasma ACTH and cortisol for 2 hrs	Peak plasma cortisol > 120% and/or ACTH > 150% of basal values suggests pituitary-dependent disease; lesser responses suggest ectopic ACTH syndrome
Inferior petrosal sinus sampling	Catheters placed in both inferior petrosal sinuses and simultaneous sampling from these and peripheral blood for ACTH; may be repeated 10 minutes after peripheral CRH injection	ACTH in either petrosal sinus > 200% peripheral ACTH suggests pituitary-dependent disease; < 150% suggests ectopic ACTH syndrome

What is the cause of Cushing's syndrome?

A history of glucocorticoid therapy is usually self-evident.

Some clinical features are more common in ectopic ACTH syndrome. Unlike pituitary tumours secreting ACTH, ectopic tumours have no residual negative feedback sensitivity to cortisol, and both ACTH and cortisol levels are usually higher than with other causes. Very high ACTH levels are associated with marked pigmentation. Very high cortisol levels overcome the barrier of 11β-HSD in the kidney and cause hypokalaemic alkalosis. Hypokalaemia aggravates both myopathy and hyperglycaemia (by inhibiting insulin secretion). When the tumour secreting ACTH is malignant (e.g. pancreatic or small-cell lung carcinomas) then the onset is usually rapid and may be associated with cachexia. For these reasons, the classical features of Cushing's syndrome are less common in ectopic ACTH syndrome, and if present suggest that a benign tumour (e.g. bronchial carcinoid) is responsible.

In Cushing's disease the pituitary tumour is almost always a microadenoma (less than 10 mm in diameter) so that other features of a pituitary macroadenoma (hypopituitarism, visual failure or disconnection hyperprolactinaemia) are rare.

Investigations

The investigation of Cushing's syndrome has confused students and postgraduates alike. The large number of tests available reflect the fact that no single test is infallible.

A recommended sequence of investigations is shown in Figure 8.21 and the interpretation of these tests is shown in Table 8.14. Some additional tests are useful in all cases of Cushing's syndrome, including plasma electrolytes, glucose, glycosylated haemoglobin and bone mineral density measurement.

Does the patient have Cushing's syndrome?

Cushing's syndrome is differentiated from normality and primary obesity by the demonstration of increased secretion of cortisol which fails to suppress with relatively low doses of dexamethasone. Increased secretion of cortisol can be detected in either plasma or urine. Plasma cortisol measured in the daytime is highly variable in healthy people, and often within this wide normal range in Cushing's syndrome. For this reason, there is no place for a random measurement of plasma cortisol in the clinic in either supporting or refuting a diagnosis of Cushing's syndrome. By contrast, plasma cortisol at midnight is low in all healthy people unless they have been stressed by venepuncture or recent admission (< 48 hours) to hospital. Evening plasma cortisol or 24-hour urine cortisol is therefore a useful measure to confirm Cushing's syndrome. However, both of these samples are awkward to obtain.

Dexamethasone is used for suppression testing because, unlike prednisolone, it does not cross-react in radioimmunoassays for cortisol. However, metabolism of dexamethasone may be altered by drugs, e.g. enzyme-inducers such as oestrogen or phenytoin. Also, the hypothalamic-pituitary-adrenal axis may 'escape' from suppression by

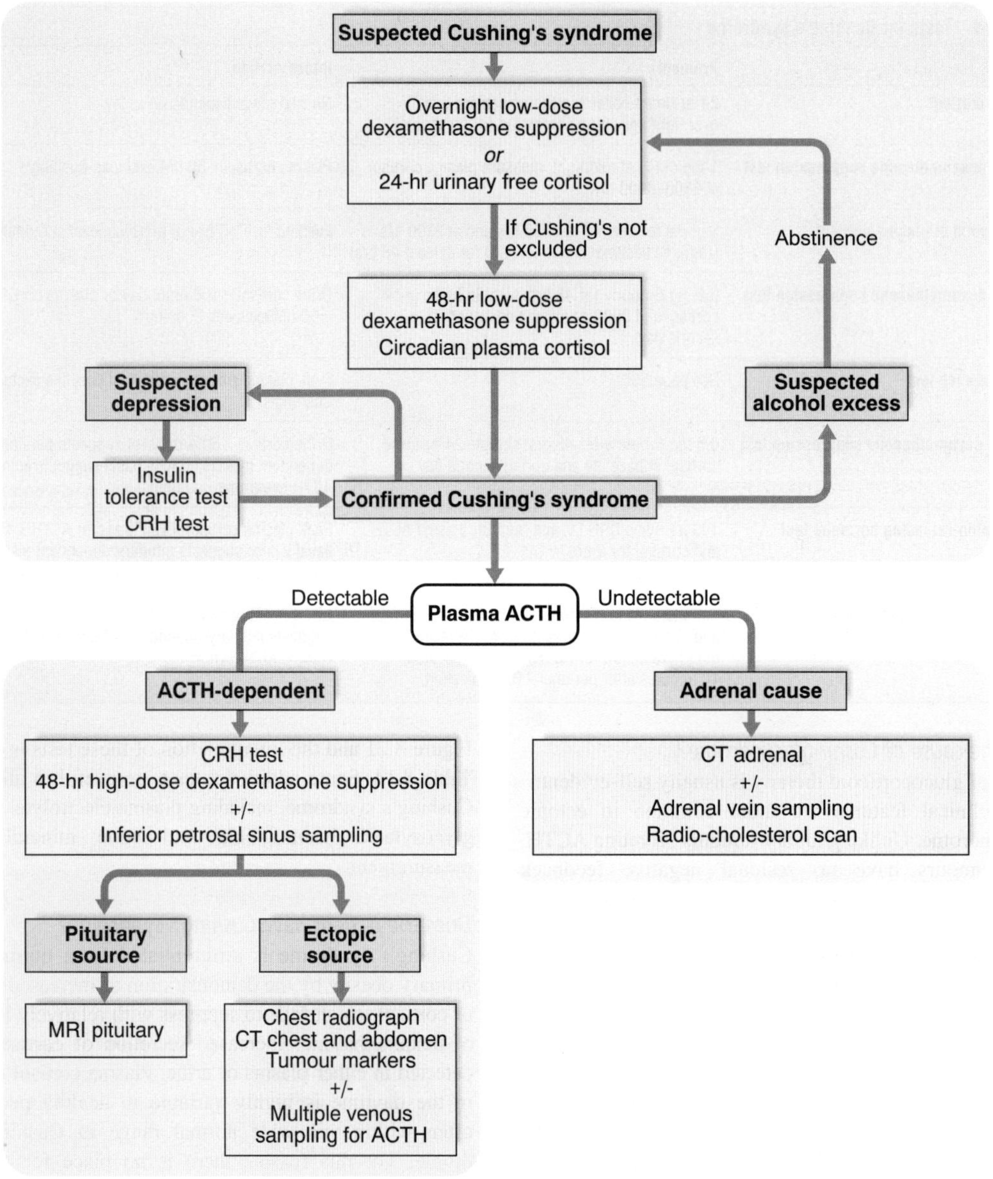

Fig. 8.21 Sequence of investigations in suspected Cushing's syndrome. (CRH = corticotrophin-releasing hormone)

dexamethasone if a more potent influence such as psychological stress supervenes.

There is a rare syndrome of *cyclical Cushing's syndrome* in which the excessive secretion of cortisol is episodic. If there is a strong clinical suspicion of Cushing's syndrome but initial screening tests are normal, then weekly 24-hour urine cortisol measurements are sometimes justified. The longest reported interval between episodes of hypercortisolaemia is 84 days.

What is the cause of the Cushing's syndrome?

Once the presence of Cushing's syndrome is established, measurement of plasma ACTH is a key step in establishing the differential diagnosis. In the presence of excess cortisol secretion an undetectable ACTH value indicates an adrenal tumour and any detectable ACTH in a random sample is pathological. Although ACTH levels above 300 ng/l suggest ectopic ACTH syndrome due to malignancy, further investigation is always necessary to discriminate pituitary from ectopic sources of ACTH. There is a small minority of patients in whom it is impossible to establish the cause of ACTH-dependent cortisol excess. These patients are usually treated medically and investigations repeated at a later date.

Tests which differentiate pituitary-dependent from ectopic ACTH production rely on the fact that pituitary tumours, but not ectopic tumours, retain some features of normal regulation of ACTH secretion. Thus, in Cushing's disease ACTH secretion is suppressed by dexamethasone, albeit at a higher dose than in normals, and ACTH is stimulated by corticotrophin-releasing hormone (CRH). Another test for this purpose which antedates the CRH test, involving administration of metyrapone, is now obsolete.

Techniques for localisation of tumours secreting ACTH or cortisol are shown in Figure 8.21. MRI with gadolinium contrast enhancement detects around 70% of pituitary microadenomas secreting ACTH (see Fig. 8.6, p. 550). Venous catheterisation with measurement of inferior petrosal sinus ACTH (i.e. draining directly from the pituitary) may be helpful in confirming Cushing's disease if the MRI scan does not show a microadenoma.

CT scanning detects most adrenal adenomas. Adrenal carcinomas are usually large (> 10 cm). If CT scanning does not demonstrate a unilateral tumour then lateralisation may be possible with either selective adrenal vein catheterisation and sampling for cortisol, or by functional adrenal scanning using ^{75}selenium-labelled cholesterol.

Management

This is essential, as untreated Cushing's syndrome has a 50% 5-year mortality. Most patients are prepared for surgery with medical therapy for a few weeks. Definitive surgery depends on the cause.

Medical therapy

A number of drugs inhibit corticosteroid biosynthesis. Metyrapone inhibits 11β-hydroxylase and increases 11-deoxycorticosterone levels, which causes hypokalaemia. Aminoglutethimide inhibits multiple enzymes including side-chain cleavage of cholesterol and is useful in combination with metyrapone. The dose of these agents is best titrated against 24-hour urine free cortisol.

Adrenal tumours

Adrenal adenomas should be surgically removed via laparoscopy or a loin incision. It may take several months for the contralateral adrenal and the hypothalamus and pituitary to recover from suppression. During this time suboptimal replacement therapy is required (0.5 mg dexamethasone in the morning). Adrenal carcinomas should also be resected if possible, the tumour bed irradiated and the patient given the adrenolytic drug o',p'-DDD. This may produce nausea and ataxia.

Cushing's disease

Trans-sphenoidal surgery with selective removal of the adenoma is the treatment of choice. Experienced surgeons can identify microadenomas which were not detected by MRI and cure about 80% of patients. Hypopituitarism and recurrence are rare. If no tumour is found and the diagnosis is definitely pituitary-dependent Cushing's, then a radical hypophysectomy may be required. If the diagnosis is not certain then bilateral adrenalectomy is an alternative.

If bilateral adrenalectomy is used in patients with pituitary-dependent Cushing's syndrome, then there is a risk that the pituitary tumour will grow in the absence of the negative feedback suppression previously provided by the elevated cortisol levels. This can result in *Nelson's syndrome*, with an aggressive pituitary macroadenoma and very high ACTH levels causing pigmentation. Nelson's syndrome can be prevented by pituitary irradiation.

External pituitary irradiation alone is of little value in adults but is surprisingly effective in children with Cushing's disease.

Following successful selective adenomectomy, plasma cortisol should be undetectable as the ACTH-producing cells around the adenoma are suppressed. The rest of the pituitary function will also need to be assessed (see p. 549). The patient should be given dexamethasone 0.5 mg daily in the morning and plasma cortisol measured (just before the dexamethasone dose) at monthly intervals. When cortisol is detectable, a short synacthen test can be performed to establish whether the hypothalamic-pituitary-adrenal axis has recovered, and dexamethasone stopped if appropriate. This recovery may take up to 18 months.

Ectopic ACTH syndrome

Benign tumours causing this syndrome (e.g. bronchial carcinoid) should be removed. Malignancies such as small-cell carcinoma of bronchus may initially respond to radiotherapy and chemotherapy. When they recur, medical therapy to inhibit cortisol synthesis may help to control severe hypokalaemia and hyperglycaemia.

MINERALOCORTICOID EXCESS

Aetiology

Causes of excessive activation of mineralocorticoid receptors are shown in the left-hand column of Table 8.15. Secondary hyperaldosteronism is described in Chapter 5 and is not dealt with here.

Clinical features

Mineralocorticoid receptor activation causes sodium retention and kaliuresis. Increased potassium excretion alters proton exchange in the distal nephron and at all cell

Table 8.15 Differential diagnosis of mineralocorticoid excess

	Plasma renin activity	Plasma aldosterone at 0900 hrs supine	Plasma aldosterone at 1200 hrs standing, relative to 0900 hrs supine	18-hydroxycortisol	Comments
Primary hyperaldosteronism					
Conn's adenoma	↓	↑	↓ (ACTH-responsive)	↑	
Bilateral adrenal hyperplasia	↓	↑	↑ (Angiotensin II-responsive)	→	
Glucocorticoid-suppressible hyperaldosteronism	↓	↑	↓ (ACTH-responsive)	↑↑	Chronic response to dexamethasone
Secondary hyperaldosteronism (see Ch. 5)	↑	↑		→	
Non-aldosterone mineralocorticoid excess					
Ectopic ACTH syndrome	↓	↓			Cortisol ↑
Liquorice or carbenoxolone administration/11β-hydroxysteroid dehydrogenase deficiency	↓	↓			↑ Ratio of metabolites of cortisol to cortisone in urine
Rare congenital adrenal hyperplasias (17α-hydroxylase and 11β-hydroxylase deficiencies)	↓	↓			↑ 11-deoxycorticosterone
11-deoxycorticosterone-secreting tumours	↓	↓			↑ 11-deoxycorticosterone
Liddle's syndrome	↓	↓			Response to amiloride but not spironolactone

membranes and causes an associated metabolic alkalosis with elevated plasma bicarbonate concentrations. Many patients are asymptomatic, but they may present with the symptoms of hypokalaemia (muscle weakness or even paralysis, especially in Chinese; polyuria secondary to renal tubular damage which produces nephrogenic diabetes insipidus; and occasionally tetany because of the metabolic alkalosis with low ionised calcium). In addition, peripheral oedema may occur both in primary hyperaldosteronism and in some forms of secondary hyperaldosteronism (e.g. hypoalbuminaemia or heart failure).

Hypertension is almost invariable in primary hyperaldosteronism and is the most common presenting feature. Indications for investigating the renin-angiotensin-aldosterone axis in hypertensive patients are given in Chapter 3. Not uncommonly, treatment with a thiazide diuretic produces marked hypokalaemia. Conversely, a low salt intake decreases the sodium available for exchange in the distal nephron and elevates plasma potassium. This might explain why as many as 70% of patients with primary hyperaldosteronism are normokalaemic.

The prevalence of primary hyperaldosteronism has been the subject of considerable debate. If only hypertensive patients with hypokalaemia are investigated then fewer than 1% of patients with hypertension will be found to have primary hyperaldosteronism. However, recent studies in which hypertensive patients have been investigated using aldosterone/renin profiling (see below) have suggested that the prevalence is about 5%. Of these about 70% have normal plasma potassium. In this larger group identified by screening, the prevalence of idiopathic bilateral adrenal hyperplasia is higher than that of adrenal adenoma (Conn's syndrome). Another group of hypertensive patients (~ 20%) have normal aldosterone levels but undetectable plasma renin activity. This is especially common in African populations, and may represent a subtle form of bilateral adrenal hyperplasia.

Investigations

Biochemical

Plasma electrolytes may show hypokalaemia and elevated bicarbonate. Plasma sodium is usually towards the upper end of the normal range in primary hyperaldosteronism but is characteristically low in secondary hyperaldosteronism (because low plasma volume stimulates ADH release and angiotensin II stimulates thirst).

To establish the presence of mineralocorticoid excess and to elucidate the cause, the key measurements are plasma renin activity and aldosterone (see Fig. 8.22). Almost all antihypertensive drugs interfere with these hormones (e.g. β-adrenoceptor antagonist drugs inhibit whilst thiazide diuretics stimulate renin secretion), so these should be stopped for at least 6 weeks beforehand. If this is not possible then the adrenergic neuron-blocking drug bethanidine (10 mg 8-hourly), which has minimal effect on the renin-angiotensin system, should be employed. Also, hypokalaemia suppresses aldosterone secretion so that

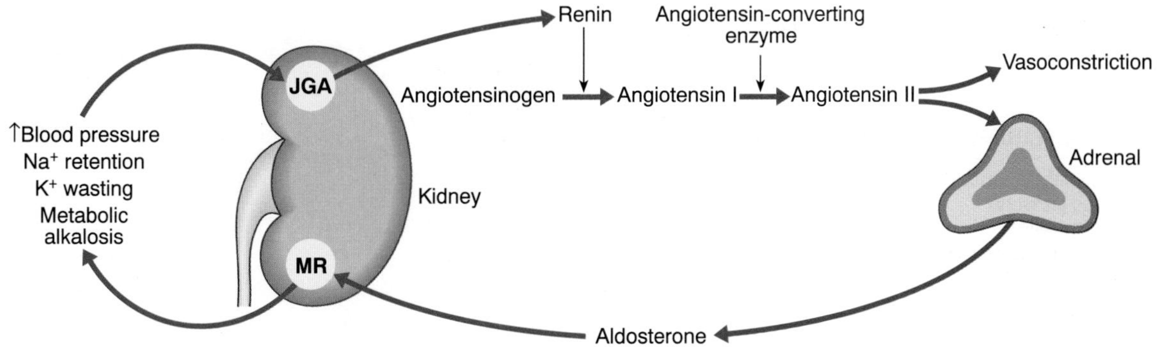

Fig. 8.22 The renin-angiotensin-aldosterone system. (JGA = juxtaglomerular apparatus; MR = mineralocorticoid receptor)

potassium supplementation may be required before the test. Similarly, an adequate sodium intake (> 100 mmol/day) is required to allow interpretation of plasma renin activity.

Given the special circumstances required to measure plasma renin activity and aldosterone, it is usually worth while performing tests which establish the diagnosis of mineralocorticoid excess and tests which identify its cause simultaneously. Thus, a 24-hour urine collection is analysed for sodium, potassium (to confirm that any hypokalaemia is due to kaliuresis) and 18-hydroxycortisol, and a sample stored for cortisol and corticosteroid metabolites if appropriate later. Blood for measurement of plasma renin activity, aldosterone and cortisol is withdrawn at 0800–0900 hrs after 30 minutes lying supine, and again at midday after 30 minutes standing. The interpretation of these tests is shown in Table 8.15. This manoeuvre allows the differentiation of excessive aldosterone secretion which is dependent on angiotensin II (rises on standing; e.g. normals and idiopathic adrenal hyperplasia) from that which is dependent on ACTH (falls from 0800 hrs to midday, confirmed by a fall in cortisol values; e.g. Conn's adenoma or glucocorticoid-suppressible hyperaldosteronism).

Localisation

The only cause of primary hyperaldosteronism which is usually treated by surgery is Conn's adenoma. Abdominal CT scanning is often the only test required to localise the tumour, but it is important to recognise that non-functioning adrenal adenomata are present in about 20% of patients with essential hypertension, and adrenal CT scans should only be performed when the biochemistry supports the diagnosis of adrenal tumour.

Sometimes the biochemistry and CT scan are not clear-cut. Adrenal vein catheterisation with measurement of aldosterone (and cortisol to confirm positioning of the catheters) is a difficult investigation to perform but may be necessary to establish whether aldosterone is unilateral or bilateral. Seleno-cholesterol scanning may also be helpful in demonstrating an adenoma. Unlike its use in the investigation of Cushing's syndrome (see p. 583), when localising a Conn's adenoma the test is performed with the patient on dexamethasone to suppress synthesis of other corticosteroids and so decrease uptake by the rest of the adrenal.

Management

The mineralocorticoid receptor antagonist spironolactone is valuable in treating both hypokalaemia and hypertension in all forms of mineralocorticoid excess. High doses (up to 400 mg/day) may be required. Up to 20% of males develop gynaecomastia on spironolactone. Amiloride (10–40 mg/day), which blocks the sodium–potassium channel regulated by aldosterone, can then be substituted.

In patients with Conn's adenoma, spironolactone is usually given for a few weeks to normalise whole-body electrolyte balance before unilateral adrenalectomy. Surgery cures the biochemical abnormality but hypertension remains in as many as 70% of cases, probably because of irreversible damage to the microcirculation.

Idiopathic hyperplasia may respond to spironolactone but often requires additional therapy for the hypertension. Adrenalectomy is not indicated.

In glucocorticoid-suppressible hyperaldosteronism, aldosterone is suppressed in a similar way to treatment of androgen excess in congenital adrenal hyperplasia (see p. 591).

CATECHOLAMINE EXCESS: PHAEOCHROMOCYTOMA

This is a rare tumour of chromaffin tissue which secretes catecholamines and is responsible for less than 0.1% of cases of hypertension. There is a useful 'rule of tens' in this condition: ~ 10% are malignant; ~ 10% are extra-adrenal (i.e. elsewhere in the sympathetic chain); and ~ 10% are familial.

Clinical features

These depend on the pattern of catecholamine secretion and are listed in the information box.

CLINICAL FEATURES OF PHAEOCHROMOCYTOMA

- Hypertension (usually paroxysmal; often postural drop of blood pressure)
- Attacks with
  - Pallor (occasionally flushing)
  - Palpitations
  - Sweating
  - Headache
  - Anxiety (fear of death—angor animi)
- Abdominal pain, vomiting
- Constipation
- Weight loss
- Glucose intolerance

Some patients may present with a complication of the hypertension, e.g. stroke, myocardial infarction, left ventricular failure or hypertensive retinopathy. Occasionally the patients may be hypotensive (especially those with dopamine-secreting tumours). There may be features of the familial syndromes associated with phaeochromocytoma including neurofibromatosis, von Hippel–Lindau syndrome, and multiple endocrine neoplasia type II (see p. 598).

Investigations

Biochemical

Excessive secretion of catecholamines can be confirmed by measuring the hormones (adrenaline, noradrenaline and dopamine) in plasma or their metabolites (e.g. vallinylmandelic acid, VMA; conjugated metanephrine and normetanephrine) in urine. However, catecholamine secretion is usually paroxysmal, so that measurements in a 24-hour urine collection are more useful than single plasma measurements for screening. Sometimes, the paroxysms are infrequent; in a patient with classical symptoms, phaeochromocytoma can only be excluded if the 24-hour urinary catecholamine excretion is normal on a day on which symptoms have occurred.

Increased urinary catecholamine excretion occurs in stressed patients (e.g. after myocardial infarction or major surgery) and is induced by some drugs (notably β-blockers and antidepressants). For this reason, a suppression test may be valuable. Normal adrenomedullary secretion is suppressed by administration of drugs which interfere with sympathetic outflow, such as clonidine or pentolinium. In phaeochromocytoma these drugs do not suppress plasma catecholamines. Provocative tests of catecholamine release should not be used.

Localisation

Once the biochemistry confirms a phaeochromocytoma, then the tumour must be localised. The biochemistry may help; only small adrenal tumours secrete large amounts of adrenaline (because of induction of phenylethanolamine-N-methyltransferase by cortisol—see p. 581). Large adrenal tumours which have outgrown the normal cortical supply, or extra-adrenal tumours, produce almost entirely noradrenaline.

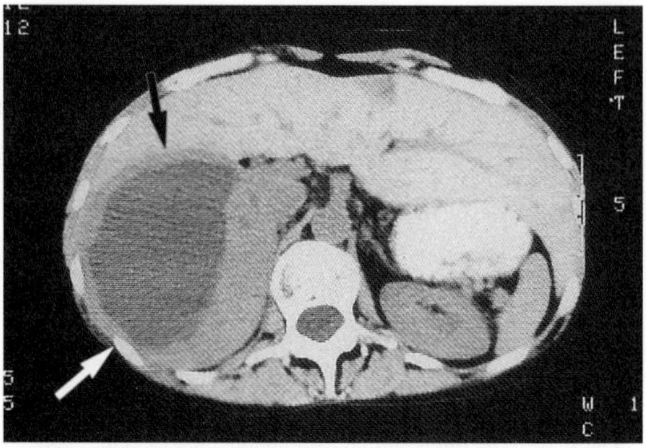

Fig. 8.23 CT scan of abdomen showing large right phaeochromocytoma (arrows).

Phaeochromocytomas are usually identified by CT scanning (see Fig. 8.23). Difficulty can arise with extra-adrenal tumours. Scintigraphy using meta-iodobenzyl guanidine (MIBG) can be useful; MIBG labelled with radioactive iodine is taken up by both benign and malignant phaeochromocytomas. If the tumour cannot be localised, then selective venous sampling with measurement of plasma noradrenaline may be required.

Management

Medical therapy is used to prepare the patient for surgery, preferably for a minimum of 6 weeks to allow restoration of normal plasma volume. The most useful drug in the face of very high circulating catecholamines is the α-blocker phenoxybenzamine (10–20 mg orally 3–4 times daily) because it is a non-competitive antagonist, unlike prazosin or doxazosin. If α-blockade produces a marked tachycardia then a β-antagonist drug such as propranolol (10–20 mg 3 times daily) should be added. On no account should the β-antagonist be given before the α-antagonist as vasoconstriction due to unopposed α-adrenoceptor activity may occur with a further increase in blood pressure.

During surgery sodium nitroprusside and the short-acting α-antagonist phentolamine are useful in controlling hypertensive episodes which may result from anaesthetic induction or tumour mobilisation. Post-operative hypotension may occur and require volume expansion and very occasionally noradrenaline. This is uncommon if the patient has been prepared with phenoxybenzamine for at least 6 weeks.

ADRENAL ANDROGEN EXCESS

Excess production of adrenal androgens may occur in ACTH-dependent Cushing's syndrome (see p. 581), with adrenal tumours (see description of hirsutism on p. 594), and in congenital defects in corticosteroid biosynthesis (see p. 591).

HYPOFUNCTION OF THE ADRENALS

Insufficiency of catecholamine secretion from the adrenal medulla is of no clinical importance unless it is accompanied by generalised autonomic neuropathy (see Ch. 14).

Adrenocortical failure can be divided into primary and secondary causes, as shown in the information box. Secondary adrenocortical insufficiency is discussed on pages 554 (hypopituitarism) and 591 (chronic glucocorticoid therapy).

CAUSES OF ADRENOCORTICAL INSUFFICIENCY

Primary (↑ ACTH)

Addison's disease

Common
- Autoimmune
  - Sporadic
  - Polyglandular syndromes (see p. 597)
- Tuberculosis
- Bilateral adrenalectomy

Rare
- Metastatic carcinoma, lymphoma
- Intra-adrenal haemorrhage (Waterhouse–Friedrichsen syndrome following meningococcal septicaemia)
- Amyloidosis
- Haemochromatosis
- Adrenal infarction or infection other than tuberculosis (esp. AIDS)

Corticosteroid biosynthetic enzyme defects
- Congenital adrenal hyperplasias
- Drugs
  - Aminoglutethimide, metyrapone, ketoconazole, etomidate etc.

Secondary (↓ ACTH)
- Hypothalamic or pituitary disease
- Glucocorticoid therapy

ADDISON'S DISEASE

Aetiology

This is a rare condition with an estimated incidence in the developed world of 8 cases per million population. However, adrenal insufficiency is a well-recognised complication in patients with AIDS and may result from a variety of causes including tuberculosis, fungal and cytomegalovirus infections. Thus, this figure is likely to be a significant underestimate.

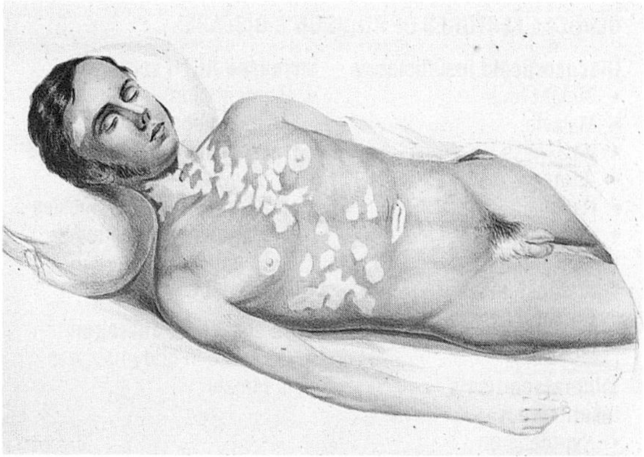

Fig. 8.24 Vitiligo in a patient with Addison's disease. This illustration was drawn by Addison in his original description in 1855 when he was an Edinburgh medical student.

Addison described the disease when he was a medical student in Edinburgh. His classic book *Diseases of the Suprarenal Capsules*, published in 1855, included detailed drawings of caseating adrenal tuberculosis. However, in one case in which the patient had gross vitiligo (a marker of autoimmune disease) he was unable to get an autopsy (see Fig. 8.24). Most likely this patient had autoimmune adrenalitis, now the most common cause of primary adrenal failure in the UK. As with other autoimmune diseases, this is more common in females than males (2:1).

Clinical features

These are listed in the information box. Deficiency of either glucocorticoids or mineralocorticoids may come first, but eventually all patients fail to secrete corticosteroids of any class. The patient may present with an acute, chronic, or acute on chronic illness.

Chronic presentation

With a chronic presentation, initial symptoms are often misdiagnosed (e.g. as chronic fatigue syndrome or depression) and it is the pigmentation that commonly raises suspicion.

The blood pressure may be normal with the patient lying down. Hence, the pressure should also be measured after standing for 1 minute. Postural hypotension (i.e. a fall in systolic pressure of at least 20 mmHg) is almost invariably present.

Vitiligo is present in 10–20% (see Fig. 8.24). Other autoimmune diseases which may be present are listed on page 597.

Acute presentation

Many patients are not diagnosed during the chronic phase and present with an acute adrenal crisis. Features include

CLINICAL FEATURES OF ADDISON'S DISEASE

Glucocorticoid insufficiency
- Weight loss
- Malaise
- Weakness
- Anorexia
- Nausea
- Vomiting
- Gastrointestinal—diarrhoea or constipation
- Postural hypotension
- Hypoglycaemia

Mineralocorticoid insufficiency
- Hypotension

Increased ACTH secretion
- Pigmentation
  - Sun-exposed areas
  - Pressure areas, e.g. elbows, knees
  - Palmar creases, knuckles
  - Mucous membranes
  - Conjunctivae
  - Recent scars

Loss of adrenal androgen
- Decrease in body hair, esp. in female

circulatory shock with severe hypotension, hyponatraemia, hyperkalaemia and, in some instances, hypoglycaemia. Muscle cramps, nausea, vomiting, diarrhoea and unexplained fever may be present. Intercurrent disease, surgery or infection may be the precipitating cause.

Investigations

The strategy for confirming the diagnosis depends upon the mode of presentation. In patients presenting with chronic illness, the investigations below should be performed before any treatment. In patients with suspected acute adrenal crisis treatment should not be delayed pending results of investigations. A random blood sample should be stored for measurement of cortisol, and it may be appropriate to spend 30 minutes performing a short ACTH stimulation test, but investigations may need to be performed after recovery.

Assessment of glucocorticoids

In health, plasma cortisol is highest in the morning, so that it is at this time that one would hope to be able to discriminate between normal and inadequate cortisol secretion. However, although in Addison's disease basal 0800 hr plasma cortisol is usually low, it may be within the normal reference range but inappropriately low for a seriously ill patient. Random measurement of plasma cortisol cannot therefore be used to confirm or refute a diagnosis of Addison's disease unless the value is high, i.e. > 550 nmol/l.

More useful is the short ACTH stimulation test (also called the tetracosactrin or short synacthen test) described in the information box on page 555. Patients with secondary adrenocortical insufficiency may also show a subnormal cortisol rise. They can be distinguished from primary adrenal failure either by measurement of ACTH (which is low in ACTH deficiency and high in Addison's disease) or by performing a long ACTH stimulation test (1 mg depot tetracosactrin intramuscularly daily for 3 days). In secondary insufficiency there is a progressive increase in plasma cortisol whereas in Addison's disease it is less than 700 nmol/l at 8 hours after the last injection.

If the patient is so ill that glucocorticoids have to be given prior to testing the adrenal response to ACTH, then the treatment should be changed to a synthetic steroid such as dexamethasone (0.75 mg/day), which does not cross-react in the plasma cortisol radioimmunoassay, prior to further investigation.

Assessment of mineralocorticoids

Patients with a combination of hyponatraemia and hyperkalaemia should always be investigated for Addison's disease. In secondary adrenocortical failure, when aldosterone secretion is intact, plasma sodium is often low but potassium is normal. Plasma renin activity and aldosterone should be measured in the supine position. In Addison's disease, plasma renin activity is nearly always high, with plasma aldosterone being either low or normal.

Other tests to establish the cause

Blood glucose (which may be low in hypocortisolaemia or high in associated diabetes mellitus) should be measured in all patients. In those who have autoimmune adrenal failure, antibodies can often be measured against steroid-secreting cells (adrenal and gonad), thyroid antigens, pancreatic β cells and parietal cells. Thyroid function tests, full blood count (for pernicious anaemia), and tests of gonadal function and serum calcium should be performed.

Other causes of adrenocortical disease are usually obvious clinically, particularly if health is not fully restored by corticosteroid replacement therapy. Tuberculosis causes adrenal calcification, visible on plain radiograph or ultrasound scan. A chest radiograph should also be taken.

Management

Patients with Addison's disease always need glucocorticoid replacement therapy and usually, but not always, mineralocorticoid. If the Addison's disease results from tuberculosis then this will need to be treated appropriately (see Ch. 4).

Glucocorticoid replacement

Cortisol (hydrocortisone) is the drug of choice. In the past, cortisone acetate was given but this has to be converted to cortisol by the liver and in some patients this process may be impaired. In someone who is not critically ill cortisol should be given by mouth, 15 mg on waking and 5 mg at 1800 hrs. The precise dose may need to be adjusted for the individual patient, but this is subjective. Excess weight gain usually indicates over-replacement, whilst persistent lethargy may be due to an inadequate dose. Measurement of plasma cortisol levels is unhelpful, because the dynamic interaction between cortisol and glucocorticoid receptors is not predicted by measurements such as the maximum or minimum plasma cortisol level after each dose. Advice to patients dependent on glucocorticoid replacement is given in the information box.

ADVICE TO PATIENTS ON GLUCOCORTICOID REPLACEMENT
Intercurrent stress
• e.g. Febrile illness—double dose of hydrocortisone
Surgery
• Minor operation—hydrocortisone 100 mg i.m. with premedication • Major operation—hydrocortisone 100 mg 6-hourly for 24 hours then 50 mg i.m. 6-hourly until ready to take tablets
Gastroenteritis
• Must have parenteral hydrocortisone if unable to take by mouth
Steroid card
• Patient should carry this at all times. Should give information regarding diagnosis, steroid, dose and doctor
Bracelet
• Patients should be encouraged to buy one of these and have it engraved with the diagnosis and a reference and phone number for a centrally held database

These are physiological replacement doses which do not cause Cushingoid side-effects.

The adrenal crisis is a medical emergency and requires intravenous hydrocortisone succinate 100 mg and intravenous fluid (normal saline and 10% dextrose for hypoglycaemia). Parenteral hydrocortisone should be continued (100 mg intramuscularly 6-hourly) until the gastrointestinal symptoms abate before starting oral therapy. The precipitating cause should be sought and, if possible, treated.

Mineralocorticoid replacement

Aldosterone is not readily available and *fludrocortisone* (i.e. 9α-fluoro-hydrocortisone) is the mineralocorticoid used. The halogen group prevents fludrocortisone from being metabolised by 11β-hydroxysteroid dehydrogenase and thereby confers a longer half-life and access to mineralocorticoid receptors. The usual dose is 0.05–0.1 mg daily. Adequacy of replacement can be assessed objectively by measurement of blood pressure, plasma electrolytes and plasma renin activity.

CONGENITAL DEFECTS IN CORTICOSTEROID BIOSYNTHESIS

Aetiology and clinical features

Defects in the cortisol biosynthetic pathway result in increased ACTH secretion via negative feedback. ACTH then stimulates the production of steroids up to the enzyme block. This produces adrenal hyperplasia. The most common enzyme defect is of 21-hydroxylase (see Fig. 8.19, p. 580). In about one-third of cases this defect affects both mineralocorticoid (aldosterone) and glucocorticoid (cortisol) production. This results in severe salt-wasting, which may be fatal in the first few weeks of life if untreated. In the other two-thirds, mineralocorticoid secretion is not affected but there may be features of cortisol insufficiency.

The increased ACTH drive results in high levels of 17OH-progesterone and androgens. The latter produce ambiguous genitalia or clitoromegaly in girls, accelerated growth and premature fusion of the epiphyses. In boys there may be enlargement of the penis and pubic hair development but without testicular enlargement (precocious pseudopuberty). Patients with mild impairment of 21-hydroxylase may present for the first time with hirsutism as adults ('late-onset'; see p. 595).

Defects of all the other enzymes have been described but are much rarer. 17-hydroxylase and 11β-hydroxylase deficiency may produce hypertension due to excess production of 11-deoxycorticosterone, a mineralocorticoid. All of these enzyme abnormalities are inherited as autosomal recessive traits. There is therefore a 1:4 chance that the sibling of an affected child will also have the disease, but a low risk of passing the disease to the next generation.

Investigations

High levels of plasma 17OH-progesterone are found in 21-hydroxylase deficiency. In late-onset cases this may only be demonstrated after ACTH administration. 17OH-progesterone can be measured in blood spot samples taken in the first week of life from heel pricks for phenylketonuria testing. Specific antenatal diagnosis can now be made by amniocentesis. Plasma electrolytes, renin activity and aldosterone should be measured. In children, bone age should be carefully followed by wrist radiographs.

Management

The aim is to suppress ACTH and hence adrenal androgen production by glucocorticoid therapy. In contrast with replacement therapy in other forms of cortisol deficiency, it is usual to give reverse replacement therapy, i.e. a larger dose of a long-acting synthetic glucocorticoid just before going to bed to suppress the nocturnal ACTH rise and a smaller dose in the morning. Treatment can be monitored by measuring profiles of ACTH and 17OH-progesterone through the day and aiming for levels within the normal range. However, complete suppression of the biochemical abnormalities carries a risk of inducing features of Cushing's syndrome. In adult women, a normal menstrual cycle is a guide to successful treatment. In children, growth velocity is the most useful measurement; either under- or over-replacement with glucocorticoids suppresses growth. Glucocorticoid treatment of an affected female can be started in utero if the diagnosis is made and hence virilisation prevented.

In 21-hydroxylase deficiency, fludrocortisone therapy may be required according to blood pressure and plasma renin activity.

Patients with late-onset 21-hydroxylase deficiency may not require glucocorticoid treatment. If hirsutism is the main problem, anti-androgen therapy may be just as effective (see p. 596).

USE OF CORTICOSTEROIDS IN THE TREATMENT OF DISEASE

The anti-inflammatory actions of glucocorticoids have led to their use in a wide variety of clinical conditions. Doses are listed in the information box.

EQUIVALENT DOSES OF GLUCOCORTICOIDS: ANTI-INFLAMMATORY POTENCY

- Hydrocortisone: 20 mg
- Cortisone acetate: 25 mg
- Prednisolone: 5 mg
- Dexamethasone: 0.75 mg

SIDE-EFFECTS OF GLUCOCORTICOID THERAPY

The side-effects are identical to the features of spontaneous Cushing's syndrome (see Fig. 8.20, p. 582). In addition, glucocorticoids cause insomnia. The effects are dose-related and hence, if possible, the dose should be kept to a minimum. Some patients will have pre-existing disease which is exacerbated by glucocorticoid therapy; particular care is required in patients with diabetes mellitus or previous episodes of glucose intolerance, to avoid symptomatic hyperglycaemia.

Even though the drug is being used for its anti-inflammatory effect this may produce problems. Thus signs of perforation of a viscus may be masked and the patient may show no febrile response to an infection. Gastric erosions are more common probably because of impaired prostaglandin synthesis. Hence the combination of corticosteroid with analgesic drugs such as aspirin may lead to haemorrhage from the stomach or duodenum. Latent tuberculosis may be reactivated and patients on corticosteroids should be advised to avoid contact with varicella zoster if they are not immune.

Osteoporosis is a particularly difficult problem in post-menopausal women who require long-term corticosteroids. There is some evidence that both sex hormone replacement therapy and bisphosphonates protect the bones in this setting.

WITHDRAWAL OF GLUCOCORTICOID THERAPY

All glucocorticoid therapy, even inhaled or topical treatment, can suppress the hypothalamic-pituitary-adrenal axis (HPA). In practice, this only leads to a risk of a hypo-adrenal crisis if glucocorticoids have been administered orally or systemically for longer than 10 days. In these circumstances, the drug must be withdrawn slowly when it is no longer required for the underlying condition, and the rate of withdrawal depends on the duration of treatment. If glucocorticoid therapy has been prolonged, then it may take many months for the HPA to recover. All patients must be advised to avoid sudden drug withdrawal. They should be issued with a steroid card or wear an engraved bracelet.

It should help the axis to recover if there is no exogenous glucocorticoid present during the nocturnal surge in ACTH secretion, i.e. if the glucocorticoid is given in the morning or even on alternate days. Giving ACTH to stimulate adrenal recovery is of no value as the hypothalamus and pituitary remain suppressed.

In patients who have received glucocorticoids for longer than a few weeks, it is valuable to confirm that the HPA is recovering during glucocorticoid withdrawal. Once the dose of glucocorticoid is reduced to a minimum (e.g. 4 mg prednisolone or 0.5 mg dexamethasone per day) then measure plasma cortisol at 0900 hrs before the next dose. If this is detectable, then perform an ACTH stimulation test (see p. 555) to confirm that glucocorticoids can be withdrawn safely.

FURTHER INFORMATION ON THE ADRENAL GLANDS

Bravo E L 1994 Evolving concepts in the pathophysiology, diagnosis and treatment of phaeochromocytoma. Endocrine Reviews 15: 356–368

Edwards C R W 1995 Adrenocortical diseases. In: Oxford textbook of medicine, 3rd edn. Oxford University Press, Oxford

Trainer P J, Grossman A 1991 The diagnosis and differential diagnosis of Cushing's syndrome. Clinical Endocrinology 34: 317–330

THE REPRODUCTIVE SYSTEM

FUNCTIONAL ANATOMY AND PHYSIOLOGY

In the male, the testis subserves two principal functions: synthesis of testosterone by the interstitial Leydig cells under the control of LH, and spermatogenesis by Sertoli cells under the control of FSH (but also requiring adequate testosterone).

In the female, physiology is complicated by variations in function during the normal menstrual cycle. FSH produces growth and development of ovarian follicles during the first 14 days after the menses. This leads to a gradual increase in oestradiol production from granulosa cells, which initially suppresses FSH secretion (negative feedback) but then, above a certain level, stimulates an increase in both the frequency and amplitude of GnRH pulses, resulting in a marked increase in LH secretion (positive feedback). The mid-cycle peak of LH (the LH surge) induces ovulation. After release of the ovum the follicle differentiates into a corpus luteum which secretes progesterone (the luteal phase). Withdrawal of progesterone results in menstrual bleeding. Circulating levels of oestrogen and progesterone in pre-menopausal women are, therefore, critically dependent on the time of the cycle. The most useful test of ovarian function is a careful menstrual history. In addition, ovulation can be confirmed by measuring progesterone during the luteal phase. Disorders of the female reproductive tract are usually treated by gynaecologists and are described here only in brief.

CLINICAL SYNDROMES IN THE MALE

HYPOGONADISM

Causes of hypogonadism are listed in the information box. The clinical features of primary (failure of the testis) and secondary (failure of the hypothalamus or anterior pituitary) hypogonadism are identical, and are described in the section on hypopituitarism (see p. 554). Patients commonly present with gynaecomastia, erectile impotence, infertility or delayed puberty (see short stature, p. 558).

Hypogonadism is confirmed by demonstrating a low random serum testosterone level. Testosterone is largely bound in plasma to sex hormone-binding globulin, and this can also be measured to confirm that the free androgen level is low. The distinction between primary and secondary hypogonadism is made by measurement of random LH and FSH. Patients with hypogonadotrophic hypogonadism should be investigated as described on page 549. Patients with hypergonadotrophic hypogonadism should have the testes examined for cryptorchidism or tumours, have measurement of serum ferritin (to exclude haemochromatosis), and a karyotype (to identify Klinefelter's syndrome). If there is no obvious cause, then no further investigations are necessary.

Treatment for androgen deficiency is described on pages 558 (short stature) and 556 (hypopituitarism).

GYNAECOMASTIA

Gynaecomastia is the presence of glandular breast tissue in males. Normal breast development in women is oestrogen-dependent but androgens oppose this effect. Gynaecomastia results from an imbalance between androgen and oestrogen activity, which may reflect androgen deficiency or oestrogen excess. Prolactin stimulates milk production in breast tissue which has been primed with oestrogen, but hyperprolactinaemia is rarely associated with gynaecomastia and galactorrhoea in men; if present, it is explained by the androgen deficiency which results from suppression of LH and FSH by prolactin, and not by the prolactin excess itself.

CAUSES OF GYNAECOMASTIA
Idiopathic
Physiological/Peripubertal
Drug-induced
• Cimetidine • Digoxin • Spironolactone • Anti-androgen therapies for prostatic carcinoma • Some exogenous anabolic steroids, e.g. stilboestrol
Hypogonadism
Primary • Klinefelter's syndrome • Autoimmune gonadal failure • Mumps orchitis • Haemochromatosis • Tuberculosis • Chemotherapy or irradiation • Rare forms of congenital adrenal hyperplasia Secondary • Hypopituitarism • Kallmann's syndrome (GnRH deficiency) • Hyperprolactinaemia Androgen resistance syndromes • Testicular feminisation syndrome • 5α-reductase deficiency
Oestrogen excess
• Liver failure (impaired steroid metabolism) • Oestrogen-secreting tumour • Human chorionic gonadotrophin (hCG)-secreting tumour

Clinical assessment

A drug history is important. Palpation allows gynaecomastia to be distinguished from the prominent soft tissue around the nipple often seen in obesity. Unilateral gynaecomastia should be treated as breast carcinoma unless proved otherwise. Features of hypogonadism should be sought (lethargy, less frequent shaving, loss of libido, erectile impotence and soft small testes).

Investigations and management

A random blood sample should be taken for testosterone, LH, FSH, oestradiol, prolactin and human chorionic gonadotrophin. If these tests are normal, and no drug is responsible, then there is no useful endocrine therapy. Surgical excision may be justified by cosmetic appearance, except in young boys with a short history in whom gynaecomastia may resolve. The surgical approach should be through a small incision around the nipple, and is best performed by a specialist in plastic surgery.

ERECTILE IMPOTENCE

Aetiology and clinical features

Causes of erectile failure are shown in the information box. With the exception of diabetes mellitus, endocrine causes are relatively uncommon, and vascular and psychosexual causes are common. Judging from experience in diabetic clinics, impotence is a markedly under-diagnosed problem. It is important to be able to discuss things frankly with the patient, establish whether there are associated features of hypogonadism (loss of libido, lethargy, less frequent shaving and soft small testes), and whether erections occur at any other time (i.e. whether the patient ever has an erection on wakening in the morning, making vascular and neuropathic causes much less likely).

CAUSES OF IMPOTENCE
With reduced libido
• Hypogonadism (see the information box, p. 593)
With intact libido
• Psychosexual • Vascular insufficiency (atheroma) • Neuropathic (e.g. diabetes mellitus, alcohol excess, multiple sclerosis)

Investigations

Blood should be taken for glucose, glycated haemoglobin, prolactin, testosterone, LH and FSH. Nocturnal tumescence monitoring (using a plethysmograph placed around the shaft of the penis overnight) is useful to establish whether blood supply and nerve function are sufficient to allow erections to occur during sleep. Intracavernosal injection (with papaverine or prostaglandin E_1) tests the adequacy of the blood supply. If it is deficient, then angiography may be performed to examine the internal pudendal arteries, but this is rarely indicated since there are few patients who are suitable for surgical intervention to these vessels. Tests of autonomic and peripheral sensory nerve conduction may be relevant.

Management

Specific causes should be treated as described elsewhere. Psychotherapy which includes the sexual partner is most useful for psychosexual problems. Neuropathy and vascular disease are unlikely to improve, but several manoeuvres may be useful. These include self-administered intracavernosal injections with prostaglandin E_1; vacuum devices which achieve an erection which is maintained by a tourniquet around the base of the penis; and prosthetic implants, either of a fixed rod or of an inflatable reservoir. Many patients elect not to use these methods, but unfortunately even more are unaware of their availability.

MALE INFERTILITY

Around 10% of couples have difficulty in conceiving children. This is attributable in roughly equal thirds to infertility in the female, infertility in the male, and idiopathic cases. Although it is common for women to present the problem to their doctor, the male should not be excluded from the assessment. He should be examined for varicocele or other testicular abnormality. A semen analysis should be performed. If he has oligospermia, then blood should be taken for prolactin, testosterone, FSH and LH. If the only biochemical abnormality is a high FSH, then an irreversible failure of spermatogenesis is likely. (The FSH rises because of lack of β-inhibin.) Testicular biopsy is rarely indicated.

In patients with gonadotrophin deficiency, fertility can be induced over several months, as described on page 556. This is usually performed once, and sperm stored for subsequent artificial insemination.

CRYPTORCHIDISM

Cryptorchidism (undescended testis) usually occurs in otherwise normal boys but may be the presenting feature of hypogonadotrophic hypogonadism. Highly retractile testes, particularly in an obese boy, may be mistaken for cryptorchidism. If the testes remain in the inguinal canal they are more liable to trauma than if situated in the scrotum. The seminiferous tubules will fail to develop in an undescended gland and, if the condition is bilateral, sterility will follow. Even in testes which remain undescended into adult life the interstitial cells function normally, so that the secondary sex characteristics develop in the usual way. In maldescent the testis takes an abnormal route and is liable to develop malignancy.

Human chorionic gonadotrophin or intranasal GnRH can induce descent in about 40% of children, but if this fails, or the condition is discovered in adulthood, then the testis or testes should either be removed or placed in the scrotum surgically.

CLINICAL SYNDROMES IN THE FEMALE

HIRSUTISM

Hirsutism is the excessive growth of thick terminal hair in an androgen-dependent distribution in women (upper lip, chin, chest, back, lower abdomen, thigh, forearm) and should be distinguished from hypertelorism, which is generalised excessive growth of vellus hair. The aetiology of androgen excess is shown in Table 8.16.

Clinical features and diagnosis

The severity of hirsutism is subjective. Some women suffer

Table 8.16 Causes of hirsutism

	Clinical features	Investigation findings	Treatment
Idiopathic	Often familial Mediterranean or Asian background	Normal	Cosmetic measures Anti-androgens
Polycystic ovarian syndrome	Obesity Oligomenorrhoea or 2° amenorrhoea Infertility ± Glucose intolerance ± Dyslipidaemia ± Hypertension	LH:FSH ratio > 2.5:1 Minor elevation of androgens* Elevated oestrone Mild hyperprolactinaemia	Weight loss Cosmetic measures Anti-androgens (Insulin sensitising drugs may be useful)
Congenital adrenal hyperplasia (95% 21-hydroxylase deficiency)	Pigmentation History of salt-wasting in childhood, ambiguous genitalia, or adrenal crisis when stressed Jewish background	Elevated androgens* which suppress with dexamethasone Abnormal rise in 17OH-progesterone with ACTH	Glucocorticoid replacement administered in reverse rhythm to suppress ACTH
Exogenous androgen administration	Athletes Virilisation	Low LH and FSH Androgens depend on which steroid is being taken	Stop steroid abuse
Androgen-secreting tumour of ovary or adrenal cortex	Rapid onset Virilisation: clitoromegaly, deep voice, balding, breast atrophy	High androgens* which do not suppress with dexamethasone or oestrogen CT scan shows a tumour	Surgical excision
Cushing's syndrome	Clinical features of Cushing's syndrome (see p. 582)	Normal or mild elevation of adrenal androgens*	Treat the cause

* e.g. Serum testosterone levels in women: < 2 nM is normal; 2–4 nM is mild elevation; > 4 nM is high and requires further investigation.

profound embarrassment from a degree of hair growth which others would not consider remarkable. Other important observations are a drug and menstrual history, calculation of body mass index, measurement of blood pressure, examination for virilisation (see Table 8.16), and associated features including acne vulgaris or Cushing's syndrome (see Fig. 8.20, p. 582). Hirsutism of recent onset associated with virilisation is suggestive of an androgen-secreting tumour, but these are rare.

Investigations

A random blood sample should be taken for testosterone, prolactin, LH and FSH. Measurement of adrenal androgens (dehydroepiandrosterone sulphate and androstenedione) may be helpful in localising the source of androgen excess, but are no more helpful than testosterone alone in diagnosing androgen excess. Oestrone is an oestrogen produced from oestradiol by 17β-hydroxysteroid dehydrogenase in adipose tissue, which is characteristically elevated in polycystic ovarian syndrome, but few laboratories provide oestrone assays. If there are clinical features of Cushing's syndrome, an overnight 1 mg dexamethasone suppression test should be performed (see p. 583).

If testosterone levels are elevated above twice the upper limit of the normal female range, especially if this is associated with low LH and FSH, then idiopathic hirsutism and polycystic ovarian syndrome are less likely, and the source of the androgen excess should be established. Congenital adrenal hyperplasia due to 21-hydroxylase deficiency is diagnosed by a short ACTH stimulation test with measurement of 17OH-progesterone (see p. 591). In patients with androgen-secreting tumours, serum testosterone does not suppress following dexamethasone (either as an overnight or 48-hour low-dose suppression test) or oestrogen (30 μg daily for 7 days). The tumour should then be sought by CT scans of adrenals and ovaries.

Management

Most patients will have used cosmetic measures such as bleaching and waxing before consulting a doctor. Electrolysis is effective for small areas, e.g. upper lip and chest hair, but is expensive. The pathophysiology of the common causes of hirsutism is poorly understood, but insulin resistance may be an important mediator in polycystic ovarian syndrome. Weight loss is a vital step to enhance insulin sensitivity and reduce the peripheral conversion of oestrogen to androgen (by aromatase) and oestradiol to oestrone in adipose tissue. In addition, insulin-sensitising drugs such as the thiazolidinediones and biguanides (see Ch. 7) may prove to have a role.

If these conservative measures have been tried and have failed, then anti-androgen therapy may be employed, as shown in Table 8.17. The life cycle of each hair follicle is at least 3 months so that no improvement is likely to be noticed before this time, when previous follicles have all

Table 8.17 Anti-androgen therapy

Mechanism of action	Drug	Dose	Hazards
Androgen receptor antagonists	Cyproterone acetate	2, 50 or 100 mg on days 1–11 of 28-day cycle with ethinyloestradiol 30 μg on days 1–21	Hepatic dysfunction Feminisation of male fetus Progesterone receptor agonist Dysfunctional uterine bleeding
	Spironolactone	100–200 mg daily	Electrolyte disturbance Carcinogenic in rats
	Flutamide	Not recommended	Hepatic dysfunction
5α-reductase inhibitors (prevent conversion of testosterone to active dihydrotestosterone)	Finasteride	Not recommended	Unproven efficacy
Suppression of ovarian steroid production	Oestrogen	See combination with cyproterone acetate above OR Conventional oestrogen-containing contraceptive	Venous thromboembolism Hypertension Weight gain Dyslipidaemia Increased breast and endometrial carcinoma
Suppression of adrenal androgen production	Exogenous glucocorticoid to suppress ACTH	e.g. Hydrocortisone 5 mg at 0900 hrs and dexamethasone 0.5 mg at 2200 hrs	Cushing's syndrome

shed their hair and replacement hair growth has been suppressed. Unless the patient has lost weight, the hirsutism will return if therapy is discontinued. The patient should be aware that prolonged exposure to some of these agents may not be desirable, and the prescription should be reviewed at least every 6 months.

SECONDARY AMENORRHOEA

The causes of this common problem are shown in the information box.

SECONDARY AMENORRHOEA

Hypothalamic dysfunction

- See page 557; also anorexia nervosa, excessive exercise, psychogenic

Pituitary disease

- See page 554; especially hyperprolactinaemia

Ovarian dysfunction

- Polycystic ovary syndrome
- Androgen-secreting tumours
- Autoimmune (premature menopause)
- Turner mosaic
- Menopause (see below)

Adrenal disease

- Cushing's syndrome, congenital adrenal hyperplasia, androgen-secreting tumours

Thyroid disease

- Hypo- and hyperthyroidism

Other conditions

- Severe systemic disease, e.g. renal failure, endometrial tuberculosis

Clinical features

These will depend on the condition. If there is weight loss then this may be primary as in anorexia nervosa, or secondary to an underlying disease such as tuberculosis, malignancy or hyperthyroidism. Weight gain may suggest Cushing's syndrome, hypothyroidism or, very rarely, a hypothalamic lesion. Hirsutism, obesity and long-standing irregular periods suggest the polycystic ovary syndrome and should be assessed as described above. The breasts need to be carefully examined for milk. The presence of other autoimmune disease should raise the possibility of autoimmune ovarian failure.

Investigations

Blood should be taken for LH, FSH, oestradiol, prolactin and TSH. In the absence of a menstrual cycle these can be taken at any time. High levels of LH and FSH with low or low-normal oestradiol suggest primary ovarian failure. Elevated LH with normal oestradiol is common in the polycystic ovary syndrome. Investigation of hyperprolactinaemia is described on page 551. Low levels of LH, FSH and oestradiol suggest hypothalamic or pituitary disease. Assessment of bone mineral density is appropriate in patients with low androgens and oestrogens.

Management

This depends on the cause.

THE MENOPAUSE

The cessation of menstruation in Western women occurs at a median age of 50.8 years. In the 5 years before there is a gradual increase in the number of anovulatory cycles. This period is referred to as the climacteric. Oestrogen and inhibin secretion falls and negative feedback results in increased pituitary secretion of LH and FSH.

Clinical features

Irregular periods commonly precede the menopause and hence the exact timing of it can only be recognised in retrospect (e.g. 6 months after the last period).

Menopausal symptoms relate to oestrogen deficiency. In some patients they are relatively minor but in others they are a major problem. The flushes may start when the patient still has regular periods and in about 25% of women they go on for more than 5 years. Their precise cause remains unknown but they are associated with an LH pulse.

MENOPAUSAL SYMPTOMS

Vasomotor effects
- Hot flushes
- Sweating

Psychological
- Anxiety
- Emotional lability
- Irritability

Genitourinary
- Dyspareunia ('senile vaginitis')
- Vaginal infections ↑
- Urgency of micturition

In the longer term, the fall in oestrogen secretion is associated with increased bone resorption and a risk of *osteoporosis* (see Ch. 12). Before the menopause, women have lower rates of cardiovascular disease than men, but this advantage is substantially reduced after the menopause.

Management

Many women seek explanation and reassurance rather than treatment.

Oestrogen replacement therapy (usually called HRT) is effective for menopausal symptoms and prevents osteoporosis. There is some evidence of benefit for cardiovascular disease. However, there is a small increase in risk of breast and endometrial cancer and of venous thromboembolism. Unlike the higher doses of oestrogen used for contraception, HRT probably has no adverse effect on blood pressure. The decision on whether to use HRT must be made on an individual basis, weighing up risk factors for these various benefits and complications, especially family history. Patients with a premature menopause (< 45 years) should be encouraged to take HRT.

Oestrogen should not be given 'unopposed' (i.e. without progesterone) in women who have not had a hysterectomy as there is then a high risk of endometrial cancer. However, although theoretically better, it is no longer considered essential to induce withdrawal bleeds, and combined oestrogen and progesterone can be given continuously. Both oestrogen and progesterone can be given either orally or by topical patches.

It is often difficult to say how long to continue HRT, but as a rough guide patients should be offered treatment for 10 years or until the age of 60 years, whichever comes sooner.

In patients who decide against oestrogen replacement (e.g. strong family history of breast cancer) vasomotor symptoms may be helped by clonidine 50 μg 12-hourly. Vaginal and urinary symptoms may be helped by topical oestrogen cream.

FURTHER INFORMATION ON THE REPRODUCTIVE SYSTEM

Conway G S 1996 Polycystic ovary syndrome: clinical aspects. Baillière's Clinical Endocrinology and Metabolism 10: 263–279

Lindsay R, Bush T L, Grady D, Speroff L, Lobo R A 1996 Estrogen replacement in menopause. Journal of Clinical Endocrinology and Metabolism 81: 3829–3838

ENDOCRINE SYNDROMES AFFECTING MULTIPLE GLANDS

There are two pathologies which can affect multiple glands: organ-specific autoimmune diseases and neoplasia.

AUTOIMMUNE DISEASE

Mechanisms of autoimmunity are discussed in Chapter 1. From an endocrinology perspective, these disorders cluster into two syndromes, as shown in the information box. In patients who present with one gland affected, the likelihood of developing further endocrine deficiency is variable, and can be predicted only in part by the detection of circulating antibodies against the different antigens in each gland. The only one of these disorders which is sufficiently prevalent to justify routine screening when antibodies are detected in the absence of any other affected gland is primary hypothyroidism. The annual incidence of hypothyroidism

AUTOIMMUNE 'POLYGLANDULAR' SYNDROMES

Type 1	Type 2
• Addison's disease	• Primary hypothyroidism
• Chronic mucocutaneous candidiasis	• Primary hypogonadism
• Hypoparathyroidism	• Diabetes mellitus type I
	• Pernicious anaemia
	• Addison's disease
	• Vitiligo

in patients with circulating antimicrosomal and anti-thyroglobulin antibodies is ~ 2%.

MULTIPLE ENDOCRINE NEOPLASIA (MEN)

A small number of patients with some of the disorders described in this chapter come from families in which multiple glands are susceptible to hyperplasia and formation of adenomas or malignant tumours. These autosomal dominant syndromes fall into two groups, as shown in the information box. In addition, there are families in which single tumours are more prevalent, e.g with acromegaly or phaeochromocytoma.

MEN syndromes should be considered in all patients with two or more of the relevant disorders (e.g. hypercalcaemia and pituitary tumour) or in those with single abnormalities who report other endocrine tumours in their family.

Important advances have been made in recent years to establish the genetic cause of these syndromes. The gene which is abnormal in MEN I has recently been cloned. Its product is called 'MENIN' but its function is not established. In MEN II, mutations in an area encoding a cysteine-rich sequence of the product of the RET proto-oncogene cause constitutive activation of a membrane-associated tyrosine kinase. RET is thought to control development of cells which migrate from the neural crest, and loss of function of the RET kinase is associated with Hirschsprung's disease.

As with all autosomal dominant disorders, there is a 50% chance that first-degree relatives will carry the affected gene. Previously, relatives of index cases had to be screened by biochemical tests (MEN I: plasma calcium, prolactin and gastrin; MEN II: plasma calcium, urinary metanephrines, and calcium-pentagastrin test with calcitonin measurements). Tumours could occur at any time of life so that these tests had to be repeated, usually annually. Now, accurate genetic diagnosis is available for both syndromes. Genetic counselling is required. Unaffected relatives not only avoid biochemical screening, but also know that they will not pass the condition to their children. In affected relatives with MEN II, prophylactic thyroid-ectomy is recommended at an early age to prevent medullary carcinoma of thyroid, and biochemical screening for the other manifestations is performed.

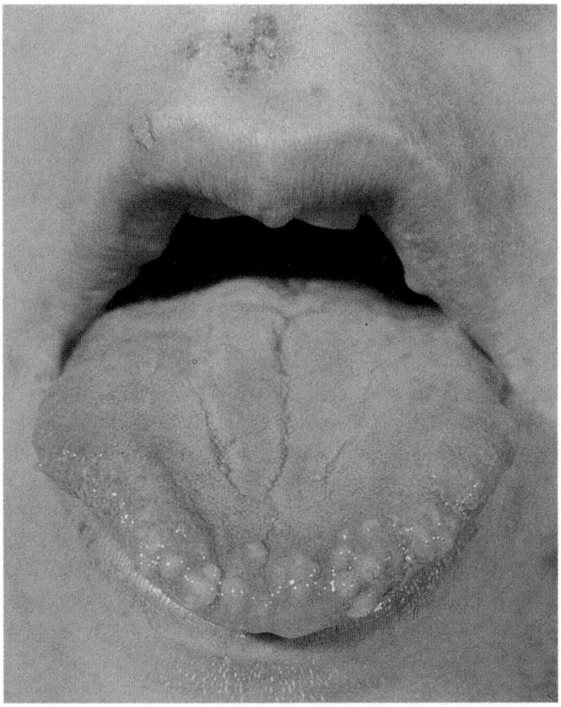

Fig. 8.25 Bumpy lips and tongue neuromas in patient with multiple endocrine neoplasia type IIb. The patient presented with vomiting and paroxysmal hypertension, and was found to have bilateral phaeochromocytomas and medullary carcinoma of thyroid.

MULTIPLE ENDOCRINE NEOPLASIA (MEN) SYNDROMES

MEN I (Wermer's syndrome)

- Primary hyperparathyroidism
- Functioning pituitary tumours
- Pancreatic tumours (e.g. insulinoma, gastrinoma)

MEN II (Sipple's syndrome)

- Primary hyperparathyroidism
- Medullary carcinoma of thyroid
- Phaeochromocytoma

In addition, in MEN IIb syndrome there are phenotypic changes (incl. marfanoid habitus, skeletal abnormalities, abnormal dental enamel, multiple mucosal neuromata; see Fig. 8.25)

FURTHER INFORMATION ON ENDOCRINE SYNDROMES AFFECTING MULTIPLE GLANDS

Jones D E J, Diamond A G 1995 The basis of autoimmunity: an overview. Baillière's Clinical Endocrinology and Metabolism 9: 1–24
Wick M J 1997 Clinical and molecular aspects of multiple endocrine neoplasia. Clinics in Laboratory Medicine 17: 39–57

Diseases of the alimentary tract and pancreas

9

K.R. PALMER • I.D. PENMAN

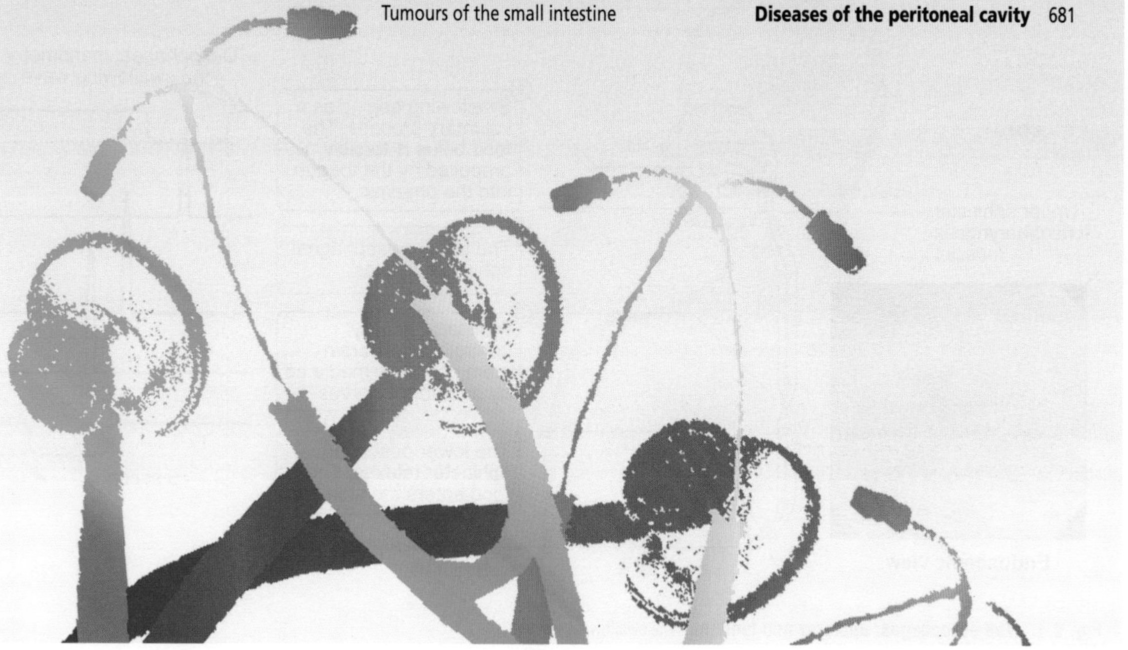

Diseases of the gastrointestinal tract are a major cause of morbidity and mortality. Approximately 10% of all general practitioner consultations in the United Kingdom are for indigestion, and 1 in 14 is for diarrhoea. Infective diarrhoea is responsible for much ill health and many deaths in the underdeveloped world. The gastrointestinal tract is the most common site for cancer development.

There have been great advances in the understanding, diagnosis and management of gastrointestinal diseases. We now realise that peptic ulcer disease is largely an infective condition due to *Helicobacter pylori*; we are aware of the molecular events in colon cancer development. Endoscopy has transformed diagnostic capability whilst therapeutic endoscopy has replaced much of operative surgery for gastrointestinal bleeding, tumour palliation and a range of biliary diseases. Powerful drugs alleviate dyspepsia and improve the lot of patients suffering from inflammatory bowel disease.

FUNCTIONAL ANATOMY, PHYSIOLOGY AND INVESTIGATIONS

FUNCTIONAL ANATOMY

OESOPHAGUS

The oesophagus is a muscular tube 25 cm long which extends from the cricoid cartilage to the cardiac orifice of the stomach. It has an upper and lower sphincter. A peristaltic swallowing wave propels the food bolus into the stomach (see Fig. 9.1).

STOMACH AND DUODENUM (see Fig. 9.2)

The stomach acts as a 'hopper', retaining and grinding food, then actively propelling the contents into the upper small bowel.

Gastric secretion (see Fig. 9.3)

Hydrogen ions, accompanied by chloride ions, are secreted in response to the activity of the hydrogen-potassium ATPase ('proton pump') from the apical membrane of the parietal cells. Acid sterilises the upper gastrointestinal tract and converts pepsinogen to pepsin. Pepsinogen is secreted by chief cells. The glycoprotein intrinsic factor, secreted in parallel with acid, is necessary for vitamin B_{12} absorption.

Gastrin and somatostatin

The hormones gastrin, derived from G cells in the antrum, and somatostatin, secreted from D cells throughout the stomach, interact to modulate gastric secretion and motility. Gastrin stimulates, whilst somatostatin suppresses acid secretion.

Protective factors

Bicarbonate ions and mucus together protect the gastroduodenal mucosa from the ulcerative properties of acid and pepsin.

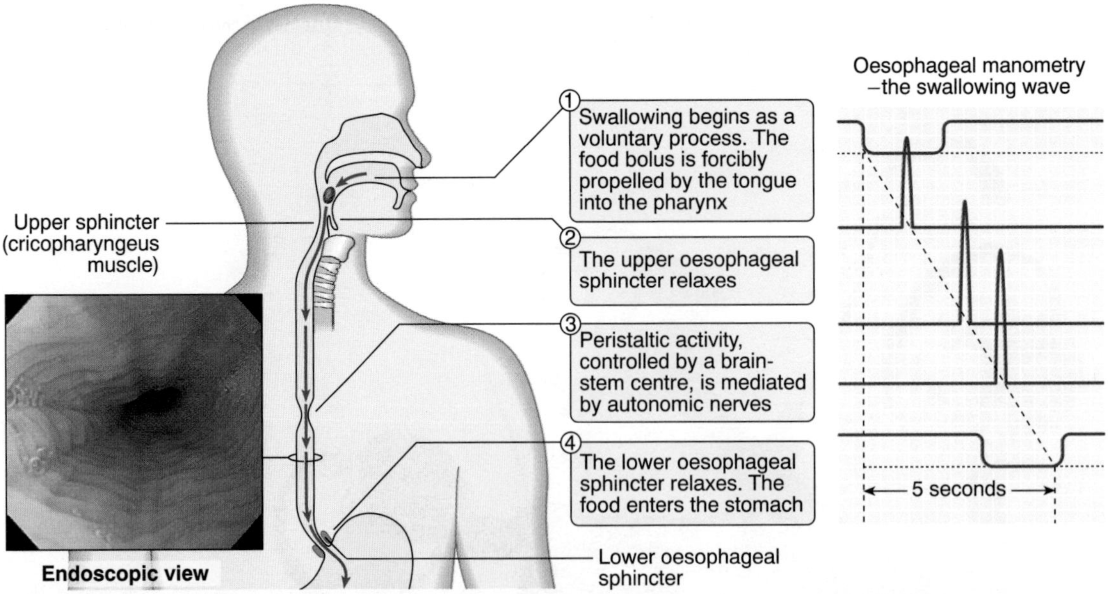
Upper sphincter (cricopharyngeus muscle)
Endoscopic view
1 Swallowing begins as a voluntary process. The food bolus is forcibly propelled by the tongue into the pharynx
2 The upper oesophageal sphincter relaxes
3 Peristaltic activity, controlled by a brain-stem centre, is mediated by autonomic nerves
4 The lower oesophageal sphincter relaxes. The food enters the stomach
Lower oesophageal sphincter
Oesophageal manometry –the swallowing wave
5 seconds

Fig. 9.1 The oesophagus: anatomy and function. The swallowing wave.

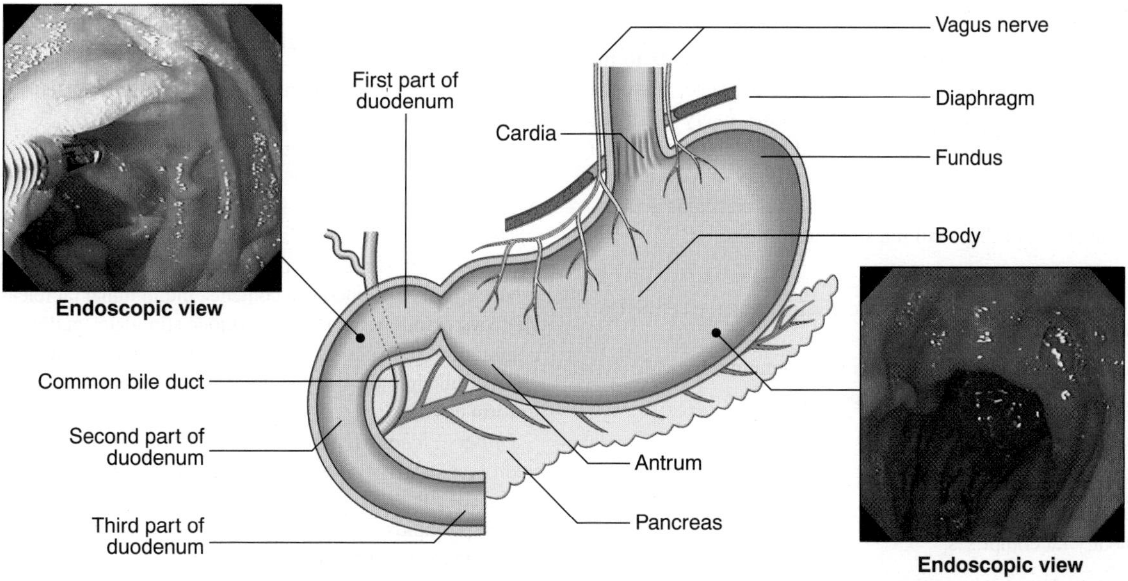

Fig. 9.2 Normal gastric and duodenal anatomy.

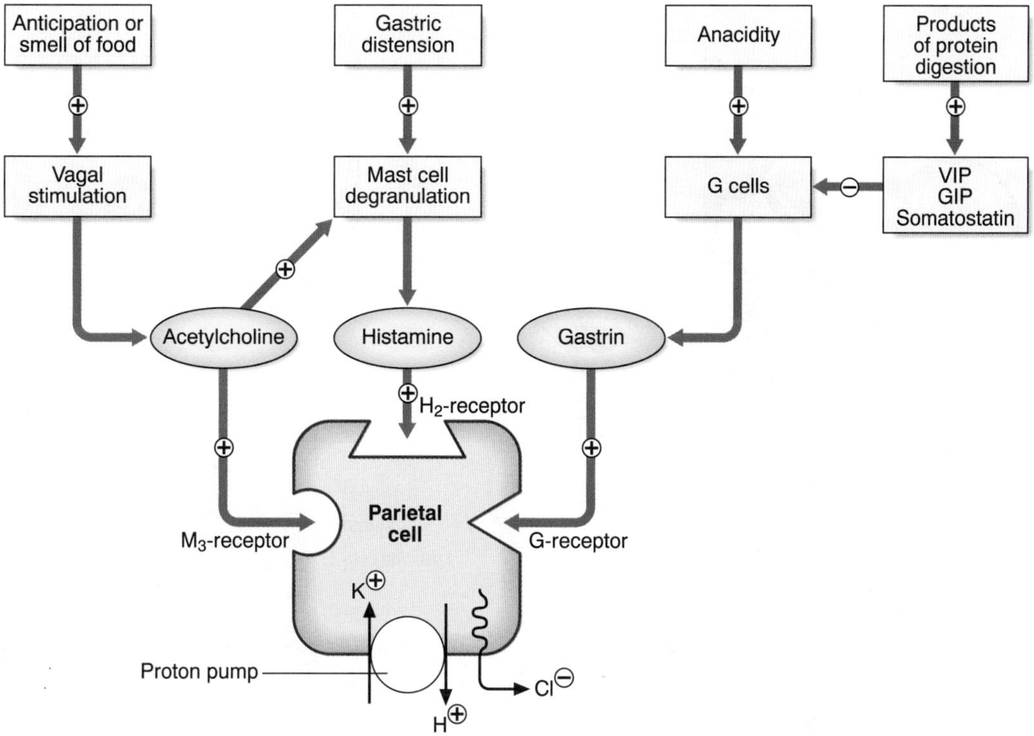

Fig. 9.3 Control of acid secretion. The parietal cell secretes acid in response to cholinergic activity, histamine and gastrin. Hydrogen ions are secreted in exchange from the apical membrane of the cell and chloride ions passively diffuse to maintain electroneutrality. (VIP = vasoactive intestinal polypeptide; GIP = gastric inhibitory polypeptide)

SMALL INTESTINE

The small bowel extends from the ligament of Treitz to the ileocaecal valve (see Fig. 9.4). In the fasted state, muscular activity is absent for at least 80% of the time. Every 1–2 hours a wave of peristaltic activity, called the migrating motor complex, passes down the small bowel. Entry of food into the gastrointestinal tract stimulates small bowel peristaltic activity.

Functions of the small intestine are:

- digestion
- absorption—the products of digestion, water, electrolytes and vitamins
- protection against ingested toxins—immunological, mechanical, enzymatic and peristaltic.

Digestion and absorption

Fat

Dietary fat comprises:

- long-chain triglycerides (a glycerol 'backbone' bound to three fatty acid molecules)
- cholesterol esters
- fat-soluble vitamins (A, D, K and E).

Digestion and absorption involve multiple, interrelated steps as food passes through the gastrointestinal tract.

Stomach. Churning activity emulsifies the fat. Limited hydrolysis of triglycerides to diglycerides and fatty acid occurs due to the activity of swallowed, lingual lipase.

Duodenum. Secretin is released in response to acid exposure. This stimulates pancreatic bicarbonate secretion, producing alkaline duodenal contents. Intraluminal fat releases cholecystokinin (CCK). This hormone stimulates gallbladder contraction and relaxes the sphincter of Oddi, resulting in entry of bile into the duodenum. Bile further emulsifies lipids to form chyme.

Upper jejunum. Pancreatic lipase and colipase hydrolyse triglycerides to monoglycerides and free fatty acids (see Fig. 9.5).

Phospholipids and cholesterol esters are hydrolysed by other pancreatic enzymes.

The lipid mixture is now emulsified by the bile acids as 'mixed micelles'.

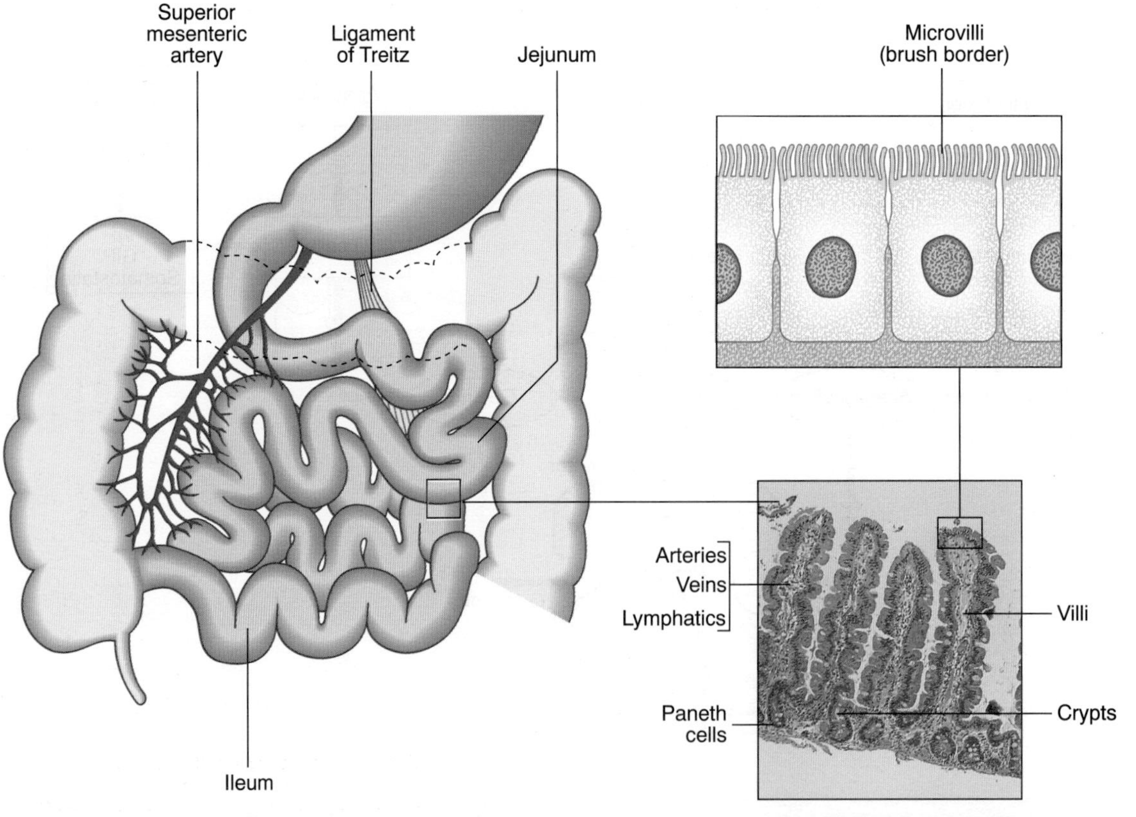

Fig. 9.4 Small intestine: anatomy. Epithelial cells are formed in crypts and differentiate as they migrate to the tip of the villi to form enterocytes (absorptive cells) and goblet cells.

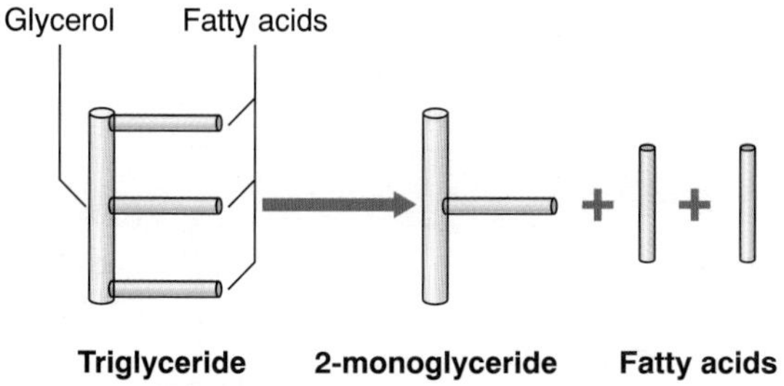

Fig. 9.5 Hydrolysis of triglycerides to monoglycerides and free fatty acids—the jejunal phase of fat digestion.

Distal small intestine. The lipid contents of the mixed micelles pass across cell membranes into enterocytes. Bile salts remain in the lumen and are absorbed in the terminal ileum, pass via the portal vein back to the liver and are then recycled (the enterohepatic circulation).

Within enterocytes, fatty acids, monoglycerides and diglycerides are re-esterified to form triglycerides. These are coated with apoproteins, phospholipids and cholesterol in the endoplasmic reticulum to form chylomicrons which leave the cells by exocytosis and eventually enter the portal circulation via lymphatics.

Carbohydrates

Dietary carbohydrate largely comprises the polysaccharide starch, some sucrose and lactose. Starch is hydrolysed by salivary and pancreatic amylases to alpha-limit dextrins containing 4–8 glucose molecules; to the disaccharide maltose; and to the trisaccharide maltotriose.

Disaccharides are digested by enzymes fixed to the microvillous membrane to form the monosaccharides glucose, galactose and fructose. Glucose and galactose enter the cell by an energy-requiring process involving a carrier protein. Fructose enters by simple diffusion.

Protein

Intragastric digestion by pepsin is quantitatively modest but nevertheless important because the resulting polypeptides and amino acids are sufficient to stimulate CCK release from the mucosa of the proximal jejunum. CCK stimulates secretion of pancreatic trypsinogen into the duodenum.

Trypsinogen is activated by enterokinase, a hormone fixed to the duodenal mucosa, to produce the active proteolytic enzyme, trypsin. Trypsin subsequently activates a range of other pancreatic proenzymes and these digest proteins to form small polypeptides and amino acids. The enzymes comprise the endopeptidases trypsin, chymotrypsin and elastase, which hydrolyse bonds within proteins, and exopeptidases, which hydrolyse the carboxyl terminus. Peptidases on the microvilli then digest polypeptides to form dipeptides and amino acids, which are absorbed by sodium-dependent active transport systems. Within the enterocytes, cytosolic peptidases further digest dipeptides to amino acids.

Water and electrolytes

Both absorption and secretion of electrolytes and water occur throughout the intestine. Net transport is the difference between absorption and secretion; in health, absorption predominates.

Electrolytes and water are transported by two pathways (see Fig. 9.6):

- the paracellular route, in which flow through tight junctions between cells is a consequence of osmotic, electrical or hydrostatic gradients
- the transcellular route across apical and basolateral membranes by energy-requiring specific active transport carriers (pumps)

Vitamins and trace elements

Water-soluble vitamins are absorbed throughout the intestine. The absorption of folic acid (see p. 522), vitamin B_{12} (see p. 522), calcium (see p. 517) and iron (see p. 518) is described elsewhere.

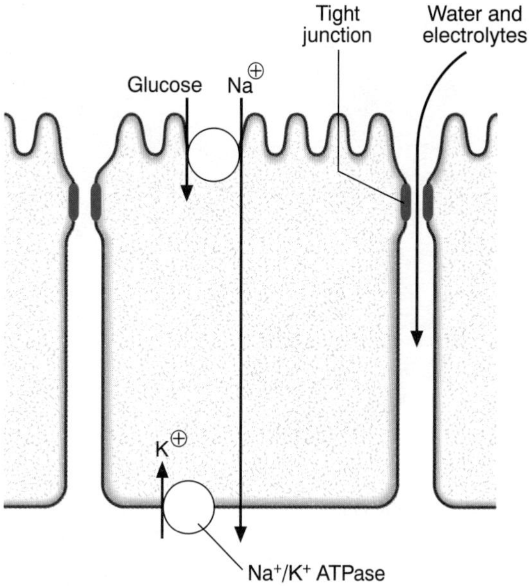

Fig. 9.6 Glucose/sodium cotransport. Glucose/sodium cotransport across the apical membrane of the enterocyte involving an energy-dependent pump on the basolateral membrane and a carrier for glucose and sodium on the apical membrane. Passive movement of water and electrolytes through tight junctions occurs as a consequence of electrochemical gradients.

Protective function of the small intestine

Immunology

B and T lymphocytes, macrophages and mast cells are found throughout the gastrointestinal mucosa. Mucosa-associated lymphoid tissue (MALT) constitutes 25% of the total lymphatic tissue of the body.

Luminal macromolecules and viral particles are transported by specialised (M) cells to Peyer's patches. These comprise lymphoid follicles with a well-defined structure. B lymphocytes within Peyer's patches differentiate to plasma cells following exposure to the antigens, and these cells migrate to mesenteric lymph nodes, thence to the blood stream via the thoracic duct and then return to the lamina propria of the gut, bronchial tree and other lymph nodes. They subsequently release the humoral antibody, IgA, which is transported into the lumen of the intestine after linkage to secretory piece. This neutralises the antigen (see Fig. 9.7).

The role of T lymphocytes is less clear, but these cells probably help localise the plasma cells to the site of antigen exposure as well as producing inflammatory mediators. Macrophages phagocytose foreign materials and secrete a

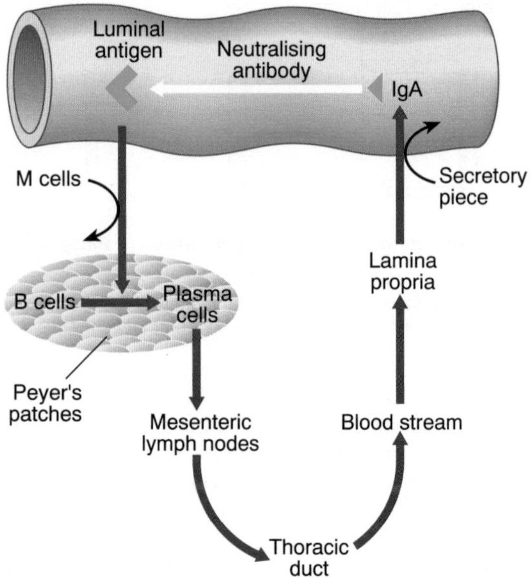

Fig. 9.7 Migration of gut lymphoid tissue in response to antigen exposure.

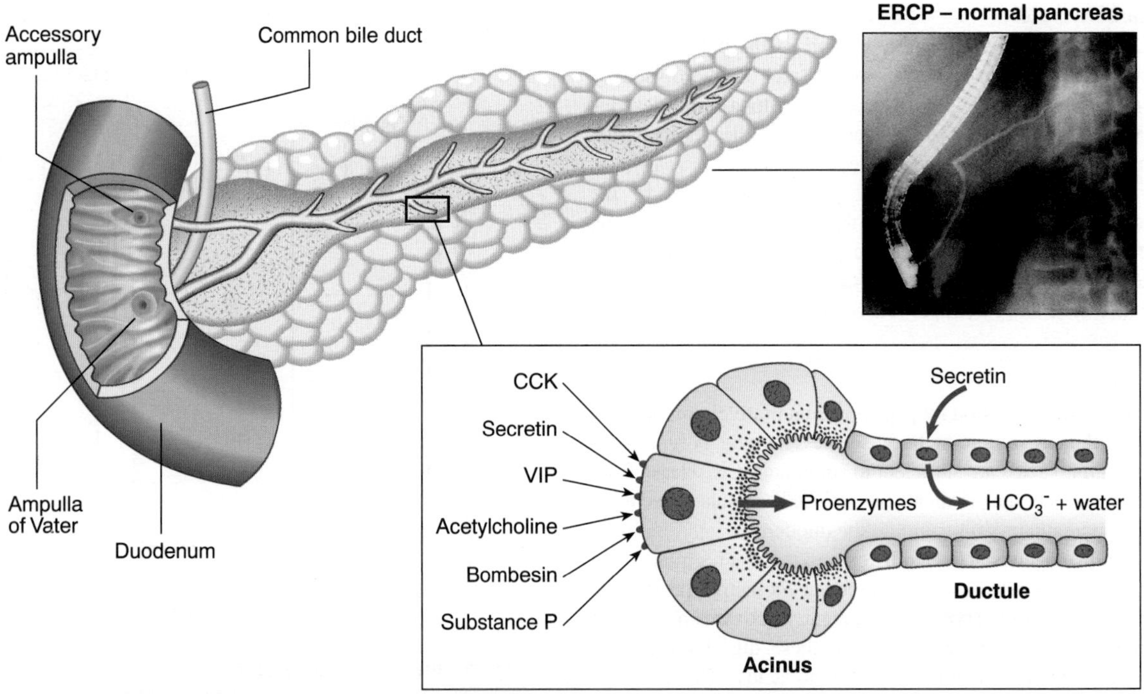

Fig. 9.8 Pancreatic structure and function. Ductular cells secrete alkaline fluid in response to secretin. Acinar cells secrete digestive enzymes from zymogen granules in response to a range of secretagogues. The photograph shows a normal pancreatic duct and side branches as defined at endoscopic retrograde cholangiopancreatography (ERCP).

range of cytokines which mediate inflammation. Activation of mast cell surface IgE receptors leads to degranulation and release of other molecules involved in inflammation.

Mucosal barrier

The epithelium of the gastrointestinal tract constitutes a barrier to luminal contents. This barrier comprises mucus, secreted by goblet cells, the membranes of the enterocytes and the tight junctions between them. These cells are constantly renewed; those of the small intestine are replaced every 48 hours.

PANCREAS

The exocrine pancreas is necessary for the digestion of fat, protein and carbohydrate. Inactive proenzymes are secreted from acinar cells in response to circulating gastrointestinal hormones (see Fig. 9.8) and are then activated by trypsin. Bicarbonate-rich fluid is secreted from ductular cells to produce an optimum, alkaline pH for enzyme activity (see Table 9.1).

Table 9.1 Pancreatic enzymes

Enzyme	Substrate	Product
Amylase	Starch and glycogen	Limit dextrans Maltose Maltriose
Lipase **Colipase**	Triglycerides	Monoglycerides and free fatty acids
Proteolytic enzymes Trypsinogen Chymotrypsinogen Proelastase Procarboxypeptidases	Proteins and polypeptides	Short polypeptides

COLON (see Fig. 9.9)

The colon absorbs water and electrolytes. It also acts as a storage organ and has contractile activity. Two types of contraction occur. The first of these is segmentation (ring contraction), which leads to mixing but not propulsion; this facilitates absorption of water and electrolytes. Propulsive (peristaltic contraction) waves cause mass movement several times a day and propel the faecal bolus to the rectum. All activity is stimulated after meals, probably in response to release of motilin and CCK.

Faecal continence depends upon maintenance of the ano-rectal angle and tonic contraction of the external anal

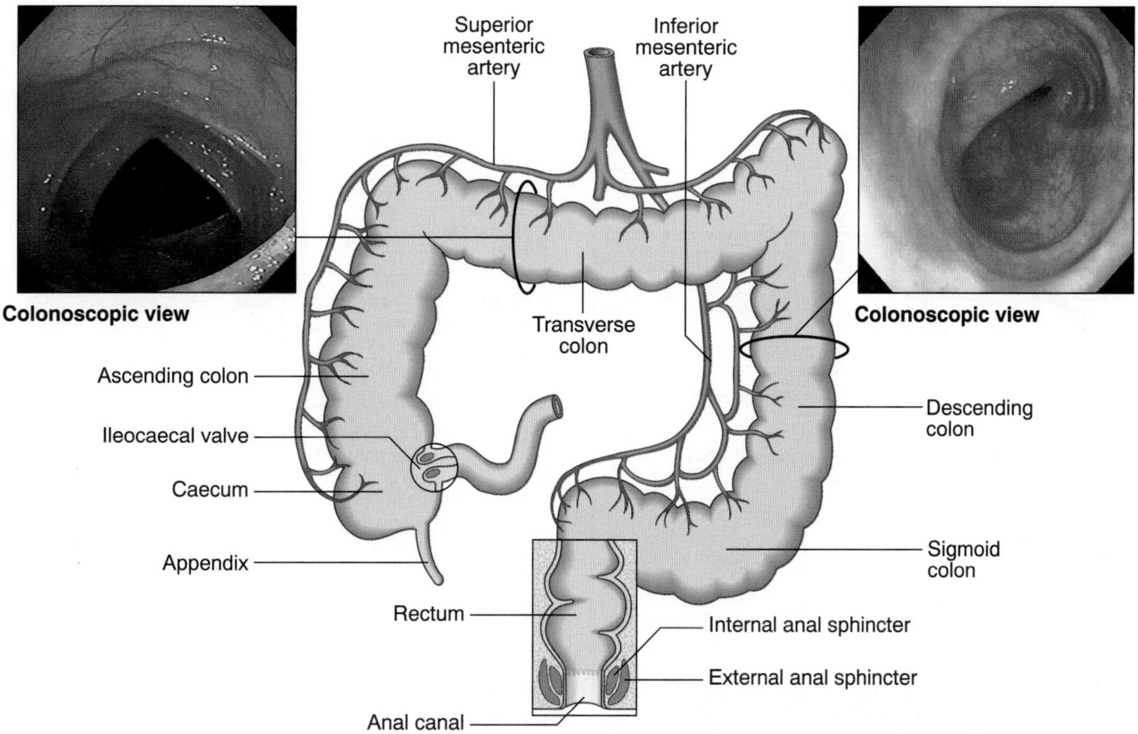

Fig. 9.9 The normal colon, rectum and anal canal.

sphincters. Relaxation of these muscles, increased intra-abdominal pressure from a Valsalva manoeuvre and contraction of abdominal muscles, with relaxation of the anal sphincters, result in defaecation.

CONTROL OF GASTROINTESTINAL FUNCTION

Secretion, absorption, motor activity, growth and differentiation are modulated by nervous and hormonal factors.

THE ENTERIC NERVOUS SYSTEM

Extrinsic innervation is provided by sympathetic nerves which release noradrenaline, and by parasympathetic, vagal nerves which release acetylcholine. In general, sympathetic pathways stimulate contraction and secretion, whilst parasympathetic pathways are inhibitory.

Extrinsic nerves interact with the intrinsic plexuses of the gastrointestinal tract (Auerbach's and Meissner's plexuses). Neuropeptides produced by these nerves exert a wide range of activities (see Table 9.2) through neurocrine, paracrine and autocrine mechanisms; some (e.g. VIP, CCK) also have endocrine actions.

GUT HORMONES

The origin, action and control of the major gut hormones are summarised in Table 9.3.

Table 9.2 Gut neuropeptides

Neuropeptide	Action
Opioids	Pain perception Decrease motility; regulate sphincter activity Increase acid secretion Modulate electrolyte and water absorption
Substance P	Propagates peristaltic activity Stimulates lower oesophageal sphincter Pain modulation
Vasoactive intestinal polypeptide (VIP)	Smooth muscle relaxation Vasodilatation
Gastrin-releasing polypeptide **Bombesin**	Mediate gastrin release
Cholecystokinin (CCK)	Controls satiety Release of acetylcholine and γ-amino butyric acid (GABA) from myenteric plexus
Neuropeptide Y	Vasocontraction of splanchnic circulation Reduces small bowel secretions

Table 9.3 Gut hormones

Hormone	Origin	Stimulus	Action
Gastrin	Stomach (G cell)	Products of protein digestion Suppressed by acid and somatostatin	Gastric acid secretion Growth of gastrointestinal mucosa
Somatostatin	Throughout GI tract (D cell)	Fat ingestion	Inhibits gastrin and insulin secretion Decreased acid secretion Decreased absorption
Cholecystokinin	Duodenum and jejunum	Products of protein digestion Fat and fatty acids Suppressed by trypsin	Stimulates pancreatic enzyme secretion Gallbladder contraction Sphincter of Oddi relaxation Satiety Decreased gastric acid secretion Reduced gastric emptying Regulates pancreatic growth
Secretin	Duodenum and jejunum	Duodenal acid Fatty acids	Pancreatic fluid and bicarbonate secretion Decreased acid secretion Reduced gastric emptying
Motilin	Duodenum and jejunum	Fasting Dietary fat	Regulates peristaltic activity
Gastric inhibitory polypeptide (GIP)	Duodenum and jejunum	Nutrients	Stimulates insulin release Inhibits acid secretion
Pancreatic polypeptide	Duodenum and jejunum	Protein digestive products Gastric distension	Inhibits pancreatic secretions
Enteroglucagon	Ileum and colon	Unknown	Modulates insulin release Trophic effect
Neurotensin	Ileum and colon	Unknown	May regulate ileal motility in response to fat
Peptide Y	Ileum and colon	Intestinal fat	Decreases pancreatic and gastric secretion
Vasoactive intestinal polypeptide (VIP)	Nerve fibres throughout gastrointestinal tract	Unknown	Regulates blood flow

INVESTIGATION OF GASTROINTESTINAL DISEASE

A wide range of tests are available for the investigation of patients with gastrointestinal symptoms. These can be classified broadly into tests of structure, tests of infection and tests of function.

TESTS OF STRUCTURE: IMAGING

Plain radiographs

Plain radiographs of the abdomen show the distribution of gas within the small and large intestines and are useful in the diagnosis of intestinal obstruction where dilated loops of bowel and (in the erect position) fluid levels are seen. The outlines of soft tissues such as liver, spleen and kidneys are usually visible, and calcification of these organs as well as pancreas, blood vessels, lymph nodes and calculi may be detected. Abdominal radiographs do not help in cases of gastrointestinal bleeding. A chest radiograph shows the diaphragm, and erect films may detect subdiaphragmatic free air in cases of perforation. Unexpected pulmonary problems such as pleural effusions will also be revealed.

Contrast studies

These provide more information than plain films. Barium sulphate is inert and provides good mucosal coating and excellent opacification. It can, however, solidify and impact proximal to an obstructive lesion. Water-soluble contrast is used to opacify bowel prior to abdominal computed tomography and in cases of suspected perforation but is less radio-opaque and is also irritant if aspirated into the lungs. Contrast studies are carried out under fluoroscopic control, which allows assessment of motility and correct patient positioning. The double contrast technique improves mucosal visualisation by using gas to distend the barium-coated intestinal surface.

Although the wall of the gut itself is not seen, barium studies are useful for detecting filling defects, which may be intraluminal (e.g. food or faeces), intramural (e.g. carcinoma) or extramural (e.g. lymph nodes). Strictures, erosions, ulcers and motility disorders can all be detected.

The major uses and limitations of various contrast studies are shown in Table 9.4.

Ultrasound, computed tomography (CT) and magnetic resonance imaging (MRI)

These are increasingly used in the evaluation of intra-abdominal disease. They are non-invasive and offer detailed images of the abdominal contents. Table 9.5 summarises their main applications in gastroenterology.

Table 9.4 Contrast radiology in the investigation of gastrointestinal disease

Indications	Major uses	Limitations
Barium swallow		
Dysphagia Heartburn Chest pain Possible motility disorder	Strictures Hiatus hernia Gastro-oesophageal reflux and motility disorders, e.g. achalasia	Risk of aspiration Poor mucosal detail Unable to biopsy
Barium meal		
Dyspepsia Epigastric pain Anaemia Vomiting Possible perforation (non-ionic contrast)	Gastric, duodenal ulcers Gastric cancer Outlet obstruction Gastric emptying disorders	Low sensitivity for early cancer Unable to biopsy or assess *Helicobacter pylori*
Barium follow-through		
Diarrhoea and abdominal pain of small bowel origin Possible obstruction by strictures etc.	Malabsorption Crohn's disease	Time-consuming Radiation exposure
Barium enema		
Altered bowel habit Rectal bleeding Anaemia Abdominal pain	Neoplasia Diverticulosis Strictures, e.g. ischaemic, megacolon	Difficult in elderly or incontinent Discomfort Less useful in inflammatory bowel disease Sigmoidoscopy to show rectum Possibly misses polyps < 1 cm

Endoscopy

Fibreoptic endoscopy is used to examine the oesophagus, stomach, duodenum and colon. Originally, light was passed down flexible quartz fibres and the reflected light passed back up to the investigator by thousands of bundles. In recent years video endoscopy has replaced fibreoptic endoscopes and the images are displayed on a colour television monitor. Endoscopes have controls to allow steering of the tip and also possess channels for suction and insufflation of air and water. An increasing array of instruments can be passed down the endoscope to allow both diagnostic and therapeutic procedures, some of which are illustrated in Figure 9.10.

Upper gastrointestinal endoscopy

After the patient has fasted for at least 4 hours, this is performed under light intravenous benzodiazepine sedation, or using only local anaesthetic throat spray. With the patient in the left lateral position the entire oesophagus (excluding pharynx), stomach and first two parts of duodenum can be seen. Indications, contraindications and complications are given in the information box on page 609.

Table 9.5 Ultrasound, CT and MRI scanning in gastroenterology

Investigation	Major uses	Limitations
Ultrasound	Abdominal masses, e.g. cysts, tumours, abscesses Organomegaly Ascites Biliary tract dilatation Gallstones Guided needle aspiration and biopsy of lesions	Low sensitivity for small lesions Little functional information Operator-dependent Gas and obesity may obscure view
CT	Assessment of pancreatic disease Hepatic tumour deposits Tumour staging Assessment of vascularity of lesions	Expensive High radiation dose May understage some tumours, e.g. oesophagogastric
MRI	Tumour staging MRCP* Pelvic/perianal Crohn's fistulae	Role in GI disease not fully established Limited availability Time-consuming 'Claustrophobic' for some

* MRCP = magnetic resonance cholangiopancreatography.

Enteroscopy

Using a longer endoscope (enteroscope) it is possible to visualise a large portion of the small intestine. Enteroscopy is of special value in the assessment of obscure, recurrent gastrointestinal bleeding.

Sigmoidoscopy and colonoscopy

Sigmoidoscopy can be carried out either in the outpatient clinic using a 20 cm rigid plastic sigmoidoscope or in the endoscopy suite using a 60 cm flexible instrument following a disposable enema for bowel preparation. When sigmoidoscopy is combined with proctoscopy, accurate detection of haemorrhoids, ulcerative colitis and distal colorectal neoplasia is possible. After full bowel cleansing it is possible to examine the entire colon and often the terminal ileum using a longer colonoscope. The information box lists the indications, contraindications and complications of colonoscopy.

Endoscopic retrograde cholangiopancreatography (ERCP)

Using a side-viewing duodenoscope, it is possible to cannulate the main pancreatic duct and common bile duct. The procedure is valuable in defining the ampulla of Vater,

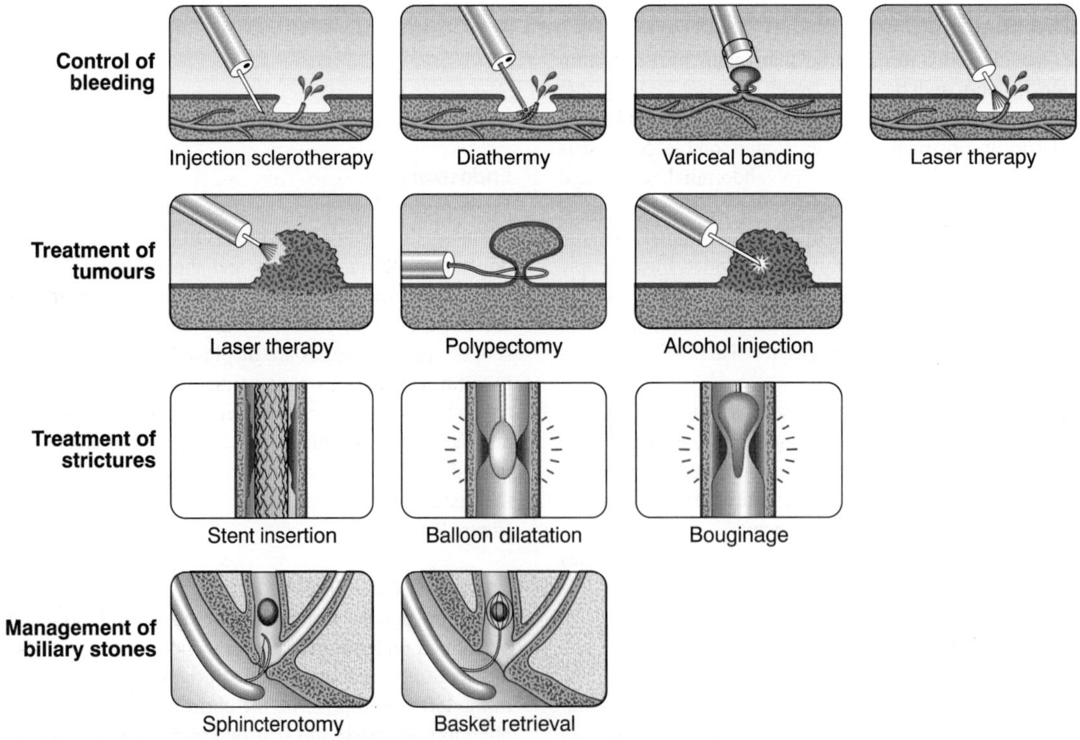

Fig. 9.10 Examples of therapeutic techniques in endoscopy.

UPPER GASTROINTESTINAL ENDOSCOPY
Indications
• Dyspepsia (especially aged over 45 years) • Abdominal pain • Atypical chest pain • Dysphagia • Vomiting • Weight loss • Acute or chronic gastrointestinal bleeding • Suspicious barium meal
Contraindications
• Severe shock • Recent myocardial infarction, unstable angina, cardiac arrhythmia* • Severe respiratory disease* • Atlanto-axial subluxation* • Possible visceral perforation * These are 'relative' contraindications; in experienced hands, endoscopy can be safely performed.
Complications
• Cardiorespiratory depression due to sedation • Aspiration pneumonia • Perforation • Bleeding • Infective endocarditis (use antibiotic prophylaxis in patients at risk—see p. 286)

biliary tree and pancreas. Its main uses include investigation of obstructive jaundice, biliary pain and suspected pancreatic disease, such as chronic pancreatitis and pancreatic cancer. Obstruction of the common bile duct by stones can be treated by stone extraction after sphincterotomy, and strictures may be stented. The procedure is technically demanding and carries a significant risk of pancreatitis (3–5%), haemorrhage (4% after sphincterotomy) and perforation (1%).

COLONOSCOPY
Indications
• Suspected inflammatory bowel disease • Altered bowel habit • Rectal bleeding or anaemia • Assessment of abnormal barium enema • Colorectal cancer surveillance • Therapeutic procedures
Contraindications
• Severe shock • Recent myocardial infarction, unstable angina, cardiac arrhythmia* • Severe respiratory disease • Possible visceral perforation • Severe, active ulcerative colitis * These are 'relative' contraindications; in experienced hands, colonoscopy can be safely performed.
Complications
• Cardiorespiratory depression due to sedation • Perforation • Bleeding • Infective endocarditis (use antibiotic prophylaxis in patients at risk—see p. 286)

Histology

Biopsy material obtained during endoscopy or percutaneously can provide useful information (see the information box).

REASONS FOR BIOPSY OR CYTOLOGICAL EXAMINATION
• Brush cytology of suspected malignant lesions • Histological assessment of mucosal abnormalities • Diagnosis of infection (e.g. *Candida, Helicobacter pylori, Giardia lamblia*) • Measurement of enzyme contents (e.g. disaccharidases) • Analysis of genetic mutations (e.g. oncogenes, tumour suppressor genes)

TESTS OF INFECTION

Bacterial cultures

Stool cultures are essential in the investigation of diarrhoea, especially when it is acute or bloody, to identify pathogenic organisms. Common pathogens are listed in Table 9.6.

Serology

Detection of antibodies plays a limited role in the diagnosis of gastrointestinal infection caused by organisms such as *Helicobacter pylori*, *Salmonella* species and *Entamoeba histolytica*.

Breath tests

Non-invasive breath tests for *H. pylori* infection are discussed

Table 9.6 Infective agents commonly responsible for infective diarrhoea

Agent type	Agent	Comments
Viruses	Rotavirus Adenoviruses Enteroviruses	Requires electron microscopy and/or viral culture methods
Bacteria	*Campylobacter jejuni*	
	Escherichia coli	Especially 0:157
	Salmonella	Phage typing
	Clostridium difficile	Also requires toxin isolation
Protozoa	*Giardia lamblia**	Microscopy of duodenal biopsy also used
	*Entamoeba histolytica**	Serological complement-fixation test also used
	Cryptosporidium *Microsporidium*	

* Fresh stool needed

below (see p. 611). Breath tests for suspected small intestinal bacterial overgrowth are discussed on page 645.

TESTS OF FUNCTION

A number of dynamic tests can be used to investigate aspects of gut function, including digestion, absorption, inflammation and epithelial permeability. Some of those more commonly used are listed in Table 9.7. In the assessment of suspected malabsorption, blood tests (full blood count, erythrocyte sedimentation rate (ESR), folate, B_{12}, iron status, albumin, calcium and phosphate) are essential. Endoscopy with distal duodenal biopsy is also indicated in most cases.

Gastrointestinal motility

Many diverse radiological, manometric and radioisotopic tests exist for investigation of gut motility but many are still research tests of limited value in daily clinical practice.

Oesophageal motility

A careful barium swallow can give useful information about oesophageal motility and videofluoroscopy, and is useful in suspected swallowing disorders. Oesophageal manometry (see Fig. 9.1, p. 600), often in conjunction with 24-hour pH measurements, is of value in diagnosing cases of refractory gastro-oesophageal reflux, achalasia and other causes of non-cardiac chest pain.

Gastric emptying

Delayed gastric emptying (gastroparesis) may be responsible for some cases of persistent nausea, vomiting, bloating or early satiety. Endoscopy and barium studies are often normal. Plotting a graph of the amount of radioisotope retained in the stomach against time is carried out after a test meal containing solids and liquids labelled with different isotopes (see Fig. 9.11).

Small intestinal transit

This is much more difficult to quantify and is seldom necessary in clinical practice. Barium follow-through examination can give a rough estimate by noting the time taken for contrast to reach the terminal ileum (normally 90 minutes or less). Orocaecal transit can be assessed by the lactulose-hydrogen breath test. Lactulose is a disaccharide which normally reaches the colon intact; here, breakdown by colonic bacteria results in hydrogen production. The time at which this occurs, as measured in expired air, is a measure of oral-caecal transit.

Table 9.7 Dynamic tests of gastrointestinal function

Process	Test	Principle	Comments
Absorption			
Fat	^{14}C-triolein breath test	Measurement of $^{14}CO_2$ in breath after oral ingestion of radio-labelled fat	Fast and non-invasive but not quantitative
	3-day faecal fat	Quantification of stool fat while patient ingests 100 g/day fat. Normally < 20 mmol/day	Non-invasive but slow and unpleasant for all
Lactose	Lactose H_2 breath test	Measurement of breath H_2 content after 50 g oral lactose. Undigested sugar is metabolised by colonic bacteria in hypolactasia	Non-invasive and accurate; may provoke pain and diarrhoea in sufferers
Bile acids	$^{75}SeHCAT$ test	Isotopic quantification of 7-day whole-body retention of oral dose ^{75}Se-labelled homocholyltaurine (> 15% = normal, < 5% = abnormal)	Accurate and specific but requires two visits and involves radiation. Can be equivocal
Pancreatic exocrine function			
	Pancreolauryl test	Pancreatic esterases cleave fluoroscein dilaurate after oral ingestion. Fluoroscein is absorbed and quantified in urine	Accurate and avoids duodenal intubation. Takes 2 days. Accurate urine collection essential
	Faecal chymotrypsin or elastase	Immunoassay of pancreatic enzymes on stool sample	Simple, quick and avoids urine collection. May not detect mild disease
Mucosal inflammation/permeability			
	^{51}Cr-EDTA	Urinary quantification of label after oral dose. More is absorbed through 'leaky' mucosa	Relatively non-invasive and accurate but involves radioactivity. Limited availability.
	Sugar tests (lactulose: rhamnose)	Small intestine absorbs mono- but not disaccharides unless inflamed. Urinary excretion of oral dose of two sugars expressed as ratio (normal < 0.04)	Non-invasive test of small bowel mucosal integrity (e.g. coeliac, Crohn's). Accurate urine collection essential
	Whole gut lavage	Patient drinks non-absorbable, inert cleansing agent until clear rectal fluid obtained for analysis.	Sensitive for gut inflammation (IgG, α_1-antitrypsin), blood loss (Hb) and protein loss (albumin). Some find it unpalatable.

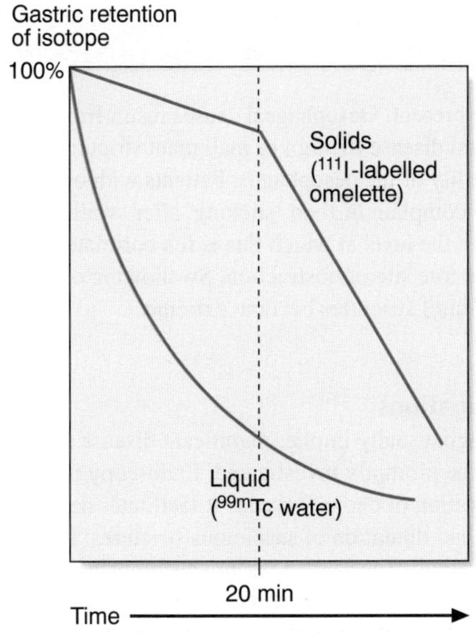

Fig. 9.11 Gastric emptying study. The body of the stomach churns solids into small particles which are then actively expelled by antral peristaltic activity. Gastric emptying is decreased by (a) fats, (b) high osmolality and (c) acid.

Colonic and anorectal motility

A plain abdominal radiograph taken on day 5 after ingestion of different-shaped inert plastic pellets on days 1–3 gives an estimate of whole gut transit time. The test is useful in the evaluation of chronic constipation when the position of any retained pellets can be observed, and helps to differentiate cases of slow transit from those due to obstructed defaecation. The mechanism of defaecation and anorectal function can be assessed by a variety of tests such as anorectal manometry, electrophysiological tests and defaecating proctography.

RADIOISOTOPE TESTS

Many different radioisotope tests are used (see Table 9.8). In some, structural information is obtained, e.g. localisation of a Meckel's diverticulum or distribution of activity in inflammatory bowel disease. Others use radioisotopes for functional information, e.g. rates of gastric emptying, ability to reabsorb bile acids. Yet others are tests of infection and rely on the presence of bacteria to hydrolyse a radio-labelled test substance followed by detection of the radioisotope in expired air (e.g. urea breath test for *H. pylori*).

Table 9.8 Commonly used radioisotope tests in gastroenterology

Test	Isotope	Major uses and principle of test
Gastric emptying study	^{99m}Tc-sulphur ^{111}In-DTPA	Used in assessment of gastric emptying, particularly for possible gastroparesis
Urea breath test	^{14}C- or ^{13}C-urea	Used in non-invasive diagnosis of *Helicobacter pylori*. Bacterial urease enzyme splits urea to ammonia and CO_2 which is detected in expired air
Meckel's scan	^{99m}Tc-pertechnetate	Diagnosis of Meckel's diverticulum in cases of obscure GI bleeding. Isotope is injected i.v. and localises in ectopic parietal mucosa within diverticulum
Labelled red cell scan	^{51}Cr-labelled erythrocytes	Diagnosis of obscure and recurrent GI bleeding. Labelled erythrocytes seen extravasating into intestine from bleeding vessel
Labelled leucocyte scan	^{111}In- or ^{99m}Tc-HMPAO -labelled leucocytes	Localisation of abscess collections and distribution of activity in inflammatory bowel disease. Patient's white cells are labelled in vitro, are reinfused and migrate to site of inflammation or infection
SeHCAT scan	^{75}Se-homo-cholyltaurine	Used in diagnosis of bile acid-related diarrhoea and terminal ileal disease. Patient's 7-day whole-body retention of oral dose of labelled bile acid is measured. Tests ability of terminal ileum to reabsorb bile acids
Triolein test	^{14}C-triolein	Diagnosis of fat malabsorption. Tests ability to digest oral dose of labelled fat by measurement of $^{14}CO_2$ in expired breath
Epithelial permeability test	^{51}Cr-albumin	Investigation of protein-losing enteropathy. Faecal excretion of labelled albumin after i.v. injection is quantified

FURTHER INFORMATION ON FUNCTIONAL ANATOMY, PHYSIOLOGY AND INVESTIGATIONS

Cook I J S 1991 Normal and disordered swallowing: new insights. Baillière's Clinical Gastroenterology 5: 245–280

Köhne G, Schneider T, Zeilz S 1996 Special features of the intestinal lymphocytic system. Baillière's Clinical Gastroenterology 10: 427–442

Taourel P, Pradel J, Bruel J-M 1994 Current CT/MRI examinations of the upper gastrointestinal tract. Baillière's Clinical Gastroenterology 8: 743–763

MAJOR MANIFESTATIONS OF GASTROINTESTINAL DISEASE

DYSPHAGIA

Dysphagia is defined as difficulty in swallowing. It may coexist with heartburn or vomiting but should be distinguished from both globus sensation (in which anxious people feel a lump in the throat without organic cause) and odynophagia (which refers to pain with swallowing, usually resulting from oesophagitis due to gastro-oesophageal reflux or candidiasis).

Dysphagia can be classified into *oropharyngeal* and *oesophageal* causes (see Fig. 9.12). Oropharyngeal disorders result from neuromuscular dysfunction affecting the initiation of swallowing by the pharynx and upper oesophageal sphincter (e.g. bulbar or pseudobulbar palsy and myasthenia gravis). Patients with oropharyngeal dysphagia have difficulty initiating swallowing and complain of choking, nasal regurgitation or tracheal aspiration. On examination, drooling, dysarthria, hoarseness and cranial nerve or other neurological signs may be present. Oesophageal causes result from either structural disease (benign or malignant strictures) or dysmotility of the oesophagus. Patients with oesophageal disease complain of food 'sticking' after swallowing, although the level at which this is felt correlates poorly with the true site of obstruction. Swallowing of liquids is normal until strictures become extreme.

Investigations

Dysphagia usually implies significant disease and should always be promptly investigated. Endoscopy is the investigation of choice because it facilitates detection, biopsy and dilatation of suspicious strictures. If no abnormality is found then barium swallow, possibly with videofluoroscopic swallowing assessment, will detect most motility disorders. In a few cases oesophageal manometry is required. The algorithm (see Fig. 9.12) summarises an approach to patients with dysphagia and lists the major causes.

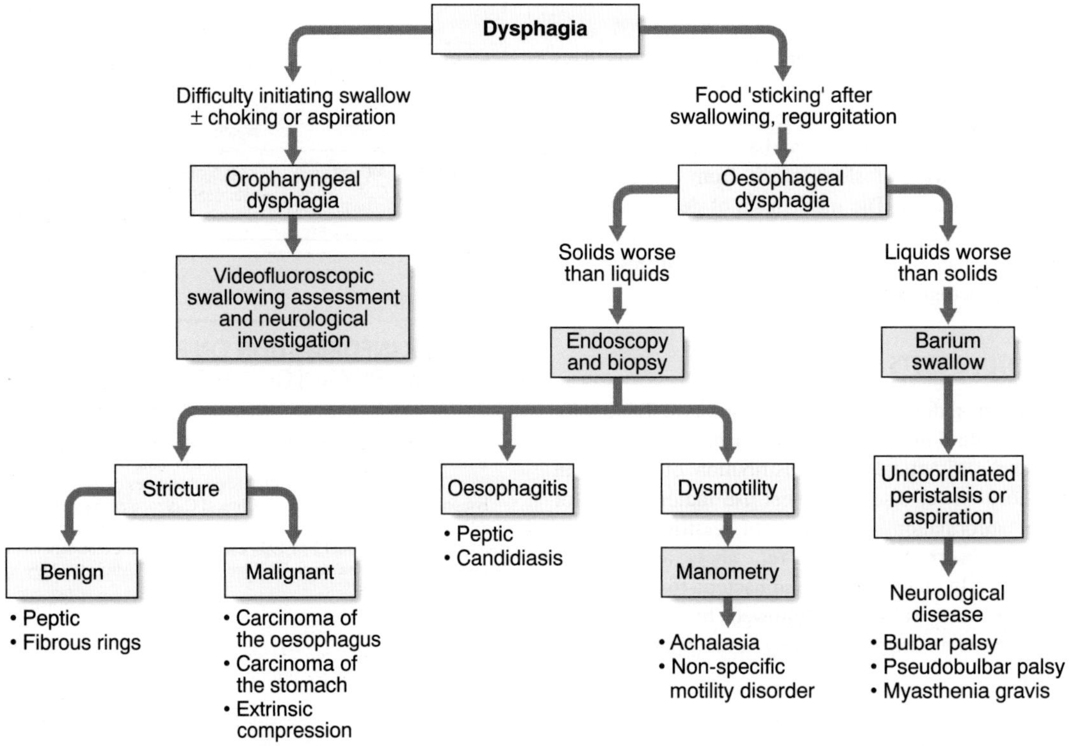

Fig. 9.12 Investigation of dysphagia.

DYSPEPSIA

Dyspepsia ('indigestion') is a collective term for non-specific symptoms thought to originate from the upper gastrointestinal tract. It encompasses many different symptoms and disorders (see the information boxes), including some arising outside the digestive system.

CAUSES OF DYSPEPSIA

Upper gastrointestinal disorders
- Peptic ulcer disease
- Gastro-oesophageal reflux disease (with or without hiatus hernia)
- Acute gastritis
- Gallstones
- Motility disorders, e.g. oesophageal spasm
- 'Functional' or non-ulcer dyspepsia

Other gastrointestinal disorders
- Irritable bowel syndrome
- Pancreatic disease (cancer, chronic pancreatitis)
- Hepatic disease (hepatitis, metastases)
- Colonic carcinoma

Systemic disease
- Myocardial ischaemia
- Renal failure
- Hypercalcaemia

Drugs
- NSAIDs
- Iron and potassium supplements
- Corticosteroids
- Digoxin

Others
- Alcohol
- Pregnancy
- Psychological, e.g. anxiety, depression

Although symptoms often correlate poorly with the underlying diagnosis, a careful history is important to:

- elicit symptoms classical of specific disorders, e.g. peptic ulcer
- detect 'alarm' features requiring urgent investigation (see the information box)
- detect atypical symptoms more suggestive of other disorders, e.g. myocardial ischaemia.

Dyspepsia is extremely prevalent, affecting up to 80% of the population at some time, and very often no abnormality is discovered during investigation, especially in younger patients. Patients with 'alarm' symptoms, those over 45 years old with new dyspepsia and younger patients unresponsive to 4 weeks of empirical treatment require prompt investigation to exclude serious gastrointestinal disease.

DEFINITIONS OF DYSPEPSIA
- Upper abdominal/lower chest pain with or without relationship to food
- Regurgitation, heartburn and waterbrash
- Anorexia, nausea, vomiting
- Bloating, belching, flatulence

'ALARM' FEATURES IN DYSPEPSIA
- Weight loss
- Anaemia
- Haematemesis and/or melaena
- Dysphagia
- Palpable abdominal mass

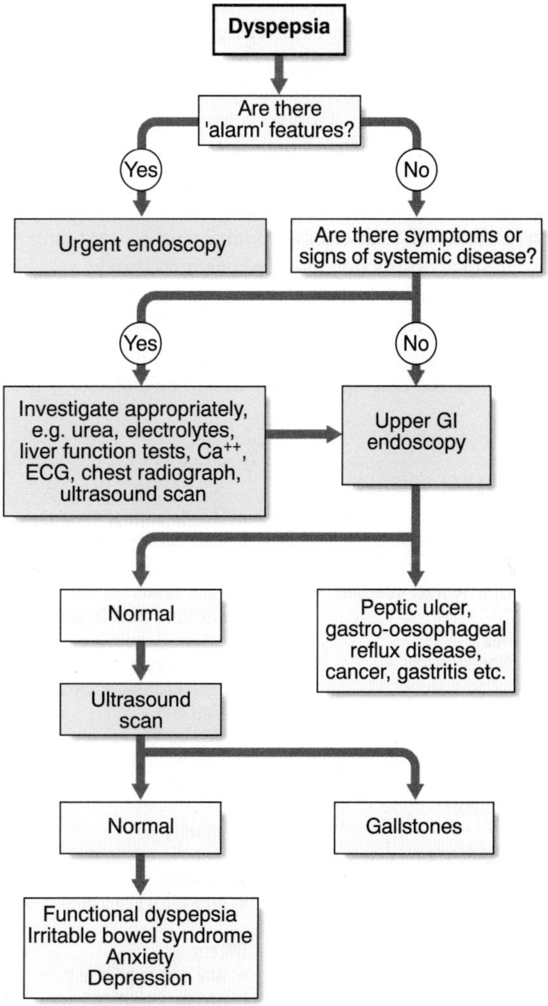

Fig. 9.13 Investigation of dyspepsia.

Examination may reveal important findings such as evidence of anaemia, weight loss, lymphadenopathy, abdominal masses or signs of liver disease. An algorithm for the investigation of dyspepsia is outlined in Figure 9.13.

VOMITING

Vomiting is a highly integrated and complex reflex involving both autonomic and somatic neural pathways. Synchronous contraction of the diaphragm, intercostal muscles and abdominal muscles raises intra-abdominal pressure and, combined with relaxation of the lower oesophageal sphincter, results in forcible ejection of gastric contents.

Vomiting is usually associated with nausea, retching, salivation, anorexia or dyspepsia. It is important to distinguish true vomiting from regurgitation and to elicit whether the vomiting is acute or chronic (recurrent), as the underlying causes may differ. Associated symptoms of abdominal pain, fever, diarrhoea, relationship to food, drug ingestion, headache, vertigo and weight loss should be sought.

Examination may reveal signs of dehydration, fever and infection. Evidence of abdominal masses, peritonitis or intestinal obstruction must be sought, as should neurological signs including papilloedema, nystagmus, photophobia and neck stiffness. Other findings may suggest alcoholism, pregnancy or bulimia as the underlying diagnosis. The diagnostic approach will be dictated by the history and examination. The major causes of vomiting are listed in the information box.

CAUSES OF VOMITING

Infections
- Gastroenteriti
- Hepatitis
- Urinary tract infection

Drugs
- Non-steroidal anti inflammatory drugs (NSAIDs)
- Antibiotics
- Opiates
- Digoxin
- Cytotoxic drugs

Gastroduodenal disease
- Chronic peptic ulcer disease (+/– gastric outlet obstruction)
- Gastric cancer
- Gastroparesis, e.g. diabetes, scleroderma, drugs

Acute abdominal disorders
- Appendicitis
- Cholecystitis
- Pancreatitis
- Intestinal obstruction

CNS disorders
- Vestibular neuronitis
- Migraine
- Meningitis
- Raised intracranial pressure

Metabolic
- Diabetic ketoacidosis
- Uraemia
- Addison's disease

Others
- Any severe pain, e.g. myocardial infarction
- Psychogenic
- Alcoholism

GASTROINTESTINAL BLEEDING

ACUTE UPPER GASTROINTESTINAL HAEMORRHAGE

This is the most common gastrointestinal emergency, accounting for 50–120 admissions to hospital per 100 000 of the population each year in the United Kingdom. Common causes are listed in Table 9.9.

Table 9.9 Causes of acute upper gastrointestinal haemorrhage

Diagnosis	%	Comments
Peptic ulcer	35–50	Dyspepsia or history of previous ulcer not invariable. Bleeding may be precipitated by NSAIDs or alcohol
Gastric erosions	10–20	Associated with NSAIDs and alcohol
Oesophagitis	10	Heartburn not invariable and bleeding usually not severe
Mallory–Weiss tear	5	Follows vomiting and retching, e.g. after alcoholic binge
Vascular malformations	5	Associated with aortic valve disease or hereditary haemorrhagic telangiectasia
Varices	2–4	Usually with evidence of liver disease
Carcinoma (oesophagus or stomach)	2	Chronic blood loss is usually present
Aorto-enteric fistula	1	Consider in any patient who presents after aortic graft surgery

Clinical features

Haematemesis may be red with clots when bleeding is profuse, or black ('coffee grounds') when less severe. Syncope may occur and is due to hypotension from intravascular volume depletion. Symptoms of anaemia suggest chronic bleeding.

Melaena is the term used to describe the passage of black, tarry stools containing altered blood; this is usually due to bleeding from the upper gastrointestinal tract, although haemorrhage from the right side of the colon is occasionally responsible. The characteristic appearance is the result of the action of digestive enzymes and of bacteria upon haemoglobin. Severe acute upper gastrointestinal bleeding can sometimes cause maroon or bright red stool.

Management

1. *Intravenous access.* The first step is to gain intravenous access using at least one large-bore cannula.
2. *Initial clinical assessment.*

- Define circulatory status. Severe bleeding causes tachycardia with hypotension and oliguria. The patient is cold, is sweating and may be agitated.
- Seek evidence of liver disease. Jaundice, cutaneous stigmata, hepatosplenomegaly and ascites may be present in decompensated cirrhosis.
- Define comorbidity. The presence of cardiorespiratory, cerebrovascular or renal disease is important, because these may be worsened by acute bleeding and because these diseases increase the hazards of endoscopy and surgical operations.

3. *Blood tests.* These include:

- A full blood count. Chronic or subacute bleeding leads to anaemia, but the haemoglobin concentration may be normal after sudden, major bleeding until haemodilution occurs.
- Urea and electrolytes. This may show evidence of renal failure. The blood urea rises as the absorbed products of luminal blood are metabolised by the liver.
- Liver function tests.
- Prothrombin time, if there is clinical suggestion of liver disease or in anticoagulated patients.
- Cross-matching of at least 2 units of blood.

4. *Resuscitation* (see p. 1033). Intravenous crystalloid fluids or colloid are given to restore the blood pressure. Blood is transfused when the patient is shocked or when the haemoglobin concentration is less than 100 g per litre.

Normal saline should be avoided in patients with liver disease because it can cause ascites.

Central venous pressure (CVP) monitoring is used in severe bleeding, particularly in patients who have cardiac disease, to assist in defining the volume of fluid replacement and in identification of rebleeding.

5. *Oxygen.* This should be given by face mask to all shocked patients.

6. *Endoscopy.* This should be carried out after adequate resuscitation. A diagnosis will be achieved in 80% of cases. Patients who are found to have major endoscopic stigmata of recent haemorrhage (see Fig. 9.14) are treated endoscopically using a thermal modality such as a 'heater probe', or by injection of dilute adrenaline into the bleeding point. Endoscopic therapy is also used for varices (see p. 695), vascular malformations and occasionally for Mallory–Weiss tears.

Visceral angiography is advisable when endoscopy is normal and the patient is actively bleeding by at least 1 ml per minute. For bleeding of lesser severity, colonoscopy is the best option; vascular malformations are the most common cause. In young patients, a ^{99}Tc-sulphur colloid scan may show bleeding from a Meckel's diverticulum.

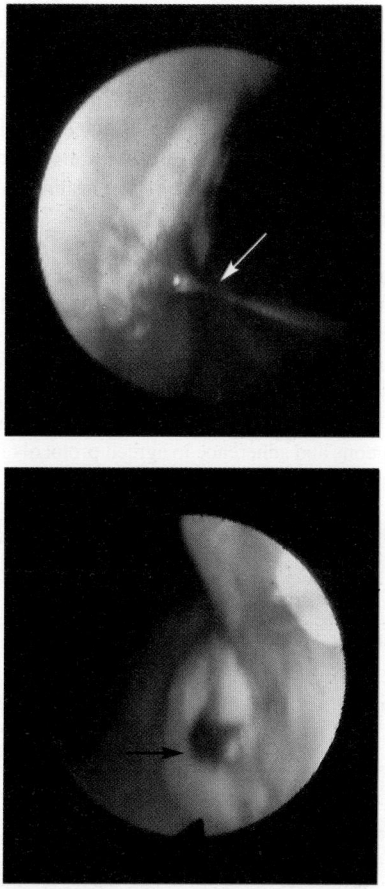

Fig. 9.14 Major stigmata of recent haemorrhage. A Active spurting haemorrhage (arrow) from a duodenal ulcer. When associated with shock, 80% of cases will continue to bleed or rebleed. B 'Visible vessel' (arrow). In reality, this is a pseudoaneurysm of the feeding artery seen here in a prepyloric peptic ulcer. It carries a 50% chance of rebleeding.

7. *Monitoring.* Patients are closely observed with hourly pulse, blood pressure and urine output measurements.

8. *Surgical operation.* An urgent surgical operation is undertaken when:

- endoscopic haemostasis fails to stop active bleeding
- rebleeding occurs on one occasion in an elderly or frail patient, or twice in younger, fitter patients.

The choice of operation depends on the site and diagnosis of the bleeding lesion. Duodenal ulcers are treated by undersewing and pyloroplasty. In contrast, gastric ulcers are treated by partial gastrectomy or simple excision. Following successful surgery for ulcer bleeding, all patients should be treated with *H. pylori* eradication therapy if positive and should avoid non-steroidal anti-inflammatory drugs (NSAIDs) in the future.

Patients who have had documented ulcer bleeding should undergo repeat upper gastrointestinal endoscopy after 6 weeks to ensure adequate ulcer healing has occurred.

Prognosis

The mortality of patients admitted to hospital following a diagnosis of acute upper gastrointestinal bleeding is approximately 10%. Risk factors for death are shown in Table 9.10. Improved mortality can be achieved by specialised units in which joint management by physicians and surgeons and adherence to agreed protocols for transfusion and surgery are applied.

Table 9.10 Risk factors for death in patients who present with acute upper gastrointestinal haemorrhage

Factor	Comments
Increasing age	Risk increases over age 60 and especially in very elderly
Comorbidity	Advanced malignancy, renal and hepatic failure are associated with particularly high mortality
Shock	Defined as pulse > 100/min, BP < 100 mmHg
Diagnosis	Varices and cancer have the worst prognosis
Endoscopic findings	Active bleeding and a non-bleeding visible vessel at endoscopy are associated with a high risk of continuing bleeding
Rebleeding*	Associated with 10-fold rise in mortality

* Defined as fresh haematemesis or melaena associated with shock or a fall of Hb > 20 g/l over 24 hours.

OVERT LOWER GASTROINTESTINAL BLEEDING

This may be due to haemorrhage from the small bowel, colon or anal canal. It is useful to distinguish those patients who present with profuse, acute bleeding from those who present with chronic or subacute bleeding of lesser severity.

CAUSES OF LOWER GASTROINTESTINAL BLEEDING

Severe acute

- Diverticular disease
- Angiodysplasia
- Ischaemia
- Meckel's diverticulum

Moderate, chronic/subacute

- Anal disease, e.g. fissure, haemorrhoids
- Inflammatory bowel disease
- Carcinoma
- Large polyps
- Angiodysplasia
- Radiation enteritis
- Solitary rectal ulcer

Severe acute lower gastrointestinal bleeding

This is an unusual medical emergency. Patients present with profuse red or maroon diarrhoea and with shock.

Diverticular disease is the most common cause. Acute bleeding is due to erosion of an artery within the mouth of a diverticulum and bleeding almost always stops spontaneously.

Angiodysplasia is a disease of the elderly in which vascular malformations develop in the proximal colon. The condition is associated with aortic valve disease and often presents after aortic valve replacement. Bleeding tends to be acute and profuse, and usually stops spontaneously but commonly recurs. Diagnosis is often difficult. Colonoscopy reveals characteristic vascular spots which are reminiscent of spider naevi. In acute bleeding, visceral angiography shows bleeding into the intestinal lumen and an abnormal large, draining vein. In some patients diagnosis is only achieved by laparotomy with on-table colonoscopy. The treatment of choice is endoscopic laser photocoagulation but right hemicolectomy is sometimes necessary in severe cases.

Ischaemia is due to occlusion of the inferior mesenteric artery and presents with abdominal colic and rectal bleeding. It should be considered in any patient who has evidence of generalised atherosclerosis.

Meckel's diverticulum with ectopic gastric epithelium may ulcerate and erode into a major artery. The diagnosis should be considered in children or adolescents who present with profuse or recurrent lower gastrointestinal bleeding. A Meckel's scan is sometimes positive but the diagnosis is commonly made only by laparotomy, at which time the diverticulum is excised.

Subacute or chronic lower gastrointestinal bleeding

This is extremely common at all ages and is usually due to haemorrhoids or anal fissure. *Haemorrhoidal* bleeding is bright red and occurs during or after defaecation. Proctoscopy is used to make the diagnosis but in subjects who also have altered bowel habit and in all patients presenting over 40 years of age, colonoscopy or barium enema is necessary to exclude coexisting colorectal cancer. *Anal fissure* should be suspected when fresh rectal bleeding and anal pain occur during defaecation.

OCCULT GASTROINTESTINAL BLEEDING

'Occult' means that blood or its breakdown products are

present in the stool but cannot be seen. Occult bleeding may be as much as 200 ml per day, may cause iron deficiency anaemia and may signify serious gastrointestinal disease. Any cause of gastrointestinal bleeding may be responsible but the most important is colorectal cancer, particularly carcinoma of the caecum which may have no gastrointestinal symptoms.

In clinical practice, investigation of the gastrointestinal tract should be considered whenever a patient presents with unexplained iron deficiency anaemia. Testing the stool for the presence of blood is unnecessary and should not influence whether or not the gastrointestinal tract is imaged because bleeding from tumours is often intermittent and a negative faecal occult blood (FOB) test does not exclude important gastrointestinal disease. Many colorectal cancer patients are FOB negative at presentation, and the only value of FOB testing relates to screening for colonic disease in asymptomatic populations.

Patients found to have colonic cancer on the basis of population screening have earlier-stage tumours and better 5-year survival rates than those patients who present with symptoms.

DIARRHOEA

The bowel frequency of the normal population ranges from three bowel movements per day to one bowel action every third day, and a normal stool consistency ranges from

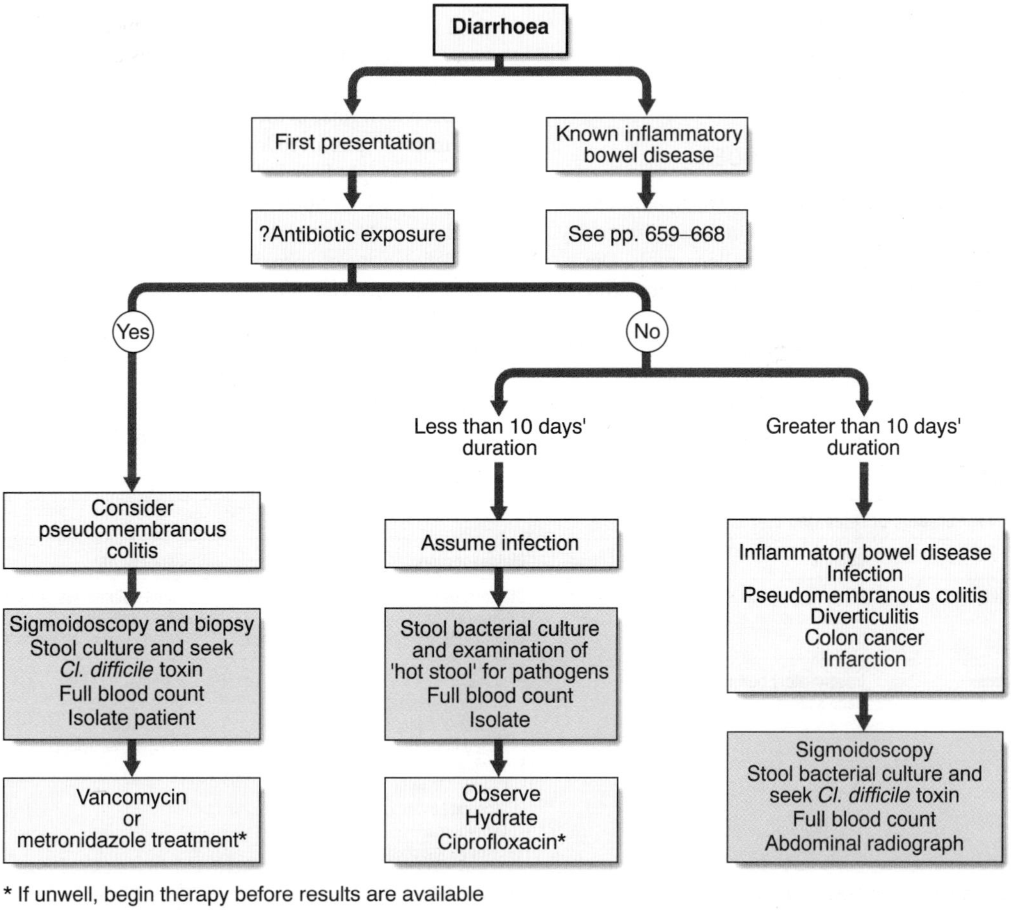

Fig. 9.15 Algorithm for the management of acute diarrhoea.

porridge-like to hard and pellety. The term 'diarrhoea' means different things to different people. Many patients and doctors think of diarrhoea in terms of increased stool frequency, and loose or watery stools. Gastroenterologists define diarrhoea as the passage of more than 200 g of stool daily, and the measurement of stool volume is sometimes helpful in patient evaluation. The most severe symptom in many patients is urgency of defaecation, and faecal incontinence is a common event in acute and chronic diarrhoeal illnesses.

ACUTE DIARRHOEA

This is extremely common and usually due to faecal-oral transmission of bacterial toxins, viruses, bacteria or protozoan organisms (see Ch. 2). Infective diarrhoea is usually short-lived and patients who present with a history of diarrhoea lasting more than 10 days rarely have an infective cause. A variety of drugs, including antibiotics, cytotoxic drugs and NSAIDs, may be responsible for acute diarrhoea. An approach to the diagnosis of patients presenting with acute diarrhoea is shown in Figure 9.15.

CHRONIC OR RELAPSING DIARRHOEA

The most common cause is irritable bowel syndrome (see p. 668), which can present with increased frequency of defaecation and loose, watery or pellety stools. Diarrhoea rarely occurs at night and is most severe before and after breakfast. At other times the patient is constipated and there are other characteristic symptoms of irritable bowel syndrome. The stool often contains mucus but never blood, and 24-hour stool volume is less than 200 g.

Chronic diarrhoea can be categorised as disease of the colon or small bowel, or malabsorption (see Table 9.11). Clinical presentation, examination of the stool, routine blood tests and imaging reveal a diagnosis in many cases. A series of negative investigations usually implies irritable bowel syndrome but some patients clearly have organic disease and need more extensive investigations.

MALABSORPTION

Digestion and absorption of nutrients is a complex, highly coordinated and extremely efficient process: normally less than 5% of ingested carbohydrate, fat and protein is excreted in the faeces. Diarrhoea and weight loss in patients with a normal diet should always lead to the suspicion of malabsorption.

The symptoms of malabsorption are diverse in nature and variable in severity. A few patients have apparently normal bowel habit but diarrhoea is usual and may be watery and voluminous. Bulky, pale and offensive stools which float in the toilet (steatorrhoea) signify fat malabsorption. Abdominal distension, borborygmi, cramps, weight loss and undigested food in the stool may be present. Some patients complain only of malaise and lethargy. In others, symptoms related to deficiencies of specific vitamins, trace elements and minerals (e.g. calcium, iron, folic acid) may occur (see Fig. 9.16).

Aetiology and pathogenesis

Malabsorption results from abnormalities of the three processes which are essential to normal digestion:

Table 9.11 Chronic or relapsing diarrhoea

	Colonic	Malabsorption	Small bowel
Clinical features	Blood and mucus in stool Cramping lower abdominal pain	Steatorrhoea Undigested food in the stool Weight loss and nutritional disturbances	Large-volume, watery stool Abdominal bloating Cramping mid-abdominal pain
Some causes	Inflammatory bowel disease Neoplasia	Pancreatic Chronic pancreatitis Cancer of pancreas Cystic fibrosis Enteropathy Coeliac disease Tropical sprue Lymphoma Lymphangiectasia	VIPoma Drug-induced NSAIDs Aminosalicylates
Investigations	Flexible sigmoidoscopy with biopsies and barium enema, or colonoscopy with biopsies	Ultrasound, CT and ERCP Small bowel biopsy Barium follow-through	Stool volume Gut Hormone profile Barium follow-through

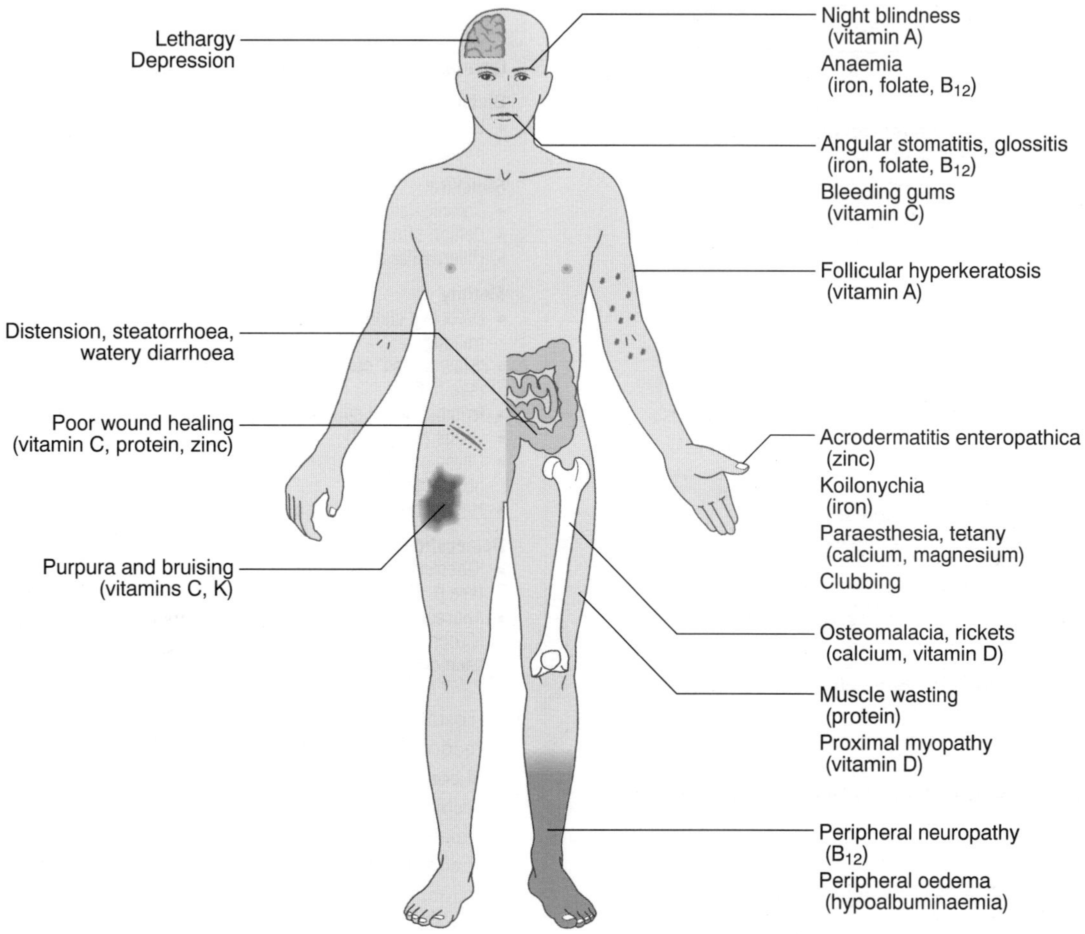

Fig. 9.16 Physical consequences of malabsorption.

ROUTINE BLOOD TESTS IN MALABSORPTION
Haematology
• Microcytic anaemia (iron deficiency) • Macrocytic anaemia (folate or B_{12} deficiency) • Increased prothrombin time (vitamin K deficiency)
Biochemistry
• Hypoalbuminaemia • Hypocalcaemia and vitamin D deficiency • Hypomagnesaemia • Deficiencies of phosphate, zinc

1. *Intraluminal maldigestion* occurs when deficiency of bile or pancreatic enzymes results in inadequate solubilisation and hydrolysis of nutrients. Fat and protein malabsorption results.
2. *Mucosal malabsorption* results from small bowel resection or conditions which damage the small intestinal epithelium, thereby diminishing the surface area for absorption and depleting brush border enzyme activity.
3. *'Postmucosal' lymphatic obstruction* prevents the uptake and transport of absorbed lipids into lymphatic vessels. Increased pressure in these vessels results in leakage into the intestinal lumen, leading to protein-losing enteropathy.

Diagnosis and investigations

Investigations are performed to confirm that malabsorption is present and then to determine the cause. Routine blood tests may show one or more of the abnormalities listed in the information box. Tests to confirm fat and protein malabsorption are performed as described on page 610.

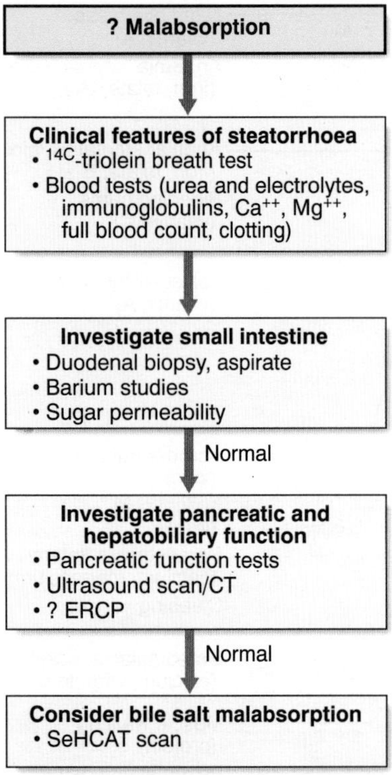

Fig. 9.17 Investigation for suspected malabsorption.

An approach to the investigation of malabsorption is shown in Figure 9.17.

CONSTIPATION

Constipation is defined as infrequent passage of hard stools. Patients may also complain of straining, a sensation of incomplete evacuation and either perianal or abdominal discomfort. Constipation may be the end result of many gastrointestinal and other medical disorders (see the information box).

The onset, duration and characteristics are important, e.g. a neonatal onset suggests Hirschsprung's disease, while a recent change in bowel activity in middle age should raise the suspicion of organic disorders such as colonic carcinoma. The presence of symptoms such as rectal bleeding, pain and weight loss are important, as are excessive straining, symptoms suggestive of irritable bowel syndrome, a history of childhood constipation and emotional distress.

Careful examination contributes more to the diagnosis than does extensive investigation. A search should be made for general medical disorders as well as signs of bloating, obstruction or masses. Neurological disorders, especially spinal cord lesions, should be sought. Perineal inspection and rectal examination are essential and may reveal abnormalities of the pelvic floor (e.g. abnormal descent, impaired sensation), anal canal or rectum (masses, faecal impaction, prolapse).

It is neither possible nor appropriate to investigate every person with this very common complaint. Most will respond to dietary fibre supplementation and the judicious use of laxatives. Middle-aged or elderly patients with a short history or worrying symptoms (rectal bleeding, pain or weight loss) must be investigated promptly, either by barium enema or colonoscopy. For those with simple constipation, investigation will usually proceed along the following lines.

CAUSES OF CONSTIPATION	
Gastrointestinal disorders	**Non-gastrointestinal disorders**
Dietary • Lack of fibre and/or fluid intake **Structural** • Colonic carcinoma • Benign strictures • Diverticular disease **Motility** • Defective childhood bowel training • 'Slow transit' constipation (see p. 677) • Irritable bowel syndrome • Drugs (see right) • Chronic intestinal pseudo-obstruction • Hirschsprung's disease **Defaecation** • 'Obstructed defaecation' (see p. 677) • Anorectal disease (Crohn's, fissures, haemorrhoids)	**Drugs** • Opiates • Anticholinergics • Calcium antagonists • Iron supplements • Aluminium-containing antacids **Metabolic/endocrine** • Diabetes mellitus • Hypercalcaemia • Hypothyroidism • Pregnancy **Neurological** • Multiple sclerosis • Spinal cord lesions • Cerebrovascular accidents • Parkinsonism **Others** • Any serious illness with immobility, especially in the elderly

Initial visit

Digital rectal examination, proctoscopy and sigmoidoscopy (to detect anorectal disease); routine biochemistry, including serum calcium and thyroid function tests; and a full blood count should be carried out. If these are normal, a 1-month trial of dietary fibre and/or laxatives is justified.

Next visit

If symptoms persist, then examination of the colon by barium enema or colonoscopy is indicated to look for structural disease.

Further investigation

If no cause is found and disabling symptoms are present, then specialist referral for investigation of possible dysmotility may be necessary. The problem may be one of infrequent desire to defaecate ('slow transit') or else may result from excessive straining ('obstructed defaecation', see p. 677). Intestinal marker studies, scintigraphy, anorectal manometry, electrophysiological studies and defaecating proctography can all be used to define the problem.

ABDOMINAL PAIN

There are several types of abdominal pain:

- *Visceral*. Gut organs are insensitive to stimuli such as burning and cutting but are sensitive to distension, contraction, torsion and stretching. Pain from unpaired structures is usually but not always felt in the midline.
- *Parietal*. Parietal peritoneum is innervated by somatic nerves, and its involvement by disease processes, e.g. inflammation, infection or neoplasia, tends to produce sharp, well-localised and lateralised pain.
- *Referred pain*. (For example, gallbladder pain is referred to the back or shoulder tip.)
- *Psychogenic*. Cultural, emotional and psychosocial factors influence everyone's experience of pain. In some patients, no organic cause can be found despite investigation, and psychogenic causes may be responsible, e.g. depression or somatisation disorder.

ACUTE ABDOMINAL PAIN

This usually presents as an emergency and may be accompanied by other features such as fever, vomiting or shock. On examination, patients may be febrile, pale and sweaty and in considerable distress. Abdominal tenderness is often accompanied by signs of peritoneal irritation, including guarding, rebound tenderness and rigidity. Bowel sounds are high-pitched and frequent in intestinal obstruction, when there will also be signs of gaseous distension and possibly visible peristalsis. Bowel sounds are absent in established generalised peritonitis. The causes of acute abdominal pain are listed in the first information box and the reader is referred to textbooks of surgery for further discussion of the acute abdomen.

CHRONIC OR RECURRENT ABDOMINAL PAIN

At the outpatient clinic a careful and detailed history is essential, with particular attention to the features of the pain and any associated symptoms (see the information boxes).

CAUSES OF ACUTE ABDOMINAL PAIN ('SURGICAL')

Inflammation
- Appendicitis
- Diverticulitis
- Cholecystitis
- Salpingitis
- Pelvic inflammatory disease
- Pancreatitis
- Pyelonephritis
- Intra-abdominal abscess

Perforation/rupture
- Peptic ulcer
- Diverticular disease
- Ovarian cyst

Vascular/ischaemia
- Ruptured aortic aneurysm
- Mesenteric infarction
- Haemorrhage or torsion (ovarian cyst, testicular)

Obstruction
- Intestinal obstruction
- Biliary colic
- Ureteric colic

Other (rare)
- See 'extraintestinal' causes below

'EXTRAINTESTINAL' CAUSES OF CHRONIC OR RECURRENT ABDOMINAL PAIN

Neurological
- Spinal cord lesions
- Radiculopathy

Locomotor
- Vertebral compression
- Abdominal muscle strain

Retroperitoneal
- Aortic aneurysm
- Malignancy
- Lymphadenopathy
- Abscess

Metabolic/endocrine
- Diabetes mellitus
- Addison's disease
- Acute intermittent porphyria
- Hypercalcaemia

Drugs/toxins
- Corticosteroids
- Azathioprine
- Lead
- Alcohol

Haematological
- Sickle-cell disease
- Haemolytic disorders

Psychogenic
- Depression
- Anxiety
- Hypochondriasis
- Somatoform pain disorder
- Somatisation disorder

IMPORTANT FACTORS IN THE ASSESSMENT OF ABDOMINAL PAIN

- Duration
- Site and radiation
- Severity
- Precipitating and relieving factors (food, drugs, alcohol, posture, movement, defaecation)
- Nature (colicky, constant, sharp or dull, wakening at night)
- Pattern (intermittent or continuous)
- Associated features (vomiting, dyspepsia, altered bowel habit)

Note should be made of the patient's general demeanour, mood and emotional state, signs of weight loss, fever, jaundice or anaemia. If thorough abdominal and rectal examination are normal, a careful search should be made for evidence of disease affecting other structures, particularly the vertebral column, spinal cord, lungs and cardiovascular system.

The initial choice of investigations will obviously depend on the clinical features elicited during the history and examination:

- Epigastric pain, dyspepsia and relationship to food suggest gastroduodenal or biliary disease. Endoscopy and ultrasound are indicated.
- Altered bowel habit, rectal bleeding or features of obstruction suggest colonic disease. Barium enema and sigmoidoscopy, or colonoscopy are indicated.
- Pain provoked by food in a patient with widespread atherosclerosis may indicate mesenteric ischaemia. Mesenteric angiography may be necessary.
- Young patients with a long history of pain relieved by defaecation, bloating and alternating bowel habit are likely to have irritable bowel syndrome (see p. 668). Simple investigations (bloods and sigmoidoscopy) may be sufficient, but persistent symptoms require exclusion of colonic or small bowel disease by radiology or endoscopy.
- Upper abdominal pain radiating to the back, a history of alcohol abuse, weight loss and diarrhoea suggest chronic pancreatitis. Ultrasound, ERCP, CT scans and pancreatic function tests are required.
- Recurrent attacks of pain in the loins or radiating to the flanks with urinary symptoms should prompt investigation for renal or ureteric stones by ultrasound and intravenous urography.
- A past history of psychiatric disturbance, repeated negative investigations or vague symptoms which do not fit any particular disease or organ pattern may point to a psychological origin for the patient's pain. Careful review of case notes and previous investigations, along with open and honest discussion with the patient may reduce the need for further cycles of unnecessary and invasive tests. Care must always be taken, however, not to miss rare causes or atypical presentations of common diseases.

CONSTANT PAIN

Patients with chronic pain which is constant or nearly always present will usually have features to suggest the underlying diagnosis, e.g. malignancy (gastric, pancreatic, colonic), hepatic metastases, chronic pancreatitis or intra-abdominal abscess. In other patients the diagnosis is not initially obvious but will become so after appropriate investigation. In a minority no cause will be found despite thorough investigation. Once unusual or rare conditions and atypical presentations of common diseases have been ruled out, the diagnosis of 'chronic idiopathic abdominal pain' is made. In these patients a psychological cause is highly likely and the most important task is to provide symptom control, if not relief, and to minimise the effects of the pain on their social, personal and occupational life. This may involve detailed psychological evaluation.

FURTHER INFORMATION ON MAJOR MANIFESTATIONS OF GASTROINTESTINAL DISEASE

Mandel J S, Bond J H, Church T R et al 1993 Reduced mortality from colorectal cancer by screening for faecal occult blood. New England Journal of Medicine 328: 1365–1371

DISEASES OF THE MOUTH AND SALIVARY GLANDS

APHTHOUS ULCERATION

Aphthous ulcers are superficial, painful ulcers which occur in any part of the mouth. Recurrent aphthous ulcers afflict up to 30% of the population and are particularly common in women prior to menstruation. The aetiology is unknown, but in severe cases other causes of oral ulceration must be considered (see the information box). Occasionally, biopsy is necessary to define the diagnosis.

Topical corticosteroids, chlortetracycline mouthwashes or a paste of betamethasone can effect healing. Symptomatic relief is achieved using local anaesthetic mouthwashes or salicylate paste. A few patients have very severe, recurrent aphthous ulcers and need oral steroids.

VINCENT'S ANGINA

This is characterised by painful, deep, sloughing ulcers which principally affect the gums. It is due to invasion of the mucous membranes by organisms such as *Borrelia vincenti* and other commensals. Invasion occurs when host resistance is low and oral hygiene is poor. Malnutrition, general debility and AIDS predispose. The illness is associated with halitosis and many patients are feverish and systemically unwell. Local treatment with hydrogen peroxide mouthwashes and broad-spectrum antibiotics are required.

CANDIDIASIS

The fungus *Candida albicans* is a normal mouth commensal but it may proliferate to cause thrush. This occurs in babies, debilitated patients, patients receiving corticosteroid or antibiotic therapy and immunosuppressed patients, especially those receiving cytotoxic therapy and patients with AIDS. White patches are seen on the tongue and buccal mucosa. Painful swallowing (odynophagia) or dysphagia suggests pharyngeal and oesophageal candidiasis. A clinical diagnosis is sufficient to instigate therapy, although brushings or biopsies can be obtained for mycological examination.

CAUSES OF ORAL ULCERATION
Aphthous
Infection • Fungal, e.g. candidiasis • Bacterial, e.g. Vincent's angina, syphilis • Viral, e.g. herpes simplex
Gastrointestinal diseases
• Crohn's disease • Coeliac disease
Dermatological conditions
• Lichen planus • Pemphigoid • Pemphigus
Drugs
• Hypersensitivity, e.g. Stevens–Johnson syndrome • Cytotoxics
Systemic diseases
• Systemic lupus erythematosus • Behçet's syndrome
Neoplasia
• Carcinoma • Leukaemia • Kaposi's sarcoma

Oral thrush is treated using nystatin or amphotericin suspensions or lozenges. Resistant cases or immunosuppressed patients may require oral fluconazole.

PAROTITIS

Parotitis is due to viral or bacterial infection. Mumps causes a self-limiting acute parotitis (see p. 85). Bacterial parotitis usually occurs as a complication of major surgery. It is a consequence of dehydration and poor oral hygiene and can be avoided by good post-operative care. Patients present with painful parotid swelling and this can be complicated by abscess formation. Broad-spectrum antibiotics are required, whilst surgical drainage is necessary for abscesses. Other causes of salivary gland enlargement are listed in the information box.

CAUSES OF SALIVARY GLAND SWELLING
Infection • Mumps • Bacterial (post-operative)
Calculi
Tumours • Benign: pleomorphic adenoma (95% of cases) • Intermediate: mucoepidermoid tumour • Malignant: carcinoma
Sjögren's syndrome (see p. 861)
Sarcoidosis

DISEASES OF THE OESOPHAGUS

GASTRO-OESOPHAGEAL REFLUX DISEASE

Gastro-oesophageal reflux is the most common cause of indigestion, affecting up to 30% of the general population.

Pathophysiology

Occasional episodes of gastro-oesophageal reflux are common in health. Reflux is followed by oesophageal peristaltic waves which efficiently clear the gullet, alkaline saliva neutralises residual acid, and symptoms do not occur. Gastro-oesophageal reflux disease develops when the oesophageal mucosa is exposed to gastric contents for prolonged periods of time, resulting in symptoms and, in a proportion of cases, to oesophagitis. Several factors are known to be involved (see Fig. 9.18).

Abnormalities of the lower oesophageal sphincter

In health, the lower oesophageal sphincter is tonically contracted, relaxing only during swallowing (see p. 600).

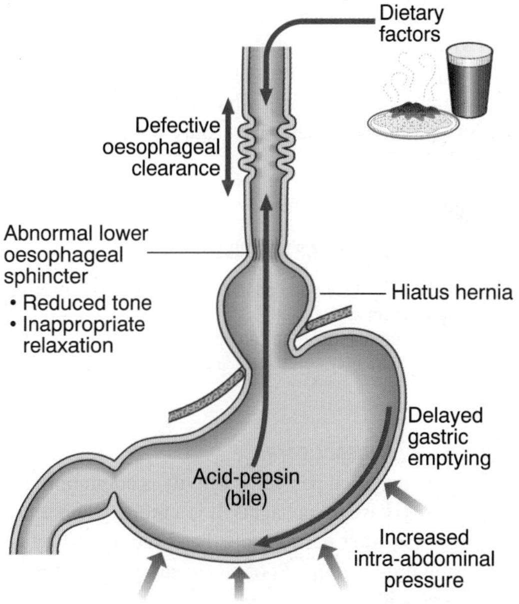

Fig. 9.18 Factors associated with the development of gastro-oesophageal reflux disease.

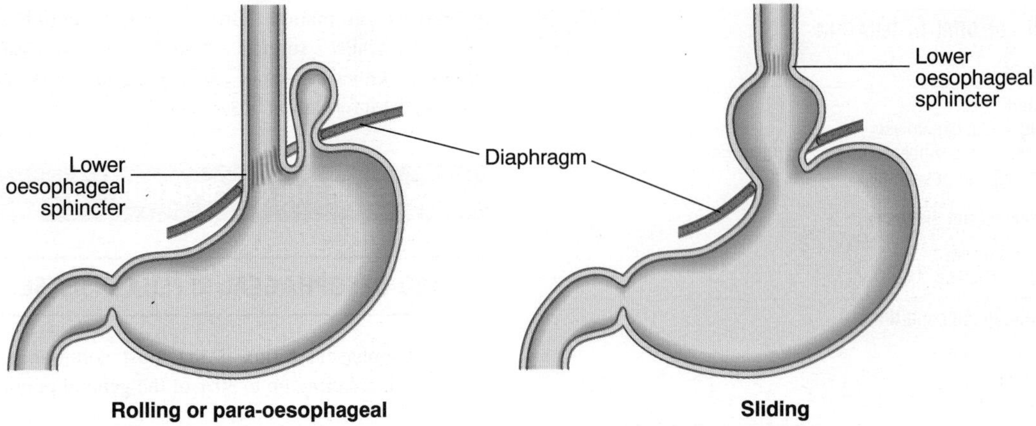

Fig. 9.19 Types of hiatus hernia.

Some patients with gastro-oesophageal reflux disease have reduced lower oesophageal sphincter tone, permitting reflux when intra-abdominal pressure rises. In others, basal sphincter tone is normal but reflux occurs in response to frequent episodes of inappropriate sphincter relaxation.

Hiatus hernia (see Fig. 9.19)

Hiatus hernia causes reflux because the pressure gradient between the abdominal and thoracic cavities, which normally pinches the hiatus, is lost. In addition, the oblique angle between the cardia and oesophagus disappears. Many patients who have large hiatus hernias develop reflux symptoms, but the relationship between the presence of a hernia and symptoms is poor. Hiatus hernia is very common in individuals who have no symptoms, and some symptomatic patients have only a very small or no hernia.

IMPORTANT FEATURES OF HIATUS HERNIA

- Occurs in 30% of the population over the age of 50 years
- Often asymptomatic
- Heartburn and regurgitation can occur
- Gastric volvulus may complicate large hernias

Delayed oesophageal clearance

Defective oesophageal peristaltic activity is commonly found in patients who have oesophagitis. It is a primary abnormality, since it persists after oesophagitis has been healed by acid-suppressing drug therapy. Poor oesophageal clearance leads to increased acid exposure time.

Gastric contents

Gastric acid is the most important oesophageal irritant and there is a close relationship between acid exposure time and symptoms. Alkaline reflux, due to bile reflux following gastric surgery, is of uncertain importance.

Defective gastric emptying

Gastric emptying is delayed in patients with gastro-oesophageal reflux disease. The reason for this is unknown.

Increased intra-abdominal pressure

Pregnancy and obesity are established predisposing causes. Weight loss commonly improves symptoms.

Dietary and environmental factors

Dietary fat, chocolate, alcohol and coffee relax the lower oesophageal sphincter and may provoke symptoms. There is little evidence to incriminate smoking or NSAIDs as causes of gastro-oesophageal reflux disease.

Clinical features

The major symptoms are heartburn and regurgitation, often provoked by bending, straining or lying down. 'Waterbrash', which is salivation due to reflex salivary gland stimulation as acid enters the gullet, is often present. A history of weight gain is common. Some patients are woken at night by choking as refluxed fluid irritates the larynx. Others develop odynophagia or dysphagia. A few present with atypical chest pain which may be severe, can mimic angina, and is probably due to reflux-induced oesophageal spasm.

Complications

Oesophagitis (see Fig. 9.20)

A range of endoscopic findings, from mild redness to severe, bleeding ulceration with stricture formation, is recognised. There is a poor correlation between symptoms and histological

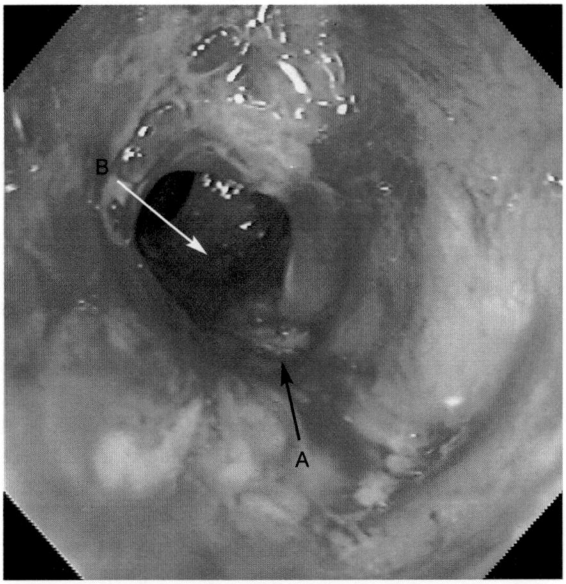

Fig. 9.20 Reflux oesophagitis. The lower gullet is ulcerated (arrow A) and bleeds easily, and an early stricture (arrow B) is present.

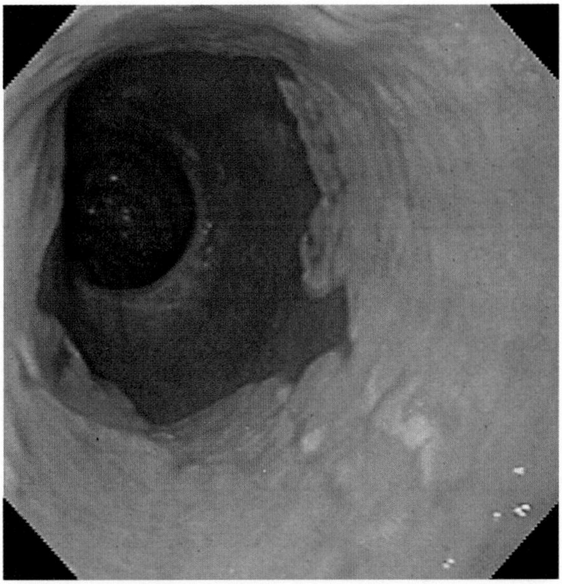

Fig. 9.21 Barrett's oesophagus. Pink columnar mucosa extending from the cardia into the lower oesophagus.

and endoscopic findings. A normal endoscopy and normal oesophageal histology are perfectly compatible with significant gastro-oesophageal reflux disease.

Barrett's oesophagus

Metaplasia of the normal squamous epithelium of the oesophagus to form columnar epithelium is known as Barrett's oesophagus and is a consequence of chronic gastro-oesophageal reflux. Almost all patients have hiatus hernia. Barrett's oesophagus is recognised endoscopically as confluent areas or fingers of pink, gastric-like mucosa extending from the cardia into the oesophagus (see Fig. 9.21). Islands of residual squamous oesophageal mucosa may be seen within areas of Barrett's metaplasia.

The risk of adenocarcinoma is increased 90–150-fold by Barrett's oesophagus and is particularly high in the presence of intestinal metaplasia with goblet cells. Consequently, patients discovered to have Barrett's change during endoscopy are considered for endoscopic surveillance programmes. Patients found to have no or minimal dysplasia are at low risk of cancer and surveillance is not cost-effective in this situation. Patients with moderate dysplasia should undergo repeated biopsies at 6–12-monthly intervals. Patients found to have severe dysplasia often have associated cancer and are usually referred for oesophageal surgery.

There is little evidence to show that medical therapy (with powerful acid-suppressing drugs) or antireflux surgery causes Barrett's oesophagus to regress.

Anaemia

Iron deficiency anaemia occurs as a consequence of chronic, insidious blood loss from long-standing oesophagitis. Almost all such patients have a large hiatus hernia. Nevertheless, hiatus hernia is very common and other causes of blood loss, particularly colorectal cancer, must be considered in anaemic patients, even when endoscopy reveals oesophagitis and a hiatus hernia.

Benign oesophageal stricture

Fibrous strictures develop as a consequence of long-standing oesophagitis. Most patients are elderly and have poor oesophageal peristaltic activity. They present with dysphagia which is worse for solids than liquids. Bolus obstruction following ingestion of meat can lead to absolute dysphagia. A history of heartburn is common but not invariable, particularly in the elderly.

Diagnosis is made by endoscopy, and biopsies of the stricture are taken to exclude malignancy. Endoscopic balloon dilatation or bouginage is undertaken. Subsequently, long-term therapy with a proton pump inhibitor drug (omeprazole 20–40 mg or lansoprazole 30 mg daily) should be started to reduce the risk of recurrent oesophagitis and stricture formation. The patient should be advised to chew food thoroughly, and it is important to ensure adequate dentition.

Investigations

Young patients who present with typical symptoms of gastro-oesophageal reflux, without worrying features such as dysphagia, weight loss or anaemia, can be treated empirically.

Investigation is advisable if patients present in middle or late age, if symptoms are atypical or if a complication is suspected. Endoscopy is the investigation of choice. This is done to exclude other upper gastrointestinal diseases which can mimic gastro-oesophageal reflux, and to identify complications. A normal endoscopy in a patient with compatible symptoms should not preclude treatment for gastro-oesophageal reflux disease.

When, despite endoscopy, the diagnosis is unclear or if surgical intervention is under consideration, 24-hour pH monitoring is indicated. This involves tethering a slim catheter with a terminal radiotelemetry pH-sensitive probe above the gastro-oesophageal junction. The intraluminal pH is recorded whilst the patient undergoes normal activities, and episodes of pain are noted and related to pH. A pH of less than 4 for more than 4% of the study time is diagnostic of reflux disease.

Management

A stepwise approach, as shown in Figure 9.22, is appropriate. The pragmatic clinician is aware that advice to alter lifestyle is rarely heeded. However, potentially useful changes include weight loss, avoidance of dietary items which the patient finds worsens symptoms, elevation of the bed head in those who experience nocturnal symptoms, avoidance of late meals and giving up smoking.

Proprietary antacids and alginates, which are said to produce a protective mucosal 'raft' over the oesophageal mucosa, are taken with considerable symptomatic benefit by most patients. H_2-receptor antagonist drugs (see p. 636) help symptoms without healing oesophagitis. They are well tolerated and the timing of medication and dosage should be tailored to individual need.

Proton pump inhibitors (see p. 636) are the treatment of choice for severe symptoms and for complicated reflux disease. Symptoms almost invariably resolve and oesophagitis heals in the majority of patients. Recurrence of symptoms is almost inevitable when therapy is stopped and some patients require life-long treatment.

Patients who fail to respond to medical therapy, those who are unwilling to take long-term proton pump inhibitors and those whose major symptom is severe regurgitation should be considered for antireflux surgery. This can be undertaken by an open approach or by laparoscopy. Although heartburn and regurgitation are alleviated in most patients, a proportion develop complications such as inability to vomit and abdominal bloating ('gas-bloat syndrome').

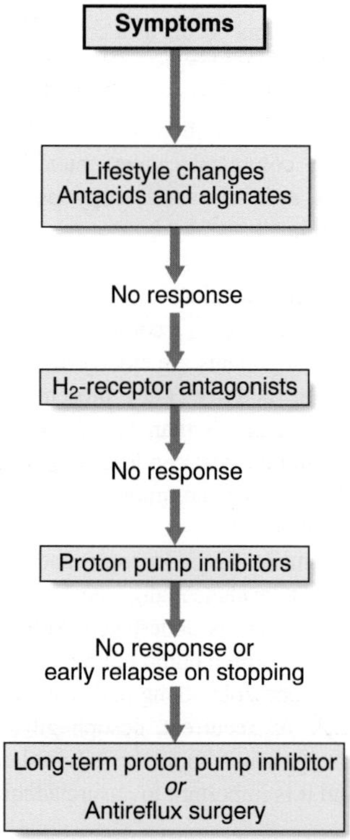

Fig. 9.22 Treatment of gastro-oesophageal reflux disease: a stepwise approach.

OTHER CAUSES OF OESOPHAGITIS

Infection

Oesophageal candidiasis occurs in debilitated patients, and those taking broad-spectrum antibiotics or cytotoxic drugs. It is a particular problem in AIDS patients, who are also susceptible to a spectrum of oesophageal infections (see p. 102).

Corrosives

Suicide attempt by household bleach is followed by painful burns of the mouth and pharynx and by extensive erosive oesophagitis. This is complicated by oesophageal perforation leading to mediastinitis and by stricture formation. At the time of presentation, treatment is conservative, based upon analgesia and nutritional support. Vomiting should be avoided and endoscopy should not be carried out at this stage because of the high risk of oesophageal perforation. Following the acute phase, a barium swallow is performed to demonstrate the extent of stricture formation. Endoscopic dilatation is usually necessary, although it is difficult and hazardous because strictures are often long, tortuous and easily perforated.

Drugs

Potassium supplements and NSAIDs may cause oesophageal ulcers when the tablets are trapped above an oesophageal stricture. Liquid preparations of these drugs should be used in such patients.

MOTILITY DISORDERS

PHARYNGEAL POUCH

Incoordination of swallowing within the pharynx leads to herniation through the cricopharyngeus muscle and formation of a pouch. Most patients are elderly and have no symptoms, although regurgitation, halitosis and dysphagia can occur. Some notice gurgling in the throat after swallowing. A barium swallow demonstrates the pouch and reveals incoordination of swallowing, often with pulmonary aspiration. Endoscopy may be hazardous since the instrument may enter and perforate the pouch. Surgical myotomy and resection of the pouch are indicated in symptomatic patients.

ACHALASIA OF THE OESOPHAGUS

Pathophysiology

Achalasia is characterised by a hypertonic lower oesophageal sphincter which fails to relax in response to the oesophageal swallowing wave. As the disease progresses the obstructed lower oesophagus dilates and peristalsis within the body of the gullet becomes less powerful.

The cause is unknown, although failure of non-adrenergic, non-cholinergic (NANC) innervation related to abnormal nitric oxide synthesis within the lower oesophageal sphincter has been found. Degeneration of ganglion cells within the sphincter and the body of the oesophagus occurs. Loss of the dorsal vagal nuclei within the brain stem can be demonstrated in later stages.

Chagas disease (see p. 162) is a disease endemic in South America in which infestation with the protozoan organism *Trypanosoma cruzi* leads to myocarditis and a range of motility disorders of the gastrointestinal tract. Destruction of the myenteric plexus causes a syndrome which is clinically indistinguishable from achalasia.

Clinical features

Achalasia is an unusual disease affecting 1:100 000 of Western populations. It usually develops in middle life, but can occur at any age. Dysphagia develops slowly, and is initially intermittent. It is worse for solids and is eased by drinking liquids, standing and moving around after eating. Heartburn does not occur, since the closed oesophageal sphincter prevents gastro-oesophageal reflux. Some patients experience episodes of severe chest pain due to oesophageal spasm ('vigorous achalasia'), although this disappears as the body of the oesophagus loses peristaltic activity. As the disease progresses dysphagia worsens, the oesophagus empties poorly and nocturnal pulmonary aspiration develops. Achalasia predisposes to squamous carcinoma of the oesophagus.

Investigations

A chest radiograph may be abnormal in late disease, with widening of the mediastinum from gross oesophageal dilatation and features of aspiration pneumonia. A barium swallow shows tapered narrowing of the lower oesophagus. In late disease the oesophageal body is dilated, aperistaltic and food-filled (see Fig. 9.23). Endoscopy must always be carried out to distinguish the radiological appearances from

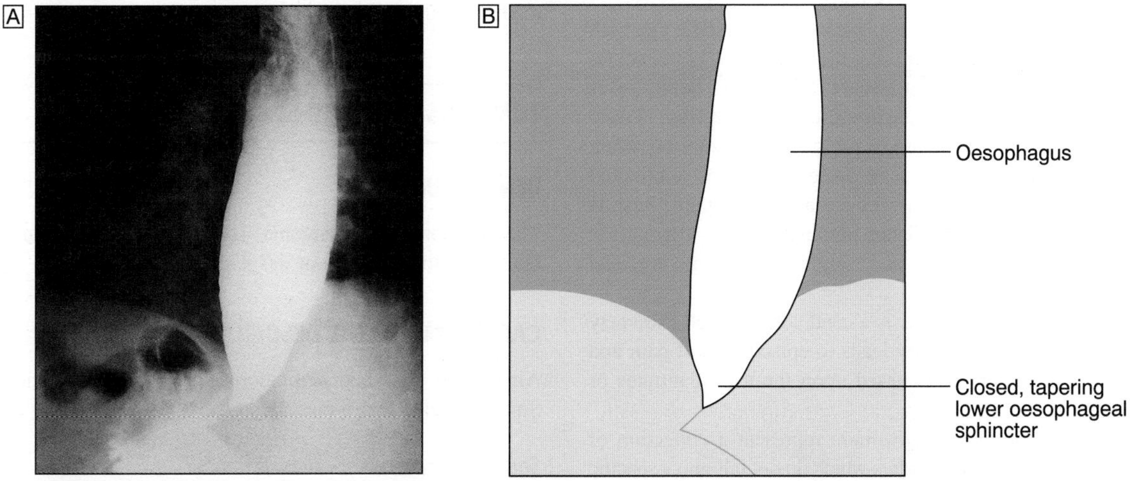

Fig. 9.23 Barium swallow showing achalasia. A Radiograph showing a dilated, barium-filled oesophagus with tapering, closed lower oesophageal sphincter. B Line diagram illustrating major structures.

carcinoma. A strategically placed carcinoma of the cardia can mimic the presentation and radiological and manometric features of achalasia ('pseudo-achalasia'). Manometry confirms the high-pressure, non-relaxing lower oesophageal sphincter with poor contractility of the oesophageal body.

Management

Endoscopic

Forceful pneumatic dilatation using a 30–35 mm-diameter endoscopically positioned balloon disrupts the oesophageal sphincter and improves symptoms in 80% of patients. Some patients require more than one dilatation but those requiring frequent dilatation are best treated surgically. Endoscopically directed injection of botulinum toxin into the lower oesophageal sphincter induces clinical remission, but late relapse is common.

Surgical

Surgical myotomy ('Heller's operation') is done by open operation or by a laparoscopic approach and is an extremely effective, although more invasive option. Both pneumatic dilatation and myotomy may be complicated by gastro-oesophageal reflux, and this can lead to severe oesophagitis because oesophageal clearance is so poor in these patients. For this reason Heller's myotomy is sometimes accompanied by an antireflux operation. Acid-suppressing drug therapy, using a proton pump inhibitor, is often necessary following surgical or endoscopic intervention for achalasia.

OTHER OESOPHAGEAL MOTILITY DISORDERS

Diffuse oesophageal spasm presents in late middle age with episodic chest pain which may mimic angina, but is sometimes accompanied by transient dysphagia. Some cases occur in response to gastro-oesophageal reflux. Treatment is based upon the use of proton pump inhibitors when gastro-oesophageal reflux is present. Oral or sublingual nitrates or nifedipine may relieve attacks of pain. Results of therapy are often disappointing and the alternatives of pneumatic dilatation and surgical myotomy are also poor.

'Nutcracker' oesophagus is a condition in which extremely forceful peristaltic activity leads to episodic chest pain and dysphagia. Treatment is based upon the use of nitrates or nifedipine.

Non-specific motility disorders represent a collection of oesophageal motility disorders which do not fall into a specific disease entity. Patients are usually elderly and present with dysphagia and chest pain. A range of manometric abnormalities from poor peristalsis to spasm occur.

SECONDARY CAUSES OF OESOPHAGEAL DYSMOTILITY

In systemic sclerosis the muscle of the oesophagus is replaced by fibrous tissue. Consequently, oesophageal peristalsis fails and this leads to heartburn and dysphagia. Oesophagitis is often severe, and benign fibrous strictures occur. Such patients require long-term therapy with proton pump inhibitor drugs. Dermatomyositis, rheumatoid arthritis and myasthenia gravis are other causes of dysphagia.

BENIGN OESOPHAGEAL STRICTURE

Benign oesophageal stricture is usually a consequence of gastro-oesophageal reflux disease and occurs most often in elderly patients who have poor oesophageal clearance. Rings, due to submucosal fibrosis, occur at the oesophago-gastric junction ('Schatzki ring') and cause intermittent dysphagia, often starting in middle age. A post-cricoid web is a rare complication of iron deficiency anaemia (Paterson–Kelly or Plummer–Vinson syndrome), and may be complicated by development of squamous carcinoma.

CAUSES OF OESOPHAGEAL STRICTURE

- Gastro-oesophageal reflux disease
- Webs and rings
- Carcinoma of the oesophagus or cardia
- Extrinsic compression from bronchial carcinoma
- Corrosive ingestion
- Post-operative scarring following oesophageal resection
- Post-radiotherapy
- Following long-term nasogastric intubation

Benign strictures are treated by endoscopic dilatation, in which wire-guided bougies or balloons are used to disrupt the fibrous tissue of the stricture.

TUMOURS OF THE OESOPHAGUS

BENIGN TUMOURS

The commonest is leiomyoma. This is usually asymptomatic but may cause bleeding or dysphagia.

CARCINOMA OF THE OESOPHAGUS

Almost all are adenocarcinoma or squamous cancers. Small-cell cancer is a rare third type.

Squamous cancer

In Western populations squamous oesophageal cancer is relatively rare (approximately 4 cases per 100 000), whilst in Iran, South Africa and China it is common (200 per

SQUAMOUS CARCINOMA: AETIOLOGICAL FACTORS

- Smoking
- Chewing betel nuts or tobacco
- Alcohol abuse
- Coeliac disease
- Achalasia of the oesophagus
- Post-cricoid web
- Post-caustic stricture
- Tylosis (familial hyperkeratosis of palms and soles)

100 000). Squamous cancer can arise in any part of the oesophagus from the post-cricoid region to the cardia. Almost all tumours above the lower third of the oesophagus are squamous cancers.

Adenocarcinoma

This arises in the lower third of the oesophagus from Barrett's oesophagus or from the cardia of the stomach. The incidence of this tumour is increasing, possibly because of the high prevalence of gastro-oesophageal reflux and Barrett's oesophagus in Western populations.

Clinical features

Most patients have a history of progressive, painless dysphagia for solid foods. Others present acutely because of food bolus obstruction. In late stages weight loss is often extreme; chest pain or hoarseness suggest mediastinal invasion. Fistulation between the oesophagus and the trachea or bronchial tree leads to coughing after swallowing, pneumonia and pleural effusion. Physical signs may be absent but even at initial presentation cachexia, cervical lymphadenopathy or other evidence of metastatic spread is common.

Investigations

The investigation of choice is upper gastrointestinal endoscopy (see Fig. 9.24) with cytology and biopsy. A barium swallow demonstrates the site and length of the stricture but adds little useful information.

Once a diagnosis has been achieved, investigations are done to stage the tumour and define operability. A chest radiograph and abdominal ultrasound may show obvious metastases. If these are negative, thoracic and abdominal CT scans are carried out to identify metastatic spread and local invasion. Invasion of the aorta and other local structures may preclude surgery. Unfortunately, the CT scan tends to understage tumours and the most sensitive modality is endoscopic ultrasound (EUS), in which an ultrasound transducer is incorporated into the tip of a modified endoscope (see Fig. 9.25).

Management

Despite modern treatment, the overall 5-year survival of patients presenting with oesophageal cancer is 6–9%, whilst that of disease which has not spread to structures outside the oesophagus is 15–20%. For disease confined to the oesophagus, surgery should be considered in fit patients. Surgery alone cures only 5–10%, but a combination of preoperative radiotherapy, chemotherapy using regimens including cisplatinum and 5-fluorouracil, and radical surgery is associated with 5-year survival of 30–50% in selected patients. Although squamous carcinomas are radiosensitive, radiotherapy alone is associated with a 5-year survival of only 5%.

Approximately 90% of patients have extensive disease at presentation; in these, treatment is palliative and based upon relief of dysphagia and pain. Endoscopically directed

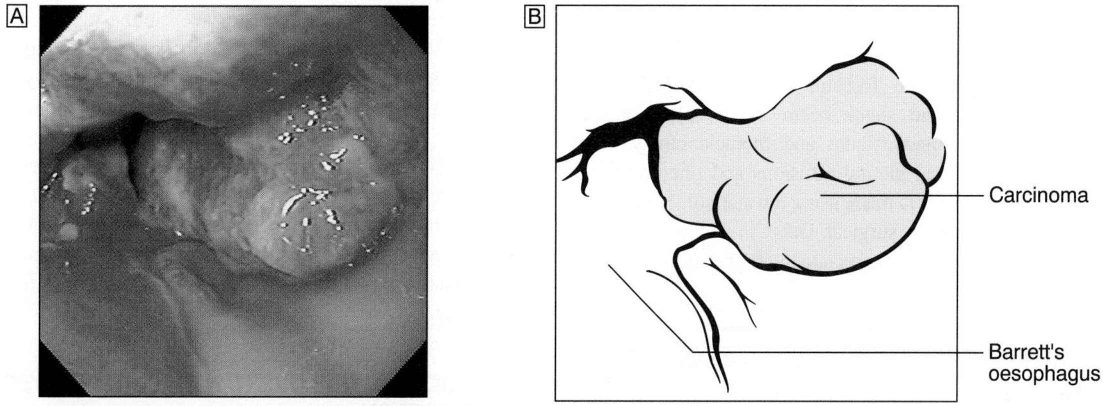

Fig. 9.24 Adenocarcinoma of the lower oesophagus in association with Barrett's oesophagus. [A] Endoscopic view. [B] Line diagram illustrating major structures.

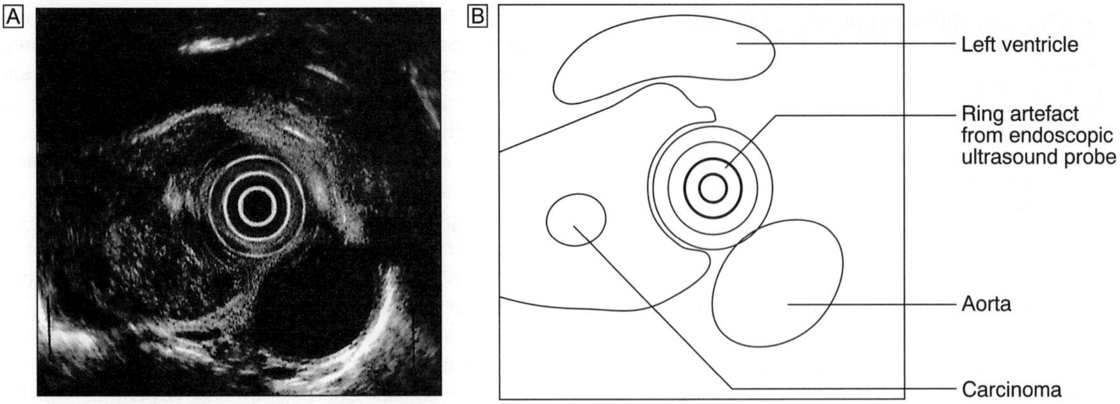

Fig. 9.25 Endoscopic ultrasound: identification of oesophageal carcinoma. A Ultrasound image. B Line diagram illustrating major structures.

tumour ablation using laser therapy or alcohol injection and insertion of stents are the major methods of improving swallowing. Palliative radiotherapy may induce shrinkage of both squamous cancers and adenocarcinomas but risks worsening stricture formation and exacerbating dysphagia. Quality of life can be improved by nutritional support and appropriate analgesia.

PERFORATION OF THE OESOPHAGUS

The most common cause is iatrogenic perforation at the time of dilatation or intubation. Malignant, corrosive or post-radiotherapy strictures are more likely to be perforated than peptic strictures. A perforated peptic stricture is usually managed conservatively using broad-spectrum antibiotics and parenteral nutrition; most heal within days. Malignant, caustic and radiotherapy stricture perforations require surgical resection or intubation.

Spontaneous oesophageal perforation ('Boerhaave's syndrome') results from forceful vomiting and retching. Severe chest pain and shock occur as oesophago-gastric contents enter the mediastinum and thoracic cavity. Subcutaneous emphysema, pleural effusions and pneumothorax develop. The diagnosis is made using a water-soluble contrast swallow and treatment is surgical. Delay in diagnosis is a key factor in the high mortality associated with this condition.

FURTHER INFORMATION ON DISEASES OF THE OESOPHAGUS

Holloway R H, Dent J 1990 Pathophysiology of gastroesophageal reflux: lower esophageal sphincter dysfunction in gastroesophageal reflux disease. Gastroenterology Clinics of North America 19: 517–536

McCord G S, Staiano A, Clouse R E 1991 Achalasia, diffuse spasm and non-specific motility disorders. Baillière's Clinical Gastroenterology 5: 307–325

Peters J H, Hoeft S, Heimbucher J 1994 Selection of patients for curative or palliative resection of oesophageal cancer based on preoperative endoscopic ultrasonography. Archives of Surgery 129: 534–539

DISEASES OF THE STOMACH AND DUODENUM

GASTRITIS

Gastritis is a histological diagnosis, although it can sometimes be recognised at endoscopy.

ACUTE GASTRITIS

Acute gastritis is often erosive and haemorrhagic. Neutrophils are the predominant inflammatory cell in the superficial epithelium. Many cases result from aspirin or NSAID ingestion. Acute gastritis often produces no symptoms but may cause dyspepsia, anorexia, nausea or vomiting, haematemesis or melaena. Many cases resolve quickly and do not merit investigation; in others, endoscopy and biopsy may be necessary to exclude peptic ulcer, cancer or bleeding. Treatment should be directed to the underlying cause. Short-term symptomatic therapy with antacids, acid suppression (e.g. H_2-receptor antagonists) or antiemetics (e.g. metoclopramide) may be necessary.

CHRONIC GASTRITIS DUE TO *HELICOBACTER PYLORI* (HP) INFECTION

The most common cause of chronic gastritis is *H. pylori*. The predominant inflammatory cells are lymphocytes and

COMMON CAUSES OF GASTRITIS
Acute gastritis (often erosive and haemorrhagic)
• Aspirin, NSAIDs • *H. pylori* (initial infection) • Alcohol • Drugs, e.g. iron preparations • Severe physiological stress, e.g. burns, multi-organ failure, CNS trauma • Bile reflux, e.g. following gastric surgery • Viral infections, e.g. cytomegalovirus (CMV), herpes simplex virus in AIDS (see p. 102)
Chronic non-specific gastritis
• *H. pylori* infection • Autoimmune (pernicious anaemia) • Post-gastrectomy
Chronic 'specific' forms (rare)
• Infections, e.g. CMV, tuberculosis • Gastrointestinal diseases, e.g. Crohn's disease • Systemic diseases, e.g. sarcoidosis, graft-versus-host disease • Idiopathic, e.g. granulomatous gastritis

plasma cells. Correlation between symptoms and endoscopic or pathological findings is poor. Most patients are asymptomatic and do not require any treatment. At present there is no indication for widespread use of HP eradication therapy in patients with chronic gastritis but without evidence of peptic ulcer disease.

AUTOIMMUNE CHRONIC GASTRITIS

This involves the body of the stomach, spares the antrum and results from autoimmune activity against parietal cells. The histological features are diffuse chronic inflammation, atrophy and loss of fundic glands, intestinal metaplasia and sometimes hyperplasia of enterochromaffin-like (ECL) cells. Parietal cell and intrinsic factor antibodies may be present. In some patients the degree of gastric atrophy is severe, and loss of intrinsic factor secretion leads to pernicious anaemia. The gastritis itself is usually asymptomatic but some patients have evidence of other organ-specific autoimmunity, particularly thyroid disease. There is a four-fold increase in the risk of gastric cancer development (see also p. 639).

MÉNÉTRIER'S DISEASE

In this rare condition the gastric pits are elongated and tortuous, with replacement of the parietal and chief cells by mucus-secreting cells. As a result, the mucosal folds of the body and fundus are greatly enlarged. Most patients are hypochlorhydric. Whilst some patients have upper gastrointestinal symptoms, the majority present in middle or old age with protein-losing enteropathy (see p. 649) due to protein leakage from the gastric mucosa. Barium meal shows enlarged, nodular and coarse folds which are also seen at endoscopy, although biopsies may not be deep enough to show all the histological features. Treatment with anti-secretory drugs may reduce protein loss but unresponsive patients require partial gastrectomy.

PEPTIC ULCER DISEASE

The term 'peptic ulcer' refers to an ulcer in the lower oesophagus, stomach or duodenum, in the jejunum after surgical anastomosis to the stomach, or, rarely, in the ileum adjacent to a Meckel's diverticulum. Ulcers in the stomach or duodenum may be acute or chronic; both penetrate the muscularis mucosae but the acute ulcer shows no evidence of fibrosis. Erosions do not penetrate the muscularis mucosae.

GASTRIC AND DUODENAL ULCER

Although the prevalence of peptic ulcer is decreasing in many Western communities, it still affects approximately 10% of all adults at some time in their lives. The male to female ratio for duodenal ulcer varies from 5:1 to 2:1, whilst that for gastric ulcer is 2:1 or less.

Aetiology

Helicobacter pylori

In the industrialised world the prevalence of *H. pylori* infection in the general population rises steadily with age, and in the UK approximately 50% of those over the age of 50 years are infected. In many parts of the underdeveloped world infection is much more common and is often acquired in childhood. Up to 90% of the population are infected by adult life in some countries. The vast majority of colonised people remain healthy and asymptomatic and only a minority develop clinical disease. Around 90% of duodenal ulcer patients and 70% of gastric ulcer patients are infected with HP (see Table 9.12).

Pathogenesis and pathophysiology of infection. The organism's motility allows it to localise and live deep beneath the mucus layer closely adherent to the epithelial surface. Here the surface pH is close to neutral and any

Table 9.12 Consequences of *H. pylori* infection

Clinical associations of HP infection	Strength of association
Duodenal ulcer	+++++
Gastric ulcer	++++
Gastric cancer	+++
Gastric B-cell lymphoma	+++
Non-ulcer dyspepsia	+
Gastro-oesophageal reflux/oesophagitis	–

acidity is buffered by the organism's production of the enzyme urease. This produces ammonia from urea and raises the pH around the bacterium. Although it is non-invasive, the bacterium stimulates chronic gastritis by provoking a local inflammatory response in the underlying epithelium due to release of a range of cytotoxins (see Fig. 9.26). HP exclusively colonises gastric-type epithelium and is only found in the duodenum in association with patches of gastric metaplasia.

Once infection in the antrum is established, there is depletion of antral somatostatin and stimulation of gastrin release from G cells. The subsequent hypergastrinaemia stimulates acid production by the parietal cells, leading to duodenal mucosal damage. Continuing damage at this site stimulates the development of patches of gastric metaplasia in the duodenum, which in turn are colonised by HP, thereby allowing further damage and eventual ulceration (see Fig. 9.27). The role of HP in the pathogenesis of gastric ulcer is less clear but HP probably reduces gastric mucosal resistance to attack from acid and pepsin.

Diagnosis. Many different diagnostic tests for HP infection are available (see Table 9.13). Some are invasive and require endoscopy; others are non-invasive. They vary in sensitivity and specificity.

Non-steroidal anti-inflammatory drugs (NSAIDs)

These damage the gastric mucosal barrier and are an important aetiological factor in up to 30% of gastric ulcers. These drugs also reduce the integrity of the duodenal mucosa but are probably responsible for only a small proportion of duodenal ulcers. They greatly increase the risk of bleeding or perforation from pre-existing gastric and duodenal ulcers.

Mechanisms of NSAID toxicity. NSAIDs are effective anti-inflammatory agents which act by inhibiting cyclo-oxygenase activity, thereby reducing the formation of pro-inflammatory prostaglandins at the site of inflammation. Prostaglandins of the E series also play a major role in the maintenance of gastroduodenal defence mechanisms (see Fig. 9.28). By depleting mucosal prostaglandin levels,

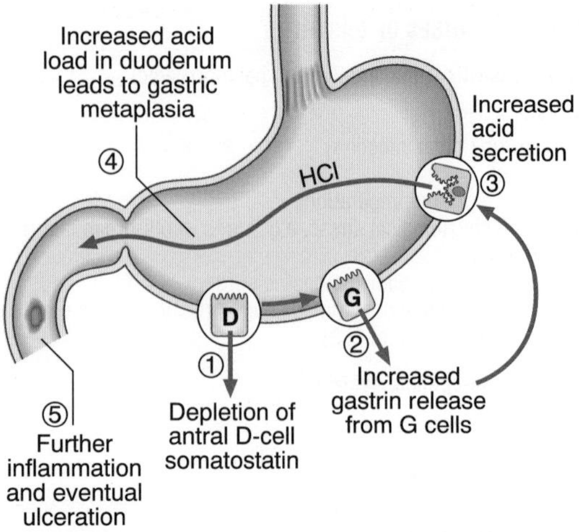

Fig. 9.27 Sequence of events in the pathophysiology of duodenal ulceration.

Table 9.13 Methods for the diagnosis of *Helicobacter pylori* infection

Test	Advantages	Disadvantages
Non-invasive		
Serology	Rapid office kits available Good for population studies	Lacks sensitivity and specificity Cannot differentiate current from past infection
Urea breath tests	High sensitivity and specificity	^{14}C uses radioactivity ^{13}C requires expensive mass spectrometer
Invasive (antral biopsy)		
Histology	Sensitive and specific Cheap	False negatives occur Takes several days to process
Rapid urease tests, e.g. CLO, Pyloritek	Cheap, quick Specific	Lack sensitivity
Microbiological culture	'Gold standard', defines antibiotic sensitivity	Slow and laborious culture Lacks sensitivity

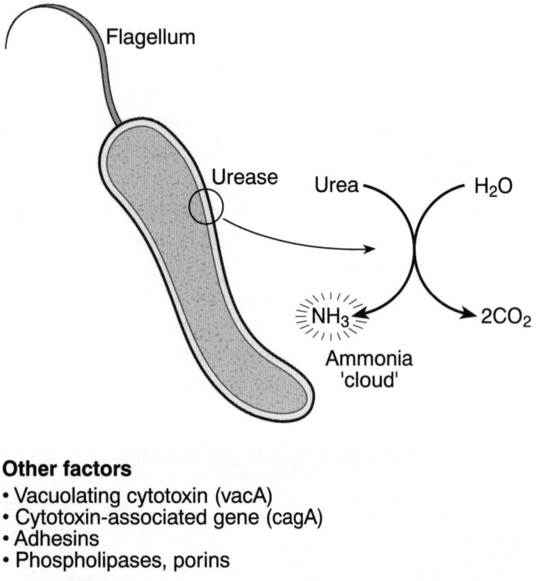

Fig. 9.26 Some factors which may influence the virulence of *Helicobacter pylori*.

aspirin and NSAIDs impair this 'cytoprotection', resulting in mucosal injury, erosions and ulceration.

A number of risk factors for NSAID-induced ulcers have been identified (see the information box) and should be considered when prescribing these drugs.

RISK FACTORS FOR NSAID-INDUCED ULCERS

- Age > 60 years
- Past history of peptic ulcer
- Past history of adverse event with NSAIDs
- Concomitant corticosteroid use
- High-dose or multiple NSAIDs
- Individual NSAID—highest with azapropazone, piroxicam; lower with ibuprofen

Management of NSAID-induced ulcers. Where possible, the offending drug should be stopped. If an NSAID must be continued then one with a lower risk of complications, e.g. ibuprofen or diclofenac, should be used at the lowest effective dose. Co-prescription of a proton pump inhibitor (e.g. omeprazole 40 mg daily) will heal most, but not all, ulcers.

The cyclo-oxygenase enzyme (COX) exists in two isoforms (COX-1 and COX-2). Current NSAIDs are non-specific inhibitors of both isoenzymes, and the development of newer, selective COX-2 inhibitors may allow effective anti-inflammatory activity with less gastrointestinal (and renal) toxicity.

Heredity

Patients with peptic ulcer often have a family history of ulcer; this is particularly so with duodenal ulcers that develop below the age of 20 years. Reasons for this familial predisposition are unclear but may reflect either intrafamilial clustering of HP infection or a true genetic risk. Links with blood group O and non-secretor status have been observed but the pathogenic significance of these findings is uncertain.

Smoking

Smoking confers an increased risk of gastric ulcer and, to a lesser extent, duodenal ulcer. Once the ulcer has formed it is more likely to cause complications and less likely to heal on standard treatment regimens if the patient continues to smoke.

Acid-pepsin versus mucosal resistance (see Fig. 9.28)

An ulcer forms when there is an imbalance between aggressive factors, i.e. the digestive power of acid and pepsin, and defensive factors, i.e. the ability of the gastric and duodenal mucosa to resist this digestive power. This mucosal resistance constitutes the gastric mucosal barrier.

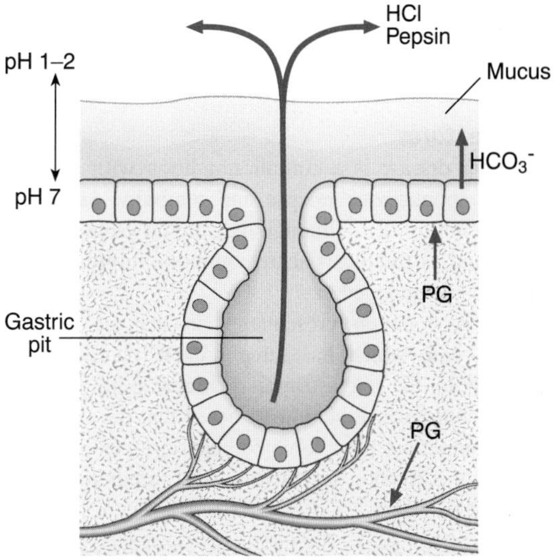

Fig. 9.28 Gastroduodenal mucosal protection. Prostaglandins (PG) stimulate bicarbonate and mucus secretion and increase mucosal blood flow. Bicarbonate ions are secreted into the unstirred mucus layer, neutralising hydrogen ions as they back-diffuse towards the epithelium. Rapid cell turnover and a rich mucosal blood supply are important protective elements.

Ulcers occur only in the presence of acid and pepsin; they are never found in achlorhydric patients such as those with pernicious anaemia. On the other hand, severe intractable peptic ulceration nearly always occurs in patients with the Zollinger–Ellison syndrome (see p. 638), which is characterised by very high acid secretion.

Until recently, it was thought that acid secretion in most duodenal ulcer patients was within normal limits, but using newly developed tests of acid secretion, it has been established that most patients do actually have markedly exaggerated acid secretion in response to stimulation by gastrin. This is the key factor in duodenal ulcer development, but in gastric ulcer patients the effects of HP are more complex, and impaired mucosal defence resulting from a combination of HP infection, NSAIDs and smoking may have a more important role.

Pathology

Chronic gastric ulcer is usually single; 90% are situated on the lesser curve within the antrum or at the junction between body and antral mucosa. Chronic duodenal ulcer usually occurs in the first part of the duodenum just distal to the junction of pyloric and duodenal mucosa; 50% are on the anterior wall. Gastric and duodenal ulcers coexist in 10% of patients and more than one peptic ulcer is found in 10–15% of patients. A chronic ulcer extends to below the muscularis mucosa and the histology shows four layers: surface debris, an infiltrate of neutrophils, granulation tissue and collagen.

Clinical features

Peptic ulcer disease is a chronic condition with a natural history of spontaneous relapse and remission lasting for decades, if not for life. Although they are different diseases, duodenal and gastric ulcers share common symptoms which will be considered together.

The most common presentation is that of recurrent abdominal pain which has three notable characteristics: localisation to the epigastrium, relationship to food and episodic occurrence. It should be noted that the diagnostic value of individual symptoms for peptic ulcer disease is poor, and the history is often a poor predictor of the presence of an ulcer.

Epigastric pain

Pain is referred to the epigastrium and is often so sharply localised that the patient can indicate its site with two or three fingers (the 'pointing sign').

Hunger pain

Pain occurs intermittently during the day, often when the stomach is empty, so that the patient identifies it as 'hunger pain' and obtains relief by eating.

Night pain

Pain wakes the patient from sleep and may be relieved by food, a drink of milk or antacids; this symptom is very characteristic of duodenal ulcer.

Pain relief

Pain is relieved by food, milk or antacids and by belching and vomiting. Relief by vomiting is more typical of gastric ulcer than of duodenal ulcer; some patients learn to induce vomiting to gain pain relief.

Episodic pain ('periodicity')

Pain is episodic and may last for several weeks at a time. Between episodes the patient feels perfectly well.

Other symptoms

Other symptoms that occur, especially during episodes of pain, include waterbrash, heartburn, loss of appetite and vomiting. Occasional vomiting occurs in about 40% of ulcer subjects; persistent vomiting occurring daily suggests gastric outlet obstruction. In a third of patients the history is less characteristic. This is especially true in elderly subjects under treatment with NSAIDs. In these patients pain may be absent or so slight that it is experienced only as a vague sense of epigastric unease. Occasionally, the only symptoms are anorexia and nausea, or a sense of undue repletion after meals. In some patients the ulcer is completely 'silent', presenting for the first time with anaemia from chronic undetected blood loss, as an abrupt haematemesis or as acute perforation; in others there is recurrent acute bleeding without ulcer pain between the attacks.

Investigations

The diagnosis can be made by double-contrast barium meal examination or by endoscopy. Endoscopy is the preferred investigation because it is more accurate and has the enormous advantage that suspicious lesions and HP status can be evaluated by biopsy. For those with a duodenal ulcer seen at barium meal, urea breath testing will accurately define the HP status. Very occasionally, a gastric ulcer may be malignant; therefore endoscopy and biopsy are mandatory when a gastric ulcer is detected on barium examination. Moreover, in gastric ulcer disease endoscopy must be repeated after suitable treatment to confirm that the ulcer has healed and to obtain further biopsies if it has not. In contrast, it is not necessary to repeat endoscopy after treating duodenal ulcers.

Management

The aims of modern management are to relieve symptoms and induce ulcer healing in the short term, and to cure the ulcer in the long term. HP eradication is the cornerstone of therapy for peptic ulcers, as this will successfully prevent relapse and eliminate the need for long-term therapy in the majority of patients.

Helicobacter pylori eradication

All patients with proven acute or chronic duodenal ulcer disease and those with gastric ulcers who are HP-positive should be offered eradication therapy as primary therapy. Treatment is based upon a proton pump inhibitor (either omeprazole or lansoprazole) taken simultaneously with two antibiotics (from amoxycillin, clarithromycin and metronidazole) for 7–10 days (see Table 9.14). Compliance, side-effects and metronidazole-resistance influence the success of therapy (see the information box).

COMMON SIDE-EFFECTS OF *HELICOBACTER PYLORI* ERADICATION THERAPY

- Diarrhoea
  30–50% of patients; usually mild but *Clostridium difficile*-associated colitis can occur
- Metronidazole
  Metallic taste (common), peripheral neuropathy (rare)
  Flushing and vomiting when taken with alcohol
- Nausea, vomiting
- Abdominal cramp
- Headache
- Rash

Table 9.14 Antibiotic regimens for *Helicobacter pylori* eradication

	OCM/LCM	OAC/LAC	OAM/LAM	BAM
Regimen	Omeprazole 40 mg once daily *or* Lansoprazole 30 mg 12-hourly *and* Clarithromycin 500 mg 12-hourly Metronidazole 400 mg 12-hourly	Omeprazole 40 mg once daily *or* Lansoprazole 30 mg 12-hourly *and* Amoxycillin 500 mg 12-hourly Clarithromycin 500 mg 12-hourly	Omeprazole 40 mg once daily *or* Lansoprazole 30 mg 12-hourly *and* Amoxycillin 500 mg 12-hourly Metronidazole 400 mg 12-hourly	Bismuth (CBS) 125 mg 6-hourly *and* Amoxycillin 500 mg 12-hourly Metronidazole 400 mg 12-hourly
1st/2nd line	1st	1st	2nd	2nd
Duration	7 days	7 days	7–10 days	14 days
Efficacy	90%	85–90%	*c.*85%*	*c.*80%
Cost	+++	+++	++	+
Comments	Effective but costly	Avoids side-effects of metronidazole	* Depends on local rates of metronidazole resistance	Cheap but longer duration of therapy

(CBS = colloidal bismuth subcitrate)

Second-line therapy should be offered to those patients who remain infected after initial therapy once the reasons for failure of first-line therapy (e.g. compliance) have been established. For those who are still colonised after two treatments, the choice lies between a third attempt with quadruple therapy (bismuth, proton pump inhibitor and two antibiotics) or simple maintenance therapy with acid suppression.

General measures

Cigarette smoking, aspirin and NSAIDs should be avoided. Alcohol in moderation is not harmful and no special dietary advice is required.

Short-term management

Many different drugs are available for the short-term management of peptic ulcer symptoms and other dyspeptic disorders (see Table 9.15).

Antacids. These are widely available for self-medication and are used for relief of minor dyspeptic symptoms. The majority are based on combinations of calcium, aluminium and magnesium salts, all of which have individual side-effects. Calcium compounds cause constipation, while magnesium-containing agents cause diarrhoea. Aluminium compounds block absorption of digoxin, tetracycline and dietary phosphates. Most have a high sodium content and can exacerbate congestive heart failure.

Table 9.15 Drugs commonly used in peptic ulcers and other acid dyspeptic disorders

Drugs	Short term	Maintenance	Side-effects
Drugs which inhibit acid secretion			
H_2-antagonists			
Cimetidine	400 mg 12-hourly or 800 mg at night	400 mg at night	Confusion, diarrhoea, interaction with elimination of warfarin, phenytoin, theophylline
Ranitidine	150 mg 12-hourly or 300 mg at night	150 mg at night	Reversible confusion
Famotidine	20 mg 12-hourly or 40 mg at night	20 mg at night	Headache, dizziness, dry mouth
Nizatidine	150 mg 12-hourly or 300 mg at night	150 mg at night	Rarely sweating, urticaria, somnolence
H+/K+ ATPase inhibitors (proton pump inhibitors)			
Omeprazole	20–40 mg once daily	20 mg at night	Hypergastrinaemia, diarrhoea, interactions with warfarin, phenytoin
Lansoprazole	30 mg once daily	15 mg at night	(as Omeprazole)
Pantoprazole	40 mg once daily	Not recommended	Hypergastrinaemia; fewer drug interactions, headache, diarrhoea, rashes
Drugs which enhance mucosal defence and prokinetic agents			
Colloidal bismuth	125 mg 6-hourly	Not recommended	Blackens tongue, teeth and faeces; rarely, bismuth toxicity with prolonged use
Misoprostol	200 µg 6-hourly	200 µg 6-hourly	Abortifacient, contraindicated in women of childbearing age; diarrhoea in up to 20%
Sucralfate	2 g 12-hourly	Not recommended	May bind and reduce absorption of digoxin, warfarin, tetracycline, phenytoin; cramps, diarrhoea, extrapyramidal effects
Cisapride	10 mg 8-hourly	10 mg 12-hourly or 20 mg at night	May cause prolonged QT interval and ventricular arrhythmias

Histamine H_2-receptor antagonist drugs. These are competitive inhibitors of histamine at the H_2-receptor on the parietal cell. Dyspeptic symptoms remit promptly, usually within days of starting treatment, and 80% of duodenal ulcers will heal after 4 weeks. These drugs do not inhibit acid secretion to the same degree as the proton pump inhibitors but are useful for the short-term management of acid dyspeptic symptoms prior to investigation. They are moderately effective for the management of reflux oesophagitis. They have a proven safety record. Several can now be purchased in the UK without prescription.

H^+/K^+ATPase ('proton pump') inhibitors. These are substituted benzimidazole compounds that specifically and irreversibly inhibit the proton pump hydrogen/potassium ATPase in the parietal cell membrane. They are the most powerful inhibitors of gastric secretion yet discovered, with maximal inhibition occurring 3–6 hours after an oral dose. They have an excellent safety profile. After a few days of treatment virtual achlorhydria is achieved and rapid healing of both gastric and duodenal ulcers follows. Omeprazole and lansoprazole are important components of HP eradication regimens. Proton pump inhibitors are also much more effective than H_2-antagonists for healing and maintenance of reflux oesophagitis.

Colloidal bismuth compounds. Colloidal bismuth subcitrate (CBS) is an ammoniacal suspension of a complex colloidal bismuth salt. It has little, if any, effect on gastric acid secretion and its ulcer-healing effect is probably due to a combination of activity against HP and enhancement of mucosal defence mechanisms.

Sucralfate. This is a basic aluminium salt of sucrose octasulphate. It has no effect on acid secretion but probably acts to protect the ulcer base from peptic activity in a number of ways. It binds to fibroblast growth factor and to the ulcer base, reducing the access of pepsin and acid. It may also enhance epithelial cell turnover. It should be taken 30–60 minutes before meals.

Synthetic prostaglandin analogues (misoprostol). Prostaglandins exert complex effects on the gastroduodenal mucosa. In low doses they protect against injury induced by aspirin and NSAIDs by enhancing mucosal blood flow, and by stimulating mucus and bicarbonate secretion and epithelial cell proliferation. At high doses acid secretion is inhibited. Misoprostol is effective for the prevention and treatment of NSAID-induced ulcers, but in clinical practice proton pump inhibitors are preferred, since they are at least as effective and have fewer side-effects.

Maintenance treatment

Continuous maintenance treatment should not be necessary after successful HP eradication. For the minority who require maintenance treatment, the lowest effective dose should be used.

Surgical treatment

The cure of most peptic ulcers by HP eradication therapy and the availability of safe, potent acid-suppressing drugs has made elective surgery for peptic ulcer disease a rare event. The indications are listed in the information box.

INDICATIONS FOR SURGERY IN PEPTIC ULCER
Emergency
• Perforation • Haemorrhage
Elective
• Complications, e.g. gastric outflow obstruction • Recurrent ulcer following gastric surgery

The operation of choice for a gastric ulcer is partial gastrectomy, preferably with a Billroth I anastomosis, in which the ulcer itself and the ulcer-bearing area of the stomach are resected. For duodenal ulcer the acid-secretory capacity of the stomach may be reduced by vagotomy; because this retards gastric emptying, a drainage operation such as pyloroplasty or gastroenterostomy is included. Highly selective vagotomy denervates only the acid-producing area of the stomach and so a drainage procedure is not required. This reduces the incidence of postcibal syndromes but the risk of ulcer recurrence is greater.

Complications of gastric resection

Some degree of disability is seen in up to 50% of patients following peptic ulcer surgery. In most, the effects are minor but in 10% of cases they significantly impair quality of life.

Early satiety and vomiting. Rapid gastric emptying leads to distension of the proximal small intestine as the hypertonic contents draw fluid into the lumen. This leads to abdominal discomfort and diarrhoea after eating. Autonomic reflexes release a range of gastrointestinal hormones which lead to vasomotor features such as flushing, palpitations, sweating, tachycardia and hypotension ('early dumping'). Patients should therefore avoid large meals with high carbohydrate content.

Bile reflux gastritis. Duodeno-gastric bile reflux leads to chronic gastritis. This is usually asymptomatic but dyspepsia can occur. Symptomatic treatment with aluminium-containing antacids or sucralfate may be effective. A few patients require revisional surgery with creation of a Roux en Y loop to prevent bile reflux into the stomach.

Late dumping syndrome. Symptoms of dumping occur 90–180 minutes after eating. The pathogenesis is broadly similar to early dumping, but in addition reactive hypoglycaemia occurs and may cause mental confusion. Rapid emptying of carbohydrates into the proximal small intestine results in an exaggerated release of insulin with subsequent reactive hypoglycaemia. Other gut hormones and enteric peptides may also be involved. Treatment is similar to that of early dumping syndrome.

Diarrhoea and maldigestion. Diarrhoea may develop after any peptic ulcer operation and usually occurs 1–2 hours after eating. Poor mixing of food in the stomach, with rapid emptying, inadequate mixing with pancreatic biliary secretions, reduced small intestinal transit times and bacterial overgrowth, may lead to malabsorption.

Diarrhoea often responds to dietary advice to eat small, dry meals with a reduced intake of refined carbohydrates. Antidiarrhoeal drugs such as codeine phosphate (15–30 mg 4–6 times a day) or loperamide (2 mg after each loose stool) are often helpful.

Weight loss. Most patients lose weight shortly after surgery and 30–40% are unable to regain all the weight which is lost. The usual cause is reduced intake because of a small gastric remnant, but diarrhoea and mild steatorrhoea also contribute.

Anaemia. Anaemia is common many years after subtotal gastrectomy. Although iron deficiency is the most common cause, folic acid and B_{12} deficiency are also seen. Inadequate dietary intake of iron and folate, lack of acid and intrinsic factor secretion, mild chronic low-grade blood loss from the gastric remnant and recurrent ulceration are responsible.

Metabolic bone disease. Both osteoporosis and osteomalacia occur as a consequence of calcium and vitamin D malabsorption.

Gastric cancer. An increased risk of gastric cancer has been reported from several epidemiological studies. The risk is highest in those with hypochlorhydria, duodeno-gastric reflux of bile, smoking and HP infection. Although the relative risk is increased, the absolute risk of cancer remains low and endoscopic surveillance is not indicated following gastric surgery.

Complications of peptic ulcer disease

These are perforation, gastric outlet obstruction and bleeding.

Perforation

When free perforation occurs, the contents of the stomach escape into the peritoneal cavity, leading to peritonitis. Perforation occurs more commonly in duodenal than in gastric ulcers, and usually in ulcers on the anterior wall. About one-quarter of all perforations occur in acute ulcers and NSAIDs are often incriminated.

Clinical features. Although perforation may be the first sign of ulcer, there is commonly a history of recurrent epigastric pain. The most striking symptom is sudden, severe pain; its distribution follows the spread of the gastric contents over the peritoneum. Pain initially develops in the upper abdomen and rapidly becomes generalised; shoulder tip pain is due to irritation of the diaphragm. The pain is accompanied by shallow respiration due to limitation of diaphragmatic movements, and by shock. The abdomen is held immobile and there is generalised 'board-like' rigidity. Intestinal sounds are absent and liver dullness to percussion decreases due to the presence of gas under the diaphragm. Vomiting is common. After some hours, symptoms improve although abdominal rigidity remains. Later, the patient's condition deteriorates as general peritonitis develops.

A radiograph of the upper abdomen in the erect position shows free air under the diaphragm. A water-soluble contrast swallow will confirm leakage of gastroduodenal contents. Radiological procedures should not be allowed to delay resuscitation or surgery based on the clinical findings.

Management and prognosis. After resuscitation, the acute perforation is treated surgically, either by simple closure, or by closure combined with vagotomy and drainage. More than half of the patients who have a simple closure will eventually require a further elective operation for recurrence of ulcer symptoms, and for this reason the second option is usually taken. Patients who are HP-positive should undergo eradication therapy.

Perforation carries a mortality of approximately 10%. The outlook is worst in elderly patients with large perforations.

Gastric outlet obstruction

The causes are shown in Table 9.16. The most common is an ulcer in the region of the pylorus.

Clinical features. Nausea, vomiting and abdominal distension are the cardinal features of gastric outlet obstruction. Large quantities of gastric content are often vomited, and food eaten 24 hours or more previously may be recognised.

Physical examination frequently shows evidence of wasting and dehydration. A succussion splash may be elicited 4 hours or more after the last meal or drink. Visible gastric peristalsis is diagnostic of gastric outlet obstruction.

Investigations. Loss of gastric contents leads to dehydration with low serum sodium, chloride and potassium, and raised bicarbonate and urea concentrations. This results in enhanced renal absorption of Na^+ in exchange for H^+ and paradoxical aciduria. Nasogastric aspiration of food residue

Table 9.16 Differential diagnosis and management of gastric outlet obstruction

Cause	Management
Fibrotic stricture from duodenal ulcer, i.e. 'pyloric stenosis'	Balloon dilatation or surgery
Oedema from pyloric channel or duodenal ulcer	Medical therapy
Carcinoma of antrum	Surgery
Adult hypertrophic pyloric stenosis	Surgery
Gastroparesis	Investigate cause, prokinetic drugs

or at least 200 ml of fluid from the stomach after an overnight fast suggests the diagnosis.

Endoscopy should be performed after the stomach has been emptied by a wide-bore nasogastric tube in order to confirm or refute organic obstruction. Endoscopic balloon dilatation of benign stenoses may be possible in some patients. In gastroparesis the pylorus is normal and the endoscope can be passed easily into the duodenum.

Barium studies are rarely advisable because they cannot usually distinguish between peptic ulcer and cancer. Moreover, barium remains in the stomach and is difficult to remove.

Management. Nasogastric suction and intravenous correction of dehydration and metabolic acidosis are undertaken. In severe cases, at least 4 litres of isotonic saline and 80 mmol of potassium may be necessary during the first 24 hours. In some patients ulcer healing with proton pump inhibitors relieves pyloric oedema and surgery is not required. In others vagotomy and gastroenterostomy are necessary, although they are best done after 7 days of gastric aspiration, which enables the stomach to return to normal size.

Bleeding

See pages 614–617.

ZOLLINGER–ELLISON SYNDROME

This is a rare disorder characterised by the triad of severe peptic ulceration, gastric acid hypersecretion and a non-beta cell islet tumour of the pancreas ('gastrinoma'). It probably accounts for about 0.1% of all cases of duodenal ulceration. The syndrome occurs in either sex at any age, although it is most common between 30 and 50 years of age.

Pathophysiology

The gastrinoma secretes large amounts of gastrin (G17 and G34), which stimulates the parietal cells of the stomach to secrete acid to their maximal capacity and increases the parietal cell mass three- to six-fold. Pentagastrin does not increase the secretory rate much above basal values because the stomach is maximally secreting. The acid output may be so great that it reaches the upper small intestine, reducing the luminal pH to 2 or less. Pancreatic lipase is inactivated and bile acids are precipitated. Diarrhoea and steatorrhoea result.

Pathology

Around 90% of tumours occur in the pancreatic head or proximal duodenal wall, the latter being more common. At least half are multiple, and tumour size can vary from 1 mm to 20 cm. Approximately one-half to two-thirds are malignant but are often slow-growing. Of these patients, 20–60% also have adenomas of the parathyroid and pituitary glands (multiple endocrine neoplasia, type MEN I; see p. 598).

Clinical features

Peptic ulcers are multiple, severe and may occur in unusual sites such as the post-bulbar duodenum, jejunum or oesophagus. There is a poor response to standard ulcer therapy. The history is usually short; bleeding and perforations are common. The syndrome may present as severe recurrent ulceration following a standard operation for peptic ulcer. Diarrhoea is seen in one-third or more of patients and can be the presenting feature. The diagnosis should be suspected in all patients with unusual or severe peptic ulceration, especially if a barium meal shows abnormally coarse gastric mucosal folds.

Investigations

Hypersecretion of acid under basal conditions with little increase following pentagastrin may be confirmed by gastric aspiration. Serum gastrin levels are grossly elevated (10–1000-fold). Injection of the hormone secretin normally causes no change or a slight decrease in circulating gastrin concentrations, but in Zollinger–Ellison syndrome there is a paradoxical dramatic increase in gastrin. Tumour localisation is often attempted using CT and selective arteriography with sampling from portal vein tributaries, but accurate preoperative localisation is impossible in up to 40% of cases.

Management

Approximately 30% of small and single tumours can be localised and resected but many tumours are multifocal. Some patients present with metastatic disease and surgery is inappropriate. Proton pump inhibitors have made total gastrectomy unnecessary and in the majority of patients continuous therapy with omeprazole heals ulcers and alleviates diarrhoea. Larger doses (60–80 mg daily) than those used to treat duodenal ulcer are required. The synthetic somatostatin analogue, octreotide, given by subcutaneous injection, reduces gastrin secretion and is sometimes of value. Overall 5-year survival is 60–75% and all patients should be monitored for the later development of other manifestations of MEN I.

FUNCTIONAL DISORDERS

NON-ULCER DYSPEPSIA (FUNCTIONAL DYSPEPSIA)

In this common condition the patient complains of dyspepsia and other ulcer-like symptoms but investigation fails to detect an ulcer. A minority of patients will actually have peptic ulcer disease which is in remission at the time of investigation.

Aetiology

The condition of non-ulcer dyspepsia probably covers a spectrum of mucosal, motility and psychiatric disorders. The symptoms caused by motor dysfunction are analogous to the motility disturbances that occur in the irritable bowel syndrome; indeed, these disorders commonly occur together.

Clinical features

Patients are usually young (< 40 years) and women are affected twice as commonly as men. Abdominal pain is associated with a variable combination of other 'dyspeptic' symptoms, the commonest being nausea and bloating after meals. Morning symptoms are characteristic and pain or nausea may occur on waking. Direct enquiry may elicit symptoms suggestive of colonic dysmotility, such as pellet-like stools or a sense of incomplete rectal evacuation on defaecation. Peptic ulcer disease must be considered, whilst in older subjects intra-abdominal malignancy is a prime concern.

There are no diagnostic signs, apart perhaps from inappropriate tenderness on abdominal palpation. Symptoms may appear disproportionate to clinical well-being and there is no weight loss. Patients often appear anxious and distraught and it is sometimes possible to detect psychological symptoms.

A drug history should be taken and the possibility of a depressive illness should be considered. Pregnancy should be ruled out in young women before radiological studies are undertaken. Alcohol abuse should be suspected when early morning nausea and retching are prominent.

Investigations

The history will often suggest the diagnosis but in older subjects an endoscopy is necessary to exclude mucosal disease. While an ultrasound scan may detect gallstones, these are rarely responsible for dyspeptic symptoms.

Management

The most important element is explanation and reassurance. Possible psychological factors should be explored and the concept of psychological influences on gut function should be explained. Cigarette smoking and alcohol abuse should be discouraged; idiosyncratic and restrictive diets are of little help.

Drug treatment is not especially successful but merits trial. Antacids are sometimes helpful. Prokinetic drugs such as metoclopramide (10 mg 8-hourly), domperidone (10–20 mg 8-hourly) or cisapride (10 mg 6-hourly or 8-hourly) may be given before meals if nausea, vomiting or bloating are prominent. Metoclopramide may induce extrapyramidal side-effects, including tardive dyskinesia in young subjects. H_2-receptor antagonist drugs may be tried if night pain or heartburn is troublesome.

Symptoms which can be associated with an identifiable cause of stress (impending marriage or divorce, or financial or employment difficulties, for example) resolve with appropriate counselling. Some patients have major chronic psychological disorders resulting in persistent or recurrent symptoms and need formal psychotherapy.

PSYCHOGENIC VOMITING

Psychogenic vomiting may occur in anxiety neurosis. It starts usually on wakening, or immediately after breakfast; only rarely does it occur later in the day. The disorder is probably a reaction to facing up to the worries of everyday life; in the young it can be due to school phobia. There may be retching alone or the vomiting of gastric secretions or food. Although psychogenic vomiting may occur regularly over long periods, there is little or no weight loss. Early morning vomiting also occurs in pregnancy, alcohol abuse and depression.

In all patients it is essential to address any underlying psychological disturbance. Tranquillisers and antiemetic drugs (e.g. metoclopramide 10 mg 8-hourly, domperidone 10 mg 8-hourly, prochlorperazine 5–10 mg 8-hourly) have only a secondary place in management.

TUMOURS OF THE STOMACH

GASTRIC CARCINOMA

Although the incidence of gastric cancer in the UK has fallen markedly in recent years, it remains the leading cause of cancer death world-wide. There is marked geographical variation in incidence. It is extremely common in China, Japan and parts of South America (mortality rate 30–40 per 100 000), less common in the UK (12–13 deaths per 100 000) and uncommon in the USA. Studies of Japanese migrants to the USA have revealed a much lower incidence in second-generation migrants, confirming the importance of environmental factors. Gastric cancer is more common in men and the incidence rises sharply after 50 years of age.

Aetiology (see Fig. 9.29)

Helicobacter pylori is associated with chronic atrophic gastritis and gastric cancer. HP infection may be responsible for 60–70% of cases and acquisition of infection at an early age may be important. Although the majority of HP-infected individuals have normal or increased acid secretion, a few become hypo- or achlorhydric and these people are thought to be at greatest risk. Chronic inflammation with generation of reactive oxygen species and depletion of the normally abundant antioxidant ascorbic acid are also important.

Diets rich in salted, smoked or pickled foods and the consumption of nitrites and nitrates are associated with cancer risk. Carcinogenic N-nitroso-compounds are formed from nitrates by the action of nitrite-reducing bacteria which colonise the achlorhydric stomach. Diets lacking fresh fruit and vegetables as well as vitamins C and vitamin A may also contribute.

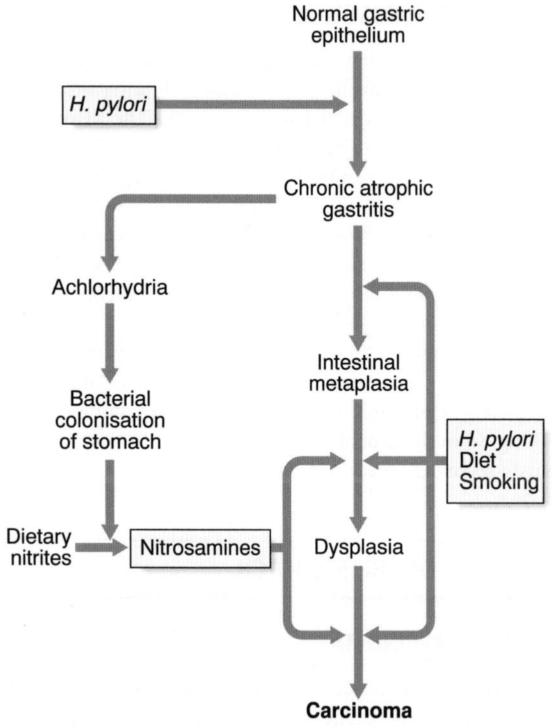

Fig. 9.29 Gastric carcinogenesis: a possible mechanism.

Other recognised risk factors include *smoking*, heavy *alcohol* intake and a number of less common factors (see the information box).

FACTORS PREDISPOSING TO GASTRIC CANCER

- Smoking
- Alcohol
- *H. pylori*
- Dietary associations (see text)
- Autoimmune gastritis (pernicious anaemia)
- Adenomatous gastric polyps
- Previous partial gastrectomy
- Ménétrier's disease
- Familial adenomatous polyposis

No predominant genetic abnormality has been identified, although cancer risk is increased two- to three-fold in first-degree relatives of patients, and links with blood group A have been reported. Rare 'gastric cancer families' have also been described.

Pathology

Virtually all tumours are adenocarcinomas arising from mucus-secreting cells in the base of the gastric crypts. Most develop upon a background of chronic atrophic gastritis with intestinal metaplasia and dysplasia. Cancers are 'intestinal', arising from areas of intestinal metaplasia with histological features reminiscent of intestinal epithelium; or 'diffuse', arising from normal gastric mucosa. Intestinal carcinomas are more common, and arise on a background of chronic mucosal injury. Diffuse cancers tend to be poorly differentiated and occur in younger patients.

Of gastric cancers, 50% occur in the antrum and 20–30% are situated in the gastric body, often on the greater curve. About 20% occur in the cardia and this type of tumour is becoming more common. Diffuse submucosal infiltration by a scirrhous cancer (linitis plastica) is uncommon. Macroscopically, tumours may be classified as polyploid, ulcerating, fungating or diffuse.

Early gastric cancer is defined as cancer confined to the mucosa or submucosa, regardless of lymph node involvement (see Fig. 9.30). It is often recognised in Japan, where widespread use of endoscopic screening is practised. Over 80% of patients in the West present with *advanced gastric cancer.*

Clinical features

Early gastric cancer is usually asymptomatic but may occasionally be discovered during endoscopy for investigation of dyspepsia. Two-thirds of patients with advanced cancers have weight loss and 50% have ulcer-like pain. Anorexia and nausea occur in one-third, while early satiety, haematemesis, melaena and dyspepsia alone are less common features. Dysphagia occurs in tumours of the gastric cardia which obstruct the gastro-oesophageal junction. Anaemia from occult bleeding is also common.

Examination may reveal no abnormalities, but signs of weight loss, anaemia or a palpable epigastric mass are not infrequent. Jaundice or ascites may signify metastatic spread. Occasionally, tumour spread occurs to the supraclavicular lymph nodes (Troisier's sign), umbilicus ('Sister Joseph's nodule') or ovaries (Krukenberg tumour). Paraneoplastic phenomena, such as acanthosis nigricans, thrombophlebitis (Trousseau's sign) and dermatomyositis, occur rarely. Metastases occur most commonly in the liver, lungs, peritoneum, bone and marrow.

Diagnosis and staging

There are no laboratory markers of sufficient accuracy for the diagnosis of gastric cancer. Upper gastrointestinal endoscopy is the investigation of choice and should be performed promptly in any dyspeptic patient with 'alarm features' (see p. 613). Multiple biopsies from the edge and base of a gastric ulcer are required and exfoliative brush cytology also improves the diagnostic yield. Barium meal is an alternative approach but any abnormalities must be followed by endoscopy to obtain biopsy. Once the diagnosis is made, further imaging is necessary for accurate staging and assessment of resectability. Endoscopic

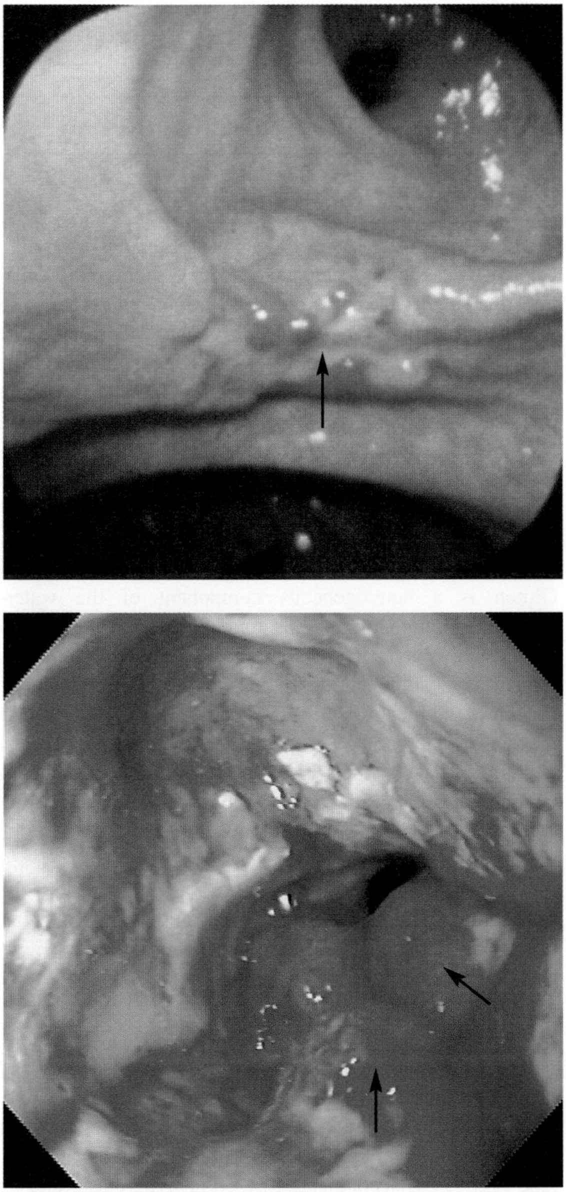

Fig. 9.30 Gastric cancer. A Endoscopic view of early cancer showing subtle mucosal irregularity of the incisura (arrow).
B Endoscopic view of late cancer showing polypoid, irregular mucosa with deep ulceration of the gastric antrum (arrows).

ultrasound will demonstrate whether the lesion has penetrated the submucosa or not and will also visualise perigastric lymph nodes. CT scans may not demonstrate small involved lymph nodes, but will show evidence of intra-abdominal spread or liver metastases. Even with these techniques, laparoscopy may be required to determine whether the tumour is resectable.

Management

Surgery

Resection offers the only hope of cure, which can be achieved in 80–90% of patients with *early* gastric cancer. For the majority who have locally advanced disease, tumours of the distal stomach require partial gastrectomy, while cancers of the proximal body or cardia may require oesophagogastrectomy. Extensive lymph node resection may also increase survival rates but carries greater morbidity. Even for those who cannot be cured, palliative resection may be safely performed in patients with low morbidity and may be necessary if features such as gastric outlet obstruction are present. Between 80 and 85% of tumours will recur, however, if serosal penetration has occurred. Post-operative radiotherapy is of no benefit. Trials of adjuvant chemotherapy following surgery have been disappointing, but the results of pre-operative neo-adjuvant chemotherapy are more encouraging.

Unresectable tumours

The management of inoperable, locally advanced cancer is unsatisfactory. Modest palliation of symptoms is observed in some patients with chemotherapy using FAM (5-fluorouracil, adriamycin and mitomycin C). Endoscopic laser ablation of tumour tissue for control of dysphagia or recurrent bleeding benefits some patients. Carcinomas at the cardia may require endoscopic dilatation, laser therapy or insertion of expandable metallic stents to allow adequate swallowing.

Prognosis

Apart from patients with early gastric cancer the prognosis remains very poor, with less than 10% surviving 5 years. Even after an apparently curative resection, 5-year survival is only around 20%. Thus the best hope for improved survival lies in greater detection of tumours at an earlier stage. The low incidence of gastric carcinoma in many Western countries makes widespread endoscopic screening impractical but urgent referral and investigation of patients with new-onset dyspepsia over the age of 45, or those with 'alarm' features, is essential. If the important association with HP proves to be causal, this offers the possibility of gastric cancer prevention by widespread eradication of the infection.

GASTRIC LYMPHOMA

Primary gastric lymphoma accounts for less than 5% of all gastric malignancies. The stomach is, however, the most common site for extranodal non-Hodgkin's lymphoma and 60% of all primary GI lymphomas occur at this site. Lymphoid tissue is not found in the normal stomach but lymphoid aggregate develops in the presence of HP infection. Indeed, HP infection is closely associated with the development of a low-grade lymphoma ('MALToma'). Preliminary reports have documented regression of this tumour after eradication of the infection.

The clinical presentation is similar to that of gastric cancer and endoscopically the tumour appears as a polyploid or ulcerating mass. While initial treatment of low-grade MALTomas consists of *Helicobacter* eradication and close observation, more aggressive lymphomas are treated by surgical resection with adjuvant chemotherapy and radiotherapy. The prognosis depends on the stage at diagnosis. Features predicting a favourable prognosis are stage I or II disease, small resectable tumours and those with low-grade histology.

OTHER TUMOURS OF THE STOMACH

Leiomyomas are occasionally found at upper gastrointestinal endoscopy. They are benign and usually asymptomatic but may occasionally be responsible for dyspepsia; they can also ulcerate and can cause gastrointestinal bleeding. A variety of different types of polyp are occasionally found. Hyperplastic polyps and fundic cystic gland polyps are of no consequence. *Adenomatous polyps*, however, may be premalignant and should be removed endoscopically.

Occasionally, gastric *carcinoid tumours* are seen in the fundus and body in patients with long-standing pernicious anaemia. These benign tumours arise from enterochromaffin-like (ECL) cells or other endocrine cells, and are often multiple but rarely invasive. Unlike carcinoid tumours arriving elsewhere in the gastrointestinal tract, they usually run a benign and favourable course. However, large (> 2 cm) carcinoids may metastasise and should be removed. Rarely, small nodules of *ectopic pancreatic exocrine tissue* are found. These 'pancreatic rests' may be mistaken for gastric neoplasms and usually cause no symptoms.

FURTHER INFORMATION ON DISEASES OF THE STOMACH AND DUODENUM

Atherton J C 1997 The clinical relevance of strain types of *Helicobacter pylori*. Gut 40: 701–703

Maton P N 1993 The management of Zollinger–Ellison syndrome. Alimentary Pharmacology and Therapeutics 7: 467–475

Nomura A, Stemmerman G N, Chyou P H, Kato I, Perez-Perez G I, Blazer M J 1991 *Helicobacter pylori* infection and gastric cancer amongst Japanese Americans in Hawaii. New England Journal of Medicine 325: 1132–1136

Parsonnet J, Hansen S, Rodriguez L et al 1994 *Helicobacter pylori* infection and gastric lymphoma. New England Journal of Medicine 330: 1267–1271

Wallace J L, Tigley A W 1995 New insights into prostaglandins and mucosal defence. Alimentary Pharmacology and Therapeutics 9: 222–235

DISEASES OF THE SMALL INTESTINE

DISORDERS CAUSING MALABSORPTION

COELIAC DISEASE (GLUTEN-SENSITIVE ENTEROPATHY)

Coeliac disease is characterised by abnormal small intestinal mucosa which returns to normal in response to a gluten-free diet. The condition occurs world-wide but is more common in northern Europe. The prevalence in the UK is 1 in 2000–8000 but reaches 1 in 300 of the population in parts of Ireland. Many mild cases are probably undiagnosed, and screening studies of asymptomatic populations suggest a prevalence of 1 in 300 throughout northern Europe.

Aetiology

Gluten is a heterogeneous component of the water-insoluble fraction of proteins found in wheat, barley, rye and possibly oats. Alcohol solubilisation of gluten produces numerous gliadin peptides (α, β, γ and o), of which α-gliadin is the most toxic to the small intestine. The precise mechanism of damage is unclear but an immunological reaction is likely (see Fig. 9.31). The jejunal mucosa contains an excess of IgA-secreting cells, and circulating antibodies to gliadin and endomysium are found in the majority of patients. Evidence for disordered T-cell function is also present and a strong association with the histocompatibility antigens HLA-B8, DR17 and DQ2 has been demonstrated. The disease may occur in up to 10% of first-degree relatives.

Pathology

Pathological changes vary considerably in both severity and extent. The disease begins in the proximal small intestine. In severe cases the mucosa looks flat with complete loss of surface villi. Histology shows 'subtotal villous atrophy' (see Fig. 9.32), accompanied by crypt hyperplasia and an accumulation of plasma cells and lymphocytes in the lamina propria. The number of intraepithelial lymphocytes is increased and these T cells differ from normal in their increased expression of the γ/δ T-cell receptor phenotype. In less severe cases the changes are milder, with blunting and widening of the villi ('partial villous atrophy'), and a few patients may show normal villous morphology with an increase in the intraepithelial lymphocyte count.

Clinical features and associations

Coeliac disease presents at any age, although it is most common in young adults. In infancy it occurs after weaning on to cereals. The presentation is highly variable, depending

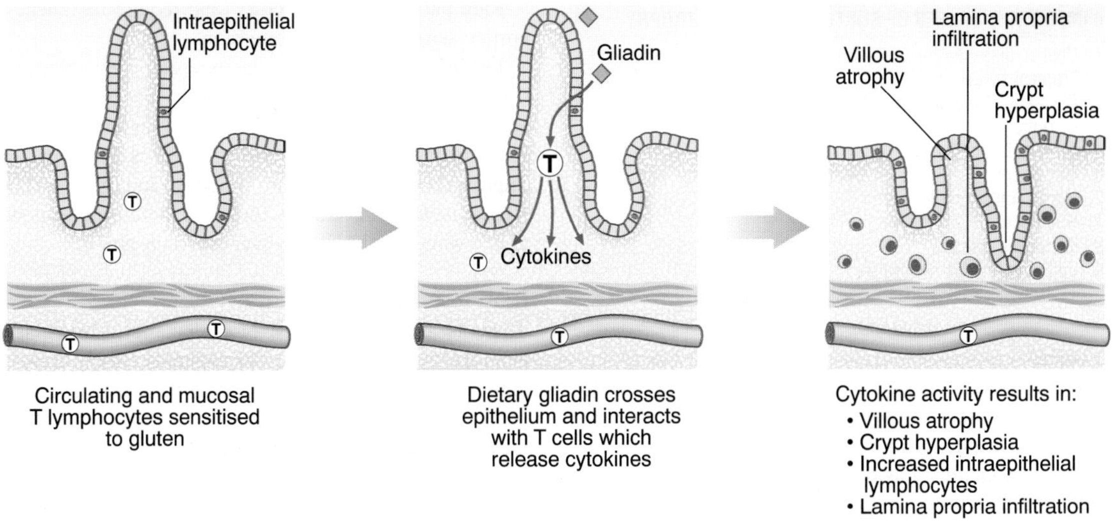

Fig. 9.31 Pathophysiology of coeliac disease.

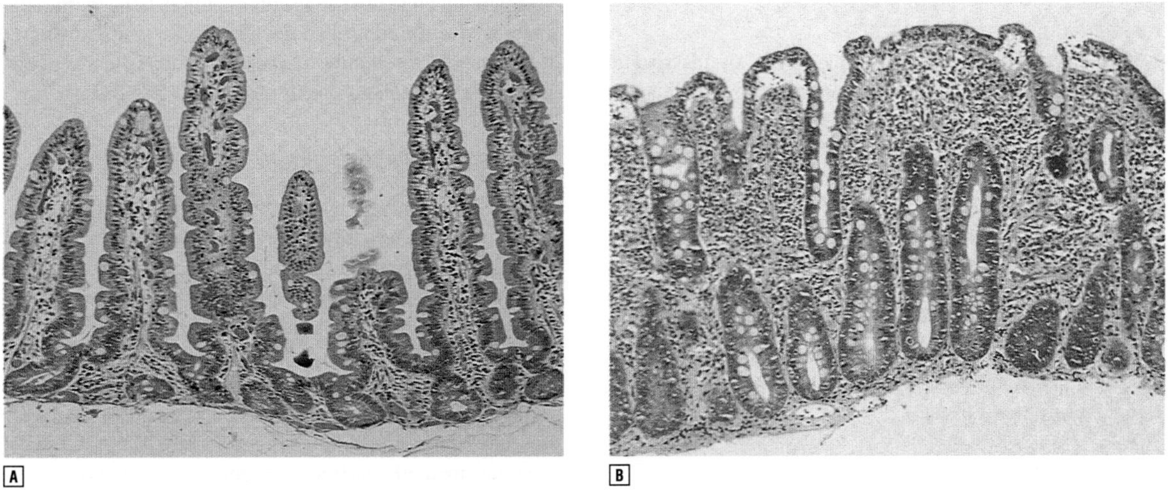

Fig. 9.32 Jejunal mucosa. A Normal. B Jejunum in coeliac disease showing subtotal villous atrophy and marked inflammatory infiltrate.

on the severity and extent of small bowel involvement. Some patients have florid malabsorption while others develop tiredness, weight loss or anaemia. On examination, features of malnutrition are common and mild abdominal distension may be present. Affected children fail to thrive and have both growth and pubertal delay, leading to short stature in adulthood.

Coeliac disease is associated with autoimmune disorders (thyroid disease, insulin-dependent diabetes mellitus and primary biliary cirrhosis), splenic atrophy, IgA deficiency, Down's syndrome and inflammatory bowel disease.

Investigations

These are performed to confirm the diagnosis and to look for consequences of malabsorption.

Jejunal biopsy

Small bowel biopsy is the gold standard. Endoscopic biopsies from the distal duodenum are usually adequate and have largely replaced peroral 'Crosby' capsule biopsies. The histological features are usually characteristic but other causes of villous atrophy should also be considered (see the information box).

10 IMPORTANT CAUSES OF SUBTOTAL VILLOUS ATROPHY

1. Coeliac disease
2. Tropical sprue
3. Dermatitis herpetiformis
4. Lymphoma
5. AIDS enteropathy
6. Giardiasis
7. Hypogammaglobulinaemia
8. Radiation
9. Whipple's disease
10. Zollinger–Ellison syndrome

Antibodies

Serum antigliadin (especially IgA) and antiendomysium antibodies are detectable in most untreated cases. The component of endomysium to which antibodies react has recently been identified as tissue transglutaminase enzyme. These antibodies are a valuable 'screening' test in patients with diarrhoea but they are not a substitute for small bowel biopsy and become negative with successful treatment. Antibodies are absent in patients with coexisting IgA deficiency.

Haematology and biochemistry

A full blood count may show microcytic or macrocytic anaemia from iron or folate deficiency and features of hyposplenism (target cells, spherocytes and Howell–Jolly bodies). Biochemical tests may reveal reduced concentrations of calcium, magnesium, total protein, albumin or vitamin D.

Other investigations

These are usually unnecessary. Barium follow-through radiographs show dilated loops of bowel, coarse or diminished folds and sometimes flocculation of contrast. Sugar tests of intestinal permeability are abnormal and a modest degree of fat malabsorption is usual.

Management

A gluten-free diet must be taken indefinitely. This requires the exclusion of wheat, rye, barley and oats and imposes severe restrictions which must be fully explained to the patient. Some patients are able to tolerate reintroduction of oats later. Rice, maize and potatoes are satisfactory sources of complex carbohydrate. Booklets produced by coeliac societies in many countries, containing diet sheets and recipes for the use of gluten-free flour, are of great value. Initially, frequent dietary counselling is required to make sure the diet is being observed, as the most common reason for failure to improve with dietary treatment is accidental or unrecognised gluten ingestion. Mineral and vitamin supplements are also given when indicated but are seldom necessary when a strict gluten-free diet is adhered to.

Rare patients are 'refractory' and require treatment with corticosteroids to induce remission.

Ideally, patients should undergo repeat jejunal biopsy after 6 months of gluten-free diet to ensure that the small bowel lesion has returned to normal, but this may not be necessary in the majority of patients in whom there is a prompt clinical improvement and a fall in antibody titre with treatment. Repeat biopsies must be performed if there is no response to gluten withdrawal or if the diagnosis is uncertain.

Prognosis and complications

There is an increased risk of malignancy, particularly of enteropathy-associated T-cell lymphoma, small bowel carcinoma and squamous carcinoma of the oesophagus. A few patients develop ulcerative jejunoileitis characterised by deep ulcers in the jejunum with malabsorption. Fever, pain, obstruction or perforation may supervene. The diagnosis is made by barium studies or enteroscopy but sometimes laparotomy and full-thickness biopsy are necessary. Treatment is difficult. Steroids are used with mixed success and some patients require surgical resection and parenteral nutrition. The course is often progressive and relentless.

Metabolic bone disease is common in patients with long-standing, poorly controlled coeliac disease and is a source of considerable morbidity. This complication is less common in patients who adhere strictly to a gluten-free diet.

DERMATITIS HERPETIFORMIS

This is characterised by crops of intensely itchy blisters over extensor surfaces of the limbs and back. Immunofluorescence shows granular or linear IgA deposition at the dermo-epidermal junction. Almost all patients have partial villous atrophy on jejunal biopsy, even though they usually have no gastrointestinal symptoms. In contrast, less than 10% of coeliac patients have evidence of dermatitis herpetiformis although both disorders are associated with the same histocompatibility antigen groups. The rash usually responds to a gluten-free diet but some patients require additional treatment with dapsone (100–150 mg daily).

TROPICAL SPRUE

Tropical sprue is defined as chronic, progressive malabsorption in a patient in or from the tropics, associated with abnormalities of small intestinal structure and function.

Aetiology

The disease occurs mainly in the West Indies and in Asia, including southern India, Malaysia and Indonesia. The epidemiological pattern and occasional epidemics suggest that an infective agent or agents may be involved. Although no single bacterium has been isolated, the condition often begins after an acute diarrhoeal illness. Small bowel overgrowth with *E. coli*, *Enterobacter* and *Klebsiella* is frequently seen.

Pathology

The changes closely resemble those of coeliac disease. Partial villous atrophy is more common than subtotal villous atrophy.

Clinical features

There is diarrhoea, abdominal distension, anorexia, fatigue and weight loss. In visitors to the tropics the onset of severe diarrhoea may be sudden and accompanied by fever. When the disorder becomes chronic, the features of megaloblastic anaemia from folic acid malabsorption and other deficiencies are common. Remissions and relapses may occur. There may be oedema, glossitis and stomatitis.

The differential diagnosis in the indigenous tropical population is an infective cause of diarrhoea. The important differential diagnosis in visitors to the tropics is giardiasis (see p. 155).

Management

Tetracycline 250 mg 6-hourly for 28 days is the treatment of choice and brings about long-term remission or cure. In most patients pharmacological doses of folic acid (5 mg daily) improve symptoms and jejunal morphology. In some cases treatment must be prolonged before improvement occurs, and occasionally patients must leave the tropics.

SMALL BOWEL BACTERIAL OVERGROWTH ('BLIND LOOP SYNDROME')

The normal duodenum and jejunum contain less than 10^4/ml organisms which are usually derived from saliva. The count of coliform organisms never exceeds 10^3/ml. In bacterial overgrowth there may be 10^8–10^{10} organisms/ml, and these are bacteria which are normally found only in the colon. Disorders which impair the normal physiological mechanisms controlling bacterial proliferation in the intestine predispose to bacterial overgrowth (see Table 9.17).

Table 9.17 Causes of small bowel bacterial overgrowth

Mechanism	Examples
Hypo- or achlorhydria	Pernicious anaemia Partial gastrectomy Long-term proton pump inhibitor therapy
Impaired intestinal motility	Scleroderma Diabetic autonomic neuropathy Chronic intestinal pseudo-obstruction
Structural abnormalities	Gastric surgery (blind loop after Billroth II operation) Jejunal diverticulosis Enterocolic fistulae (e.g. Crohn's disease) Extensive small bowel resection Strictures (e.g. Crohn's disease)
Impaired immune function	Hypogammaglobulinaemia

The most important are loss of gastric acidity, impaired intestinal motility and structural abnormalities which allow colonic bacteria to gain access to the small intestine or provide a secluded haven from the peristaltic stream.

Clinical features

The patient presents with watery diarrhoea and/or steatorrhoea with anaemia due to B_{12} deficiency. These arise because of deconjugation of bile acids, which impairs micelle formation, and because of bacterial utilisation of vitamin B_{12}. There may also be symptoms from the underlying intestinal cause.

Investigations

Serum vitamin B_{12} concentration is low, whilst folate levels are normal or elevated because the bacteria produce folic acid. Barium follow-through or small bowel enema reveals blind loops or fistulae. Endoscopic duodenal biopsies exclude mucosal disease such as coeliac disease. During endoscopy, aspiration of jejunal contents for bacteriological examination is carried out; the laboratory analysis requires anaerobic and aerobic culture techniques. The diagnosis can often be made non-invasively using the glucose hydrogen or ^{14}C-glycocholic acid breath tests. In these tests breath samples are serially measured after oral ingestion of the test material. Bacteria within the small bowel cause an early rise in breath hydrogen from glucose (see Fig. 9.33) or ^{14}C from ^{14}C-glycocholate.

Management

The underlying cause of small bowel bacterial overgrowth should be addressed. Tetracycline 250 mg 6-hourly for

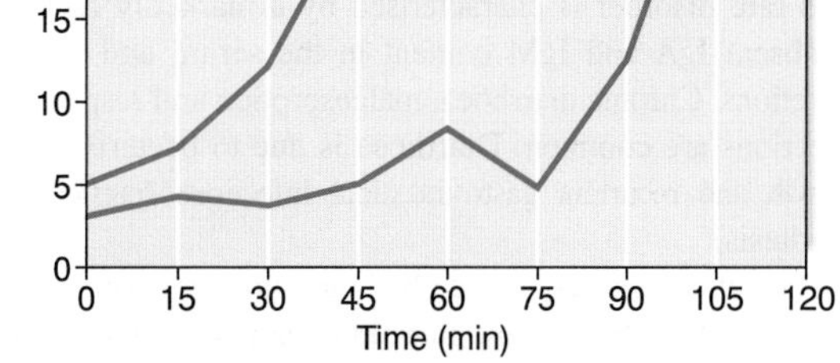

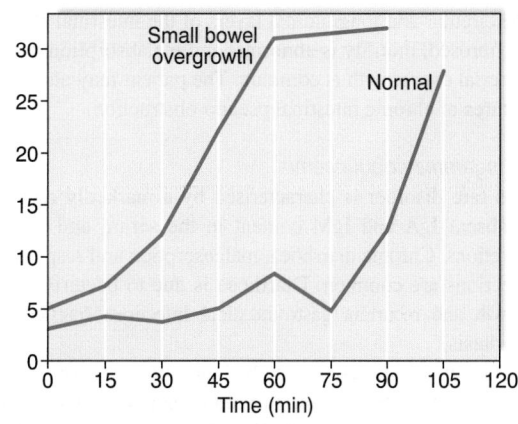

Fig. 9.33 Early rise in breath hydrogen in small bowel bacterial overgrowth. Breath samples are analysed after ingestion of glucose. Bacteria within the small bowel release hydrogen as the glucose is digested.

7 days is the treatment of choice, although up to 50% of patients do not respond adequately. Metronidazole 400 mg 8-hourly or ciprofloxacin 250 mg 12-hourly are alternatives. Some patients require up to 4 weeks of treatment and, in a few, continuous rotating courses of antibiotics are necessary. Intramuscular vitamin B_{12} supplementation is needed in chronic cases.

Some specific causes of bacterial overgrowth

(see Table 9.17)

Jejunal diverticulosis

This is often seen on barium follow-through examinations in patients over the age of 50 years. The diverticula are usually asymptomatic but predispose to bacterial overgrowth and subsequent malabsorption. Rarely they may cause acute or chronic gastrointestinal bleeding, obstruction or perforation.

Diabetic diarrhoea

This results from diabetic autonomic neuropathy (see p. 502), which reduces small bowel motility and affects enterocyte secretion. In some diabetic patients coexisting pancreatic insufficiency or coeliac disease may be responsible. The diarrhoea is watery. It may be continuous or interrupted by bouts of constipation. It is often worse at night, frequently associated with faecal incontinence and may be refractory to antidiarrhoeal drugs. Treatment with antibiotics may be helpful but antidiarrhoeal drugs (diphenoxylate 5 mg 8-hourly orally or loperamide 2 mg 4–6-hourly orally) or opiates are usually needed. The α_2-adrenergic agonist clonidine (50–100 μg 8-hourly) or octreotide may benefit some patients.

Progressive systemic sclerosis (scleroderma)

The circular and longitudinal layers of the intestinal muscle are fibrosed, motility is abnormal and malabsorption due to bacterial overgrowth is common. The patient may also have features of chronic intestinal pseudo-obstruction.

Hypogammaglobulinaemia

This rare disorder is characterised by a markedly reduced or absent IgA and IgM content in the serum and jejunal secretions. Chronic diarrhoea, malabsorption and respiratory infections are common. Diarrhoea is due to bacterial overgrowth and recurrent gastrointestinal infections (particularly giardiasis).

The diagnosis is made by measurement of serum immunoglobulins and by intestinal biopsy which shows reduced or absent plasma cells and nodules of lymphoid tissue (nodular lymphoid hyperplasia). Some patients have the histological features of coeliac disease. Treatment involves control of giardiasis (see p. 155) and, if necessary, regular parenteral replacement of immunoglobulins.

WHIPPLE'S DISEASE

This rare condition is characterised by infiltration of small intestinal mucosa by 'foamy' macrophages which stain positive with periodic acid-Schiff (PAS) reagent. The disease is a multisystem one and almost any organ can be affected, sometimes long before gastrointestinal involvement becomes apparent.

CLINICAL FEATURES OF WHIPPLE'S DISEASE
Gastrointestinal
• Diarrhoea, steatorrhoea, weight loss, bloating, protein-losing enteropathy, ascites, hepatosplenomegaly (< 5%)
Musculoskeletal
• Seronegative large joint arthropathy, sacroiliitis
Cardiac
• Pericarditis (10%), myocarditis, endocarditis, coronary arteritis
Neurological
• Apathy, fits, dementia, myoclonus, meningitis, cranial nerve lesions
Pulmonary
• Chronic cough, pleurisy, pulmonary infiltrates
Haematological
• Anaemia, lymphadenopathy
Other
• Fever, pigmentation

Electron microscopy reveals small Gram-positive bacilli (*Tropheryma whippelli*) within the macrophages. Villi are widened and flattened; densely packed macrophages occur in the lamina propria. These may obstruct lymphatic drainage, causing fat malabsorption.

Clinical features

Middle-aged men are most commonly affected and the presentation depends on the pattern of organ involvement. Low-grade fever is common and most patients have joint symptoms to some degree. Occasionally, neurological manifestations may predominate.

Management

Whipple's disease is often fatal if untreated but responds well, at least initially, to penicillin, tetracycline or sulphonamides. Symptoms resolve within a week and biopsy changes revert to normal in a few weeks. Long-term follow-up is essential, as relapse occurs in up to one-third of patients. This often occurs within the central nervous system, in which case 2 weeks of parenteral penicillin and co-trimoxazole, followed by 6–12 months of oral co-trimoxazole, are necessary.

INTESTINAL RESECTION

The long-term effects of small bowel resection depend on the site and the amount of intestine resected, and vary from trivial to life-threatening.

Ileal resection (see Fig. 9.34)

This usually occurs following surgery for Crohn's disease. Vitamin B_{12} and bile salt malabsorption develops. Unabsorbed bile salts pass into the colon, stimulating water and electrolyte secretion and resulting in diarrhoea. If hepatic synthesis of new bile salts cannot keep pace with faecal losses, then fat malabsorption occurs. Another consequence is the formation of lithogenic bile, leading to gallstones. Renal calculi, rich in oxalate, develop. Normally, oxalate in the colon is bound to and precipitated by calcium. Unabsorbed bile salts preferentially bind calcium, leaving free oxalate to be absorbed with subsequent development of urinary oxalate calculi.

Patients have urgent watery diarrhoea or mild steatorrhoea. Contrast studies of the small bowel and tests of B_{12} and bile acid absorption (see p. 610) are useful investigations. Parenteral vitamin B_{12} supplementation is necessary. Diarrhoea usually responds well to cholestyramine, a resin which binds bile salts in the intestinal lumen. Aluminium hydroxide may also do this in those unable to tolerate cholestyramine.

Massive resection (short bowel syndrome)

Short bowel syndrome is defined as malabsorption resulting from extensive small intestinal resection. Many factors determine the severity, including the extent and site of resection, the presence of underlying disease in the remaining intestine, the presence of the ileocaecal valve and the ability of the remaining small intestine to undergo 'adaptation'.

Aetiology and pathogenesis

The syndrome has many causes (see the information box) but in adults it usually results from Crohn's disease or mesenteric infarction.

AETIOLOGY OF SHORT BOWEL SYNDROME
Children
• Congenital anomalies (e.g. mid-gut volvulus, atresia) • Necrotising enterocolitis
Adults
• Crohn's disease • Mesenteric infarction • Radiation enteritis • Volvulus

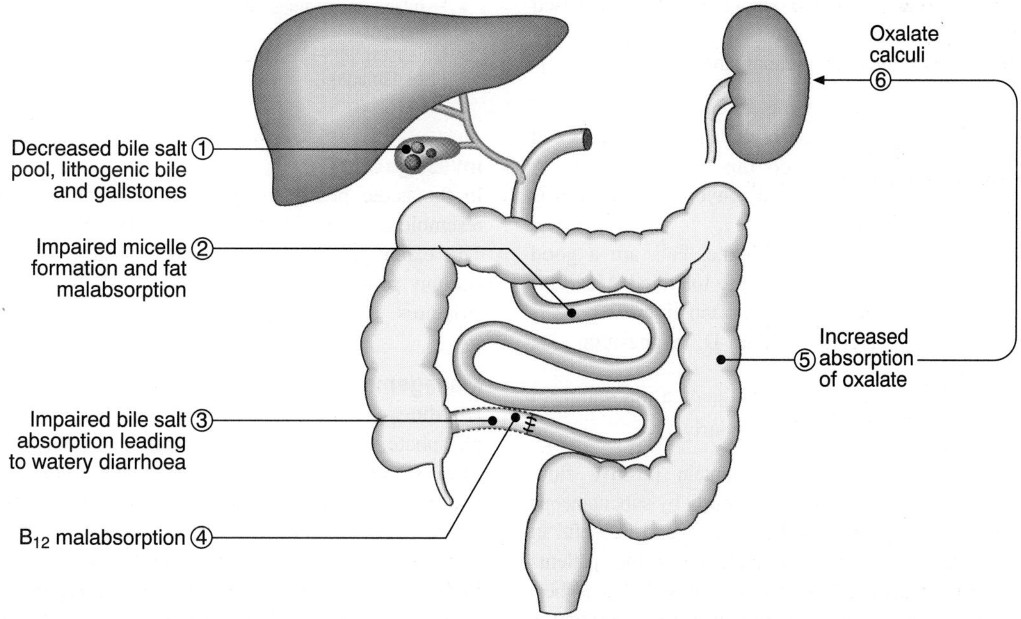

Fig. 9.34 Consequences of ileal resection.

Loss of surface area for digestion and absorption is the key problem. These processes are normally completed within the first 100 cm of jejunum, and enteral feeding is usually possible if this amount of small intestine remains. The proximal small bowel normally reabsorbs around 8 of the 9 litres of fluid it receives daily, and patients with a high jejunostomy are at great risk of hypovolaemia, dehydration and electrolyte losses. The presence of some or all of the colon may markedly improve these losses by increased water reabsorption. The presence of an intact ileocaecal valve ameliorates the clinical picture by slowing small intestinal transit and reducing bacterial overgrowth. The remaining small bowel mucosa undergoes 'adaptation', whereby mucosal hyperplasia over months or years increases the effective surface area for absorption.

Clinical features

Severely affected patients have large volumes of jejunostomy fluid losses or, if the colon is preserved, diarrhoea and steatorrhoea. Dehydration and signs of hypovolaemia are common, as are weight loss, loss of muscle bulk and malnutrition. Some patients remain in satisfactory, but precarious, fluid balance until a minor intercurrent illness or intestinal upset occurs, when they can rapidly become dehydrated.

Management

In the immediate post-operative period, total parenteral nutrition (TPN) is started. Proton pump inhibitor therapy is given to reduce gastric secretions. Enteral feeding is cautiously introduced under careful supervision and is slowly increased as tolerated.

The principles of long-term management are:

- Detailed nutritional assessments at regular intervals.
- Monitoring of fluid and electrolyte balance. Patients can usually be taught how to do this for themselves. A readily available supply of oral rehydration solution is useful for intercurrent illness.
- Adequate calorie and protein intake. Fats are a good energy source and should be taken as tolerated. Medium-chain triglyceride supplements are often given.
- Replacement B_{12}, calcium, vitamin D, magnesium, zinc and folic acid.
- Antidiarrhoeal agents, e.g. loperamide (2–4 mg 6-hourly) or codeine phosphate (30 mg 4–6-hourly).

Some patients are unable to maintain positive fluid balance. Octreotide (50–200 μg 8–12-hourly by subcutaneous injection) reduces gastrointestinal secretions and is useful in such individuals. Despite these measures some patients require long-term home TPN for survival and this is best managed in specialist centres. Small bowel transplantation is an option in some patients but rejection and 'graft-versus-host' disease remain significant hurdles to be overcome.

RADIATION ENTERITIS AND PROCTOCOLITIS

Intestinal damage occurs in up to 10–15% of patients undergoing radiotherapy for abdominal or pelvic malignancy. The risk varies with total dose, dosing schedule and the use of concomitant chemotherapy.

Pathology

The rectum, sigmoid colon and terminal ileum are most frequently involved. Radiation causes acute inflammation, shortening of villi, oedema and crypt abscess formation. This usually resolves completely but in some patients an obliterative endarteritis affecting the endothelium of submucosal arterioles develops over 2–12 months. Fibroblastic proliferation produces progressive ischaemic fibrosis over years and may lead to adhesions, ulceration, strictures, obstruction or fistula to adjacent organs.

Clinical features

In the acute phase there is nausea, vomiting, cramping abdominal pain and diarrhoea. When the rectum and colon are involved, rectal mucus, bleeding and tenesmus occur. The chronic phase develops after 5–10 years in some patients and produces one or more of the problems listed in the information box.

CHRONIC COMPLICATIONS OF INTESTINAL IRRADIATION

- Proctocolitis
- Small bowel strictures
- Fistulae—rectovaginal, colovesical, enterocolic
- Adhesions
- Malabsorption—bacterial overgrowth, bile salt malabsorption (ileal damage)

Investigations

In the acute phase the rectal changes at sigmoidoscopy resemble those of ulcerative proctitis (see Fig. 9.42, p. 664). The extent of the lesion is determined by colonoscopy. Barium follow-through examination shows small bowel strictures, ulcers and fistulae.

Management

Diarrhoea in the acute phase is treated with codeine phosphate, diphenoxylate or loperamide in standard dosage. Local steroid enemas help proctitis, and antibiotics may be required for bacterial overgrowth. Nutritional supplements are necessary when malabsorption is present. Cholestyramine (4 g as a single sachet) is useful for bile salt malabsorption. Endoscopic laser therapy may reduce bleeding from proctitis. Surgery should be avoided, if possible, because the injured intestine is difficult to resect and anastomose, but may be necessary for obstruction, perforation or fistula.

ABETALIPOPROTEINAEMIA

This rare autosomal recessive disorder results from deficiency of apolipoprotein B and subsequent failure of chylomicron formation. It leads to fat malabsorption and deficiency of fat-soluble vitamins. Jejunal biopsy reveals enterocytes distended with resynthesised triglyceride and normal villous morphology. Serum cholesterol and triglyceride levels are low. A number of other abnormalities occur in this syndrome, including acanthocytosis, retinitis pigmentosa and a progressive neurological disorder with cerebellar and dorsal column signs. Symptoms may be improved by a low-fat diet supplemented with medium-chain triglycerides and vitamins A, D, E and K.

MOTILITY DISORDERS

CHRONIC INTESTINAL PSEUDO-OBSTRUCTION

Small intestinal motility is disordered in conditions which affect the smooth muscle or nerves of the intestine. Many cases are 'primary' (idiopathic), while others are 'secondary' to a variety of disorders or drugs (see the information box).

COMMON CAUSES OF CHRONIC INTESTINAL PSEUDO-OBSTRUCTION
Primary or idiopathic
• Rare familial visceral myopathies or neuropathies • Congenital aganglionosis
Secondary
• Drugs, e.g. opiates, tricyclic antidepressants, phenothiazines • Smooth muscle disorders, e.g. scleroderma, amyloidosis, mitochondrial myopathies • Myenteric plexus disorders, e.g. paraneoplastic syndrome in small-cell lung cancer • CNS disorders, e.g. Parkinsonism, autonomic neuropathy • Endocrine and metabolic disorders, e.g. hypothyroidism, phaeochromocytoma, acute intermittent porphyria

Clinical features

There are recurrent episodes of nausea, vomiting, abdominal discomfort and distension, often worse after food. Alternating constipation and diarrhoea occur and weight loss results from malabsorption (due to bacterial overgrowth) and fear of eating. There may also be symptoms of dysmotility affecting other parts of the gastrointestinal tract, e.g. dysphagia, and, in primary cases, features of bladder dysfunction.

Investigations

The diagnosis is often delayed and a high index of suspicion is needed. Plain radiographs show distended loops of bowel and air-fluid levels but barium studies demonstrate no mechanical obstruction. Laparotomy is sometimes performed to exclude obstruction and to obtain full-thickness biopsies of the intestine. Electron microscopy, histochemistry and special stains define rare, specific syndromes.

Management

This is often difficult. Underlying causes should be addressed and further surgery avoided if at all possible. Prokinetic agents (cisapride or domperidone) may enhance motility, and antibiotics are given for bacterial overgrowth. Nutritional and psychological support are also necessary.

MISCELLANEOUS DISORDERS OF THE SMALL INTESTINE

PROTEIN-LOSING ENTEROPATHY

This term is used when there is excessive loss of protein into the gut lumen, sufficient to cause hypoproteinaemia. Less than 10% of plasma protein is normally lost from the gastrointestinal tract. Protein-losing enteropathy occurs in many gut disorders but is most common in those where ulceration occurs. In other disorders protein loss results from increased mucosal permeability or obstruction of intestinal lymphatic vessels.

Patients present with peripheral oedema and hypoproteinaemia in the presence of normal liver function and without proteinuria. There may also be features of the underlying cause.

CAUSES OF PROTEIN-LOSING ENTEROPATHY
With mucosal erosions or ulceration
• Crohn's disease • Ulcerative colitis • Oesophageal, gastric or colonic cancer • Lymphoma • Radiation damage
Without mucosal erosions or ulceration
• Ménétrier's disease • Bacterial overgrowth • Coeliac disease • Tropical sprue • Eosinophilic gastroenteritis • Systemic lupus erythematosus
With lymphatic obstruction
• Intestinal lymphangiectasia • Constrictive pericarditis • Lymphoma • Whipple's disease

The diagnosis is confirmed by measurement of faecal clearance of α_1-antitrypsin or ^{51}Cr-labelled albumin after intravenous injection. Other investigations are performed to determine the underlying cause. Treatment is that of the underlying disorder, nutritional support and measures to control peripheral oedema.

INTESTINAL LYMPHANGIECTASIA

This may be primary, resulting from congenital malunion of lymphatics, or secondary to lymphatic obstruction due to lymphoma, filariasis or constrictive pericarditis. Impaired drainage of intestinal lymphatic vessels leads to discharge of protein and fat-rich lymph into the gastrointestinal lumen. The condition presents with peripheral lymphoedema, pleural effusions or chylous ascites, and steatorrhoea. Investigations reveal hypoalbuminaemia, lymphocytopenia and reduced serum immunoglobulin concentrations. Jejunal biopsies show greatly dilated lacteals and lymphangiography shows lymphatic obstruction. Treatment consists of a low-fat diet with medium-chain triglyceride supplements.

ULCERATION OF THE SMALL INTESTINE

Small bowel ulcers are uncommon and are either idiopathic or secondary to underlying intestinal disorders (see the information box).

CAUSES OF SMALL INTESTINAL ULCERS

- Idiopathic
- Inflammatory bowel disease, e.g. Crohn's
- Drugs, e.g. NSAIDs, enteric-coated potassium tablets
- Ulcerative jejunoileitis
- Lymphoma and carcinoma
- Infections, e.g. tuberculosis, typhoid, yersinia
- Others, e.g. radiation, vasculitis

Ulcers are more common in the ileum, and cause bleeding, perforation, stricture formation or obstruction. Barium studies and enteroscopy confirm the diagnosis.

EOSINOPHILIC GASTROENTERITIS

This rare disorder of unknown aetiology can affect any part of the gastrointestinal tract and is characterised by eosinophil infiltration affecting the gut wall in the absence of parasitic infection or eosinophilia of other tissues. Peripheral blood eosinophilia is present in 80% of cases.

Inflammation and destruction affect mucosal, muscular and/or serosal layers.

Clinical features

There are features of obstruction and inflammation, such as colicky pain, nausea and vomiting, diarrhoea and weight loss. Protein-losing enteropathy occurs and up to 50% of patients have a history of other allergic disorders. Serosal involvement may produce eosinophilic ascites.

Diagnosis and management

The diagnosis is made by histological assessment of multiple endoscopic biopsies, although full-thickness biopsies are occasionally required. Other investigations are performed to exclude parasitic infection and other causes of eosinophilia. A raised serum IgE concentration is often seen.

Dietary manipulations are rarely effective although elimination diets, especially of milk, may benefit a few patients. Severe symptoms are treated with prednisolone 20–40 mg daily and/or disodium cromoglycate, which stabilises mast cell membranes. The prognosis is good in the majority of patients.

MECKEL'S DIVERTICULUM

This is the commonest congenital anomaly of the gastrointestinal tract and occurs in 0.3–3% of people. Most patients are asymptomatic. The diverticulum results from failure of closure of the vitelline duct, with persistence of a blind-ending sac arising from the antimesenteric border of the ileum, usually occurs within 100 cm of the ileocaecal valve, and is up to 5 cm long. Approximately 50% contain ectopic gastric mucosa; rarely, colonic, pancreatic or endometrial tissue is present.

Complications most commonly occur in the first 2 years of life but are occasionally seen in young adults. Bleeding results from ulceration of ileal mucosa adjacent to the ectopic parietal cells and presents as recurrent melaena or altered blood per rectum. Diagnosis can be made by scanning the abdomen using a gamma counter following an intravenous injection of ^{99M}-technetium pertechnetate, which is concentrated by ectopic parietal cells. Other complications include intestinal obstruction, diverticulitis, intussusception and perforation. Intervention is unnecessary unless complications occur. The vast majority of patients remain asymptomatic throughout life.

ADVERSE FOOD REACTIONS

Adverse food reactions are common and are subdivided into food intolerance and food allergy, the former being much more common.

FOOD INTOLERANCE

This involves adverse reactions to food which are not immune-mediated and result from a wide range of mechanisms. Contaminants in food, preservatives and lactase deficiency may all be involved.

LACTOSE INTOLERANCE

Human milk contains around 200 mmol/l of lactose which is normally digested to glucose and galactose by the brush border enzyme lactase prior to absorption. In most populations enterocyte lactase activity declines throughout childhood. The enzyme is deficient in up to 90% of adult Africans, Asians and South Americans, but only 5% of northern Europeans.

In cases of racially determined (primary) lactase deficiency, jejunal morphology is normal. 'Secondary' lactase deficiency occurs as a consequence of disorders which damage the jejunal mucosa, e.g. coeliac disease and viral gastroenteritis. Unhydrolysed lactose enters the colon, where bacterial fermentation produces volatile short-chain fatty acids, hydrogen and carbon dioxide.

Clinical features

In most people lactase deficiency is completely asymptomatic. However, some complain of colicky pain, abdominal distension, increased flatus, borborygmi and diarrhoea after ingesting milk or milk products. Irritable bowel syndrome is often suspected but the diagnosis is suggested by clinical improvement on lactose withdrawal. The lactose hydrogen breath test is a useful non-invasive confirmatory test.

Dietary exclusion of lactose is recommended, although most sufferers are able to tolerate small amounts of milk without symptoms. Addition of commercial lactase preparations to milk has been effective in some studies but is costly.

DIARRHOEA DUE TO OTHER SUGARS

'Osmotic' diarrhoea can be caused by sorbitol, an unabsorbable carbohydrate which is used as an artificial sweetener. Fructose may also cause diarrhoea if consumed in greater quantities (e.g. in fruit juices) than can be absorbed.

FOOD ALLERGY

Food allergies are immune-mediated disorders due to IgE antibodies and type I hypersensitivity reactions. Up to 20% of the population perceive themselves to suffer from food allergy but only 1–2% of adults have genuine food allergies. The most common culprits are peanuts, milk, eggs, soya and shellfish.

Clinical manifestations occur immediately on exposure and range from trivial to life-threatening or even fatal anaphylaxis. In the '*oral allergy syndrome*' contact with certain fresh fruit juices results in urticaria and angio-oedema of the lips and oropharynx. '*Allergic gastroenteropathy*' has features similar to eosinophilic gastroenteritis, while '*gastrointestinal anaphylaxis*' consists of nausea, vomiting, diarrhoea and sometimes cardiovascular and respiratory collapse. Fatal reactions to trace amounts of peanuts are well documented.

The diagnosis of food allergy is difficult to prove or refute. Skin prick tests and measurements of antigen-specific IgE antibodies in serum have limited predictive value. Double-blind placebo-controlled food challenges are the gold standard, but are laborious and are not readily available. In many cases clinical suspicion and trials of elimination diets are used.

Treatment of proven food allergy consists of detailed patient education and awareness, strict elimination of the offending antigen and in some cases antihistamines or disodium cromoglycate. Anaphylaxis should be treated as a medical emergency with resuscitation, airway support and intravenous adrenaline. Subsequently, patients should wear an information bracelet and be taught to carry and use a preloaded adrenaline syringe.

INFECTIONS OF THE SMALL INTESTINE

TRAVELLERS' DIARRHOEA

See page 65.

GIARDIASIS

See page 155.

AMOEBIASIS

See page 153.

ABDOMINAL TUBERCULOSIS

Mycobacterium tuberculosis is a rare cause of abdominal disease in Caucasians but must be considered in immigrants from the underdeveloped world and in AIDS patients. Gut infection usually results from human *Mycobacterium tuberculosis* which is swallowed after coughing. Many patients have no pulmonary symptoms and a normal chest radiograph.

The area most commonly affected is the ileocaecal region; presentation and radiological findings may be very similar to those of Crohn's disease. Abdominal pain can be acute or of several months' duration, but diarrhoea is less common in tuberculosis (TB) than in Crohn's disease. Low-grade fever is common but not invariable. Like Crohn's disease, TB can affect any part of the gastrointestinal tract, and perianal disease with fistula is recognised. Peritoneal TB may result in peritonitis with exudative ascites, associated with abdominal pain and fever. Granulomatous hepatitis occurs.

Diagnosis

Abdominal TB causes an elevated erythrocyte sedimentation rate (ESR); a raised serum alkaline phosphatase concentration suggests hepatic involvement. Histological confirmation is sought by endoscopic or liver biopsy. Caseation of granulomata is unusual and acid- and alcohol-fast bacteria are often scanty. Culture may be helpful but identification of the organism may take 6 weeks. Newer serological tests may prove valuable.

Management

When the presentation is very suggestive of abdominal tuberculosis, triple chemotherapy (see p. 352) should be commenced even if bacteriological or histological proof is lacking.

CRYPTOSPORIDIOSIS

Cryptosporidiosis and other protozoal infections, including isosporiasis *(Isospora belli)* and microsporidiosis, are dealt with on page 102.

TUMOURS OF THE SMALL INTESTINE

The small intestine is rarely affected by neoplasia, and less than 5% of all gastrointestinal tumours occur here.

Benign tumours

The most common are adenomas, leiomyomas, lipomas and hamartomas. Adenomas are most often found in the periampullary region and are usually asymptomatic, although occult bleeding or obstruction due to intussusception may occur. Transformation to adenocarcinoma is rare. Multiple adenomas are common in the duodenum of patients with familial adenomatous polyposis (FAP), who merit regular endoscopic surveillance. Hamartomatous polyps with almost no malignant potential occur in Peutz–Jeghers syndrome (see p. 673).

Malignant tumours

These are rare and include, in decreasing order of frequency, adenocarcinoma, carcinoid tumour, leiomyosarcoma and lymphoma. The majority occur in middle age or later. Kaposi's sarcoma is seen in patients with AIDS.

Adenocarcinomas occur with increased frequency in patients with familial adenomatous polyposis, coeliac disease and Peutz–Jeghers syndrome. The non-specific presentation and rarity of these lesions often leads to delay in diagnosis. Barium follow-through examination or small bowel enema studies will demonstrate most lesions. Enteroscopy, mesenteric angiography and computed tomography also play a role in investigation.

CARCINOID TUMOURS

These are derived from enterochromaffin cells and are most common in the ileum. Localised spread and the potential for metastasis to the liver increase with primary lesions over 2 cm in diameter. Carcinoid tumours also occur in the rectum and in the appendix; those in the latter are usually benign. Overall, these tumours are less aggressive than carcinomas and their growth is usually slow.

The term *'carcinoid syndrome'* refers to the systemic symptoms produced when secretory products of the neoplastic enterochromaffin cells reach the systemic circulation. When produced by the primary tumour they are usually metabolised in the liver and do not reach the systemic circulation. The syndrome is therefore only seen when 5-hydroxytryptamine (5-HT, serotonin), bradykinin and other peptide hormones are released by hepatic metastases.

Management

The treatment of a carcinoid tumour is surgical resection. The treatment of carcinoid syndrome is palliative because hepatic metastases have occurred, although prolonged survival is common. Surgical removal of the primary tumour is usually attempted and the hepatic metastases are often excised as reduction of tumour mass improves symptoms. Hepatic artery embolisation retards growth of hepatic deposits. A variety of pharmacological agents are available to block some of the effects of 5-HT, kinins and other secretory products. The most useful is octreotide 200 μg 8-hourly by subcutaneous injection. Cytotoxic chemotherapy has only a minor role.

CLINICAL FEATURES OF THE CARCINOID SYNDROME

- Small-bowel obstruction due to the tumour mass
- Intestinal ischaemia (due to mesenteric infiltration or vasospasm)
- Hepatic metastases causing pain, hepatomegaly and jaundice
- Flushing and wheezing
- Diarrhoea
- Cardiac involvement (tricuspid regurgitation, pulmonary stenosis, right ventricular endocardial plaques) leading to heart failure
- Facial telangiectasia

The diagnosis is made by detecting excess levels of the 5-HT metabolite, 5-HIAA, in a 24-hour urine collection.

LYMPHOMA

Non-Hodgkin's lymphoma may involve the gastrointestinal tract as part of more generalised disease or may rarely arise in the gut, with the small intestine being most commonly affected. Lymphomas occur with increased frequency in patients with coeliac disease, AIDS and other immunodeficiency states. Most are of B-cell origin, although that associated with coeliac disease is derived from T cells (enteropathy-associated T-cell lymphoma).

Colicky abdominal pain, obstruction and weight loss are the usual presenting features and perforation is also occasionally seen. Malabsorption is only a feature of diffuse bowel involvement and hepatosplenomegaly is rare.

The diagnosis is made by small bowel biopsy, radiological contrast studies and CT scan. Staging investigations are performed. Surgical resection where possible is the treatment of choice, with radiotherapy and combination chemotherapy reserved for those with advanced disease. The prognosis depends largely on the stage at diagnosis, cell type, patient age and the presence of 'B' symptoms (see p. 780).

IMMUNOPROLIFERATIVE SMALL INTESTINAL DISEASE (IPSID)

Also known as 'alpha heavy chain disease', this rare condition occurs mainly in the Mediterranean, Middle East and North America. The aetiology is unknown but it may be a response to chronic stimulation by bacterial antigens. The condition varies in severity from relatively benign to frankly malignant.

The small intestinal mucosa is diffusely affected, especially proximally, by a dense lymphoplasmacytic infiltrate. Enlarged mesenteric lymph nodes are also common. Most patients are young adults who present with malabsorption, anorexia and fever. Serum electrophoresis confirms the presence of alpha heavy chains (from the Fc portion of IgA). Prolonged remissions can be obtained with long-term antibiotic therapy but chemotherapy is required for those who fail to respond or who have aggressive disease.

FURTHER INFORMATION ON DISEASES OF THE SMALL INTESTINE

Lennard-Jones J E 1994 Practical management of the short bowel. Alimentary Pharmacology and Therapeutics 8: 563–570

Marsh M N 1992 Coeliac and allied sprue syndromes. In: Turnberg L A (ed) Absorption and malabsorption. Seminars in Gastrointestinal Diseases 4: 214–223

DISEASES OF THE PANCREAS

ACUTE PANCREATITIS

Acute pancreatitis affects 10–28 per 100 000 of the population. In survivors, pancreatic function and structure recover completely.

Pathophysiology

Acute oedematous pancreatitis is characterised by interstitial inflammation and oedema with peripancreatic fat necrosis but sparing of the acinar cells. Oedematous pancreatitis may resolve or progress to *necrotising pancreatitis* in which acinar cells are destroyed. This can progress further to *acute haemorrhagic pancreatitis*, characterised by bleeding into the pancreas and retroperitoneum.

Acute pancreatitis is a consequence of premature activation of zymogen granules, releasing proteases which digest the pancreas and surrounding tissue (see Fig. 9.35). The normal pancreas has only a poorly developed capsule, and adjacent structures, including the common bile duct, duodenum, splenic vein and the transverse colon, are commonly involved in the inflammatory process. The severity of acute pancreatitis is dependent upon the balance between activity of released proteolytic enzymes and antiproteolytic factors. The latter comprise an intracellular pancreatic trypsin inhibitor protein and circulating α_2-macroglobulin, α_1-antitrypsin and C1-esterase inhibitors. Causes of acute pancreatitis are given in the information box.

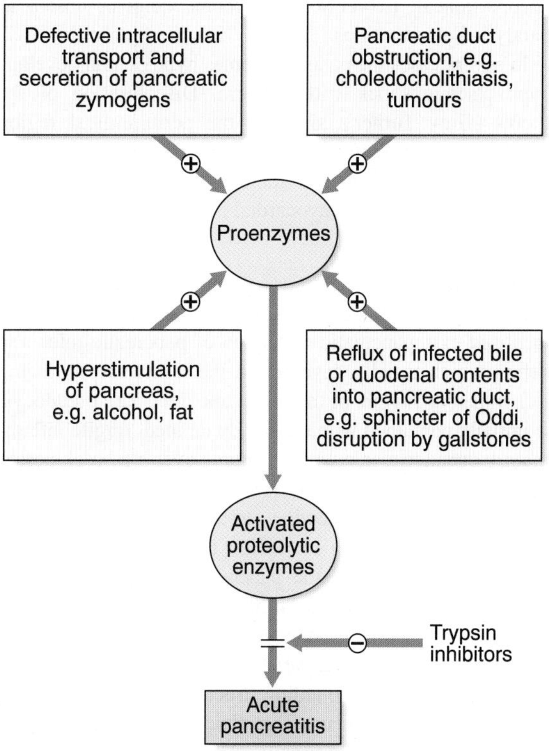

Fig. 9.35 Pathophysiology of acute pancreatitis.

CAUSES OF ACUTE PANCREATITIS
Common (90% of cases)
• Gallstones • Alcohol • Idiopathic
Rare
• Post-ERCP • Post-surgical (abdominal, cardiopulmonary bypass) • Trauma • Drugs (azathioprine, thiazide diuretics, sodium valproate) • Metabolic (hypercalcaemia, hypertriglyceridaemia) • Pancreas divisum (see p. 657) • Infection (mumps, Coxsackie virus) • Hereditary • Renal failure • Organ transplantation (kidney, liver)

Clinical features

Severe, constant upper abdominal pain which radiates to the back in 65% of cases builds up over 15–60 minutes. Nausea and vomiting are common. There is marked epigastric tenderness but in the early stages (and in contrast to a perforated peptic ulcer), guarding and rebound tenderness are absent because the inflammation is principally retroperitoneal. Bowel sounds become quiet or absent as paralytic ileus develops.

In severe cases the patient becomes hypoxic and develops hypovolaemic shock with oliguria. Discoloration of the flanks (Grey Turner's sign) or the periumbilical region (Cullen's sign) are features of haemorrhagic pancreatitis. The differential diagnosis includes a perforated viscus, acute cholecystitis and myocardial infarction.

Complications

These are listed in Table 9.18. A pancreatic pseudocyst is a localised extrapancreatic collection of pancreatic juice and debris which usually develops in the lesser sac following inflammatory rupture of the pancreatic duct. The pseudocyst is initially contained within a poorly defined, fragile inflammatory pseudocapsule which matures over a 6-week period to form a fibrous capsule (see Fig. 9.36). Small intrapancreatic cysts and pseudocysts are common features of both acute and chronic pancreatitis; they are usually asymptomatic and resolve as the pancreatitis recovers. Pseudocysts greater than 6 cm in diameter seldom disappear spontaneously. Large pseudocysts cause constant abdominal pain, can produce a palpable abdominal mass and may compress or erode surrounding structures.

Pancreatic ascites occurs when fluid leaks from a disrupted pancreatic duct into the peritoneal cavity. Leakage into the thoracic cavity can result in a pleural effusion or a bronchopancreatic fistula.

Table 9.18 Complications of acute pancreatitis

Complication	Cause
Systemic	
Shock and renal failure	Increased vascular permeability from kinin release, paralytic ileus, vomiting
Hypoxia	Acute respiratory distress syndrome (ARDS) due to microthrombi in pulmonary vessels
Hyperglycaemia	Disruption of islets of Langerhans with altered insulin/glucagon axis
Hypocalcaemia	Sequestration of calcium in fat necrosis, fall in ionised calcium (? cause)
Reduced serum albumin concentration	Increased capillary permeability
Pancreatic	
Abscess	Infection of necrotic pancreatic tissue
Pseudocyst	Disruption of pancreatic ducts
Pancreatic ascites or pleural effusion	Disruption of pancreatic ducts
Gastrointestinal	
Upper gastrointestinal bleeding	Gastric or duodenal erosions
Variceal haemorrhage erosion into colon	Splenic or portal vein thrombosis
Duodenal obstruction	Compression by pancreatic mass
Obstructive jaundice	Compression of common bile duct by pancreatic mass

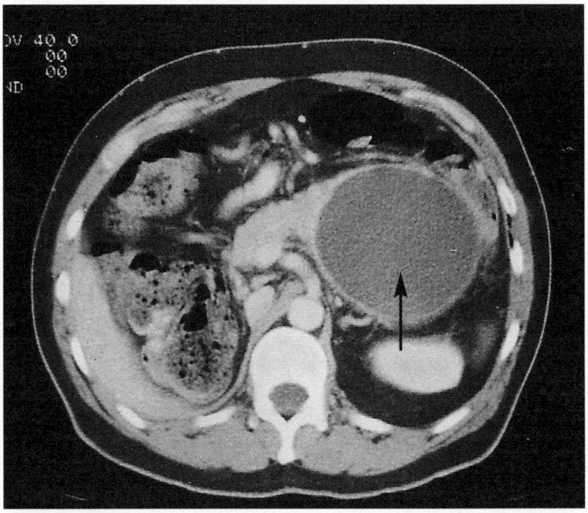

Fig. 9.36 CT scan showing large pancreatic pseudocyst (arrow) developing from the body of the pancreas.

Diagnosis

The diagnosis of acute pancreatitis is based upon elevation of serum amylase or lipase concentrations and ultrasound evidence of pancreatic swelling.

Amylase is efficiently excreted by the kidneys, and concentrations may have returned to normal if measured 24–48 hours after the onset of pancreatitis. In this situation the diagnosis can be made by demonstrating an elevated urinary amylase:creatinine ratio. A persistently elevated serum amylase concentration suggests pseudocyst formation. Peritoneal amylase concentrations are massively elevated in pancreatic ascites. Serum amylase concentrations are also elevated (but to a lesser extent) in intestinal ischaemia, perforated peptic ulcer and ruptured ovarian cyst, and the salivary isoenzyme of amylase is elevated in parotitis.

Ultrasound scanning confirms the diagnosis, although in the earlier stages the gland may not be grossly swollen. The ultrasound scan is also useful because it may show gallstones, biliary obstruction or pseudocyst formation.

CT scanning is used to define the viability of the pancreas. Necrotising pancreatitis is associated with decreased pancreatic enhancement following intravenous injection of contrast material. The presence of gas within necrotic material suggests infection and impending abscess formation, in which case percutaneous aspiration of material for bacterial culture should be carried out. Involvement of the colon, blood vessels and other adjacent structures by the inflammatory process is best seen by CT.

Certain investigations have important prognostic value at the time of presentation (see the information box). In addition, serial assessment of C-reactive protein (CRP) is a useful indicator of progress. It is worth noting that the serum amylase concentration has no prognostic value.

ADVERSE PROGNOSTIC FACTORS IN ACUTE PANCREATITIS (GLASGOW CRITERIA)*

- $PO_2 < 8$ kPa
- White blood cell count (WBC) > 15×10^9/litre
- Albumin < 30 g/l
- Serum calcium < 2 mmol/l (corrected)
- Glucose > 10 mmol/l
- Urea > 16 mmol/l (after rehydration)
- Alanine aminotransferase (ALT) > 200 U/l
- Lactate dehydrogenase (LDH) > 600 U/l

* Severity and prognosis worsen as the number of these factors increases.

Management

The initial management is based upon analgesia using pethidine and correction of hypovolaemia using normal saline and/or colloids. A central venous line and urinary catheter are used to monitor shocked patients. Hypoxic patients need oxygen, although patients who develop acute respiratory distress syndrome (ARDS) may require ventilatory support. Hyperglycaemia is corrected using insulin, but it is not necessary to correct hypocalcaemia by intravenous calcium injection unless tetany occurs.

Nasogastric aspiration is only necessary if paralytic ileus is present. Enteral feeding is withheld until clinical and biochemical improvement occurs, but parenteral nutrition should be started at an early stage in severe cases because such patients are in a severely catabolic state and often have a prolonged illness. Prophylaxis of thrombo-embolism with low-dose subcutaneous heparin is also advisable.

Patients who present with cholangitis or jaundice in association with severe acute pancreatitis should undergo urgent ERCP to diagnose and treat choledocholithiasis. In less severe cases of gallstone pancreatitis, ERCP may be carried out after the acute phase has resolved.

Management of complications

Patients who have developed necrotising pancreatitis or pancreatic abscess require urgent surgical débridement of the pancreas, followed by drainage of the pancreatic bed. Pancreatic pseudocysts are treated by drainage into the stomach or duodenum. This is usually done after at least 6 weeks, once a pseudocapsule has matured, using open surgery or endoscopic methods. Pancreatic ascites is an indication for distal pancreatectomy.

Prognosis

The overall mortality of acute pancreatitis is approximately 10%. Patients with necrotising pancreatitis and pancreatic abscess have a mortality of at least 50% and should be managed in specialist hepatobiliary/pancreatic surgical units.

CHRONIC PANCREATITIS

Chronic pancreatitis is a chronic inflammatory disease characterised by fibrosis and destruction of exocrine pancreatic tissue. Diabetes mellitus occurs in advanced cases because the islets of Langerhans are involved.

Pathophysiology

Between 70 and 80% of cases result from alcohol abuse (see Fig. 9.37). Other causes are listed in the information box.

Clinical features

Chronic pancreatitis predominantly affects middle-aged alcoholic men. Almost all present with abdominal pain. In 50% this occurs as episodes of 'acute pancreatitis', although each attack results in a degree of permanent

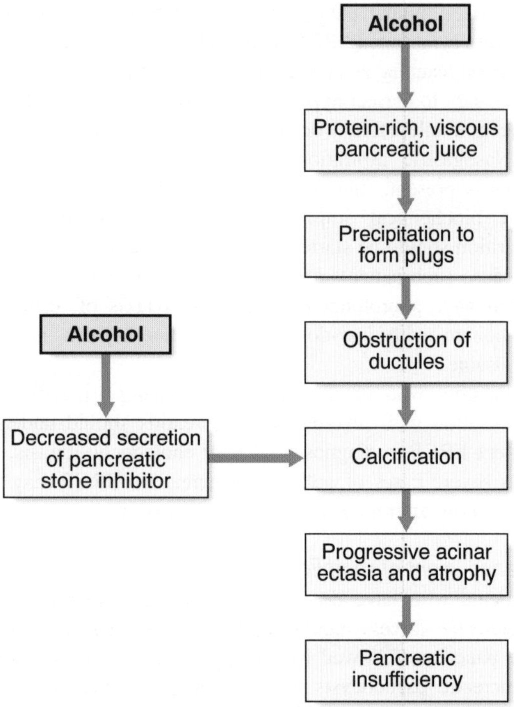

Fig. 9.37 Pathophysiology of chronic pancreatitis.

CAUSES OF CHRONIC PANCREATITIS

• Calcific
  Alcoholism
  Tropical (? related to malnutrition or dietary toxins)
• Obstructive
  Stenosis of the ampulla of Vater
• Pancreas divisum (see p. 657)
• Cystic fibrosis
• Hereditary
• Idiopathic

N.B. Many patients have gallstones but these do not cause chronic pancreatitis.

pancreatic damage. Relentless, slowly progressive chronic pain without acute exacerbations affects 35% of patients, whilst the remainder have no pain but present with diarrhoea. Pain is due to a combination of increased pressure within the pancreatic ducts and direct involvement of pancreatic and peripancreatic nerves by the inflammatory process. Pain may be relieved by leaning forwards or by drinking alcohol. Approximately one-fifth of patients chronically consume opiate analgesics.

Weight loss is common and results from a combination of anorexia, avoidance of food because of postprandial pain, malabsorption and/or diabetes. Steatorrhoea occurs when more than 90% of the exocrine tissue has been destroyed; protein malabsorption only develops in the most advanced cases. Overall, 30% of patients are diabetic, but this figure rises to 70% in those with chronic calcific pancreatitis.

COMPLICATIONS OF CHRONIC PANCREATITIS
• Pseudocysts and pancreatic ascites, which occur in both acute and chronic pancreatitis • Extrahepatic obstructive jaundice due to a benign stricture of the common bile duct as it passes through the diseased pancreas • Duodenal stenosis • Portal or splenic vein thrombosis leading to segmental portal hypertension and gastric varices • Peptic ulcer

Physical examination reveals a thin, malnourished patient with epigastric tenderness. Skin pigmentation over the abdomen and back is common and results from chronic use of a hot water bottle *(erythema ab igne)*. Many patients have features of other alcohol- and smoking-related diseases.

Investigations (see the information box)

These are done to:

- make a diagnosis of chronic pancreatitis
- define pancreatic function
- demonstrate anatomical abnormalities prior to surgical intervention.

INVESTIGATIONS IN CHRONIC PANCREATITIS
Tests to establish the diagnosis
• Ultrasound • CT scan (may show atrophy, calcification or ductal dilatation) • Abdominal radiograph (may show calcification) • ERCP only if non-invasive tests are negative or equivocal (see Fig. 9.38) • Endoscopic ultrasound
Tests of pancreatic function
• Collection of pancreatic juice after secretion injection (gold standard but invasive and seldom used) • Pancreolauryl or PABA test (see p. 610) • Faecal pancreatic chymotrypsin or elastase • Oral glucose tolerance test
Tests of anatomy prior to surgery
• ERCP (see Fig. 9.38)

Management

Alcohol abuse

Alcohol avoidance is crucial in halting the progression of the disease and reducing pain. Unfortunately, counselling and psychiatric intervention are rarely successful and the majority of patients continue to drink alcohol.

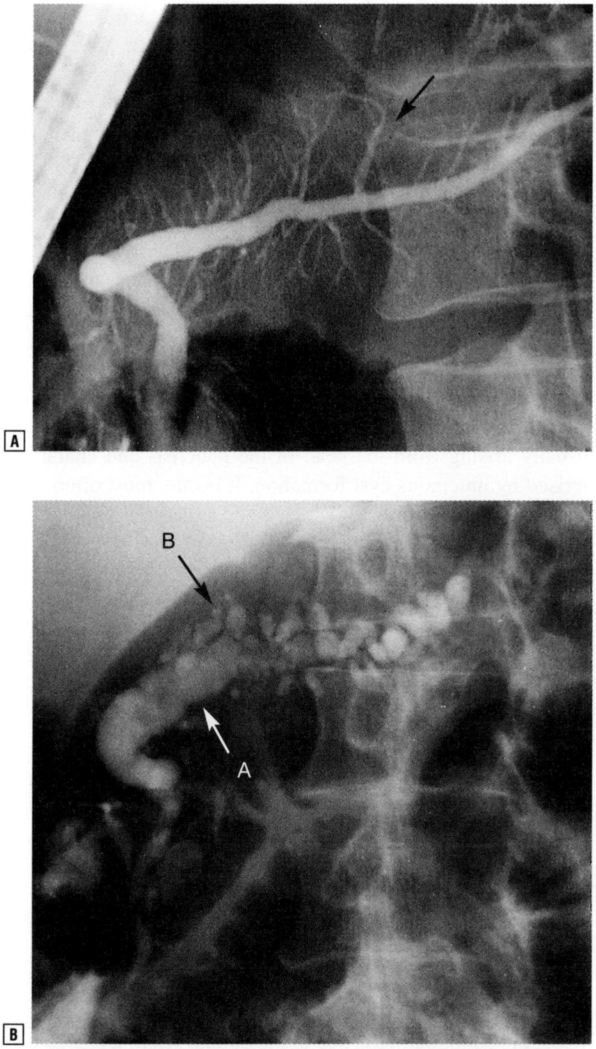

Fig. 9.38 ERCP in chronic pancreatitis. A Early pancreatitis. Irregular dilated side branches (arrow). B Advanced disease. Dilated, irregular main duct (arrow A), with obstructed abnormal side branches (arrow B).

Pain relief

A range of analgesic drugs, particularly non-steroidal anti-inflammatory agents, are valuable but the severe and unremitting nature of the pain often leads to opiate use with the risk of addiction. Oral pancreatic enzyme supplements suppress pancreatic secretion and their regular use reduces analgesic consumption in some patients.

Patients who are abstinent from alcohol and who have severe chronic pain which is resistant to conservative measures are considered for surgical or endoscopic pancreatic therapy (see the information box).

INTERVENTION IN CHRONIC PANCREATITIS
Endoscopic therapy
• Dilatation or stenting of main pancreatic duct • Removal of calculi (mechanical or shock wave lithotripsy)
Surgical methods
• Partial pancreatic resection • Pancreatico-jejunostomy

In some patients ERCP does not show a surgically or endoscopically correctable abnormality and in these patients the only surgical approach is total pancreatectomy. Unfortunately, some patients will continue to experience pain. Moreover, the procedure causes diabetes which may be difficult to control, with a high risk of hypoglycaemia (since both insulin and glucagon release are absent), and is a cause of significant morbidity and mortality.

Steatorrhoea

This is treated by oral fat restriction (with supplementary medium-chain triglyceride therapy in malnourished patients) and oral pancreatic enzyme supplements. A proton pump inhibitor is added to optimise duodenal pH for pancreatic enzyme activity.

Diabetes

Diabetes requires carbohydrate restriction and insulin therapy.

Management of complications

Surgical or endoscopic therapy may be necessary for the management of pseudocysts, pancreatic ascites, common bile duct or duodenal stricture and the consequences of portal hypertension. Many patients also require treatment for other alcohol- and smoking-related diseases and for the consequences of self-neglect and malnutrition.

CONGENITAL ABNORMALITIES OF THE PANCREAS

PANCREAS DIVISUM

This is due to failure of the primitive dorsal and ventral ducts to fuse during embryonic development of the pancreas. As a consequence, most of the pancreatic drainage occurs through the smaller accessory ampulla rather than through the major ampulla.

Pancreas divisum occurs in 7–10% of the normal population and is usually asymptomatic. Some patients develop acute pancreatitis, chronic pancreatitis or atypical abdominal pain, possibly because drainage through the accessory papilla is restricted.

ANNULAR PANCREAS

In this congenital anomaly, the pancreas encircles the second/third part of the duodenum, leading to gastric outlet obstruction. Annular pancreas is associated with malrotation of the intestine, with atresias and with cardiac anomalies.

CYSTIC FIBROSIS

This disease is considered in detail on page 337. The gastrointestinal manifestations of cystic fibrosis are pancreatic insufficiency and meconium ileus. Peptic ulcer, and hepatic and biliary disease also occur.

Pancreatic secretions are protein- and mucus-rich. The resultant viscous juice forms plugs which obstruct the pancreatic ductules, leading to progressive destruction of acinar cells. Steatorrhoea is universal and the large-volume bulky stools predispose to rectal prolapse. Malnutrition is compounded by the metabolic demands of respiratory failure and by diabetes which develops in 40% of patients by adolescence.

The majority of patients survive well into adulthood and heart/lung transplantation can further prolong life. Optimal treatment of the cystic fibrosis patient depends upon an assiduous team approach to respiratory, nutritional and hepatobiliary complications. Nutritional counselling and supervision are important to ensure intake of high-energy foods, providing 120–150% of the recommended intake for normal subjects. Fats are an important calorie source and, despite the presence of steatorrhoea, fat intake should not be restricted. Supplementary fat-soluble vitamins are also necessary.

High-dose oral pancreatic enzymes are necessary, in doses sufficient to control steatorrhoea and stool frequency. A proton pump inhibitor aids fat digestion by producing an optimal duodenal pH. Diabetic patients usually require insulin injections rather than oral hypoglycaemic agents.

Meconium ileus

Mucus-rich plugs within intestinal contents can obstruct the small or large intestine. Meconium ileus is treated by the mucolytic agent N-acetylcysteine given orally, by Gastrografin enema or by gut lavage using polyethylene glycol. In resistant cases of meconium ileus surgical resection may be necessary.

TUMOURS OF THE PANCREAS

Pancreatic carcinoma affects 10–15 per 100 000 in Western populations, rising to 100 per 100 000 in those over the age of 70. Men are affected twice as often as women. The disease is associated with smoking and chronic pancreatitis.

Pathology

Approximately 90% of pancreatic neoplasms are adenocarcinomas which arise from the pancreatic ducts. These tumours involve local structures and metastasise to regional lymph nodes at an early stage. The majority of patients have advanced disease at the time of presentation.

Ampullary or periampullary adenocarcinomas are rare neoplasms which arise from the ampulla of Vater or adjacent duodenum. These tumours are often polypoid and ulcerated; they infiltrate the duodenum but behave less aggressively than pancreatic adenocarcinoma.

Cystadenocarcinoma is a very rare, slowly growing tumour, usually arising from the head of the pancreas and characterised by mucinous cyst formation. It occurs most often in middle-aged women.

Clinical features

The clinical features of pancreatic cancer are pain, weight loss and obstructive jaundice. The pain results from invasion of the coeliac plexus and is characteristically incessant and boring. It often radiates from the upper abdomen through to the back and may be eased a little by bending forwards. Almost all patients lose weight and many are cachectic. Weight loss is the consequence of anorexia, steatorrhoea and metabolic effects of the tumour. Around 60% of tumours arise from the head of the pancreas, and involvement of the common bile duct results in the development of obstructive jaundice, often with severe pruritus.

A few patients present with diarrhoea, vomiting from duodenal obstruction, diabetes mellitus, recurrent venous thrombosis, acute pancreatitis or depression.

Physical examination reveals clear evidence of weight loss. An abdominal mass due to the tumour itself, a palpable gallbladder or hepatic metastasis is commonly found. A palpable gallbladder in a jaundiced patient is usually the consequence of distal biliary obstruction by a pancreatic cancer (Courvoisier's sign).

Investigations

When a patient presents with biochemically confirmed cholestatic jaundice the diagnosis is usually made by ultrasound and CT scans (see Fig. 9.39). Diagnosis in non-jaundiced patients is often delayed because presenting symptoms are relatively non-specific.

Fit patients with small localised tumours should undergo staging to define operability. Laparoscopy with laparoscopic ultrasound will define tumour size, involvement of blood vessels and metastatic spread. In patients unsuitable for surgery because of advanced disease, frailty or comorbid disease, ultrasound or CT-guided cytology or biopsy may be used to confirm the diagnosis.

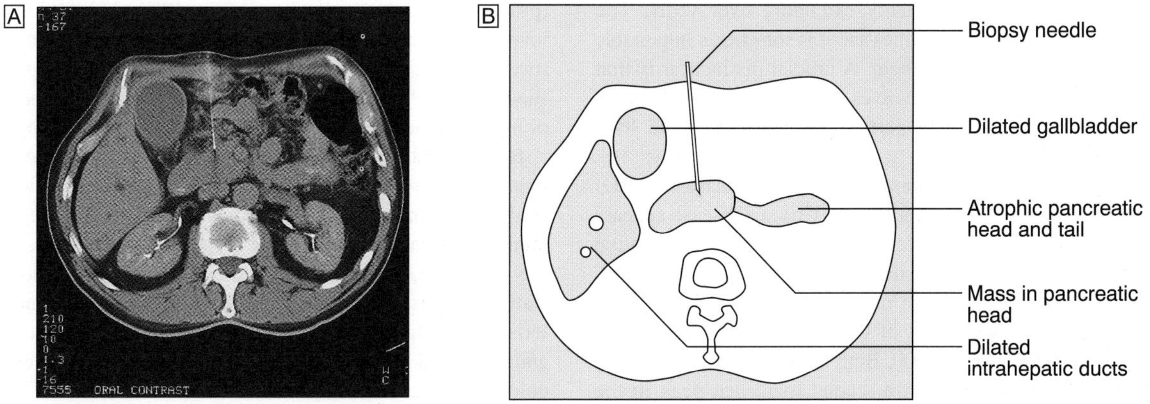

Fig. 9.39 Carcinoma of the pancreatic head. A CT scan obtained during biopsy of mass in pancreatic head. B Line diagram illustrating major structures.

ERCP is a sensitive method of diagnosing pancreatic cancer and is valuable when the diagnosis is in doubt, although differentiation between cancer and localised chronic pancreatitis can be difficult. The main role of ERCP is to insert a stent into the common bile duct to relieve obstructive jaundice.

Management

Surgical resection is the only method of effecting cure; adjuvant chemotherapy or radiotherapy confers no clear additional benefits. Unfortunately, a mere 15% of tumours are amenable to curative resection since most neoplasms are locally advanced at the time of diagnosis.

For the vast majority of patients therapy is based on palliation of pain and obstructive jaundice. Pain relief is achieved using analgesic drugs and, in some patients, coeliac plexus block by a percutaneous phenol injection. Jaundice is relieved by choledochojejunostomy in fit patients; percutaneous or endoscopic stenting may be useful in the elderly or in patients who have very advanced disease.

A total of 25% of patients undergoing resection of ampullary or periampullary tumours survive for 5 years and this contrasts with negligible survival in patients who present with pancreatic ductal cancer.

ENDOCRINE TUMOURS

These arise from neuro-endocrine tissue within the pancreas. They may occur in association with parathyroid and pituitary adenomas (MEN I, see p. 598). The majority of endocrine tumours are non-secretory and, although malignant, grow slowly and metastasise late. Other tumours secrete hormones and present because of their endocrine effects (see Table 9.19). Neuro-endocrine pancreatic tumours may be single, but are frequently multifocal and arise from other clusters of neuro-endocrine cells derived from neural crest tissues. They are localised by CT scanning, angiography and by estimation of hormone concentrations in blood derived from draining veins.

Table 9.19 Endocrine pancreatic tumours

Tumour	Hormone	Effects
Gastrinoma	Gastrin	Peptic ulcer and steatorrhoea
Insulinoma	Insulin	Recurrent hypoglycaemia
VIPoma	VIP	Watery diarrhoea and hypokalaemia
Glucagonoma	Glucagon	Diabetes mellitus, necrolytic migratory erythema
Somatostatinoma	Somatostatin	Diabetes mellitus and steatorrhoea

FURTHER INFORMATION ON DISEASES OF THE PANCREAS

Evans J D, Wilson P G, Carver C et al 1997 Outcome of surgery for chronic pancreatitis. British Journal of Surgery 84: 624–629
Heath D I, Imrie C W 1991 The diagnosis and assessment of severity in acute pancreatitis. In: Johnson C D, Imrie C W (eds) Pancreatic disease: progress and prospects. Springer-Verlag, Berlin
Rode J 1990 The pathology of pancreatic cancer. Baillière's Clinical Gastroenterology 4: 793–814

INFLAMMATORY BOWEL DISEASE

Ulcerative colitis and Crohn's disease are chronic inflammatory bowel diseases which pursue a protracted relapsing and remitting course, usually extending over years. The diseases have many similarities and it is sometimes impossible to differentiate between them. A crucial distinction is that ulcerative colitis only involves the colon, while Crohn's disease can involve any part of the gastrointestinal tract from mouth to anus.

The incidence of inflammatory bowel disease (IBD) varies widely between populations; Crohn's disease appears to be very rare in the underdeveloped world yet ulcerative colitis, although still unusual, is becoming more common. In the West, the incidence of ulcerative colitis is stable at 10 per 100 000 while that of Crohn's disease is increasing and is now 5–7 per 100 000. Both diseases most commonly start in young adults with a second incidence peak in the seventh decade.

Pathogenesis

Both genetic and environmental factors are implicated (see the information box). The cellular events involved in the pathogenesis of Crohn's disease and ulcerative colitis involve activation of macrophages, lymphocytes and polymorphonuclear cells with release of inflammatory mediators, and these events represent targets for future therapeutic intervention (see Fig. 9.40).

FACTORS ASSOCIATED WITH THE DEVELOPMENT OF INFLAMMATORY BOWEL DISEASE

Genetic

- More common in Jewish people
- 10% have a first-degree relative or at least one close relative with inflammatory bowel disease
- High concordance between identical twins
- Associated with autoimmune thyroiditis and SLE
- Ulcerative colitis—HLA genes are important
- Crohn's—non-HLA genes may be important
- Ulcerative colitis and Crohn's patients with HLA-B27 commonly develop ankylosing spondylitis

Environmental

- Associated with low-residue, high refined sugar diet
- Ulcerative colitis—commoner in non-smokers and ex-smokers
- Crohn's—most patients are smokers
- Possible associations with measles virus and atypical mycobacterial infection

Pathology

In both diseases the intestinal wall is infiltrated with acute and chronic inflammatory cells. There are important differences in the distribution of disease and in histological features (see Fig. 9.41 on p. 662).

Ulcerative colitis

Inflammation invariably involves the rectum (proctitis). It may spread proximally to involve the sigmoid colon (proctosigmoiditis) and in a minority the whole colon is involved (pancolitis). Inflammation is confluent and is more severe distally. In long-standing pancolitis the bowel becomes shortened and 'pseudopolyps' develop; these represent normal or hypertrophied residual mucosa within areas of atrophy.

Histologically, the inflammatory process is limited to the mucosa and spares the deeper layers of the bowel wall. Both acute and chronic inflammatory cells infiltrate the lamina propria and the crypts ('cryptitis'). Crypt abscesses are typical. Goblet cells lose their mucus and in long-standing cases glands become distorted. Dysplasia, characterised by heaping of cells within the crypts, nuclear atypia and increased mitotic rate, may herald the development of colon cancer.

Crohn's disease

The sites most commonly involved, in order of frequency, are terminal ileum and right side of colon, colon alone, terminal ileum alone, ileum and jejunum. Characteristically, the entire wall of the bowel is oedematous and thickened. There are deep ulcers which often appear as linear fissures; thus the mucosa between them is described as 'cobblestone'. Deep ulcers may penetrate through the bowel wall to initiate abscesses or fistulae. Fistulae may develop between adjacent loops of bowel or between affected segments of bowel and the bladder, uterus or vagina and may appear in the perineum.

Characteristically, the changes are patchy. Even when a relatively short segment of bowel is affected, the inflammatory process is interrupted by islands of normal mucosa and the change from the affected part is abrupt. A small lesion separated in this way from a major area of involvement is referred to as a 'skip' lesion. The mesenteric lymph nodes are enlarged and the mesentery thickened.

Histologically, chronic inflammation is seen through all the layers of the bowel wall, which is thickened as a result. There are focal aggregates of epithelioid histiocytes, which may be surrounded by lymphocytes and contain giant cells. Lymphoid aggregates or microgranulomas are also seen, and when these are near to the surface of the mucosa they often ulcerate to form tiny aphthous-like ulcers.

Clinical features

Ulcerative colitis

The first attack is usually the most severe and thereafter the disease is followed by relapses and remissions. Only a minority of patients have chronic, unremitting symptoms. Emotional stress, intercurrent infection, gastroenteritis, antibiotics or NSAID therapy may provoke a relapse. The clinical features depend upon the site and activity of the disease.

Proctitis causes rectal bleeding and mucus discharge, sometimes accompanied by tenesmus. Some patients pass frequent, small-volume fluid stools, while others are

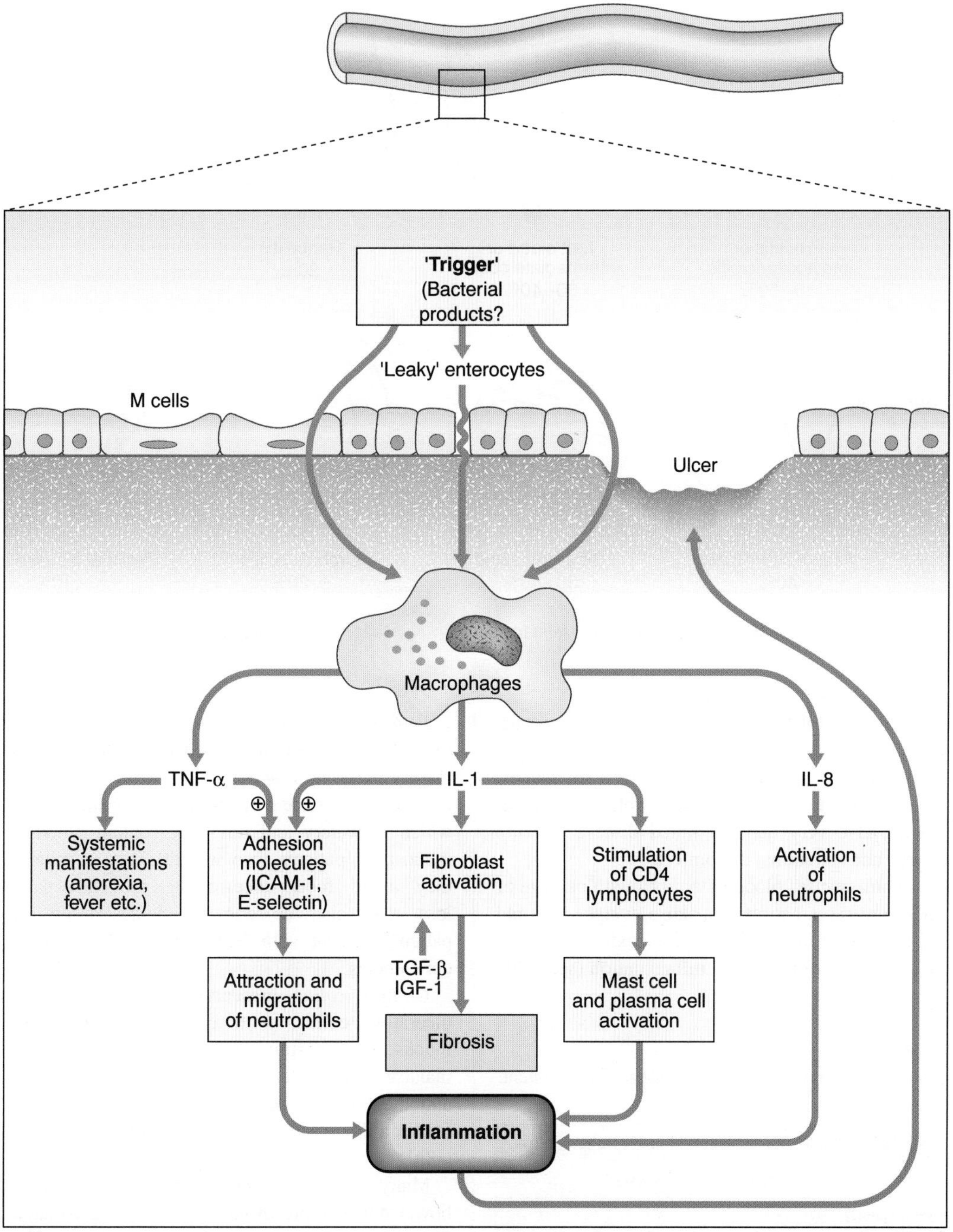

Fig. 9.40 Pathogenesis of inflammatory bowel disease. Dietary or bacterial antigens are either taken up by specialised M cells, pass between leaky epithelial cells in genetically predisposed individuals, or enter the lamina propria through ulcerated mucosa. Macrophages within Peyer's patches process the antigen and then secrete a series of cytokines. **Tumour necrosis factor alpha (TNF-α)** upregulates adhesion molecules (E-selectin and ICAM-1). These are localised on the vascular endothelium and cause circulating neutrophils to adhere to the endothelium and then pass through into the bowel wall. TNF-α is also largely responsible for the anorexia, malaise, fever and metabolic bone disease which characterise inflammatory bowel disease. **Interleukin-1 (IL-1)** also upregulates adhesion molecules, thereby aiding neutrophil recruitment. In addition, IL-1 activates CD4 lymphocytes. These in turn secrete interleukins 3 and 4, which activate mast cells and plasma cells. Mast cells secrete molecules (platelet activating factor and leucotrienes), which are necessary for inflammation; plasma cells secrete IgG and IgE. IL-1 stimulates other CD4 cells to secrete gamma interferon (IFN-γ) and this results in expression of HLA-DR antigens on the intestinal mucosa. Lastly, in Crohn's disease, but not ulcerative colitis, IL-1, TGF-β and IGF-1 (secreted from various sources) activate fibroblasts, thereby stimulating collagen metabolism, fibrosis and stricture formation. **Interleukin-8 (IL-8)** attracts, activates and degranulates neutrophils. Toxic proteases and reactive oxygen species are released; these are cytotoxic and cause ulceration.

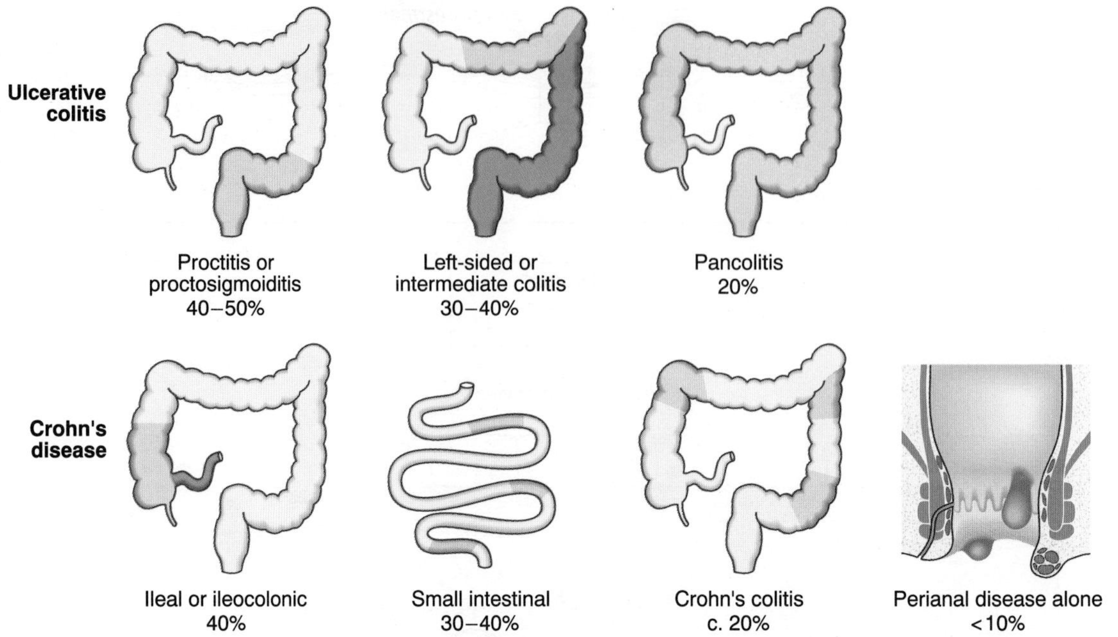

Fig. 9.41 Common patterns of disease distribution in inflammatory bowel disease. Overlap of distribution is common in Crohn's disease.

constipated and pass pellety stools. Constitutional symptoms do not occur.

Proctosigmoiditis causes bloody diarrhoea with mucus. Almost all patients are constitutionally well but a small minority who have very active, limited disease develop fever, lethargy and abdominal discomfort.

Extensive colitis causes bloody diarrhoea with passage of mucus. In severe cases anorexia, malaise, weight loss and abdominal pain occur, and the patient is toxic with fever, tachycardia and signs of peritoneal inflammation (see Table 9.20).

Crohn's disease

Presentation depends on the major site of disease involvement.

Table 9.20 Disease severity assessment in ulcerative colitis

	Mild	Severe
Daily bowel frequency	< 4	> 6
Blood in stools	+/–	+++
Stool volume (g/24 hours)	< 200	> 400
Pulse (bpm)	< 90	> 90
Temperature (°C)	Normal	> 37.5, 2 days out of 4
Sigmoidoscopy	Normal or granular mucosa	Blood in lumen
Abdominal radiograph	Normal	Dilated bowel and/or mucosal islands
Haemoglobin (g/L)	Normal	< 100
ESR (mm/hr)	< 30	> 30
Serum albumin (g/L)	> 35	< 30

Ileal disease causes abdominal pain, principally due to subacute intestinal obstruction, although an inflammatory mass, intra-abdominal abscess or acute obstruction may be responsible. Pain is often associated with diarrhoea which is watery and does not contain blood or mucus. Almost all patients lose weight. This is usually because they avoid food since eating provokes pain. Weight loss may also be due to malabsorption, and some patients present with features of fat, protein or vitamin deficiencies.

Crohn's colitis presents in an identical manner to ulcerative colitis, with bloody diarrhoea, passage of mucus and constitutional symptoms including lethargy, malaise, anorexia and weight loss. Rectal sparing and the presence of perianal disease are features which favour a diagnosis of Crohn's disease rather than ulcerative colitis.

Many patients present with symptoms of both small bowel and colonic disease. A few have isolated perianal disease, vomiting from jejunal strictures or severe oral ulceration.

Physical examination often reveals evidence of weight loss, anaemia with glossitis and angular stomatitis. There is abdominal tenderness, most marked over the inflamed area. An abdominal mass due to matted loops of thickened bowel or an intra-abdominal abscess may occur. Perianal skin tags, fissures or fistulae are found in at least 50% of patients.

Complications

Intestinal

- *Severe, life-threatening inflammation of the colon.* This occurs in both ulcerative colitis and Crohn's disease. In the most extreme cases the colon dilates (toxic megacolon) and bacterial toxins pass freely across the diseased mucosa into the portal, then systemic circulation. This complication occurs most commonly during the first attack of colitis and is recognised by the features described in Table 9.20. An abdominal radiograph should be taken daily because when the transverse colon is dilated to more than 6 cm (see Fig. 9.46, p. 666) there is a high risk of colonic perforation and subsequent generalised peritonitis and death.
- *Perforation of the small intestine or colon.* This can occur without the development of toxic megacolon.
- *Life-threatening acute haemorrhage.* Haemorrhage due to erosion of a major artery is a rare complication of both conditions.
- *Fistula and perianal disease.* Fistulous connections between loops of affected bowel, or between bowel and bladder or vagina are specific complications of Crohn's disease and do not occur in ulcerative colitis. Entero-enteric fistulae cause diarrhoea and malabsorption due to blind loop syndrome. Enterovesical fistulation causes recurrent urinary infections and pneumaturia. An enterovaginal fistula causes a feculent vaginal discharge. Fistulation from the bowel may also cause perianal or ischiorectal abscesses, fissures and fistulae. These may sometimes be extremely severe and can be the source of great morbidity.
- *Cancer.* Patients with extensive active colitis of more than 8 years' duration are at increased risk of colon cancer. The cumulative risk for ulcerative colitis may be as high as 20% after 30 years but is probably less for Crohn's colitis. Tumours develop in areas of dysplasia and may be multiple. Small bowel adenocarcinoma is a rare complication of long-standing small bowel Crohn's disease.

Patients with long-standing, extensive colitis are therefore entered into surveillance colonoscopy programmes beginning 8–10 years after diagnosis. Multiple random biopsies are taken every 10 cm throughout the colon and additional biopsies are taken from raised or ulcerated areas. Dysplastic changes are graded by histopathologists as mild, moderate or severe. Assessment of biopsies is subjective and the presence of active inflammation makes analysis of dysplasia very difficult. Patients who have no evidence of dysplasia or only mild dysplasia are screened biannually while those with moderate dysplasia undergo more frequent colonoscopy. Patients with severe dysplasia should be considered for panproctocolectomy because of the high risk of colon cancer development.

Extraintestinal

Inflammatory bowel disease can be considered as a systemic illness and in some patients extraintestinal complications dominate the clinical picture. Some of these occur during relapse of intestinal disease; others appear unrelated to intestinal disease activity (see the information box).

SYSTEMIC COMPLICATIONS OF INFLAMMATORY BOWEL DISEASE
Seronegative arthritis
• Acute arthritis affecting medium-sized joints* • Sacroiliitis • Ankylosing spondylitis (HLA-B27)
Dermatological
• Erythema nodosum* • Pyoderma gangrenosum* • Oral aphthous ulcers*
Ocular
• Conjunctivitis* • Iritis* • Episcleritis*
Hepatic and biliary
• Primary sclerosing cholangitis (ulcerative colitis only) • Gallstones • Autoimmune hepatitis • Fatty liver • Portal pyaemia and liver abscess* • Amyloidosis • Cholangiocarcinoma
Renal
• Oxalate calculi (small bowel Crohn's) • Amyloidosis • Ureteric obstruction (Crohn's)
Vascular
• Deep vein thrombosis* • Portal or mesenteric vein thrombosis*
* Tend to occur during acute relapse of bowel disease.

Differential diagnosis (see the information boxes)

Ulcerative colitis

The major diagnostic difficulty is to distinguish the first attack of acute colitis from infection. In general, diarrhoea lasting longer than 10 days in Western countries is unlikely to be the result of infection. A history of foreign travel, antibiotic exposure (pseudomembranous colitis) or homosexual contact suggest infection. Stool microscopy, culture and examination for *Clostridium difficile* toxin plus biopsies of rectum for ova and cysts, blood cultures and serological tests for infection are useful.

CONDITIONS WHICH CAN MIMIC ULCERATIVE OR CROHN'S COLITIS

Infective	Non-infective
Bacterial • *Salmonella* • *Shigella* • *Campylobacter jejuni* • Enteropathic *E. coli* • Gonococcal proctitis • Pseudomembranous colitis	**Vascular** • Ischaemic colitis • Radiation proctitis **Idiopathic** • Collagenous colitis • Behçet's disease
Viral • Herpes simplex proctitis • *Chlamydia* proctitis	**Drugs** • NSAIDs **Neoplastic** • Colonic carcinoma
Protozoal • Amoebiasis	**Other** • Diverticulitis

Small bowel Crohn's disease

Crohn's disease can usually be diagnosed with confidence without histological confirmation in the appropriate clinical setting. In atypical cases biopsy or surgical resection are necessary to exclude other diseases (see the information box). This can often be done endoscopically by ileal intubation at colonoscopy, but sometimes laparotomy or laparoscopy with resection or full-thickness biopsy is necessary.

DIFFERENTIAL DIAGNOSIS OF SMALL BOWEL CROHN'S DISEASE

- Other causes of right iliac fossa mass
  - Caecal carcinoma*
  - Appendix abscess*
  - Infection (tuberculosis, *Yersinia*, actinomycosis)
- Mesenteric adenitis
- Pelvic inflammatory disease
- Lymphoma

* Common; other causes are rare.

Investigations

These confirm the diagnosis, define disease distribution and activity, and identify specific complications.

Blood tests

Anaemia results from bleeding or malabsorption of iron, folic acid or vitamin B_{12}. Serum albumin concentration falls as a consequence of protein-losing enteropathy, reflecting active and extensive disease, or because of poor nutrition. The ESR is raised in exacerbations or because of abscess. Elevation of C-reactive protein and orosomucoid concentrations is helpful in monitoring Crohn's disease activity.

Bacteriology

Stool cultures are performed to exclude superimposed enteric infection in patients who present with exacerbations of inflammatory bowel disease. Blood cultures are also advisable in patients with known colitis or Crohn's disease who develop fever.

Endoscopy

Sigmoidoscopy with biopsies is a simple and essential investigation in all patients who present with diarrhoea (see Fig. 9.42). Rectal sparing, perianal disease and discrete ulcers suggest Crohn's disease rather than ulcerative colitis.

Colonoscopy may show active inflammation with pseudopolyps or a complicating carcinoma. Biopsies are taken to define disease extent, as this is underestimated by endoscopic appearances alone, and to seek dysplasia in patients with long-standing colitis. In ulcerative colitis the macroscopic and histological abnormalities are confluent and most severe in the distal colon and rectum. Stricture formation does not occur in the absence of a carcinoma. In Crohn's colitis the endoscopic abnormalities are patchy, with normal mucosa between the areas of abnormality. Aphthoid or deeper ulcers and strictures are common.

Barium studies

Barium enema is a less sensitive investigation than colonoscopy for the investigation of colitis. In long-standing ulcerative colitis the colon is shortened and loses haustra to become tubular, and pseudopolyps are seen (see Fig. 9.43). In Crohn's colitis a range of abnormalities occur.

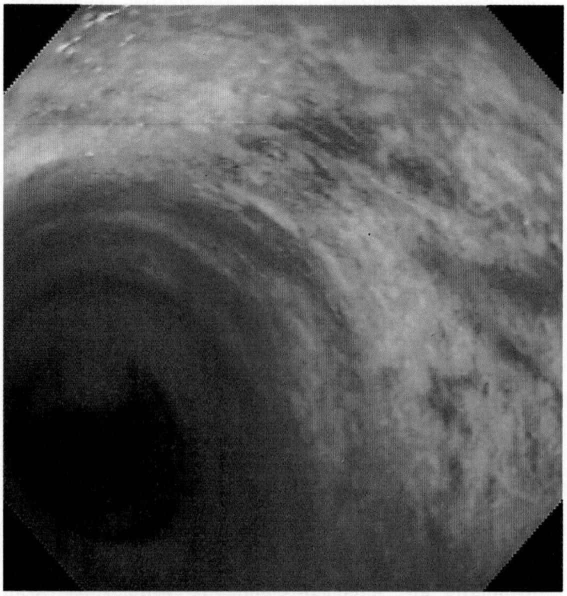

Fig. 9.42 Sigmoidoscopic view of moderately active ulcerative colitis. Mucosa is erythematous and friable (with contact bleeding). Submucosal blood vessels are no longer visible.

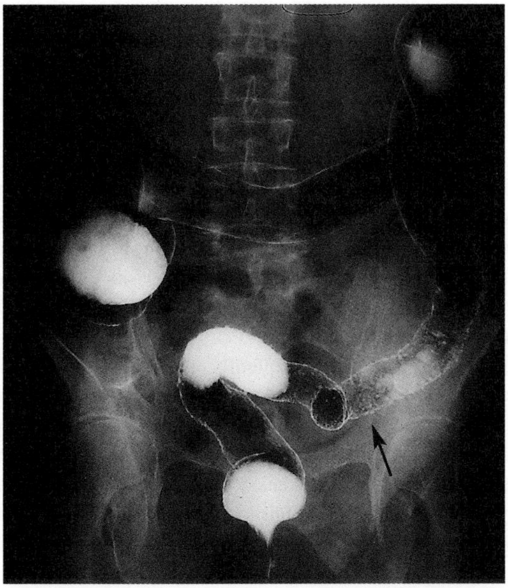

Fig. 9.43 Barium enema showing shortened colon, loss of haustra, pseudopolyps and fine ulceration (arrow).

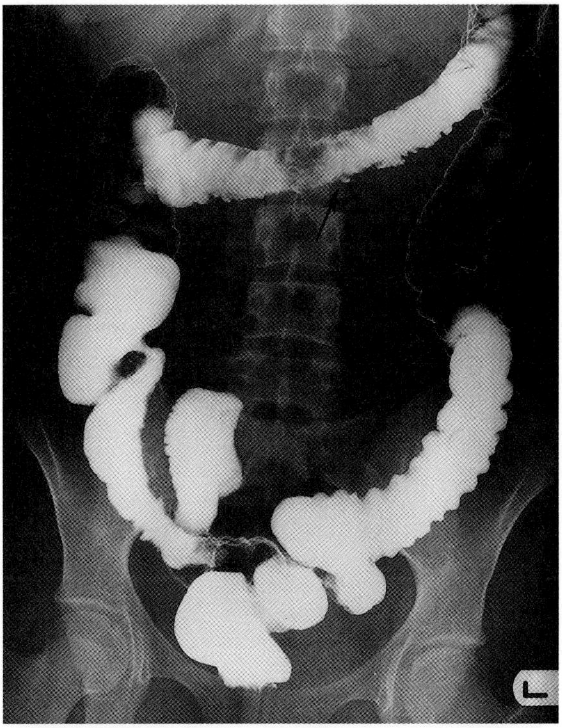

Fig. 9.44 Ileocolonic Crohn's disease. Barium enema showing normal rectum and sigmoid colon, typical aphthous ulceration in the descending colon, ulceration (arrow) and lack of haustra in the transverse colon. The ascending colon and caecum are normal and there is typical Crohn's disease affecting the terminal ileum, with coarse ulceration, rigidity and lack of mucosal folds.

The appearances may be identical to those of ulcerative colitis but skip lesions, strictures and deeper ulcers are characteristic (see Fig. 9.44). Reflux into the terminal ileum may show stricture and ulcers.

Contrast studies of the small bowel are normal in ulcerative colitis, but in Crohn's disease affected areas are narrowed and ulcerated; multiple strictures are common (see Fig. 9.45).

Plain radiographs

A straight abdominal radiograph is essential in the management of patients who present with severe active disease. In colitis dilatation of the colon (see Fig. 9.46), mucosal oedema ('thumb-printing') or evidence of perforation may be found. In small bowel Crohn's disease there may be evidence of

A B
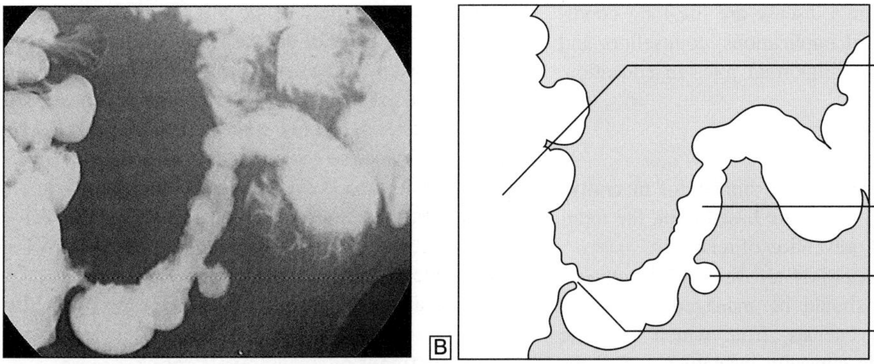

Fig. 9.45 Barium follow-through showing terminal ileal Crohn's disease. A Radiograph. B Line drawing to illustrate major structures.

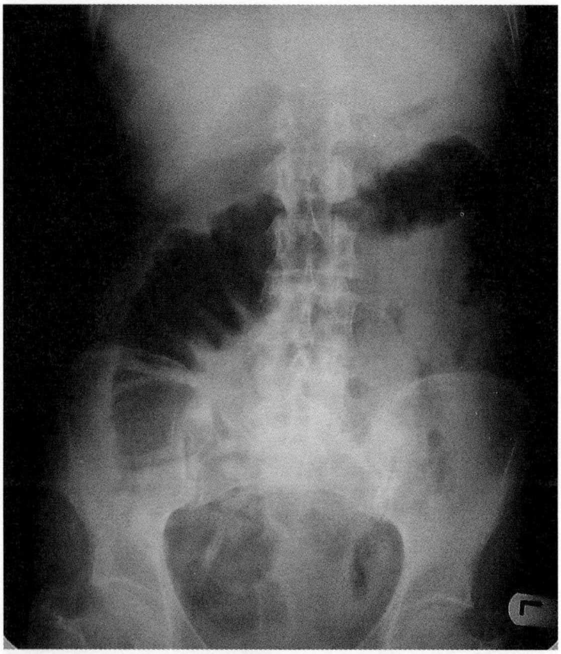

Fig. 9.46 Plain abdominal radiograph showing a grossly dilated colon due to severe ulcerative colitis.

intestinal obstruction or displacement of bowel loops by a mass.

Radionuclide scans

Radio-labelled white cell scans show areas of active inflammation. This is less sensitive than other imaging modalities but is useful in severely ill patients in whom invasive tests are best avoided.

Management

Best treatment depends upon a team approach involving physicians, surgeons, radiologists and dietitians. Both ulcerative colitis and Crohn's disease are life-long conditions and have psychosocial implications; counsellors and patient support groups have important roles in education, reassurance and coping.

Drug treatment of colitis

The principles of drug treatment are similar for ulcerative colitis and Crohn's colitis. These are based upon the treatment of active disease and prevention of relapse.

Active colitis. Corticosteroids are first-line treatment. Active proctosigmoiditis should be managed by steroid foam or liquid retention enemas, from which systemic corticosteroid absorption is clinically insignificant. Patients with very active proctosigmoiditis, those who are unable to retain enemas, and patients who have active, extensive colitis need oral corticosteroids. Prednisolone (30–40 mg/day orally) is given for 2 weeks and then reduced slowly over 8 weeks. Severe active colitis can be treated with intravenous methylprednisolone (60 mg daily by infusion). Once improvement occurs, the patient is converted to a reducing regimen of oral prednisolone.

Systemic steroid complications, such as mood changes, acne, weight gain and dyspepsia, are common but these resolve as the dose is reduced. Long-term, high-dose therapy must be avoided because of risks of the more severe steroid complications such as metabolic bone disease and infection.

Patients who relapse frequently after courses of steroids or who require maintenance steroid therapy may be considered for azathioprine treatment (1.5–2 mg per kg body weight daily). This immunosuppressant drug exerts its maximal effect only after 6–12 weeks, and corticosteroid therapy may have to be continued until this time. Treatment is sometimes complicated by bone marrow suppression, nausea, vomiting, myalgia and acute pancreatitis.

Antidiarrhoeal agents (codeine phosphate, loperamide or diphenoxylate) are sometimes useful but should be avoided in severe active disease.

Maintenance of remission. This is based upon the use of aminosalicylates (5-ASA). Sulphasalazine is a dimer comprising 5-aminosalicylic acid bound by an azo bond to sulphapyridine. The parent molecule is poorly absorbed by the small intestine but colonic bacteria break the azo bond to release 5-ASA which enters the colonic mucosa where it exerts its anti-inflammatory effects. Sulphapyridine has no anti-inflammatory activity but ensures 5-ASA delivery to the colon. Sulphasalazine (2–3 g daily in divided doses) has beneficial effects in mildly active colitis but its main role is to prevent relapse. The drug has no proven benefit in small bowel disease. Side-effects occur in 20% of patients, half of whom are intolerant of the drug. The major side-effects are nausea and vomiting, headache, rashes, reversible azoospermia, haemolytic anaemia and agranulocytosis. These complications are dose-related and are due to the sulphapyridine moiety.

Alternative ways of delivering 5-ASA to the colon which avoid sulphapyridine complications have been developed. Mesalazine is an enteric-coated form in which 5-ASA is slowly released from a cellulose-based or pH-dependent coating. Olsalazine comprises two molecules of 5-ASA bound by an azo bond to optimise delivery to the colon. These newer aminosalicylates are as effective as sulphasalazine but have fewer side-effects. 5-ASA liquid or foam retention enemas are also available and are as effective as steroid enemas for treating active proctitis.

Drug treatment of small bowel Crohn's disease

Drug treatment for active disease is based upon the use of oral corticosteroids (prednisolone 30–40 mg daily), reducing over 6–8 weeks. Patients who respond yet frequently relapse after stopping steroids, or who are steroid-dependent, are usually treated with azathioprine (1.5–2 mg per kg body weight daily). Steroid side-effects can be overcome by using budesonide; this is a potent synthetic corticosteroid which reduces mucosal inflammation. (9 mg is equivalent to 30 mg of prednisolone.) Following absorption, the drug undergoes extensive first-pass metabolism in the liver; adrenocortical suppression is minimised and steroid side-effects are reduced.

Some patients respond inadequately to steroids and azathioprine and in these, other immunosuppressive drugs such as methotrexate or immunomodulatory agents such as cyclosporin or antibodies to tumour necrosis factor α (TNF-α) may have a role.

There is no evidence that drug therapy is useful in maintaining remission.

Nutritional therapy

Many patients embark upon 'elimination diets' in which specific foods are avoided. Although some colitic patients do improve on a milk-free diet and a few others respond to avoidance of wheat, the best advice for the majority of patients is to eat a well-balanced, healthy diet and to avoid only those foods which, by experience, are poorly tolerated. Exceptions include patients with small bowel strictures, who should avoid nuts, pulses, raw fruit and vegetables which may precipitate intestinal obstruction, and patients with a combination of proctitis and constipation who benefit from increased dietary fibre.

Many patients who have severe chronic inflammatory bowel disease are undernourished. They require dietary assessment and appropriate calorie, protein, vitamin and mineral supplements. This is particularly important in children.

Specific nutritional therapy can induce remission in active Crohn's disease but not ulcerative colitis. Elemental diets which contain simple sugars, triglycerides, amino acids, vitamins and trace elements, and polymeric diets which contain oligopeptides rather than amino acids, are both effective. Normal food is avoided for the 2–4 weeks of treatment. Possible modes of action include improved nutrition, exclusion of dietary antigens and avoidance of dietary fibre. Unfortunately, nutritional therapy is expensive, is often poorly tolerated, and is usually followed by disease relapse on return to a normal diet.

Surgical treatment

Ulcerative colitis. Up to 60% of patients with extensive ulcerative colitis eventually require surgery. The indications are listed in the information box. Impaired quality of life, with impact upon occupation and on social and family life, is the most important of these.

Surgery involves removal of the entire colon and rectum and cures the patient. Before surgery, patients must be counselled by doctors, stoma nurses and by patients who have undergone similar surgery. The choice of procedure is either panproctocolectomy with ileostomy or proctocolectomy with ileal-anal pouch anastomosis. Surgical textbooks should be consulted for further details.

INDICATIONS FOR SURGERY: ULCERATIVE COLITIS
Impaired quality of life
• Loss of occupation or education • Disruption of family life
Failure of medical therapy
• Dependence upon oral corticosteroids • Complications of drug therapy
Fulminant colitis
Disease complications, unresponsive to medical therapy
• Arthritis • Pyoderma gangrenosum
Colon cancer or severe dysplasia

Crohn's disease. The indications for surgery are similar to those for ulcerative colitis. Operations are often necessary to deal with fistulae, abscesses and perianal disease and may also be required to relieve small or large bowel obstruction.

Up to 80% of patients eventually need some form of surgical intervention, but unlike ulcerative colitis, surgery does not cure the patient and disease recurrence is the rule. Surgical intervention should therefore be as conservative as possible in order to minimise loss of viable intestine and to avoid creation of a short bowel syndrome.

Patients who have localised segments of Crohn's colitis may be managed by segmental resection. Others who have extensive colitis require total colectomy but ileal-anal pouch formation should be avoided because of the high risk of disease recurrence within the pouch and subsequent fistula, abscess formation and pouch failure.

Patients who have perianal Crohn's disease are managed as conservatively as possible by drainage of abscess and avoidance of resection or reconstructive procedures. Obstructing or fistulating small bowel disease may require resection of affected tissue. Patients who have multiple or recurrent strictures are considered for strictureplasty in which the stricture is not resected but instead incised in its longitudinal axis and sutured transversely.

Management of complications

Fulminant colitis. This is a life-threatening complication which demands intensive medical and surgical management. Patients should be monitored frequently for clinical signs of peritonitis, fever and tachycardia. Stool frequency and volumes are documented and abdominal radiographs are taken daily to seek evidence of toxic dilatation or perforation. The patient must also be counselled about the possibility of surgery.

If improvement has not occurred within 5–7 days, or if the patient deteriorates, urgent colectomy should be undertaken. The lower rectum can be left in situ for subsequent ileo-anal pouch reconstruction. Key steps in the management of fulminant ulcerative colitis are listed in the information box.

MANAGEMENT OF FULMINANT ULCERATIVE COLITIS

- Intravenous fluids
- Transfusion if Hb < 100 g/L
- I.v. methylprednisolone infusion (60 mg daily)
- Antibiotics for proven infection
- Nutritional support
- Subcutaneous heparin for prophylaxis of venous thromboembolism
- Avoidance of opiates and antidiarrhoeal agents

Perianal disease. The treatment of perianal disease, including fissure, fistula and abscess formation, is based upon a conservative approach. For many patients symptoms are few, even when the visible disease is apparently severe. In these the benefits of medical or surgical intervention are few and the relative risks of complications are high. Patients who have painful or discharging perineal disease are managed jointly by surgeons and physicians. Metronidazole or ciprofloxacin therapy may relieve pain and eliminate sepsis. Abscesses require drainage but radical procedures risk damage to the anal sphincters and faecal incontinence.

Inflammatory bowel disease in special circumstances

Childhood

Ulcerative colitis and Crohn's disease can develop before adolescence. Chronic ill health results in growth failure, metabolic bone disease and delayed puberty. Loss of schooling and social contact, as well as frequent hospitalisation, can have important psychosocial consequences. Treatment is similar to that described for adults and may require use of corticosteroids, immunosuppressive drugs and surgery. Monitoring of height, weight and sexual development is important.

Pregnancy

The activity of inflammatory bowel disease is not usually affected by pregnancy although relapse may be more common after parturition. Drug therapy including aminosalicylates, corticosteroids and azathioprine can be safely continued throughout the pregnancy.

Prognosis

Life expectancy in patients with inflammatory bowel disease is now similar to that of the general population. Although many patients require surgery and admission to hospital for other reasons, the majority have an excellent work record and pursue a normal life.

MICROSCOPIC COLITIS

Some patients experience watery diarrhoea as a consequence of microscopic *('lymphocytic')* colitis. The colonoscopic appearances are normal but histological examination of biopsies shows a range of abnormalities.

Collagenous colitis is characterised by the presence of a thick submucosal band of collagen; a chronic inflammatory infiltrate is usually seen. The disease is more common in women and is associated with rheumatoid arthritis, diabetes and coeliac disease. Patients have a history of intermittent watery diarrhoea and treatment is based upon the use of antidiarrhoeal drugs, aminosalicylates and topical steroid enemas.

FURTHER INFORMATION ON INFLAMMATORY BOWEL DISEASE

Elton E, Hanauer S B 1996 The medical management of Crohn's disease. Alimentary and Pharmacological Therapeutics 10: 1–22

Hyde G M, Jewell D P 1997 The management of severe ulcerative colitis. Alimentary and Pharmacological Therapeutics 11: 419–424

Pemberton J H, Kelly K A, Beart R W J 1987 Ileal pouch–anal anastomosis for chronic ulcerative colitis: long-term results. Annals of Surgery 206: 504–513

Shanahan F, Targan S 1994 Mechanisms of tissue injury in inflammatory bowel disease. In: Targan S, Shanahan F (eds) Inflammatory bowel disease: from bench to bedside. Williams & Wilkins, Baltimore

Travis S P L, Farrant J M, Ricketts C et al 1996 Predicting outcome in severe ulcerative colitis. Gut 38: 905–910

IRRITABLE BOWEL SYNDROME

Irritable bowel syndrome (IBS) is a functional bowel disorder in which abdominal pain is associated with defaecation or a change in bowel habit with features of disordered defaecation and distension.

Epidemiology

Approximately 20% of the general population fulfil diagnostic criteria for irritable bowel syndrome but only 10% of these consult their doctors because of gastrointestinal symptoms. Nevertheless, IBS is the most common cause of gastrointestinal referral and accounts for frequent absenteeism from work and impaired quality of life. Young, white women are most often affected. There is wide overlap with functional dyspepsia, chronic fatigue syndrome, dysmenorrhoea and urinary frequency. A significant proportion of these patients have a history of physical or sexual abuse.

Aetiology

Irritable bowel syndrome encompasses a wide range of symptoms and a single cause is unlikely. It is generally believed that most patients develop symptoms in response to psychosocial factors, altered gastrointestinal motility, altered visceral sensation or luminal factors.

Psychosocial factors

About 50% of patients meet criteria for a psychiatric diagnosis. A range of disturbances are identified, including anxiety, depression, somatisation and neurosis. Panic attacks are also common. Acute psychological stress and overt psychiatric disease are known to alter gastrointestinal motility in both irritable bowel patients and healthy people.

Altered gastrointestinal motility

A range of motility disorders are found but none is diagnostic. Patients with diarrhoea as a predominant symptom exhibit clusters of rapid jejunal contraction waves, rapid intestinal transit and an increased number of fast and propagated colonic contractions. Those who are predominantly constipated have decreased orocaecal transit and a reduced number of high-amplitude, propagated colonic contraction waves.

Abnormal visceral perception

Irritable bowel syndrome is associated with increased sensitivity to intestinal distension induced by inflation of balloons in the ileum, colon and rectum.

Luminal factors

Some patients develop irritable bowel syndrome following an episode of gastroenteritis, while others may be intolerant of specific dietary components, particularly dairy products and wheat.

Clinical features

The most common presentation is that of abdominal pain. This is usually colicky or 'cramping', is felt in the lower abdomen and is relieved by defaecation. Abdominal bloating worsens throughout the day; the cause is unknown but it is not due to excessive intestinal gas. The bowel habit is variable. Most patients alternate between episodes of diarrhoea and constipation but it is useful to classify patients as having predominantly constipation or predominantly diarrhoea. The constipated type tend to pass infrequent pellety stools, usually in association with abdominal pain or proctalgia. Those with diarrhoea have frequent defaecation but produce low-volume stools and rarely have nocturnal symptoms. Passage of mucus is common but rectal bleeding does not occur.

FEATURES OF IRRITABLE BOWEL SYNDROME

- Altered bowel habit
- Colicky abdominal pain
- Abdominal distension
- Rectal mucus
- Feeling of incomplete defaecation

Despite apparently severe symptoms, patients do not lose weight and are constitutionally well. Many have other 'functional' symptoms including dyspepsia, urinary frequency, headaches, backache and chronic fatigue syndrome. Physical examination does not reveal any abnormalities, although abdominal bloating and variable tenderness to palpation are common.

Diagnosis

Investigations are normal. A positive diagnosis can confidently be made in patients under the age of 40 years without resort to complicated tests. Full blood count, ESR and sigmoidoscopy are usually done routinely, but barium enema or colonoscopy should only be undertaken in older patients to exclude colorectal cancer. Those who present atypically require investigations to exclude organic gastrointestinal disease. Diarrhoea-predominant patients justify investigations to exclude microscopic colitis (see p. 668), lactose intolerance (see p. 651) and bile acid malabsorption (see p. 610). All patients who give a history of rectal bleeding should undergo colonoscopy or barium enema to exclude colonic cancer or inflammatory bowel disease.

Management

The most important step is reassurance. Many patients are concerned that they have developed cancer, and a cycle of anxiety leading to colonic symptoms, which further heighten anxiety, can be broken by explanation that symptoms are not due to organic disease but are the result of altered bowel motility and sensation. In patients who fail to respond to reassurance, treatment is tailored to the predominant symptoms (see Fig. 9.47).

Patients with intractable symptoms sometimes benefit from several months of therapy with amitriptyline. This is given in doses (10–25 mg at night) which are much lower than those used to treat depression. Side-effects include dry mouth and drowsiness but these are usually mild and the drug is well tolerated. It may act by reducing visceral sensation and by altering gastrointestinal motility. Hypnotherapy is reserved for the most difficult cases.

Most patients have a relapsing and a remitting course. Exacerbations often follow stressful life events, occupational dissatisfaction and difficulties with interpersonal relationships.

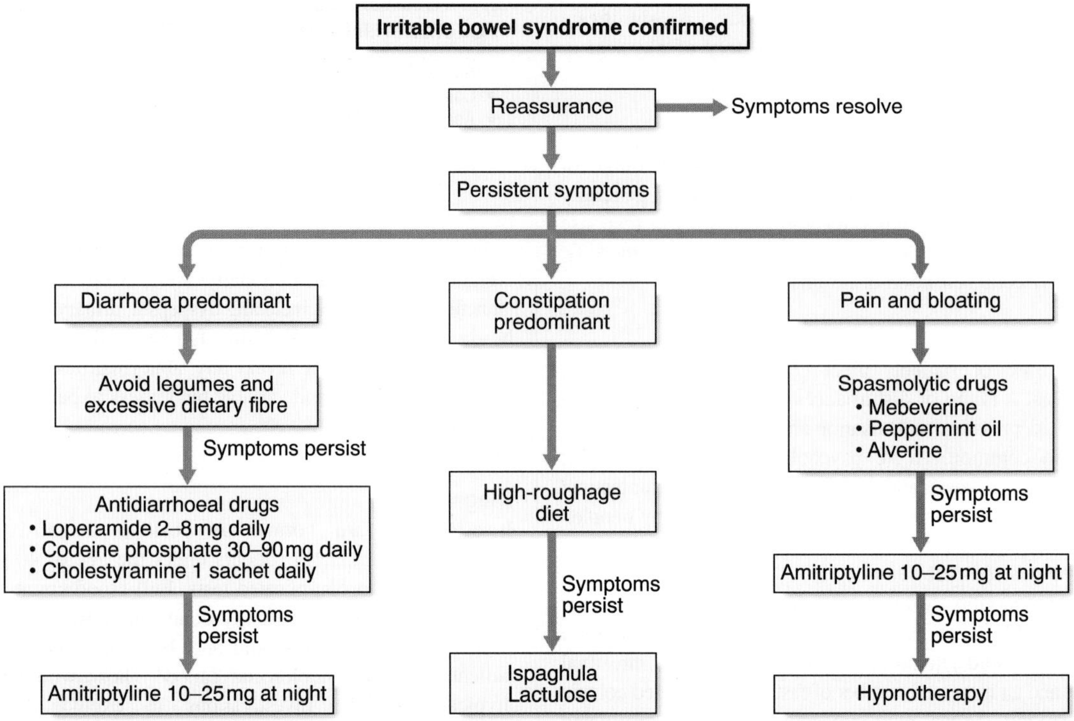

Fig. 9.47 Management of irritable bowel syndrome.

FURTHER INFORMATION ON IRRITABLE BOWEL SYNDROME

Camilleri M, Choi M-G 1997 Irritable bowel syndrome. Alimentary and Pharmacological Therapeutics 11: 3–15

AIDS AND THE GASTROINTESTINAL TRACT

See page 101.

ISCHAEMIC GUT INJURY (see Fig. 9.48)

This is usually the result of arterial occlusion. Severe hypotension and venous insufficiency are less frequent causes.

ACUTE SMALL BOWEL ISCHAEMIA

An embolus from the heart to the superior mesenteric artery is responsible for 40–50% of cases. Non-occlusive ischaemia following hypotension results from myocardial infarction, heart failure, arrhythmias or sudden blood loss. The pathological spectrum ranges from a transient alteration of bowel function to transmural haemorrhagic necrosis and gangrene.

Patients usually have evidence of cardiac disease and arrhythmia. Almost all develop abdominal pain and this is characteristically more impressive than the physical findings. In the early stages the only physical sign is abdominal distension, and signs of peritonitis develop at a late stage as a consequence of necrotic intestine.

Leucocytosis, metabolic acidosis, hyperphosphataemia and hyperamylasaemia are typical. Plain abdominal radiographs show 'thumb-printing' due to mucosal oedema. Mesenteric angiography reveals an occluded or narrowed major artery with spasm of arterial arcades, although most patients undergo laparotomy on the basis of a clinical diagnosis without undergoing angiography.

The key steps in treatment are resuscitation, correction of cardiac disease and intravenous antibiotic therapy, followed by laparotomy, at which embolectomy, thrombectomy and resection of non-viable bowel are carried out. A 'second look' laparotomy 24–48 hours later is sometimes undertaken to resect any further necrotic intestine. The results of therapy are dependent upon early intervention; patients treated at a late stage have a 75% mortality rate.

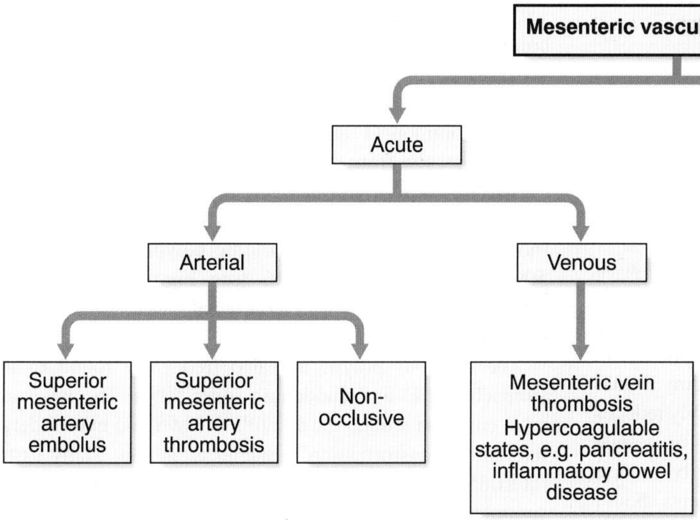

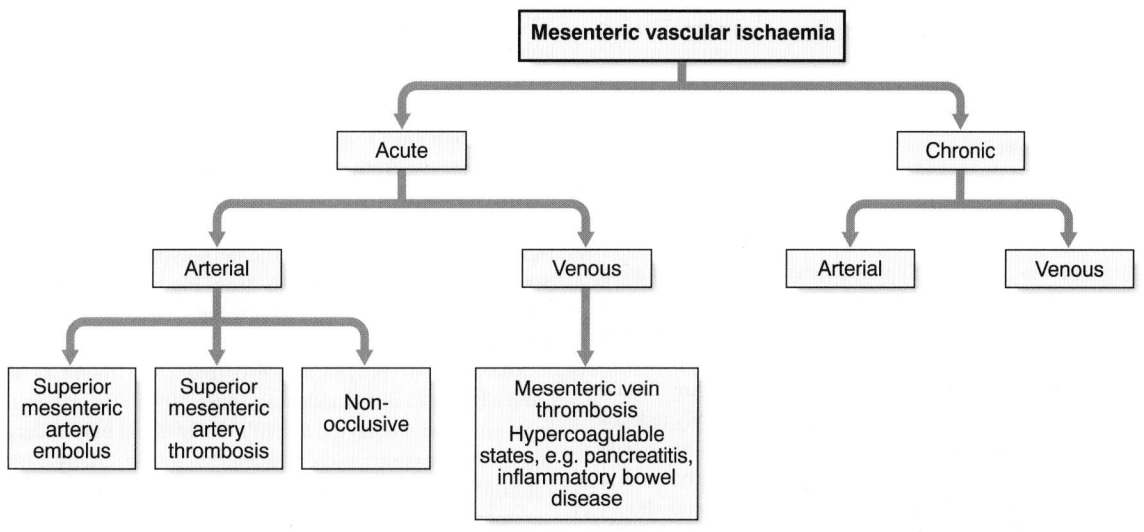

Fig. 9.48 Types of mesenteric vascular ischaemia.

ACUTE COLONIC ISCHAEMIA

The splenic flexure and descending colon have little collateral circulation and lie in 'watershed' areas of arterial supply. A spectrum of injury ranging from reversible colopathy, through transient colitis, colonic stricture, gangrene and fulminant pancolitis can occur. Arterial thromboembolism is usually responsible but colonic ischaemia can also occur following severe hypotension, colonic volvulus, strangulated hernia, systemic vasculitis or hypercoagulable states.

The patient is usually elderly and presents with sudden onset of cramping left-sided lower abdominal pain and rectal bleeding. In the majority of cases symptoms resolve spontaneously over 24–48 hours and healing occurs within 2 weeks. Some are left with a residual fibrous stricture or a segment of colitis. A minority develop gangrene and peritonitis. The diagnosis is established by colonoscopy or barium enema which should be performed within 48 hours of presentation because mucosal ulceration and oedema may have otherwise resolved.

CHRONIC MESENTERIC ISCHAEMIA

This results from atherosclerotic stenosis affecting at least two of the coeliac axis, superior mesenteric and inferior mesenteric arteries. The patient develops dull but severe mid- or upper abdominal pain approximately 30 minutes after eating. Patients lose weight because of reluctance to eat, and a proportion experience diarrhoea. Physical examination invariably shows evidence of generalised arterial disease. An abdominal bruit is sometimes audible but is a non-specific finding. Mesenteric angiography confirms at least two affected mesenteric arteries. Vascular reconstruction is sometimes possible. Left untreated, many patients eventually develop intestinal infarction.

DISORDERS OF THE COLON AND RECTUM

TUMOURS OF THE COLON AND RECTUM

SPORADIC POLYPS

Polyps may be neoplastic or non-neoplastic. The latter include hamartomas, metaplastic ('hyperplastic') polyps and inflammatory polyps. These have no malignant potential. Polyps may be single or multiple and vary from a few millimetres to several centimetres in size.

Colorectal adenomas are extremely common in the Western world and the prevalence rises with age; 50% of people over 60 years of age have adenomas, and in half of these the polyps are multiple. They are more common in the rectum and distal colon and are either pedunculated or sessile. Histologically, they are classified as either tubular, villous or tubulovillous, according to the glandular architecture.

Adenomas are usually asymptomatic and discovered incidentally. Occasionally, they cause bleeding and anaemia. Villous adenomas sometimes secrete large amounts of mucus, causing diarrhoea and hypokalaemia. The majority of cancers arise from adenomas ('adenoma-carcinoma sequence') over 5–10 years, although not all polyps carry the same degree of risk. Features associated with a higher risk of subsequent

RISK FACTORS FOR MALIGNANT CHANGE IN COLONIC POLYPS

- Large size (> 2 cm)
- Multiple polyps
- Villous architecture
- Dysplasia

malignancy in colonic polyps are listed in the information box.

Discovery of a polyp at sigmoidoscopy is an indication for colonoscopy because proximal polyps are present in 40–50% of such patients. Colonoscopic polypectomy should be carried out wherever possible, as this considerably reduces subsequent colorectal cancer risk. Very large or sessile polyps which cannot be removed endoscopically require surgery. Once all polyps have been removed, patients should undergo surveillance colonoscopy at 3–5-year intervals, as new polyps develop in 50% of patients. Patients over 75 years of age do not require repeated colonoscopies, as their lifetime cancer risk is low.

Between 10 and 20% of polyps show histological evidence of malignancy. When cancer cells are found within 2 mm of the resection margin of the polyp, when the polyp cancer is poorly differentiated or when lymphatic invasion is present, segmental colonic resection is recommended. Malignant polyps without these features can be followed up by surveillance colonoscopy.

POLYPOSIS SYNDROMES

Polyposis syndromes are classified by histopathology (see Table 9.21). It should be noted that, while the hamartomatous polyps in Peutz–Jeghers syndrome and juvenile polyposis are not themselves neoplastic, these disorders are associated with an increased risk of certain malignancies, e.g. breast, colon, ovary and thyroid.

Familial adenomatous polyposis (FAP)

This uncommon (1 in 8000–14 000) autosomal dominant disorder results from germ line mutation of the APC gene on the long arm of chromosome 5. One-third of cases arise as new mutations and have no family history. Hundreds to thousands of adenomatous colonic polyps will develop in 50% of patients by age 16 (see Fig. 9.49). Of those affected, 90% will develop colorectal cancer by the age of 45 years.

Adenomatous polyps are also frequently found in the stomach (50%) and duodenum (over 90%). The latter are most common around the ampulla of Vater and may undergo malignant transformation to adenocarcinoma. Many extra-intestinal features are also seen in FAP and these are summarised in the information box.

Desmoid tumours occur in 10% of patients and usually arise in the mesentery or abdominal wall. Although benign, they may become very large, may cause compression of adjacent organs and are difficult to remove. Congenital hypertrophy of the retinal pigment epithelium can be seen as dark, round, pigmented retinal lesions. When present in an at-risk individual they are 100% predictive of the presence of FAP.

EXTRAINTESTINAL FEATURES OF FAMILIAL ADENOMATOUS POLYPOSIS

- Subcutaneous epidermoid cysts (extremities, face, scalp)
- Lipomas
- Benign osteomas, especially skull and angle of mandible
- Desmoid tumours
- Dental abnormalities (15–20%)
- Congenital hypertrophy of the retinal pigment epithelium (CHRPE)

Table 9.21 Gastrointestinal polyposis syndromes

	Neoplastic	Non-neoplastic			
	Familial adenomatous polyposis	**Peutz–Jeghers syndrome**	**Juvenile polyposis**	**Cronkhite–Canada syndrome**	**Cowden's disease**
Inheritance	Autosomal dominant	Autosomal dominant	Autosomal dominant in 1/3	None	Autosomal dominant
Oesophageal polyps	–	–	–	+	+
Gastric polyps	+	++	+	+++	+++
Small bowel polyps	++	+++	++	++	++
Colonic polyps	+++	++	++	+++	+
Other features	See text	See text	See text	Hair loss, pigmentation, nail dystrophy, malabsorption	Many congenital anomalies, oral and cutaneous hamartomas, thyroid and breast tumours

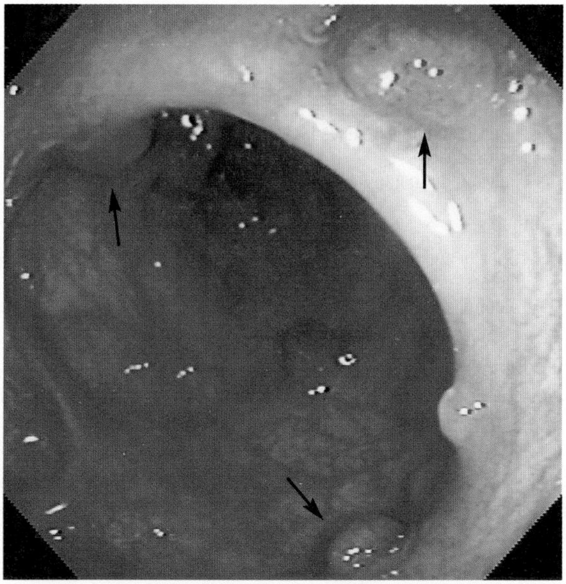

Fig. 9.49 Colonoscopic view in familial adenomatous polyposis. There are multiple small polyps throughout (arrows).

Clinically, several variants of FAP exist, including Gardner's syndrome, Turcot's syndrome and 'attenuated FAP', in which far fewer polyps are found and cancer development is delayed. In Gardner's syndrome, benign extraintestinal features are prominent, notably epidermoid cysts and osteomas. Turcot's syndrome was formerly thought to be a distinct genetic entity but the majority of patients also have APC mutations. The syndrome is characterised by FAP with brain tumours (astrocytoma or medulloblastoma).

Diagnosis and management

In newly diagnosed cases with new mutations, genetic testing by DNA linkage analysis confirms the diagnosis, and all first-degree relatives should also undergo testing. In families with known FAP, at-risk family members should undergo sigmoidoscopy starting at 10–12 years of age and repeated every 1–2 years. Genetic linkage analysis is also performed and can accurately detect over 95% of those at risk of FAP. Affected individuals should undergo colectomy after school or college education has been completed. The operation of choice is ileal pouch-anal anastomosis. Periodic upper gastrointestinal endoscopy is recommended to detect duodenal adenomas.

Peutz–Jeghers syndrome

This is characterised by multiple hamartomatous polyps in the small intestine and colon, as well as melanin pigmentation of the lips, mouth and digits (see Fig. 9.50). Most cases are asymptomatic, although chronic bleeding, anaemia or intussusception are seen. There is a small but significant risk of small bowel adenocarcinoma, cancer of the pancreas, ovary, breast and endometrium.

Juvenile polyposis

Tens to hundreds of mucus-filled hamartomatous polyps are found in the colon and rectum. One-third of cases are inherited in an autosomal dominant manner and up to 20% of patients develop colorectal cancer before the age of 40.

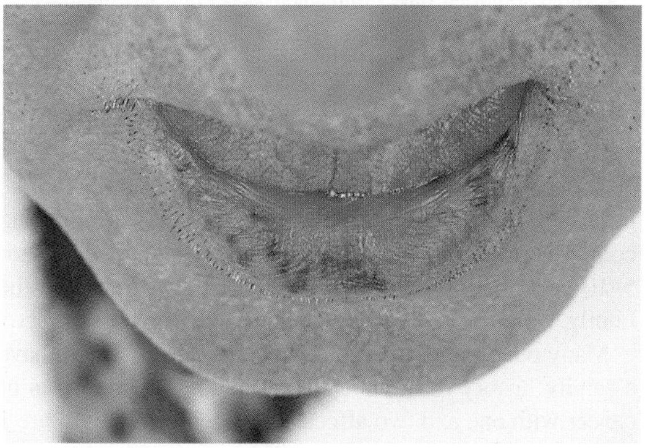

A

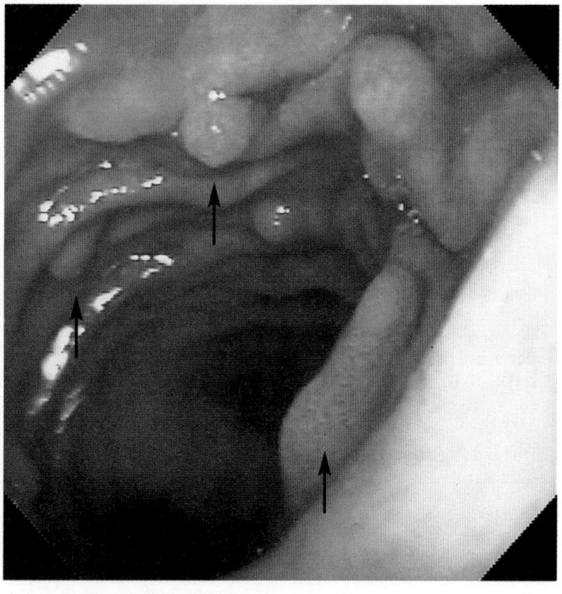

B

Fig. 9.50 Peutz–Jeghers syndrome. A Typical lip pigmentation. B Endoscopic view of multiple hamartomatous polyps in the duodenum (arrows).

Colonoscopy with biopsies should be performed every 1–3 years.

COLORECTAL CANCER

Although relatively rare in the underdeveloped world, colorectal cancer is the second most common internal malignancy and the second leading cause of cancer deaths in Western countries. In the UK, the incidence is 60 per 100 000. The condition becomes increasingly common over the age of 50.

Aetiology

Both environmental and genetic factors are important in colorectal carcinogenesis.

Environmental factors

Environmental factors probably account for 80–90% of all colorectal cancers. This figure is based on the wide geographic variation in incidence and the decrease in risk seen in migrants who move from high- to low-risk countries. Dietary factors are believed to be most important and these are summarised in Table 9.22; other recognised risk factors are listed in the information box.

Genetic factors

Colorectal cancer development results from the accumulation of multiple genetic mutations (see Fig. 1.18, p. 21). Several important hereditary forms of colon cancer are recognised, as described below.

Hereditary non-polyposis colon cancer and familial risk of colorectal cancer

Familial adenomatous polyposis (FAP) accounts for only 1% of cases of colonic cancer. In a further 10% there is a strong family history of colorectal cancer at an early age.

Table 9.22 Dietary risk factors for colorectal cancer development

Risk factor	Comments
Increased risk	
Red meat	High saturated fat and protein content Carcinogenic amines formed during cooking
Saturated animal fat	High faecal bile acid and fatty acid levels May affect colonic prostaglandin turnover
Decreased risk	
Dietary fibre	Effects vary with fibre type. Shortened transit time, binding of bile acids and effects on bacterial flora proposed
Fruit and vegetables	Green vegetables contain anticarcinogens, e.g. glucosinolates and flavonoids. Little evidence for protection from vitamins A, C, E
Calcium	Binds and precipitates faecal bile acids
Folic acid	Reverses DNA hypomethylation

NON-DIETARY RISK FACTORS IN COLORECTAL CANCER

Medical conditions

- Colorectal adenomas (see p. 671)
- Long-standing extensive ulcerative colitis (see p. 663)
- Acromegaly
- Pelvic radiotherapy

Others

- Obesity and sedentary lifestyle—may be related to dietary factors
- Alcohol and tobacco (weak association)

Pedigrees of these families with 'hereditary non-polyposis colon cancer' (HNPCC, also known as Lynch syndrome) indicate an autosomal dominant pattern of inheritance.

These patients have germ-line mutations in one or more genes (designated hMSH2, hMLH1, hPMS1 and hPMS2) involved in the repair of errors which normally occur during DNA replication (see Fig. 1.7, p. 7). Failure of this DNA 'mismatch repair' system results in a genetically unstable phenotype and accumulation of multiple somatic mutations throughout the genome.

The four criteria necessary for diagnosing this condition are given in the information box. The lifetime risk of colorectal cancer in affected individuals is 80%. The mean age of cancer development is 45 years, and two-thirds of tumours occur proximally, in contrast to sporadic colon cancer. In a subset of patients, there is also an increased incidence of cancers of the endometrium, urinary tract, stomach and pancreas.

CRITERIA FOR THE DIAGNOSIS OF HEREDITARY NON-POLYPOSIS COLON CANCER

- Three or more relatives with colon cancer (at least one first-degree)
- Colorectal cancer in two or more generations
- At least one member affected under 50 years of age
- Familial adenomatous polyposis (FAP) excluded

Those who fulfil the criteria for diagnosis should be referred for pedigree assessment, genetic testing and colonoscopy. This should begin around 25 years of age or 5–10 years earlier than the youngest case of cancer in the family. Colonoscopy needs to be repeated every 1–2 years.

Many other patients, who do not have HNPCC, still have a family history of colorectal cancer. The relative risks of cancer with one and two affected first-degree relatives are 1 in 12 and 1 in 6, respectively. The risk is even higher if relatives were affected at an early age. The genes mediating this increased risk are unknown.

Pathology

Most tumours arise from malignant transformation of a benign adenomatous polyp. Over 50% occur in the rectosigmoid and synchronous tumours are present in 2–5% of patients. Macroscopically, the majority are either polypoid and 'fungating', or annular and constricting. Spread occurs through the bowel wall. Rectal cancers may invade the pelvic viscera and side walls. Lymphatic invasion is common at presentation, as is spread through both portal and systemic circulations to reach the liver and, less commonly, the lungs. Tumour stage at diagnosis is the most important determinant of prognosis (see p. 1050).

Clinical features

Symptoms vary depending on the site of the carcinoma. In tumours of the left colon, fresh rectal bleeding is common and obstruction occurs early. Tumours of the right colon present with anaemia from occult bleeding, or altered bowel habit but obstruction is a late feature. Colicky lower abdominal pain is present in two-thirds of patients and rectal bleeding occurs in 50%. A minority present with features of either obstruction or perforation, leading to peritonitis, localised abscess or fistula formation. Carcinoma of the rectum usually causes early bleeding, mucus discharge or a feeling of incomplete emptying. Between 10 and 20% of all patients present solely with iron deficiency anaemia or weight loss.

On examination there may be a palpable mass, signs of anaemia or hepatomegaly from metastases. Low rectal tumours may be palpable on digital examination.

Investigations

Rigid sigmoidoscopy will detect approximately one-third of tumours. Colonoscopy (see Fig. 9.51) is the investigation of choice because it is more sensitive and specific than barium enema. Furthermore, lesions can be biopsied and polyps removed. Endoanal ultrasound is increasingly used for pre-operative staging of rectal cancers. Computed tomography is valuable for detecting hepatic metastases, although intra-operative ultrasound is being used increasingly for this purpose. A proportion of patients have raised serum carcinoembryonic antigen (CEA) concentrations but this is variable and so of little use in diagnosis. Measurements of CEA are valuable, however, during follow-up and can help to detect early recurrence.

Management

Surgery

The tumour is removed, along with adequate resection margins and pericolic lymph nodes. Continuity is restored by direct anastomosis wherever possible. Carcinomas within 5 cm of the anal verge may require abdominoperineal resection and formation of a colostomy. All patients should be counselled pre-operatively about the possible need for a stoma. Solitary hepatic metastases are sometimes resected at a later stage.

Post-operatively, patients should undergo colonoscopy after 6–12 months and periodically thereafter to search for local recurrence or development of new 'metachronous' lesions, which occur in 6% of cases.

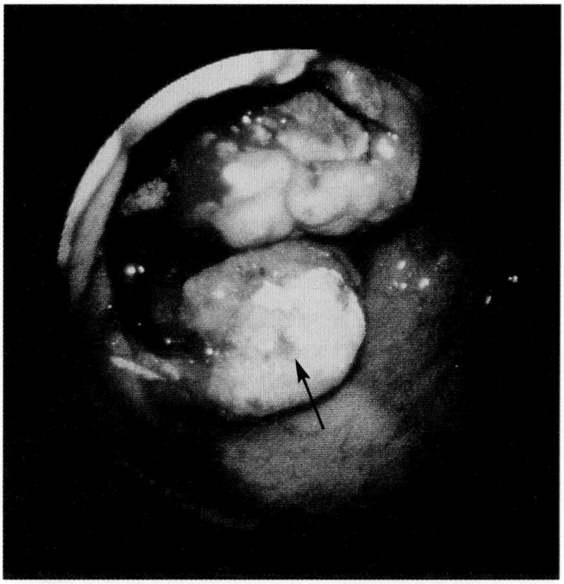

Fig. 9.51 Colonoscopic view of a polypoid colonic carcinoma (arrow).

Adjuvant therapy

Two-thirds of patients have lymph node or distant spread (Dukes stage C or D—see Table 9.23) at presentation and are, therefore, beyond cure with surgery alone. Most recurrences are within 3 years of diagnosis.

Colonic cancers recur in lymph nodes, liver and peritoneum. Adjuvant chemotherapy with 5-fluorouracil and folinic acid (to reduce toxicity) improves both disease-free and overall survival in patients with Dukes C colon cancer. This combination also provides useful palliation for patients with metastatic disease and is usually well tolerated. In patients with Dukes B or C rectal tumours, post-operative radiotherapy, in combination with 5-fluorouracil, reduces local recurrence and mortality.

Table 9.23 Dukes staging of colorectal cancer (Astler–Coller modification)

Stage	Tumour spread	5-year survival rate (%)
A	Mucosa only	> 95
B1	Submucosa or muscularis propria	90
B2	Subserosa or mesorectum	75
C1	Muscularis + lymph node involvement	75
C2	Subserosa or mesorectum + nodal involvement	25–50

Prevention and screening

Evidence suggests that colorectal cancer is preventable. At present there are no guidelines in the UK for primary prevention by dietary or lifestyle changes. Regular ingestion of aspirin or NSAIDs may reduce future risk of colonic polyps and cancer but their routine use in asymptomatic people is not yet recommended.

Secondary prevention aims to detect and remove lesions at an early or premalignant stage. Several potential methods exist:

- Widespread screening by regular *faecal occult blood (FOB) testing* reduces colorectal cancer mortality by 15–20% and increases the proportion of early cancers detected. These tests currently lack sensitivity and specificity and need to be improved. In the USA, annual FOB screening is recommended after the age of 50 years.
- *Colonoscopy* remains the gold standard but requires expertise, is expensive and carries risks, and most countries lack the resources to offer this form of screening.
- *Flexible sigmoidoscopy* is an alternative option and has been shown to reduce overall colorectal cancer mortality by approximately 35% (70% for cases arising in the rectosigmoid). It is recommended in the USA every 3–5 years after 50 years of age.
- Screening by *molecular genetic analysis* is an exciting prospect but is not yet available.

DIVERTICULOSIS

Diverticula are acquired and are most common in the sigmoid and descending colon of middle-aged people. Diverticulosis is present in over 50% of people above the age of 70 and is usually asymptomatic. Symptomatic or complicated diverticulosis ('diverticulitis') is much less common.

Aetiology

A life-long refined diet with a relative deficiency of fibre is widely thought to be responsible and the condition is rare in populations with a high dietary fibre intake, particularly in Africa and parts of Asia. It is postulated that small-volume stools require high intracolonic pressures for propulsion and this leads to herniation of mucosa between the taeniae coli (see Fig. 9.52).

Pathology

Diverticula consist of protrusions of mucosa covered by peritoneum. There is commonly hypertrophy of the circular muscle coat. Inflammation is thought to result from impaction of diverticula with faecaliths. This may resolve spontaneously or progress to cause perforation, local abscess formation, fistula and peritonitis. Repeated attacks of inflammation lead to thickening of the bowel wall, narrowing of the lumen and eventual obstruction.

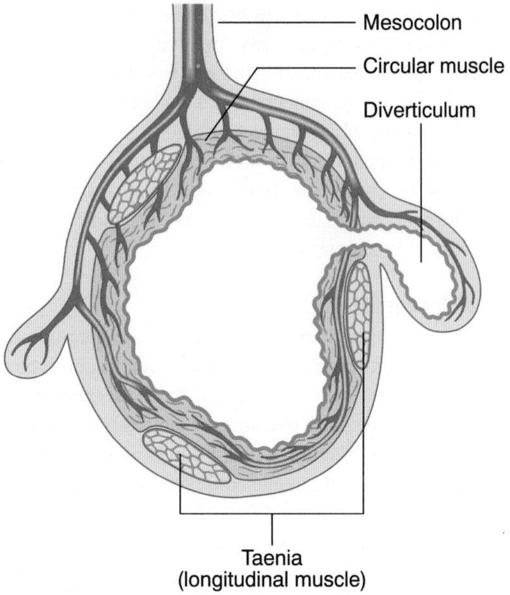

Fig. 9.52 The human colon in diverticulosis. The colonic wall is weak between the taeniae. The blood vessels that supply the colon pierce the circular muscle and weaken it further by forming tunnels. Diverticula usually emerge through these points of least resistance.

Clinical features

Symptoms are usually the result of associated constipation or spasm. Colicky pain is usually suprapubic or felt in the left iliac fossa. The descending colon may be palpable and, in attacks of diverticulitis, there is local tenderness, guarding, rigidity and a palpable mass. During these episodes there may also be diarrhoea, rectal bleeding or fever. Diverticular disease is complicated by perforation, pericolic abscess and acute rectal bleeding. These complications are more common in patients who take NSAIDs or aspirin.

Investigations

These are usually performed to exclude colorectal neoplasia. Barium enema confirms the presence of diverticula (see Fig. 9.53). Strictures and fistula may also be seen. Flexible sigmoidoscopy is performed to exclude a coexisting neoplasm which is easily missed radiologically. Colonoscopy requires expertise and carries a risk of perforation. Computed tomography is used to assess complications.

Management

Diverticulosis which is asymptomatic and discovered coincidentally requires no treatment. Constipation can be relieved by a high-fibre diet with or without a bulking laxative (ispaghula husk, 1–2 sachets daily) taken with plenty of fluids. Stimulants should be avoided.

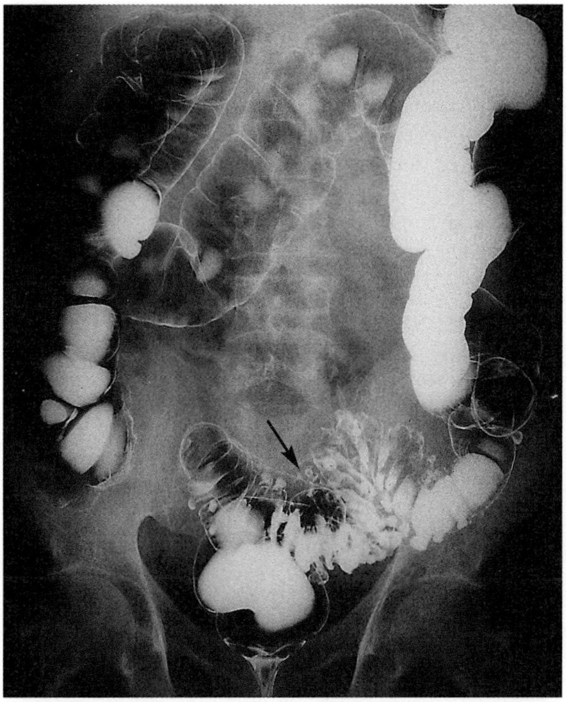

Fig. 9.53 Barium enema showing severe diverticular disease. There is tortuosity and narrowing of the sigmoid colon with multiple diverticula (arrow).

An acute attack of diverticulitis requires 7 days of metronidazole (400 mg 8-hourly orally) along with either a cephalosporin or ampicillin (500 mg 6-hourly orally). Severe cases require intravenous fluids, analgesia and nasogastric suction. Emergency surgery is reserved for severe haemorrhage or perforation. Elective surgery is performed in patients after recovery from repeated acute attacks of obstruction, and resection of the affected segment with primary anastomosis is the procedure of choice.

CONSTIPATION AND DISORDERS OF DEFAECATION

The clinical approach to patients with constipation and its aetiology have been described on page 620.

SIMPLE CONSTIPATION

This is extremely common and does not imply underlying organic disease. It usually responds to increased dietary fibre or the use of bulking agents; an adequate fluid intake is also essential. Many types of laxative are available, and these are listed in Table 9.24.

Table 9.24 Laxatives

Class	Examples
Bulk-forming	Ispaghula husk Methylcellulose
Stimulants	Bisacodyl Danthron Docusate Senna
Faecal softeners	Docusate Arachis oil enema
Osmotic laxatives	Lactulose Lactitol Magnesium salts
Others	Polyethylene glycol (PEG)* Phosphate enema*

* Used mainly for bowel preparation prior to investigation or surgery.

SEVERE IDIOPATHIC CONSTIPATION

This occurs almost exclusively in young women and often begins in childhood or adolescence. The cause is unknown but some have 'slow transit' with reduced motor activity in the colon. Others have 'obstructed defaecation' resulting from inappropriate contraction of the external anal sphincter and puborectalis muscle (anismus).

The condition is often resistant to treatment. Bulking agents may exacerbate symptoms but prokinetic agents (cisapride 10 mg 8-hourly) benefit some patients with slow transit. Glycerol suppositories and biofeedback techniques are used for those with obstructed defaecation. Rarely, subtotal colectomy is necessary as a last resort.

FAECAL IMPACTION

In faecal impaction a large, hard mass of stool fills the rectum. This tends to occur in disabled, immobile or institutionalised patients, especially the elderly or demented. Constipating drugs, autonomic neuropathy and painful anal conditions also contribute. Megacolon, intestinal obstruction and urinary tract infections may supervene. Perforation and bleeding from pressure-induced ulceration are occasionally seen. Treatment involves adequate hydration and careful digital disimpaction after softening the impacted stool with arachis oil enemas. Stimulants should be avoided.

MELANOSIS COLI AND LAXATIVE ABUSE SYNDROMES

Long-term consumption of stimulant laxatives leads to

accumulation of lipofuscin pigment in macrophages in the lamina propria. This imparts a brown discoloration to the colonic mucosa, often described as resembling 'tiger skin'. The condition is benign and resolves when the laxatives are stopped.

Prolonged laxative use may rarely result in megacolon or 'cathartic colon', in which barium enema demonstrates a featureless mucosa, loss of haustra and shortening of the bowel.

Surreptitious laxative abuse is a psychiatric condition seen in young women, some of whom have a history of bulimia or anorexia nervosa. They complain of refractory watery diarrhoea. Laxative use is usually denied and may continue even when patients are undergoing investigation. Screening of urine for laxatives may reveal the diagnosis.

MEGACOLON

Megacolon is characterised by dilatation of the colon and refractory constipation. It may be congenital (Hirschsprung's disease) or develop in later life (acquired megacolon).

Hirschsprung's disease

This is a congenital aganglionosis of the large intestine, with an incidence of 1 in 5000. It may be local or diffuse and a family history is present in one-third of all cases. The condition results from failure of migration of neuroblasts into the gut wall during embryogenesis. Ganglion cells are absent from nerve plexuses, most commonly in a short segment of the rectum and/or sigmoid colon. As a result, the internal anal sphincter fails to relax. Constipation, abdominal distension and vomiting usually develop immediately after birth but a few cases do not present until childhood or adolescence. The rectum is empty on digital examination.

Barium enema shows a small rectum and colonic dilatation above the narrowed segment. Full-thickness biopsies are required to demonstrate nerve plexuses and confirm the absence of ganglion cells. Histochemical stains for acetylcholinesterase are also used. Anorectal manometry demonstrates failure of the rectum to relax with balloon distension. Treatment involves resection of the affected segment.

Acquired megacolon

This may develop in childhood as a result of voluntary withholding of stool during toilet training. In such cases it presents after the first year of life and is distinguished from Hirschsprung's disease by the urge to defaecate and the presence of stool in the rectum. It usually responds to osmotic laxatives.

In adults, acquired megacolon has several causes. It is seen in depressed or demented patients, either as part of the condition or as a side-effect of antidepressant drugs. Prolonged abuse of stimulant laxatives may cause degeneration of the myenteric plexus, while interruption of sensory or motor innervation may be responsible in a number of neurological disorders. Scleroderma and hypothyroidism are other recognised causes.

Most patients can be managed conservatively by treatment of the underlying cause, high-residue diets, laxatives and the judicious use of enemas. Cisapride is helpful in a minority of patients. Subtotal colectomy is a last resort for the most severely affected patients.

ACUTE COLONIC PSEUDO-OBSTRUCTION (OGILVIE'S SYNDROME)

This condition has many causes (see the information box) and is characterised by relatively sudden onset of painless, massive enlargement of the proximal colon accompanied by distension; there are no features of mechanical obstruction. Bowel sounds are normal or high-pitched rather than absent. Left untreated, it may progress to perforation, peritonitis and death.

Plain abdominal radiographs show colonic dilatation with air extending to the rectum. A caecal diameter greater than 10–12 cm is associated with a high risk of perforation. Single-contrast or water-soluble barium enemas demonstrate the absence of mechanical obstruction.

CAUSES OF ACUTE COLONIC PSEUDO-OBSTRUCTION

- Trauma, burns
- Recent surgery
- Drugs, e.g. opiates, phenothiazines
- Respiratory failure
- Electrolyte and acid-base disorders
- Diabetes mellitus
- Uraemia

Management consists of treating the underlying disorder and correcting any biochemical abnormalities. Decompression either with a rectal tube or by careful colonoscopy may be effective but needs to be repeated until the condition resolves. In severe cases, surgical or fluoroscopic defunctioning caecostomy is necessary.

CLOSTRIDIUM DIFFICILE INFECTION

Antibiotic-associated diarrhoea, antibiotic-associated colitis and pseudomembranous colitis are part of the same disease spectrum which results from disturbance of the normal intestinal flora. *C. difficile* can be isolated from a variable proportion of patients and is thought to be the cause in most cases.

Pathogenesis

Around 5% of healthy adults and up to 20% of elderly patients in long-term care carry *C. difficile*. Infection is usually hospital-acquired and becomes established when the normal colonic bacterial flora is disrupted by antibiotic treatment. It can also occur, however, in debilitated patients who have not been exposed to antibiotics. Although almost any antibiotic may be responsible, the most commonly implicated are cephalosporins, ampicillin, amoxycillin and clindamycin.

The organism produces two exotoxins (A and B), both of which contribute to virulence; it is not known, however, why toxin production only occurs at certain times and under certain conditions.

Pathology

Initially the mucosa shows focal areas of inflammation and ulceration. In severe cases the ulcers become covered by a creamy-white adherent 'pseudomembrane' composed of fibrin, debris and polymorphs.

Clinical features

These usually begin in the first week of antibiotic therapy but can occur at any time up to 6 weeks after treatment has finished. The onset is often insidious, with lower abdominal pain and diarrhoea which may become profuse and watery. The presentation may resemble acute ulcerative colitis with bloody diarrhoea, fever and even toxic dilatation and perforation. Ileus is also seen in pseudomembranous colitis.

Diagnosis

The diagnosis should be suspected in any patient who is currently taking or has recently taken antibiotics. The rectal appearances at sigmoidoscopy may be characteristic, with erythema, white plaques or an adherent pseudomembrane. At other times the appearances resemble those of ulcerative colitis. In some cases the rectum is spared and the changes predominantly affect the proximal colon. Biopsies are done routinely.

Stool cultures isolate *C. difficile* in 30% of patients with antibiotic-associated diarrhoea and over 90% of those with pseudomembranous colitis. As some healthy people may harbour *C. difficile*, isolation of toxins A and B by cell cytotoxicity assays is required to prove the diagnosis. Culture and toxin isolation can be difficult and may take up to 72 hours.

Management

The offending antibiotic should be stopped and the patient should be isolated. Supportive therapy with intravenous fluids and bowel rest is often needed. Ill patients and those with evidence of ileus, dilatation or pseudomembranous colitis should be treated with antibiotics. These are most effective when given orally and there is little to choose between metronidazole 400 mg 8-hourly and vancomycin 125 mg 6-hourly. Seven to ten days of therapy are usually effective, although relapses occur in 5–20% and require repeated treatment. Preventive measures include the responsible use of antibiotics and improved ward hygiene, hand-washing and disinfection policies.

ENDOMETRIOSIS

Ectopic endometrial tissue can become embedded on the serosal aspect of the intestine, most frequently in the sigmoid and rectum. The overlying mucosa is usually intact. Cyclical engorgement and inflammation result in pain, bleeding, diarrhoea, constipation and adhesions or obstruction. Low backache is frequent. The onset is usually between 20 and 45 years and is more common in nulliparous women. Bimanual examination may reveal tender nodules in the pouch of Douglas. Endoscopic studies only reveal the diagnosis if carried out during menstruation, when a bluish mass with intact overlying mucosa is apparent. In some patients laparoscopy is required. Treatment options include laparoscopic diathermy and hormonal therapy with gonadotrophin-releasing hormone analogues or danazol.

PNEUMATOSIS CYSTOIDES INTESTINALIS

In this rare condition multiple gas-filled submucosal cysts line the colonic and small bowel walls. The cause is unknown but the condition may be seen in patients with chronic cardiac or pulmonary disease, pyloric obstruction, scleroderma or dermatomyositis. Most patients are asymptomatic, although there may be abdominal cramp, diarrhoea, tenesmus, rectal bleeding and mucus discharge. The cysts are recognised on sigmoidoscopy, plain abdominal radiographs or barium enema. Fasting breath hydrogen levels are elevated and fall with treatment. Therapies reported to be effective include prolonged high-flow oxygen, elemental diets and antibiotics.

FURTHER INFORMATION ON DISORDERS OF THE COLON AND RECTUM

Kinzler K W, Vogelstein B 1996 Lessons from hereditary colorectal cancer. Cell 87: 159–170

Lynch H T, Smyrk T C, Watson P et al 1993 Genetics, natural history, tumour spectrum and pathology of hereditary non-polyposis colorectal cancer: an updated review. Gastroenterology 104: 1535–1549

ANORECTAL DISORDERS

FAECAL INCONTINENCE

The normal control of anal continence is described on page 605. Common causes of incontinence are listed in the information box.

CAUSES OF FAECAL INCONTINENCE

- Obstetric trauma—childbirth, hysterectomy
- Severe diarrhoea, faecal impaction
- Congenital anorectal anomalies
- Anorectal disease—haemorrhoids, rectal prolapse, Crohn's disease
- Neurological disorders—spinal cord or cauda equina lesions, senile dementia

Patients are often embarrassed to admit incontinence and may complain only of 'diarrhoea'. A careful history and examination, especially of the anorectum and perineum, may help to establish the underlying cause. Endoanal ultrasound is valuable for defining the integrity of the anal sphincters, while anorectal manometry and electrophysiology are also useful investigations if available.

Management

This is often very difficult. Underlying disorders should be treated and diarrhoea managed with loperamide, diphenoxylate or codeine phosphate. Pelvic floor exercises and biofeedback techniques help some patients, and those with confirmed anal sphincter defects may benefit from sphincter repair operations.

HAEMORRHOIDS ('PILES')

Haemorrhoids arise from congestion of the internal and/or external venous plexuses around the anal canal. They are extremely common in adults. The aetiology is unknown, although they are associated with constipation and straining and may develop for the first time during pregnancy. First-degree piles bleed, while second-degree piles prolapse but retract spontaneously. Third-degree piles are those which require manual placement after prolapsing. Bright red rectal bleeding occurs after defaecation. Other symptoms include pain, pruritus ani and mucus discharge. Treatment involves measures to prevent constipation and straining. Injection sclerotherapy, infrared coagulation or band ligation are effective for most, but a minority of patients require haemorrhoidectomy, which is usually curative.

PRURITUS ANI

This is common and can result from many causes (see the information box), most of which result in contamination of the perianal skin with faecal contents.

Itching may be trivial or severe and results in an itch-scratch-itch cycle which exacerbates the problem. When no underlying cause is found, all local barrier ointments and creams must be stopped. Good personal hygiene is essential, with careful washing after defaecation. The perineal area must be kept dry and clean. Bulk-forming laxatives may reduce faecal soiling.

CAUSES OF PRURITUS ANI

Local anorectal conditions
- Haemorrhoids
- Fistula, fissures
- Poor hygiene

Skin disorders
- Contact dermatitis
- Psoriasis
- Lichen planus

Infections
- Threadworms
- Candidiasis

Other
- Diarrhoea or incontinence of any cause
- Irritable bowel syndrome
- Anxiety

SOLITARY RECTAL ULCER SYNDROME

This is most common in young adults and occurs on the anterior rectal wall. It is thought to result from localised chronic trauma and/or ischaemia associated with disordered puborectalis function and mucosal prolapse. The ulcer is seen at sigmoidoscopy and biopsies show a characteristic accumulation of collagen.

Symptoms include minor bleeding and mucus per rectum, tenesmus and perineal pain. Treatment is often difficult but avoidance of straining at defaecation is important and treatment of constipation may help. Marked mucosal prolapse is treated surgically.

ANAL FISSURE

In this common problem traumatic or ischaemic damage to the anal mucosa results in a superficial mucosal tear, most commonly in the midline posteriorly. Spasm of the internal anal sphincter exacerbates the condition. Severe pain occurs on defaecation and there may be minor bleeding, mucus discharge and pruritus. The skin may be indurated and an oedematous skin tag, or 'sentinel pile', adjacent to the fissure is common.

Avoidance of constipation with bulk-forming laxatives is important. Relaxation of the internal sphincter is normally mediated by nitric oxide, and glyceryl trinitrate ointment, which donates nitric oxide, is effective in a proportion of patients. Manual dilatation under anaesthesia leads to long-term incontinence and has been superseded by lateral anal sphincterotomy for those requiring surgery.

ANORECTAL ABSCESSES AND FISTULAE

Perianal abscesses develop between the internal and external anal sphincters and may point at the perianal skin. Ischiorectal abscesses occur lateral to the sphincters in the ischiorectal fossa. They usually result from infection of anal glands by normal intestinal bacteria. Crohn's disease (see p. 662) is sometimes responsible.

Patients complain of extreme perianal pain, fever and/or discharge of pus. Spontaneous rupture may also lead to the development of fistulae. These may be superficial or may track through the anal sphincters to reach the rectum.

Abscesses are drained surgically and fistulae are laid open with care to avoid sphincter damage.

DISEASES OF THE PERITONEAL CAVITY

PERITONITIS

Surgical peritonitis occurs as the result of a ruptured viscus (see surgical textbooks). Peritonitis may also complicate ascites (spontaneous bacterial peritonitis) or may occur in children in the absence of ascites, due to infection with pneumococci or β-haemolytic streptococci.

Chlamydial peritonitis is a complication of pelvic inflammatory disease. The affected woman presents with right upper quadrant abdominal pain, pyrexia and a hepatic rub (the Fitz-hugh–Curtis syndrome).

TUMOURS

The most common is secondary adenocarcinoma from the ovary or gastrointestinal tract.

Mesothelioma is a rare tumour complicating asbestos exposure. It presents as a diffuse abdominal mass, due to omental infiltration, and with ascites. The prognosis is extremely poor.

Diseases of the liver and biliary system 10

N.D.C. FINLAYSON • P.C. HAYES • K.J. SIMPSON

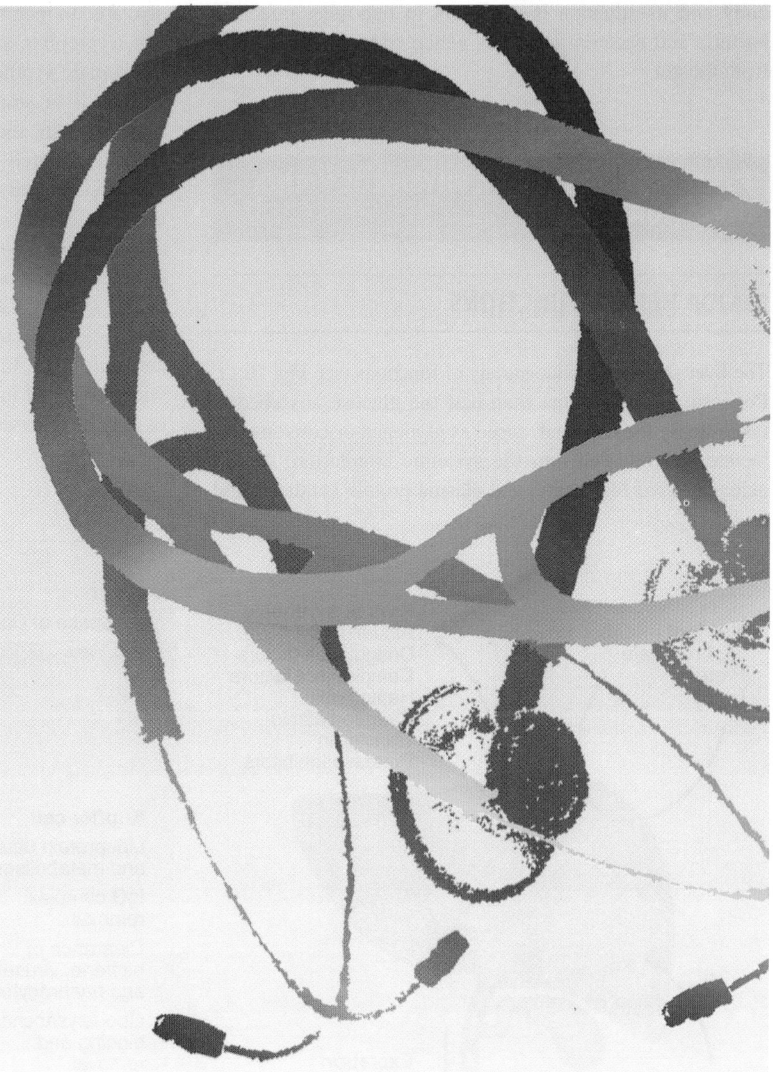

The liver is one of the heaviest organs in the body (1.2–1.5 kg) and serves the principal function of maintaining the body's internal milieu. The anatomical position of the liver is key to fulfilling this function as almost all absorption of foreign material into the body takes place in the gut and the portal blood draining the gut flows to the liver, which subsequently controls the release of absorbed nutrients into the systemic circulation. In addition to its function in metabolising nutrients, the liver is able to store and release a variety of substrates, vitamins and minerals and plays a crucial role in drug and bilirubin metabolism. The liver is also the largest reticulo-endothelial organ in the body and its situation is important in removing infecting bacteria and bacterial products, which often enter the body from the gut.

FUNCTIONAL ANATOMY, PHYSIOLOGY AND INVESTIGATIONS

MAJOR HEPATIC FUNCTIONS

The liver performs a wide variety of functions (see Fig. 10.1). Following a meal, more than half the glucose absorbed is taken up by the liver and stored as glycogen or converted to lactate and released into the systemic circulation. Amino acids are used for hepatic and plasma protein synthesis and excess amino acids are catabolised to urea. In contrast, during fasting the liver releases glucose, derived either from the breakdown of glycogen or from gluconeogenesis using amino acids released from extrahepatic tissues such as muscle. Synthesis of urea, and endogenous protein and hepatic amino acid release are suppressed during fasting.

The liver plays a central role in the metabolism of bilirubin and bile salts, drugs and alcohol (discussed on p. 689). Some vitamins, such as A, D and B_{12}, are stored by the liver in large amounts, while others, such as vitamin K and folate, are stored in smaller concentrations and disappear rapidly if dietary intake is deficient. The liver is also able to metabolise vitamins to more active compounds, e.g. tryptophan and vitamin D. Vitamin K is essential for the hepatic synthesis of coagulation factors II, VII, IX and X. The liver stores minerals such as iron, in ferritin and haemosiderin, and copper.

Approximately 15% of the liver is composed of cells other than hepatocytes (see Fig. 10.2). Foremost among these are the Kupffer cells, derived from blood monocytes. These cells constitute the largest single mass of tissue-resident monocytes in the body and account for 80% of the phagocytic capacity of this system. Kupffer cells remove aged and damaged red blood cells, bacteria, viruses, antigen-antibody complexes and endotoxin. In addition, these cells are able to produce a wide variety of inflammatory mediators that may act locally or may be released into the systemic circulation.

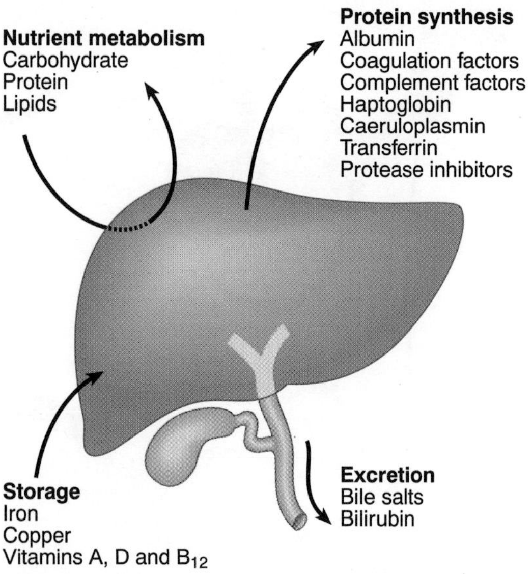

Fig. 10.1 Important liver functions.

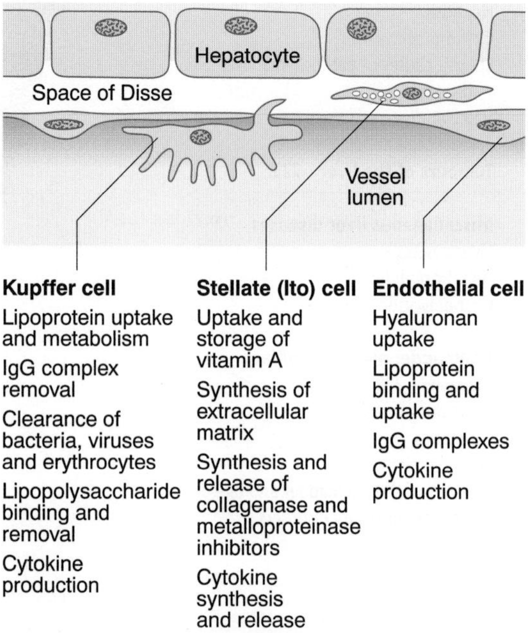

Fig. 10.2 Function of non-parenchymal liver cells.

FUNCTIONAL ANATOMY

The liver has traditionally been divided into the left and right lobes, by the falciform ligament, fissure of the ligamentum teres and fissure of the ligamentum venosum. Advances in hepatic surgery, however, have indicated a more useful division into right and left hemilivers based on the hepatic blood supply (see Fig. 10.3). The right and left hemilivers are further divided into a total of eight segments in accordance with subdivisions of the hepatic and portal veins. Each segment is made up of multiple smaller units known as lobules, comprised of a central vein, radiating sinusoids separated from each other by single liver cell (hepatocyte) plates and peripheral portal tracts. However, the hepatic lobule has no functional significance. The functional unit of the liver is the hepatic acinus (see Fig. 10.4), which is anatomically almost the reverse of the hepatic lobule. Blood flows into the hepatic acinus via the single terminal branches of the portal vein and hepatic artery located in the portal tracts, and along the hepatic sinusoids, then drains into several hepatic venous tributaries at the periphery of the acinus. In contrast, the flow of bile is in the opposite direction along the biliary canaliculi into terminal bile ductules (cholangioles) and subsequently into the interlobular bile ducts located in the portal tracts. The hepatocytes in each acinus can be divided functionally into three different zones, in accordance with their position relative to the terminal portal tract. The hepatocytes in zone 1 are closest to the terminal branches of the portal vein and hepatic artery and therefore are supplied first with oxygenated blood, and with blood containing the highest concentration of nutrients and toxins. The hepatocytes in zone 3 are furthest from the portal tracts and closest to the hepatic veins and are therefore relatively hypoxic compared with the hepatocytes in zone 1.

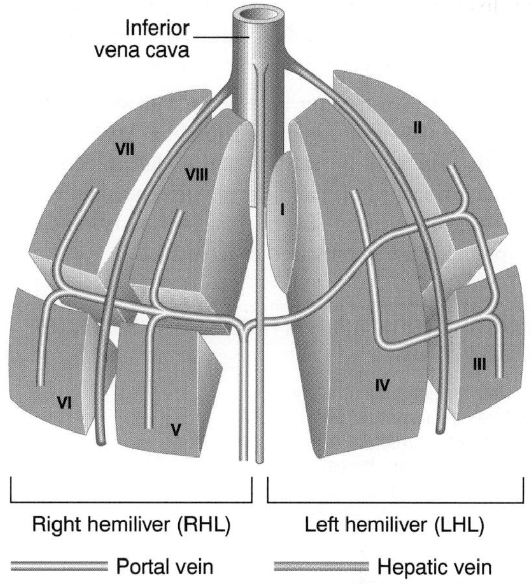

Fig. 10.3 Schematic representation of the liver.

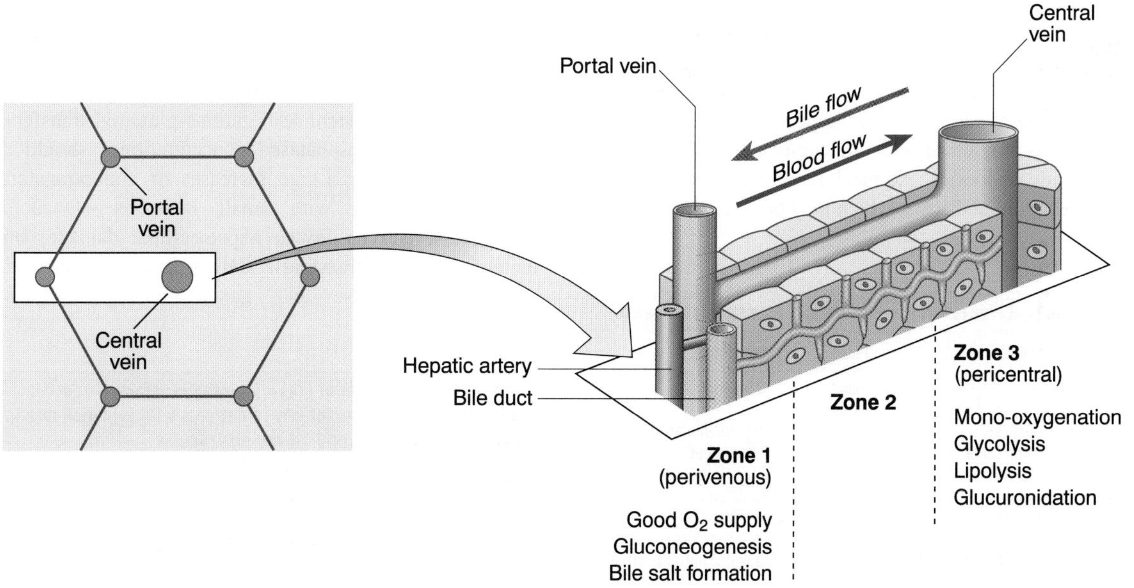

Fig. 10.4 Hepatic acinus. Functional unit of the liver.

INVESTIGATION OF HEPATOBILIARY DISEASE

The aims of investigation in patients with suspected liver disease are shown in the information box. Investigation of liver disease usually starts with a full blood count, coagulation screen, urea and electrolyte concentrations, and liver function tests. Liver function tests and their interpretation are summarised in Table 10.1.

AIMS OF INVESTIGATIONS IN PATIENTS WITH SUSPECTED LIVER DISEASE

- Detect hepatic abnormality
- Measure severity of liver damage
- Define the structural effects on the liver
- Identify the specific cause
- Investigate possible complications

TESTS OF FUNCTION

Full blood count

The haemoglobin concentration, and white cell and platelet count may be normal. A normochromic normocytic anaemia can reflect acute upper gastrointestinal haemorrhage from oesophago-gastric varices or peptic ulcer disease, the latter being more common in liver disease than the general population. Chronic blood loss from peptic ulcers or portal hypertensive gastropathy may produce a chronic hypochromic microcytic anaemia secondary to iron deficiency. A high erythrocyte mean cell volume (macrocytosis) is associated with alcohol abuse, but target cells in any jaundice patient also result in a macrocytosis. Rarely, an erythrocytosis occurs in hepatocellular carcinoma due to ectopic secretion of erythropoietin. Leucopenia and thrombocytopenia may complicate portal hypertension and hypersplenism. In contrast, leucocytosis may occur with cholangitis, alcoholic hepatitis and hepatic abscesses. Atypical lymphocytes are seen in infectious mononucleosis, which may be complicated by an acute hepatitis. Thrombocytosis may occur in those with active gastrointestinal haemorrhage and, rarely, in association with hepatocellular carcinoma.

Coagulation tests

The liver synthesises most coagulation factors, and requires vitamin K to activate factors II, VII, IX and X. Severe liver damage and prolonged biliary obstruction, which reduces vitamin K absorption, are associated with a reduced plasma fibrinogen concentration and prolongation of the prothrombin time. The prothrombin time depends on factors I, II, V, VII and X, and is prolonged when the plasma concentration of any of these factors falls below 30% of normal. The normal half-lives of the vitamin K-dependent coagulation factors in the blood are short (5–72 hours). Therefore changes in the prothrombin time occur relatively quickly following liver damage, and provide valuable prognostic information in patients with acute severe or fulminant hepatitis. An increased prothrombin time is evidence of severe liver damage in chronic liver disease, provided that vitamin K (10 mg by slow i.v. injection) is given to exclude deficiency. Hypercoagulation can cause hepatic venous thrombosis and the Budd–Chiari syndrome (see p. 722).

Biochemical tests

Hyponatraemia occurs in severe liver disease and is multifactorial in aetiology. Serum urea may be reduced due to impaired hepatic synthesis. Increased urea may occur following gastrointestinal haemorrhage, but when associated with a high serum creatinine and low urinary sodium excretion is indicative of hepatorenal failure, which carries a grave prognosis.

The 'liver function tests', or 'liver tests', do not indicate a specific diagnosis but point to underlying pathological processes. The transaminase, gamma-glutamyl transferase, and alkaline phosphatase concentrations should be considered together. Large increases of aminotransferase activity associated with small increases of alkaline phosphatase activity favour hepatocellular damage; small increases of aminotransferase activity and large increases of alkaline phosphatase and gamma-glutamyl transferase

Table 10.1 Liver function tests used to assess liver disease

Measurement	Fluid	Assessment
Bilirubin[1]	Plasma Urine	Transport
Aminotransferases[2]	Plasma	Hepatocellular damage
Alkaline phosphatase	Plasma	Biliary obstruction
Gamma-glutamyl transferase	Plasma	Enzyme induction
Proteins (total and albumin)	Plasma	Synthesis
Coagulation tests	Plasma	Synthesis

[1] Bilirubin detected in the urine identifies conjugated hyperbilirubinaemia and indicates hepatobiliary disease.
[2] Alanine aminotransferase is more specific for liver damage than aspartate aminotransferase.

Table 10.2 Relation of plasma aminotransferase and alkaline phosphatase activity in patients with jaundice due to acute viral hepatitis and biliary obstruction

Enzyme combination		Diagnostic likelihood	
Aminotransferase	**Alkaline phosphatase**	**Viral hepatitis**	**Biliary obstruction**
$> \times 6$	$< \times 2.5$	90%	10%
$< \times 6$	$> \times 2.5$	10%	80%
Other combinations		No clear separation	

DRUGS CAUSING HEPATIC MICROSOMAL ENZYME INDUCTION AND INCREASED PLASMA GAMMA-GLUTAMYL TRANSFERASE ACTIVITY

- Barbiturates
- Carbamazepine
- Ethanol
- Glucocorticoids
- Griseofulvin
- Isoniazid
- Meprobamate
- Phenytoin
- Primidone
- Rifampicin

(GGTP) activity favour biliary obstruction (see Table 10.2). Unfortunately, these patterns do not absolutely separate the two diagnostic groups and further investigation with hepatic imaging is essential. Isolated elevation of the serum GGTP is relatively common and may occur during ingestion of microsomal enzyme-inducing drugs (see the information box). The serum bilirubin and albumin concentrations reflect hepatic transport and synthetic function.

Specific aetiological investigations

A variety of blood tests are available to determine the aetiology of hepatic disease (see Table 10.3), and are discussed under specific diseases.

IMAGING TECHNIQUES

Several complementary imaging techniques can be used to determine the site and general nature of structural lesions in the liver and biliary tree. Oral cholecystography, opacifying the gallbladder with contrast, is rarely used now due to the availability and reliability of ultrasound. Ultrasound requires a skilled operator but is safe and comfortable for the patient. Its most frequent use is the identification of gallstones (see Fig. 10.5) and biliary obstruction. Ultrasound is often used in the initial assessment of patients with liver disease to determine further investigation. However, it is often difficult to identify diffuse parenchymal diseases, and focal lesions, such as tumours or metastatic disease, may not be resolved unless they are more than about 2 cm in diameter and have echogenic characteristics sufficiently different from normal liver tissue. The advent of colour Doppler ultrasound has allowed blood flow in the hepatic artery, portal vein and hepatic veins to be investigated. Endoscopic and laparoscopic ultrasound provide high-resolution images of the pancreas, biliary tree and liver.

Table 10.3 Specific aetiological investigations

Disease	Test
Haemochromatosis	Serum ferritin Serum iron, iron-binding capacity, saturation Polymerase chain reaction (PCR) for genetic abnormality
Wilson's disease	Serum caeruloplasmin Serum, urine, liver copper estimations
Hepatitis A infections	IgM anti-hepatitis A virus
Hepatitis B infections	Hepatitis B surface antigen (HBsAg) Hepatitis Be antigen (HBeAg) Hepatitis B viral DNA (HBV-DNA) Anti-hepatitis-B core (anti-HBc) Anti-hepatitis-B surface (anti-HBs) Anti-hepatitis Be (anti-HBe)
Hepatitis C	Anti-HCV antibodies (various) PCR for hepatitis C viral RNA
Hepatitis D	Anti-hepatitis D (IgM and IgG)
Hepatitis E	Anti-hepatitis E (anti-HEV)
Autoimmune chronic active hepatitis	Serum immunoglobulins Serum antinuclear factor, anti-smooth muscle and liver, kidney, microsomal (LKM) antibodies
Primary biliary cirrhosis	Serum immunoglobulins Serum antimitochondrial antibodies

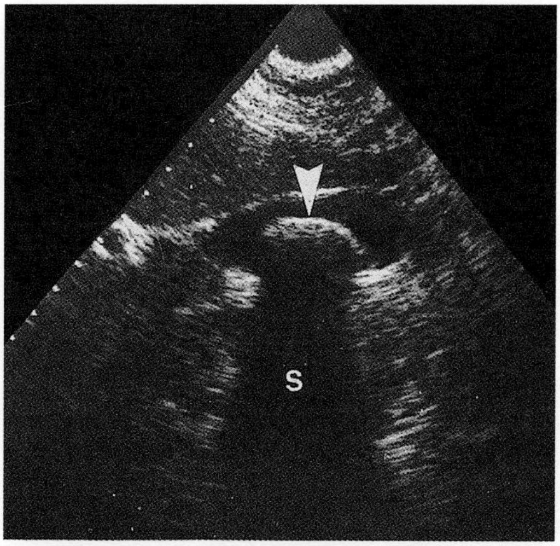

Fig. 10.5 Ultrasound of the gallbladder showing stone in the gallbladder. Stone (arrow) with acoustic shadow (S).

Computed tomography (CT) can be used for the same purposes as ultrasound, but detects smaller focal lesions in the liver, especially when combined with portography, in which contrast material is injected into the splenic or superior mesenteric artery. Magnetic resonance imaging (MRI) can also be used to study focal liver lesions and biliary disease, but is often not available and its place relative to ultrasonography and CT remains to be defined.

Cholangiography can also be undertaken via an endoscopic (endoscopic retrograde cholangiopancreatography, ERCP) or percutaneous approach (percutaneous transhepatic cholangiogram, PTC) (see Fig. 10.6). The latter does not

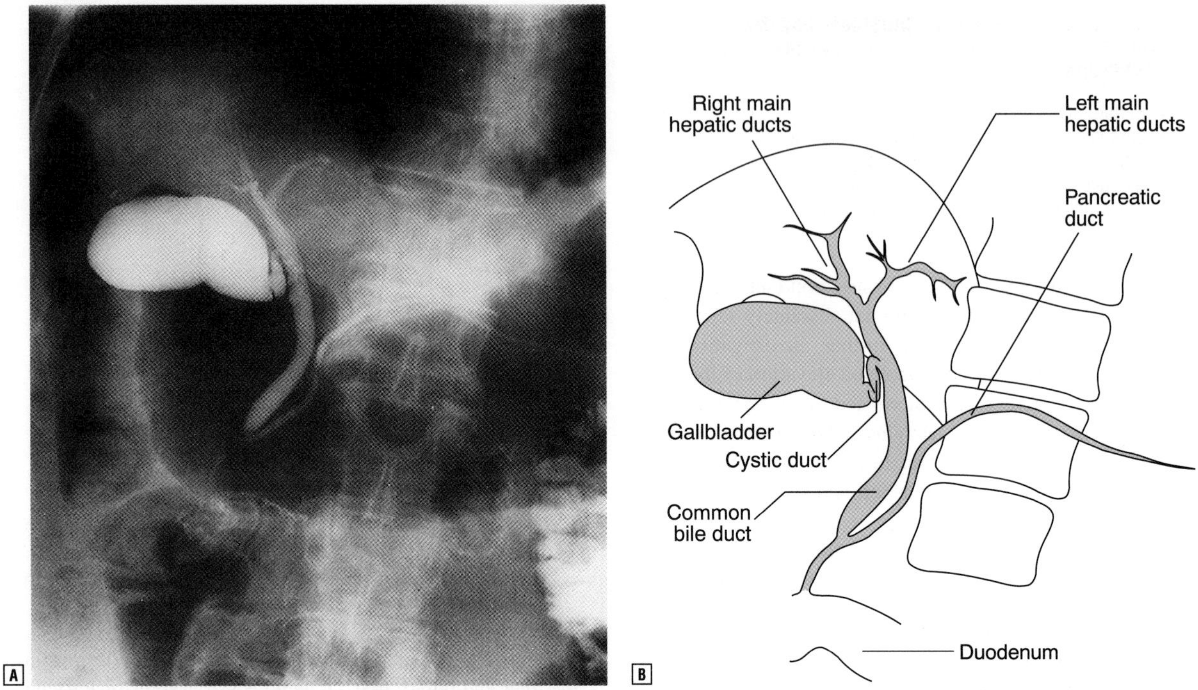

Fig. 10.6 ERCP showing normal biliary and pancreatic duct system.

allow the ampulla of Vater or pancreatic duct to be imaged. Both endoscopic and percutaneous approaches allow therapeutic interventions such as the insertion of biliary stents across malignant bile duct strictures.

Hepatic arteriography is most useful for localising focal liver lesions, particularly primary and secondary tumours, and is necessary in planning hepatic surgery. Hepatic portal venography is rarely performed, but imaging of the hepatic veins is necessary in patients with suspected Budd–Chiari syndrome.

Plain abdominal radiographs and radionucleotide liver scanning are now rarely employed to investigate liver diseases.

SPECIAL TESTS

Liver biopsy

This is performed with a Trucut or Menghini needle, usually through an intercostal space, using local analgesia. Liver biopsy is a relatively safe procedure, if the conditions detailed in the information box are met, but should never be undertaken lightly as the mortality rate is about 0.05%. The main complications are abdominal and/or shoulder pain, bleeding and, rarely, biliary peritonitis which usually occurs when a biopsy is performed in a patient with obstruction of a large

Table 10.4 Investigation of complications of hepatic cirrhosis

Complication	Investigations
Hepatic encephalopathy	Investigation for any precipitating cause Psychometric tests Electroencephalogram (EEG) Sensory evoked potentials
Portal hypertension	Upper GI endoscopy Barium swallow and meal Liver ultrasound Abdominal CT Wedge hepatic pressure Venography of hepatic veins
Ascites	Ascitic fluid sampling (for protein concentration, white blood cell count, bacterial culture, cytological examination) Liver ultrasound Laparoscopy
Renal failure	Urine analysis Renal ultrasound Central venous pressure recording Renal biopsy
Hepatocellular carcinoma	Alpha-fetoprotein Liver ultrasound Abdominal CT Hepatic angiogram Laparoscopy and biopsy of lesion

CONDITIONS REQUIRED FOR SAFE LIVER BIOPSY

- Cooperative patient
- Prothrombin time < 4 seconds prolonged
- Platelet count >100 × 10^9/l
- Exclusion of bile duct obstruction, localised skin infection, advanced chronic obstructive pulmonary disease, marked ascites and severe anaemia

bile duct. Liver biopsies can be carried out in patients with defective haemostasis after correction with fresh frozen plasma and platelet transfusion or, if the biopsy is obtained by the transjugular route or percutaneously under ultrasound control, with subsequent plugging of the needle track with procoagulant material. Operative or laparoscopic liver biopsy may sometimes be valuable, as in the staging of lymphoma.

Investigation of the potential complications of liver disease

Investigation of patients for specific complications is especially important in those who have cirrhosis of the liver. The investigations employed are summarised in Table 10.4 and are discussed in more detail in the relevant sections.

FURTHER INFORMATION ON FUNCTIONAL ANATOMY, PHYSIOLOGY AND INVESTIGATIONS

Gebhardt R 1992 Metabolic zonation of the liver. Pharmacology Therapeutics 53: 275–354

Hegarty J R, Williams R 1984 Liver biopsy. British Medical Journal 288: 1254–1256

Lautt W W 1997 Hepatic vasculature: a conceptual review. Gastroenterology 73: 1163–1169

MAJOR MANIFESTATIONS OF LIVER DISEASE

Liver disease produces a wide range of clinical manifestations. Acute liver disease is most common and jaundice is its main manifestation, usually in association with systemic features of an acute illness. Severe acute liver disease can give rise to neuropsychiatric symptoms (encephalopathy) which characterise the rare syndrome of fulminant or acute hepatic failure. Chronic liver disease causes manifestations resulting from damage to the liver itself and from portal hypertension. Fluid retention (ascites and oedema) and hepatic encephalopathy are due mainly to a combination of these two processes and are features of chronic liver failure (or hepatic decompensation). The main manifestation of portal hypertension is bleeding from varices or gastropathy. In most countries the dominant cause of portal hypertension is hepatic cirrhosis, and though the underlying liver disease is always advanced, liver failure may or may not be present.

Investigation of patients with abnormal liver function tests

The almost universal availability of automated biochemical analysis and the frequency of insurance, employment and health screening examinations have led increasingly to the identification of abnormal biochemical liver tests in asymptomatic people. Whilst the finding of abnormal biochemical liver tests may be indicative of a severe underlying liver disease, it is important to note that chronic liver disease may be associated with normal liver function tests; hence approximately 10% of patients with cirrhosis are identified unexpectedly at laparotomy or autopsy.

Investigation of patients with abnormal liver function tests starts with a clinical history and physical examination. In particular, clinical features of jaundice, pruritus, ascites, gastrointestinal bleeding and hepatic encephalopathy are sought. Fatigue, tiredness and weakness are also common features in patients with chronic liver disease. The physical examination specifically addresses whether or not there are cutaneous manifestations of chronic liver disease such as palmar erythema, spider telangiectasia and other skin changes. Abdominal examination may reveal hepatosplenomegaly and ascites. Features of hepatic encephalopathy, such as flapping tremor (asterixis) and constructional apraxia, should be sought. In the absence of specific features in the history or physical examination, further investigation of abnormal liver function tests may suggest a cholestatic or hepatitic abnormality. Further investigation proceeds as illustrated in the investigation algorithm (see Fig. 10.7, p. 690).

JAUNDICE

Jaundice refers to the yellow appearance of the skin, sclerae and mucous membranes resulting from an increased bilirubin concentration in the body fluids. It is detectable clinically when the plasma bilirubin exceeds 50 μmol/l (3 mg/dl). Internal tissues and body fluids are coloured yellow but not the brain, as bilirubin does not cross the blood–brain barrier other than in the immediate neonatal period. Mechanisms leading to jaundice are shown in the information box on page 690.

Bilirubin metabolism

Unconjugated bilirubin is produced (425–510 mmol, 250–300 mg daily) from the catabolism of haem after removal of its iron component. The sources of

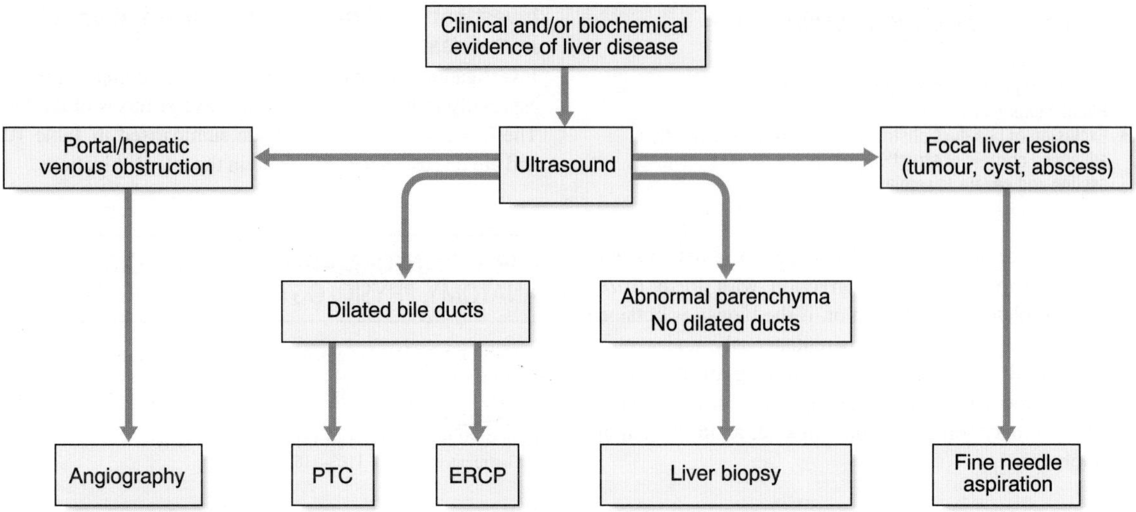

Fig. 10.7 Investigative procedures in liver disease. Suggested sequence for identifying structural lesions in the liver and biliary tract. (ERCP = endoscopic retrograde cholangiopancreatography; PTC = percutaneous transhepatic cholangiography)

MECHANISMS PRODUCING JAUNDICE

Increased production

- Haemolysis

Impaired excretion

- Congenital non-haemolytic hyperbilirubinaemia
  - Gilbert's syndrome
  - Crigler–Najjar type I and type II
  - Dubin–Johnson syndrome
  - Rotor's syndrome
- Hepatocellular jaundice
  - Acute parenchymal liver disease
  - Chronic parenchymal liver disease
- Cholestasis

unconjugated bilirubin are detailed in the information box top right. Bilirubin in the blood is normally almost all unconjugated and, as it is not water-soluble, it is bound to albumin and does not pass into the urine. Further metabolism of bilirubin is shown in Figure 10.8. Unconjugated bilirubin is conjugated by the endoplasmic reticulum enzyme, glucuronyl transferase, into bilirubin mono- and diglucuronide. These bilirubin conjugates are water-soluble and exported into the bile via specific carriers on the hepatocyte membrane. Conjugated bilirubin is metabolised by colonic bacteria forming stercobilinogen, which may be further oxidised to stercobilin. Both stercobilinogen and stercobilin are then excreted in the stool. A small amount of stercobilinogen (4 mg/day) is absorbed from the bowel, passes through the liver and excreted in the urine, where it is known as urobilinogen, or, following further oxidisation, urobilin.

SOURCES OF UNCONJUGATED BILIRUBIN

- Haemoglobin breakdown
- Catabolism of other haem-containing proteins, e.g. myoglobin and cytochrome enzymes
- Ineffective erythropoiesis

HAEMOLYTIC JAUNDICE

This results from increased destruction of red blood cells, or their precursors in the marrow, causing increased bilirubin production (see p. 761). Jaundice due to haemolysis is usually mild because a healthy liver can excrete a bilirubin load six times greater than normal before unconjugated bilirubin accumulates in the plasma. Exceptions to this occur in the newborn when the hepatic bilirubin transport mechanism is immature, and in patients with liver disease.

Clinical features

These are detailed on page 761. There are often no stigmata of chronic liver disease other than jaundice. Increased excretion of bilirubin and hence stercobilinogen leads to normal-coloured or dark stools, and increased urobilinogen excretion causes the urine to turn dark on standing as urobilin is formed. Pallor due to anaemia and splenomegaly due to excessive reticulo-endothelial activity are usually present.

Investigations

The plasma bilirubin is usually less than 100 μmol/l (6 mg/dl) and the liver function tests are otherwise normal.

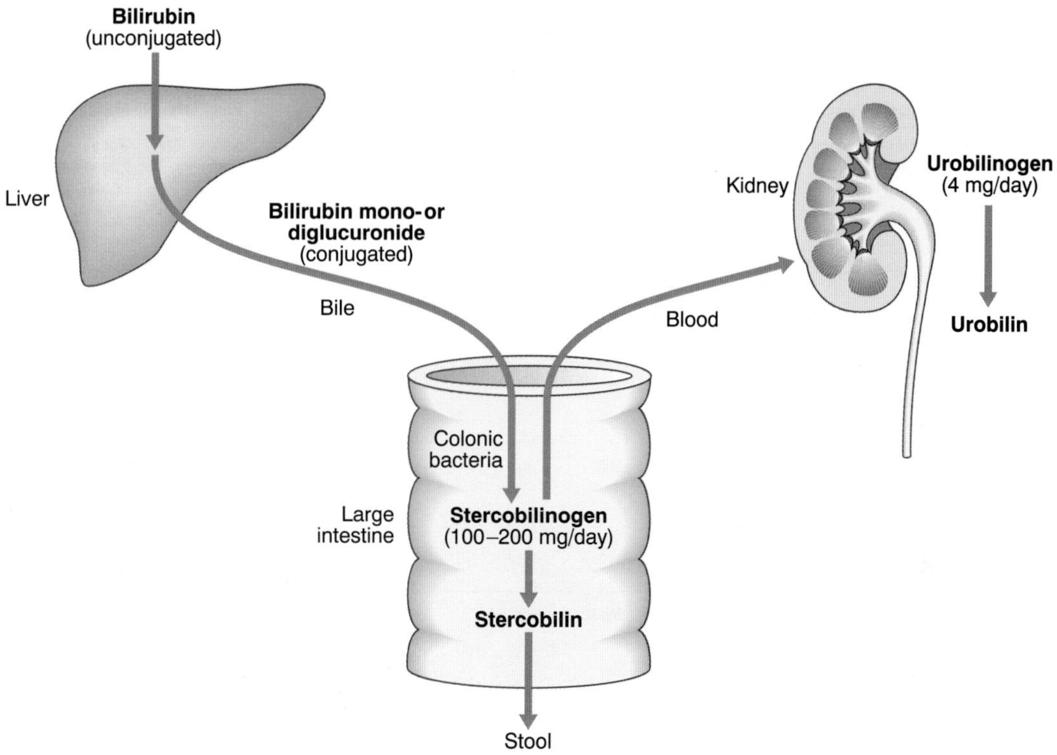

Fig. 10.8 Pathway of bilirubin excretion.

There is no bilirubinuria because the hyperbilirubinaemia is dominantly unconjugated. The blood count and film may show evidence of haemolytic anaemia (see p. 761).

CONGENITAL NON-HAEMOLYTIC HYPERBILIRUBINAEMIA

Gilbert's syndrome is the only common form of congenital non-haemolytic hyperbilirubinaemia. All other forms are very rare (see Table 10.5, p. 692). In adults this condition has an excellent prognosis, needs no treatment, and is clinically important only because it may be mistaken for more serious liver disease.

HEPATOCELLULAR JAUNDICE

Hepatocellular jaundice results from an inability of the liver to transport bilirubin into the bile, occurring as a result of parenchymal liver disease. Bilirubin transport across the hepatocytes may be impaired at any point between uptake of unconjugated bilirubin into the cells and transport of conjugated bilirubin into the canaliculi. In addition, swelling of cells and oedema resulting from the disease itself may cause obstruction of the biliary canaliculi. In hepatocellular jaundice the concentrations in the blood of both unconjugated and conjugated bilirubin increase, perhaps because of the variable way in which bilirubin transport is disturbed. The severity of jaundice, the other clinical features, and the investigation and treatment vary with the underlying disease and are considered later in this chapter.

CHOLESTATIC JAUNDICE

In unrelieved cholestasis jaundice tends to become progressively severe because conjugated bilirubin is unable to enter the bile canaliculi and passes back into the blood, and also because there is a failure of clearance of unconjugated bilirubin arriving at the liver cells.

Aetiology

The causes of cholestatic jaundice are listed in the information box on page 692. Cholestasis may be due to failure of the hepatocytes to generate bile flow, to obstruction to bile flow in the bile ducts in the portal tracts, or to obstruction to bile flow in the extrahepatic bile ducts between the porta hepatis and the papilla of Vater. Causes of cholestasis can operate at more than one of these levels, and those confined

Table 10.5 Congenital non-haemolytic hyperbilirubinaemia

Syndrome	Inheritance	Age of presentation	Hyperbilirubinaemia Type	Severity	Bilirubinuria	Liver defect(s)	Prognosis	Management
Gilbert's	Autosomal dominant	Young adult (any)	Unconjugated	Mild	No	Glucuronyl transferase reduced Occasional mild haemolysis Defective bilirubin uptake	Normal life-span	None Phenobarbitone occasionally
Crigler–Najjar								
Type I	Autosomal recessive	Neonate	Unconjugated	Very severe	No	Glucuronyl transferase absent	Rapid death (kernicterus)	None
Type II	Autosomal dominant	Neonate	Unconjugated	Severe	No	Glucuronyl transferase greatly reduced	Can survive to adulthood	Phenobarbitone Ultraviolet light Liver transplant
Dubin–Johnson	Autosomal recessive	Any	Conjugated	Mild	Yes	Canalicular excretion of organic anions (e.g. bilirubin, cholecystographic contrast agents) reduced	Normal life-span	None
Rotor	Autosomal dominant	Any	Conjugated	Mild	Yes	Defective bilirubin uptake Reduced intrahepatic binding	Normal life-span	None

CAUSES OF CHOLESTATIC JAUNDICE

Intrahepatic
- Primary biliary cirrhosis
- Primary sclerosing cholangitis
- Alcohol
- Drugs
- Viral hepatitis
- Autoimmune hepatitis
- Severe bacterial infections
- Post-operative
- Hodgkin's lymphoma
- Pregnancy
- Idiopathic recurrent cholestasis

Extrahepatic
- Choledocholithiasis
- Carcinoma
  - Ampullary
  - Pancreatic
  - Bile duct (cholangiocarcinoma)
  - Secondary
- Cystic fibrosis
- Parasitic infection
- Traumatic biliary structures

CLINICAL FEATURES IN CHOLESTATIC JAUNDICE

Cholestasis

Early features
- Jaundice
- Dark urine
- Pale stools
- Pruritus

Late features
- Xanthelasma and xanthomata
- Malabsorption
  - Weight loss
  - Steatorrhoea
  - Osteomalacia
  - Bleeding tendency

Cholangitis
- Fever
- Rigors
- Pain
- Hepatic abscess

to the extrahepatic bile ducts may be amenable to surgical correction.

Clinical features

Clinical features in cholestatic jaundice include those due to cholestasis itself and to the development of cholangitis consequent to biliary obstruction. These features are listed in the information box top right. Clinical features in cholestatic jaundice also include those which point to a likely cause for the condition (see Table 10.6) and are discussed in greater detail in the relevant sections. None of the clinical features noted in the table is pathognomonic of a particular cause, but each is more likely in some diseases than in others.

Investigations

Investigations in individual patients are determined by the history and clinical findings. Usually, biochemical tests show greater elevation of the alkaline phosphatase and GGTP compared with the aminotransferases and an ultrasound is performed to identify any biliary dilatation. Subsequent investigation is shown in Figure 10.7, page 690.

Management

This depends on the underlying cause of the cholestasis and is discussed in detail in the relevant sections.

Table 10.6 Underlying causes of cholestatic jaundice related to clinical features*

Clinical feature	Causes
Jaundice	
Static or increasing	Carcinoma
Fluctuating	Stone Stricture Pancreatitis Choledochal cyst
Abdominal pain	Stone Pancreatitis Choledochal cyst
Cholangitis	Stone Stricture Choledochal cyst
Abdominal scar	Stone Stricture
Irregular hepatomegaly	Hepatic carcinoma
Palpable gallbladder	Carcinoma below cystic duct (usually pancreas)
Abdominal mass	Carcinoma Pancreatitis (cyst) Choledochal cyst
Occult blood in stools	Papillary tumour

* Each of the diseases listed here can give rise to almost any of the clinical features shown. The more likely causes of each clinical feature are given.

UNUSUAL FORMS OF CHOLESTASIS

Cholestasis of pregnancy
This is probably caused by an inherited susceptibility of the patient's liver cells to oestrogens; this condition may also be precipitated by oral contraceptives. Pruritus is the dominant symptom and jaundice occurs in about half of the patients. Itching almost always starts in the third trimester of pregnancy and remits within about 2 weeks of delivery. Pruritus can be relieved with cholestyramine (see p. 720). No harm comes to the fetus, but the condition tends to recur in subsequent pregnancies.

Benign recurrent intrahepatic cholestasis
This is a rare condition in which episodes of cholestasis lasting from 1–6 months occur, starting in adolescence or early adult life. Genetic factors are probably important as more than one family member may be affected. Episodes start with pruritus, and painless jaundice develops later. Liver function tests show the pattern of cholestasis (see p. 686); liver biopsy shows cholestasis during an episode but is normal between episodes. Treatment is required to relieve pruritus and the long-term prognosis is good.

PORTAL HYPERTENSION

Portal hypertension is characterised by prolonged elevation of the portal venous pressure (normally 2–5 mmHg). Patients developing clinical features or complications of portal hypertension usually have portal venous pressures above 12 mmHg.

Aetiology and pathogenesis
Portal venous pressure is determined by the portal blood flow and by the portal vascular resistance. Increased vascular resistance is usually the main factor producing portal hypertension, irrespective of its cause, and consequently the causes of portal hypertension are classified in accordance with the main sites of obstruction to blood flow in the portal venous system (see Fig. 10.9, p. 694 and the information box).

CAUSES OF PORTAL HYPERTENSION ACCORDING TO THE SITE OF PORTAL VENOUS OBSTRUCTION

Common causes

- Extrahepatic
  - Sepsis (umbilical, portal pyaemia)
  - Unknown (most cases of extrahepatic obstruction)
- Intrahepatic pre-sinusoidal
  - Schistosomiasis
- Intrahepatic parenchymal
  - Cirrhosis

Other causes

- Extrahepatic
  - Umbilical vein transfusion
  - Thrombosis
    - Thrombotic diseases
    - Oral contraceptives
    - Pregnancy
    - Secondary (cirrhosis)
  - Abdominal trauma
  - Biliary surgery
  - Malignant disease
    - Pancreas or liver
  - Pancreatitis
  - Congenital
- Intrahepatic pre-sinusoidal
  - Myeloproliferative/lymphoproliferative disease
  - Congenital hepatic fibrosis
  - Drugs
  - Vinyl chloride
  - Sarcoidosis
  - Idiopathic
- Intrahepatic parenchymal
  - Budd–Chiari syndrome
  - Veno-occlusive disease
  - Cystic liver disease
  - Partial nodular transformation of the liver (see p. 727)
  - Metastatic malignant disease

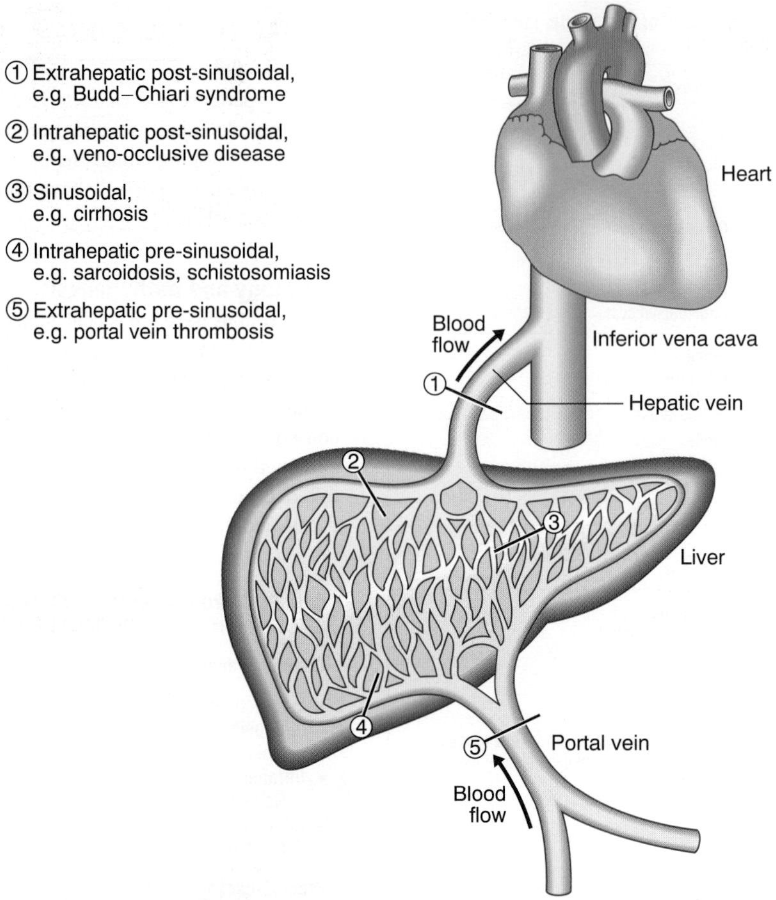

Fig. 10.9 Classification of portal hypertension according to site of vascular obstruction.

Extrahepatic portal vein obstruction is frequently the cause of portal hypertension in childhood and adolescence, while cirrhosis causes 90% or more of portal hypertension in adults in Western countries. Schistosomiasis is the most common cause of portal hypertension world-wide but it is infrequent outside endemic areas. Increased portal vascular resistance leads to a gradual reduction in the flow of portal blood to the liver and simultaneously to the development of collateral vessels, allowing portal blood to bypass the liver and enter the systemic circulation directly. Increased portal blood flow may contribute to portal hypertension but is not the dominant factor. Collateral vessel formation is widespread but occurs particularly in the gastrointestinal tract, especially the oesophagus, stomach and rectum, in the anterior abdominal wall, and in the renal, lumbar, ovarian and testicular vasculature. Normally, virtually all the portal blood flows through the liver but, as collateral vessel formation progresses, half or more, and occasionally almost all, of the portal blood flow can be shunted directly to the systemic circulation.

Clinical features

The clinical features of portal hypertension result principally from portal venous congestion and from collateral vessel formation. Splenomegaly is a cardinal finding, and a diagnosis of portal hypertension is unlikely when splenomegaly cannot be detected clinically or by ultrasonography. The spleen is rarely enlarged more than 5 cm below the left costal margin in adults, but more marked splenomegaly can occur in childhood and adolescence. Hypersplenism is common and frequently results in thrombocytopenia. Platelet counts are usually around 100×10^9/l; values below 50×10^9/l are rare. Leucopenia occurs occasionally, but anaemia can hardly ever be attributed to hypersplenism. Collateral vessels may be visible on the anterior abdominal wall and occasionally several radiate from the umbilicus to form a caput medusae. Rarely, a large umbilical collateral vessel has a blood flow sufficient to give a venous hum on auscultation (Cruveilhier–Baumgarten syndrome). The most important collateral vessels occur in the oesophagus and stomach, where they can cause severe bleeding (see p. 695). Rectal varices also cause bleeding and are often mistaken for haemorrhoids, which are no more common in portal hypertension than in the general population. Fetor hepaticus results from portasystemic shunting of blood which allows mercaptans to pass directly to the lungs.

Investigations

Radiological and endoscopic examination of the upper gastrointestinal tract can show varices. This establishes the presence of portal hypertension but not its cause (see Fig. 10.10). Imaging, particularly ultrasonography, can show features of portal hypertension, such as splenomegaly and collateral vessels, and can sometimes indicate the cause, such as liver disease or portal vein thrombosis. Portal venography demonstrates the site and often the cause of portal venous obstruction and is performed prior to surgical intervention. Portal venous pressure measurements are rarely needed but can be used to confirm portal hypertension and to differentiate sinusoidal and pre-sinusoidal forms.

Complications

Gastrointestinal bleeding from varices or from congestive gastropathy is the main complication (see the information box). Hypersplenism is rarely severe enough to be clinically significant and portal hypertension is only one factor contributing to the development of ascites (see p. 698), renal failure (see p. 704) and hepatic encephalopathy (see p. 700).

COMPLICATIONS OF PORTAL HYPERTENSION

- Variceal bleeding
  Oesophageal, gastric, other (rare)
- Congestive gastropathy
- Hypersplenism
- Ascites
- Renal failure
- Hepatic encephalopathy

VARICEAL BLEEDING

Variceal bleeding occurs from oesophageal varices that are usually located within 3–5 cm of the oesophago-gastric junction or from gastric varices. The size of the varices, endoscopic variceal stigma such as red spots and red stripes, high portal pressure and liver failure are all general factors that predispose to bleeding. Drugs capable of causing mucosal erosion, such as salicylates and other non-steroidal anti-inflammatory drugs, can also precipitate bleeding. Variceal bleeding is often severe, and recurrent bleeding occurs if preventive treatment is not given.

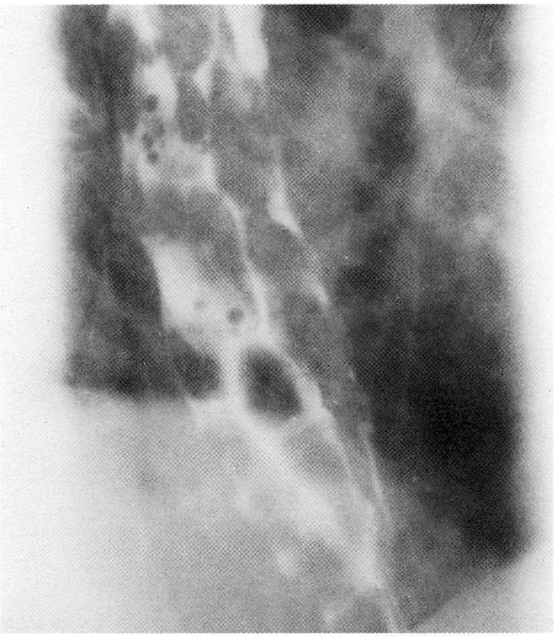

A

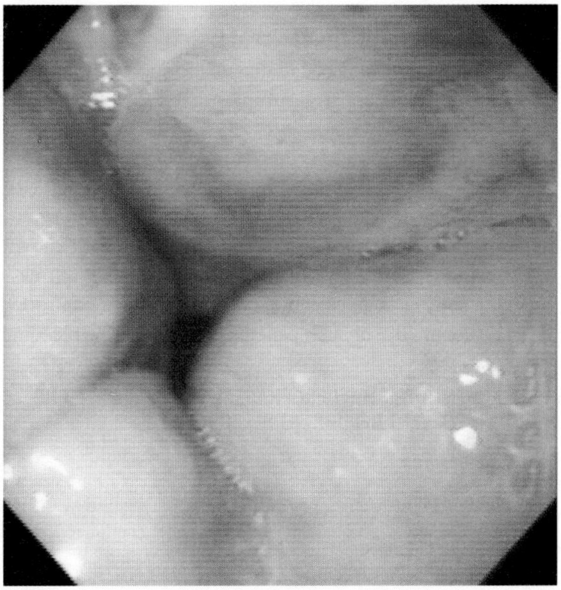

B

Fig. 10.10 Oesophageal varices. A Barium swallow. B Endoscopic view showing four large varices encroaching on the oesophageal lumen.

Bleeding from varices at other sites is comparatively uncommon but most often occurs from varices in the rectum or associated with intestinal stomas.

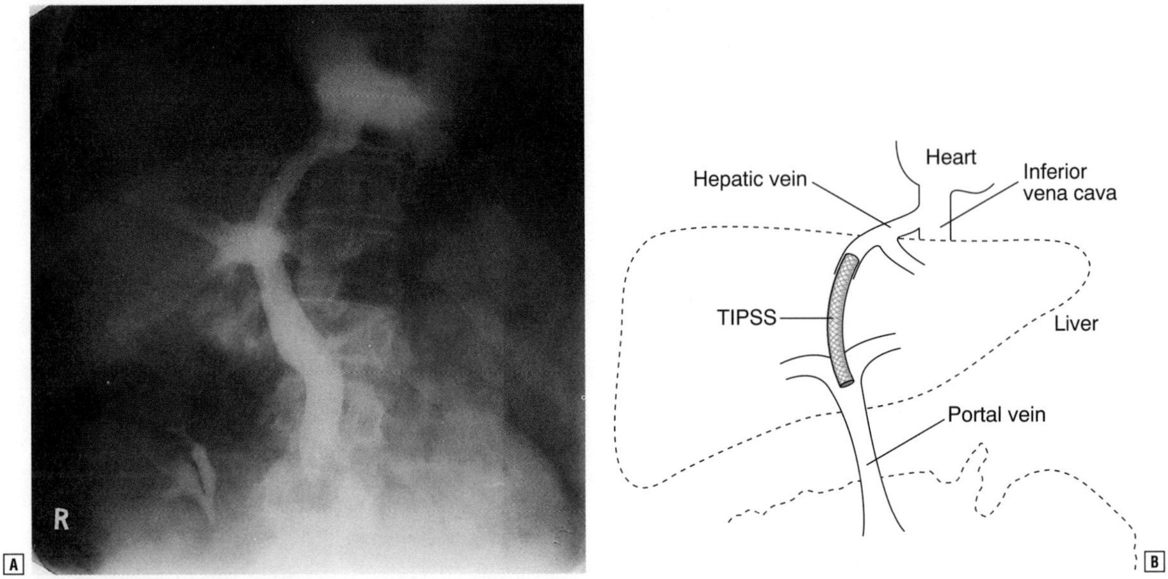

Fig. 10.11 Transjugular intrahepatic portasystemic stent shunt (TIPSS). [A] A TIPSS radiograph showing placement of TIPSS within the portal vein allowing blood to flow from the right hepatic vein into the inferior vena cava. Note contrast within the superior mesenteric vein but not the splenic vein which has collapsed with the reduction in portal pressure. [B] Explanatory diagram.

Management of acute variceal bleeding

The differential diagnosis and diagnostic approach in patients with acute upper gastrointestinal haemorrhage are detailed on page 614.

The priority in acute bleeding from oesophageal varices is to restore the circulation with blood and plasma, not least because shock reduces liver blood flow and causes further deterioration of liver function. Even in patients with known varices, the source of bleeding should always be confirmed by endoscopy as soon as acute bleeding has been controlled because about 20% of such patients are found to be bleeding from some other lesion, especially acute gastric erosions. Several treatments are available to stop acute variceal bleeding and to prevent its recurring (see the information box). Sclerotherapy and banding are the preferred initial means for treating variceal bleeding (see p. 697).

TREATMENTS TO STOP OESOPHAGEAL VARICEAL BLEEDING AND TO PREVENT RECURRENT BLEEDING
Local measures
• Sclerotherapy • Banding • Balloon tamponade • Oesophageal transection
Reduction of portal venous pressure
• Somatostatin (octreotide) • Vasopressin • Terlipressin
Prevention of recurrent bleeding
• Sclerotherapy/banding • Transjugular intrahepatic portasystemic stent shunt • Portasystemic shunt surgery (unselective or selective) • Propranolol

Reduction of portal venous pressure

Pharmacological reduction of portal pressure is less important than sclerotherapy or banding, is expensive, and is not always used. Octreotide is probably the drug of choice currently. Transjugular intrahepatic portasystemic stent shunts (TIPSS) are increasingly being used for reducing portal pressure (see below and Fig. 10.11).

Pharmacological treatment. Octreotide, the synthetic form of somatostatin, reduces the portal pressure and can stop variceal bleeding. It has few side-effects and is given in a dose of 50 μg intravenously, followed by an infusion of 50 μg hourly.

Vasopressin constricts the splanchnic arterioles and reduces portal blood flow and hence portal pressure. It is best given by intravenous infusion 0.4 U/min until bleeding stops or for 24 hours, and then 0.2 U/min for a further 24 hours. Vasoconstriction also occurs in other vascular beds and can cause angina, arrhythmia and even myocardial infarction. Nitroglycerin should be given transdermally or intravenously to combat these side-effects. Vasopressin should not be used in patients with ischaemic heart disease. Terlipressin is an alternative to vasopressin with certain advantages, since vasopressin is released from it over several hours in amounts sufficient to reduce the portal pressure without producing systemic effects. It is given in a dose of 2 mg i.v. 6-hourly until bleeding stops and then 1 mg 6-hourly for a further 24 hours.

Transjugular intrahepatic portasystemic stent shunting (TIPSS). This technique, described below, can be used for acute bleeding not responding to sclerotherapy or banding. Emergency portasystemic shunt surgery has a mortality of 50% or more and is now virtually never used for treating active variceal bleeding.

Local measures

The measures used to control acute variceal bleeding include sclerotherapy, banding, balloon tamponade and oesophageal transection.

Sclerotherapy or banding. This is the most widely used initial treatment and is undertaken if possible at the time of diagnostic endoscopy. It stops variceal bleeding in 80% of patients and can be repeated if bleeding recurs. Active bleeding at endoscopy may make sclerotherapy hazardous, and in such circumstances bleeding should be controlled by balloon tamponade prior to sclerotherapy. Banding can be used to stop acute variceal bleeding but it is less easy to apply than sclerotherapy in this situation (see Fig. 10.12).

Balloon tamponade. This technique employs a Sengstaken–Blakemore tube possessing two balloons which exert pressure in the fundus of the stomach and in the lower oesophagus, respectively. Current modifications, such as the Minnesota tube, incorporate sufficient lumens to allow material to be aspirated from the stomach and from the oesophagus above the oesophageal balloon. The tube should be passed through the mouth and its presence in the stomach should be checked by auscultating the upper abdomen while injecting air into the stomach and by radiology. Gentle traction is used to maintain pressure on the varices. The gastric balloon only should be inflated initially as this alone will usually control bleeding, and if the oesophageal balloon needs to be used it should be deflated for about 10 minutes every 3 hours to avoid oesophageal mucosal damage. Balloon tamponade will almost always stop oesophageal and gastric fundal variceal bleeding, but it only allows time for the use of more definitive therapy.

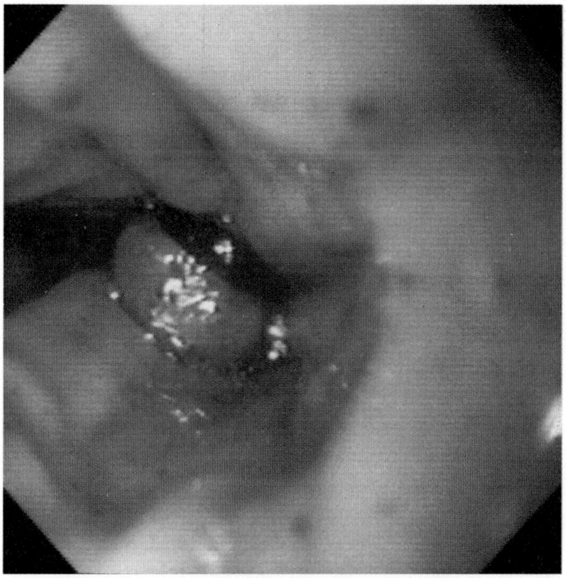

Fig. 10.12 Appearances of oesophageal varices following application of strangulating bands (band ligation).

Oesophageal transection. Transection of the varices can be performed relatively easily with a stapling gun though it carries some risk of subsequent oesophageal stenosis. The operation is used when TIPSS is not available and when bleeding cannot be controlled by the other therapies described.

Prevention of recurrent bleeding

Recurrent bleeding is the rule rather than the exception in patients who have previously bled from oesophageal varices, and treatment to prevent this is needed.

Sclerotherapy

This is the most widely used method for preventing recurrent oesophageal variceal bleeding. Varices are injected with a sclerosing agent as soon as practicable after bleeding, and injections are repeated every 1–2 weeks thereafter until the varices are obliterated. Regular follow-up endoscopy is necessary to allow treatment of any recurrence of varices. The treatment is not free of risk as injections can cause transient chest or abdominal pain, fever, transient dysphagia and occasionally oesophageal perforation. Oesophageal strictures may develop. However, mortality is low even in those with poor liver function, and recurrent bleeding is largely prevented. Prolongation of life has been claimed but this remains to be proven.

Banding

This is a technique in which varices are sucked into an endoscope accessory allowing them to be occluded with a tight rubber band. The occluded varix subsequently sloughs with variceal obliteration. The technique is applied in the same way as sclerotherapy, is generally more effective, and has fewer side-effects.

Transjugular intrahepatic portasystemic stent shunting (TIPSS)

This is a technique in which a stent is placed between the portal vein and the hepatic vein in the liver to provide a portasystemic shunt to reduce portal pressure. The procedure is carried out under radiological control via the internal jugular vein; prior patency of the portal vein must be determined angiographically, coagulation deficiencies may require correction with fresh frozen plasma and antibiotic cover is provided. Successful shunt placement stops and prevents variceal bleeding. Further bleeding necessitates investigation and treatment (angioplasty) of shunt occlusion. Hepatic encephalopathy may occur following TIPSS and requires that the shunt diameter be reduced. The long-term value of the technique remains to be assessed.

Portasystemic shunt surgery

This was previously the treatment of choice because such shunts effectively prevented bleeding, provided the shunt remained patent. However, the mortality associated with this procedure is high, especially where liver function is poor, and follow-up of patients has shown that they often suffered troublesome hepatic encephalopathy. Furthermore, survival is not prolonged, as death from liver failure occurs. In practice, portasystemic shunts are now reserved for patients in whom other treatments have not been successful and are offered only to those with good liver function.

Propranolol

Propranolol (80–160 mg/day) reduces the portal venous pressure in portal hypertension and has been used to prevent recurrent variceal bleeding; however, it has not yet been accepted generally in treatment.

Prophylaxis of initial variceal bleeding

In view of the mortality and morbidity associated with variceal haemorrhage, portasystemic shunts, sclerotherapy and propranolol have all been used to try to prevent initial bleeding from varices. Propranolol in a dose of 80–160 mg daily has given beneficial results and can be used to prevent initial variceal bleeding.

CONGESTIVE GASTROPATHY

Long-standing portal hypertension causes chronic gastric congestion recognisable at endoscopy as multiple areas of punctate erythema. Similar lesions occur rarely more distally in the gastrointestinal tract. These areas may become eroded, causing bleeding from multiple sites. Acute bleeding can occur, but repeated minor bleeding causing iron-deficiency anaemia is more common. Anaemia may be prevented by oral iron supplements but repeated blood transfusions can become necessary. Reduction of the portal pressure using propranolol 80–160 mg/day is the best initial treatment, and if this is ineffective a TIPSS procedure can be undertaken.

ASCITES

Ascites refers to the accumulation of free fluid in the peritoneal cavity. While cirrhosis is a common cause of ascites, there are many other causes, and these need to be considered even in a patient with chronic liver disease (see the information box).

CAUSES OF ASCITES

Common causes	Other causes
• Malignant disease Hepatic, peritoneal • Cardiac failure • Hepatic cirrhosis	• Hypoproteinaemia Nephrotic syndrome, protein-losing enteropathy, malnutrition • Hepatic venous occlusion Budd–Chiari syndrome, veno-occlusive disease • Infection Tuberculosis, spontaneous bacterial peritonitis • Pancreatitis • Lymphatic obstruction • Rare Meigs' syndrome, vasculitis, hypo-thyroidism, renal dialysis

Pathogenesis

Liver failure and portal hypertension in cirrhosis cause general sodium and water retention in the body, with localisation of fluid in the peritoneum occurring due to the high venous pressure in the mesenteric circulation. The means whereby sodium and water retention occurs are unknown, and two general theories have been put forward. One explanation postulates that following the loss of fluid into the peritoneum there is compensatory renal retention of sodium and water ('underfilling theory'), while the other postulates a primary renal retention of sodium and water with eventual overspill of fluid into the peritoneum ('overflow theory'). The mechanisms for renal sodium retention remain poorly understood but include activation of the renin-angiotensin system with secondary aldosteronism, increased sympathetic nervous activity, alteration of atrial natriuretic hormone secretion and altered activity of the kallikrein-kinin system.

Clinical features

Ascites causes abdominal distension with fullness in the flanks, shifting dullness on percussion, and a fluid thrill when the ascites is marked (see Fig. 10.13). These signs do not appear until the ascites volume exceeds a litre even in thin patients, and much larger volumes can be hard to detect in the obese. Associated features consequent on ascites include distortion or eversion of the umbilicus, herniae, abdominal striae, divarication of the recti and, occasionally, meralgia paraesthetica (see p. 995) and scrotal oedema. Pleural effusions can be found in about 10% of patients, usually on the right side. Most are small and only

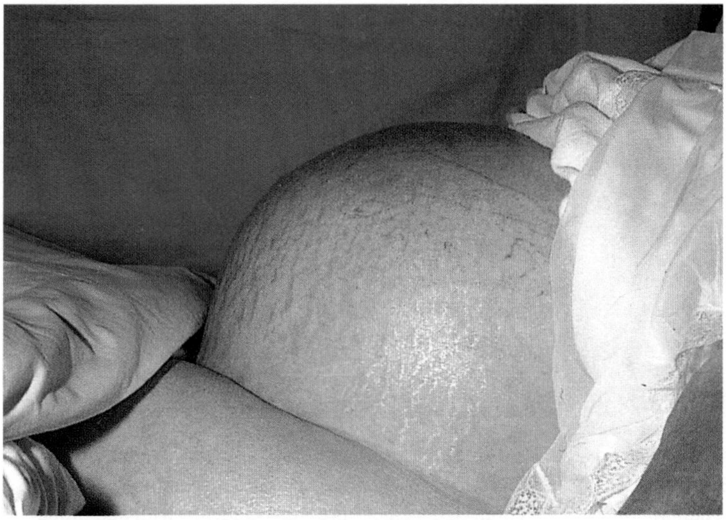

Fig. 10.13 Abdominal swelling in ascites.

identified on chest radiographs, but occasionally a massive hydrothorax occurs. Pleural effusions, particularly on the left side, should not be assumed to be due to the ascites.

Investigations

Ultrasonography is the best means of confirming ascites, demonstrating ascites in the obese, or detecting small volumes of fluid. Abdominal radiographs can show ascites, but they are insensitive and non-specific. Paracentesis can also be used to confirm the presence of ascites, but is most useful in obtaining ascitic fluid for analysis, if necessary under ultrasonic guidance. The appearance of the ascites may point to the underlying cause (see Table 10.7). The ascites protein concentration and the serum-ascites albumin gradient are used to separate ascites due to transudation from ascites due to exudation. Ascites protein concentrations below 25 g/l or serum-ascites albumin gradients above 1.5 are usually found in ascites due to cirrhosis. Ascites amylase activity above 1000 U/l identifies pancreatic ascites, and low ascites glucose concentrations suggest malignant disease or tuberculosis. Cytological examination can reveal malignant cells, and polymorphonuclear leucocyte counts above 250/mm^3 strongly suggest infection. Laparoscopy can be valuable in detecting peritoneal disease.

Table 10.7 Appearances and causes of ascites

Cause	Appearance*
Cirrhosis	Clear, straw-coloured or light green
Malignant disease	Bloody
Infection	Cloudy
Biliary communication	Heavy bile staining
Lymphatic obstruction	Milky-white (chylous)

* Milky-white chylomicrons pass into supernatant on centrifugation.

Diagnosis

In the great majority of patients ascites is caused by malignant disease, cirrhosis or cardiac failure; however, the presence of cirrhosis does not necessarily mean that this is the cause of the ascites. This is particularly so when liver function is good or when there is no evidence of portal hypertension, and in such patients a complication of cirrhosis, such as hepatocellular carcinoma or portal vein thrombosis, should be sought or an independent cause of ascites considered. Ascites with a protein concentration above 25 g/l raises the possibility of infection (especially tuberculosis), malignancy, hepatic venous obstruction, pancreatic ascites or, rarely, hypothyroidism.

Management

Successful treatment of ascites relieves discomfort but does not prolong life, and if over-vigorous can produce serious disorders of fluid and electrolyte balance, and precipitate hepatic encephalopathy (see p. 700). Conventional treatment aims to reduce body sodium and water by restricting intake, promoting urine output and, if necessary, removing ascites directly. The rate of loss of sodium and water is most easily measured by regular weighing, and as no more than 900 ml can be mobilised from the peritoneum daily if fluid depletion in the rest of the body is to be avoided, the body weight should not fall by more than 1 kg daily.

Sodium and water restriction

Restriction of dietary sodium intake is essential to achieving negative sodium balance in patients with ascites. Restriction to 80 mmol/day ('no added salt diet') may be adequate, but restriction to 40 mmol/day is necessary in more severe ascites and this requires close dietetic supervision. Drugs containing relatively large amounts of sodium and those promoting sodium retention such as non-steroidal analgesic agents must be avoided. Restriction of water intake to 0.5–1.0 litre/day is necessary only if the plasma sodium falls below 125 mmol/1. A few patients will have a satisfactory diuresis on this treatment alone.

Diuretic drugs

Most patients require diuretic drugs in addition to sodium restriction. Spironolactone (100–400 mg/day) is the drug of choice for long-term therapy because it is a powerful aldosterone antagonist, but it can cause painful gynaecomastia and hyperkalaemia. Some patients will also require powerful loop diuretics (e.g. frusemide), though these can cause fluid, electrolyte and renal function disorders. Diuresis is improved if patients are rested in bed while the diuretics are acting, perhaps because renal blood flow increases in the horizontal position.

Paracentesis

Paracentesis of 3–5 litres over 1–2 hours has always been used for immediate relief of cardiorespiratory distress due to gross ascites, but large paracentesis alone has previously been regarded as a hazardous treatment for ascites. Paracentesis to dryness or the removal of 3–5 litres daily is now recognised as a safe treatment, provided the circulation is supported by giving a colloid such as human albumin solutions (6–8 g/l ascites removed) or other plasma expanders as required. Total paracentesis can be used as an initial therapy or when other treatments fail.

LeVeen shunt

The LeVeen shunt is a long tube with a non-return valve running subcutaneously from the peritoneum to the internal jugular vein in the neck, which allows ascitic fluid to pass directly into the systemic circulation. It is effective in ascites resistant to conventional treatment, but complications including infection, superior vena caval thrombosis, pulmonary oedema, bleeding from oesophageal varices and disseminated intravascular coagulopathy limit its use.

Transjugular intrahepatic portasystemic stent shunting (TIPSS)

TIPSS (see p. 697) can relieve resistant ascites but does not prolong life. It can be used where liver function is reasonable or in patients awaiting liver transplantation. It should not be used in the terminally ill.

Prognosis

Ascites is a serious development in cirrhosis as only 10–20% of patients survive 5 years from its appearance. The outlook is not universally poor, however, and is best in those with well-maintained liver function and where the response to therapy is good. The prognosis is also better where a treatable cause for the underlying cirrhosis is present (see p. 707) or where a precipitating cause for ascites such as excess salt intake is found.

Complications

Ascites may be complicated by infections which may be spontaneous (see below) or, more commonly, precipitated by invasive investigations or treatment, such as upper gastrointestinal endoscopy and injection sclerotherapy. Ascites can also be complicated by renal failure. Both of these complications have adverse prognostic significance.

SPONTANEOUS BACTERIAL PERITONITIS (SBP)

Patients with cirrhosis are very susceptible to infection of ascitic fluid as part of their general susceptibility to infection. SBP usually presents suddenly with abdominal pain, rebound tenderness, absent bowel sounds and fever in a patient with obvious features of cirrhosis and ascites. Abdominal signs are mild or absent in about one-third of patients, and in these patients hepatic encephalopathy and fever are the main features. Paracentesis may show cloudy fluid, and an ascites neutrophil count above $250/mm^3$ almost invariably indicates infection. The source of infection cannot usually be determined, but most organisms isolated from ascitic fluid or blood cultures are of enteric origin and *Escherichia coli* is the organism isolated most frequently. Ascites culture in blood culture bottles gives the highest yield of organisms. SBP needs to be differentiated from other intra-abdominal emergencies, and the finding of multiple organisms on culture should arouse suspicion of a perforated viscus. Treatment is started immediately with a broad spectrum of antibiotics such as cefotaxime (1 g i.v. 8-hourly) and metronidazole (1 g rectally 8-hourly). Recurrence of SBP is common and may be reduced by norfloxacin (400 mg daily). Infection of other fluid collections that may occur in patients with cirrhosis, such as pleural and pericardial effusions, have been reported.

HEPATIC (PORTASYSTEMIC) ENCEPHALOPATHY

Hepatic encephalopathy is a neuropsychiatric syndrome caused by liver disease. It occurs most often in patients with cirrhosis but is seen in acute form in acute hepatic failure.

Aetiology

Hepatic encephalopathy is generally regarded as being due to a biochemical disturbance of brain function because it is reversible and rarely shows marked pathological changes in the brain. Liver failure and portasystemic shunting of blood are two important factors underlying hepatic encephalopathy and the balance between these varies in different patients. Some degree of liver failure is a constant factor as portasystemic shunting of blood hardly ever causes encephalopathy if the liver function is normal. Little is known of the biochemical 'neurotoxins' causing the encephalopathy, but they are thought to be mainly nitrogenous substances produced in the gut, at least in part by bacterial action, which are normally metabolised by the healthy liver so that they do not enter the systemic circulation. Ammonia has long been considered an important factor and much interest has centred recently on the false neurotransmitter gamma-aminobutyric acid; both are produced in the intestine. Additional putative substances include other false neurotransmitters such as octopamine, amino acids, mercaptans and fatty acids. Some factors appear to precipitate hepatic encephalopathy by increasing the availability of these substances; in addition, the brain in cirrhosis may be sensitised to other factors such as drugs that are able to precipitate hepatic encephalopathy (see the information box). Disruption of the function of the blood–brain barrier is more a feature of acute hepatic failure where it leads to cerebral oedema.

FACTORS PRECIPITATING HEPATIC ENCEPHALOPATHY

- Uraemia
  Spontaneous, diuretic-induced
- Drugs
  Sedatives, antidepressants, hypnotics
- Gastrointestinal bleeding
- Excess dietary protein
- Constipation
- Paracentesis (volumes > 3–5 litres)
- Hypokalaemia
- Infection
- Trauma (including surgery)
- Portasystemic shunts
  Surgical, spontaneous (large)

Clinical features

The clinical features include changes of intellect, personality, emotions and consciousness with or without neurological signs. When an episode develops acutely a precipitating factor may be found (see the information box). The earliest features are very mild, but as the condition becomes more severe, apathy, inability to concentrate, confusion, disorientation, drowsiness, slurring of speech and eventually coma develop. Convulsions sometimes occur. Examination usually shows a flapping tremor (asterixis), inability to perform simple mental arithmetic tasks (see Fig. 10.14) or draw objects such as a star (constructional apraxia), and, as the condition progresses, hyper-reflexia and bilateral extensor plantar responses. Hepatic encephalopathy should not be diagnosed when focal neurological signs are found, though these can

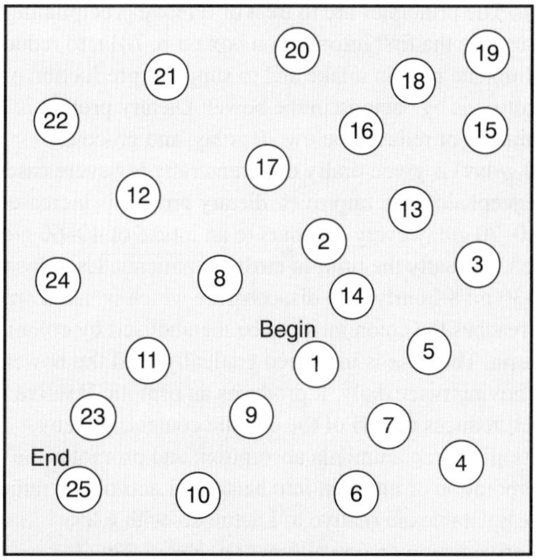

Fig. 10.14 Number connection test used in assessing encephalopathy.

DIFFERENTIAL DIAGNOSIS OF HEPATIC ENCEPHALOPATHY

- Subdural haematoma
- Drug or alcohol intoxication
- Delirium tremens
- Wernicke's encephalopathy
- Primary psychiatric disorders
- Hypoglycaemia
- Neurological Wilson's disease

occur. Fetor hepaticus, a sweet musty odour to the breath, is usually present but is more a sign of liver failure and portasystemic shunting than of hepatic encephalopathy. Rarely, chronic hepatic encephalopathy (hepatocerebral degeneration) gives rise to variable combinations of cerebellar dysfunction, Parkinsonian syndromes, spastic paraplegia and dementia.

Investigations

The diagnosis can usually be made clinically, but when doubt exists an electroencephalogram (EEG) shows diffuse slowing of the normal alpha waves with eventual development of delta waves. The arterial ammonia is usually increased but this investigation is of little or no diagnostic value as increased concentrations occur in the absence of hepatic encephalopathy. Other clinical conditions that may be confused with hepatic encephalopathy are listed in the information box.

Management

Episodes of encephalopathy are common in cirrhosis and are usually readily reversible until the terminal stages occur. The principles are to treat or remove precipitating causes (see the first information box on p. 701), to reduce or eliminate protein intake and to suppress production of neurotoxins by bacteria in the bowel. Dietary protein is eliminated or reduced below 20 g/day, and glucose (300 g/day) is given orally or parenterally in severe cases. As encephalopathy improves, dietary protein is increased by 10–20 g/day every 48 hours to an intake of 40–60 g/day, which is usually the limit in cirrhotic patients. Lactulose (15–30 ml 8-hourly) is a disaccharide which is taken orally and reaches the colon intact to be metabolised by colonic bacteria. The dose is increased gradually until the bowels are moving twice daily. It produces an osmotic laxative effect, reduces the pH of the colonic content, thereby limiting colonic ammonia absorption, and promotes the incorporation of nitrogen into bacteria. Lactitol is a rather more palatable alternative to Lactulose, with a less explosive action on bowel function. Neomycin (1–4 g 4–6-hourly) is an antibiotic which acts by reducing the bacterial floral content of the bowel. It can be used in addition to, or as an alternative to, Lactulose if diarrhoea becomes troublesome. Neomycin is poorly absorbed from the bowel but sufficient gains access to the body to contraindicate its use when uraemia is present; it is less desirable than Lactulose for long-term use. Ototoxicity is the main deleterious effect.

HEPATOPULMONARY SYNDROME

Many patients with cirrhosis are hypoxaemic due to a variety of causes including pulmonary hypertension, pleural effusions and the hepatopulmonary syndrome. This latter is characterised by resistant hypoxaemia and intrapulmonary vascular dilatation. Clinical features include digital clubbing, cyanosis and spider naevi, and a typical feature is a reduction in arterial oxygen saturation on standing. The hepatopulmonary syndrome is now considered an indication for liver transplantation.

ACUTE (FULMINANT) HEPATIC FAILURE

Acute or fulminant hepatic failure is a rare syndrome in which hepatic encephalopathy, characterised by mental changes progressing from confusion to stupor and coma, results from a sudden severe impairment of hepatic function. The syndrome is defined further as occurring within 8 weeks of onset of the precipitating illness, in the absence of

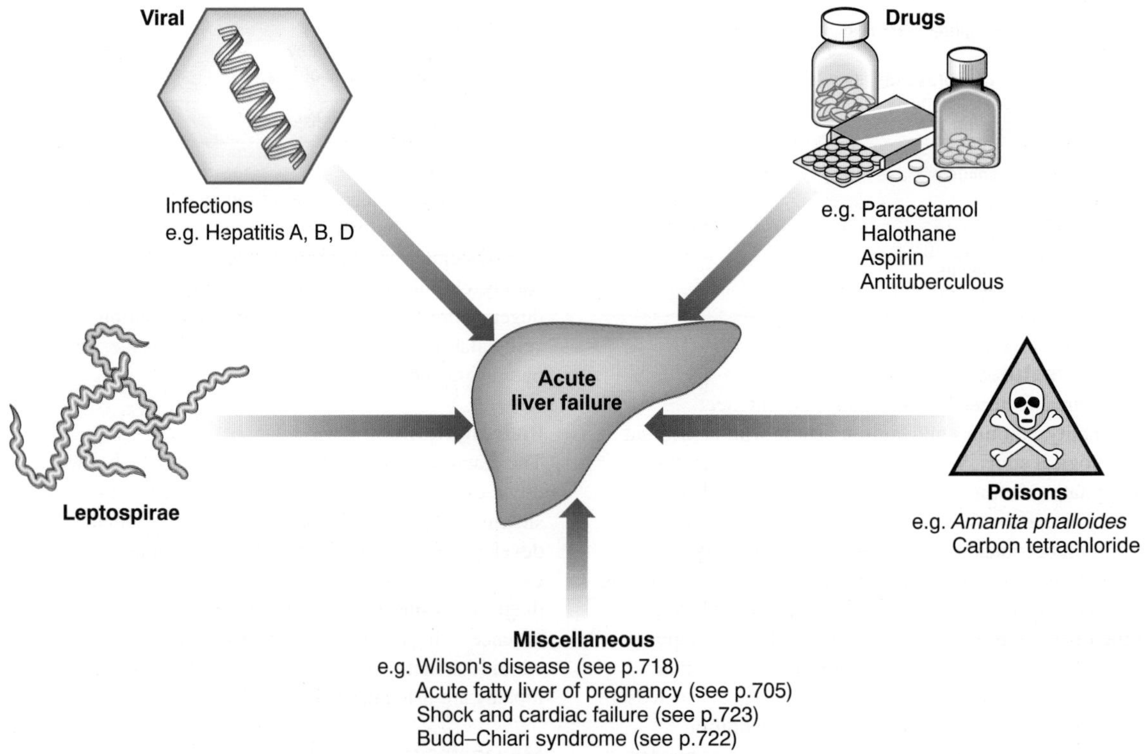

Fig. 10.15 Causes of acute liver failure.

evidence of pre-existing liver disease, to distinguish it from those instances in which hepatic encephalopathy represents a deterioration in chronic liver disease.

Aetiology

Any cause of liver damage can produce acute hepatic failure provided it is sufficiently severe (see Fig. 10.15). Acute viral hepatitis is the most common cause worldwide; paracetamol toxicity (see p. 1119) is the most frequent cause in the UK. Otherwise acute liver failure occurs occasionally with other drugs, or from *Amanita phalloides* (mushroom) poisoning, in pregnancy, in Wilson's disease, following shock and, rarely, in extensive malignant disease in the liver.

Pathology

Extensive parenchymal necrosis is the most common histological appearance. In fatal cases, less than 30% of the liver cells appear viable and often few such cells are seen. Severe fatty degeneration is characteristic of fulminant hepatic failure caused by drugs such as tetracycline, pregnancy and Reye's syndrome.

Clinical features

Cerebral disturbance (hepatic encephalopathy) is the cardinal manifestation of acute hepatic failure, but in the early stages this can be mild and episodic. The earliest clinical features are often subtle and include reduced alertness and poor concentration, progressing through behavioural abnormalities such as restlessness, aggressive outbursts and mania, to drowsiness and coma (see Table 10.8). Confusion, disorientation, inversion of sleep rhythm, slurred speech, yawning, hiccup and convulsions may also occur. A flapping 'hepatic' tremor (asterixis) of the extended hands is characteristic, but may be absent. Cerebral oedema can produce increased intracranial pressure causing unequal or abnormally reacting pupils, fixed pupils with spontaneous respiration, hypertensive episodes and bradycardia, hyperventilation, profuse sweating, local or general myoclonus, focal fits or decerebrate posturing. Papilloedema occurs rarely and is a late sign. More general symptoms include weakness, nausea and vomiting. Right hypochondrial pain is only an occasional feature.

Examination shows jaundice, which develops rapidly and is usually deep in subsequently fatal cases. Jaundice is not seen in Reye's syndrome, and death in other causes of acute hepatic failure occasionally occurs before jaundice develops. Fetor hepaticus can be present. The liver may be enlarged initially but later becomes impalpable. Splenomegaly is uncommon and never prominent. Ascites and oedema are late developments and may be a consequence of fluid therapy. Other features are related to the development of complications (see the first information box) which are considered below in the management of the condition.

Table 10.8 Clinical grading of hepatic encephalopathy

Clinical grade	Clinical signs
Grade 1	Poor concentration, slurred speech, slow mentation, disordered sleep rhythm
Grade 2	Drowsy but easily rousable, occasional aggressive behaviour, lethargic
Grade 3	Marked confusion, drowsy, sleepy but responds to pain and voice, gross disorientation
Grade 4	Unresponsive to voice, may or may not respond to painful stimuli, unconscious

Investigations

Investigations are used to determine the cause of the liver failure and the prognosis (see the information boxes). The prothrombin time rapidly becomes prolonged as coagulation factor synthesis fails; this is the laboratory test of greatest prognostic value and it should be measured at least twice daily. The plasma bilirubin reflects the degree of jaundice. Plasma aminotransferase activity is particularly high after paracetamol overdose, reaching 100 to 500 times the normal activity, but falls as liver damage progresses and is not helpful in determining prognosis. Plasma albumin concentration remains normal unless the course is prolonged. Percutaneous liver biopsy is contraindicated because of the severe coagulopathy, but can be undertaken by the transjugular route. Liver biopsy is particularly helpful in patients with suspected malignancy.

COMPLICATIONS OF ACUTE HEPATIC FAILURE

- Encephalopathy
- Cerebral oedema
- Respiratory failure
- Hypotension
- Hypothermia
- Infection
- Bleeding
- Pancreatitis
- Renal failure
- Metabolic
  - Hypoglycaemia
  - Hypokalaemia
  - Hypocalcaemia
  - Hypomagnesaemia
  - Acid-base disturbance

INVESTIGATIONS TO DETERMINE THE CAUSE OF ACUTE LIVER FAILURE

- Toxicology screen of blood and urine
- IgM anti-HBs
- IgM anti-HAV
- Anti-HEV, cytomegalovirus (CMV), herpes simplex, Epstein–Barr virus (EBV)
- Caeruloplasmin, serum copper, urinary copper
- Autoantibodies: ANF, AMA, ASMA, LKM
- Ultrasound of liver and Doppler of hepatic veins
- Chest radiograph

PROGNOSTIC CRITERIA IN ACUTE HEPATIC FAILURE*
Paracetamol overdose
• pH < 7.3 at or beyond 24 hours following the overdose *or* • Serum creatinine > 300 μmol/l, prothrombin time > 100 seconds and encephalopathy grade 3 or 4
Non-paracetamol cases
• Prothrombin time > 100 seconds *or* • Any three of the following: Jaundice to encephalopathy > 7 days Age < 10 or > 40 years Indeterminate or drug-induced causes Bilirubin > 300 μmol/l Prothrombin time > 50 seconds
* Predict a mortality rate of ≥ 90%.

OBSERVATIONS IN FULMINANT HEPATIC FAILURE
Neurological
• Conscious level • Pupils—size, equality, reactivity • Fundi—papilloedema • Plantar responses
Cardiorespiratory
• Pulse • Blood pressure • Central venous pressure • Respiratory rate
Fluid balance
• Input—oral, intravenous • Output Hourly urine output, 24-hour sodium output Vomiting, diarrhoea
Blood analyses
• Peripheral blood count (including platelets) • Creatinine, urea • Sodium, potassium, HCO_2^-, calcium, magnesium • Glucose (2-hourly in acute phase) • Prothrombin time
Infection surveillance
• Cultures—blood, urine, throat, sputum, cannula sites • Chest radiograph • Temperature

Complications

Life-threatening complications, some amenable to conservative therapy, can arise during management (see the information box).

Management

A patient with acute hepatic damage should be observed in a high-dependency or intensive care unit as soon as a progressively prolonging prothrombin time or hepatic encephalopathy is identified (see the information box) so that prompt treatment of complications can be initiated. Conservative treatment aims to maintain life in the hope that hepatic regeneration will occur, but early transfer to a specialised unit should always be considered. Liver transplantation is an increasingly important treatment for acute hepatic failure, and criteria have been developed to identify patients unlikely to survive without a transplant. Patients should, wherever possible, be transferred to a transplant centre before these criteria are met to allow time for assessment of the patient and maximise the time for a donor liver to become available. Survival following liver transplantation for acute liver failure is improving with increasing experience and 1-year survival rates of about 60% can be expected. Survival without transplantation is under 10%. N-acetylcysteine (at the same dose as is administered following paracetamol overdosage—see p. 1119—but continuing the infusion at 6.25 mg/kg hourly) is given from the outset in many specialist units, as its use has been reported to improve survival, regardless of aetiology. The reasons for this are unknown but may include improved oxygen delivery to peripheral tissues.

CHRONIC LIVER FAILURE

Chronic liver disease and chronic liver failure are not synonymous terms, although the former can eventually lead to the latter. Chronic liver disease causes many clinical features, such as are seen in cirrhosis (see p. 707), and chronic liver failure develops when liver function can no longer maintain normal physiological conditions. The term 'hepatic decompensation' is often used when chronic liver failure occurs and may be precipitated by a number of events including infection or variceal haemorrhage. Chronic liver failure is a syndrome characterised by clinical and laboratory features including ascites and oedema due to sodium retention by the kidneys, the normal function of which is dependent on liver function; hepatic encephalopathy due to brain dysfunction consequent on liver failure; jaundice due to inadequate hepatic bilirubin transport; and hypoalbuminaemia and coagulation abnormality due to deficient hepatic protein synthesis.

RENAL FAILURE

Renal failure consequent on liver failure can occur in cirrhosis. The kidneys themselves are intrinsically normal and renal failure is thought to result from altered systemic blood flow including diminished renal blood flow. The condition is called 'functional renal failure of cirrhosis' or the 'hepatorenal syndrome'. It occurs in advanced cirrhosis, almost always with ascites, and uraemia is characterised by the absence of proteinuria or abnormal urinary sediment, a urine sodium excretion below 10 mmol/day, and a urine/plasma osmolality ratio greater than 1.5. It is important to exclude hypovolaemia by measuring the central venous pressure and giving colloidal solutions such as human albumin solutions to maintain the pressure at 0–5 cm of water. The treatment of hepatorenal syndrome includes giving dopamine (1–2 μg/kg/min) to maximise renal blood flow and thereafter diuretics. Uraemia and endogenous protein breakdown should be limited by restricting protein intake to 20 g/day and giving 300 g of carbohydrate daily. Recovery depends ultimately on improvement of liver function but in chronic liver disease this seldom occurs. Accordingly, the prognosis is very poor unless liver transplantation can be undertaken.

FURTHER INFORMATION ON MAJOR MANIFESTATIONS OF LIVER DISEASE

Cordoba J, Blei A T 1997 Treatment of hepatic encephalopathy. American Journal of Gastroenterology 92: 1429–1439
Grace N D 1997 Diagnosis and treatment of gastrointestinal bleeding secondary to portal hypertension. American Journal of Gastroenterology 92: 1081–1091
Jalan R, Hayes P C 1997 Hepatic encephalopathy and ascites. Lancet 350: 1309–1315
Lee W M 1996 Management of acute liver failure. Seminars in Liver Disease 16: 369–378
Record C O 1991 Neurochemistry of hepatic encephalopathy. Gut 32: 1261–1263
Riordan S M, Williams R 1997 Treatment of hepatic encephalopathy. New England Journal of Medicine 337: 473–479
Runyon B A 1994 Care of patients with ascites. New England Journal of Medicine 330: 337–342
Stanley A J, Hayes P C 1997 Portal hypertension and variceal haemorrhage. Lancet 350: 1235–1239

PARENCHYMAL LIVER DISEASE

Parenchymal liver disease may be classified clinically as acute (< 6 months) or chronic (> 6 months), or on a histological basis. The histological features of liver disease are often diverse and variable, with several features occurring together. Broadly, however, parenchymal liver disease can be classified into fatty liver (steatosis), hepatitis and cirrhosis.

STEATOSIS

Mild steatosis involving less than 10% of hepatocytes is normal; more severe steatosis is seen in a number of other conditions (see the information box). It is often detected incidentally, and its clinical manifestations are very variable.

CAUSES OF STEATOSIS (FATTY LIVER) AND STEATOHEPATITIS

Macrovesicular steatosis/ steatohepatitis	Microvesicular steatosis
• Alcohol • Obesity • Diabetes mellitus • Rapid weight reduction • Starvation (kwashiorkor) • Malabsorption • Parenteral nutrition • Intestinal bypass operations • Drugs (amiodarone, minocycline, iron)	• Fatty liver of pregnancy • Reye's syndrome • Inherited metabolic disorders (e.g. urea cycle defect, fatty acid oxidation defects, Wolman's disease, Alpers' syndrome) • Drugs (e.g. sodium valproate, ketoprofen, aspirin, didanosine)

Pathology

Steatosis may be macrovesicular where a single fat globule fills the liver cell and pushes the nucleus to the periphery, or microvesicular where small fat vacuoles give the liver cell a foamy appearance and the nucleus remains central. Macrovesicular steatosis, with or without some microvesicular steatosis, is common and generally benign. Microvesicular steatosis occurs in more serious conditions and can be associated with mitochondrial damage which causes impaired oxidative metabolism. Steatosis is usually not associated with any inflammatory infiltrate or fibrosis within the liver. However, in some patients macrovesicular steatosis occurs with associated neutrophilic infiltrate, liver cell death and, rarely, Mallory's hyaline. This histological change has been termed steatohepatitis. Steatohepatitis may be caused by alcohol abuse; however, in some patients with other causes (see the information box) there is no history of excessive alcohol consumption. Such patients have so-called non-alcoholic steatohepatitis or NASH.

Clinical features and management

Macrovesicular steatosis is often asymptomatic or is associated with the clinical features of its cause, such as diabetes mellitus. It is therefore often found incidentally. Hepatomegaly sometimes with hepatic tenderness is the only clinical feature. Liver function tests usually show mild non-specific abnormalities and ultrasonography shows generally increased echogenicity (bright liver). The treatment is that of the underlying disorder. Ursodeoxycholic acid may improve the liver function tests and the histological appearances in patients with non-alcoholic steatohepatitis (NASH).

Microvesicular steatosis may be associated with the acute onset of fatigue and vomiting, progressing if severe to encephalopathy and coma. Jaundice occurs with fatty liver of pregnancy, alcohol and sometimes drug-induced steatosis, but is typically absent in Reye's syndrome. Acute hepatic failure due to microvesicular steatosis may require intensive care support or emergency liver transplantation.

Prognosis

The outlook for most patients with steatosis is excellent, although a few deaths have been reported. In patients with alcoholic steatosis, the severity of the fatty change can predict the eventual progression to cirrhosis. Previously, the prognosis of patients with acute fatty liver of pregnancy was considered poor. However, milder forms of this condition are now more frequently recognised.

HEPATITIS

In this disorder there is inflammation of the liver which results in damage to hepatocytes with subsequent cell death. Acute injury is generally followed by complete recovery. Prolonged inflammation may be accompanied by fibrosis and progression to cirrhosis. The most common causes of hepatitis are listed in the information box.

CAUSES OF HEPATITIS

Viral infections
- Hepatitis A virus
- Hepatitis B virus
- Hepatitis C virus
- Hepatitis D virus
- Hepatitis E
- EBV, CMV, herpes simplex

Autoimmune disorders
- Autoimmune chronic hepatitis
- Toxins
- Alcohol
- Drugs, e.g. isoniazid, rifampicin, halothane, chlorpromazine

Miscellaneous
- Wilson's disease
- α_1-antitrypsin deficiency

Pathology

The histological appearances in hepatitis are generally classified as acute or chronic but they are not always readily separable and areas of overlap occur.

Acute hepatitis

The pathology of acute hepatitis depends on the cause of the damage. Lesions in acute viral hepatitis and most instances of acute damage due to drugs are similar. Cell damage occurs throughout the liver, particularly in centrilobular areas, though individual lobules are variably affected. Damaged hepatocytes are swollen and granular, while dead ones become shrunken and deeply stained acidophilic bodies. These changes, originally described in yellow fever (Councilman bodies), are strong indicators of acute hepatitis. The lobules may be infiltrated with mononuclear cells (lobulitis). Polymorphonuclear leucocytes and fatty change are not seen except in occasional cases of tetracycline or carbon tetrachloride poisoning. The portal tracts are enlarged and contain a predominantly mononuclear cell infiltrate (triaditis). More severe damage is accompanied by collapse of the reticulin framework, particularly between the central veins and portal tracts, which become linked to one another; this is known as bridging or subacute hepatic necrosis. Very severe damage destroys whole lobules (massive necrosis) and is the lesion underlying most instances of acute hepatic failure. Cholestasis is occasionally prominent.

Chronic hepatitis

Chronic hepatitis is characterised by a mononuclear inflammatory cell infiltrate of the portal tracts (see Fig. 10.16). When this infiltrate is confined to the portal tract and is associated with a normal lobular architecture, the condition is regarded as mild and progression to cirrhosis is uncommon. Invasion of inflammatory cells into the periportal parenchyma with loss of definition of the portal-periportal interface (limiting plate), damage to the periportal hepatocytes and formation of hepatocyte 'rosettes' is termed interface hepatitis. Interface hepatitis is often associated with progressive parenchymal damage and fibrosis leading to cirrhosis. Histological or immunohistochemical staining of liver tissue may help in confirming the specific aetiology of a chronic hepatitis, such as with hepatitis B.

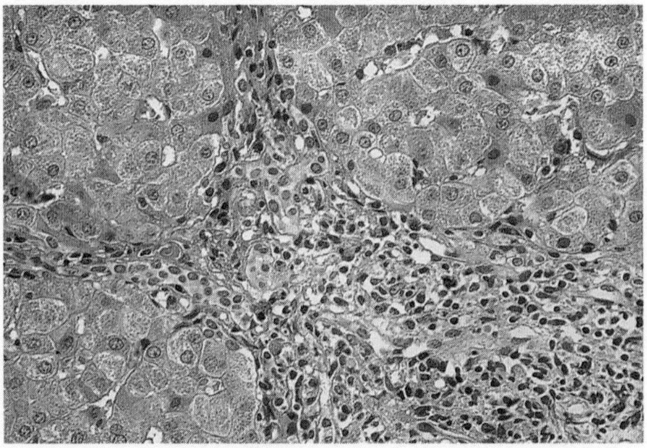

Fig. 10.16 Chronic active hepatitis.

Clinical features and management

The clinical manifestations of acute and chronic hepatitis are discussed in more detail within the specific aetiological sections. However, patients with either acute or chronic hepatitis often initially develop non-specific symptoms such as fatigue, nausea, anorexia and difficulty in concentrating. Jaundice is not always present. Upper abdominal discomfort and pain may occur with active hepatitis. Severe hepatitis may be associated with acute liver failure manifest by encephalopathy, increasing jaundice and prolongation of the prothrombin time. Treatment depends on the specific aetiology of the hepatitis and is discussed below in the appropriate section.

Prognosis

The prognosis of acute hepatitis depends on the aetiology and is discussed below in the specific sections. Prognostic factors requiring consideration of liver transplantation in acute hepatic failure are discussed above (see p. 704). The prognosis of chronic hepatitis also depends on its aetiology and, more importantly, on the efficacy of any treatment in the prevention of progression to cirrhosis. Specific treatments are discussed below in the appropriate sections.

CIRRHOSIS OF THE LIVER

Hepatic cirrhosis can occur at any age and often causes prolonged morbidity. It frequently manifests itself in younger adults and is an important cause of premature death. Causes are listed in the information box.

CAUSES OF CIRRHOSIS

- Any cause of chronic hepatitis
- Alcohol
- Primary biliary cirrhosis
- Primary sclerosing cholangitis
- Secondary biliary cirrhosis (stones, strictures)
- Haemochromatosis
- Wilson's disease
- α_1-antitrypsin deficiency

Pathology

The changes in cirrhosis affect the whole liver but not necessarily every lobule (see Fig. 10.17). They include progressive and widespread death of liver cells associated with inflammation and fibrosis leading to loss of the normal lobular liver architecture. Destruction of the liver architecture causes distortion and loss of the normal hepatic vasculature with the development of portal-systemic vascular shunts, and the formation of nodules rather than lobules due to the proliferation of surviving hepatocytes. The evolution of cirrhosis is gradual and progressive, and consequently cirrhotic livers have an infinitely variable appearance, limiting the usefulness of anatomical classifications. The current classification includes micronodular cirrhosis, characterised by regular connective tissue septa, regenerative nodules approximating in size to the original lobules (1 mm in diameter) and involvement of every lobule; and macronodular cirrhosis, in which the connective tissue septa vary in thickness and the nodules show marked differences in size, with large ones containing histologically normal lobules. Micronodular cirrhosis tends to evolve gradually into macronodular cirrhosis, and intermediate mixed forms are seen.

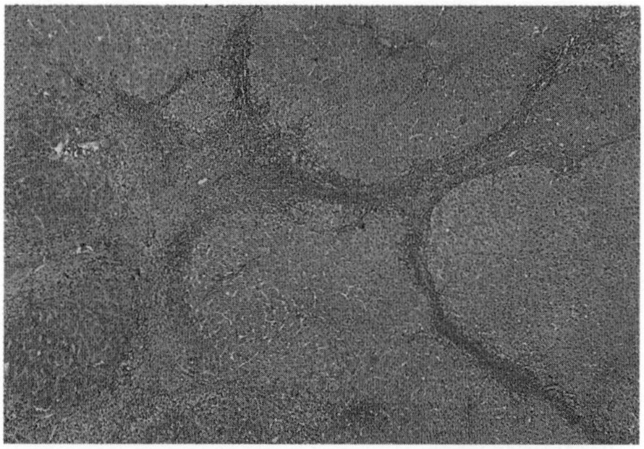

Fig. 10.17 Histology of cirrhosis of the liver revealing regeneration nodules surrounded by dense connective tissue.

Clinical features

These vary greatly and include any combination of the manifestations described below. Autopsy series have highlighted the fact that cirrhosis may be entirely asymptomatic, and in life may be found incidentally at surgery or may be associated with minimal features such as isolated hepatomegaly. Frequent complaints include weakness, fatigue, muscle cramps, weight loss and non-specific digestive symptoms such as anorexia, nausea, vomiting, upper abdominal discomfort and gaseous abdominal distension. Otherwise, clinical features are due mainly to hepatic insufficiency and portal hypertension (see the information box).

Hepatomegaly is common, but progressive hepatocyte destruction and fibrosis gradually reduce liver size as the disease progresses. The liver is often hard, irregular and painless. Jaundice is usually mild when it first appears and is due primarily to a failure to excrete bilirubin. Mild haemolysis occurs in cirrhosis but is not important in the development of jaundice. Palmar erythema can be seen early in the disease, but it is of limited diagnostic value as it occurs in many other conditions associated with a hyperdynamic circulation as well as in some normal

CLINICAL FEATURES OF HEPATIC CIRRHOSIS

Hepatomegaly

Jaundice

Ascites

Circulatory changes
- Spider telangiectasia, palmar erythema, cyanosis

Endocrine changes
- Loss of libido, hair loss
- Men: gynaecomastia, testicular atrophy, impotence
- Women: breast atrophy, irregular menses, amenorrhoea

Haemorrhagic tendency
- Bruises, purpura, epistaxis, menorrhagia

Portal hypertension
- Splenomegaly, collateral vessels, variceal bleeding, fetor hepaticus

Hepatic (portasystemic) encephalopathy

Other features
- Pigmentation, digital clubbing, low-grade fever

people. Spider telangiectasia are due to associated arteriolar changes and comprise a central arteriole (which occasionally raises the skin surface) from which small vessels radiate. They vary in size from 1–2 mm to 1–2 cm in diameter, are usually found only above the nipples, and can occur early in the disease. One or two small spider telangiectasia are found in about 2% of healthy people and they can occur transiently in greater numbers in the third trimester of pregnancy, but otherwise are a strong indicator of liver disease. Florid spider telangiectasia, gynaecomastia and parotid enlargement are most common in alcoholic cirrhosis. Pigmentation is most striking in haemochromatosis and in any cirrhosis associated with prolonged cholestasis. Pulmonary arteriovenous shunts also develop, leading to hypoxaemia and eventually to central cyanosis, but this is a late feature.

Endocrine changes are noticed more readily in men, who show loss of male hair distribution and testicular atrophy. Gynaecomastia is infrequent and can be due to drugs such as spironolactone. Easy bruising becomes more frequent as cirrhosis advances, and epistaxis is common and sometimes severe; it can mimic upper gastrointestinal bleeding if the blood is swallowed. Splenomegaly, collateral vessel formation and fetor hepaticus are features of portal hypertension, which occurs in more advanced disease (see p. 693). Haemorrhoids are often said to be more common in patients with portal hypertension but there is no evidence for this. Ascites is due to a combination of liver failure and portal hypertension (see p. 698) and signifies advanced disease. Evidence of hepatic encephalopathy also becomes increasingly common with advancing disease (see p. 700). Non-specific features of chronic liver disease include pigmentation, clubbing of the fingers and toes, and low-grade fever. Dupuytren's contracture is traditionally regarded as being associated with cirrhosis, especially that due to alcohol, but the evidence for this association is weak.

Management

This includes the treatment of any known cause (discussed below), the maintenance of nutrition, and treatment of the complications of cirrhosis (discussed above). Chronic liver failure due to cirrhosis can also be treated by orthotopic liver transplantation which currently accounts for about three-quarters of all liver transplant operations. Liver transplantation is most commonly undertaken in patients with cholestatic forms of cirrhosis, especially primary biliary cirrhosis, alcoholic cirrhosis and cirrhosis due to hepatitis C virus. Patients with alcoholic cirrhosis need to show a capacity for abstinence. Rarer indications include metabolic diseases such as α_1-antitrypsin deficiency and haemochromatosis. Signs of liver failure pointing to the need for transplantation include sustained or increased jaundice (bilirubin > 100 mmol/l in cholestatic diseases such as primary biliary cirrhosis), ascites or hepatic encephalopathy not responding readily to medical therapy, and hypoalbuminaemia (< 30 g/l). Fatigue and lethargy affecting the quality of life, intractable itching in cholestatic disease, and recurrent variceal bleeding are additional indications. The main contraindications are sepsis, the acquired immunodeficiency syndrome (AIDS), extrahepatic malignancy, active alcohol or other substance abuse and marked cardiorespiratory or renal dysfunction not attributable to hepatic disease. Survival at 1 year after transplantation is about 80%, and the prognosis thereafter is good.

Prognosis

The overall prognosis in cirrhosis is poor. Many patients present with advanced disease and/or serious complications that carry a high mortality. Overall, only 25% of patients survive 5 years from diagnosis, but where liver function is good, 50% survive for 5 years and 25% for up to 10 years. The prognosis is more favourable where the underlying cause of the cirrhosis can be corrected, as in alcohol abuse, haemochromatosis and Wilson's disease.

Laboratory tests give only a rough guide to prognosis in individual patients. Deteriorating liver function as evidenced by jaundice, ascites or encephalopathy indicates a poor prognosis unless a treatable cause such as infection is found. Increasing plasma bilirubin, falling plasma albumin or an albumin concentration < 30 g/l, marked hyponatraemia (< 120 mmol/l not due to diuretic therapy), and a prolonged prothrombin time are all bad prognostic signs (see Table 10.9). The course of cirrhosis is uncertain, as unforeseen complications such as variceal bleeding may lead to death unexpectedly.

Table 10.9 Child–Pugh classification of prognosis in cirrhosis

Score	1	2	3
Encephalopathy	None	Mild	Marked
Bilirubin (μmol/l)	< 34	34–50	> 50
Albumin (g/l)	> 35	28–35	< 28
Prothrombin time (s prolonged)	< 4	4–6	> 6
Ascites	None	Mild	Marked
Bilirubin (in primary biliary cirrhosis and sclerosing cholangitis)	< 68	68–170	> 170

Add the individual scores: < 7 = Child's A; 7–9 = Child's B; and > 9 = Child's C. The survival for Child's C, the poorest prognostic group, is less than 12 months.

SPECIFIC CAUSES OF PARENCHYMAL LIVER DISEASE

VIRAL HEPATITIS

Viral hepatitis is almost always caused by one or other of the specific hepatitis viruses; hepatitis due to other viruses accounts for only about 1–2% of cases (see the information box). All these viruses give rise to illnesses which are similar in their clinical and pathological features and which are frequently anicteric or asymptomatic. Table 10.10 summarises the features of the major hepatitis viruses.

CAUSES OF VIRAL HEPATITIS

- Hepatitis A virus
- Hepatitis B virus
- Hepatitis C virus
- Hepatitis D virus
- Hepatitis E virus
- Non-A non-B non-C viral hepatitis
- Cytomegalovirus
- Epstein–Barr virus
- Herpes simplex virus
- Yellow fever virus

Virology

The hepatitis viruses (A–E) all cause primarily hepatic illness in humans but otherwise are quite distinct and belong to separate virus groups.

Hepatitis A

The hepatitis A virus (HAV) belongs to the picornavirus group of enteroviruses and, although it can be cultured, this is only done for research purposes. HAV is highly infectious and is spread by the faecal-oral route by persons incubating or suffering from the disease. Infected persons excrete viruses in the faeces for about 2–3 weeks before the onset of the illness and for up to 2 weeks thereafter. Children are most commonly affected and conditions of overcrowding and poor sanitation facilitate spread. In occasional outbreaks water, milk and shellfish have been the vehicles of transmission. Though faeces are the usual source, a transient viraemia in the incubation period occasionally allows infection to be spread by blood and by homosexual activity, especially in men. A chronic carrier state, analogous to that for hepatitis B virus, does not occur.

Hepatitis B

The hepatitis B virus (HBV) is the only hepadna virus causing infection in humans. It cannot yet be grown but can be transmitted to certain primates, such as the chimpanzee, in which it replicates. It comprises a capsule and a core containing DNA and a DNA polymerase enzyme (see Fig. 10.18). The virus and an excess of its capsular material circulate in the blood, where it can be identified (see

Table 10.10 Features of the main hepatitis viruses

	Hepatitis A	Hepatitis B	Hepatitis C	Hepatitis D	Hepatitis E
Virus					
Group	Enterovirus	Hepadna	Flavivirus	Incomplete virus	Caliciviruses
Nucleic acid	RNA	DNA	RNA	RNA	RNA
Size (diameter)	27 nm	42 nm	30–38 nm	35 nm	27 nm
Incubation (weeks)	2–4	4–20	2–26	6–9	3–8
Spread					
Faeces	Yes	No	No	No	Yes
Blood	Uncommon	Yes	Yes	Yes	No
Saliva*	Yes	Yes	Yes	?	?
Sexual	Uncommon	Yes	Uncommon	Yes	?
Vertical	No	Yes	Uncommon	Yes	No
Chronic infection	No	Yes (5–10%)	Yes (> 50%)	Yes	No
Prevention					
Active	Vaccine	Vaccine	No	Prevented by prevention of hepatitis B virus infection	No
Passive	Immune serum globulin	Hyperimmune serum globulin	No		No

* All body fluids are potentially infectious, though some (e.g. urine) are less infectious.

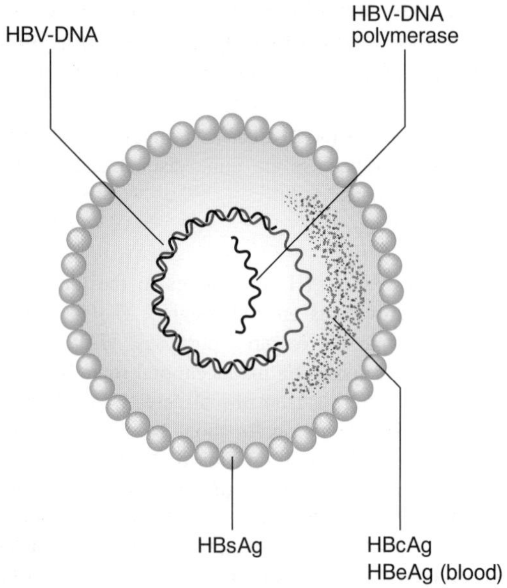

Fig. 10.18 Schematic diagram of hepatitis B virus.

p. 712). Humans are the only source of infection. Individuals incubating or suffering from acute hepatitis are highly infectious for at least as long as the HBsAg is in the blood. Patients with chronic infections may be asymptomatic or have chronic liver failure. These individuals are most infectious when markers of continuing viral replication such as HBeAg, HBV-DNA or DNA polymerase are present in the blood, and are least infectious when these are absent and only anti-HBe is present.

Blood is the main source of infection and spread may follow transfusion of infected blood or blood products or result from injections with contaminated needles, a mode of spread most common among parenteral drug abusers who share needles. Blood and blood products used for transfusion are no longer a major source of infection, provided that donor blood is tested for the virus, and less than 10% of all post-transfusion hepatitis is now attributable to the HBV. Only products such as albumin solutions and gammaglobulin which are pasteurised are wholly free of risk. Tattooing or acupuncture can also spread this disease if inadequately sterilised needles are used.

HBV can also cause sporadic infections which cannot be attributed to parenteral modes of spread. The means of non-parenteral transmission are uncertain, but the discovery of the HBsAg or HBV-DNA in body fluids such as saliva, urine, semen and vaginal secretions suggests many mechanisms. Close personal contact seems necessary for transmission of infection, and sexual intercourse, especially in male homosexuals, is an important route. The virus may be spread vertically from mother to child in the immediate perinatal period.

Hepatitis C

The hepatitis C virus (HCV) is an RNA-containing flavivirus which cannot yet be grown but which can infect primates (see Fig. 10.19). Humans seem to be the sole source of infection, and inoculation with blood or blood products is the best-recognised mode of transmission. HCV caused over 90% of post-transfusion hepatitis before serological tests allowed the screening of blood donors, and accounted for the high incidence of chronic hepatitis in patients with haemophilia. Screening of blood donors and heat treatment of coagulation factor concentrates should prevent infection in future. Parenteral drug abusers continue to be at high risk of HCV infection. Sporadic HCV infection also occurs but the modes of transmission are unknown. Sexual and vertical spread may occur but are less common than in HBV infection. Chronic infection occurs in about 70–80% of patients and this is usually life-long. Most never suffer an acute illness. Lifelong preventive measures are required to limit infection of other individuals.

Hepatitis D

The hepatitis D virus (HDV) is an RNA defective virus which has no independent existence; it requires the HBV

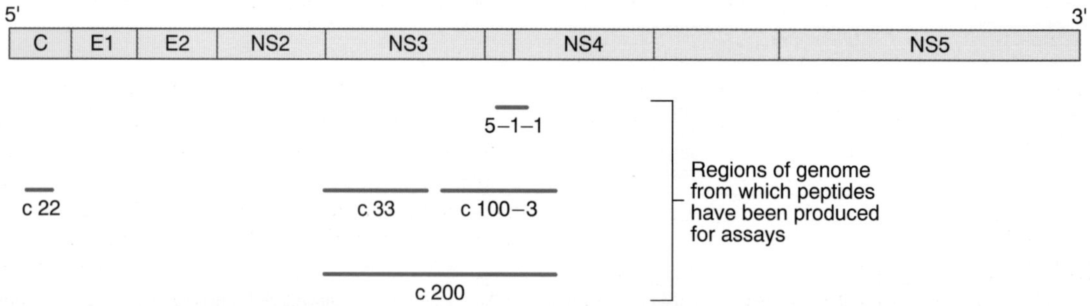

Fig. 10.19 Schematic diagram of hepatitis C virus. RNA coding regions. (C = core protein; E = envelope proteins; NS = non-structural proteins)

for replication and has the same sources and modes of spread as HBV. It can infect individuals simultaneously with HBV, or it can superinfect those who are already chronic carriers of HBV. Simultaneous infections give rise to acute hepatitis which is often severe but is limited by recovery from the HBV infection. Infections in individuals who are chronic carriers of the HBV can cause acute infection with spontaneous recovery, and occasionally simultaneous cessation of the chronic HBV infection occurs. Chronic infection with the HBV and the HDV can also occur, and this frequently causes more rapidly progressive chronic hepatitis and eventually cirrhosis. HDV has been reported recently in the absence of HBV following liver transplantation; how the HDV maintains itself in such instances is unknown.

HDV has a world-wide distribution. It is endemic in parts of the Mediterranean basin, Africa and South America where transmission is mainly by close personal contact, and occasionally by vertical transmission from mothers who also carry the hepatitis B virus. In non-endemic areas, transmission is mainly a consequence of parenteral drug abuse.

Hepatitis E

The hepatitis E virus (HEV) is an RNA virus which is excreted in the stools and spreads by the faecal-oral route. It is found in countries where sanitation is poor and causes large epidemics of water-borne hepatitis. Occasional cases are recognised in patients in developed countries following a visit to an area where infection is endemic. The clinical illness resembles acute HAV infection and recovery is the rule, but pregnant women have a high risk of acute hepatic failure. Chronic infection does not occur.

Other (non-A, non-B, non-C) hepatitis

Non-A, non-B (NANB) hepatitis was the term used previously to describe hepatitis thought to be due to a virus but not HAV or HBV. HCV and HEV are the main hepatitis viruses to emerge from this group. Further such viruses do exist, but the hepatitis viruses described above now account for the majority of hepatitis virus infections. Cytomegalovirus and Epstein–Barr virus infection causes abnormal liver function tests in most patients, and occasionally icteric hepatitis occurs. Herpes simplex is a rare cause of hepatitis in adults, most of whom are immunocompromised, and yellow fever virus causes hepatitis in parts of the world where it is endemic. Abnormal liver function tests are also common in chickenpox, measles, rubella and acute HIV infection.

Clinical features

Prodromal symptoms usually precede the development of jaundice by a few days to 2 weeks. They are the common manifestations of an acute infectious disease and include chills, headache and malaise. Gastrointestinal symptoms may be prominent; anorexia and distaste for cigarettes are frequent, and nausea, vomiting and diarrhoea may follow. A steady upper abdominal pain, occasionally severe, occurs as a result of stretching of the peritoneum over the enlarged liver. Initially physical signs are scanty; the liver is usually tender though not readily palpable, enlarged cervical lymph nodes may be found, and splenomegaly may occur, particularly in children. Patients with HBV infection often have arthralgia during the prodrome, and occasionally a 'serum sickness syndrome' with skin rashes (including urticaria) and polyarthritis occurs.

Dark urine and a yellow tint to the sclerae herald the onset of jaundice. As obstruction to the biliary canaliculi develops, the jaundice deepens, the stools become paler, the urine darker, and the liver more easily palpable. At this time the appetite often improves and gastrointestinal symptoms diminish in intensity. Thereafter the jaundice recedes, the stools and urine regain their normal colour, the liver enlargement regresses, and in the course of 3–6 weeks the majority of patients recover. Mild illnesses may run an anicteric course recognised only because of known contact with a definite case or by the association of vague gastrointestinal complaints or malaise with bilirubinuria and biochemical evidence of hepatic dysfunction.

Investigations

A plasma aminotransferase activity exceeding 400 U/l, even before jaundice develops, is the most striking abnormality. The plasma bilirubin reflects the severity of the jaundice. The alkaline phosphatase activity rarely exceeds 250 U/l unless marked cholestasis develops, and the albumin concentration is normal. Prolongation of the prothrombin time is a reliable indication of severe liver damage (see p. 686). Bilirubinuria is an early finding, occurring in the prodromal phase and usually continuing into the convalescent period. Mild proteinuria may be present. The white cell count is normal or low in uncomplicated cases, sometimes with a relative lymphocytosis; this is of some value in differentiation from Weil's disease (see p. 137). Serological tests can identify HAV, HBV, HEV, cytomegalovirus and Epstein–Barr infection but are unreliable in acute HCV infection. Differential diagnosis is discussed on page 706.

Specific virological tests

Hepatitis A. Only one hepatitis A virus (HAV) antigen has been found, and individuals infected with the HAV make an antibody to this antigen (anti-HAV). Anti-HAV is important in diagnosis as the HAV is only present in the blood transiently during the incubation period. Excretion in the stools occurs for only 7–14 days after the onset of the clinical illness and the virus cannot be grown readily. Anti-HAV of IgM type, indicating a primary immune response, is already present in the blood at the onset of the clinical illness and is diagnostic of an acute HAV infection. Titres of this antibody fall to low levels within about 3 months of

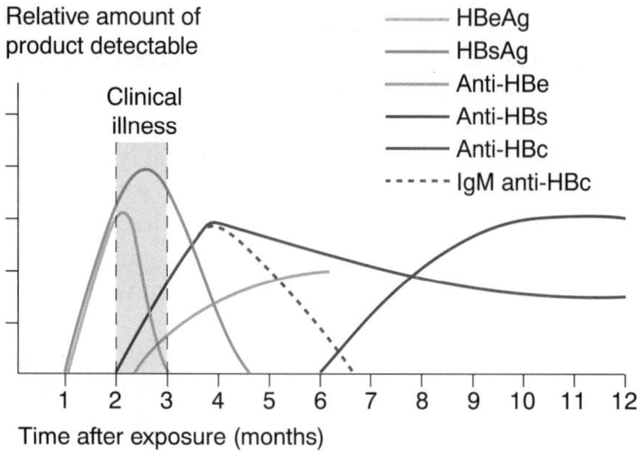

Fig. 10.20 Serological responses to hepatitis B virus infection. (HBsAG = hepatitis B surface antigen; anti-HBs = antibody to HBsAg; HBeAg = hepatitis B e antigen; anti-HBe = antibody to HBeAg; anti-HBc = antibody to hepatitis B core antigen)

recovery. Anti-HAV of IgG type is of no diagnostic value as HAV infection is common and this antibody persists for years after infection, but it can be used to measure the prevalence of HAV infection. Its presence indicates immunity to HAV.

Hepatitis B. The hepatitis B virus (HBV) contains several antigens to which infected persons can make immune responses (see Fig. 10.20); these antigens and their antibodies are important in identifying HBV infection (see Table 10.11).

In acute infection the hepatitis B surface antigen (HBsAg) is a reliable marker of HBV infection, and a negative test for the HBsAg makes HBV infection very unlikely but not impossible (see Fig. 10.20). HBsAg appears in the blood late in the incubation period and before the prodromal phase of acute type B hepatitis; it may be present for only a few days, disappearing even before jaundice has developed, but usually lasts for 3–4 weeks and can persist for up to 5 months. Antibody to HBsAg (anti-HBs) usually appears after about 3–6 months and persists for many years or perhaps permanently. Anti-HBs implies either a previous infection, in which case anti-HBc (see below) is usually also present, or previous vaccination if anti-HBc is not present. The hepatitis B core antigen (HBcAg) is not found in the blood, but antibody to it (anti-HBc) appears early in the illness and rapidly reaches a high titre which then subsides gradually and persists. Anti-HBc is initially of IgM type with IgG antibody appearing later. Anti-HBc (IgM) can sometimes reveal an acute HBV infection when the HBsAg has disappeared and before anti-HBs has developed (see Fig. 10.20). The hepatitis Be antigen (HBeAg) appears only transiently at the outset of the illness and is followed by the production of antibody (anti-HBe). The HBeAg reflects active replication of the virus in the liver.

Table 10.11 Interpretation of main investigations used in the serological diagnosis of hepatitis B virus infection

		Anti-HBc		
Interpretation	**HBsAg**	**IgM**	**IgG**	**Anti-HBs**
Incubation period	+	+	–	–
Acute hepatitis				
Early	+	+	–	–
Established	+	+	+	–
Established (occasional)	–	+	+	–
Convalescence				
(3–6 months)	–	±	+	±
(6–9 months)	–	–	+	+
Post-infection				
> 1 year	–	–	+	+
Uncertain	–	–	+	–
Chronic infection				
Usual	+	–	+	–
Occasional	–	–	+	–
Immunisation without infection	–	–	–	+

* Very variable.
+ = positive; – = negative; ± = present at low titre or absent. (HBsAg = surface antigen; anti-HBc = antibody to core antigen;anti-HBs = antibody to surface antigen)

Chronic HBV infection (see p. 714) is marked by the presence of the HBsAg and anti-HBc (IgG) in the blood (see Table 10.11). Rarely, anti-HBc (IgG) alone is the sole evidence of chronic infection. Usually, the HBeAg or anti-HBe is also present; the HBeAg indicates continued active replication of the virus in the liver while anti-HBe implies that replication is occurring at a much lower level or that HBV-DNA has become integrated into host hepatocyte DNA. Polymerase chain reactions (PCR) can show HBV-DNA in the blood, implying that viral replication is occurring. This is rarely needed for diagnosis but can be useful in selecting for, and measuring response to, therapy. Rarely, mutant forms of the virus cannot synthesise the 'e' antigen and HBV-DNA is necessary for their detection.

Hepatitis C. The HCV contains several antigens giving rise to antibodies in infected individuals and these are used in diagnosis. Previously, diagnosis depended on identifying antibody to a single viral antigen (C100), but this test gave false-positive reactions, especially in conditions such as autoimmune hepatitis associated with hyperglobulinaemia, and false-negative reactions. Current laboratory diagnosis depends on identifying antibodies to several viral antigens. These tests generally identify chronic HCV infection as the diagnostic antibodies appear irregularly in the blood during the first 3 months of illness. PCR can show HCV-RNA in the blood, but they are not used routinely for diagnosis. They can be used where antibody tests give equivocal results and in selecting for, and measuring response to, therapy.

Hepatitis D. The HDV contains a single antigen to which infected individuals make an antibody (anti-HDV). Delta antigen appears in the blood only transiently, and in practice diagnosis depends on detecting anti-HDV. Simultaneous infection with the HBV and HDV followed by full recovery is associated with the appearance of low titres of anti-HDV of IgM type occurring within a few days of the onset of the illness. This antibody generally disappears within 2 months but persists in a few patients. Superinfection of patients with chronic hepatitis B virus infection leads to the production of high titres of anti-HDV, initially IgM and later IgG. Such patients may then develop chronic infection with both viruses, in which case anti-HDV titres plateau at high levels.

Hepatitis E. Individuals infected with the hepatitis E virus (HEV) produce anti-HEV which is used in diagnosis. Routine assays for the serological identification of HEV infection should be available in the near future.

Complications

While many complications of acute viral hepatitis are recognised (see the information box), in practice serious complications are uncommon. Fatalities are rare and are usually attributable to acute hepatic failure (see p. 702). The return of symptoms and signs of acute hepatitis during recovery is characteristic of relapsing hepatitis and occurs in 5–15% of patients. Asymptomatic 'biochemical' relapses with increases of plasma aminotransferase activity are even more common. Relapsing hepatitis resolves spontaneously and does not imply a worse prognosis. Cholestasis can develop at any stage during the course of the illness, causing more severe jaundice of a clinically and biochemically obstructive type which may follow a prolonged course. Liver biopsy shows the features of hepatitis with prominent cholestasis and no evidence of chronic liver damage. This cholestatic illness may continue for many months; however, the prognosis is good.

Debility for 2–3 months is common following clinical and biochemical recovery. Sometimes, particularly in anxious patients, there may be prolonged malaise, anorexia, nausea and right hypochondrial discomfort without clinical or biochemical evidence of liver disease. This syndrome is known as the post-hepatitis syndrome.

Chronic hepatitis and cirrhosis develop when chronic HBV infection occurs, with or without HDV superinfection, or HCV infection. These chronic viral infections also predispose to hepatocellular carcinoma. Unconjugated hyperbilirubinaemia is sometimes found after acute viral hepatitis. Most instances are probably due to pre-existing Gilbert's syndrome.

Systemic complications are rare but include aplastic anaemia. This seems most common after HCV and HEV infection and may not become apparent for up to a year after the hepatic illness. Other complications are mostly related to HBV infection and include connective tissue disease, particularly polyarteritis nodosa, and renal damage such as glomerulonephritis. Henoch–Schönlein purpura and papular acrodermatitis have been reported in children.

COMPLICATIONS OF ACUTE VIRAL HEPATITIS

- Acute hepatic failure
- Relapsing hepatitis
  - Biochemical
  - Clinical
- Cholestatic hepatitis
- Post-hepatitis syndrome
- Hyperbilirubinaemia (Gilbert's syndrome)*
- Aplastic anaemia
- Connective tissue disease
- Renal failure
- Henoch–Schönlein purpura
- Papular acrodermatitis
- Chronic hepatitis
- Cirrhosis (hepatitis B, C and D viruses)
- Hepatocellular carcinoma

*Gilbert's syndrome may be brought to light by follow-up of viral hepatitis.

Management

There is no specific treatment for acute viral hepatitis. Only the more severely affected patients require care in hospital, principally to allow early detection of developing acute hepatic failure. The post-hepatitis syndrome is treated by reassurance.

Diet

A nutritious diet containing 2–3000 kcal daily is given. This is often not tolerated initially owing to anorexia and nausea, in which case a light diet supplemented by fruit drinks and glucose is usually acceptable. The content of the diet is dictated largely by the patient's wishes; however, a good protein intake should be encouraged. If vomiting is severe, intravenous fluid and glucose may be required.

Drugs

Drugs should be avoided, especially in severe hepatitis, because many are metabolised in the liver. This applies especially to sedative and hypnotic agents. Alcohol must be avoided during the illness but can be taken once clinical and biochemical recovery have occurred. Oral contraceptives may be resumed after clinical and biochemical recovery.

Interferon. Treatment of chronic hepatitis B is limited and currently interferon is the only licensed drug. It is most effective in patients with high serum transaminase concentrations and active hepatitis on biopsy, who have not acquired infection at birth and those who are HIV-negative. A response to interferon is characterised by an increase in serum aminotransferases after 6–8 weeks of therapy. Great care is necessary, therefore, in treating patients with cirrhosis as liver failure may be induced. Treatment is generally unsuccessful in those infected at birth and in immunodeficient patients.

Interferon is the only drug available for the treatment of HCV infection; elimination of the HCV-RNA from the blood after 6–12 months' treatment is achieved in only about 15% of cases. Combination therapy with interferon and ribavirin is currently being evaluated.

Surgery

Surgery during acute viral hepatitis carries a significant risk of post-operative liver failure. Only life-saving operations should be carried out.

Liver transplantation

Liver transplantation may be required for acute or chronic liver failure due to hepatitis viruses.

Prognosis

The overall mortality of acute viral hepatitis is about 0.5% in otherwise well patients under 40 years of age, but mortality reaches about 3% in patients over 60 years. Mortality may be much higher in patients with other serious diseases, such as chronic liver disease, carcinoma or lymphoma. Acute hepatic failure is rare in HAV infection and chronic infection does not occur. Pregnant women with HEV infection are particularly liable to acute hepatic failure which is associated with a high mortality but again chronic infection does not occur. Full recovery occurs in 90–95% of adults following acute HBV infection. The remaining 5–10% develop a chronic infection which usually continues for life, though later recovery occurs occasionally. Infection passing from mother to child at birth leads to chronic infection in the child in 95% of cases and recovery is rare. Chronic infection is also common in immunodeficient individuals such as those with Down's syndrome or human immunodeficiency virus (HIV) infection. Recovery from acute HBV infection occurs within 6 months and is characterised by the appearance of antibody to viral antigens. Persistence of HBeAg beyond this time indicates chronic infection. Most patients acquiring HCV infections (80%) develop a chronic infection. Chronic HBV and HCV usually remain asymptomatic for years and are not associated with an early increase in mortality. However, many patients eventually develop cirrhosis and some progress to hepatocellular carcinoma. Combined HBV and HDV cause more aggressive disease.

Prevention

Hepatitis A. Infection in the community is best prevented by improving social conditions, especially overcrowding and poor sanitation. Individuals can be given substantial protection from infection by active immunisation with an inactivated virus vaccine (Havrix). Immediate protection can be provided by immune serum globulin if this is given soon after exposure to the virus. This can be considered for those at particular risk such as close contacts, the elderly, those with other major disease and perhaps pregnant women. Immune serum globulin can be effective in an outbreak of hepatitis, in a school or nursery, as injection of those at risk prevents secondary spread to families. Persons travelling to endemic areas are protected best by vaccination, but where time is limited vaccine and immune serum globulin can be injected in separate sites to provide immediate and longer- term protection. The protective effect of immune serum globulin is attributed to its anti-HAV content and those with anti-HAV in the blood are protected naturally.

Hepatitis B. A recombinant hepatitis B vaccine containing HBsAg is available (Engerix) and is capable of producing active immunisation in 95% of normal individuals. The vaccine gives a high degree of protection and should be used particularly in those at special risk of infection who are not already immune, as evidenced by anti-HBs in the blood (see the information box). The vaccine is ineffective in those already infected by the HBV. Type B hepatitis can be prevented or minimised by the intramuscular injection of hyperimmune serum globulin prepared from blood containing anti-HBs. This should be given within 24 hours, or at most a week, of exposure to infected blood in circumstances likely to cause infection; these include accidental needle puncture, gross personal contamination with infected blood, oral ingestion or contamination of mucous membranes, or exposure to infected blood in the presence of cuts and grazes. Vaccine can be given together with hyperimmune globulin (active-passive immunisation).

Hepatitis C. There is no available active or passive protection against HCV infection.

AT-RISK GROUPS MERITING HEPATITIS B VACCINATION IN LOWLY ENDEMIC AREAS

Parenteral drug abusers

Homosexuals (male)

Close contacts of infected individuals
- Newborn of infected mothers
- Regular sexual partners

Patients on chronic haemodialysis

Medical/nursing personnel
- Dentists
- Surgeons/obstetricians
- Accident and emergency departments
- Intensive care
- Liver units
- Endoscopy units
- Oncology units

Laboratory staff handling blood

Hepatitis D. Hepatitis D is effectively prevented by preventing hepatitis B.

Hepatitis E. There is no available active or passive protection against HEV infection.

AUTOIMMUNE HEPATITIS

This form of chronic hepatitis occurs most often in women, particularly in the second and third decades of life.

Aetiology and pathology

The cause of autoimmune hepatitis remains to be identified. Several subtypes of this disorder have been proposed with differing immunological markers. Classical (type I) autoimmune hepatitis is characterised by a high frequency of other autoimmune disorders such as Graves' disease. Type I autoimmune hepatitis is associated with HLA-DR3 and DR4, particularly HLA-DRB3*0101 and HLA-DRB1*0401. These patients have high titres of antinuclear and anti-smooth muscle antibodies but none of these antibodies are cytotoxic. A suggested hypothesis for the development of type I autoimmune hepatitis is the aberrant expression on the hepatocyte of HLA antigen, influenced by viral, genetic and environmental factors. Type II autoimmune hepatitis is characterised by the presence of anti-LKM (liver–kidney microsomal) antibodies and lack of antinuclear and anti-smooth muscle antibodies. Anti-LKM antibodies recognise cytochrome P450-IID6, which is expressed on the hepatocyte membrane. The pathological features of both forms of autoimmune hepatitis are similar and are described on page 706.

Clinical features

The onset is usually insidious, with fatigue, anorexia and jaundice. In about one-quarter of patients the onset is acute, resembling viral hepatitis, but resolution does not occur. Other features include fever, arthralgia, vitiligo and epistaxis. Amenorrhoea is the rule. On examination, the general health is at first good. Jaundice is mild to moderate or occasionally absent, but signs of chronic liver disease, especially spider telangiectasia and hepatosplenomegaly, are usually present. Sometimes a 'Cushingoid' face with acne, hirsutism and pink cutaneous striae, especially on the thighs and abdomen, are present. Bruises may be seen. Though liver disease usually dominates the clinical syndrome, in florid autoimmune hepatitis many associated conditions occur, emphasising its essentially systemic nature (see the information box).

Investigations

Liver function tests vary with the activity of the disease. Active inflammation is reflected by the plasma aminotransferase activity, and the severity of liver damage by the plasma albumin concentration and prothrombin time. Aminotransferase activity is often increased more than 10-fold in relapses occurring in patients with florid disease, and hypoalbuminaemia and marked hyperglobulinaemia are common. Hyperglobulinaemia is polyclonal and due mainly to marked increases in IgG. The plasma bilirubin reflects the degree of jaundice but usually does not exceed 100 μmol/l (6 mg/dl). The plasma alkaline phosphatase activity reflects the degree of intrahepatic cholestasis.

Serological testing for specific autoantibodies may suggest autoimmune hepatitis (see Table 10.12). However, these autoantibodies are all heterogenous and can be found in apparently healthy people, particularly in women and in older people. Antinuclear antibodies occur in about 5% of healthy people and anti-smooth muscle antibody in 1.5%, but antimitochondrial antibody is rare, being found in about 0.01%. Autoantibody titres in such healthy people are usually low. Antinuclear and antimitochondrial antibodies also occur in connective tissue diseases and in autoimmune diseases, including various thyroid disorders and pernicious anaemia, while anti-smooth muscle antibody has been reported in infectious mononucleosis and a variety of malignant diseases. Antinuclear antibodies are found in half the patients with autoimmune hepatitis, smooth muscle antibodies in two-thirds, and antimitochondrial antibodies in 15% (see Table 10.12). Antimicrosomal antibodies (anti-LKM) occur particularly in children and adolescents.

Liver biopsy shows interface hepatitis with or without cirrhosis.

SYSTEMIC COMPLICATIONS OF AUTOIMMUNE HEPATITIS

- Migrating polyarthritis
- Urticarial skin rashes
- Lymphadenopathy
- Hashimoto's thyroiditis
- Thyrotoxicosis
- Myxoedema
- Coombs positive haemolytic anaemia
- Pleurisy
- Transient pulmonary infiltrates
- Ulcerative colitis
- Glomerulonephritis
- Nephrotic syndrome

Table 10.12 Approximate occurrence of antinuclear, anti-smooth muscle and antimitochondrial antibodies in chronic liver diseases not associated with chronic hepatitis virus infection

Disease	Antinuclear antibody (%)	Anti-smooth muscle antibody (%)	Antimitochondrial antibody* (%)
Autoimmune hepatitis	80	70	15
Primary biliary cirrhosis	25	35	95
Cryptogenic cirrhosis	40	30	15

* Patients with antimitochondrial antibody frequently have cholestatic liver function tests and may have primary biliary cirrhosis (see text).

Management

Treatment with corticosteroids is life-saving in autoimmune hepatitis, particularly during exacerbations of active and symptomatic disease. Initially, prednisolone 30 mg/day is given orally and the dose reduced gradually as the patient and liver function tests improve. Maintenance therapy is required for at least 2 years after liver function tests have become normal, and withdrawal of treatment should not be considered unless a liver biopsy is also normal. Side-effects from prednisolone are uncommon at a maintenance dose of 10 mg/day or less; azathioprine 50–100 mg/day orally may be added to the therapy to allow the dose of prednisolone to be reduced to this level. Corticosteroids treat and prevent acute exacerbations rather than prevent cirrhosis and are less important in asymptomatic autoimmune hepatitis with mild biochemical and histological activity.

Prognosis

The disease occurs in exacerbations and remissions, and most patients eventually develop cirrhosis and its complications (see p. 707). Hepatocellular carcinoma is uncommon. About half of patients with symptoms die of liver failure within 5 years if no treatment is given, but this falls to about 10% with therapy.

DRUGS, TOXINS AND THE LIVER

The liver is the main organ in which drugs are metabolised and consequently is important in determining the effects of drugs in the body. Liver disease may alter the capacity of the liver to metabolise drugs and unexpected toxicity may occur when patients with liver disease are given drugs in normal doses (see p. 1104).

Drugs themselves can damage the liver and there is increasing recognition of the many forms of hepatic damage attributable to them (see the information boxes).

MANIFESTATIONS OF DRUG HEPATOTOXICITY

Acute hepatic damage
- Acute hepatitis
- Cholestatic hepatitis
- Cholestasis

Abnormal liver function tests

Hepatic fibrosis

Chronic hepatitis

Cirrhosis

Hepatic vascular damage
- Budd–Chiari syndrome
- Veno-occlusive disease
- Hepatoportal sclerosis

Neoplasia
- Adenoma
- Hepatocellular carcinoma
- Haemangioma/haemangiosarcoma

THE DIAGNOSIS OF ACUTE DRUG-INDUCED LIVER DISEASE

- Consider the possibility of a drug-induced problem
- Tabulate drugs taken
  - Prescribed
  - Self-administered
- Relate drugs to the onset of the illness
- Look for pre-existing liver disease
  - Clinical examination
  - Previous liver investigations
- Consider alternative causes
  - Viral hepatitis—serological tests
  - Biliary disease—ultrasound
- Observe the effects of stopping the suspected drugs
- Liver biopsy
  - Suspected pre-existing liver disease
  - Failure to improve

N.B. Challenge tests with drugs virtually never performed.

ALCOHOLIC (ETHANOLIC) LIVER DISEASE

In many societies alcohol is the most common cause of chronic liver disease.

Aetiology and pathology

Alcohol is metabolised almost exclusively in the liver. It is first converted to acetaldehyde, mainly by the mitochondrial enzyme alcohol dehydrogenase but also by the mixed-function oxidase enzymes of the smooth endoplasmic reticulum. Alcohol is a powerful inducer of the mixed-function oxidases, thereby increasing the ability of the liver to metabolise alcohol and many drugs metabolised by these enzymes. Acetaldehyde is converted to acetate by acetaldehyde dehydrogenase, and acetate is metabolised by the Krebs cycle enzymes.

The hepatic lesions of alcoholic liver disease (see below) are attributable directly to alcohol. The risk of developing alcoholic liver disease is related directly to the amount of alcohol (any kind) ingested but is more likely to be clinically apparent at daily intakes above 30 g (3 units) in men and 20 g (2 units) in women. More than 5 years of drinking, and usually more than 10 years, are required to produce alcoholic cirrhosis, and a steady daily intake is more hazardous than intermittent drinking.

The mechanism or mechanisms underlying the ability of alcohol to produce individual liver lesions are poorly understood. Fatty change is attributed to an impaired excretion and enhanced synthesis of triacylglycerol by hepatocytes. The development of alcoholic hepatitis, fibrosis and cirrhosis is much more obscure. Biochemical mechanisms involving the production of toxic metabolites, called adducts, during the conversion of acetaldehyde to

PATHOLOGICAL FEATURES OF ALCOHOLIC LIVER DISEASE
• Mitochondrial swelling* • Proliferation of endoplasmic reticulum* • Macrovesicular or microvesicular steatosis • Lipogranulomas • Mallory's hyaline • Siderosis • Autoimmune (interface) hepatitis • Central hyaline sclerosis • Fibrosis • Cirrhosis • Hepatocellular carcinoma
* Visible on electron microscopy.

acetate and an immune reaction to liver cells altered by alcohol may be involved in these forms of liver damage. Alcohol causes several different lesions in the liver which can occur together in any combination (see the information box).

Clinical features

Alcoholic liver disease manifests as a clinical spectrum ranging from non-specific symptoms, with few or no physical abnormalities, to advanced cirrhosis. The ready availability of laboratory investigations can reveal alcoholic liver damage in patients with other diseases or in asymptomatic people undergoing medical examination. This spectrum is often divided into four syndromes (see the information box), but in reality these overlap considerably and the various pathological changes can coexist in the same liver.

CLINICAL SYNDROMES OF ALCOHOLIC LIVER DISEASE	
Fatty liver • Non-specific symptoms • Hepatomegaly **Hepatitis** • Severe illness • Malnutrition • Jaundice • Hepatomegaly • Ascites • Encephalopathy	**Cholestasis** • Jaundice • Abdominal pain • Hepatomegaly (often tender) **Cirrhosis**

Investigations

Investigations aim to establish alcohol abuse, exclude alternative causes of liver disease, and assess the severity of liver damage. The clinical history from the patient, relatives and friends is most important in establishing alcohol abuse, its duration and, in particular, severity. Biological markers of alcohol abuse suggest and support a history of alcohol abuse; the most universally used indicators are a peripheral blood macrocytosis in the absence of anaemia and increased

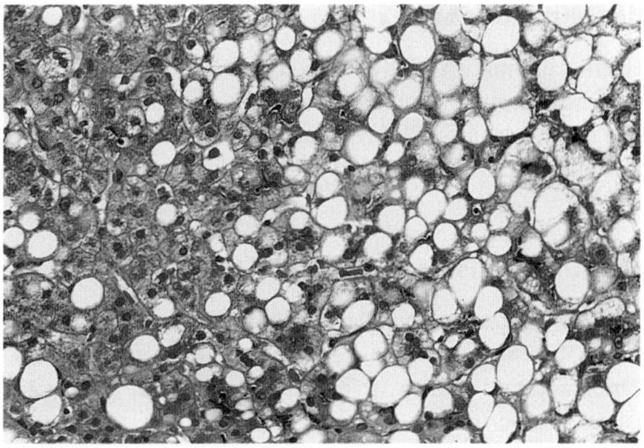

Fig. 10.21 Histology of alcoholic fatty liver. The fatty change (steatosis) is evident as fat globules within the cytoplasm of the liver cells.

plasma gamma-glutamyl transferase. Absence of these markers does not exclude alcohol abuse. Unexplained rib fractures on a chest radiograph are also associated with alcohol abuse. Investigation of the extent of liver damage often requires a liver biopsy (see Fig. 10.21), which may reveal an alternative cause for hepatic cirrhosis.

Management

Cessation of alcohol intake is the single most important treatment and without this all other therapies are of limited value. Life-long abstinence is the best advice and is essential for those with more severe liver damage. Good nutrition is also important and feeding via a fine-bore nasogastric tube may be needed in severely ill patients. Treatment for complications such as encephalopathy (see p. 700), ascites (see p. 698) and variceal bleeding (see p. 695) may be required. Corticosteroid therapy may be of some value in patients with severe alcoholic hepatitis.

Prognosis

The most important prognostic factor is the patient's ability to stop drinking alcohol. General health and longevity are improved when this occurs, irrespective of the form of alcoholic liver disease. Alcoholic fatty liver generally has a good prognosis and usually disappears after about 3 months of abstinence. Alcoholic hepatitis has a significantly worse prognosis because about one-third of patients die in the acute episode if liver function is poor, as evidenced by a prothrombin time sufficiently prolonged to preclude liver biopsy. Patients may progress to cirrhosis after recovery, particularly if drinking continues. Alcoholic cirrhosis often presents with a serious complication such as variceal bleeding or ascites, and only about one-half of such patients survive 5 years from presentation. However, most who survive the initial illness and who become abstinent survive beyond 5 years.

HAEMOCHROMATOSIS

Haemochromatosis is a condition in which the amount of total body iron is increased; the excess iron is deposited in and causes damage to several organs including the liver. It may be primary, or secondary to other diseases.

HEREDITARY (PRIMARY) HAEMOCHROMATOSIS

This is a disease in which the total body iron reaches 20–60 g (normally 4 g). Iron is deposited widely in the body. The important organs involved are the liver, pancreatic islets, endocrine glands and heart. In the liver, iron deposition occurs first in the periportal hepatocytes, extending later to all hepatocytes. The gradual development of fibrous septa leads to the formation of irregular nodules, and finally regeneration results in macronodular cirrhosis. An excess of liver iron can occur in alcoholic cirrhosis but this is mild by comparison with haemochromatosis.

Aetiology

Hereditary haemochromatosis is caused by an increased absorption of dietary iron. This inability to limit iron absorption is inherited as an autosomal recessive gene located on chromosome 6. Most patients have a single-point mutation resulting in a cysteine to tyrosine substitution at position 282 (C282Y) in a protein with structural and function similarity to the HLA proteins. Only homozygotes develop the disease, but other factors must also be important as at least 90% of patients are male. Iron loss in menstruation and pregnancy may protect females.

Clinical features

The disease usually presents in men aged 40 years or over with signs of hepatic cirrhosis (especially hepatomegaly), diabetes mellitus or heart failure. Leaden-grey skin pigmentation due to excess melanin occurs especially in exposed parts, axillae, groins and genitalia, hence the term 'bronzed diabetes'. Impotence, loss of libido, testicular atrophy and arthritis with chondrocalcinosis secondary to calcium pyrophosphate deposition are also common. Increasingly, early clinical features are being recognised, particularly tiredness, fatigue and arthropathy.

Investigations

The serum ferritin is greatly increased; the plasma iron is also increased, with a highly saturated plasma iron binding capacity. Computed tomography may show features suggesting excess hepatic iron. The diagnosis is confirmed by liver biopsy, which shows heavy iron deposition and hepatic fibrosis which may have progressed to cirrhosis. The iron content of the liver can be measured directly. The abnormal gene can now be detected; a single gene mutation accounts for about 90% of cases, and homozygotes and heterozygotes can be differentiated.

Management

Treatment consists of weekly venesection of 500 ml (250 mg iron) until the serum iron is normal; this may take 2 years or more. Thereafter, venesection is continued as required to keep the serum ferritin normal. Other therapy includes that for cirrhosis and diabetes mellitus. Other first-degree family members should be investigated, preferably by genetic screening and also by checking the plasma ferritin and iron-binding saturation. Asymptomatic disease should be treated.

Prognosis

Hereditary haemochromatosis has a good prognosis compared with other forms of cirrhosis, as three-quarters of patients are alive 5 years after the diagnosis. This is probably because liver function is usually well preserved at diagnosis and improves with therapy. Hepatocellular carcinoma is the main cause of death occurring in about one-third of patients with cirrhosis irrespective of therapy.

SECONDARY HAEMOCHROMATOSIS

Many conditions, including chronic haemolytic disorders, sideroblastic anaemia, other conditions requiring multiple blood transfusion (generally over 50 litres), porphyria cutanea tarda, dietary iron overload and occasionally alcoholic cirrhosis, are associated with widespread secondary siderosis. The features are similar to haemochromatosis, but the history and clinical findings point to the true diagnosis. Some patients are heterozygotes for the primary haemochromatosis gene and this may contribute to the development of iron overload.

WILSON'S DISEASE (HEPATOLENTICULAR DEGENERATION)

This is a rare but important condition in which the total body copper is increased with excess copper deposited in, and causing damage to, several organs.

Aetiology and pathology

Wilson's disease is inherited as an autosomal recessive disorder that results in abnormal copper metabolism. The gene responsible is on chromosome 13 and has been designated ATP7B, with multiple genome mutations identified. Normally, dietary copper is absorbed from the stomach and proximal small intestine and is rapidly taken into the liver, where it is stored and incorporated into caeruloplasmin, which is secreted into the blood. The accumulation of excessive copper in the body is ultimately prevented by its excretion, the most important route being via the bile. The precise nature of the metabolic defect in Wilson's disease is unknown, but it results in a failure of biliary copper excretion causing accumulation in the body. There is almost always a failure of synthesis of caeruloplasmin also, though some 5% of patients with Wilson's disease have a normal plasma caeruloplasmin concentration. The amount of copper in the body at birth is normal, but thereafter it increases steadily and the organs most affected are the liver, basal ganglia of the brain, eyes, kidneys and skeleton.

Clinical features

Symptoms usually arise between the ages of 5 and 30 years. Hepatic disease occurs predominantly in childhood and early adolescence, while neurological damage causes basal ganglion syndromes and dementia in later adolescence. These manifestations can occur alone or simultaneously. Other manifestations include haemolysis, renal tubular damage and osteoporosis, but these are virtually never presenting features.

Kayser–Fleischer rings

These are the most important single clinical clue to the diagnosis and they can be seen in most patients presenting in or after adolescence, albeit sometimes only by slit-lamp examination. Appearances indistinguishable from Kayser–Fleischer rings are found rarely in other forms of chronic hepatitis and cirrhosis. Kayser–Fleischer rings are characterised by greenish-brown discoloration of the corneal margin appearing first at the upper periphery (see Fig. 10.22). They eventually disappear with treatment.

Liver disease

This can manifest in many ways which are not specific. Episodes of acute hepatitis which are sometimes recurrent can occur, especially in children, and may progress to acute hepatic failure. Chronic persistent hepatitis and chronic active hepatitis can also develop, and eventually cirrhosis with liver failure and portal hypertension. Recurrent acute hepatitis of unknown cause, especially accompanied by haemolysis, or chronic liver disease of unknown cause in a patient under 40 years old suggests Wilson's disease.

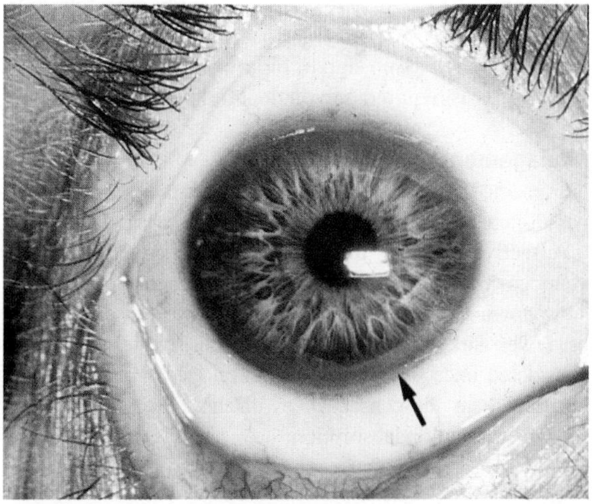

Fig. 10.22 Kayser–Fleischer rings at the junction of the cornea and sclera (arrow) in a patient with Wilson's disease.

Neurological disease

Clinical features include a variety of extrapyramidal features, particularly tremor, choreoathetosis, dystonia, parkinsonism and dementia.

Investigations

A low serum caeruloplasmin is the best single laboratory clue to the diagnosis. However, advanced liver failure from any cause can reduce the serum caeruloplasmin, and occasionally the serum caeruloplasmin is normal in Wilson's disease. Other features of disordered copper metabolism should therefore be sought; these include a low serum copper concentration, a high urine copper excretion, and a very high hepatic copper content. Patients with Wilson's disease fail to incorporate radioactive copper into caeruloplasmin, but this test is almost never needed. Gene detection in diagnosis is limited by the existence of several defects.

Management

The copper-binding agent penicillamine is the drug of choice in Wilson's disease. The dose given must be sufficient to produce cupriuresis and most patients require 1.5 g/day (range 1–4 g). The dose can be reduced once the disease is in remission, but treatment must continue for life and care must be taken to ensure that reaccumulation of copper does not occur. Young women should continue to take the drug during pregnancy. Serious toxic effects of penicillamine are rare in Wilson's disease. If they do occur, trientine dihydrochloride (1.2–2.4 g/day) is the next drug of choice. Liver transplantation may be needed for acute hepatic failure or for advanced cirrhosis with liver failure.

Prognosis

The prognosis of Wilson's disease is excellent provided treatment is started before there is irreversible damage; the long-term complication of hepatocellular carcinoma does not occur. Siblings and children of patients with Wilson's disease must be investigated and treatment should be given to any who have the disease even if it is asymptomatic.

ALPHA$_1$-ANTITRYPSIN DEFICIENCY

Alpha$_1$-antitrypsin (α_1-AT) is a serine protease inhibitor (Pi) produced by the liver. The form of α_1-AT is genetically determined, and one of these forms (PiZ) cannot be secreted into the blood by the liver cells owing to polymerisation within the endoplasmic reticulum of the hepatocyte. Homozygous individuals (PiZZ) have low plasma α_1-AT concentrations, though globules containing α_1-AT are found in the liver, and this form of α_1-AT deficiency is associated with hepatic and pulmonary disease. Liver disease includes cholestatic jaundice in the neonatal period (neonatal hepatitis) which can resolve spontaneously, chronic hepatitis and cirrhosis in adults, and in the long term the development of hepatocellular carcinoma. There are no clinical features distinguishing liver disease due to α_1-AT deficiency from other causes of liver disease, and the diagnosis is made from the low plasma α_1-AT concentration and the PiZZ phenotype. α_1-AT-containing globules can be demonstrated in the liver but this is not necessary for making the diagnosis. Occasionally, patients with liver disease and minor reductions of plasma α_1-AT concentrations have α_1-AT phenotypes other than PiZZ, such as PiMZ or PiSZ, but the relationship of these genotypes to liver disease is uncertain. No specific treatment is available; the concurrent risk of severe and early-onset emphysema dictates that all patients are strongly advised to abandon cigarette smoking.

BILIARY CIRRHOSIS

Biliary cirrhosis results from destruction of intrahepatic bile ducts in cases of primary biliary cirrhosis or primary sclerosing cholangitis, or secondary to prolonged obstruction.

PRIMARY BILIARY CIRRHOSIS

Primary biliary cirrhosis (PBC) affects predominantly women who usually present clinically in middle age. The ready availability of diagnostic tests has revealed asymptomatic disease which can remain quiescent for years, and has shown that PBC is a relatively common form of cirrhosis.

Aetiology and pathology

The cause of PBC is unknown but immune reactions causing liver damage are suspected. Autoantibodies and immune complexes are found in the blood, cellular immunity is impaired, and abnormal cellular immune reactions have been described. The primary pathological lesion is a chronic granulomatous inflammation damaging and destroying the interlobular bile ducts, and progressive inflammatory damage with fibrosis spreading from the portal tracts to the liver parenchyma which eventually leads to cirrhosis.

Clinical features

Non-specific symptoms such as lethargy, fatigue and arthralgia are common and may precede diagnosis for a long time. Pruritus is the most common initial complaint pointing to hepatobiliary disease and it may precede jaundice by months or years. Bile acids have been suggested as the cause of pruritus but this remains unproven. Jaundice is occasionally a presenting feature but pruritus is usually also present. Although there may be abdominal discomfort, the abdominal pain, fever and rigors which are often features of large bile duct obstruction do not occur. Diarrhoea from malabsorption of fat, and pain and tingling in the hands and feet due to lipid infiltration of peripheral nerves occasionally occur. Bone pain or fractures resulting from osteomalacia from malabsorption or osteoporosis (hepatic osteodystrophy) can be prominent and distressing features in advanced disease.

Initially patients are well nourished but considerable weight loss can occur as the disease progresses. Scratch marks may be found. Jaundice is only prominent late in the disease and can become intense. Xanthomatous deposits occur in a minority, especially around the eyes, in the hand creases and over the elbows, knees and buttocks. Hepatomegaly is virtually constant, and splenomegaly becomes increasingly common as portal hypertension develops. Liver failure and portal hypertension arise as the disease progresses.

Associated diseases

Autoimmune and connective tissue diseases occur with increased frequency in primary biliary cirrhosis, particularly the sicca syndrome (see p. 861) and thyroid diseases. Hypothyroidism should always be considered in patients with fatigue.

Investigations

Liver function tests show the pattern of cholestasis (see p. 686). The antimitochondrial antibody is present in over 95% of patients, and when it is absent histological evidence for the diagnosis is needed together with cholangiography by endoscopic retrograde cholangiopancreatography (ERCP, see pp. 687–688) to exclude other biliary disease. Antinuclear and smooth muscle antibodies may be present (see Table 10.12, p. 715) and autoantibodies found in associated diseases may also be found. Ultrasound examination shows no sign of biliary obstruction. As noted, liver biopsy is required only in doubtful cases.

Management

No specific therapy is available. Corticosteroids, azathioprine, penicillamine and cyclosporin have all been tried, but none is effective and all may have serious adverse effects. Ursodeoxycholic acid improves liver function tests, may slow down histological progression and has the advantage of fewer side-effects. Transplantation should always be considered once liver failure has developed. Treatment may be needed for the consequences of cholestasis, particularly for pruritus and malabsorption.

Pruritus

This is the main symptom demanding relief. It is achieved best with the anion-binding resin cholestyramine, which reduces the concentration of bile acids in the body by binding them in the intestine and increasing their excretion in the stool. A dose of 4–16 g/day orally is used. The powder is mixed in orange juice and the main dose (8 g) is taken with breakfast when maximal duodenal bile acid concentrations occur. Cholestyramine may bind other drugs in the gut (e.g. anticoagulants), which should therefore be taken 1 hour before the binding agent. Cholestyramine is sometimes ineffective, especially in complete biliary obstruction. Rifampicin or ultraviolet light may help in such patients.

Malabsorption

Prolonged cholestasis is associated with steatorrhoea and malabsorption of fat-soluble vitamins and calcium. Steatorrhoea can be reduced by limiting fat intake to 40 g/day. Monthly injections of vitamin K_1 (10 mg), vitamin D (calciferol 1 mg/day; alfacalcidol 1 mg/day orally) and calcium supplements should also be given, the last as effervescent calcium gluconate (2–4 g/day). The effervescent preparation, however, contains significant amounts of sodium, and where there is fluid retention calcium gluconate alone should be used. Associated coeliac disease requires exclusion.

SECONDARY BILIARY CIRRHOSIS

This develops after prolonged large duct biliary obstruction due to gallstones, bile duct strictures or sclerosing cholangitis (see below). Carcinomas rarely cause secondary biliary cirrhosis as survival is limited. There is chronic cholestasis with episodes of ascending cholangitis or even liver abscess (see p. 725). Digital clubbing is common and xanthomata and bone pain may develop. Cirrhosis, ascites and portal hypertension are late features. Cholangitis requires treatment with antibiotics, which can be given continuously if attacks occur frequently.

PRIMARY SCLEROSING CHOLANGITIS

This condition, which is being increasingly diagnosed, refers to fibrotic obliteration of the intra- and/or extrahepatic bile duct system, which may be primary or secondary in type. Primary sclerosing cholangitis has no known cause but is often associated with ulcerative colitis and occasionally with retroperitoneal fibrosis, HIV infection or a variety of autoimmune disorders. There is an association between primary sclerosing cholangitis and the HLA haplotypes B8, DR2 and DR3. In secondary sclerosing cholangitis there is an underlying disorder of the biliary tree causing the fibrotic state—for example, retained bile duct stones or strictures following surgery.

Clinical features

The patient presents with jaundice, which may fluctuate, intermittent fever, pruritus and right upper quadrant pain. Eventually hepatic cirrhosis, i.e. secondary biliary cirrhosis (see above) develops. There is a high frequency of cholangiocarcinoma, and progressive jaundice, anorexia and weight loss are suggestive of this complication.

Investigations

Liver function tests demonstrate cholestasis with elevation of the serum bilirubin, gamma-glutamyl transferase and alkaline phosphatase. These abnormalities may fluctuate. The prothrombin time may be prolonged if cholestasis is long-standing or hepatic cirrhosis and liver failure have developed. Perinuclear antineutrophil cytoplasmic antibodies (p-ANCA, see p. 808) have been found in this disease, especially where it is associated with ulcerative colitis. Ultrasonography may not show biliary abnormality as the thickened fibrotic ducts are not dilated, and diagnosis is best made by ERCP, which typically shows narrowed, irregular obstruction and 'beading' of the extra- and intrahepatic bile ducts (see Fig. 10.23). The disease may affect the whole of the biliary system or may be confined to the extra- or intrahepatic portion of the bile ducts. The diagnosis may also be made by a percutaneous transhepatic cholangiogram. At liver biopsy a typical whorled appearance of bile ducts may be seen. Bile duct tissue obtained at laparotomy may demonstrate the characteristic lymphocytic cell infiltrate with plasma cells and giant cells. The main differential diagnosis is cholangiocarcinoma.

Management

There is no specific treatment, but antibiotics are needed during episodes of cholangitis. Ursodeoxycholic acid has

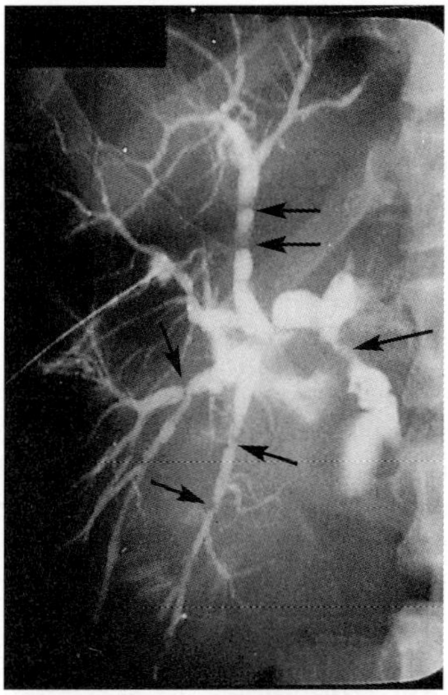

Fig. 10.23 A percutaneous cholangiogram in sclerosing cholangitis showing the irregularity in the biliary tree.

been used but its efficacy is in doubt. Corticosteroids and other immunosuppressive drugs are of no value. Biliary drainage may be attempted using stents placed at ERCP, but this is only reasonable where a single dominant stricture is present. Liver transplantation is the only effective therapy in patients with advanced disease.

VASCULAR DISEASE OF THE LIVER

HEPATIC ARTERIAL DISEASE

Hepatic arterial disease is rare and difficult to diagnose, but it can cause serious liver damage. Hepatic artery occlusion may be caused by emboli, neoplasms, polyarteritis nodosa or blunt trauma. It usually causes severe upper abdominal pain with or without signs of circulatory shock. Liver function tests show a high transaminase activity as in other causes of acute liver damage. Patients usually survive if the liver and portal blood supply are otherwise normal.

Hepatic artery aneurysms are extrahepatic in three-quarters of cases and intrahepatic in one-quarter. Atheroma, vasculitis, bacterial endocarditis, and surgical or biopsy trauma are the main causes. They usually cause bleeding into the biliary tree, peritoneum or intestine and are diagnosed best by arteriography. Treatment is surgical. Any of the vasculitides can affect the hepatic artery, but this rarely causes symptoms.

PORTAL VENOUS DISEASE

Portal venous thrombosis is rare but can occur in any condition predisposing to thrombosis. It also occurs with local intra-abdominal inflammatory or neoplastic disease and is a recognised complication of portal hypertension. Acute portal venous thrombosis causes abdominal pain and diarrhoea and may lead to bowel infarction. Treatment is surgical. Less acute thrombosis can be asymptomatic and may later give rise to extrahepatic portal hypertension (see p. 693).

HEPATIC VENOUS OUTFLOW OBSTRUCTION

Obstruction to hepatic venous blood flow can occur in the small central hepatic veins, in the large hepatic veins, in the inferior vena cava or in the heart. The clinical features depend on the cause and on the speed with which obstruction develops, but congestive hepatomegaly and ascites are features in all patients.

BUDD–CHIARI SYNDROME

Aetiology and pathology

This is an uncommon condition in which obstruction occurs in the larger hepatic veins and sometimes the inferior vena cava. The cause cannot be found in about half of patients. In the others, thrombosis may be due to haematological diseases including primary proliferative polycythaemia, paroxysmal nocturnal haemoglobinuria and antithrombin III, protein C or protein S deficiencies. Pregnancy and oral contraceptive use, obstruction due to tumours, particularly carcinomas of the liver, kidneys or adrenals, congenital venous webs and occasionally inferior vena caval stenosis are the other main causes. Hepatic congestion affecting the centrilobular areas is the initial consequence; centrilobular fibrosis develops later and eventually cirrhosis in those who survive long enough.

Clinical features

Sudden venous occlusion causes the rapid development of upper abdominal pain, marked ascites and occasionally acute hepatic failure. More gradual occlusion causes gross ascites and often upper abdominal discomfort. Hepatomegaly, often with tenderness over the liver, is almost always present. Peripheral oedema occurs only when there is inferior vena cava obstruction. Features of cirrhosis and portal hypertension develop in those who survive the acute event.

Investigations

Liver function tests vary considerably depending on the presentation and can show the features of acute hepatitis (see p. 686) when the onset is rapid. Ascitic fluid analysis typically shows a protein concentration above 25 g/l in the early stages but is often lower later in the disease. Ultrasound examination may reveal obliteration of the hepatic veins and reversed flow in the portal vein. Isotope imaging may show preservation of the caudate lobe, as it often has a separate venous drainage system not involved in the disease. Hepatic venography shows occlusion of the hepatic veins and any inferior vena cava involvement, and liver biopsy demonstrates centrilobular congestion with fibrosis depending upon the duration of the illness.

Management

Predisposing causes should be treated as far as possible, and where recent thrombosis is suspected treatment with streptokinase followed by heparin and oral anticoagulation are considered. Ascites is treated medically initially but this often has limited success, in which case a LeVeen shunt (see p. 699) or a portal-systemic shunt can be used. Direct surgical treatment of the venous obstruction is rarely possible but occasionally a web can be resected or an inferior caval stenosis dilated. Some patients may be successfully managed by insertion of a transjugular intrahepatic portasystemic stent shunt. Progressive liver failure is an indication for liver transplantation.

Prognosis

The prognosis is generally poor, particularly when the onset is sudden; one-third to two-thirds of patients die within a year and few live more than 5 years. Some patients survive to develop cirrhosis.

VENO-OCCLUSIVE DISEASE

Widespread occlusion of central hepatic veins is the characteristic of this condition. Pyrrolizidine alkaloids in *Senecio* and *Heliotropium* plants used to make teas are the best known causes, but cytotoxic drugs and hepatic irradiation are increasingly recognised causes. The clinical features, investigation and management of veno-occlusive disease are similar to those of the Budd–Chiari syndrome (see above).

CARDIAC DISEASE

Hepatic damage due primarily to congestion is always present in cardiac failure from any cause, but the clinical features are usually dominated by the cardiac disease. Occasionally the hepatic features are more prominent.

Acute hepatitis

Rapidly developing cardiac failure sometimes causes a syndrome suggesting an acute hepatitis. This occurs most often following myocardial infarction, decompensation of any chronic myocardial disease or respiratory condition associated with cor pulmonale, or rapidly developing cardiac tamponade. The patient is generally very ill with an enlarged tender liver, with or without jaundice, and liver function tests showing an acute hepatitis. The correct diagnosis is made by recognising that the cardiac output is low, the jugular venous pressure is high, and that other signs of cardiac disease are present.

Ascites

Cardiac failure sometimes causes hepatomegaly and ascites disproportionate to the degree of peripheral oedema, and hence can mimic ascites due to liver disease. A high ascites protein concentration may suggest hepatic venous outflow obstruction. Constrictive pericarditis (see p. 301) is particularly likely to mislead, as a normal heart size points away from heart disease. A raised jugular venous pressure is the most important single clue to the diagnosis. Rarely, long-standing cardiac failure and hepatic congestion cause cardiac cirrhosis, and this is suggested by hard irregular hepatomegaly or a palpable spleen due to portal hypertension.

Management

The treatment of these patients is that of the underlying causative disease.

FURTHER INFORMATION ON PARENCHYMAL LIVER DISEASE

Bacon B R 1997 Diagnosis and management of hemochromatosis. Gastroenterology 113: 995–999

Dusheiko G M 1996 New treatments for chronic viral-hepatitis-B and viral-hepatitis-C. Baillière's Clinical Gastroenterology 10: 299–333

Elder G H, Worwood M 1998 Mutations in the hemochromatosis gene, porphyria cutanea tarda and iron overload. Hepatology 27: 289–291

French S W 1995 Rationale for therapy for alcoholic liver disease. Gastroenterology 109: 617–620

Hoofnagle J H, DiBisceglie A M 1997 The treatment of chronic viral hepatitis. New England Journal of Medicine 336: 347–356

Jones D E J, Bassendine M F 1997 Primary biliary cirrhosis. Journal of Internal Medicine 241: 345–348

Kaplan M M 1997 Toward better treatment of primary sclerosing cholangitis. New England Journal of Medicine 336: 719–721

Krawitt E L 1996 Medical progress—autoimmune hepatitis. New England Journal of Medicine 334: 897–903

Lee W M 1995 Drug-induced hepatotoxicity. New England Journal of Medicine 333: 1118–1127

Lemon S M, Thomas D L 1997 Vaccines to prevent viral hepatitis. New England Journal of Medicine 336: 196–204

Lumeng L, Crabb D W 1994 Genetic aspects and risk factors in alcoholism and alcoholic liver disease. Gastroenterology 107: 572–578

Sherlock S 1995 Alcoholic liver disease. Lancet 345: 227–229

Sherman D, Williams R 1995 Liver transplantation for alcoholic liver disease. Journal of Hepatology 23: 474–479

Sjogren M H 1996 Serologic diagnosis of viral-hepatitis. Medical Clinics of North America 80: 929

Yarze J C, Martin P, Munoz S J, Friedman L S 1992 Wilson's disease: current status. American Journal of Medicine 92: 643–654

TUMOURS OF THE LIVER

HEPATOCELLULAR CARCINOMA (HEPATOMA)

Hepatocellular carcinoma is the principal primary malignant liver tumour. Its incidence shows great geographic variation, being common in Africa and South-east Asia but rare in temperate climates.

Aetiology

Chronic hepatitis B virus infection has emerged as the most important cause world-wide, but chronic hepatitis C virus infection is becoming increasingly important. Aflatoxin contamination of foods may be important in tropical countries. Cirrhosis and male sex are the main factors related to hepatocellular carcinoma in temperate climates. Cirrhosis is present in 80% of cases and may be of any type; however, hepatocellular carcinoma appears most commonly in haemochromatosis and alcoholic cirrhosis, predominantly male diseases, and rarely in primary biliary cirrhosis, which mainly affects women. Exposure to toxins such as thorotrast and arsenic usually produce angiosarcomas but may also cause hepatocellular carcinomas. Oestrogens, androgens and anabolic steroids may cause adenomas or, rarely, hepatocellular carcinomas.

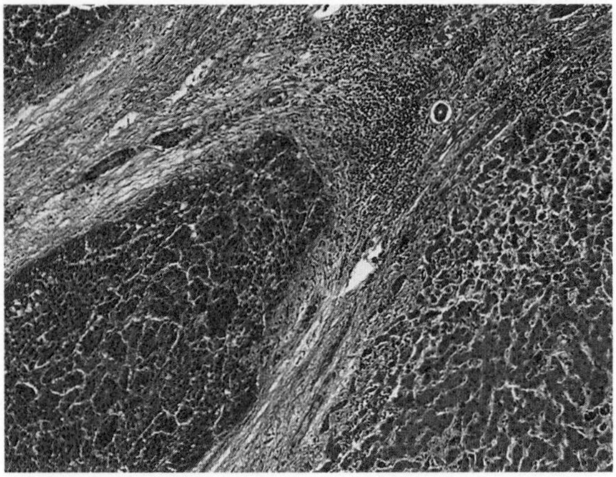

Fig. 10.24 Histology of hepatocellular carcinoma (left) arising within cirrhotic liver (right).

Pathology

Macroscopically, the tumour may comprise a single mass or multiple nodules or occasionally be diffusely invasive. Microscopically, the tumour is made up of trabeculae of well-differentiated malignant cells resembling hepatocytes (see Fig. 10.24). Bile secretion by tumour cells is diagnostic. Intravascular invasion and growth are often features and may result in tumour spread into the portal vein or inferior vena cava. The tumour metastasises mainly to regional lymph nodes, the lungs and bones. Clinical deterioration in a patient with cirrhosis should always lead to suspicion of hepatocellular carcinoma.

Clinical features

These include weakness, anorexia, weight loss, fever, abdominal pain, a large irregular liver or an abdominal mass, and ascites. Hepatocellular carcinomas are vascular and a bruit may be heard over the liver or intra-abdominal bleeding may occur.

Screening

Hepatocellular carcinoma is most common in patients with cirrhosis, especially if associated with HCV infection, haemochromatosis, or alcohol. Treatment can only be curative if small asymptomatic tumours are removed by resection or liver transplantation. Such tumours can be detected by regular serum alpha-fetoprotein measurements and ultrasound examinations undertaken at 6-monthly intervals.

Investigations

A greatly increased or rising serum alpha-fetoprotein is virtually diagnostic (see p. 1051). Imaging usually reveals one or more filling defects, laparoscopy may reveal the tumour and the diagnosis can be confirmed by liver aspiration or biopsy which risks 'seeding' the tumour along the biopsy tract. Liver function tests give variable non-specific results. Metabolic abnormalities include polycythaemia, hypercalcaemia, hypoglycaemia and porphyria cutanea tarda.

Management

Surgical removal requires a tumour confined to one lobe in the absence of cirrhosis and is rarely feasible, but the possibility should always be considered. Arterial embolisation with or without local injection of chemotherapeutic agents (chemoembolisation) can provide palliation for hepatic pain. Chemotherapy has been disappointing. Liver transplantation can be considered for small tumours not amenable to local resection.

Prognosis

The outlook is very poor. Surgery alone gives prolonged survival, but only about 10% of patients are suitable for this therapy. Few patients survive beyond a year.

FIBROLAMELLAR HEPATOCELLULAR CARCINOMA

This rare variant differs from other hepatocellular carcinomas in that it occurs in young adults, equally in males and females, and is not associated with cirrhosis or hepatitis B or C virus infection. It usually presents with pain due to bleeding into the tumour, which may later cause intrahepatic or intraperitoneal calcification. The serum alpha-fetoprotein is usually normal, and biopsy shows large polygonal malignant hepatocytes in a dense fibrous tissue stroma. Two-thirds of tumours are resectable and transplantation is worth-while where there is no spread beyond the liver. Two-thirds of patients survive beyond 5 years.

OTHER PRIMARY MALIGNANT TUMOURS

These are rare but include haemangio-endothelial sarcomas and cholangiocarcinoma (see p. 735).

SECONDARY MALIGNANT TUMOURS

These are common and usually originate from carcinomas in the lung, breast, abdomen or pelvis. They may be single or multiple. Peritoneal dissemination frequently results in ascites.

Clinical features

The primary neoplasm is asymptomatic in about half the patients. Hepatomegaly may suggest cirrhosis, but splenomegaly is rare. There is usually rapid liver enlargement with fever, weight loss and jaundice.

Investigations

A raised alkaline phosphatase activity is the most common biochemical abnormality but the liver function tests may be normal. Ascitic fluid has a high protein content and may be blood-stained, and cytology sometimes reveals malignant cells. Imaging (see p. 687) usually reveals filling defects (see Fig. 10.25), laparoscopy may reveal the tumour (see Fig. 10.26), and the diagnosis can be confirmed by liver aspiration or biopsy.

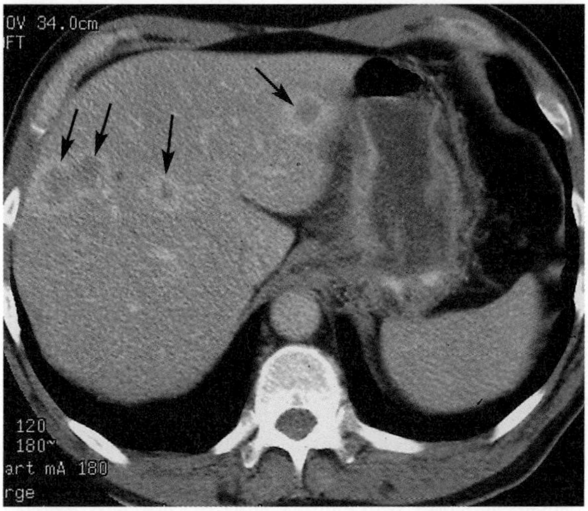

Fig. 10.25 CT showing multiple liver metastases (arrows).

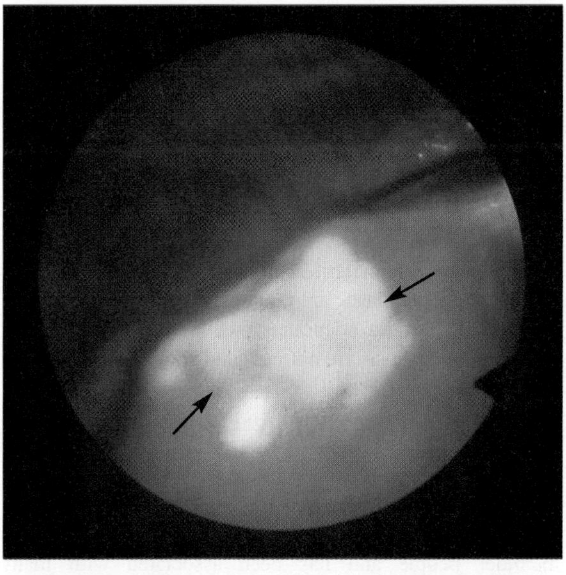

Fig. 10.26 Laparoscopic appearance of a hepatic metastasis from colonic carcinoma.

Management

Every effort should be made to detect resectable secondary tumours, as improvements in hepatic resection can improve survival and give the best palliation, particularly for relatively slow-growing tumours such as colonic carcinomas. Patients with hormone-producing tumours, such as gastrinomas, insulinomas and glucagonomas, and lymphomas may benefit from chemotherapy. Unfortunately, palliative treatment to relieve pain is all that is available for most patients; this may include arterial embolisation of the tumour masses.

BENIGN TUMOURS

Hepatic adenomas are rare vascular tumours which may present as an abdominal mass or with abdominal pain or intraperitoneal bleeding. They are more common in women and may be caused by oral contraceptives, androgens and anabolic steroids. Haemangiomas are the most common benign liver tumours but rarely cause symptoms.

FURTHER INFORMATION ON TUMOURS OF THE LIVER

Trinchet J C, Beaugrand M 1997 Treatment of hepatocellular carcinoma in patients with cirrhosis. Journal of Hepatology 27: 756–765

Zuckerman A J 1997 Prevention of primary liver cancer by immunization. New England Journal of Medicine 336: 1906–1907

MISCELLANEOUS LIVER DISEASES

LIVER ABSCESS

Liver abscesses are either pyogenic or amoebic; the two have similar clinical features.

PYOGENIC ABSCESS

Pyogenic liver abscesses are uncommon but important because they are potentially curable, inevitably fatal if untreated, and readily overlooked.

Aetiology and pathology

Infection can reach the liver in several ways (see the information box). Abscesses are most common in older patients and usually result from ascending infection due to biliary obstruction (cholangitis), whereas abscesses in young adults consequent on suppurative appendicitis, which were previously common, are now rare. Immunocompromised patients are particularly likely to develop liver abscesses. Abscesses

SOURCES OF BACTERIAL INFECTION OF THE LIVER

• Biliary obstruction (cholangitis)
• Haematogenous
    Portal vein (mesenteric infections)
    Hepatic artery (bacteraemia)
• Direct extension
• Trauma
    Penetrating or non-penetrating
• Infection of liver tumour or cyst

vary greatly in size, single lesions are more common in the right liver, and multiple abscesses are usually due to infection secondary to biliary obstruction. *E. coli* and various streptococci are the most common organisms, anaerobes including streptococci and *Bacteroides* can often be found, and multiple organisms are present in one-third of patients.

Clinical features

Patients are generally ill with fever, sometimes rigors, and weight loss. Abdominal pain is the most common symptom and is usually in the right upper quadrant, sometimes with radiation to the right shoulder. The pain may be pleuritic in nature. Hepatomegaly is found in more than half the patients and tenderness can usually be elicited by gentle percussion over the organ. Mild jaundice may be present but is severe only when large abscesses cause biliary obstruction. Abnormalities are present at the base of the right lung in about one-quarter of patients. Atypical presentations are common and explain the frequency with which the diagnosis is made only at autopsy. This is a particular problem in patients with gradually developing illnesses which may not include abdominal pain, with pyrexia of unknown cause, and in patients with clinical features pointing to an underlying cause such as colonic diverticular disease or to metastatic abscesses.

Investigations

Liver imaging is the most revealing investigation and shows 90% or more of symptomatic abscesses. Needle aspiration under ultrasound guidance confirms the diagnosis and provides pus for culture. A leucocytosis is frequent, plasma alkaline phosphatase activity is usually increased, and the serum albumin is often low. The chest radiograph may show a raised right diaphragm and lung collapse or an effusion at the base of the right lung. Blood culture should always be carried out as it may reveal the causative organism.

Management

This includes antibiotics and drainage of the abscess. Pending the results of culture of blood and pus from the abscess, treatment should commence with a combination of antibiotics such as ampicillin, gentamicin and metronidazole. Aspiration or drainage with a catheter placed

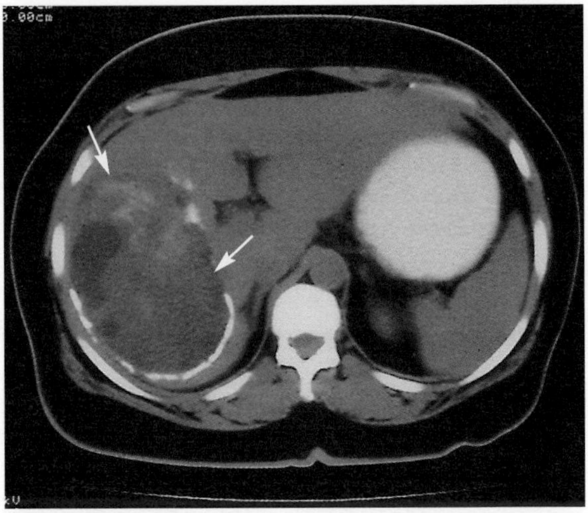

Fig. 10.27 Hydatid cyst of the liver on CT (arrows).

in the abscess under ultrasound guidance is required, with surgical drainage needed for those which fail to respond.

Prognosis

The mortality of liver abscesses is 20–40%; failure to make the diagnosis is the most common cause of death. Older patients and those with multiple abscesses also have a higher mortality.

AMOEBIC ABSCESS

Amoebic liver abscesses occur particularly in endemic areas, but they can occur anywhere in the world (see Fig. 10.27). Amoebic infections are considered elsewhere (see p. 153).

HEPATIC NODULES

Liver diseases characterised primarily by hepatic nodules which are not neoplastic are rare, and three types are usually recognised. Hepatic adenomas (see p. 725) and nodules occurring in cirrhosis are not included with these diseases.

NODULAR REGENERATIVE HYPERPLASIA OF THE LIVER

This disease is characterised by small hepatocyte nodules throughout the liver not associated with fibrosis. It occurs in older people and has been associated with many conditions such as connective tissue disease, haemato-logical diseases and with immunosuppressive and cortico-steroid drugs. The condition usually presents as an abdominal mass or occasionally because of portal hypertension. Diagnosis is made by liver biopsy. Liver function is good and the prognosis is very favourable, but hepatocellular carcinoma occurs occasionally.

FOCAL NODULAR HYPERPLASIA OF THE LIVER

This usually takes the form of a single subcapsular liver nodule, yellow-brown in colour and with central fibrosis. It is almost always asymptomatic and found by chance. Intraperitoneal bleeding is a rare complication.

PARTIAL NODULAR TRANSFORMATION OF THE LIVER

Nodules in this condition are restricted to the perihilar region of the liver where they can cause portal hypertension. The rest of the liver is normal and liver function is excellent. The diagnosis can be made finally by pathological examination of the liver only as needle liver biopsy is normal.

FIBROPOLYCYSTIC DISEASE

Fibropolycystic diseases of the liver and biliary system constitute a heterogeneous group of rare disorders, some of which are inherited. They are not distinct entities, as combined lesions occur.

ADULT HEPATORENAL POLYCYSTIC DISEASE

The kidneys are predominantly affected in this condition, which is inherited as an autosomal dominant trait (see p. 452). Hepatic cysts which do not communicate with the biliary system are present in over half the patients with renal cysts, and cysts can also be found in other organs. Cerebrovascular aneurysms sometimes develop too. Cysts restricted to the liver constitute a separate rare genetic disorder.

Hepatic cysts are often discovered by chance; complications are rare, but include pain or jaundice from cyst enlargement, haemorrhage into cysts, or cyst infection. Portal hypertension and bleeding from varices are very rare.

Diagnosis is made best by ultrasonography. Resection of a large cyst or groups of cysts is only required if symptoms are troublesome, and the prognosis is excellent as liver function is good. Cholangiocarcinoma is a rare complication.

CONGENITAL HEPATIC FIBROSIS

This is characterised by broad bands of fibrous tissue linking the portal tracts in the liver, abnormalities of the interlobular bile ducts, and sometimes a lack of portal venules. The renal tubules may show cystic dilatation (medullary sponge kidney, see p. 453), and eventually renal cysts may develop. The condition can be inherited as an autosomal recessive trait. Liver involvement causes portal hypertension with splenomegaly and bleeding from oesophageal varices that usually presents in adolescence or in early adult life. The prognosis is good because liver function remains good. Treatment is required for variceal bleeding and occasionally cholangitis (see p. 734). Patients can present during childhood with renal failure if the kidneys are severely affected.

CHOLEDOCHAL CYSTS

This term applies to cysts anywhere in the biliary tree (see Fig. 10.28). The great majority cause diffuse dilatation of the

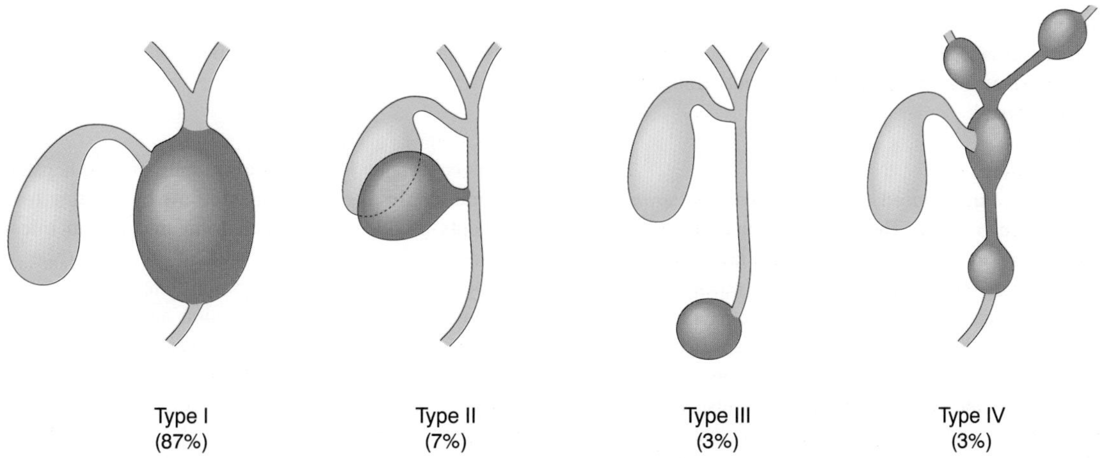

Fig. 10.28 Classification and frequency of choledochal cysts.

common bile duct (type I), but others take the form of biliary diverticula (type II), dilatation of the intraduodenal bile duct (type III) and multiple biliary cysts (type IV). The last type merges with Caroli's syndrome (see below). Recurrent jaundice and abdominal pain, and an abdominal mass are typical but these occur together in only a minority of patients. Prolonged biliary obstruction predisposes to cholangitis, liver abscess and eventually biliary cirrhosis, and there is an increased incidence of cholangiocarcinoma. Excision is the treatment of choice if this is possible; otherwise a biliary bypass operation is performed.

CAROLI'S SYNDROME

This is very rare and is characterised by segmental saccular dilatations of the intrahepatic biliary tree. The whole liver is usually affected, and extrahepatic biliary dilatation occurs in about one-quarter of patients. Recurrent attacks of cholangitis (see p. 734) occur and may cause hepatic abscesses. Complications include biliary stones and cholangiocarcinoma. Antibiotics are required for episodes of cholangitis, and occasionally localised disease can be treated by segmental liver resection.

OTHER HEPATIC CYSTS

Isolated single cysts in the liver are quite common. They rarely cause symptoms and are usually found incidentally when imaging is performed.

Non-parasitic cysts

Most non-parasitic liver cysts are congenital in origin and the majority are solitary. They rarely communicate with the biliary tree. They are usually asymptomatic but can cause abdominal pain, nausea or vomiting, and if the cysts become big enough, they may be palpable. Jaundice occasionally results from biliary compression, and infection, haemorrhage and rupture are other rare complications. Other non-parasitic hepatic cysts include traumatic and neoplastic cysts.

Parasitic cysts

These cysts are caused by *Echinococcus granulosus* infection (see p. 171). They have an outer layer derived from the host, an intermediate laminated layer, and an inner germinal layer. They can be single or multiple. Chronic cysts become calcified. The cysts may be asymptomatic or may cause abdominal pain or a mass. There is a peripheral blood eosinophilia, radiographs may show calcification, imaging shows the cyst(s), and serological tests are positive. Rupture or secondary infection of cysts can occur, and other organs may be involved. Surgical removal of the intact cyst after sterilisation with alcohol or formalin is necessary.

FURTHER INFORMATION ON MISCELLANEOUS LIVER DISEASES

Caroli J 1973 Diseases of the intrahepatic biliary tree. Clinics in Gastroenterology 2: 147–161

Pinzani M, Lannoy N, Peres D et al 1996 Isolated polycystic liver disease as a distinct genetic disease unlinked to polycystic kidney disease 1 and 2. Hepatology 23: 249–252

Rosen C B, Nagorney D M 1997 Hepatic tumours and nodules. In: Shearman D J C, Finlayson N, Camilleri M Diseases of the gastrointestinal tract and liver. Churchill Livingstone, Edinburgh

GALLBLADDER AND OTHER BILIARY DISEASES

FUNCTIONAL ANATOMY

BILIARY SYSTEM

The biliary tract begins in the biliary canaliculi, which are integral parts of the hepatocytes, and the intrahepatic bile ducts derived from them join progressively to form the right and left hepatic ducts. These ducts join as they emerge from the liver to form the common hepatic duct, which forms the common bile duct after joining the cystic duct (see Fig. 10.29). The common bile duct is approximately 5 cm long and has a thin-walled wide-lumened proximal part and a thick-walled narrow-lumened distal part surrounded by the choledochal sphincter. The distal common bile duct usually joins the pancreatic duct before it enters the duodenum. The gallbladder is a pear-shaped sac lying under the right hemiliver with its fundus located anteriorly behind the tip of the 9th costal cartilage. Its body and neck pass posteromedially towards the porta hepatis and the cystic duct then joins it to the common hepatic duct. The cystic duct mucosa has prominent crescentic folds (valves of Heister), giving it a beaded appearance on cholangiography.

BILE

The liver secretes 1–2 litres of bile daily, and the hepatocytes provide the driving force for bile flow by creating osmotic gradients of bile acids which form micelles in bile (bile acid-dependent bile flow) and of sodium (bile acid-independent bile flow). Common bile duct pressure is maintained by rhythmic contraction and relaxation of the choledochal sphincter and this pressure exceeds gallbladder pressure in the fasting state so that bile normally flows into the gallbladder where it is concentrated some 10-fold by resorption of water and electrolytes. Cholecystokinin released from the duodenal mucosa during feeding causes gallbladder contraction and reduces choledochal sphincter pressure and consequently bile flows into the duodenum.

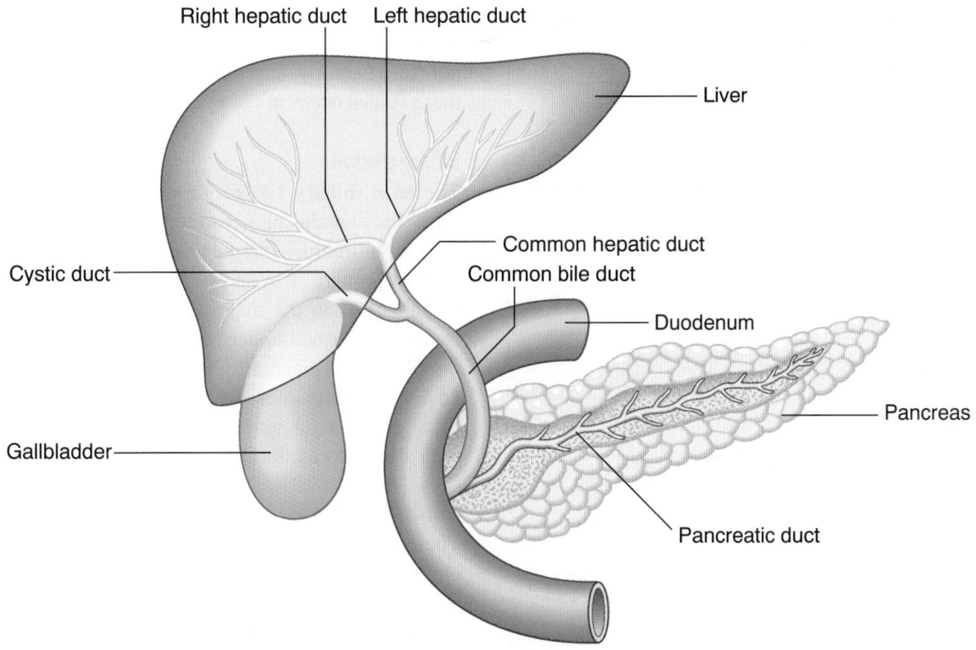

Fig. 10.29 Functional anatomy of the biliary tree.

Vagal activity maintains gallbladder tone, but sympathetic activity has little or no effect on the gallbladder.

GALLSTONES

Gallstone formation is the most common disorder of the biliary tree and it is unusual for the gallbladder to be diseased in the absence of gallstones.

Pathology

Gallstones are conveniently classified into cholesterol or pigment stones. Cholesterol stones are most common in industrialised countries whereas pigment stones are more frequent in developing countries. Gallstones contain varying quantities of calcium salts including calcium bilirubinate, carbonate, phosphate and palmitate, which are radio-opaque.

Epidemiology

Gallstones are common and occur in 7% of males and 15% of females aged 18–65 years, with an overall prevalence of 11%. In those under 40 years there is a 3:1 female preponderance whereas in the elderly the sex ratio is about equal. Gallstones are common in North America, Europe and Australia and are less frequent in India, the Far East and Africa. In developed countries the incidence of symptomatic gallstones appears to be increasing and they occur at an earlier age.

The most important risk factors for cholesterol and pigment gallstones are shown in Tables 10.13 and 10.14. There has been much debate over the role of diet in cholesterol gallstone disease, and an increase in dietary cholesterol, fat, total calories and refined carbohydrate or lack of dietary fibre have all been implicated. At present the best data support an association between simple refined sugar in the diet and gallstones. There is a negative association between a moderate alcohol intake (2–3 units daily) and gallstones.

Table 10.13 Risk factors and mechanisms for cholesterol gallstones

Factor	Mechanism
Age	↑ Cholesterol secretion
Female	↑ Cholesterol secretion
Pregnancy	↑ Cholesterol secretion ↓ Bile salt secretion Impaired gallbladder motility
Obesity	↑ Cholesterol secretion
Rapid weight loss	↑ Cholesterol secretion
Racial	↑ Cholesterol secretion
Gallbladder stasis **Brief fast** **TPN therapy** **Spinal cord injury**	Impaired gallbladder emptying

(TPN = total parenteral nutrition)

Table 10.14 Composition and risk factors for pigment stones

	Black	Brown
Composition	Polymerised calcium bilirubinates⁺⁺ Mucin glycoprotein⁺ Calcium phosphate Calcium carbonate Cholesterol	Calcium bilirubinate crystals⁺⁺ Mucin glycoprotein⁺ Cholesterol⁺ Calcium palmitate/stearate⁺
Risk	Haemolysis Age Hepatic cirrhosis Ileal resection/disease	Infected bile Stasis

⁺⁺ Major component
⁺ Lesser component

Aetiology

Gallstone formation is multifactorial, and the factors involved are related to the type of gallstone.

Cholesterol gallstones

Cholesterol is held in solution in bile by its association with bile acids and phospholipids in the form of micelles and vesicles. Biliary lipoproteins may also have a role in solubilising cholesterol. In gallstone disease the liver produces bile which contains an excess of cholesterol either because there is a relative deficiency of bile salts or a relative excess of cholesterol. Such bile, which is supersaturated with cholesterol, is termed 'lithogenic'. Disorders with the potential to induce the production of lithogenic bile are shown in the information box. Factors initiating crystallisation of cholesterol in lithogenic bile (nucleation factors) are also important; patients with cholesterol gallstones have gallbladder bile which forms cholesterol crystals more rapidly than equally saturated bile from patients who do not form gallstones. Factors favouring nucleation (mucus, calcium, fatty acids, other proteins) and antinucleating factors (apolipoproteins) have been described.

PATHOGENIC FACTORS LEADING TO THE PRODUCTION OF LITHOGENIC BILE

- Defective bile salt synthesis
- Excessive intestinal loss of bile salts
- Over-sensitive bile salt feedback
- Excessive cholesterol secretion
- Abnormal gallbladder function

Pigment stones

Brown crumbly pigment stones are almost always the consequence of bacterial or parasitic infection in the biliary tree. They are found commonly in the Far East where infection of the biliary tree allows bacterial β-glucuronidase to hydrolyse conjugated bilirubin to its free form, which then precipitates as calcium bilirubinate. The mechanism of black pigment gallstone formation in developed countries is not satisfactorily explained. Haemolysis is important as these stones occur in chronic haemolytic disease.

Biliary sludge

The term 'biliary sludge' describes bile which is in a gel form that contains numerous crystals or microspheroliths of calcium bilirubinate granules and cholesterol crystals as well as glycoproteins. It is an essential precursor to the formation of gallstones in the majority of patients. Biliary sludge is frequently formed under normal conditions, but then either dissolves or is cleared by the gallbladder and only in about 15% of patients does it persist to form cholesterol stones. Fasting, parenteral nutrition and pregnancy are also associated with sludge formation.

Clinical features

The majority of gallstones are asymptomatic and remain so. Only about 10% of those with gallstones develop clinical evidence of gallstone disease.

Symptomatic gallstones (see the information box) manifest either as biliary pain ('biliary colic') or as a consequence of cholecystitis. If a gallstone becomes acutely impacted in the cystic duct the patient will experience pain. The term 'biliary colic' is a misnomer because the pain does not rhythmically increase and decrease in intensity as in colic experienced in intestinal and renal disease. Instead the pain is typically of sudden onset and is sustained for about 2 hours; its continuation for more than 6 hours suggests that a complication such as cholecystitis or pancreatitis has developed. Pain is felt in the epigastrium (70% of patients) or right upper quadrant (20% of patients) and radiates to the interscapular region or the tip of the right scapula, but other sites include the left upper quadrant, the epigastrium and the lower chest, and can be confused with intrathoracic disease, oesophagitis, myocardial infarction or dissecting aneurysm.

Combinations of fatty food intolerance, dyspepsia and flatulence not attributable to other causes have been referred

CLINICAL FEATURES AND COMPLICATIONS OF GALLSTONES

Clinical features	Complications
• Asymptomatic • Biliary colic • Acute cholecystitis • Chronic cholecystitis	• Empyema of the gallbladder • Porcelain gallbladder (see p. 731) • Choledocholithiasis • Pancreatitis • Fistulae between the gallbladder and duodenum or colon • Mirizzi's syndrome (see p. 732) • Gallstone ileus • Cancer of the gallbladder

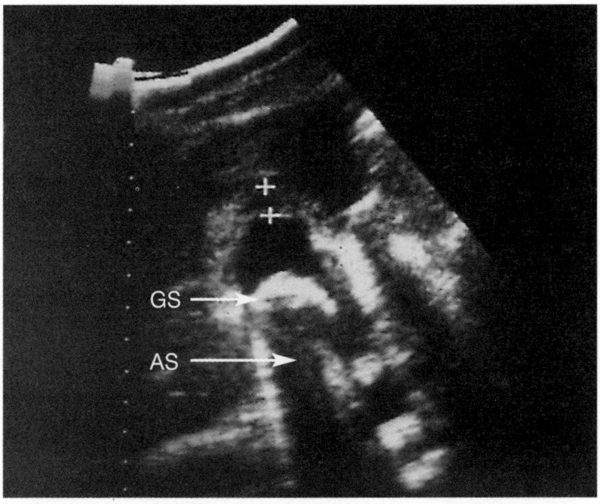

Fig. 10.30 Ultrasound showing gallstones (GS) with an acoustic shadow (AS) behind the stone.

to as 'gallstone dyspepsia'. These symptoms are not now recognised as caused by gallstones and are best regarded as non-ulcer dyspepsia (see p. 638).

Investigations

A plain abdominal radiograph will demonstrate calcified gallstones in 20% of patients. Ultrasonography is the method of choice to diagnose gallstones (see Fig. 10.30) but oral cholecystography and CT can also be used. Oral cholecystectomy shows whether or not the gallbladder is functioning, and this is useful if oral dissolution therapy is being considered (see under Management below).

Complications

Occlusion of the cystic duct for any prolonged period of time results in acute cholecystitis. Other complications include chronic cholecystitis, and hydrops of the gallbladder, in which there is slow distension of the gallbladder from continuous secretion of mucus. If this material becomes infected an empyema develops. Calcium may be secreted into the lumen of the hydropic gallbladder causing limy bile, and if calcium salts are precipitated in the gallbladder wall the radiological appearance of 'porcelain' gallbladder results.

Gallstones (cholecystolithiasis) migrate to the common bile duct in 10–20% of patients and cause biliary colic, but choledocholithiasis may be asymptomatic. Rarely, fistulae develop between the gallbladder and the duodenum, colon or stomach, and a fistulous tract may arise between the common bile duct and adjacent organs. Air will be seen in the biliary tree on plain abdominal radiographs. If a stone larger than 2.5 cm in diameter has migrated into the gut it may impact either at the terminal ileum or occasionally in the duodenum or sigmoid colon. The resultant intestinal obstruction may be followed by 'gallstone ileus'. Rarely, gallstones impacted in the cystic duct cause stricturing in the common hepatic duct (Mirizzi's syndrome).

Cancer of the gallbladder is rare, although it is recognised more frequently in an ageing population and in a 'porcelain' gallbladder. In over 95% of patients with gallbladder cancer there are accompanying gallstones. Cancer is usually diagnosed only at cholecystectomy for gallstone disease.

Management

Asymptomatic gallstones found incidentally are not usually treated because the majority will never give symptoms. Symptomatic gallstones are best treated surgically, but they can also be dissolved, fragmented in the gallbladder or removed mechanically from the common bile duct (see the information box).

TREATMENT OF GALLSTONES

- Cholecystectomy—open or laparoscopic
- Bile acids—chenodeoxycholic or ursodeoxycholic
- Contact dissolution
- Lithotripsy
- Endoscopic sphincterotomy

Medical dissolution of gallstones can be achieved by oral administration of the bile acid ursodeoxycholic acid. Radiolucent gallstones, a gallbladder that opacifies on oral cholecystography, stones not larger than 15 mm in diameter, moderate obesity and no or at most mild symptoms are the features which suggest that drug therapy may be feasible. Success can be expected in approximately 75% of patients who are not obese. Non-responders are patients who have radiolucent pigment stones which do not dissolve with ursodeoxycholic acid. Extracorporeal shock wave lithotripsy has recently been introduced, with the advantage of being non-invasive and safe, but at present it is expensive and not widely available. Bile salt therapy is necessary following lithotripsy to dissolve the gallstone fragments within the gallbladder. As in the case of oral bile salt therapy, only 30% of all patients with gallbladder disease are suitable for lithotripsy. All therapeutic regimens which retain the gallbladder have a 50% recurrence of stones after 5 years.

CHOLECYSTITIS

ACUTE CHOLECYSTITIS

Aetiology and pathology

Acute cholecystitis is almost always associated with obstruction of the gallbladder neck or cystic duct by a gallstone.

Occasionally obstruction may be by mucus, parasitic worms or a tumour. The pathogenesis is unclear, but the initial inflammation is possibly chemically induced. This leads to gallbladder mucosal damage which releases phospholipase, converting biliary lecithin to lysolecithin, a recognised mucosal toxin. At the time of surgery approximately 50% of cultures of the gallbladder contents are sterile. Infection occurs eventually and in elderly patients or those with diabetes mellitus a severe infection with gas-forming organisms can cause emphysematous cholecystitis. Acalculous cholecystitis can occur, especially following trauma.

Clinical features

The cardinal feature is pain in the right upper quadrant but also in the epigastrium, the right shoulder tip or interscapular region. It usually lasts for more than an hour but differentiation between biliary colic (see p. 730) and acute cholecystitis may be difficult; features suggesting cholecystitis include severe and prolonged pain, fever and leucocytosis.

Examination shows right hypochondrial tenderness, rigidity worse on inspiration (Murphy's sign), and occasionally a gallbladder mass. Fever is present and rigors may occur. Leucocytosis is common except in the elderly patient where the signs of inflammation may be minimal. Jaundice occurs in 20–25% of patients even if there are no stones in the common bile duct, and may represent oedematous pressure on or stricturing of the common hepatic duct (Mirizzi's syndrome). Minor increases of plasma transaminase and amylase activity may be encountered.

Cholecystitis usually resolves with medical treatment, but the inflammation may progress to an empyema or perforation and peritonitis. Acute cholecystitis in elderly people is a particular hazard as the disease tends to be severe, may have few localising clinical signs, and is associated with a high frequency of empyema and perforation (see p. 731). The mortality rate in elderly patients may reach 10%.

Investigations

Plain radiographs of the abdomen and chest may show gallstones, subdiaphragmatic gas (due to perforation of a viscus), and intrabiliary gas due to fistulation of a gallstone into the intestine (see p. 731), and are important in excluding lower lobe pneumonia. Ultrasonography detects gallstones and gallbladder thickening due to cholecystitis, and cholescintigraphy, if available, shows cystic duct obstruction. The plasma amylase should be measured to detect pancreatitis (see p. 653), which may be a complication of gallstones. The peripheral blood count often shows a leucocytosis.

Management

Medical

This consists of bed rest, pain relief, antibiotics and maintenance of fluid balance. Severe pain is relieved using morphine and the increased tone of the choledochal sphincter may be minimised by the concurrent use of atropine. Less severe pain can be relieved by pethidine, pentazocine or diclofenac. Antibiotics are required. A cephalosporin (such as cefuroxime) is the antibiotic of choice, and metronidazole is usually added in severely ill patients. Fluid balance is maintained by intravenous therapy and nasogastric aspiration is only needed for persistent vomiting.

Surgical

Emergency surgery is required when cholecystitis progresses in spite of medical therapy and in patients with a severe systemic illness and the development of complications such as empyema or perforation. Otherwise operations should be carried out after 2–3 days of medical therapy. Laparoscopic surgery can be used. Delayed surgery after 2–3 months is no longer favoured. Recurrent biliary colic or cholecystitis is frequent if the gallbladder is not removed.

POST-CHOLECYSTECTOMY SYNDROME

Dyspeptic symptoms following cholecystectomy (post-cholecystectomy syndrome) occur in about 30% of patients depending on how the condition is defined, how actively symptoms are sought, and the indications for cholecystectomy. When cholecystectomy is performed for acute calculous cholecystitis at least 70% of patients remain symptom-free. Post-cholecystectomy symptoms occur most frequently in women, in patients who have a history longer than 5 years

CAUSES OF POST-CHOLECYSTECTOMY SYMPTOMS
Immediate post-surgical
• Biliary injury • Bleeding • Biliary peritonitis • Abscess • Fistula
Biliary
• Common bile duct stones • Benign stricture • Tumour • Cystic duct stump syndrome • Papillary disorders Dysfunction, stenosis
Extrabiliary
• Flatulent dyspepsia • Peptic ulcer • Pancreatic disease • Gastro-oesophageal reflux • Irritable bowel syndrome • Functional abdominal pain

prior to cholecystectomy, and in patients in whom the operation was undertaken for non-calculous gallbladder disease (see the information box). Severe post-cholecystectomy syndrome occurs in only 2–5% of patients.

The usual complaints include right upper quadrant abdominal pain, flatulence, fatty food intolerance, and occasionally jaundice and cholangitis. Liver function tests may be abnormal and sometimes show cholestasis. Ultrasonography is used to detect biliary obstruction, and retrograde cholangiopancreatography is usually needed to detect common bile duct stones. Other investigations which may be required include upper gastrointestinal endoscopy, barium examination of the small intestine, pancreatic function tests, cholescintigraphy and a liver biopsy. The question of a functional illness should also be considered.

Treatment of any cause such as residual stones should be carried out. Where no cause is found, reassurance that no serious abnormality has been found may be sufficient. Features at ERCP suggesting biliary dyskinesia should prompt consideration of endoscopic sphincterotomy, and where no abnormality is found treatment for irritable bowel syndrome (see p. 668) can be tried.

CHRONIC CHOLECYSTITIS

Chronic inflammation of the gallbladder is almost invariably associated with gallstones. The condition may be asymptomatic. The usual symptoms are those of recurrent attacks of upper abdominal pain, often at night and following a heavy meal. The clinical features are similar to those of acute calculous cholecystitis but milder. The patient may recover spontaneously or following analgesia and antibiotics. Patients are advised to undergo a cholecystectomy.

CHOLEDOCHOLITHIASIS

Stones in the common bile duct occur in 10–15% of patients with gallstones. These stones account for more than 80% of common bile duct stones; they migrate from the gallbladder, and are similar in appearance and chemical composition to the stones found elsewhere. Primary bile duct stones may develop within the common bile duct many years after a cholecystectomy and represent the accumulation of biliary sludge consequent upon dysfunction of the sphincter of Oddi. In Far Eastern countries, where bile duct infection is common, primary common bile duct stones are thought to follow bacterial infection secondary to parasitic infections with *Clonorchis sinensis*, *Ascaris lumbricoides* or *Fasciola hepatica*. Common bile duct stones can cause partial or complete bile duct obstruction and may be complicated by stricture, cholangitis due to secondary bacterial infection, liver abscess and septicaemia.

Clinical features

Choledocholithiasis may be asymptomatic or manifest as recurrent abdominal pain with or without jaundice. The pain is usually in the right upper quadrant and fever, pruritus and dark urine may be present. Painless jaundice is uncommon. Physical examination may show the scar of a previous cholecystectomy; if the gallbladder is present it is usually small, fibrotic and impalpable.

Investigations

Liver function tests show a cholestatic pattern and bilirubinuria is present. If cholangitis is present the patient usually has a leucocytosis. The most convenient method of demonstrating obstruction to the common bile duct is by ultrasonography which shows dilated extra- and intrahepatic bile ducts together with gallbladder stones, but it is not always successful in indicating the cause of the obstruction in the common bile duct (see Fig. 10.31). Endoscopic retrograde cholangiography has the advantage that not only can a diagnosis be made of obstruction and its cause, but common bile duct stones can be removed. Percutaneous transhepatic cholangiography may also be used.

Management

Cholangitis requires analgesia for pain, intravenous fluids and broad-spectrum antibiotics such as cefuroxime and metronidazole. Blood cultures should be taken before the antibiotics are administered. Patients require stone removal

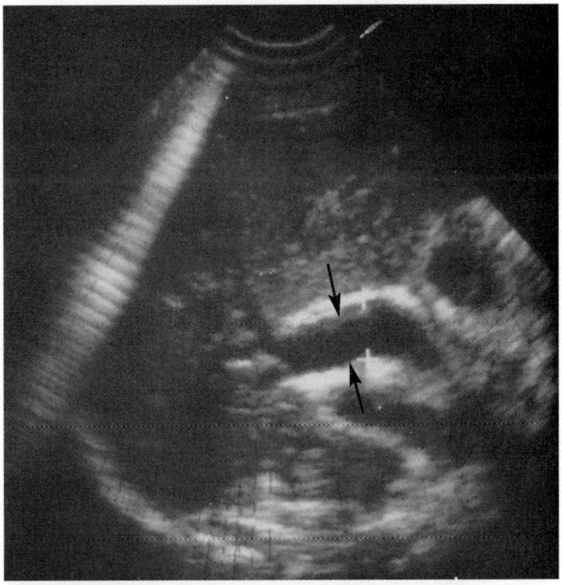

Fig. 10.31 Ultrasound showing dilated bile ducts (between arrows) in obstructive jaundice secondary to obstruction of the common bile duct.

either surgically or by endoscopic sphincterotomy via ERCP. The latter is increasingly used as the first approach for the removal of bile duct stones, particularly in patients over the age of 60 years. Endoscopic sphincterotomy and stone extraction is successful in about 90% of patients and has a low morbidity and mortality. Less commonly used techniques include extracorporeal lithotripsy.

Surgical treatment of choledocholithiasis is performed less frequently because of the higher morbidity and mortality compared with an endoscopic sphincterotomy. Before exploring the common bile duct an accurate diagnosis of choledocholithiasis should be confirmed by intraoperative cholangiography or choledochoscopy. If gallstones are found, the bile duct is explored, all stones are removed, stone clearance is checked by cholangiography or choledochoscopy, and a T-tube is inserted into the common bile duct.

RECURRENT PYOGENIC CHOLANGITIS (ASIATIC CHOLANGIOHEPATITIS)

This disease occurs in South-east Asia. Biliary sludge, calcium bilirubinate concretions and stones accumulate in the intrahepatic bile ducts with secondary bacterial infection. The patients present with recurrent attacks of upper abdominal pain, fever and cholestatic jaundice. Investigation of the biliary tree demonstrates that both the intra- and extrahepatic portions are filled with soft biliary mud. Eventually the liver becomes scarred and liver abscesses develop. The condition is difficult to manage and requires drainage of the biliary tract with extraction of stones, antibiotics and, in certain patients, partial resection of damaged areas of the liver.

TUMOURS OF THE GALLBLADDER AND BILE DUCT

CARCINOMA OF THE GALLBLADDER

This is a rare tumour occurring more often in females and is usually encountered above the age of 70 years. More than 90% of such tumours are adenocarcinomas; the remainder are anaplastic or, rarely, squamous tumours. Gallstones are usually present and are thought to be important in the aetiology of the tumour.

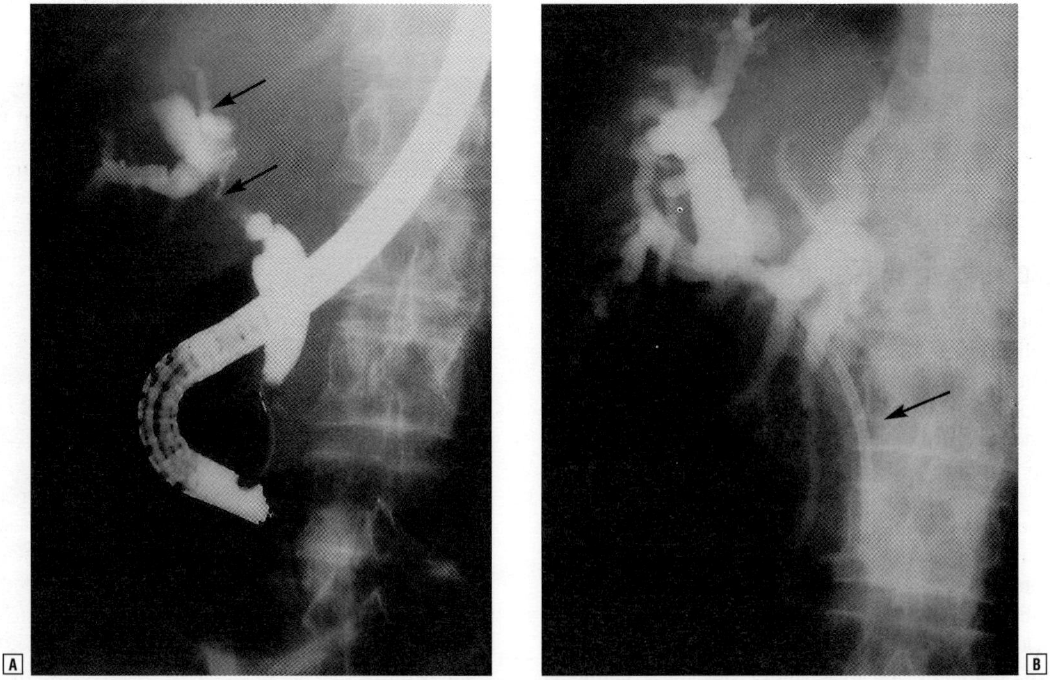

Fig. 10.32 Cholangiocarcinoma. A ERCP showing malignant biliary stricture (bottom arrow) and dilated intrahepatic bile ducts above (top arrow). B Post-ERCP stenting showing plastic endobiliary stent (arrow) which will draw bile from the dilated ducts above the stricture into the duodenum.

The condition is usually diagnosed at surgery for gallstone disease. Occasionally it may manifest as repeated attacks of biliary pain and later persistent jaundice and weight loss. A gallbladder mass may be palpable in the right hypochondrium. Liver function tests show cholestasis, and gallbladder calcification (porcelain gallbladder) may be found on radiograph. The tumour may be diagnosed on ultrasonography. The treatment is surgical excision but local extension of the tumour beyond the wall of the gallbladder into the liver and surrounding tissues is not infrequent and palliative management is usually all that can be offered. Survival is generally short.

CHOLANGIOCARCINOMA

This uncommon tumour arises anywhere in the biliary tree from the small intrahepatic bile ducts to the papilla of Vater. The cause is unknown but it is associated with gallstones and primary sclerosing cholangitis (see p. 721). Primary sclerosing cholangitis is associated with ulcerative colitis, and cholangiocarcinoma may occur some years after proctocolectomy or as a presenting feature, with ulcerative colitis being discovered only subsequently.

The patient presents with jaundice which may be intermittent. Half the patients have upper abdominal pain and weight loss. The diagnosis is made by endoscopic cholangiography or percutaneous transhepatic cholangiography but can be difficult to confirm in patients with sclerosing cholangitis. Cholangiocarcinomas can occasionally be excised surgically, but most patients are treated by inserting drainage stents across the tumour using endoscopic or transhepatic techniques (see Fig. 10.32).

CARCINOMA AT THE PAPILLA OF VATER

Nearly 40% of all adenocarcinomas of the small intestine arise in relationship to the papilla of Vater and present with pain, anaemia, vomiting and weight loss. Jaundice may be intermittent or persistent. Diagnosis is made by duodenal endoscopy and biopsy of the tumour. Ampullary carcinoma must be differentiated from carcinoma of the head of the pancreas and a cholangiocarcinoma because both these conditions have a worse prognosis.

Curative surgical treatment can be undertaken by pancreaticoduodenectomy or a segmental resection and the 5-year survival may be as high as 50%. When this is impossible a palliative bypass or insertion of a drainage stent is performed.

BENIGN GALLBLADDER TUMOURS

These are uncommon, often asymptomatic and usually found incidentally at operation or autopsy. Cholesterol polyps, sometimes associated with cholesterolosis, papillomas and adenomas, are the main types.

MISCELLANEOUS BILIARY DISORDERS

BILIARY MOTOR DISORDERS

Some patients with right upper quadrant discomfort do not have gallstones and the term 'biliary dyskinesia' has been introduced to describe this condition. The dyskinetic disorder may affect either the gallbladder or the sphincter of Oddi. Patients complain of recurrent epigastric or right upper quadrant pain.

The diagnosis is established by excluding gallstones and undertaking tests to demonstrate that contraction of the gallbladder is associated with pain or that the papilla is stenosed. ERCP, endoscopic manometry, intraoperative manometry and radiomanometry are all used in an attempt to define this disorder more clearly. Identification of biliary dyskinesia remains difficult and the treatment is uncertain. Some of these patients are being treated with a sphincterotomy at the time of endoscopic assessment of the condition.

CHOLESTEROLOSIS OF THE GALLBLADDER

In this condition lipid deposits in the submucosa and epithelium appear as multiple yellow spots on the pink mucosa, giving rise to the description 'strawberry gallbladder'. The condition is asymptomatic but may occasionally present with right upper quadrant pain. Radiologically the features are those of small fixed filling defects on cholecystography or ultrasonography and the radiologist can usually differentiate between gallstones and cholesterolosis. The condition is usually diagnosed at cholecystectomy; if the diagnosis is made radiologically, cholecystectomy is indicated.

ADENOMYOMATOSIS OF THE GALLBLADDER

In this condition there is hyperplasia of the muscle and mucosa of the gallbladder. The projection of pouches of mucous membrane through weak points in the muscle coat produces Rokitansky–Aschoff sinuses. There is much disagreement over whether adenomyomatosis is a cause of right upper quadrant pain or other gastrointestinal symptoms. It may be diagnosed by oral cholecystography when a halo or ring of opacified diverticula can be seen around the gallbladder. Other appearances include deformity of the body of the gallbladder or marked irregularity of the outline. Localised adenomyomatosis in the region of the gallbladder fundus causes the appearance of a 'Phrygian cap'. Most patients are treated by cholecystectomy but it is advisable first to exclude other diseases in the upper gastrointestinal tract.

FURTHER INFORMATION ON GALLBLADDER AND OTHER BILIARY DISEASES

Chapman R W 1991 Aetiology and natural history of primary sclerosing cholangitis: a decade of progress? Gut 32: 1433–1435
Davidson B R 1993 Progress in determining the nature of bile duct strictures. Gut 34: 725–726
Jakiche A, Carey W 1995 The tortoise and the hare—the race toward improved treatment for gallstones. Journal of Gastroenterology 90: 1915–1917
Johnston D E, Kaplan M M 1993 Pathogenesis and treatment of gallstones. New England Journal of Medicine 328: 412–421
Northfield T 1994 Management of gallstones—overview. European Journal of Gastroenterology and Hepatology 10: 849–851
Soloway R D, Crowther R S 1995 Bacteria and cholesterol gallstones—molecular biology comes to gallstone pathogenesis. Gastroenterology 108: 934–936
Toouli J 1989 What is sphincter of Oddi dysfunction? Gut 30: 753–761

Diseases of the blood 11

M.J. MACKIE • C.A. LUDLAM • A.P. HAYNES

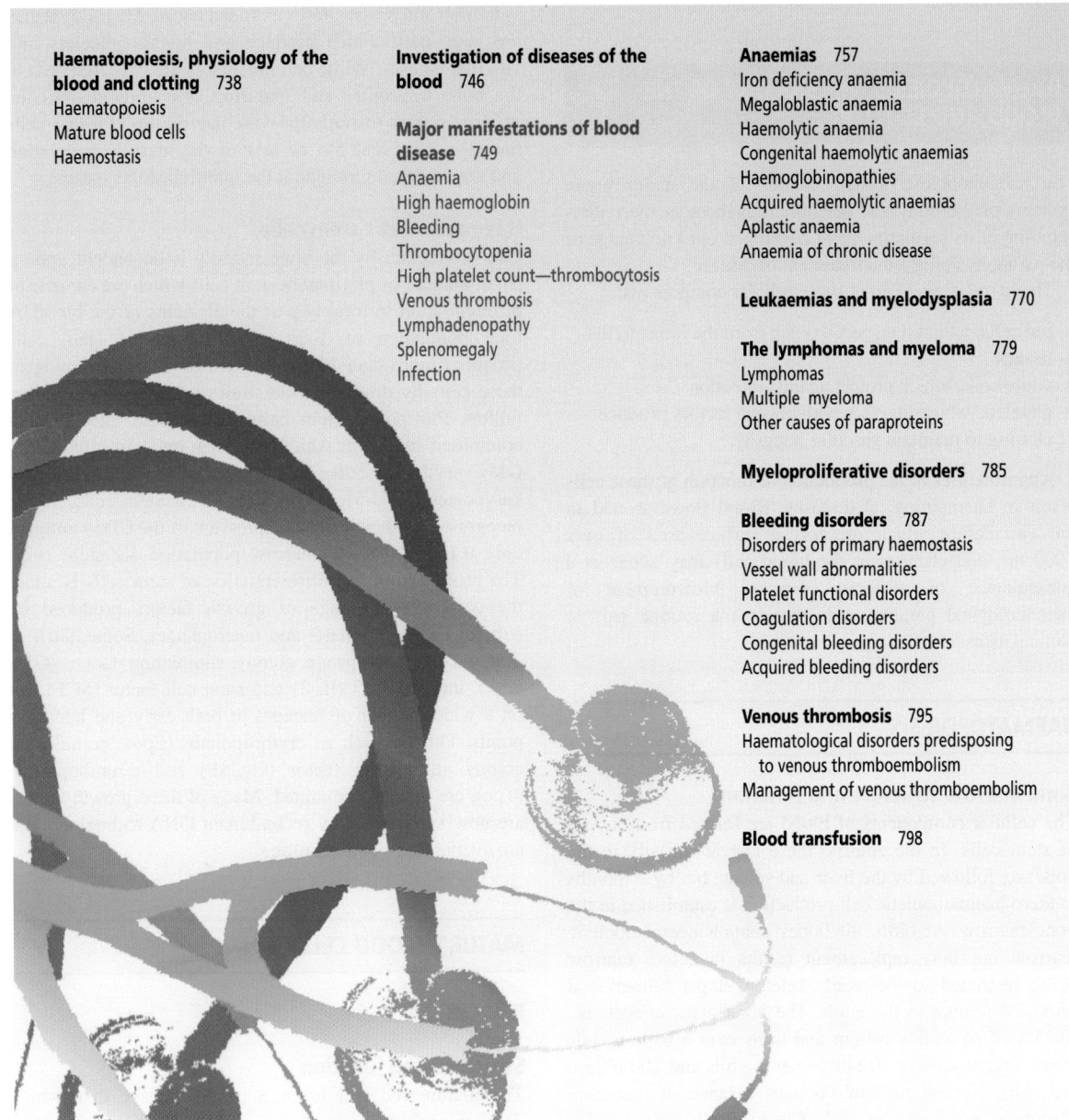

Blood diseases cover a wide spectrum of illnesses ranging from anaemias, amongst the most common disorders affecting mankind, to relatively rare conditions such as leukaemias and congenital coagulation disorders. Although the latter are uncommon, recent advances in their understanding at the cellular and molecular level are already beginning to impact on diagnosis and treatment.

Diseases affecting any system can, however, secondarily influence haematological parameters, making their study an integral part of the assessment of any medical disease. This assessment is facilitated by the ease of access to the blood and bone marrow.

HAEMATOPOIESIS, PHYSIOLOGY OF THE BLOOD AND CLOTTING

The haematopoietic system is one of the major organ systems of the body and scientific advances in the understanding of its regulation have developed our knowledge of the pathophysiology and treatment of disease.

The blood is made up of three cellular components:

- red cells, which transport oxygen from the lungs to the tissues
- white cells, which protect against infection
- platelets, which together with plasma factors produce clotting to maintain vascular integrity.

Abnormalities of the production or function of these cells result in haematological diseases. Blood flows around in the vasculature which presents a surface area of over 1000 m^2, and changes in the blood cells may occur as a consequence of systemic disease. Measurement of haematological parameters is therefore a routine part of clinical assessment.

HAEMATOPOIESIS

Bone marrow structure and function

The cellular components of blood are formed from a pool of stem cells. In the embryo these appear initially in the yolk sac, followed by the liver and spleen, but by 5 months in utero haematopoietic cell production is established in the bone marrow. At birth, all bones contain haematopoietic marrow but fatty replacement results in active marrow being restricted to the axial skeleton, upper humeri and proximal femora in the adult. The bone marrow accounts for 5% of an adult's weight and turns over a trillion cells every day, producing 70 billion neutrophils and 200 billion red cells. Normal marrow contains a range of immature precursors and a storage pool of mature cells for release at times of increased demand. Up to 10 times the circulating number of neutrophils are stored in the marrow, whilst for red cells the storage and circulating pools are equal in size. In normal marrow some 50–60% of cells are dedicated to myeloid cell production.

Bone marrow occupies the intertrabecular spaces in trabecular bone. Haematopoietic cells exist in a framework of reticular cells and collagen in intimate relationship with stromal cells, adipocytes and macrophages, which provide the necessary microenvironment. Normal marrow has a characteristic organisation (see Fig. 11.1). Nests of red cell precursors cluster around a central macrophage which provides iron and phagocytoses extruded nuclei. Megakaryocytes are large cells which produce and release platelets into vascular sinuses. White cell precursors are clustered next to the bone trabeculae and maturing cells migrate into the marrow spaces towards the vascular sinuses. Plasma cells normally represent 5% or less of the marrow population and are scattered throughout the intertrabecular spaces.

Haematopoietic stem cells

Cell production by the bone marrow is dependent upon a small number of pluripotent stem cells which are capable of differentiation to form any of the elements of the blood. A total population of 1–2 $\times$ 10^6 pluripotent stem cells produces more than 10^{11} cells each day, and poisoning of these cells by drugs or irradiation results in bone marrow failure. Pluripotent stem cells differentiate into lineage-committed stem cells which will form myeloid cells (CFU-GM), erythroid cells (BFU-E and CFU-E) and megakaryocytes (CFU-Meg) (see Fig. 11.2). Stem cells can be recognised by their surface expression of the CD34 antigen; only 0.1–0.3% of the marrow population are stem cells. The proliferation and differentiation of stem cells is under the control of a range of growth factors produced by stromal cells, fibroblasts and macrophages. Some, such as granulocyte macrophage colony stimulating factor (GM-CSF), interleukin 3 (IL-3) and stem cell factor (SCF), act on a wide number of lineages at both early and late time points. Others, such as erythropoietin (Epo), granulocyte colony stimulating factor (G-CSF) and thrombopoietin (Tpo), are lineage-committed. Many of these growth factors are now synthesised by recombinant DNA technology and are available for clinical usage.

MATURE BLOOD CELLS

RED CELLS

Structure and function

The mature red cell is an 8 μm biconcave disc which delivers oxygen to the tissues from the lungs and carbon

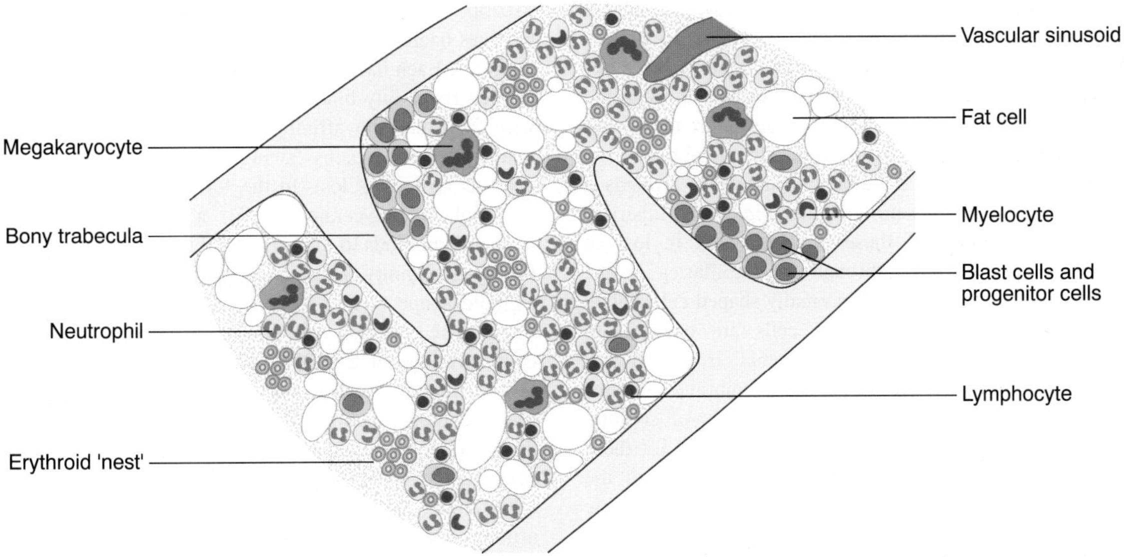

Fig. 11.1 Structural organisation of normal bone marrow.

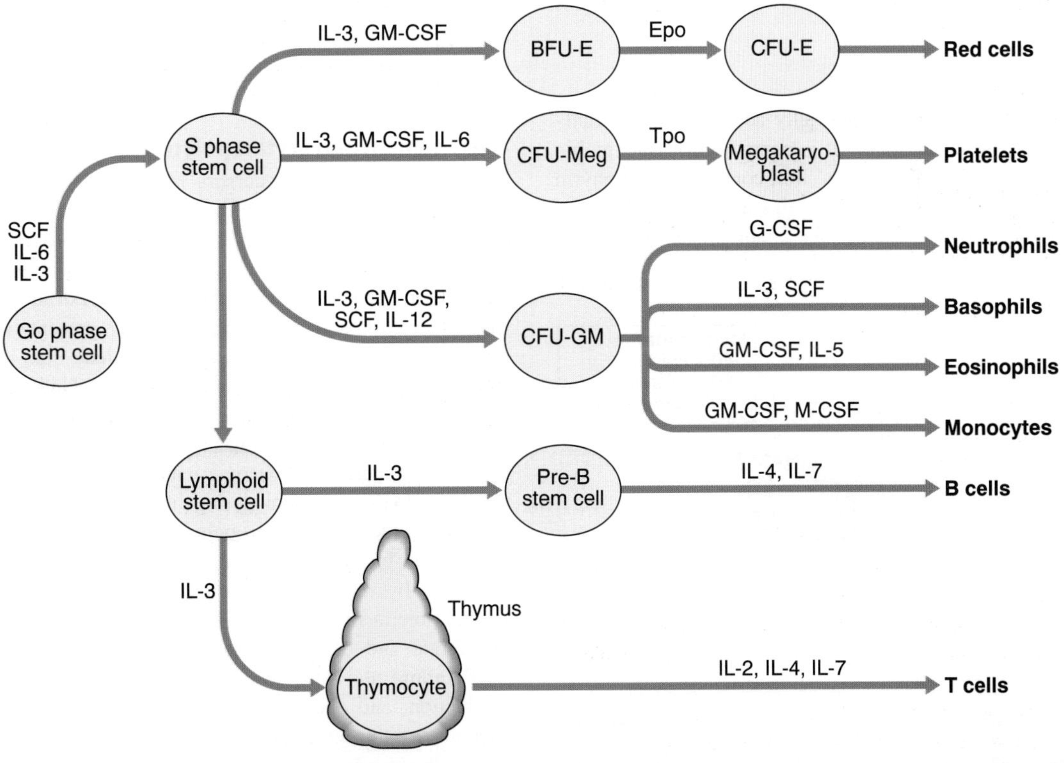

Fig. 11.2 Stem cells and growth factors in haemopoietic cell development. (BFU-E = blast forming unit-erythroid; CFU-Meg = colony forming unit-megakaryocyte; CFU-GM = colony forming unit-granulocyte macrophage; CFU-E = colony forming unit-erythroid; IL = interleukin; SCF = stem cell factor; GM-CSF = granulocyte macrophage colony stimulating factor; Epo = erythropoietin; Tpo = thrombopoietin; G-CSF = granulocyte colony stimulating factor; M-CSF = macrophage colony stimulating factor)

dioxide in the reverse direction. It is anucleate and has no mitochondria; the normal red cell lifespan is about 120 days but in this time it will travel approximately 300 miles around the circulation. Red cells have to pass through the smallest capillaries in the circulation and their membrane structure is adapted to be deformable. The membrane has a lipid bilayer to which a 'skeleton' of filamentous proteins is attached via special link proteins (see Fig. 11.3). Inherited abnormalities of any of these proteins result in loss of membrane as cells pass through the capillaries in the spleen, and the formation of abnormally shaped cells called spherocytes or elliptocytes. Red cells are exposed to osmotic stress in the pulmonary and renal circulation and, to maintain normal homeostasis, the membrane contains ion pumps which control intracellular levels of sodium, potassium, chloride and bicarbonate. The energy for these functions is provided by the metabolic pathways of the cytosol; 90% of glucose metabolism occurs via anaerobic glycolysis which produces adenosine triphosphate (ATP), and 10% via the pentose phosphate pathway which produces nicotinamide adenine dinucleotide phosphate (NADPH). Membrane proteins inserted into the lipid bilayer also form the antigens recognised by blood grouping. The ABO and Rhesus systems are the most commonly recognised but over 400 blood group antigens have been described.

Haemoglobin

Haemoglobin is a protein specially adapted for gas transport to and from the lungs. It is composed of four globin chains, each containing an iron-containing porphyrin pigment termed haem. Globin chains are a combination of two alpha and two non-alpha chains; haemoglobin A

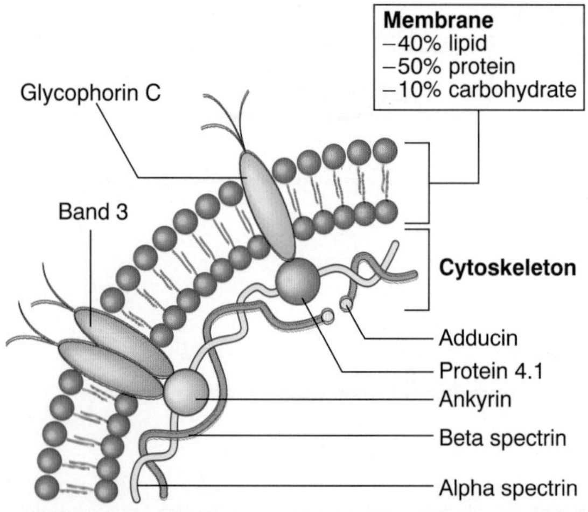

Fig. 11.3 Normal structure of red cell membrane.

($\alpha\alpha/\beta\beta$) represents over 90% of adult haemoglobin, whereas haemoglobin F ($\alpha\alpha/\gamma\gamma$) is the predominant type in the fetus. Each haem contains a ferrous ion (Fe^{++}) to which oxygen reversibly binds; the final oxygen to bind does so with 20 times the affinity of the first. When oxygen is bound, the beta chains 'swing' closer together and move apart as oxygen is lost. In the 'open' deoxygenated state, 2,3 diphosphoglycerate (DPG), a product of red cell metabolism, binds to the haemoglobin molecule and lowers its oxygen affinity. These complex interactions produce the sigmoid shape of the oxygen dissociation curve (see Fig. 11.4). The position of this curve depends upon the concentrations of 2,3 DPG, H^+ ions and CO_2; increased levels shift the curve to the right and cause oxygen to be released more readily. Tissue hypoxia increases all three and favours increased availability of oxygen from the red cell. Haemoglobin F is unable to bind 2,3 DPG and has a left-shifted oxygen dissociation curve; this increased affinity, together with the low pH of fetal blood, ensures fetal oxygenation. Amino acid mutations affecting the haem-binding pockets of globin chains or the 'hinge' interactions between globin chains result in haemoglobinopathies or unstable haemoglobins. Alpha globin chains are produced by two genes on chromosome 16 and beta globin chains by a single gene on chromosome 11; imbalance in the production of globin chains produces the thalassaemias.

Development and erythropoietin

The earliest red cell precursors in the bone marrow are nucleated. These cells divide rapidly without time for growth between divisions and produce progressively smaller daughter cells which undergo haemoglobinisation. Maturation is complete when the nucleus is extruded but at this stage, ribosomal material is still present in the cytoplasm. This can be stained by methylene blue to give the characteristic appearance of reticulocytes. Under normal staining reticulocytes are large cells with a faint blue tinge which is termed polychromasia. Reticulocytes lose their ribosomal material and become mature over 3 days, being released into the circulation during this time. A reticulocytosis will reflect increased erythropoiesis. Red cell production is controlled by erythropoietin, a polypeptide hormone produced by renal tubular cells in response to hypoxia. Erythropoietin stimulates committed erythroid stem cells to proliferate and decreases maturation time. Patients with renal failure are anaemic due to failure of erythropoietin production, and exogenous recombinant hormone can be used to treat this anaemia.

Destruction

Red cells at the end of their lifespan are phagocytosed by the reticulo-endothelial system. Amino acids from globin chains

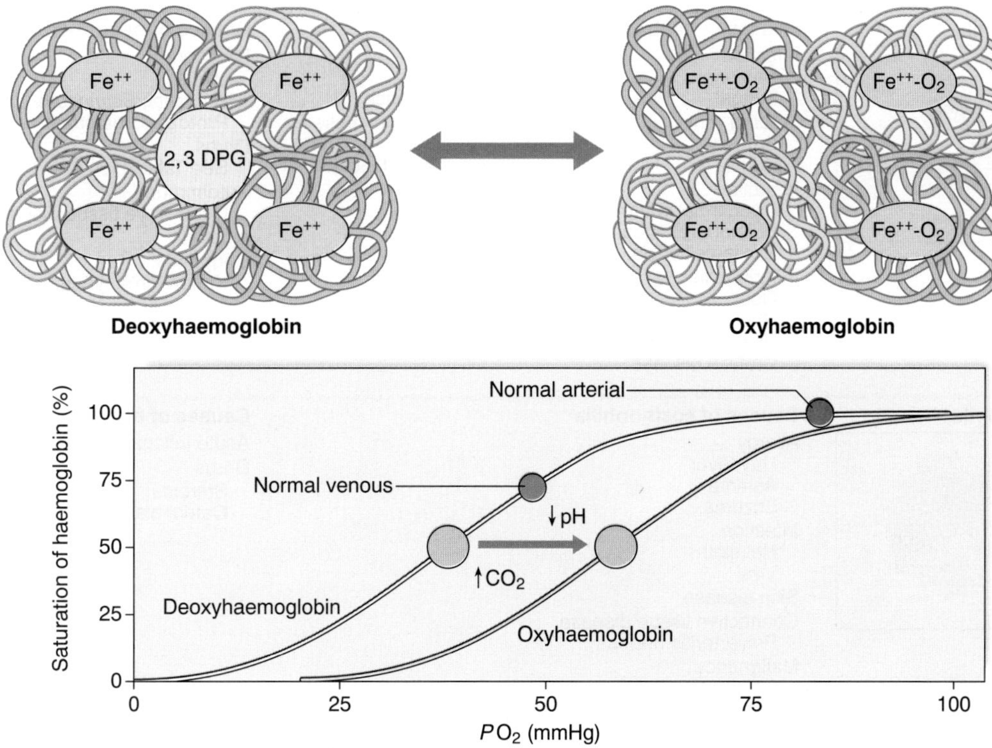

Fig. 11.4 Structure of the normal haemoglobin molecule and its relationship to the oxygen dissociation curve.

are recycled and iron is removed from haem for reuse in haemoglobin synthesis. The remnant haem structure is degraded to bilirubin and conjugated to glucuronic acid before excretion into bile. In the small bowel, bilirubin is converted to stercobilin; most of this is excreted, but a small amount is reabsorbed and excreted by the kidney as urobilinogen. Increased red cell destruction due to haemolysis or ineffective haemopoiesis will result in jaundice and increased urinary urobilinogen. Free intravascular haemoglobin is toxic and haptoglobins are plasma proteins produced by the liver which normally bind free haemoglobin in the circulation.

WHITE CELLS

Structure, function and development

Five major types of white cell are recognised: neutrophils, eosinophils, basophils, monocytes and lymphocytes. In the child up to the age of 7 years, lymphocytes are the predominant white cell type but after the age of 7 neutrophils are the most abundant type. Neutrophils, eosinophils and basophils are termed granulocytes, being distinguished by the presence of prominent cytoplasmic granulation (see Fig. 11.5).

Neutrophils

Mature cells are 10–14 μm in diameter with a multilobular nucleus containing 2–5 segments; hence the term polymorphonuclear leucocyte. Their main function is to recognise and ingest foreign particles and microorganisms, which are then destroyed without toxic effects on normal tissues. Two types of granule are recognised: primary or azurophil granules, and the more numerous secondary or specific granules. Primary granules contain myeloperoxidase and other proteins which are important for microbial killing and are released intracellularly. Secondary granules contain a number of membrane proteins such as adhesion molecules and components of the oxidase enzyme with which neutrophils produce superoxide radicals for microbial killing. These are released into the plasma membrane upon degranulation and the granule contents, such as lactoferrin, are released extracellularly. Granule staining becomes more intense in response to infection and is termed 'toxic granulation'. The degree of nuclear segmentation may vary; in megaloblastic anaemia or iron deficiency, cells with six or more nuclear segments appear and the process is termed 'right shift'. This also occurs in toxic states.

The earliest recognisable neutrophil precursor is the myeloblast, which differentiates into promyelocytes with

Neutrophils

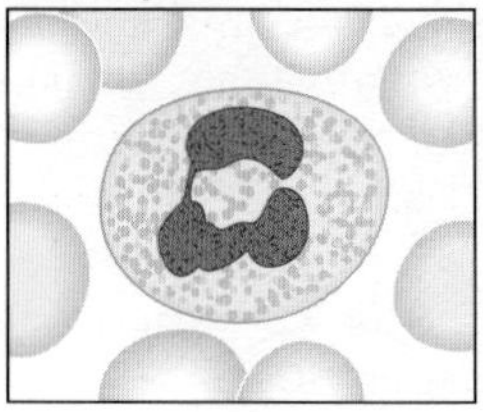

Causes of neutrophilia

Infection
- Bacterial
- Fungal

Trauma
- Surgery
- Burns

Infarction
- Myocardial infarct
- Pulmonary embolus
- Sickle-cell crisis

Inflammation
- Gout
- Rheumatoid arthritis
- Ulcerative colitis
- Crohn's disease

Malignancy
- Solid tumours
- Hodgkin's disease

Myeloproliferative disease
- Polycythaemia
- Chronic myeloid leukaemia

Physiological
- Exercise
- Pregnancy

Causes of neutropenia

Infection
- Viral
- Bacterial; *Salmonella*
- Protozoal; malaria

Drugs
- See Table 11.1

Autoimmune
- Connective tissue disease

Alcohol

Congenital
- Kostmann's syndrome

Eosinophils

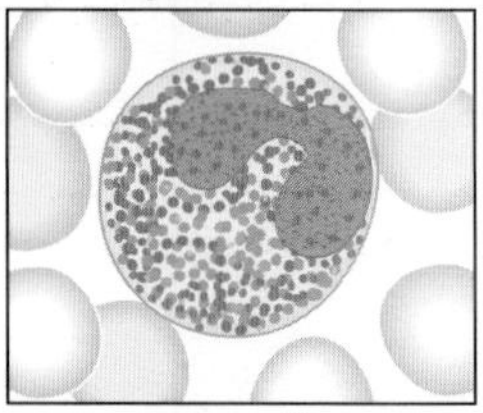

Causes of eosinophilia

Allergy
- Hay fever
- Asthma
- Eczema

Infection
- Helminths
- Viral

Skin disease

Connective tissue disease
- Polyarteritis nodosa

Malignancy
- Solid tumours
- Lymphomas

Drugs
- Gold

Causes of eosinopenia

Acute inflammation

Drugs
- Steroids
- Catecholamines

Basophils

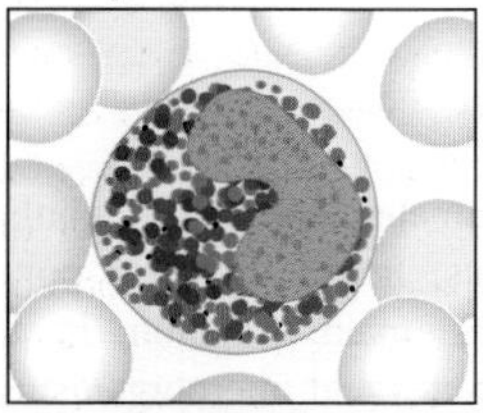

Causes of basophilia

Myeloproliferative disease
- Polycythaemia
- Chronic myeloid leukaemia

Inflammation
- Acute hypersensitivity
- Ulcerative colitis
- Crohn's disease

Iron deficiency

Causes of basopenia

Hyperthyroidism

Monocytes

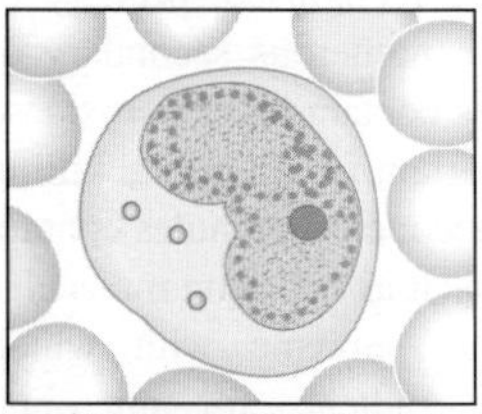

Causes of monocytosis

Infection
- Bacterial; TB

Inflammation
- Connective tissue disease
- Ulcerative colitis
- Crohn's disease

Malignancy
- Solid tumours

Lymphocytes

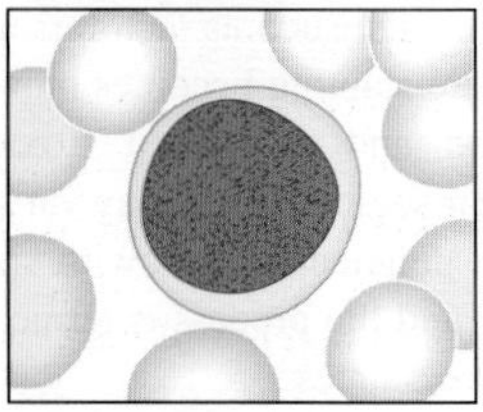

Causes of lymphocytosis

Infection
- Viral
- Bacterial, *Bordatella pertussis*

Lymphoproliferative disease
- Chronic lymphatic leukaemia
- Lymphoma

Post-splenectomy

Causes of lymphopenia

Inflammation
- Connective tissue disease

Lymphoma

Renal failure

Drugs
- Steroids
- Cytotoxics

Congenital
- Severe combined immunodeficiency

Table 11.1 Drugs associated with neutropenia

Group	Examples
Analgesics/anti-inflammatory agents	Phenylbutazone, oxyphenylbutazone, gold, diflunisal Penicillamine, naproxen
Antithyroid	Carbimazole, propylthiouracil
Anti-arrhythmics	Quinidine, procainamide, tocainide
Antihypertensives	Captopril, enalapril, nifedipine
Antidepressants/psychotropics	Amitriptyline, dothiepin, mianserin
Antimalarials	Pyrimethamine/dapsone, sulfadoxine/pyrimethamine, chloroquine
Anticonvulsants	Phenytoin, sodium valproate, carbamazepine
Antibiotics	Sulphonamides, penicillins, cephalosporins
Miscellaneous	Cimetidine, ranitidine, chlorpropamide, zidovudine

primary granules; these then become myelocytes, with primary and secondary granules; and finally maturation occurs via the metamyelocyte stage to segmented neutrophils. This process takes 17–25 days and a large storage pool of mature cells exists in the bone marrow. Every day some 1×10^{14} neutrophils enter the circulation, where cells may be freely circulating or attached to endothelium in the marginating pool. These two pools are equal in size and factors such as exercise or catecholamines increase the cells flowing in the blood, so increasing the white cell count. Neutrophils spend 6–10 hours in the circulation and 1–2 days after passing into the tissues before being consumed in the inflammatory process or phagocytosed by macrophages. Myelocytes or metamyelocytes are normally only found in the marrow but may appear in the circulation in infection or toxic states. The appearance of more primitive myeloid precursors in the blood is often associated with the presence of nucleated red cells and is termed a 'leucoerythroblastic' picture, which indicates a serious disturbance of marrow function.

Eosinophils

Eosinophils are a similar size to neutrophils but usually only represent 1–6% of the circulating white cells. They have bilobed nuclei and have prominent orange granules on H and E staining, which are larger than those seen in the neutrophil. Eosinophils are phagocytic and their granules contain a peroxidase capable of generating reactive oxygen species and proteins involved in the intracellular killing of protozoa and helminths.

Basophils

Basophils are the same size as neutrophils but are less common than eosinophils, representing less than 1% of circulating white cells. They contain dense black granules which usually obscure the nucleus. Mast cells resemble basophils but are only found in the tissues. Basophils bind IgE antibody on to their surface, and exposure to specific antigen results in degranulation with release of histamine, leucotrienes and heparin. These cells are involved in hypersensitivity reactions.

Monocytes

Monocytes are the largest of the white cells, with a diameter of 12–20 μm and an irregular nucleus in abundant pale blue cytoplasm containing occasional cytoplasmic vacuoles. These cells migrate into the tissues where they become macrophages, Kupffer cells or antigen-presenting dendritic cells. The former phagocytose debris, apoptotic cells and microorganisms. They produce a variety of cytokines when activated, such as interleukin-1, tumour necrosis factor and GM-CSF. Monocytes are long-lived cells.

Lymphocytes

These are heterogeneous, with the smaller cells being equal in size to red cells and the largest to neutrophils. Small lymphocytes are circular with scanty cytoplasm but the larger cells are more irregular with abundant blue cytoplasm. The majority of lymphocytes in the circulation are T cells (80%), which can be recognised by their expression of the CD antigens CD1, 2, 3, 4, 5, 7 and 8. The T cells mediate cellular immunity and two major types are recognised: CD4 positive helper cells and CD8 positive suppressor cells (see p. 28). The B cells mediate humoral immunity and can be recognised by their expression of immunoglobulin light chains (kappa or lambda in a ratio of 2:1). Lymphocyte subpopulations can be defined with specific functions and their lifespan can vary from several days to many years.

HAEMOSTASIS

With the evolution of the circulation as a transport system, an efficient mechanism developed, not only to prevent blood loss from a damaged vessel to secure haemostasis but also to prevent the inappropriate cessation of flow. Haemostasis depends upon interactions between the vessel wall, platelets and clotting factors. Two phases of haemostasis can be recognised: primary and secondary. In the initial primary phase, the damaged vessel contracts and activated platelets aggregate at the site of damage to form a plug to arrest haemorrhage. This occurs over a number of minutes

Fig. 11.5 ***(Opposite page)*** **Normal white blood cells.**

and is subsequently followed by the secondary deposition of a fibrin mesh to secure the platelet plug. These two processes are interlinked; damaged endothelium activates platelets, which then provide the optimal surface for the enzymatic generation of insoluble fibrin.

PLATELETS

Structure, function and development

Resting platelets are discoid-shaped, with a diameter of 2–4 μm (see Fig. 11.6). The surface membrane invaginates to form a tubular network, the canalicular system. This provides a large surface area of phospholipid on to which clotting factors can absorb. Three types of granule are present in the cytoplasm:

- alpha granules contain fibrinogen and von Willebrand factor
- dense (delta) granules store adenosine diphosphate (ADP) and 5-hydroxytryptamine (5-HT, serotonin)
- lysosomes contain acid hydrolases.

When platelets are activated by ADP, thrombin or collagen they contract to become spherical and extend pseudopodia which adhere to the subendothelium and other platelets. Upon activation, platelet granules discharge their contents, which encourage further platelet aggregation and fibrin formation. At the same time, arachidonic acid is released from the platelet membrane and converted by cyclo-oxygenase to endoperoxides and the powerful platelet aggregating agent, thromboxane A2. Aspirin and non-steroidal anti-inflammatory drugs irreversibly inhibit platelet cyclo-oxygenase and impair platelet function. Platelet-binding to subendothelium is dependent on high molecular weight von Willebrand factor released from endothelial cells, which bridges the gap between platelet membrane glycoproteins and subendothelial collagen. Interplatelet aggregation is dependent upon fibrinogen binding to platelet glycoproteins.

Platelets are derived from megakaryocytes, each of which sheds several thousand platelets directly into the circulation in the marrow sinusoids. Megakaryocytes are derived from lineage-committed stem cells, the CFU-Meg, and their proliferation and ploidy are controlled by a newly described growth factor termed thrombopoietin (Tpo). Platelets circulate for 8–14 days before they are destroyed in the reticulo-endothelial system. Some 30% of peripheral platelets are normally pooled in the spleen and not circulating.

CLOTTING FACTORS

The clotting system consists of a series of soluble inactive zymogens designated by roman numerals. When proteolytically cleaved and activated, each is capable of activating one or more components of the cascade. Activated factors are designated by the suffix ‘a’. These reactions usually require a source of appropriate phospholipid and calcium. Two pathways of activation are recognised (see Fig. 11.7).

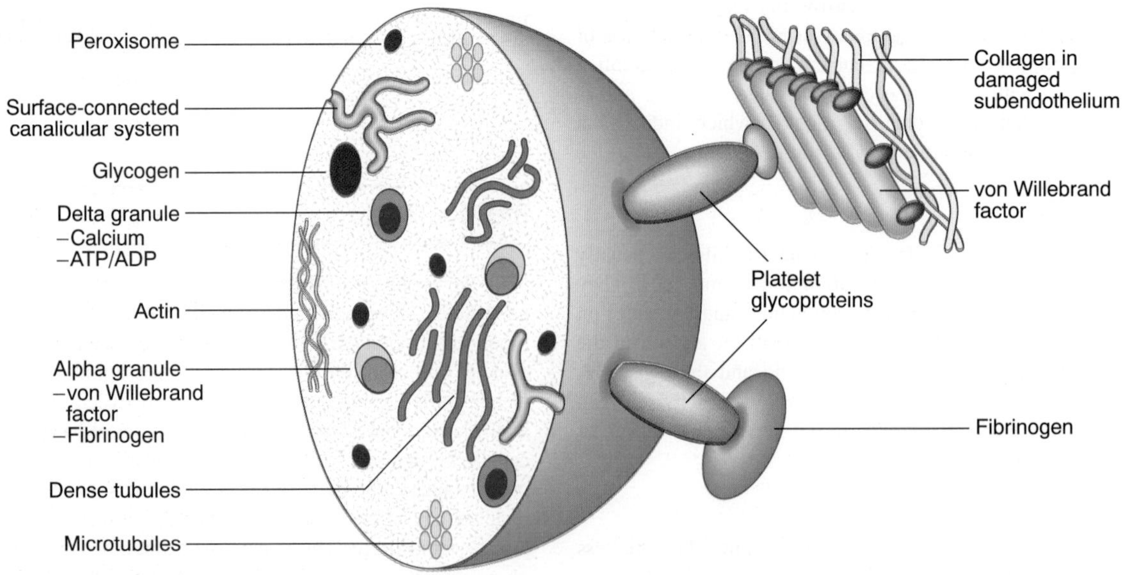

Fig. 11.6 Normal platelet structure.

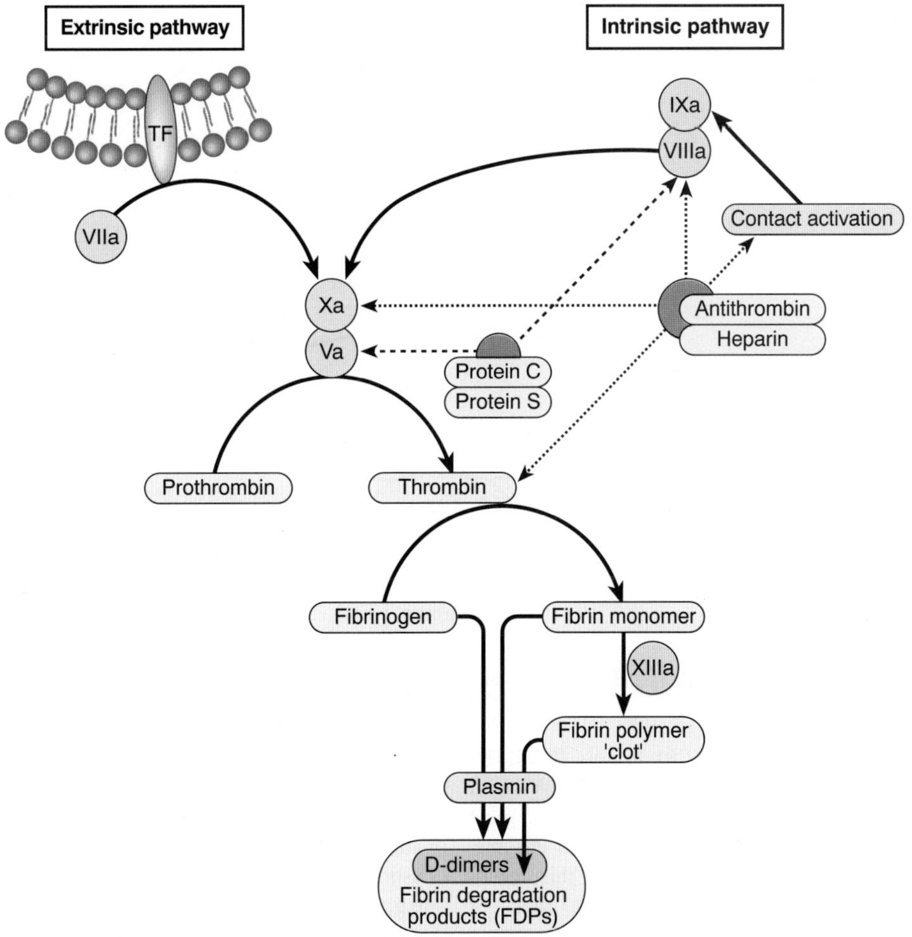

Fig. 11.7 Normal haemostatic mechanisms: clotting factors of the intrinsic and extrinsic pathways. Broken lines signify inhibitory activity. (See p. 794 for an explanation of D-dimers.)

The 'extrinsic' pathway is the principal physiological haemostatic mechanism in vivo. When vessels are damaged, subendothelial cells are exposed. All cells not exposed to the circulation express a 100 kDa transmembrane protein termed tissue factor (TF); the brain, uterus and tumour tissues are particularly rich in this factor. Tissue factor can also be expressed by damaged endothelial cells and activated monocytes. Tissue factor activates factor VII, which in turn activates factor X. In the 'intrinsic' pathway, the negatively charged subendothelial surface and collagen exposed by vessel damage activate the 'contact system', which in turn activates the complex of factors VIII and IX. This complex then activates factor X. Activated factor X forms a complex with factor V on the surface of activated platelets and this complex converts prothrombin to thrombin. Thrombin converts fibrinogen to fibrin monomer, which polymerises and is cross-linked by factor XIII to form stable clot. Thrombin plays a crucial role in this 'final common pathway'; platelets, factors V, VIII and XI are activated by thrombin, which generates a positive feedback loop. Congenital deficiencies of any of these factors will result in a bleeding diathesis.

The extrinsic pathway is assessed by the 'prothrombin time' (PT). The intrinsic pathway is assessed by the 'activated partial thromboplastin time' (APTT).

Clotting factors are synthesised by the liver but factor V is also produced in platelets and endothelial cells. Factors II, VII, IX and X are produced as inactive proteins. These factors are rich in glutamic acid (Gla) residues, which must be carboxylated to permit calcium-binding and association with phospholipid to generate an active catalytic site. The carboxylase enzyme responsible for this in the liver uses

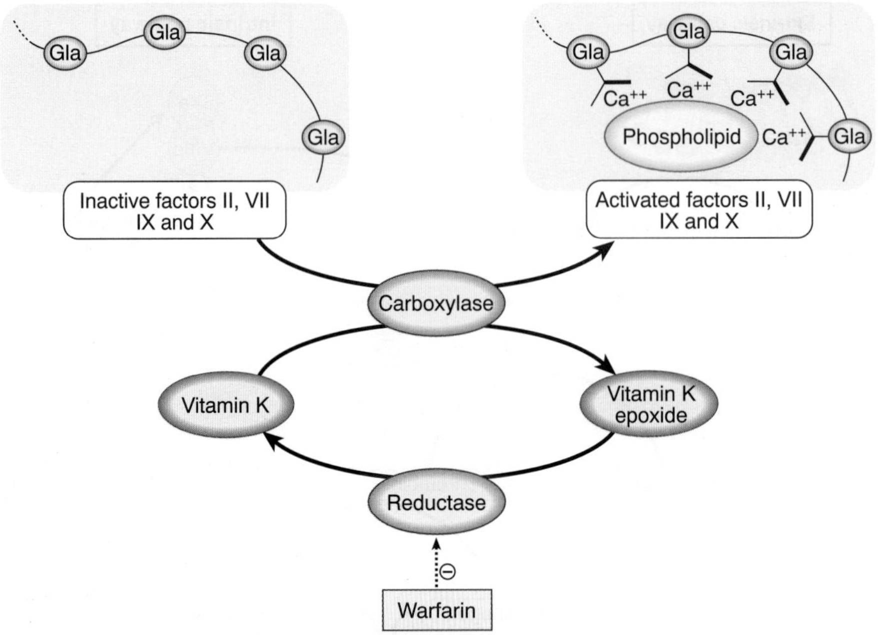

Fig. 11.8 The role of vitamin K in clotting and the mechanism of action of warfarin.

vitamin K as a cofactor (see Fig. 11.8). Factors II, VII, IX and X are therefore termed vitamin K-dependent. Vitamin K is converted to an epoxide in this reaction and must be regenerated to its active form by a reductase enzyme. This reductase is inhibited by warfarin and this mechanism forms the basis of the anticoagulant effect of coumarins.

To prevent inappropriate activation of the clotting cascade, natural inhibitors of the clotting systems are present (see Fig. 11.7). Antithrombin III is a protein produced by the liver which has weak inhibitory activity against thrombin and factor Xa. When antithrombin binds to heparin, however, this inhibitory activity is markedly accelerated and this forms the basis of the anticoagulant action of heparin. Protein C is a vitamin K-dependent factor produced by the liver; when activated by interaction with protein S, it inhibits factor Va. These natural inhibitors are powerful control points in the positive feedback cascade of clotting, and abnormalities in their function result in a tendency to thrombosis.

INVESTIGATION OF DISEASES OF THE BLOOD

THE FULL BLOOD COUNT (FBC)

This is the haematology test which is requested most frequently by clinicians. Blood anticoagulated with ethylenediaminetetraacetic acid (EDTA) is rapidly processed through an automatic analyser. A variety of technologies (particle-sizing, radio frequency and laser instrumentation) are used to measure the haemoglobin, count the red cells, estimate the haematocrit and measure red cell parameters, e.g. mean cell volume (MCV), mean cell haemoglobin content and mean cell haemoglobin concentration. The absolute white count is measured and a differential count performed. The most modern version of analysers has the ability to provide a full five-part differential. A platelet count is also measured. Thus a wealth of information is provided by what can be regarded as a simple test. It is important to appreciate that a number of conditions can lead to spurious results (see Table 11.2). The reference

Table 11.2 Causes of spurious results from automatic full blood count analysers

Result	Explanation
Increased haemoglobin	Lipaemia, jaundice, very high white cell count
Reduced haemoglobin	Improper sample mixing, blood taken from a vein into which an infusion is flowing
Increased mean red cell volume	Cold agglutinins, non-ketotic hyperosmolarity
Increased white cell count	Nucleated red cells
Reduced platelet count	Clots in the sample, platelet clumping or satellitism

Table 11.3 Reference range for haematological parameters

Parameter	Female	Male	Male and female
Haemoglobin (Hb) g/l	115–165	130–180	
Haematocrit (Hct)	0.37–0.47	0.4–0.54	
Red blood cells (RBC) $\times 10^9$/l	3.8–5.8	4.5–6.5	
Erythrocyte sedimentation rate (ESR) mm in 1 hour	0–7	0–5	
Mean cell volume (MCV) fl			76–98
Mean corpuscular haemoglobin (MCH) pg			27–35
Mean corpuscular haemoglobin concentration (MCHC) g/dl			31–35
Red cell distribution width (RDW)			11–16
Platelets $\times 10^9$/l			150–400
White blood cells $\times 10^9$/l			4.0–11.0
Differential WBC			
Neutrophils			2.0–7.5 $\times 10^9$/l (40–75%)
Lymphocytes			1.5–4.0 $\times 10^9$/l (20–45%)
Monocytes			0.2–0.8 $\times 10^9$/l (2–10%)
Eosinophils			0.04–0.4 $\times 10^9$/l (1–6%)
Basophils			0.01–0.1 $\times 10^9$/l (0–1%)
Reticulocytes			10–100 $\times 10^9$/l (0.2–2%)
Serum ferritin	14–150 µg/l	17–300 µg/l	
Serum vitamin B_{12}			140–725 ng/l
Serum folate			1.9–9.0 µg/l
Red cell folate			118–450 µg/l
Red cell mass	20–30 ml/kg	25–35 ml/kg	
Plasma volume			40–50 ml/kg

Table 11.4 Terms describing abnormal blood film appearances and their meaning

Term	Meaning
Microcytosis	The average size of the red cells is reduced. The mean cell volume will be reduced. It is commonly found in iron deficiency anaemia and other disorders of haemoglobin synthesis (thalassaemias)
Macrocytosis	The average size of red cells is greater than normal. The mean cell volume will be increased. It is seen, for instance, in megaloblastic anaemias but its occurrence does not necessarily mean a megaloblastic change in the marrow. A common cause is excessive alcohol consumption
Hypochromia	The red cells contain less than the normal amount of haemoglobin and they stain less deeply. They show greater than normal central pallor. Hypochromia is commonly associated with microcytosis and is a characteristic feature of disorders of haemoglobin synthesis, most commonly iron deficiency
Anisocytosis	Inequality in the size of the red cells. It is found in many forms of anaemia but is very prominent in megaloblastic anaemia
Poikilocytosis	Marked irregularity in the shape of the red cells. It is never present without anisocytosis and usually reflects dyserythropoiesis
Target cells	Abnormally flat red cells with a central mass of haemoglobin surrounded by a ring of pallor and an outer ring of haemoglobin. They are commonly associated with liver disease, impaired or absent splenic function (hyposplenism) and haemoglobinopathies
Polychromasia and reticulocytosis	Young red cells when stained by the Romanowsky method have a faint bluish colour (basophilia) due to residual ribosomal material. A blood film in which such cells are present in increased numbers along with those of normal orange colour is said to show polychromasia. This, like reticulocytosis, indicates increased production of new red cells by the bone marrow
Punctate basophilia (basophilic stippling)	Abnormally damaged young red cells may show scattered deep-blue dots in the cytoplasm with Romanowsky staining. Such punctate basophilia may be found in any severe anaemia but the presence of many of these cells is most commonly seen in beta-thalassaemia and chronic lead poisoning, where it may occur when the anaemia is slight
Howell–Jolly bodies	Remnants of nuclear material left in the erythrocyte after the nucleus is extruded. They are normally removed by the spleen and their presence usually indicates a non-functioning or absent spleen. Their numbers are greatly increased in certain erythropoietic disorders, e.g. megaloblastic anaemia
Pappenheimer bodies	Iron-protein complexes (sideroblastic granules) found in red cells in certain iron overload states and increased when the spleen is non-functioning or absent
Nucleated red cells	Usually normoblasts, found in the blood when erythropoiesis is very vigorous or when there is irritation of the bone marrow, as in leukaemia or infiltration by secondary tumour
Hypersegmented polymorphs	Present when more than 3% of the polymorphs have five or more lobes or there are any with six lobes. B_{12} or folate deficiency is a common cause
Leucoerythroblastic	A blood picture in which primitive granulocytes and erythroblasts are simultaneously present in the peripheral blood. It is usually, but not necessarily, associated with anaemia and reflects bone marrow irritation, as in malignant infiltration of the marrow, or disordered haemopoiesis, as in myelofibrosis. It can occur as a reaction to severe haemolysis or bleeding

values for a number of common haematological parameters in adults are given in Table 11.3.

BLOOD FILM EXAMINATION

Although the technical advances of modern full blood count analysers have resulted in fewer blood films requiring examination, scrutiny of the blood film can often yield invaluable information (see Table 11.4). Analysers, in the main, are not able to recognise abnormal white cells such as blast cells or identify abnormalities of red cell shape and content (Howell–Jolly bodies, basophilic stippling, malarial parasites etc.).

BONE MARROW EXAMINATION

Bone marrow examination is performed in adults either from the posterior iliac crest or, rarely, the sternum. Marrow may be simply aspirated or a bone marrow biopsy (trephine) performed. The latter cannot be obtained safely from the sternum and increasingly both aspirate and biopsy are performed from the posterior iliac crest. A biopsy is superior for assessing marrow cellularity and infiltration. Bone marrow examination is performed under local anaesthesia and can easily be undertaken as an outpatient procedure. Both aspiration and trephine biopsy can be carried out by the same needle but often separate needles are used.

Marrow is examined not only for its morphological appearances but increasingly cell marker studies, karyotyping and molecular biology studies are undertaken, as appropriate, for the accurate diagnosis and assessment of malignant disease. Marrow can also be sent for culture in cases of suspected tuberculosis. The main indications for a bone marrow examination are shown in the information box.

MAIN INDICATIONS FOR BONE MARROW EXAMINATION

Marrow disorders

- Leukaemias
- Lymphomas
- Secondary carcinoma
- Myeloproliferative disorders

Cytopenia(s)

- Neutropenia
- Thrombocytopenia
- Anaemia—complex cases or aplasia

INVESTIGATION OF THE COAGULATION SYSTEM

Bleeding disorders

The investigation of a patient with a possible bleeding disorder is directed by the clinical circumstances. The initial screening tests are usually a platelet count, prothrombin time (PT), activated partial thromboplastin time (APTT) and fibrinogen concentration (see Table 11.5).

Table 11.5 Screening tests for assessing a patient for a bleeding disorder

Investigation	Normal range	Situations in which the test is abnormal
Platelet count	150–350 × 10^9/l	Thrombocytopenia Congenital Acquired
Bleeding time	Less than 8 minutes	Thrombocytopenia Thrombopathy Congenital Acquired, e.g. aspirin, von Willebrand disease
Prothrombin time	12–14 seconds	Deficiency of factors II, V, VII, X Liver disease Warfarin therapy DIC*
Activated partial thromboplastin time	30–40 seconds	Deficiency of factors II, V, VIII, IX, X, XI, XII Haemophilia A and B Von Willebrand disease DIC*
Fibrinogen concentration	1.5–3.0 g/dl	Congenital hypofibrinogenaemia

* Disseminated intravascular coagulation.

The extrinsic system (see Fig. 11.7) is assessed with the PT, in which the patient's plasma is incubated with tissue factor and calcium. The reaction proceeds with the activation by factor VIIa of factor X and to a lesser extent factor IX. Thus the prothrombin time is particularly sensitive to a deficiency of factors VII, X and V. The APTT is determined by adding an activator to plasma—for instance, a suspension of kaolin—along with an extract of phospholipid (to mimic the platelet membrane). The APTT is prolonged with a deficiency of factor II, V, VIII, IX, X, XI or XII. Neither the PT nor the APTT is sensitive to minor deficiencies of fibrinogen or a lack of factor XIII, an enzyme which cross-links molecules of fibrin to enhance the strength of the polymerising fibrin; both these factors therefore need to be measured by specific assays. It is possible to measure the plasma concentration of all of the other coagulation factors by relatively simple clotting assays.

Platelet function can be assessed by performing a standardised template bleeding time test. In this investigation a small incision is made on the forearm below a sphygmomanometer cuff inflated up to 40 mmHg. The bleeding time is prolonged in those with platelet functional defects, thrombocytopenia and von Willebrand disease. Platelet function can be further assessed by measuring aggregation in response to various agents, e.g. adrenaline and collagen, or measuring the constituents of the intracellular granules, e.g. ATP/ADP.

Thrombotic disorders

As for a patient with a possible bleeding disorder, the history is of crucial importance in deciding which investigations should be undertaken (see the first information box). The available investigations to assess thrombophilia, i.e. the propensity to (particularly venous) thrombosis, are set out in the second information box. Anticoagulants can alter either the concentration or the activity of several of the plasma factors and, if possible, blood samples should therefore be collected before, or after discontinuation of, anticoagulant therapy. On occasion this is not possible and the result has to be interpreted in the knowledge of the effect of the prevailing anticoagulant.

INDICATIONS FOR THROMBOPHILIA SCREEN

Patients with any of the following features should be screened for thrombophilia:

- Venous thrombosis < 45 years
- Recurrent venous thrombosis
- Family history of venous thrombosis
- Venous thrombosis at an unusual site
  e.g. Cerebral venous thrombosis
  Hepatic vein (Budd–Chiari syndrome)
  Portal vein
- Arterial and venous thrombosis

INVESTIGATION OF THROMBOPHILIA

- Antithrombin
- Protein C
- Protein S
- Factor II Leiden
- Factor V Leiden
- Thrombin/reptilase time (for dysfibrinogenaemia)
- Antiphospholipid antibody
  Lupus anticoagulant
  Anticardiolipin antibody
- Homocysteine

FURTHER INFORMATION ON INVESTIGATION OF DISEASES OF THE BLOOD

Dacie J V, Lewis S M 1995 Practical haematology, 8th edn. Churchill Livingstone, Edinburgh

MAJOR MANIFESTATIONS OF BLOOD DISEASE

ANAEMIA

Clinical features of anaemia reflect the diminished oxygen-carrying capacity of the blood. The severity depends on the degree of the anaemia and the rapidity of its development but is independent of its cause. The general features of anaemia are listed in the first information box.

The classification of anaemias outlined in the second information box helps to guide the clinician in planning investigations as it reflects the underlying mechanisms. The most common cause of anaemia is iron deficiency and the most common reason for this is blood loss. However, anaemia is often multifactorial.

An alternative classification of anaemia is based on the size of the red cell, which is most accurately indicated by the MCV. In the presence of anaemia:

- a normal MCV suggests either acute blood loss or the anaemia of chronic disease (ACD)
- a low MCV suggests iron deficiency or thalassaemia
- a high MCV suggests B_{12} or folate deficiency.

Flow charts can be developed indicating the pattern of

SYMPTOMS AND SIGNS OF ANAEMIA

Symptoms	Signs
• Lassitude • Fatigue • Breathlessness on exertion • Palpitations • Throbbing in head and ears • Dizziness • Tinnitus • Headache • Dimness of vision • Insomnia • Paraesthesia in fingers and toes • Angina	• Pallor of: Skin Mucous membranes Palms of hands Conjunctivae • Tachycardia • Cardiac dilatation • Systolic flow murmurs • Oedema

CAUSES OF ANAEMIA

Decreased or ineffective marrow production

- Lack of iron, B_{12} or folate
- Hypoplasia
- Invasion by malignant cells

Peripheral causes

- Blood loss
- Haemolysis
- Hypersplenism

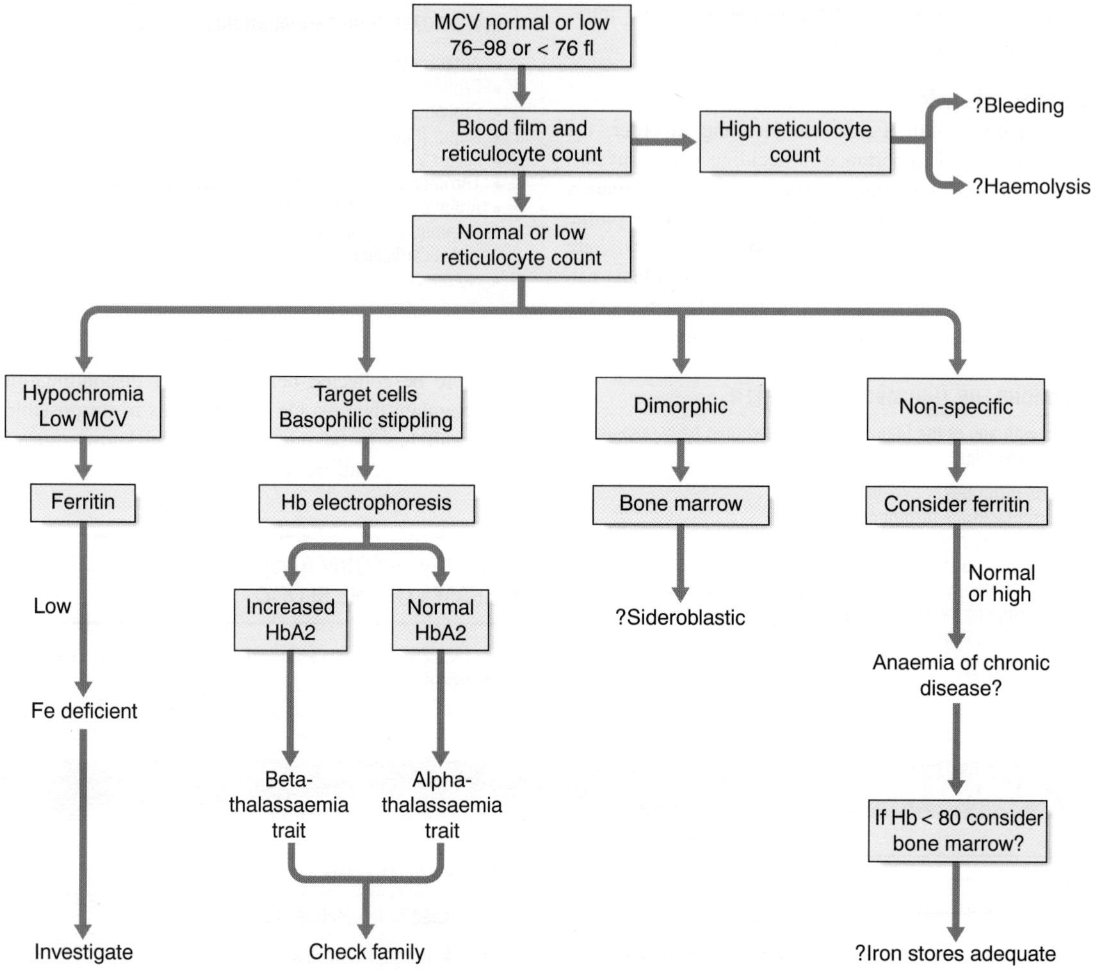

Fig. 11.9 Investigation of anaemia: MCV normal or low.

investigation in an anaemic patient based on the MCV (see Figs 11.9 and 11.10).

Clinical clues as to the cause of the anaemia are obtained from the history and examination of the patient:

- As the most common type of anaemia world-wide is iron deficiency, enquiry as to the symptoms of gastrointestinal disease is very important. This should be particularly directed towards establishing whether there is any likely source of blood loss. However, lack of specific complaints does not rule out silent pathology.
- Females still menstruating should be asked in detail about their periods.
- A dietary history is very important, particularly as regards the intake of iron and folate. Dietary deficiency of B_{12} is unusual unless the patient excludes all animal products (i.e. is a vegan). Surgical resection of the stomach or small bowel may lead to malabsorption of iron and/or B_{12}.
- Previous medical history may reveal a disease which is known to be associated with anaemia (the anaemia of chronic disease).
- Family history and ethnic background of the patient are important. Haemolytic anaemias such as the haemoglobinopathies and hereditary spherocytosis may be suspected from the family history. Pernicious anaemia may also run in the family.
- Drug history may reveal the ingestion of drugs which can be associated with blood loss but drugs may also cause haemolysis or aplasia (e.g. aspirin and other non-steroidal anti-inflammatory drugs—see pp. 768–769).

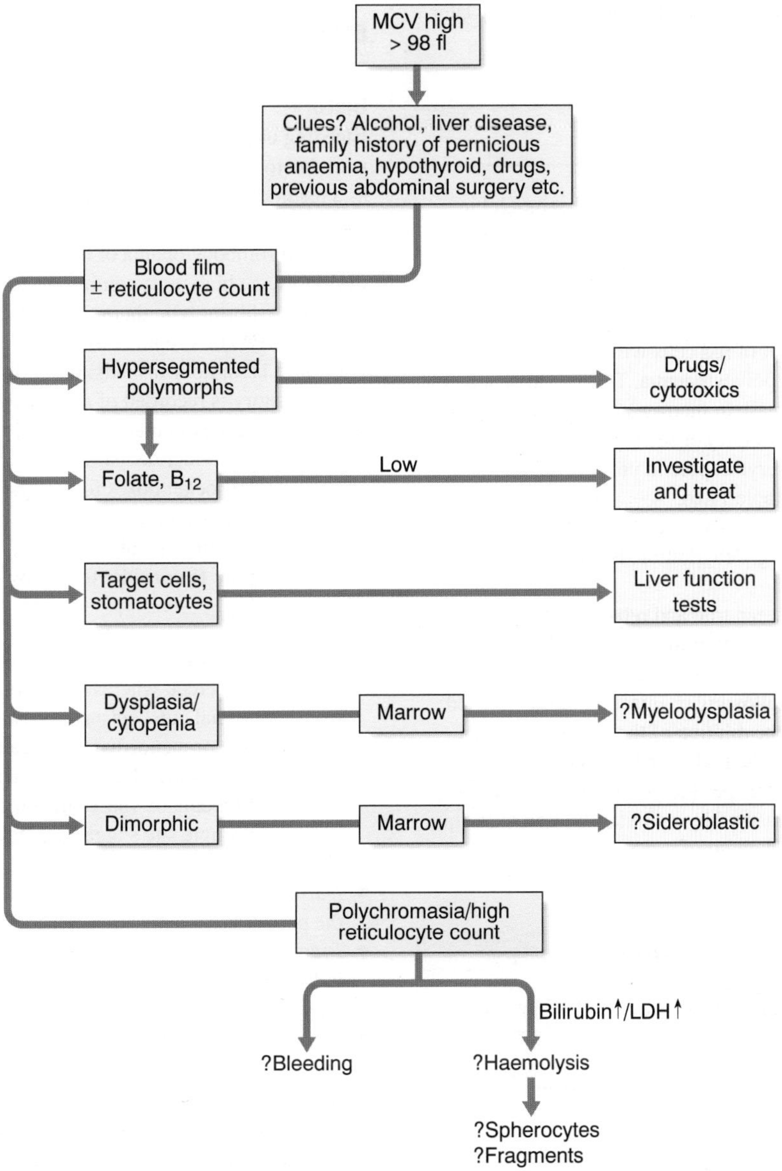

Fig. 11.10 Investigation of anaemia: high MCV. (LDH = lactate dehydrogenase)

As well as the general physical findings of anaemia shown in the information box on page 749, there may be specific findings related to the aetiology of the anaemia; for example, a patient may be found to have a right iliac fossa mass due to an underlying caecal carcinoma or a bulky uterus due to fibroids. The presence of jaundice should alert the physician to the possibility of a haemolytic disease. Sickle-cell anaemia (see p. 764) not only results in symptoms of anaemia, but microvascular occlusion due to the abnormal red cell also results in organ damage and pain. These painful crises may be acute, presenting with, for example, chest symptoms or long bone pain. However, there may be chronic pain from avascular necrosis and leg ulcers.

Vitamin B_{12} deficiency may be associated with signs of subacute combined degeneration of the cord and also is a cause of optic atrophy and dementia.

Specific types of anaemia are dealt with separately later in this chapter (see pp. 757–770).

HIGH HAEMOGLOBIN

It is essential to determine whether a high haemoglobin is due to true or relative polycythaemia because their further investigation and management are quite different.

A raised haemoglobin is usually due to an absolute increase in the number of red cells within the circulation; this is known as true polycythaemia. This can arise either due to a primary increase in marrow activity (primary proliferative polycythaemia) or secondary to hypoxia or excess inappropriate erythropoietin production, e.g. lung or renal disorders (see Table 11.6).

The haemoglobin can also be raised due to a reduction in the plasma volume, e.g. dehydration, leading to relative polycythaemia.

To distinguish between true and relative polycythaemia it is necessary to measure the circulating red cell mass by labelling an aliquot of the patient's erythrocytes with a tracer dose of ^{51}Cr. Following re-injection of the labelled cells and measuring the dilution of the isotope, the total volume of red cells in the body can be assessed; the result is expressed in millilitres per kilogram body weight. The plasma volume is measured by a similar dilution technique using homologous ^{125}I albumin.

Table 11.6 Classification of polycythaemia

Red cell mass	Plasma volume	Cause
True polycythaemia		
Raised	Normal	Primary
		Primary proliferative polycythaemia
		Secondary
		Hypoxia
		High altitude
		Lung disease
		Cyanotic heart disease
		Smoking
		High-affinity haemoglobins
		Inappropriate erythropoietin production
		Renal
		Hydronephrosis
		Cysts
		Carcinoma
		Tumours
		Liver
		Uterus
		Cerebellum
Relative polycythaemia		
Normal	Decreased	Dehydration

BLEEDING

History

Bleeding usually results from either a breach of the vessel wall due to a specific insult, e.g. peptic ulcer, or trauma, or as a result of generalised haemostatic failure. This arises secondary to deficiency of one or more of the coagulation factors, thrombocytopenia or occasionally excessive fibrinolysis, which most commonly arises following therapeutic fibrinolytic therapy with tissue plasminogen activator (tPA) or streptokinase.

Prior to laboratory investigation it is important that a careful history is recorded of all bleeding episodes as well as a full clinical examination. A history of bleeding is often remarkably reproducible, particularly after dental extraction; if a socket oozes for 2 days after removal of a tooth on one occasion, this is likely to occur again following each subsequent extraction.

It is important to consider the following points when taking a history:

- *Site of bleeds*. Muscle and joint bleeds indicate a coagulation defect, whereas purpura, prolonged bleeding from superficial cuts, epistaxis, gastrointestinal haemorrhage or menorrhagia indicate a failure of primary haemostasis due to a platelet disorder, thrombocytopenia or von Willebrand disease. Recurrent bleeds at a single site suggest a local structural abnormality.
- *Duration of history*. It may be possible to assess whether the patient has a congenital or acquired disorder.
- *Precipitating causes*. Bleeding arising spontaneously indicates a more severe defect than if haemorrhage arises only after trauma.
- *Surgery*. Enquiry about all operations is useful but particularly about dental extractions, tonsillectomy and circumcision, as these are all stressful tests of the haemostatic system. Bleeding that starts immediately after surgery indicates defective platelet plug formation, whereas that which comes on after several hours is more indicative of failure of platelet plug stabilisation by fibrin due to a coagulation defect.
- *Family history*. Absence of relatives with clinically significant bleeding does not exclude a hereditary bleeding diathesis; about one-third of cases of haemophilia, for example, arise in individuals without a family history.
- *Systemic illnesses*. Many diseases, or their treatment, may be associated with bleeding but it is particularly important to consider the possibility of hepatic or renal failure, paraproteinaemia or a collagenosis.
- *Drugs*. Almost any medicine can potentially produce bleeding, either by depressing marrow function with

consequent thrombocytopenia or by interacting with warfarin. Non-steroidal anti-inflammatory drugs inhibit platelet function; the effect of aspirin may last for up to 10 days after a single tablet.

Examination

Superficial examination may reveal bruises and purpura or scars due to poor healing following prolonged superficial bleeding. Telangiectasia of lips and tongue point to hereditary haemorrhagic telangiectasia. Joints should be carefully scrutinised for evidence of haemarthroses. A full general medical examination is important because it may give clues of systemic illness—for example, stigmata of liver disease; splenomegaly may cause thrombocytopenia due to hypersplenism.

Investigations

Screening investigations and their interpretation are described on page 748 and in Table 11.5. If the patient has a history strongly suggestive of a bleeding disorder and all the preliminary screening tests give normal results, it may be appropriate to perform further investigations. The clinical history may be a useful guide as to whether attention should be directed to platelet function (or von Willebrand disease) or coagulation disturbance, e.g. haemophilia.

THROMBOCYTOPENIA

A reduced platelet count may arise by one of three mechanisms:

- failure of megakaryocyte maturation
- excessive platelet consumption after their release into the circulation
- their sequestration in an enlarged spleen.

The common causes of thrombocytopenia are listed in the information box.

Spontaneous bleeding does not usually occur until the platelet count falls below about 30×10^9/l unless their function is also compromised—for example, following aspirin ingestion. Purpura and spontaneous bruising are characteristic but there may also be oral, nasal, gastrointestinal or genitourinary bleeding. Severe thrombocytopenia results in optic fundal haemorrhage (see Fig. 11.11), which may be a prelude to a rapidly fatal intracranial bleed.

Investigations to determine the possible cause of thrombocytopenia should be directed towards the conditions listed in the information box. A blood film may give diagnostic information, e.g. acute leukaemia. Examination of the bone marrow will reveal whether there is an infiltrate such as carcinoma, a reduced number of megakaryocytes, e.g. hypoplastic anaemia, or an increased number of megakaryocytes indicating excessive peripheral destruction, e.g. idiopathic thrombocytopenic purpura.

CAUSES OF THROMBOCYTOPENIA
Marrow disorders
• Hypoplasia Idiopathic Drug-induced—cytotoxic, antimetabolite, thiazides • Infiltration Leukaemia Myeloma Carcinoma Myelofibrosis Osteopetrosis • B_{12}/folate deficiency
Increased consumption of platelets
• Disseminated intravascular coagulation (DIC) • Idiopathic thrombocytopenic purpura (ITP) • Viral infections—e.g. Epstein–Barr virus, HIV • Bacterial infections—e.g. Gram-negative septicaemia
Hypersplenism
• Lymphomas • Liver disease

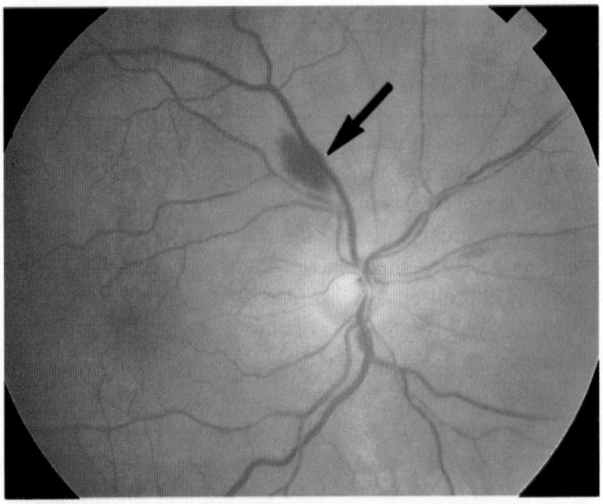

Fig. 11.11 Superficial fundal haemorrhage (arrow). The haemorrhage is in a patient with a platelet count of 5×10^9/l.

HIGH PLATELET COUNT—THROMBOCYTOSIS

The platelet count is most commonly raised as part of the

secondary response to infection, collagenosis, malignancy or gastrointestinal bleeding (see the information box). In these circumstances the presenting clinical features are those of the underlying disorder. Thrombosis or bleeding secondary to a reactive increase in platelet count is rare.

CAUSES OF A RAISED PLATELET COUNT
Reactive thrombocytosis
• Chronic inflammatory disorders • Malignant disease • Tissue damage • Haemolytic anaemias • Post-splenectomy • Post-haemorrhage
Malignant thrombocytosis
• Essential thrombocythaemia • Polycythaemia rubra vera • Myelofibrosis • Chronic myeloid leukaemia

In essential thrombocythaemia, in which there is primary proliferation of megakaryocytes in the marrow, the patient may have haemorrhagic features secondary to platelet dysfunction, e.g. mucocutaneous or gastrointestinal haemorrhage. Alternatively, the patient may present with occlusion of a major artery, e.g. thrombotic stroke or venous thrombosis. Occlusion of smaller vessels may result in transient ischaemic attacks, amaurosis fugax, or distal ischaemia or gangrene (see Fig. 11.12). A high platelet count is also a feature of other myeloproliferative disorders such as primary proliferative polycythaemia or chronic myeloid leukaemia.

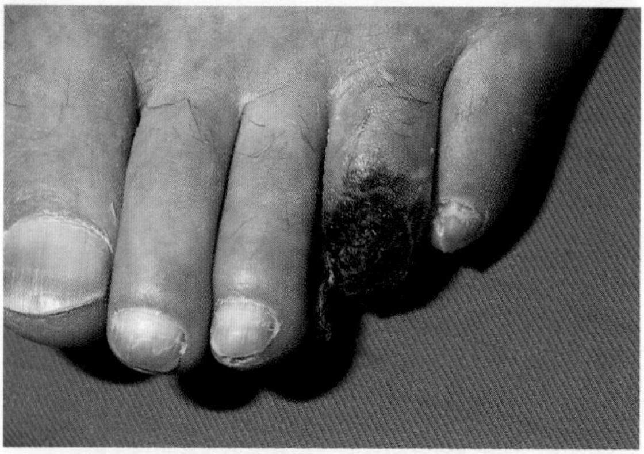

Fig. 11.12 Thrombocytosis causing vessel occlusion and gangrene.

VENOUS THROMBOSIS

Swelling of either leg or both legs is a common presenting symptom. Deep venous thrombosis (DVT) in the leg characteristically causes pain, swelling, increase in temperature and dilatation of the superficial veins. Often, however, there are only minimal symptoms and DVT cannot be excluded without appropriate investigations.

Unilateral leg swelling may also result from a spontaneous or post-traumatic calf haematoma, cellulitis or a ruptured Baker's cyst (see the information box). This latter condition usually arises in individuals with pre-existing rheumatoid disease of the knee. The leak of synovial fluid into the calf is accompanied by a decrease in the size of the cyst in the popliteal fossa and an intense pain in the calf due to the irritant synovial fluid.

CAUSES OF SWOLLEN LEG
• Venous thrombosis • Calf haematoma • Skin inflammation, including cellulitis • Baker's cyst • Pelvic disease obstructing venous or lymphatic return • Right-sided cardiac failure • Hypoalbuminaemia

When both legs are swollen, the likely cause is either impaired venous or lymphatic return due to obstruction in the pelvis or above, or impaired cardiac function resulting in right-sided heart failure. Hypoalbuminaemia often results in bilateral pitting leg oedema.

Investigation of swollen leg

For unilateral leg swelling the initial assessment is usually to establish whether or not a DVT is present. DVTs are usually unilateral but may be bilateral when they are extensive and extend into the pelvic veins and inferior vena cava (IVC). For bilateral leg swelling it may be appropriate to exclude pelvic, retroperitoneal and cardiac pathology as well as hypoalbuminaemia.

Venography is the most reliable technique for assessing the presence of venous thrombosis. Radio-opaque dye is injected into a vein on the dorsum of the foot and the deep veins are visualised by dynamic X-ray imaging, with appropriate static films being taken to provide a permanent record of the thrombus. Venography for more proximal thrombosis can be performed by catheterisation of the femoral vein to visualise the pelvic veins and IVC.

Doppler ultrasound is a reliable, non-invasive method for detecting venous thrombosis. The technique depends upon demonstrating non-compressibility of the vein in the presence of thrombus. This technique can only detect thrombus in larger veins and is therefore only reliable for assessing veins at or above the popliteal fossa as far as the inguinal ligament. In some patients it can identify major thrombus in the IVC.

Once a patient has a proven venous thrombosis it is necessary to consider whether he or she may have a thrombophilic condition. Those individuals fulfilling the clinical criteria set out in the first information box on page 749 should be investigated as in the second information box on that page.

LYMPHADENOPATHY

Enlarged lymph glands may be an important indicator of haematological disease but they are not uncommon in reaction to infection or inflammation (see the information box). Some features may help to identify the likely cause of lymphadenopathy. Reactive nodes usually expand rapidly and are painful but those due to haematological disease are more often painless. Nodes may be localised or generalised. Localised nodes should elicit a search for a source of inflammation in the appropriate drainage area: the scalp, ear, mouth, face or teeth for the neck; the breast for the axilla; and the perineum or external genitalia for inguinal nodes. Generalised lymphadenopathy may be secondary to infection, connective tissue disease or extensive skin disease but is more likely to signify underlying haematological malignancy. Weight loss and drenching night sweats which may require a change of night clothes are associated with haematological malignancies, particularly lymphoma. Initial investigations may include a full blood count (to detect neutrophilia in infection or evidence of haematological disease), an erythrocyte sedimentation rate (ESR) and a chest radiograph (to exclude mediastinal lymphadenopathy). If the findings are suspicious of malignancy, a formal excision biopsy of a representative node is indicated to confirm a histological diagnosis.

CAUSES OF LYMPHADENOPATHY
Infective
• Bacterial Streptococcal, tuberculosis • Viral Epstein–Barr, HIV • Protozoal Toxoplasmosis, brucellosis • Fungal Histoplasmosis, coccidioidomycosis
Neoplastic
• Primary Leukaemias, lymphomas • Secondary e.g. Lung, breast, thyroid, stomach
Connective tissue disorders
• Rheumatoid arthritis, systemic lupus erythematosus (SLE)
Sarcoidosis
Amyloidosis
Drugs
• Phenytoin

SPLENOMEGALY

The spleen may be enlarged by involvement by lymphoproliferative disease, by the resumption of extramedullary haemopoiesis in myeloproliferative disease, or by enhanced reticulo-endothelial activity in autoimmune haemolysis. A list of the causes of splenomegaly is given in the information box on p. 756. Massive splenomegaly occurs in chronic myeloid leukaemia, myelofibrosis, malaria or kala-azar. Hepatosplenomegaly is more suggestive of lympho- or myeloproliferative disease, liver disease and infiltration such as amyloid. The additional presence of lymphadenopathy makes a diagnosis of lymphoproliferative disease more likely. An enlarged spleen may cause abdominal discomfort, with back pain and abdominal bloating due to stomach compression. Splenic infarction may occur and produce severe abdominal pain radiating to the left shoulder tip, associated with a splenic rub on auscultation. Rarely, spontaneous or traumatic rupture may occur.

Investigation will centre on the suspected cause. Imaging of the spleen by ultrasound or computed tomography (CT) will detect variations in density in the spleen which may be a feature of lymphoproliferative disease; it also allows visualisation of the liver or abdominal lymph nodes. Biopsy of the latter or superficial nodes may provide the diagnosis. A chest radiograph to exclude hilar nodes may be helpful. An FBC may show pancytopenia secondary to hypersplenism and if other abnormalities are present, such as abnormal lymphocytes or a leucoerythroblastic blood film, a bone marrow examination may be helpful. Screening for liver or infectious disease may be appropriate. If all investigations are unhelpful, splenectomy may be diagnostic.

CAUSES OF SPLENOMEGALY

Congestive
- Intrahepatic portal hypertension
  - Cirrhosis
  - Hepatic vein occlusion
- Extrahepatic portal hypertension
  - Thrombosis, stenosis or malformation of the portal or splenic vein
- Cardiac
  - Chronic congestive cardiac failure

Infective
- Bacterial
  - Endocarditis
  - Septicaemia
  - Tuberculosis
  - Brucellosis
  - Salmonella
- Viral
  - Hepatitis
  - Epstein–Barr
  - Cytomegalovirus
- Protozoal
  - Malaria, leishmaniasis
  - Trypanosomiasis
- Fungal
  - Histoplasmosis

Inflammatory/granulomatous disorders
- Felty's syndrome, SLE
- Sarcoidosis

Haematological
- Red cell disorders
  - Megaloblastic anaemia
  - Haemoglobinopathies
- Autoimmune haemolytic anaemias
- Myeloproliferative disorders
  - Chronic myeloid leukaemia
  - Myelofibrosis, primary polycythaemia, essential thrombocythaemia
- Neoplastic
  - Leukaemias, lymphomas

Other malignancies
- Secondary—rare

Storage disease
- Gaucher's disease
- Niemann–Pick disease

Miscellaneous
- Cysts, amyloid, hyperthyroidism

INFECTION

Infection is a major complication of haematological disorders. The cause relates to the immune deficit caused by the disease itself (see Table 11.7), to the treatment, e.g. chemotherapy, or commonly in practice to a combination of both.

The type of infection is related to the immune deficit produced by the disease and/or its treatment (see Table 11.8).

Table 11.7 Examples of potential pathogens occurring in particular defects of the host's defences in patients with primary haematological disease

Deficit	Disease	Likely organisms	
Neutropenia	Acute leukaemia	Bacteria	
		Gram +	*Staphylococcus aureus* *Staphylococcus albus* Streptococci
		Gram −	*Escherichia coli* *Haemophilus influenzae* *Klebsiella* *Pseudomonas*
		Fungi	*Candida* *Aspergillus, Mucormycosis*
Immunoglobulin	Multiple myeloma Chronic lymphatic leukaemia Congenital agammaglobulinaemia	Bacteria Gram + and − (as above)	
Cellular immunity	Hodgkin's disease Non-Hodgkin's lymphoma	Viruses	Herpes simplex and zoster, cytomegalovirus
		Protozoa	*Pneumocystis carinii* and *Toxoplasma gondii*
		Fungi	*Cryptococcus neoformans, Candida*
		Bacteria	*Mycobacteria, Salmonella, Legionella, Streptococcus pneumoniae, Haemophilus influenzae, Staphylococcus aureus*
	Haemophilia (HIV-positive)	Parasites	*Pneumocystis carinii* *Toxoplasma gondii* *Cryptosporidium*
		Fungus	*Candida*

Organ/system involved	Disease	Likely organisms
Table 11.8 Likely organisms causing organ infections in various haematological disorders		
Chest	Acute non-lymphoblastic leukaemia	Bacteria, fungi
	Acute lymphoblastic leukaemia	Bacteria *Pneumocystis carinii*
	Bone marrow transplant	
	Early	Bacteria, fungi
	Later	*Pneumocystis carinii* Cytomegalovirus
CNS	Hodgkin's	*Listeria monocytogenes* *Cryptococcus neoformans* *Toxoplasma gondii*
Mouth	Acute leukaemia	*Candida* Herpes simplex Anaerobic bacteria
Perianal area	Acute leukaemia	Gram-negative bacteria and anaerobes
Skin	Acute leukaemia	*Staphylococcus* *Pseudomonas* *Candida*
	Lymphoproliferative disorders	Herpes zoster
	Infected central line	*Staphylococcus epidermidis*

Infection related to neutropenia is a particularly common and potentially very severe complication. Fever is the first and may be the only manifestation of infection. The lack of neutrophils allows the patient to become septicaemic and shocked within hours if immediate antibiotic therapy is not commenced. The management of such patients is discussed later in the chapter (see p. 773). The signs associated with the focus of infection are often minimal because of the neutropenia, and minor sore throats or perianal discomfort may well indicate the focus of any infection.

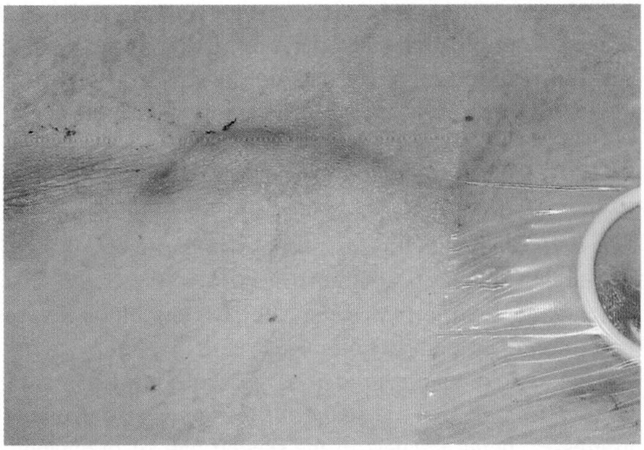

Fig. 11.13 Hickman line. Central line-infected tunnel.

In recent years the administration of chemotherapy has been facilitated by the insertion of a central line. Unfortunately, these may get infected (see Fig. 11.13). Usually Gram-positive organisms are involved.

FURTHER INFORMATION ON MAJOR MANIFESTATIONS OF BLOOD DISEASE

Jandl J H 1996 Blood: textbook of haematology, 2nd edn. Little Brown, London

ANAEMIAS

Anaemia may be defined as a state in which the blood haemoglobin is below the normal range for the patient's age and sex. As many as 30% of the world's population may be affected at some time. The most common cause world-wide is iron deficiency and it is estimated that half a billion people are affected.

IRON DEFICIENCY ANAEMIA

Aetiology

The aetiology of iron deficiency anaemia varies with the age, sex and country of residence of the patient. Iron deficiency usually results from loss of iron because of bleeding, an inadequate diet or malabsorption (see p. 749). Occasionally, iron may be lost in the urine in the form of haemosiderin. Loss due to bleeding in greater amounts than can be balanced in absorption is by far the most common cause.

There are periods in life when iron deficiency may be regarded as almost physiological. At birth the normal infant has a store in the form of a very high haemoglobin level and in addition some iron is available in the liver. This is adequate for erythropoietic requirements in the first few months of life. Thereafter a mild degree of deficiency appears because milk is a very poor source of iron. If weaning is delayed for 1 or 2 years, as is the custom in certain parts of the world, deficiency may become marked. The deficiency is fairly quickly corrected when the child is weaned to a good diet. Prematurity and haemorrhage from the cord at birth deprive the infant of the normal store of iron and deficiency may appear sooner and be more severe. Adolescents have a marked growth spurt and iron requirements may outstrip absorption. Food fads are not uncommon at this age, which may contribute to the problem.

Menstruation causes an average loss of 30 mg of iron per month, requiring increased absorption of approximately 1 mg daily. Although this loss disappears during pregnancy, the mother requires additional iron for the fetus, the placenta, her own increased red cell mass and blood loss at parturition. The daily requirements will be about 2.5 mg plus the basic requirement of 1 mg per day, giving a total of 3.5 mg. This increased demand for iron rises as pregnancy progresses, being greatest in the second half of pregnancy. Thus iron deficiency is more common in females than males during the reproductive years.

In post-menopausal women and adult men the most common cause of iron deficiency is gastrointestinal bleeding—for example, from gastric erosions associated with anti-inflammatory drugs, neoplastic disease and peptic ulcers. In tropical and subtropical areas, infestation with hookworm and *Schistosoma* is also very common and is the main cause of iron deficiency. A diet containing inadequate iron can cause or contribute to iron deficiency anaemia at all ages. The elderly, particularly men living alone, are susceptible.

Investigations (see Table 11.9)

The haematological findings are a reduced haemoglobin with normal or slightly reduced red cell count and a low mean cell volume (MCV) of less than 76 fl. The white cell and differential counts are usually normal. A raised platelet count may suggest that bleeding is the cause of the deficiency. Bone marrow iron stores stained by the Prussian blue technique are found to be empty.

Table 11.9 Diagnostic features of iron deficiency

Investigation	Result
Haemoglobin	Variably reduced
Mean cell volume	Reduced
Erythrocyte count	Normal or reduced to less than Hb level would suggest
Blood film	Hypochromia, microcytosis, oval and elliptical cells, poikilocytes in more severe cases
Leucocyte count differential	Normal
Platelet count	Normal or raised
Bone marrow iron stores	Empty
Plasma transferrin	Raised
Plasma iron	Reduced
Serum ferritin	Reduced

Iron deficiency suspected because of the finding of a low MCV is best confirmed by measuring the ferritin. However, inflammatory conditions such as rheumatoid arthritis and certain tumours raise the ferritin level and patients with these conditions who have iron deficiency may have a ferritin in the low/normal range. Unfortunately, the serum iron is subject to considerable diurnal variation and low levels are found in the presence of inflammation or infection. Iron absorption is increased in iron deficiency and the total iron-binding capacity rises. Thus a low serum iron associated with a high total iron-binding capacity is much more specific for iron deficiency. However, the total iron-binding capacity may be reduced by poor nutrition.

Diagnosis of the cause of iron deficiency

The direction of the investigations will obviously be influenced by the age and sex of the patient, the history and the findings on examination. Excessive menstrual loss and repeated pregnancy are common causes. In the absence of any clear lead, evidence of gastrointestinal blood loss should first be sought using faecal occult blood tests, barium meal, enema and upper and lower gastrointestinal tract endoscopy. In the face of unexplained iron deficiency anaemia negative barium studies or occult blood tests cannot be accepted as evidence of the absence of lesions. Chromium-labelled red cells may be used to measure blood loss into the gut. The level of radioactivity in the stool provides an accurate measurement of the amount of blood lost. Coeliac disease may present in adults as an isolated iron deficiency. The stools and urine should be examined in tropical countries for hookworm infestation and schistosomiasis. Patients in whom there is a known cause of intravascular red cell destruction, such as a prosthetic heart valve, should have urine tested for haemosiderin.

Management

Most patients can be treated orally and the cheapest preparation is dried ferrous sulphate given as a tablet containing 200 mg of the salt (60 mg elemental iron) 8-hourly. A small proportion of patients develop dyspepsia, constipation or diarrhoea. If this occurs, more expensive proprietary preparations may be tried. Delayed-release preparations are to be avoided as they release little iron in the upper jejunum where absorption is best. Proprietary liquid preparations may be used.

A response to oral medication usually appears in under 2 weeks. The haemoglobin should rise by 10 g/l every 7–10 days. If no response is seen, it may be that the patient is not taking the tablets. A check may be made by examining the stool, which will be grey or black if the patient is ingesting iron. Failure to respond to iron therapy may be due to poor compliance, continued blood loss, severe malabsorption or the wrong diagnosis. Iron should be continued for 3–6 months after the haemoglobin level has returned to normal, to replenish iron stores. Continuous oral therapy may be required or the iron may be given parenterally to patients with malabsorption, or chronic loss as in haemosiderinuria.

Parenteral iron therapy

This is suitable for those very few patients who are genuinely unable to take iron by mouth because of pain, vomiting or diarrhoea, who are unable to absorb iron because of some disorder of the gastrointestinal tract or who are unreliable in taking oral preparations. Iron given by injection has also been used for the treatment of anaemia of rheumatoid arthritis, for the correction of severe anaemia in the late stages of pregnancy and following major operations. The recommended single dose of iron-sorbitol is 1.5 mg of iron per kg of body weight given daily. The number of injections given depends on the severity of the anaemia and the manufacturer's dosage guidelines should be followed. Iron-sorbitol should be given by deep intramuscular injection, never intravenously.

MEGALOBLASTIC ANAEMIA

Haematopoietic tissue is one of a number of rapidly proliferating tissues in which DNA synthesis is intense. Both vitamin B_{12} and folate are essential for DNA synthesis, and deficiency of either or both causes a failure of DNA synthesis and disordered cell proliferation. Haematopoiesis is particularly susceptible and division of cells is delayed and eventually halted. Morphological changes appear in the marrow cells. In the erythrocyte series these changes are described as megaloblastic because the cells appear abnormally large. Changes also occur in the granulocyte precursors (giant metamyelocytes) and megakaryocytes, and disordered morphology can be seen in other rapidly dividing cells such as those of the gastrointestinal tract.

The massive destruction of marrow cells from dyserythropoiesis liberates large quantities of enzymes including lactate dehydrogenase (LDH), which rises to very high levels in the blood. Eventually, in the absence of treatment, cell production fails. Excessive doses of antimetabolites, such as those used in the treatment of cancer which interfere with DNA synthesis, have similar effects, and may induce severe dysplasia and morphological changes in the marrow and blood very similar to those produced by vitamin B_{12} and folate deficiency.

The findings on investigation of a megaloblastic anaemia, whatever the cause, are given in Table 11.10. Most patients with megaloblastic anaemia suffer from deficiency of either vitamin B_{12} or folate, which is demonstrated by deficient blood levels of these vitamins.

Table 11.10 Diagnostic features of a megaloblastic anaemia

Investigation	Result
Haemoglobin	Often reduced, may be very low
Mean cell volume	Usually raised, commonly > 120 fl
Erythrocyte count	Low for degree of anaemia
Blood film	Oval macrocytosis, poikilocytosis, red cell fragmentation, neutrophil hypersegmentation
Reticulocyte count	Low for degree of anaemia
Leucocyte count	Low, normal or reduced
Platelet count	Low, normal or reduced
Bone marrow	Increased cellularity, megaloblastic changes in erythroid series, giant metamyelocytes, dysplastic megakaryocytes, increased iron in stores, pathological non-ring sideroblasts
Serum iron	Elevated
Iron-binding capacity	Increased saturation
Serum ferritin	Elevated
Plasma LDH	Elevated, often markedly

MEGALOBLASTIC ANAEMIA DUE TO VITAMIN B_{12} DEFICIENCY

Absorption of vitamin B_{12}

Vitamin B_{12} is a cobalt-containing porphyrin, termed cobalamin. The absorption of vitamin B_{12} from the lower ileum is facilitated by gastric intrinsic factor, a glycoprotein synthesised by gastric parietal cells, which complexes with ingested vitamin B_{12} in the stomach. The complex is taken up at special binding sites in the ileum, where the vitamin B_{12} is released to the ileal cells. Intrinsic factor is not absorbed. After absorption vitamin B_{12} is bound to a carrier protein in the plasma (transcobalamin II), transported to the tissues and taken up by cells as required. Vitamin B_{12} is stored in the liver, where there may be up to 3 years' supply.

Deficiency of vitamin B_{12}

This vitamin is obtained mainly from animal foodstuffs. Vegetables alone are an inadequate source. Normal requirements of vitamin B_{12} are 1–2 µg daily. Deficiency takes at least 3 years to appear and occurs because of the factors listed in the information box below. A low serum B_{12} concentration may be secondary to a low serum folate level.

CAUSES OF VITAMIN B_{12} DEFICIENCY

- Inadequate diet (true vegans)
- Intrinsic factor deficiency
  - Pernicious anaemia, gastrectomy
  - Congenital deficiency without gastric atrophy (rare)
- Disease of the terminal ileum
  - e.g. Crohn's disease
- Vitamin B_{12} may be removed from the gut by:
  - Bacterial proliferation in stagnant loops
  - Parasites such as the fish tapeworm

Dietary insufficiency. This is rare unless meat and other animal foodstuffs are not eaten (e.g. in vegans). The deficiency is readily corrected by the parenteral administration of vitamin B_{12}. Thereafter the vitamin should be given by mouth.

Gastrectomy. Total resection of the stomach results in a complete loss of intrinsic factor production and failure to absorb vitamin B_{12}. The patient requires life-long vitamin B_{12} injections. Partial gastrectomy reduces vitamin B_{12} absorption, in some cases to the point that deficiency occurs. Gastritis may, in part, be responsible. The Schilling test often demonstrates reduced absorption. One annual injection of 1000 μg of hydroxocobalamin is adequate prophylaxis for a patient who has had a partial gastrectomy.

Disease of the terminal ileum. This should be suspected if the Schilling test is not corrected by the addition of adequate amounts of intrinsic factor.

Bacterial colonisation of the small intestine. This results in an abnormal Schilling test, both without and with intrinsic factor; this is corrected by the administration of tetracycline.

Prevalence

The majority of patients with vitamin B_{12} deficiency have Addisonian pernicious anaemia. This appears to be relatively uncommon in tropical countries.

ADDISONIAN PERNICIOUS ANAEMIA

The term Addisonian pernicious anaemia should be limited to megaloblastic anaemia due to a failure of secretion of intrinsic factor by the stomach other than from total gastrectomy. It is an autoimmune disease and in about 50% of patients antibodies to intrinsic factor can be demonstrated. The disease is rare before the age of 30, occurs mainly between 45 and 65 years, and affects females more frequently than males.

Pathology

There is evidence of increased blood destruction, including unconjugated hyperbilirubinaemia and increased deposition of iron (haemosiderin) in the liver, spleen, kidneys and bone marrow. The gastric mucosa is thin and atrophic.

DIAGNOSTIC FEATURES OF ADDISONIAN PERNICIOUS ANAEMIA
Diagnostic findings
• Very low serum vitamin B_{12}, often less than 50 ng/l • Anti-intrinsic factor antibodies in serum (present in 50%)
Corroborative findings
• Macrocytic dysplastic blood picture • Megaloblastic marrow • Abnormal vitamin B_{12} absorption test corrected by addition of intrinsic factor (Schilling test)

Investigations

Helpful findings in the diagnosis of Addisonian pernicious anaemia are given in the information box.

MEGALOBLASTIC ANAEMIA DUE TO FOLATE DEFICIENCY

Folic acid and interaction with vitamin B_{12}

Folic acid (pteroylglutamic acid) and related compounds are known as folates. The body obtains folates by the breakdown of food polyglutamates to monoglutamates in the small intestine or mucosal cell. Folic acid as such is available only as a medicinal compound. In the plasma, folate appears as methyl tetrahydrofolate which is changed to tetrahydrofolate (THF) by a pathway for which vitamin B_{12} is essential. Without this, active folate coenzymes are poorly formed. 5,10 methylene THF is the form essential for the synthesis of DNA. Dihydrofolate from this step is reconverted to THF by dihydrofolate reductase, an enzyme inhibited by the folate antagonist, methotrexate. Formyl THF (folinic acid) will bypass both the metabolic blocks created by vitamin B_{12} deficiency or methotrexate and acts as an antidote to this drug. Clinically, folinic acid or folic acid must not be used to treat vitamin B_{12} deficiency or severe neurological damage may result, although the anaemia may be corrected. The daily requirement of folate for a normal healthy adult is 100 μg.

Folate deficiency

Folate occurs mainly in the form of polyglutamates in both vegetable and animal foodstuffs. Much is destroyed by cooking. Body stores are relatively small, lasting only a few weeks. Folate is absorbed mainly in the jejunum. The causes of folate deficiency are shown in the information box.

CAUSES OF FOLATE DEFICIENCY
Diet
• Poor intake of vegetables
Malabsorption
• e.g. Coeliac disease
Increased demand
• Pregnancy • Cell proliferation, e.g. haemolysis
Drugs*
• Certain anticonvulsants (e.g. phenytoin) • The contraceptive pill • Certain cytotoxic drugs (e.g. methotrexate)
* Usually only a problem in patients deficient in folate from another cause.

Prevalence

Approximately 60% of all megaloblastic anaemias in Britain are due to folate deficiency. In tropical countries most megaloblastic disease is due to folate deficiency associated with malnutrition, infection and pregnancy.

Investigations

Diagnostic features of a folic acid deficiency anaemia are given in the information box.

DIAGNOSTIC FEATURES OF FOLIC ACID DEFICIENCY
Diagnostic findings
• Low serum folate levels (fasting blood sample) • Red cell folate levels low (but may be normal if folate deficiency is of very recent onset)
Corroborative findings
• Macrocytic dysplastic blood picture • Megaloblastic marrow

Management of megaloblastic anaemia

The decision to give a blood transfusion in a patient with a megaloblastic anaemia is based on general principles concerning the clinical state of the patient. It should be seriously considered when the haemoglobin level is so low as to endanger life—for example, under 40 g/l. In all types of chronic anaemia of sufficient severity to require transfusion the blood should be given very slowly, preferably as red cell concentrate, because of the danger of producing cardiac failure. A diuretic is given simultaneously (frusemide 40–80 mg).

Vitamin B_{12} deficiency

Hydroxocobalamin is given parenterally in a dosage of 1000 µg. After an initial dose injections are given every 2–3 days for a further five doses. Maintenance therapy consists of 1000 µg parenterally every 3 months.

Within 48 hours of the first injection the bone marrow shows a striking change from a megaloblastic to a normoblastic state. The serum iron drops precipitously and hypokalaemia may be a problem sufficient to require replacement therapy. Within 2–3 days the reticulocyte count begins to rise, reaching a maximum between the 5th and 10th days. The response may be delayed if there is coexisting inflammatory disease or if the patient has been transfused. There is a brief peak of erythrocyte output due to the maturation of the large number of cells held in maturation arrest by the vitamin B_{12} deficiency. Depending on the initial erythrocyte count, the proportion of reticulocytes may rise above 50% but soon falls to below 10% as more normal production is resumed.

In some patients the rapid regeneration of the blood depletes the iron reserves of the body and recovery is halted. To prevent this, ferrous sulphate 200 mg daily should be given soon after the commencement of treatment. A combined deficiency of vitamin B_{12} and iron is recognised by the presence of macrocytosis and hypochromia—a dimorphic blood picture. The correctly treated patient has a normal life expectancy with the maintenance of a normal blood count by adequate specific treatment. There is, however, a statistically significant increase in death from gastric carcinoma in patients with pernicious anaemia. Patients with subacute combined degeneration of the cord receive monthly hydroxocobalamin injections.

If a patient with pernicious anaemia fails to respond to parenteral administration of adequate doses of hydroxocobalamin, it suggests that the diagnosis is wrong. The patient may be suffering from another type of megaloblastic anaemia which may be partially or completely refractory to hydroxocobalamin. Such patients respond to folic acid. An unsustained response may indicate depletion of iron stores and the need for oral iron therapy.

Folate deficiency

Treatment with a daily dose of 5 mg of folic acid by mouth is sufficient; 5 mg once weekly is always adequate for maintenance therapy. Folic acid must never be given, other than with vitamin B_{12}, in Addisonian pernicious anaemia or other vitamin B_{12} deficiency anaemias, because of the risk of aggravating or precipitating neurological features of vitamin B_{12} depletion.

Megaloblastic change due to vitamin B_{12} deficiency is very rare in pregnancy. It is therefore reasonable to give folate supplements (350 µg daily) to all pregnant women. When a drug such as methotrexate inhibits dihydrofolate reductase, it is possible to employ folinic acid to overcome the metabolic block. Folinic acid may be given as tablets, 15 mg daily orally, or as an injection intravenously or intramuscularly at a dose of 3 mg/ml. Folinic acid mouthwashes are used to counteract the oral side-effects of folate antagonist drugs. Megaloblastic disorder caused by other cytotoxic drugs which inhibit DNA synthesis is not reversed by either vitamin B_{12} or folate administration.

HAEMOLYTIC ANAEMIA

Various abnormalities may shorten the normal red cell lifespan of 120 days, and anaemia develops when marrow output no longer compensates. The increased output of new erythrocytes is reflected in a raised reticulocyte count, which gives an indication of the severity of the process. Normoblasts may be released under extreme stress. The catabolic pathways for haemoglobin degradation are overloaded and there is a modest increase in unconjugated bilirubin in the blood and increased re-absorption of urobilinogen from the gut, which is excreted in the urine in increased amounts. Bilirubin does not appear in the urine. Jaundice is mild.

Haemolysis may occur intravascularly or extravascularly. Haemoglobin liberated into the plasma is bound mainly by the α_2 globulin, haptoglobin, to form a complex too large to be lost in the urine. It is taken up by the liver and degraded. Some haemoglobin is partially degraded and bound to albumin to form methaemalbumin. If all the haptoglobin has been consumed, free haemoglobin may be lost in the urine. In small amounts this is re-absorbed by the renal tubules, where the haemoglobin is degraded and the iron stored as haemosiderin. Sloughing of the renal tubular cells gives rise to haemosiderinuria which, if found, always indicates intravascular haemolysis. Haemoglobinuria occurs when greater amounts of haemoglobin are lost, giving the urine a black appearance ('black water').

Extravascular haemolysis occurs in the phagocytic cells of the spleen, liver, bone marrow and other organs and there may be little or no depletion of haptoglobin. Estimation of the haptoglobin level in the blood is not always easily interpreted. Inflammatory disease and steroid therapy both increase haptoglobin levels. Ahaptoglobinaemia may occur as an inherited disorder. Nevertheless, absence of haptoglobin is usually a strong indicator of haemolytic disease. Its presence does not exclude haemolysis.

Blood and marrow findings

The peripheral blood shows a moderate macrocytosis and polychromasia from reticulocytosis, while specific red cell abnormalities may give a clue to the type of haemolytic disease. There may be a polymorphonuclear leucocytosis. The marrow shows erythroid hyperplasia. A megaloblastic change usually reflects depletion of folate reserves. Increased erythropoietic turnover in the marrow is associated with increased serum lactate dehydrogenase levels which, in the absence of folate deficiency, closely follows the severity of the haemolytic disorder. Red cell survival can be measured crudely using radioactive chromium (^{51}Cr). Surface counting performed at the same time over liver and spleen may give an indication of the site of haemolysis. If transfusion has been given, the patient's blood will contain a mixed cell population which is not suitable for ^{51}Cr studies. In these circumstances cross-matched donor cells should be used for labelling.

Aetiology

The causes of haemolytic anaemias are classified as congenital or acquired and are listed in the information box.

CAUSES OF HAEMOLYTIC ANAEMIA

Congenital

Membrane abnormalities
- Hereditary spherocytosis
- Hereditary elliptocytosis

Haemoglobinopathies
- Lack of haemoglobin chain synthesis
  Thalassaemias
- Amino acid substitution on the haemoglobin chain
  Haemoglobin S, C, D

Red cell enzyme defects
- Glucose-6-phosphate dehydrogenase deficiency

Acquired

Immune
- Isoimmune
- Autoimmune
  Warm antibody
  Cold antibody
- Alloimmune

Non-immune
- Mechanical
  Artificial cardiac valves
  Burns
  Microangiopathic
  March haemoglobinuria
- Infections
- *Clostridium perfringens*, malaria
- Drugs, chemicals
- Dyserythropoietic
  Paroxysmal nocturnal haemoglobinuria

CONGENITAL HAEMOLYTIC ANAEMIAS

The principal disorders are hereditary spherocytosis, glucose-6-phosphate dehydrogenase (G6PD) deficiency and the haemoglobinopathies (e.g. sickle-cell disease and thalassaemia). G6PD deficiency and haemoglobinopathies are most common in Black Africans; thalassaemia is most frequent in the Mediterranean area.

HEREDITARY SPHEROCYTOSIS

This is an autosomal dominant disorder in which the principal abnormality appears to be a deficiency of spectrin, a red cell membrane protein. Approximately 25% of patients have no family history. The erythrocyte envelope is abnormally permeable and the sodium pumps are overworked. The exact nature of the red blood cell defect may vary from family to family. The erythrocytes lose their biconcave shape, become spherical and are more susceptible to osmotic lysis. These spherocytes are destroyed almost exclusively by the spleen. The severity of the disorder is very variable even within an affected family. Haemolysis is mainly extravascular.

Investigations

The diagnosis is made by demonstrating a haemolytic state together with spherocytes in the blood film, increased osmotic fragility reflecting the spherocytes and the demonstration of the same disorder in other members of the family. The Coombs test is negative. There is an increased loss of urobilinogen in the urine. Red cell survival studies with ^{51}Cr show destruction of red cells almost exclusively in the spleen. The differential diagnosis is from other causes of spherocytosis, particularly the various forms of immune haemolysis.

Management

Splenectomy results in striking and usually permanent improvement both in the symptoms and in the anaemia and should be advised when:

- the anaemia causes persistent impairment of health
- severe haemolytic or aplastic crises have occurred
- other members of the family have died from the disease
- evidence of cholecystitis and cholelithiasis is present.

Opinion differs as to the desirability of operation for patients with no disability. The operation should be performed during a period of remission; in young children it should be deferred until they are as old as possible and should be preceded by vaccination against pneumococcal and *Haemophilus influenzae* infection. Those patients who live in areas where the likelihood of meningococcal infection is high should receive vaccination against meningococci. Following splenectomy, resistance to some infections is impaired and daily penicillin V, 250 mg 12-hourly, should be prescribed.

Severe haemolytic crises require treatment by blood transfusion. Blood must be matched very carefully and administered very slowly, as gross haemolytic transfusion reactions are common in this disease. Folic acid, 5 mg daily orally, is prescribed to support the increased erythropoiesis.

GLUCOSE-6-PHOSPHATE DEHYDROGENASE DEFICIENCY

Glucose-6-phosphate dehydrogenase (G6PD) is the first enzyme in the hexose monophosphate shunt of the Embden–Meyerhof glycolytic pathway from which red cells derive most of their metabolic energy. The function of this shunt is to service the enzymes glutathione reductase and glutathione peroxidase, which protect the red cells against damage due to oxidation. This protective mechanism is crippled in the absence of G6PD and certain drugs in sufficient concentration can seriously injure the erythrocyte.

The deficiency is inherited as an X-linked disorder with a high frequency among Black Africans who possess an electrophoretic enzyme polymorphism with A and B type enzymes. The enzyme is A type (A-) in deficient Black Africans. In Caucasians only the normal B type enzyme is found and the deficient type is also B (B-). In West and East Africa about 20% of males (hemizygotes) and about 4% of females (homozygous for the abnormal gene) are affected and the enzyme activity is about 15% of normal. Heterozygous females have two populations of red cells, one deficient and the other normal. A total of 100 million persons are affected by this disorder world-wide. The deficiency in Caucasian and Oriental populations is more severe, enzyme activity being less than 1% of normal. Favism (haemolytic anaemia from the ingestion of the broad bean, *Vicia faba*) is due to deficiency of G6PD of the severe variety (B-). Some cases of haemolytic disease of the newborn are caused by this deficiency. Other rare types of G6PD, biochemically different from the above, may be associated with congenital non-spherocytic haemolytic disease and occur sporadically in all races.

Many drugs in common clinical use—for example, some antimalarials (dapsone) and sulphonamides—are capable of precipitating haemolysis in individuals with G6PD deficiency. Infections may also potentiate the haemolytic action of drugs such as aspirin, chloramphenicol and chloroquine.

Investigations

The diagnosis can be confirmed by estimating the G6PD activity of the red cell but this may not be entirely accurate if there is considerable reticulocytosis. A number of screening tests are also available. The characteristics of intravascular haemolysis are usually present: haemoglobinaemia, methaemalbuminaemia, haemoglobinuria, ahaptoglobinaemia and later haemosiderinuria.

Management

This is by removal of the toxic agent. Recovery is usually rapid but if the anaemia is severe, transfusion of red cells with a normal enzyme complement may be required. Thereafter, the patient should be advised to avoid drugs which may precipitate the disorder. Splenectomy is without value.

HAEMOGLOBINOPATHIES

The haemoglobinopathies can be classified into two subgroups:

- where there is an alteration in the amino acid structure of the polypeptide chains of the globin fraction of haemoglobin, commonly called the abnormal haemoglobins; the best-known example is haemoglobin S, found in sickle-cell anaemia
- where the amino acid sequence is normal but polypeptide chain production is impaired or absent for a variety of reasons; these are the thalassaemias.

Abnormal haemoglobins are caused by amino acid substitutions in their polypeptide chains. These in turn reflect

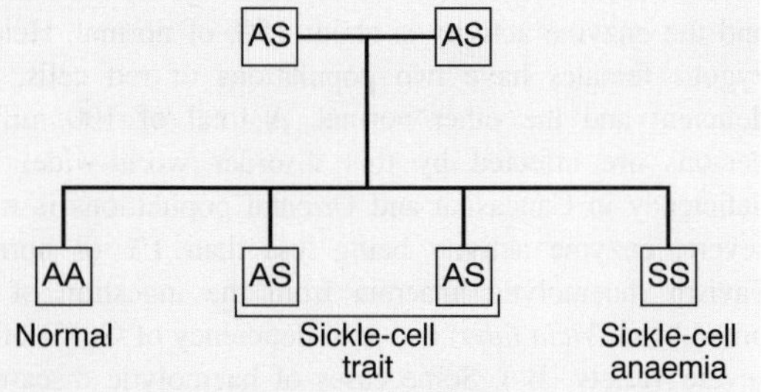

Fig. 11.14 Possible genotype of offspring of parents with sickle-cell trait.

mutations in the structural genes controlling the production of these chains. Several hundred haemoglobin variants are known, some functionally normal, most not. Originally they were designated by letters of the alphabet, e.g. S, C, E and so on. Now this does not suffice and for some years new variants have been given names, often of the towns or districts in which they were discovered. Sickle-cell haemoglobin or haemoglobin S is the most important but haemoglobin C, D and E are also significant in some parts of the world, particularly when inherited along with haemoglobin S or with beta-thalassaemia.

Control of haemoglobin synthesis is inherited from both parents. Thus a normal adult can be depicted as having the haemoglobin genotype AA, sickle-cell trait by AS and sickle-cell anaemia or homozygous S disease by SS. The inheritance when both parents have sickle-cell trait can be shown as in Figure 11.14. There is a 1:4 chance with each pregnancy that the offspring will have sickle-cell anaemia.

SICKLE-CELL ANAEMIA

Epidemiology

The patient with sickle-cell trait is relatively resistant to the lethal effects of falciparum malaria in early childhood. The high incidence of this deleterious gene in Equatorial Africa is thus explained by the selective advantage for survival it confers in an environment of endemic falciparum malaria. Patients with sickle-cell anaemia do not have correspondingly greater resistance to falciparum malaria. The geographical distribution of sickle-cell anaemia and other haemoglobinopathies is shown in Figure 11.15. The greatest prevalence of haemoglobinopathies occurs in tropical Africa, where the heterozygote frequency is over 20%. In American Black populations sickle-cell trait has a frequency of 8%.

Pathogenesis

When haemoglobin S is deoxygenated, the molecules of haemoglobin polymerise to form pseudocrystalline structures known as 'tactoids'. These distort the red cell membrane and produce characteristic sickle-shaped cells. The polymerisation is reversible when re-oxygenation occurs. The distortion of the red cell membrane, however, may become permanent and the red cell 'irreversibly sickled'. The greater the concentration of sickle-cell

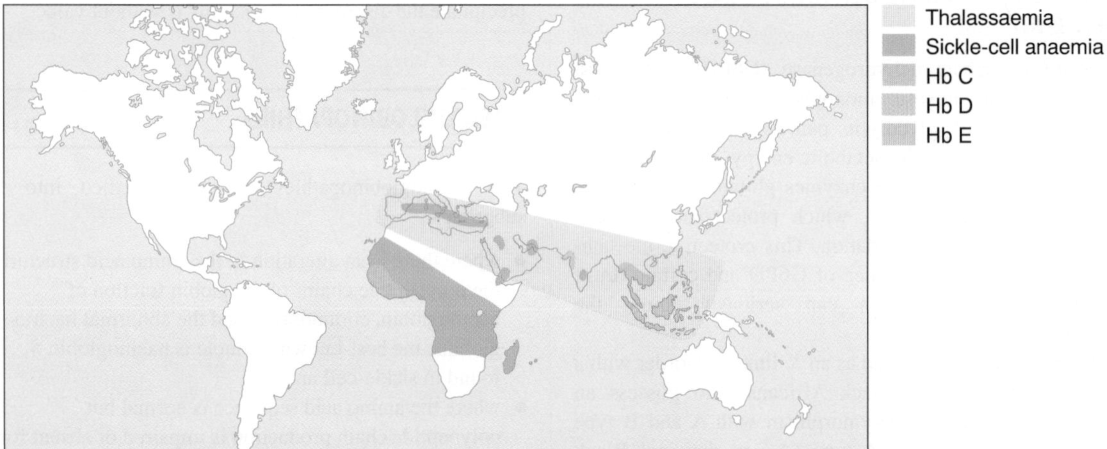

Fig. 11.15 The geographical distribution of the haemoglobinopathies.

haemoglobin in the individual cell, the more easily tactoids are formed, but this process may be enhanced or retarded by the presence of other haemoglobins. Thus haemoglobin C participates in the polymerisation more readily than haemoglobin A, whereas haemoglobin F strongly inhibits polymerisation.

Clinical features

Most of the red cells in sickle-cell anaemia contain haemoglobin S and little else. They are very prone to sickle even in vivo under normal conditions. This happens particularly in those parts of the microvasculature which are sinusoidal and where the flow is sluggish. Sickled cells increase blood viscosity, traverse capillaries poorly and tend to obstruct flow, thereby increasing the sickling of other cells and eventually stopping the flow (see Fig. 11.16). Thrombosis follows and an area of tissue infarction results, causing severe pain, swelling and tenderness (infarction crisis). In addition these cells are phagocytosed in large numbers by the mononuclear-phagocyte system, which reduces their lifespan considerably and gives rise to haemolysis.

Investigations

Diagnosis is based on the patient's race, history, clinical findings and investigations which demonstrate the presence of Hb S and no other major abnormal haemoglobin in the blood. The haematological features in SS patients are anaemia with reticulocytosis, the blood film showing sickle cells, target cells and, in patients over the age of 7, features of hyposplenism. Rapid screening tests are available to demonstrate the presence of sickle-cell haemoglobin but it is important to remember that these will be positive in both sickle-cell disease and trait. A family study should reveal that both parents carry the abnormal gene for Hb S. In this way true sickle-cell anaemia can be differentiated from other diseases in which haemoglobin S is combined with thalassaemia or some other abnormal haemoglobin such as C or D.

Management

Preliminary experience with allogeneic transplantation has introduced the prospect of cure for the first time in the management of sickle-cell patients. However, its exact role remains to be defined and benefits must be balanced against

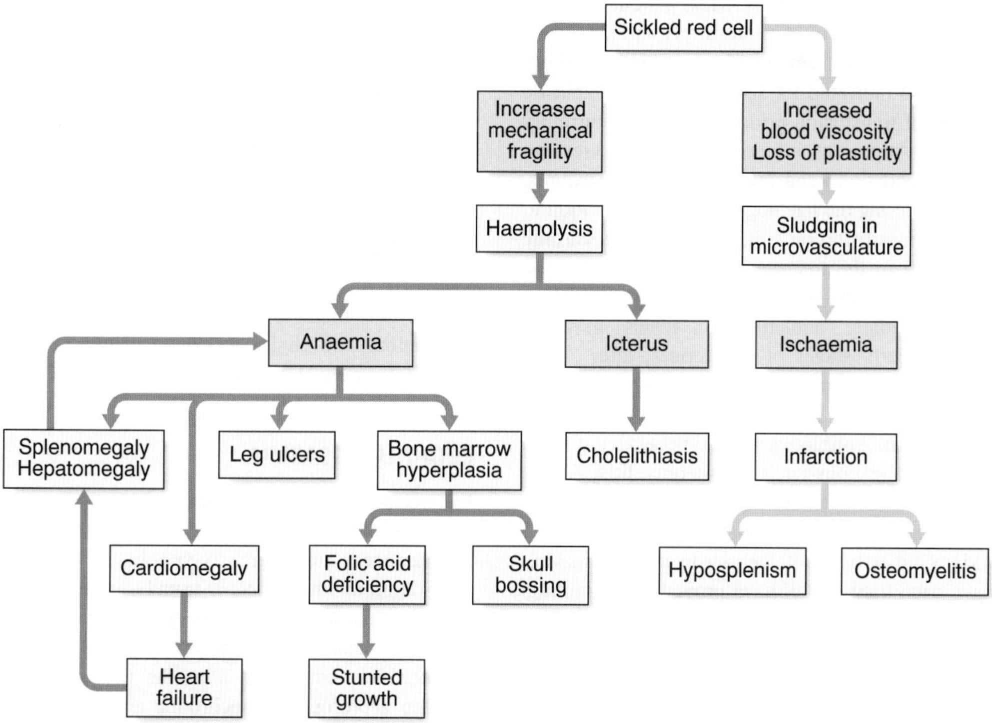

Fig. 11.16 Clinical effects of sickled red cells.

the morbidity and mortality of the procedure. There are obvious economic implications, especially as the disease is most prevalent in areas of the world where money for high-technology medicine is limited.

General management is aimed at alleviation of the symptoms and the promotion of a lifestyle that will minimise the ill effects of the disorder. Regular folic acid supplements (5 mg daily) are prescribed to support the greatly increased erythropoietic activity. Exacerbation of the chronic haemolytic anaemia is commonly associated with infections, which should be treated promptly and prevented—for example, life-long antimalarials taken where appropriate. Young patients with hyposplenism should receive phenoxymethylpenicillin and be vaccinated (see p. 763). Patients should avoid becoming chilled, dehydrated or exposed to hypoxia—for example, at high altitudes. An acute exacerbation of the anaemia may have no obvious precipitating cause. The spleen and liver may enlarge rapidly and the haemoglobin drops, sometimes with alarming speed (sequestration crisis). Parents should be taught to examine affected children for an enlarging spleen. Transfusion with red cell concentrate is urgently required.

The patient should be adequately hydrated in less severe illness and transfusion with red cell concentrate is used only if essential because of the risk of alloantibody formation and subsequent reactions. Most patients become used to a haemoglobin level of about 80 g/l and should be transfused only when the haemoglobin drops below 50 g/l. Transfusion is also indicated for sequestration and aplastic crises. The role of transfusion prior to surgery is currently under evaluation. At present, it seems reasonable to reserve transfusion for ophthalmic and major surgical procedures, with a view to lowering the haemoglobin S concentration to 30%. Exchange transfusion on either an acute or a chronic basis is employed in the management of cerebrovascular disease and the acute chest syndrome.

Powerful, potentially addictive analgesics may be necessary in the early stages of pain crises; after 24–48 hours they should be replaced by milder non-addictive preparations. The prompt correction of dehydration often helps to relieve pain. Antibiotics will be necessary if there are infective complications such as osteomyelitis. At the end of pregnancy these episodes may precipitate a pseudotoxaemia syndrome that requires heparin therapy and no sedation. Many other types of therapy to prevent in vivo sickling have been tried but all have proved disappointing. Recently, however, the administration of hydroxyurea, which can elevate haemoglobin F, has been shown to reduce the incidence of painful crises.

Prognosis

It is probable that in Africa few children with sickle-cell anaemia will survive to adult life without medical attention. With standard medical care 15% will die by the age of 20 years and 50% by the age of 40.

HAEMOGLOBIN SC DISEASE

This disorder behaves like a mild variety of sickle-cell anaemia. Episodes of infarction are less frequent and anaemia is either absent or less severe. Aseptic necrosis of the femoral head, retinal vein thrombosis and painless haematuria are not uncommon complications. Pregnancy is the main hazard because the same complications occur as in sickle-cell anaemia, particularly fat and bone marrow embolisation of the lungs and pseudotoxaemia.

HAEMOGLOBIN C DISEASE

This is a benign haemoglobinopathy which, in its homozygous form, is not associated with much morbidity. It may cause megaloblastic anaemia in pregnancy and considerable splenomegaly in adult life. No specific treatment is required other than folic acid supplements in pregnancy.

THE THALASSAEMIAS

Thalassaemia is an inherited impairment of haemoglobin production, in which there is partial or complete failure to synthesise a specific type of globin chain. The exact nature of the defect varies and it is probable that a number of different faults occur along the pathway which translates the genetic information into a polypeptide chain. The gene itself may be deleted; it usually is in alpha-thalassaemia. When the abnormality is heterozygous, synthesis of haemoglobin is only mildly affected and little disability occurs. Synthesis is grossly impaired when the patient is homozygous and there is an imbalance in polypeptide chain production. The chains produced in excess precipitate in the cell, forming Heinz bodies.

BETA-THALASSAEMIA

Failure to synthesise beta chains (beta-thalassaemia) is the most common type and is seen in highest frequency in the Mediterranean area. Heterozygotes have thalassaemia minor, a condition in which there is usually mild anaemia and little or no clinical disability. Homozygotes (thalassaemia major) either are unable to synthesise haemoglobin A or at best produce very little and, after the first 4 months of life, develop a profound hypochromic anaemia. The diagnostic features are listed in the information box.

Beta-thalassaemia minor is often detected only when iron therapy for a mild microcytic anaemia fails. The diag-

DIAGNOSTIC FEATURES OF BETA-THALASSAEMIA
Major
• Profound hypochromic anaemia • Evidence of severe red cell dysplasia • Erythroblastosis • Absence or gross reduction of the amount of haemoglobin A • Raised levels of haemoglobin F • Evidence that both parents have thalassaemia minor
Minor
• Mild anaemia • Microcytic hypochromic erythrocytes (not iron-deficient) • Some target cells • Punctate basophilia • Raised resistance of erythrocytes to osmotic lysis • Raised haemoglobin A2 fraction • Evidence that one parent has thalassaemia minor

nostic features are also summarised in the information box. Symptoms are absent or mild. Intermediate grades of severity occur.

Management

The treatment of beta-thalassaemia major is given in Table 11.11. Cure is now a possibility for selected children, with allogeneic bone marrow transplantation.

Prevention

It is possible to identify a fetus with homozygous beta-thalassaemia by obtaining chorionic villus material for DNA analysis sufficiently early in pregnancy to allow termination of pregnancy. This examination is appropriate if both parents are known to be carriers (beta-thalassaemia minor) and will accept a termination.

ALPHA-THALASSAEMIA

The reduction or absence of alpha chain synthesis is common in South-east Asia. There are two alpha gene loci on chromosome 16 and therefore four alpha genes. If one is deleted there is no clinical effect. If two are deleted there may be a mild hypochromic anaemia. If three are deleted the patient has haemoglobin H disease and if all four are deleted the baby is stillborn (hydrops fetalis). Haemoglobin H is a beta-chain tetramer formed from the excess of chains. It is functionally useless. Treatment of haemoglobin H disease is similar to that of beta-thalassaemia of intermediate severity. In some patients the disorder is due to a combination of alpha-thalassaemia genes with genes which produce a functionally useless globin chain, Hb Constant Spring. The combinations are shown in the information box.

Table 11.11 Treatment of beta-thalassaemia major

Problem	Management
Erythropoietic failure	Allogeneic bone marrow transplantation from human leucocyte antigen (HLA)-compatible sibling Transfusion to maintain Hb > 100 g/l Folic acid 5 mg daily
Iron overload	Iron therapy forbidden Desferrioxamine therapy
Splenomegaly causing mechanical problems, excessive transfusion required	Splenectomy

ALPHA-THALASSAEMIA
Cause
• Failure of production of haemoglobin chain due to gene deletion
Age and sex
• Both sexes from birth onward
Genetics
• 2 alpha chain genes from each parent
Presentation
• Hydrops fetalis: all genes deleted • Haemoglobin H: three genes deleted • Mild hypochromic microcytic anaemia: two genes deleted
Treatment
• Hydrops fetalis: none available • Haemoglobin H: no specific therapy required; avoid iron therapy; folic acid if necessary

ACQUIRED HAEMOLYTIC ANAEMIAS

IMMUNE–AUTOIMMUNE HAEMOLYTIC ANAEMIA

In this disorder antibodies are formed against red cell antigens and cause inappropriate destruction of cells. The two main types are categorised on the basis of the thermal characteristics of the antibody:

- 'Warm' antibodies have a thermal optimum of 37°C and account for 80% of cases. The majority are IgG. A specificity, if it can be demonstrated, is usually to the Rhesus system.
- 'Cold' antibodies have a thermal optimum of 4°C but sometimes a thermal range of up to 37°C. These antibodies are IgM and bind complement. Cold antibodies are found in approximately 20% of autoimmune haemolytic anaemias.

WARM AUTOIMMUNE HAEMOLYTIC ANAEMIA

Many cases are idiopathic but some occur in association with chronic lymphatic leukaemia, lymphoma, systemic lupus erythematosus (SLE) or certain drugs (e.g. methyldopa).

Investigations

The diagnosis is suggested by finding spherocytes and increased polychromasia on the blood film. It is established by demonstrating evidence of antibody on the red cells by the direct antiglobulin test (Coombs test). This test detects the presence of antibodies on the surface of erythrocytes using an antihuman globulin (AHG) antiserum. As antibodies are human globulin, they are recognised by the AHG, which attacks them and causes agglutination of the erythrocytes. This is the 'direct' test. When antibodies are present in serum they must first be attached to red cells with the appropriate antigen before their presence can be detected as described above. This is known as the 'indirect' test. Elution of antibody from the red cells allows investigation of specificity against a panel of cells. The majority of these antibodies can be shown to have anti-Rhesus specificity. Of these, anti-e is the most common. Identification of specificity, if possible, is useful, as blood for transfusion which does not carry the specific antigen can be chosen.

Management

This is with prednisolone 40 mg daily for 3–4 weeks; thereafter the dose is slowly reduced. Response to treatment can be monitored with reticulocyte counts and haemoglobin estimations. The dose should be increased if relapse occurs and maintained for a further 2–3 weeks, when reduction may be tried again. Blood transfusion is avoided unless an antibody specificity has clearly been identified and antigen-free blood is available. In life-threatening situations, the least incompatible blood available can be given, covered by high doses of prednisolone. Splenectomy should be considered if treatment fails from the beginning, or if there is a fall in the haemoglobin following reduction/cessation of steroids.

COLD AGGLUTININ DISEASE

Idiopathic cold agglutinin disease occurs mainly in the elderly. Symptoms reflect a tendency of the red cells to agglutinate and sludge in the microvasculature of the extremities where the blood is cooled. Raynaud's phenomenon (see p. 268) is usually present and also acrocyanosis. A low-grade chronic haemolytic anaemia occurs. All these problems are worse in cold weather. Characteristic haematological features are a very high MCV and agglutination on the blood film; these features are reversed if the blood is warmed to 37°C. 'Cold' antibody is present in enormously high titres with anti-I or i specificity. The antiglobulin test is almost always positive and demonstrates complement-binding.

Treatment consists of keeping the extremities warm. Transfusion is possible but the specimen collected for transfusion must be kept warm during transport to the laboratory; the cross-matched blood should be transfused via a blood-warmer. Steroids and splenectomy are of little value but immunosuppressive therapy may decrease antibody levels in severe cases.

Cold antibody-type disease may also occur in association with *Mycoplasma pneumoniae* infection and infectious mononucleosis, when the haemolysis is usually self-limiting. If found in lymphoma the haemolysis tends to be more chronic.

Paroxysmal cold haemoglobinuria is a rare cause of haemolysis in children. It can be associated with syphilis. It is characterised by the Donath–Landsteiner IgG antibody which may be found, and has anti-P specificity.

NON-IMMUNE HAEMOLYTIC ANAEMIA

Mechanical trauma

Shearing of red cells may occur as a result of incompetent heart valves and when cells are forced through fibrin deposited in the vasculature. The latter may be deposited by a number of processes resulting in microangiopathic haemolysis. This may occur in disseminated malignancy, toxaemia of pregnancy, the accelerated phase of hypertension and in the haemolytic uraemic syndrome. Direct mechanical trauma has been associated with vigorous contact activities such as karate or prolonged marching (march haemoglobinuria). Thermal injury in severe burns may result in haemolysis, in which characteristic small spherocytes can be seen in the film. An important laboratory finding in the majority of mechanically induced haemolytic anaemias is the demonstration of red cell fragmentation on the blood film. As the haemolysis is mainly intravascular, haemosiderin may be found in the urine.

Infections

Malarial infection, usually with *Plasmodium falciparum*, often results in a mild degree of haemolysis. Less frequently there is severe intravascular haemolysis: blackwater fever. The parasites should be seen in the red blood cells on the blood film and the management is discussed on page 152. *Clostridium perfringens* septicaemia may cause devastating intravascular haemolysis characterised by spherocytosis. The mechanism is thought to be the production of lecithinase activity. The organism is sensitive to penicillin.

Drugs and chemicals

Dapsone and salazopyrin may result in haemolysis in patients who are not G6PD-deficient. The mechanism is oxidant and individual variation in drug metabolism is an important factor. Dapsone is acetylated and slow acetylators are much more prone to haemolysis. The demonstration of Heinz bodies is a strong pointer to the diagnosis. Haemolysis has been described following exposure to arsenic gas, copper, chlorate, nitrites and nitrobenzene derivatives. Anaemia is a feature of lead poisoning but this is not predominantly haemolytic. Several enzymes of haem synthesis are inhibited and basophilic stippling is a characteristic finding on the blood film due to pyrimidine-5′-nucleotidase inhibition.

APLASTIC ANAEMIA

PRIMARY IDIOPATHIC ACQUIRED APLASTIC ANAEMIA

The annual prevalence in the United States and United Kingdom is approximately 3–6 cases per million; the disease is much more common in certain other parts of the world—for example, China. The basic problem is failure of the stem cells to a varying degree, producing hypoplasia of the marrow elements. An autoimmune mechanism may be responsible in a proportion of cases.

Investigations

Known causes of hypoplastic and aplastic anaemia must first be excluded. A careful inquiry into exposure to drugs, chemicals and radiation should be made. A history of viral illness, particularly hepatitis, may be important. A full blood count demonstrates a pancytopenia. Neutropenia is the most marked aspect of the leucopenia, although leucopenia may not be the first abnormality. The anaemia is normocytic, normochromic and often marked. Platelet production is often the most severely affected and the last to recover. The bone marrow should be examined by aspiration and trephine. The latter provides a better assessment of cellularity and an aspirate may be difficult to obtain (dry tap).

Management

All patients will require blood product support and aggressive management of infection. The curative treatment for young (< 20 year-old) patients with severe idiopathic aplastic anaemia is allogeneic bone marrow transplantation if there is an available donor. Those with a compatible sibling donor should proceed to transplantation as soon as possible. Successful pre-transplant conditioning can be achieved with cyclophosphamide alone. In older patients, immunosuppressive therapy gives equivalent results.

A number of drugs have been investigated for older patients and those without a donor, including androgens, steroids, cyclosporin and antilymphocyte/antithymocyte globulin. These approaches, in the main, reflect the likelihood that an immunological mechanism is involved in a significant proportion of cases. Antilymphocyte globulin has been the most successful agent, although haematological responses are often incomplete and long-term follow-up has revealed a proportion of cases developing myelodysplasia. Short-term toxicity is in the form of serum sickness. More recently there has been an interest in combination therapy; females with severe aplastic anaemia appear to benefit particularly from a combination of antilymphocyte globulin, androgens and steroids.

Prognosis

The prognosis of severe aplastic anaemia managed with supportive therapy only is poor and more than 50% of patients die, usually in the first year. However, the survival of over 60% has been reported after bone marrow transplantation in young patients and similar results can be achieved with immunosuppressive regimens involving antithymocyte globulin.

SECONDARY APLASIA

Causes of this condition are listed in the information box. It is not practical to list all the drugs which have been suspected of causing aplasia but it is important to investigate the reported side-effects of all drugs taken over the preceding months. In some instances the cytopenia is more selective and affects only one cell line, most often the neutrophils. Frequently this is an incidental finding unassociated with ill health. It probably has an immune basis but this is difficult to prove.

CAUSES OF ACQUIRED APLASTIC ANAEMIA

- Drugs—cytotoxic drugs, idiosyncratic
  - Antibiotics—chloramphenicol, sulphonamides
  - Antirheumatic agents—penicillamine, gold, phenylbutazone, indomethacin
  - Antithyroid drugs
  - Anticonvulsants
  - Immunosuppressives—azathioprine
- Chemicals
  - Benzene toluene solvent abuse—glue-sniffing
  - Insecticides—chlorinated hydrocarbons (DDT), organophosphates and carbonates
- Radiation
- Viral hepatitis
- Pregnancy
- Paroxysmal nocturnal haemoglobinuria

The clinical features and methods of diagnosis are the same as for primary idiopathic aplastic anaemia. An underlying cause should be treated or removed but otherwise the management is as for the idiopathic form. Bone marrow transplantation may have to be considered in young patients who have HLA-matched sibling donors.

ANAEMIA OF CHRONIC DISEASE

This is a common type of anaemia, particularly in hospital populations. Characteristic features are as follows:

- The anaemia occurs in the setting of chronic infections, chronic inflammation, or neoplasia.
- The anaemia is not related to bleeding, haemolysis or marrow infiltration.
- The anaemia is generally mild, in the range 85–115 g/l, and is usually associated with a normal MCV (normocytic normochromic), but up to 25% may have a reduced MCV.
- The serum iron is low but iron stores are normal or increased, as indicated by the ferritin or stainable marrow iron.

Pathogenesis

The pathogenesis of this type of anaemia is thought to involve abnormalities of iron metabolism and erythropoiesis. Recent interest has been centred on the role of erythropoietin and the inhibitory effect of various cytokines (interleukin-1 and tumour necrosis factor alpha) on erythropoiesis. Erythropoietin levels appear to be lower than would be expected for the degree of anaemia. Administration of erythropoietin to patients with rheumatoid arthritis has a beneficial effect on the anaemia.

Management

A particular problem is to distinguish the anaemia of chronic disease (ACD) associated with a low MCV from iron deficiency. The ferritin level is elevated in inflammatory conditions and the serum iron is low in both the ACD and iron deficiency. A ferritin in the low/normal range (up to 100 μg/1) in the setting of disorders associated with the ACD may indicate iron deficiency. Examination of the marrow is useful to assess iron stores. A trial of oral iron could be given in difficult situations. A positive response occurs in true iron deficiency but not in ACD. Measures which reduce the severity of the underlying disorder generally help to improve the ACD.

FURTHER INFORMATION ON ANAEMIAS

Hoffbrand V, Provan D 1997 Macrocytic anaemias. British Medical Journal 314: 430–433

Smith A G 1997 Prescribing iron. Prescribers' Journal 37: 82–87

Weatherall D J 1997 The hereditary anaemias. British Medical Journal 314: 492–496

LEUKAEMIAS AND MYELODYSPLASIA

Leukaemias are a group of malignant disorders of the haematopoietic tissues characteristically associated with increased numbers of primitive white cells (blasts) in the bone marrow. The course of leukaemia may vary from a few days or weeks to many years, depending on the type.

Epidemiology

The incidence of leukaemia of all types in the population is approximately 10 per 100 000 per annum, of which just under half are acute leukaemia. Males are affected more frequently than females, the ratio being about 3:2 in acute leukaemia, 2:1 in chronic lymphocytic leukaemia, and 1.3:1 in chronic myeloid leukaemia. Geographic variation in incidence does occur, the most striking being the rarity of chronic lymphocytic leukaemia in the Chinese and related races. Acute leukaemia occurs at all ages. Acute lymphoblastic leukaemia shows a peak of incidence in the 1–5 age group. All forms of acute myeloid leukaemia have their lowest incidence in young adult life and there is a striking rise over the age of 50. Chronic leukaemias occur mainly in middle and old age.

Aetiology

The cause of the leukaemia is unknown in the majority of patients. Several factors, however, are associated with the development of leukaemia and these are listed in the information box.

FACTORS ASSOCIATED WITH THE DEVELOPMENT OF LEUKAEMIA
Ionising radiation
• A significant increase in myeloid leukaemia followed the atomic bombing of Japanese cities • An increase in leukaemia was observed after the use of radiotherapy for ankylosing spondylitis and diagnostic radiographs of the fetus in pregnancy
Cytotoxic drugs
• These, particularly alkylating agents, may induce myeloid leukaemia, usually after a latent period of several years
Exposure to benzene in industry
Retroviruses
• One rare form of T cell leukaemia/lymphoma appears to be associated with a retrovirus similar to the viruses causing leukaemia in cats and cattle
Genetic
• There is a greatly increased incidence of leukaemia in the identical twin of patients with leukaemia • Increased incidence occurs in Down's syndrome and other genetic disorders
Immunological
• Immune deficiency states are associated with an increase in haematological malignancy

Terminology and classification

The terms 'acute' and 'chronic', when applied to leukaemia, refer to the clinical behaviour of the disease. In acute leukaemia the history is usually brief and life expectancy, without treatment, short. In chronic leukaemias the patients may have been unwell for months and survival is measured in years. A significant number of chronic leukaemias are discovered incidentally.

Not all leukaemias are associated with an increased leucocyte count or even the appearance of abnormal cells in the blood. The diagnosis is made from an examination of the bone marrow.

The classification of leukaemia is given in the information boxes.

A CLASSIFICATION OF LEUKAEMIA

Acute	Chronic
• Lymphoblastic • Myeloid	• Lymphatic • Myeloid

Although leukaemias are divided into lymphoid and myeloid varieties, recent advances have shown that this division may be artificial because in acute leukaemias the two types may coexist in the same patient. Nevertheless there is a value in maintaining the distinction, as the drug therapy of the two main types is substantially different.

The subclassification of the lymphoblastic varieties is possibly of greater value, for the subtype dictates greater variation in treatment. The 'common' type which constitutes 70% of all patients responds well to treatment and carries the best chance of long-term remission. The classification of acute myeloblastic leukaemia into eight varieties reflects the variable degree of maturation of the granulocyte series, the common involvement of the monocyte series with the granulocyte series, and also the involvement of erythrocytic and megakaryocytic elements.

SUBCLASSIFICATIONS OF LEUKAEMIA

Acute lymphoblastic
- Common type (pre-B)
- T cell
- B cell
- Undifferentiated

Acute myeloid
FAB[1] classification
- M0 undifferentiated
- M1 minimal differentiation
- M2 differentiated
- M3 promyelocytic
- M4 myelomonocytic
- M5 monocytic
- M6 erythrocytic
- M7 megakaryocytic

Chronic lymphatic
- Common B cell
- Rare T cell

Chronic myeloid
- Ph[2] positive
- Ph[2] negative, BCR[3] positive
- Ph[2] negative, BCR[3] negative
- Eosinophilic leukaemia

[1] FAB = French, American, British.
[2] Ph = Philadelphia chromosome.
[3] BCR = breakpoint cluster region.

ACUTE LEUKAEMIA

There is a failure of cell maturation in acute leukaemia. Proliferation of cells which do not mature leads to an increasing accumulation of useless cells which take up more and more marrow space at the expense of the normal haematopoietic elements. Eventually this proliferation spills into the blood. The evolution of acute leukaemia is illustrated schematically in Figure 11.17. Acute myeloblastic leukaemia is about four times more common than acute lymphoblastic leukaemia in adults. In children the lymphoblastic variety is more common. The clinical features are usually those of bone marrow failure (anaemia, bleeding or infection) and these are discussed in the section on major manifestations.

Investigations

Blood examination usually shows anaemia with a normal or raised MCV. The leucocyte count may vary from as low as $1 \times 10^9/l$ to as high as $500 \times 10^9/l$ or more. In the majority of patients the count is below $100 \times 10^9/l$. The blood film appearance of blast cells and other primitive cells is usually diagnostic. Sometimes the blast cell count may be very low in the peripheral blood and a bone marrow examination is necessary to establish the diagnosis. Severe thrombocytopenia is usual but not invariable.

The bone marrow is the most valuable diagnostic investigation and will provide material for cytology, cytogenetics and immunological phenotyping. A trephine biopsy should be taken if no marrow is obtained (dry tap). The marrow is

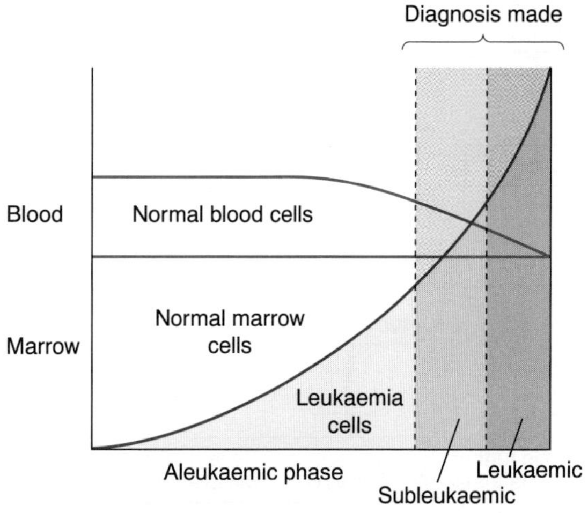

Fig. 11.17 The development of leukaemia.

INVESTIGATIONS FOR THE ASSESSMENT OF ACUTE LEUKAEMIA

Haemostatic function
- Coagulation screen
- Fibrinogen
- D-dimers (see p. 794)

Renal function
- Plasma urea
- Plasma creatinine

Hepatic function
- Total protein
- Albumin
- Bilirubin
- Alkaline phosphatase
- Alanine aminotransferase (ALT)

Cellular proliferation
- Plasma LDH
- Plasma urate

usually hypercellular, with replacement of normal elements by leukaemic blast cells in varying degrees (but more than 30% of the cells). The presence of Auer rods in the cytoplasm of blast cells indicates a myeloblastic type of leukaemia.

Other basic investigations required at diagnosis are given in the information box .

Management

The general strategy for acute leukaemia is given in Figure 11.18. The first decision must be whether or not to give specific treatment. However, specific treatment is generally aggressive and has a number of side-effects. It may not be appropriate for the following groups of patients:

- the very elderly (over 80 years of age)
- patients with other serious disorders
- patients who decline specific therapy
- patients with types of leukaemia known to be very unresponsive to specific treatment (secondary leukaemias, patients with multiple chromosome abnormalities).

In these patients supportive treatment only should be offered; this can effect considerable improvement in well-being. These decisions must, if possible, be made with the understanding and cooperation of patient and relatives.

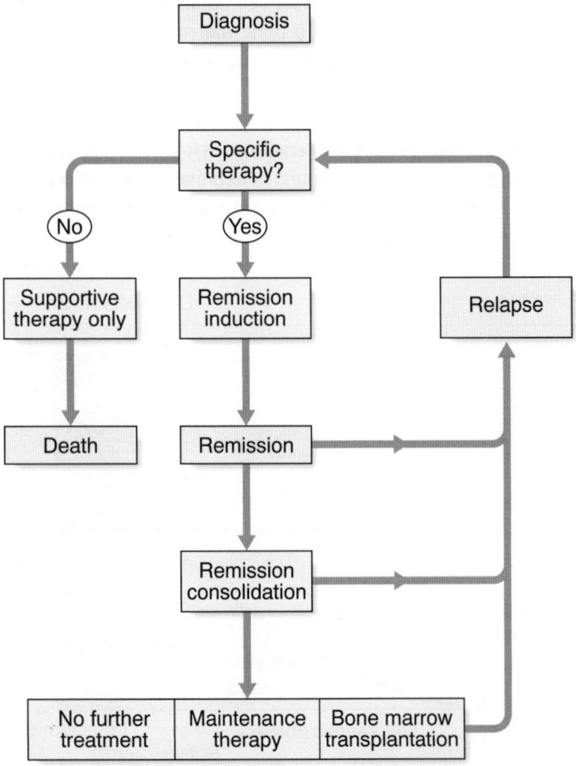

Fig. 11.18 Treatment strategy in acute leukaemia.

Specific therapy

If a decision to embark on specific therapy has been taken, the patient should be prepared in the ways listed in the information box. It is unwise to attempt aggressive management of acute leukaemia unless adequate services are available for the provision of supportive therapy. Such treatment should only be directed by physicians experienced in the management of leukaemic patients.

MANAGEMENT OF ACUTE LEUKAEMIA: SPECIFIC THERAPY

- Existing infections identified and treated (e.g. urinary tract infection, oral candidiasis, dental, gingival and skin infections)
- Anaemia corrected with red cell concentrate infusion
- Thrombocytopenic bleeding controlled with platelet transfusion
- If possible, central venous catheter (e.g. Hickman line) inserted to facilitate access to the circulation for delivery of chemotherapy
- Therapeutic regimen carefully explained to the patient

The aim of treatment is to destroy the leukaemic clone of cells without destroying the residual normal stem cell compartment from which repopulation of the haematopoietic tissues will occur. There are three phases:

- *Remission induction.* In this phase the bulk of the tumour is destroyed by combination chemotherapy. The patient goes through a period of severe bone marrow hypoplasia, requiring intensive support and inpatient care from specially trained medical and nursing staff.
- *Remission consolidation.* If remission has been achieved by induction therapy, residual disease is attacked by therapy during the consolidation phase. This consists of a number of courses of chemotherapy, again resulting in periods of marrow hypoplasia. In cases of acute lymphoblastic leukaemia it is necessary to give therapy to the central nervous system. This usually consists of a combination of cranial irradiation and intrathecal methotrexate.
- *Remission maintenance.* If the patient is still in remission after the consolidation phase for acute lymphoblastic

Table 11.12 Drugs commonly used in the treatment of acute leukaemia

Phase	Lymphoblastic	Myeloid
Induction	Vincristine (i.v.) Prednisolone (oral) L-asparaginase (i.v.) Daunorubicin (i.v.) Methotrexate (intrathecal)	Daunorubicin (i.v.) Cytosine arabinoside (i.v.) Etoposide (i.v. and oral) Thioguanine (oral)
Consolidation	Daunorubicin (i.v.) Cytosine arabinoside (i.v.) Etoposide (i.v.)	Cytosine arabinoside (i.v.) Amsacrine (i.v.) Mitozantrone (i.v.)
Maintenance	Prednisolone (oral) Vincristine (i.v.) Mercaptopurine (oral) Methotrexate (oral)	

leukaemia, a period of maintenance therapy is given, consisting of a repeating cycle of drug administration. This may extend for up to 2 years if relapse does not occur and is usually given on an outpatient basis. Thereafter, specific therapy is discontinued and the patient observed. This phase is not thought to be of benefit in patients with acute myeloblastic leukaemia who have been brought into complete remission by induction and consolidation therapy.

The detail of the schedules for these treatments will be found in specialist texts. The drugs most commonly employed for the two main varieties of acute leukaemia are given in Table 11.12. If a patient fails to go into remission with induction treatment, alternative drug combinations may be tried but generally the outlook is poor. Alternatively, a decision may be taken not to give any further specific therapy and to provide supportive treatment only. Disease which relapses during treatment or soon after the end of treatment carries a poor prognosis and is difficult to treat. The longer after the end of treatment that relapse occurs, the more likely it is that further treatment will be effective.

Supportive therapy

Aggressive and potentially curative therapy which involves periods of severe bone marrow failure would not be possible without adequate and skilled supportive care. The following problems commonly arise.

Anaemia. Anaemia is treated with red cell concentrate infusion to maintain a haemoglobin above 100 g/l.

Bleeding. Thrombocytopenic bleeding requires platelet transfusions unless the bleeding is trivial. Freshly harvested platelets from five donors are pooled and provided as a pack. One or two packs daily may be required if bleeding is severe. Coagulation abnormalities occur and need accurate diagnosis and treatment as appropriate, usually with fresh frozen plasma. The role of prophylactic platelet transfusion is controversial. However, many units give platelets in an attempt to keep the count above 10×10^9/l.

Infection. Fever (greater than 38°C) lasting over 1 hour in a neutropenic patient (absolute neutrophil count < 1.0×10^9/l) indicates possible septicaemia. Parenteral broad-spectrum antibiotic therapy is essential. Empirical therapy with a combination of an aminoglycoside (e.g. gentamicin) is given with a broad-spectrum penicillin (e.g. piperacillin/tazobactam). This combination is synergistic and bacteriocidal and should be continued for at least 5 days after the fever has resolved. The organisms most commonly associated with severe neutropenia are Gram-positive bacteria such as *Staphylococcus aureus* and *Staphylococcus epidermidis*. The Gram-negative infections with organisms such as *Escherichia coli*, *Pseudomonas* and *Klebsiella* are more likely to cause rapid clinical deterioration and these organisms must be covered with the initial empirical therapy. Gram-positive infection, particularly when the patient has an indwelling intravenous catheter, may require vancomycin. Patients with lymphoblastic leukaemia are susceptible to infection with *Pneumocystis carinii*, which causes a severe pneumonia. Diagnosis may be difficult and is obtained either from bronchial washings or open lung biopsy. Treatment is with high-dose co-trimoxazole, initially intravenously with change to oral treatment as soon as possible.

Oral and pharyngeal monilial infection is common. Prophylaxis with fluconazole is often considered and this drug is effective for treatment of established local infection.

For systemic fungal infection with *Candida* or pulmonary aspergillosis, intravenous amphotericin is required: 0.5–1 mg/kg per day for at least 3 weeks. Amphotericin is nephrotoxic and hepatotoxic. Renal and hepatic function should be monitored closely, particularly if the patient is receiving antibiotics which are also nephrotoxic. Potassium supplementation is usually required. For patients who experience nephrotoxicity with standard amphotericin, newer lipid formulations of amphotericin can be administered without further deterioration of renal function.

Herpes simplex infection occurs frequently round the lips and nose during ablative therapy for acute leukaemia. Aciclovir (200 mg 5 times per day) may be prescribed prophylactically to patients with a history of cold sores or elevated titres to herpes simplex. The intravenous dose is 5 mg/kg over 1 hour, repeated 8-hourly. Herpes zoster can also be treated in the early stage with aciclovir at a dose of 10 mg/kg 8-hourly intravenously for 5 days. Cytomegalovirus infection has become a problem in some leukaemia units. Treatment is difficult but a combination of ganciclovir and immunoglobulin can be tried.

The value of isolation facilities, such as laminar flow rooms, is debatable but may contribute to staff awareness of careful barrier nursing practice. The isolation is often psychologically stressful for the patient.

Metabolic problems. Continuous monitoring of renal, hepatic and haemostatic function is necessary, together with fluid balance measurements. Patients are often severely anorexic and may find drinking difficult. The necessary fluids and electrolytes often must be given intravenously for as long as necessary. Renal toxicity occurs with some antibiotics (e.g. aminoglycosides) and antifungal agents (amphotericin).

Psychological support. Psychological support of the patient is very important. Patients should be kept informed, and their questions answered and fears allayed as far as possible. An optimistic attitude from the staff is vital. Delusions, hallucinations and paranoia are not uncommon during periods of severe bone marrow failure and septicaemic episodes, and should be met with patience and understanding.

Alternative chemotherapy. Gentle chemotherapy not designed to achieve remission may be used to curb excessive leucocyte proliferation. Drugs used for this purpose include hydroxyurea up to 4 g daily and mercaptopurine up to 150 mg daily. The effect is to reduce the leucocyte count without inducing bone marrow failure.

Prognosis

Without treatment the median survival of patients with acute leukaemia is about 5 weeks. This may be extended to a number of months with supportive treatment. Patients who achieve remission with specific therapy have a better outlook. Around 80% of adult patients under 60 years of age with acute lymphoblastic leukaemia and acute myeloblastic leukaemia achieve remission. Remission rates are lower for older patients. However, the relapse rate continues to be high. Median survival for acute lymphoblastic leukaemia patients is about 30 months; patients with acute myeloblastic leukaemia under 55 have a 40% 5-year survival with the best modern chemotherapy. Poor prognostic factors for survival are given in the information box.

POOR PROGNOSTIC FEATURES IN ACUTE LEUKAEMIA

- Increasing age
- Male sex
- High leucocyte levels at diagnosis
- Cytogenetic abnormalities
- CNS involvement at diagnosis

Allogeneic bone marrow transplantation (BMT)

This until recently has been the only therapeutic measure which held out the hope of 'cure' for persons with a variety of haematological disorders, particularly those listed in the information box top right.

Healthy marrow from a donor is injected intravenously into a recipient who has been suitably 'conditioned'. The conditioning therapy used most frequently is high-dose cyclophosphamide and total body irradiation. Conditioning ablates the recipient's haematopoietic and immunological tissues. The injected cells 'home' to the marrow and produce enough erythrocytes, granulocytes and platelets for the patient's needs in about 3–4 weeks. It takes up to 3 or more years to regain good lymphocyte function and immunological stability. During this period, particularly in the first year, the patient is at great risk from opportunistic infections.

GENERAL INDICATIONS FOR ALLOGENEIC BONE MARROW TRANSPLANTATION

- Neoplastic disorders affecting the totipotent or pluripotent stem cell compartment (e.g. leukaemias)
- Those with a failure of haematopoiesis (e.g. aplastic anaemia)
- A major inherited defect in blood cell production (e.g. thalassaemia, immunodeficiency diseases)
- Inborn errors of metabolism with missing enzymes or cell lines

The preferred donors are histocompatible siblings and the best results are obtained in patients aged under 20. Older patients can be transplanted, but results become progressively worse with age. The patient must be sufficiently stable psychologically to contend with the period of illness during the transplantation process. The patient should be free of other disorders which might seriously limit lifespan. Bone marrow transplantation requires specialised supervision and supportive facilities with fully trained staff. It is best performed in units established for the care of acute leukaemias under the primary care of haematologists, with the cooperation of immunologists, microbiologists, radiotherapists and full laboratory services.

Bone marrow transplantation may be syngeneic (identical twin donor) or allogeneic (non-identical donor). Disorders for which allogeneic transplantation is currently considered are shown in the information box.

HAEMATOLOGICAL INDICATIONS FOR ALLOGENEIC BONE MARROW TRANSPLANTATION

- Acute myeloblastic leukaemia in first remission
- Chronic myeloid leukaemia in chronic phase
- T and B cell lymphoblastic leukaemia in first remission
- Acute lymphoblastic leukaemia (common pre-B type) in second remission
- Severe aplastic anaemia
- Acute myelofibrosis
- Severe immunodeficiency syndromes

Transplantation is also a possibility for resistant acute leukaemia and selected patients with lymphoma. The role of allogeneic BMT in patients with haemoglobinopathies such as sickle-cell disease is controversial.

The main complications of allogeneic bone marrow transplantation are outlined in the information box.

The long-term survival for patients undergoing allogeneic bone marrow transplantation in acute leukaemia is around 50%. A total of 30% succumb to procedure-related morbidity (graft-versus-host disease, pneumonitis) and in 20% the disease relapses.

COMPLICATIONS OF ALLOGENEIC BONE MARROW TRANSPLANTATION

- Mucositis
- Infection
- Acute graft-versus-host disease
- Pneumonitis
- Chronic graft-versus-host disease
- Infertility
- Cataract formation
- Secondary malignant disease

Graft-versus-host disease (GVHD)

Problems of GVHD and interstitial pneumonitis may cause serious morbidity and death if the graft is successful. Even low-grade GVHD, which is probably advantageous in terms of survival, can reduce the quality of life. GVHD is due to the cytotoxic activity of donor T lymphocytes which become sensitised to their new host, regarding it as foreign. This may cause either an acute or a chronic form of GVHD.

Acute GVHD. The acute GVHD usually appears 14–21 days after the graft, although it may appear earlier or up to 70 days later. It can affect the skin, liver and gut, and may vary from being mild to lethal. It appears to be associated with infection, although the relationship is not fully understood. Methotrexate, cyclosporin, anti-thymocyte globulin, high-dose corticosteroids and T cell depletion of the donor marrow have all been used to try to prevent the disorder. The more severe forms prove very difficult to control; high-dose steroids may be helpful.

Chronic GVHD. This may follow acute GVHD or arise independently; it occurs later than acute GVHD. It often resembles a connective tissue disorder, although in mild cases a rash may be the only manifestation. Chronic GVHD is usually treated with steroids. Cyclosporin can be used in cases associated with thrombocytopenia. Associated with chronic GVHD is a graft-versus-leukaemia effect, which results in a lower relapse rate.

Infection

Infection is the other major problem during recovery from BMT. Details are given in Table 11.13.

Table 11.13 Infection during recovery from bone marrow transplant (BMT)

Infection	Period after BMT	Treatment
Herpes simplex	0–4 weeks	Aciclovir
Bacterial, fungal	0–4 weeks	As for acute leukaemia (see p. 773)
Cytomegalovirus	7–21 weeks	If patient is CMV-negative, use CMV-negative blood products Hyperimmune immunoglobulin and ganciclovir for documented infections
Varicella zoster	After 13 weeks	Aciclovir, 10 mg/kg per day for 1–2 weeks i.v.
Pneumocystis carinii	8–26 weeks	Co-trimoxazole
Interstitial pneumonitis (non-infective)	6–18 weeks	No specific therapy Prednisolone, 60 mg daily orally, may be tried

Autologous bone marrow transplantation—peripheral blood stem cell transplantation

In this procedure the patient's own marrow is harvested, to be given back again after intensive therapy. It may be used for disorders which do not primarily involve the haematopoietic tissues or in patients in whom very good remissions have been achieved in conditions such as acute leukaemias and high-grade lymphomas. In acute leukaemias the procedure carries a lower procedure-related mortality rate than with allogeneic bone marrow transplantation but there is a high relapse rate (50%). However, there is some data to suggest that in certain patients with acute leukaemia autologous transplantation might confer a modest advantage over chemotherapy, although the results from further trials are required to substantiate this. The issue of whether the stem cells should be treated (purged) in an attempt to remove any residual leukaemia cells is controversial. Stem cells were originally always obtained by harvesting them from the marrow. More recently, stem cells have been collected from the peripheral blood during the recovery phase following a period of chemotherapy-induced marrow hypoplasia. Infusion of stem cells from the peripheral blood results in significantly faster engraftment compared with those obtained from the marrow.

CHRONIC MYELOID LEUKAEMIA

Chronic myeloid leukaemia is a disorder of proliferation which is unrestrained and excessive. Maturation proceeds fairly normally. The disease occurs chiefly between the ages of 30 and 80 years, with a peak at 55 years. It is rare, with an annual incidence in the UK of 1 per 100 000. The disease is found in all races. The aetiology is unknown.

Cytogenetic and molecular aspects

Approximately 90% of patients with chronic myeloid leukaemia have a chromosome abnormality known as the Philadelphia (Ph) chromosome. This is a shortened chromosome 22 and is the result of a reciprocal translocation of material with chromosome 9. The break on chromosome 22 occurs in the breakpoint cluster region (BCR). The fragment from chromosome 9 that joins the BCR carries the Abelson (ABL) oncogene, which forms a chimeric gene with the remains of the BCR. This chimeric gene codes for 210 kDa protein with tyrosine kinase activity, which plays a causative role in the disease. Some Ph-negative patients also have evidence of the same molecular abnormality.

Natural history

The disease has three phases: a chronic phase, in which the disease is responsive to treatment, is easily controlled and is essentially a benign neoplasm; an accelerated phase (not always seen), in which disease control becomes more difficult; and a blast crisis phase, in which the disease transforms into an acute leukaemia, either myeloid (70%) or lymphoblastic (30%), which is relatively refractory to treatment. Blast crises occur randomly and are the cause of death in the majority of patients. Patient survival is therefore dictated by the timing of blast crises, which cannot be predicted.

Clinical features

The frequency of the more common symptoms at presentation is given in Table 11.14. About 25% of patients are asymptomatic at diagnosis. On examination the principal clinical finding is splenomegaly, which is present in 90% of patients. In about 10% the enlargement is massive, extending to over 15 cm below the costal margin. The spleen is usually firm, smooth and painless but occasionally infarction may occur, giving rise to exquisite tenderness. A friction rub may be heard in cases of splenic infarction. Other causes of massive splenomegaly apart from chronic myeloid leukaemia are myelofibrosis, lymphoma and malaria. Hepatomegaly occurs in about 50% of patients. Lymphadenopathy is unusual. A list of causes of splenomegaly is shown in the information box on page 756.

Investigations

Examination of the blood usually shows a normocytic normochromic anaemia. The mean haemoglobin is 105 g/l with a range of 70–150 g/l. The mean leucocyte count is 220×10^9/l with a range of 9.5–600. The mean platelet count is 445×10^9/l with a range of 162–2000. In the blood film the full range of granulocyte precursors from myeloblasts to mature neutrophils is seen, with peaks at the myelocyte and mature granulocyte stage of maturation. Myeloblasts are usually less than 10%. There is often an absolute increase in eosinophils and basophils, and nucleated red cells are common. If the disease progresses through an accelerated phase the percentage of the more primitive cells increases. There is a dramatic increase in the number of circulating myeloblasts as the disease enters blast transformation. In about one-third of patients very high platelet counts are seen during treatment, both in chronic and accelerated phases, but these usually drop dramatically at blast transformation. Basophilia tends to increase as the disease progresses.

The peripheral blood is the most useful diagnostically but bone marrow material should be obtained for chromosome analysis to demonstrate the presence of the Philadelphia chromosome. Increasingly, DNA analysis is being undertaken to demonstrate the presence of the chimeric Abelson-BCR gene. Other characteristic findings on investigation include a very low neutrophil alkaline phosphatase score and very high vitamin B_{12} levels in the plasma. Lactate dehydrogenase levels are also substantially elevated.

Table 11.14 Symptoms at presentation of chronic myeloid leukaemia

Symptom	Present (%)
Tiredness	37
Weight loss	26
Breathlessness	21
Abdominal pain and discomfort	21
Lethargy	13
Anorexia	12
Sweating	11
Abdominal fullness	10
Bruising	7
Vague ill health	7

Management

No specific therapy is required if the patient is asymptomatic and the leucocyte count not greatly elevated. In the majority of patients, however, treatment is necessary.

Chemotherapy

Hydroxyurea is currently the most widely used oral agent to provide initial control of the disease. A daily dose of around 2–4 g is used initially and the dose is tailored to maintain the white count in the normal range. Treatment with hydroxyurea alone, however, does not diminish the frequency of the Philadelphia chromosome or affect the onset of blast cell transformation. Two types of treatment given in chronic phase can affect survival and result in the loss of the Philadelphia chromosome.

Alpha interferon

This is given intramuscularly or subcutaneously at 3–9 mega units daily. It can induce and maintain control of this disease in chronic phase in about 70% of patients. In addition, however, reduction in the percentage of Ph-positive cells is seen in about 20% and apparent elimination of the Ph chromosome in about 5%. There is evidence that interferon prolongs survival in those who achieve a significant reduction in Ph-positive cells. Only prolonged follow-up will determine whether such patients are cured. Interferon therapy causes 'flu-like' symptoms initially, tiredness, somnolence, weight loss, dizziness, nausea, vomiting, loss of taste, diarrhoea and headache. Some of these side-effects may be controlled with paracetamol; others such as severe bone pain and severe weight loss are reasons for discontinuation. The majority of patients tolerate the therapy well, particularly if the dose can be reduced to 3 mega units 3 times per week. It is probably unwise to use interferon therapy in patients over 75 years of age because of neurotoxicity. During treatment the aim should be to maintain the leucocyte count at low levels between 2 and 5×10^9/l.

Allogeneic or syngeneic bone marrow transplant from a matched sibling donor

This provides the only means of obtaining long-term remission in this disease. It is available to those under the age of 40 years who have a suitable donor. The best results are obtained in patients in early chronic phase when about 60% can expect prolongation of survival and possible cure. The results of transplantation in accelerated and blast transformation phases are poor. As only a few patients have matched family donors available, there is increasing interest in transplantation using matched unrelated volunteer donors. Such a transplant carries higher morbidity and mortality but may offer up to 40% the prospect of long-term survival. Various autografting approaches are also under evaluation.

Treatment of the accelerated phase and blast crisis of the disease is more difficult. In accelerated phase, hydroxyurea can be an effective single agent; low-dose cytosine arabinoside can also be tried. When blast transformation occurs, the type of blast cell should be ascertained by cytochemical and immunological techniques. If lymphoblastic, the response to appropriate treatment (see p. 773) is better than if myeloblastic. Response to treatment for the latter is very poor. There is a strong case for supportive therapy only, particularly in older patients.

Prognosis

Patients treated conventionally have a 15% risk of death in the first 12 months, and thereafter an annual risk of 20–25%. Median survival is about 45 months with chemotherapy, but is 65 months with interferon; patients who have a significant reduction in the Philadelphia chromosome with interferon do best. Patients receiving an allograft from a sibling early in chronic phase have a 60% chance of prolonged survival.

Philadelphia chromosome-negative chronic myeloid leukaemia

About half of these patients have the classical molecular abnormality (BCR-positive) without a demonstrable Ph chromosome. They behave as Ph chromosome-positive patients and they should be managed in the same way. The remainder (BCR-negative) tend to be older, mostly males, with lower platelet counts and higher absolute monocyte counts, and respond poorly to treatment. Median survival is less than 1 year.

CHRONIC LYMPHOCYTIC LEUKAEMIA

This is the most common variety of leukaemia. The male to female ratio is 2:1 and the majority of patients are over the age of 45, with a peak at 65. The disease is very rare in the Chinese and related races. In this disease B lymphocytes, which would normally respond to antigens by transformation and antibody formation, fail to do so. An ever-increasing mass of immuno-incompetent cells accumulate, to the detriment of immune function and normal bone marrow haemopoiesis. The receptor profile of the lymphocytes almost always demonstrates a B-cell type of disease. T-cell disease occurs rarely (5%). The light chains of immunoglobulins produced by these B cells tend to be either kappa or lambda in type, indicating in the majority of cases a monoclonal expansion of cells. The B cells of chronic lymphatic leukaemia characteristically express a T-cell antigen, CD5.

Clinical features

The onset is very insidious. Indeed in around 25% of patients the diagnosis is made incidentally. Presenting problems may be anaemia or painful lymphadenopathy; infections may be present at the time of diagnosis but often occur later in the progress of the disease (see p. 778).

Investigations

Peripheral blood examination usually shows a mild but gradually increasing anaemia. Haemolytic anaemia may occur and is usually warm autoimmune in type. In the majority of patients the leucocyte count is between 50 and 200×10^9/1, although it may occasionally be greatly increased, up to 1000×10^9/1. About 95% or more of these cells are lymphocytes which are predominantly of the small variety. Bone marrow examination by aspirate and trephine may be helpful not only in the diagnosis of cases with a low white count but also for prognosis. Cases with diffuse marrow involvement tend to do worst. Chromosome analysis can be helpful, cases with trisomy 12, the most common abnormality, again having a poorer prognosis. The platelet count is either low, normal or only mildly reduced. Estimations of total proteins and immunoglobulin levels should be undertaken to establish the degree of immunosuppression which is common and progressive. In some patients immunoglobulin levels may be raised and there may be a monoclonal band. Urate levels are seldom raised because cell turnover is low.

Staging

The disease may be staged according to the criteria of the widely accepted international classification which is given in the information box.

STAGING OF CHRONIC LYMPHOCYTIC LEUKAEMIA
Clinical stage A
• No anaemia or thrombocytopenia and less than three areas of lymphoid enlargement
Clinical stage B
• No anaemia or thrombocytopenia, with three or more involved areas of lymphoid enlargement
Clinical stage C
• Anaemia and/or thrombocytopenia regardless of the number of areas of lymphoid enlargement

Management

Treatment depends upon the stage of the disease:

- *Clinical stage A.* No specific treatment required. Life expectancy is normal in older patients. The patient should be reassured.
- *Clinical stage B.* No treatment may be required if asymptomatic. Chemotherapy with chlorambucil may be initiated in symptomatic patients. Local radiotherapy to lymph nodes which cause discomfort may be given.
- *Clinical stage C.* Anaemia may require transfusion with red cell concentrate. Bone marrow failure, if present, is treated initially with prednisolone, 40 mg daily for 2–4 weeks. A degree of bone marrow recovery is usually achieved.

Cytotoxic therapy

Chlorambucil, 5 mg orally daily, over long periods with dose adjustment according to blood counts, will reduce the abnormal lymphocyte mass and produce symptomatic improvement in most patients. Alternatively, chlorambucil may be given as intermittent high-dose therapy, 0.4 mg/kg every 2 weeks incrementing by 0.1 mg/kg until the maximum tolerated dose is reached. This is continued until the desired therapeutic effect is obtained. In stage C disease there is some evidence that more aggressive combination chemotherapy might be beneficial but this is controversial. Fludarabine, a synthetic nucleoside, appears to be the most active drug and is undergoing intensive evaluation.

Radiotherapy

Total body irradiation using very small doses spread over 5 weeks in 10 fractions is effective and well tolerated, especially by the elderly. Local radiotherapy may be used to reduce spleen size or treat local problems due to the disease.

Infections

These must be vigorously treated with antibiotics as appropriate. Recurrent viral or non-specific infections (often respiratory) sometimes respond to immunoglobulin replacement therapy. Aciclovir is indicated for herpetic infections.

Splenectomy

This may be required to treat autoimmune haemolytic anaemia or gross splenic enlargement.

Prognosis

The overall median survival is about 6 years. Clinical stage A patients have a median survival of over 12 years and stage C patients between 2 and 3 years. Approximately 50% of patients die of infection and 30% of causes unrelated to chronic lymphocytic leukaemia. Unlike chronic myeloid leukaemia, chronic lymphocytic leukaemia rarely transforms to an acute phase.

HAIRY CELL LEUKAEMIA

This is a rare lymphoproliferative chronic B cell disorder.

Clinical features

The male to female ratio is 6:1 and the median age is 50. Presenting symptoms are generally those of ill health and recurrent infections. Splenomegaly occurs in 90% but lymph node enlargement is unusual.

Investigations

Severe neutropenia, monocytopenia and the characteristic hairy cells in blood and bone marrow are typical. These cells usually type as B lymphocytes but characteristically express CD25 and FMC7. A characteristic test is the demonstration that the acid phosphatase staining reaction in the cells is resistant to the action of tartrate. The neutrophil alkaline phosphatase score is almost always very high.

Management

Over recent years a number of treatments have been shown to produce long-lasting remissions. Cladribine and deoxycoformycin are effective in producing long periods of disease control.

PROLYMPHOCYTIC LEUKAEMIA

This is another variant of chronic lymphatic leukaemia found mainly in males over the age of 60; 25% of cases are of the T cell variety. There is massive splenomegaly with little lymphadenopathy and a very high leucocyte count, often in excess of 400×10^9/l. The characteristic cell is a large lymphocyte with a prominent nucleolus. Treatment is generally unsuccessful and the prognosis very poor. Leucophoresis for very high white counts, splenectomy and chemotherapy may be tried.

MYELODYSPLASTIC SYNDROME (MDS)

This syndrome consists of a clonal group of disorders which represent steps in the progression to the development of leukaemia. It is characterised by variable cytopenia, hypogranular neutrophils with nuclear hyper- or hypo-segmentation and hypercellular marrow with dysplastic changes in all three cell lines. The syndrome is being recognised more frequently; its exact incidence is uncertain but it is thought to be more common than acute leukaemia. Usually the disease presents as a primary problem in elderly patients, although it may occur as a secondary complication of treatment for malignant disease in younger patients. The syndrome comprises the following conditions:

- refractory anaemia
- refractory anaemia with ring sideroblasts (sideroblastic anaemia)
- chronic myelomonocytic leukaemia
- refractory anaemia with excess of blasts (RAEB)
- refractory anaemia with excess of blasts in transformation (RAEB-t).

Diagnosis

The diagnosis should be considered in a patient with a cytopenia with the dysplastic features indicated above. A marrow aspiration should be performed, which is usually hypercellular with evidence of dysplasia. Blast cells may be increased but do not reach the 30% level which indicates acute leukaemia. Chromosome analysis frequently reveals abnormalities, particularly of chromosomes 5 or 7.

Management

Treatment is unsatisfactory. Transfusion of blood and platelets and treatment of infection are required for all. Aggressive antileukaemic therapy is not generally successful. Differentiating agents such as retinoic acid have not fulfilled their promise. Low-dose cytosine arabinoside (20 mg subcutaneously, twice daily) produces occasional remission but this is short-lived. Allogeneic transplantation should be considered in younger patients who have a donor, but results indicate only a 30% success rate.

Prognosis

The first two conditions listed above are relatively chronic disorders while the latter three show a more aggressive course with a tendency to terminate as acute myeloid leukaemia. Thus patients with refractory and sideroblastic anaemia may survive for years but prognosis in the other three conditions is measured usually in months.

FURTHER INFORMATION ON LEUKAEMIAS AND MYELODYSPLASIA

Leisner R J, Goldstone A H 1997 The acute leukaemias. British Medical Journal 314: 733–736

Mead G M 1997 Malignant lymphomas and chronic lymphocytic leukaemia. British Medical Journal 314: 1103–1106

Oscier D G 1997 The myelodysplastic syndromes. British Medical Journal 314: 883–886

THE LYMPHOMAS AND MYELOMA

LYMPHOMAS

These neoplasms are divided clinically and histologically into Hodgkin's and non-Hodgkin's lymphoma. The majority are of B cell origin. Non-Hodgkin's lymphomas are divided into low-grade and high-grade tumours on the basis of their proliferation rate. High-grade tumours are dividing rapidly, have only been present for a matter of weeks before diagnosis and may be life-threatening. Low-grade tumours are dividing slowly, may have been present for many months before diagnosis and behave in an indolent fashion.

HODGKIN'S DISEASE

EPIDEMIOLOGY AND AETIOLOGY OF HODGKIN'S DISEASE
Incidence
• Approximately 4 new cases/100 000 population/year
Sex ratio
• Slight male excess overall (1.5:1)
Age
• Median age 31 years; first peak in 20–35s and second peak in 50–70s age group
Aetiology
• Unknown. More common in patients from well-educated backgrounds and small families. Three times more likely with a past history of glandular fever but no causal link to Epstein–Barr virus infection proven

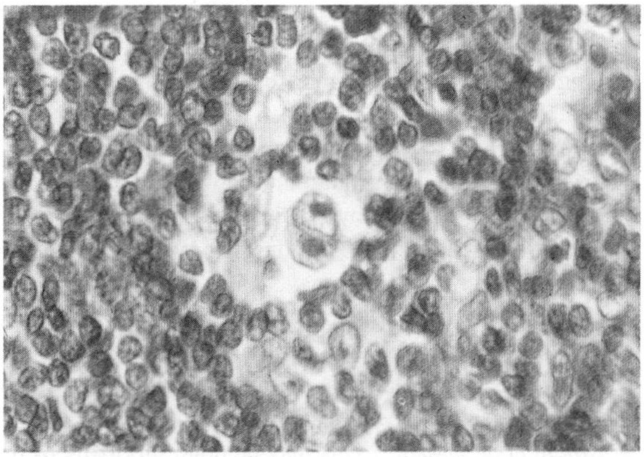

Fig. 11.19 Hodgkin's disease. Reed–Sternberg cell.

PATHOLOGICAL CLASSIFICATION OF HODGKIN'S LYMPHOMA

- Lymphocyte-predominant
- Nodular sclerosing
- Mixed cellularity
- Lymphocyte-depleted

The histological hallmark is the presence of Reed–Sternberg cells, which are large malignant lymphoid cells of uncertain origin (see Fig. 11.19). They are often present in only small numbers but surrounded by large numbers of reactive normal T cells, plasma cells and eosinophils. Four types of Hodgkin's disease are recognised from the appearance of the Reed–Sternberg cells and surrounding reactive cells (see the information box). The nodular sclerosing type accounts for the initial peak in young patients and is more common in women. Mixed cellularity is more common in the elderly peak. Lymphocyte-predominant Hodgkin's disease is now recognised as a low-grade B-cell non-Hodgkin's lymphoma. Lymphocyte-depleted Hodgkin's disease is rare and probably represents a T-cell non-Hodgkin's lymphoma.

Clinical features

There is painless rubbery lymphadenopathy, usually in the neck or supraclavicular fossae, which may fluctuate in size. Young patients with nodular sclerosing disease may have large mediastinal masses which are surprisingly asymptomatic but may cause dry cough and some breathlessness. Isolated subdiaphragmatic nodes occur in less than 10% at diagnosis. Hepatosplenomegaly may be present but does not always indicate disease. Spread is contiguous from one node to the next and extranodal disease, such as bone, brain or skin involvement, is rare.

Investigations

- *Full blood count.* This may be completely normal. Normochromic, normocytic anaemia may be present and, together with lymphopenia, is a bad prognostic factor. An eosinophilia or a neutrophilia may be present.
- *ESR.* This may be raised.
- *Renal function.* Investigate to ensure normal prior to treatment.
- *Liver function.* This may be abnormal in the absence of disease or due to hepatic infiltration. An obstructive pattern may be caused by nodes at the porta hepatis.
- *LDH.* Raised levels are an adverse prognostic factor.
- *Chest radiograph.* This may show a mediastinal mass.
- *CT scan.* Scan chest and abdomen to permit staging (see Table 11.15). CT scanning has replaced laparotomy. Bulky disease greater than 10 cm in a single node mass is an adverse prognostic feature.
- *Lymph node biopsy.* This may be done surgically or by percutaneous needle biopsy under radiological guidance (see Fig. 11.20).

Table 11.15 Clinical stages of Hodgkin's disease (Ann Arbor classification)

Stage	Definition
I	Involvement of a single lymph node region (I) or extra-lymphatic site (IE)
II	Involvement of two or more lymph node regions (II) or an extralymphatic site and lymph node regions on the same side of (above or below) the diaphragm (IIE)
III	Involvement of lymph node regions on both sides of the diaphragm with (IIIE) or without (III) localised extralymphatic involvement or involvement of the spleen (IIIS) or both (IIISE)
IV	Diffuse involvement of one or more extralymphatic tissues, e.g. liver or bone marrow
A	No systemic symptoms
B	Weight loss, drenching sweats

The lymphatic structures are defined as the lymph nodes, spleen, thymus, Waldeyer's ring, appendix and Peyer's patches

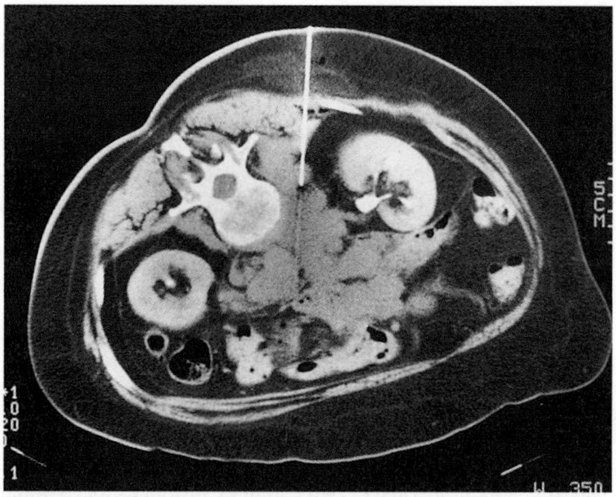

Fig. 11.20 CT-guided percutaneous needle biopsy of retroperitoneal nodes involved by lymphoma.

Management

Treatment options include radiotherapy, chemotherapy or a combination of the two (see the information box).

THERAPEUTIC GUIDELINES FOR HODGKIN'S LYMPHOMA

Indications for radiotherapy

- Stage I disease
- Stage IIA disease with three or fewer areas of involvement
- After chemotherapy to sites where there was originally bulk disease
- To lesions causing serious pressure problems

Indications for chemotherapy

- All patients with B symptoms
- Stage II disease with more than three areas of involvement
- Stage III and stage IV disease

Table 11.16 The ChlVPP regimen

Drug	Dose
Chlorambucil	6 mg/m^2 (up to 10 mg total) days 1–14 orally
Vinblastine	6 mg/m^2 (up to 10 mg total) days 1 and 8 i.v.
Procarbazine	100 mg/m^2 days 1–14 orally
Prednisolone	40 mg/m^2 days 1–14 orally

Radiotherapy

Good results are obtained in localised stage IA or stage IIA disease with no adverse prognostic features. Fertility is usually preserved after radiotherapy. Careful planning is required to limit doses delivered to normal tissues. Women receiving breast irradiation during the treatment of chest disease have an increased risk of breast cancer and should be placed on a screening programme. Patients continuing to smoke after lung irradiation are at risk of lung cancer.

Chemotherapy

All other patients are treated initially with chemotherapy. The regimen in Table 11.16 is widely used in the UK. This regimen was developed from the MOPP regimen (nitrogen mustard, vincristine, prednisolone and procarbazine) but drugs were substituted to reduce vomiting, alopecia and long-term toxicity. Over 80% of patients will respond to this combination therapy with drugs delivered on an outpatient basis every 3–4 weeks for a total of 6–8 cycles. Routine support with growth factors such as G-CSF is not required. Treatment response is assessed clinically and by repeat CT scanning. This type of chemotherapy carries a high risk of inducing permanent infertility in men; adequate counselling and sperm storage must be offered at diagnosis. The risk of infertility is lower for women but advice concerning the obtaining of ovarian tissue before the start of treatment should be discussed as appropriate. Premature menopause may result from the treatment and hormone replacement therapy should be discussed with the patient. Steroids can cause avascular necrosis of bone, particularly the femoral head. Myelodysplasia and acute leukaemia can occur 5–10 years after alkylating therapy but the incidence is less than 5%.

Combined modality therapy

Radiotherapy may be given to original sites of bulky disease after treatment by chemotherapy to reduce the risk of relapse. This form of treatment carries the greatest risk of long-term complications.

Prognosis

Over 90% of patients with stage IA disease are cured by radiotherapy alone. Patients with stage IIA disease have a reduced cure rate from radiotherapy. Approximately 70% of patients treated with chemotherapy are cured. The 15% of patients who fail to respond to initial chemotherapy have a poor prognosis but some may achieve long-term survival after high-dose therapy and autologous stem cell rescue.

Relapse

Patients relapsing after local radiotherapy have a good cure rate after subsequent chemotherapy but with an increased risk of long-term toxicity. Patients relapsing within a year of initial chemotherapy have a good salvage rate by high-dose therapy and autologous stem cell rescue. Patients relapsing after 1 year may obtain long-term survival by further chemotherapy.

NON-HODGKIN'S LYMPHOMA

Non-Hodgkin's lymphomas (NHLs) are monoclonal proliferations of lymphoid cells and may be of B cell (70%) or T cell (30%) origin. The incidence of these tumours has increased by 50% in the last 10–20 years in the Western world. At the same time treatment outcomes have not improved and mortality rates from NHL have increased.

The difficulties of establishing a reproducible and clinically useful histological classification of NHLs have been reflected in the large number of classification systems to date. A recently developed system, the REAL classification, has introduced phenotypic, molecular and cytogenetic information which, together with morphology, has allowed reproducible definition of clinical disease entities. Clinically, the most important factor is grade, which is a

EPIDEMIOLOGY AND AETIOLOGY OF NON-HODGKIN'S LYMPHOMA

Incidence

- 12 new cases/100 000 people/year

Sex ratio

- Slight male excess

Age

- Median age 65–70 years

Aetiology

No single causative abnormality described

- Viruses: Lymphoma is a late manifestation of human immunodeficiency virus (HIV) infection. Specific lymphoma types are associated with EBV, human herpes-virus 8 (HHV8) and human T lymphotrophic virus (HTLV) infection
- Bacteria: The development of gastric lymphoma can be associated with *Helicobacter pylori* infection
- Genetics: Some lymphomas are associated with specific chromosome lesions; the t(14:18) translocation in follicular lymphoma results in the dysregulated expression of the bcl-2 gene product which inhibits apoptotic cell death
- Immune: Lymphoma occurs in congenital immunodeficiency states and in immunosuppressed patients post-organ transplantation

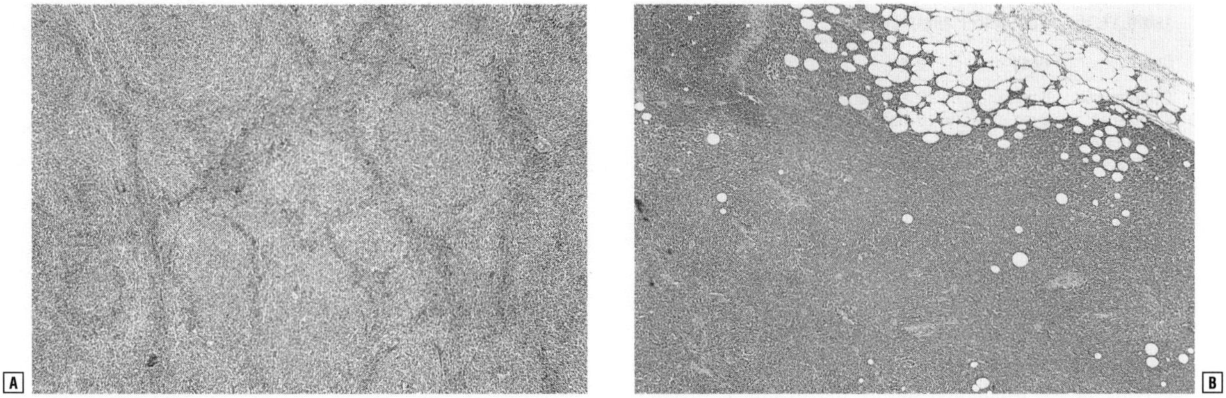

Fig. 11.21 Non-Hodgkin's lymphoma. A (Low-grade) follicular or nodular pattern. B (High-grade) diffuse pattern of histology.

reflection of proliferation rate. High-grade NHLs have high proliferation rates, rapidly produce symptoms, are fatal if untreated but are potentially curable. Low-grade NHLs have low proliferation rates, may be asymptomatic for many months before presentation, run an indolent course but are not curable by conventional therapy. Overall, about one-third of cases are high-grade diffuse large-cell NHL and a further third are low-grade follicular NHL (see Fig. 11.21).

Clinical features

NHLs are widely disseminated at presentation more commonly than Hodgkin's disease, presenting with lymph node enlargement which may be associated with systemic upset: weight loss, sweats, fever and itching. Hepatosplenomegaly may be present. Extranodal disease is more common in NHLs, with involvement of the bone marrow, gut, thyroid, lung, skin, testis, brain and, more rarely, bone. Extranodal disease is more common in T cell disease whilst bone marrow involvement is more common in low-grade (50–60%) rather than high-grade (10%) disease. The same staging system is used for both Hodgkin's disease and NHLs but NHLs are more likely to be stage III or IV at presentation. Compression syndromes may occur; gut obstruction, ascites, superior vena caval obstruction and spinal cord compression may all be presenting features.

Investigations

These are as for Hodgkin's disease but in addition the following should be performed:

- *Routine bone marrow aspirate and trephine.*
- *Immunophenotyping of surface antigens to distinguish T and B cell tumours.* This may be done on blood, marrow or nodal material.
- *Immunoglobulin determination.* Some lymphomas are associated with IgG or M paraproteins which serve as markers for treatment response.
- *Uric acid levels.* Some very aggressive high-grade NHLs are associated with very high urate levels, which can precipitate renal failure when treatment is started.
- *Human immunodeficiency virus (HIV) testing.* This may be appropriate if risk factors are present.

Management

The factors listed in the information box will influence the choice of therapy in NHLs.

FACTORS DETERMINING MANAGEMENT STRATEGY IN NON-HODGKIN'S LYMPHOMA

- Age of the patient
- Degree of ill health (concomitant disease)
- Histological grade
- Staging of the disease
- HIV status
- Patient's wishes

Low-grade NHL

Asymptomatic patients may not require therapy. Indications for treatment include: marked systemic symptoms, lymphadenopathy causing discomfort or disfigurement, bone marrow failure or compression syndromes. The options are:

- *Radiotherapy.* This can be used for localised stage I disease, which is rare.
- *Chemotherapy.* This is the mainstay of therapy. Most patients will respond to oral therapy with chlorambucil, which is well tolerated. More intensive intravenous chemotherapy in younger patients produces better quality of life but no survival benefit. Neither therapy will cure patients.
- *Transplantation.* Studies of autologous stem cell transplantation are in progress. Such high-dose therapy

improves disease-free survival but longer follow-up is awaited before conclusions can be made about cure.

High-grade NHL

These patients need treatment at initial presentation:

- *Chemotherapy.* The majority (> 90%) will need intravenous combination chemotherapy. The CHOP regimen (cyclophosphamide, adriamycin, vincristine and prednisolone) remains the mainstay of therapy.
- *Radiotherapy.* A very few stage I patients with no bulky disease may be suitable for radiotherapy. Radiotherapy is indicated to a residual localised site of bulk disease after chemotherapy, for spinal cord and other compression syndromes.
- *Transplantation.* Autologous stem cell transplantation appears to benefit some patients at relapse. Lymphoblastic lymphoma is a very aggressive lymphoma which predominantly affects young adults, who should be considered candidates for allogeneic or autologous transplantation after response to initial chemotherapy.

Prognosis

Low-grade NHL

These tumours run an indolent remitting and relapsing course with an overall median survival of 10 years.

Death occurs after transformation to a higher-grade NHL, which is associated with poor survival.

High-grade NHL

Some 80% of patients respond initially but only 35% will have disease-free survival at 5 years. Relapse is associated with a poor response to further chemotherapy (< 10% 5-year survival), but in patients under 65 stem cell transplantation improves survival.

Increasing age, advanced stage, concomitant disease, a raised LDH and T cell phenotype predict poor outcome.

MULTIPLE MYELOMA

This is a malignant proliferation of plasma cells.

Normal plasma cells are derived from B cells and produce immunoglobulins which contain heavy and light chains. Normal immunoglobulins are polyclonal, which means that a variety of heavy chains are produced and each may be of kappa or lambda light chain type. In myeloma plasma cells produce immunoglobulin of a single heavy and light chain, a monoclonal protein commonly referred to as a paraprotein. In some cases only light chain is produced and this appears in the urine as Bence Jones proteinuria. The frequency of different paraprotein types in myeloma is shown in Table 11.17.

EPIDEMIOLOGY AND AETIOLOGY OF MULTIPLE MYELOMA

Incidence

- 4 new cases/100 000 population/year

Sex ratio

- 2 males:1 female

Age

- Median age 60–70 years. More common in Afro-Caribbeans

Aetiology

- Unknown

Table 11.17 Classification of multiple myeloma

Type of paraprotein	Relative frequency (%)
IgG	55
IgA	21
Light chain only	22
Others (D, E, non-secretory)	2

Pathology

Although a small number of malignant plasma cells are present in the circulation, the majority are present in the bone marrow. The malignant plasma cells produce cytokines, which stimulate osteoclasts and result in net bone absorption (see Fig. 11.22). The resulting lytic lesions cause bone pain, fractures and hypercalcaemia. Marrow involvement can result in anaemia or pancytopenia (see Table 11.18).

Clinical features

These are listed in the first information box on page 784.

Investigations

The diagnosis of myeloma requires two of the following criteria:

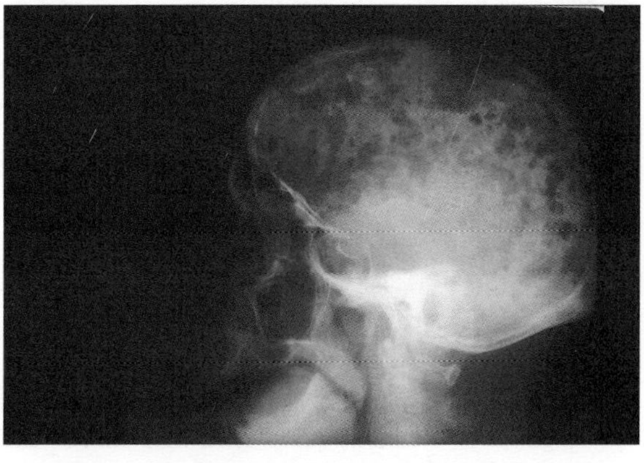

Fig. 11.22 Translucencies in skull radiograph—multiple myeloma.

Table 11.18 Multiple myeloma: the relationship between pathology, the effect of the disease process and symptoms

Pathology	Effect	Symptoms
Marrow involvement with malignant plasma cells	Bone erosion due to stimulation of osteoclasts Pathological fracture Hypercalcaemia Bone marrow failure: anaemia	Pain Severe local pain Lethargy, thirst Tiredness
Excess production of paraprotein and light chains	Renal damage Increased blood viscosity Amyloidosis—renal damage	None until uraemic None until severe, then blurred vision, headache, vertigo, stupor, coma Of nephrotic syndrome
Reduction in number of normal plasma cells	Impaired immune function	Susceptibility to infection, particularly respiratory

CLINICAL FEATURES OF MULTIPLE MYELOMA

- Weight loss, malaise and fatigue occur
- 60% present with bone pain, particularly back and rib pain
- Anorexia, vomiting, diarrhoea or constipation and polyuria occur with hypercalcaemia, which is present in 30%
- Hypercalcaemia and dehydration contribute to renal impairment, which is present in 50% at diagnosis
- Pneumococcal, chest and urinary tract infections are common due to failure of production of normal immunoglobulins
- Headache, confusion, breathlessness, visual disturbance and bleeding can occur secondary to hyperviscosity, which is particularly associated with IgA proteins
- Some 5% present with paralysis secondary to spinal cord compression by an extradural plasma cell mass
- Carpal tunnel syndrome, nephrotic syndrome, cardiac failure and neuropathy can occur secondary to amyloid deposition

POINTS TO NOTE IN THE DIAGNOSIS OF MYELOMA

- In the absence of fractures or bone repair the plasma alkaline phosphatase and the bone scan are normal
- Serum β_2-microglobulin estimations may provide a useful assessment of prognosis
- The absence of immune paresis (reduction of normal immunoglobulins below normal levels) should cast doubt on the diagnosis
- Only about 5% of patients with ESRs persistently above 100 mm in the first hour have myeloma

- marrow plasmacytosis
- serum and/or urinary paraprotein
- skeletal lesions.

Investigations are listed in Table 11.19.

Management

If patients are asymptomatic, treatment may not be required. Otherwise, treatment consists of the following:

- *Immediate support.*
  —High fluid intake to treat renal impairment and hypercalcaemia
  —Analgesia for bone pain
  —Biphosphonates for hypercalcaemia

Table 11.19 Rationale for investigations in multiple myeloma

Problem	Investigations
Renal function	Urea and electrolytes, creatinine, urate
Presence of hypercalcaemia	Blood calcium Albumin
Presence of bone fractures	Radiographs Blood alkaline phosphatase Isotope bone scan
Degree of immune paresis	Plasma immunoglobulin
Degree of bone marrow failure	Blood counts Reticulocyte count
Degree of haemostasis	Bleeding time Coagulation screen
Blood viscosity	Plasma viscosity
Disease activity	Serum β_2-microglobulin

  —Allopurinol to prevent urate nephropathy
  —Plasmapheresis, which may be necessary for hyperviscosity.
- *Chemotherapy.* In older patients, melphalan is an effective oral therapy, whilst in younger patients treatment with intravenous agents may improve response.

Treatment is administered until the measured paraprotein levels have stopped falling. This is termed 'plateau phase' and may last for weeks or years. Successive relapses respond less well to treatment.

- *Radiotherapy.* This is effective for localised bone pain not responding to simple analgesia and for pathological fractures. Chronic bisphosphonate therapy may reduce bone pain and skeletal events. Alpha interferon may prolong the plateau phase.
- *Transplantation.* Standard treatment does not cure myeloma. Stem cell autotransplants may improve quality of life and prolong survival. Allogeneic bone marrow transplantation may offer the prospect of cure for some patients.

Prognosis

The median survival of patients receiving standard treatment is approximately 40 months. Autotransplantation improves survival and quality of life by slowing the rate of progression of bone disease.

POOR PROGNOSTIC FEATURES AT DIAGNOSIS IN MULTIPLE MYELOMA
• A haemoglobin concentration of less than 70 g/l • Severe hypoalbuminaemia • Intractable renal failure • Thrombocytopenia • High β_2-microglobulin levels • Plasma cell leukaemia

OTHER CAUSES OF PARAPROTEINS

Although there are a number of causes of a paraprotein apart from myeloma, two require particular consideration: monoclonal gammopathy of uncertain significance and an IgM paraprotein occurring in the context of a non-Hodgkin's lymphoma (still commonly called Waldenström's macroglobulinaemia).

MONOCLONAL GAMMOPATHY OF UNCERTAIN SIGNIFICANCE (MGUS)

A paraprotein is present in the blood but with no other features of myeloma.

EPIDEMIOLOGY AND AETIOLOGY OF MONOCLONAL GAMMOPATHY OF UNCERTAIN SIGNIFICANCE (MGUS)
Incidence
• 3% of the over-70s and up to 8% of the population in hospital inpatients
Sex ratio
• Equal
Age
• Elderly
Aetiology
• Unknown

Clinical features

Patients are usually asymptomatic.

Investigations

- Routine blood count and biochemistry are normal.
- The paraprotein is usually present in a small amount with no associated immune paresis.
- There are no lytic lesions on the bones.
- The bone marrow may have increased plasma cells but these are usually less than 10%.

Management

There is a need to follow up to monitor clinical symptoms and paraprotein levels, and if these change, further investigation is warranted. It should be remembered that paraproteins may be associated with connective tissue disease, lymphomas, amyloidosis, chronic lymphatic leukaemia and solid tumours.

Prognosis

With long-term follow-up, approximately 30% of patients develop other problems; 20% develop myeloma and the remainder solid tumours.

WALDENSTRÖM'S MACROGLOBULINAEMIA

This is a low-grade lymphoplasmacytoid lymphoma associated with an IgM paraprotein causing clinical features of hyperviscosity syndrome.

It is a rare tumour occurring in the elderly and in a slight excess of males.

Patients classically present with features of hyperviscosity such as nosebleeds, bruising, confusion and visual disturbance. However, presentation may be with anaemia, systemic symptoms, splenomegaly or lymphadenopathy.

Patients are found on investigation to have an IgM paraprotein associated with a raised plasma viscosity. The bone marrow has a characteristic appearance, with infiltration with lymphoid cells and in addition many mast cells.

Management

Severe hyperviscosity and anaemia may necessitate plasmapheresis to remove IgM and make blood transfusion possible. Treatment with oral agents such as chlorambucil is effective but rather slow.

Prognosis

Median survival is 5 years.

FURTHER INFORMATION ON THE LYMPHOMAS AND MYELOMA

Singer C R J 1997 Myeloma and related conditions. British Medical Journal 314: 960–963

MYELOPROLIFERATIVE DISORDERS

These make up a group of chronic interrelated conditions characterised by clonal proliferation of marrow erythroid precursors (primary proliferative polycythaemia, PPP), megakaryocytes (essential thrombocythaemia and myelofibrosis) or myeloid cells (chronic myeloid leukaemia). Although the majority of patients are classifiable as having one of these disorders, occasionally some have features of two of these conditions. Furthermore, there is often progression from one to another; particularly common is the transformation from PPP to myelofibrosis.

Chronic myeloid leukaemia, although usually classified as a myeloproliferative condition, has many characteristics of a leukaemic condition and is considered in detail elsewhere (see p. 775).

MYELOFIBROSIS

In myelofibrosis the bone marrow is initially hypercellular, particularly with an excess of abnormal megakaryocytes. These poorly functioning cells fail to package growth factors, e.g. platelet-derived growth factor, within the developing platelet granules, and instead these factors diffuse into the intercellular milieu, resulting in stimulation and proliferation of fibroblasts. As the disease progresses, the marrow becomes heavily infiltrated with fibroblasts.

Clinical features

Most patients with myelofibrosis present over the age of 50 years with lassitude, weight loss, night sweats and some intolerance of heat. The spleen may be greatly enlarged and splenic infarcts may occur.

Investigations

Anaemia, sometimes macrocytic, is common. The leucocyte count varies, with an increase in granulocytes and usually a leucoerythroblastic blood picture. The erythrocytes show very characteristic teardrop poikilocytes. The platelet count may be very high, normal or low and giant forms are seen in the blood film. The neutrophil alkaline phosphatase score is frequently raised, as is the urate level. The marrow is often difficult to aspirate and a trephine biopsy shows an excess of megakaryocytes and increased reticulin and fibrous tissue replacement. Folate deficiency is very common.

Management

Treatment is largely supportive with blood transfusion. Folic acid (5 mg daily) should be given. Cytotoxic therapy with drugs such as hydroxyurea up to 2 g daily can be used cautiously to try to reduce the spleen size or a very high white cell count. Splenectomy may be required if the grossly enlarged spleen is causing distress or because transfusion requirements are excessive. Prognosis is variable and survival may exceed 10 years. The disease is progressive with steady deterioration. Bone marrow transplantation should be considered for young patients.

ESSENTIAL THROMBOCYTHAEMIA

The malignant proliferation of megakaryocytes results in a raised level of circulating platelets which may, in addition, have aberrant function. Prior to making a diagnosis of essential thrombocythaemia it is important to consider whether the raised platelet count is a feature of one of the other myeloproliferative disorders or is reactive to an inflammatory condition (see p. 754).

Clinical features

Often patients are asymptomatic and the diagnosis is made following a routine full blood count. Some present with excessive bruising and bleeding, venous or arterial thrombosis, occlusion of the small vessels in digits (see Fig. 11.12, p. 754) or transient ischaemic attacks. Splenomegaly may be present. In some patients, however, the blood film reveals changes due to splenic atrophy—for example, Howell–Jolly bodies—as a result of asymptomatic splenic infarction. In most individuals the condition is chronic, with the platelet count only gradually increasing.

Management

If the patient is less than 40 years old, has a platelet count less than 1000×10^9/l and is clinically asymptomatic, i.e. there is absence of bleeding and thrombosis, no active treatment to reduce the platelet count may be indicated. The patient should be kept under regular review with serial platelet counts; daily aspirin therapy is often recommended. For those with a platelet count over 1000×10^9/l or those with symptoms, treatment is with oral hydroxyurea or intravenous radioactive phosphorus (^{32}P). Aspirin is particularly useful therapy for those with digital ischaemia. On rare occasions the platelet count rises rapidly, sometimes accompanied by blast cells in the peripheral blood, and this condition of megakaryocytic leukaemia should be treated like acute myeloid leukaemia.

PRIMARY PROLIFERATIVE POLYCYTHAEMIA (PPP)

Clinical features

PPP occurs mainly in patients over the age of 40 years and is more common in males than females. There may be no symptoms and the disorder is diagnosed incidentally. Common complaints are lassitude, loss of concentration, headaches, dizziness, blackouts, pruritus, epistaxis and 'indigestion'. Some patients present with manifestations of arterial peripheral vascular disease or a cerebrovascular accident. The patients often have a high colour with suffused conjunctivae; retinal vein engorgement may be found. The spleen is palpable in 75% of patients at diagnosis. Thrombotic complications may occur and peptic ulceration is common, sometimes complicated by bleeding.

Investigations

Diagnosis is made by finding true polycythaemia by red cell mass/plasma volume determination and clinical features of splenomegaly, raised serum urate (due to increased marrow cell turnover) and the absence of secondary causes, e.g. lung or renal disease (see Table 11.6 on p. 752 and the information box below). As well as the haemoglobin being raised, in many cases of PPP the neutrophil and platelet counts are also raised, whereas in secondary polycythaemia these latter parameters are usually normal. In difficult diagnostic cases, in vitro culture of the marrow may be helpful; in PPP it grows autonomously in the absence of added growth factors.

DIAGNOSIS OF PRIMARY PROLIFERATIVE POLYCYTHAEMIA: POSITIVE FEATURES

- Elevated red cell mass
- Splenomegaly
- An associated elevation of white cell and platelet counts
- Hypercellular marrow with hyperplasia of erythropoiesis/granulopoiesis and megakaryocytes
- Absent iron stores
- Elevated neutrophil alkaline phosphatase score
- Elevated serum B_{12} levels
- Absence of secondary causes of erythrocytosis

Management

Venesection is the simplest therapeutic measure and the best to use if the diagnosis is in doubt; 500 ml of blood (less if the patient is elderly) is removed and the venesection repeated within a day or two if necessary until the haematocrit reading is reduced to <45% or an Hb of 120 g/l. Clinical improvement occurs rapidly with the reduction of blood viscosity. The haemoglobin will eventually remain reduced because of iron deficiency. If the platelet count rises this can be controlled by hydroxyurea. Radioactive phosphorus (5 mCi of ^{32}P i.v.) is an effective form of treatment for older patients when the diagnosis is certain. The full effect on the haemoglobin will not appear for 3 months but the white cell count and platelet count respond more quickly. Further doses may be required but often there is good disease control for periods of up to 18 months. The major problem with radioactive phosphorus is that it is leukaemogenic but actual acute leukaemia only develops in a small minority after 10 years.

Prognosis

The median lifespan after diagnosis in treated patients exceeds 10 years. Some patients survive more than 20 years. The disease may convert to another myeloproliferative disorder—for example, essential thrombocythaemia, and about 15% develop myelofibrosis. Acute leukaemia develops principally in those patients who have been treated with radioactive phosphorus. Despite more efficient treatment, deaths still occur because of thrombotic events.

FURTHER INFORMATION ON MYELOPROLIFERATIVE DISORDERS

Messinezy M, Pearson T C 1997 Polycythaemia, primary (essential) thrombocythaemia and myelofibrosis. British Medical Journal 314: 587–590

BLEEDING DISORDERS

DISORDERS OF PRIMARY HAEMOSTASIS

Platelet functional disorders, thrombocytopenia and von Willebrand disease, along with diseases affecting the vessel wall, may all result in failure of the initial platelet plug formation in primary haemostasis.

VESSEL WALL ABNORMALITIES

Abnormalities of the vessel walls, both congenital and acquired—for example, vasculitis, may result in a propensity to purpuric lesions which are often slightly raised. Causes of non-thrombocytopenic purpura are listed in the information box.

CAUSES OF NON-THROMBOCYTOPENIC PURPURA

- Senile purpura
- Factitious purpura
- Henoch–Schönlein purpura
- Vasculitis
- Paraproteinaemias
- Purpura fulminans
- Embolic purpura

HEREDITARY HAEMORRHAGIC TELANGIECTASIA

Hereditary haemorrhagic telangiectasia is a dominantly inherited condition in which telangiectasia and small aneurysms are found on the fingertips, face, nasal passages, tongue and gastrointestinal tract. A small group of these patients also develop pulmonary arteriovenous malformation. Patients present either with recurrent bleeds, particularly epistaxis, or iron deficiency due to occult gastrointestinal bleeding. Treatment can be difficult because of the multiple bleeding points but regular iron therapy often allows the marrow to compensate for blood loss. Local cautery or laser therapy may prevent single lesions from bleeding. A variety of medical therapies have been tried—for example, oestrogens—but none has been found to be effective.

EHLERS–DANLOS DISEASE

Ehlers–Danlos disease is a congenital disorder of collagen synthesis in which the capillaries are poorly supported by subcutaneous collagen and ecchymoses are commonly observed.

PLATELET FUNCTIONAL DISORDERS

Even in the presence of a normal platelet count an individual may bleed if the function of the platelets is reduced. Congenital abnormalities include rare disorders of the membrane glycoproteins—for example, thrombasthenia and Bernard–Soulier syndrome, or the presence of defective platelet granules—for example, a deficiency of dense granules giving rise to storage pool disorders. Such patients exhibit bleeding of platelet type which varies in severity between patients, some presenting with frequent recurrent bleeds whilst others are only diagnosed because of excessive post-operative haemorrhage. Mild functional disorders, which only cause excessive bleeding after trauma or surgery, are often not diagnosed and are probably relatively common.

Many drugs inhibit platelets. Aspirin and other non-steroidal drugs inhibit platelet cyclo-oxygenase, preventing the conversion of arachidonic acid to the potent platelet aggregator thromboxane B_2. Other drugs which inhibit platelet function are listed in the information box.

DRUGS INHIBITING PLATELET FUNCTION

Non-steroidal anti-inflammatory drugs
- Aspirin
- Indomethacin
- Phenylbutazone
- Sulphinpyrazone

Antibiotics
- Penicillins
- Cephalosporins

Dextran

Heparin

β-blockers

THROMBOCYTOPENIA

Thrombocytopenia causing clinically significant bleeding constitutes a haematological emergency which should be promptly investigated and appropriately treated. Treatment should be directed at the underlying condition as well as including specific treatment to raise the platelet count when appropriate. In general, platelet transfusions should be given only if the platelet count is less than 10×10^9/l, or to treat troublesome bleeding such as persistent epistaxis, or to treat potentially life-threatening bleeding—for example, gastrointestinal haemorrhage. Such transfusions provide only temporary relief because the survival of the platelets in the circulation is only a few days at most, and in many instances may be only a matter of minutes or hours if the thrombocytopenia is due to increased platelet consumption, as in idiopathic thrombocytopenic purpura or disseminated intravascular coagulation.

IDIOPATHIC THROMBOCYTOPENIC PURPURA (ITP)

The presence of autoantibodies, often directed against platelet membrane glycoprotein IIb-IIIa, causes the premature removal of platelets by the monocyte-macrophage system. Occasionally, antigen-antibody immune complexes adhere to platelets at their Fc receptor, resulting in their premature removal from the circulation.

Clinical features

In children, ITP often presents 2–3 weeks after a viral illness, with the sudden onset of purpura and sometimes oral and nasal bleeding. The peripheral blood film is normal, apart from a greatly reduced platelet number, whilst the bone marrow reveals an obvious increase in megakaryocytes. It is important to ascertain that the child does not have any other systemic illness and in particular disseminated intravascular coagulation.

In adults, ITP more commonly affects females and has an insidious onset. It is unusual for there to be a history of a preceding viral infection. At presentation some cases may be associated with symptoms or signs of a collagenosis or rheumatoid arthritis, whilst in others these disorders may become apparent several years later. The condition is likely to become chronic, with remissions and relapses.

Management

Children

If the child has only mild bleeding symptoms it is usual to withhold any specific treatment, as the condition in the majority of instances is self-limiting within a few weeks. The presence of moderate to severe purpura, bruising or epistaxis and a platelet count less than 10×10^9/l is an indication for prednisolone 2 mg/kg daily. The platelet count usually rises promptly within 1–3 days. Persistent epistaxis, gastrointestinal bleeding, retinal haemorrhages or any suggestion of intracranial bleeding should be treated immediately by a platelet transfusion. If fresh bleeding persists for more than a few days following the introduction of steroids, intravenous immunoglobulin should be given.

Adults

Treatment with prednisolone 1 mg/kg daily is less rewarding than in children; often the platelet count rises in response to therapy but falls again when the dose is reduced or stopped. As with children, persistent or potentially life-threatening bleeding should be treated with platelet transfusion. Intravenous immunoglobulin (IVIgG) (1 g/kg) should be given if the patient is very haemorrhagic or the bleeding is immediately life-threatening. The mechanism by which IVIgG raises the platelet count remains uncertain, although increasing evidence indicates that it may be due to blocking of monocyte-macrophage Fc receptors.

Relapses should be treated by increasing the dose of prednisolone. If a patient has two relapses it is customary to consider splenectomy. This should be preceded by pneumococcal, meningococcal and *Haemophilus influenzae* vaccination. As so many adults with ITP eventually require splenectomy it is prudent to vaccinate all patients at presentation (subcutaneously—if vaccination is given by the customary intramuscular route it may result in a haematoma) before they become immunosuppressed with a prolonged course of steroids. Splenectomy is curative in about 70% of patients and in the remainder the aim should be to keep the patient free of symptoms rather than treat the platelet count alone. Often such patients have counts of 20–30 × 10^9/l without symptoms; some require long-term maintenance with prednisolone at 5 mg/day. If significant bleeding persists despite splenectomy and a small dose of steroids, vincristine, immunosuppressive therapy—for example, cyclophosphamide, or repeated infusions of intravenous immunoglobulin should be considered.

COAGULATION DISORDERS

Coagulation factor disorders can either arise from a single factor, usually congenital, deficiency—for example, factor VIII, resulting in haemophilia A—or from multiple factor deficiencies which are often acquired—for example, secondary to liver disease or warfarin therapy. Of the single congenital deficiencies haemophilia A and B are the most common although, rarely, any of the coagulation factors may be reduced. The congenital disorders almost exclusively arise as a result of an abnormality in gene coding for the coagulation factor.

CONGENITAL BLEEDING DISORDERS

HAEMOPHILIA A

Of the various congenital disorders of coagulation a reduction of factor VIII resulting in haemophilia A, which affects 1/10 000 individuals, is the most common. Factor VIII is primarily synthesised by the liver but other organs such as the spleen, kidney and placenta may also contribute. Plasma factor VIII has a half-life of about 12 hours and is carried non-covalently bound to the von Willebrand factor (vWF). The very large 286 kilobase factor VIII gene is located on the X chromosome and consists of 26 exons. Many different defects in the gene have been identified—for example, single base changes resulting in amino acid substitutions or nonsense codons (causing premature chain termination), deletions or inversions. The normal factor VIII gene has been cloned and recombinant factor VIII is available to treat patients.

Genetics

The factor VIII gene is localised on the X chromosome, making haemophilia A a sex-linked disorder. Thus on pedigree grounds all daughters of haemophiliacs are obligate carriers and sisters have a 50% chance of being a carrier. If a carrier has a son, he has a 50% chance of having haemophilia, and a daughter has a 50% chance of being a carrier. Haemophilia 'breeds true' within a family. All members will have the same abnormality of the factor VIII gene; thus if one individual has severe haemophilia, all others affected will also have a severe form of the disorder. Female carriers of haemophilia tend to have reduced factor VIII levels because of random inactivation of the X chromosome in the developing fetus (lyonisation). An indication of carriership can be ascertained by measurement of the factor VIII/vWF ratio, which is reduced in carriers compared with normal individuals.

The use of molecular genetic techniques has revolutionised the identification of carriers and the antenatal diagnosis of haemophilia. If the mutation giving rise to the haemophilia is known, this can be sought in the potential carrier or used for antenatal diagnosis. Tracing of the haemophilia gene within families can also be accomplished using gene probes which detect restriction fragment length polymorphisms (RFLPs). The most useful probes are those that detect an endonuclease restriction site within the gene and these are known as 'genomic' probes. Other probes detect endonuclease sites close to the gene and these 'linked' probes are less reliable because recombination between the factor VIII gene and the endonuclease site may occur during meiosis. Antenatal diagnosis can be undertaken in a female who has a high probability of being a carrier. This is accomplished by chorion villus sampling (CVS), usually after 11 weeks' gestation, sexing the fetus and using informative factor VIII probes. Alternatively, the fetus can be sexed at 16 weeks' gestation by amniocentesis and, if male, a fetal blood sample obtained at about 19–20 weeks. The CVS technique is preferable because it allows for the possibility of therapeutic termination at about 12 weeks compared with 20 weeks following fetal blood sampling.

Clinical features

Although haemophilia A is a congenital disorder it is unusual for excessive bleeding to be noticed until babies are about 6 months old, when superficial bruising or a haemarthrosis may occur. This apparent delay in presentation is due to the relative inactivity of babies in the first few months of life and it is only when they begin to move about that more trauma results in bleeding. It is not uncommon for children to be initially classified as having non-accidental injury unless all such children are appropriately investigated for the presence of a bleeding disorder (see Table 11.5, p. 748).

The normal factor VIII level is 50–150% and is usually measured by a clotting assay. In haemophilia the propensity to bleeding is related to the plasma factor VIII level. The severity of haemophilia is set out in Table 11.20.

Individuals with severe haemophilia (factor VIII < 2%) experience recurrent haemarthroses in large joints (see Fig. 11.23). These usually begin spontaneously without apparent trauma and the joints most commonly affected are knees, elbows, ankles and hips. A typical severe haemophiliac may have one or two bleeds each week. The patient is aware that bleeding has started because he experiences an abnormal sensation in the joint. If treatment is not given at this stage bleeding continues, resulting in a hot, swollen and very painful joint. Without treatment severe pain and swelling may last for many days before gradually subsiding. Recurrent bleeds into joints lead to synovial hypertrophy, destruction of the cartilage and secondary osteoarthrosis (see Fig. 11.24). The resultant limitation of movement may greatly reduce the function of joints, making walking difficult.

Table 11.20 Severity of haemophilia

Degree of severity	Factor VIII or IX level	Clinical presentation
Severe	< 2%	Spontaneous haemarthroses and muscle haematomas
Moderate	2–10%	Mild trauma or surgery cause haematomas
Mild	10–50%	Major injury or surgery results in excess bleeding

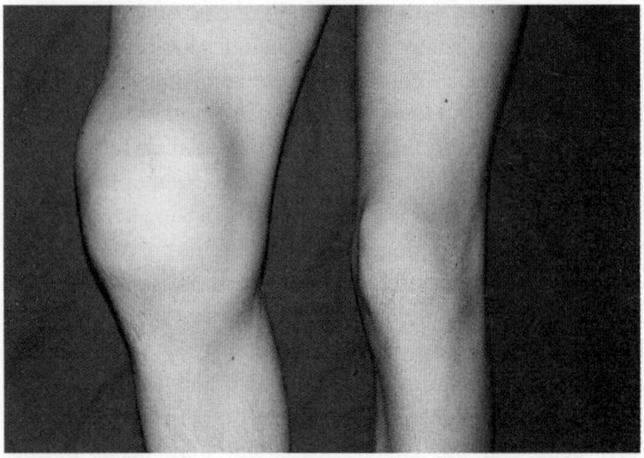

Fig. 11.23 Large haemarthrosis in the right knee of a boy with haemophilia A.

Muscle haematomas are also characteristic of haemophilia. These occur most commonly in the calf and psoas muscles but they can arise in almost any muscle. Although less common than haemarthroses, a single episode can leave severe lasting damage if not effectively treated. A large psoas bleed, for example, may extend to press on the femoral nerve with consequent paraesthesia in the thigh and weakness of the quadriceps; although some of this injury may be reversible, the patient is often left with some weakness in the leg. Furthermore, if the bleed does not resolve completely, recurrences at the same site may occur, leading to progressive muscle and nerve damage. Calf haematomas are also serious because of the inflexible fascial sheath surrounding the soleus and gastrocnemius muscles. Untreated haemorrhage causes a rise in pressure with eventual ischaemia, necrosis, fibrosis and subsequent contraction and shortening of the Achilles tendon (see Fig. 11.25).

Although joint and muscle bleeds are the most common sites for haemorrhage, bleeding can occur at almost any site. It is particularly serious if it takes place in a confined anatomical space associated with vital structures. The intracranial area is one such site and unless it is treated very promptly, haemorrhage here is often fatal (see Fig. 11.26).

Individuals with moderate haemophilia usually only experience haemorrhage after minor trauma and those with the mild form of the disorder, following more major trauma or surgery. Whereas severe haemophilia is usually diagnosed within the first 2 years of life, individuals with moderate and mild forms may escape diagnosis until adulthood.

Management

Bleeding episodes should be treated early by raising the factor VIII level. This is most commonly accomplished by intravenous infusion of factor VIII concentrate. Such concentrates are freeze-dried and stable at 4°C and can therefore be stored in domestic refrigerators. This facility, which allows many patients to treat themselves at home, revolutionised haemophilia care in the 1970s; prior to this,

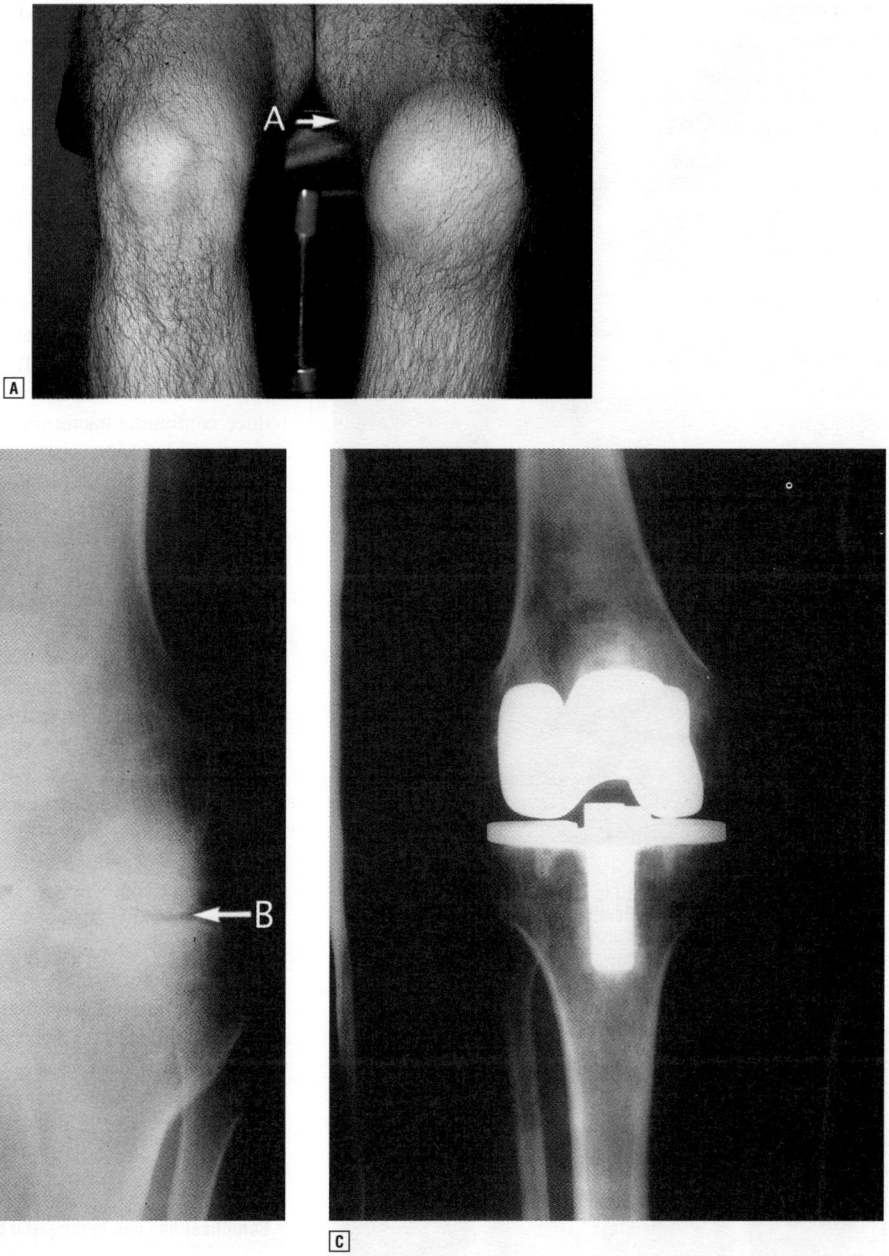

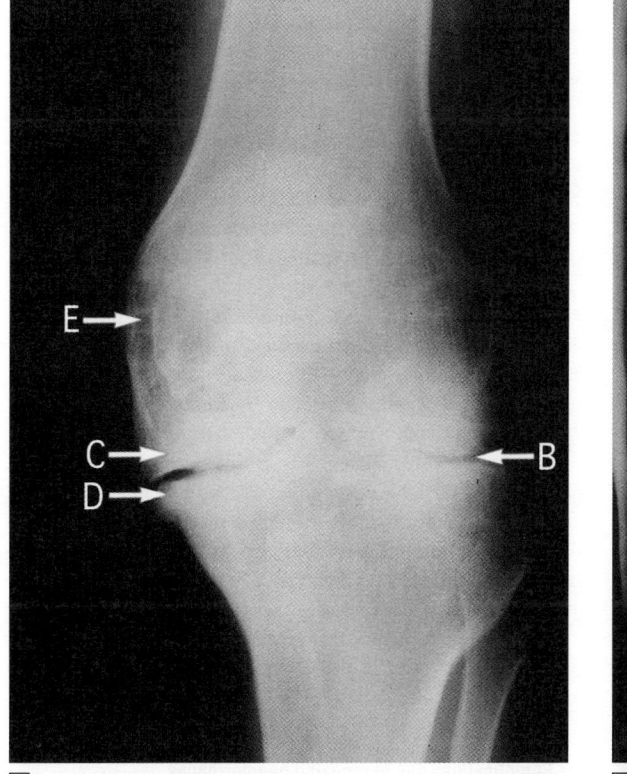

Fig. 11.24 Chronic haemophilic arthropathy of the left knee. [A] Repeated bleeds have led to broadening of the femoral epicondyles. Unilateral atrophy of the quadriceps (A) is easily seen. [B] Radiograph confirms broadening of femoral epicondyles. There is no cartilage present, as evidenced by the close proximity of the femur and tibia (B); sclerosis (C), osteophyte (D) and bony cysts (E) are present. [C] A haemophiliac's stiff joint with minimal flexion has been replaced by a prosthesis. This enabled the joint to have a greatly extended range of motion which very markedly improved the patient's mobility.

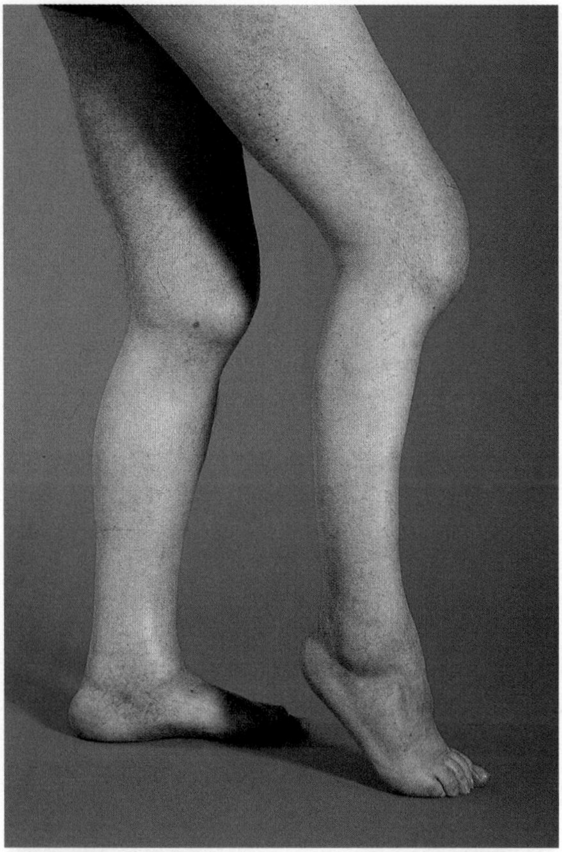

Fig. 11.25 Atrophy of the calf in an adult following an inadequately treated gastrocnemius haematoma as a child. The increased pressure of the haematoma caused ischaemia of the muscle, this being followed by necrosis, fibrosis and subsequent contraction to give the equinus deformity.

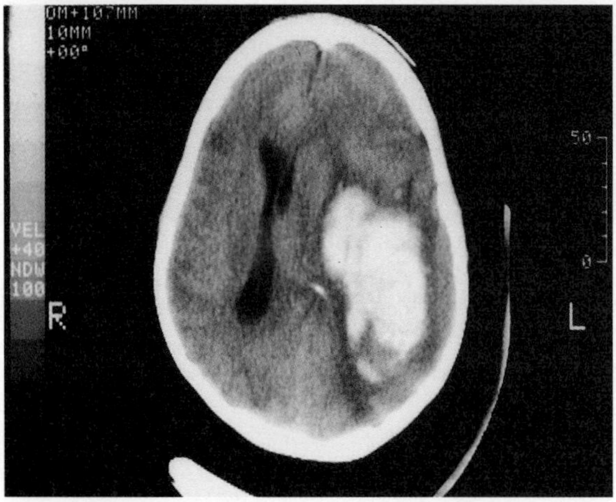

Fig. 11.26 CT scan revealing a major intracerebral haematoma. This apparently arose spontaneously in a severe haemophiliac.

patients had to travel to hospital to receive treatment for each bleed with fresh frozen plasma or cryoprecipitate. All plasma-derived factor VIII concentrates are now prepared from donors who are perceived as having a low risk of viral carriage—for example, of HIV. The plasma is screened for the presence of antibodies to hepatitis B and C viruses and HIV and the final product is treated either by heat or chemicals in an attempt to inactivate any residual viruses. Concentrates prepared with these precautions have a good safety record. However, factor VIII prepared by recombinant DNA technology is now available and this is likely to replace the use of plasma-derived concentrates.

In addition to factor VIII concentrate therapy, resting either in bed or with a splint of the bleeding site helps reduce continuing haemorrhage. Once bleeding has settled, the patient should be mobilised and given physiotherapy to restore strength to the surrounding muscles.

Complications of therapy

Although factor VIII concentrates have transformed the lives of haemophiliacs by allowing many to lead near-normal lives, this freedom has been bought at the cost of side-effects from repeated injections of concentrate (see the information box). Many patients treated before 1985, when concentrates were first treated with heat or chemicals to destroy viruses, became infected by the hepatitis and human immunodeficiency viruses. As a result most severe haemophiliacs have been exposed to hepatitis B virus and have developed immunity, as evidenced by the development of anti-HBs. A small number become chronic HBsAg carriers and may infect sexual partners, who should therefore be offered hepatitis B immunisation. They are also at risk of delta virus infection. All potential recipients of pooled blood products should be offered hepatitis A and B immunisation because it will protect against hepatitis A, B and D infection. Hepatitis C virus was ubiquitously transmitted by concentrates prior to 1985, resulting in virtually all recipients becoming infected. It is clear that

LONG-TERM SEQUELAE OF HAEMOPHILIA

Complications due to repeated haemorrhages

- Arthropathy of large joints, e.g. knees, elbows
- Atrophy of muscles secondary to haematomas
- Mononeuropathy resulting from pressure by haematomas

Complications due to therapy

- Anti-factor VIII antibody development
- Virus transmission
  - Hepatitis A virus—acute self-limiting illness
  - Hepatitis B virus—5–10% become chronic HBsAg carriers
  - Hepatitis C virus—chronic progressive liver disease
  - Hepatitis D virus—only arises in those with HBsAg
  - Human immunodeficiency virus—AIDS
  - Parvovirus—acute systemic self-limiting illness

many of these patients have hepatitis, and a significant proportion are progressing to cirrhosis and hepatocellular carcinoma. Interferon therapy benefits a proportion of patients. Patients with clinically severe liver disease or liver cancer should be considered for transplantation.

Prior to 1985, HIV was transmitted to haemophiliacs by concentrates, resulting in approximately 60% of severe haemophiliacs becoming infected. The clinical consequences are very similar to those for other individuals who have become infected with HIV (see p. 105), although their clinical course is perhaps more like that of those who become infected intravenously—for example, drug abusers—than those who become infected sexually. Kaposi's sarcoma, for example, is rare in haemophiliacs compared with homosexuals.

The other serious consequence of factor VIII infusion is the development of anti-factor VIII antibodies, which arises in about 10–30% of severe haemophiliacs. Such antibodies rapidly neutralise therapeutic infusions, making treatment relatively ineffective. Individuals may be treated with porcine factor VIII because the antibody may have lower activity against the animal factor VIII than against human. Alternatively, infusions of activated clotting factors, e.g. VIIa or Feiba (factor eight inhibitor bypassing activity—an activated concentrate of factors II, IX and X) may stop bleeding.

In individuals with a basal factor VIII level of 10% or greater it may be possible to raise the level approximately three- to five-fold with intravenous desmopressin (0.3 μg/kg). This is often sufficient to treat a mild bleed or cover minor surgery such as dental extraction. Injections can be repeated 6–8-hourly, although the response to second and subsequent infusions is not as good due to the development of tachyphylaxis. Desmopressin is an important form of therapy because it may avoid patients being exposed to blood products.

Surgery in haemophiliacs can be safely performed provided the patient does not have an inhibitor to factor VIII and receives appropriate doses of concentrate. A single infusion of factor VIII is usually adequate for simple dental extractions in an individual with severe haemophilia, along with a 10-day course of tranexamic acid (a fibrinolytic inhibitor) and antibiotic. Major surgery—for example, orthopaedic surgery—requires twice-daily therapy for 14 days or longer.

HAEMOPHILIA B (CHRISTMAS DISEASE)

Aberrations of the factor IX gene, which is also present on the X chromosome, result in a reduction of the plasma factor IX level, giving rise to haemophilia B. This disorder is clinically indistinguishable from haemophilia A and is less common. The frequency of bleeding episodes is related to the severity of the deficiency of the plasma factor IX level. Treatment is with a factor IX concentrate; it is used in much the same way as factor VIII for haemophilia A. Carrier identification and antenatal diagnosis can be accomplished if the specific mutation is known or with gene probes, although different ones from those used for the factor VIII gene.

VON WILLEBRAND DISEASE

Genetics

The gene for von Willebrand factor (vWF) is located on chromosome 12 and therefore the disorder is inherited in an autosomal fashion. In most families it has the appearance of being inherited in a dominant manner; rarely it appears in a clinically severe form with almost undetectable levels of vWF. In these circumstances the patient usually inherits a different abnormal vWF gene from each parent and is thus a compound heterozygote. Probes are available to trace the gene in a family, although in most instances antenatal diagnosis is not indicated because of the relatively mild nature of the disorder.

The vWF is a protein, synthesised by endothelial cells and megakaryocytes, that performs two principal functions. It acts as carrier protein for factor VIII, to which it is non-covalently bound. A deficiency of vWF therefore results in a secondary reduction in the plasma factor VIII level. Its other function is to form bridges between platelets and subendothelial components—for example, collagen, allowing platelets to adhere to damaged vessel walls (see Fig. 11.6, p. 744). A deficiency of vWF therefore also leads to prolonged primary haemorrhage after trauma.

Clinical features

As vWF participates, along with platelets, in primary haemostasis, patients present with haemorrhagic manifestations which are similar to individuals with reduced platelet function. Superficial bruising, epistaxis, menorrhagia and gastrointestinal haemorrhage are common. Bleeding episodes are usually much less common than in severe haemophilia and excessive haemorrhage may only be observed after trauma or surgery. Within a single family the disease is of very variable expression so that some members may have quite severe and frequent bleeds, whereas others are relatively little troubled.

Investigations

The disorder is characterised by finding a reduced level of vWF, which is often accompanied by a secondary reduction in factor VIII and a prolongation of the bleeding time.

Management

Many episodes of mild haemorrhage can be successfully

treated with desmopressin, which raises the vWF level, resulting in a secondary increase in factor VIII. For more serious or persistent bleeds haemostasis can be achieved with some factor VIII concentrates which contain considerable quantities of vWF in addition to factor VIII.

ACQUIRED BLEEDING DISORDERS

DISSEMINATED INTRAVASCULAR COAGULATION (DIC)

Clinical features

Disseminated intravascular coagulation can be initiated by a variety of different mechanisms in a number of diverse but distinct clinical situations, as set out in the information box. Endothelial damage, due to many causes—for example, endotoxin produced during Gram-negative septicaemia—may activate endothelial cells to produce tissue factor, which leads to activation of the coagulation cascade through the extrinsic pathway. The presence of thromboplastin from damaged tissues, placenta, fat embolus or following brain injury may also activate coagulation. Intravascular coagulation takes place with consumption of platelets, factors V and VIII and fibrinogen. This results in a potential haemorrhagic state, due to the depletion of haemostatic components, which may be exacerbated by activation of the fibrinolytic system secondary to the deposition of fibrin.

CAUSES OF DISSEMINATED INTRAVASCULAR COAGULATION

Infections
- *Escherichia coli*
- *Neisseria meningitidis*
- *Streptococcus pneumoniae*
- Malaria

Cancers
- Lung
- Pancreas
- Prostate

Obstetric
- Abruptio placentae
- Retained dead fetus
- Pre-eclampsia
- Amniotic fluid embolism

Investigations

DIC should be suspected when any of the conditions in the information box above are encountered. Definitive diagnosis depends on the finding of thrombocytopenia, prolongation of the prothrombin time (due to factor V and fibrinogen deficiency) and activated partial thromboplastin time (due to factors V, VIII and fibrinogen deficiency), a low fibrinogen concentration and increased levels of D-dimer (which is cleaved from fibrin by plasmin, establishing evidence of fibrin lysis).

Management

Therapy should be aimed at treating the underlying condition causing the DIC—for example, intravenous antibiotics for suspected septicaemia. Exacerbating factors such as acidosis, dehydration, renal failure and hypoxia should be corrected. If the patient is bleeding, blood products to correct identified abnormalities such as platelets and/or cryoprecipitate (which is enriched in factor VIII and fibrinogen) should be given. It may also be reasonable to treat severe coagulation abnormalities in the absence of frank bleeding to prevent sudden catastrophic haemorrhage—for example, intracranial bleed or massive gastrointestinal haemorrhage.

LIVER DISEASE

In severe parenchymal liver disease bleeding may arise from many different causes. Local anatomical abnormalities are often the site of major bleeding—for example, oesophageal varices or peptic ulcer, and this may be difficult to arrest because of deficiencies in components of the haemostatic system. These may arise because of reduced hepatic synthesis—for example, factors II, VII, IX, X and fibrinogen, DIC, reduced clearance of plasminogen activator, or thrombocytopenia secondary to hypersplenism. Treatment should be reserved for acute bleeds or to cover interventional procedures—for example, liver biopsy.

Cholestatic jaundice reduces vitamin K absorption and leads to a deficiency of function of factors II, VII, IX and X due to reduced gamma carboxylation. This deficiency can be readily and effectively treated with vitamin K_1 1 mg daily parenterally for several days.

RENAL FAILURE

The severity of the haemorrhagic state in renal failure is proportional to the plasma urea concentration. Bleeding manifestations are of platelet type, with gastrointestinal haemorrhage being particularly common. The causes are multifactorial, including anaemia, mild thrombocytopenia and the accumulation of low molecular waste products, normally excreted by the kidney, that inhibit platelet function. Treatment is by dialysis to reduce the urea concentration, and platelet concentrate infusions; red cell transfusions raise the haemoglobin and decrease the propensity to bleed. Increasing the concentration of vWF, either by cryoprecipitate or desmopressin, may promote haemostasis.

FURTHER INFORMATION ON BLEEDING DISORDERS

Forbes C D, Aledort L, Madhok R 1997 Haemophilia. Chapman & Hall, London

Lee C A 1996 Haemophilia. Baillière's Clinical Haematology 9, 2

VENOUS THROMBOSIS

Both arterial and venous thrombosis may arise either because of damage to vessels—for instance, atheroma or varicose veins, or as a result of changes in the plasma or cellular elements. Predisposing conditions for venous thromboembolism are listed in the information box.

FACTORS PREDISPOSING TO VENOUS THROMBOSIS

Patient factors
- Age greater than 40 years
- Obesity
- Varicose veins
- Previous deep venous thrombosis
- Oral contraceptive
- Pregnancy/puerperium
- Dehydration
- Immobility

Surgical conditions
- Surgery especially if
  > 30 minutes' duration
  Abdominal or pelvic
  Orthopaedic to lower limb

Medical conditions
- Myocardial infarction/ heart failure
- Inflammatory bowel disease
- Malignancy
- Nephrotic syndrome
- Behçet's syndrome
- Homocystinaemia

Haematological disorders
- Primary proliferative polycythaemia
- Essential thrombocythaemia
- Myelofibrosis
- Paroxysmal nocturnal haemoglobinuria

Deficiency of anticoagulants
- Antithrombin
- Protein C
- Protein S
- Factor II or V Leiden

Antiphospholipid antibody
- Lupus anticoagulant
- Anticardiolipin antibody

HAEMATOLOGICAL DISORDERS PREDISPOSING TO VENOUS THROMBOEMBOLISM

When a thrombotic event arises in an individual under the age of 40 years, particularly if there is a family history of thrombosis, investigations should be undertaken to assess whether there is a predisposing plasma abnormality (see the information box on p. 749). Often several risk factors are present when an acute deep venous thrombosis (DVT) occurs. Thus an obese patient over the age of 40 years, with factor V Leiden, may undergo abdominal surgery and develop a post-operative DVT.

ANTITHROMBIN DEFICIENCY

Antithrombin is a protease inhibitor which inactivates factors IIa, VIIa, IXa, Xa and XIa, especially in the presence of heparin (which greatly potentiates its activity). Congenital deficiency of antithrombin is associated with a predisposition to venous thromboembolism. Such patients may be relatively resistant to anticoagulation with heparin because of the low level of antithrombin which is necessary for heparin to produce its anticoagulant effect.

PROTEIN C AND S DEFICIENCIES

Protein C is a vitamin K-dependent protein which, when activated by traces of thrombin in the presence of protein S, inactivates factors Va and VIIIa. Thus a deficiency of either protein C or S results in a prothrombotic state due to reduced inhibition of activated factor V and VIII. A deficiency of either factor is usually inherited in an autosomal fashion.

FACTOR II LEIDEN

This genetic polymorphism in the prothrombin gene is associated with an increased plasma level of prothrombin and venous thromboembolism. It is present in about 2% of the normal population and about 6% of those with venous thrombus.

FACTOR V LEIDEN

This common disorder is associated with venous thrombosis. It was originally characterised as an inability of the patient's plasma clotting time to lengthen in the presence of activated protein C (APC). Further investigation revealed that the abnormality resided in the substrate for APC, namely factor Va; a substitution of arginine by glutamine at position 506 prevents its cleavage and hence inactivation. Factor Va will therefore tend to persist, resulting in a tendency to venous thrombosis.

The mutation has been identified in about 3–5% of healthy individuals in Western Europe and North America and about 20–40% of those with a history of venous thrombosis at a young age. The risk of venous thrombosis in individuals with this mutation is substantially increased if the patient has a second plasma abnormality, e.g. a lupus anticoagulant (see below).

ANTIPHOSPHOLIPID ANTIBODY SYNDROME

In the recently recognised antiphospholipid antibody syndrome an antibody in the patient's plasma has activity against enzymic reactions in the coagulation cascade that are enhanced by platelet membranes (or in vitro by phospholipid). The antibody, in vitro, has the effect of prolonging the APTT because it interacts with the phospholipid in the reaction tube and inhibits the binding or enzymic interactions of the coagulation components. It is most sensitively diagnosed by prolongation of the Russell viper venom time of plasma, an effect that can be neutralised by adding platelet membranes. When the antibody inhibits coagulation in these ways it is known as the lupus anticoagulant. In some individuals the antibody can be detected because it binds to cardiolipin in an in vitro test system, when it is known as an anticardiolipin antibody. The term antiphospholipid antibody encompasses both a lupus anticoagulant and anticardiolipin antibody; some individuals are only positive for one of these activities, whereas in others both activities are present.

Clinical features

The antiphospholipid antibody is associated with a constellation of clinical conditions (see the information box) found to be associated with a history of thromboembolism. The antibody has now been found in some individuals with a history of arterial or venous thromboembolism, often at a young age but without features of SLE; in this case it is known as the primary antiphospholipid antibody syndrome. The antibody is also associated with recurrent spontaneous abortions as well as intrauterine fetal growth retardation. The mechanism by which the antibody predisposes to thrombosis is unclear but it may be related to either maintaining platelets in an activated state within the circulation or possibly inhibiting the fibrinolytic activity of endothelial cells.

ANTIPHOSPHOLIPID SYNDROME

The clinical features are mainly related to arterial or venous occlusion which may affect one or several organs.

Haematological
- Thrombocytopenia
- Autoimmune haemolytic anaemia

Cardiac
- Myocardial infarction
- Pulmonary hypertension
- Valvular disease, e.g. mitral

Neurological
- Cerebral ischaemia
  Single lesions
  Multi-infarct dementia
- Migraine
- Epilepsy
- Chorea
- Transverse myelopathy

Renal
- Renal vein thrombosis
- Glomerular thrombosis

Endocrine
- Adrenal thrombosis—Addison's disease

GI tract
- Bowel ischaemia
- Budd–Chiari syndrome

Skin
- Livedo reticularis
- Recurrent skin ulcers

Obstetric
- Recurrent spontaneous abortions
- Intrauterine growth retardation

MANAGEMENT OF VENOUS THROMBO-EMBOLISM

The treatment of a thrombosis depends upon its site and extent and on the age of the thrombus. Prior to any antithrombotic therapy it is essential to consider whether the patient has a significant contraindication to anticoagulant therapy. On occasions antithrombotic therapy may have to be given to a patient who has a contraindication and in this instance the potential benefits have to be weighed against the risk of serious haemorrhage. Indications and contraindications to anticoagulation are given in the information boxes.

INDICATIONS FOR ANTICOAGULATION

Heparin
- Treatment and prevention of deep venous thrombosis
- Pulmonary embolism
- Myocardial infarction, to prevent:
  1. Coronary re-occlusion after thrombolysis
  2. Mural thrombosis
- Unstable angina pectoris
- Acute peripheral arterial occlusion

Warfarin

• Prophylaxis against deep venous thrombosis	therapeutic corrected prothrombin ratio (INR) 2.0
• Treatment of deep venous thrombosis and pulmonary embolism • Arterial embolism • Mitral stenosis with atrial fibrillation • Transient ischaemic attacks	INR 2.0–3.0
• Recurrent deep venous thrombosis • Mechanical prosthetic cardiac valves	INR 3.0–4.5

(INR = international normalised ratio)

CONTRAINDICATIONS TO ANTICOAGULATION

- Recent surgery, especially to eye or CNS
- Pre-existing haemorrhagic state
  e.g. Liver disease
  Renal failure
  Haemophilia
  Thrombocytopenia
- Pre-existing structural lesions
  e.g. Peptic ulcer
- Recent cerebral haemorrhage
- Uncontrolled hypertension

Anticoagulant therapy

Heparin

Standard or unfractionated heparin (SH) produces its anticoagulant effect by potentiating the activity of antithrombin which inhibits the procoagulant enzymic activity of factors IIa, VIIa, IXa, Xa and XIa (see Fig. 11.7, p. 745).

The more recently developed low molecular weight heparins (LMWH) augment antithrombin activity preferentially against factor Xa. LMWH does not prolong the APTT, unlike SH, and if its plasma level needs to be measured this is accomplished by use of a specific anti-Xa-based assay. LMWH, because of its high bioavailability after subcutaneous injection, is given either as a fixed or weight-related dose. Normally, therefore, the plasma LMWH level does not need to be measured. LMWHs are now licensed for the treatment of both DVT and pulmonary embolism; they are now replacing standard heparin as the initial treatment of choice.

The therapeutic indications for heparin use are listed in the information box above.

The treatment of established venous thrombosis can be with either subcutaneous LMWH or intravenous SH. LMWH is probably the treatment of choice because it is easy to administer as a daily subcutaneous injection and is as effective and safe as SH. If SH is to be used it should be started with a loading dose of 5000 Units intravenously, followed by a continuous infusion of 20 U/kg hourly initially. The level of anticoagulation should be assessed after 6 hours and then, if satisfactory, daily by use of a coagulation test which is appropriately sensitive to heparin—for example, APTT. It is usual to aim for a patient time which is 1.5–2.5 times the control time of the test. Treatment with either LMWH or SH should continue for 6–8 days, depending upon the extent of the thrombus. In most patients it is appropriate to start warfarin therapy at the same time as heparin, as it takes several days to decrease the concentration of the vitamin K-dependent clotting factors. Heparin should be continued until the 'international normalised ratio' (INR) is > 2.0 for 2 consecutive days.

Warfarin

Warfarin inhibits the vitamin K-dependent carboxylation of factors II, VII, IX and X in the liver (see Fig. 11.8, p. 746). Carboxylation of glutamyl residues of these coagulation factors increases their negative charge and allows them to maintain their active three-dimensional structure. The recognised indications for warfarin therapy are listed in the information box above.

Therapy with warfarin must be initiated with a loading dose—for example, 10 mg orally—on the first day, and subsequent daily doses depending on the INR. This should be in the range 2.0–4.5; the degree of anticoagulation depends on the clinical circumstances and the appropriate prothrombin ratio is given in the information box above. The prothrombin time ratio of patients' clotting time to that of the control is adjusted to give a standardised INR so that results from different laboratories are comparable. Following a single episode of venous thromboembolism it is usual to continue oral anticoagulation for 3–6 months, but if the patient has a thrombophilic condition warfarin may need to be continued on a long-term basis. If a patient has had two episodes of venous thromboembolism life-long warfarin is often considered appropriate. It is important to remember that nearly all drugs, such as non-steroidal anti-inflammatories, can potentially modify the degree of warfarin therapy, and therefore the INR should be checked 2 or 3 days after stopping or starting any other medicine.

If the patient bleeds, the anticoagulant effect of warfarin may be reversed by vitamin K_1, 1 mg slowly intravenously; the effect becomes apparent within about 6 hours, although it may not fully reverse anticoagulation for 1 or 2 days. The INR should be repeated after 6 hours and a further dose of vitamin K_1 given if appropriate. If the patient has a serious haemorrhage, reversal can be effected quickly by giving coagulation concentrate containing factors II, IX and X (50 U/kg) or, if this is unavailable, fresh frozen plasma.

Prevention of venous thrombosis

All patients admitted to hospital should be assessed for their risk of venous thromboembolism. A summary of the risk categories is given in the information boxes on page 795 and below. Early mobilisation of all patients is important to prevent DVTs. Patients at medium or high risk may require additional antithrombotic measures. Knee-length graduated compression (TED) stockings are effective in medium-risk individuals. In medium-risk patients SH can also be used; the usual dose is 5000 U 12-hourly subcutaneously and should be started pre-operatively and continued until the patient is fully mobile. High-risk individuals should receive SH and TED stockings or LMWH in a prophylactic dose. Routine monitoring of SH or LMWH for prophylaxis is not necessary. Any individual who has any of the additional risk factors in the information box is also at increased likelihood of thrombosis and every care should be taken to ensure that, as far as possible, the risk can be lessened prior to surgery—for instance, the haemoglobin reduced in polycythaemia.

ANTITHROMBOTIC PROPHYLAXIS

Patients in the following categories should be considered for specific antithrombotic prophylaxis:

Moderate risk of DVT

- Major surgery in patients > 40 years or with other risk factor (see the information box on p. 795)
- Major medical illness
  e.g. Heart failure
  Chest infection
  Malignancy
  Inflammatory bowel disease

High risk of DVT

- Hip or knee surgery
- Major abdominal or pelvic surgery for malignancy or with history of DVT or known thrombophilia (see the first information box on p. 749)

FURTHER INFORMATION ON VENOUS THROMBOSIS

Hampton K K, Preston F E 1997 Bleeding disorders, thrombosis and anticoagulation. British Medical Journal 314: 1026–1029

Pineo G F, Hall R D 1998 Prevention, diagnosis and management of venous thromboembolism. Baillière's Clinical Haematology II, I

Verstraete M 1997 Prophylaxis of venous thromboembolism. British Medical Journal 314: 123–125

BLOOD TRANSFUSION

The modern transfusion service is able to prepare a number of components from each donated unit of blood; very little whole blood is used in adult practice. This enables each product to be stored under ideal conditions, prolonging its life and making available the appropriate product for a particular clinical situation. Red cell concentrates are prepared by removing the plasma, which is further processed, and substituting additive electrolyte solutions to maintain the functions of the red cells and ensure that the viscosity of the product allows rapid transfusion where necessary. The decision to transfuse red cells is made on clinical grounds. Patients with chronic anaemias may be relatively asymptomatic. The loss of approximately 20% of the whole blood volume can be corrected by crystalloid solutions. The transfusion of one unit of red cells generally raises the haemoglobin by 10 g/l.

The use of products for haemostatic disorders has already been discussed.

THE ABO BLOOD GROUP SYSTEM

A large number of blood group antigens have been identified. The ABO system is particularly important, as naturally occurring antibodies are found in the plasma of patients who lack the appropriate antigen. The antibodies to the other blood group antigens (Rhesus, Duffy, Kell, Kidd etc.) only develop in individuals who lack the particular antigen and who are exposed to the antigen, either by transfusion or during pregnancy. The frequency of the ABO blood groups in the United Kingdom is given in Table 11.21. If blood taken from a group A individual is given to a group B patient, a severe, possibly fatal, haemolytic reaction will result.

THE RHESUS (RH) SYSTEM

This system consists of three sets of antigen: Ee, Ce and Dd (d denotes absence of D). A particular set (e.g. CDe) is inherited from each parent. Antibodies to the Rh system rarely occur naturally and arise because of exposure during pregnancy or transfusion. In routine clinical transfusion practice individuals are typed as Rh D positive (85% of the UK population) or negative. The D antigen is the most immunogenic and anti-D is responsible for most of the clinical problems which arise with the Rh system.

Table 11.21 The ABO system

Phenotype	Antigens	Naturally occurring antibodies	Frequency (%)
O	O	Anti-A, anti-B	46
A	A	Anti-B	42
B	B	Anti-A	9
AB	AB	Nil	3

PRINCIPLES OF THE CROSS-MATCH

In order to ensure that no antibody/antigen reaction leads to haemolysis, blood is firstly selected for a patient on the basis of his or her ABO and Rh D group. However, it is possible that the patient could have an antibody to any of the other groups. The cross-match procedure is basically a check to see that there is compatibility between the patient's serum and the red cells from the potential donor units. Donor cells and patient's serum are reacted together under conditions which would result in agglutination of cells which have reacted with an antibody. If such a reaction occurs, blood cannot be issued. The nature of the antibody has to be determined and donor units have to be selected that lack the antigen to which the particular antibody is directed. The grouping and cross-matching of blood on a routine basis when no incompatibility is found should be accomplished in under 40 minutes. Blood should not be issued if an incompatibility is found until a full explanation for the incompatibility has been determined and compatible blood identified. Most hospitals have available group O negative blood for use in extreme emergency situations, in which there is judged, on clinical grounds, to be no time for formal grouping and matching.

HAZARDS OF TRANSFUSION

The transfusion of blood products is not without its complications and about 5% of patients receiving a transfusion will have a reaction. Most of the reactions are relatively mild but they can be severe, even fatal. The symptoms related to transfusion reactions are non-specific (see Table 11.22).

It is often very difficult to distinguish on clinical grounds between a transfusion reaction and other complications which may occur during a patient's hospitalisation. The appreciation of these symptoms may obviously be extremely

Table 11.22 Transfusion reactions

Symptom	Frequency (%)
Chills	55
Fever	47
Urticaria	35
Tachycardia	28
Chest tightness	7
Breathlessness	7
Nausea, vomiting	7
Lumbar pain	5
Haemoglobinuria	5
Hypotension	2
Jaundice	1

difficult in the anaesthetised patient. The safest approach is to assume that the event is transfusion-related, stop the transfusion and begin the appropriate investigations (see the information box). Transfusion reactions can be classified as acute, if they occur within 72 hours, or delayed (see Table 11.23).

ACUTE HAEMOLYTIC TRANSFUSION REACTIONS

Aetiology

- Haemolysis due to antibody destruction of incompatible red cells, usually involving the ABO system

Clinical features

- Usually commence within minutes of the infusion of the incompatible unit
- Chills/rigors and fever
- Lumbar pain and/or chest tightness
- Burning sensation at infusion site
- Development of shock and/or bleeding
- In anaesthetised patients—hypotension, bleeding and pyrexia

Management

- Stop the transfusion
- Check the identity of the patient and the blood unit
- Monitor patient's pulse, blood pressure and urine output
- Send unit(s) of blood back to the laboratory
- Check full blood count, bilirubin and coagulation screen
- Regroup and cross-match patient's samples and units of blood
- Support patient's circulatory volume and haemostatic status

N.B. Rarely, blood may be bacterially contaminated, producing a similar shock-like picture. Take blood cultures.

Table 11.23 Classification of transfusion reactions

Acute (during or within 72 hours)	Delayed (after 72 hours)
Immunological	
Haemolytic: haemolytic transfusion reactions	Haemolytic: delayed haemolytic transfusion reactions
Non-haemolytic	Post-transfusion purpura
Febrile non-haemolytic reactions	Graft-versus-host disease
Allergic reactions	Allo-immunisation (particularly HLA)
Urticarial	
Anaphylactoid	
Non-cardiac pulmonary oedema	
Non-immunological	
Circulatory overload	Iron overload
Physical damage	Viral hepatitis (A, B, C)
Overheating	HIV/AIDS
Freezing	Other transmissible diseases
Incompatible solutions	Syphilis
Bacterial contamination	Malaria
Metabolic effects of stored blood	Cytomegalovirus etc.
Hypothermia	
Increased O_2 affinity	
Potassium changes	
Microaggregates	
Dilutional coagulation defects	

A detailed discussion of all the complications listed should be sought in specialist texts. Certain conditions, such as the various types of viral hepatitis, HIV infection and iron overload, are discussed elsewhere in this book. The signs and symptoms, causation and management of haemolytic reactions (acute and delayed), and febrile non-haemolytic reactions are considered in the information boxes.

FEBRILE NON-HAEMOLYTIC TRANSFUSION REACTIONS

Aetiology

- Anti-white cell or anti-HLA antibodies reacting with white cells in the unit. Occurs in 1% of transfusions but especially in multitransfused or multiparous individuals

Clinical features

- Reaction usually occurs after more than 1 Unit has been transfused
- Fever/chills
- Urticaria

Management

- Stop the transfusion
- Exclude a haemolytic reaction
- Give symptomatic treatment for pyrexia
- Consider premedication with antihistamines and/or steroids if further blood required
- Use leuco-depleted blood in patients who have more than two consecutive febrile, non-haemolytic transfusion reactions

DELAYED HAEMOLYTIC TRANSFUSION REACTIONS

Aetiology

- Reaction occurs 5–7 days after transfusion. The transfusion has stimulated the production of an antibody which was not detected at the initial cross-match

Clinical features

- Anaemia
- Jaundice

Management

- A diagnosis suggested by the finding of polychromasia and spherocytes on the blood film
- Serological investigation to demonstrate a blood group antibody which previously had not been detected
- Compatible blood made available using serological findings

SAFE TRANSFUSION PRACTICE

The clinician expects to be supplied with high-quality blood products. In many parts of the world the responsibility for selecting and testing donors, and the preparation, quality control and storage of blood products are the responsibility of a specially organised blood transfusion service. Transfusion laboratories based in local hospitals will match the product with the patient and the clinician exerts little control over these areas. However, the cause of the majority of fatal haemolytic transfusion reactions is a clerical error due to faulty labelling of the specimen and/or a failure to identify the recipient correctly. This type of error can be minimised by following the procedures outlined in principle below. Individual hospitals will frequently have their own policies for ordering and administering blood for transfusion and blood products, which should be followed.

A clinician drawing blood for cross-matching should:

- positively identify the patient at the bedside
- label the tubes and request form after identifying the patient
- ensure that all the information requested by the transfusion laboratory is given on both the tube and request form. This information must match!

The person administering blood should:

- positively identify the patient at the bedside
- ensure that the patient identification and the identification of the units match
- check that the ABO and Rh D groups of the patient and units are identical
- inspect the units for evidence of damage
- ensure that the checking procedures are validated by another member of the nursing or medical staff
- complete the necessary documentation, indicating the detailed identification of the units transfused.

FURTHER INFORMATION ON BLOOD TRANSFUSION

Mollison P L, Engelfreit C P, Contreras M 1997 Blood transfusion and clinical medicine, 10th edn. Blackwell Science, Oxford

Diseases of the connective tissues, joints and bones

12

G. NUKI • S.H. RALSTON • R. LUQMANI

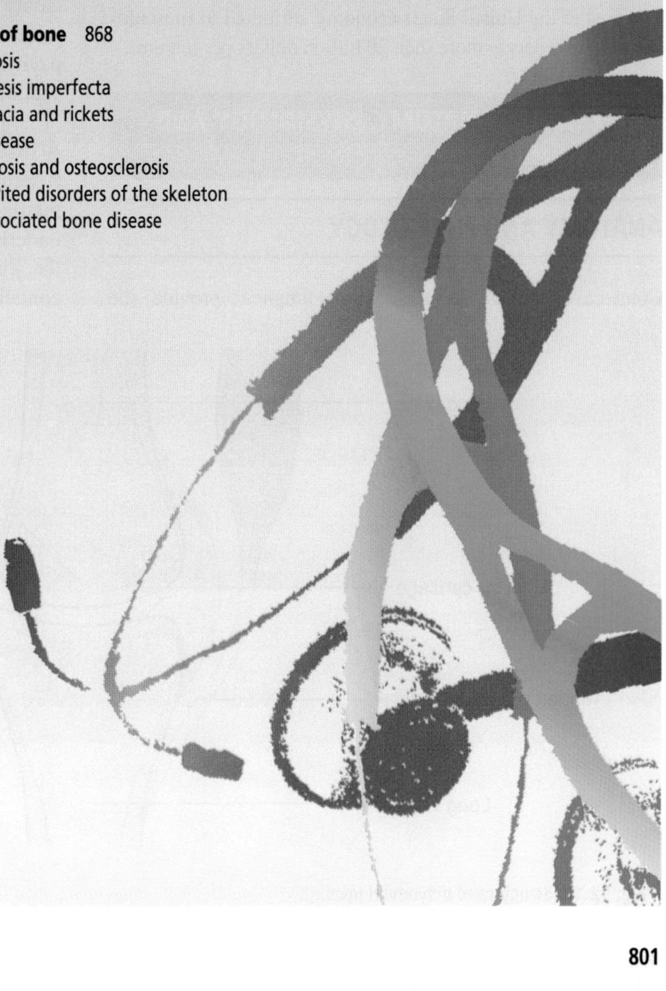

Diseases of the musculoskeletal system and connective tissues comprise a heterogeneous group of disorders in which musculoskeletal pain and stiffness are prominent.

Rheumatic diseases affect people of all ages and ethnic groups. Their frequency increases with age; as many as 40% of people over the age of 65 years in the United Kingdom have had some kind of rheumatic disorder and 20 million people experience a rheumatic complaint each year. Five million suffer from osteoarthritis, 500 000 have rheumatoid arthritis and there are 12 000 children with juvenile idiopathic arthritis. Each year back pain results in more than 2 million general practitioner consultations and more than one-third of all post-menopausal women suffer an osteoporosis-related fracture. Rheumatic complaints account for 20–25% of all consultations in general practice and 15% of all those on a GP's list in the UK consult their doctor each year with a musculoskeletal problem. In Europe rheumatic diseases are the most common cause of physical impairment in the community and about one-third of all people with physical disabilities have a rheumatic disease as the primary cause of their disability. In the UK about a quarter of a million people are severely disabled by a rheumatic disease and no other group of disorders is responsible for greater loss of earnings. The cost to the United States economy attributed to musculoskeletal disorders is more than 20 billion dollars per annum.

FUNCTIONAL ANATOMY, PHYSIOLOGY AND INVESTIGATIONS

ANATOMY AND PHYSIOLOGY

Connective tissues, as their name implies, provide the structural framework for the body and all its organs. Connective tissues are composed of cells of mesenchymal origin that synthesise and secrete an extracellular matrix consisting of variable amounts of collagens, proteoglycans and elastin as well as glycoproteins such as laminin and fibronectin. Fibronectin, laminin, collagen and some other glycoproteins act as ligands for transmembrane adhesion proteins called integrins, that regulate cell-matrix interactions by linking the extracellular matrix proteins with the cytoskeleton. Early in embryonic development connective tissues differentiate to form the specialised tissues required for musculoskeletal function, such as muscles, tendons, ligaments, cartilage and bone.

Bones are joined to each other at joints. These may be *fibrous*, as in the symphysis pubis; *cartilagenous*, as in the costochondral joints and intervertebral discs; or *synovial*, as in the more complex joints of the limbs where greater movement is required.

SYNOVIAL JOINTS (see Fig. 12.1)

In the freely movable synovial joints the ends of the bones are covered with articular cartilage and separated by a joint cavity filled with clear, viscous synovial fluid. A fibrous joint capsule holds the bones together and encloses the joint cavity. The capsule is lined by synovial membrane which produces the synovial fluid.

Articular cartilage (see Fig. 12.2)

Articular cartilage consists of chondrocytes embedded in a matrix which is calcified in its deeper layer adjacent to the underlying bone. The hyaline articular cartilage provides the joints with low-friction surfaces. It is avascular and contains no nerves. The collagen fibre framework which

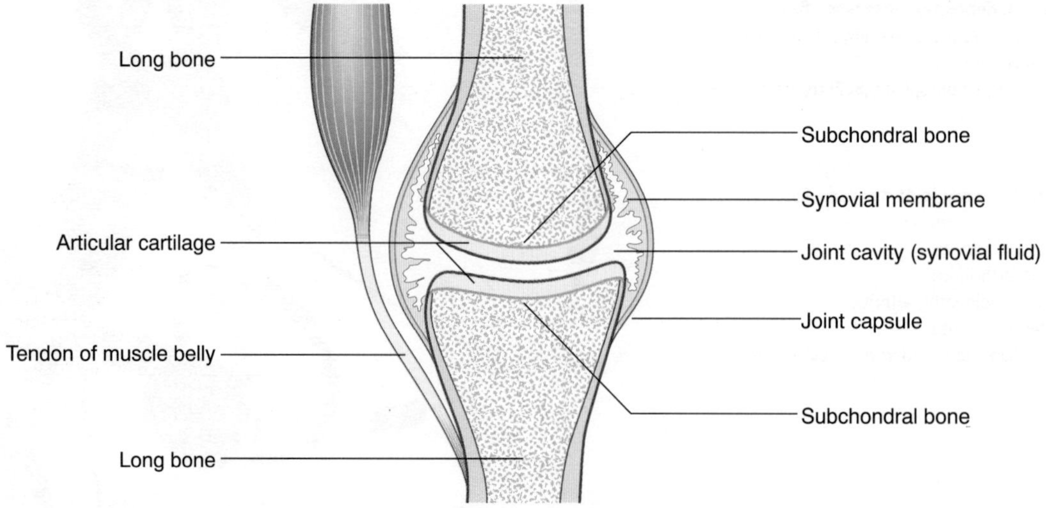

Fig. 12.1 Structure of a synovial joint.

gives the cartilage its tensile strength is composed principally of type II collagen with small amounts of other collagens. The collagen meshwork entraps the proteoglycans to create a fibre-reinforced hydrated gel which resists compression. Aggrecan is the principal proteoglycan in articular cartilage. It consists of a protein core with side-chains of chondroitin sulphate and keratan sulphate. Aggrecan molecules are joined by link proteins to hyaluronic acid, and cartilage also contains small amounts of other glycoproteins. Articular cartilage matrix integrity and proteoglycan synthesis are critically dependent on movement and mechanical stimulation of chondrocytes. Aggrecan and collagen turnover depends on a balance between degradative enzymes (aggrecanase, collagenase, stromelysin and gelatinase) and a tissue inhibitor of metalloproteinases (TIMP). Aggrecan turnover is much faster than that of collagen, and the collagen fibre network in cartilage has a very limited capacity for repair.

The synovial membrane

The synovial membrane lines the capsule of synovial joints, bursae and tendon sheaths. It consists of type A macrophage-like phagocytic cells and type B fibroblast-like cells which are responsible for secretion of the synovial

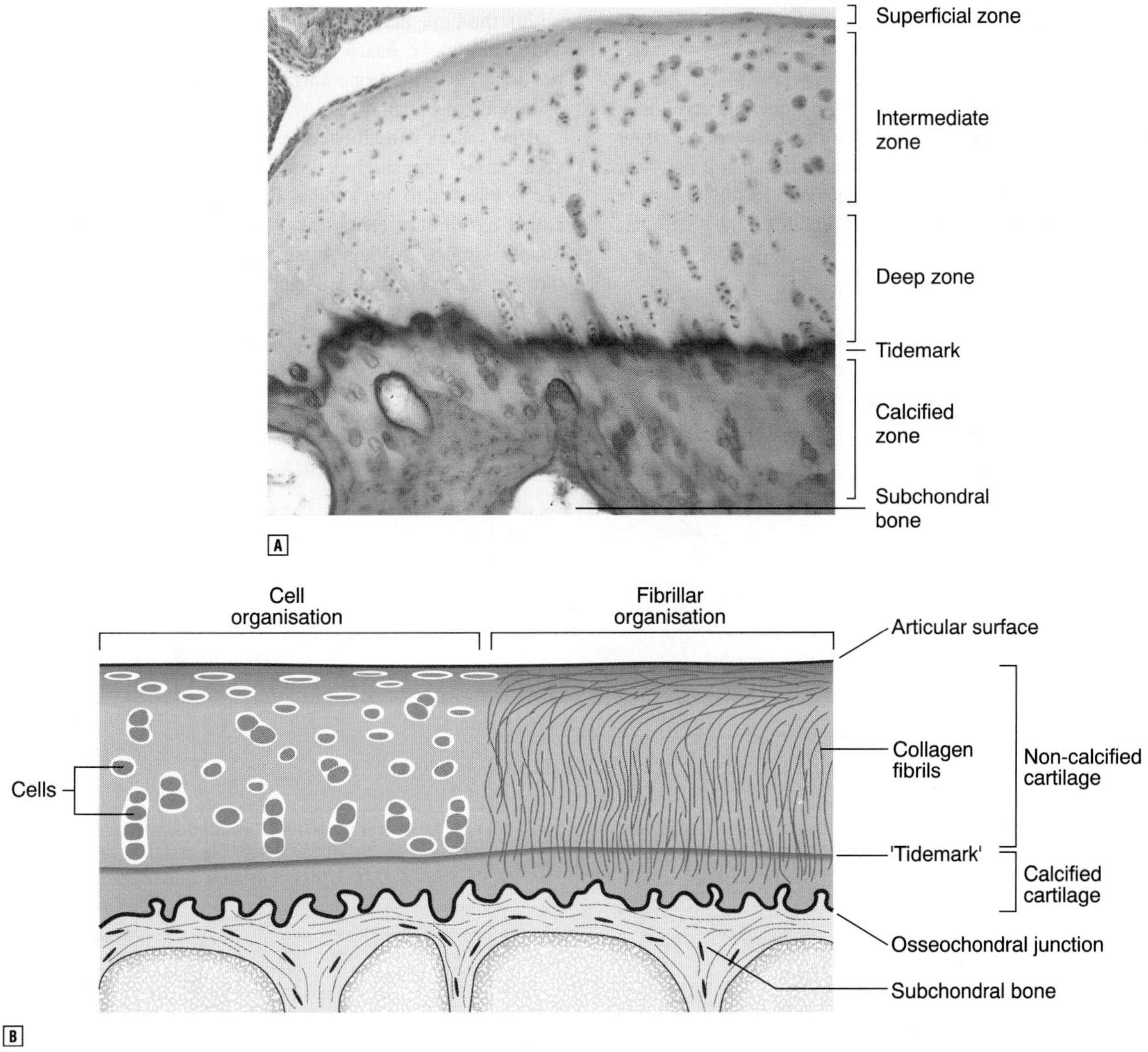

Fig. 12.2 The structure of articular cartilage. A Histological section of normal articular cartilage from a knee showing the different cartilage layers. B Line diagram illustrating the cellular and matrix components.

fluid. The intercellular matrix contains secreted hyaluronan, type VI collagen, chondroitin sulphate and tenascin. The synovial cells interdigitate without tight intercellular junctions and the lining is rich in fenestrated capillaries, allowing diffusion of fluid and plasma proteins between the circulation and the joint.

The synovial fluid

The synovial fluid plays an important role in the nutrition of the avascular articular cartilage and in the lubrication of joints. It consists of an ultrafiltrate of plasma, to which locally secreted hyaluronan and lubricin have been added. The hyaluronan gives the fluid remarkable viscoelastic properties which are important for lubrication during joint movement, while the lubricin is a glycoprotein that acts as a lubricant during static loading of joints.

The capsule, ligaments and periosteum

These contain sensory afferent fast-conducting myelinated nerve fibres which are responsible for proprioception. Slow-conducting, unmyelinated c-fibres which transmit pain sensation are also found in these tissues and in the synovium, where they regulate microvascular function.

BONE

Bone provides mechanical support for joints, tendons and ligaments which are attached at entheses. It also acts as a reservoir for calcium and phosphate in the preservation of normal mineral homeostasis.

Two types of bone are found in the normal skeleton: cortical bone, which predominates in the shafts (diaphyses) of the long bones, and trabecular bone, which predominates in the ends of the long bones (epiphyses) and vertebral bodies (see Fig. 12.3). Because of its greater surface area, trabecular bone is remodelled more quickly than cortical bone and, as a result, is subject to more rapid bone loss under conditions of increased bone turnover. Cortical bone is composed of Haversian systems, which in turn consist of a series of concentric lamellae of collagen fibres surrounding a central canal that contains blood vessels. Nutrients reach the central parts of the bone via an interconnecting system of canaliculi which run between osteocytes buried deep within the bone matrix and lining cells on the bone surface. Trabecular bone has a similar structure, but the lamellae run parallel to the bone surface, rather than concentrically as in cortical bone.

Bone matrix is mainly composed of type I collagen. After collagen is deposited in bone matrix, the protein chains become linked to one another by specialised covalent bonds called pyridinium cross-links, which help to give bone its tensile strength. When bone is formed rapidly in high-turnover disorders such as Paget's disease or bone metastases, the lamellae are laid down in a disorderly fashion, giving rise to 'woven bone' which is mechanically weaker than normal bone. Bone matrix also contains small amounts of

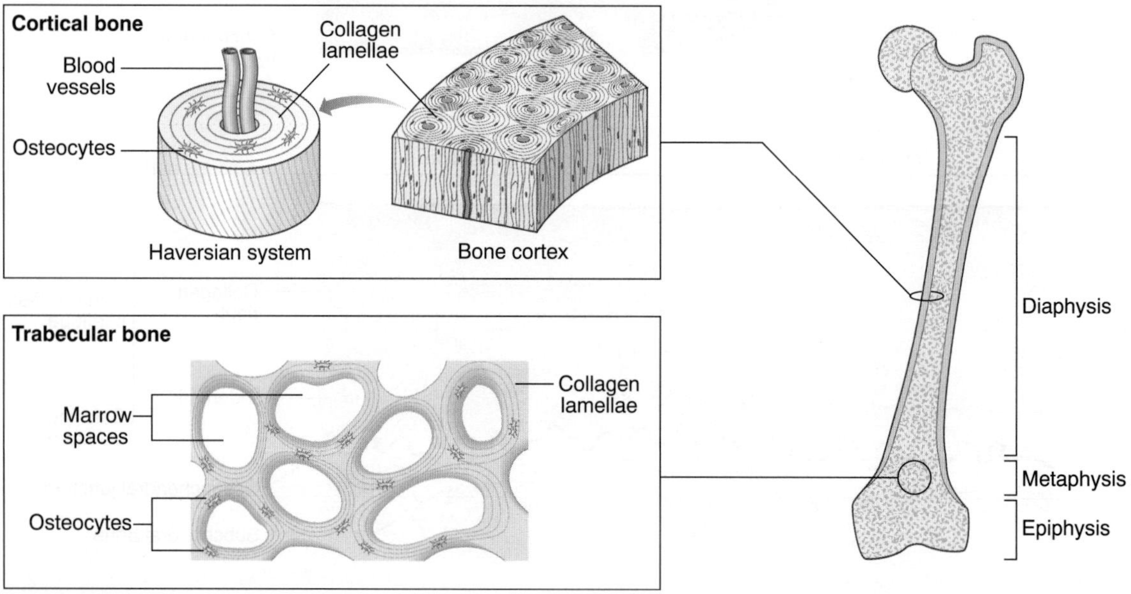

Fig. 12.3 Organisation of bone. Cortical bone predominates in the shafts of the long bones, whereas trabecular bone predominates at the ends of the long bones and vertebrae. Flat bones, such as the pelvis and skull, have approximately equal amounts of cortical and trabecular bone.

other collagens and several non-collagenous proteins and glycoproteins. Some of these, such as osteocalcin, are specific to bone, whereas others, such as osteopontin, fibronectin and growth factors, are also found in other connective tissues. Non-collagenous bone proteins are probably involved in mediating attachment of bone cells to bone matrix, and in regulating bone-cell activity during bone remodelling. The organic component of bone forms a framework upon which mineralisation occurs. During bone formation, osteoblasts lay down uncalcified bone matrix which contains all the components described above and small amounts of other proteins which are adsorbed from extracellular fluid. After a lag phase of about 10 days, the matrix becomes mineralised, as hydroxyapatite (Ca_{10} $(PO_4)_6$ OH_2) is deposited in spaces between collagen fibrils. Mineralisation provides bone with mechanical rigidity.

BONE REMODELLING

The mechanical integrity of the skeleton is maintained by the process of bone remodelling, which occurs throughout life to allow damaged bone to be replaced by new bone (see Fig. 12.4). Approximately 10% of bone surface in the adult skeleton is being remodelled at any one time. Remodelling commences with attraction of osteoclasts to the site which is to be resorbed. Osteoclasts are multinucleated phagocytic cells, rich in the enzyme tartrate-resistant acid phosphatase, which are formed by fusion of precursors derived from cells of the monocyte/macrophage lineage. Osteoclasts form a tight seal over the bone surface and resorb bone by secreting hydrochloric acid and proteolytic enzymes, which dissolve hydroxyapatite and degrade bone matrix, respectively. When resorption is complete, osteoclasts undergo programmed cell death (apoptosis), in the so-called reversal phase which heralds the start of bone formation. Bone formation begins with the attraction of osteoblast precursors, derived from marrow stromal cells, to the bone surface. These cells differentiate into mature osteoblasts rich in the enzyme alkaline phosphatase. Osteoblasts lay down bone matrix which is initially unmineralised (osteoid), but which subsequently becomes calcified after about 10 days to form mature bone. During bone formation, some osteoblasts become trapped within the matrix and differentiate into osteocytes, which connect with one another and with flattened lining cells on the bone surface by an intricate network of cytoplasmic processes, running through canaliculi in bone matrix. Osteocytes probably act as sensors of mechanical strain, and secrete signalling molecules such as prostaglandins and nitric oxide (NO), which modulate the function of neighbouring bone cells.

Bone remodelling is a highly organised process, but the mechanisms which determine where and when remodelling occurs are poorly understood. Mechanical stimuli and areas of microdamage are likely to be important determinants. Local increases in remodelling occur in association with the secretion of inflammatory cytokines such as interleukin-1 (IL-1) and tumour necrosis factor (TNF) in diseases such as rheumatoid arthritis. Calciotropic hormones such as para-

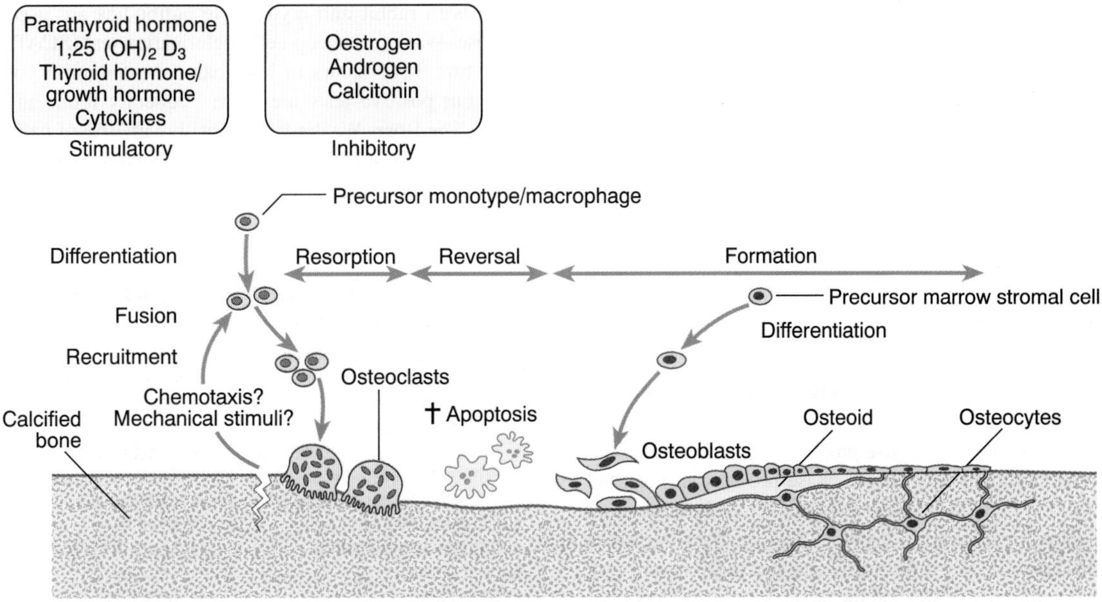

Fig. 12.4 The bone remodelling cycle. ($1,25\ (OH)_2\ D$ = 1,25 dihydroxyvitamin D)

thyroid hormone (PTH) and 1,25 dihydroxyvitamin D_3 act together to increase bone remodelling on a systemic basis, allowing skeletal calcium to be mobilised for the maintenance of plasma calcium homeostasis (see p. 575). Bone remodelling is also increased by thyroid hormone and growth hormone, but suppressed by oestrogen, androgens and calcitonin.

INVESTIGATION OF RHEUMATIC AND BONE DISEASE

INVESTIGATION OF RHEUMATIC DISEASES

Diagnosis in patients with arthritis and connective tissue diseases is usually established from a detailed history and careful physical examination. Laboratory tests and imaging can be helpful in confirming a clinical diagnosis and in assessing the activity and progression of disease, but few of the tests available are specific.

Haematology

Patients with active inflammatory rheumatic diseases often have a moderate normochromic, normocytic anaemia with a raised platelet count. A mixed or microcytic picture with a low mean cell volume may indicate superadded iron deficiency due to gastrointestinal blood loss from treatment with non-steroidal anti-inflammatory drugs (NSAIDs). Serum ferritin measurements are not a reliable indication of iron stores in patients with chronic inflammatory diseases, as the serum ferritin fluctuates with the activity of the systemic inflammation.

A *polymorphonuclear leucocytosis* may occur in patients with septic arthritis, acute gouty arthritis, systemic juvenile idiopathic arthritis or systemic vasculitis, as well as in patients receiving high-dosage corticosteroid therapy. *Eosinophilia* may be associated with a drug hypersensitivity reaction, the Churg–Strauss syndrome and Wegener's granulomatosis. *Leucopenia* or *thrombocytopenia* can be seen in patients with Felty's syndrome or systemic lupus erythematosus (SLE); or as a manifestation of bone marrow suppression in patients receiving treatment with cytotoxic or disease-modifying antirheumatic drugs.

Erythrocyte sedimentation rate, plasma viscosity and acute-phase reactants

Hepatic synthesis of *c-reactive protein* (CRP), *serum amyloid A* (SAA) and many other acute-phase proteins is increased in response to IL-6 in patients with active inflammation while albumin concentrations fall. These changes in plasma proteins are indirectly reflected by changes in the *erythrocyte sedimentation rate* (ESR) and the *plasma viscosity*. A normal CRP, ESR or plasma viscosity can be helpful in excluding active systemic inflammation in most clinical situations but the ESR may not be raised as expected in patients with cardiac failure or polycythaemia, and in some patients with active SLE or seronegative arthritis. Conversely, the ESR may be persistently raised in patients with chronic rheumatoid arthritis and hypergammaglobulinaemia, and in such patients the ESR cannot be used to follow the activity of the inflammatory joint disease.

Biochemical tests

The plasma *uric acid* level may be raised in patients with gout and is used to monitor the efficacy of hypouricaemic drug therapy. *Serum aldolase* and *creatinine phosphokinase* levels can be used to follow the activity of inflammatory muscle diseases. The plasma *urea* or *creatinine* may be raised in systemic connective tissue diseases where there is renal involvement or as a consequence of drug toxicity in patients receiving antirheumatic drugs (NSAIDs, gold, d-penicillamine or cyclosporin A). *Liver function tests* may be abnormal as a consequence of drug hepatotoxicity and are used to monitor treatment with sulphasalazine and methotrexate.

Serological tests

Rheumatoid factors

Rheumatoid factors (RF) are immunoglobulins of the IgG, IgA or IgM class which react with the Fc portion of IgG. In clinical immunological practice RF of the IgM class is usually detected and measured semi-quantitatively by testing the ability of the patient's serum to agglutinate carrier particles coated with IgG. Polystyrene particles coated with human IgG are used in the latex slide test, and sheep erythrocytes coated with rabbit anti-erythrocyte antibodies are used in the Rose–Waaler or sheep-cell agglutination test (SCAT). A SCAT titre 1:32 occurs in less than 5% of normal young adults but positive tests are more frequently found in the elderly. The Rose–Waaler test is positive in 70% of patients with rheumatoid arthritis but it may not become positive for several months after the onset of symptoms; positive tests

DISEASES WHICH MAY BE ASSOCIATED WITH POSITIVE RHEUMATOID FACTOR TESTS

Autoimmune and connective tissue diseases
- Rheumatoid arthritis
- Sjögren's syndrome
- Systemic lupus erythematosus
- Progressive systemic sclerosis
- Polymyositis/dermatomyositis
- Fibrosing alveolitis
- Chronic active hepatitis
- Liver cirrhosis
- Sarcoidosis
- Waldenström's macroglobulinaemia

Chronic infections
- Infectious mononucleosis
- Infectious hepatitis
- Bacterial endocarditis
- Tuberculosis
- Syphilis
- Yaws
- Leprosy
- Kala-azar
- Schistosomiasis
- Filariasis

are also found in other autoimmune diseases and chronic infections listed in the information box.

Antinuclear antibodies

Antinuclear antibodies (ANA) are detected by indirect immunofluorescence. The ANA is a good screening test for SLE as more than 90% of patients have positive tests, but positive tests are also found in many other conditions (see the information box). Low-titre ANA has no clinical significance and is frequently found in normal elderly people. The *lupus erythematosus (LE) cell test* is less sensitive, very time-consuming and hardly more specific. Radioimmunoassays and enzyme-linked immunosorbent assays (ELISA) for anti-DNA antibodies to undenatured double-stranded DNA have much greater specificity for the diagnosis of SLE but *anti-DNA antibodies* are present in the serum in significant amounts in only about half the patients with SLE at any one time.

ANTINUCLEAR ANTIBODIES: DISEASE ASSOCIATIONS

- Systemic lupus erythematosus
- Juvenile idiopathic arthritis
- Mixed connective tissue disease
- Polymyositis
- Systemic sclerosis
- Sjögren's syndrome
- Rheumatoid arthritis
- Fibrosing alveolitis
- Chronic liver disease
- Thyroiditis
- Myasthenia gravis
- Leukaemia
- Transient viral infections

Antiphospholipid antibodies

Antiphospholipid antibodies are a group of heterogeneous autoantibodies which are primarily directed against a complex antigen, of which β2-glycoprotein-1 is an essential component. Antiphospholipid (anticardiolipin) antibodies detected by solid-phase immunoassays occur in many patients with SLE, 'lupus-like' disease and a number of other autoimmune disorders, as well as in the *primary antiphospholipid syndrome* which is characterised by arterial and venous thrombosis, thrombocytopenia and recurrent fetal loss in pregnant women. Antiphospholipid antibodies can be associated with recurrent cerebral ischaemia, livedo reticularis and hypertension *(Sneddon's syndrome)* or a *catastrophic antiphospholipid syndrome* characterised by multiple organ infarction, acute respiratory distress syndrome (ARDS), pulmonary hypertension, renal failure and major central nervous system dysfunction. Antiphospholipid antibodies may also give rise to false positive serological tests for syphilis. In such patients the Venereal Disease Research Laboratory (VDRL) and Wassermann complement fixation tests may be positive but the more specific fluorescent treponemal antibody absorption test is negative. Antiphospholipid antibodies can also inhibit in vitro blood coagulation tests and 'lupus anticoagulant' activity can be detected by a prolongation of the activated partial thromboplastin time (APTT) or the diluted Russell viper venom time but there is no direct correlation between such circulating anticoagulant antibodies and antiphospholipid antibodies detected by ELISA.

Other autoantibodies which can be useful in the diagnosis of connective tissue diseases are listed in Table 12.1.

Immune complexes and complement activation

Elevated levels of circulating immune complexes occur in many autoimmune diseases, infections and malignancies, and detection of circulating immune complexes is seldom useful for diagnosis or monitoring the progress of patients with connective tissue diseases or systemic vasculitides.

Measurements of total haemolytic complement (CH_{50}) and C_3 and C_4 complement components can, however, be useful in the diagnosis and management of SLE. Low levels indicate activation of the classical complement pathway by immune complexes. A low CH_{50} in the presence of normal values of C_3 and C_4 suggests the possibility of inherited C_2 complement deficiency or other rarer inherited deficiencies of complement components.

There are no reliable blood tests that will make a diagnosis of *vasculitis*. Complement activation with reduced circulating levels of C_3, C_4 and CH_{50} is typically seen in mixed essential cryoglobulinaemia, along with the presence of circulating cryoglobulins (immunoglobulins which precipitate at less

Table 12.1 Autoantibodies in connective tissue diseases

Antibody	Disease
RF	Rheumatoid arthritis and other disease
ANA	Systemic lupus erythematosus (SLE), systemic sclerosis, myositis, rheumatoid arthritis, juvenile idiopathic arthritis and other diseases
Anti-ds-DNA	SLE
ENA	
Anti-RNP	Mixed connective tissue disease (high titres), SLE
Anti-Sm	SLE
Anti-histone H_1, H_3, H_4	SLE
Anti-histone H_{2A}, H_{2B}	Drug-induced SLE
Anti-SSA (anti-Ro)	Sjögren's syndrome, SLE, neonatal lupus
Anti-SSB (anti-La)	Sjögren's syndrome, SLE
Anti-topoisomerase 1 (SCL 70)	Systemic sclerosis
Anti-centromere	Limited systemic sclerosis (CREST syndrome—see p. 859)
Anti-Jo-1	Polymyositis, dermatomyositis with lung disease
ANCA	
c-ANCA	Wegener's granulomatosis
p-ANCA	Systemic vasculitis and other diseases

than body temperature) and, in over 80% of cases, with evidence of hepatitis C infection. Evidence of hepatitis B infection is present in a distinct subgroup of patients with polyarteritis nodosa (PAN). High levels of von Willebrand factor and circulating anti-endothelial cell antibodies reflect endothelial cell damage in all forms of vasculitis.

Antineutrophil cytoplasmic antibodies

Antineutrophil cytoplasmic antibodies (ANCAs) are found in many forms of vasculitis. Antibodies to proteinase 3 result in granular staining of the neutrophil cytoplasm. This cytoplasmic or c-ANCA is found in about 80% of patients with Wegener's granulomatosis and some patients with microscopic polyangiitis and rapidly progressive idiopathic glomerulonephritis. Antibodies to myeloperoxidase are associated with perinuclear staining (p-ANCA). They are found in about 40–50% of patients with microscopic polyangiitis and other types of systemic vasculitis but not all patients with a positive ANCA have vasculitis.

Synovial fluid analysis

Analysis of synovial fluid is essential for the immediate diagnosis of joint infections and crystal arthropathies. Synovial fluid analysis can also be useful in the differential diagnosis of inflammatory and degenerative arthropathies (see Table 12.2).

Blood contamination can follow a traumatic tap but evenly blood-stained haemarthroses are characteristically associated with haemophilia, villonodular synovitis, neuropathic joints, pyrophosphate arthropathy and resolving infections, as well as with trauma.

Tissue biopsies

Synovial biopsy is an important investigation if tuberculosis or a tumour is suspected but is seldom useful in distinguishing different types of inflammatory arthritis. It can be undertaken by blind needle biopsy, arthroscopy or open surgery. *Muscle biopsies* are important in establishing the diagnosis in patients with primary muscle diseases, and biopsy of clinically involved organs or tissue such as skin, muscle, kidney, nerve or nasal mucosa is important in obtaining histological confirmation of the diagnosis in patients with systemic vasculitides. Renal biopsy can be helpful and important in establishing the diagnosis and prognosis in patients with SLE who have renal insufficiency, proteinuria or an active urinary sediment (see p. 855). Tissue evidence for immune complex deposition can also be obtained from the detection of complement components and immunoglobulins by immunofluorescence in other organ biopsies, but the finding of immune complex deposits at the dermo-epidermal junction of normal skin (the lupus 'band' test) has been largely abandoned because it is invasive, relatively non-specific and seldom helpful in practice.

Arthroscopy

This is particularly useful for excluding meniscus tears in the knee and can also be used to establish the extent of erosive cartilage damage or osteoarthritis.

Imaging

Radiographs are frequently used as aids to diagnosis in patients with arthritis and they are also used to follow the progression of osteoarthritis and inflammatory joint diseases. Radiographs of the hands and feet are particularly useful, as there are characteristic patterns of joint involvement in a number of types of osteoarthritis and metabolic disorder as well as in inflammatory joint diseases (see Table 12.3). In some patients radiographs may reveal diagnostic features even in the absence of symptoms and signs.

In osteoarthritis radiographs of affected joints show loss of joint space and marginal osteophytes with subchondral bone sclerosis, bone remodelling and cyst formation in more advanced cases (see Figs 12.5 and 12.6).

The stages of radiological progression in rheumatoid arthritis are shown in the information box.

A single anterior-posterior radiograph of the pelvis is useful in detecting sacroiliitis (see Fig. 12.7, p. 810) in

Table 12.2 Synovial fluid analysis

	Colour	Viscosity	Clarity	Cell count/mm^3	Other tests
Normal	Colourless	Very high	Clear	0–200	
Osteoarthritis	Colourless	High	Clear	200–4000	
Rheumatoid arthritis	Yellow	Low	Cloudy	2000–40 000	
Seronegative inflammatory arthritis	Yellow	Low	Cloudy	2000–40 000	
Gout-pseudogout	Variable	Low	Variable	2000–40 000	Crystals monosodium urate (MSU)/ calcium pyrophosphate dihydrate (CPPD) on polarising microscopy
Septic arthritis	Yellow	Low	Very turbid	> 50 000	Gram stain and culture

patients with spondarthritides and in the evaluation of degenerative and inflammatory diseases affecting the hips. A lateral radiograph of the lumbar spine can be useful in confirming vertebral compression fractures and diseases affecting the intervertebral discs (see Fig. 12.8).

Computed tomography (CT) and *magnetic resonance imaging* (MRI) can be useful in the further evaluation of disc prolapses (see Fig. 12.9) and other spinal disorders, and they can also be very sensitive ways of detecting avascular necrosis and osteomyelitis. MRI is increasingly used to evaluate meniscus tears and other internal derangements of the knees as well as details of articular and periarticular pathology in the shoulder, hip and other joints.

Ultrasound can be useful to detect popliteal (Baker's) cysts behind the knee and details of pathology in patients with shoulder pain. *Skeletal scintigraphy* using ^{99m}-Tc bisphosphonate can be helpful in detecting increased bone turnover in patients with fractures, bone infections or

STAGES OF RADIOLOGICAL PROGRESSION IN RHEUMATOID ARTHRITIS

I	Periarticular osteoporosis
II	Loss of articular cartilage ('joint space')
III	Erosions
IV	Subluxation and ankylosis

Table 12.3 Common patterns of joint involvement

Pattern	Inflammatory	Degenerative
Isolated distal interphalangeal joint disease	Psoriasis	Nodal osteoarthritis
Bony swelling in distal interphalangeal, proximal interphalangeal and carpometacarpal joints, thumbs	—	Primary generalised osteoarthritis
Symmetrical involvement of metacarpophalangeal and proximal interphalangeal joints	Rheumatoid arthritis, psoriatic arthritis, SLE	Metabolic osteo-arthritis (e.g. haemo-chromatosis)
Asymmetrical oligoarticular large joint involvement	Reactive, psoriatic, ankylosing spondylitis, inflammatory bowel disease-associated arthritis	Osteoarthritis
Proximal girdle joints	Rheumatoid arthritis Polymyalgia rheumatica	
Axial and sacroiliac joints	Ankylosing spondylitis	Osteoarthritis Cervical and lumbar spondylosis, diffuse idiopathic skeletal hyperostosis
Monoarticular	Infection, gout, pseudogout, psoriatic arthritis	Primary osteo-arthritis of hip or knee, post-traumatic osteoarthritis

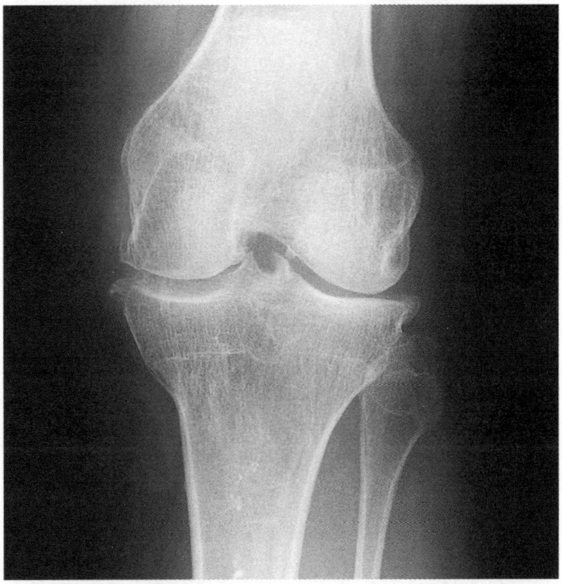

Fig. 12.5 Osteoarthritis of the knee. Weight-bearing radiograph showing joint space narrowing with osteophyte formation and early subchondral bone sclerosis.

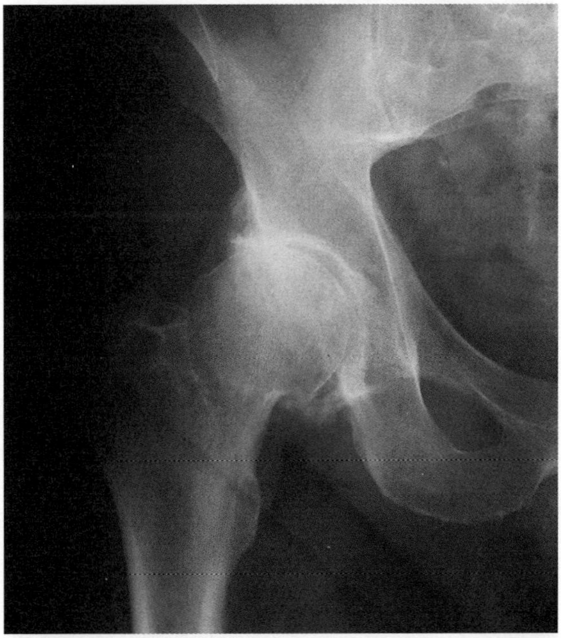

Fig. 12.6 Osteoarthritis of the hip. Radiograph showing loss of articular cartilage, bone sclerosis and remodelling of the femoral head.

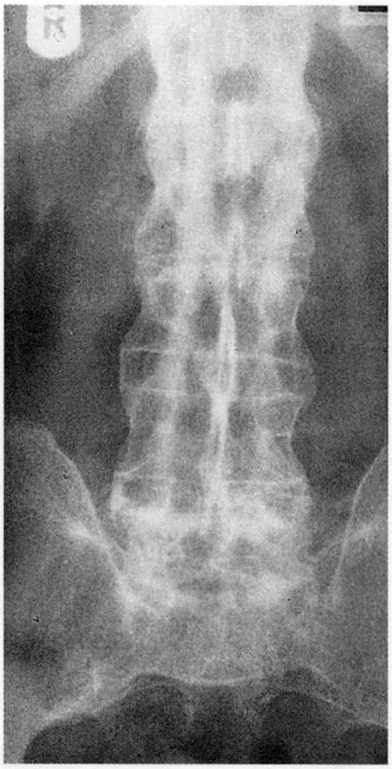

Fig. 12.7 Advanced ankylosing spondylitis. Radiograph of spine showing obliteration of sacroiliac joint and 'bamboo' appearance due to ligamentous ossification.

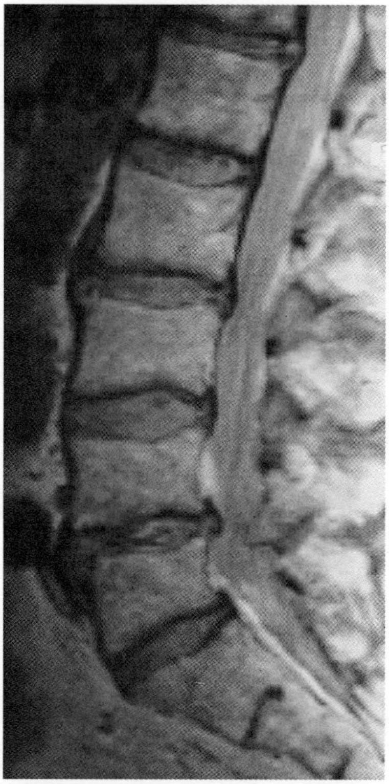

Fig. 12.9 Prolapsed L4/5 lumbar intervertebral disc. Sagittal MRI shows loss of disc height with anterior and posterior disc protrusion.

metastases (see Fig. 12.11, p. 812) when radiographs are negative, but isotope uptake is also increased in joints in patients with inflammatory and degenerative arthritis.

^{67}-Gallium and ^{111}-indium scans are occasionally used to localise infections, and *single photon emission* CT (SPECT) and *positron emission tomography* (PET) are being developed to detect abnormalities in brain blood flow and metabolism in patients with cerebral lupus and vasculitis.

Renal or coeliac-axis *angiography* is rarely used to reveal evidence of segmental artery narrowing and aneurysm formation in patients with systemic necrotising vasculitis when there is no clear evidence of specific organ pathology from other tests.

INVESTIGATION OF BONE DISEASES

Biochemical tests

Some metabolic diseases, such as Paget's disease and os-

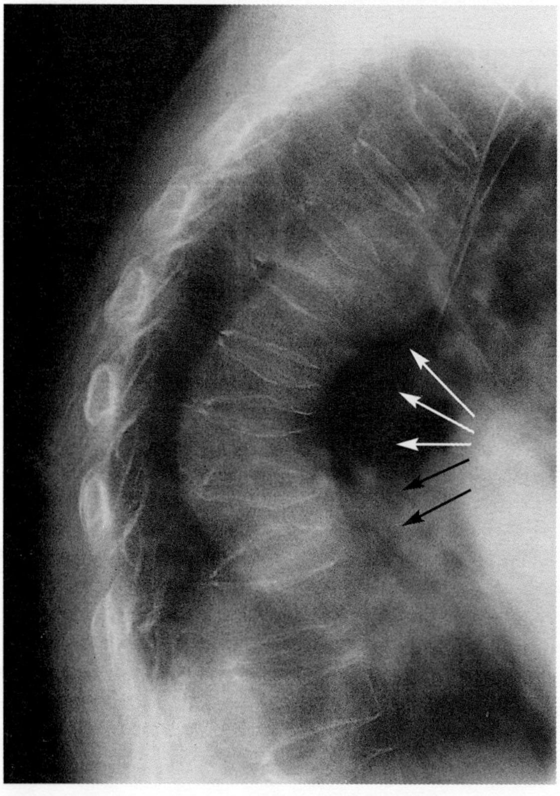

Fig. 12.8 Lateral radiograph of patient with osteoporotic vertebral fractures. The radiograph shows typical appearances of osteoporotic vertebral fractures with kyphosis and multiple wedge deformities (arrows).

Table 12.4 Biochemical features of various metabolic bone diseases

	Serum calcium	Serum phosphate	Serum alkaline phosphatase (sAP)	Comment
Osteoporosis	Normal	Normal	Normal	sAP may be slightly raised after a healing fracture
Paget's disease	Normal	Normal	High/very high	Hypercalcaemia can occur after immobilisation in Paget's
Osteomalacia	Low/normal	Low/normal	High	Osteomalacia can be present with a normal sAP value

teomalacia, have characteristic abnormalities on biochemical testing which are useful in diagnosis and monitoring response to treatment (see Table 12.4). Specific biochemical markers of collagen breakdown (urine pyridinium cross-links or urinary hydroxyproline) and osteoblast function (serum osteocalcin, collagen propeptides) can be used to assess bone turnover, but these assays are not widely available in routine practice.

Imaging

Radiographs are valuable in the diagnosis and assessment of bone structure, suspected fractures and bone deformity. They are of limited value, however, in the detection of early osteolytic lesions and osteoporosis as a large amount of bone mineral (30%) must be lost from the skeleton before it can be detected by radiography.

Bone mineral density (BMD) measurements are invaluable for the assessment of patients with suspected osteoporosis. Although there are several ways of measuring BMD, *dual energy X-ray absorptiometry* (DXA) is currently the method of choice because of its sensitivity, precision and low radiation dose. DXA scanning is based on the fact that mineralised bone impedes the passage of X-rays through bone tissue. Differences between patients are analysed by computer in relation to known standards to give BMD readings in the spine, hip or forearm. DXA machines plot the results as absolute bone density (in grams of hydroxyapatite/cm^2) and in relation to reference ranges

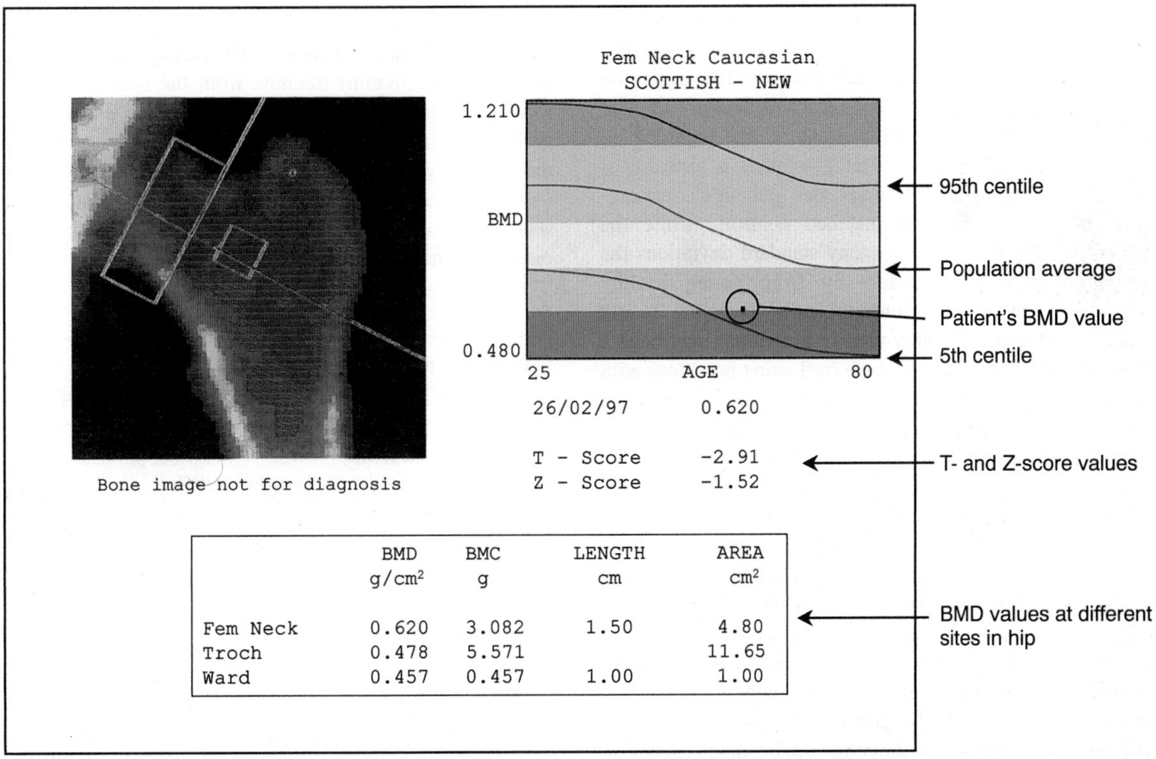

Fig. 12.10 Dual-energy X-ray absorptiometry scan. The DXA scan of the hip in an asymptomatic 58-year-old woman shows a reduction in bone mineral density compared with the value in young healthy individuals. This is reflected by the T-score value of -2.91. The BMD is also reduced when compared with the population average value in a woman of this age, reflected by the Z-score of -1.52. According to WHO criteria, this woman would be classified as having osteoporosis.

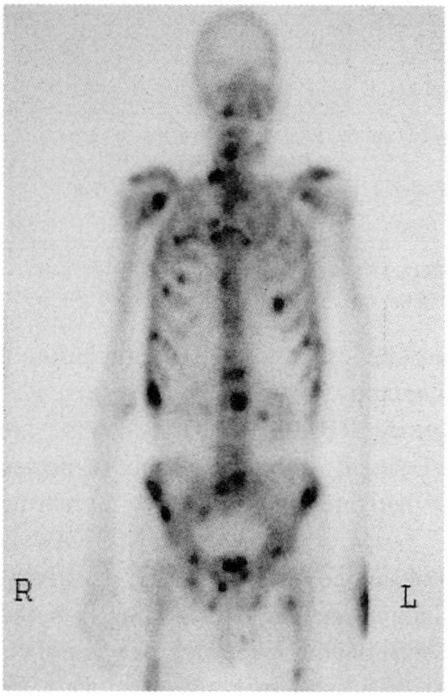

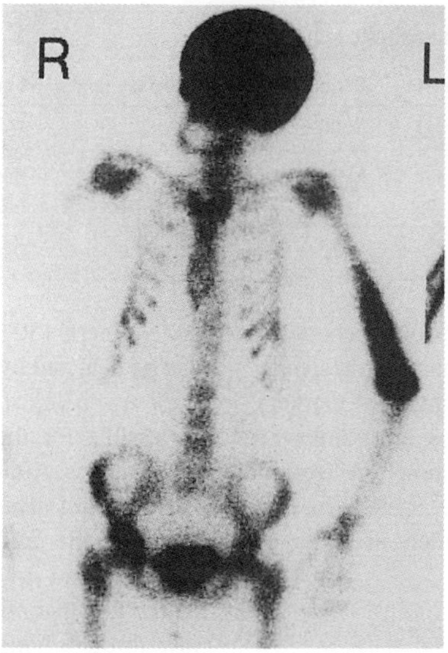

Fig. 12.11 Radioisotope bone scans in metastatic bone disease and Paget's disease. Sites of increased tracer uptake are shown as black areas on the scan. A Note the multiple hot spots, typical of metastatic disease. B Compare with the intense homogeneous uptake in the skull, humerus, pelvis and femorae, typical of Paget's disease.

giving 'Z-score' and 'T-score' values (see Fig. 12.10). By World Health Organization (WHO) criteria, individuals with a T-score between –1.0 and –2.5 are regarded as having *osteopaenia* (slightly reduced bone mass), whereas those with a T-score below –2.5 are regarded as having *osteoporosis*. Individuals with T-scores of below –2.5 who have also suffered a fragility fracture are regarded as having *severe osteoporosis*. The Z-score is a measure of how many standard deviations the patient's measurement differs by from age-matched controls, while the T-score is a measure of how many standard deviations the patient's measurement differs by from young healthy controls. Osteoporotic patients typically have low T- and Z-scores, whereas a healthy elderly individual may have a normal Z-score but a low T-score (reflecting bone loss with age).

Quantitative ultrasound examination provides an alternative to bone densitometry in the assessment of patients with osteoporosis and fracture risk, but at present this is mainly being used as a research tool.

Radionuclide bone scanning is of value in the diagnosis of metastatic bone disease and Paget's disease. The technique is based on the incorporation of radio-labelled bisphosphonate within newly formed bone at sites of active remodelling, with imaging of tracer uptake ('hot spots') by a gamma camera. Although the incorporation of isotope is not specific to a particular disease, the patterns of uptake in different diseases usually allow a diagnosis to be made (see Fig. 12.11). Bone scans are generally more sensitive than radiographs in detecting metastatic disease but negative results can occur in multiple myeloma where the osteoblastic response is often suppressed.

Bone biopsy

Bone biopsy is helpful in establishing the diagnosis in selected patients with metabolic bone disease when other tests have proved inconclusive. The biopsy is taken using a large-diameter (8 mm) trephine from the iliac crest under local anaesthetic and the sample is processed for histology, preferably without decalcification. The biopsy sample can then be analysed for the presence of mineralisation defects (osteomalacia) or marrow infiltrates (e.g. mastocytosis, secondary tumour), and to determine the extent of osteoblast and osteoclast activity.

FURTHER INFORMATION ON FUNCTIONAL ANATOMY, PHYSIOLOGY AND INVESTIGATIONS

Bird H A, Dougados M (eds) 1996 Imaging techniques, part II: modern methods. Baillière's Clinical Rheumatology 10: 561–734

Compston J E, Cooper C, Kanis J A 1995 Bone densitometry in clinical practice. British Medical Journal 310: 1507–1510

Henderson B, Edwards J C W 1987 The synovial lining in health and disease. Chapman & Hall, London

Kaye J J 1990 Arthritis: roles of radiography and other imaging techniques in evaluation. Radiology 177: 601–608

Levick J R, McDonald J N 1995 Fluid movement across synovium in healthy joints: role of synovial fluid macromolecules. Annals of the Rheumatic Diseases 54: 417–422

Parfitt A M, Mundy G R, Roodman G D et al 1996 A new model for the regulation of bone resorption, with particular reference to the effects of bisphosphonates. Journal of Bone and Mineral Research 11: 150–159

Silman A J, Symmons D P M (eds) 1995 Classification and assessment of rheumatoid diseases. Baillière's Clinical Rheumatology 9: 253–432

Stockwell R A 1991 Cartilage failure in osteoarthritis: relevance of normal structure and function. Clinical Anatomy 4: 161–191

MAJOR MANIFESTATIONS OF JOINT DISEASE

ACUTE MONOARTHRITIS

Four main common diagnoses need to be considered in patients who present with a single hot, painful, tender and swollen joint:

- bacterial infection
- crystal arthritis
- reactive arthritis
- trauma.

The differential diagnosis is, however, potentially very wide (see the information box) and includes many conditions such as rheumatoid arthritis or psoriatic arthritis that more commonly present as a polyarthritis. It is important to remember that atypical presentations of common disorders are always more likely than rare diseases.

DIFFERENTIAL DIAGNOSIS OF ACUTE MONOARTHRITIS

Infection • Bacterial • Viral • Fungal • Spirochaetal	**Traumatic** • Haemarthrosis • Internal derangement • Loose body • Fracture
Crystal arthropathy • Gout • Pseudogout	**Degenerative** • Primary osteoarthritis • Secondary osteoarthritis
Inflammatory • Rheumatoid arthritis • Juvenile idiopathic arthritis • Reactive • Psoriatic • Inflammatory bowel disease • Erythema nodosum • Palindromic • Plant thorn synovitis • Paraneoplastic	**Bone disease** • Osteomyelitis • Osteonecrosis **Blood disorders** • Leukaemia • Haemophilia • Anticoagulants **Other** • Villonodular synovitis • Tumours

Age and sex can be helpful indicators. A *reactive arthritis* following an enteric infection is the most common cause of an acute monoarthritis in young adults in the UK. *Disseminated gonococcal infection* is more frequent in the USA, and in females, but needs to be considered in all sexually active young people presenting with an acute monoarthritis or oligoarthritis. An associated tenosynovitis or pustular rash can be a useful additional pointer and diagnosis is based on the history, physical findings and culture of blood, synovial fluid and skin lesions as well as cultures from the cervix, urethra, throat and rectum.

Osteomyelitis and *leukaemia* are important causes of hot painful joints in children but *pauciarticular juvenile idiopathic arthritis* (see p. 852) and *septic arthritis* are more common. *Acute gouty arthritis* is seen more often in men and 70% of first attacks occur in the metatarsal joint of the great toe (see p. 832). Acute *pseudogout* seldom occurs before middle age. The typical presentation is in an elderly hospitalised patient recovering from another acute illness or major surgery. The patient may develop a single acutely painful swollen knee or ankle and the concern is whether or not he or she has developed septic arthritis or gout.

ACUTE SEPTIC ARTHRITIS

The priority is always to exclude infection and if there is any doubt the joint must be aspirated so that the synovial fluid can be examined for microorganisms. A history of fever, rigors or a polymorphonuclear leucocytosis may be important clues to the diagnosis but their absence does not exclude bacterial infection. Microorganisms usually reach the joint by haematogenous spread following bacteraemia so it is important to look for evidence of septic skin lesions, abrasions, or throat or urinary tract infection. Direct entry of organisms into joints following penetrating wounds or joint injections is much less common, as is direct spread from local osteomyelitis.

Management

Blood and synovial fluid should be cultured, and treatment started on a 'best guess' policy, using the antibiotics most likely to be effective, until the results of cultures are available. In adults, *Staphylococcus aureus* and *Streptococcus pyogenes* are the most common infecting organisms, but others are possible. In prosthetic joints, and in heavily immunosuppressed patients, more unusual organisms may be found. High-dose parenteral antibiotics for 2–3 weeks, followed by 9–10 weeks of oral antibiotics, are often required. The joint should be rested, usually in hospital, and regular joint aspiration is performed to remove pus. Once pain has reduced, gentle physiotherapy to maintain muscle strength and range of movement should be encouraged. It is important to be vigilant for the presence or development of infection elsewhere (e.g. lung, subphrenic abscess, pericardium or other joints). Outcome for the individual joint is recovery in about 70% of cases, with chronic disability affecting the remainder. If a prosthetic joint is infected, it will usually need to be removed. In practice, most patients with acute septic arthritis will have thick pus in the joint, rather than cloudy fluid which is typical of any inflammatory arthritis, and infection is most likely to occur in patients with a pre-existing arthritis such as rheumatoid arthritis. In such patients and in other immunosuppressed patients systemic features of infection may be absent and the joint itself may not be very acutely painful or inflamed.

CHRONIC INFLAMMATORY MONOARTHRITIS

Chronic inflammatory monoarthritis of more than 4 weeks' duration must raise the suspicion of infection with a slow-growing organism such as *Mycobacterium tuberculosis*, atypical mycobacteria or fungi, especially in immunosuppressed patients. Synovitis resulting from a plant thorn or other foreign body is a possibility if there has been a penetrating injury; villonodular synovitis and tumours may need to be considered. Arthroscopy, and synovial biopsy and culture are usually required in such cases.

POLYARTHRALGIA AND POLYARTHRITIS

Polyarthralgia (joint pain without clinical evidence of arthritis) is a frequent reason for consultation in primary care. The list of common causes is broad and ranges from trivial, self-limiting illnesses to potentially serious life-threatening, disabling diseases (see the information box).

A careful history and examination may be all that is needed to establish a diagnosis of bursitis, tendonitis, fibromyalgia or depression, but hypothyroidism and metabolic bone disease will require confirmation with thyroid function tests and plasma biochemical assays (see Fig. 12.12).

IMPORTANT CAUSES OF POLYARTHRALGIA

- Viral infections
- Depression
- Soft tissue rheumatism/fibromyalgia
- Bursitis/tendonitis at multiple sites
- Early systemic rheumatic diseases
- Hypothyroidism
- Metabolic bone disease

A number of viral infections are commonly associated with arthralgia and transient polyarthritis. These include parvovirus B19, hepatitis B and C, mumps, chickenpox, infectious mononucleosis, and adenoviral, enteroviral and arboviral infections. Hepatitis-associated arthritis occurs in up to 30% of patients with hepatitis B. Typically it is associated with fever and rash and precedes the onset of jaundice. Rubella arthritis follows 1–7 days after the rash or 2–6 weeks after vaccination in 30–40% of adults. A symmetrical inflammatory polyarthritis may be associated with symptoms of carpal tunnel compression or tenosynovitis. Joint pain, stiffness and swelling, which may be severe,

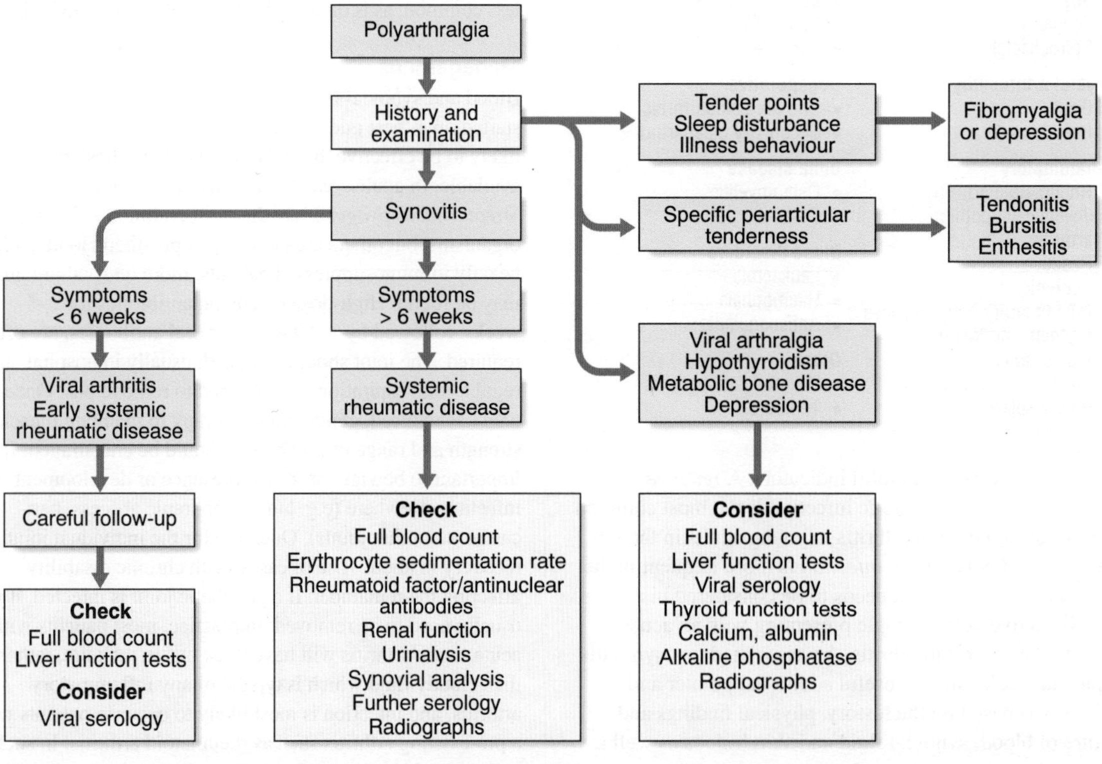

Fig. 12.12 An approach to the differential diagnosis of polyarthralgia. The algorithm illustrates guidelines for assessment of patients presenting with multiple joint pains.

usually settle in 1–4 weeks but the condition may persist with intermittent arthralgia for some months. Posterior cervical lymphadenopathy and a high lymphocyte count in the synovial fluid may be helpful in diagnosis.

At onset, it can be impossible to distinguish acute viral polyarthritis from persistent inflammatory joint disease. If viral titres confirm the diagnosis, then an optimistic prognosis and reassurance can be given that most cases will have resolved within 12 months of onset.

POLYARTHRITIS

The differential diagnosis of polyarthritis (arthritis affecting four or more joints) includes a wide range of systemic, inflammatory, metabolic and degenerative diseases (see the information box). A careful clinical history and general medical examination are mandatory, with particular attention being given to the onset, chronology and pattern of joint involvement. A definitive diagnosis may not be possible with polyarthritis of less than 6 weeks' duration.

Important diagnostic clues may be obtained from:

- the past medical history:
  - —previous episodes of characteristic arthritis in rheumatoid arthritis, reactive arthritis or gout
  - —low back pain and inactivity stiffness in ankylosing spondylitis
  - —extra-articular symptoms and signs (see Table 12.5)
- the family history:
  - —spondarthritis
  - —psoriasis
  - —gout
  - —nodal osteoarthritis
- the social and occupational history:
  - —heavy alcohol intake in gout
  - —intravenous drug abuse in septic arthritis or HIV infection
  - —sexual promiscuity in reactive or gonococcal arthritis
  - —occupational chemical exposure, e.g. vinyl chloride and Raynaud's phenomenon
  - —occupational trauma, e.g. farming and osteoarthritis in hips and knees.

CAUSES AND PATTERNS OF POLYARTHRITIS

Symmetrical inflammatory
- Viral arthritis
- Rheumatoid arthritis
- Juvenile idiopathic arthritis
- Systemic lupus erythematosus

Asymmetrical pauciarticular
- Psoriatic arthritis
- Reiter's syndrome
- Enteropathic arthritis
- Ankylosing spondylitis
- Behçet's disease
- Bacterial endocarditis
- Sarcoidosis
- Septic arthritis
- Pauciarticular juvenile idiopathic arthritis

Additive
- Gonococcal arthritis

Flitting
- Rheumatic fever
- Septicaemia

Metabolic
- Polyarticular gout
- Pyrophosphate arthropathy
- Acromegalic arthritis
- Haemochromatosis
- Hyperlipidaemia

Osteoarthritis
- Nodal osteoarthritis
- Non-nodal generalised osteoarthritis

Table 12.5 Common extra-articular features in rheumatic diseases

Disease	Extra-articular feature
Rheumatoid arthritis	Nodules, episcleritis, keratoconjunctivitis sicca, pleurisy, fibrosing alveolitis, pericarditis, neuropathies, nail fold vasculitis, Raynaud's phenomenon
Psoriatic arthritis	Psoriasis, nail changes
Reactive arthritis/Reiter's disease	Diarrhoea, urethritis, conjunctivitis, iritis, mouth ulcers, balanitis, keratoderma blennorrhagica, enthesitis
Ankylosing spondylitis	Iritis, enthesitis
Colitic arthritis	Ulcerative colitis, Crohn's disease, erythema nodosum
Sarcoidosis	Erythema nodosum, hilar lymphadenopathy
Gouty arthritis	Tophi, obesity, hypertension
Systemic lupus erythematosus	Raynaud's phenomenon, photosensitivity, rashes, alopecia, fever, pleurisy, pericarditis, renal disease, CNS disorders

LOW BACK PAIN

Non-specific low back pain of mechanical origin is second only to the common cold as a cause of self-limiting symptoms and disability in the community.

RHEUMATIC COMPLAINTS: WORLD HEALTH ORGANIZATION (WHO) CLASSIFICATION

- Back pain
- Regional periarticular or 'soft tissue' disorders
- Osteoarthritis and related disorders
- Inflammatory arthropathies

Epidemiology

It has been calculated that more than three-quarters of the world's population experience back pain at some time in their lives, and in developed Western countries low back pain is the most common cause of sickness-related absence from work. In the UK approximately 10% of people who suffer episodes of low back pain consult their general practitioner annually, more than 2 million consultations and more than 50 million days lost from work each year.

More than 90% of episodes of low back pain are of mechanical origin and most resolve spontaneously within 1–2 weeks. In about 30% of patients episodes can last as long as a month but chronic low back pain of more than 3 months' duration accounts for less than 3% of all cases.

Mechanical low back pain is particularly associated with occupations that involve heavy lifting, bending or twisting such as manual labouring or nursing, but people whose jobs involve awkward static posture or prolonged driving are also at increased risk. Episodes of occupationally related low back pain are twice as common in adults over the age of 40 years. The overall prevalence is similar in both sexes but recurrences are more common in men (20% in 1 year). Job dissatisfaction, depression, obesity, smoking, alcohol and socio-economic deprivation have also been implicated.

Aetiology

The common type of short-lived mechanical low back pain is not associated with a definable aetiology or spinal pathology. The causes of rarer but more serious chronic back pain are listed in the information box.

CAUSES OF BACK PAIN

Mechanical
- Prolapsed intervertebral disc
- Lumbar spondylosis
- Spondylolysis/ spondylolisthesis
- Spinal stenosis
- Congenital abnormalities
- Non-specific

Inflammatory
- Infections
- Sacroiliitis
- Ankylosing spondylitis
- Arachnoiditis

Metabolic
- Osteoporosis
- Osteomalacia
- Hyperparathyroidism
- Paget's disease

Neoplastic
- Metastases
- Myeloma
- Reticuloses
- Osteoid osteoma
- Intrathecal tumours

Referred pain
- Peptic ulcer
- Pancreas
- Bowel
- Kidney
- Aortic aneurysm
- Endometriosis
- Ovary
- Retroperitoneal fibrosis
- Herpes zoster
- Hip disease
- Polymyalgia rheumatica

Other
- Scheuermann's osteochondritis
- Diffuse idiopathic skeletal hyperostosis (DISH)
- Fibromyalgia

Clinical features

Mechanical low back pain is characteristically acute in onset and frequently associated with a definite history of lifting or bending (see the information box).

Radiation of pain to the thighs can be associated with sprains of muscles, ligaments and apophyseal joints as well as with nerve root irritation. However, pain which radiates down the back of the leg beyond the knee and pain which is aggravated by coughing, sneezing and straining at stool is usually associated with disc protrusion or other causes of nerve root compression. Radicular pain is frequently sharp and lancinating in quality and associated with signs of lumbar nerve root irritation (see Table 14.35, p. 1004).

Other medical and systemic causes of low back pain are usually more insidious in onset, more prolonged in duration and not so obviously influenced by posture and movement (see the information box).

SIMPLE MECHANICAL LOW BACK PAIN

History
- Sudden onset
- Precipitated by lifting or bending
- Recurrent episodes; age 20–50
- Pain limited to back or upper leg
- No clear-cut nerve root distribution
- Improved by resting
- General health good

Examination
- Asymmetrical movements of lumbar spine
- Asymmetrical straight leg raising
- Pain aggravated by movements
- No neurological deficit
- No back pain on axial loading or simulated rotation

Investigations
- No blood tests or radiograph required

Management
- Reassurance and positive approach
- Encourage normal physical activity
- Limit bed rest to 1–2 days in severe cases
- Simple analgesics
- Patient education
- Consider physical therapy

Outcome
- Recovery in 1–2 weeks

POINTERS TO BACK PAIN WITH SERIOUS PATHOLOGY
- Insidious onset
- Severe and progressive pain not relieved by rest
- Unremitting night pain
- Localisation to multiple spinal levels
- Age < 20 years or > 55 years
- Systemic illness, e.g. weight loss, night sweats
- Pain in thoracic spine
- Relevant medical history, e.g. malignancy, steroid treatment etc.

RED FLAGS FOR EMERGENCY INVESTIGATION
- Loss of bowel or bladder control
- Saddle area sensory disturbance or loss of sphincter tone
- Sensory level on neurological examination
- Bilateral leg pain with bilateral neurological deficit

Back pain due to sacroiliitis or spondylitis is typically ameliorated by physical activity and exercise as well as being associated with prolonged early morning and inactivity stiffness.

Systematic enquiry may give important clues to rarer causes of back pain. Anorexia, weight loss or dyspepsia may point to a penetrating peptic ulcer, or gastric or pancreatic tumour, while changes in bowel habit, prostatism or gynaecological symptoms can be clues to colon cancer, prostatic metastases, endometriosis or uterine/ovarian malignancies.

A history of intermittent claudication may be an indication of severe peripheral vascular disease, spinal stenosis or lateral canal stenosis.

Social and psychiatric assessment is also important, as primary and secondary illness behaviour is relatively frequent in patients with chronic low back pain, particularly when litigation or insurance claims are pending.

Local tenderness over the spine, loss of lumbar lordosis and postural changes associated with muscle spasm and an uncompensated non-structural scoliosis are common physical signs associated with all causes of mechanical low back pain. Disc prolapse and other causes of nerve root compression can frequently be established by careful neurological assessment, and the diagnosis of early sacroiliitis and spondylitis may be entirely dependent on physical assessment (see p. 849) in the early stages.

Clinical tests that help to identify individuals with functional, non-organic back pain are shown in the information box.

TESTS FOR FUNCTIONAL LOW BACK PAIN

- Tenderness to superficial touch
- Simulation tests, e.g. pain on axial loading or spinal rotation in one plane
- Distraction tests, e.g. limited straight leg raising but able to sit with legs flexed to 90°
- Regional inconsistencies, e.g. symptoms and sensory loss that fail to follow neuro-anatomy
- Over-reaction to examination with illness behaviour

N.B. Three out of five positive tests strongly suggest a non-organic cause for symptoms.

Investigations

Blood tests and radiographs are rarely helpful in patients with acute low back pain.

A low haemoglobin and raised CRP or ESR may augment a clinical suspicion of inflammation or malignancy. A raised acid phosphatase or prostate-specific antigen (PSA) is associated with metastatic carcinoma of the prostate, and raised alkaline phosphatase with other bone metastases and Paget's disease. Myelomatosis is associated with a monoclonal band on immunoelectrophoresis and the presence of urine light chains (Bence Jones proteinuria).

Plain radiographs are indicated in all patients whose pain has not resolved spontaneously within 1 month, but are only of clear diagnostic value in a minority of patients with sacroiliitis, ankylosing spondylitis, Paget's disease, lytic or sclerotic metastases, myelomatosis, osteoporotic crush fractures or spinal infections. Disc degeneration can be associated with loss of disc height and gas formation in the nucleus pulposus as well as with vertebral sclerosis and osteophyte formation but radiological signs of lumbar spondylosis are common in middle-aged and elderly people in the absence of symptoms. Minor congenital abnormalities, such as spina bifida occulta and transitional vertebrae, are not associated with low back pain. Bone scintigraphy with ^{99m}-Tc bisphosphonate is the imaging technique of choice for detecting the presence and extent of metastases and Paget's disease, and can also be useful for the identification of fractures and bone infection when plain radiographs are negative. MRI is rapidly becoming the imaging modality of choice for defining most difficult spinal pathology where surgery is being considered (see Fig. 12.9, p. 810). CT is, however, superior for detection of subtle abnormalities of the bony architecture of the spine and sacroiliac joints in patients with back pain and normal plain radiographs. Myelography and CT myelography are particularly useful for the pre-operative assessment of the site of tumours, disc herniation and nerve root entrapment and are also employed when MRI is contraindicated because of the presence of a cardiac pace-maker or ferromagnetic clips. EMG and nerve conduction studies, with or without measurement of somatosensory evoked responses, are occasionally required to confirm the localisation of nerve root lesions.

Even the most sophisticated investigation techniques seldom reveal treatable new pathology in patients with chronic low back pain of more than a year's duration.

Management

Most episodes of mechanical low back pain settle spontaneously in 1–2 weeks with explanation, reassurance and simple analgesics without the need for bed rest. In more severe cases short-term home help or nursing services may be required and mobilisation can be facilitated by provision of a temporary lumbar corset and/or exercise physiotherapy. The McKenzie technique of passive extension and postural correction can speed up return to work, as can manipulation in some cases.

Chiropractic manipulation has also been shown to be superior to hydrotherapy and traction in patients with chronic low back pain but controlled clinical trials have failed to show that treatment with short-wave diathermy, ultrasound, acupuncture or transcutaneous nerve stimulation (TENS) have anything more than a placebo effect.

Epidural corticosteroid injections are occasionally used in patients with nerve root compression that has failed to respond to more conservative treatment, and facet joint injections of steroid and/or local anaesthetic are sometimes used under fluoroscopic control in patients with apophyseal joint pathology simulating nerve root irritation, but the efficacy of such injections remains uncertain.

Intractable low back pain may be helped by the judicious use of tricyclic antidepressants to augment analgesia or relieve depression while psychological counselling and social support are indicated in selected cases. Surgery is required in less than 1% of patients with low back pain.

LUMBAR SPONDYLOSIS

Degenerative changes in the discs and lumbar spine are almost universal in the elderly.

Aetiology

Disc degeneration is age-related and starts in the third decade. Reduction in the molecular size of the proteoglycans of the nucleus pulposus is associated with loss of viscoelastic properties. Increased load-bearing by the annulus is followed by focal damage and disc herniation in some cases (see Fig. 12.13). Simultaneously, the development of osteoarthritic changes in the spinal apophyseal joints leads to increases in sheer stress and disc damage with cleft formation and osteophyte formation around the vertebral margins. The combination of disc prolapse and osteophytosis can result in direct nerve root compression and indirect ischaemic neuronal damage.

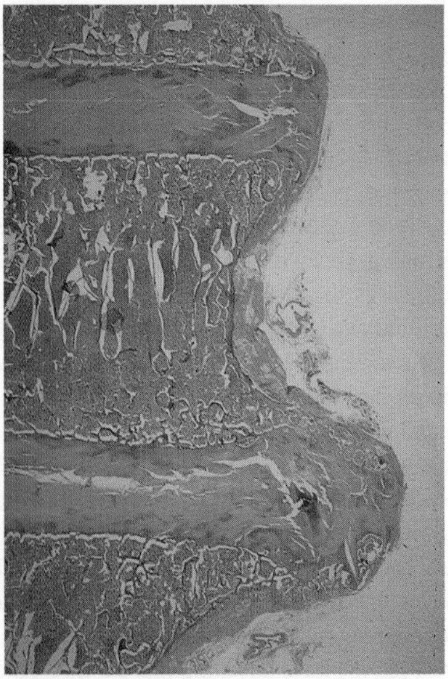

Fig. 12.13 Lumbar spondylosis. Low-power cross-section of vertebral column showing disc degeneration and osteophytosis.

Clinical features

Advanced lumbar spondylosis is frequently associated with low back pain but the clinical features are very variable and there is a poor correlation between symptoms and radiographic changes. Postural low back pain is often provoked by prolonged sitting, standing, bending or lifting. Acute episodes with symptoms and signs of nerve root compression are similar to those following acute disc prolapse (see p. 1001), and investigation and management follow the same lines.

SPONDYLOLYSIS AND SPONDYLOLISTHESIS

Spondylolysis describes a simple defect in the pars interarticularis. In spondylolisthesis a vertebra slips forward on the one below and this is usually associated with spondylolysis (see Fig. 12.14).

Aetiology

Spondylolisthesis may be congenital, post-traumatic or degenerative. Rarely, it can result from metastatic destruction of the posterior elements.

Clinical features

Uncomplicated spondylolysis is not associated with symptoms but spondylolisthesis is variably associated with low back pain aggravated by standing and walking. More severe cases can result in nerve root compression or a lumbar stenosis syndrome and the vertebral slip is occasionally palpable.

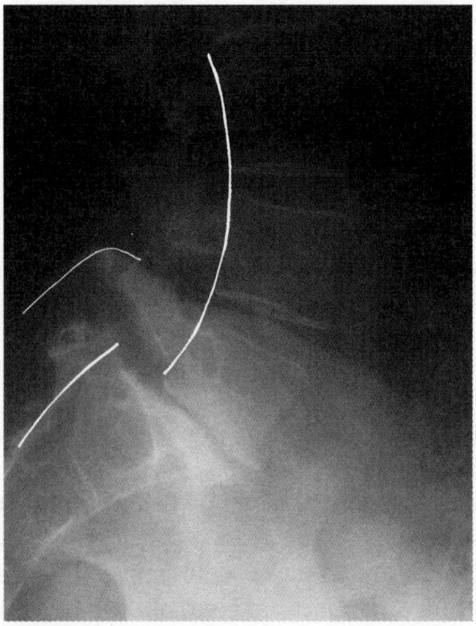

Fig. 12.14 Lumbar spondylolisthesis. Lateral radiograph showing L5/S1 spondylolisthesis with disc space narrowing, sclerosis and a defect in the posterior element (spondylolysis).

Investigations

Spondylolysis and spondylolisthesis can be easily diagnosed with lateral or oblique radiographs of the lumbar spine (see Fig. 12.14). MRI may be required if there is nerve root involvement.

Management

Postural advice and muscle-strengthening exercises are all that are required in milder cases. Surgical fusion is indicated in patients with severe and recurrent low back pain, and surgical decompression is mandatory prior to fusion in patients with significant lumbar stenosis or symptoms of cauda equina compression.

ARACHNOIDITIS

Severe low back pain with or without nerve root symptoms can be associated with chronic inflammation of the nerve root sheaths in the spinal canal. Chronic arachnoiditis may be a complication of meningitis or spinal surgery but is seen most frequently as a late complication of myelography with oil-based contrast agents. The diagnosis can be confirmed by MRI or radiculography but no satisfactory treatment is available.

SCHEUERMANN'S OSTEOCHONDRITIS

This disorder of unknown aetiology is seen predominantly in male adolescents who develop a painless dorsal kyphosis in association with irregular ossification of the vertebral end plates. Back pain, aggravated by exercise and relieved by rest, occurs if the vertebrae of the upper lumbar spine are affected and secondary spondylosis can follow in middle age. Excessive exercise and heavy manual labour before epiphyseal fusion has occurred may aggravate the problem. Treatment is with rest and protective postural exercises. The deformity is seldom severe enough to warrant corrective surgery.

DIFFUSE IDIOPATHIC SKELETAL HYPEROSTOSIS (DISH)

DISH, also known as *Forrestier's disease* and *ankylosing hyperostosis*, is a chronic age-related disorder characterised by exuberant new bone formation. The condition is defined radiologically by the presence of flowing ossification along the anterolateral aspect of at least four contiguous vertebral bodies (see Fig. 12.15). It is distinguished from lumbar spondylosis by the preservation of disc height and the absence of the vacuum phenomenon or marginal sclerosis of the vertebral bodies; and from ankylosing spondylitis by the absence of sacroiliitis or apophyseal joint fusion.

Epidemiology

DISH is a common disorder in the elderly, seen in 10% of males and 8% of females over the age of 65 years. It is seldom seen below the age of 45. The prevalence in male Pima Indians is greater than 50% and this may reflect their high prevalence of obesity and diabetes mellitus.

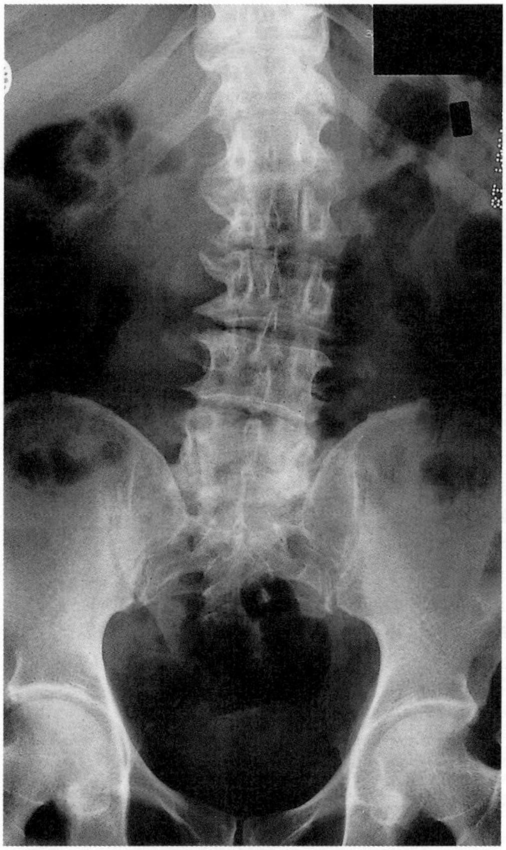

Fig. 12.15 Diffuse idiopathic skeletal hyperostosis (DISH). Radiograph of thoracolumbar spine showing typical appearances of flowing ossification of more than four contiguous vertebrae. The disc spaces are preserved and the sacroiliac joints are normal.

Aetiology and pathogenesis

DISH appears to be the consequence of a systemic disturbance which results in excessive proteoglycan production at entheses prior to ossification and hyperostosis. It occurs more frequently in association with gout, obesity, hypertension, type II diabetes mellitus and hyperinsulinaemia, but growth hormone and somatomedin levels are not increased. Hyperostosis occurs predominantly on the right side of the thoracolumbar spine, except in patients with situs inversus, suggesting that the presence of the aorta influences the development of ossification in some way. Hyperostosis can also be a complication of systemic therapy with retinoids (see p. 903).

Clinical features

The development of DISH can be associated with restriction of movements of the neck and spine or it may be detected as an asymptomatic radiographic finding. It is seldom associated with pain in the axial skeleton. Heel pain can occur in association with calcaneal spur formation and DISH may be associated occasionally with a form of hypertrophic hip osteoarthrosis. Extraspinal ossification at other sites such as the olecranon and patella is seldom associated with symptoms. Dysphagia, cervical myelopathy and lumbar stenosis are rare complications.

Investigations

The diagnosis is established with simple radiographs. MRI, CT or myelography is only required if lumbar stenosis is suspected.

Management

In the absence of any specific therapy, management involves general advice with regard to weight loss and the maintenance of musculoskeletal fitness. Heel pads and suitable footwear are generally more effective than steroid injections for patients with heel pain and calcaneal spurs.

NECK PAIN

Neck pain, stiffness and restriction of movements are frequent consequences of trauma and degenerative disorders of the cervical spine.

Epidemiology

Transient episodes of acute neck pain and stiffness occur in 40–50% of all adults, with an increasing incidence in those over the age of 45 years. Many attacks appear to be precipitated by awkward sleeping posture and most resolve spontaneously within 1–4 days.

Neck pain of mechanical origin is less common than low back pain as a cause of industrial disability but assembly line workers and heavy manual labourers are at particular risk. Violinists and other performing artists are prone to recurrent neck pain of postural origin.

More prolonged neck pain and stiffness lasting up to 2–3 months is a frequent sequel of 'whiplash' flexion/hyperextension injuries in up to 50% of all serious car collisions, even in the absence of fracture or nerve root injury. More protracted disability in such patients is often associated with compensation claims and secondary psychological problems.

Aetiology

The common types of transient acute neck pain and stiffness are not associated with definable aetiology or spinal pathology. Other causes of neck pain are listed in the information box.

CAUSES OF NECK PAIN

Mechanical
- Postural
- Whiplash injury
- Disc prolapse
- Cervical spondylosis
- Thoracic outlet/neurovascular syndromes

Inflammatory
- Infections
- Ankylosing spondylitis
- Juvenile idiopathic arthritis
- Rheumatoid arthritis
- Polymyalgia rheumatica

Metabolic
- Osteoporosis
- Osteomalacia
- Paget's disease
- Crystal arthropathies

Neoplastic
- Metastases
- Myeloma
- Reticulosis
- Intrathecal tumours

Other
- Torticollis
- Fibromyalgia

Referred pain
- Angina pectoris
- Aortic aneurysm
- Pancoast tumour
- Diaphragm
- Pharynx
- Cervical lymph nodes
- Teeth
- Acromioclavicular joints
- Shoulder

Clinical features

Mechanical neck pain is characteristically acute in onset and associated with restriction of neck movements and a history of awkward posture or trauma. The pain is frequently referred to the occiput or shoulders as well as the nuchal muscles, and neck pain associated with acute disc prolapse may be aggravated by coughing and sneezing. Occipital, retro-orbital and temporal referral of pain suggests pathology in the atlas, axis or 3rd cervical vertebra while interscapular pain and anterior chest wall pain masquerading as angina may be associated with lesions of the lower cervical spine (C6 and C7). Neck pain associated with disc protrusions or cervical spondylosis is frequently complicated by cervical radiculopathy with characteristic radiation of pain, paraesthesiae, sensory loss, muscle weakness, wasting and reflex changes in the arm (see p. 1001).

Inflammatory, metabolic and neoplastic diseases are associated with neck pain that is more insidious in onset, more prolonged in duration and usually not so obviously influenced by posture and movement.

Investigations

Blood tests, radiography, CT, bone scintigraphy and nerve conduction studies are selectively employed as in patients with low back pain (see p. 817).

MRI has become the imaging modality of choice for detecting minor disc prolapse as well as spinal cord pathology (see Fig. 12.16). Lumbar puncture and CSF examination are essential in patients with suspected meningitis or subarachnoid haemorrhage.

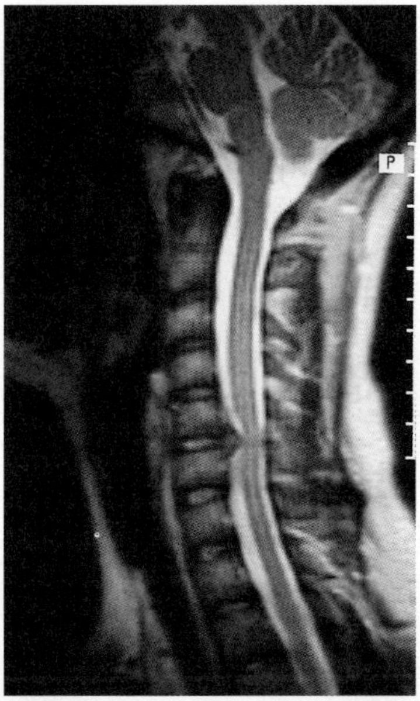

Fig. 12.16 Cervical disc prolapse. MRI of cervical spine showing disc prolapse at C5/6.

Management

Most episodes of mechanical and postural acute neck pain will resolve in less than a week with nothing more than simple analgesics, a soft collar and strong reassurance. Traction can be effective in patients with more severe and more prolonged acute neck pain associated with disc prolapse and radiculopathy. Traction can rarely be associated with vertebral artery damage or neurological complications and should never be used in patients with radiographic evidence of advanced cervical spondylosis or other pathology. Chronic cervical pain syndromes are best treated conservatively with postural advice, muscle-strengthening exercises, judicious use of analgesics and a cervical collar during acute exacerbations. Surgery is only rarely required in patients with symptoms and neurological signs of radiculopathy or progressive cervical myelopathy.

CERVICAL SPONDYLOSIS

Disc degeneration with associated osteophyte formation and osteoarthritis of the spinal apophyseal joints, collectively termed cervical spondylosis, is almost universal in elderly people.

Aetiology and pathogenesis

See lumbar spondylosis, page 818.

Clinical features

Two-thirds of patients over the age of 65 years experience neck pain in association with cervical spondylosis but there is a poor correlation between symptoms and radiographic signs. Cervical radiculopathy is associated with characteristic radiation of pain, paraesthesiae, sensory loss, muscle weakness, wasting and reflex changes in the arm (see p. 1001). Drop attacks and vertigo precipitated by neck extension are common consequences of vertebro-basilar ischaemia, while visual disturbance, unsteadiness, nausea, dyspnoea and cardiac arrhythmias are rarely the result of sympathetic nerve stimulation. Dysphagia is occasionally caused by massive osteophyte formation.

FIBROMYALGIA (FIBROSITIS, MYOFASCIAL PAIN SYNDROME)

This is a very common but poorly defined syndrome of chronic musculoskeletal pain that affects about 2% of all patients seen in general practice and as many as 20% of patients referred to rheumatologists in the USA. It usually occurs between the ages of 20 and 60 and is 10 times more frequent in women.

Clinical features

The syndrome is characterised by diffuse muscle pain, stiffness and fatigue in association with sleep disturbance and focal point tenderness. Additional features frequently include tension headaches, dysmenorrhoea and symptoms of an irritable bowel syndrome suggesting a strong psychosomatic component. A proportion of patients have features of anxiety and depression.

Investigations

Radiographs and laboratory investigations (full blood count, ESR, creatine kinase and serological tests for RF and ANA) are only helpful in excluding other more serious pathology. EMG and nerve conduction studies are normal but most patients have a disturbance of stage IV non-rapid eye movement sleep on EEG.

Management

Strong medical reassurance, coupled with advice from a physiotherapist about posture and improving physical fitness, can sometimes be helpful. A small evening dose of a tricyclic antidepressant may improve sleep but the condition tends to have a chronic and protracted course in most patients.

SHOULDER PAIN

Shoulder pain is the most common musculoskeletal complaint in men and women over the age of 40 years. It is

COMMON CAUSES OF SHOULDER PAIN
Extracapsular
• Rotator cuff lesions Supraspinatus tendonitis or tear Calcific tendonitis Subacromial bursitis Infraspinatus tendonitis Subscapularis lesions • Bicipital tendonitis or tear
Acromioclavicular
• Arthritis
Glenohumeral
• Arthritis • Capsulitis • Bone disease
Referred
• Cervical nerve root • Ischaemic heart disease • Subdiaphragmatic pathology • Reflex sympathetic dystrophy • Polymyalgia rheumatica

most frequently associated with extracapsular traumatic, inflammatory or degenerative lesions of the tendons of the rotator cuff. Other important causes are listed in the information box.

Most painful shoulders can be diagnosed without the need for imaging. Radiographs are required, however, if shoulder pain persists, and ultrasound or MRI is occasionally used to localise rotator cuff tears and distinguish tears from tendonitis.

Supraspinatus tendonitis results from impingement of the tendon on the acromion (see Fig. 12.17). It is

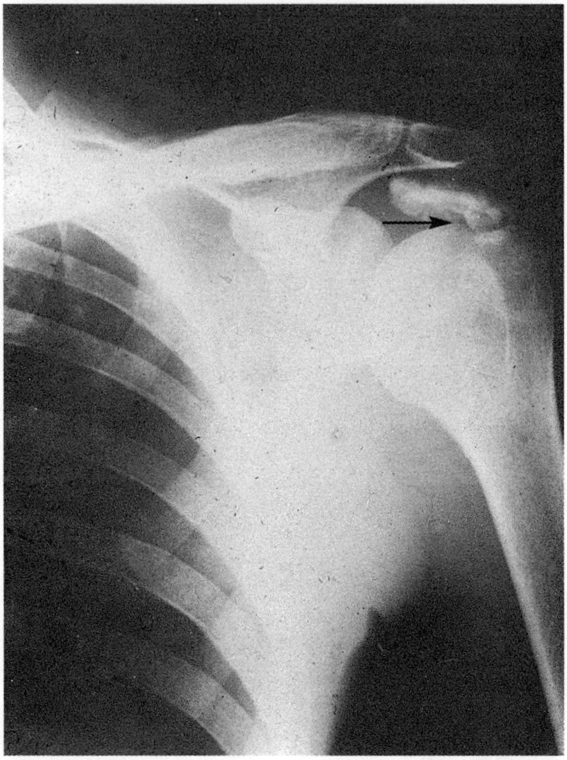

Fig. 12.18 Supraspinatus tendonitis. Radiograph showing soft tissue calcification in the subacromial space (arrow).

characterised by a 'painful arc' on abduction of the arm which can be abolished by external rotation, as well as by local tenderness over the greater tuberosity and pain on resisted abduction. *Partial tears* are associated with identical symptoms and signs. In some cases there is

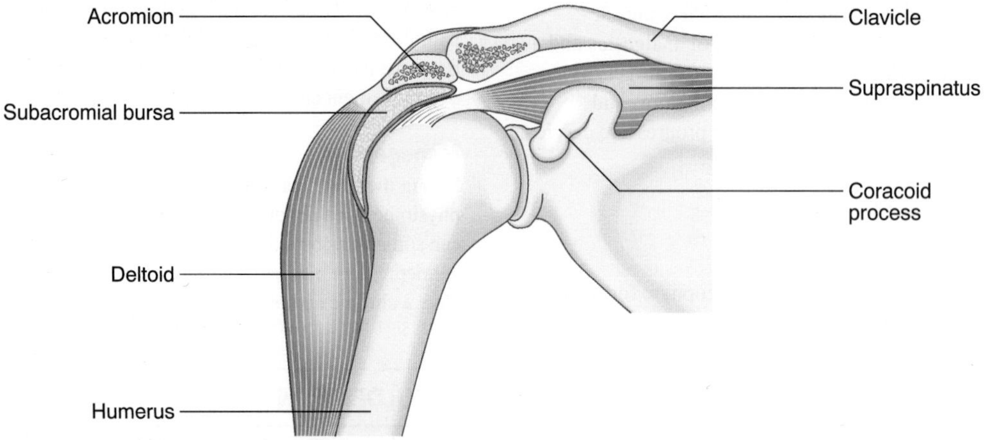

Fig. 12.17 Cross-section of shoulder joint showing relationships of rotator cuff tendons.

radiographic evidence of calcific deposits *(calcific tendonitis)* (see Fig. 12.18). Rupture of calcific material into the subacromial bursa occasionally results in acutely painful gout-like attacks of inflammatory *subacromial bursitis*. Fluid aspirated from the bursa contains crystals of calcium hydroxyapatite. Treatment is with local injection of steroid.

Bicipital tendonitis can be recognised by pain and tenderness in the bicipital groove aggravated by resisted flexion of the elbow.

Infraspinatus tendonitis is associated with pain on resisted external rotation, while *subscapularis lesions* cause pain on resisted internal rotation of the arm.

Capsulitis (frozen shoulder) is a common and disabling condition in which severe spontaneous shoulder pain is initially associated with capsular tenderness and painful restriction of all shoulder movements, and later with painless restriction of movements alone. A frozen shoulder may be a late consequence of a rotator cuff lesion and sometimes follows myocardial infarction, hemiplegia, herpes zoster, or breast or thoracic surgery.

Treatment is with analgesics and local corticosteroid injection in the early phase, and mobilising exercises after the pain has resolved.

The natural history is for slow but complete recovery, the complete cycle sometimes taking as long as 2 years.

SHOULDER-HAND SYNDROME

This syndrome is characterised by burning pain, vasomotor changes and severe limitation of movement of the hand in association with restriction of shoulder movements. A radiograph of the hand shows patchy osteoporosis after some weeks or months. It is a manifestation of *complex reflex sympathetic dystrophy* and may be a sequel to the same disorders that precede a frozen shoulder. Epilepsy, barbiturates and antituberculous drugs can also be predisposing factors. Exaggerated illness behaviour is a feature in some patients.

Treatment is aimed at mobilising the affected limb. Analgesics, a short course of systemic corticosteroids, sympathetic nerve block and physiotherapy each have their advocates in this difficult situation. The prognosis for recovery is less certain than in frozen shoulder.

ELBOW PAIN

Elbow pain may be referred from the shoulder, cervical spine or brachial plexus, but periarticular soft tissue lesions are common.

'Tennis elbow' is associated with mild inflammation and/or partial tears of the origin of the extensor muscles at the lateral epicondyle. Local tenderness and pain on active wrist extension are characteristic, and treatment is with local corticosteroid injection, ultrasound and/or advice concerning inappropriate use.

'Golfer's elbow' results from similar lesions in the origin of the common flexor tendon at the medial epicondyle, and treatment is also with local corticosteroid injections, ultrasound and general advice concerning musculoskeletal protection.

Olecranon bursitis can follow local trauma but infection, gout and rheumatoid arthritis are also important causes that need to be considered.

HAND AND WRIST PAIN

Non-articular causes of hand pain include:

- tenosynovitis
- median nerve compression (carpal tunnel syndrome)
- C8/T1 radiculopathy
- thoracic outlet syndrome
- algodystrophy (reflex sympathetic dystrophy)
- angina pectoris
- Raynaud's phenomenon.

Trigger finger results from stenosing tenosynovitis in the flexor tendon sheath, with intermittent locking of the finger in flexion. A local corticosteroid injection usually relieves the problem and surgical decompression is only occasionally required.

De Quervain's tenosynovitis results from traumatic or work-related tenosynovitis of the tendon sheaths of abductor pollicis longus and extensor pollicis brevis. Pain on moving the thumb and wrist is associated with tenderness in the 'anatomical snuff-box' between the tendons and pain on forced ulnar deviation of the wrist with the thumb apposed to the palm (Finkelstein's sign). Treatment is primarily with rest and splinting but local corticosteroid injection is occasionally required. Surgical decompression is very rarely necessary.

Dupuytren's contracture results from fibrosis and contracture of the superficial palmar fascia. Inability to extend the fingers is associated with puckering of the skin and the presence of palpable nodules. The fourth finger is usually the earliest to be affected. The condition is age-related and occurs four times more frequently in men. Undetermined genetic factors are clearly involved, with a dominant pattern of inheritance. An association with knuckle pads, plantar fibromatosis and Peyronie's disease in some patients suggests the possibility of a generalised susceptibility to fibrosis in connective tissues. Dupuytren's contracture can also occur in association with alcohol misuse, epilepsy and chronic pulmonary disorders but must be distinguished from cheiro-arthropathy in patients with diabetes mellitus and flexor tendon tenosynovitis in patients with rheumatoid arthritis and other types of inflammatory polyarthritis. Local protection, stretching exercises and strong reassurance are all that is required in most patients but progressive deformities with functional impairment necessitate fasciectomy in a few.

HIP PAIN

Pain in the region of the hip is frequently associated with periarticular tendonitis or bursitis as well as with bone disorders and arthritis of the hips and sacroiliac joints. Common causes of referred pain are shown in Table 12.6.

Trochanteric bursitis is associated with aching or burning pain over the lateral aspect of the hip and thigh, which is aggravated by walking, squatting and resisted abduction of the hip. There may be local tenderness and swelling over the greater trochanter.

Radiographs may show periosteal irregularity and some calcification around the trochanter. Treatment is with rest, analgesics and local corticosteroid injection.

Iliopsoas bursitis occurs in association with inflammatory or degenerative arthritis of the hip. Patients may present with a painless or painful inguinal swelling, a swollen leg or symptoms and signs of femoral nerve compression. The diagnosis can be confirmed by ultrasound, CT, MRI or arthrography. If treatment with local corticosteroid is ineffective, surgical excision is required.

Iliogluteal bursitis ('Weaver's bottom') is associated with pain and tenderness over the ischial tuberosities, which is aggravated by sitting and lying. Treatment is with local corticosteroid injection and the avoidance of local pressure.

Adductor tendonitis causes groin pain which is aggravated by abduction and resisted adduction of the hip; this is usually a sports-related problem in gymnasts or horseback riders. Treatment is with rest and analgesics, and corticosteroid injections are seldom required.

Table 12.6 Referred pain in the hip region

Source of pain	Site of pain
Sacroiliac joints	Buttock
Thoracolumbar spine	
T12–L1	Greater trochanter
L2–L4	Inguinal region + anterior thigh
Abdominal pathology	
Psoas abscess Pelvic inflammation Retroperitoneal haemorrhage	Groin + anterior thigh aggravated by resisted hip flexion
Femoral/inguinal hernias	Groin + anterior thigh
Vascular disease	
Aortic aneurysm Iliac artery thrombosis	Claudication of buttock or thigh

KNEE PAIN

Knee pain, locking and effusion commonly result from meniscus tears, loose bodies or osteochondritis dissecans in children and adolescents. Pain may be referred from pathology in the hip or spine (see Table 12.7). Periarticular causes of knee pain in adults include ligament injuries, tendonitis, enthesitis and bursitis.

Prepatellar bursitis ('housemaid's knee') most frequently follows the trauma of prolonged or unaccustomed kneeling but infection and gout need to be considered and the bursa aspirated for microscopy and culture if there is any doubt. Most cases settle solely with rest and the avoidance of kneeling.

Infrapatellar bursitis is characterised by swelling and tenderness adjacent to the insertion of the patellar tendon into the tibial tubercle when the knee is extended.

Anserine bursitis presents as pain and tenderness on the medial side of the lower femur. Women with valgus deformities of the knees are particularly susceptible but it may be hard to distinguish from *tendonitis* and *medial ligament sprains* in runners. Treatment is with rest and analgesics and local corticosteroid injection.

Impingement of a medial patellar *plica* can be associated with pain over the medial femoral condyle and a sensation of snapping. The diagnosis is confirmed by detecting an inflamed plica on arthroscopy, and the problem is relieved by arthroscopic resection.

Pellegrini–Stieda disease is a cause of pain and tenderness over the medial side of the lower femur. It follows injuries to the medial collateral ligament and is characteristically associated with calcification at the ligament insertion on radiograph. Symptoms usually settle with rest and analgesics alone.

Anterior knee pain is a common problem in adolescent girls. Characteristically, the pain is worse at night and aggravated by sporting activities. In a small proportion of

Table 12.7 Common causes of referred knee pain

Source of pain	Age group
Osteomyelitis (femur or tibia) **Acute synovitis of hip** **Perthes' disease**	Childhood
Slipped femoral epiphysis **Bone tumour** **Osteomyelitis**	Adolescence
Osteoarthritis of hip	Adult

these patients there is evidence of non-progressive fibrillation of the articular cartilage of the patella on arthroscopy—*chondromalacia patellae*. The condition is self-limiting and treatment should be conservative, with quadriceps-strengthening exercises, stretching of the hamstrings and the avoidance of high heels.

Osgood–Schlatter's disease is due to apophysitis of the tibial tubercle. Adolescents present with pain, swelling and tenderness at the patella tendon insertion, aggravated by resisted extension of the knee. Lateral radiographs show fragmentation of the tibial tubercle. In most patients symptoms settle with rest and disappear altogether following fusion of the tibial tubercle.

The *anterior tibial compartment syndrome* is characterised by severe pain in the front of the lower leg, which is aggravated by exercise and relieved by rest. Symptoms result from fascial compression of the muscles in the anterior tibial compartment and may be associated with a foot drop. Treatment is by surgical decompression.

FOOT AND ANKLE PAIN

Pes planus ('flat foot') results from loss of the longitudinal arch. Pain is only experienced following ligament sprains, excessive walking or weight gain, or if there is associated spasm of the peroneal muscles. Acquired causes of pes planus include trauma, constitutional hypermobility, rheumatoid arthritis and neuropathic arthropathies. Medial arch supports in well-fitting shoes and/or intrinsic muscle-strengthening exercises will relieve symptoms in most cases but individually moulded rigid orthotics are required for patients with hyperpronated feet, provided the foot is not rigid as a result of fusion of the tarsal bones (tarsal coalition).

Pes cavus ('claw foot') is characterised by the presence of a high medial arch and secondary metatarsal callosities with clawing of the toes. Rarely, it is associated with neurological disorders such as Friedreich's ataxia, spina bifida or poliomyelitis. Foot pain can be ameliorated with medial arch supports and metatarsal insoles in most patients, and surgical intervention with fasciectomy or osteotomy are only very rarely indicated.

Hallux valgus deformity with secondary bursitis (bunions) and osteoarthritis of the first metatarsophalangeal joints is commonly associated with local forefoot pain and flattening of the transverse metatarsal arch. The problem is more common in women as a consequence of wearing narrow high-heeled shoes. Surgical correction is required in patients with intractable pain and severe deformity but most patients respond to adjustment of footwear alone.

Hallux rigidus is associated with severe intermittent aching pain and restriction of movements of the first metatarsophalangeal joint. This is usually secondary to osteoarthritis in the elderly but occasionally occurs as a primary problem without obvious cause in young adults. Treatment is with wide-fitting shoes with rigid soles and metatarsal bars. Arthrodesis is rarely required.

Morton's neuroma is the name given to an entrapment neuropathy of the interdigital nerves which occurs most frequently between the third and fourth metatarsal heads in middle-aged women who wear ill-fitting shoes. Neuralgic, lancinating pain, which is characteristically aggravated by wearing shoes, may be associated with local sensory loss and a palpable tender mass between the metatarsal heads. Many patients respond to adjustment of footwear with or without a local corticosteroid injection but surgical excision is occasionally required.

Non-articular causes of hind foot pain in adults include *Achilles tendon tears*, *Achilles tendonitis* and *retrocalcaneal bursitis*. Pain and local tenderness at the Achilles tendon insertion in boys can be associated with *retrocalcaneal apophysitis* (Sever's disease). Achilles tendon ruptures require surgical repair, but other causes of pain behind the heel are managed conservatively with rest, local protective padding and a raised heel; corticosteroid injections are contraindicated.

Plantar fasciitis is associated with pain and tenderness under the heel on standing or walking. In some cases this results from an inflammatory enthesitis as part of a seronegative spondarthritis (see p. 849), and may or may not be associated with the presence of a calcaneal spur on radiograph. Treatment is with silicone heel pads, ultrasound or occasionally local corticosteroid injection.

FURTHER INFORMATION ON MAJOR MANIFESTATIONS OF JOINT DISEASE

American College of Rheumatology Ad-hoc Committee on Clinical Guidelines 1996 Guidelines for the initial evaluation of the adult patient with acute musculoskeletal symptoms. Arthritis and Rheumatism 39: 1–8

Baker D G, Schumacher Jnr H R 1993 Acute monoarthritis. New England Journal of Medicine 319: 1013–1015

Borenstein D G, Wiesel S W, Boden S D 1995 Low back pain: medical diagnosis and comprehensive management, 2nd edn. W B Saunders, Philadelphia, pp. 299–337

Frey C 1996 Hindfoot disorders. Current Opinion in Orthopaedics 7: 17–21

Nordin M, Cedrashi C, Vischer T L (eds) 1998 New approaches to the low back pain patient. Baillière's Clinical Rheumatology 12: 1–173

Suarez-Almazor M E, Belseck E, Russell A S et al 1997 Use of lumbar radiographs for early diagnosis of low back pain: proposed guidelines would increase utilisation. Journal of the American Medical Association 277: 1782–1786

Swezey R L 1996 Chronic neck pain. Rheumatic Disease Clinics of North America 22: 411–438

Waddell G 1982 An approach to backache. British Journal of Hospital Medicine 28: 187–219

OSTEOARTHRITIS AND RELATED DISORDERS

OSTEOARTHRITIS

Osteoarthritis (OA, osteoarthrosis or degenerative joint disease) is not a single disease. Rather it is the end result of a variety of patterns of joint failure. To a greater or lesser extent it is always characterised by both degeneration of articular cartilage and simultaneous proliferation of new bone, cartilage and connective tissue. The proliferative response results in some degree of remodelling of the joint contour. Inflammatory changes in the synovium are usually minor and secondary.

Epidemiology

Radiological and autopsy surveys show a steady rise in degenerative changes in joints from the age of 30. By the age of 65, 80% of people have some radiographic evidence of osteoarthritis, although only 25% may have symptoms. Males and females are both affected but OA is more generalised and more severe in older women. Geographical surveys show differences in both the prevalence of OA and the pattern of joint involvement. OA of the hips is much more frequent in Caucasians than in Blacks or Chinese. Twin and family studies show the importance of genetic factors, particularly in the nodal form of primary generalised osteoarthritis, and associations have been reported with the HLA-A_1B_8 and α_1-antitrypsin MZ phenotypes. Obesity and body mass index are particularly associated with knee OA, while osteoporosis and smoking appear to have a modest protective effect. Cold, damp climates are associated with more symptoms but not with greater radiological prevalence.

Aetiology and pathogenesis

OA is classified as primary if the aetiology is unknown and secondary when degenerative joint changes occur in response to a recognisable local or systemic factor. The causes of secondary osteoarthritis are listed in the information box. Developmental abnormalities are believed to be of major importance in the aetiology of OA of the hip, and collagen gene defects have been identified in a few families in whom familial, premature, polyarticular OA is associated with an epiphyseal or spondyloepiphyseal dysplasia. Epidemiological surveys suggest that physical factors involved in occupations such as farming are important determinants in hip OA. Abnormal surface contacts and weight-bearing alignments lead to increased local mechanical stress and wear. Post-traumatic malalignment and incongruity of joints are well established as important predisposing causes of premature OA.

Metabolic diseases lead to degeneration of cartilage by very different mechanisms. In alkaptonuria (ochronosis) a genetically determined defect of homogentisic acid oxidase results in the accumulation of a pigmented polymer that binds to collagen, rendering it brittle and prone to mechanical degradation. Crystal deposition of calcium pyrophosphate dihydrate or hydroxyapatite may alter the properties of cartilage matrix directly but crystal formation usually follows the matrix changes.

CAUSES OF SECONDARY OSTEOARTHRITIS

Developmental
- Perthes' disease
- Slipped capital femoral epiphysis
- Epiphysiolysis
- Hip dysplasia
- Epiphysial dysplasias
- Intra-articular acetabular labrum

Traumatic
- Intra-articular fracture
- Meniscectomy
- Occupational, e.g. elbows of pneumatic drill operators
- Hypermobility, e.g. Ehlers–Danlos syndrome
- Long leg arthropathy

Metabolic
- Alkaptonuria (ochronosis)
- Haemochromatosis
- Wilson's disease
- Chondrocalcinosis

Endocrine
- Acromegaly

Inflammatory
- Rheumatoid arthritis
- Gout
- Septic arthritis
- Haemophilia

Aseptic necrosis
- Corticosteroids
- Sickle-cell disease
- Decompression sickness
- SLE and other collagenoses

Neuropathic
- Tabes dorsalis
- Syringomyelia
- Diabetes mellitus
- Peripheral nerve lesions

Miscellaneous
- Paget's disease
- Gaucher's disease

It is uncertain whether the degenerative joint disease seen in acromegaly is a consequence of joint incongruity following cartilage overgrowth or whether the endocrine disturbance results in a mechanically defective matrix. Paget's disease, Gaucher's disease and various diseases associated with aseptic necrosis result in pathological changes in subchondral bone, with consequent altered stresses on the overlying articular cartilage. Thus OA can be the end result of disorders in which defective cartilage matrix disintegrates under the influence of normal mechanical stresses, and disorders in which normal cartilage matrix fails secondary to abnormal mechanical loads (see Fig. 12.19).

Current concepts of the pathogenesis of OA are based on the assumption that, whatever the provoking cause, the final pathway of changes in articular cartilage is identical. Two mechanical hypotheses merit consideration. The first suggests that the initiating event is fatigue fracture of the collagen fibre network, which is followed by increased hydration of the articular cartilage with unravelling of the proteoglycans and loss of proteoglycans into the synovial fluid. There is some evidence of augmented metalloproteinase activity and indirect evidence of a putative 'aggrecanase' but collagen may also be lost as a result of mechanical attrition.

The alternative hypothesis suggests that the initial lesions are microfractures of the subchondral bone following repetitive loading. Healing of these microfractures leads

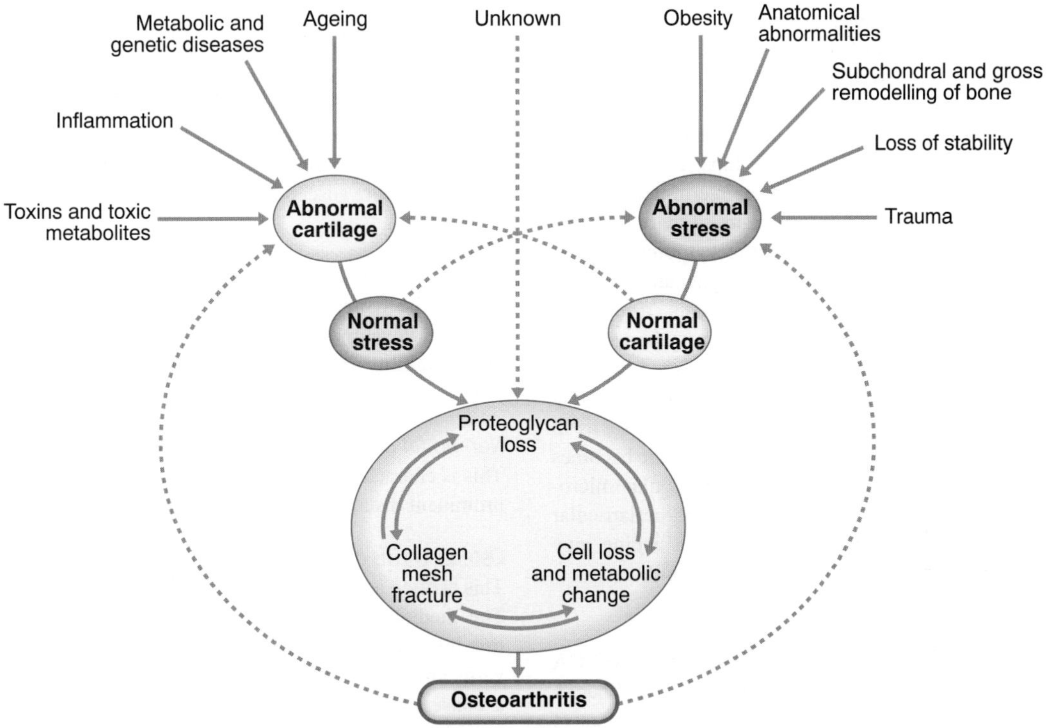

Fig. 12.19 The development of osteoarthritis. Simplified schematic outline of mechanisms of cartilage failure. Causes may be categorised as those producing either abnormal cartilage or abnormal loading. In either case there is an imbalance between tissue composition and the stress to which it is subjected which produces changes in the matrix structure and production by cells.

to significant loss of resilience of the subchondral bone, which in turn creates a sheer stress gradient in the adjacent articular cartilage. As the process evolves, the cartilage surface becomes fibrillated and deep clefts appear, with reduplication and proliferation of chondrocytes within them. Simultaneous proliferative changes commence at the joint margins, with formation of osteophytes. Eventually, articular cartilage is lost altogether in areas of maximum mechanical stress and the underlying bone becomes hardened and eburnated. Cysts may form but bony ankylosis does not occur (see Fig. 12.20). The associated biochemical changes in articular cartilage are summarised in the information box.

BIOCHEMICAL CHANGES IN OA CARTILAGE

- ↑H_2O
- ↓Collagen, proteoglycan, monomer size, hyaluronate, keratan sulphate and chondroitin sulphate
- ↑Chondroitin 4:6 ratio
- Expression of fetal chondroitin sulphate epitopes
- ↑Collagen and proteoglycan synthesis
- ↑'Aggrecanase', stromelysin and collagenase

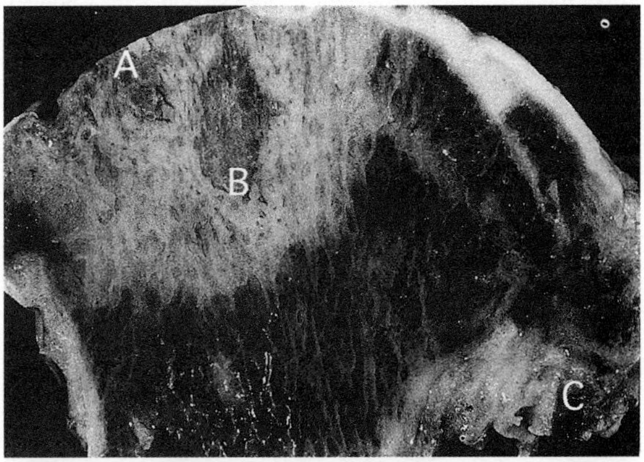

Fig. 12.20 The pathology of osteoarthritis. Cross-section of head of femur in patient with advanced OA. Note (A) loss of articular cartilage, (B) cyst formation and (C) bone sclerosis, as well as osteophyte formation and remodelling of the femoral head.

Clinical features

The joints most frequently involved are those of the spine, hips, knees and hands. The disease is confined to one or only a few joints in the majority of patients. Common patterns of joint involvement include the nodal and non-nodal types of primary generalised OA with prominent involvement of the knees and hands (distal interphalangeal joints, proximal interphalangeal joints, carpometacarpal joints of thumbs), as well as OA confined to the knees or hips. The symptoms are gradual in onset. Pain is at first intermittent and is provoked by the use of the joint and relieved by rest. As the disease progresses, movement in the affected joint becomes increasingly limited, initially as a result of pain and muscular spasm, but later because of capsular fibrosis, osteophyte formation and remodelling of bone. There may be repeated effusions into joints, especially after minor twists or injuries. Crepitus may be felt or even heard. Associated muscle wasting is an important factor in the progress of the disease, as in the absence of normal muscular control the joint becomes more prone to injury. Pain arises from trabecular microfractures, traumatic lesions in the capsule and periarticular tissues, and a low-grade synovitis. Nocturnal aching may be attributable to hyperaemia of the subchondral bone.

Nodal osteoarthritis

This is a clinically distinct form of primary generalised OA which occurs predominantly in middle-aged women. Characteristically it affects the terminal interphalangeal joints of the fingers, with the development of gelatinous cysts or bony outgrowths on the dorsal aspect of these joints (Heberden's nodes, see Fig. 12.21). The onset is sometimes acute, with considerable pain, swelling and inflammation. Although associated with a good deal of deformity, Heberden's nodes seldom cause serious disability. Similar lesions may affect the proximal interphalangeal joints (Bouchard's nodes), and the disorder also frequently involves the carpometacarpal joints of the thumbs, the spinal apophyseal joints, the hips and the knees. A strong family history of Heberden's nodes is usual in such patients and though the existence of multi-generation families with the disorder appears to suggest a single autosomal dominant gene, careful family studies reveal polygenic inheritance in both nodal and non-nodal primary generalised osteoarthritis (PGOA). Patients with nodal PGOA are more susceptible to secondary OA.

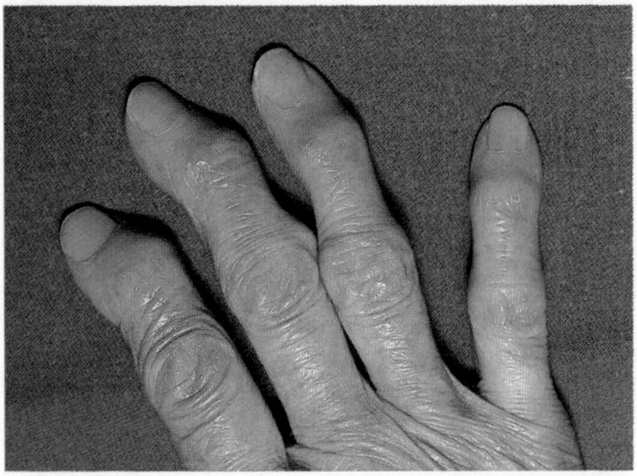

Fig. 12.21 Nodal osteoarthritis. Distal interphalangeal joint subluxation with Heberden's nodes. There are also early Bouchard's nodes at the proximal interphalangeal joints.

Erosive OA

This is a more severe form of nodal PGOA, characterised by episodic symptoms and signs of local joint inflammation, with the development of destructive subchondral erosions and instability in the proximal and distal interphalangeal joints.

Non-nodal PGOA

This is characterised by a more equal sex incidence and less prominent distal interphalangeal joint disease.

Osteoarthritis of the knees

This is often associated with obesity and hand OA in women. The medial and patellofemoral compartments are usually first involved and more advanced disease is associated with varus knee deformities. Isolated knee OA may, however, be a consequence of varus knee deformities associated with medial meniscectomy and dysplasias such as Blount's disease.

Isolated hip OA

This is frequently secondary to definable predisposing causes such as inequality of leg lengths, preceding hip disease, acetabular dysplasia or occupational trauma. The superior pole of the hip is typically affected in such cases, whereas hip disease in PGOA is usually medial or concentric.

Investigations

The blood count and ESR are characteristically normal. Synovial fluid is viscous and has a low cell count; apatite crystals can rarely be detected (see Table 12.2, p. 808). Cartilage degradation products such as keratan sulphate and pyridinoline cross-links derived from collagen are increased in the synovial fluid and urine but these are too non-specific and variable to be useful for diagnosis or following progress.

Radiographs show loss of joint space and formation of marginal osteophytes. Subchondral bone sclerosis, bone remodelling and cyst formation are seen in more advanced cases (see Figs 12.5 and 12.6, p. 809). Isotope scintigraphy with ^{99m}-Tc bisphosphonate shows increased uptake of isotope in OA joints that are destined to develop progressive damage.

Management

Treatment is directed towards relieving symptoms, maintaining and improving joint function, and minimising handicap. Patient education and the encouragement of a positive approach are particularly important in osteoarthritis. While the pathological changes of OA are irreversible, the overall prognosis for maintaining function is generally good and a great deal can be done to alleviate symptoms. Improving muscle strength and maintaining mobility are just as important as the avoidance of undue trauma and physical stress to affected joints. Simple joint protection techniques include such measures as the fitting of rubber heels to reduce jarring and minimise the risk of slipping, the provision of built-up shoes to equalise leg lengths, weight reduction in obese patients with OA of the knee or hip, and the provision of a suitable walking-stick. Occasionally, patients are advised to change their occupation, transfer to lighter work or give up unduly strenuous hobbies; more often modification of existing activities to avoid prolonged standing or walking is all that is required.

Simple non-narcotic analgesics such as paracetamol or co-proxamol are the drugs of choice for relieving pain in OA. Some patients obtain better symptom control with small, analgesic doses of NSAIDs. Larger anti-inflammatory doses are usually no more effective and carry an increased risk of causing gastric erosion or haemorrhage, particularly in elderly debilitated women. Prostaglandin synthetase inhibitors are also liable to cause impairment of renal function and fluid retention in patients with renal insufficiency and/or cardiac disease. Concerns that some NSAIDs may be associated with cartilage damage, due to inhibition of proteoglycan metabolism or the excessive use of damaged joints, are probably exaggerated.

Although some NSAIDs (diclofenac, piroxicam and tiaprofenic acid), and other agents such as glycosaminoglycan peptide complex, pentosan polyphosphate and hyaluronan, have been shown to have a chondroprotective effect in in vitro and animal experiments, there is no good clinical evidence that these or any other drugs have significant disease-modifying effects in human OA.

Intra-articular hyaluronan injections can give temporary pain relief and occasional intra-articular or periarticular corticosteroid injections can be helpful, especially in the knee. Hydrotherapy may be useful for patients with OA of the hip associated with pain and muscle spasm.

Surgery needs to be considered in patients with more advanced hip and knee disease (see Table 12.12, p. 847). Precision osteotomy can prolong the life of malaligned joints as well as relieving pain by reducing intraosseous pressure. Hip and knee arthroplasties can transform the quality of life of patients with intractable pain and disability.

FURTHER INFORMATION ON OSTEOARTHRITIS AND RELATED DISORDERS

Brandt K D, Doherty M, Lohmander L S (eds) 1998 Osteoarthritis. Oxford University Press, Oxford

Creamer P, Hochberg M C 1997 Osteoarthritis. Lancet 350: 503

Kuettner E K, Schleyerbach R, Peyron J G et al (eds) 1998 Cartilage and osteoarthritis. Raven, New York

CRYSTAL DEPOSITION DISEASES

A variety of crystals are associated with acute and chronic arthritis, periarthritis, tendonitis and deposition in connective tissues (see Table 12.8).

CALCIUM PYROPHOSPHATE DIHYDRATE (CPPD) DEPOSITION (CHONDROCALCINOSIS, PYROPHOSPHATE ARTHROPATHY)

CPPD crystals are deposited in fibrous and articular cartilage, where they are associated with degenerative changes. Shedding of crystals into the joint space provokes an attack of synovitis—*pseudogout*. Autopsy and radiological surveys indicate that chondrocalcinosis is a common age-related finding often unassociated with symptoms of articular disease. The menisci and articular cartilage of the knee are the most common sites.

Aetiology

Chondrocalcinosis and pseudogout are not the result of a single disease. The majority of cases are sporadic and no underlying cause can be found. Genetic factors are import-

Table 12.8 Crystal-associated arthropathies and deposition in connective tissue

Crystal	Associations
***Calcium pyrophosphate dihydrate (CPPD)**	Acute pseudogout Variety of patterns of chronic inflammatory/degenerative arthritis Chondrocalcinosis
***Basic calcium phosphate** **Hydroxyapatite** **Octacalcium phosphate** **Tricalcium phosphate** **Dicalcium phosphate dihydrate**	Calcific periarthritis/tendonitis Acute/chronic inflammatory arthritis Destructive arthropathy Soft tissue calcinosis
Calcium oxalate **Aluminium phosphate**	Acute arthritis in patients on renal dialysis
***Monosodium urate (MSU)**	Acute/chronic gouty arthritis Renal calculi Tophi
Xanthine	Acute arthritis (rare) Renal calculi Asymptomatic deposition in muscles
Cholesterol	Chronic synovial effusions in RA/OA
Cysteine **Cystine**	Acute arthritis
Charcot–Leyden (lysophospholipase)	Synovial fluid and tissues with eosinophilia

* Most common.

CHONDROCALCINOSIS (PYROPHOSPHATE ARTHROPATHY)	
Familial	
Sporadic	
Metabolic	
• Hyperparathyroidism	• Hypophosphatasia
• Haemochromatosis	• Gout
• Hypothyroidism	• Ochronosis
• Hypomagnesaemia	• Wilson's disease

ant in some families, with increases in intracellular pyrophosphate concentrations in some kindreds and a collagen gene defect in others. A variety of metabolic disorders have been associated with chondrocalcinosis and these are listed in the information box.

No common determinant comparable to the hyperuricaemia of gout has been identified, but pyrophosphate concentrations are increased in synovial fluids. This, coupled with the association with hypophosphatasia, has suggested that the disease may be a consequence of defective pyrophosphatase activity.

Clinical features

Pyrophosphate arthropathy can mimic many other conditions. Six clinical patterns of disease are described in the information box.

CHONDROCALCINOSIS: PATTERNS OF CLINICAL DISEASE
Type A: Pseudogout
• The affected joint becomes suddenly painful, warm, swollen and tender. The knee is the site of more than half of all attacks, the duration of which can vary from a few days to 4 weeks. Subacute or 'petite' attacks are not uncommon and there may be polyarticular clustering of acute attacks. Men are affected more frequently than women
Type B: Pseudorheumatoid arthritis
• In a few patients there is a subacute inflammatory polyarthritis which may last for several months
Type C: Pseudo-osteoarthritis with superimposed acute attacks
Type D: Pseudo-osteoarthritis without acute attacks
• Types C and D account for nearly half of patients. Women are more frequently affected. Prominent involvement of the wrists and metacarpophalangeal joints clearly distinguishes pseudo-osteoarthritic chondrocalcinosis from primary generalised osteoarthrosis
Type E: Asymptomatic
• This is the most common
Type F: Pseudoneuropathic
• Severe destructive changes resembling those of Charcot joints can occur in the knee and shoulder in the absence of any neurological defect (see Fig. 12.22)

Investigations

Radiographs show CPPD in articular cartilage, the menisci of the knees (see Fig. 12.23), the labrum of the acetabulum and glenoid cavity, the triangular cartilage of the wrist and the symphysis pubis. Examination of synovial fluid under polarising light microscopy allows CPPD crystals to be distinguished from monosodium urate crystals. X-ray diffraction techniques differentiate CPPD from calcium phosphate and calcium hydroxyapatite crystals found in synovial fluid in osteoarthritis and other forms of degenerative joint disease.

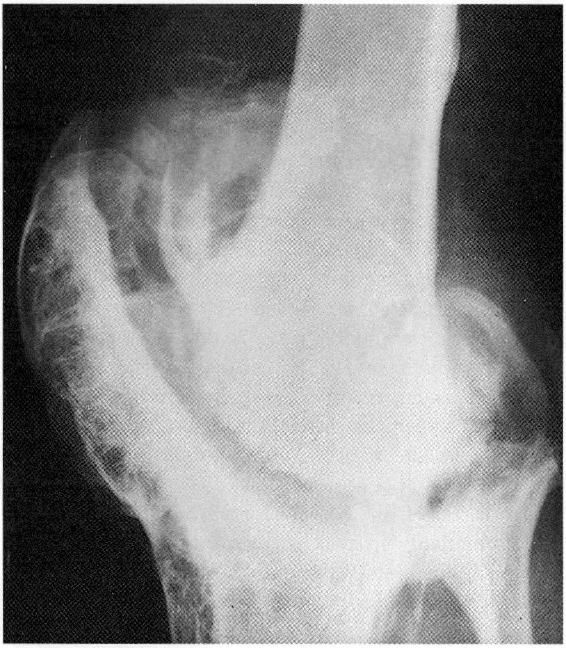

Fig. 12.22 Pseudoneuropathic calcium pyrophosphate dihydrate disease. Radiograph of knee showing severe destructive and proliferative changes.

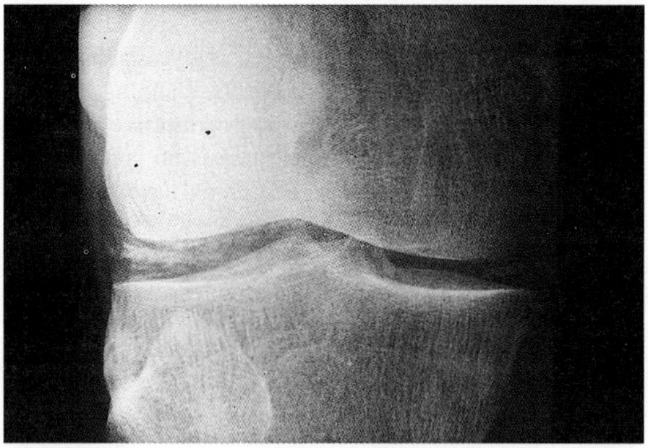

Fig. 12.23 Chondrocalcinosis. Radiograph of knee showing calcification of meniscus in patient with calcium pyrophosphate deposition disease.

Management

Joint aspiration and intra-articular injection of corticosteroids are the most effective means of treating acute attacks of pseudogout. NSAIDs and colchicine are less effective than in classical gout.

BASIC CALCIUM PHOSPHATE (BCP) CRYSTAL DEPOSITION

Controlled deposition of the BCP crystal hydroxyapatite (HA) is essential for the formation of normal bone, dentine and enamel. Deposition of HA and other BCP crystals in connective tissues occurs in a variety of disorders associated with damage to collagen (see the information box).

DISORDERS ASSOCIATED WITH CONNECTIVE TISSUE DAMAGE AND DEPOSITION OF BASIC CALCIUM PHOSPHATE

- Rotator cuff injuries
- Hip arthroplasty
- Paraplegia
- Myositis ossificans
- Prolapsed intervertebral discs
- Calcific aortic valves
- Systemic sclerosis
- Dermatomyositis
- Paget's disease
- Chronic dialysis
- Vitamin D intoxication

CALCIFIC PERIARTHRITIS

Acute calcific periarthritis is characterised by periarticular inflammation in association with juxta-articular deposition of HA crystals. The shoulder region is most frequently affected in middle-aged men or women, but monoarticular/ polyarticular attacks can also occur at the hip, knee, ankle, elbow and wrist. The cause of calcific periarthritis of the shoulder is usually unknown but the problem may be familial or secondary in patients with chronic renal failure undergoing dialysis.

Acute inflammation results from peritendonitis or bursitis following sudden release of HA crystals from a primary deposit in the tendon.

Radiographs usually show evidence of a calcinotic deposit in the supraspinatus tendon (see Fig. 12.18, p. 822), the rotator cuff or subacromial bursa and this occasionally disappears following an acute attack. Identification of the crystals from the bursal fluid requires X-ray diffraction, infrared spectroscopy or electron microscopy but is not necessary in clinical practice.

Acute attacks usually respond to treatment with NSAIDs or colchicine, and aspiration, corticosteroid injection or surgical excision is very rarely indicated.

APATITE-ASSOCIATED DESTRUCTIVE ARTHROPATHY ('MILWAUKEE' SHOULDER/KNEE SYNDROME, CUFF-TEAR ARTHROPATHY)

This is an unusual but distinctive type of destructive arthropathy seen in the elderly. Women are affected more than men. The shoulders and knees are the main joints affected but the wrists, hips and mid-tarsal joints are also rarely involved. Sudden onset of pain and swelling in the dominant shoulder is associated with the presence of a large cool effusion, variable pain on moving the joint and the rapid development of joint subluxation and destruction. Radiographs show evidence of rotator cuff defects with upward migration and destruction of the humeral head but little in the way of bone remodelling or osteophyte formation. Some cases are associated with calcific periarthritis. Synovial fluid analysis shows large volumes of relatively non-inflammatory fluid with numerous crystals of CPPD and HA, as well as elevated levels of collagenase and neutral protease activity.

Treatment is with simple analgesics, NSAIDs and supportive physiotherapy, as well as with joint aspiration and intra-articular injection of corticosteroid. Rarely, surgical intervention with a shoulder joint spacer or replacement arthroplasty is required.

GOUT

Gout describes a number of disorders in which crystals of monosodium urate monohydrate derived from hyperuricaemic body fluids give rise to inflammatory arthritis, tenosynovitis, bursitis or cellulitis, tophaceous deposits, urolithiasis and renal disease. Prolonged hyperuricaemia is necessary but not sufficient for the development of gout.

Epidemiology

Gouty arthritis is predominantly a problem of post-pubertal males and is seldom seen in women before the menopause. It is the most common cause of inflammatory joint disease in men over 40 years old. In a typical UK general practice of 2000 patients, there may be 17 men and 3 women with gouty arthritis and 10 times that number with asymptomatic hyperuricaemia. Serum uric acid concentrations are distributed in the community as a continuous variable and are determined by a number of demographic factors, of which age, sex, body bulk and genetic constitution are the most important. Serum uric acid levels are higher in urban than in rural communities and are positively correlated with intelligence, social class, weight, haemoglobin, serum proteins and a high protein diet.

Hyperuricaemia is arbitrarily defined as a serum uric acid level greater than two standard deviations from the mean, i.e. above 0.42 mmol/1 in adult males and 0.36 mmol/l in adult females.

Aetiology

The concentration of uric acid in body fluids depends on a balance between purine synthesis plus ingestion and uric

FACTORS PREDISPOSING TO HYPERURICAEMIA AND GOUT
Diminished renal excretion of uric acid
• Renal failure • Drugs Diuretics Pyrazinamide Low doses of aspirin • Lead poisoning • Hyperparathyroidism • Myxoedema • Down's syndrome • Lactic acidosis Alcohol Exercise Starvation Vomiting Toxaemia of pregnancy Type I glycogen storage disease • Unidentified inherited defect
Increased production of uric acid
• Increased turnover of purines Myeloproliferative disorders, e.g. polycythaemia vera Lymphoproliferative disorders, e.g. chronic lymphatic leukaemia Psoriasis—severe, exfoliative • Increased purine synthesis de novo Hypoxanthine-guanine phosphoribosyl transferase deficiency Phosphoribosyl pyrophosphate synthetase overactivity Glucose-6-phosphatase deficiency Idiopathic

acid elimination through the kidneys and intestine (see Fig. 12.24). Purine nucleotide synthesis and degradation are regulated by a network of enzyme pathways (see Fig. 12.25).

Various genetic and environmental factors lead to hyperuricaemia and gout by decreasing the excretion of uric acid and/or increasing its production, as shown in the information box. In more than 75% of patients with gout there appears to be a genetically determined defect in fractional urate excretion which results in an inability to increase uric acid excretion in response to a purine load. Increased production of uric acid is at least partly responsible for hyperuricaemia in 20–25% of gout patients. In the absence of significant renal impairment such patients are hyperexcretors of uric acid. Specific enzyme defects resulting in an increase in de novo purine synthesis account for less than 2% of cases. They should be suspected:

- in the absence of disorders resulting in increased turnover of purines
- if gout develops at an unusually early age
- if there is a family history of gout commencing at an early age
- if uric acid lithiasis is the first presenting feature.

Clinical features

Acute gout

The metatarsophalangeal joint of a great toe is the site of the first attack of acute gouty arthritis in 70% of patients; the ankle, the knee, the small joints of the feet and hands, and the wrist and elbow follow in decreasing order of frequency. The onset may be insidious or explosively sudden, often waking the patient from sleep. The affected joint is hot, red and swollen, with shiny overlying skin and dilated veins; it is excruciatingly painful and tender. Very acute attacks may be accompanied by fever, leucocytosis and a raised ESR and are occasionally preceded by prodromal symptoms such as anorexia, nausea or a change in mood. If untreated, the attack lasts for days or weeks but it eventually subsides spontaneously. Resolution of the acute attack may be accompanied by local pruritus and desquamation of the overlying skin.

Some patients have only a single attack, or suffer another only after an interval of many months or years. More often there is a tendency to have recurrent attacks. These increase

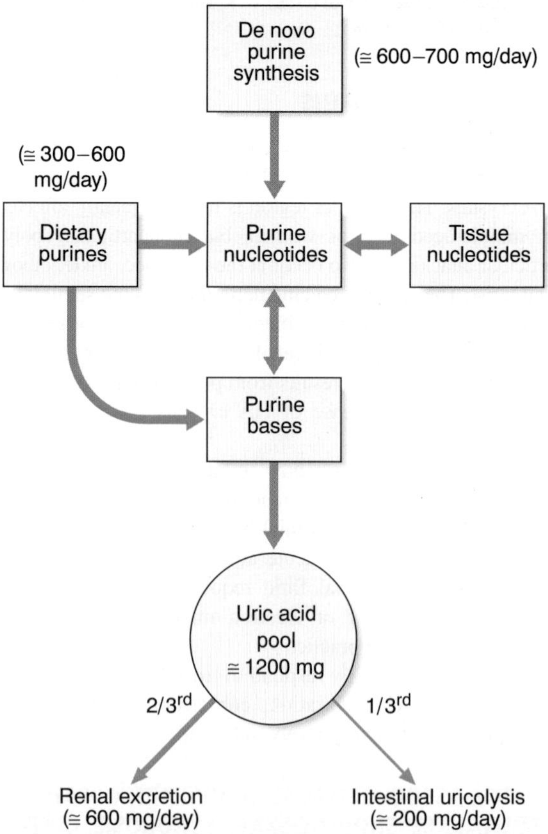

Fig. 12.24 The uric acid pool. Origins and disposal of uric acid in normal humans.

in frequency and duration so that eventually one attack may merge into another and the patient remains in a prolonged state of subacute gout. Acute attacks are occasionally polyarticular, and tenosynovitis, bursitis or cellulitis may be the presenting feature.

Acute attacks may be precipitated by sudden rises in serum urate following dietary excess, alcohol, severe dietary restriction or diuretic drugs, or by sudden falls following initiation of therapy with allopurinol or uricosuric drugs. Acute attacks may also be provoked by trauma, unusual physical exercise, surgery or severe systemic illness.

Chronic gout

First attacks of gouty arthritis are seldom associated with residual disability but recurrent acute attacks are followed by progressive cartilage and bone erosion in association with deposition of tophi and secondary degenerative changes. Severe functional impairment and gross joint deformities may occur in chronic tophaceous gout. Tophi are frequently found in the cartilage of the ear, bursae and tendon sheaths. Tophus formation is related to serum uric acid and to local factors. Tophi seldom develop in individuals with asymptomatic hyperuricaemia; however, they may develop rapidly in the feet or hands in post-menopausal women with heart failure and renal insufficiency who develop acute or subacute gouty arthritis following prolonged diuretic administration.

Urate urolithiasis

This occurs in about 10% of patients with gout attending British hospital clinics. The incidence is much higher in hot climates. The formation of urate calculi is also favoured by:

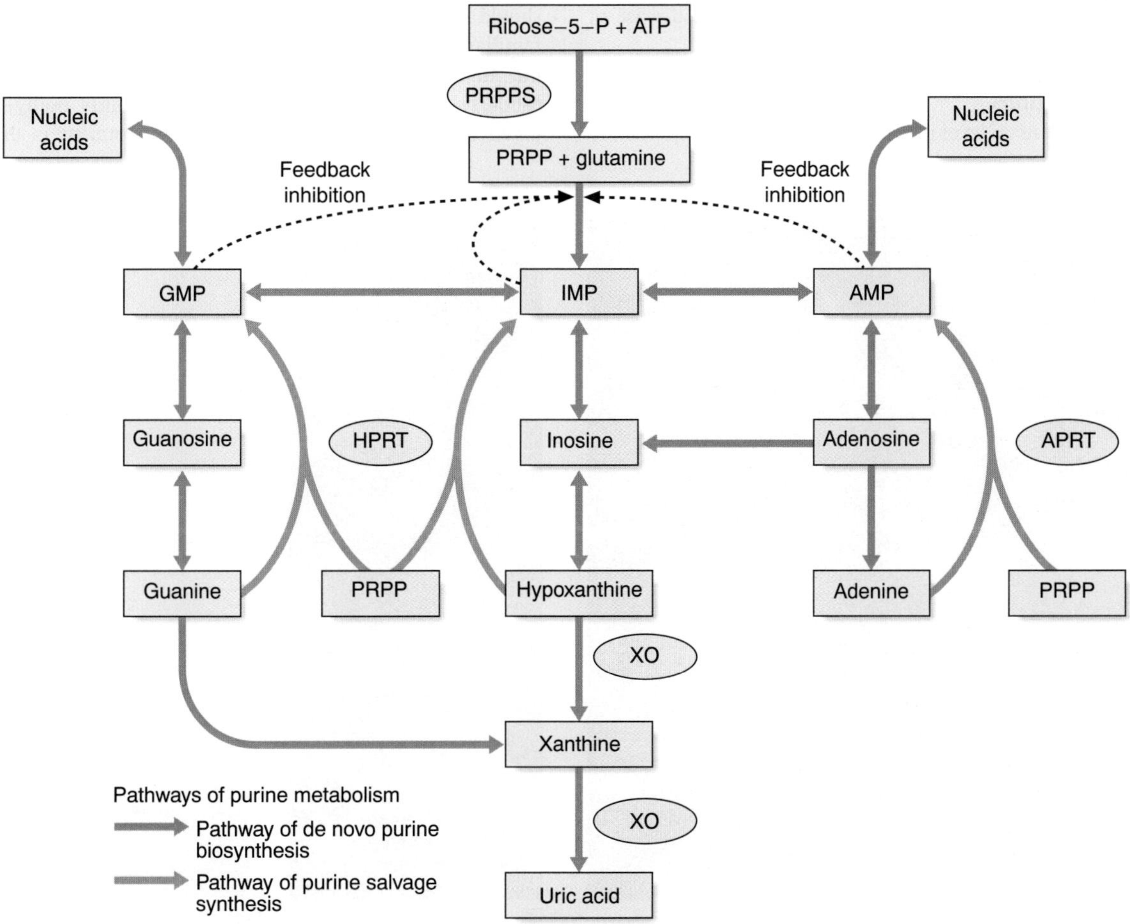

Fig. 12.25 Pathways of purine metabolism in mammalian cells. (AMP, GMP, IMP = adenosine, guanosine and inosine monophosphate; ATP = adenosine triphosphate; APRT, HPRT = adenine and hypoxanthine-guanine phosphoribosyl transferase; PRPP(S) = phosphoribosyl pyrophosphate (synthetase); XO = xanthine oxidase)

- hyperuricosuria
- purine overproduction
- excessive purine ingestion
- uricosuric drugs and defects in tubular resorption of uric acid
- low urine pH, e.g. in chronic diarrhoeal diseases or following ileostomy.

Chronic urate nephropathy

This results from a combination of renal tubular obstruction, uric acid calculi, hypertension, glomerulosclerosis and secondary pyelonephritis. It is rare in the absence of well-established chronic gouty arthritis.

Other manifestations

Gout and hyperuricaemia are frequently associated with obesity, type IV hyperlipoproteinaemia, diabetes mellitus, hypertension and ischaemic heart disease. Hyperuricaemia itself is not, however, a risk factor for vascular disease or diabetes mellitus.

Investigations

The serum urate level is usually raised but it is important to appreciate that this does not prove the diagnosis because asymptomatic hyperuricaemia is very common. Whenever possible, synovial fluid should be aspirated and examined under polarising light (see Fig. 12.26). Acute attacks of gout can occur when the serum urate level is normal. This is frequently seen in patients who have received treatment with allopurinol or a uricosuric agent.

Joint radiographs may show characteristic punched-out erosions associated with the soft tissue swelling of urate tophi, occasionally flecked with calcium. The diagnosis will be clinically apparent in such patients. In others the erosions may be indistinguishable from those seen in various forms of inflammatory arthritis.

Management

NSAIDs are the agents of choice. It is important to start treatment as early as possible, to use adequate doses and to avoid salicylates and diuretics. Patients known to have gout should keep a supply of an NSAID with which they are familiar so that an acute attack can be aborted as soon as the first symptoms are noticed. Indomethacin (50 mg 6-hourly orally) or naproxen (500 mg 8-hourly orally) is given until the acute attack subsides. Treatment is then

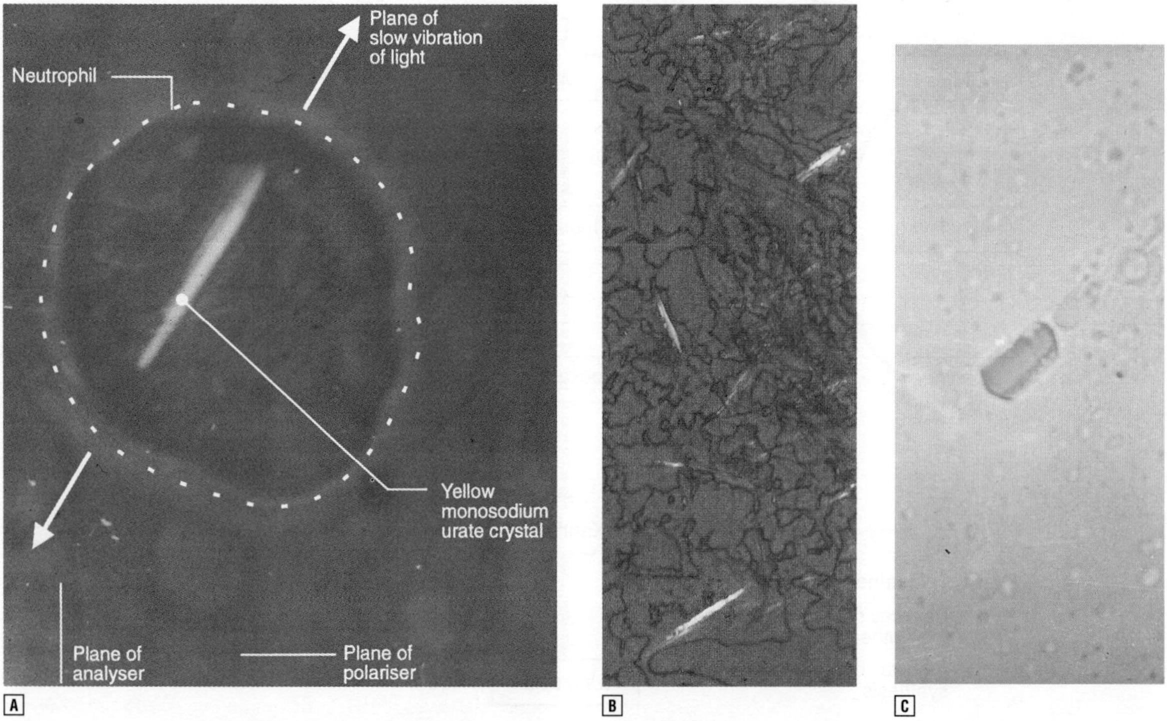

Fig. 12.26 Polarised light microscopy in the diagnosis of crystal-associated arthritis. [A] Photograph and overlying diagram of needle-shaped crystal of monosodium urate (MSU) in polymorphonuclear leucocyte from joint fluid of patient with gouty arthritis. Arrows show the plane of polarised light. [B] Negatively birefringent MSU crystal in synovial tissue. [C] Positively birefringent rhomboidal CPPD crystal.

continued with lower doses for 7–10 days. Colchicine is highly effective but causes vomiting and diarrhoea in many patients in the doses that need to be used (1 mg at once followed by 0.5 mg 2-hourly orally).

Prevention

Prolonged administration of drugs which lower the serum urate level should be considered following the resolution of the acute attack in patients with:

- recurrent attacks of gouty arthritis
- tophi or evidence of chronic gouty arthritis
- associated renal disease
- gout and markedly raised serum urate.

Allopurinol

This is the drug of choice for long-term prophylaxis because of its convenience and low incidence of side-effects. It lowers the serum urate by inhibiting xanthine oxidase, which is responsible for the conversion of xanthine and hypoxanthine to uric acid. Oral treatment is commenced with 300 mg once daily together with colchicine 0.5 mg 12-hourly to avert the acute attacks of gouty arthritis which frequently follow initiation of hypouricaemic drug therapy. It is important not to commence treatment with allopurinol until several weeks have elapsed after the last acute attack and to continue concurrent administration of colchicine for several months. The dose of allopurinol may have to be adjusted to bring the serum urate within the normal range. If renal function is impaired, lower doses (100 mg daily or less) must be used, according to the severity of the renal insufficiency.

Uricosuric agents

These can also be very effective in lowering the serum urate level, reducing the frequency of acute attacks of gout and decreasing the size of the tophi. Probenecid 0.5–1 g 12-hourly orally or sulphinpyrazone 100 mg 8-hourly is given with colchicine 0.5 mg 12-hourly orally. Salicylates must be avoided as they antagonise the uricosuric effects of these drugs. Uricosuric drug therapy is contraindicated:

- in gout with overproduction of uric acid and gross uricosuria
- in patients with renal failure (ineffective)
- in patients with urate urolithiasis.

Benzbromarone 100 mg daily can be used in patients with moderate renal impairment when other uricosuric agents are ineffective.

Diet

There is no need for severe dietary restrictions but excessive purine intake and overindulgence in alcohol should be avoided. Gradual weight loss is encouraged in obese patients and is associated with a fall in serum urate. Severe calorie restriction must be avoided as it causes lactic acidosis and a rise in serum urate.

Surgery

This is occasionally required to deal with a large or ulcerating tophus.

Asymptomatic hyperuricaemia

This does not require prophylactic treatment in the absence of a history, family history or clinical evidence of gout. A search should be made for causes of secondary hyperuricaemia (see p. 831). Obese subjects should lose weight gradually and have their blood pressure and renal function monitored annually.

FURTHER INFORMATION ON CRYSTAL DEPOSITION DISEASES

Emmerson B T 1996 The management of gout. New England Journal of Medicine 334: 445–450

Nuki G 1998 Gout. Medicine 26: 54–59

Schumacher H R 1996 Crystal-induced arthritis: an overview. American Journal of Medicine 100: 465–525

INFLAMMATORY JOINT DISEASE

RHEUMATOID ARTHRITIS

Rheumatoid arthritis (RA) is the most common form of chronic inflammatory joint disease. In its typical form RA is a symmetrical, destructive and deforming polyarthritis affecting small and large synovial joints, with associated systemic disturbance, a variety of extra-articular features and the presence of circulating antiglobulin antibodies (rheumatoid factors). Characteristically, the course of the disease is prolonged with exacerbations and remissions but atypical, asymmetrical and incomplete forms are not uncommon.

Epidemiology

Rheumatoid arthritis occurs throughout the world and in all ethnic groups. Climate, altitude and geography do not appear to influence its prevalence but a higher proportion of patients in Western and urban communities have more severe and disabling disease. The overall prevalence of RA in Caucasian populations is about 1%, with a female to male ratio of 3:1. The disease starts most commonly between the third and fifth decades but the age of onset follows a normal distribution curve and no age group is exempted. With an annual incidence of new cases of about 200 per million per

CRITERIA FOR THE DIAGNOSIS OF RHEUMATOID ARTHRITIS (American Rheumatism Association 1988 revision)

- Morning stiffness (> 1 hour)*
- Arthritis of three or more joint areas*
- Arthritis of hand joints*
- Symmetrical arthritis*
- Rheumatoid nodules
- Rheumatoid factor
- Radiological changes

* Duration of 6 weeks or more.

N.B. Diagnosis of RA made with four or more criteria.

year, 5% of women and 2% of men over the age of 55 years are affected.

A diagnosis of rheumatoid arthritis can be established in patients with clinical features of inflammatory arthritis of 6 weeks' duration. The criteria for the diagnosis of RA used for epidemiological purposes are shown in the information box.

Aetiology

Although the cause of rheumatoid arthritis remains obscure, there is evidence that the disease is triggered by Th_1 lymphocyte activation and production of proinflammatory cytokines such as IL-1, TNF-α and IL-6 in genetically predisposed individuals with defined human leucocyte antigen (HLA) class II haplotypes. HLA-DR4 is the major susceptibility haplotype in most ethnic groups but DR1 is

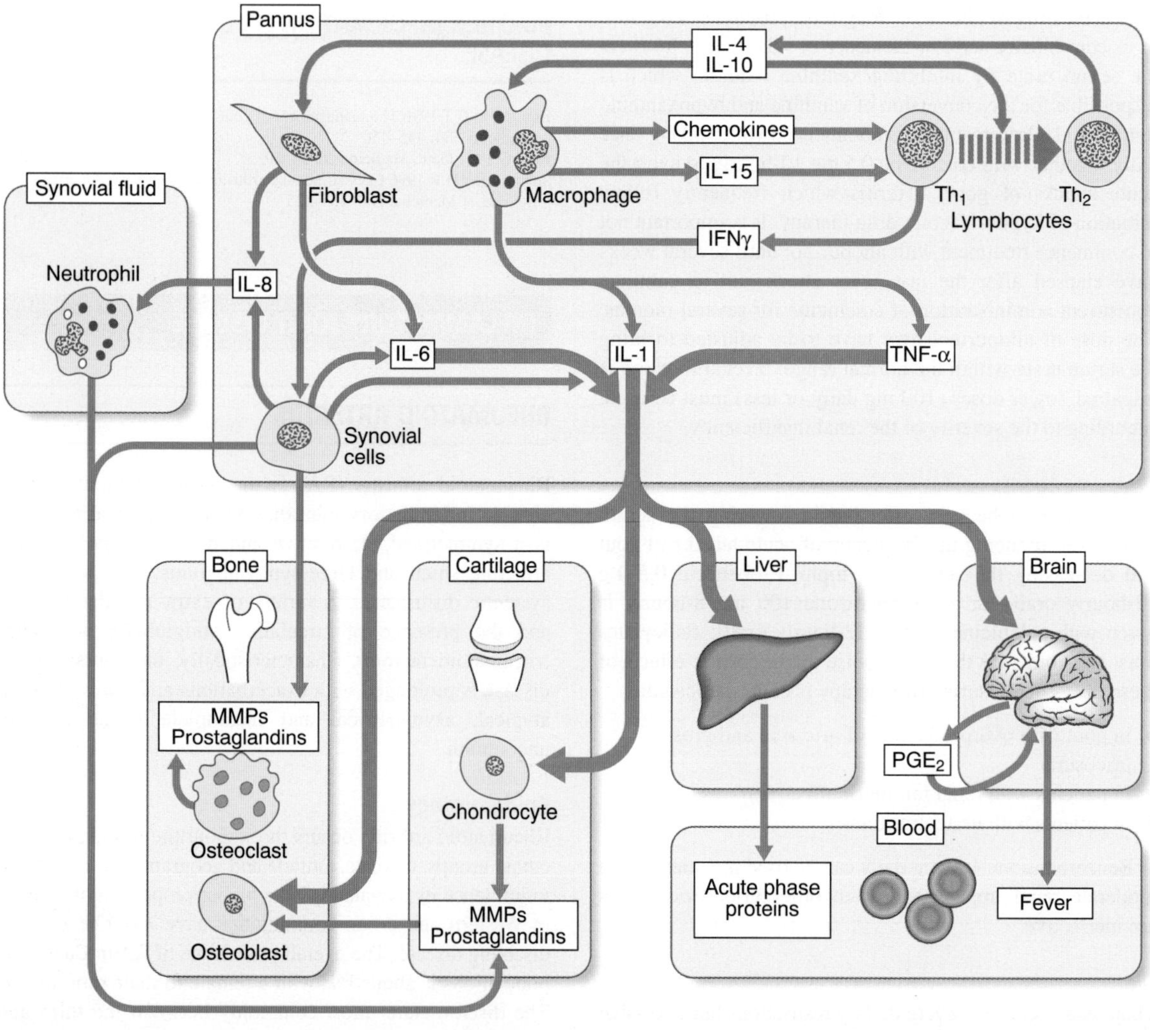

Fig. 12.27 Pathogenesis of rheumatoid arthritis. Possible sequence of events with network of cells, cytokines and mediators. (IL = interleukin; Th_1 and Th_2 = Th_1 and Th_2 lymphocyte subsets; IFN = interferon; MMPs = metalloproteinases; PGE_2 = prostaglandin E_2)

more important in Indians and Israelis and DW15 in Japanese; alleles of DW10, DW13 and DW14 have also been implicated.

The molecular basis for disease susceptibility resides in a shared epitope found in the third allelic hypervariable region of HLA-DR β_1, between amino acid residues 67 and 74 which flank the T-cell recognition site (see Fig. 1.24, p. 29). Whether or not one or more exogenous or autoantigenic peptides can bind this disease susceptibility epitope to initiate or perpetuate disease is still unclear, but it is of interest that an Epstein–Barr virus glycoprotein (GP110) contains the identical amino acid sequence. Other potential mechanisms for persistent antigenic stimulation and altered immune reactivity are shown in the information box.

POTENTIAL MECHANISMS FOR PERSISTENT ANTIGEN STIMULATION AND ALTERED IMMUNE REACTIVITY IN RA

- Retroviral or parvoviral gene products
- Degraded bacterial cell wall peptidoglycans
- Bacterial/viral antigens cross-reacting with articular components
- Superantigen-driven disorder
- Autoantigenicity following enzyme/free radical damage to IgG or type II collagen
- Anti-idiotype antibodies
- Defective glycosylation IgG

Clinical evidence for the importance of genetic factors comes from an increase in the frequency of disease in first-degree relatives of patients with RA, and a higher concordance rate of disease in identical twins (30%) compared with that in non-identical twins (5%). Between 50% and 75% of Caucasian patients with RA are HLA-DR4-positive compared with 20–25% of the normal population. However, tissue-typing studies in families with multiple cases of RA suggest that HLA genes may only account for 30% of the genetic determinants involved. Specific T-cell receptors, immunoglobulin genes and cytokine gene polymorphisms may also be involved in determining severity and/or susceptibility to RA.

Whatever the initiating stimulus, RA is characterised by persistent cellular activation, autoimmunity and the presence of immune complexes at sites of articular and extra-articular lesions (see the information box). The development of amyloidosis in some patients provides further clinical evidence for chronic immune stimulation. The striking remissions of activity that can follow lymphocyte depletion by thoracic duct drainage, lymphocytophoresis or cytotoxic drug therapy point to the importance of lymphocytes and cellular immunity. Rheumatoid arthritis is both an extravascular immune complex disease and a disorder of cell-mediated immunity in which the events depicted in Figure 12.27 lead to chronic inflammation, granuloma formation and joint destruction. The severity of tissue damage is also related to joint movement and physical stress.

EVIDENCE FOR CELLULAR ACTIVATION, AUTOIMMUNITY AND IMMUNE COMPLEX PATHOLOGY IN RA

Cellular activation

- MHC class II expression by dendritic and synovial lining cells
- Adhesion molecule expression by endothelial cells
- Leucocyte emigration and activation of CD4 lymphocytes, B lymphocytes, plasma cells and monocytes
- Production of cytokines, prostaglandins, leucotrienes, metalloproteinases, acute-phase proteins, heat shock proteins and O_2 free radicals

Autoantibodies

- Rheumatoid factors
- Antinuclear antibodies
- Anticollagen antibodies

Immune complex pathology

- IgG-IgG and IgG-IgM complexes in synovial fluid
- Complement activation with $\downarrow C_3$, C_4 and CH_{50}

Pathology (see Fig. 12.28)

The earliest change is swelling and congestion of the synovial membrane and the underlying connective tissues, which become infiltrated with lymphocytes (especially CD4 T cells), plasma cells and macrophages. Effusion of synovial fluid into the joint space takes place during active phases of the disease. Hypertrophy of the synovial membrane occurs, with the formation of lymphoid follicles resembling an immunologically active lymph node. Inflammatory granulation tissue (pannus) spreads over and under the articular cartilage, which is progressively eroded and destroyed. Later, fibrous or bony ankylosis may occur. Muscles adjacent to inflamed joints atrophy and there may be focal infiltration with lymphocytes.

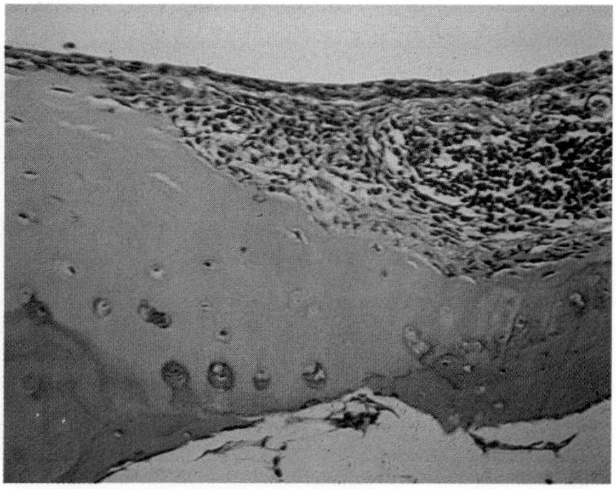

Fig. 12.28 Pathology of rheumatoid arthritis. Synovial pannus eroding articular cartilage.

Subcutaneous nodules consist of a central area of fibrinoid material surrounded by a palisade of proliferating mononuclear cells. Similar granulomatous lesions may occur in the pleura, lung, pericardium and sclera. Lymph nodes are often hyperplastic, showing many lymphoid follicles with large germinal centres and numerous plasma cells in the sinuses and medullary cords. Immunofluorescence shows that the plasma cells in the synovium and lymph nodes synthesise rheumatoid factors.

Clinical features

In the majority of patients the onset is insidious, with joint pain, stiffness and symmetrical swelling of a number of peripheral joints, but other disease patterns can occur (see the information box). Initially, pain may be experienced only on movement of joints, but rest pain and prolonged early morning stiffness are characteristic features of all kinds of inflammatory arthritis.

PATTERNS OF ONSET IN RHEUMATOID ARTHRITIS

• Insidious	70%	• Oligoarticular	45%
• Acute	15%	• Polyarticular	35%
• Systemic	10%	• Monoarticular	20%
• Palindromic	5%		

In the typical case the small joints of the fingers and toes are the first to be affected. Swelling of the proximal, but not the distal, interphalangeal joints gives the fingers a 'spindled' appearance (see Fig. 12.29), and swelling of the metatarsophalangeal joints results in 'broadening' of the forefoot. As the disease progresses with or without intervening remissions, it tends to spread to involve the wrists, elbows, shoulders, knees, ankles, subtalar and midtarsal joints. The hips become involved only in the more severely affected, but neck pain and stiffness from cervical spine disease is common. The temporomandibular, acromioclavicular, sternoclavicular and crico-arytenoid joints are sometimes affected.

In 10–15% of patients the disease starts as an acute polyarthritis with severe systemic symptoms. A systemic onset, with fever, weight loss, profound fatigue and malaise without joint symptoms, occurs less often, particularly in middle-aged men, and this can cause diagnostic confusion with malignant disease or chronic infections. The onset is palindromic in some patients, with recurrent acute episodes of joint pain and stiffness in individual joints lasting only a few hours or days. In about one-third of such cases the disease evolves into one more typical of arthritis. The onset of RA in the elderly can be indistinguishable from polymyalgia rheumatica with pain and stiffness in the region of the hip and shoulder girdles but no apparent synovitis. The presence of rheumatoid factor in such patients may be a clue to the true diagnosis before typical joint changes have developed.

Progression

As the disease advances, muscle atrophy, and tendon sheath and joint destruction result in limitation of joint motion, joint instability, subluxation and deformities. At first, deformities are correctable, but later permanent contractures develop.

Characteristic deformities include flexion contractures of the small joints of the hands and feet, the knees, hips and elbows. Anterior subluxation of the metacarpophalangeal joints is common, with ulnar deviation of the fingers (see Fig. 12.29A). Other finger deformities lead to greater loss of hand function. These include the 'swan neck' deformity (see Fig. 12.29B), the *boutonnière* or 'button-hole' deformity (fixed flexion of the proximal interphalangeal joint and

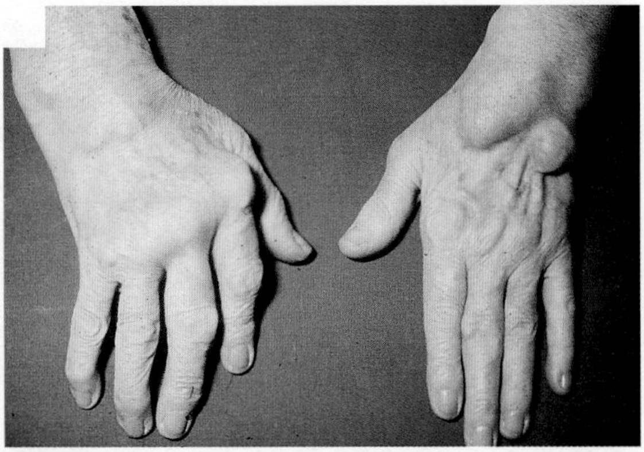

A

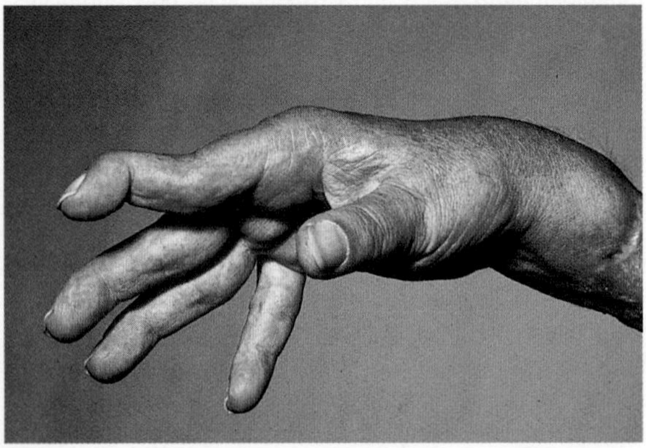

B

Fig. 12.29 The hand in rheumatoid arthritis. A Ulnar deviation of the fingers with wasting of the small muscles of the hands and synovial swelling at the wrists, the extensor tendon sheaths, the metacarpophalangeal and proximal interphalangeal joints. B 'Swan neck' deformity of the fingers.

extension of the terminal interphalangeal joint), and a Z deformity of the thumb. Dorsal subluxation of the ulnar styloid of the wrist is common and may contribute to rupture of the 4th and 5th extensor tendons when these are already the site of tenosynovitis.

In the forefoot, subluxation of the metatarsophalangeal joints is followed by clawing of the toes, callosities over the exposed metatarsal heads and a painful sensation of 'walking on pebbles'. In the hindfoot, calcaneal erosions may develop at the insertion of the Achilles tendon, and valgus deformities at the subtalar joint are common.

Tenosynovitis and *bursitis* are integral features of RA, as tendon sheaths and bursae are also lined with synovium. 'Triggering' of the fingers may be associated with nodules in the flexor tendon sheaths which can progress to permanent flexion contractures or tendon rupture if left untreated.

Popliteal cysts (Baker's cysts) communicate with the knee but fluid is prevented from returning to the joint by a valve-like mechanism. The high pressure generated by flexion of the knee, especially when effusions are present, can cause gradual extension or rupture of the cyst into the calf. Rupture is accompanied by calf pain, swelling, tenderness and pitting oedema. Diagnostic confusion with deep vein thrombosis can usually be avoided by careful consideration of the history but ultrasound examination, venogram or arthrogram is occasionally required to establish the correct diagnosis (see Fig. 12.30).

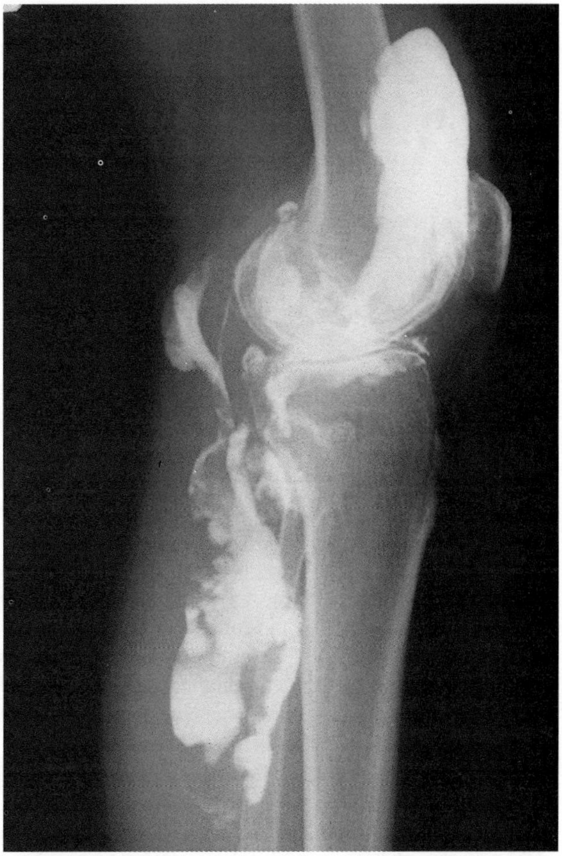

Fig. 12.30 Rupture of knee joint in rheumatoid arthritis. Arthrogram showing radio-opaque contrast medium in popliteal cyst and tissues of the calf.

EXTRA-ARTICULAR MANIFESTATIONS OF RHEUMATOID DISEASE

Systemic
- Fever
- Weight loss
- Fatigue
- Susceptibility to infection

Musculoskeletal
- Muscle wasting
- Tenosynovitis
- Bursitis
- Osteoporosis

Haematological
- Anaemia
- Thrombocytosis
- Eosinophilia

Lymphatic
- Splenomegaly
- Felty's syndrome

Nodules
- Sinuses
- Fistulae

Ocular
- Episcleritis
- Scleritis
- Scleromalacia
- Keratoconjunctivitis sicca

Vasculitis
- Digital arteritis
- Ulcers
- Pyoderma gangrenosum
- Mononeuritis multiplex
- Visceral arteritis

Cardiac
- Pericarditis
- Myocarditis
- Endocarditis
- Conduction defects
- Coronary vasculitis
- Granulomatous aortitis

Pulmonary
- Nodules
- Pleural effusions
- Fibrosing alveolitis
- Bronchiolitis
- Caplan's syndrome

Neurological
- Cervical cord compression
- Compression neuropathies
- Peripheral neuropathy
- Mononeuritis multiplex

Amyloidosis

Extra-articular features

Rheumatoid arthritis is a systemic disease. Anorexia, weight loss, lethargy, myalgia and Raynaud's phenomenon (see p. 268) occur commonly throughout its course and may precede the onset of articular symptoms by weeks or months. The many extra-articular features of the disease are listed in the information box.

Lymphadenopathy is usually found in nodes draining actively inflamed joints but more generalised lymphadenopathy can give rise to diagnostic confusion when arthritis is minimal or quiescent. The nodes are discrete and non-tender. Histology shows a reactive hyperplasia which can be mistaken for lymphoma.

Periarticular osteoporosis, muscle weakness and *wasting* are prominent adjacent to inflamed and functionally impaired joints. *Generalised osteoporosis, muscle wasting* and *skin atrophy* occur as global secondary complications of systemic inflammation and circulating Th_1 proinflammatory cytokines (IL-1, IL-6, TNF-α). Often seen early in the course of the

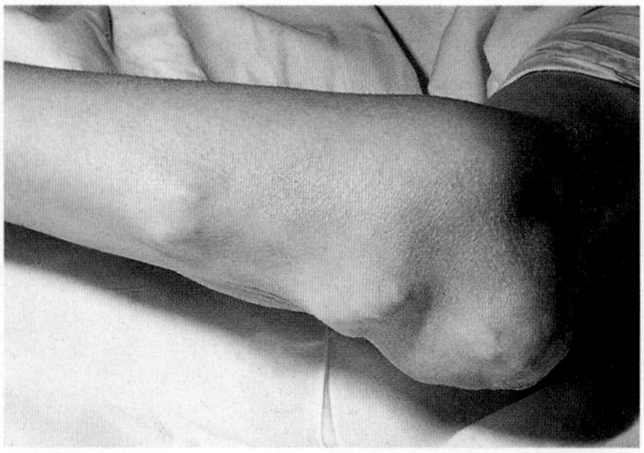

Fig. 12.31 Rheumatoid nodules.

disease, they progress to become major features in very active or advanced cases.

Subcutaneous nodules occur in about 20% of patients. They are usually seen at sites of pressure or friction, such as the extensor surfaces of the forearms below the elbow (see Fig. 12.31), the scalp, sacrum, scapula and Achilles tendon, as well as the fingers and toes. Ulceration and secondary infection are common. Nodules are almost invariably associated with the presence of rheumatoid factor.

Ocular manifestations

Episcleritis is a frequent, painless and benign feature in patients with nodular seropositive disease. It is not associated with visual disturbance and requires no specific therapy. *Scleritis* is rarer but more serious. The eye is red and painful with inflammatory changes throughout the sclera and uveal tract. The pupil may be irregular from adhesions (synechiae), which can cause secondary glaucoma and visual impairment. *Scleromalacia* may follow episodes of scleritis and is seen as a blue discoloration of the white of the eye. *Scleromalacia perforans* follows necrosis of the sclera and may require grafting or enucleation of the eye. *Keratoconjunctivitis sicca* (secondary Sjögren's syndrome) occurs in 10% of RA patients. Lack of lacrimal secretions results in grittiness, burning or itching associated with sticky mucous threads. Diagnosis can be confirmed by finding a reduction in the rate of tear secretion (Schirmer test).

Cardiovascular manifestations

Asymptomatic *pericarditis* occurs in about one-third of patients with seropositive RA. *Pericardial effusions* and *constrictive pericarditis* are rarer complications. Very rarely, granulomatous lesions lead to *heart block*, *cardiomyopathy*, *coronary artery occlusion* or *aortic regurgitation*.

Vasculitis

Diffuse *necrotising vasculitis* is seen particularly in patients with nodules and positive tests for rheumatoid factor. Clinical manifestations vary with the size and site of the vessel involved. Small-vessel disease of the terminal arterioles or capillaries is often associated with no more than nail fold infarcts, leg ulcers or purpura. Large areas of skin necrosis or digital gangrene have more serious clinical significance and may herald the onset of *malignant rheumatoid disease*. Such patients are often febrile, with severe systemic disturbance and multiple extra-articular manifestations. A medium-vessel arteritis, histologically resembling polyarteritis nodosa, may result in catastrophic mesenteric, renal, cerebrovascular or coronary artery occlusion. Such patients frequently have evidence of circulating immune complexes, hypergammaglobulinaemia, cryoglobulins and hypocomplementaemia.

Pulmonary manifestations

See page 374.

Neurological manifestations

Entrapment neuropathies result from compression of peripheral nerves by hypertrophied synovium. Median nerve compression in the carpal tunnel is the most common and may be an early clinical manifestation of the disease. Others include ulnar nerve compression at the elbow, peroneal nerve palsy at the knee and posterior tibial nerve entrapment in the flexor retinaculum at the ankle (tarsal tunnel syndrome). A more diffuse symmetrical *peripheral neuropathy* can occur and is usually limited to symptoms and signs of mild 'glove and stocking' sensory loss. *Mononeuritis multiplex* follows occlusion of vasa nervorum in patients with arteritis. *Cervical cord compression* can result from subluxation of the cervical spine at the atlantoaxial joint or at a subaxial level. Atlantoaxial subluxation is a common finding in long-standing RA and can be diagnosed from lateral radiographs of the cervical spine taken in full flexion (see Fig. 12.32). Although usually associated with no more than neck pain radiating to the occiput, it can result in cord compression and sudden death if the neck is manipulated inadvertently under an anaesthetic. Progressive cervical myelopathy may develop more insidiously with limb weakness, difficulty in holding up the head and tetraparesis. These problems occur more often following subluxation at a subaxial level and may require operative decompression and fixation.

Haematological manifestations

A *normochromic normocytic anaemia* of chronic disease which does not respond to oral iron is very common in active rheumatoid disease. The picture is frequently complicated by true iron deficiency secondary to gastrointestinal blood loss from treatment with NSAIDs. Thrombocytosis is a feature of active systemic inflammation. Much less frequently there may be a macrocytic anaemia associated with folate deficiency. *Felty's syndrome* is the association of splenomegaly

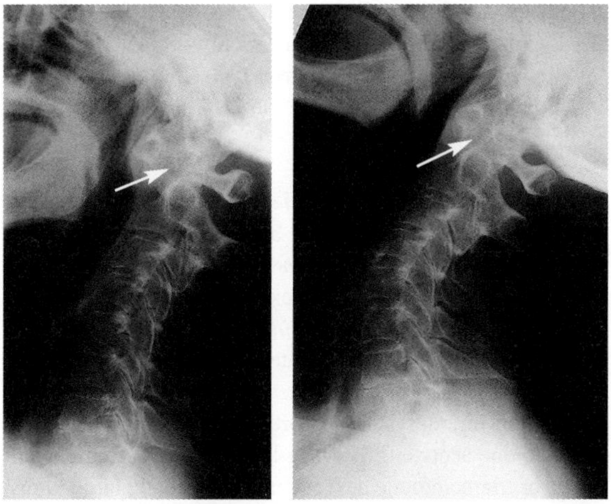

Fig. 12.32 Subluxation of cervical spine in rheumatoid arthritis: lateral radiographs. [A] Flexion. [B] Extension. Note the atlantoaxial subluxation with an increase in the pre-odontoid gap from 5 mm in extension to 12 mm on flexion.

and neutropenia with rheumatoid arthritis. The features are listed in the information box.

Complications

Septic arthritis may complicate rheumatoid arthritis, particularly in patients with long-standing nodular seropositive disease. In debilitated patients, fever and leucocytosis may be absent and the signs of infection limited to malaise and slight exacerbation of inflammation in one or more joints. *Staphylococcus aureus* is commonly implicated secondary to invasion from an ulcerated nodule or infected skin lesion. *Amyloidosis* is a complication of prolonged active disease and is found in 25–30% of patients at autopsy, making rheumatoid arthritis a leading cause of secondary amyloidosis.

FELTY'S SYNDROME

- Age of onset 50–70
- F > M
- Caucasians > Blacks
- Incidence < 1% RA patients
- Long-standing RA
- Deforming but inactive disease
- Seropositive

Common clinical features

- Splenomegaly
- Lymphadenopathy
- Weight loss
- Skin pigmentation
- Keratoconjunctivitis sicca
- Nodules
- Vasculitis
- Leg ulcers
- Recurrent infections

Laboratory findings

- Anaemia
- Neutropenia
- Thrombocytopenia
- Impaired T and B cell immunity
- Abnormal liver function

INVESTIGATIONS IN RHEUMATOID ARTHRITIS

To establish diagnosis
- Clinical criteria
- Markers of inflammation
- Serological tests
- Radiographs
- Synovial analysis

To document extent of pathological changes
- Radiographs

Occasionally:
- Arthrography
- Scintigraphy
- Ultrasound
- CT
- MRI

To monitor disease activity in response to therapy
- Clinical measures
  - Pain (visual analogue scale)
  - Early morning stiffness (minutes)
  - Joint tenderness (number of inflamed joints, articular index)
- ESR, plasma viscosity or acute-phase proteins (e.g. CRP)
- Haemoglobin

To assess progression of disease
- Radiographs
- Functional assessment

To monitor for safety of drug therapy
- Haematology
- Urinalysis
- Biochemistry
- Other tests

Investigations

These are listed in the information box and on pages 806–808.

Management

The aetiology of rheumatoid arthritis is unknown, and so treatment is empirically directed towards:

- relief of symptoms
- suppression of active and progressive disease
- conservation and restoration of function in affected joints.

To a greater or lesser extent these are achieved by combining:

- treatment of the patient—drugs, rest, physiotherapy, surgery—*with*
- modification of the environment—aids, appliances, housing, occupation, statutory social benefits.

GRADING OF FUNCTION IN RHEUMATOID ARTHRITIS

- I Fit for all activities—no handicap
- II Moderate restriction—independent despite some limitation of joint movement
- III Marked restriction—limited self-care. Some assistance required
- IV Confined to chair or bed-bound—largely incapacitated and dependent

In a chronic and frequently progressive disease characterised by exacerbations and remissions over many years, as well as by systemic, psychiatric and social complications, periodic assessment of radiological progression, disease activity and disability is required (see the information box). General practitioners and hospital physicians have a special responsibility to coordinate a team of medical specialists, orthopaedic surgeons, occupational therapists, physiotherapists, nurses, social workers and other health professionals in an integrated programme of multidisciplinary care and rehabilitation.

Patient education, counselling and continuing medical support are usually required for successful management, while physical rehabilitation, reconstructive surgery and environmental adaptation assume increasing importance when advancing joint damage and deformity are associated with functional impairment.

Repeated medical, functional and social assessment are required if patients are to maintain their maximum physical, psychological, social and vocational potential.

General treatment in the active phase

Physical rest, anti-inflammatory drug therapy and maintenance exercises are the cornerstones of treatment for exacerbations of rheumatoid arthritis. Admission to hospital is necessary in a minority of patients when widespread active polyarthritis is associated with signs of constitutional disturbance and there has been no response to rest at home and optimal doses of NSAIDs and disease-modifying antirheumatic drugs (DMARDs).

The rest from physical and emotional stress provided by 1–2 weeks in a hospital ward or day-patient unit is usually sufficient to induce a marked remission of symptoms without recourse to strict bed rest. Hospitalisation allows for detailed assessment by all members of the arthritis team followed by a programme of medical and physical rehabilitation best suited to the individual's needs.

In a few patients a period of complete bed rest may be required to induce a remission. In these circumstances it is essential to prevent the development of 'bed deformities' by ensuring appropriate positioning of joints. Foot and quadriceps exercises should be performed daily, along with maintenance exercises for muscle groups in unaffected limbs.

Anaemia of chronic disease responds best to induction of disease remission, and oral iron is only indicated in those patients with superadded true iron deficiency. Folic acid is occasionally required to treat an associated macrocytic anaemia.

Local measures in the active phase

Rest splints. These can be useful to support a particularly painful joint, such as the knee or wrist; splints are used to prevent or correct flexion deformities.

Intra-articular corticosteroid injections. These are useful for settling inflammation in isolated joints that remain painful and inflamed despite general measures. Local injection of a long-acting microcrystalline corticosteroid such as methylprednisolone acetate (20–80 mg large joints; 4–10 mg small joints) or triamcinolone hexacetonide (10–40 mg large joints; 2–6 mg small joints) can bring symptomatic relief lasting weeks or months. Repeated injections at short intervals, particularly in weight-bearing joints, should be avoided. Local injection of a corticosteroid is also the treatment of choice for bursitis, tenosynovitis and carpal tunnel syndrome when rest, splints and other general measures have not been effective.

Non-steroidal anti-inflammatory drugs

In optimal anti-inflammatory doses (see Table 12.9) NSAIDs can be very effective in relieving pain and stiffness but they do not alter the course of the disease and the margin between effective and toxic doses is often small.

Inhibition of prostaglandin synthetase is a major pharmacological action common to all these agents but simultaneous inhibition of the cytoprotective effect of prostanoids on gastric mucosa makes them liable to cause gastrointestinal side-effects such as dyspepsia, ulceration and haemorrhage. NSAID-associated upper gastrointestinal haemorrhage is the most frequent serious adverse drug-related event to be reported to the Committee on Safety of Medicines. Elderly

Table 12.9 Some commonly used non-steroidal analgesic anti-inflammatory drugs (NSAIDs)

Drug	Dose
Low risk	
Ibuprofen	< 1600 mg/day
Average risk	
Diclofenac	75–150 mg/day
Indomethacin	75–150 mg/day
Naproxen	500–1000 mg/day
Piroxicam	10–30 mg/day
High risk	
Azapropazone	1200–1800 mg/day
Partially selective cyclo-oxygenase-2 inhibitors	
Aceclofenac	100–200 mg/day
Meloxicam	7.5–15 mg/day
Nabumetone	500–1500 mg/day

women are particularly susceptible and case control studies suggest that one-fifth of all admissions to hospital in patients over the age of 60 with bleeding gastric or duodenal ulcers are directly attributable to taking NSAIDs. About 1% of RA patients receiving NSAID drugs are admitted to hospital each year with a major GI bleed. Treatment with these agents should be avoided in patients with peptic ulceration but it is important to realise that endoscopic evidence of ulcers is found in 20% of NSAID-treated patients even in the absence of symptoms. When NSAID treatment cannot be avoided, peptic ulcers can be made to heal by concomitant administration of H_2 antagonists (cimetidine, ranitidine), proton pump inhibitors (omeprazole, lansoprazole) or prostaglandin E analogues (misoprostol). The risk of NSAID-induced gastric ulceration can also be reduced by the simultaneous administration of omeprazole, ranitidine or misoprostol 100–200 μg 6-hourly to high-risk patients. These include elderly and physically disabled debilitated patients, patients receiving corticosteroids and patients with a previous history of peptic ulceration or bleed.

Other side-effects of NSAIDs include fluid retention, rashes, interstitial nephritis, occasional hepatotoxicity and, rarely, asthma and anaphylaxis.

Recent pharmaco-epidemiological studies in general practice have shown differences in the toxicity of established NSAIDs (see Table 12.9). Research has further revealed two isoforms of cyclo-oxygenase: a constitutive (COX-1) enzyme important for homeostatic protection of the gastric mucosa and kidney; and an inducible (COX-2) enzyme which generates inflammatory prostaglandins. This raises the possibility of developing selective COX-2 inhibitors free from gastric and renal toxicity.

It is advisable to start with one of the established, less expensive NSAIDs, with a low incidence of side-effects, for a trial period of about 2–3 weeks. Another NSAID can be tried if the response is not satisfactory but simultaneous administration of more than one NSAID results in an increase in the risk of adverse events without significant therapeutic benefit.

Simple analgesics

Drugs without appreciable anti-inflammatory action include peripherally acting agents such as paracetamol and centrally acting narcotic analgesics such as dextropropoxyphene, dihydrocodeine, nefopam and tramadol. Although centrally acting narcotic analgesics should generally be avoided in the management of rheumatic diseases, simple analgesics are frequently used as additions to therapy when pain relief is inadequate. Combination drugs such as co-proxamol (paracetamol and dextropropoxyphene) can be safe and effective when used in moderate doses.

Slow-acting antirheumatic drugs

The addition of a ‘disease-modifying’ antirheumatic drug (DMARD) should be considered in all patients with symptoms and signs of active inflammatory arthritis. Drugs of this type do not possess immediate anti-inflammatory effects but will improve joint pain, stiffness and swelling and reduce systemic symptoms, acute-phase proteins, sedimentation rate and rheumatoid factor titre over a period of months. If started early they may have a marginal effect in reducing the rate of radiological progression of disease but their main benefit is in inducing a symptomatic remission for 1–2 years in 40–60% of patients. They are usually introduced in a pyramidal fashion, starting with the safest agent, but the threshold for ascending the pyramid is determined by the severity of the disease (see Fig. 12.33).

Antimalarials. Hydroxychloroquine sulphate (< 6.5 mg/kg) can be used as an adjunct to basic therapy. Clinical benefit is noted in about half the patients in 4–12 weeks and the drug should be discontinued if there is no effect within 6 months. Occasional side-effects include nausea, diarrhoea, rashes, haemolytic anaemia, ototoxicity and neuromyopathy, and there is a small risk of ocular toxicity after more than a year of therapy. Deposits of the drug in the cornea may produce disturbances of vision which tend to disappear when the drug is withdrawn. Rarely, retinopathy can result in permanent visual impairment. If the drug is effective it is advisable to check visual acuity, macular function with an Amsler grid, and the ophthalmoscopic appearance of the maculae after 1 year and at 6-monthly intervals thereafter. In order to reduce the risks of ocular toxicity antimalarials are often given for only 10 months in each year. In some patients the dose can be halved without exacerbation of symptoms. Although antimalarials are generally less effective than other DMARDs, their use is associated with fewer patient dropouts for toxicity.

Sulphasalazine. This has a good benefit-to-risk profile and is frequently used as the first choice of DMARD. Approximately 50% of patients respond in 3–6 months. Nausea and vomiting can be troublesome but these symptoms can usually be avoided if treatment is started with 500 mg daily of the enteric-coated preparation, increasing to 1 g 12-hourly over a period of 4 weeks. Depression, rashes, megaloblastic anaemia and hepatitis are rarer side-effects and the full blood count and liver function tests should be monitored regularly every 1–3 months.

Methotrexate, d-penicillamine and parenteral gold. These are slow-acting, suppressive antirheumatic drugs which have been shown to decrease the progression of erosive changes as well as reduce the activity of the disease in 50–60% of patients. Due to a high incidence of toxic effects, treatment with these agents should only be considered as an addition to basic therapy when there are clear indications for the use of a disease-modifying drug and the patient has failed to respond to antimalarials or sulphasalazine. Indications for use are listed in the information box.

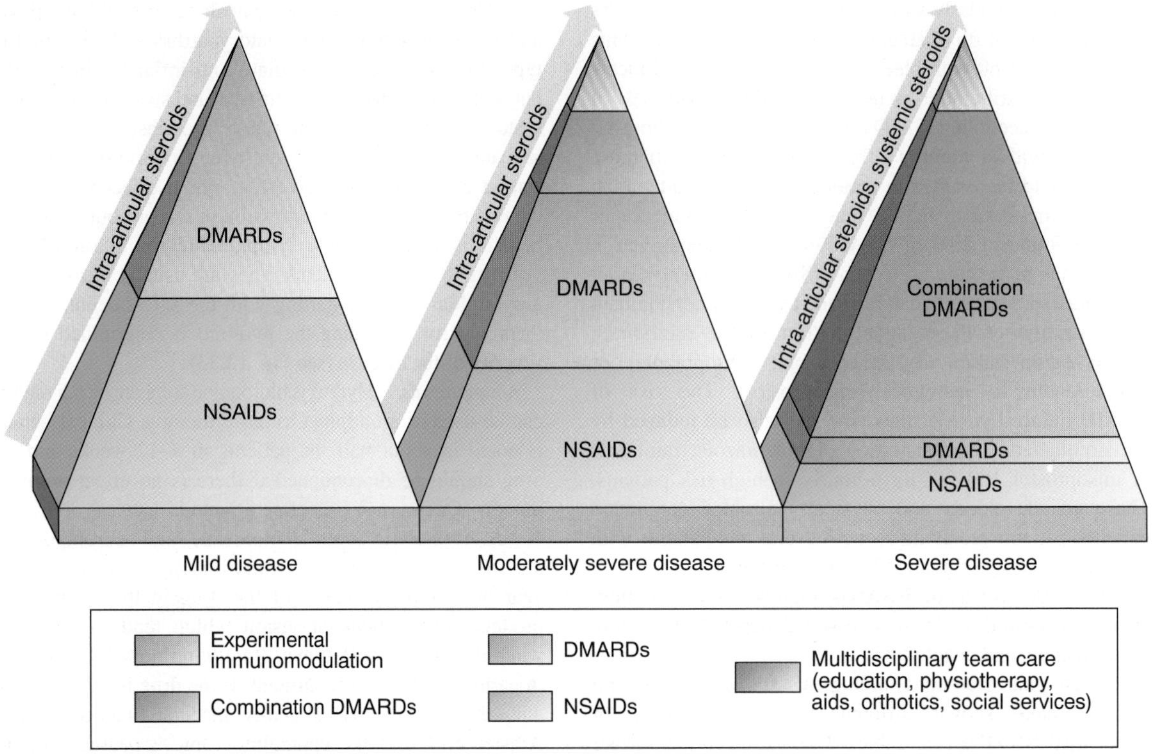

Fig. 12.33 The pyramidal approach to therapy in rheumatoid arthritis. The speed and height attained on the pyramid are determined by the severity of disease and response to treatment.

INDICATIONS FOR DISEASE-MODIFYING DRUGS
• Persistent symptoms and signs of inflammatory arthritis • Evidence of progressive radiological damage • Troublesome extra-articular manifestations • Palindromic rheumatoid arthritis

Methotrexate is now the drug of choice in patients with active or aggressive disease who have failed to respond to sulphasalazine. It works more quickly than other DMARDs, with significant improvement in symptoms in 4–6 weeks. It is administered as an oral pulse of 5–30 mg weekly with a 5 mg dose of folic acid on the day following methotrexate to reduce the incidence of adverse reactions. Methotrexate is only rarely associated with bone marrow suppression or acute disturbances of liver function, but full blood counts and liver function tests must be monitored regularly and care must be taken to avoid drug interaction with sulphonamides. Increased susceptibility to infection is important and acute pulmonary toxicity is an unpredictable problem in 5–10% of patients. The silent development of progressive hepatic fibrosis has been recorded and the drug should not be given to patients who are taking alcohol regularly.

When parenteral gold is chosen, after a test dose of 10 mg, weekly intramuscular injections of 50 mg sodium aurothiomalate are given until a response is obtained, usually by 2–3 months. The intervals between injections are progressively increased, provided the remission is maintained, and the drug is continued indefinitely. Gold injections should be stopped if there has been no clinical benefit after 6 months.

Adverse effects include pruritic rashes, exfoliative dermatitis, mouth ulcers, enterocolitis, proteinuria and the nephrotic syndrome, thrombocytopenia, agranulocytosis and aplastic anaemia. All are potentially serious and preclude further therapy. Patients who are HLA-DR3-positive are particularly at risk of developing a gold-induced immune complex glomerulonephritis. Monitoring should include a routine urinalysis and full blood counts with platelets, initially prior to each injection.

Pruritus may respond to antihistamines, and exfoliative dermatitis, thrombocytopenia, agranulocytosis and nephropathy to corticosteroids. Patients with agranulocytosis almost invariably recover if they can be protected from serious infection; those with aplastic anaemia have a more serious prognosis. Dimercaprol (BAL) combines with heavy metals to form a stable compound which is rapidly excreted in the urine; 3 mg/kg body weight should be administered intramuscularly 6-hourly for 3–4 days in patients with aplastic anaemia who have not responded to withdrawal of gold injections after 4–5 days.

Auranofin, an oral gold compound, is less toxic than parenteral preparations but short- and medium-term efficacy are also lower. The usual dose is 6 mg daily but this can be increased to 9 mg daily if there has been no response after 3–4 months. Diarrhoea is a common side-effect during the early phases of treatment. Mouth ulcers, dermatitis, proteinuria and bone marrow suppression are significantly less likely than with intramuscular gold but the full blood count and routine urinalysis need to be monitored regularly.

D-penicillamine is commenced with a single evening dose of 125 or 250 mg orally and dosage is increased by no more than 250 mg monthly to a maximum of 1 g daily. Clinical benefit is noted several weeks after an effective dose has been achieved and reaches a maximum after 4–6 months.

Rashes, loss of taste, nausea, vomiting and serious febrile reactions can occur soon after starting treatment. Later side-effects include mouth ulcers, proteinuria and the nephrotic syndrome. Very rarely, diseases resembling systemic lupus erythematosus, myasthenia gravis, pemphigus and Goodpasture's syndrome can occur. Thrombocytopenia and pancytopenia may occur at any time and are potentially the most serious toxic effects.

Patients should be monitored, initially at weekly intervals, by urinalysis and full blood counts, including platelets. Proteinuria and mild thrombocytopenia are indications for cessation of therapy, followed by re-introduction of the drug at a lower dose if the abnormalities disappear. It is advisable to withdraw d-penicillamine altogether if the side-effects recur. Febrile reactions and pancytopenia are absolute indications for drug withdrawal. The likelihood of side-effects with d-penicillamine is increased in slow sulphoxidisers.

Other disease-modifying antirheumatic drugs

Dapsone is associated with slow clinical improvement and reduction of acute-phase proteins but haemolytic anaemia can be a troublesome side-effect, particularly in slow acetylators. Other compounds which have been shown to have slow-acting antirheumatic activity include the antibacterial agent rifampicin, the antihypertensive agent captopril, some d-penicillamine analogues, the pentapeptide thymosin and the isoxazole derivative leflunamide.

Corticosteroids. These have a very potent anti-inflammatory activity but doses required to maintain adequate symptomatic relief on a long-term basis are accompanied by an unacceptable level of side-effects, and the extent to which corticosteroids possess the disease-modifying properties of the slow-acting antirheumatic agents remains uncertain. There is some recent evidence to suggest that the addition of a fixed dose of 7.5 mg prednisolone daily to NSAID and DMARD therapy can slow the rate of radiological progression over 2 years in patients with early RA. Concern about long-term side-effects means that indications for their use are usually restricted and a slow-acting antirheumatic agent is usually commenced simultaneously with a view to gradual withdrawal of corticosteroid therapy when remission has been obtained.

The main indications for the use of systemic corticosteroids are:

- in exceptionally severe exacerbations which are not remitting with rest, intra-articular injections of corticosteroids, NSAIDs and DMARDs
- when other measures fail to control persistently disabling symptoms in breadwinners or young mothers who have to return to work
- in some elderly patients when acute disease is threatening to render them bed-bound
- in life- or sight-threatening visceral disease such as severe pericarditis or scleritis.

Prednisolone is the corticosteroid of choice. It should be administered as a single morning oral dose of no more than 7.5 mg daily to minimise suppression of the hypothalamo-pituitary-adrenal axis. An evening dose of 5 mg is sometimes more useful in overcoming intractable early morning stiffness.

The potential side-effects of steroids are numerous (see the information box). Infection and osteoporosis are

SIDE-EFFECTS OF SYSTEMIC CORTICOSTEROIDS

Endocrine
- Moon face
- Truncal obesity
- Hirsutism
- Impotence
- Menstrual irregularity
- Suppression of hypothalamo-pituitary-adrenal axis
- Growth suppression

Metabolic
- Negative calcium, potassium and nitrogen balance
- Sodium and fluid retention
- Hyperglycaemia
- Hyperlipoproteinaemia

Musculoskeletal
- Myopathy
- Osteoporosis
- Avascular necrosis

Skin
- Acne, striae
- Skin atrophy
- Bruising
- Impaired wound-healing

Immunological
- Suppression of delayed hypersensitivity
- Reactivation of TB
- Susceptibility to infection

Gastrointestinal
- Peptic ulceration
- Pancreatitis

Cardiovascular
- Hypertension
- Congestive cardiac failure

Ocular
- Glaucoma
- Cataracts

CNS
- Changes in mood and personality
- Psychosis
- Benign intracranial hypertension

particularly troublesome in patients with RA, and patients commencing prolonged systemic steroid therapy should be given bone prophylaxis with calcitriol, vitamin D and calcium, or a bisphosphonate.

Immunomodulation

A number of cytotoxic and immunostimulant agents have been found to have both symptomatic and slow-acting disease-modifying activity in rheumatoid arthritis. The effects are mediated as much by anti-inflammatory as by immunoregulatory activity and their usefulness is limited by immediate and potential long-term toxicity.

The indications for use of these agents at present are limited to:

- life-threatening extra-articular manifestations which have failed to respond to corticosteroids or second-line agents
- severe active symptomatic and progressive joint disease that has failed to respond to all other forms of therapy
- patients receiving unacceptably high doses of corticosteroids in whom dose reduction has not been possible.

Mechanisms of action of commonly used agents are summarised in Table 12.10 and toxic effects in Table 12.11. Methotrexate is discussed on page 843.

Azathioprine. This has been shown to be effective in both high (2.5 mg/kg) and low (1.25 mg/kg) oral doses. Adverse effects include vomiting, stomatitis, diarrhoea, hepatitis and particularly bone marrow suppression and susceptibility to infection. Monitoring is with regular full blood counts, weekly at first and then at longer intervals.

Cyclophosphamide. This has a narrow therapeutic range but is effective in a daily oral dose of 1–2 mg/kg. Adverse effects include alopecia, azoospermia, anovulation, cystitis, nausea and vomiting, susceptibility to infection, bone marrow suppression and teratogenesis. Monitoring is by fortnightly or monthly full blood counts and routine urinalysis. Toxicity may be reduced by intermittent intravenous infusion or oral boluses (0.5–1.5 g/m^2).

Cyclosporin A. This is effective in doses of 2.5–4 mg/kg daily given in divided oral doses 12-hourly. Adverse effects include anorexia, nausea, hepatotoxicity, hypertension and dose-related impairment of glomerular filtration. The full blood count, urinalysis and plasma creatinine should be measured weekly at first and later every 2–4 weeks, and the blood pressure should be monitored.

Table 12.10 Mechanism of action of the immunomodulating drugs

Drug	Class	Effects
Azathioprine	Purine analogue	Inhibits purine synthesis of DNA and RNA
Cyclophosphamide **Chlorambucil**	Alkylating agent	Direct binding of DNA, RNA and proteins
Methotrexate	Folic acid antagonist	Binds dihydrofolate reductase Blocks de novo purine and thymidylate synthesis
Cyclosporin A	Fungal polypeptide	Cyclosporin A–cyclophyllin complex inhibits signal transduction in lymphocyte calcineurin

Novel approaches to immunotherapy

Targeted immunotherapy with a variety of mouse, chimeric and humanised monoclonal antibodies is superseding non-specific immunosuppression in the hope that the risks of infection can be reduced, but all such approaches remain experimental. Targets include CD4, CD5, CD7 and CD25 (IL-2 receptor) on lymphocytes, CDW52 on monocytes and lymphocytes, adhesion molecules (ICAM-1) and other cytokines and cytokine receptors such as TNF-α and the IL-1 receptor. Recent placebo-controlled trials of anti-TNF-α monoclonal antibody therapy have demonstrated good short-term efficacy and safety, and placebo-controlled trials of self-administered daily subcutaneous injection of a recombinant IL-1 receptor antagonist have shown modest symptomatic benefit and marginal slowing of erosions in patients with active disease.

Table 12.11 Toxic effects of immunosuppressive drugs

	Azathioprine	Methotrexate	Cyclophosphamide	Chlorambucil	Cyclosporin A
GI tract	+	++	+	+	+
Bone marrow	++	++	++	+++	+
Bladder	0	0	+++	0	0
Kidneys	0	+	0	0	+++
Liver	+	+++	0	0	++
Lungs	+	+++	+	+	0
Gonads	0	0	+++	+++	0
Fetus	±	+++	±	±	±
Neoplasia	++	+/–	++	++	+

0 to +++ = no toxicity to severe toxicity.

Other measures

Patients with Sjögren's syndrome require scrupulous oral and ocular hygiene and the instillation of artificial tears (hypromellose eye drops). Drug hypersensitivity is sometimes a problem. Corticosteroids are used in Felty's syndrome but the outcome is unsatisfactory. Splenectomy is reserved for patients with serious or life-threatening infections and is followed by remission in 60% of patients.

Medical synovectomy

Synovial obliteration can be achieved with osmic acid or a variety of radiocolloids if pain, effusion and synovitis persist despite local corticosteroid injections, systemic drug therapy and physical measures. ^{90}-Yttrium silicate is used for large joints such as the knee, and ^{159}-erbium acetate for the small joints of the hands. Joints are immobilised for 72 hours to reduce spread to regional lymph nodes. Patients under the age of 45 should not be treated in this manner.

Surgical treatment and rehabilitation

There are many circumstances in the overall management of patients with severe and progressive rheumatoid arthritis in which orthopaedic surgical procedures are required to relieve pain and conserve or restore locomotor function (see Table 12.12).

Surgical decompression and synovectomy of the wrist and tendon sheaths of the hands are often needed when other measures have failed to relieve a carpal tunnel syndrome or flexion contractures of the fingers resulting from fibrosis and nodule formation. Flexor and extensor tendon synovectomy, the latter often accompanied by resection of a subluxed ulnar styloid, can be important measures in preventing tendon ruptures. Synovectomy of joints will not prevent disease progression but may be indicated for pain relief when drug therapy, local rest, intra-articular injections and radiocolloids have failed to provide symptomatic relief.

At a later stage, when tendons, cartilage and bone have been eroded and the mechanics of joints disturbed, reconstructive tendon surgery, osteotomy, arthrodesis and a variety of arthroplasties with or without prostheses play a major part in the rehabilitation of the patient.

If surgical treatment is to be successful the aims and consequences of each operation should be carefully considered as part of an integrated programme of management and rehabilitation. This is often best achieved where physicians and surgeons with special experience work together in a combined rheumatology/orthopaedic clinic with other allied health professionals. Assessment of motivation, social support and environment are no less important than careful consideration of the patient's general health and detailed assessment of the extent of disease in other joints, the integrity of the cervical spine, and the presence or absence of infection, arteritis or osteoporosis. In particular, it must be appreciated that, whereas many patients with slowly progressive disease can be kept mobile and functionally independent by a series of major joint replacements carried out over a number of years, it is seldom possible to mobilise a patient who has been chair- or bed-bound for a long period by multiple joint replacement during a single lengthy hospital admission. In these and other circumstances pain relief and functional independence are better served by provision of a suitable wheelchair, home adjustments, physical aids and social services.

When a patient cannot return to a former occupation it may be necessary to suggest a change of employment where less strain will be thrown on the damaged joints. It should be emphasised, however, that patients have the best chance of returning to active work with their former employers. It cannot be stressed too strongly that adequate treatment in

Table 12.12 Some useful surgical procedures in RA and OA

Procedures	Indication
Soft tissue release (decompression)	
Carpal tunnel	Median nerve compression
Tarsal tunnel	Posterior tibial nerve entrapment
Flexor tendon sheaths of hand	Relief of 'trigger fingers'
Rerouting ulnar nerve at elbow	Ulnar nerve entrapment
Tendon repairs and transfers	
Extensor tendons of hands	Rupture of extensor tendons
Flexor tendon of thumbs and fingers	Rupture of flexor tendons
Synovectomy	
Wrist and extensor tendon sheaths (and excision of ulnar styloid)	Pain relief and prevention of extensor tendon rupture
Osteotomy	
Keller's operation	Correct hallux valgus
Femoral osteotomy	Pain relief Correct deformity of early OA in hip
Tibial osteotomy	Pain relief Correct deformity of unicompartmental OA in knee
Excision arthroplasty	
Radial head	Pain on subluxation of radio-ulnar joint
Lateral end of clavicle	Pain in acromioclavicular joint
Fowler's operation (metatarsal head resection)	Forefoot pain on metatarsophalangeal joint subluxation
Joint replacement	
Hip, knee, elbow, shoulder, ankle, metacarpophalangeal joints of hands	Pain relief Maintain, restore and improve function
Arthrodesis	
Interphalangeal joint of thumb or fingers	Improve hand function
Metacarpophalangeal joint of thumb	Improve pinch grip
Wrist	Pain relief, improve grip
Ankle and subtalar joints	Pain relief, stabilise hind foot

the early stages and throughout the course of the disease enables most patients to return to some form of wage-earning activity. Disabilities of all kinds can be reduced even in the 25% of patients running a severe progressive course.

Prognosis

The course and prognosis in rheumatoid arthritis are very variable. In those patients with disease of such severity as to require admission to hospital, review after 10 years shows that 25% will have a complete remission of symptoms and remain fit for all normal activities; 40% will have only moderate impairment of function despite exacerbations and remissions of disease; 25% will be more severely disabled; and 10% will be severely crippled. (This rises to 20% after 20 years.) The overall prognosis is much better if the many patients in the community are considered whose symptoms are never of such severity as to require admission to hospital. A poor prognosis may be associated with:

- high titres of rheumatoid factor
- insidious onset of disease
- more than a year of active disease without remission
- early development of nodules and erosions
- extra-articular manifestations
- severe functional impairment.

Life expectancy is reduced by 10–15 years in patients with RA, and mortality is particularly increased in RA patients with functional impairment. The 5-year survival for severely disabled RA patients is reduced by 50% and the prognosis in such patients is similar to that for patients with three-vessel coronary artery disease or stage IV Hodgkin's disease.

PSORIATIC ARTHRITIS

This is a seronegative inflammatory arthritis found in patients with psoriasis, a past or family history of psoriasis or with characteristic changes in the nails.

Epidemiology

Psoriatic arthritis occurs in about 1/1000 of the general population and in 7% of patients with psoriasis. Approximately 20% of all patients with seronegative polyarthritis have psoriasis, while the prevalence of psoriasis in seropositive rheumatoid arthritis is no higher than that in the general population, suggesting that the association of the skin disease with seronegative arthritis does not arise by chance alone. The onset is usually between the age of 25 and 40 years.

Clinical features

Five distinct clinical patterns of psoriatic arthritis are recognised and are listed in the information box. An inflammatory arthritis affecting the distal interphalangeal joints, which are typically not involved in RA, is the most characteristic form of psoriatic arthropathy and is almost invariably associated with nail changes (see Fig. 12.34). However, an asymmetrical or symmetrical seronegative arthritis resembling RA is more common.

CLINICAL PATTERNS OF PSORIATIC ARTHROPATHY	
• Asymmetrical oligoarthritis	35%
• Symmetrical seronegative arthritis	30%
• Sacroiliitis/spondylitis	15%
• Distal interphalangeal joint arthritis	15%
• Arthritis mutilans	5%

Sacroiliitis and spondylitis indistinguishable from classical ankylosing spondylitis can occur alone or in association with any of the clinical patterns of peripheral arthritis.

Extra-articular features are limited to:

- skin lesions. These may be widespread scaling lesions, typically over extensor surfaces, or insignificant and confined to such areas as the scalp, natal cleft and umbilicus, where they are easily overlooked (see p. 900).
- nail changes. These include pitting, onycholysis, subungual hyperkeratosis and horizontal ridging.
- iritis.

Investigations

The ESR is usually only moderately raised and there may be a mild normochromic normocytic anaemia in active cases. Tests for RF and ANA are negative. Radiographs showing asymmetrical disease, terminal interphalangeal joint involvement and relatively little periarticular osteoporosis may help to distinguish psoriatic arthritis from rheumatoid arthritis. The changes in the axial skeleton resemble those in ankylosing spondylitis.

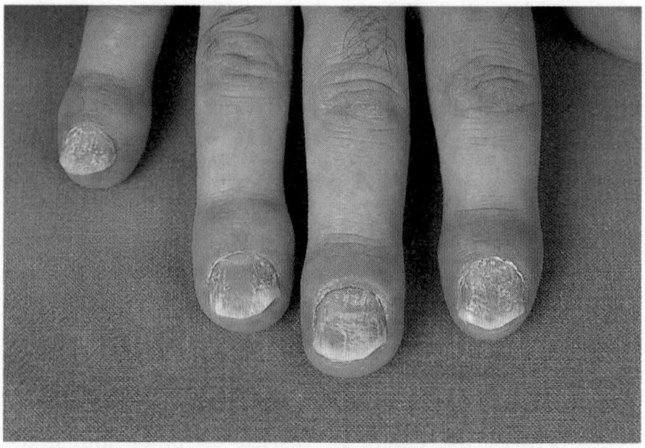

Fig. 12.34 Psoriatic arthritis. Arthritis in the distal interphalangeal joints with associated nail changes (pitting and onycholysis).

Management

NSAIDs are usually all that is required to control symptoms. Sulphasalazine and gold can be used in persistently symptomatic progressive cases without exacerbation of the psoriasis but the antimalarials chloroquine and hydroxychloroquine may give rise to exfoliative reactions. Methotrexate and other immunosuppressive drugs are used when sulphasalazine has failed, as well as to control progressive arthritis or extensive incapacitating skin disease. The retinoid acitretin (20 mg daily—see p. 903) has been shown to be effective in treating the arthritis as well as the skin lesions but it must be avoided in young women because of its teratogenicity. Its use is complicated by mucocutaneous side-effects, hyperlipidaemia, myalgias and extraspinal calcification. Photochemotherapy with methoxypsoralen and long-wave ultraviolet light (PUVA) is primarily used for patients with severe skin lesions but can also help some patients with synchronous exacerbations of inflammatory arthritis. Splints and prolonged rest are avoided because of the increased tendency to fibrous and bony ankylosis but intra-articular steroid injections can be used to good effect in persistently active and symptomatic joints.

Prognosis

This is better than for rheumatoid arthritis, with the exception of those rare patients with arthritis mutilans.

SPONDARTHRITIDES

This is a group of diseases in which an inflammatory arthritis, characterised by persistently negative tests for IgM rheumatoid factor, is variably associated with a number of other common articular, extra-articular and genetic features. These are listed in the first information box. The features held in common by the spondarthritides are shown in the second information box.

THE SPONDARTHRITIDES

- Ankylosing spondylitis
- Enteric-acquired reactive arthritis (including Reiter's disease) (EARA)
- Sexually acquired reactive arthritis (SARA)
- Enteropathic arthritis
  - Ulcerative colitis
  - Crohn's disease
- Juvenile spondylitis

FEATURES COMMON TO THE SPONDARTHRITIDES

- Sacroiliitis and/or spondylitis
- Asymmetrical oligoarthritis
- Enthesitis
- Anterior uveitis
- Familial association
- High prevalence of HLA-B27

Current concepts of the aetiology of these disorders are that they may arise as an abnormal response to infection in genetically predisposed persons carrying the HLA-B27 antigen. In some an inciting organism has been identified, as in Reiter's disease which can follow bacterial dysentery or chlamydial urethritis, or in the reactive arthritis following infection with *Yersinia enterocolitica*. In the others the infectious agent remains obscure. It is uncertain whether possession of HLA-B27 predisposes towards disease because:

- it may be merely a marker for an immune response gene
- susceptibility to arthritis is increased as a result of cross-reactivity between a B27-determined host gene product and an antigen carried by the invading organism
- the inciting organism modifies HLA-B27 positive cellular receptors in such a way as to initiate an autoimmune reaction or render the cells more susceptible to cytotoxic lymphocytes.

ANKYLOSING SPONDYLITIS

In its typical form this is a chronic inflammatory arthritis with a predilection for the sacroiliac joints and spine. It is characterised by progressive stiffening and fusion of the axial skeleton.

Epidemiology

Typically, ankylosing spondylitis is a disease with a peak onset in the second and third decades and a male to female ratio of about 4:1. More than 90% of affected persons carry the histocompatibility antigen HLA-B27. The overall prevalence varies from 0.5–1% in most communities but is much greater in the Pima and Haida Indians who have a high prevalence of HLA-B27. First-degree relatives of patients with ankylosing spondylitis have a greatly increased incidence of psoriatic arthritis, inflammatory bowel disease and Reiter's syndrome. Chronic prostatitis is more common than would be anticipated but it is not possible to isolate organisms from prostatic fluid. Faecal carriage of some *Klebsiella* species is increased in ankylosing spondylitis and this may be related to exacerbation of the disease.

Pathology

Biopsy material from peripheral joints shows changes similar to those found in rheumatoid arthritis. Bony ankylosis, however, occurs more frequently. The characteristic *enthesopathy* comprises multiple foci of inflammation with lymphocytes and plasma cells at ligamentous attachments and adjacent erosion of bone. Healing of similar lesions at the junction of the vertebral bodies and annulus fibrosus of the intervertebral discs leads to the new bone formation (syndesmophytes) which is the hallmark of the disease.

Clinical features

The onset is usually insidious, with recurring episodes of low back pain and stiffness sometimes radiating to the buttocks or thighs. Characteristically the symptoms are worse in the early morning and after inactivity. Occasionally the onset may be acute, resembling a lumbar disc protrusion. A few patients present with symptoms referable to the dorsal or cervical spine but such cases usually reveal evidence of previous sacroiliitis and lumbar spine involvement.

Chest pain aggravated by breathing results from involvement of the costovertebral joints. Plantar fasciitis, Achilles tendonitis and tenderness over bony prominences such as the iliac crest, ischial tuberosity and greater trochanter are typical. Around 25% of patients have an attack of acute anterior uveitis during the course of the disease and this may occasionally be the presenting feature. A peripheral joint is first affected in 10% and in a further 10% symptoms begin in childhood as one variety of pauciarticular juvenile idiopathic arthritis.

Early signs include failure to obliterate the lumbar lordosis on forward flexion, pain on sacroiliac compression, and restriction of movements of the lumbar spine in all directions. As the disease progresses, stiffness increases throughout the spine, and chest expansion frequently becomes restricted. Spinal fusion occurs in only a minority and in most of these is not associated with much deformity. A few develop kyphosis of the dorsal and cervical spine, which can be incapacitating, especially when associated with hip involvement.

Iritis occurs in up to 25% of patients but other extra-articular features are rare. These manifestations are listed in the information box.

EXTRA-ARTICULAR MANIFESTATIONS OF ANKYLOSING SPONDYLITIS

- Iritis
- Amyloidosis
- Aortic regurgitation
- Osteoporosis
- Cardiac conduction defects
- Myelopathy secondary to atlantoaxial subluxation
- Apical pulmonary fibrosis
- Cauda equina syndrome

Investigations

The ESR is usually raised but may be normal. Tests for rheumatoid factor are negative and synovial fluid complement levels are not depressed.

Radiological signs of sacroiliitis begin in the lower part of the joints, with irregularity and marginal sclerosis eventually progressing to fusion. In the lumbar spine there may be 'squaring' of the vertebrae owing to ossification of the anterior longitudinal ligament, syndesmophyte formation, erosion and sclerosis at the anterior corners of the vertebrae, and facetal joint changes. Progressive ossification results in the typical 'bamboo' spine (see Fig. 12.7, p. 810). Erosive changes may be seen in the symphysis pubis, the ischial tuberosities and peripheral joints. Osteoporosis and atlantoaxial dislocation can occur.

Radionuclide bone scanning may reveal evidence of sacroiliitis or spinal involvement when radiographs are negative but the increased uptake of the bone-seeking isotope is non-specific and reflects bone blood flow and turnover.

Management

The principles are to relieve pain and stiffness, maintain a maximal range of skeletal mobility and avoid the development of deformities. Early in the disease patients should be taught to perform regular exercises at home and encouraged to take up active non-contact sports like swimming. Poor bed and chair posture must be avoided.

NSAIDs are used to relieve symptoms but do not themselves alter the course of the disease. A few patients with spondylitis find phenylbutazone the most effective drug; it can usually be given safely even over prolonged periods, provided a daily oral dose of 300 mg is not exceeded.

The addition of enteric-coated sulphasalazine 500 mg 6-hourly orally can be helpful in patients with persistent peripheral arthritis and has been shown to be of marginal benefit in suppressing the axial disease.

Radiotherapy is occasionally indicated if the response to drug therapy is unsatisfactory. It does not affect the course of the disease, however, and earlier regimens of treatment, when excessive radiation was employed, were associated with a 10-fold increase in the risk of developing leukaemia.

Local corticosteroid injections can be used for plantar fasciitis and the management of other manifestations of enthesopathy. Systemic steroids are sometimes required for treatment of acute iritis.

Hip disease may require surgery, and total hip arthroplasty has largely obviated the need for difficult spinal surgery in those with advanced deformity.

Prognosis

Around 75% or more of patients with ankylosing spondylitis are able to remain in employment without significant loss of time from work. Restriction of chest movements does not predispose to pulmonary infection but systemic complications and especially hip involvement carry a worse prognosis.

REACTIVE ARTHRITIS

Reiter's disease is the triad of non-specific urethritis, conjunctivitis and reactive arthritis that follows bacterial

ARTHRITOGENIC BACTERIA IMPLICATED IN REACTIVE ARTHRITIS

EARA	SARA
• *Salmonella*	• *Chlamydia*
• *Shigella*	
• *Campylobacter*	
• *Yersinia*	

dysentery or exposure to sexually transmitted infection. Incomplete forms are frequent and include the most common variety of inflammatory arthritis seen in young men. The bacteria implicated in reactive arthritis are listed in the information box.

Epidemiology

Between 1 and 2% of patients with non-specific urethritis seen at clinics for sexually transmitted diseases have reactive arthritis and there is a similar incidence following outbreaks of shigellosis. A male with HLA-B27 runs a 20% risk of getting reactive arthritis following an attack of shigella dysentery. Although predominantly a disease of young men, the apparent 50:1 male to female ratio is spuriously high, as urethritis is frequently ignored in women and children.

Clinical features

The onset is typically acute, with the simultaneous development of urethritis, conjunctivitis (in about 50%) and an inflammatory oligoarthritis affecting the large or small joints of the lower limbs, 1–3 weeks following sexual exposure or an attack of dysentery. There may be considerable systemic disturbance with fever, weight loss and vasomotor changes in the feet.

Often the onset is insidious and many patients present with monoarthritis of a knee or an asymmetrical inflammatory arthritis of some interphalangeal joints. Symptoms and signs of urethritis or conjunctivitis may have been minimal or forgotten. In such patients heel pain, Achilles tendonitis or plantar fasciitis are a valuable clue, while the presence of circinate balanitis or the rash of keratoderma blennorrhagica can establish the diagnosis, even in the absence of the classical triad and without an overt history of sexual promiscuity or dysentery. The skin lesions vary from faint macules, vesicles and pustules on the hands and feet to marked hyperkeratosis with plaque-like lesions spreading to the scalp and trunk. These may be associated with severe nail dystrophy and massive subungual hyperkeratosis (see Fig. 12.35).

Ocular involvement is usually limited to mild bilateral conjunctivitis which subsides spontaneously within a month. Acute iritis occurs at the outset in 10% of patients. It is distinguished from simple conjunctivitis by injection of the ciliary vessels around the cornea, by a constricted, irregular or unreactive pupil and by cells in the anterior chamber on slit lamp examination. Unlike the conjunctivitis, it requires urgent treatment. Chronic iritis may lead to glaucoma and blindness.

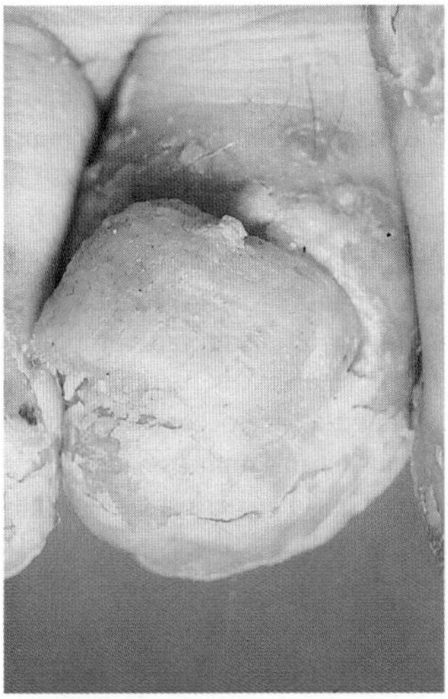

Fig. 12.35 Reiter's syndrome. Subungual hyperkeratosis and keratoderma blennorrhagica.

The urethritis is usually associated with minor dysuria and a clear sterile discharge. Sometimes it is asymptomatic and detected only by finding mucoid threads in the first voided specimen of early morning urine. Occasionally there may be severe dysuria, haematuria and suprapubic discomfort from an associated acute haemorrhagic cystitis and prostatitis.

The arthritis is usually self-limiting, with spontaneous remission of symptoms within 2–3 months of onset. There is, however, a recurrence rate of about 15% per annum, not necessarily related to further overt exposure to infection. Low back pain and stiffness from sacroiliitis are common and 15–20% of patients develop spondylitis. Iritis occurs in 30% of patients with recurring arthritis. Other extra-articular features are less common and are included in the information box.

Investigations

The ESR is often raised during the acute phase and may remain so long after joint symptoms have settled. Poly-

REITER'S SYNDROME: EXTRA-ARTICULAR FEATURES

- Conjunctivitis
- Iritis
- Urethritis
- Pericarditis/pleurisy
- Aortic incompetence
- Cardiac conduction defects
- Meningoencephalitis
- Peripheral neuropathy
- Keratoderma blennorrhagica

morphonuclear leucocytosis and an anaemia of chronic disease are further indications of active systemic disturbance. The synovial fluid has the characteristics of a low viscosity inflammatory effusion with leucocyte counts as high as 50 000/mm^3 but it is sterile on culture. Giant synovial macrophages can be seen. Serum tests for rheumatoid factor and antinuclear factor are negative. Tissue typing reveals HLA-B27 in more than 70% of cases.

In most patients there are no radiographic abnormalities but periarticular osteoporosis, reduction of joint space and erosive changes can occur when there has been prolonged or recurrent inflammatory arthritis. The changes may be accompanied by periostitis in the metatarsals, phalanges and pelvis, and there may be large, 'fluffy' calcaneal spurs. Sacroiliitis is indistinguishable from that seen in ankylosing spondylitis but the spinal changes include early isolated bony spurs and paravertebral ossification. These are also seen in psoriasis but not in ankylosing spondylitis.

Management

This is mainly symptomatic and supportive. Rest and NSAIDs are required during the acute phases, together with judicious aspiration of joints and intra-articular or other local steroid injections. Systemic corticosteroids are rarely required. Iritis is a medical emergency requiring topical, subconjunctival or systemic corticosteroids. Severe progressive arthritis and intractable keratoderma blennorrhagica occasionally warrant cytotoxic drug therapy. The non-specific urethritis is usually treated with a short course of tetracycline and there is now some evidence that it reduces the frequency of arthritis in sexually acquired cases.

Around 10% of patients have evidence of active disease 20 years after the onset. Spondylitis, chronic erosive arthritis, recurrent acute arthritis and uveitis are the major causes of long-term morbidity.

ARTHRITIS AND INFLAMMATORY BOWEL DISEASE

Two patterns of seronegative inflammatory arthritis are associated with ulcerative colitis and Crohn's disease.

Enteropathic synovitis is an acute, often migratory, non-erosive oligoarthritis which occurs in 12% of patients with ulcerative colitis and 20% of those with Crohn's disease. The knees, ankles and other weight-bearing joints are most commonly affected but the wrists and small joints of the fingers and toes can also be involved. The arthritis tends to follow exacerbations of the underlying bowel disease, sometimes in association with aphthous mouth ulcers, iritis and erythema nodosum. It ceases to be a problem following total colectomy for ulcerative colitis. The higher prevalence of arthritis in Crohn's disease may reflect the greater difficulty in eradicating the bowel problem.

Sacroiliitis (16%) and ankylosing spondylitis (6%) are also seen in the course of these disorders, but they pursue an independent course and often precede the bowel disease.

BEHÇET'S SYNDROME AND WHIPPLE'S DISEASE

See pages 868 and 646.

JUVENILE IDIOPATHIC ARTHRITIS

Inflammatory arthritis in children is much less common than in adults. It is defined as a diagnosis of exclusion, since there are no features or tests which definitely prove that a child has juvenile idiopathic arthritis (JIA). A list of some of the possible alternative diagnoses to be considered is shown in the information box and can include the widest differential diagnosis in paediatric practice. In most children, however, the diagnosis is straightforward.

DIFFERENTIAL DIAGNOSIS OF JUVENILE IDIOPATHIC ARTHRITIS

The list is not exhaustive

- **A**nxiety
- **R**ickets/metabolic
- **T**umour
- **H**aematological malignancies/haemophilia/sickle-cell disease
- **R**eactive arthritis
- **I**mmune (e.g. SLE)
- **T**rauma/hypermobility
- **I**njury (non-accidental)
- **S**epsis

Genetic and environmental factors are involved but the aetiology is still largely unknown. The pattern of onset of arthritis in the first few months is used as a basis for classification, and this serves a useful purpose in helping to guide appropriate therapy. The most recent classification agreed by the International League against Rheumatism (ILAR) is shown in Table 12.13.

The effect of the disease on growth and development may be considerable, both around the arthritic joints as well as overall.

Management

The traditional view that most children grow out of their arthritis is incorrect. Long-term follow-up data suggests that 16 years or more following diagnosis nearly half of the children are significantly disabled. Disease is active at 10 years in up to 35% of children and 30% have erosive arthritis. Reported remission rates for JIA in 5–10-year follow-up studies confirm the differential between oligo-articular (40–80% in remission), polyarticular (20–54% in remission) and systemic (0–35% in remission) JIA. In other

Table 12.13 Classification of juvenile idiopathic arthritis. Children (aged under 16 before onset of symptoms) will have had other conditions excluded, and have had persistent features of arthritis for at least 6 weeks.

Pattern	Comments	Summary of main features
Systemic arthritis	Lymphadenopathy, hepatosplenomegaly, pleurisy, pericarditis and a high intermittent fever are associated with myalgia, arthralgia and eventually polyarthritis. Weight loss and retardation of growth may be striking. The characteristic evanescent macular rash tends to appear when the temperature is raised. Remission usually occurs within 6 months but half the children have recurrent attacks and one-quarter develop a severe chronic polyarthritis. These are the children most likely to develop secondary amyloidosis	Fever > 2 weeks Evanescent rash Arthritis
Oligoarthritis—persisting	Most common form, typically affecting young girls with mono- or oligoarticular arthritis but seldom any constitutional symptoms. HLA-DR5 and positive tests for ANA are risk factors for chronic asymptomatic uveitis which can occur in up to half of this group. Regular slit lamp examinations are required if this complication is to be detected and treated early enough to preserve normal vision	Arthritis of 1–4 joints in first 6 months of disease
Oligoarthritis—extending	Spreading arthritis, as the name implies. This often carries a poor prognosis, since by definition this is an aggressive form, developing into a widespread polyarticular arthritis	Arthritis of 1–4 joints in first 6 months of disease
Polyarthritis RF-	This can occur at any age. At least five joints are commonly affected acutely or insidiously. Inflammatory arthritis near growing epiphyses may result in growth acceleration or arrest. Early fusion in the cervical spine and mandible gives rise to the short stiff neck, receding chin and dental problems very characteristic of adults who have had JIA. Two-thirds have residual problems into adult life, although only 10–15% have severe destructive arthritis	Arthritis of at least five joints in first 6 months of disease
Polyarthritis RF+	The onset is usually after the age of 8 years. The disease resembles severe adult-onset rheumatoid arthritis with progressive erosive joint changes in the majority. Extra-articular features include nodules and vasculitis. ANA tests are positive in 75%	Arthritis of at least five joints in first 6 months of disease × 2 positive RF 3 months apart
Psoriatic arthritis	Possibly one-third of all JIA is related to psoriasis in the child or his or her family	Arthritis and psoriasis *or* Arthritis and family history of psoriasis *and either* Dactylitis *or* nail abnormalities (pitting or onycholysis)
Enthesitis-related arthritis	Older boys with mono- or oligoarticular arthritis affecting hips, knees or ankles. Sacroiliitis is common and there is frequently a family history of uveitis, ankylosing spondylitis or another spondyloarthritis. 75% of these boys are HLA-B27-positive and in some the disease gradually evolves into ankylosing spondylitis in early adult life	Arthritis of at least five joints after first 6 months of disease Arthritis plus enthesitis *or* Arthritis *plus two of*: Sacroiliac joint tenderness Inflammatory spinal pain HLA-B27 Family history of uveitis or spondyloarthritis or inflammatory bowel disease Anterior uveitis
Other arthritides	Patients who either do not fit into any of the above categories, or who fit into more than one category	

words, the majority of patients with polyarticular and systemic arthritis never go into remission.

A multidisciplinary approach is recommended, involving rheumatologists, paediatricians, ophthalmologists, dentists/orthodontists, psychologists, physiotherapists, occupational therapists, nurses, social workers and teachers. Active physiotherapy is of great importance to reduce deformities and maintain muscle strength. Rest may be required when joints are acutely inflamed but care must be taken to avoid development of flexion deformities of the hips and knees, by encouraging regular prone lying and the use of appropriate lightweight splints. Whenever possible, the child should be kept mobile and ambulant, and daily physiotherapy is given to maintain a good range of joint movements and muscle strength. Hydrotherapy in a warm pool is particularly useful.

Slow-acting antirheumatic drugs should be considered early on in the disease course for all forms of polyarthritis. Previously, most rheumatologists did not start these drugs in children until 2.5 years after the onset of disease, by which time 50% of the children with systemic arthritis or polyarticular JIA will already have developed erosions. Poor prognostic features include polyarticular disease, systemic arthritis that evolves into polyarthritis, extended oligoarticular disease and polyarticular disease attributable to psoriatic arthritis. NSAIDs may be the only medication required, especially in the oligoarthritis pattern. They are, however, used at much higher doses than in adults (approximately 10–20 mg/kg/day of naproxen is a typical prescription for such a child) and are usually very well tolerated. Aspirin should be avoided because of the risk of Reye's syndrome. If NSAIDs fail to settle the arthritis, intra-articular steroid injections are used to treat resistant joints, with or without intravenous steroids if there are multiple active joints. Joint injections in children can have long-lasting benefits compared with adult joint injections. Multiple joint injections can induce remission in 20% of patients by 1 year. If patients fail to respond, methotrexate is added for at least 2 years (with additional hydroxychloroquine or cyclosporin A if methotrexate alone is not effective). Slow-acting antirheumatic drugs such as methotrexate and sulphasalazine are helpful in managing polyarticular forms of the disease but gold, d-penicillamine and hydroxychloroquine have no significant beneficial effect in these conditions. Special consideration needs to be given to maintaining the child's education and helping parents to develop a sensible, vigilant but not overprotective approach.

Long-term corticosteroids are reserved for children with severe systemic disease, for those with chronic uveitis not responding to local therapy and where very active joint disease does not respond to other measures. The use of alternate-day corticosteroids should always be considered because daily doses of prednisolone as low as 3 mg can inhibit growth in children under the age of 5 years. Corticosteroids do not arrest the progression of disease. Chlorambucil is used in children with secondary amyloidosis.

In children with systemic arthritis who have failed to respond to steroids or NSAIDs for at least 2 years, combination therapy including methotrexate, cyclophosphamide and prednisolone has been successful. The balance is swinging in favour of early aggressive treatment in children with risk factors for poor outcome with the hope that this will achieve better long-term results.

Surgery is usually limited to the rehabilitation of children with deformities. Soft tissue-release operations may be helpful in eliminating difficult flexion contractures, and osteotomies may be required when joints have been allowed to fuse in poor positions. Total hip arthroplasty can be considered for severely damaged joints as soon as growth has ceased.

INFECTIVE ARTHRITIS

SEPTIC ARTHRITIS

See page 813.

ARTHRITIS ASSOCIATED WITH OTHER SPECIFIC INFECTIONS

Gonococcal arthritis

This is more common in females than males and not infrequently commences at the time of a menstrual period within 2–3 weeks of genital infection. Joint involvement is usually asymmetrical and polyarticular with an acute, or subacute, migratory polyarthralgia or polyarthritis. Tenosynovitis, an 'additive' as opposed to a 'flitting' pattern of joint involvement, and a macular, vesicular or pustular rash are important diagnostic clues even in the absence of overt genital gonorrhoea.

The diagnosis can be established by cultures of synovial fluid, blood, skin lesions or from the genital tract. However, the organism is only identified in joint fluid in 20% of patients. Most patients respond to penicillin, 1 mega unit daily for 2 weeks, with dramatic improvement in 3–4 days.

Meningococcal infection

This can be associated with:

- an acute transient polyarthritis that is seen simultaneously with the characteristic petechial rash
- a purulent monoarthritis which usually occurs after 5 days, *or*
- a flitting polyarthralgia in patients with chronic meningococcaemia.

Penicillin is the treatment of choice.

Brucellosis

This is associated with polyarthralgia or transient polyarthritis. Rarely, there may be a septic arthritis or spondylitis. Destructive lesions in one vertebra or a number of contiguous vertebrae lead to severe pain, disc narrowing and marginal proliferation of osteophytes with early bony fusion of vertebrae. Chronic bursitis and osteomyelitis may also occur. Diagnosis is established by blood and synovial fluid cultures coupled with rising antibody titres. Management is given on page 128.

Tuberculosis of joints

This is usually secondary to an established focus in the lungs or kidneys. Articular infection is rarely seen in the UK except in malnourished or socially deprived elderly or immigrant groups, following the eradication of bovine tuberculosis. A single large joint is affected in more than three-quarters of all patients. Clinical features include joint pain, stiffness, swelling and restriction of movements associated with anorexia, weight loss and night sweats. In the early stages of the disease, radiographs show only periarticular osteoporosis and soft tissue swelling. Later, there is narrowing of the joint space, bony erosion and collapse of subchondral bone with little associated periosteal reaction. The tuberculin skin test is strongly positive and diagnosis can sometimes be made by direct bacteriological examination and culture of synovial fluid. In other patients synovial biopsy is required. After antibiotic control has been established (see p. 352), synovectomy may be required in those with extensive disease.

Leprosy
This can have a number of osteoarticular manifestations. Joint deformities of the hands and feet are common as a sequel to peripheral nerve involvement and these may be complicated by neuropathic joints. Osteomyelitis may complicate digital ulceration and hypersensitivity reactions may resemble rheumatoid arthritis.

Syphilitic arthritis
Congenital syphilis can be associated with painful para-articular swelling due to epiphyseal involvement soon after birth, or painless effusions of the knees (Clutton's joints) in adolescents. Acquired secondary syphilis may be associated with a migrating polyarthralgia resembling rheumatic fever, and neuropathic (Charcot) joints are a feature of tabes dorsalis.

Lyme arthritis
See page 138.

Fungal infections
These are rare. Blastomycosis, histoplasmosis and sporotrichosis can be associated with destructive lesions of bones and joints. Histoplasmosis and coccidioidomycosis may also be associated with erythema nodosum and a benign polyarthritis.

Viral infections
See Chapter 2.

MISCELLANEOUS DISORDERS OF SYNOVIAL JOINTS

ACROMEGALY

This is associated with a symmetrical arthropathy in 50% of patients. The small joints of the hands, wrists and knees are particularly affected, as is the spine. Hypertrophy of synovium and articular cartilage is associated with periosteal new bone formation, osteophytosis, 'tufting' of the terminal phalanges and premature osteoarthrosis and hypertrophic spondylosis.

AMYLOIDOSIS

Amyloidosis, a multisystem disease, may be generalised or localised. It may be primary, or associated with conditions such as rheumatoid arthritis, chronic suppuration, lepromatous leprosy and myelomatosis. Amyloidosis may present with carpal tunnel compression and a polyarthritis superficially resembling rheumatoid arthritis. The synovium is infiltrated with amyloid protein and the diagnosis can be made by finding fragments of amyloid tissue in the synovial fluid.

HYPERLIPIDAEMIA

Type II hyperlipidaemia can be associated with a migratory polyarthritis, and widespread xanthomas with tendon deposits. Type IV hyperlipidaemia can be associated with arthralgia and morning stiffness and also hyperuricaemia and gout.

SARCOIDOSIS

Sarcoidosis usually presents with erythema nodosum and hilar lymphadenopathy associated with a symmetrical non-destructive inflammatory arthritis especially affecting the knees, ankles and wrists. A rarer, more specific asymmetrical destructive arthritis affects similar joints and biopsy of the synovium in these patients shows evidence of non-caseating granulomas. Radiologically, there may be 'punched-out' cystic bone lesions and also 'cortical erosions' and joint destruction.

FURTHER INFORMATION ON INFLAMMATORY JOINT DISEASE

American College of Rheumatology Ad Hoc Committee 1996 Guidelines for the management of rheumatoid arthritis. Arthritis and Rheumatism 39: 713–722

Kalden J R, Manger B 1997 Biologic agents in the treatment of inflammatory rheumatic diseases. Current Opinion in Rheumatology 9: 206–212

Muller-Cadner V, Gay R E, Gay S 1997 Cellular pathways of joint destruction. Current Opinion in Rheumatology 9: 213–220

Sieger J, Kingsley G 1996 Recent advances in the pathogenesis of reactive arthritis. Immunology Today 17: 160–163

Winchester R 1995 Psoriatic arthritis. Dermatologic Clinics 13: 779–792

Wordsworth P, Brown M A 1996 The genetics of rheumatoid arthritis and allied conditions. In: Emery A, Connor M, Rimoin D (eds) Principles and practice of medical genetics. Churchill Livingstone, New York, pp. 2251–2771

CONNECTIVE TISSUE DISEASES

SYSTEMIC LUPUS ERYTHEMATOSUS (SLE)

This is a multisystem connective tissue disease characterised by the presence of numerous autoantibodies, circulating immune complexes and widespread immunologically determined tissue damage.

Epidemiology
SLE affects individuals throughout the world but occurs more frequently in the USA and the Far East. Americans of African origin are particularly susceptible, with a prevalence as high as 1/250 among females. The increasing use of sensitive tests for antinuclear antibodies suggests that mild and incomplete cases frequently occur. The onset is most

commonly in the second and third decades, with a female/male ratio of 9:1. The sex incidence is more equal in children and the elderly.

Aetiology and pathogenesis

Although the cause of SLE remains obscure, current concepts suggest that this is a multifactorial disorder in which there is profound disturbance of immune regulation. A defect of T lymphocyte function is associated with polyclonal B lymphocyte activation and the uncontrolled production of autoantibodies and immune complexes.

Evidence for genetic factors in the aetiology of the disease includes:

- its concurrence in monozygotic twin pairs
- a higher than expected prevalence of SLE, other connective tissue diseases, antinuclear antibodies and immune complexes in related family members
- inherited deficiency of isolated complement components, notably C2 in some patients
- increased prevalence of the histocompatibility antigens HLA-B8 and DR3.

Evidence for the influence of environmental factors includes:

- the provocative effect of sunlight
- the induction of lupus erythematosus by drugs
- the importance of oestrogens as determinants of disease expression. Exacerbations commonly occur in pregnancy and the puerperium and prevalence is increased in fertile women, those using oral contraceptives and men with Klinefelter's syndrome.

There is evidence of viral infection in animal models of SLE but not in humans.

Immunologically mediated tissue damage results from at least two different mechanisms in SLE:

- direct type II antibody-mediated cytotoxicity. Brain damage and abortion may be a consequence of cytotoxicity by cold reactive antibodies which cross-react with neural and trophoblast tissues.
- immune complex (and complement)-mediated type III hypersensitivity. The renal and vascular lesions of SLE appear to be a consequence of deposition of circulating DNA-anti-DNA and other complexes in tissues.

Clinical features

Arthritis, arthralgia and fever

These are the most common presenting features. Unlike other types of inflammatory arthritis, symptoms may begin during pregnancy and there may be a past history of spontaneous abortions. The arthritis can be transient and migratory or a more persistent seronegative polyarthritis. Chronic inflammatory arthritis and tenosynovitis may lead to deformities and contractures but erosive changes are very uncommon.

Skin lesions

These are seen in more than two-thirds of patients. In addition to the classical, photosensitive erythematous 'butterfly' rash (see Fig. 12.36) across the face, there may be lesions of discoid lupus or a vasculitic rash. The latter may present as purpura or periungual erythema, with 'chilblain-like' lesions or digital infarcts. Livedo reticularis and Raynaud's phenomenon (see p. 268) are common, while bullous eruptions and panniculitis ('lupus profundus') occur more rarely. Alopecia can be a useful diagnostic pointer and is seen in more than 50% of patients. Painful oral or nasopharyngeal ulcers are less common.

Cardiopulmonary features

These include pericarditis, myocarditis and endocarditis,

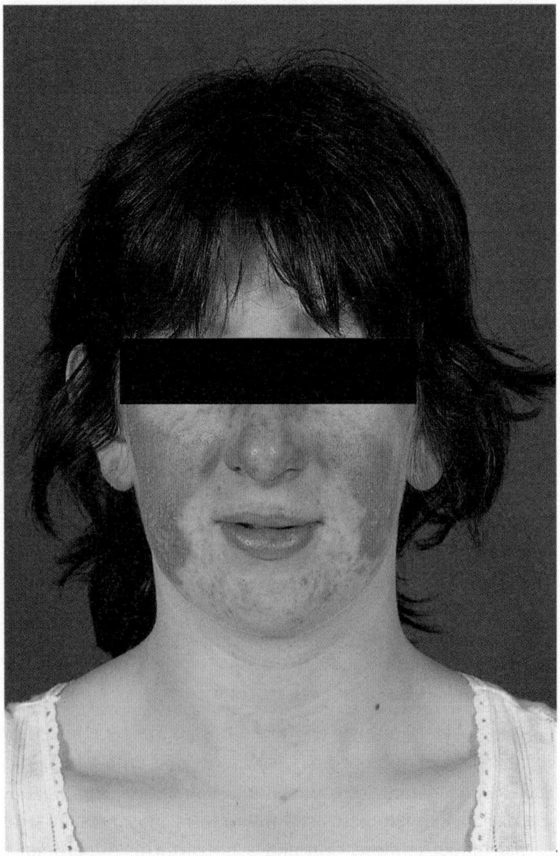

Fig. 12.36 Systemic lupus erythematosus. 'Butterfly'-distribution facial rash.

pleurisy, fibrosing alveolitis and acute lupus pneumonitis, as well as a 'shrinking lung syndrome' with progressive elevation of the diaphragms and linear scars from recurrent pulmonary infarction (see p. 374). Lung function tests reveal impairment of ventilation and diffusion in these and many patients without overt clinical or radiological evidence of pulmonary involvement. Verrucous (Libman–Sacks) endocarditis may be demonstrated by echocardiography.

Renal involvement

This carries the worst prognosis. It may result in the nephrotic syndrome and renal failure or it may be limited to insignificant proteinuria or the presence of red cells or casts (see p. 428).

Central nervous system involvement

This occurs in up to half of patients. In the majority it is limited to mild psychiatric disturbance or epilepsy but in a few there may be severe depression, dementia, organic psychosis, cranial nerve lesions, hemiplegia, transverse myelitis, chorea, cerebellar ataxia or peripheral neuropathy. Severe manifestations are associated with a poor prognosis.

Other manifestations

Gastrointestinal symptoms are frequent but non-specific. Abdominal pain can be due to peritonitis, perisplenitis, pancreatitis or vasculitis. Gastric or duodenal perforation may be a complication of corticosteroid therapy; colonic or gallbladder perforations are more likely to be a consequence of necrotising arteritis. Lymphadenopathy is found in half of patients and a moderately enlarged spleen in 20–30%. Ocular findings include keratoconjunctivitis sicca, episcleritis, retinal vasculitis and soft exudates.

Investigations

See pages 806–808.

Management

Articular symptoms and less severe inflammatory manifestations should be managed without corticosteroids whenever possible, but NSAIDs must be used with care in patients with renal disease. Antimalarials are particularly useful in the management of patients with troublesome skin and joint lesions and they can reduce the frequency of severe exacerbations of disease. Acute and life-threatening manifestations of SLE require systemic corticosteroid therapy, often initially in oral doses of 40–80 mg prednisolone or equivalent daily. With remission of disease careful attempts are made to withdraw steroids or maintain patients on very low doses or alternate-day regimens of steroid therapy.

Immunosuppressive drugs are reserved for patients with severe focal or diffuse proliferative glomerulonephritis and for those requiring maintenance steroid doses so high as to cause severe side-effects.

The combination of plasma exchange and immunosuppressive drug therapy may be useful in some patients with serious steroid-resistant exacerbations.

Patients with thrombotic problems (see p. 807) associated with the antiphospholipid antibody syndrome are managed with small doses of aspirin and anticoagulants.

Prognosis

Prognosis for life has improved dramatically over the last 30 years and the 5-year survival should now be better than 90%. Much of this apparent improvement results, however, from the detection of milder cases using highly sensitive immunological tests for diagnostic purposes. Patients with severe renal, neurological or pulmonary involvement have the worst prognosis. Renal biopsy can provide a guide to prognosis. Infection is an important cause of morbidity, particularly in patients receiving high doses of corticosteroids and immunosuppressives. Pregnancy is not contraindicated, provided the disease is in reasonable remission and renal, cardiac and cerebral functions are intact.

Drug-induced SLE

Positive tests for antinuclear factor are frequently encountered in patients receiving procainamide, hydralazine, anticonvulsants, oral contraceptives and phenothiazines. Much more rarely, a syndrome resembling SLE develops. Fever, polyarthritis, skin lesions, lymphadenopathy, serositis and pulmonary infiltrates are frequent, but renal disease and neurological manifestations are rare. Complement levels are usually normal and antibodies to double-stranded DNA absent. Slow acetylators of hydralazine and those with the HLA-DR4 histocompatibility antigen appear to be particularly at risk. Remission usually follows drug withdrawal. Occasionally a short course of corticosteroids is required.

Chronic discoid lupus erythematosus

This is more common than SLE. The skin lesions are characterised by photosensitivity, erythema, scaling, follicular plugging and telangiectasia. In most patients the disease is limited to the skin. ANA tests are positive but anti-DNA antibodies are not usually found and complement levels are normal. SLE may occasionally supervene.

MIXED CONNECTIVE TISSUE DISEASE (MCTD)

This is characterised by overlapping clinical features suggesting SLE, progressive systemic sclerosis (see below) and polymyositis in association with very high titres of a circulating antinuclear antibody with specificity for a ribonuclease-sensitive extractable nuclear antigen (ENA), identified as a nuclear ribonucleoprotein (nRNP).

Clinical features

Women are affected four times more commonly than men. The onset is usually in the third or fourth decade but may be at any age. Raynaud's phenomenon with 'sausage' swelling of the fingers, skin changes resembling dermatomyositis or scleroderma and a mild inflammatory polyarthritis are typically associated with proximal muscle weakness and tenderness and abnormal oesophageal motility. Diffuse interstitial pulmonary fibrosis is not uncommon but cardiac, renal and central nervous system involvement is very rare. The ESR and muscle enzymes are usually moderately raised. The condition is further characterised by a good response to low-dosage steroid therapy.

SYSTEMIC SCLEROSIS AND RELATED SCLERODERMA SYNDROMES

This is a heterogeneous group of disorders of connective tissue, characterised by fibrosis and degenerative changes in the skin and many internal organs (see the information box).

SYSTEMIC SCLEROSIS AND SCLERODERMA SYNDROMES

- Systemic sclerosis
  - Diffuse scleroderma
  - Limited cutaneous (CREST syndrome—see p. 859)
- Morphoea (local or widespread)
  - Linear scleroderma
- Overlap syndromes
- Undifferentiated connective tissue diseases
- Chemically induced
  - Occupational
  - Drugs
- Pseudoscleroderma syndromes

Epidemiology

The prevalence of systemic sclerosis is 10–20/100 000 population with an annual incidence of 1–2/100 000 and a 4:1 female to male ratio. HLA associations include the DR1, DR2, DR3, DR5 and DRW52 class II alleles. Environmental risk factors include exposure to silica dusts, vinyl chloride, epoxy resins and trichlorethylene.

Pathogenesis

Immunologically mediated inflammation in genetically predisposed individuals is followed by intimal thickening in small blood vessels and excessive production and cross-linking of type I collagen. There is evidence of T lymphocyte and complement activation as well as autoimmunity with the presence of autoantibodies to nuclear antigens (see Table 12.1, p. 807). Endothelial injury results in the release of the powerful vasoconstrictor endothelin as well as in secondary platelet activation with a release of other vasoconstrictor mediators (5-hydroxytryptamine, thromboxane A_2 and adenosine diphosphate—ADP).

Clinical features

The onset is most frequently in the 30–50 age group. Severe *Raynaud's phenomenon* (see p. 268) is usually the presenting complaint and may precede other features by months or years. Critical digital ischaemia leads to ulceration, infarction, pulp atrophy and gangrene.

Skin changes (see Fig. 12.37)

Initially there is often well-demarcated non-pitting oedema and induration associated with 'sausage' swelling and restriction of movement of the fingers. Later the skin becomes shiny, with atrophy and ulceration of the fingertips, with or without associated calcinosis. The skin of the face, limbs and trunk is variably affected and there may be striking pigmentation and telangiectasia. As the disease progresses, the face may become taut and mask-like, with 'beaking' of the nose and difficulty in opening the mouth. Tightening of skin over bony prominences results in flexion contractures and liability to trauma. There is often erythema and dilated capillaries of the proximal nail folds.

Musculoskeletal manifestations

These include arthralgia, a mild non-erosive inflammatory arthritis and 'leathery' crepitus in affected tendon sheaths or joints. Muscle weakness and wasting results from both disuse atrophy and low-grade myositis.

Gastrointestinal tract

This is involved in the majority of patients. Reflux oesophagitis associated with a sliding hiatus hernia is common and loss of oesophageal peristalsis can be detected on recumbent barium swallow examination even in the

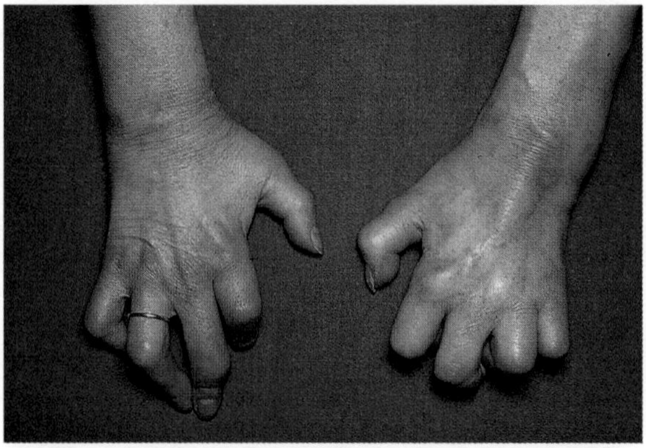

Fig. 12.37 Systemic sclerosis. Hands showing tight shiny skin, sclerodactyly, flexion contractures of the fingers and thickening of an extensor tendon sheath.

absence of dysphagia. Dilatation of segments of large and small bowel occurs less frequently, causing intermittent abdominal pain, constipation, distension and obstruction; there may be diarrhoea and malabsorption secondary to bacterial overgrowth. Systemic sclerosis may be associated with primary biliary cirrhosis and with Sjögren's syndrome.

Pulmonary fibrosis

This occurs in many patients with diffuse disease and antibodies to Scl-70 (see below). It is covered in detail on page 374.

Other manifestations

Cardiac involvement can be secondary to systemic or pulmonary hypertension, and pericarditis, cardiomyopathy, heart block and aortic valve lesions can also occur. Renal involvement with accelerated hypertension may develop at any stage in patients with diffuse systemic disease and is an important cause of morbidity and mortality. Cranial or peripheral nerve lesions occur rarely.

Investigations

The ANA is positive in about 50% of patients, with a nucleolar or speckled staining pattern. Antibodies to single-stranded RNA and to an extractable nuclear antigen anti-Scl-70 (anti-topoisomerase I) occur in 20% and may be a marker for pulmonary involvement. Anti-DNA antibodies are not detected and complement levels are normal.

If not clinically evident, dilated, tortuous and 'dropped out' capillary loops may be detected on nail-fold capillaroscopy in patients with Raynaud's phenomenon who are destined to develop a connective tissue disease.

Management

No form of drug therapy has been proved to be effective in arresting the progression of severe progressive systemic sclerosis. Corticosteroids may produce some symptomatic benefit in early disease where inflammatory oedema or associated myositis and/or arthritis are prominent features and d-penicillamine can interfere with collagen cross-linking. Nifedipine and prostacyclin infusions may occasionally be helpful in patients with severe Raynaud's phenomenon. Captopril or other angiotensin-converting enzyme (ACE) inhibitors can be dramatically effective in patients with renal crises and accelerated hypertension. Clinical trials of immunosuppressive drugs or bone marrow ablation with stem cell transplantation are underway in patients who have rapidly progressive systemic sclerosis (PSS) with lung involvement.

Attention should be paid to protecting the limbs from cold, the urgent treatment of chest infections and therapy for cardiac, respiratory and renal failure. Articular symptoms should be managed with NSAIDs. Episodes of steatorrhoea often respond to a short course of a broad-spectrum antibiotic.

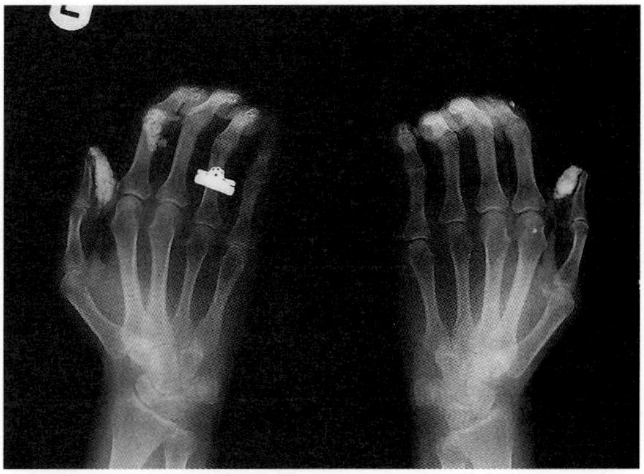

Fig. 12.38 Scleroderma. Radiograph of hands showing soft tissue calcinosis.

Prognosis

The outlook appears worse in those with late-onset disease, widespread skin involvement of the trunk, and renal, cardiac or respiratory disease. The overall 5-year survival is 70%.

LIMITED CUTANEOUS SYSTEMIC SCLEROSIS (CREST SYNDROME)

This subset of patients have skin disease limited to sites distal to the elbow and knee with only occasional involvement of the face and neck. *C*alcinosis (see Fig. 12.38), *R*aynaud's phenomenon, o*E*sophageal involvement, *S*clerodactyly and *T*elangiectasia are the features of the CREST syndrome. Severe pulmonary hypertension can be a complication in some patients. An anticentromere antinuclear antibody with specificity for a protein of the chromosomal kinetochore is present in the serum (see Table 12.1, p. 807).

MORPHOEA AND LINEAR SCLERODERMA

These are limited to characteristic, well-demarcated, pale, indurated lesions of the skin and subcutaneous connective tissues. Serological findings may be similar to those of systemic sclerosis but systemic features rarely develop.

EOSINOPHILIC FASCIITIS

This is a scleroderma-like condition characterised by pain, swelling and tenderness of the hands, forearms and feet where induration of the skin and subcutaneous tissues is not associated with Raynaud's phenomenon or systemic sclerosis. Carpal tunnel compression may be an early feature and the onset frequently follows abnormal exercise. Eosinophilia and hyperglobulinaemia are characteristic and the diagnosis is confirmed by finding an inflammatory cell infiltrate with prominent eosinophils in association with marked fibrosis of the subcutaneous fascia. Eosinophilic fasciitis responds to corticosteroids but is usually self-limiting. Excessive consumption of L-tryptophan (in some health foods) should be excluded.

PSEUDOSCLERODERMA

Other conditions which may give rise to induration or brawny oedema of the skin that must be considered in the differential diagnosis of scleroderma include scleroedema, scleromyxoedema, amyloidosis and acromegaly.

POLYMYOSITIS AND DERMATOMYOSITIS

These are diffuse connective tissue disorders in which muscle weakness and inflammatory changes in muscle and skin are the predominant features.

Epidemiology

These rare disorders (incidence 2–10/million population per annum) occur throughout the world in all races and at all ages. The aetiology is obscure but persons with HLA-B8/DR3 appear to be genetically predisposed.

Clinical features

It is possible to define five clinical subsets, which are listed in the information box.

MYOSITIS SUBSETS

- Adult polymyositis
- Adult dermatomyositis
- Adult polymyositis/dermatomyositis with malignancies
- Childhood dermatomyositis
- Polymyositis in other connective tissue diseases

Adult polymyositis

Adult polymyositis occurs three times more frequently in women than in men. The onset is usually insidious in the third to fifth decades. The patients may experience difficulty in climbing stairs or rising from a low chair, and on examination there is weakness of the pelvic and shoulder girdle muscles. Sometimes the onset is more abrupt, with rapid progression of muscular weakness. Involvement of pharyngeal, laryngeal and respiratory muscles can lead to dysphagia, dysphonia and respiratory failure within a few days. In the majority of cases progression is less rapid and profound. Spontaneous remissions are followed by some return of muscle strength but there may be atrophy, calcinosis and fibrosis in damaged muscles causing flexion contractures. Muscle pain and tenderness are unusual except in very acute illness. Mild arthralgia or inflammatory arthritis, Raynaud's phenomenon and erythematous rashes on the elbows and knuckles are frequent associated features.

Adult dermatomyositis

This is also more common in women. Acute or subacute muscle weakness is accompanied by periorbital oedema and a characteristic violet 'heliotrope' rash on the upper eyelids. In addition there may be a photosensitive, erythematous, scaling rash on the face, shoulders, upper arms and chest with red patches over knuckles, elbows and knees. Muscle pain, tenderness and weight loss are common, as are arthralgia and mild inflammatory polyarthritis.

Inflammatory myositis associated with malignancy

Less common than was previously thought, this is seen only after the age of 40 years, particularly in association with ovarian, gastric and nasopharyngeal carcinoma. The onset of symptoms is usually insidious and the clinical picture does not differ from that of typical polymyositis or dermatomyositis. The associated carcinoma may not become apparent for 2–3 years. Its resection is sometimes associated with remission of the myositis.

Childhood dermatomyositis

This most commonly affects children between the ages of 4 and 10 years. Muscle weakness is usually accompanied by the typical rash of dermatomyositis. Muscle atrophy, contractures and subcutaneous calcification may be widespread and severe. Recurrent abdominal pain due to vasculitis is also a feature.

Investigations

Serum aminotransferases, aldolase and creatinine phosphokinase are usually raised and are useful guides to the activity of the disease. Tests for rheumatoid factor and ANA are often positive and there may be antibodies to an extractable nuclear antigen (Jo-1). Electromyography may show characteristic changes which can be very helpful in distinguishing polymyositis from peripheral neuropathy. Muscle biopsy (see Fig. 12.39) shows fibre necrosis and regeneration in association with an inflammatory cell infiltrate. MRI can be used to detect active myositis non-invasively. Screening for malignancy is usually limited to relatively non-invasive investigations such as chest radiograph, mammography, pelvic/abdominal ultrasound, urinalysis and a search for tumour markers in the serum.

Management

Prednisolone 40–60 mg daily is used initially to induce a remission. Muscle enzyme levels may fall before clinical improvement is noted. The dose is then gradually reduced whilst muscle strength and serum enzyme levels continue to be monitored. Doses of 10–15 mg prednisolone daily are often needed to maintain remission. Immunosuppressive

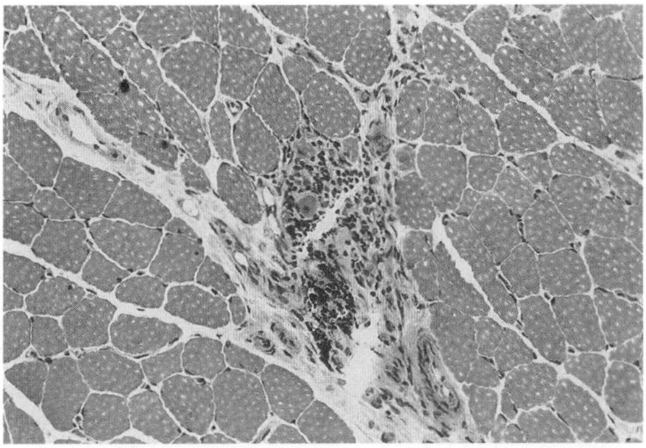

Fig. 12.39 Muscle biopsy from a patient with inflammatory myositis. The sample shows an intense inflammatory cell infiltrate in an area of degenerating and regenerating muscle fibres.

therapy is occasionally used when there is no response to corticosteroids. The use of splints and physiotherapy to prevent contractures should not be neglected. Prognosis is closely related to the presence or absence of associated malignancy and to the age of onset, being poorer in older patients.

SJÖGREN'S SYNDROME

This is an autoimmune disorder of unknown aetiology, characterised by lymphocytic infiltration of the salivary and lacrimal glands leading to xerostomia and keratoconjunctivitis sicca. In some patients sicca symptoms predominate—*primary Sjögren's (sicca) syndrome*, while in others it is associated with another connective tissue disease such as RA, SLE, PSS or MCTD—*secondary Sjögren's syndrome*. The main features of primary and secondary Sjögren's syndrome are contrasted in the information boxes.

Investigations

The salivary flow rate is reduced and reduction in lacrimal secretion can be demonstrated by use of the Schirmer tear test. If necessary, the diagnosis can be confirmed by demonstrating focal lymphocytic infiltration in the minor salivary glands in a lip biopsy. Biopsy of a major salivary gland is only necessary if there is concern that the patient may have developed a lymphoma. Patients with Sjögren's syndrome are characterised by having a wide range of autoantibodies (see the information boxes).

Management

Lacrimal substitution with hypromellose or other 'artificial teardrops' can relieve symptoms of keratoconjunctivitis sicca in mild cases. Soft contact lenses can be useful for corneal protection in patients with filamentary keratitis, and occlusion of the lacrimal ducts is occasionally needed. Treatment of xerostomia is more difficult and none of the available saliva substitutes is very effective. Vaginal dryness is treated with lubricants such as KY jelly. Systemic corticosteroids and immunosuppressive drugs are only occasionally indicated to control severe extraglandular manifestations of Sjögren's syndrome.

PRIMARY SJÖGREN'S (SICCA) SYNDROME

- Age of onset 40–60
- F > M
- HLA-B8/DR3

Common clinical features
- Keratoconjunctivitis sicca
- Xerostomia
- Salivary gland enlargement

Rarer clinical features
- Anaemia, leucopenia, thrombocytopenia, lymphadenopathy, lymphoreticular malignancy, hepatomegaly, hyperglobulinaemic purpura, vasculitis, neuropathy, myositis, fibrosing alveolitis, glomerulonephritis, renal tubular acidosis

Autoantibodies frequently detected
- Rheumatoid factor
- ANA
- SS-A (Anti-Ro)
- SS-B (Anti-La)
- Salivary duct
- Gastric parietal cell
- Thyroid

SECONDARY SJÖGREN'S SYNDROME

- Age of onset 40–60
- F > M
- HLA-B8/DR3
- Incidence 10% of RA patients

Common clinical features
- Mild keratoconjunctivitis sicca
- Dry mouth

Other associated autoimmune disorders
- Systemic lupus erythematosus
- Progressive systemic sclerosis
- Primary biliary cirrhosis
- Chronic active hepatitis
- Myasthenia gravis
- Polymyositis
- Thyroiditis

Autoantibodies frequently detected
- Rheumatoid factor
- ANA
- Salivary duct
- Gastric parietal cell
- Thyroid

RELAPSING POLYCHONDRITIS

This is an acute, systemic, episodic disorder characterised by inflammation and destruction of cartilage.

Epidemiology

Relapsing polychondritis is rare, with an estimated annual

RELAPSING POLYCHONDRITIS: CLINICAL FEATURES

Ears
- Auricular chondritis
- Conductive deafness
- Nerve deafness
- Vestibular damage

Nose
- Nasal tenderness
- Saddle nose deformity

Throat
- Hoarseness
- Stridor
- Laryngeal/tracheal stricture

Eyes
- Episcleritis/scleritis
- Uveitis/keratitis

Joints
- Seronegative arthritis

Cardiovascular features
- Conduction defects
- Valvular disease
- Small-/large-vessel vasculitis

Kidneys
- Proliferative glomerulonephritis

incidence of only 3.5/million. In 30% of patients there is an associated autoimmune or connective tissue disease.

Clinical features

Most patients present with pain and swelling of the pinna of the ear or nose with or without an associated seronegative arthritis. Other manifestations are summarised in the information box.

Investigations

Laboratory abnormalities during acute phases include non-specific indices of systemic inflammation (anaemia of chronic disease, leucocytosis, thrombocytosis, elevated ESR and acute-phase proteins) and raised levels of serum antibodies to type II collagen and a 148 kDa cartilage-specific protein. Positive tests for other autoantibodies usually reflect an associated autoimmune or connective tissue disease. Pulmonary function tests and CT scanning are used to define the extent of laryngotracheal involvement, and audiometry, ECG and echocardiography are required when there is deafness or cardiovascular disease. The tissue diagnosis can be confirmed by biopsy in patients with auricular chondritis; renal biopsy may show a proliferative glomerulonephritis in patients with proteinuria or active urinary sediments.

Management

Mild episodes of auricular and nasal chondritis and seronegative arthritis usually respond to NSAIDs with or without low-dosage corticosteroids. Other more serious manifestations require treatment with high-dosage prednisolone (1 mg/kg) and sometimes cytotoxic drugs.

FAMILIAL MEDITERRANEAN FEVER

This is a rare genetic disorder which is largely restricted to Armenians, Sephardic Jews and other ethnic groups originating from the Middle East and eastern Mediterranean. Inheritance is usually autosomal recessive but families with dominant inheritance have been described.

Clinical features

The disease is characterised by repetitive episodes of high fever, peritonitis, pleurisy and inflammatory arthritis. Typical acute attacks resolve spontaneously without residua in 12–72 hours but joint effusions and synovitis, especially in the knees and hips, may persist between febrile episodes, with progressive damage to articular cartilage. The onset of symptoms is usually in childhood or early adolescence but the frequency of attacks varies greatly from regular weekly bouts of fever to occasional, irregular episodes with months or years of intervening spontaneous remission. Myalgia, erysipelas-like skin lesions and cutaneous vasculitis can occur, while the presence of haematuria or persistent proteinuria usually signals the development of renal amyloidosis.

Investigations

Acute attacks are associated with a raised ESR and non-specific rises in acute-phase proteins such as C-reactive protein and fibrinogen as well as the serum amyloid A protein. Peritoneal, pleural and synovial aspirates are characteristically sterile exudates with a predominance of polymorphonuclear leucocytes. Chest radiographs may demonstrate small pleural effusions, and straight radiographs of the abdomen may show multiple small bowel fluid levels. Patients with protracted hip pain may show loss of articular cartilage and/or radiological evidence of osteonecrosis. Histological evidence of renal amyloidosis is established by renal biopsy.

Management

Prophylactic oral colchicine (1–2 mg daily) prevents the development of renal amyloidosis and suppresses acute attacks in two-thirds of patients. Renal transplantation and hip arthroplasty are necessary in a small minority.

SYSTEMIC VASCULITIS

Vasculitis is defined as inflammation of blood vessels leading to end-organ or tissue damage. It has been suggested that more common forms of vessel injury, such as atheroma, may have an onset triggered by an episode of vasculitis. Vasculitis is present in many types of inflammatory rheumatic disease such as SLE, progressive systemic sclerosis and childhood dermatomyositis. In these conditions, the vasculitis is regarded as a secondary manifestation of the primary disease. The primary vasculitides are less common, with an annual incidence of between 25 and 40 new cases per million. The most serious forms (such as Wegener's granulomatosis and microscopic polyangiitis) are uniformly fatal if untreated, and may cause significant morbidity even with appropriate therapy. Despite major advances in our understanding of their mechanisms, the aetiology of the primary vasculitides remains unclear, and classification is based on vessel size (see Table 12.14).

The key to recognising the presence of a vasculitis is multisystem involvement. The differential diagnosis will include sepsis, metastatic tumours and multiple emboli (cholesterol, septic and thrombotic), as well as vasculitis occurring as a manifestation of an underlying connective tissue disorder. However, the characteristic patterns of disease in vasculitis should raise suspicion of the diagnosis. Once the diagnosis is made, patients must be thoroughly

Table 12.14 The primary vasculitides

Vessel size	Summary of main features
LARGE-VESSEL ARTERITIS **Giant cell arteritis (temporal arteritis)**	Elderly predominance Unaccustomed headache; scalp tenderness; possible visual loss; constitutional features; symptoms of acute ischaemia Biopsy within 1 week of steroid therapy; skip lesions Steroids are the main form of therapy Relapse in 30%
Takayasu's arteritis (pulseless disease or aortic arch syndrome)	Young female predominance; racial variation in incidence New loss of pulses; bruits; chronic ischaemic symptoms/signs; constitutional features Angiogram demonstrates vessel narrowing with post-stenotic dilatation Steroids are the main form of therapy Good outcome in > 90%
MEDIUM-SIZE VESSEL ARTERITIS **Classical polyarteritis nodosa**	Multisystem involvement (muscle, nerve, gut and skin); constitutional features Hepatitis B-positive or hepatitis B-negative; arteritis on biopsy or aneurysms on angiography Interferon α and steroids if hepatitis B-positive; cyclophosphamide and steroids if hepatitis B-negative Mortality < 20%; relapse rate around 50%
Kawasaki disease (mucocutaneous lymph node syndrome)	Acute disease in childhood; resembles viral exanthem Associated coronary artery aneurysms with mortality if untreated Aspirin and intravenous immunoglobulin Possible link to later development of atheroma
SMALL-VESSEL DISEASE OF ARTERIOLES, CAPILLARIES AND VENULES **Microscopic polyangiitis**	Haematuria, systemic illness, lung haemorrhage Renal biopsy shows focal segmental necrotising glomerulonephritis; typically P-ANCA (myeloperoxidase) positive Cyclophosphamide and steroids +/– plasmapheresis Mortality 10–40%; relapse in 20%
Wegener's granulomatosis	Upper and lower airway disease with renal involvement; systemic features common; isolated involvement of ENT or lung well recognised Granulomatous inflammation in airways; focal segmental necrotising glomerulonephritis; typically C-ANCA (serine proteinase 3) positive Cyclophosphamide and steroids +/– plasmapheresis Mortality 10–20%; relapse in 50%
Churg–Strauss syndrome	Asthma, eosinophilia, allergic rhinitis, pulmonary infiltrates Cardiac involvement accounts for half of deaths; typically P-ANCA positive Steroids are mainstay, with additional cyclophosphamide for more serious manifestations Low mortality; high relapse
Leucocytoclastic vasculitis	Isolated skin purpura Antihistamines usually control symptoms Presence of ANCA may precede development of systemic features, requiring cyclophosphamide and prednisolone
Henoch–Schönlein purpura	Small purpuric spots associated with intra-abdominal pain, flitting arthritis; occasionally rectal bleeding and/or haematuria Usually follows respiratory infections in childhood and is self-limiting; adults suffer a more indolent course
Essential mixed cryoglobulinaemia	Type II cryoglobulinaemia Purpura, arthralgia, urticaria, ulcers Strong association with hepatitis C Antiviral therapy plus steroids/plasmapheresis

investigated to determine the exact pattern of organ or system involvement. Not only does this assist in classification, but more importantly it will determine the choice of therapy.

LARGE-VESSEL VASCULITIS

Polymyalgia rheumatica/giant cell arteritis

Polymyalgia rheumatica (PMR)

This is common in the elderly (approximately 500 new cases/million/year over the age of 50). There is a close association with giant cell arteritis, which is at least 10 times less frequent. Typical clinical features include severe pain and stiffness in the neck, back, shoulders, upper arms and thighs, often associated with profound and prolonged early morning stiffness. Physical signs are usually limited to slight tenderness of the acromioclavicular or sternoclavicular joints but occasionally there may be evidence of mild inflammatory arthritis in a more peripheral joint. There is no associated primary myositis or muscle tenderness. Although patients with cranial arteritis have arterial tenderness or absence of pulsation, the peripheral arteries are usually clinically normal in patients presenting with polymyalgia rheumatica. Approximately one-third of patients develop features of cranial arteritis at some point in the course of their disease. The risk of serious ocular complications is low, however.

The ESR is markedly raised in the majority of patients and there may be a normochromic normocytic anaemia of chronic disease. Temporal artery biopsy shows evidence of giant cell arteritis in 15–40% of patients with polymyalgia rheumatica but it is safe to assume that the true frequency of vasculitis is 100%.

The response to corticosteroid therapy is dramatic. Treatment should be commenced with oral prednisolone (15 mg daily). The diagnosis should be reviewed if there is no striking remission of symptoms within a week. It is usually possible to begin tapering the dose of prednisolone 4–8 weeks after starting treatment and most patients can be maintained in clinical remission with 5–7 mg prednisolone daily.

Nearly all patients require corticosteroid therapy for 2 years but most can be weaned from steroids by 5 years. A few patients have a more prolonged chronic illness. The need for maintenance prednisolone should be reviewed, with an attempt at gradual steroid withdrawal in all patients after 2 years, and the risks of relapse need to be balanced against the risks of steroid side-effects. Prophylactic calcium supplements should be given from the onset of therapy to all patients and the addition of a small dose of azathioprine needs to be considered as a steroid-sparing manoeuvre in patients whose disease cannot be maintained in clinical remission with less than 10 mg of prednisolone daily.

Giant cell arteritis (GCA)

The incidence is highest in the elderly (16–100 new cases/million/annum, mean age at onset 70 years (range 50–90) with a 4:1 female to male ratio).

Most patients (75%) present with severe headaches and many have scalp tenderness. The onset can be acute or insidious and is often associated with constitutional symptoms of anorexia, fatigue, weight loss, fever, depression and general malaise. Visual problems such as diplopia, scintillating scotomata, transient blindness and ptosis are common. Permanent visual loss can result from ischaemic optic atrophy secondary to vasculitis in the posterior ciliary arteries. Central retinal artery occlusion is rare. Other features include transient ischaemic attacks, brain-stem infarcts and jaw claudication. Examination may reveal thickened and tender temporal arteries. The diagnosis should be suspected in any elderly patient with visual impairment, especially if headache and malaise are present.

GCA is characterised on temporal artery biopsy by an inflammatory infiltrate of lymphocytes, plasma cells, 'giant' macrophages and eosinophils throughout the arterial wall, with predominant necrosis of the media and fragmentation of the internal elastic lamina. Affected vessels may become occluded. The pathological process is of unknown cause, but may have an autoimmune basis because it occurs more frequently in patients with other autoimmune disorders such as thyroid disease or rheumatoid arthritis. The external carotid artery and its branches are particularly susceptible; the ophthalmic, vertebral and subclavian vessels are often involved. Less commonly, the internal carotid, coronary, uterine and mesenteric arteries are affected.

The ESR is usually elevated well above 50 mm/hour. Temporal artery biopsy may confirm the diagnosis but is not always positive, due to the presence of skip lesions (areas of inflammation adjacent to normal histological appearances) or the effects of therapy (especially if the biopsy is delayed more than 1 week from starting steroids).

Systemic steroids (prednisolone 20–60 mg daily) should be started immediately if clinical suspicion is strong, because the risk of visual loss is high. Temporal artery biopsy may be delayed for up to 1 week before histological resolution is likely to occur. Steroid doses are reduced gradually over the first few weeks to a maintenance level of 10–20 mg daily, guided by symptoms and the ESR. The symptoms improve dramatically within a day or two of starting steroids but visual failure is usually permanent. Maintenance therapy is required for at least 1 year, and rarely for the rest of the patient's life. Relapse occurs in 30%, and is an indication to restart high-dose steroids with additional immunosuppressive agents, typically azathioprine or methotrexate.

Takayasu's arteritis (pulseless disease or aortic arch syndrome)

Takayasu's disease is a chronic inflammatory granulomatous panarteritis of elastic arteries (i.e. the aorta, its major branches and occasionally the pulmonary arteries). It is most common in women (female to male ratio 8:1) under the age of 40 years. Whilst rare (1–3 new cases/million/annum) in Europe and the USA it is more common in Mexico and the Far East. Twin studies and weak association with HLA-B5 suggest that genetic factors are important but little else is known about its aetiology or pathogenesis.

Constitutional symptoms are common (fever/sweats, fatigue, weight loss, arthralgia/myalgia and anaemia). Headaches, syncope, arm claudication and angina suggest vascular insufficiency. Clinical examination may reveal loss of pulses, bruits, hypertension and aortic incompetence. Rarely, patients present with myocardial infarction, pleurisy and panniculitis. In some patients there is a long phase of non-specific systemic illness prior to the development of vascular complications when examination typically reveals the presence of vascular bruits and diminished or absent pulses. The upper limbs are affected more commonly than the lower limbs.

A normocytic normochromic anaemia of chronic disease, mild leucocytosis and raised ESR are non-specific features of systemic inflammation. Chest radiographs may show widening of the aorta as well as cardiomegaly. Arch aortography or intravenous digital subtraction angiography is usually required to demonstrate stenoses in the aortic arch or its branches (type I), atypical coarctation with involvement of the descending aorta (type II) or a mixed picture (type III).

Most patients respond to high-dose oral prednisolone (1–2 mg/kg daily) but additional immunosuppressive therapy with methotrexate or cyclophosphamide may be required. Reconstructive vascular surgery is needed in a few cases. The 5-year survival in treated patients is 90%.

MEDIUM-SIZE ARTERIES

Classical polyarteritis nodosa (PAN)

Classical PAN is a necrotising vasculitis affecting medium-sized arteries. PAN is a rare disorder with an annual incidence of 2.4/million in most populations. All age groups can be affected, with a peak incidence in the fourth and fifth decades and a male to female ratio of 2:1. PAN is divided into hepatitis B-related and hepatitis B-unrelated forms. (The latter is now the most common variety as a result of increasing uptake of hepatitis B immunisation.) In 5–50%, depending on the population studied, PAN is associated with circulating immune complexes containing the hepatitis B surface antigen. The incidence of PAN is 10 times higher in the Inuit population of Alaska where hepatitis B infection is endemic.

Patients typically present with a vague systemic illness, muscle pains, mononeuritis multiplex, abdominal pains, arthritis and/or skin lesions such as ulcers, palpable purpura, cutaneous infarcts or gangrene. Mononeuritis multiplex results from arteritic involvement of the vasa nervorum. Severe hypertension and/or renal impairment usually indicate the presence of renal infarction; acute surgical presentation with abdominal pain, peritonitis, pancreatitis, major gastro-intestinal haemorrhage, and gut or gallbladder infarction are well recognised. Testicular pain, and leg and jaw claudication can occur as a result of vascular occlusion and about one-third of patients have some lung involvement, with chest pain, consolidation or variable pulmonary infiltrates.

Angiography reveals multiple aneurysms and smooth narrowing of affected vessels (typically involving the coeliac axis). Biopsy of symptomatic muscle or sural nerve confirms the presence of a necrotising vasculitis.

Antiviral therapy (for the hepatitis B-related variety) or immunosuppressive therapy with cyclophosphamide and corticosteroids leads to improvement in the majority of cases. Mortality is less than 20%, although relapse is a common feature of hepatitis B-negative PAN (around 50%).

Kawasaki disease (mucocutaneous lymph node syndrome)

Kawasaki disease (KD) is an acute systemic disorder of childhood, resembling a viral exanthem, associated with a vasculitis that characteristically involves the coronary arteries. The annual incidence in Japan is 700–800 new cases/million in children under the age of 5 but it is less common elsewhere in the world. Boys are affected three times as often as girls. The clinical picture and epidemic occurrence in Japan suggest an infective aetiology but no definite aetiological virus or bacterium has been identified.

The principal clinical features are shown in the information box. Cardiovascular complications include coronary aneurysms, transient coronary artery dilatation, myocardial infarction, pericarditis and effusions and cardiac failure.

A polymorphonuclear leucocytosis, thrombocytosis and raised acute-phase proteins are typically present. Some children have circulating antineutrophil cytoplasmic antibodies (ANCA) and most have anti-endothelial cell antibodies. Coronary vessel abnormalities can be visualised by two-dimensional echocardiography or coronary angiography.

FEATURES OF KAWASAKI DISEASE

Five out of six clinical features, or four out of six clinical features together with evidence of coronary dilatation, are required to establish the diagnosis

- Fever persisting for more than 5 days
- Bilateral conjunctival congestion
- Erythema of the lips, buccal mucosa and tongue
- Acute non-purulent cervical lymphadenopathy
- Polymorphous exanthema
- Erythema of palms and soles (oedema followed by desquamation)
- Coronary dilatation

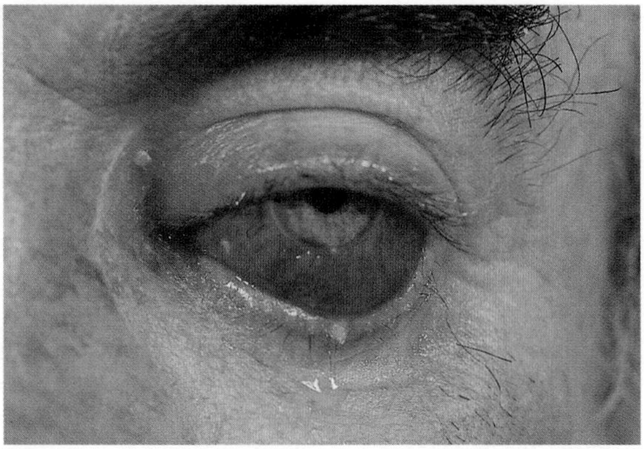

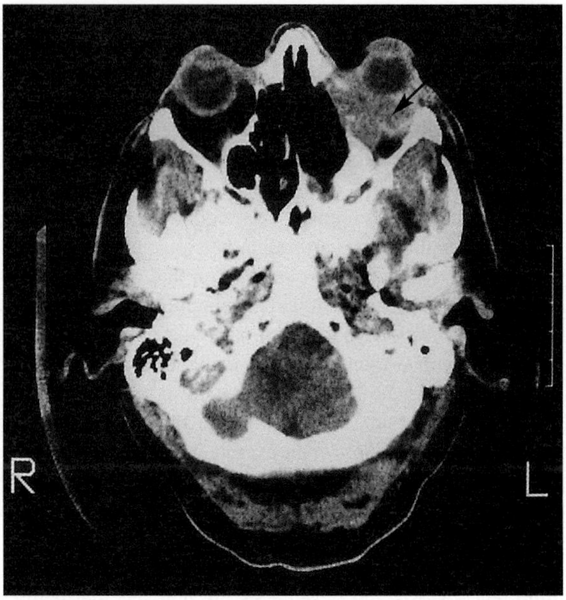

Fig. 12.40 Wegener's granulomatosis. [A] Patient with retro-orbital granuloma and proptosis. The eye is fixed, reddened and very painful. [B] CT scan showing inflammatory tissue invading the extraocular muscles (arrow).

Treatment is with aspirin (5 mg/kg daily) and high-dosage intravenous gammaglobulin (400 mg/kg daily for 4 days). Most children recover and the overall mortality is less than 2%. Relapse is rare. Steroids should be avoided because of the risk of worsening the coronary artery dilatation. It has been suggested that untreated KD may be much more common than we realise, and may be responsible for the later development of adult coronary artery atheroma and ischaemic heart disease.

SMALL-VESSEL DISEASE OF ARTERIOLES, CAPILLARIES AND VENULES

The first three forms of small-vessel vasculitis will be described as a group since they are most often associated with the presence of circulating ANCA, require similar management strategies, and together represent the most serious forms of systemic vasculitis.

Microscopic polyangiitis (MPA)

The annual incidence is 3.6/million in the UK, the disease presenting as a systemic disorder associated with a necrotising glomerulonephritis and/or lung haemorrhage. The differential diagnosis usually includes Goodpasture's syndrome from which it is distinguished by the absence of antibodies to glomerular basement membrane. Patients often present with a short history of constitutional symptoms, palpable purpura, and abdominal and musculoskeletal pain. The dominant pulmonary manifestation is alveolar haemorrhage, typically with hypertension and an active urinary sediment.

Wegener's granulomatosis (WG)

This form of systemic vasculitis has an annual incidence of 8.5/million in the UK. Characteristically, it presents with upper and lower respiratory tract lesions in association with a focal segmental necrotising glomerulonephritis. Systemic features of a major multisystem disorder may be preceded by months or years of recurrent rhinitis, epistaxis, sinusitis or serous otitis media, or a shorter history of pulmonary symptoms such as cough, haemoptysis, chest pain or dyspnoea. In some patients with limited Wegener's granulomatosis there is little in the way of systemic necrotising vasculitis, and local granuloma formation predominates, with chronic sinusitis, nasal and orbital destruction (see Fig. 12.40), or cavitating lung lesions.

Churg–Strauss syndrome (CSS)

This condition has an annual incidence of up to 3.3/million in the UK. Allergic rhinitis and nasal polyposis may have been present for years. Asthma is often a later development but typically the diagnosis is not made until 3 years after the onset of asthma, when features of a systemic vasculitis develop. Pulmonary infiltrates and eosinophilia are the major features in this syndrome, which is also associated with multisystem necrotising vasculitis. Many patients (up to 70%) develop a cutaneous nodular or papular rash, and over 60% present with accompanying mononeuritis multiplex. Sural nerve biopsy often reveals vasculitis of the vasa nervorum, together with perineural eosinophil infiltration. Cardiac manifestations account for half of deaths, and include myocardial infarction, cardiomyopathy and pericarditis.

Management of MPA, WG and CSS

MPA and WG are usually treated with high-dosage oral prednisolone (1 mg/kg daily) and cyclophosphamide (2 mg/kg daily) or fortnightly intravenous boluses of prednisolone (10 mg/kg) and cyclophosphamide (15 mg/kg) from the outset. Churg–Strauss vasculitis frequently responds to high-dosage steroids alone. Doses of prednisolone and cyclophosphamide are reduced gradually following induction of remission, and full blood counts must be carefully monitored. The dose of cyclophosphamide is reduced in the elderly; mesna is given to patients on bolus therapy to reduce the risk of haemorrhagic cystitis. Other potential side-effects are shown in Table 12.11 (see p. 846). Following successful induction of remission, patients are usually switched to a maintenance regimen of azathioprine and low-dose prednisolone. Therapy usually continues for 1–2 years before withdrawal is considered. Relapse rates are highest in C-ANCA (serine proteinase-3) positive WG. Plasma exchange is undertaken in patients with severe or resistant disease. Intravenous gammaglobulin and anti-T cell therapies are considered when other remedies have failed, or where other therapies cannot be used. Trimethoprim/sulphamethoxazole (co-trimoxazole) or methotrexate (15–25 mg/week) can be used for treating patients with more limited forms of WG. Co-trimoxazole may reduce the incidence of relapse in systemic WG.

The use of cytotoxic drugs has transformed the prognosis for patients with WG. What was once a disease with a 100% mortality in 2 years now has a better than 80% 5-year survival. The prognosis in Churg–Strauss vasculitis is similarly good but life expectancy is shorter in patients with MP.

Leucocytoclastic vasculitis

Cutaneous leucocytoclastic vasculitis affecting small and medium-sized vessels in the skin (see Fig. 12.41) can be associated with serum sickness, drug reactions, infections and malignant tumours. It is important to look for any underlying conditions, and to assess patients for evidence of internal organ involvement more typical of MPA, WG and CSS. In most cases, skin vasculitis is an isolated finding and does not necessarily mean that the patient requires aggressive systemic therapy.

Patients develop palpable purpura and/or urticaria. Hypersensitivity vasculitis is an immune complex disorder and investigations sometimes reveal evidence of circulating IgG, IgM or IgA immune complexes as well as leucocytoclasis and immune complex deposition in skin biopsies.

Treatment is with antihistamines to control symptoms associated with urticaria in mild cases. Corticosteroids and pulses of cyclophosphamide are occasionally required in patients with severe systemic disease and glomerulonephritis. Recent evidence suggests that those patients who are ANCA-positive are most likely to require immunosuppressive drugs.

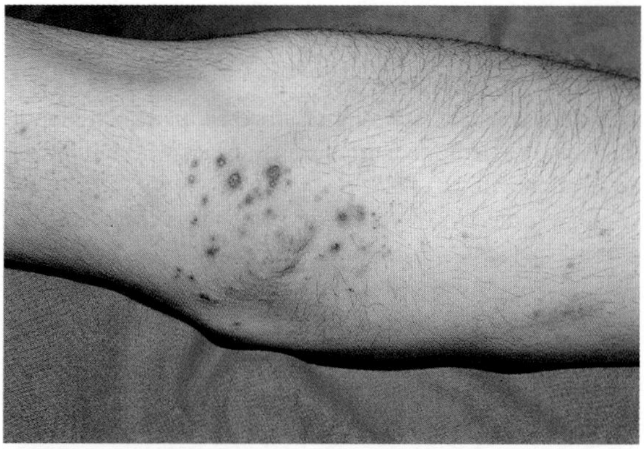

Fig. 12.41 Cutaneous vasculitis: palpable purpura. The elbow is a common site.

Henoch–Schönlein purpura

This small-vessel vasculitis is most commonly seen in children. It is associated with abdominal pain and an acute arthritis affecting one or more joints for a few days at a time. The disease frequently follows an upper respiratory infection and usually lasts for less than 3 months. Boys are affected twice as frequently as girls. Non-thrombocytopenic purpura is found characteristically over the buttocks and lower legs, and up to half the children affected have angio-oedema. Intussusception, rectal bleeding and renal involvement (see p. 428) are features of more severe cases.

Essential mixed cryoglobulinaemic vasculitis (type II cryoglobulinaemia)

Cryoglobulins are circulating immunoglobulins which precipitate out in the cold. There are three forms of cryoglobulinaemia (see Table 12.15). Typical clinical features include palpable purpura, urticaria, cutaneous ulceration, and arthralgia. Less common features include Raynaud's phenomenon, glomerulonephritis, liver dysfunction (often related to an underlying hepatitis C infection), neuropathy and lymphadenopathy. Antiviral therapy (interferon α), steroids and plasmapheresis have been used with success. Hepatitis C infection is difficult to eradicate.

Table 12.15 Classification of cryoglobulins

Cryoglobulinaemia	Antibodies	Disease
Type I	Monoclonal	Myeloma, macroglobulinaemia, some forms of lymphoma
Type II	Monoclonal IgM RF and polyclonal	Essential mixed Cryoglobulinaemia often associated with hepatitis C infection
Type III	Polyclonal antibodies	

OTHER FORMS OF SYSTEMIC VASCULITIS

Behçet's syndrome

This disease is rare in Western Europe but more common in Japan and eastern Mediterranean countries where it has an association with HLA-B5.

Major criteria are recurrent aphthous stomatitis, skin lesions (pathergy, a tendency to form sterile pustules at sites of skin trauma such as venepuncture sites), uveitis and genital ulceration. Minor criteria are inflammatory arthritis of large joints, intestinal ulceration, meningoencephalitis, epididymitis and thrombophlebitis. In the presence of all four major criteria the syndrome is said to be 'complete'; in the presence of three, 'incomplete'. The arthritis is mono-articular or oligoarticular and non-erosive. It most frequently involves the knees, ankles, wrists and elbows. Occasionally the sacroiliac joints are affected.

Treatment is symptomatic, with NSAIDs; corticosteroids and immunosuppressive therapy are reserved for the more serious systemic manifestations.

UNCLASSIFIED PRIMARY VASCULITIS

Despite our best efforts at evaluating and investigating patients, there will be a significant number (up to one-third of cases in some series) in whom a diagnosis of vasculitis is made, but who do not clearly fit into one of the above categories. The usual difficulty arises from trying to distinguish microscopic polyangiitis from Wegener's granulomatosis, or Wegener's granulomatosis from Churg–Strauss syndrome. These patients should be labelled as having an unclassified vasculitis. In terms of therapy and prognosis, the diagnostic label is not as important as the pattern of involvement. For example, if there is significant glomerulonephritis, the patients require immunosuppressive therapy with cyclophosphamide and steroids.

FURTHER INFORMATION ON CONNECTIVE TISSUE DISEASES

Alarcon-Segovia D, Cabral A 1996 Autoantibodies in systemic lupus erythematosus. Current Opinion in Rheumatology 8: 403–407

Lahita R G (ed) 1992 Systemic lupus erythematosus, 2nd edn. Churchill Livingstone, New York

Steen V D (ed) 1996 Scleroderma. Rheumatic Disease Clinics of North America 22: 647–931

Yazici H, Husby G (eds) 1997 Vasculitis. Baillière's Clinical Rheumatology 11: 2

DISEASES OF BONE

OSTEOPOROSIS

Osteoporosis is characterised by reduced bone mass, micro-architectural deterioration of bone tissue and an increased risk of fracture. Fractures related to osteoporosis are a major public health problem in all developed countries; in the UK alone they affect over 150 000 individuals annually at a cost of over £750 million.

Pathogenesis

The most important risk factor for osteoporotic fractures is reduced bone mass. Bone mass increases during growth to reach a peak between the ages of 25 and 35 and falls thereafter in both sexes, with an accelerated phase of more rapid loss in women, due to oestrogen deficiency at the menopause (see Fig. 12.42). Genetic factors are important in the pathogenesis of osteoporosis and family studies suggest that genetic influences account for 70–85% of individual variance in bone mass. The molecular-genetic basis by which bone mass is regulated is incompletely defined, but may involve subtle variations in the structure or regulation of genes which are involved in forming bone matrix and regulating bone turnover. Of the environmental

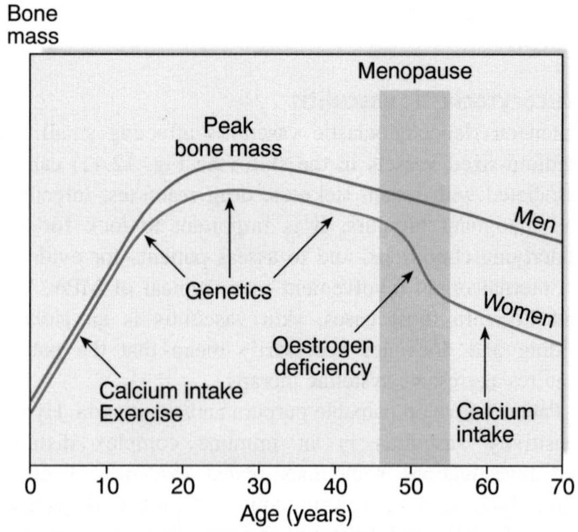

Fig. 12.42 Changes in bone loss with age in men and women. Bone mass increases with growth to reach a peak between 25 and 35 years. Thereafter there is gradual bone loss in both sexes, with an accelerated phase of bone loss in women after the menopause due to oestrogen deficiency. Exercise and calcium intake during childhood, coupled with genetic factors, are important in determining peak bone mass, while calcium intake during later life is important in determining age-related bone loss.

CAUSES OF OSTEOPOROSIS

Genetic
- Race
- Low body weight
- Family history

Endocrine
- Hypogonadism
- Early menopause
- Thyrotoxicosis
- Hyperparathyroidism

Gastrointestinal disease
- Inflammatory bowel disease
- Malabsorption
- Chronic liver disease

Inflammatory disease
- Ankylosing spondylitis
- Rheumatoid arthritis

Drugs
- Corticosteroids

Substance abuse
- Alcohol*
- Smoking

Lifestyle
- Diet/calcium intake
- Exercise/immobility
- Highly trained athletes*

Inherited
- Osteogenesis imperfecta
- Homocystinuria
- Gaucher's disease

Other
- Anorexia nervosa*
- Myeloma
- Neoplasia
- Mastocytosis
- Pregnancy-associated
- Juvenile

* Low body weight, poor diet, low calcium intake and hypogonadism contribute significantly to osteoporosis in anorexia and alcoholics, and hypogonadism to osteoporosis in athletes.

factors known to influence bone mass in normal individuals, the most important are exercise and calcium intake during growth and adolescence. Calcium intake is also important in determining the rate of post-menopausal bone loss. Osteoporosis may also occur as a complication of endocrine, inflammatory and neoplastic conditions, and as a complication of certain drug treatments and substance abuse (see the information box).

Clinical features

Most individuals who have osteoporosis on the basis of bone densitometry are asymptomatic. The importance of osteoporosis lies in the fact that it is associated with an increased risk of fracture which is proportionate to the reduction in bone mass. These fractures typically affect the forearm (Colles fracture), spine (vertebral fracture) and femur (hip fracture). Colles fractures and vertebral fractures most often occur in women aged 55 and above, whereas hip fractures affect older individuals (aged 70+). Osteoporotic limb fractures are usually precipitated by falls, whereas the precipitating factor in vertebral fracture is often being lifted or lifting a heavy weight. The clinical presentation of vertebral fracture is highly variable; in some cases the onset is sudden, with acute back pain so severe as to mimic myocardial infarction, whereas in others the presentation is insidious, with gradual loss of height and chronic back pain. The pain of osteoporotic fracture often radiates anteriorly with a nerve root distribution and may be made worse by back movements. Percussion over affected vertebrae is often painful. Thoracic kyphosis is typical in patients with multiple vertebral fractures. Since low bone density alone does not cause symptoms, many patients with quite advanced osteoporosis remain asymptomatic until a fracture occurs.

Diagnosis

Osteoporotic spinal fractures can be confirmed by the typical wedge appearances of affected vertebrae on a lateral radiograph (see Fig. 12.8, p. 810). Plain radiographs are often normal in patients with osteoporosis who do not have fractures and BMD measurements are necessary to make the diagnosis in such cases. BMD measurements should be reserved for patients where there is reason to suspect the diagnosis on clinical grounds (see the information box). Biochemical measurements are not usually helpful in the diagnosis of osteoporosis; serum alkaline phosphatase may be transiently raised following a fracture but a sustained elevation suggests an alternative diagnosis such as osteomalacia. Bone biopsy is not routinely required, except to exclude other pathology.

INDICATIONS FOR BONE DENSITOMETRY

- Early menopause (< 45 years)
- Hypogonadism
- Family history of osteoporosis
- Radiological evidence of osteoporosis
- Previous fracture after minimal trauma
- Strong risk factors
  - Low body weight
  - Smoking/alcohol abuse
  - Immobility/poor diet
  - Steroid therapy
- Co-existing disease
  - Endocrine
  - Gastrointestinal
  - Inflammatory

Management

Lifestyle changes

Patients with mild to moderate reductions in BMD (T-score values of between –1.0 and –2.5) who do not have fractures should be given general advice on lifestyle factors such as smoking (stop), alcohol (limit to < 20 units/week for men and < 15 units/week for women), dietary calcium intake (aim for 1500 mg daily) and exercise (encourage). In patients with greater reductions in bone density (T-score values of –2.5 and below) specific drug therapy should be considered (see the information box).

Hormone replacement therapy

Hormone replacement therapy (HRT) with oestrogen is the treatment of choice for prevention of osteoporosis. Progestogens should be added to oestrogen in women with

AGENTS USED IN THE PREVENTION AND TREATMENT OF OSTEOPOROSIS

- Hormone replacement therapy
- Bisphosphonates
  - Etidronate
  - Alendronate
- Calcium
- Calcitonin
- Vitamin D and analogues
- Sodium fluoride
- Anabolic steroids

an intact uterus to reduce the risk of endometrial carcinoma. A history of hypertension, stroke and ischaemic heart disease are not contraindications to HRT and, indeed, women on HRT may have a reduced risk of cardiovascular arterial disease. HRT is generally contraindicated in patients with a history of breast cancer and endometrial cancer and there is evidence to suggest that the risk of breast carcinoma may be slightly increased in healthy women who are long-term users of HRT (> 10 years). Previous venous thrombosis is a relative contra-indication to HRT. Many women are unable to tolerate HRT because of side-effects such as weight gain, fluid retention, menstrual bleeding and breast tenderness. The beneficial effects of HRT in patients with established osteoporosis with fractures are less marked than those in whom it is used for osteoporosis prevention, but HRT will increase bone mass even in patients with advanced disease and should also be considered in this situation. Androgen replacement is indicated in males with osteoporosis due to hypogonadism, although its role is unclear in men with idiopathic osteoporosis.

Bisphosphonates

Bisphosphonates provide an alternative to HRT for the prevention and treatment of osteoporosis. Bisphosphonates are synthetic analogues of pyrophosphate that adsorb on to bone surfaces and become incorporated within bone matrix. When bone which contains bisphosphonate is ingested by resorbing osteoclasts, the drug is released within the cell at high concentration and exerts a toxic effect, leading to cell death and thus inhibiting bone resorption. In clinical practice, treatment with bisphosphonate is usually accompanied by a modest increase in bone mass (5–10%) which is thought to be due to continued bone formation in the face of suppressed bone resorption.

Alendronate (10 mg daily, with calcium supplements) is effective in both the prevention of osteoporosis and the treatment of established osteoporosis in post-menopausal women, in whom it increases bone mass and reduces fracture risk. Etidronate (400 mg daily for 2 weeks, followed by 13 weeks' calcium supplements) has similar effects and has also been found to be helpful in the treatment of osteoporosis in men and in corticosteroid-induced osteoporosis. Bisphosphonates are generally well tolerated, but alendronate can cause upper gastrointestinal upset and should be avoided in patients with dyspepsia, hiatus hernia and peptic ulceration.

Calcium

Calcium supplements are widely used as an adjunct to other treatments in the prevention and treatment of osteoporosis. When used alone, calcium supplements do not increase bone mass but they do slow bone loss in post-menopausal women. The effect of calcium supplementation is greatest in those with a low dietary calcium intake, and calcium supplements should be considered in all post-menopausal women with osteoporosis who are taking less than the recommended intake of 1500 mg daily. Calcium supplements are also indicated in male osteoporosis and in steroid-induced osteoporosis.

Other treatments

Calcitonin prevents bone loss in osteoporosis, but it is not widely used because of side-effects such as flushing and nausea, relatively high cost and availability of other agents with equal or greater efficacy. Anabolic steroids such as stanozolol have similarly been shown to increase bone mass in osteoporosis but there is no data on fracture prevention, and tolerability is poor due to side-effects such as hirsutism, weight gain, fluid retention and disturbance of liver function. Vitamin D and active vitamin D metabolites may have a role in the treatment of established osteoporosis and in the prevention of hip fracture. Low-dose vitamin D (1000 i.u. daily) and calcium supplements have been found to reduce the risk of hip fracture in elderly institutionalised patients. Calcitriol, the active metabolite of vitamin D, has been found to be effective in secondary prevention of vertebral fractures in some studies, but not in others. Calcitriol therapy must be closely monitored in view of the risk of hypercalcaemia and hypercalciuria. Sodium fluoride differs from most of the other agents discussed so far in having a specific stimulatory effect on bone formation. Sodium fluoride can give impressive increases in bone mass (30% or more), but the therapeutic window is narrow since fluoride can promote formation of woven bone with reduced mechanical strength. In view of this, the role of fluoride in the treatment of osteoporosis is controversial.

OSTEOGENESIS IMPERFECTA

Osteogenesis imperfecta (OI) is a rare disease which presents with severe osteoporosis and multiple fractures in infancy and childhood. Other clinical features include blue sclerae and abnormal dentition but these abnormalities are not seen in all patients. Osteogenesis imperfecta is due to mutations affecting the protein-coding regions of the type I collagen genes (COLIA1 and COLIA2), which cause a reduction in the amount of collagen produced and/or prevent the collagen molecules from folding normally into a triple helix. Severity of the disease is highly variable, depending on where the mutation occurs. The clinical picture ranges from the very severe, in which multiple fractures occur in infancy and childhood, to the relatively mild, which can first present in adulthood and mimic osteoporosis. The diagnosis of OI is suspected on the basis of a clinical history of frequent fractures in childhood and may be confirmed by analysis of the collagen protein chains extracted from cultured skin fibroblasts. There is no specific treatment for OI, although recent studies with the bisphosphonate pamidronate have demonstrably reduced fracture rates in affected children.

Table 12.16 Causes of osteomalacia and rickets

Predisposing factor/cause	Mechanism
Lack of sunlight exposure; dietary lack of meat and dairy products	Failure of vitamin D precursor synthesis in the skin/low levels of vitamin D in diet
Gastrointestinal disease/chronic liver disease	Malabsorption of vitamin D and calcium
Aluminium toxicity/bisphosphonate	Direct inhibition of bone mineralisation
Chronic renal failure	Reduced conversion of 25 (OH) D_3 to 1,25 $(OH)_2$ D_3
Vitamin D-dependent rickets type I (autosomal recessive)	Mutation in renal 1-α-hydroxylase which converts 25 (OH) D_3 to 1,25 $(OH)_2$ D_3
Vitamin D-dependent rickets type II (autosomal recessive)	Mutation in vitamin D receptor
Hypophosphataemic rickets (X-linked dominant)	Inherited defect in renal tubular phosphate reabsorption leading to hypophosphataemia
Hypophosphatasia (autosomal recessive)	Defect/mutation in bone alkaline phosphatase which normally degrades inhibitors of bone mineralisation at the calcification front

HRT therapy is indicated to prevent post-menopausal bone loss in women with OI.

OSTEOMALACIA AND RICKETS (see Table 12.16)

Osteomalacia and rickets are now rare in the UK except in certain high-risk groups including Asian immigrants, elderly housebound individuals, institutionalised patients, and patients with gastrointestinal disease, chronic liver disease and chronic renal failure.

Pathogenesis

Osteomalacia and rickets are characterised by increased bone turnover with failure of bone mineralisation. Vitamin D deficiency is the most common cause of rickets and osteomalacia, either as the result of reduced dietary intake or reduced sunlight exposure (see Fig. 12.43). The calcium malabsorption which results from vitamin D deficiency triggers an increase in PTH secretion, which in turn increases bone turnover but which also stimulates phosphaturia, thus causing phosphate deficiency. It is this combination of calcium deficiency and phosphate deficiency which causes osteomalacia. Other causes of osteomalacia include failure of conversion of 25 hydroxyvitamin D (25 (OH) D) to 1,25 dihydroxyvitamin D (1,25 $(OH)_2$ D) because of renal failure, aluminium toxicity (see p. 437), and bisphosphonate (usually etidronate) therapy. Rare causes include:

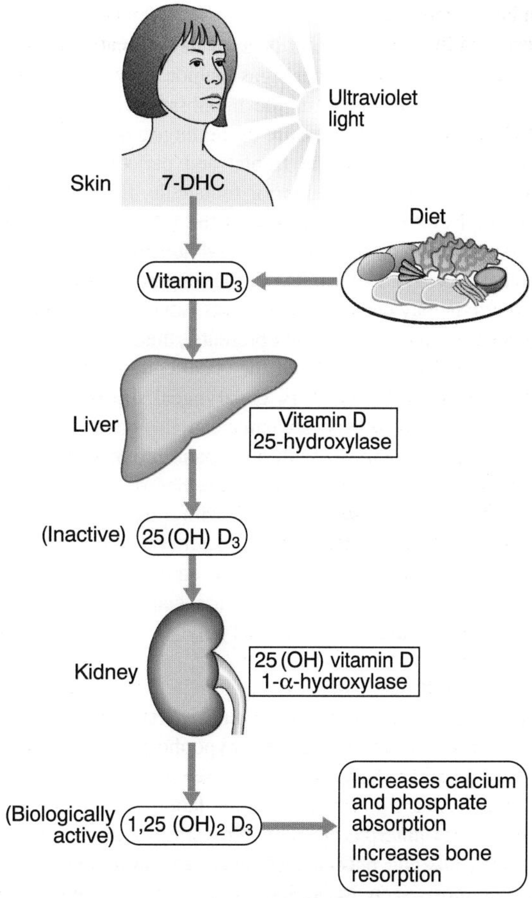

Fig. 12.43 Vitamin D metabolism in humans. Vitamin D is derived from the diet (20%) and the action of UV light on the skin (80%), which converts 7-dehydrocholesterol (7-DHC) to vitamin D. The vitamin then undergoes hydroxylation steps in the liver and kidney to yield the active metabolite 1,25 $(OH)_2$ D_3 which acts on the gut to increase calcium and phosphate absorption and on bone to increase bone resorption.

- hypophosphataemic rickets—an X-linked dominant condition caused by an inherited defect in renal tubular phosphate reabsorption
- an inherited defect in the renal 1-α-hydroxylase enzyme, which is necessary for conversion of 25 (OH) D to 1,25 $(OH)_2$ D (vitamin D-dependent rickets type I)
- end-organ resistance to 1,25 $(OH)_2$ D due to inherited mutations in the vitamin D receptor (vitamin D-dependent rickets type II)
- an inherited deficiency in alkaline phosphatase (hypophosphatasia). Osteomalacia occurs in hypophosphatasia because an important function of alkaline phosphatase is to metabolise phosphate-containing compounds which act as inhibitors of bone mineralisation.

Clinical features

Infants with rickets exhibit delayed development and have muscular hypotonia. Other signs include craniotabes (small round unossified areas in the membranous bones of the skull, yielding to the pressure of the finger, with a cracking feeling); 'bossing' of the frontal and parietal bones; and delayed closure of the anterior fontanelle. Enlargement of the epiphyses at the lower end of the radius occurs, along with swelling of the costochondral junctions of the ribs (rickety rosary). Deformities of the long bones, chest spine and pelvis may occur. Severe rickets can be associated with hypocalcaemic tetany, which presents clinically with spasm of the hands and feet and of the vocal cords, resulting in a high-pitched distressing cry or laryngeal stridor. Epileptic seizures related to hypocalcaemia can also occur. In adults, osteomalacia manifests with bone pain, proximal muscular weakness and severe malaise. Muscular weakness is prominent and the patient may walk with a waddling gait and experience difficulty in climbing stairs or getting out of a chair. Bone and muscular tenderness on pressure is common and focal bone pain may occur in association with fractures or pseudofractures of the ribs and pelvis.

Investigations

The diagnosis of osteomalacia and rickets is supported by the finding of hypocalcaemia, hypophosphataemia and a raised alkaline phosphatase level (see Table 12.4, p. 811), although the significance of the latter finding is more difficult to interpret in children, since, due to skeletal growth, alkaline phosphatase levels are normally elevated above those seen in adults. Radiological examination in children with rickets may show characteristic changes in the epiphyses at the lower ends of the radius; the zones of epiphyseal cartilage are thickened and the distal ends of the shafts are widened, leading to 'saucer' deformity. In adults, bone radiographs may be normal or show only the presence of osteoporosis with vertebral crush fractures. In more advanced cases, focal radiolucent bands (pseudofractures or Looser's zones) may be seen affecting the ribs, the axillary border of the scapula, the pubic rami and the medial cortex of the upper femur. These are a late feature, however, and are absent in many cases.

The most common differential diagnosis of osteomalacia in adults is osteoporosis, which is also characterised by bone pain and fractures, and which can be associated with slightly raised alkaline phosphatase levels in the context of a healing fracture. In cases where there is any doubt, transiliac bone biopsy is indicated, which will show the pathognomonic features of increased thickness and extent of osteoid seams.

Management

Rickets and osteomalacia respond rapidly to vitamin D and calcium supplementation, but in severe cases where there is hypocalcaemic tetany, urgent treatment with intravenous calcium gluconate (10 ml/10%) may also be required. Daily doses of between 25 and 50 μg (1000–2000 i.u.) of vitamin D (cholecalciferol), combined with 500–1000 mg calcium, are sufficient to heal most cases of osteomalacia and rickets, but higher doses of vitamin D or parenteral vitamin D therapy may be necessary in intestinal malabsorption and liver disease. Since there is a risk of vitamin D toxicity with the high doses required to treat these conditions, many clinicians favour use of the active vitamin D metabolites (1-α-hydroxyvitamin D or 1,25 dihydroxyvitamin D, 0.5–2.5 μg daily). Although these agents also carry a risk of toxicity, it is reversed much more rapidly on stopping treatment (days) than with cholecalciferol (weeks or months).

Healing of rickets and osteomalacia is accompanied by improvement in radiological appearances. Serum calcium and phosphorus return to within the normal range soon after commencing treatment, whereas alkaline phosphatase levels often increase at the start of treatment, before falling to within the normal range as the bone disease heals. The dose of vitamin D and the need for continuing therapy should be assessed by regular biochemical monitoring. When alkaline phosphatase levels fall to normal, the dose of vitamin D can be stopped or dropped to a maintenance prophylactic level (10 μg/400 i.u. daily). Recurrence can be prevented by regular sunlight exposure and maintenance of a diet containing dairy products and meat, or by administration of low-dose vitamin D supplements (10 μg/400 i.u. daily). Patients with osteomalacia due to malabsorption or chronic liver disease may need higher maintenance doses of vitamin D or its active metabolites to prevent recurrence.

Special measures are required to treat the rare cases of osteomalacia and rickets which are not due to simple vitamin D deficiency. Indeed, these conditions often first come to light when the patient fails to respond to vitamin D. Hypophosphataemic rickets respond to phosphate supplementation and active vitamin D metabolites, which are needed to offset the hypocalcaemic effect of the phosphate. Patients with vitamin D-dependent rickets type I respond to 'physiological' doses of active vitamin D metabolites (1-α-hydroxyvitamin D or 1,25 dihydroxyvitamin D, 0.5–2.5 μg daily). Patients with vitamin D-dependent rickets type II are more difficult to treat, but sometimes the receptor defect can be partially overcome by high doses of active metabolites and/or by enteral or parenteral calcium and phosphate supplementation. There is no effective treatment for hypophosphatasia. Management of osteomalacia in renal disease and aluminium toxicity is discussed elsewhere (see p. 437).

PAGET'S DISEASE

Paget's disease of bone is characterised by increased and disorganised bone resorption and bone formation on a focal or multifocal basis throughout the skeleton. The pelvis, femur, tibia, lumbar spine, skull and scapula are commonly affected, whereas involvement of the small bones of the hands and feet is rare. It is of interest that Paget's disease rarely spreads to new bones after diagnosis, which possibly suggests that the bones are 'imprinted' to be affected at an early stage in life. Paget's disease is uncommon before the age of 40 years but increases in incidence with age to affect 10% of the population in the UK by the age of 85. Although Paget's is common in the USA and Western Europe, it is rare in Orientals, Asians and Scandinavians. The common occurrence of Paget's disease in Western Europeans who have emigrated to Australia, New Zealand and South Africa, compared with a low incidence in the indigenous population, suggests that genetic factors are important in aetiology. Clinically, Paget's disease is associated with bone deformity, bone pain and increased susceptibility to pathological fracture. Paget's disease also predisposes to the development of osteoarthritis in joints adjacent to affected bones.

Pathogenesis

The dramatic increase in bone resorption and bone formation in Paget's disease disrupts normal bone architecture and compromises mechanical strength, resulting in bone deformity and an increased risk of fracture (see Fig. 12.44). Bone blood flow is increased, and the affected bones enlarge and become deformed. Although the cause of Paget's disease is unknown, there is much evidence to suggest that the primary abnormality is in cells of the osteoclast lineage. Osteoclasts in Paget's disease are much larger than normal, containing up to 100 nuclei, and have been found to contain microcylindrical inclusions. This led to the hypothesis that Paget's disease may be due to a 'slow-virus' infection of osteoclasts, but no virus has ever been recovered from Pagetic bone and this theory remains unproven. Genetic factors are important in the pathogenesis of Paget's disease. This is reflected by the striking racial differences in incidence referred to previously and the occurrence of a positive family history in up to 15% of patients. Many families have been described in whom Paget's is inherited as an autosomal dominant trait, and molecular-genetic studies have suggested the presence of a susceptibility locus for the disease on chromosome 18q in some families.

Clinical features

Paget's disease is often discovered as an incidental finding

A

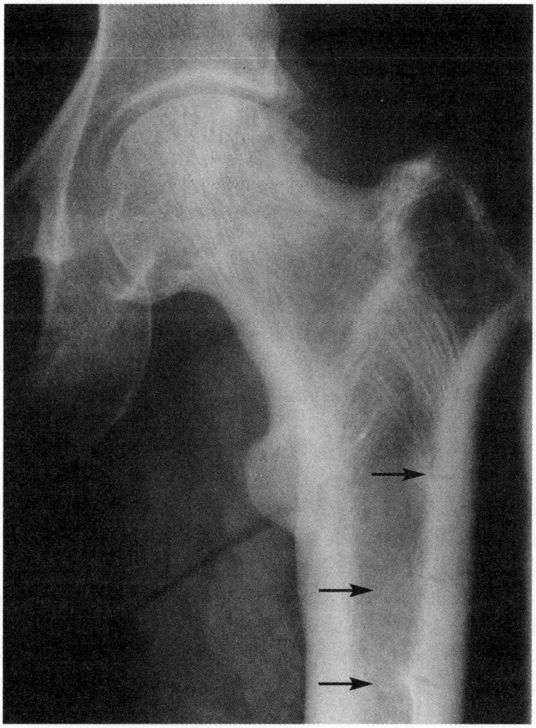

B

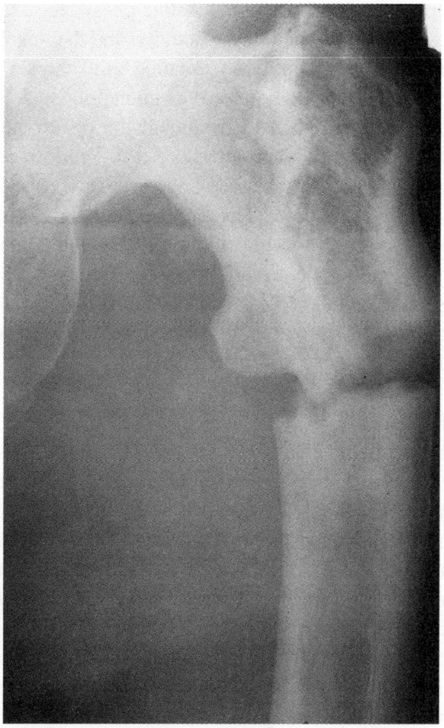

Fig. 12.44 Radiograph of Paget's disease. A Several pseudofractures (arrows) in a deformed Pagetic femur with cortical expansion and osteosclerosis. B The patient presented with an aching pain in the leg, but suffered a spontaneous fracture of the femoral shaft while walking before treatment could be commenced.

in patients who are under investigation for another disorder, but may also present with bone deformity, pain or pathological fracture. Clinical signs include bone deformity, warmth of the skin over affected bones and pathological fracture. Bone deformity is usually evident in weight-bearing bones such as the femur and tibia, but may also occur in the spine, pelvis and skull. The incidence of osteoarthritis is increased in Paget's disease and, rarely, increased vascularity of Pagetic bone can precipitate high-output cardiac failure in elderly patients with limited cardiac reserve. Skull involvement is a particularly serious complication of Paget's disease, since it can progress insidiously in the absence of symptoms to cause deafness and other cranial nerve lesions by encroaching on the foramina in the base of the skull. Other neurological lesions such as spinal cord compression and nerve root compression syndromes may also occur when Paget's disease affects the spine. Osteosarcoma is a rare but serious complication of Paget's disease and has a poor prognosis. It should be suspected in a patient with established Paget's who suffers a sudden increase in pain or swelling of an affected bone.

Diagnosis

Paget's disease is characterised by raised serum alkaline phosphatase levels in the presence of normal serum calcium and phosphate levels. The raised alkaline phosphatase levels reflect an increase in osteoblastic activity, and the degree of elevation provides an approximate guide as to the severity and extent of disease. Radiological examination is useful to confirm the diagnosis and to document the occurrence of bone deformity, coexisting arthritis and pseudofractures (see Fig. 12.44), but radionuclide bone scan examination is a more sensitive means of detecting and assessing overall extent of the disease (see Fig. 12.11, p. 812). Although the biochemical, radiographic and bone scan appearances are usually pathognomonic, osteosclerotic metastases can occasionally enter into the differential diagnosis, and in such cases bone biopsy may be required.

Management

Medical treatment should be offered in painful Paget's disease and when Paget's disease affects a weight-bearing long bone or the skull. Therapy of Paget's disease is based on giving drugs which inhibit osteoclast activity. Although the primary effect of these agents is on bone resorption, treatment is accompanied by a reduction in bone formation, reflecting the fact that the processes of resorption and formation are closely coupled in Pagetic bone. Bisphosphonates are now the treatment of choice. These drugs reduce bone turnover in Pagetic lesions and can help partially to restore normal bone architecture. Three bisphosphonates are currently licensed in the UK for treatment of Paget's disease. Etidronate (400 mg daily for 3–6 months) is effective and well tolerated but it should be avoided in patients with pseudofractures and deformities of weight-bearing limb bones, since it can cause osteomalacia. Pamidronate is more potent than etidronate, and is the drug of choice for severe Paget's disease. Pamidronate does not cause problems with osteomalacia but must be given intravenously. A typical regimen for a patient with severe disease would consist of an initial treatment with 2–3 60 mg infusions, followed by 60 mg at 3-month intervals, depending on the response of alkaline phosphatase. A further alternative is oral tiludronate (400 mg daily for 3–6 months), a sulphur-containing bisphosphonate which is more potent than etidronate and has no adverse effect on mineralisation. Calcitonin is less effective than bisphosphonates for the treatment of Paget's disease and is now seldom used.

The effectiveness of anti-Pagetic therapy should be monitored by regular measurement of serum levels of alkaline phosphatase (every 2–3 months), with the aim of restoring values to within the normal range. Pain does not provide a good guide to efficacy of treatment since it can persist even after biochemical remission has been achieved. Here, other causes should be sought for the pain. Secondary osteoarthritis of the hip or knee may require joint replacement, which should be preceded with a course of medical therapy to reduce disease activity and bone blood flow.

OSTEOPETROSIS AND OSTEOSCLEROSIS

These compose a heterogeneous group of conditions characterised by increased bone density secondary to defective resorption of bone by osteoclasts. The clinical phenotype is highly variable and ranges from a severe disorder which presents with bone marrow failure in childhood to a milder, often asymptomatic form, which presents in adults. In the severe childhood form there is failure to thrive, delayed eruption of dentition and cranial nerve palsies due to failure of cranial foramina formation. Bone marrow failure occurs due to replacement of the marrow cavity with bone. This condition can be successfully treated by marrow transplantation in infancy, implying a defect in the genes which control osteoclast formation and activity. The adult-onset type may present with bone pain, cranial nerve palsies and osteoarthritis or may be asymptomatic, only to be discovered by the finding of increased bone density on skeletal radiographs taken for other reasons.

The molecular defects in most forms of human osteopetrosis have not yet been defined. One type of osteopetrosis is associated with renal tubular acidosis and deficiency of the enzyme carbonic anhydrase II, responsible for acid production in osteoclasts. In this disorder osteoclasts form normally, but they are unable to resorb bone because of their inability to produce acid which is responsible for dissolution of bone mineral. Another form of osteopetrosis (pycnodysostosis) has been found to be due to deficiency of cathepsin K, a protease which is necessary for degradation of bone matrix. Acquired forms of osteosclerosis have been described in intravenous drug abusers with hepatitis C infection, in patients with lymphoma, myelosclerosis, systemic mastocytosis and in the rare condition of *fibrogenesis imperfecta ossium*. This is an acquired disorder of unknown cause characterised by intractable bone pain, mixed osteosclerotic/osteolytic lesions on radiograph and multiple fractures. Electron microscopy studies of affected bone show a disorganised pattern of collagen fibril deposition, with abnormal mineralisation, although the cause is unknown. There is no specific treatment.

RARE INHERITED DISORDERS OF THE SKELETON

Marfan's syndrome is characterised by skeletal disproportion (arm span greater than height), arachnodactyly, sternal depression, lens dislocation and a high arched palate, due to mutations in the fibrillin gene, a component of extracellular matrix. The most serious complications of this disease are in the cardiovascular system where mitral valve prolapse, aortic incompetence and dissection of the aorta occur. *Ehlers–Danlos syndrome* is characterised by skin laxity, hypermobility of joints, scoliosis, short stature, ocular fragility, skin bruising and visceral vascular catastrophes. The disease is genetically heterogeneous and may occur as the result of mutations in several genes including type II collagen, lysyl oxidase deficiency, fibronectin and elastin. Osteoporosis and Marfan-like appearances occur in *homocystinuria*, which is due to deficiency of the enzyme cystathionine synthetase. Other features include mental retardation, and venous and arterial thrombosis. The diagnosis is made by finding homocystine in the urine, and patients respond to treatment with pyridoxine. The *chondrodystrophies* are a related group of inherited disorders characterised by abnormal growth and development of bone and cartilage. Various clinical subtypes are recognised due to mutations in a variety of genes. Some are due to mutations in extracellular matrix genes including collagens type II, IX and X and cartilage oligomatrix protein, whereas other subtypes are due to mutations in other molecules involved in cartilage growth and differentiation, including fibroblast growth factor receptor 3 and PTH-related protein. The *mucopolysaccharidoses* form another group of inborn errors of metabolism in which lysosomal enzyme defects lead to abnormal accumulation of glycosaminoglycans. All are associated with stiff joints and short stature, except for the Morquio syndrome, which is associated with hypermobility and atlantoaxial subluxation. The diagnoses are confirmed by identification of the urinary glycosaminoglycan metabolites and detection of the enzyme defects in fibroblast cultures.

CANCER-ASSOCIATED BONE DISEASE

Bone disease is a frequent complication of malignancy. Hypercalcaemia is probably the most common metabolic complication of malignancy, which in most cases is due to excessive release of PTH-related protein (PTHrP) by solid tumours such as carcinoma of the lung, breast and genitourinary system. The mechanisms and treatment of this condition are discussed in more detail on page 576. Less commonly, osteomalacia can occur as a complication of malignancy, particularly in association with mesenchymal tumours. In this case, it is thought that the tumour releases a factor which promotes renal phosphate wasting.

Bone metastases are common in patients with tumours of the bronchus, breast and prostate, and with multiple myeloma. Metastatic bone disease typically presents with bone pain, pathological fracture or neurological symptoms due to nerve root compression or spinal cord compression. The diagnosis is suspected on the basis of clinical history and typical appearances of local osteolytic lesions on radiological examination of affected bones. Radionuclide bone scan examination is a more sensitive means of detecting bone metastases but osteolytic lesions in myeloma can occur in the absence of new bone formation, leading to a false negative result. Osteosclerotic metastases also occur and are particularly characteristic of prostatic carcinoma.

The treatment of metastatic bone disease is interdisciplinary, but four broad approaches can be identified and must often be used in combination for effective symptom control (see the information box). The most effective means of controlling bone metastases is to treat the primary tumour with chemotherapy or hormone therapy, but in many cases the tumour may have become resistant to these measures, necessitating an alternative approach. In this case, efforts should focus on control of pain with analgesics/NSAIDs,

MANAGEMENT OF BONE METASTASES
Treatment of the primary tumour
• Chemotherapy • Hormone therapy
Treatment of local lesions
• Fixation of fractures • Spinal cord decompression • Radiotherapy
Inhibition of osteoclastic bone resorption
• Bisphosphonates
Treatment of pain
• Analgesics/NSAIDs • Nerve blocks • Radiotherapy

nerve blockade or local radiotherapy. Orthopaedic surgery may also be required to treat pathological fractures or to stabilise local osteolytic lesions which seem destined to result in pathological fractures if left untreated. Finally, surgical decompression may be indicated as a palliative manoeuvre in the treatment of spinal metastases which are encroaching on the spinal cord.

Recent research has shown that bisphosphonates are effective in the secondary prevention of osteolytic disease due to breast cancer and multiple myeloma. The bisphosphonates work in this situation by virtue of the fact that most tumours cause osteolytic lesions by the release of local factors which increase osteoclast formation and activity, leading to local increases in bone destruction in areas of the skeleton which are involved by tumour. Since bisphosphonates inhibit osteoclast activity, the bone surrounding tumour deposits is protected from further damage and the formation of new lesions is inhibited. Oral clodronate and intravenous pamidronate have been most widely studied in this situation and have been shown to prevent the development of pathological fractures, to improve bone pain and to reduce skeletal morbidity in patients with breast carcinoma, multiple myeloma and other tumour types. Most experience has been obtained with intermittent intravenous pamidronate (90 mg i.v. once monthly) or oral clodronate (up to 3.2 g daily). The effects in myeloma are particularly good and it is currently recommended that all patients with myeloma should be treated with adjuvant bisphosphonate therapy, along with standard chemotherapy.

Primary bone tumours are less common than secondary bone tumours. The presentation is with local pain and swelling, and treatment is primarily surgical. The reader is referred to textbooks of orthopaedic surgery for a more detailed discussion on presentation, clinical features and management.

FURTHER INFORMATION ON DISEASES OF BONE

Compston J E 1994 The therapeutic use of bisphosphonates. British Medical Journal 309: 711–716

Delmas P D, Meunier P J 1997 The management of Paget's disease of bone. New England Journal of Medicine 336: 558–566

Houler M R, McCaine T A 1992 Basic and clinical concepts related to vitamin D metabolism. New England Journal of Medicine 297: 974–982

Ralston S H 1997 Science medicine and the future: osteoporosis. British Medical Journal 315: 469–472

Diseases of the skin

13

O.M.V. SCHOFIELD • J.A.A. HUNTER

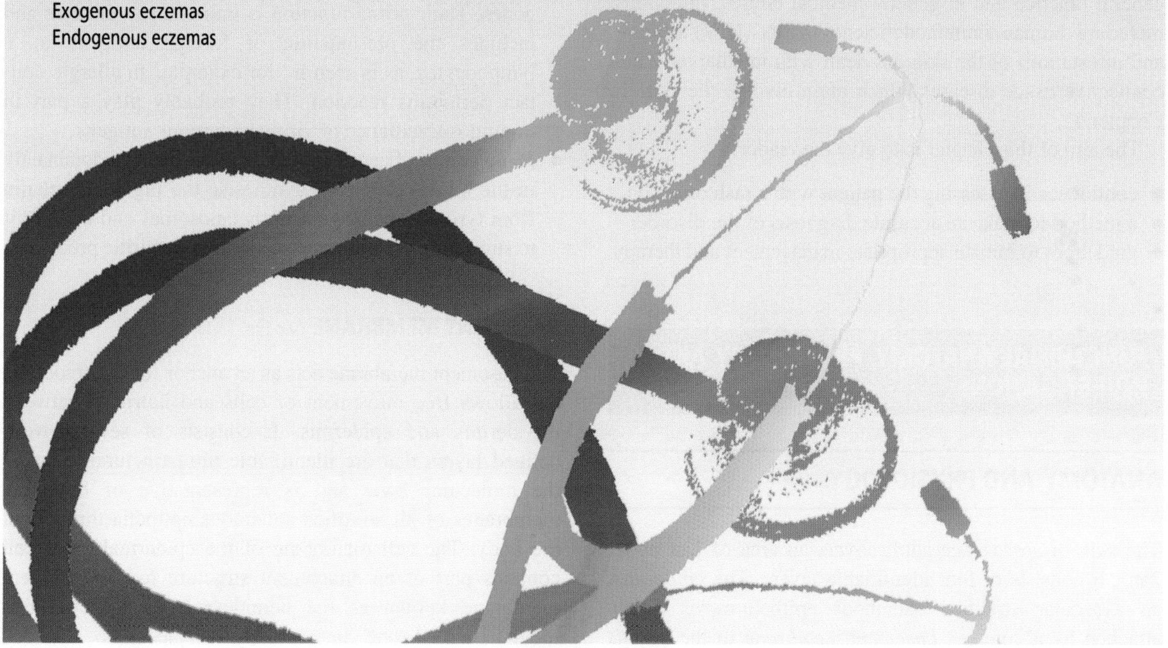

Large community prevalence studies in the United Kingdom and United States of America have demonstrated that between 20 and 30% of the population have a skin disease requiring attention but only 1 person in 5 seeks medical help. Skin cancers are the most common tumours world-wide and at present in the UK their annual incidence is increasing at a rate of around 7% per annum. Skin complaints affect all ages from the neonate to the elderly and cause harm in a number of ways, as shown in the information box.

THE FOUR Ds
Discomfort
• Most often itching or pain (e.g. eczema, post-herpetic neuralgia)
Disfigurement
• Leading to embarrassment and withdrawal from society (e.g. birth marks, acne vulgaris and psoriasis)
Disability
• Leading to loss of work and wages (e.g. dermatitis of the hands and feet)
Death
• Rare but still seen (e.g. angioedema, metastatic skin cancer and widespread blistering)

Every clinician has ample opportunity to look at the skin when listening to or examining a patient and should be able to identify important and common skin disorders. This chapter emphasises those skin conditions that are frequently seen in general practice and in general medical clinics. Infections, including human immunodeficiency virus (HIV) disease, and infestations of the skin are dealt with in Chapter 2 and connective tissue diseases which often involve the skin, in Chapter 12.

The aim of this chapter is to give the reader:

- confidence in assessing the patient with a rash or lesion
- a method to make an accurate diagnosis of the disorder
- guidelines to initiate appropriate management and therapy.

FUNCTIONAL ANATOMY, PHYSIOLOGY AND INVESTIGATIONS

ANATOMY AND PHYSIOLOGY

The skin of an average adult covers an area of just under 2 m^2. It consists of four identifiable layers. The *epidermis*, an avascular stratified squamous epithelium, is firmly attached by a complex *basement membrane* to the *dermis* (see Fig. 13.1). The dermis contains and supports blood vessels, nerves and adnexal structures such as hair follicles and sweat glands. Below the dermis is the subcutis or *hypodermis*, which consists predominantly of fat.

EPIDERMIS (see Fig. 13.1)

Keratinocytes comprise 95% of epidermal cells. They synthesise insoluble proteins known as keratins of two main types: basic (type I) and acidic (type II). Individual keratins of each type pair up to form intermediate filaments (tonofilaments) which provide the basic cytoskeleton of the cell. Keratinocytes also synthesise the lipid-rich cornified envelope in the stratum corneum and this superficial horny layer is primarily responsible for the protective barrier function of skin. Keratinocytes are generated by division of stem cells in the basal layer of the epidermis and move outwards. They die in the granular layer and become flattened anucleate cells (bricks) in the most superficial horny layer, surrounded by the hydrophobic cornified envelope (mortar); they are finally shed at the surface. In normal skin this process takes about 4 weeks but in conditions such as psoriasis it is greatly accelerated. Keratinocytes are attached to each other by complex adhesion structures known as desmosomes.

A few *Merkel cells* are found in the basal layer of the epidermis and are thought to arise embryologically from keratinocytes; they act as transducers for fine touch.

Two main types of dendritic cell make up most of the remaining 5% of the epidermal cells:

- *Langerhans cells* are dendritic bone-marrow-derived cells that circulate between the epidermis and the local lymph nodes. Their prime function is immune surveillance and includes the presentation of foreign antigens to T lymphocytes, as is seen in, for example, an allergic contact dermatitis reaction. They probably play a part in immunosurveillance of viral and tumour antigens.
- *Melanocytes*, of neural crest origin, are found predominantly in the basal layer; they synthesise the pigment melanin from tyrosine, package it in melanosomes and transfer it to surrounding keratinocytes via their dendritic processes.

BASEMENT MEMBRANE (see Fig. 13.1)

The basement membrane acts as an anchor for the epidermis but allows free movement of cells and nutrients between the dermis and epidermis. It consists of several well-defined layers that are identifiable ultrastructurally and at the molecular level and is representative of basement membranes of all stratified squamous epithelia throughout the body. The cell membrane of the epidermal basal cell contains part of an attachment structure to the basement membrane known as the hemidesmosome. The lamina lucida is the zone immediately subjacent to the cell

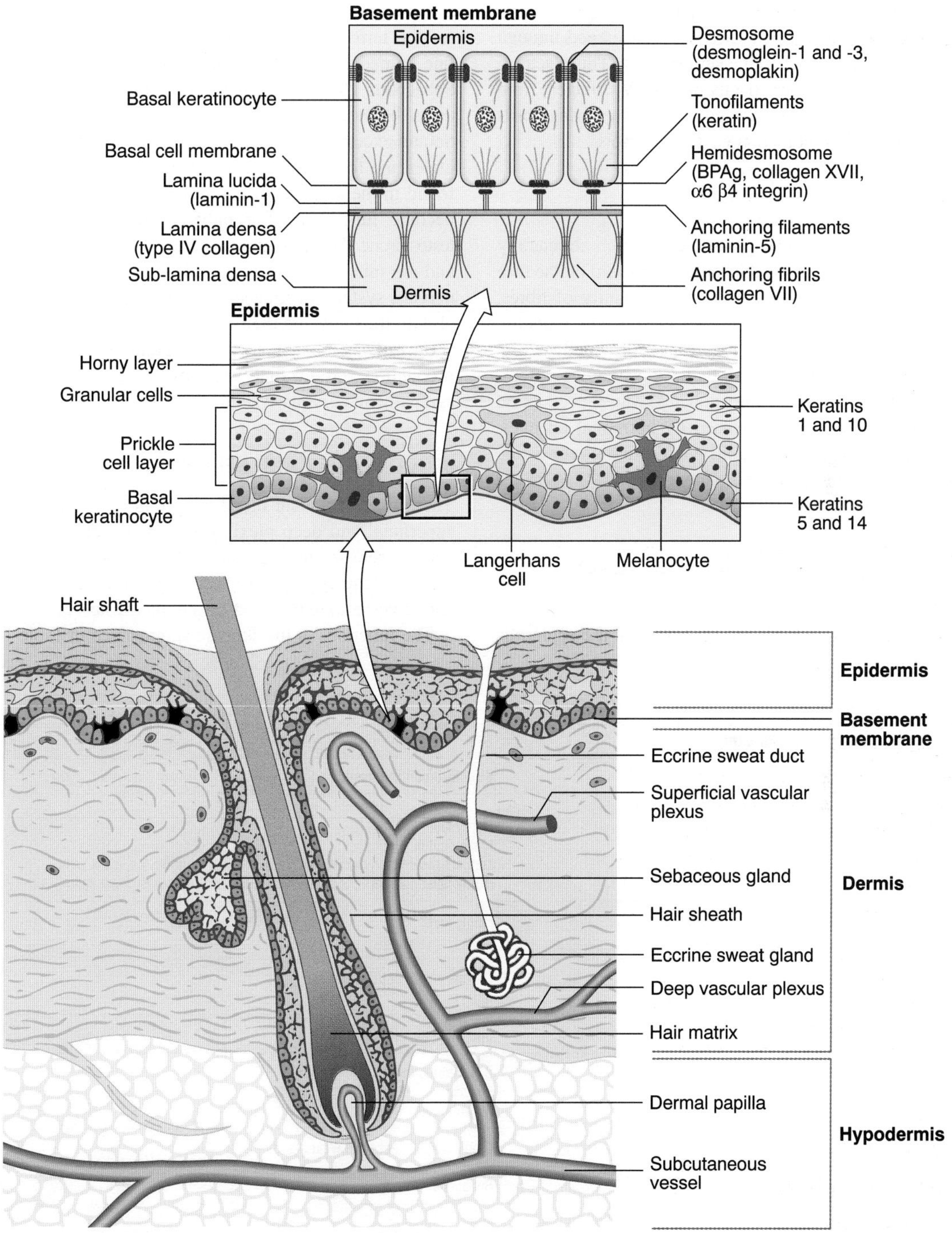

Fig. 13.1 Structure of normal skin.

membrane of the basal cell which is composed predominantly of laminin. Anchoring filaments extend through the lamina lucida to attach to the lamina densa. This electron-dense layer consists predominantly of type IV collagen; from it extend loops of type VII collagen forming anchoring fibrils that fasten the basement membrane to the dermis.

DERMIS

The dermis is vascular and supports the epidermis structurally and nutritionally. It varies in thickness from 1 mm on the face to 4 mm on the back. It consists predominantly of fibres, mostly collagens I and III but also elastin and reticulin, synthesised by fibroblasts. Support is provided by an amorphous ground substance (mostly the glycosaminoglycans, hyaluronic acid and dermatan sulphate), whose production and catabolism may be influenced by hormonal changes. Finally, there is a cellular component to the dermis consisting of many fibroblasts, mast cells, mononuclear phagocytes, lymphocytes and Langerhans cells.

EPIDERMAL APPENDAGES: HAIR AND SWEAT GLANDS

Hair, nails and sweat glands are derived from the epidermis at various stages in gestation. Coarse, medullated hair accounts for the terminal hair of the scalp and pubic areas. Short, fine unmedullated hairs make up the remaining body hair. Sebaceous glands arise from these hair follicles and their ducts discharge sebum into the upper part of the hair follicle. Sebum excretion is under the control of testosterone in both males and females. Apocrine glands are those sweat glands found in the axillae, perineum, genitalia and areolae which become functional after puberty under the influence of testosterone. Apocrine glands secrete sweat via the hair follicle and are innervated by adrenergic fibres of the sympathetic nervous system. Eccrine sweat glands are found everywhere else on the body and their ducts open directly on to the skin surface. They are responsible for thermoregulation by sweat production and are innervated by cholinergic fibres of the sympathetic nervous system.

BLOOD VESSELS AND NERVES

There is an abundant blood supply in the skin arranged in superficial and deep plexi. The skin is well supplied with nerves; sensory nerves end in the dermis and, to a much lesser extent, the epidermis associated with Merkel cells. Blood vessels are supplied by autonomic nerves.

The functions of the skin are summarised in Table 13.1.

Table 13.1 Functions of the skin

Function	Structure/cell involved
Protection against:	
Chemicals, particles	Horny layer
Ultraviolet radiation	Melanocytes
Antigens, haptens	Langerhans cells, lymphocytes, mononuclear phagocytes, mast cells
Microbes	Horny layer, Langerhans cells, mononuclear phagocytes, mast cells
Preservation of a balanced internal environment Prevents loss of water, electrolytes and macromolecules	Horny layer
Shock absorber Strong, yet elastic and compliant covering	Dermis and subcutaneous fat
Sensation	Specialist nerve endings
Calorie reserve	Subcutaneous fat
Vitamin D synthesis	Keratinocytes
Temperature regulation	Blood vessels, eccrine sweat glands
Lubrication and waterproofing	Sebaceous glands
Protection and prising	Nails
Hormonal Testosterone synthesis from inactive precursors and testosterone conversion to other androgenic steroids	Hair follicles Sebaceous glands
Body odour (more important in animals)	Apocrine sweat glands
Psychosocial	Hair, nails

Table 13.2 Terms used to describe skin lesions

Term	Definition	Term	Definition
PRIMARY LESIONS		**SECONDARY LESIONS** (which evolve from primary lesions)	
Macule	Small flat area of altered colour or texture	**Scale**	A flake arising from the horny layer
Papule	Small solid elevation of skin, less than 0.5 cm in diameter	**Crust**	Looks like a scale, but is composed of dried blood or tissue fluid
Nodule	A solid mass in the skin, usually greater than 0.5 cm in diameter	**Ulcer**	An area of skin from which the whole of the epidermis and at least the upper part of the dermis have been lost
Plaque	Elevated area of skin greater than 2 cm in diameter but without substantial depth	**Excoriation**	An ulcer or erosion produced by scratching
Vesicle	Circumscribed elevation of skin, less than 0.5 cm in diameter, and containing fluid	**Erosion**	An area of skin denuded by a complete or partial loss of the epidermis
Bulla	Circumscribed elevation of skin, over 0.5 cm in diameter, and containing fluid	**Fissure**	A slit in the skin
Pustule	A visible accumulation of pus in the skin	**Sinus**	A cavity or channel that permits the escape of pus or fluid
Abscess	A localised collection of pus in a cavity, more than 1 cm in diameter	**Scar**	The result of healing, in which normal structures are permanently replaced by fibrous tissue
Wheal	An elevated, white, compressible, evanescent area produced by dermal oedema	**Atrophy**	Thinning of skin due to diminution of the epidermis, dermis, subcutaneous fat
Papilloma	A nipple-like mass projecting from the skin	**Stria**	A streak-like, linear, atrophic, pink, purple or white lesion of the skin due to changes in the connective tissue
Petechiae	Pinhead-sized macules of blood in the skin		
Purpura	A larger macule or papule of blood in the skin		
Ecchymosis	A larger extravasation of blood into the skin		
Haematoma	A swelling from gross bleeding		
Burrow	A linear or curvilinear papule, caused by a burrowing scabies mite		
Comedo	A plug of keratin and sebum wedged in a dilated pilosebaceous orifice		
Telangiectasia	The visible dilatation of small cutaneous blood vessels		

DIAGNOSIS AND INVESTIGATION OF SKIN DISORDERS

The key to successful treatment is accurate diagnosis. This requires a careful history, thorough examination of the skin, hair and nails, and the judicious use of the laboratory. Often it is best to have a quick look at the skin before obtaining a full history as this should prompt the right questions.

HISTORY

The principles of a general medical history should be followed, with emphasis on the events surrounding the onset of the skin lesions and the progression of the disease. A careful inquiry into drugs, a past or family history of skin disorders, and details of the patient's occupation and any hobbies are important. The more difficult the diagnosis, the more important the history.

EXAMINATION

To examine the skin properly the lighting must be uniform and bright, the patient undressed (if necessary), and make-up and dressings removed. The signs to note are shown in the information box.

A magnifying lens is essential; rashes and lesions cannot often be diagnosed at arm's length.

Most investigative tests in the assessment of a rash can be performed in the clinic, often with immediate results.

SIGNS OF RASH TO NOTE

Distribution

- Is it symmetrical or asymmetrical? Is it dermatomal? Are any areas spared?

Morphology of individual lesions

- Appreciation of the definitions in Table 13.2 will save much time in describing lesions. The colour, surface contour, geometric shape, texture, temperature and even smell of lesions often warrant further description

Configuration of lesions

- Are the lesions discrete, confluent, grouped, circinate or linear?

DIASCOPY

The use of a glass slide pressed firmly on a skin lesion can distinguish a pink lesion due to vasodilatation, which blanches, from a pink lesion due to leakage of blood into the skin (purpura), which does not blanch. Identification of a granulomatous lesion by this method reveals the characteristic 'apple jelly nodule'.

EPILUMINESCENCE MICROSCOPY (DERMATOSCOPY)

This is a non-invasive method of examining pigmented lesions using an illuminated magnification lens with oil immersion directly on the lesion. With training and experience it is possible to identify features that are indicative of malignancy.

WOOD'S LIGHT

This involves ultraviolet radiation (wavelength 360 nm) from a light source which has a nickel oxide filter (Wood's filter) to eliminate visible light. This causes green fluorescence in scalp ringworm when it is due to *Microsporum canis*, a sporadic ectothrix infection. It evokes coral pink fluorescence of flexural skin in erythrasma, caused by the bacterium *Corynebacterium minutissimum*. Wood's light also enhances examination of cutaneous pigmentary abnormalities.

MYCOLOGY SAMPLES

Cutaneous scale, nail clippings and plucked hairs can be examined by light microscopy when mounted in 20% potassium hydroxide. This allows the keratin to be dissolved and fungal hyphae can be identified. If the potassium hydroxide solution contains indian ink, the typical 'spaghetti and meatballs' hyphae and spores of the yeast *Pityrosporum orbiculare* can be readily identified in pityriasis versicolor. In addition, samples are sent for identification by culture.

SWABS

Bacterial swabs

Bacterial swabs taken into bacterial culture medium are very useful in dermatology. It is important to identify a culprit organism and also obtain sensitivities for appropriate antibiotic use.

Viral swabs

Blister or pustule samples for herpes simplex and varicella zoster can be visualised within a few hours, either by electron microscopy or indirect immunofluorescence. Samples are also cultured for identification when conserved in viral culture medium.

PRICK TESTS

Prick tests are an intracutaneous way of detecting type I hypersensitivity (immediate) to various antigens such as pollen, house dust mite and various foods. The skin is pricked with a size 25 gauge needle through a commercially prepared antigen solution. After 10 minutes the resulting wheal is carefully recorded. As an alternative, specific IgE levels to antigens can be measured on a sample of serum by a specific radioallergosorbent test (RAST).

PATCH TESTS

Patch tests detect type IV hypersensitivity (delayed). A standard European battery of common allergens such as nickel and chromate is applied to the skin of the back under aluminium discs for 48 hours. The sites are then examined for a positive reaction and then again at 96 hours. Any evidence at this time of an eczematous reaction is suggestive of a type IV hypersensitivity to that particular allergen.

BIOPSY

Skin biopsies are taken under local anaesthetic. It is best to select an early or typical lesion on a non-exposed site. They are either elliptical or taken with a 'punch biopsy' that removes a cylindrical portion of skin (between 2 mm and 6 mm in diameter). Sutures are generally removed from the face after 1 week; the back and arms, after 10 days; and the legs after 2 weeks.

HISTOLOGY

Skin biopsies are fixed in 10% formalin for histological examination and routine staining with haematoxylin and eosin. Immunocytochemistry is also performed on formalin fixed sections using antibodies that recognise specific cell markers, e.g. T cell subset markers.

IMMUNOFLUORESCENCE

A portion of the skin biopsy can be frozen in liquid nitrogen for direct immunofluorescence (IF). This involves visualising antigens that are present in the skin by identifying them with fluorescein-labelled antibodies. The fluorescence can then be seen under a fluorescence microscope. Similarly, indirect immunofluorescence can identify circulating antibodies in the serum by an additional step of adding the serum to a section of normal skin.

ELECTRON MICROSCOPY

This is a useful investigation performed on skin samples in some rare blistering disorders, such as epidermolysis bullosa acquisita, and in many of the genodermatoses to elucidate the ultrastructural abnormalities.

PHOTOTESTING

Exposure of the skin to known wavelengths of light can reproduce the skin changes in the photodermatoses. Such action spectroscopy can only be performed in specialised centres.

FURTHER INFORMATION ON FUNCTIONAL ANATOMY, PHYSIOLOGY AND INVESTIGATIONS

Christiano A M, Uitto J 1996 Molecular complexity of the cutaneous basement membrane zone—revelations from the paradigms of epidermolysis bullosa. Experimental Dermatology 5: 1–11

Eady R A J, Leigh I M, Pope F M 1998 Anatomy and organisation of human skin. In: Champion R H, Burton J L, Burns D A, Breathnach S M (eds) Textbook of dermatology, 6th edn, 37–113. Blackwell Scientific, Oxford

MAJOR MANIFESTATIONS OF SKIN DISEASE

THE CHANGING MOLE

Recently there has been much publicity on the early recognition of cancer, to allow treatment when it can be curative. Self-examination of the skin is easy and free; campaigns which encourage this monthly routine are beginning to meet with some success. Consultations in both general practice and hospital about a changing mole (a lay term for a long-standing pigmented spot) are common, and more superficial malignant melanomas are removed nowadays than 20 years ago.

Many algorithms have been designed to distinguish a malignant melanoma from a benign pigmented lesion but none is foolproof. The general approach listed below should bring some order to handling this major manifestation and, if followed, should at least allow the doctor to have a reasonable idea of whether a changing pigmented spot is a malignant melanoma or not and to determine the course of action to take.

History

- Determine the precise nature of the change (see p. 911). Is it due to the development of itch, inflammation, bleeding or ulceration or changes in the colour, size, shape or surface of the lesion? Alarm bells should ring if the change has persisted for longer than a month. Subtle changes should not be ignored, as many patients are good observers and get to know their own moles well. If the change has settled, could it have been due to a common insult such as nicking a facial naevus when shaving, plucking hairs from a naevus or the irritant effect of a depilatory?
- Is the patient worried about change in one or many moles? Paradoxically, concern about many moles should not alert the doctor so much as anxiety over a solitary lesion.
- Assess the patient's threshold for concern, but remember that patients with cancerophobia are not immune to cancer. At the other end of the spectrum, don't be hoodwinked by a patient's denial of possible cancer—'I don't think that the change I have noted is anything to worry about, doctor, but ...'. Listen and listen, more so if the patient has never consulted you before about a changing mole.

Examination

Examine the changing pigmented lesion *carefully*; this means with the help of a magnifying lens. A dermatologist will also use a dermatoscope (see p. 882). Usually, the big question is whether the lesion is a benign melanocytic naevus (see p. 911) or a malignant melanoma (see p. 914). Before trying to answer this, exclude the possibility that it is another type of pigmented lesion:

- *Lentigo* (see p. 908).
- *Ephelis (freckle)* (see p. 908).
- *Seborrhoeic wart* (see p. 912).
- *Dermatofibroma*. Lightly pigmented firm dermal nodules, these are common on extremities in young adults. They have an iceberg effect and feel larger than they look. There is dimpling when the skin is squeezed on both sides.
- *Pigmented basal cell carcinoma* (see p. 913). These are usually found on the face of the elderly, slowly growing. They have a blue-brown hue with an opalescent look. There may be a rolled edge around an ulcer.
- *Subungual haematoma* (see p. 910 and Fig. 13.24).

Melanocytic naevus versus malignant melanoma

Here the ABCDE rule (see the information box) is very helpful, providing the fine skin markings are assessed

ABCDE FEATURES OF MALIGNANT MELANOMA

- **A**symmetry
- **B**order irregular
- **C**olour irregular
- **D**iameter often greater than 0.5 cm
- **E**levation irregular

(+ Loss of skin markings)

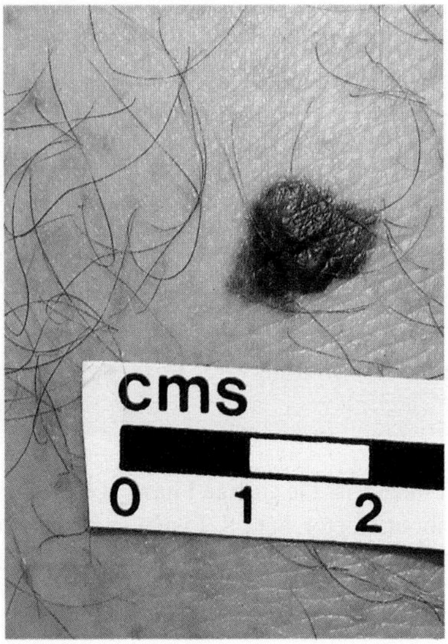

Fig. 13.2 Malignant melanoma. A changing mole which fails the ABCDE test.

afterwards (see Fig. 13.2). Loss of normal skin markings is not diagnostic but is suggestive of melanoma. Conversely, normal skin markings and the presence of fine hairs dispersed evenly over a lesion, though reassuring, are not certain signs of benignity.

Does the patient have other pigmented lesions?

Ask and examine. Seborrhoeic warts are usually multiple. Some patients have multiple benign melanocytic naevi with unusual features (e.g. lightly pigmented haloes, rosette-like flecks of darker pigmentation within the lesion) which could alter the interpretation of change in a solitary naevus which has been examined. If a naevus, especially a changing one, appears significantly different (colour, shape, size etc.) from others, then it should be treated with suspicion.

Management

- Any changing lesion which is suspected of being a malignant melanoma should be excised without delay, with a 2 mm margin of normal skin for histological confirmation.
- If there is even a low index of suspicion of a malignant melanoma, then the lesion should be reviewed 1 month and maybe 3 months later with the help of a careful record (measurements and description) or, even better, a close-up photograph. Continuing change demands excision.
- If the lesion is considered benign, then the patient is reassured *but* advised to report back without delay if the change and concern continue, so that the lesion may be reassessed. Too many melanomas are still seen in patients who have taken a doctor's reassurance as gospel and who do not return for further advice, even though the change has become more pronounced and even accelerated.
- Malignant melanoma can break most rules. Listen, look and think. If in doubt, cut out and then check the histology.

ITCH (PRURITUS)

Pruritus is defined as a sensation that provokes the desire to scratch. It is a phenomenon attributable to both central and peripheral neural mechanisms. Nerve endings in the region of the dermo-epidermal junction transmit the sensation of itch via slow-conducting C fibres and it is probably modulated centrally. Scratching, transmitted via fast-conducting A fibres, temporarily suppresses the sensation of itch by down-regulating the peripheral input (Wall's 'gate' mechanism). Pruritus is a common presenting symptom of both primary skin diseases and underlying medical disorders.

History

The main details to elicit from the history of a patient with pruritus are:

- *The time course* of the itching. This should be carefully defined as to whether it is sudden, as in infestations and urticaria, or chronic, as in chronic skin diseases such as eczema.
- *Localisation* of the pruritus, including the site of onset. For example, in an infant with atopic eczema the cheeks are the usual site to be first affected, whereas scabies almost never affects the face or scalp. Is the itch confined to certain sites, as in localised skin disease such as lichen planus and lichen simplex chronicus, or generalised, as in eczema and scabies?
- *Exacerbating factors*, such as heat and exercise in cholinergic urticaria, water in aquagenic pruritus and creams in certain forms of eczema.
- *Alleviating factors*, such as topical antipruritic treatments which ease itching in post-scabetic pruritus, tepid showering and ice packs in urticaria, and centrally acting sedative antihistamines which help in urticaria, and intermittently in eczema.
- *Involvement of other family members*, as in a scabetic infestation. Insect bites usually only affect one member of the family.
- *General health* of the patient. Has it changed, suggesting an underlying medical disorder?

Examination

Decide by examining the skin whether there is a primary skin condition or whether the only clinical features are excoriations, perhaps with some secondary eczematisation or infection. This approach in taking a history and

PRURITUS
Skin diseases associated with generalised pruritus
• Eczema • Scabies • Urticaria/dermographism • Senile pruritus
Skin diseases associated with localised pruritus
• Eczema • Lichen planus • Dermatitis herpetiformis • Pediculosis
Pruritus with no evidence of skin disease

examining a patient with pruritus will lead to one of three diagnostic groups (see the information box).

1. *Generalised pruritus associated with skin disease.* The most common causes of a widespread itchy rash are eczema, usually atopic, and scabies infestation. These can be difficult to distinguish clinically, particularly in children. Secondary eczematisation occurs in scabies, giving rise to eczema-like lesions all over the body. Examine carefully for scabetic burrows, particularly in the finger and toe webs, along the borders of both the hands and the feet and at the wrists, and extract the mite (see p. 183) to make a definite diagnosis. After treatment pruritus may continue for several weeks but may be helped by topical crotamiton and emollients. Pruritus is a common skin complaint in pregnancy and may be due to several causes (see Table 13.3).
2. *Localised pruritus associated with skin disease.* In these cases a careful examination with a hand-held magnifying glass and sometimes a skin biopsy of the rash will elicit the diagnosis.
3. *Pruritus with no evidence of skin disease.* Table 13.4 lists the medical conditions that are associated with pruritus. A complete physical examination should be performed to assess any evidence of underlying disease, including a careful search for lymphadenopathy. Appropriate investigations would include a full blood count, serum ferritin, urea and electrolytes, liver function tests, thyroid function and a chest radiograph. The physical examination and investigations should be repeated annually in cases of pruritus of unknown cause.

Management of pruritus of no known cause

Treatment for those patients with pruritus of unknown cause with no evidence of skin disease is:

1. topical antipruritic creams including crotamiton, emollients containing menthol and phenol, capsaicin 0.025%
2. UVB phototherapy
3. naloxone (opioid antagonist) for intractable cases of unidentified aetiology.

Table 13.3 Causes of pruritus in pregnancy

Condition	Gestation	Treatment
Obstetric cholestasis	3rd trimester Associated with abnormal liver function tests	Emollients Chlorpheniramine Cholestyramine Early delivery
Pemphigoid gestationis	3rd trimester Pruritus followed by blistering Starts around the umbilicus	Topical or oral steroids
Polymorphic eruption (papular urticaria) of pregnancy	3rd trimester—after delivery Polymorphic lesions with urticaria	Chlorpheniramine
Prurigo gestationis	2nd trimester Excoriated papules	Emollients Topical steroids Chlorpheniramine
Pruritic folliculitis	Aseptic pustules on trunk	Topical steroids

Table 13.4 Medical conditions that cause pruritus

Medical condition	Cause of pruritus	Treatment (Added to that of primary condition)
Liver disease		
Cholestasis	Elevated bile salts	Cholestyramine Rifampicin Antihistamines UVB
	Central opioid effect	Naloxone
Hepatitis C	Unknown	
Chronic renal disease	Multifactorial including: Secondary hyper-parathyroidism Elevated plasma histamine	UVB Oral activated charcoal Capsaicin
Blood disease		
Anaemia	Iron deficiency	Iron replacement
Polycythaemia rubra vera	Unknown	
Lymphoma, leukaemia, myeloma	Unknown	
Thyroid disease		
Thyrotoxicosis and hypothyroidism	Generalised due to dry skin Localised may be due to *Candida*	Emollients
HIV infection	Infection, infestation	Treatment of opportunistic infection
	Eosinophilic folliculitis	Local steroids, UVB
	Unknown	UVB
Malignancy	Unknown	
Psychogenic	Neuropeptides	Psychotherapy Anxiolytics Antidepressives

THE SUDDEN WIDESPREAD SCALY RASH (PAPULOSQUAMOUS ERUPTIONS)

A common presenting complaint in general practice is an eruptive scaly rash sometimes associated with itching. The main causes are listed in the information box. These can usually be distinguished by a discriminating history and examination. Secondary syphilis is an extremely rare cause of an eruptive scaly rash in current medical practice in the UK.

SUDDEN WIDESPREAD SCALY RASHES
• Eczema (see p. 896) • Psoriasis (see p. 900) • Pityriasis rosea • Lichen planus (see p. 903) • Drug eruption (see p. 919) • Pityriasis versicolor

History

How long has the rash been present?

Atopic eczema often starts within the first 2 years of life and fluctuates in extent and severity subsequently. *Psoriasis* can start at any age but usually does so between the ages of 15 and 40 years. *Pityriasis rosea* affects a similar age group and tends to occur in the autumn and spring. Both *pityriasis rosea* and *drug eruptions* have an acute onset, drug eruptions starting within a few days or weeks of taking the drugs. *Pityriasis versicolor* is a common yeast infection of the body and scalp. It can be acute in onset or persist for many years in the same individual.

Where on the body did it start?

Atopic eczema starts most commonly on the face in infants and then spreads to involve the flexures. However, it can sometimes just affect the extensor surfaces or may be present in coin-like lesions (discoid eczema). *Psoriasis* is classically present on the extensor surfaces—that is, the elbows and knees. Psoriasis can appear anywhere on the body in small (guttate), medium and large plaques all over the torso and limbs. *Lichen planus* usually presents as an intensely itchy localised papular eruption with a characteristic colour and morphology (see p. 903). Less commonly, it can be widespread and often exhibits the Köbner phenomenon (see Fig. 13.17, p. 904). *Pityriasis rosea* starts as a single herald patch that can occur anywhere on the body but usually is present on the trunk. This is a solitary erythematous lesion which starts as a papule and enlarges rapidly over a few days. *Pityriasis versicolor* usually affects the trunk and outer upper arms.

How has the rash evolved?

In *pityriasis rosea* the herald patch is followed in a few days by the appearance of many smaller plaques present mostly on the torso in a 'fir tree' distribution but it can also occur on the neck, extremities and flexures (inverse pityriasis rosea). The herald patch tends to persist throughout the eruption and the whole eruption can last for up to 3 months. *Atopic eczema* can, at varying stages, be localised or generalised but is a chronic disorder that fluctuates in severity throughout childhood. *Psoriasis* in the classical form tends to involve the elbows, knees, lower back and scalp. In the guttate (small plaque) variety many small red scaly plaques appear on the trunk and may persist for several months. Some cases subsequently develop chronic plaque psoriasis. *Macular-papular drug eruptions* evolve with exfoliation (a shedding of the most superficial portion of the skin) and may leave post-inflammatory hyperpigmentation. *Pityriasis versicolor* can be very chronic and is often exacerbated by sun exposure; it also becomes more obvious in the tanned individual because of its hypopigmentation and therefore patients often present after their summer holidays. On the other hand, it appears as light brown scaly patches on untanned Caucasoid skin.

Is it itchy?

Atopic eczema is extremely itchy and this is invariably the presenting complaint. Itching is exacerbated by changes in temperature, e.g. undressing, and contact with irritants such as wool. It is not known why atopic eczema is so itchy and antihistamines have little effect. *Drug eruptions* are usually pruritic. *Psoriasis* and *pityriasis rosea* are not usually so itchy. The rash of *pityriasis versicolor* is asymptomatic.

Was there a preceding illness?

Guttate psoriasis is often preceded by a β-haemolytic streptococcal sore throat. A small percentage of people with *pityriasis rosea* have a prodromal illness with malaise, headache and arthralgia. A patient who develops a morbilliform *drug eruption* will usually have the same reaction to that specific drug or to chemically related ones on each challenge. Rashes in response to drugs are not common; however, most patients with infectious mononucleosis treated with amoxycillin will develop an erythematous macular-papular rash. It is essential therefore to take a careful history of medications and preceding illnesses at least 4 weeks prior to the onset of the rash.

Is it associated with any systemic symptoms?

Certain *drug eruptions* can cause systemic upset with fever, malaise and joint pains and are associated with an eosinophilia. In *eczema*, superinfection can be associated with systemic symptoms of fever and malaise. *Staphylococcus aureus* causing secondary impetiginisation is the most common, but a streptococcus can cause similar features. Herpes simplex virus type I causes a widespread severe painful erosive skin eruption in patients with atopic eczema *(eczema herpeticum)*, which is a medical emergency requiring inpatient treatment with intravenous antiviral therapy and medical support. Arthritis occurs in 7% of patients with *psoriasis* (see p. 848).

Examination

The distribution of the rash can be very useful in discriminating between the various causes of a scaly rash: flexural, extensor surfaces, truncal, palms and soles, scalp involvement. Morphologically, these conditions are distinguishable by careful assessment with the use of a magnifying lens. Associated skin features that give useful diagnostic clues can be found by complete skin examination (see Table 13.5).

ERYTHRODERMA

Eczema, psoriasis, drug eruptions and lichen planus rarely progress to erythroderma, defined as erythema with or without scaling of almost all the body surface. Other causes include cutaneous T-cell lymphoma (Sézary syndrome), the psoriasis-like condition pityriasis rubra pilaris, and rare types of ichthyosis. Erythroderma may occur at any age and is associated with extreme morbidity and appreciable mortality. It may appear suddenly or evolve slowly.

Erythrodermic patients may be systemically unwell with shivering, due to loss of temperature control, and pyrexia. The pulse rate may be elevated and the blood pressure low due to volume depletion. Careful examination of the cardiovascular and respiratory systems is essential. Peripheral oedema is a common finding consequent on the erythroderma, low albumin and high-output cardiac failure. Lymph nodes may be enlarged, either reactively, caused by the skin inflammation, or secondary to lymphomatous infiltration.

URTICARIA (NETTLE RASH, HIVES)

Urticaria is a common reaction pattern characterised by the presence of itchy or 'burning' oedematous swellings (wheals) occurring anywhere on the body and lasting for less than 24 hours. Acute urticaria may be associated with more diffuse swelling (angioedema) of the lips, face and throat and, rarely, wheezing, abdominal pain, headaches and even anaphylactic shock (see p. 1032). Severe angioedema can be life-threatening due to respiratory obstruction. The symptoms of urticaria and angioedema are due to mast cell degranulation with release of histamine. There are a number of ways in which this can happen (see Fig. 13.3). Causes are listed in the information box.

CAUSES OF URTICARIA

Acute and chronic urticaria

- Allergens (in foods, inhalants and injections)
- Drugs (see Table 13.15, p. 920)
- Contact (e.g. animal saliva, latex)
- Physical (e.g. heat, cold, pressure, sun, exercise, water)
- Infection (e.g. viral hepatitis, infectious mononucleosis, HIV infection during seroconversion)
- Other conditions (e.g. systemic lupus erythematosus, autoimmunity, pregnancy, intestinal parasites)
- Idiopathic

Urticarial vasculitis

- Hepatitis B
- Systemic lupus erythematosus
- Idiopathic

Table 13.5 Clinical features of common eruptive scaly rashes

Type of rash	Distribution	Morphology	Associated clinical signs
Eczema	Face/flexures	Poorly defined erythema and scaling Lichenification	Shiny nails Infraorbital crease 'Dirty neck'
Psoriasis	Extensor surfaces	Well-defined plaques with a silvery scale	Nail pitting and onycholysis Scalp involvement Axillae and genital areas often affected
Pityriasis rosea	'Fir tree' pattern on torso	Well-defined erythematous papules and plaques with collarette of scale	
Drug eruption	Widespread	Macular-papular erythematous scaly areas which merge and are followed by exfoliation	
Pityriasis versicolor	Upper torso and upper shoulders	Hypo- and hyperpigmented scaly patches	
Lichen planus	Distal limbs, esp. volar aspect of wrists Lower back	Shiny, flat-topped violaceous papules with Wickham's striae	White lacy network buccal mucosa Rarely, nail changes

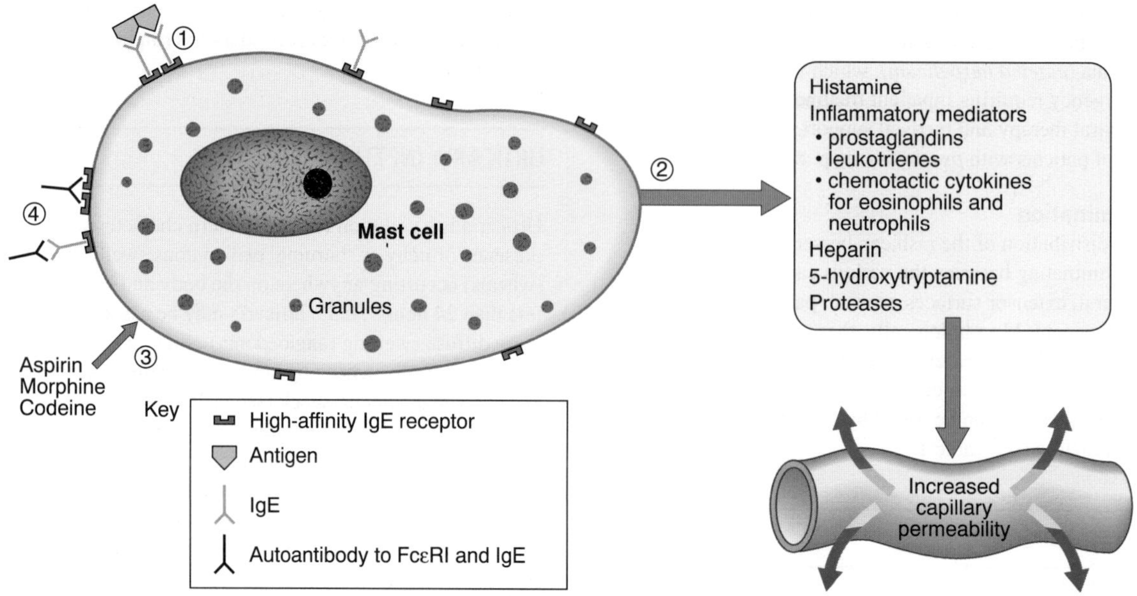

Fig. 13.3 Pathogenesis of urticaria. Mast cell degranulation occurs in a variety of ways. (1) Type I hypersensitivity causing massive degranulation and sometimes anaphylaxis. (2) Spontaneous mast cell degranulation in chronic urticaria. (3) Chemical mast cell degranulation. (4) Autoimmunity, which accounts for 30% of chronic urticaria.

Clinical features

Two important questions are:

1. *How long does the individual lesion last?*
   < 24 hours (urticaria)
   > 24 hours (urticarial vasculitis)
2. *How long has the condition been present?*
   < 6 weeks (acute urticaria)
   > 6 weeks (chronic urticaria)

First of all, one must establish whether the patient has acute or chronic urticaria or urticarial vasculitis by the questions listed above. Then, the doctor should check whether there are any features of angioedema or any associated systemic symptoms which would imply a more serious condition. A careful history is the best way to elicit the probable cause of the urticaria. A record of possible allergens, particularly drugs (see Table 13.15, p. 920) must be elicited. The physical urticarias can be identified by appropriate questions (see the information box). A family history must be sought in cases of angioedema. Examination may reveal nothing, as this is a transient eruption, or may uncover the classical wheals, which can vary from papules to large extensive plaques (see Fig. 13.4).

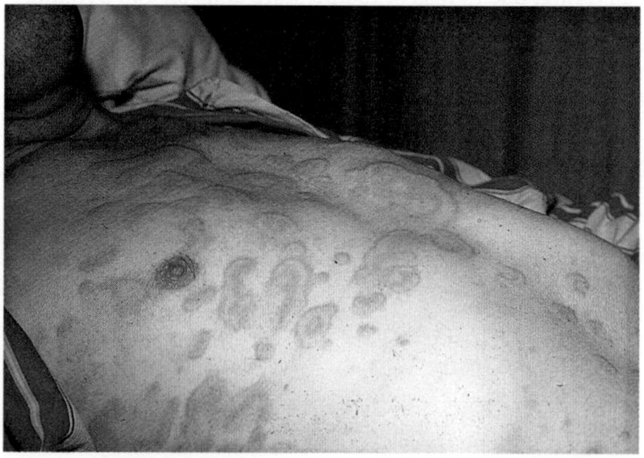

Fig. 13.4 Widespread acute urticaria. In this case urticaria was due to penicillin allergy.

Investigations

These need to be directed at the possible underlying cause as elicited from the clinical history:

- full blood count including eosinophil count in cases of underlying parasites

- erythrocyte sedimentation rate, which would be elevated in cases of vasculitis
- urea and electrolytes and liver function tests, which might reveal an underlying disorder
- total IgE and specific IgE to possible allergens, e.g. foods such as shellfish and peanuts
- antinuclear factor in chronic urticaria or urticarial vasculitis
- CH50 as a general guide to complement activation and C_3 and C_4 levels as evidence of complement consumption via both the classical and alternative pathways.

C_1 esterase inhibitor may be quantitatively reduced or more rarely functionally deficient in hereditary angioedema. In some laboratories serum protease is available as a useful investigation to confirm anaphylaxis when estimated within 24 hours of the reaction. A skin biopsy is confirmatory in the relatively rare cases of urticarial vasculitis. Physical urticarias can be confirmed by the appropriate physical challenge. Frequently no cause can be found for chronic urticaria.

Management

Antihistamines can alleviate symptoms of acute widespread urticaria. Most chronic cases respond to a non-sedative antihistamine (cetirizine 10 mg once daily, loratadine 10 mg once daily and acrivastine 8 mg 8-hourly), given alone or in combination with a sedative antihistamine. H_2-antagonists such as cimetidine can be a useful adjunct, as can mast cell stabilisers—for example, ketotifen 1 mg 12-hourly. It may be necessary to give a short reducing course of oral prednisolone up to 40 mg per day in severe acute urticaria. Patients with a history of life-threatening angioedema or anaphylaxis should carry a self-administered injection kit of epinephrine (adrenaline). If treatment is early enough, tracheostomy should be avoidable. The management of anaphylactic shock is described on page 1033.

The avoidance of precipitants, e.g. aspirin, is mandatory in all cases of urticaria. In those cases where a specific precipitant is identified, this must be carefully avoided.

PHOTOSENSITIVITY

Sunlight is a causative or exacerbating factor in many skin diseases. Photosensitisation is limited to exposure from ultraviolet radiation (UVR) and visible light. A diagram of the electromagnetic spectrum is shown in Figure 13.5 (see also Fig. 1.8, p. 8).

Clinical features

The clinical history may give a clear indication that the rash is temporally related to sun exposure, whereas in other cases there is no indication of light aggravation.

When a rash is related to sunshine then the sites affected tend to be light-exposed sites: the face, particularly the nose and the cheeks but excluding the eyelids, an area under the

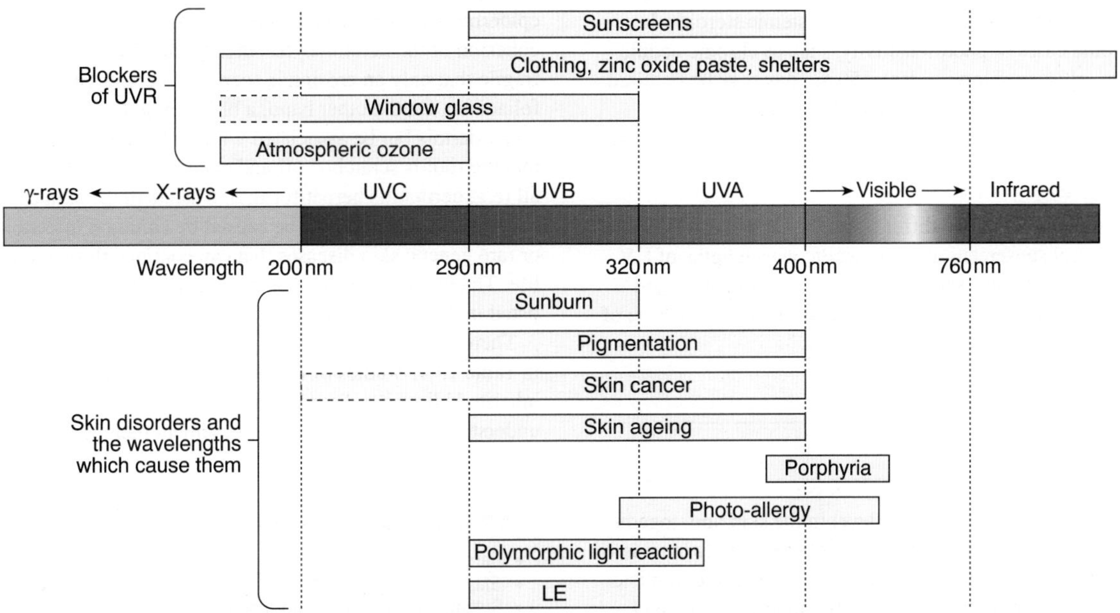

Fig. 13.5 The electromagnetic spectrum. (LE = lupus erythematosus)

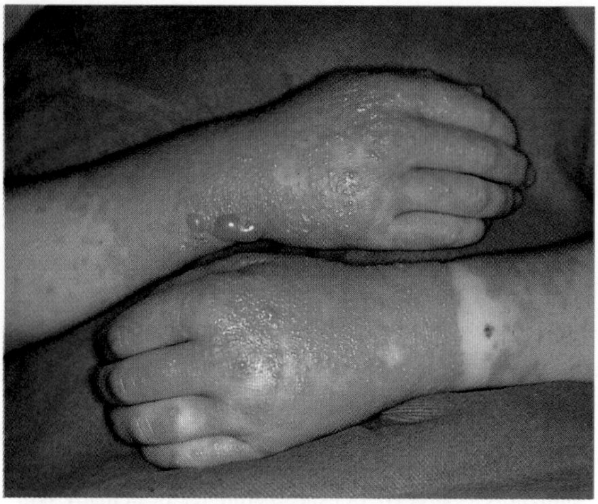

Fig. 13.6 Bullous photosensitive eruption. Note sharp cut-off at wrists, due to protection by shirt sleeves and sparing of skin under watch and strap.

chin and an area in the shadow of the nose; the dorsae of the forearms and hands, with sparing of the finger webs and palms (see Fig. 13.6).

There are four main groups of photosensitive dermatoses and these are listed in Table 13.6.

Table 13.6 The photosensitive dermatoses

Cause	Condition	Clinical features
Drugs	Phototoxic drug eruption	Common, exaggerated sunburn occurs minutes after sun exposure Caused by phenothiazines, amiodarone, tetracyclines
	Photo-allergic drug eruption	Occurs more than 24 hours after sun exposure; causes a dermatitis or lichen planus-like reaction Caused by thiazides, enalapril, hydroxychloroquine, phenothiazines, or topical, e.g. fragrances Can become permanent (persistent light reactor)
Metabolic	Porphyrias	Particularly porphyria cutanea tarda (see p. 917)
	Pellagra	Diarrhoea, dementia, dermatitis due to dietary lack of tryptophan
Exacerbation of pre-existing conditions	Lupus erythematosus	See page 855
	Erythema multiforme	See page 917
	Herpes simplex	See page 108
Idiopathic	Polymorphic light eruption	Itchy papulo-vesicular eruption on exposed sites within hours of UV exposure
	Solar urticaria	Urticaria after 1-hour exposure
	Chronic actinic dermatitis	Disabling, itchy dermatitis on exposed sites in elderly men

Management

Once a photosensitive eruption is identified on clinical grounds, it can be confirmed by phototesting. Treatment is often with topical or occasionally systemic steroids. In chronic cases of photosensitivity, such as chronic actinic dermatitis, azathioprine 100–150 mg/day may be required as further immunosuppression. The main preventive treatment for the photosensitive dermatoses is sunscreens.

Sunscreens

Sunscreens act in two different ways: chemical or physical. Chemical sunscreens absorb specific wavelengths of UV radiation. Physical sunscreens reflect UV radiation and visible light. Most available products are a combination of UVA and UVB chemical sunscreens.

BLISTERS

The skin can separate at any level in the skin and, together with the accumulation of fluid, this causes the formation of vesicles (< 0.5 cm) or bullae (> 0.5 cm). The site of blister formation within the skin depends on the aetiology and underlying pathogenesis. In certain conditions, the blisters may only rarely be seen. If a blister occurs high up in the epidermis (intraepidermal) and is due to a defect in cohesion of the keratinocytes, then the blister may be so fragile that only an erosion is seen (e.g. pemphigus foliaceus). On the other hand, a blister might occur in the upper dermis but be associated with such intense pruritus that the roof is scratched off and one rarely sees a blister at all (e.g. dermatitis herpetiformis). Blisters in the skin can occur at any age and may be caused by common infections or rare genetic skin diseases that can continue throughout life. The main causes of blistering presenting at birth are listed in the information box.

There are several types of epidermolysis bullosa, as seen in Table 13.7. Studies of the pathogenesis of these rare inherited blistering disorders have increased our understanding of the cutaneous basement membrane.

CAUSES OF BLISTERING AT BIRTH

- Herpes simplex
- *Staphylococcus aureus*
- Bullous ichthyosiform erythroderma
- Epidermolysis bullosa (see Table 13.7)
- Incontinentia pigmenti

Table 13.7 Different types of epidermolysis bullosa

Type	Mode of inheritance	Level of blister	Abnormal protein	Clinical features
Simple	Autosomal dominant	Epidermal basal cell	Keratins 5 and 14	Usually just blisters on palms and soles No scarring; nails normal; no oral involvement Rare recessive type associated with muscular dystrophy (plectin mutation)
Junctional	Autosomal recessive	Lamina lucida	Laminin-5 and α_6 β_4 integrin	Large, raw areas and flaccid blisters at birth Common around mouth and anus; heal slowly Nails and oral mucosa involved Often lethal May be diagnosed prenatally by chorionic villus sampling
Dystrophic	Autosomal dominant	Dermis below lamina densa	Collagen VII	Blisters on knees, elbows and fingers Healing with scarring and milia Nails may be involved Mouth seldom affected
	Autosomal recessive	Dermis below lamina densa	Collagen VII	Blisters often present at birth; seen on hands, feet, elbows and knees Heal with scarring which is so severe that digits may be lost Milia present Oral and oesophageal blistering followed by scarring/stricture Abnormal teeth Increased incidence of cutaneous squamous cell carcinoma in early adulthood

Table 13.8 Causes of acquired blisters

		Generalised	
	Localised	**With mucosal involvement**	**With no mucosal involvement**
Vesicular	Herpes simplex Herpes zoster Impetigo		Eczema herpeticum Dermatitis herpetiformis Epidermolysis bullosa acquisita
Bullous	Impetigo Bullous cellulitis Bullous stasis oedema Acute eczema Insect bites Fixed drug eruptions	Pemphigus Bullous erythema multiforme/Stevens–Johnson syndrome Toxic epidermal necrolysis	Acute eczema Erythema multiforme Bullous pemphigoid Epidermolysis bullosa acquisita Bullous lupus erythematosus Pseudoporphyria Porphyria cutanea tarda Drug eruptions, e.g. barbiturates

Adults who present with a blistering skin condition need to be assessed according to Table 13.8.

Management

It is important to exclude both viral and bacterial infection as a cause of blistering and this is easily done by taking a swab from the blister fluid for bacterial assessment by both microscopy and culture. A similar sterile swab can be placed in viral culture medium and, in the case of the herpes virus, immediate electron microscopy or immunofluorescence performed on a sample of the blister fluid smeared on to a slide. If there is no evidence of infection and the diagnosis is not apparent from the more common conditions listed in Table 13.8, then a skin biopsy should be taken for histological assessment and a frozen sample for indirect immunofluorescence. The clinical and immunopathological findings for the immunobullous disorders are documented in Table 13.9. In the case of the rare genetic skin diseases a portion of the skin biopsy is processed for electron microscopy to enable a more accurate assessment to be made of the site of blistering and the ultrastructural abnormalities. Further investigation is necessary for certain blistering conditions:

- *Pemphigus*. This is associated with underlying malignancy including lymphoma in a small proportion of patients ('paraneoplastic pemphigus'). Therefore a complete physical examination is mandatory and investigations including full blood count, erythrocyte sedimentation rate, urea and electrolytes, liver function tests, chest radiograph and any other directed scans should be performed.
- *Dermatitis herpetiformis*. This is associated with coeliac disease and therefore all patients with this diagnosis should have blood taken for an anti-endomysial and anti-gliadin antibody screen and a jejunal biopsy should be performed if indicated.

Table 13.9 Clinical features and skin biopsy findings in some immune-mediated blistering skin conditions

Disease	Age	Site of blisters	Nature of blisters	Mucous membrane involvement	Antigen	Circulating antibody (indirect IF)	Fixed antibody (direct IF)	Treatment
Pemphigus vulgaris	40–60 yrs	Torso, head	Flaccid and fragile, many erosions	100%	Desmoglein-3 (120kD)	IgG	IgG, C_3 intercellular (epidermal)	Steroids Cyclophosphamide
Bullous pemphigoid (see Fig. 13.7)	60s and over	Trunk (esp. flexures) and limbs	Tense	Occasionally	BP-220 (part of hemidesmosome)	IgG (70%)	IgG, C_3 at BMZ	Steroids Azathioprine
Dermatitis herpetiformis	Young, associated with coeliac disease	Elbows, lower back, buttocks	Excoriated and often not present	No	Unknown	None	Granular IgA in papillary dermis	Dapsone Gluten-free diet
Pemphigoid gestationis	Young pregnant female	Periumbilical and limbs	Tense	Rare	Collagen XVII (part of hemidesmosome BP-180)	IgG	C_3, C_5 at BMZ	Steroids
Epidermolysis bullosa acquisita	All ages	Widespread	Tense, scarring	Common (50%)	Type VII collagen	IgG (anti-type VII collagen)	IgG at BMZ	Poor response to steroids Cyclophosphamide Methotrexate Azathioprine
Bullous lupus erythematosus	Young, black female	Widespread	Tense	Rare	Type VII collagen	Anti-type VII collagen	IgG, IgA, IgM at BMZ	Dapsone

Note Pemphigus is characterised by an intraepidermal level of blistering (superficial). All the other conditions above have a subepidermal level of blistering. (BMZ = basement membrane zone)

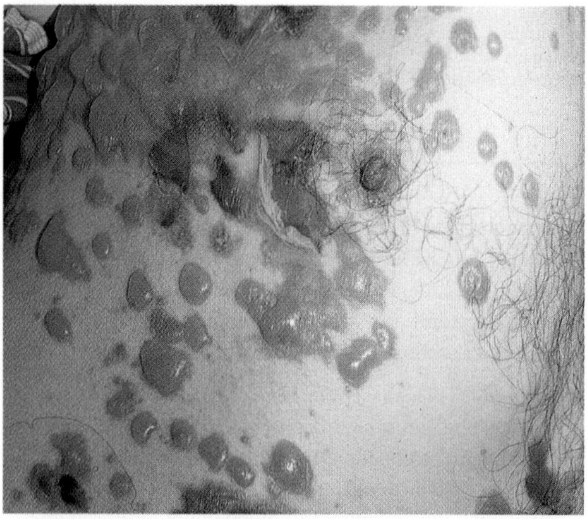

Fig. 13.7 Bullous pemphigoid. Large tense and unilocular blisters clustered in and around the axilla.

- *Epidermolysis bullosa acquisita* (EBA). This is associated with inflammatory bowel disease, multiple myeloma and lymphoma and these conditions should therefore be excluded.
- *Bullous lupus erythematosus*. It is important to follow patients with bullous lupus erythematosus for activity of their systemic disease. There is a high incidence of clinically significant glomerulonephritis (> 90%).
- *Porphyria cutanea tarda and pseudoporphyria* (see p. 917).

LEG ULCERS

Ulceration of the skin is the complete loss of the epidermis and part of the dermis. When present on the lower leg, it is usually due to vascular disease and the vast majority (75%) of cases are due in part to venous hypertension. The site of ulceration on the lower leg can give a good indication of the underlying cause (see Fig. 13.8), although this is not an absolute guide. For each cause of leg ulceration there are several different underlying pathologies that have to be considered (see the information box).

Management

When the doctor is faced with a patient with leg ulceration, the history of the onset of the disorder and any underlying predisposing conditions should be sought. Then the site and

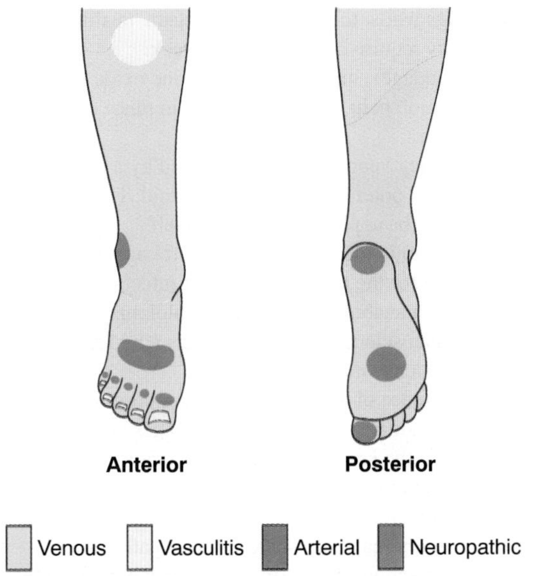

Fig. 13.8 Causes of lower leg ulceration.

MAIN CAUSES OF LEG ULCERATION

Venous hypertension
- See text

Arterial disease
- Atherosclerosis
- Vasculitis
- Buerger's disease

Small vessel disease
- Diabetes mellitus
- Vasculitis

Abnormalities of blood
- Sickle-cell disease
- Cryoglobulinaemia
- Spherocytosis
- Immune complex disease

Neuropathy
- Diabetes mellitus
- Leprosy
- Syphilis

Tumour
- Squamous cell carcinoma
- Basal cell carcinoma
- Malignant melanoma
- Kaposi's sarcoma

Trauma
- Injury
- Artefact

surrounding skin should be carefully assessed. The appropriate investigations should include:

- *Urinalysis* for glycosuria.
- *Full blood count* to detect anaemia and blood dyscrasias.
- *Bacterial swab* to detect pathogens. Systemic antibiotics are only required if there is a purulent discharge, rapid extension, cellulitis, lymphangitis or septicaemia.
- *Doppler ultrasound* to assess arterial circulation if the peripheral pulses cannot be felt. If the ankle systolic pressure divided by the brachial systolic pressure is > 0.8 then there is insignificant arterial disease. (An exception to this rule occurs in some patients with peripheral vascular disease associated with diabetes, in whom arterial calcification of the lower limb vessels produces a spuriously high ankle/brachial index.)
- *Venography*, which is occasionally useful in detecting surgically remediable venous incompetence.

The main conditions and the differences between them are discussed below.

LEG ULCERATION DUE TO VENOUS DISEASE

Damage to the venous system of the leg results in oedema, haemosiderin deposition, eczema, fibrosis and ulceration.

Aetiology

In the normal leg there is a superficial low-pressure venous system connected to the deep, high-pressure veins by perforating veins. Muscular activity, aided by valves in the veins, pumps blood from the superficial to the deep system and towards the heart. Incompetent valves in the deep and perforating veins result in the retrograde flow of blood to the superficial system ('venous hypertension'), causing a rise in capillary hydrostatic pressure. Fibrinogen is forced out through the capillary walls and fibrin is deposited as a pericapillary cuff blocking the diffusion of oxygen and nutrients to the skin. The skin ulcerates when a critical degree of hypoxia is reached.

Incompetent veins leading to venous hypertension may be due to previous deep vein thrombosis (see pp. 754 and 795), congenital or familial valve incompetence, infection or deep venous obstruction (e.g. from a pelvic tumour).

Clinical features

The problem usually starts in middle age. Leg ulcers are more likely to occur and to persist in obese people. Varicose veins, although often present, are not inevitable. The first symptom is frequently heaviness of the legs, followed by the development of oedema. Haemosiderin pigmentation and ivory-coloured scarring may then be seen, sometimes associated with venous eczema (see p. 899). The signs progress to lipodermatosclerosis, firm induration due to fibrosis of the dermis and subcutis, which may produce the well-known 'inverted champagne bottle' appearance. Ulceration, often precipitated by minor trauma or infection, soon occurs. Ulcers are seen typically around the medial malleolus but may encircle the ankle (see Fig. 13.9). If conditions are favourable, the ulcers will heal by granulation and small epithelial islands at the base and with epithelial growth from the edges. Healing is often slow and may never be complete. Recurrent ulceration is common even after good healing.

Complications

Chronic venous ulcers are invariably colonised by bacteria. Only if infection becomes overt (see above) is systemic

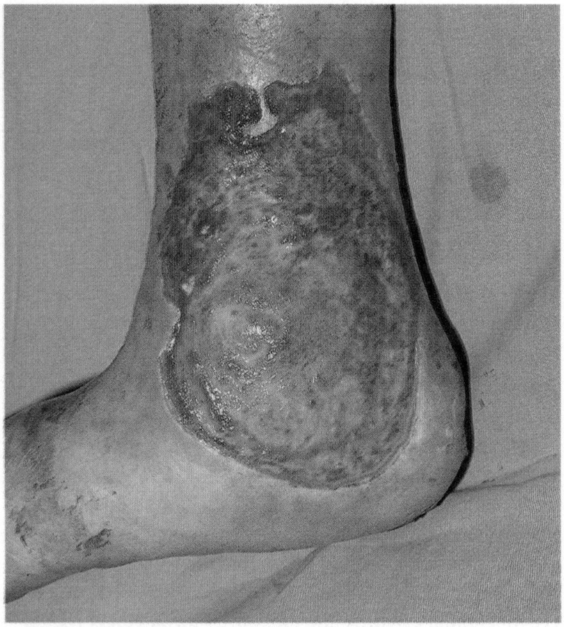

Fig. 13.9 A large venous ulcer overlying the medial malleolus.

antibiotic treatment required. Contact dermatitis to an ointment, dressing or bandage is not uncommon. The usual culprits are preservatives, lanolin and neomycin. Lipodermatosclerosis may cause lymphoedema, leading to hyperkeratosis and the so-called 'mossy foot'. A squamous cell carcinoma developing in a venous ulcer (Marjolin's ulcer) is rarely responsible for its failure to heal.

Diagnosis

See above.

Management

- General management includes dietary advice for the obese and encouragement to take gentle exercise.
- Oedema should be reduced by the regular use of compression bandages, keeping the legs elevated when sitting and the judicious use of diuretics.
- The exudate and slough should be removed with normal saline solution or 0.5% aqueous silver nitrate or 5% aqueous hydrogen peroxide. If the ulcer is very purulent, soaking the leg for 15 minutes in 1:10 000 dilution of aqueous potassium permanganate may be helpful.
- Dressings commonly used for venous ulceration include antibiotic-impregnated tulle dressings, non-adhesive absorbent dressings (alginates, charcoals, hydrogels or hydrocolloids) and dry non-adherent dressings.
- The frequency of dressings depends on the state of the ulcer. Very purulent and exudative ulcers may need daily dressings whilst the dressing on a clean, healing ulcer may only require changing every week.
- Paste bandages, impregnated with zinc oxide or ichthammol, help to keep dressings in place and provide protection.
- Surrounding venous eczema is treated by a mild or moderately potent topical corticosteroid. The steroid should not be applied to the ulcer itself.
- Oral antibiotic therapy, given in short course, is only necessary for the treatment of overt infection (see above). An anabolic steroid, stanozolol, may help lipodermatosclerosis, but side-effects (fluid retention, hepatotoxicity) may limit its use.
- In the absence of any evidence of compromised arterial supply, graduated compression bandages applied from the toes to the knees enhance venous return and have been shown to be most beneficial in the healing of venous leg ulcers.
- Vein surgery may help some younger patients with persistent venous ulcers. Pinch grafts may hasten the healing of clean ulcers but do not influence their rate of recurrence.

LEG ULCERATION DUE TO ARTERIAL DISEASE

Deep, painful and punched-out ulcers on the lower leg, especially if they occur on the shin and foot and are preceded by a history of intermittent claudication, are likely to be due to arterial disease (see the information box, p. 893). Risk factors include smoking, hypertension, diabetes mellitus and hyperlipidaemia. The foot is cyanotic and cold and the skin surrounding the ulcer is atrophic and hairless. The peripheral arterial pulses are absent or reduced. Doppler studies are required and then, if arterial insufficiency is confirmed, compression bandaging should be prohibited and advice from a vascular surgeon sought.

LEG ULCERATION DUE TO VASCULITIS

These ulcers start as painful, palpable, purpuric lesions turning into small punched-out ulcers. The involvement of larger vessels is heralded by painful nodules which may ulcerate. The intractable, deep, sharply demarcated ulcers of rheumatoid arthritis are due to an underlying vasculitis (see p. 862). Management includes treatment of the underlying disorder as well as immunosuppression with, for example, steroids or cyclophosphamide.

LEG ULCERATION DUE TO NEUROPATHY

The most common cause of a neuropathic ulcer is diabetes. The ulcer occurs over weight-bearing areas such as the heel. Microangiopathy also contributes to ulceration in diabetes. This is discussed in detail on page 502.

TOO LITTLE OR TOO MUCH HAIR

A patient who complains of too little or too much hair should be treated with sensitivity. These complaints may cause genuine morbidity. The causes are numerous and varied but a systematic approach to the history and examination can easily be used to elicit the correct diagnosis. Hair undergoes a regular cycle of growth. Each cycle is independent of its neighbours in humans, whereas, for instance, moulting animals have hairs in a synchronous cycle. At any one time and depending on the age and sex of the person, up to 90% of hair follicles can be in anagen, the growing phase, and only 10% in telogen, the resting phase when hairs are normally shed. An alteration in this ratio can lead to an increased rate of hair loss and thus an impression of impending baldness.

ALOPECIA

The term means nothing more than loss of hair. There are many causes and patterns (see Table 13.10).

A detailed history, careful scalp examination and complete physical examination should enable a confident diagnosis to be made.

Alopecia areata

This non-scarring condition appears as sharply defined non-inflamed bald patches, usually on the scalp. During the active stage of hair loss pathognomonic 'exclamation mark' hairs are seen (broken-off hairs of 3–4 mm long, which taper off towards the scalp—see Fig. 13.10). An uncommon diffuse pattern on the scalp is recognised. The condition may affect the eyebrows, eyelashes and beard. Pitting and longitudinal wrinkling of the nail may be seen. The hair usually regrows spontaneously in small bald patches, but the outlook is less good with larger patches and when the alopecia appears early in life or is associated with atopy. Alopecia totalis describes complete loss of scalp hair and alopecia universalis complete loss of all hair. There is an association of alopecia areata with autoimmune disorders, atopy and Down's syndrome.

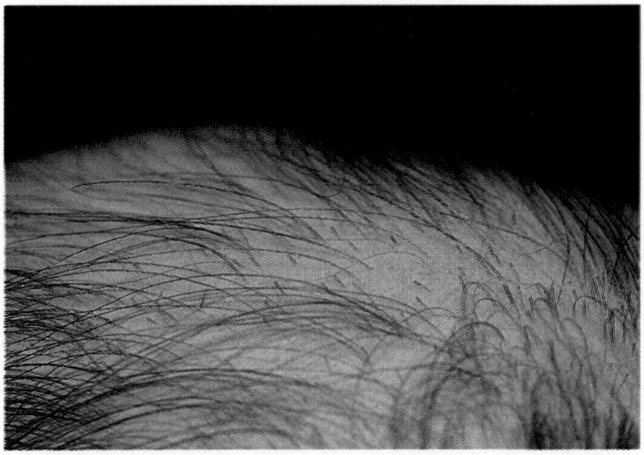

Fig. 13.10 Alopecia areata. Marked hair loss with diagnostic exclamation mark hairs.

Table 13.10 Classification of alopecia

Localised	Diffuse
Non-scarring	
Tinea capitis	Androgenetic alopecia
Alopecia areata	Telogen effluvium
Androgenetic alopecia	Metabolic
Traumatic (trichotillomania, traction, cosmetic)	Hypothyroidism
	Hyperthyroidism
	Hypopituitarism
	Diabetes mellitus
	HIV disease
	Nutritional deficiency
	Liver disease
	Post-partum
	Alopecia areata
Scarring	
Idiopathic	Discoid lupus erythematosus
Developmental defects	Radiotherapy
Discoid lupus erythematosus	Folliculitis decalvans
Herpes zoster	Lichen planus pilaris
Pseudopelade	
Tinea capitis/kerion	

Androgenetic alopecia

Male-pattern baldness is physiological in men over 20 years old, though rarely it may be extensive and develop at an alarming pace in the late teens. It also occurs in females, most obviously after the menopause. The well-known distribution (bitemporal recession and then crown involvement) is described as 'male-pattern' but this type of hair loss in females is often diffuse.

Investigations

Laboratory tests, including a full blood count, erythrocyte sedimentation rate, urea and electrolytes, liver and thyroid function tests, an autoantibody profile and *Treponema pallidum* haemagglutination (TPHA) test should help determine the cause of non-scarring alopecia. More specialised tests, including the hair pluck test where up to 50 hairs are removed with epilating forceps to determine the anagen:telogen ratio, are seldom necessary. Mycological assessment is advisable in cases of localised hair loss with scaling. A scalp biopsy, with direct immunofluorescence, may help to confirm a diagnosis of lichen planus of the scalp or discoid lupus erythematosus.

Treatment

Successful treatment of alopecia is difficult and management of these patients includes support and reassurance. Any underlying condition should be treated. Alopecia areata sometimes responds to topical or intralesional steroids such as 0.3 ml of triamcinolone (10 mg/ml). A few patients with androgenetic alopecia may be helped by topical 2% minoxidil solution. In females, anti-androgen therapy such as cyproterone acetate is used. A wig may be the most appropriate treatment for extensive alopecia. Scalp surgery and autologous hair transplants are expensive but sometimes effective in androgenetic alopecia.

HIRSUTISM

Hirsutism is the growth of terminal hair in a male pattern in a female. It should be distinguished from hypertrichosis, which describes the excessive growth of terminal hair in either sex in a non-androgenic distribution.

Hirsutism is often racial (e.g. Mediterranean Caucasians and Asians) and familial. Some degree of hirsutism is common after the menopause. The cause of most cases of hirsutism is unknown and only a small minority have a demonstrable hormonal abnormality.

Investigations

Full endocrinological investigations are required if hirsutism:

- occurs in childhood
- is of sudden onset
- is accompanied by signs of virilisation
- is associated with menstrual irregularity or cessation.

In addition to the screening tests for hyperandrogenism (see p. 905), Cushing's syndrome needs to be excluded by diurnal cortisol levels, adrenocorticotrophic hormone (ACTH) level and, if implicated, a dexamethasone suppression test.

Management

Depilatory creams, waxing, electrolysis, bleaching and shaving are often used for physiological hirsutism.

Any remediable cause should be corrected by medical and surgical methods, sometimes with the help of the endocrinologist or gynaecologist. Oral anti-androgens may be helpful.

FURTHER INFORMATION ON MAJOR MANIFESTATIONS OF SKIN DISEASE

González E, González S 1996 Drug photosensitivity, idiopathic photodermatoses and sunscreens. Journal of the American Academy of Dermatology 35: 871–885

Greaves M W 1993 New pathophysiological and clinical insights into pruritus. Journal of Dermatology 20: 735–740

Margolis D J 1993 The healing of recalcitrant leg ulcers. Current Opinion in Dermatology 31–36

Sawaya M E, Hordinsky M K 1992 Advances in alopecia areata and androgenetic alopecia. Advances in Dermatology 7: 211–227

Wakelin S H, Black M M 1997 The autoimmune bullous diseases. Journal of the Royal College of Physicians 31(4): 364–368

THE ECZEMAS

The terms 'eczema' and 'dermatitis' are synonymous. They refer to distinctive reaction patterns in the skin, which can be either acute or chronic and are due to a number of causes.

Histopathology

In the acute stage oedema of the epidermis (spongiosis) progresses to the formation of intraepidermal vesicles, which may enlarge and rupture. In the chronic stage there is less oedema and vesiculation but more thickening of the epidermis (acanthosis); this is accompanied by a variable degree of vasodilatation and T-helper lymphocytic infiltration in the upper dermis.

Classification

There are two groups of eczemas: exogenous and endogenous. While overlap between the two groups is common, distinction between them is critical for treatment because avoidance of incriminating contactants takes precedence over other measures in the management of exogenous eczema. The information box shows the classification of the eczemas.

CLASSIFICATION OF THE ECZEMAS
Exogenous
• Irritant • Allergic
Endogenous
• Atopic • Seborrhoeic • Discoid • Asteatotic • Gravitational • Localised neurodermatitis • Pompholyx

Clinical features

The clinical signs are similar in all types of eczema but vary according to the duration of the rash. The features of acute and chronic eczema are listed in the information box.

THE ECZEMA REACTION
Acute
• Redness and swelling, usually with ill-defined margin • Papules, vesicles and, more rarely, large blisters • Exudation and cracking • Scaling
Chronic
• May show all of the above features, though it is usually less vesicular and exudative • Lichenification, a dry leathery thickening with increased skin markings, is secondary to rubbing and scratching • Fissures and scratch marks • Pigmentation

EXOGENOUS ECZEMAS

IRRITANT ECZEMA

Detergents, alkalis, acids, solvents and abrasive dusts are common causes. There is a wide range of susceptibility to weak irritants. Irritant eczema accounts for the majority of industrial cases and work loss. The elderly, those with fair and dry skin, and those with an atopic background (personal or family history of asthma, hay fever or eczema) are especially vulnerable. Napkin eczema in babies is common and due to irritant ammoniacal urine and faeces.

Strong irritants elicit an acute reaction at the site of contact whereas weak irritants most often cause chronic eczema, especially of the hands, after prolonged exposure.

CONTACT ALLERGIC ECZEMA

This is due to a delayed hypersensitivity reaction (see p. 33) following contact with antigens or haptens. Previous exposure to the allergen is required for sensitisation and the reaction is specific to the allergen or closely related chemicals. Common allergens and their origin are listed in Table 13.11.

Table 13.11 Some common allergens

Allergen	Present in
Nickel	Jewellery, jean studs, bra clips
Dichromate	Cement, leather, matches
Rubber chemicals	Clothing, shoes, tyres
Colophony	Sticking plaster, collodion
Paraphenylenediamine	Hair dye, clothing
Balsam of Peru	Perfumes, citrus fruits
Neomycin, benzocaine	Topical applications
Parabens	Preservative in cosmetics and creams
Wool alcohols	Lanolin, cosmetics, creams
Epoxy resin	Resin adhesives

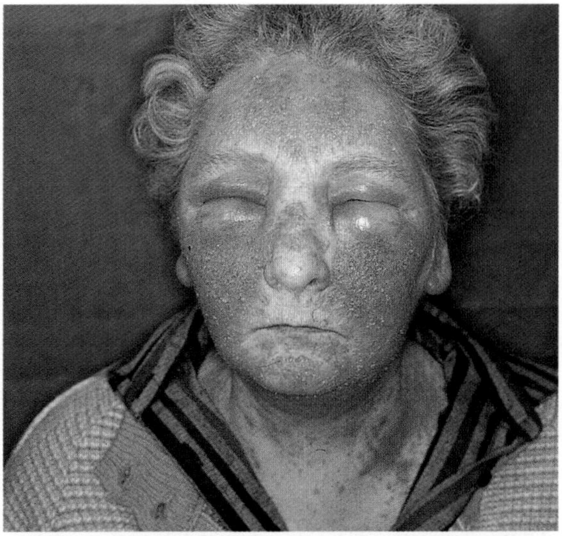

Fig. 13.11 Allergic contact eczema. This was caused by the application of an antihistamine cream. The acute eczematous reaction and bilateral periorbital oedema are typical.

The eczema reaction occurs wherever the allergen contacts the skin and sensitisation persists indefinitely. It is important to determine the original site of the rash before secondary spread obscures the picture, as this often provides the best clue to the contactant. There are many easily recognisable patterns, e.g. eczema of the earlobes, wrists and back due to contact with nickel in costume jewellery, watches and bra clips; or eczema of the hands and wrists due to rubber gloves. Oedema of the lax skin of the eyelids and genitalia is a frequent concomitant of allergic contact eczema (see Fig. 13.11).

ENDOGENOUS ECZEMAS

ATOPIC ECZEMA

Atopy is a genetic predisposition to form excessive IgE which leads to a generalised and prolonged hypersensitivity to common environmental antigens, including pollen and the house dust mite. Atopic individuals manifest one or more of a group of diseases that includes asthma, hay fever, urticaria, food and other allergies, and this distinctive form of eczema. These atopic conditions tend to run true to type within each family. Atopic eczema has clear diagnostic criteria which are listed in the information box.

Aetiology

The inheritance of atopic eczema is controversial. The disorder is concordant in 86% of monozygotic twins but only in 21% of dizygotes. Atopic diseases show maternal imprinting—that is, they are inherited more often from the mother than

DIAGNOSTIC CRITERIA FOR ATOPIC ECZEMA
Itchy skin and at least three of the following: • History of itch in skin creases (or cheeks if < 4 years) • History of asthma/hay fever (or in a first-degree relative if < 4 years) • Dry skin • Visible flexural eczema (cheeks, forehead, outer limbs if < 4 years) • Onset in first 2 years of life

from the father. A polygenic mode of inheritance is likely. More than one genetic locus has been identified that might play a role in the inheritance of atopy and more specifically atopic eczema.

The prevalence of atopic eczema is increasing and has increased between two- and five-fold over the last 30 years. It now affects 1 in 10 schoolchildren. Environmental factors, such as exposure to allergens either in utero or during childhood, have been shown to have a role in the aetiology of atopic eczema.

The pathogenesis of atopic eczema is complex and still incompletely understood. It is best considered as an interplay of genetic susceptibility that causes epidermal barrier dysfunction and abnormal immune responses, which are then stimulated by different environmental factors.

Clinical features

The cardinal feature of atopic eczema is itch, and scratching may account for many of the signs. Widespread dryness of the skin is another feature. The distribution and character of the rash vary with age, as shown in the first information box opposite. Complications are listed in the second box.

SEBORRHOEIC ECZEMA

The name is a poor one because this condition is unrelated to seborrhoea but it remains in common usage. Its cause is unknown but the yeast-like fungus, *Pityrosporum orbiculare*, appears to be a perpetuating factor. Seborrhoeic eczema is a commonly presenting feature of HIV disease and can be very severe in this condition.

This type of eczema affects the scalp, with marked scaling (dandruff), and the ears, central face and nasolabial folds, and eyebrows. On the body it is found in the flexures: the axillae, umbilicus, breasts and groin, and the pre-sternal and interscapular skin.

DISCOID ECZEMA

This is a common form of eczema recognised by discrete coin-shaped lesions of eczema seen on the limbs of young men, associated with alcohol excess, and of elderly men. It can occur in children with atopic eczema and tends to be more stubborn to treat.

ATOPIC ECZEMA: DISTRIBUTION AND CHARACTER OF RASH
Infancy
• The eczema is often acute and involves the face and trunk • The napkin area is frequently spared
Childhood
• The rash settles on the backs of the knees, fronts of the elbows, wrists and ankles (see Fig. 13.12)
Adults
• The face and trunk are once more involved; lichenification is common

COMPLICATIONS OF ATOPIC ECZEMA
• Superinfection most often with bacteria *(Staph. aureus)* but also importantly with viruses. *Herpes simplex* virus causes a widespread severe eruption—eczema herpeticum. *Papillomavirus* and *Molluscum contagiosum* superinfections are also more common and are encouraged by use of local steroids • Irritant reactions due to defective barrier function • Poor growth due to chronic disease and sleep disturbance • Children with atopic eczema have an increased incidence of food allergy, particularly to eggs, cow's milk, protein, fish, wheat and soya. These foods cause an immediate urticarial eruption rather than exacerbating their eczema • Psychological factors for patients and their family

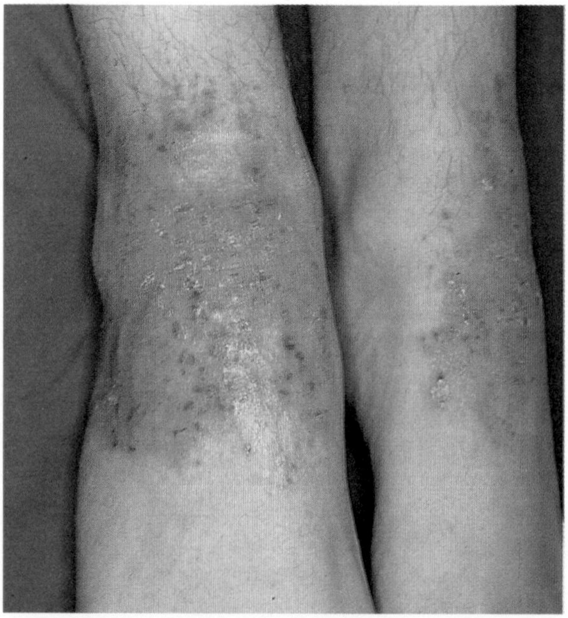

Fig. 13.12 Atopic subacute eczema on the fronts of the ankles of a teenager. These are sites of predilection, along with the cubital and popliteal fossae, in atopic eczema.

ASTEATOTIC ECZEMA

This is frequently seen in the hospitalised elderly, especially when the skin is dry; low humidity caused by central heating, overwashing and diuretics are contributory factors. It occurs most often on the lower legs as a rippled or 'crazy paving' pattern of fine fissuring on an erythematous background.

GRAVITATIONAL (STASIS) ECZEMA

This occurs on the lower legs and is often associated with signs of venous insufficiency (oedema, red or bluish discoloration, loss of hair, induration, haemosiderin pigmentation and ulceration).

LOCALISED NEURODERMATITIS (LICHEN SIMPLEX)

This describes a plaque of lichenified eczema due to repeated rubbing or scratching, as a habit or in response to stress. Common sites include the nape of the neck, the lower legs and the anogenital area.

POMPHOLYX (DYSHIDROTIC ECZEMA)

Recurrent vesicles and bullae occur on the palms, palmar surface of the fingers and soles and are excruciatingly itchy. This form of eczema can occur in atopic eczema and in the exogenous eczemas. It can be provoked by heat, stress and nickel ingestion in a nickel-sensitive patient but is often idiopathic.

Investigation of eczema (for details of tests see pp. 881–882)

Patch tests

These are performed in suspected cases of contact allergic dermatitis (see p. 882).

IgE and specific IgE

These are occasionally performed to support the diagnosis of atopic eczema and to determine specific environmental allergens, e.g. pet dander, horse hair, house dust mite, pollens and foods.

Prick tests

The indications are the same as for specific IgE but are less commonly performed.

Bacterial and viral swabs for microscopy and culture

These are extremely useful tests to exclude secondary infection. In addition, in the case of recurrent impetigo in a child with atopic eczema, bacterial swabs should be taken from carrier sites (nares, axillae and groin) from the affected individual and all household members.

General management of eczema

The main points are listed in the information box.

GENERAL MANAGEMENT FOR ALL TYPES OF ECZEMA

- Explanation, reassurance and encouragement
- Avoidance of contact with irritants
- Regular use of greasy emollients
- Careful use of topical steroids

Lotions and creams are preferable in acute eczema and ointments in chronic cases; they are usually applied twice daily. Only 1% hydrocortisone should be used on the face and in infancy. Even in adults it is seldom necessary to prescribe more than 200 g of a low-potency steroid (e.g. 1% hydrocortisone), 50 g of a moderately potent steroid (e.g. 0.05% clobetasone butyrate) or 30 g of a potent steroid (e.g. 0.1% betamethasone valerate, 0.1% mometasone furoate) per week. Very potent topical steroids (e.g. 0.05% clobetasol proprionate) should not be used long-term. The side-effects of strong or extensive local steroid therapy should always be borne in mind when patients are applying these preparations for years on end. They include skin thinning (with striae, fragility and purpura), enhanced or disguised infections, and systemic absorption (causing suppression of the hypothalamic-pituitary-adrenal axis and even Cushingoid features).

Bland emollients (e.g. emulsifying ointment) are used regularly, either directly on the skin or in the bath. They not only prevent excessive water loss from an already dry skin, but also help to reduce the amount of local steroid used. Emollient soap substitutes (e.g. aqueous cream) are also helpful. Sedative antihistamines (e.g. trimeprazine tartrate) are of value if sleep is interrupted.

Specific measures (for certain types of eczema) additional to general treatment

Irritant eczema

This is best treated by the regular use of barrier creams both to cleanse and to protect. In addition, protective clothing has to be used, e.g. gloves.

Contact allergic eczema

Avoidance of the culprit allergen is the most important treatment for this form of eczema and may involve lifestyle changes such as a new job or giving up hobbies. Measures used for irritant eczema are also helpful.

Atopic eczema

Explanation and patient support are increasingly provided for these patients through general practice, dermatology clinics, community liaison nurses and patient support groups such as the National Eczema Society in the UK. Treatment involves the regular use of emollients (moisturisers) and the least possible use of topical steroids. These topical treatments can be used with a variety of bandaging such as 'wet wraps', tar and ichthammol paste bandages. Allergen avoidance has a role in selected patients. Routine inoculations are allowed during quiescent phases of eczema. An egg-free measles vaccine is available for children who have severe egg allergy.

Seborrhoeic eczema

Local antiseptic, mild topical steroids and antifungal treatments are useful in this condition. Ketoconazole shampoo is an effective treatment for all areas.

Gravitational eczema

Local steroids (see above) should only be applied to eczematous areas and ulcers should be avoided. Sensitisation to topical antibiotics (neomycin) and preservatives (e.g. chlorocresol) is common in this form of eczema. Associated peripheral oedema should be eliminated by elevation of the leg and graded compression bandages.

FURTHER INFORMATION ON THE ECZEMAS

McHenry P M, Williams H C, Bingham E A 1995 Management of atopic eczema. British Medical Journal 310: 845–847

Scheffer H 1996 Search for genes predisposing to atopic disease. Lancet 348: 560–561

Williams H 1995 Atopic eczema: we should look to the environment. British Medical Journal 311: 1241–1242

ERYTHEMATOUS SCALY ERUPTIONS

Psoriasis and lichen planus will be described here in detail though other conditions were covered on pages 886–887.

PSORIASIS

Psoriasis is a non-infectious, inflammatory disease of the skin, characterised by well-defined erythematous plaques with large, adherent, silvery scales.

The main abnormality in psoriasis is increased epidermal proliferation due to excessive division of cells in the basal layers. The transit time of keratinocytes through the epidermis is shortened and the epidermal turnover time falls from 28 to 5 or 6 days.

Between 1% and 3% of most populations has psoriasis. It is most common in Europe and North America. It may start at any age but is rare under 10 years and often seen between 15 and 40 years. The course of disease is unpredictable but is usually chronic with exacerbations and remissions.

Aetiology

Basic defect

This remains unknown but the following factors are involved.

Genetic. There is frequently a genetic predisposition. A child with one affected parent has a 15% chance of developing the disease and this rises to 50% if both parents are affected. If non-psoriatic parents have a child with psoriasis, the risk for subsequent children is about 10%. Psoriasis is a genetically complex disease trait. There is wide clinical and genetic heterogeneity. Linkages have been demonstrated to different loci, including chromosomes 6p (Cw6 region), 17q, 4q and 2q.

Biochemical. It is not known if biochemical abnormalities are the cause or result of increased epidermal proliferation. There are increased levels of prostaglandins, leukotrienes and hydroxyeicosatetraenoic (HETE) acids in the epidermis. These may cause both the increased cellular proliferation seen in psoriasis and the inflammatory changes. Increased activity of phospholipase A_2 appears to be primarily responsible for these changes.

Decreased cyclic adenosine monophosphate (cAMP) and increased cyclic guanosine monophosphate (cGMP) are found in lesions, and β-adrenoceptor antagonist drugs may exacerbate psoriasis by inhibiting cAMP formation. Polyamines are elevated in lesional skin, due to increased activity of ornithine decarboxylase, and may be intimately associated with cellular proliferation. Plasminogen activator is greatly increased in the lesions of psoriasis and its level parallels the epidermal mitotic rate.

The level of calmodulin, a calcium-binding protein, is also raised in lesions and falls with successful treatment. The calcium-calmodulin complex may regulate epidermal cell proliferation by influencing phospholipase A_2 and cAMP phosphodiesterase (catalyses cAMP conversion to AMP) activity.

Immunopathological. The inflammatory reaction may be part of an immunological response to as yet unknown antigens. Immune complexes to epidermal antigens have been detected in damaged skin and may activate complement, thereby attracting neutrophils to the area. Certain interleukins (IL-1, IL-2, IL-6 and IL-8), interferon γ, and growth factors (TNFα and TGFα) are elevated, and adhesion molecules are expressed or upregulated in lesions of psoriasis. The mononuclear infiltrate is mainly of T lymphocytes, most of which are of the helper type (Th-1) in the dermis and of the cytotoxic type in the epidermis. The beneficial effect of cyclosporin A in psoriasis may be due to its anti-T helper cell effect. Streptococcal superantigens, from the throat, appear to be responsible for T-cell activation in guttate psoriasis.

Dermal. There is substantial evidence to suggest that the increased epidermal cell proliferation of psoriasis is also related to the increased replication and metabolism of dermal fibroblasts. Both dermal and epidermal abnormalities appear to be necessary for the sustenance of psoriasis.

Given the basic defect, an individual may not inevitably develop psoriasis but certain precipitating factors make this more likely.

Precipitating factors

Although there appears to be no obvious precipitating factor in about 70% of exacerbations of psoriasis, the factors shown in the information box are responsible for the minority of flare-ups.

Pathology

The histology of psoriasis is depicted in Figure 13.13.

Clinical features

Stable plaque psoriasis

This is the most common type. Individual lesions are well demarcated and range from a few millimetres to several centimetres in diameter (see Fig. 13.14). The lesions are red with dry, silvery-white scaling, which may be obvious only after scraping the surface. The elbows, knees and lower back are commonly involved.

Other sites of predilection include:

- *Scalp*. This site is often involved, presumably due to repeated trauma from brushing and combing. Areas of marked scaling are interspersed with normal skin, producing a lumpiness which is more easily felt than seen. Significant hair loss occurs only if there is gross involvement.

FACTORS CAUSING FLARE-UPS OF PSORIASIS
Trauma
• When the condition is erupting lesions appear in areas of skin damage such as scratches or surgical wounds (Köbner phenomenon)
Infection
• β-haemolytic streptococcal throat infections often precede guttate psoriasis
Sunlight
• Rarely, ultraviolet radiation may worsen psoriasis
Drugs
• Antimalarials, β-adrenoceptor antagonists and lithium may worsen psoriasis and the rash may 'rebound' after stopping systemic corticosteroids or potent local corticosteroids
Emotion
• Anxiety precipitates some exacerbations

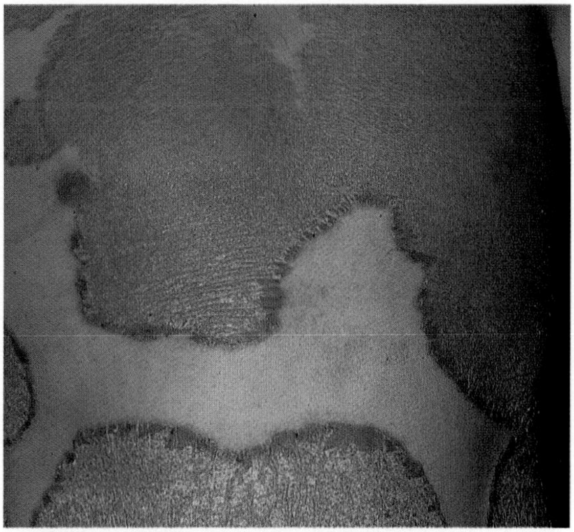

Fig. 13.14 Large, sharply circumscribed plaques of psoriasis. The silvery scaling of the lower (untreated) plaque is typical.

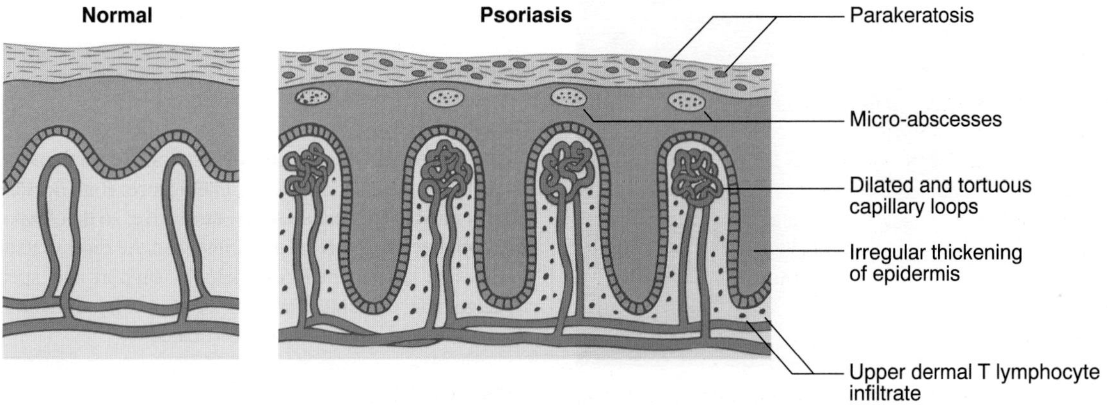

Fig. 13.13 The histology of psoriasis.

- *Nails*. Involvement of the nails is common, with 'thimble pitting', onycholysis (separation of the nail from the nail bed) (see Fig. 13.15) and subungual hyperkeratosis. It often reflects the severity of the psoriasis elsewhere.
- *Flexures*. Psoriasis involving the natal cleft, submammary and axillary folds is not scaly but red, glistening and symmetrical (see Fig. 13.16).
- *Palms*. Psoriasis here is often difficult to recognise, as individual plaques may be poorly demarcated and barely erythematous.
- *Napkin area*. This may give the first hint of a psoriatic tendency in an infant.

Guttate psoriasis

This is usually seen in children and adolescents and may be the first sign of psoriasis. The rash often appears rapidly and individual lesions are droplet-shaped, small (seldom greater than 1 cm in diameter) and scaly. Bouts of guttate psoriasis usually clear in a few months, but patients may develop the plaque pattern later.

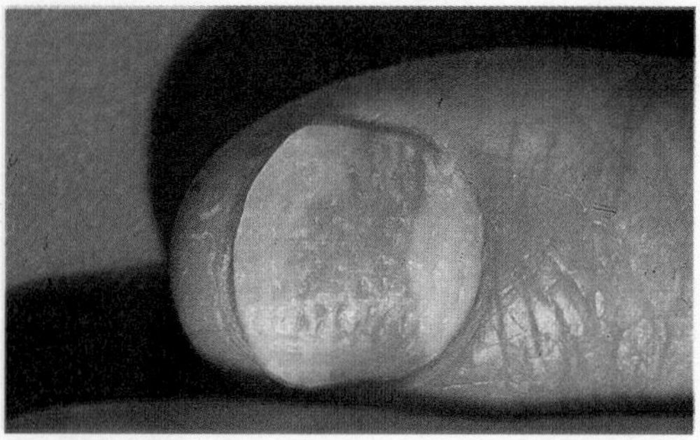

Fig. 13.15 Coarse pitting of the nail and separation of the nail from the nail bed (onycholysis). These are both classic features of psoriasis.

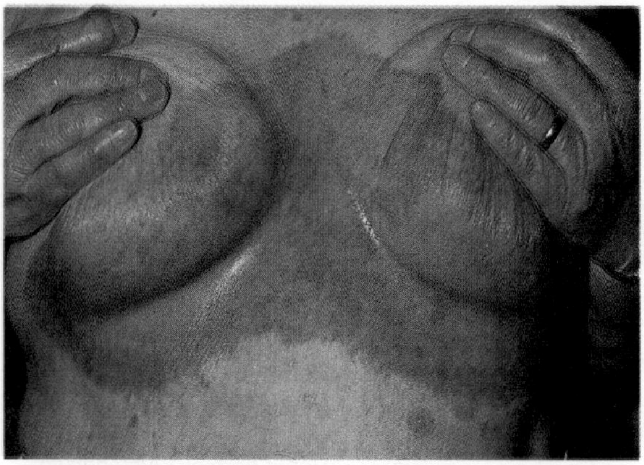

Fig. 13.16 Flexural psoriasis. Note the glistening but not scaly rash.

Erythrodermic psoriasis

The skin becomes universally red and scaly. Shivering compensates for the considerable heat loss. This unpleasant variant may be initiated by the irritant effect of tar or dithranol or the withdrawal of systemic or potent topical corticosteroids.

Pustular psoriasis

The generalised form is a rare but serious type of psoriasis. The onset is sudden, with myriads of small sterile pustules erupting on an erythematous base. The patient is ill with a swinging pyrexia, coinciding with the appearance of new pustules, and requires hospital admission.

The localised form is more common. It most often involves the palms and soles. The eruption consists of numerous small sterile pustules lying on an erythematous base, which leave brown macules or scaling in their wake. Some regard this as a separate disease entity.

Complications

Psoriatic arthropathy is a possible complication (see p. 848), occurring in about 5% of psoriatics. Distal arthritis involves the terminal interphalangeal joints of the toes and fingers, especially those with marked nail changes. Other patterns include: involvement of a single large joint, a variety which mimics rheumatoid arthritis and which may be destructive; and one involving the sacroiliac joints and lumbar spine (associated with HLA-B27). Tests for rheumatoid factor are usually negative in true psoriatic arthropathy and rheumatoid nodules are absent.

Investigations

Few are indicated. Biopsy is seldom necessary because the clinical picture is usually characteristic. Throat swabbing for β-haemolytic streptococci should be performed in guttate psoriasis and an ASO titre or DNAase B may be helpful. Skin scrapings and nail clippings may have to be examined to exclude tinea. Radiology and tests for rheumatoid factor are important in assessing arthritis.

Management

General measures

Explanation, reassurance and instruction are vital and must relate to the patient's or parent's intelligence. Both doctor and patient must keep the disease in perspective, so that treatment does not become more troublesome than the disease itself.

Physical and mental rest help to support the specific management of acute flare-ups of psoriasis. Concomitant depression and anxiety should be treated.

Local measures

Coal tar preparations. Crude coal tar and its distillation products have been used to treat psoriasis for many years.

Their main mode of action is probably by inhibiting DNA synthesis.

Many products are available; in general the messier, less refined preparations (e.g. 10% strong coal tar solution and 4% tar paste) are more effective than the more refined and cleaner proprietary ointments. They are applied to the patches of psoriasis once or twice daily. Salicylic acid (1–2%), sometimes added to tar preparations to remove scaling, is useful in the management of scalp psoriasis.

Dithranol. This also inhibits DNA synthesis. Although it is irritant and more tricky to use than coal tar, its use has become widespread. The most popular regimen is short contact therapy in which the cream is applied to lesions for no longer than 30 minutes and then washed off. Initially 0.1% dithranol cream is used but, depending on the response, the strength may be increased stepwise to 2% over a few weeks. Dithranol stains normal skin purple-brown but the discoloration peels off after a few days.

Eruptive and unstable patches of psoriasis are unsuitable for treatment with coal tar or dithranol and those with limited experience of their use should select test patches of psoriasis for initial treatment. Coal tar preparations and dithranol are best avoided on the face, genitalia and body folds because they are irritating.

Calcipotriol. This recently introduced vitamin D analogue reduces epidermal proliferation and restores a normal horny layer. It is applied twice daily and, providing no more than 100 g is used each week, it does not cause hypercalcaemia and hypercalciuria. Patients like calcipotriol because it is odourless, colourless and does not stain. Irritation, which is usually transient, is the main side-effect.

Retinoids. Topical preparations have become available recently. They are most useful for localised plaques. Significant systemic absorption is avoided by limiting the amount applied.

Corticosteroids. These are liked by patients and some doctors because they are clean and effective initially. However, there are few indications for their long-term use as, on their withdrawal, psoriasis may relapse rapidly or even change to an unstable phase which is more difficult to manage than previously. Their use should be limited as shown in the information box.

Only mild steroids should be used on the face but moderately potent ones are suitable for elsewhere. Tar-steroid combinations are a useful stepping stone to pure tar preparations, while steroid-antifungal combinations are helpful for flexural psoriasis.

Ultraviolet radiation. Most patients improve with natural sunlight and many clear their psoriasis by sunbathing during holiday periods. During the winter 6-week courses of medium-wave or narrow-band ultraviolet radiation (UVB) given in specialist centres 2–3 times weekly are often helpful. In the majority of patients sunbeds (emitting long-wave ultraviolet waves—UVA) are not beneficial. Combination therapies with UVB, coal tar preparations and dithranol are used to clear psoriasis more quickly than can be achieved by monotherapies.

LIMITATIONS ON USE OF TOPICAL CORTICOSTEROIDS FOR PSORIASIS

- The face, ears, genitalia and flexures where tar and dithranol are seldom tolerated
- Patients who cannot use alternative local preparations because of allergic or irritant reactions
- Unresponsive psoriasis of the scalp, palms and soles

Systemic treatment

This will be considered by a dermatologist if extensive psoriasis fails to respond to the local measures outlined above. The most commonly used systemic treatments are photochemotherapy with PUVA (psoralen + UVA), retinoids (acitretin), methotrexate and cyclosporin A. All of these treatments have potential side-effects and patients receiving them require regular, specialist supervision.

LICHEN PLANUS

Lichen planus is a condition characterised by intensely itchy papules involving the flexor surfaces, genitalia and mucous membranes.

Aetiology

The cause is unknown but an immune pathogenesis is suspected as there is an association with some autoimmune diseases such as myasthenia gravis, and with thymoma and graft-versus-host disease. Rashes with clinical and histological features of lichen planus can occur in chronic active hepatitis, hepatitis B and C infections, and patients taking drugs, the most common culprits being gold and other heavy metals, sulphonamides, penicillamine, antimalarials, antituberculous drugs and thiazide diuretics. It also occurs in those handling colour developers.

Pathology

There is hyperkeratosis, a prominent granular layer, basal cell degeneration and a heavy T lymphocyte infiltration in the upper dermis. Degenerating basal cells may form colloid (apoptotic) bodies. The T cell-basal cell interaction leaves a 'sawtooth' dermo-epidermal junction. The picture suggests an immune reaction to an unknown epidermal antigen.

Clinical features

Lichen planus tends to start on the distal limbs, most commonly the volar aspects of the wrists (see Fig. 13.17), and the lower back. Intensely itchy, flat-topped, pink-purplish papules appear and some develop a characteristic fine white network on their surface (Wickham's striae). New lesions may appear at the site of trauma (Köbner phenomenon) and

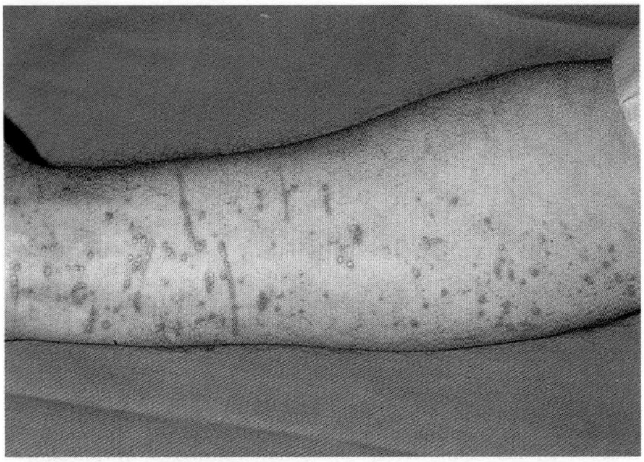

Fig. 13.17 Lichen planus. Glistening discrete papules involving the volar aspects of the forearm and wrist. Note the lesions along scratch marks (Köbner phenomenon).

the rash may spread rapidly to become generalised. Individual lesions may last for many months and the eruption as a whole tends to last about 1 year, often leaving marked post-inflammatory pigmentation. Mucous membrane involvement, comprising an asymptomatic fine white lacy network or pinhead-sized white papules, occurs in about two-thirds of patients. The nails are usually normal but in 10% they may be affected, with changes ranging from longitudinal grooving to destruction of the nail fold and bed. Variants of the classic picture are rare and often challenging diagnostically. They include annular, atrophic, bullous, follicular, hypertrophic and ulcerative types.

Diagnosis

This is usually clear-cut clinically but a skin biopsy can be helpful. Other erythematous scaly conditions should be considered in the differential diagnosis, including guttate psoriasis, pityriasis rosea, pityriasis lichenoides and drug eruptions.

Management

The condition is self-limiting. Moderately potent or potent local corticosteroids may be required for the intense itch. Systemic corticosteroid courses of up to 3 months may be required for acute widespread disease, ulcerative oral lesions and nail destruction. Acitretin, an oral retinoid, may help some patients with stubborn lichen planus.

FURTHER INFORMATION ON ERYTHEMATOUS SCALY ERUPTIONS

Barker J N W N 1991 The pathophysiology of psoriasis. Lancet 338: 227–230

Barker J N W N 1997 Psoriasis. Journal of the Royal College of Physicians 31(3): 238–240

Farr P M 1997 Ultraviolet phototherapy. Journal of the Royal College of Physicians 31(3): 250–253

DISORDERS OF THE PILOSEBACEOUS UNIT

ACNE VULGARIS

This affects many teenagers. Its prevalence is similar in both sexes but the peak age of severity in females is 16–17 years and in males 17–19 years. Acne clears by the age of 23–25 years in 90% of patients but 5% of women and 1% of men still need treatment in their thirties or even forties.

Aetiology

Many factors, rather than a single one, combine to cause chronic inflammation of blocked pilosebaceous follicles (see Fig. 13.18).

Sebum secretion is increased, but this alone need not cause acne; for example, patients with acromegaly or Parkinson's disease have high sebum secretion rates but no acne. The sebum secretion rate may remain high after acne has healed.

Hormones are another factor; androgens from the testes, ovaries and adrenals are the main ones which stimulate sebum secretion. In acne the sebaceous glands appear to be unduly sensitive to normal levels of these hormones.

Increased and abnormal keratinisation at the exit of the pilosebaceous follicle obstructs the flow of sebum. Bacteria play a pathogenic role. *Proprionobacterium acnes* is a normal skin commensal. It colonises the pilosebaceous ducts, breaks down triglycerides releasing free fatty acids, produces substances chemotactic for inflammatory cells, and induces the ductal epithelium to secrete pro-inflammatory cytokines. Rupture of the follicle is associated with intense inflammation.

Acne is often familial. The inheritance pattern is probably polygenic.

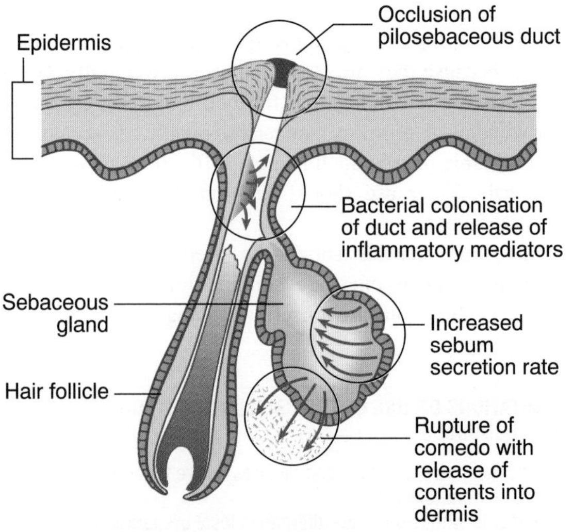

Fig. 13.18 The pathogenesis of acne.

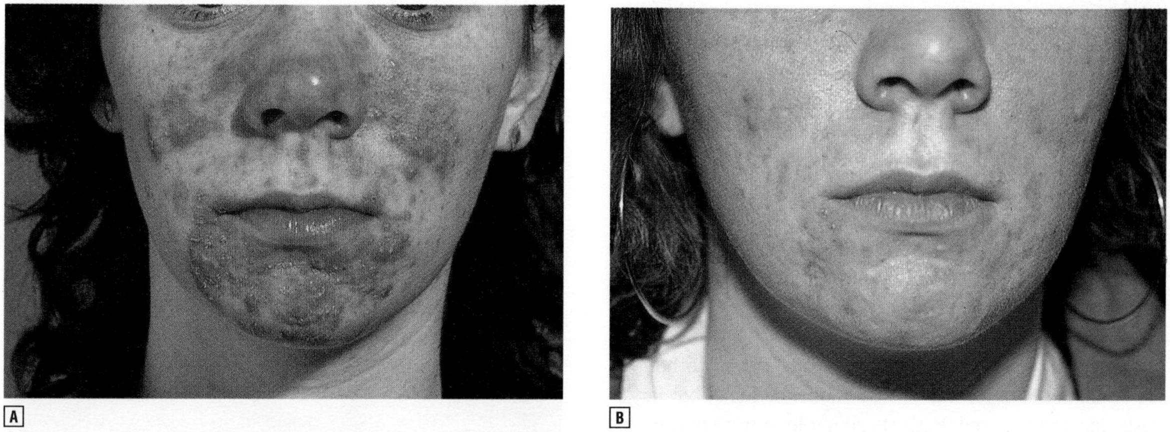

Fig. 13.19 **Unpleasant cystic acne in a teenager.** A Before treatment. B After prolonged systemic antibiotic treatment.

Clinical features

Lesions are limited to the face, shoulders, upper chest and back. Seborrhoea (greasy skin) is often present. Open comedones (blackheads) due to plugging by keratin and sebum of the pilosebaceous orifice, or closed comedones (whiteheads) due to accretions of sebum and keratin deeper in the pilosebaceous ducts, are always evident. Inflammatory papules, nodules and cysts occur (see Fig. 13.19A), with one or two types of lesion predominating. Scarring may follow.

There are less common variants of acne:

- Conglobate acne is severe, with many abscesses and cysts, often connected by intercommunicating sinuses; scarring is marked.
- Acne fulminans is a conglobate acne accompanied by fever, joint pains and a high erythrocyte sedimentation rate.
- Excoriated acne manifests as discrete denuded areas caused by picking and is seen most often in early teenage girls.
- Infantile acne is rare and is due to transplacental stimulation of the infant's adrenals. It may last up to 3 years and may be the forerunner of severe acne in adolescence.
- Exogenous acne may be caused by tars, chlorinated hydrocarbons, oils and oily cosmetics; comedones dominate the clinical picture.
- Drug-induced acne may result from treatment with corticosteroids, androgenic steroids, lithium, oral contraceptives and anticonvulsant therapy.
- Polycystic ovarian syndrome is characterised by menstrual irregularities and/or infertility, hirsutism, acne and male-pattern alopecia.
- Acne associated with virilisation, including clitorimegaly, may be due to an androgen-secreting tumour of the adrenals, ovaries or testes or, rarely, late-onset congenital adrenal hyperplasia due to 21-hydroxylase deficiency. The gene frequency for this condition is very high in Ashkenazi Jews (19%), inhabitants of the former Yugoslavia (12%) and Italians (6%).

Investigations

Swabs may be necessary to exclude a pyogenic infection, anaerobic infection, and Gram-negative folliculitis. In cases where there is a history of menstrual disturbance or clinical evidence of virilisation, it is necessary to exclude the polycystic ovarian syndrome, an androgen-secreting tumour and congenital adrenal hyperplasia (see p. 591). In such cases serum testosterone, sex hormone-binding globulin (SHBG), luteinising hormone (LH) and follicle-stimulating hormone (FSH), androstenedione (A4), dehydroepiandrostenedione sulphate (DHEA[S]) and 17-hydroxyprogesterone levels should be measured. Polycystic ovarian syndrome is characterised by modestly elevated testosterone, A4 and DHEA[S] levels, a reduced SHBG level and an LH:FSH ratio of greater than 3:1. Pelvic ultrasound may reveal multiple small ovarian cysts. An appreciable number of patients with acne have ultrasound evidence of ovarian cysts without biochemical evidence of polycystic ovarian syndrome. Congenital adrenal hyperplasia is associated with high levels of 17-hydroxyprogesterone and androgen-secreting tumours, with marked elevation in serum androgen levels.

Management

Comedo-papular acne is managed by local treatment alone; pustular-cystic and scarring acne require local and systemic treatment.

Local measures

Regular washing with soap and water is essential. Antibacterial skin cleansers containing chlorhexidine are also useful. Preparations containing benzoyl peroxide and retinoic acid are the cornerstone of local treatment and many proprietary products are available. They are irritant and drying and although some care is required to gauge an appropriate and regular regimen of application, most are applied once daily at night. Local clindamycin and erythromycin are helpful. The beneficial effect of ultraviolet B is usually short-lived.

Systemic measures

Antibiotics are used initially. They should not be used for less than 3 months and may even be necessary for 2 or 3 years. Oxytetracycline (up to 250 mg 6-hourly), minocycline (100 mg daily) and erythromycin (up to 250 mg 6-hourly) are suitable doses for adults with moderate acne, but larger doses may be required. Patients taking long-term antibiotics should be reviewed regularly for side-effects, which fortunately are rare, though they include potentially dangerous benign intracranial hypertension (with tetracyclines) and autoimmune hepatitis (minocycline).

Isotretinoin (13-cis-retinoic acid) is a very valuable addition to the list of drugs used for treating severe acne. It reduces sebum secretion dramatically and is given in a 4-month course. Although sebum secretion eventually rebounds to its former level after the drug is stopped, the acne does not usually recur. Side-effects, especially drying of the skin and mucous membranes, are common but well tolerated. Rarely, abnormalities of liver function occur and limit treatment. Depression, sometimes leading to suicide, is also a rare accompaniment of treatment and patients should be warned about this before starting a course of isotretinoin. The main problem is that the drug is highly teratogenic and females requiring it must have a negative pregnancy test before treatment and take an oral contraceptive for at least a month before the course of isotretinoin, during the course and for 3 months after. Pregnancy tests at monthly reviews are also advisable.

Hormonal treatment in the form of a combined anti-androgen (cyproterone acetate) oestrogen pill, taken in courses as an oral contraceptive, is available in many countries and may help women with persistent acne resistant to treatment with antibiotics or those with 'polycystic ovarian syndrome'. Monitoring is as for any female on an oral contraceptive.

Physical measures

Cysts can be incised and drained under local anaesthetic. Intralesional injections of triamcinolone acetonide (0.1–0.2 ml of a 10 mg/ml solution) hasten the resolution of stubborn cysts.

ROSACEA

Rosacea is a persistent facial eruption of unknown cause characterised by erythema and pustules. Sebum secretion is normal though sebaceous gland hyperplasia and associated inflammation are seen histologically.

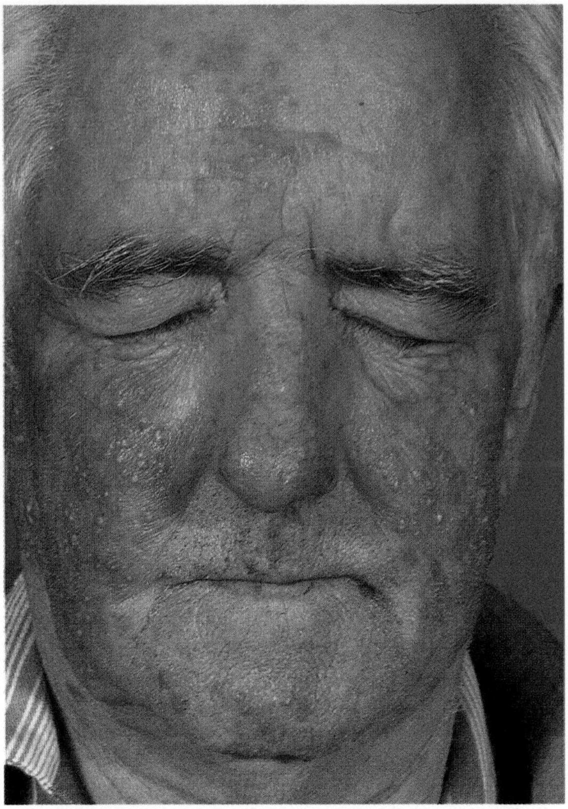

Fig. 13.20 Rosacea. The colour is distinctive and the papulo-pustular rash involves the cheeks, centre of forehead and chin.

Clinical features

The disorder is most common in middle age. The cheeks, chin and central forehead are affected (see Fig. 13.20). Intermittent blushing is followed by fixed erythema and telangiectasia. Dome-shaped papules and pustules but no comedones occur. Rhinophyma, with erythema, sebaceous gland hyperplasia and overgrowth of the soft tissues of the nose, is sometimes associated. Blepharitis and conjunctivitis are complications.

Diagnosis

This is often obvious on clinical grounds but acne, seborrhoeic eczema, photosensitivity and systemic lupus erythematosus must be distinguished.

Management

Mild cases may respond to local metronidazole gel. Usually an 8–10-week course of a tetracycline or erythromycin is required (dose as for acne) and repeat courses are often necessary. Plastic surgery may be required for rhinophyma.

FURTHER INFORMATION ON DISORDERS OF THE PILOSEBACEOUS UNIT

Bork K 1993 Drug-induced acne. Current Opinion in Dermatology 85–90
Cunliffe W 1989 Acne. Martin Dunitz, London
Greaves M W 1998 Flushing and flushing syndromes, rosacea and perioral dermatitis. In: Champion R H, Burton J L, Burns D A, Breathnach S M (eds) Textbook of dermatology, 6th edn, pp. 2099–2112. Blackwell Scientific, Oxford
Leyden J J 1997 Drug therapy: therapy for acne vulgaris. New England Journal of Medicine 336: 1156–1162

PRESSURE SORES

Pressure sores are caused by ischaemia due to sustained or repeated pressure on skin overlying bony prominences. Up to one-third of patients over 70 years old in hospital develop pressure sores, especially those with a fractured neck of femur. The morbidity and mortality of those with deep ulcers are high.

Aetiology

The main factors responsible for pressure sores are:

- prolonged immobility and recumbency, e.g. paraplegia, arthritis and apathy
- diminished sensation, e.g. neurological disease
- vascular disease, e.g. atherosclerosis
- malnutrition, general debility and severe systemic illness, e.g. alcoholism and malignant cachexia.

Clinical features

The sore starts as a localised area of erythema and progresses to a superficial blister or erosion. If the cause is not corrected, deeper damage occurs, with the development of a black eschar which, when removed or shed, leaves a deep and penetrating ulcer, often colonised by *Pseudomonas aeruginosa*. The skin overlying the sacrum, greater trochanter, ischial tuberosity, tuberosity of calcaneus and lateral malleolus is especially susceptible.

Management

This is not easy but the following are important:

- prevention by regular turning of recumbent patients and the use of antipressure mattresses in susceptible patients
- treatment of malnutrition and the general condition
- débridement: regular cleansing with normal saline or 0.5% aqueous silver nitrate; an appropriate systemic antibiotic if there is spreading infection; antibacterial preparations locally; absorbent dressings (see leg ulcers, p. 894); semi-permeable dressings such as Opsite
- plastic surgical reconstruction, which may be indicated in the young when the ulcer is clean.

FURTHER INFORMATION ON PRESSURE SORES

Kanj L F, Van B Wilking S, Phillips T 1998 Pressure ulcers. Journal of the American Academy of Dermatology 38: 517–536

DISORDERS OF PIGMENTATION

DECREASED PIGMENTATION

OCULOCUTANEOUS ALBINISM

Little or no melanin is made in the skin and eyes in this disorder. There are two main types, tyrosinase negative and tyrosinase positive, distinguished by the hair bulb test. Both are inherited as autosomal recessive traits, the abnormal gene for each type being found on different chromosomes.

Clinical features

At birth the whole skin is white and pigment is also deficient in the hair, iris and retina. Albinos have poor vision, photophobia and rotatory nystagmus. Sunburn is common. As tyrosinase-positive albinos grow older they gain a little pigment so that their hair becomes straw-coloured, their irides less translucent and their skin slightly freckled. As melanocytes are present, albinos have non-pigmented melanocytic naevi and may develop amelanotic malignant melanomas. Other skin tumours are also common in albinos living in the tropics.

Management

Avoidance of sun exposure, and the use of sun blocks and protective clothing are essential, especially in the tropics. Termination of affected pregnancies, diagnosed by fetal biopsy at 20 weeks' gestation, may also be considered, especially for those living in sunny climates.

VITILIGO

Vitiligo is an acquired condition affecting 1% of all races, in which circumscribed depigmented patches develop.

Aetiology

There is complete loss of melanocytes from affected patches. There may be a positive family history of the disorder in those with generalised vitiligo and this type is associated with autoimmune diseases such as diabetes, thyroid and adrenal disorders, and pernicious anaemia. Trauma and sunburn may precipitate the appearance of vitiligo.

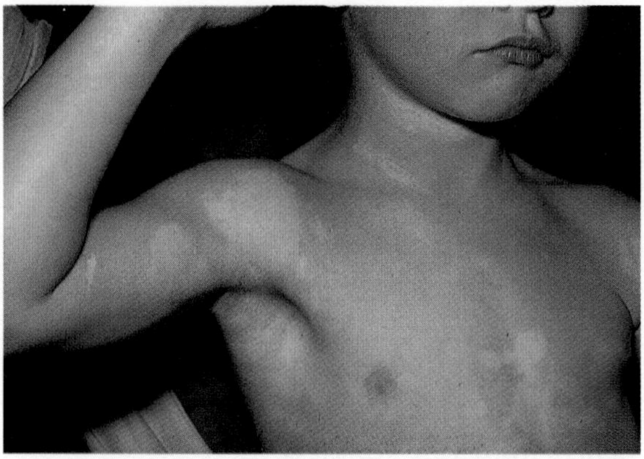

Fig. 13.21 Vitiligo. Widespread patches in a youngster with a strong family history of autoimmune diseases.

Clinical features

Segmental vitiligo is restricted to one part of the body, but not necessarily a dermatome. Generalised vitiligo (see Fig. 13.21) is often symmetrical and frequently involves the hands, wrists, knees and neck as well as the area around the body orifices. The hair of the scalp and beard may also depigment. The patches of depigmentation are sharply defined and, in Caucasians, may be surrounded by 'café au lait'-coloured hyperpigmentation. Some spotty perifollicular pigment may be seen within the depigmented patches and is sometimes the first sign of repigmentation. Sensation in the depigmented patches is normal (cf. tuberculoid leprosy, p. 131). The course is unpredictable but most patches remain static or enlarge; a few repigment spontaneously.

Management

This is unsatisfactory. It is important to protect the patches from excessive sun exposure by clothing or sunscreen preparations. Camouflage cosmetics may be helpful, especially in black people. Photochemotherapy with PUVA (see p. 903) is rarely helpful. Open studies of the efficacy of topical catalase and UVB have been encouraging but the results of controlled trials are awaited.

PHENYLKETONURIA (see p. 532)

This rare metabolic cause of hypopigmentation has a prevalence of about 1:25 000.

HYPOPITUITARISM

The hypopigmentation is due to a decreased production of pituitary melanotrophic hormones (see p. 554). The complexion has a pale, yellow tinge; there is skin atrophy and thinning or loss of the sexual hair.

INCREASED PIGMENTATION

This is mostly due to hypermelanosis but other pigments may occasionally be deposited in the skin so that orange discoloration may suggest carotenaemia; a bronze colour, haemochromatosis (see p. 718); and other hues, drug eruptions (see Table 13.12).

LOCALISED HYPERMELANOSIS

Freckles

These lesions, also known as ephelides, are sharply demarcated light brown-ginger macules of up to 5 mm in diameter. They are most prominent on exposed sites; they multiply and become darker with sun exposure. The melanin in the basal cell layer of the epidermis is increased without melanocytic proliferation.

Lentigines

These are dark brown macules ranging from 1 mm to 1 cm across. Although discrete, their outline may be irregular. Lentigines occur in childhood but are most common after middle age on the backs of the hands ('liver spots') and on the face. Lentigines have an increased number of melanocytes which produce excessive melanin.

Multiple lentigines are seen on and around the lips, buccal mucosa and fingers in the Peutz–Jeghers syndrome (associated with small intestinal polyposis and intussusception).

DIFFUSE HYPERMELANOSIS

Endocrine pigmentation

Chloasma describes discrete patches of facial pigmentation which occur in pregnancy and in some women taking oral contraceptives. Diffuse pigmentation, sometimes worse in the skin creases, may be a feature of Addison's disease (see p. 589), Cushing's syndrome (see p. 581), Nelson's

Table 13.12 Drug-induced pigmentation

Drug	Appearance
Amiodarone	Slate-grey, exposed sites
Arsenic	Diffuse bronze pigmentation with superimposed 'raindrop' depigmentation
Bleomycin	Often flexural, brown
Busulphan	Diffuse brown
Chloroquine	Blue-grey, exposed sites
Clofazimine	Red
Mepacrine	Yellow
Minocycline	Slate-grey, scars, temples, shins and sclera
Phenothiazines	Slate-grey, exposed sites
Psoralens	Brown, exposed sites

syndrome, and chronic renal failure (see p. 433). In all of these cases it is due to an increase in the levels of pituitary melanotrophic peptides (see p. 554).

Drug-induced pigmentation

Table 13.12 lists some drugs which may cause hyperpigmentation, not invariably due to hypermelanosis alone but sometimes due to deposition of the drug or its metabolite, either of which may be complexed with melanin.

FURTHER INFORMATION ON DISORDERS OF PIGMENTATION

Bolognia J, Pawelek J M 1988 Biology of hypopigmentation. Journal of the American Academy of Dermatology 19: 217–255
Orlow S J 1993 Recent advances in oculocutaneous albinism. Current Opinion in Dermatology 73–77

DISORDERS OF THE NAILS

The condition of the nails may reflect both local and systemic disease, and omission of this part of the general examination could result in some important diagnostic clues being overlooked.

The nail plate arises from the nail matrix and lies on the nail bed (see Fig. 13.22). The keratinous plate is produced by cells of the matrix and, to a much lesser extent, the bed. Finger nails grow about 1 cm every 3 months and toe nails at about one-third of this rate.

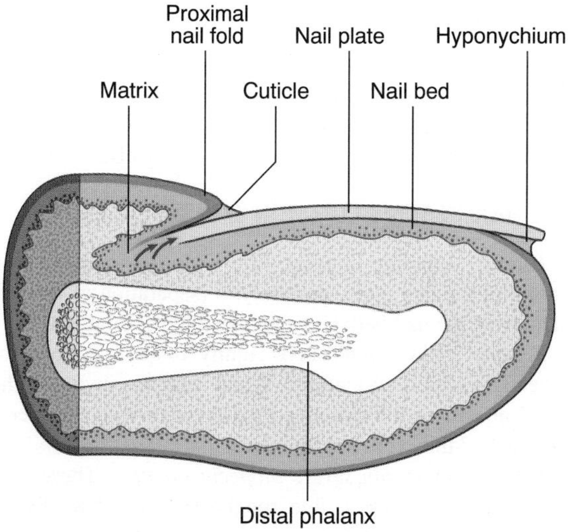

Fig. 13.22 The nail plate and bed.

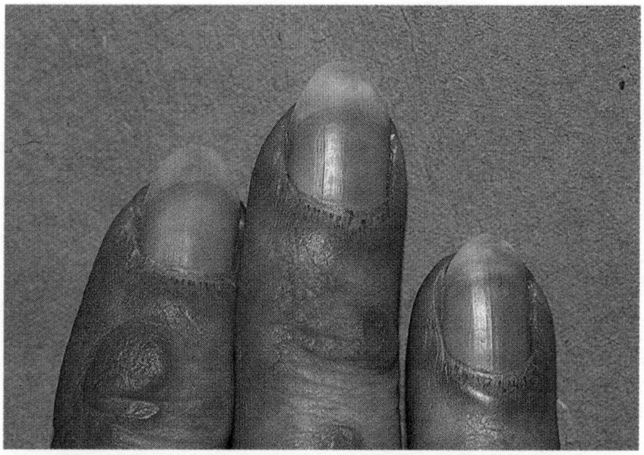

Fig. 13.23 Dermatomyositis. The erythema, dilated and tortuous capillaries in the proximal nail fold and the Gottron's papules on the digits are important diagnostic features.

NAIL FOLD DISORDERS

Examination of the nail folds should accompany examination of the nails. Paronychia describes inflamed and swollen nail folds. Chronic paronychia is seen most commonly in those with a poor peripheral circulation, in those involved in wet work, in diabetics and those who are over-enthusiastic when manicuring their cuticles. Ragged cuticles and dilated or thrombosed capillaries in the proximal nail folds are important pointers to connective tissue disease (see Fig. 13.23).

NAIL PLATE DISORDERS

These may be isolated abnormalities due to congenital disease or trauma or reflect other diseases, either systemic or those just involving the skin. Longitudinal ridging and beading of the nail plate is not abnormal and increases with age. Similarly, occasional white transverse flecks (striate leuconychia) are seen frequently in normal nails and are due to airspaces within the plate and not, contrary to popular belief, to insufficient calcium.

CONGENITAL DISEASE

Pachyonychia congenita is a rare autosomal dominant condition. Some families have been shown to have mutations in keratins. The nails are grossly thickened, especially at the free edge, and discoloured from birth.

TRAUMA

Splinter haemorrhages. These are fine linear dark brown flecks running longitudinally in the plate. They are most commonly due to trauma but may be seen in nail psoriasis. They are also a sign of subacute bacterial endocarditis (see p. 286).

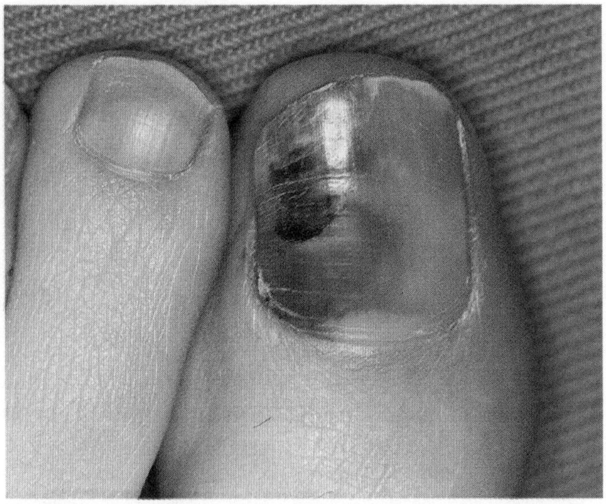

Fig. 13.24 Subungual haematoma.

Subungual haematomas (see Fig. 13.24). These may appear as a crimson, purple or grey-brown discoloration of the nail plate, most frequently that of the big toe. Sometimes, but not always, there is a history of trauma. The abnormality appears suddenly and the nail folds remain uninvolved (cf. subungual malignant melanoma, p. 915). As the nail grows out, a normally coloured band develops proximally.

Habit-tic dystrophy. This is common, and is due to the habit of picking or fiddling with the proximal nail fold of the thumb. This produces a ladder pattern of transverse ridges and furrows up the centre of the nail.

Chronic trauma. Chronic trauma from ill-fitting shoes and from sport may cause malalignment and thickening of the nails, known as onychogryphosis, and lead to ingrowing toe nails.

THE NAIL IN SYSTEMIC DISEASE

Koilonychia (see Fig. 13.25A). This is a concave or spoon-shaped deformity of the plate which is a sign of iron deficiency. It is seen most often in countries where malnutrition is prevalent.

Beau's lines (see Fig. 13.25B). These are transverse grooves which appear at the same time on all nails, a few weeks after an acute illness, and which move out to the free margins as the nails grow.

Digital clubbing. In its most gross form this is seen as a bulbous swelling of the tip of the finger (see Figs 13.25C and D) or toe. The normal angle between the proximal part of the nail and the skin is lost. Causes include:

- *respiratory*—bronchogenic carcinoma, asbestosis (especially with mesothelioma), suppurative lung disease (empyema, bronchiectasis, cystic fibrosis), fibrosing alveolitis

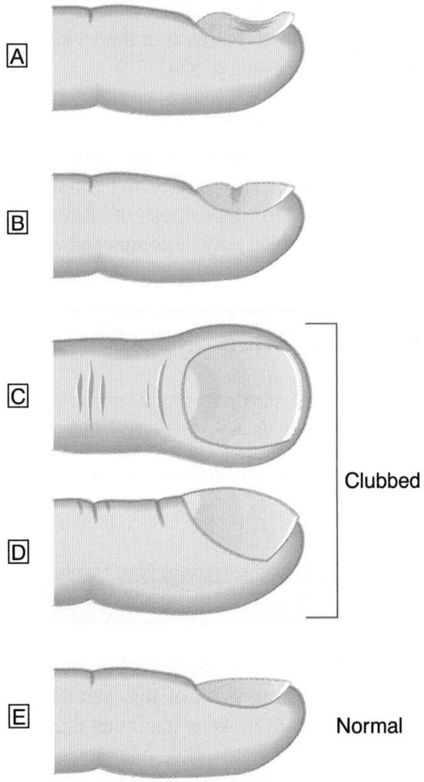

Fig. 13.25 The nail in systemic disease. A Koilonychia. B Beau's lines. C and D Digital clubbing. E Normal nail.

- *cardiac*—cyanotic congenital heart disease, subacute bacterial endocarditis
- *other*—inflammatory bowel disease, biliary cirrhosis, thyrotoxicosis, familial.

Whitening of the nails. This is a rare sign of hypoalbuminaemia. 'Half and half' nails (white proximally and red-brown distally) are seen in some patients with renal failure. Rarely, drugs (e.g. antimalarials) may discolour nails.

THE NAIL IN SOME COMMON SKIN DISEASES

Psoriasis (see Fig. 13.15, p. 902). This may cause coarse pitting of the nail plate, onycholysis (separation of the nail plate from the nail bed) and subungual hyperkeratosis.

Eczema. Shiny nails may signify frequent rubbing of eczematous skin elsewhere. When eczema involves the distal phalanges the nail may be deformed, with transverse ridging and thickening of the plate.

Lichen planus and severe alopecia areata. These may cause trachyonychia, a fine roughness and white discoloration of the nail plate.

Dermatophyte infection. This causes yellow-brown discoloration and crumbling of the plate which starts at the

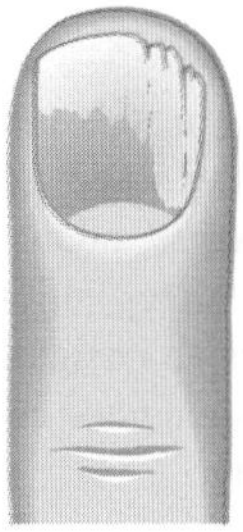

Fig. 13.26 Dermatophyte infection. This causes discoloration and crumbliness of the nail plate.

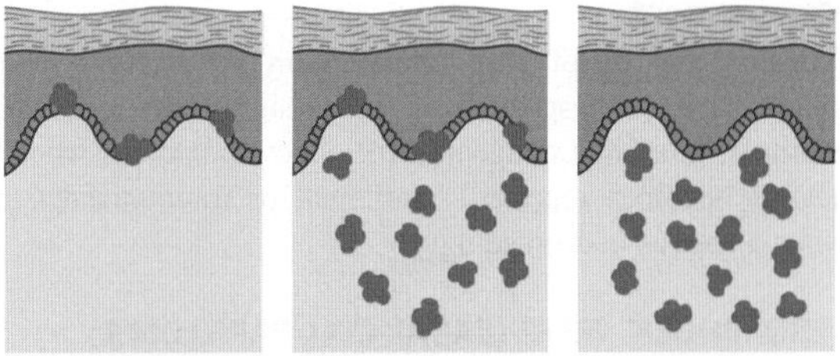

Fig. 13.27 Classification of melanocytic naevi. Classification is based on microscopic location of the clumps of naevus cells.

free margins and spreads proximally (see Fig. 13.26). Usually only a few nails are infected and frequently only on one foot or hand.

FURTHER INFORMATION ON DISORDERS OF THE NAILS

Baran R, Dawber R P R 1994 Diseases of the nails and their management. Blackwell Scientific, Oxford

SKIN TUMOURS

The increasing number of patients over 70 years old is paralleled by an increasing incidence of skin cancer. Only the most common benign tumours and a few malignant ones will be described in this section.

BENIGN TUMOURS

MELANOCYTIC NAEVI

Melanocytic naevi (moles) are localised benign proliferations of melanocytes. Their cause is unknown but they are often familial. They are very common, the average number on the skin in different populations ranging from 15 to 40. They are more profuse in Caucasians living in sunny climates. With the exception of congenital melanocytic naevi (which are present at birth or appear shortly after birth), most melanocytic naevi appear in early childhood, at adolescence, and during pregnancy or oestrogen therapy. New lesions appear less often after the age of 20.

Clinical features

Acquired melanocytic naevi are classified according to the microscopic location of the clumps of melanocytes in the skin (see Fig. 13.27). Junctional naevi are usually circular and macular; their colour ranges from mid- to dark brown and may vary within a single lesion. Compound and intradermal naevi are similar to one another in appearance; both are nodules of up to 1 cm in diameter, though intradermal naevi are usually less pigmented than compound naevi. Their surface may be smooth, cerebriform or even hyperkeratotic and papillomatous, and they are often hairy.

Clinically and histologically atypical melanocytic naevi (also known as dysplastic naevi) may run in some families in which cases of malignant melanoma are seen. These profuse, large and irregularly pigmented naevi are most obvious on the trunk. Their edges are irregular and they vary greatly in size, often being over 1 cm in diameter. Some are pinkish and an inflamed halo may surround them.

Whereas about 30–50% of malignant melanomas develop from melanocytic naevi, the converse is far from true and only a minute percentage of melanocytic naevi become malignant. Malignant change is most likely in large congenital melanocytic naevi (risk estimated around 6%) and in atypical (dysplastic) melanocytic naevi (precise risk still unclear). However, as the skin can be so easily seen, there is an unrivalled opportunity to observe and report change which might signify early and curable malignancy. Any change (see the information box) in a mole deserves attention, even though the reason for it is often not sinister.

Such changing lesions should be examined carefully remembering the 'ABCDE' features of malignant melanoma listed in the information box on page 883.

SIGNIFICANT CHANGES IN MELANOCYTIC NAEVI

- Itch
- Enlargement
- Increased or decreased pigmentation
- Alteration in shape
- Irregularity of surface or edge
- Inflammation
- Ulceration
- Bleeding

Management
Excision and histological examination are needed when malignancy is suspected or is a significant risk—for example, in a large congenital melanocytic naevus, when a naevus becomes repeatedly inflamed or traumatised, and when a naevus is deemed ugly.

SEBORRHOEIC WART (BASAL CELL PAPILLOMA)

These common benign epidermal tumours are unrelated to sebaceous glands. Their appearance is usually unexplained but multiple lesions may be inherited as an autosomal dominant trait. Occasionally they appear in the wake of an inflammatory dermatosis and, very rarely, a sudden eruption of multiple itchy lesions may be associated with an internal tumour.

Clinical features
Seborrhoeic warts appear usually after the age of 50 years but flat inconspicuous lesions may be visible earlier. They are most commonly found on the trunk and face. The sexes are equally affected. The lesions vary in colour from yellow to dark brown and have a distinctive, raised and 'stuck-on' appearance. They are sometimes pedunculated. Their surface may have greasy scaling and scattered pinpoint keratin plugs. They become more profuse with age but remain benign (see Fig. 13.28).

Investigation
Biopsy is necessary only in dubious cases, most often to exclude malignant melanoma.

Management
Seborrhoeic warts may be left alone but unsightly or easily traumatised lesions are simply removed by curettage under local anaesthetic or by cryotherapy.

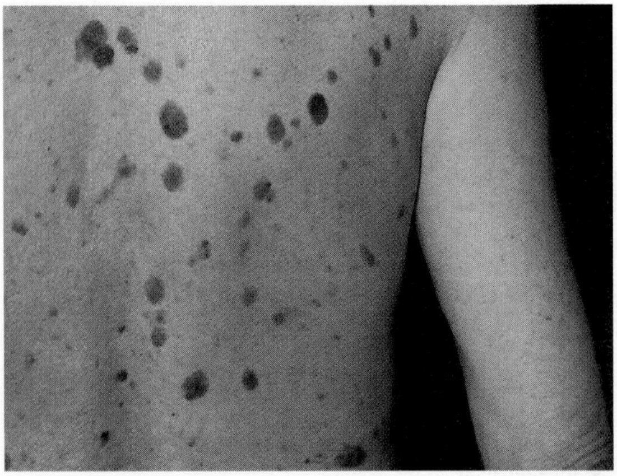

Fig. 13.28 Multiple seborrhoeic warts.

KERATOACANTHOMA

Usually considered benign, this rapidly growing tumour is seen most often on sun-exposed skin. It grows over a few weeks into a dome-shaped nodule, often with a central keratin plug. Spontaneous resolution will occur but it often takes months and leaves an unsightly scar. The histology is very similar to that of squamous cell carcinoma. Treatment is by excision or curettage.

PRE-MALIGNANT TUMOURS

ACTINIC KERATOSIS

These discrete, rough-surfaced lesions occur on light-exposed areas. They are caused by cumulative sun exposure. Caucasians living near the equator are most at risk and invariably develop them, although they also affect the middle-aged and elderly in temperate climates. Actinic keratoses are not seen in black people. They are pre-malignant, though only a few turn into squamous cell carcinomas.

Clinical features
The multiple pink or grey hyperkeratotic lesions seldom exceed 1 cm in diameter and are most common on the backs of the hands, the face and bald scalp (see Fig. 13.29). Many resolve spontaneously. Transition to squamous cell carcinoma, although rare (about 1/1000 per year), should be suspected if a lesion becomes thickened and palpable, enlarges, ulcerates or bleeds.

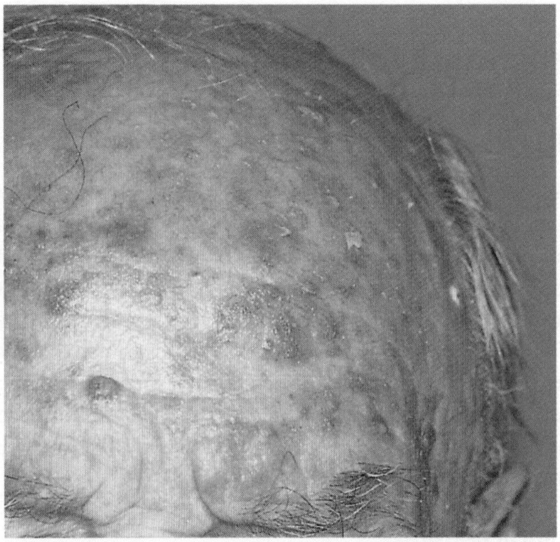

Fig. 13.29 Numerous actinic keratoses in a white patient who had lived for years in the tropics.

Management

Cryotherapy with liquid nitrogen is effective, though multiple lesions may be treated with 5% 5-fluorouracil cream under specialist guidance. Lesions which do not respond to treatment should be regarded with suspicion and biopsied.

INTRAEPIDERMAL CARCINOMA

Clinical features

A slow-growing pink/red scaly plaque is suggestive of intraepidermal carcinoma (see Fig. 13.30). These lesions are characteristically seen on the lower legs of elderly women but can occur anywhere on the body. They are occasionally misdiagnosed as psoriasis or discoid eczema. Important distinguishing features include the fact that they are often single; if multiple, they are not symmetrical. They are chronic and asymptomatic, and show no response to topical steroids.

Investigations

An incisional biopsy will confirm the diagnosis. Dysplastic keratinocytes are seen confined within the epidermis.

Treatment

Treatment is local destruction with cryotherapy or topical 5-fluorouracil.

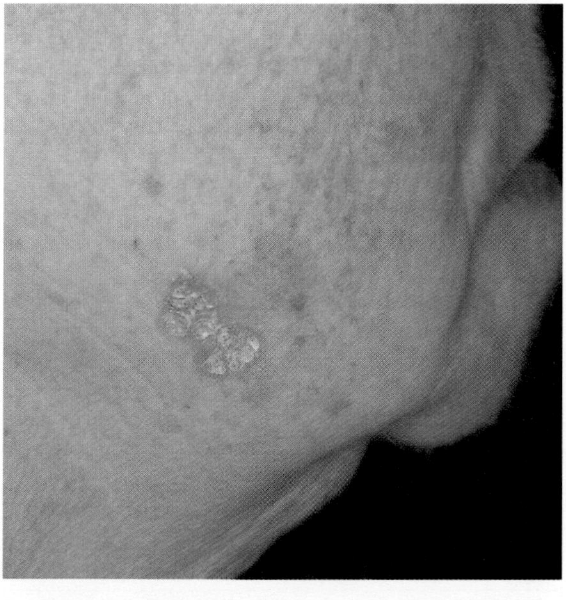

Fig. 13.30 Intraepidermal carcinoma (right cheek). This persistent psoriasis-like plaque recurred after the original (anterior) lesion was treated by freezing.

MALIGNANT TUMOURS

BASAL CELL CARCINOMA (BCC)

This is the most common form of skin cancer and is usually found on the face of the middle-aged or elderly. The tumour invades locally but rarely metastasises. 'Rodent ulcer' is a term commonly used for slowly expanding ulcerative basal cell carcinoma. The malignant cells resemble basal keratinocytes.

Aetiology

Cumulative sun exposure is the most important factor in the development of these tumours and they are more common in Caucasians living near the equator (see Fig. 1.8, p. 8). They may also occur in scars following vaccination and trauma or appear on skin previously treated with X-rays.

Clinical features

The most common type is the *nodulo-ulcerative form*. The earliest lesion is a small, glistening, skin-coloured papule, often with fine telangiectatic vessels on the surface, which slowly enlarges. Central necrosis may occur, which leaves an ulcer surrounded by a rolled pearly edge (see Fig. 13.31). Without treatment lesions may reach 1–2 cm in diameter over 5–10 years. Slow but relentless growth causes local tissue destruction. Sometimes this type of tumour becomes *cystic* or *pigmented*. The *cicatricial* variant of basal cell carcinoma is a slowly expanding, yellow or grey waxy plaque with an ill-defined edge. Fibrosis often follows ulceration and crusting and the lesion may appear as an enlarging scar. The *superficial* (multifocal) variant is seen most often on the trunk; it appears as a slowly enlarging pink or brown scaly plaque with a fine 'whipcord' edge. If left, it may grow to 10 cm in diameter.

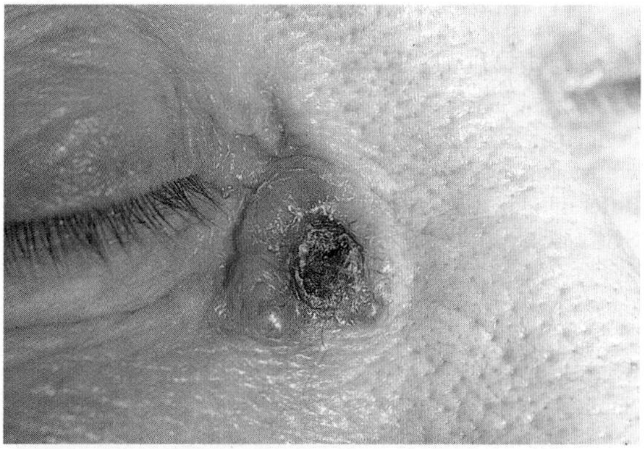

Fig. 13.31 Basal cell carcinoma. A slowly growing pearly nodule just below the inner canthus. The central crust overlies an ulcerated area.

Management

If the diagnosis is uncertain an incision biopsy or a scraping for cytology can be confirmatory. Excision, with 0.5 cm of normal skin, is the treatment of choice for most patients. Lesions with an ill-defined edge are best excised by specialist surgeons, who might take advantage of microscopic examination of clearance *during* the operation (Mohs' technique). Radiotherapy is effective and should be reserved for biopsy-proven lesions when surgery is contraindicated. Superficial BCCs can be treated with curettage and cautery, cryotherapy or topical 5-fluorouracil. A more recent treatment available in some centres is photodynamic therapy, which relies on the ability of BCC cells to take up a photosensitiser, haematoporphyrin. The tumour cells can then be selectively destroyed by monochromatic laser light. The cure rate for all types of BCC is over 95% but regular follow-up for at least 3 years is required to detect local recurrence.

SQUAMOUS CELL CARCINOMA (SCC)

Squamous cell carcinoma is the second most common skin cancer after BCC and is increasing in incidence worldwide. The mean age of presentation is in the seventh decade.

Aetiology

Skin type is the most important risk factor in the development of SCC. Long-term ultraviolet radiation is an immunosuppressant in the skin and is the main aetiological factor in these malignant tumours of keratinocytes (see Fig. 1.8, p. 8). There is an increased risk of SCC in renal transplant patients, particularly with multiple human papillomavirus (HPV)-induced warts. Certain HPV types are implicated as having an oncogenic role in cutaneous SCC. Other risk factors include arsenic ingestion, chronic cutaneous ulcers, chronic radiodermatitis and rare genetic disorders such as xeroderma pigmentosum and epidermodysplasia verruciformis.

Clinical features

Squamous cell carcinoma is a proliferative tumour that has a history of growth over a few months. Varying clinical presentations include keratotic nodules (see Fig. 13.32), exophytic erythematous nodules, infiltrating firm tumours and ulcers with an indurated edge. Histology also varies from well-differentiated tumours to anaplastic. Approximately 50% of SCCs occur on the head and neck. SCCs are common on the lip and pinnae and are more likely to metastasise from these sites.

Management

Surgical excision with a 3–4 mm margin is the treatment of choice and has a cure rate of 90%. As with BCC, radiotherapy can be used in selected cases. Follow-up for 5 years is necessary to examine for local recurrence, evidence of metastases and second primaries.

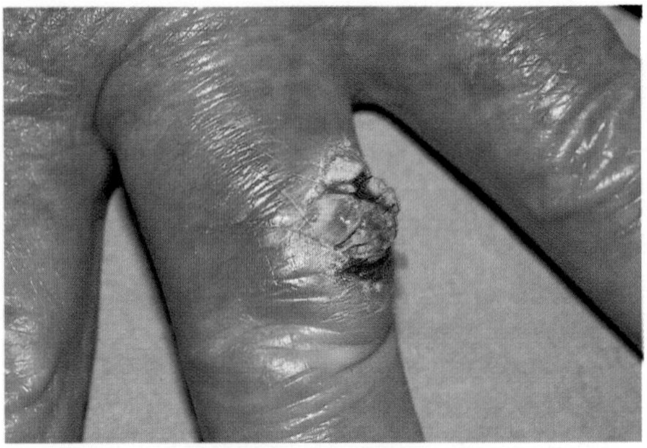

Fig. 13.32 Squamous cell carcinoma. A warty nodule with induration of the adjacent skin.

MALIGNANT MELANOMA

Malignant melanoma attracts a disproportionate amount of attention because it is so lethal; prevention, early diagnosis and treatment are by far the best ways of combatting its dangers. It is rarely seen in black people but its incidence in Caucasians in the UK and USA is doubling, approximately every 10 years. Sunlight is the most important cause (see Fig. 1.8, p. 8). There is a higher incidence in Caucasians living near the equator (over 40 per 100 000 per annum) than those living in temperate zones (10 per 100 000 per annum). The tumour is rare before puberty, and in areas of low incidence (including the UK) the tumour is twice as common in females. Those with blond or red hair, fair skin which tans poorly, many freckles and melanocytic naevi, atypical melanocytic naevi and a family or personal history of a previous melanoma have an increased risk of developing the tumour.

Clinical features

The classification of invasive malignant melanomas is seen in Table 13.13.

Two-thirds of invasive melanomas are preceded by a superficial and radial growth phase characterised by an expanding, irregularly pigmented macule or plaque. Its margin is usually irregular with reniform projections (see Fig. 13.33). Lentigo maligna (in situ changes of malignancy only) and lentigo maligna melanoma occur most often on

Table 13.13 Classification of cutaneous malignant melanoma

Type of invasive melanoma	Presence of preceding in situ/radial growth phase
Superficial spreading	+
Lentigo maligna	+
Nodular	–
Acral lentiginous	+

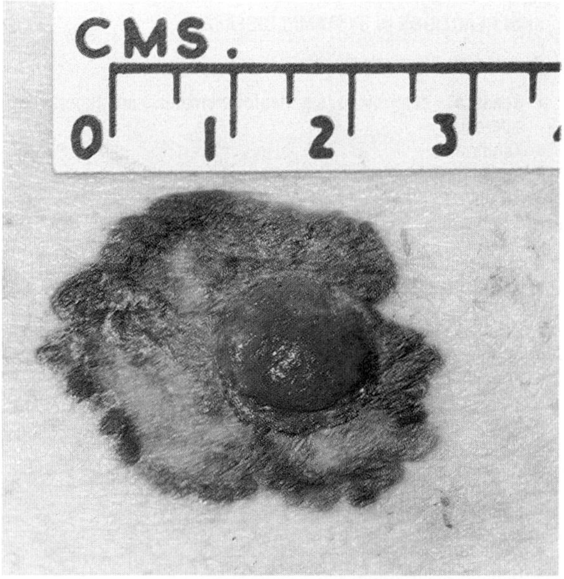

Fig. 13.33 Superficial spreading melanoma. The radial growth phase was present for about 3 years before the invasive amelanotic nodule developed within it. Note irregular outline, asymmetrical shape and different hues, including depigmented areas signifying spontaneous regression.

the exposed skin of the elderly. A speckled macular lentigo maligna may have been present for many years before a nodule of invasive melanoma appears within it. The in situ phase of superficial spreading melanoma, the most common type in Caucasians, seldom lasts for longer than 2 years, usually shows much colour variation and is often palpable. Acral lentiginous melanoma occurs on the palms and soles and is the most common type in the Chinese and Japanese. Nodular melanoma develops as a pigmented nodule with no preceding in situ phase. All changing pigmented lesions deserve careful examination remembering the 'ABCDE' features of malignant melanoma (see p. 883). About 30–50% of melanomas appear to develop in a preceding melanocytic naevus (see p. 911). A change in any naevus should raise suspicion of malignant transformation.

True amelanotic melanomas occur but are rare; flecks of pigmentation can usually be seen with a lens. Subungual melanomas present as painless, expanding areas of pigmentation under a nail and usually involve the nail fold.

The clinical stages of malignant melanoma are shown in the information box.

CLINICAL STAGES OF MALIGNANT MELANOMA	
• Stage I	Primary lesion only
• Stage II	Regional nodal disease
• Stage III	Distant disease (nodal or visceral)

The diagnosis should be established by local excision biopsy of the suspected lesion with 2 mm lateral clearance and with a cuff of subcutaneous fat deep to the tumour. Incisional biopsies are not recommended as a routine but may be unavoidable with some large and doubtful lesions and at certain sites.

Management

Only *surgical excision* is effective. A 3 cm clearance is at present recommended for tumours greater than 1 mm thick. Direct closure, without grafting, may be possible. Tumours less than 1 mm thick are removed with a 1 cm clearance; direct closure is nearly always possible. Elective (prophylactic) local node dissection may benefit some patients with tumours of intermediate depth (2.0–3.5 mm). Palpable local nodes in stage II patients should always be removed by radical block dissection. Chemotherapy, rarely curative, is palliative in 25% of patients with stage III melanoma.

Prevention and early diagnosis are best achieved by education of those at highest risk who live or holiday in sunny climates. Successful campaigns have focused on regular self-examination and the ways in which sun exposure can be reduced by avoidance, clothing and sunscreen preparations. Public awareness and compliance have been encouraged by imaginative and gimmicky slogans like the Australian 'Slip, slap and slop' advice (slip on the shirt, slap on the hat and slop on the sunscreen) and 'sunsmart' campaigns. All physicians have a duty to increase public awareness of the dangers of ultraviolet exposure.

Prognosis

The prognosis of patients with a malignant melanoma can be determined with reasonable accuracy. Those with clinical stage III disease fare least well (less than 10% survive 2 years); patients with stage II disease have a 20–30% chance; and those with stage I disease a 70% chance of surviving 5 years. The thickness of the tumour (measured microscopically by Breslow's method, which gives the distance between the granular cell layer and the deepest part of the tumour) is a reliable predictor of the prognosis for patients with stage I disease. The prognosis is excellent for those with tumours less than 1 mm thick (over 90% survive 5 years), but becomes less good with thicker tumours. The 5-year survival of patients with tumours greater than 3.5 mm thick is about 50%. In general, females fare better than males and tumours at certain sites (e.g. lower leg) are less aggressive.

CUTANEOUS T-CELL LYMPHOMA (MYCOSIS FUNGOIDES)

Lymphomas of the skin are rare. In contrast to B-cell lymphomas (sudden appearance of skin tumours) cutaneous

T-cell lymphoma usually evolves slowly, often over many years. A plaque stage (resembling psoriasis) is followed by skin tumour and systemic phases.

FURTHER INFORMATION ON SKIN TUMOURS

Goldberg L H 1996 Skin cancer quartet: basal cell carcinoma. Lancet 347: 663–667

Mankin R 1996 Skin cancer quartet: squamous cell carcinoma. Lancet 347: 735–738

NIH Consensus Development Panel on Early Melanoma 1992 Diagnosis and treatment of early melanoma. Journal of the American Medical Association 268: 1314–1319

Rivers J K 1996 Skin cancer quartet: melanoma. Lancet 347: 803–806

THE SKIN AND SYSTEMIC DISEASE

Skin reactions can be linked with an underlying systemic disease in a number of ways, as shown in the information box. Only common or important associations will be discussed below.

SKIN REACTIONS IN SYSTEMIC DISEASE
Part of a multisystem disease
• Genetically determined (e.g. neurofibromatosis and tuberous sclerosis) • Xanthomas • Amyloidosis • Porphyria • Sarcoidosis
A non-specific and not invariable reaction pattern to a systemic disease
• Urticaria • Erythema multiforme • Annular erythemas • Erythema nodosum • Pyoderma gangrenosum • Sweet's syndrome • Generalised pruritus
A sign of internal malignancy
• Dermatomyositis • Generalised pruritus • Acanthosis nigricans • Superficial thrombophlebitis
A sign of internal organ failure
• Liver—generalised pruritus, pigmentation, spider naevi and palmar erythema • Kidney—generalised pruritus and pigmentation • Pancreas (diabetes mellitus)—necrobiosis lipoidica
A result of a common genetic link with the systemic disorder
• Dermatitis herpetiformis and gluten-sensitive enteropathy • Psoriasis and some types of arthropathy
The cause of the systemic disease
• Exfoliative dermatitis causing high-output cardiac failure
A result of treatment of the systemic disease
• Drug eruptions

NEUROFIBROMATOSIS: TYPE 1

Light brown (café au lait) macules can be seen in healthy people and are also a feature of:

- Albright's syndrome (polyostotic fibrous dysplasia), where the margins are very irregular
- Bloom's syndrome.

The skin markers of von Recklinghausen's type of neurofibromatosis include scattered and discrete café au lait macules, axillary freckling and a variable number of cutaneous neurofibromata (see p. 1020). The tumours may be small and superficial or large and deep. Small circular pigmented hamartomas of the iris (Lisch nodules) appear in early childhood.

NEUROFIBROMATOSIS: TYPE 2

See page 1020.

SEGMENTAL NEUROFIBROMATOSIS: TYPE 5

The cutaneous features of café au lait macules and neurofibromata are found in a dermatomal distribution. This is due to mosaicism of the NF-1 gene. So far there have been no reported cases of an affected offspring with NF-1 from a patient with NF-5.

TUBEROUS SCLEROSIS

This is an autosomal dominant condition with hamartomas affecting many systems.

The classic triad of clinical features is mental retardation, epilepsy and skin lesions but not all are invariably present. The skin signs include small white oval (ash leaf) macules, pink or yellowish papules on the centre of the face (adenoma sebaceum), peri- and subungual fibromata and connective tissue naevi (cobblestone-like plaques at the base of the spine, sometimes called shagreen patches).

XANTHOMAS

These deposits of fatty material in the skin, subcutaneous fat and tendons may be the first clue to primary or secondary hyperlipidaemia (see p. 534).

Various clinical patterns are seen which correlate well with the underlying cause. They include:

- eruptive yellow papules on the buttocks (eruptive xanthomas)
- yellowish macules or plaques (plane xanthomas)
- small yellow-grey plaques around the eyes (xanthelasma palpebrarum)
- nodules over the elbows and knees (tuberous xanthomas)
- subcutaneous nodules attached to tendons, especially those on the dorsal aspect of the fingers and the Achilles tendons (tendinous xanthomas).

When xanthomas are detected the fasting blood lipids and the electrophoretic pattern of plasma lipoproteins must be measured, though abnormalities will not always be detected.

AMYLOIDOSIS

This is described on page 541. Skin lesions are uncommon in systemic amyloidosis secondary to rheumatoid arthritis or other chronic inflammatory diseases.

Deposits of amyloid in the skin, appearing often as waxy plaques around the eyes, are prominent in primary systemic amyloidosis and in amyloid associated with multiple myeloma. 'Pinch purpura', appearing where the skin is traumatised, is due to amyloid infiltration of blood vessels and may also be a striking feature.

PORPHYRIA

The classification and metabolic abnormalities of the porphyrias are found on page 541. Certain porphyrias can affect the skin.

Porphyria cutanea tarda

This porphyria usually starts in adulthood and can be inherited and precipitated by alcohol, iron overload, oestrogens, hepatitis C and HIV disease. Some cases are acquired and are associated with underlying liver disease such as cirrhosis and hepatic tumours. The cutaneous features are increased skin fragility, blistering (see Fig. 13.34A), erosions and milia occurring on light-exposed areas such as the backs of the hands. Facial hypertrichosis and hyperpigmentation may also be seen. Diagnosis is made by demonstrating coral pink fluorescence of the urine by Wood's light (see Fig. 13.34B). Characteristic faecal, plasma and urinary porphyrin abnormalities are confirmatory.

Erythropoietic protoporphyria

This is a rare porphyria that starts in childhood, with burning and pain on light-exposed areas. Scars occur, particularly on the nose. Examination of the red cells, plasma and stool for raised protoporphyrins is confirmatory.

Variegate porphyria

Cutaneous features are similar to those of porphyria cutanea tarda. Systemic features are the same as those of acute intermittent porphyria.

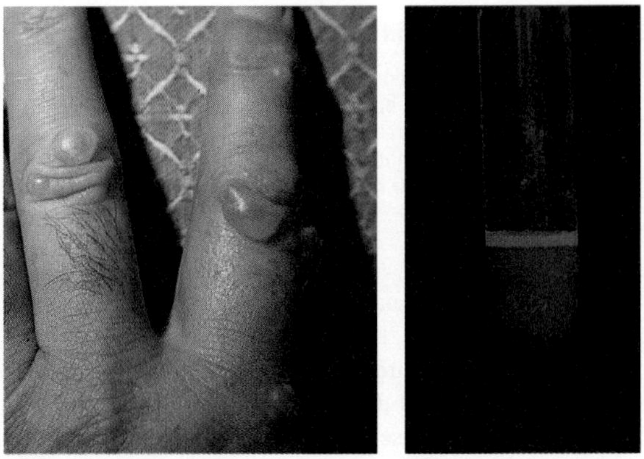

A B

Fig. 13.34 Cutaneous hepatic porphyria. A Recent skin fragility and blistering on the backs of the fingers. B The urine of this patient contained excessive uroporphyrins fluorescing under long-wave ultraviolet when extracted.

Hereditary coproporphyria

Around 30% of these patients are photosensitive. Systemic features are the same as those of acute intermittent porphyria.

Pseudoporphyrias

Sun-bed usage, non-steroidal anti-inflammatory drugs (particularly naproxen) and renal failure can give rise to skin lesions that mimic the photosensitive porphyrias, particularly porphyria cutanea tarda. The pathogenesis is as yet unclear.

SARCOIDOSIS

This is covered in detail on page 367.

Skin lesions are seen in about one-third of patients with systemic sarcoidosis. The clinical features include erythema nodosum, granulomatous deposits in long-standing scars, dusky infiltrated plaques on the nose and fingers (lupus pernio), and scattered brownish-red, violaceous or hypopigmented papules or nodules which vary in number, size and distribution.

ERYTHEMA MULTIFORME

As its name implies, this is a reaction pattern of multiform erythematous lesions. The precipitating factor may not be found in some cases but attacks are provoked by the factors listed in the information box.

PROVOKING FACTORS IN ERYTHEMA MULTIFORME
• Herpes simplex infections • Other viral infections, e.g. orf, and mycoplasma • Bacterial infections • Drugs, especially sulphonamides, penicillins and barbiturates • Internal malignancy or its treatment with radiotherapy

Clinical features

The multiform erythematous lesions may be urticaria-like and some have obvious 'bull's-eye' or 'target' lesions. Blisters may be seen in the centre or around the edges of the lesions. In some cases blisters dominate the picture; the Stevens–Johnson syndrome is severe bullous erythema multiforme with emphasis on mucosal involvement including the mouth, eyes and genitals, with accompanying constitutional disturbance.

Management

Severe cases are usually managed with tapering courses of systemic corticosteroids after treatment, if possible, of the primary cause.

ERYTHEMA NODOSUM

This characteristic reaction pattern is due to a vasculitis in the deep dermis and subcutaneous fat.

Erythema nodosum may be provoked by the factors listed in the information box.

PROVOKING FACTORS IN ERYTHEMA NODOSUM
Infections
• Bacteria (streptococci, tuberculosis, brucellosis and leprosy), viruses, mycoplasma, rickettsia, chlamydia and fungi
Drugs
• e.g. Sulphonamides and oral contraceptives
Systemic disease
• e.g. Sarcoidosis, ulcerative colitis and Crohn's disease

Clinical features

Painful, palpable, dusky blue-red nodules are most commonly seen on the lower legs. Malaise, fever and joint pains are common. The lesions resolve slowly over a month, leaving bruise-like marks in their wake.

Management

The underlying cause should be determined and treated. Bed rest and oral non-steroidal anti-inflammatory drugs may hasten resolution. Tapering systemic corticosteroid courses may be required in stubborn cases.

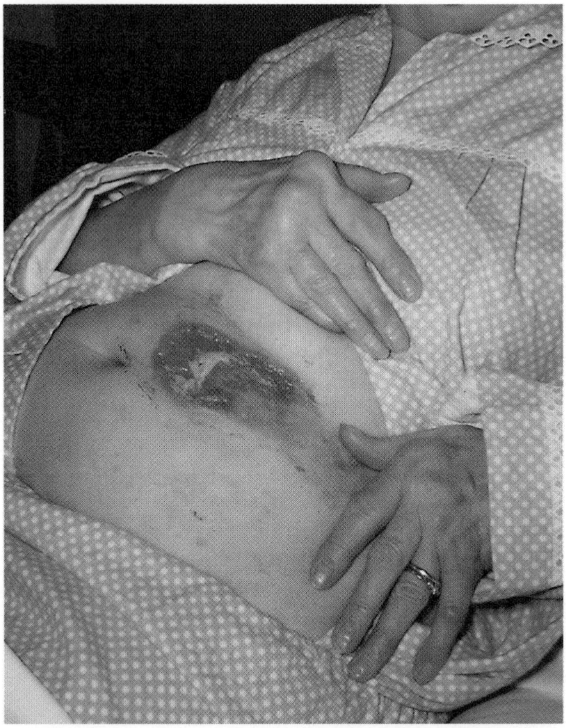

Fig. 13.35 Pyoderma gangrenosum. A large indolent ulcer in a patient with rheumatoid arthritis. Note healing in one part.

PYODERMA GANGRENOSUM

Pyoderma gangrenosum (PG) predominantly occurs in adults between the ages of 25 and 54 years. It is an eruption that starts as an inflamed nodule or pustule which breaks down centrally and rapidly progresses to an ulcer with an indurated or undermined purplish or pustular edge (see Fig. 13.35). Lesions may be single or multiple and are classified as ulcerative, pustular, bullous and vegetative. Although PG may arise in the absence of any underlying disease, it is usually associated with a systemic disease, such as inflammatory bowel disease, arthritis (both rheumatoid arthritis and sero-negative arthropathies), immunodeficiency and immunosuppression including HIV disease, monoclonal gammopathies and leukaemia. The management of PG includes investigations for possible associated systemic disease. There are no diagnostic features on biopsy and therefore the diagnosis is primarily clinical. Local therapy includes pain relief, prevention of secondary

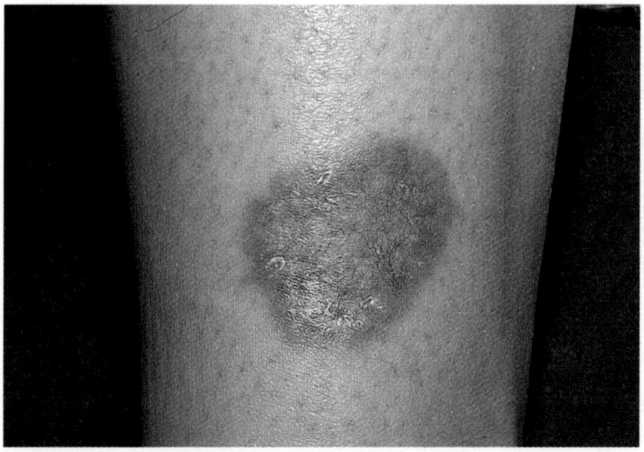

Fig. 13.36 Necrobiosis lipoidica. An atrophic yellowish plaque on the skin of a diabetic.

bacterial infection and dressings. Systemic therapy includes oral steroids in a tapering dose, dapsone 50–150 mg/day, minocycline 100 mg/day and cyclosporin (5 mg/kg); once the patient is clear of disease recurrences are only intermittent.

ACANTHOSIS NIGRICANS

This is a velvety thickening and pigmentation of the major flexures, particularly the axillae. There are several types of acanthosis nigricans. The most common form is a weight-dependent mild acanthosis nigricans (obesity-associated). When the patient loses weight the cutaneous features regress. Secondly, acanthosis nigricans can be associated with various syndromes, some of which have insulin resistance as a feature. Finally, acanthosis nigricans can be associated with malignancy, particularly gastric (60%). Pruritus is a feature of malignancy-associated acanthosis and regression occurs after the tumour is excised. Acanthosis nigricans sometimes recurs with metastatic disease.

NECROBIOSIS LIPOIDICA

This condition is important to recognise because of its association with diabetes mellitus. Less than 1% of diabetics have necrobiosis, but more than 85% of patients with necrobiosis will have or will develop diabetes.

Typically, the lesions appear as shiny, atrophic and slightly yellow plaques on the shins (see Fig. 13.36). Underlying telangiectasia is easily seen. Minor knocks may precipitate slow-healing ulcers. No treatment is very effective. Topical and intralesional steroids are used, as is long-term PUVA.

GRANULOMA ANNULARE

This is a common cutaneous condition of uncertain aetiology. Dermal nodules occur singly or in an annular configuration. They are asymptomatic but cause consternation because they commonly occur on highly visible sites such as the hands and feet. Histologically, palisading granulomata are found in the dermis. Intralesional steroids can be helpful, but the natural history is spontaneous resolution after a few months to a couple of years.

DRUG ERUPTIONS

Cutaneous drug reactions are common and almost any drug can cause them. Drug reactions may reasonably be included

Table 13.14 Drug eruptions and their mechanisms

Mechanism	Example
Non-immunological (non-allergic)	
Unwarranted pharmacological effect	Striae due to corticosteroids; mouth ulcers due to methotrexate
Drug overdosage or failure to metabolise or excrete the drug	Morphine rashes in patients with liver disease
Drug interaction	Warfarin toxicity when coadministered with aspirin or phenylbutazone
Idiosyncratic reaction (an odd reaction which may be genetically determined and is peculiar to an individual)	Drug-induced variegate porphyria
Phototoxic reaction	Chlorpromazine-induced light reactions
Altered skin ecology	Tetracyclines causing vaginal candidiasis
Exacerbation of pre-existing skin condition	Lithium and β-adrenoceptor antagonist worsening of psoriasis
Immunological (allergic)	
Immediate hypersensitivity	Penicillin-induced urticaria
Immune complex reaction	Drug-induced vasculitis or erythema multiforme
Delayed hypersensitivity	Drug-induced exfoliative dermatitis or photo-allergic reactions

Table 13.15 Drug eruptions and some drugs which may cause them		
Name of reaction pattern	**Clinical features**	**Drugs which commonly cause reaction**
Toxic erythema	Erythematous plaques Morbilliform, sometimes with urticarial or erythema multiforme-like elements	Antibiotics (especially ampicillin) Sulphonamides, thiazide diuretics, phenylbutazone, para-aminosalicylic acid (PAS)
Urticaria	Itchy wheals, sometimes accompanied by angioedema	Salicylates, codeine, antibiotics, dextran and ACE inhibitors
Erythema and scaling	Small, scaly, pink papules to large, scaly, red papules	Antibiotics (especially penicillins and sulphonamides), anticonvulsants, ACE inhibitors, barbiturates, gold and penicillamine
Allergic vasculitis	Painful, palpable purpura followed by necrotic ulcers	Sulphonamides, phenylbutazone, indomethacin, phenytoin and oral contraceptives
Erythema multiforme	Target-like lesions and bullae on the extensor aspects of the limbs	Sulphonamides, phenylbutazone and barbiturates
Purpura	Widespread purpura not due to thrombocytopenia or a coagulation defect	Thiazides, sulphonamides, phenylbutazone, sulphonylurea, barbiturates and quinine
Bullous eruptions	May be associated with erythema and purpura. May occur at pressure sites in drug-induced coma	Barbiturates, penicillamine, nalidixic acid
Exfoliative dermatitis	Universal redness and scaling, shivering	Phenylbutazone, para-aminosalicylic acid (PAS), isoniazid and gold
Fixed drug eruptions	Round, erythematous and sometimes bullous plaques develop at the same site every time the drug is given. Pigmentation left in wake	Tetracyclines, quinine, sulphonamides and barbiturates
Acneiform eruptions	Rash resembles acne (see p. 904)	Lithium, oral contraceptive, androgenic or glucocorticoid steroids. Antituberculosis and anticonvulsant drugs
Toxic epidermal necrolysis	Rash resembles that of scaled skin (see Fig. 13.37)	Barbiturates, phenytoin, phenylbutazone and penicillin
Hair loss	Diffuse	Cytotoxic agents, acitretin, anticoagulants, antithyroid drugs and oral contraceptives
Hypertrichosis		Diazoxide, minoxidil and cyclosporin A
Photosensitivity	Rash limited to exposed skin	Thiazides, tetracyclines, phenothiazines, sulphonamides, nalidixic acid and psoralens
Pigmentation	Irregular melanin pigmentation on face Slate-grey colour of exposed skin Diffuse yellow coloration of skin Streaky depigmentation of hair	Oral contraceptives Phenothiazines Mepacrine Chloroquine

in the differential diagnosis of most skin diseases. Although the mechanisms are poorly understood, drug eruptions may be classified as shown in Table 13.14.

Clinical features

The most common types of drug eruption and their cause are listed in Table 13.15. It is important not to forget the possibility of a drug eruption when faced with a rash which is atypical of a known skin disease (see Fig. 13.38). Further clues to make the diagnosis are included in the information box.

DIAGNOSTIC CLUES TO DRUG ERUPTIONS

- Past history of reaction to suspected drug
- Introduction of suspected drug a few days before onset of rash
- Recent prescription of a drug commonly associated with rashes (e.g. penicillin, sulphonamide, thiazide, allopurinol, phenylbutazone)
- A symmetrical eruption which may fit with a well-recognised pattern caused by one of the current drugs

Investigations

There are no specific investigations which help. Prick tests and in vitro tests for allergy are too unreliable for routine use. Readministration, as a diagnostic test, is usually unwise unless the reaction is mild and there is no suitable alternative drug.

Management

The first step is to withdraw the suspected drug(s). This may not be easy, or even possible, if there is no alternative

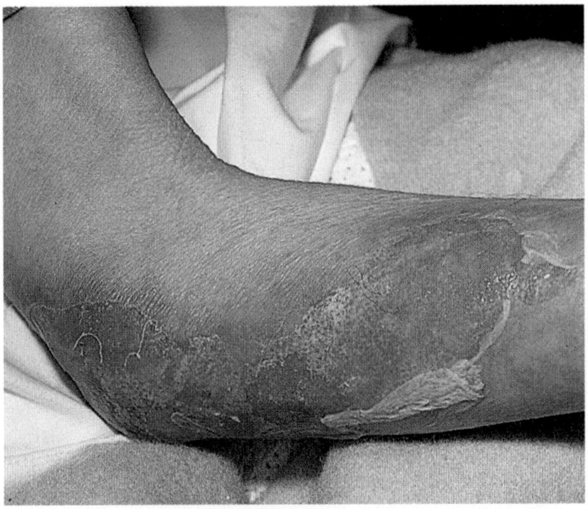

Fig. 13.37 Toxic epidermal necrolysis. In this case it was due to an anticonvulsant.

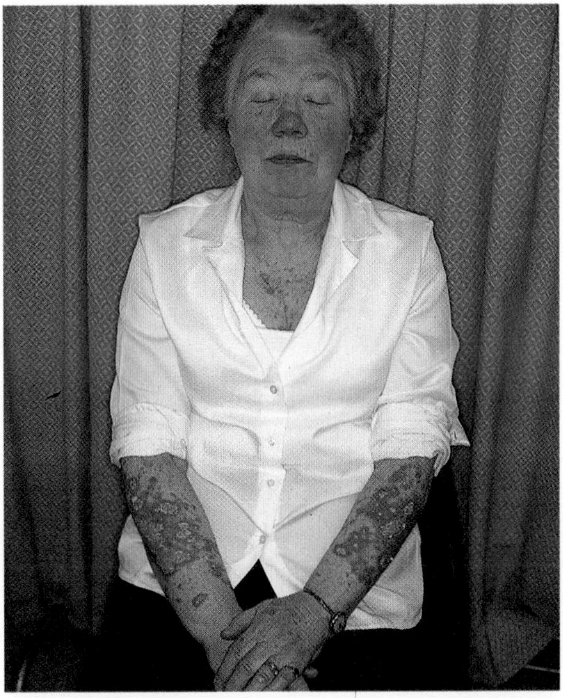

Fig. 13.38 Drug eruption. A weird but symmetrical erythematous scaly rash with a distribution suggesting a degree of photosensitivity. The rash persisted until the recently prescribed sulphonylurea was withdrawn.

available. The decision will depend on many factors, including the severity and nature of the drug reaction, its potential reversibility and the probability that the drug caused the reaction. Supportive treatment with antihistamines or a tailored course of systemic corticosteroids may be indicated, depending on the type of skin reaction. The emergency treatment of anaphylactic shock is described on page 1033.

FURTHER INFORMATION ON THE SKIN AND SYSTEMIC DISEASE

Powell F C, Su D, Perry H O 1996 Pyoderma gangrenosum: classification and management. Journal of the American Academy of Dermatology 34: 395–409

Schwartz R A 1994 Acanthosis nigricans. Journal of the American Academy of Dermatology 31: 1–19

Weissman K, Graham R M 1998 Systemic disease and the skin. In: Champion R H, Burton J L, Burns D A, Breathnach S M (eds) Textbook of dermatology, 6th edn, pp. 2703–2757. Blackwell Scientific, Oxford

FURTHER INFORMATION: THE SKIN AND SYSTEMIC DISEASE

Diseases of the nervous system 14

C.M.C. ALLEN • C.J. LUECK

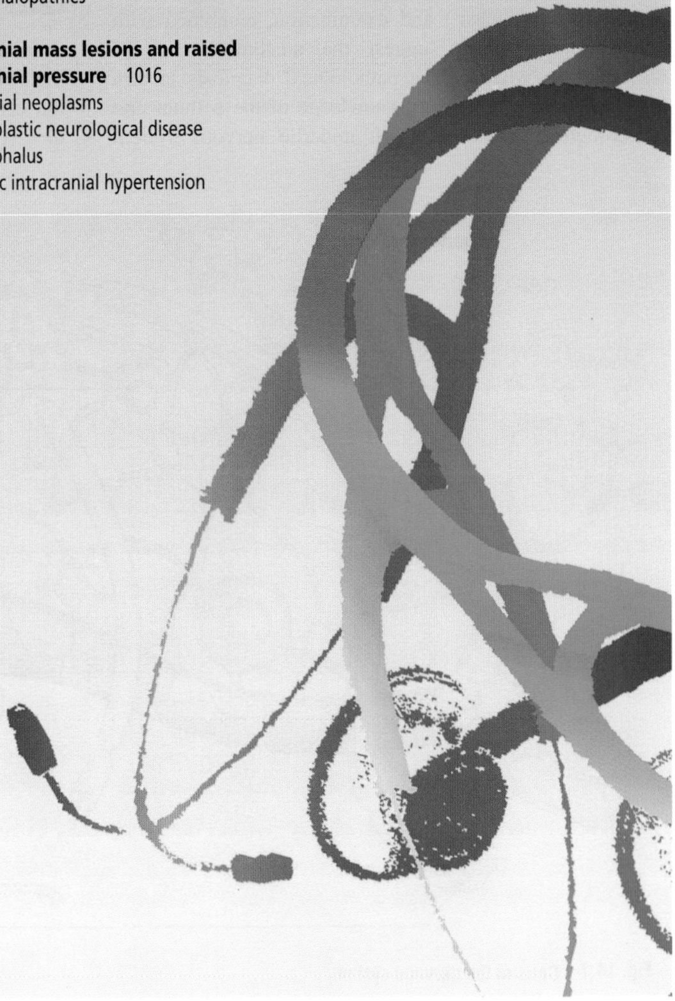

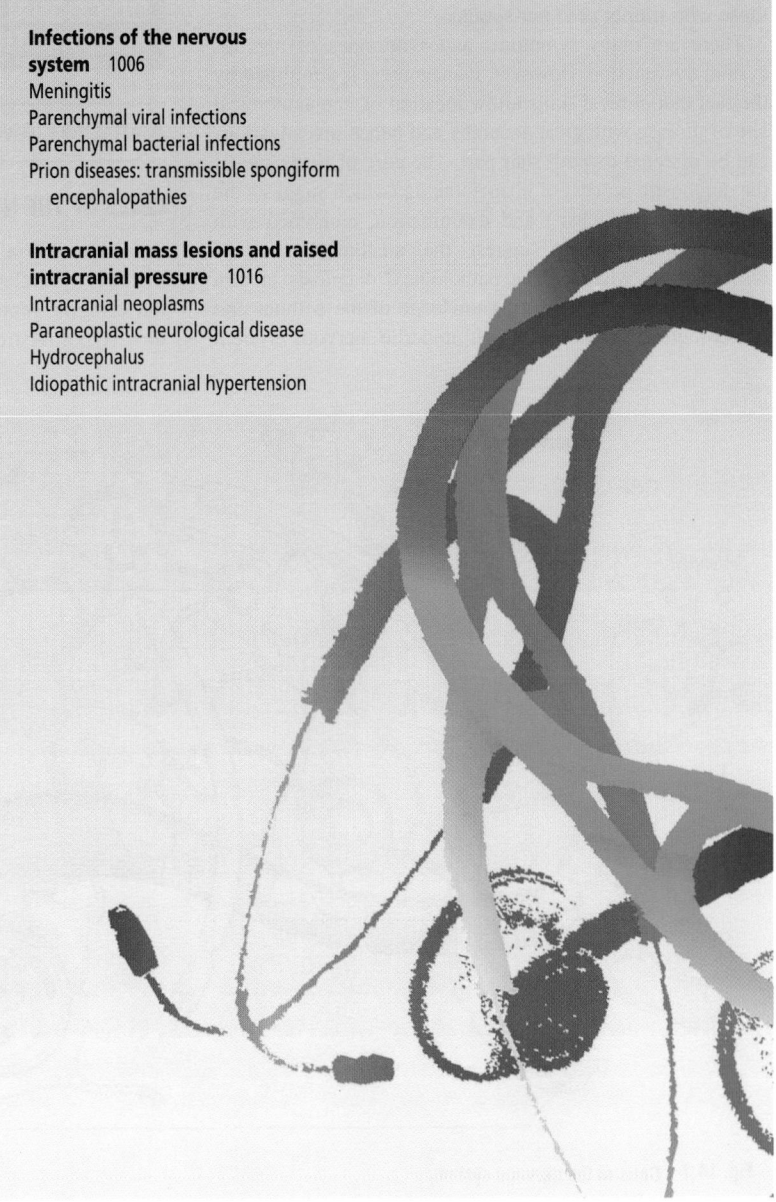

The brain, spinal cord and peripheral nerves constitute an organ responsible for perception of the environment, a person's behaviour within it and maintenance of the body's internal milieu in readiness for this behaviour. Disorders of the nervous system are responsible for about one-fifth of acute medical admissions and are also responsible for a large proportion of chronic physical disability. In the United Kingdom it has been estimated that nearly 10% of the population consult their general practitioner each year with a neurological symptom. Often such symptoms, whilst generating anxiety in the patient, are not associated with neurological disease and considerable clinical skill may be needed to distinguish those with significant disease from those who simply need reassurance.

There are many symptoms and syndromes of nervous system dysfunction. However, management is simplified by the fact that clinical skills allow location of the anatomical site of disease with great accuracy and hence investigations can be directed towards that part. The core of neurology is the diagnostic process of history-taking (which suggests the pathology—the 'what') and examination, combined with investigations (which suggest the anatomical site of disease—the 'where'). The pathological diagnosis in turn leads to therapy. Increasing knowledge of the cellular and physiological processes which underlie nervous system function provides the basis for the growing number of pharmacological interventions now available.

Once the patient's deficit is identified (the neurological diagnosis), the clinician needs to assess what impact this deficit has had on the patient's functioning (disability) and, in turn, how this is affecting his or her life (handicap). An increasing number of effective treatments are available for nervous system diseases, but management needs to be directed at correcting the patient's disability (and hence handicap), even if the pathological process cannot be corrected.

FUNCTIONAL ANATOMY, PHYSIOLOGY AND INVESTIGATIONS

ANATOMY AND PHYSIOLOGY

CELLS OF THE NERVOUS SYSTEM

In addition to a variety of neurons, the nervous system includes specialised blood vessels, ependymal cells lining the cerebral ventricles and glial cells, of which there are three types. Astrocytes form the structural framework for

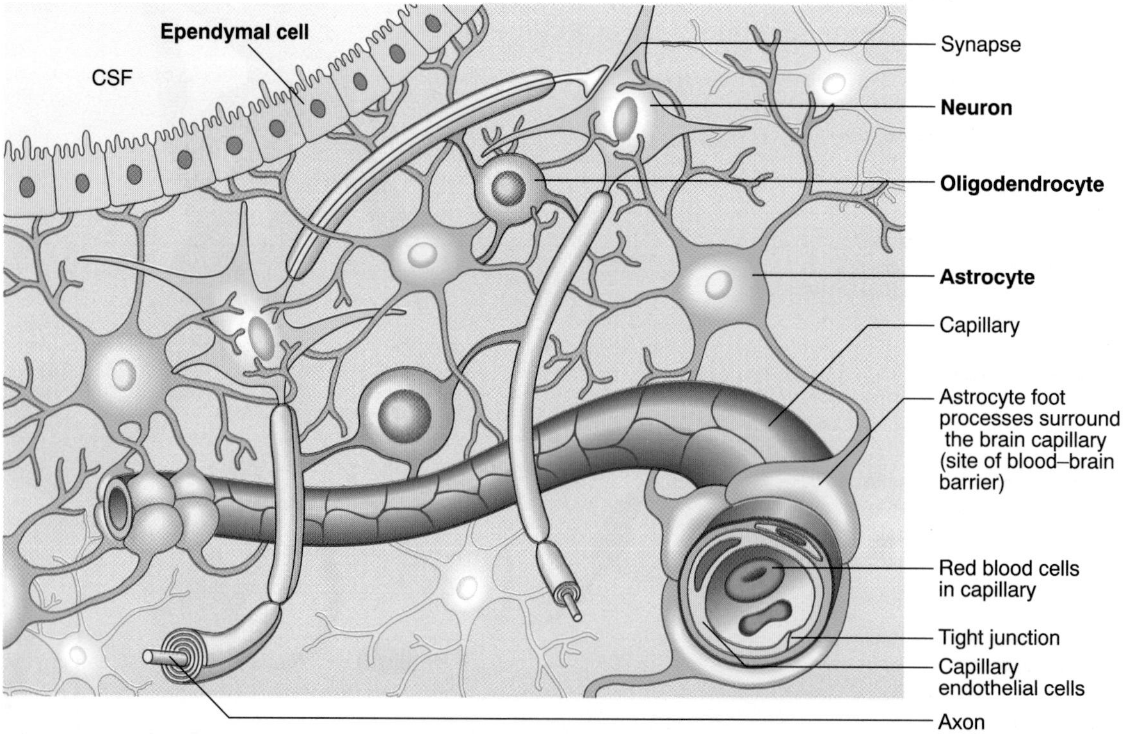

Fig. 14.1 Cells of the nervous system.

the neurons and control their biochemical environment. Astrocyte foot processes are closely associated with the blood vessels to form the blood–brain barrier (see Fig. 14.1). Oligodendrocytes are responsible for the formation and maintenance of the myelin sheath, which surrounds axons and is essential for the fast transmission of action potentials by saltatory conduction. Microglia are blood-derived mononuclear macrophages.

THE GENERATION AND TRANSMISSION OF THE NERVOUS IMPULSE

The functioning of the nervous system rests upon two physiological principles: the generation of an action potential with its conduction down axons, and the synaptic transmission of these impulses between neurons and/or muscle cells. Synaptic transmission involves the release from a neuron of neurotransmitter molecules which bind to specific receptors on the membrane of the receptor cell. These molecules alter either that cell's membrane potential (via effects, direct and indirect, upon ion channel permeability) or its metabolic function (see Fig. 14.2). There are over 20 different neurotransmitters known to act at different sites in the nervous system, all potentially amenable to pharmacological manipulation (see Table 14.1, p. 926).

The cell bodies of neurons are acted upon by synapses, both inhibitory and excitatory, with large numbers of other neurons. Each neuron therefore acts as a microprocessor, reacting to the influences upon it by changes to its cell membrane potential, causing it to be more or less ready to discharge an impulse down its axon(s). The synapsing neuron terminals are also subject to regulation by receptor sites on their pre-synaptic membrane, which modify the release of transmitter across the synaptic cleft. The effect of some neurotransmitters may be to produce long-term modulation of metabolic function or gene expression rather than simply to change the membrane potential. This effect probably underlies more complex processes in cognition, such as long-term memory.

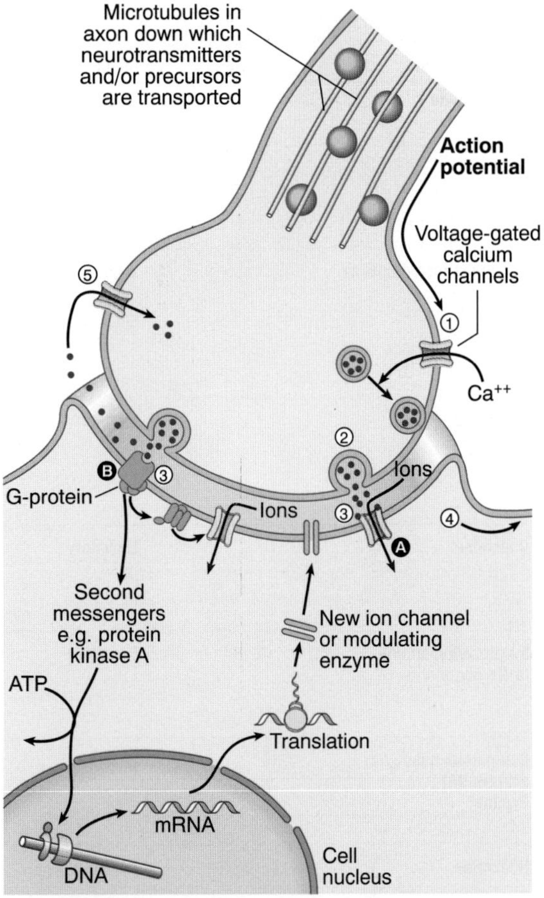

Fig. 14.2 Neurotransmission and neurotransmitters. (1) An action potential arriving at the nerve terminal depolarises the membrane and this opens voltage-gated calcium channels. (2) Entry of calcium causes the fusion of synaptic vesicles containing neurotransmitters with the pre-synaptic membrane and release of the neurotransmitter across the synaptic cleft. (3) The neurotransmitter binds to receptors on the post-synaptic membrane to either (A) open ligand-gated ion channels which, by allowing ion entry, depolarise the membrane and initiate an action potential (4), or (B) bind to metabotrophic receptors, which activate an effector enzyme (e.g. adenylyl cyclase) and thus via the intracellular second messenger system modulate gene transcription, leading to changes in synthesis of ion channels or modulating enzymes. (5) Neurotransmitters are taken up at the pre-synaptic membrane and/or metabolised.

MAJOR ANATOMICAL DIVISIONS OF THE NERVOUS SYSTEM (see Fig. 14.3, p. 927)

Cerebral hemispheres

The cerebral cortex constitutes the highest level of nervous function, the anterior half dealing with executive functions and the posterior half constructing a perception of the environment. Collections of cells in the depths of the hemispheres deal with motor control (the basal ganglia), the appropriate attention to sensory perception (the thalamus), emotion and memory (the limbic system) and control over internal bodily functions (the hypothalamus). The cerebral ventricles contain the choroid plexus; this produces the cerebrospinal fluid (CSF), which cushions the brain within the cranium. From the fourth ventricle the CSF leaves through foramina in the brain stem to circulate down around the spinal cord and over the surface of brain, where it is reabsorbed into the cerebral venous system (see Fig. 14.49, p. 1022).

The brain stem

In addition to containing all the sensory and motor

Table 14.1 Neurotransmitters

Neurotransmitter	Effect	Clinical relevance	Pharmacology
Acetylcholine	Excitatory	Alzheimer's disease Myasthenia Parkinson's disease Huntington's chorea Motion sickness Bladder control Vomiting	Donepezil Acetylcholinesterase inhibitors Anticholinergics
Noradrenaline/adrenaline	Excitatory	Migraine Mood disorders Cardiovascular control Bladder control Appetite Sleep disorders	α-blockers Clonidine Antidepressants Dexamphetamine β-blockers
Glutamate **Aspartate**	Excitatory	Cerebral ischaemia Epilepsy Memory Degenerative diseases (motor neuron disease)	Lamotrigine Riluzole
Dopamine	Excitatory	Parkinson's disease Schizophrenia Vomiting	L-dopa Dopamine agonists Major tranquillisers Metoclopramide
5-hydroxytryptamine (5-HT, serotonin)	Excitatory	Migraine Depression Pain Sleep	Pizotifen, sumatriptan Antidepressants
Gamma-aminobutyric acid (GABA) **Glycine**	Inhibitory	Epilepsy Spasticity	Phenobarbitone Anticonvulsants Benzodiazepines Baclofen
Histamine	Inhibitory	Uncertain	
Neuropeptides Vasopressin Adrenocorticotrophic hormone (ACTH) Melanocyte-stimulating hormone (MSH) Substance P Opioid peptides (> 20) e.g. endorphins, enkephalins, dynorphins	Excitatory and inhibitory	 Memory Uncertain Pain	
Purines Adenosine triphosphate/diphosphate (ATP/ADP) Adenosine monophosphate (AMP) Adenosine	Excitatory and modulation of neurotransmission	Uncertain	
Nitric oxide	Modulation of neurotransmission	Memory Cerebral ischaemia	

pathways entering and leaving the hemispheres, the brain stem houses the nuclei of the cranial nerves and other important collections of neurons. These are involved in the control of conjugate eye movements, the maintenance of balance, cardiorespiratory control and the maintenance of arousal.

The spinal cord

The spinal cord contains not only the afferent and efferent fibres arranged in functionally discrete bundles but also, in the grey matter, collections of cells which are responsible for lower-order motor reflexes and the primary processing of sensory information, including pain.

The peripheral nervous system

Afferent and efferent connections with the central nervous system are made by axons, which may be invested in myelin sheaths consisting of the wrapped membranes of the Schwann cells. The sensory cell bodies are situated in the dorsal root ganglia in the spinal exit foramina, whilst

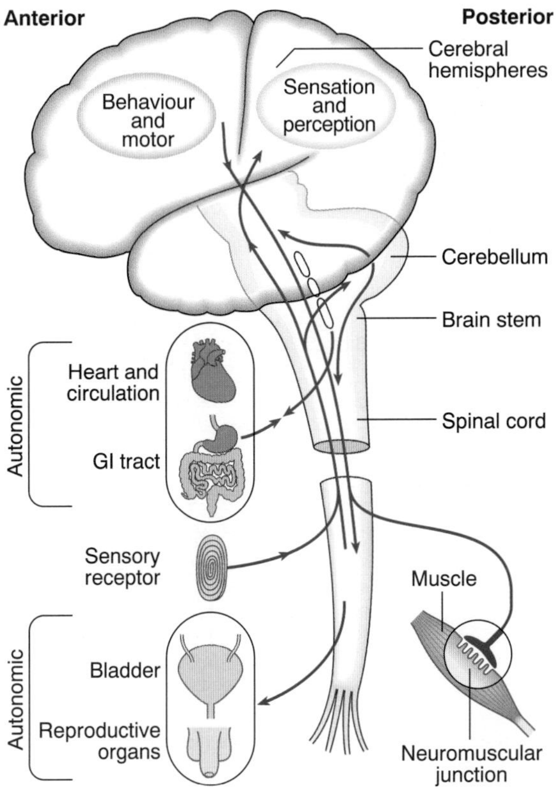

Fig. 14.3 The major anatomical components of the nervous system.

the distal ends of their neurons are invested with various specialised endings for the transduction of external stimuli into nervous impulses. The motor cell bodies are in the anterior horns of the spinal cord. Motor neurons initiate muscle contraction by the release of acetylcholine across the neuromuscular junction, with the resultant change in potential in the muscle end plate.

The autonomic system

The unconscious neural control of the body's physiology is effected through the autonomic system. This innervates the cardiovascular and respiratory systems, smooth muscle of the gastrointestinal tract, and glands throughout the body. The autonomic system is controlled centrally by diffuse modulatory systems in the brain stem, limbic system and frontal lobes, which are concerned with arousal and background behavioural responses to threat. The output of the autonomic system is divided functionally and pharmacologically into two divisions: the parasympathetic and sympathetic systems.

INVESTIGATION OF NEUROLOGICAL DISEASE

TESTS OF FUNCTION (CLINICAL NEUROPHYSIOLOGY)

In the investigation of neurological disease, tests of function have a somewhat more restricted application than tests of structure (i.e. imaging). Nevertheless, recording of electrical activity over the brain and assessment of nerve and muscle function are essential in certain conditions. The major tests are electroencephalography (EEG), evoked potentials (EPs), and nerve conduction studies/electromyography (NCS/EMG).

Electroencephalography

Electrical activity arising in the cerebral cortex can be detected using electrodes placed on the scalp, although this is estimated to detect only 0.1–1% of the brain's electrical activity at any one time. An array of electrodes provides spatial information. Rhythmical wave-forms can be detected and are distinguished by their frequency. When the eyes are shut, the most obvious frequency over the occipital cortex is 7–13/s; this is known as alpha rhythm, and disappears when the eyes are opened. Other frequency bands seen over different parts of the brain in different circumstances are beta (faster than 13/s), theta (4–6/s), and delta (slower than 4/s). Lower frequencies predominate in the very young, and during sleep.

Various diseases result in abnormalities of the EEG. These may be continuous or episodic, focal or diffuse. Examples of continuous abnormalities include a global increase in fast frequencies (beta) seen with sedating drugs (e.g. benzodiazepines), or marked slowing seen over a structural lesion such as a tumour or an infarct. With the advent of modern neuro-imaging, EEG has lost its use in localising lesions (except in the management of epilepsy—see below), but it is still useful in the management of patients who have disturbance of consciousness or disorders of sleep, in the diagnosis of cerebral diseases such as encephalitis and in certain dementias (e.g. Creutzfeldt–Jakob disease).

The most important use of EEG is in the management of epilepsy. It must be stressed, however, that only in rare circumstances will an EEG provide unequivocal evidence of epilepsy, and it is therefore not useful as a diagnostic test for the presence of epilepsy. Its use is predominantly to distinguish the type of epilepsy present, and whether there is an epileptic focus, particularly if surgery for epilepsy is contemplated.

During an epileptic seizure, high-voltage 'transients' can be recorded. These may be generalised, as in the 3 cycle/s 'spike and wave' of childhood absence epilepsy (petit mal), or more focal in partial epilepsies (see Fig. 14.4). However, it is unusual to record a seizure itself, except in the case of childhood absence epilepsy. Nevertheless, it is often

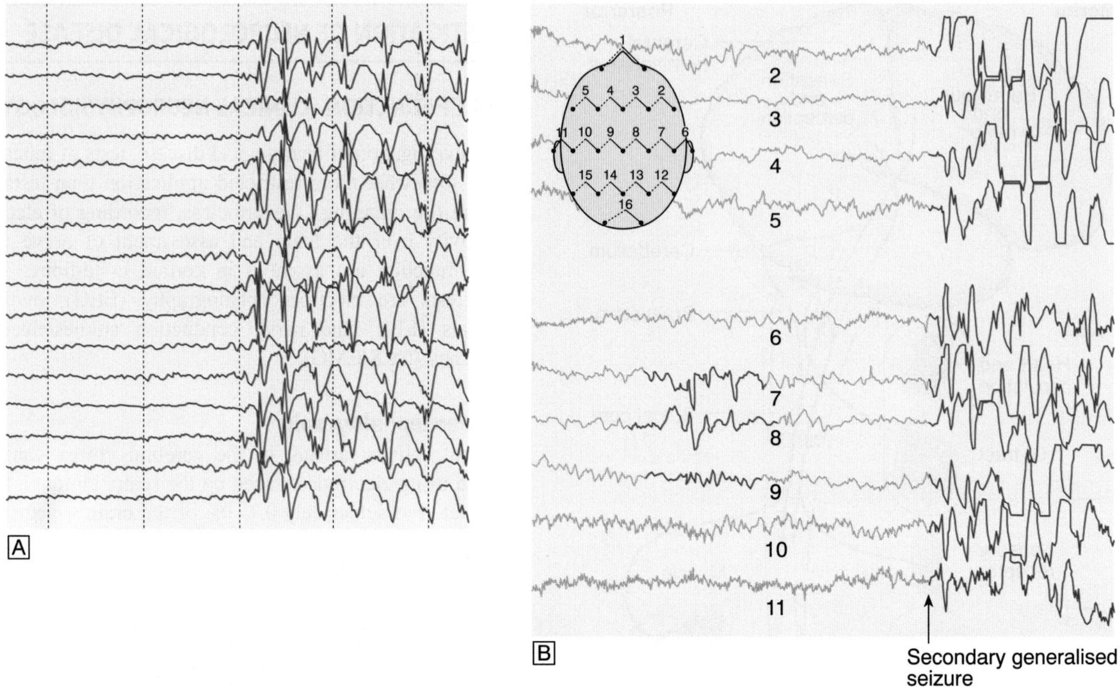

Fig. 14.4 EEGs in epilepsy. A Primary generalised epileptic discharge. B Focal sharp waves over the right parietal region (between electrodes 7 and 8—shown in purple) with secondary generalised discharge.

possible to detect 'epileptiform' abnormalities in between seizures in the form of 'spikes' and 'sharp waves' which lend support to a clinical diagnosis. The likelihood of detecting these abnormalities is enhanced by hyperventilation, photic flicker, sleep and some drugs. Note that even so, some 50% of patients with proven epilepsy will have a normal 'routine' EEG, and, conversely, the presence of features often seen in association with epilepsy does not, of itself, make a diagnosis (although the false positive rate for clear-cut epileptiform features is < 1/1000).

It is possible to enhance the information provided by a variety of means. For example, the usual 30-minute recording session can be lengthened to 24 hours by the use of a light-weight tape recorder. The addition of video information to the EEG allows comparison of behaviour with cerebral activity. In special circumstances, electrodes can be surgically positioned, e.g. through the foramen ovale, to record from the inferior temporal surface.

Evoked potentials

If a stimulus is provided—for example, to the eye—it would normally be impossible to detect the small EEG response evoked over the occipital cortex as the signal would be lost in background noise. However, if the EEG data from 100–1000 repeated stimuli are averaged electronically, this noise is removed and an evoked potential recorded whose latency and amplitude can be measured.

Evoked potentials can be measured following visual, auditory or somatosensory stimuli if electrodes are appropriately positioned, though visual evoked potentials are by far the most commonly used (see Fig. 14.5). Abnormalities of the evoked potential indicate damage to the relevant pathway, either in the form of a conduction delay (increased latency), or reduced amplitude, or both.

With the advent of magnetic resonance imaging (MRI), the use of evoked potentials is becoming much more restricted to specialised indications, such as providing a semi-objective measure of visual function.

Nerve conduction studies and electromyography

Using surface or needle electrodes, it is possible to record action potentials from nerves which lie close to the skin surface, as well as from muscles. If a nerve trunk is stimulated with a small electric potential, it is possible to record the resulting compound action potential (the sum of all the individual nerves' action potentials) as it travels down the nerve. A normal compound action potential would have an amplitude of 5–30 microvolts, depending upon the nerve. If the recorded potential is smaller than expected, this provides evidence of a reduction in the overall number of functioning axons. Central conduction times can be measured using electromagnetic induction of

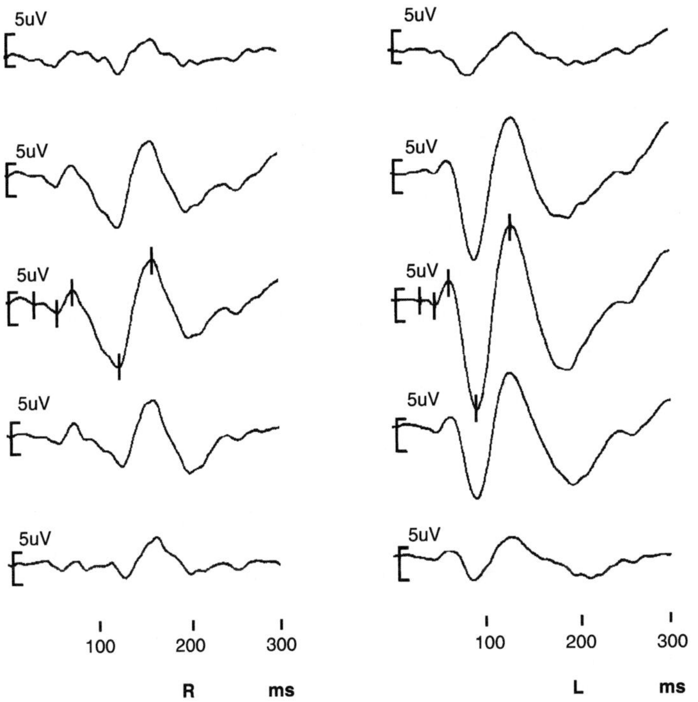

Fig. 14.5 Visual evoked responses (VER) recording showing delay on right.

action potential in the cortex or spinal cord by the local application of specialised coils.

Compound action potentials (CMAPs) can also be recorded over muscles in response to motor nerve stimulation. These are easier to record because the muscle amplifies the response, typical amplitudes being 1–20 millivolts. By measuring the response latency to stimulation of a nerve at two different points along its length, it is possible to calculate nerve conduction velocities (NCVs). This can be done for both sensory and motor nerves, and typical values are 50–60 m/s. Slowing of conduction velocity is suggestive of peripheral nerve demyelination which may be either diffuse (as in a demyelinating peripheral neuropathy) or focal (as in pressure palsies or conduction block).

The principal use of nerve conduction studies is to identify damage to peripheral nerves, and to determine whether the pathological process is focal or diffuse and whether the damage is principally axonal or demyelinating. It is also possible to obtain some information about nerve roots by more sophisticated analysis of responses to impulses initially conducted antidromically to the spinal cord, and then returning orthodromically to the stimulation point (F waves).

Fine concentric needle electrodes can be inserted into muscle bellies themselves and the potentials from individual motor units recorded. It is possible to record abnormal spontaneous activity arising from muscles at rest, such as fibrillations (a sign of denervation) or myotonic discharges. Abnormalities in the shape and size of muscle potentials can help in the differential diagnosis of denervation and structural muscle diseases. Myopathies caused by metabolic abnormalities (causing electromechanical dissociation rather than loss of fibre structure) show no changes on needle EMG.

Electromyography can also be used to investigate the neuromuscular junction. Repetitive stimulation of a nerve with trains of electrical impulses at 3–15/s does not normally result in a significant fall-off in the amplitude of the resulting muscle action potential. However, such a decrement is seen in myasthenia gravis (see p. 997), and provides one of the key diagnostic features. Augmentation of the response to repetitive stimulation is seen in the Lambert–Eaton myasthenic syndrome, though usually at higher stimulation frequencies.

Imaging

Imaging is crucial to the identification of lesions of the nervous system in disease. There are various techniques, based on the use of X-rays (plain radiographs, computed tomography (CT), myelography and angiography), magnetic resonance (MR imaging—MRI—or MR angiography), ultrasound (Doppler imaging of blood vessels), and radioisotopes (single photon emission computerised tomography (SPECT) and positron emission tomography (PET)). The indications, usefulness and limits of each technique are listed in Table 14.2 on page 930. The application of various techniques depends upon the area of the neuraxis which is being investigated.

Table 14.2 Techniques available for imaging the nervous system

Technique	Principle	Applications	Advantages	Disadvantages	Comments
X-ray	Attenuation of X-ray beam by radio-opaque substances (calcium, metal, contrast etc.)	Plain radiographs CT Radiculography Myelography Contrast angiography	Widely available Relatively cheap Relatively quick	Ionising radiation Reactions to contrast Myelography and angiography are invasive and therefore carry risks	In neurology, plain radiographs only demonstrate fracture or foreign bodies CT is investigation of choice for trauma and stroke Intra-arterial X-ray contrast angiography still 'gold standard'
Magnetic resonance imaging (MRI)	Magnetic resonance of different tissues depends on free hydrogen/water content. Signals changed by movement (e.g. flowing blood)	Structural imaging MR angiography (MRA) Functional MR MR spectroscopy	High-quality soft tissue delineation Better views of posterior fossa and temporal lobes No ionising radiation Non-invasive	Expensive Not yet widely available Angiography looks at blood flow, not anatomy Scans uncomfortable/claustrophobic	Increasing application Functional MR and MR spectroscopy still research tools
Ultrasound	Echoes from high-frequency sound source localise structure Doppler phenomenon used to measure rate of flow	Doppler Duplex scans	Cheap Quick Non-invasive	Operator-dependent Poor anatomical definition	Useful as screening tool
Radioisotope imaging	Radio-labelled isotopes bind to structure(s) of interest, or used to assess relative blood flow	Isotope brain scan SPECT PET	In vivo demonstration of functional anatomy (e.g. ligand binding, blood flow)	Poor spatial resolution Ionising radiation Expensive, especially PET Not widely available	Isotope scans now obsolete SPECT and PET largely research tools

(CT = computerised tomography; PET = positron emission tomography; SPECT = single photon emission computerised tomography)

Head and orbit

The use of plain skull radiographs is largely restricted to the diagnosis of fractures and sinus disease. CT or MRI is needed to image pathology inside the skull. Which of these two scans is used depends on what information is being sought and, to some extent, how urgently it is required, as CT is often more easily available than MRI. CT will show bone and calcium well, and will easily image collections of blood. It will also detect abnormalities of the brain and ventricles, such as atrophy, tumours, cysts, abscesses, vascular lesions and hydrocephalus. Diagnostic yield is often improved by the use of intravenous contrast and spiral CT methods. It is, however, limited in its ability to image the posterior fossa (because of the surrounding bone density), and it is poor at detecting abnormalities of white matter and at allowing detailed analysis of grey matter.

MRI is much more useful in the investigation of posterior fossa disease as it is not affected by the surrounding bone. It is much more sensitive than CT to abnormalities of white and grey matter, and is therefore useful in the investigation of inflammatory conditions such as multiple sclerosis, and in investigating epilepsy. MRI can also provide additional information about structural brain lesions which may complement that available from CT. It is also useful in imaging the orbits, where special imaging sequences can be used to compensate for orbital fat, and thereby allow clear views of extraocular muscles, optic nerve and other orbital structures.

Standard isotope brain scans are of little value in assessing structure if other imaging facilities are available. However, the blood flow and function of the cerebral hemispheres can be assessed by using either SPECT or PET. Examples of brain imaged by the various techniques are shown in Figure 14.6.

The neck

Plain radiographs of the neck are useful in the investigation of structural damage to vertebrae, such as that resulting from trauma or inflammatory damage (e.g. rheumatoid arthritis). They can also provide implicit information about intervertebral disc disease, but not detailed information about the cervical cord or nerve roots, for which myelography or MRI is needed.

Myelography is invasive. Potential complications include headache, seizures and meningitis. With the advent of MRI its use is declining. Nevertheless, it is still of value if MRI is not available, or the patient cannot tolerate lying within an MRI scanner. Radio-opaque contrast is injected into the lumbar theca and then moved up to the cervical region by tilting the patient. The contrast outlines the nerve roots and spinal cord, thereby providing information about abnormal structure. Examples of the neck imaged by plain radiographs, myelography and MRI are shown in Figure 14.7 on page 932.

Lumbo-sacral region

Imaging of this region is similar to imaging the neck and plain radiographs are of limited use. Contrast can be injected into the lumbar thecal space and used to outline the lower nerve roots only (radiculography), or it can be run up

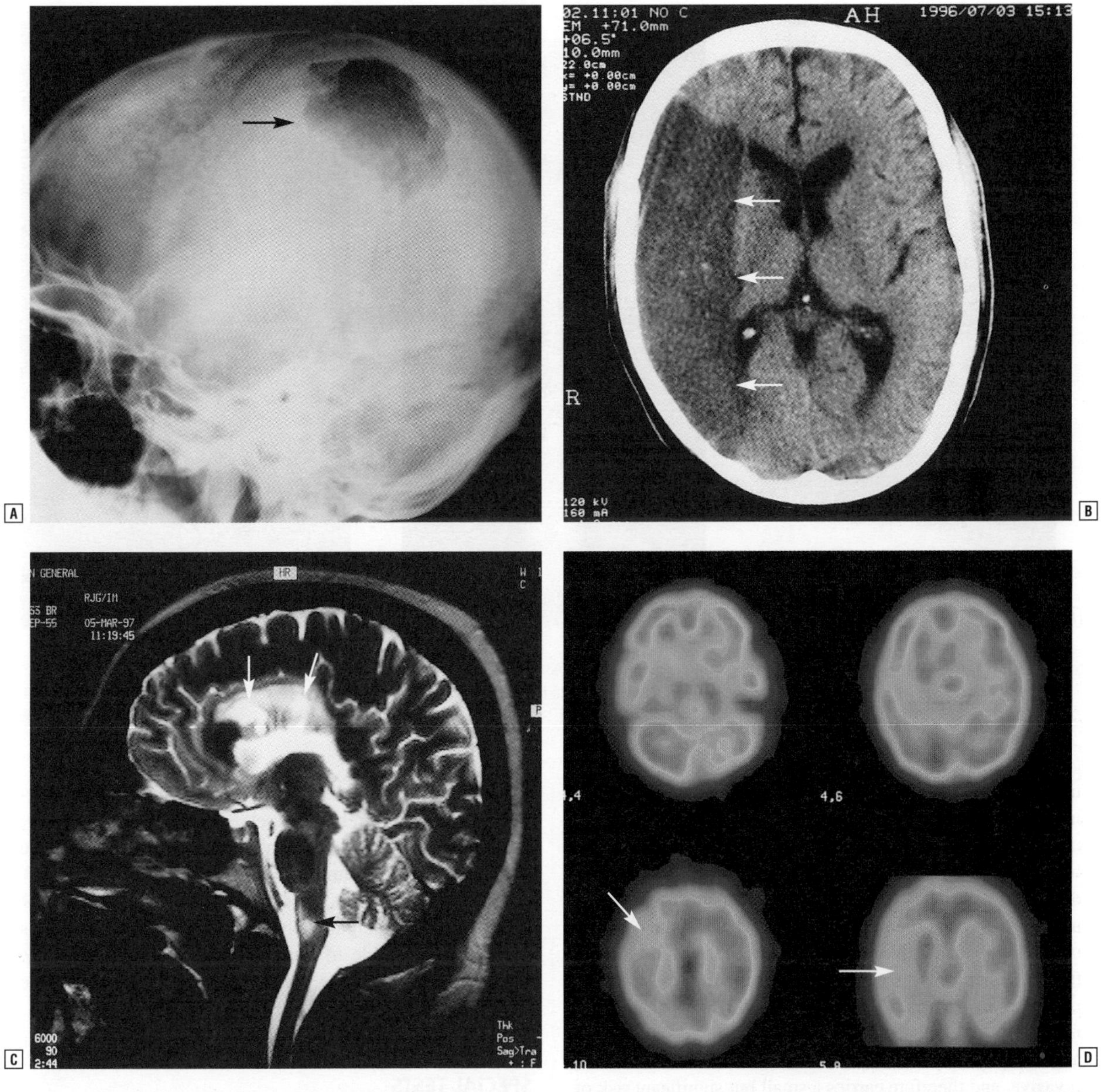

Fig. 14.6 Different techniques of imaging head and brain. A Skull radiograph showing lytic vault lesion (eosinophilic granuloma—arrow). B CT showing complete middle cerebral artery infarct (arrows). C MRI showing widespread areas of high signal in multiple sclerosis (arrows). D SPECT after caudate infarct shows relative hypoperfusion of overlying right cerebral cortex (arrows).

to outline the conus and spinal cord (myelography). The information obtained may be enhanced by the additional use of CT following myelography. Non-contrast CT of the lumbar spine can be used to image the vertebrae and discs, but nervous tissue cannot be distinguished from CSF, although the addition of contrast by myelography allows individual nerve roots to be seen. As with the cervical spine, MRI provides a non-invasive way of obtaining high-resolution images of both the vertebral column and the relevant neural structures.

Blood vessels

Various techniques are available to investigate extracranial and intracranial blood vessels. The least invasive is that of

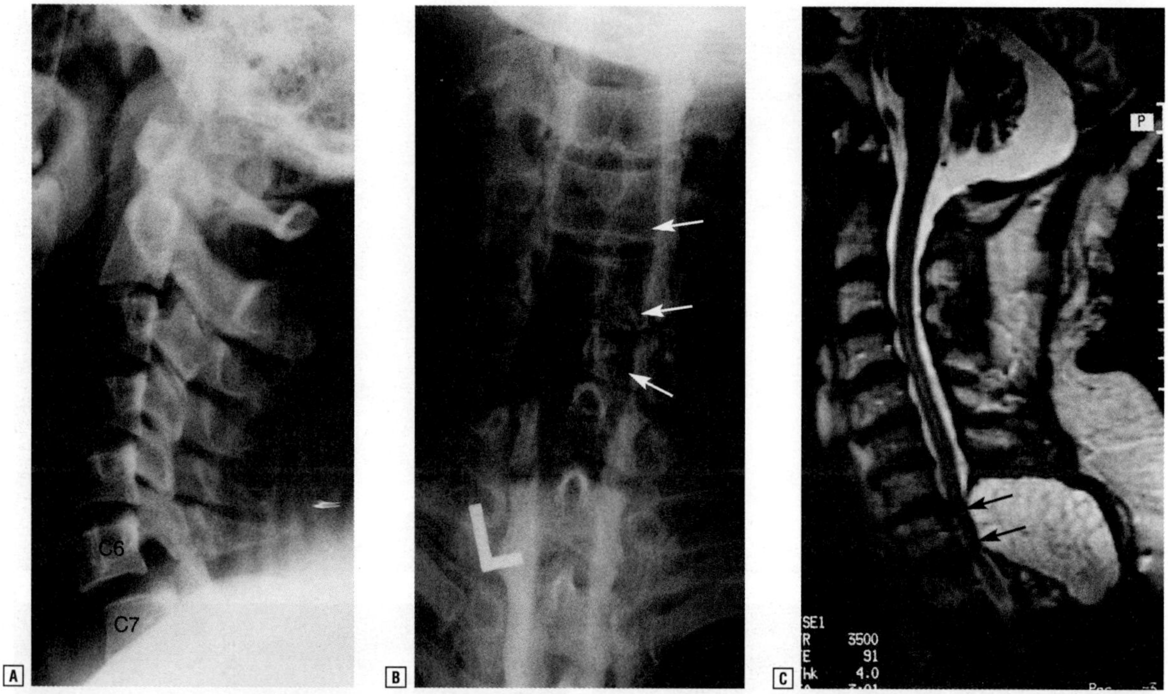

Fig. 14.7 Different techniques of imaging cervical spine. A Lateral radiograph showing bilateral C6/7 facet dislocation. B Myelogram showing widening of cervical cord due to astrocytoma (arrows). C MRI showing posterior epidural compression from adenocarcinomatous metastasis to the posterior arch of T1 (arrows).

ultrasound (Doppler or duplex scanning), which is used to investigate the carotid and the vertebral arteries in the neck, usually as part of the investigation of stroke. In skilled hands, reliable information can be provided about the degree of arterial stenosis, and the technique often gives useful anatomical information, e.g. whether there is an ulcerating plaque. Information concerning the blood flow in the intracerebral vessels is also becoming increasingly possible using transcranial Doppler. The anatomical resolution of Doppler imaging is limited, and formal angiography may still be required. The latter is, however, invasive, and therefore carries a small but significant risk of stroke, or even death. Thus, the major role of Doppler imaging is as a screening test to determine whether invasive angiography is indicated.

Blood vessels can be outlined by the injection of radio-opaque contrast. The X-ray images obtained can be enhanced by the use of computer-assisted digital subtraction, or by the use of spiral CT. Contrast may be injected intravenously or intra-arterially. The former requires a much higher total dose of contrast, and the images obtained are not as good, but the latter involves feeding catheters up through the arterial tree, and is thus associated with a higher complication rate. Formal intra-arterial angiography is required to delineate lesions of the extracranial carotid artery prior to endarterectomy, and is also used to investigate abnormalities of intracerebral vessels such as arterial (berry) aneurysms or arteriovenous malformations, or to delineate the blood supply of tumours prior to surgery.

Flowing blood can be detected by specialised MR sequences in MR angiography. The anatomical resolution is still not comparable to that of intra-arterial angiography, but the investigation is non-invasive. Examples of these different techniques are given in Figure 14.8.

SPECIAL TESTS

Blood tests

Many systemic conditions affect the nervous system and these can often be diagnosed with the help of blood tests: for example, confusion due to hypothyroidism, a stroke due to systemic lupus erythematosus, ataxia due to vitamin B_{12} deficiency, or myelopathy due to syphilis. The blood tests relating to general medical conditions which affect the nervous system are dealt with in the sections dealing with the conditions themselves.

There are, however, a number of blood tests which are used in investigating specific neurological diseases. These include haematological tests (e.g. looking for acanthocytes

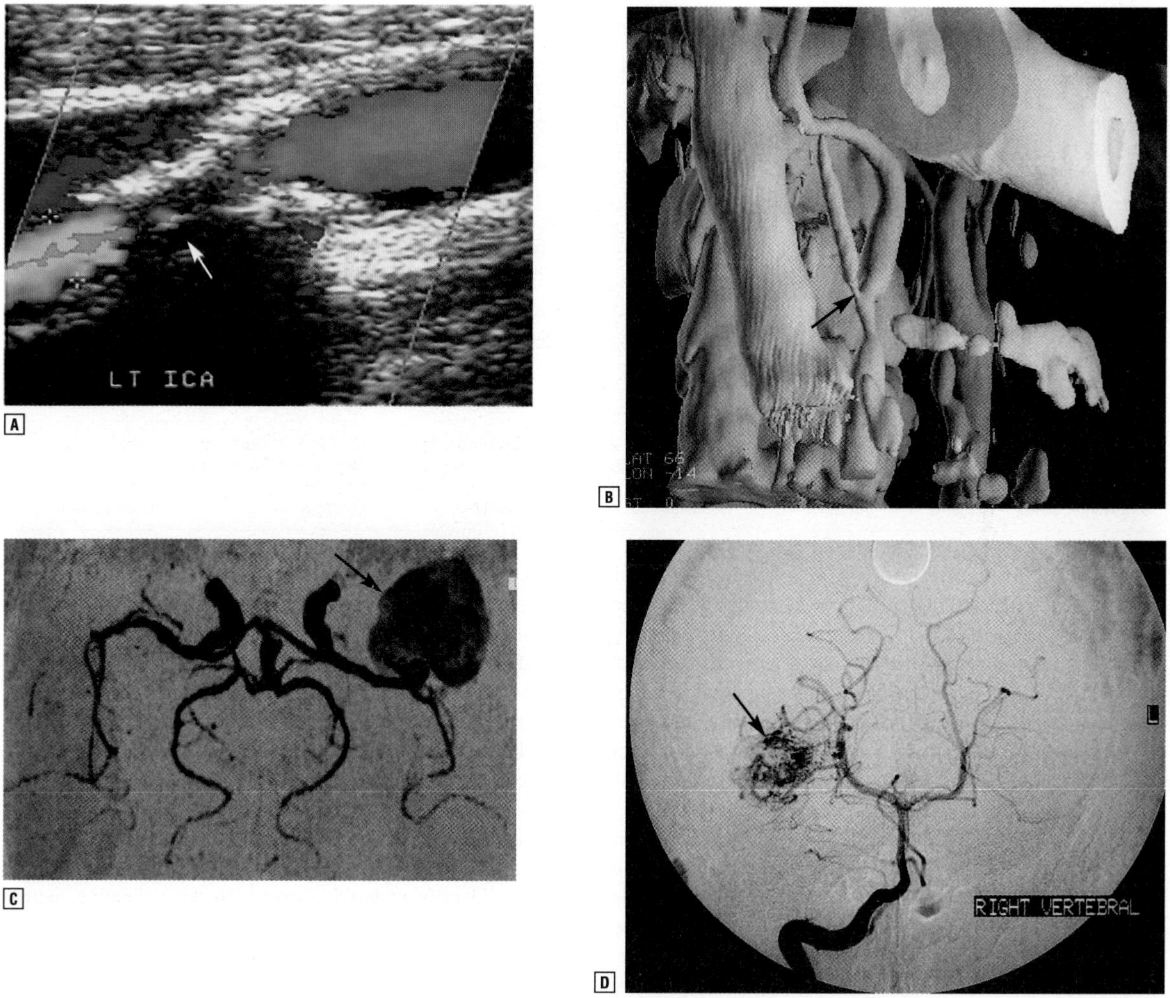

Fig. 14.8 Different techniques of imaging blood vessels. A Doppler scan showing 80% stenosis of internal carotid artery (arrow). B 3-D reconstruction of CT angiogram showing stenosis at the carotid bifurcation (arrow). C MR angiogram showing giant aneurysm at the middle cerebral artery bifurcation (arrow). D Intra-arterial angiography showing arteriovenous malformation (arrow).

to diagnose neuroacanthocytosis), biochemical tests (e.g. creatine kinase in muscle diseases, copper studies to diagnose Wilson's disease) or tests to help diagnose innumerable infections of the nervous system. In addition, there are a number of specific antibodies which are useful diagnostically. These include antibodies to acetylcholine receptors and skeletal muscle, seen in myasthenia gravis, and to voltage-gated calcium channels in Lambert–Eaton myasthenic syndrome. Antibodies to different types of ganglioside (glycoproteins expressed on nerve membranes) can be seen in various types of neuropathy including multifocal motor neuronopathy, and the Guillain–Barré syndrome (particularly the Miller Fisher variant). Also, antineuronal antibodies provide markers of paraneoplastic cerebellar or neuropathic syndromes.

An increasing number of inherited neurological conditions can now be diagnosed by DNA analysis. These include diseases caused by increased numbers of trinucleotide repeats, such as Huntington's disease, myotonic dystrophy and some types of spinocerebellar ataxia. Also, defects of mitochondrial DNA can be detected in many conditions including Leber's hereditary optic neuropathy, and some syndromes causing epilepsy or stroke-like syndromes.

Lumbar puncture

This involves the insertion of a needle between lumbar spinous processes, through the dura and into the cerebrospinal fluid (CSF) under local anaesthetic. The intracranial pressure can be measured and CSF removed for analysis. CSF is normally clear and colourless. Tests usually per-

Table 14.3 CSF parameters in health and some common disorders

	Normal	Subarachnoid haemorrhage	Acute bacterial meningitis	Viral meningitis	Tuberculous meningitis	Multiple sclerosis
Pressure	50–180 mm	Increased	Normal/increased	Normal	Normal/increased	Normal
Colour	Clear	Blood-stained Xanthochromic	Cloudy	Clear	Clear/cloudy	Clear
Red cell count	0–4/mm^3	Raised	Normal	Normal	Normal	Normal
White cell count	0–4/mm^3	Normal/slightly raised	1000–5000 polymorphs	10–2000 lymphocytes	50–5000 lymphocytes	0–50 lymphocytes
Glucose	> 60% of blood level	Normal	Decreased	Normal	Decreased	Normal
Protein	< 0.5 g/l	Increased	Increased	Normal/increased	Increased	Normal/increased
Microbiology	Sterile	Sterile	Organisms on Gram stain and/or culture	Sterile/virus detected	Ziehl–Neelsen/auramine stain or TB culture positive	Sterile
Oligoclonal bands	Negative	Negative	Not measured	Not measured	Not measured	Often positive

formed on CSF include centrifuging to determine the colour of the supernatant (which is yellow or xanthochromic some hours after subarachnoid haemorrhage), biochemistry (glucose, total protein, and protein electrophoresis to detect oligoclonal bands), microbiology, immunology (e.g. Venereal disease reference laboratory (VDRL) test—see p. 184, paraneoplastic antibodies) and cytology (to detect malignant cells). Normal values for these tests, and various abnormalities found in diseases are shown in Table 14.3.

Lumbar puncture is indicated in the investigation of infections (e.g. meningitis or encephalitis), subarachnoid haemorrhage, inflammatory conditions (e.g. multiple sclerosis, sarcoidosis and cerebral lupus) and some neurological malignancies (e.g. carcinomatous meningitis, lymphoma and leukaemia), and to measure CSF pressure (e.g. in idiopathic intracranial hypertension). It is, of course, part of the procedure of myelography, and can be part of therapeutic procedures, either to lower CSF pressure, or to administer drugs.

If there is a space-occupying lesion in the head, lumbar puncture can result in a shift of intracerebral contents downwards, towards and into the spinal canal. This process is known as coning, and is potentially fatal (see p. 1017). Consequently, lumbar puncture is contraindicated if there is any suggestion of raised intracranial pressure (e.g. papilloedema), depressed level of consciousness, or focal neurological signs suggesting a cerebral lesion, until imaging of the head (by CT or MRI) has excluded a space-occupying lesion or hydrocephalus.

About 30% of lumbar punctures are followed by low-pressure headache, which can be severe. Other minor complications involve transient radicular pain during the procedure, and pain over the lumbar region. Provided the test is performed under sterile conditions, infections such as meningitis are extremely rare. Lumbar puncture is contraindicated in anticoagulated patients but not in those on aspirin.

Biopsies

Nerve and muscle are occasionally biopsied to assist in the diagnosis and management of a number of neurological conditions. Likewise, it is occasionally necessary to biopsy brain or meninges.

Nerve is biopsied as part of the investigation of peripheral neuropathies. Usually, the sural nerve is sampled at the ankle or the radial nerve at the wrist. Histology is often able to help identify underlying causes in demyelinating neuropathies (e.g. vasculitic) or, occasionally, infiltration with abnormal substances such as amyloid. However, nerve biopsy is not performed unless it is reasonably likely to diagnose a potentially treatable condition such as an inflammatory neuropathy, since there is an appreciable morbidity risk.

Skeletal muscle biopsy is performed more frequently. The quadriceps muscle is often sampled, though this depends somewhat on which muscles are affected. Indications include the investigation of primary muscle disease, as muscle histology can be used to distinguish neurogenic wasting, myositis and myopathy, which may be difficult to distinguish clinically. Histology and enzyme histochemistry can also be helpful in the diagnosis of more widespread metabolic disorders, such as mitochondrial and some storage diseases. Though pain and infection can follow the procedure, these are much less of a problem than following nerve biopsy.

The nature of lesions demonstrated by brain imaging can often be inferred from the appearances as well as the history, examination and other, less invasive, investigations. However, there are situations in which the nature of lesions is not clear, and it is important to obtain tissue for histological examination. Likewise, it is sometimes necessary to biopsy the brain parenchyma itself in unexplained degenerative diseases (e.g. unusual dementias) so as not to miss potentially treatable disease.

Brain biopsy used to require full craniotomy. However, owing to the increased availability and sophistication of cerebral imaging, it is now possible to biopsy most lesions stereotactically through a burr hole in the skull. The complication rate of such stereotactic biopsies is much lower than that of open craniotomy, but haemorrhage, infection and death still occur. Hence, brain biopsy is only considered if diagnosis cannot be reached in any other way.

FURTHER INFORMATION ON FUNCTIONAL ANATOMY, PHYSIOLOGY AND INVESTIGATIONS

Aminoff M J 1992 Electrodiagnosis in clinical neurology, 3rd edn. Churchill Livingstone, New York

Bear M F, Connors B W, Paradiso M A 1996 Neuroscience: explaining the brain. Williams & Wilkins, Baltimore

Nolte J, Angevine J B 1995 The human brain: in photographs and diagrams. Mosby, St Louis

Yock D H 1995 Magnetic resonance imaging of CNS disease: a teaching file. Mosby, St Louis

MAJOR MANIFESTATIONS OF NERVOUS SYSTEM DISEASE

HEADACHE AND FACIAL PAIN

Headache is one of the most frequent neurological symptoms encountered in primary care and hospital practice, and yet is seldom associated with significant neurological disease unless accompanied by other symptoms or neurological signs. Nevertheless, patients suffering from headaches frequently fear serious brain disease. In order to manage patients effectively, it is important to be aware of this mismatch between a patient's fear of disease and its actual likelihood. Careful clinical assessment will usually allow the identification of one of a limited number of headache or facial pain syndromes (see the information box). After taking a careful history and performing the appropriate neurological examination, it is often not necessary to perform further investigations. The patient can be reassured and provided with symptomatic treatment.

COMMON HEADACHE AND FACIAL PAIN SYNDROMES

- Tension headache
- Migraine
- Cluster headache
- Raised intracranial pressure
- Benign paroxysmal headaches (see Table 14.4, p. 938)
- Trigeminal neuralgia
- Atypical facial pain
- Post-herpetic neuralgia

Pathophysiology

It is often difficult to explain the pain of headaches, especially in those not caused by serious disease, by reference to current neurobiological understanding of the mechanisms of pain. Within the skull the dura (including the dural sinuses and falx cerebri) and the proximal parts of the large pial blood vessels are the main structures sensitive to pain. The brain parenchyma, pial arteries over the convexities, and the cerebral ventricles and choroid plexus are known to be insensitive to pain. The pain-sensitive intracranial structures are mostly innervated by branches of the trigeminal nerve and some by branches of the upper cervical nerves. This probably accounts for the patterns of pain referral seen in intracranial disease when these pain-sensitive parts of the intracranial contents are stretched, distended or otherwise irritated.

A DIAGNOSTIC APPROACH TO THE PATIENT WITH HEADACHE

Unless the history is suggestive of structural disease, patients with headache who are normal on neurological examination are unlikely to have a serious disorder, however distressing their symptoms. The features of a patient's history which are helpful in making a clear diagnosis of the cause of a headache are shown in the information box.

IMPORTANT POINTS IN THE HEADACHE HISTORY

- The tempo of onset
- The time of day of onset of maximal pain
- The effect of posture, coughing and straining
- The location of the pain
- Any associated symptoms

Patients can be divided into those with chronic headache (a duration of several weeks or more) and those with more acute headache. Serious acute neurological disease should always be considered in patients with headaches of very sudden onset. Subarachnoid haemorrhage (see p. 978) causes a very sudden headache which may or may not be localised, although only one person in eight who has such a 'thunderclap' headache will have had a subarachnoid haemorrhage. A patient with subarachnoid haemorrhage almost invariably develops other symptoms including vomiting and neck stiffness, though the latter may take some hours to develop. The main differential diagnosis in a patient with a sudden severe headache is between subarachnoid haemorrhage and a migraine variant. Meningitis occasionally presents apoplectically, but the headache is usually less dramatic in onset.

Headache coming on over a matter of hours is less likely to be associated with structural disease and more likely to be due to migraine, unless accompanied by other significant symptoms or signs. Patients with bacterial meningitis are usually generally ill and pyrexial, and exhibit meningism. Patients with viral meningitis may present with a pyrexia and quite sudden and severe headache coming on over an hour or so but are less likely to have neck stiffness or other signs of meningism. Migraine headaches (see below) may be accompanied or preceded by vomiting and focal neurological symptoms (usually in the form of zigzag 'fortification spectra' or tingling moving slowly over part of the body).

When headaches are intermittent rather than continuous over a period of days or weeks they are most likely to be migrainous but it is worth while paying attention to the time of day they occur and the presence or absence of precipitating factors. The headache of raised intracranial pressure is present on waking and often resolves or improves as the patient becomes upright (reducing the intracranial pressure) or takes simple analgesia (see the information box). It is unusual for a patient to present with such a headache alone since it is usually not sufficiently severe to cause alarm, the presentation of the causative mass lesion being provoked by a seizure or by focal neurological dysfunction (aphasia, hemiplegia etc.). The exceptions to this are patients with acute hydrocephalus who present with a more severe headache. As with other causes of raised intracranial pressure, this is worse when lying, bending forward or coughing, and frequently causes vomiting in the morning (especially in children). Hydrocephalus may cause no other symptoms except gait ataxia, though examination may reveal papilloedema.

Headaches that persist for weeks, are present all day, and are poorly responsive to simple analgesia are very likely to be tension headaches, whatever their other characteristics. Headaches so well localised by the patient that a finger is used to locate the exact spot on the skull are never associated with significant disease.

HEADACHE OF RAISED INTRACRANIAL PRESSURE

- Worse in morning, improves through the day
- Associated with morning vomiting
- Worse bending forward
- Worse with cough and straining
- Relieved by analgesia
- Dull ache, often mild

In a patient over 60 years with a head pain localised to one or both temples, giant cell arteritis (see p. 864) should be considered, especially if the temporal pulses are not palpable and/or the arteries are enlarged and tender.

TENSION HEADACHE

Clinical features

This is the most common type of headache and may be experienced at some time by the majority of the population in some form. The pain is usually constant and generalised but often radiates forward from the occipital region. It is described as 'dull', 'tight' or like a 'pressure', and there may be a sensation of a band round the head or pressure at the vertex. In contrast to migraine, the pain may continue for weeks or months without interruption, although the severity may vary, and there is no associated vomiting or photophobia. The patient can usually continue normal activities and the pain may be less noticeable when the patient is occupied. The pain is characteristically less severe in the early part of the day and becomes more troublesome as the day goes on. Local tenderness may be present over the skull vault or in the occiput but this should be distinguished from the acute pain precipitated by skin contact in trigeminal neuralgia and the exquisite tenderness of temporal arteritis. Typically, the headache is reported to be poorly responsive to ordinary analgesia.

Pathogenesis

The cause of tension headaches is obscure. There is little evidence for the hypothesis that it is caused by excessive contraction of the muscles of the head and neck. Emotional strain or anxiety are common precipitants to tension headache and there is sometimes an underlying depressive illness. Anxiety about the headache itself may lead to continuation of symptoms, and patients often become convinced of a serious underlying condition.

Management

Careful assessment, and explanation of likely precipitants and that the symptoms are not due to any sinister underlying pathology are more likely to be beneficial than analgesics. There is evidence that patients with this syndrome benefit from a perception that their problem has been taken seriously and rigorously assessed, but over-extensive investigations can worsen a patient's anxiety. Courses of muscle relaxation and stress management may help.

MIGRAINE

Clinical features

Patients may refer to any episodic paroxysmal headache as migraine. However, it is best to look upon migraine as a triad of paroxysmal headache, vomiting and focal neurological events (usually visual). Patients with all three of these features are said to have classical migraine. Those with just paroxysmal headache with or without vomiting but no classical focal events are said to have common migraine. It has been estimated that the lifetime prevalence of migraine is about 20% of females and 6% of males. Over 90% of migraine sufferers will have their first attack by the time they are 40 years old. Typically, a classical migraine attack starts with a non-specific prodrome of malaise and irritability followed by the 'aura' of a focal neurological event, a severe throbbing hemicranial headache, photophobia and vomiting. During the headache phase patients prefer to be in a quiet, darkened room and go to sleep. The headache may persist for several days.

The aura of migraine is most often in the form of 'fortification spectra', shimmering silvery zigzag lines which march across the visual fields over 20 minutes, sometimes leaving a trail of visual field loss. In some patients there is a spreading front of tingling followed by numbness which moves, over 20–30 minutes, from one part of the body to another, or even aphasia when the dominant side is involved. Weakness rather than sensory symptoms in migraine is distinctly unusual and 'hemiplegic migraine' should be diagnosed with extreme caution. In some patients the focal events may occur by themselves ('migraine equivalent') but other, structural disorders of the brain, or focal epilepsy, need then to be considered in the differential diagnosis.

Aetiology and pathogenesis

The aetiology of migraine is largely unknown. There is often a family history of migraine, suggesting a genetic predisposition. The great female preponderance and the tendency for some women to have migraine attacks at certain points in their menstrual cycle hint at hormonal influences. The relevance of the contraceptive pill in this context is difficult to establish. In some patients there are identifiable dietary precipitants such as cheese, chocolate or red wine. When psychological stress is involved, the migraine attack often occurs after the period of strain so that some patients tend to have attacks at weekends or at the beginning of a holiday.

The 'aura' of classical migraine probably represents a spreading front of excitation followed by a depression of activity of cortical cells. The cause of this is not understood but probably represents a paroxysmal alteration in cortical modulation pathways from the brain stem (especially serotoninergic projections). The headache is caused by vasodilatation of extracranial vessels and may, like the headache following an epileptic seizure, be a non-specific effect of intracranial metabolic disturbance.

Management

Identification and avoidance of precipitants may prevent attacks. Treatment of an acute attack consists of simple analgesia with aspirin or paracetamol with an antiemetic such as metoclopramide. This is best in the form of effervescent combined preparations which enable better absorption. Severe attacks can be treated with sumatriptan, a 5-HT agonist which is a potent vasoconstrictor of the extracranial arteries, given either by subcutaneous injection or orally. Ergotamine preparations, whilst effective in some patients, should be avoided since they easily lead to a situation where headaches occur due to withdrawal of the ergotamine, establishing a vicious circle. This seems less likely to occur with sumatriptan. If attacks are frequent, prevention of migraine can be effected by propranolol (80–160 mg daily, preferably in a sustained-release preparation), pizotifen (a 5-HT antagonist, 1.5–3.0 mg daily) or a tricyclic such as amitriptyline (10–50 mg at night).

MIGRAINOUS NEURALGIA (CLUSTER HEADACHE)

Clinical features

This is a migraine variant, some 10–50 times less common than migraine. There is 5:1 predominance of males, with the onset usually in the third decade. The characteristic syndrome comprises periodic, severe unilateral periorbital pain, often accompanied by a Horner's syndrome (including conjunctival injection), unilateral lacrimation and nasal congestion. The pain, whilst being very severe, is characteristically brief (30–90 minutes). Typically, the patient develops these symptoms at a particular time of day (often in the early hours of the morning). The syndrome may occur repeatedly for a number of weeks, followed by a respite for a number of months before another cluster occurs.

Pathogenesis

There is little genetic predisposition and no provoking dietary factors which, along with the male predominance, suggest a different aetiology from that of classical migraine. Patients are usually heavy smokers with a higher than average alcohol consumption.

Management

Acute attacks may be reliably halted with subcutaneous injections of sumatriptan; other migraine therapies are ineffective, probably because of the brevity of the individual attacks. Preventive therapy with the agents used for migraine is often ineffective but attacks can be prevented in some patients with verapamil (80–120 mg 8-hourly), methysergide (4–10 mg daily, for a maximum of 3 months only), or short courses of corticosteroids. Patients with severe and debilitating clusters can be helped with lithium therapy although the usual precautions concerning the use of this drug should be observed (see p. 1081).

COITAL AND EXERCISE-INDUCED CEPHALGIA

Clinical features

Patients are almost exclusively middle-aged men who develop a sudden, often very severe, headache at the climax of sexual intercourse. There is usually no vomiting and no neck stiffness, and the severe headache does not persist for more than 10–15 minutes, though a less severe dull headache may persist for some hours. This type of paroxysmal headache often needs to be distinguished, by CT scan and/or CSF examination, from the thunderclap headache of a subarachnoid haemorrhage. A very similar headache may occur during physical exertion, especially if this is attempted with unaccustomed vigour in an unfit person.

Management

Coital or exertional cephalgia is usually brief though frightening and may not need more than ordinary analgesia for the residual headache. The syndrome may not recur and may be prevented with propranolol (as for migraine) or indomethacin (75 mg daily).

Other paroxysmal headaches are described in Table 14.4.

A DIAGNOSTIC APPROACH TO PATIENTS WITH FACIAL PAIN

Pain in and around the eye, when not caused by ocular disease, should be considered as a headache (above). This includes the dramatic pain of migrainous neuralgia or cluster headache. Rarely, pain in or around the eye may be caused by inflammatory or infiltrative lesions at the apex of the orbit or the cavernous sinus behind but tell-tale signs from involvement of the ocular motor nerves usually accompany this. Pain in the eye may accompany disorders of the carotid artery, particularly dissections, and may then be accompanied by a Horner's syndrome.

Pain in the other parts of the face can be due to problems with the teeth or the temporo-mandibular joint. Inflamed nasal sinuses are seldom the cause of lasting facial pain in the absence of obvious nasal congestion. The very rare but serious condition of subdural empyema needs to be considered if 'sinusitis' is followed by very severe unilateral facial pain and signs of cerebral irritation (seizures and/or obtundation). Destructive lesions of the trigeminal nerve causing pain are extremely rare since such lesions usually cause loss of sensation in the nerve's territory rather than pain.

Most patients with persisting pain in the face have trigeminal neuralgia, atypical facial pain or post-herpetic neuralgia. The main distinction between these is in the nature of the pain. In trigeminal neuralgia the pain is very brief, though severe and recurrent, described as 'like sheet lightning', most frequently in the second division of the nerve. Atypical facial pain, on the other hand, is continuous and unremitting, centred over the maxilla, usually on the left side, and occurs most frequently in middle-aged women. Post-herpetic neuralgia is continuous and is felt as a burning pain throughout the affected territory which is often very sensitive to light touch. The cause is usually obvious from a history of 'shingles' in the ophthalmic division of the trigeminal nerve.

TRIGEMINAL NEURALGIA

Clinical features

This condition causes very sharp lancinating pains in the second and third divisions of the trigeminal nerve territory, usually in middle-aged or elderly patients. The pain is severe and very brief, but repetitive, causing the patient to flinch as if with a motor tic, hence the French term for the condition, 'tic douloureux'. The pain may be precipitated by touching trigger zones within the trigeminal territory or by eating etc. Usually there are no other signs, although trigeminal neuralgia may occur in advanced multiple sclerosis or, rarely, with other lesions, in which case there may be sensory changes in the trigeminal nerve territory or other brain-stem symptoms and signs. There is a tendency for the condition to remit and relapse over many years.

Pathogenesis

The current hypothesis as to aetiology suggests that the neuralgia is most commonly caused by compression of the

Table 14.4 Benign paroxysmal headaches

Headache type	Character of pain	Duration	Location	Comment
Ice pick	Stabbing	Very brief (split-second)	Variable, usually temporal or parietal	Benign, more common in migraineurs
Ice cream	Sharp, severe	30–120 seconds	Bitemporal/occipital	Obvious trigger by cold stimuli
Exertional	Bursting	Minutes to hours	Generalised	Intracranial pathology needs excluding
Cough	Bursting	Seconds to minutes	Occipital or generalised	Intracranial pathology needs excluding (especially cranio-cervical junction)

trigeminal nerve rootlets at their entry to the brain stem by aberrant loops of the cerebellar arteries. Other compressive lesions, usually benign, are occasionally found in this site. When trigeminal neuralgia occurs in multiple sclerosis there is a plaque of demyelination in the trigeminal root entry zone.

Management

The pain usually responds to carbamazepine, in doses of up to 1200 mg daily. It is wise to start with much lower doses and escalate the dose according to effect, as one might when using this drug for epilepsy. In patients who cannot tolerate carbamazepine, phenytoin may be effective, but other anticonvulsants are not. If drug treatment fails and/or when the condition does not remit, various surgical treatments are available. The simplest is the injection of alcohol or phenol into a peripheral branch of the nerve. Probably more effective is the percutaneous placing of a radiofrequency lesion in the nerve near the Gasserian ganglion. Care has to be taken not to cause excessive damage to sensation in the face to prevent the complication of neurogenic pain ('anaesthesia dolorosa') which is worse than the neuralgia. Alternatively, the vascular compression of the trigeminal nerve can be relieved through a small posterior craniotomy, often with substantial success. This latter approach is usually favoured in younger patients in whom the other injection treatments may have to be repeated and become less effective.

DIZZINESS, BLACKOUTS AND 'FUNNY TURNS'

Episodes of lost or altered consciousness are a frequent symptom in primary care and in hospital practice, especially in the elderly (see p. 1070). A patient may complain of 'blacking out', 'going dizzy', 'coming over queer', 'having a funny turn' or other local variants. The first task is to discover exactly what the patient means by the terms used. Some patients, for example, mean by 'blackout' that their vision darkens without alteration in consciousness (defined here as an awareness of the environment and ability to respond to it). More often 'blackout' is used to describe an episode of lost consciousness with or without falling down. The terms 'blackout' or 'funny turn' can also be used to refer to transient periods of amnesia, when the patient loses memory for a period of time. 'Dizziness' is used frequently to describe an abnormal perception of movement of the environment (vertigo), but may be used to mean a feeling of faintness, some other alteration of consciousness, or unsteadiness.

After a careful history from the patient, supplemented by a witness account, it should be clear whether the patient is describing an episode of loss of consciousness, altered consciousness, vertigo, transient amnesia or something else. The former two symptoms suggest a problem in mechanisms maintaining normal awareness. Vertigo is caused by an alteration in function of the peripheral vestibular organs or the central control mechanisms of balance and posture.

A DIAGNOSTIC APPROACH TO THE PATIENT WITH VERTIGO

Abnormal perception of movement of the environment occurs as a result of a mismatch of the information about a person's position in the environment reaching the brain from the eyes, the limb proprioceptive apparatus, and the vestibular system. Vertigo arising from inappropriate input from the labyrinthine apparatus is within the experience of most people, since this is the 'dizziness' which occurs after someone has spun round vigorously and then stops. Vertigo caused by labyrinthine disorders is usually short-lived, though it may recur, whilst vertigo arising from central disorders (of the brain stem) is often persistent and accompanied by other signs of brain-stem dysfunction. A careful analysis of the history will reveal the likely cause in most patients. Figure 17.4 (see p. 1071) outlines the assessment of dizziness in elderly patients.

VERTIGO CAUSED BY LABYRINTHINE DISTURBANCES

Labyrinthitis ('vestibular neuronitis')

This is the most common cause of severe vertigo, assumed to be due to a self-limiting infection of the labyrinth, presenting usually in the third or fourth decade as severe vertigo, with vomiting and ataxia, often coming on when waking. The vertigo is most severe at onset and settles down over the next few days, though afterwards vertigo may be provoked by head movement (positional vertigo) for some time. During the attack nystagmus will be present but does not persist for long.

Benign paroxysmal positional vertigo

In older patients paroxysms of vertigo occurring with certain head movements may be due to the presence of degenerative material obstructing the free flow of endolymph in the labyrinth (cupulolithiasis). Each attack of vertigo lasts seconds but the patient often becomes very distressed and reluctant to move the head, which can in turn produce a muscle tension type of headache. Positional vertigo may also occur after concussive head injuries.

Ménière's disease

This is a cause of labyrinthine vertigo which is probably diagnosed too readily. Patients usually present first with tinnitus and distorted hearing, and then develop paroxysmal attacks of vertigo preceded by a sense of fullness in the ear. Examination in this circumstance shows sensorineural hearing loss on the affected side.

Symptomatic relief of labyrinthine causes of vertigo can be achieved with 'vestibular sedatives' (e.g. cinnarizine, prochlorperazine, betahistine). Positional vertigo can be improved with exercises which are designed to habituate the central mechanisms to the inappropriate signals from the labyrinth. Patients with intractable symptoms should be referred to an ENT specialist for assessment.

CENTRAL CAUSES OF VERTIGO

Any disease that affects the vestibular nucleus in the brain stem or its connections can cause vertigo. This can be distinguished from peripheral causes of vertigo by its persistence, and the usual association of other signs. Positionally induced central vertigo persists for as long as the position is maintained, unlike the common peripheral positional vertigo which fatigues quite quickly if the inducing position is maintained. The same is true of any accompanying nystagmus. Transient causes such as brain-stem ischaemia can be recognised by the association with other symptoms of brain-stem dysfunction such as dysarthria or diplopia. If deafness is present and the history is not suggestive of Ménière's disease, extra-axial compression of the 8th cranial nerve by a lesion such as an acoustic neuroma (see p. 1020) should be suspected. Rarely, vertigo originating from the cerebral cortex may be a manifestation of a partial seizure in the temporal lobe.

A DIAGNOSTIC APPROACH TO THE PATIENT WITH EPISODIC LOSS OF CONSCIOUSNESS

Loss of consciousness, other than in sleep, suggests a global dysfunction of the brain. As a transient phenomenon, this most commonly comes about because of a recoverable loss of adequate blood supply to the brain, i.e. syncope (see below). Alternatively, loss of consciousness occurs from sudden dysfunction of the electrical control mechanisms of the brain during a seizure (fit). Episodes of loss of consciousness are therefore either fits or faints. This clear categorisation is confused by some patients who have various types of psychogenic blackout or non-epileptic seizure.

The distinction of a seizure from a faint can only be made from an analysis of the history from the patient and from someone who witnessed the attack. No amount of investigation can replace a clear history in these circumstances. Features in the history useful in distinguishing a seizure from a faint are shown in Table 14.5.

Table 14.5 Features helpful in distinguishing seizures from faints

	Seizure	Faint
Aura (e.g. olfactory)	+	–
Cyanosis	+	–
Tongue-biting	+	–
Post-ictal confusion	+	–
Post-ictal amnesia	+	–
Post-ictal headache	+	–

SYNCOPE

A faint is often preceded by a brief feeling of 'light-headedness'; vision then darkens and there may be a ringing in the ears. Vasovagal syncope (see p. 225) may be provoked by some emotionally charged event (e.g. venepuncture) and almost always occurs from the standing position. Cardiac syncope (see p. 225), caused by a sudden decline in cardiac output and hence cerebral perfusion, may be provoked by exertion (e.g. with severe aortic stenosis), or occur completely 'out of the blue' (as in heart block). The loss of consciousness is brief, and the patient recovers quickly as long as he or she has assumed the horizontal position. In vasovagal syncope the loss of consciousness is gradual and rarely associated with injury. There is no amnesia for events that occur after regaining awareness. During a syncopal attack incontinence of urine can occur and there may be some stiffening of the limbs and even some brief twitching of the limbs, but tongue-biting never occurs.

SEIZURES

A seizure is any abnormal clinical event caused by an electrical discharge from the brain, whilst epilepsy is a tendency to have seizures (see p. 942). Major seizures cause loss of consciousness, with the patient falling to the ground and presenting with a history of 'blackouts'. Minor seizures causing alteration of consciousness, without the patient falling to the ground, may also be described as 'blackouts'.

Pathophysiology

In the normally functioning cortex, synchronous discharge amongst neighbouring groups of neurons is limited by recurrent and collateral inhibitory circuits. The inhibitory transmitter gamma-aminobutyric acid (GABA) is particularly important in this role and drugs which block GABA receptors provoke seizures. There are also a large number of excitatory neurotransmitters, of which acetylcholine and the amino acids glutamate and aspartate are examples (see

Table 14.1, p. 926). 'Epileptic' cerebral cortex exhibits hypersynchronous repetitive discharges involving large groups of neurons. Intracellular recordings show bursts of rapid-action potential firing, with reduction of the transmembrane potential (paroxysmal depolarisation shift). It is likely that both reduction in inhibitory systems and excessive excitation play a part in the genesis of seizure activity. Cells undergoing repetitive 'epileptic' discharges undergo morphological and physiological changes which make them more likely to produce subsequent abnormal discharges ('kindling').

The chief division of seizure types on physiological grounds is between partial (focal) seizures in which paroxysmal neuronal activity is limited to one part of the cerebrum, and generalised seizures where the electrophysiological abnormality involves both hemispheres simultaneously and synchronously (see Fig. 14.9). If partial seizures remain localised, the symptomatology depends on the cortical area affected. If consciousness (the awareness of, and ability to respond to, the environment) is preserved, the attack is termed 'simple'. If, however, the activity involves some parts of the brain dealing with awareness (such as the temporal or frontal lobes), then consciousness is affected and a 'complex partial seizure' results. Further spread into the diencephalon and thence throughout the remainder of the cortex leads to a secondarily generalised seizure.

In primary generalised seizures, the abnormal activity is seen to begin synchronously throughout the cortex without an initial partial onset. It probably originates in the central diencephalic mechanisms controlling cortical activation (see Fig. 14.9). This is recognisable on an EEG which shows spikes and waves of abnormal activity (see Fig. 14.4, p. 928) and quite often provocation of abnormalities with hyperventilation and/or photic stimulation. This may cause a major seizure identical to a secondarily generalised seizure, or a more restricted clinical manifestation if the abnormal electrical activity fails to affect muscle tone. In this case there is an 'absence', in which consciousness is lost but the patient remains standing or sitting in an attack which may be difficult to distinguish clinically from a complex partial seizure in the temporal lobe.

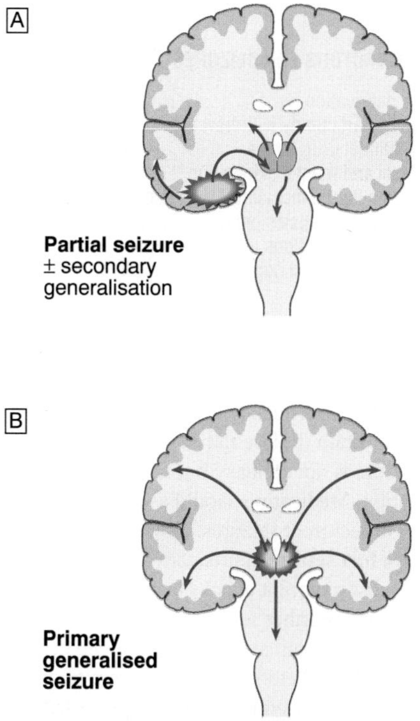

Fig. 14.9 The pathophysiological classification of seizures. A A partial seizure originates from a paroxysmal discharge in a focal area of the cerebral cortex (often the temporal lobe); the seizure may subsequently spread to the rest of the brain (secondary generalisation) via diencephalic activating pathways. B In primary generalised seizures the abnormal electrical discharges originate from the diencephalic activating system and spread simultaneously to all areas of the cortex.

Clinical features

Tonic clonic seizures

A tonic clonic seizure may be preceded by a partial seizure (the 'aura') which can take various forms, described below. However, a history of such an 'aura' is commonly not obtained, probably because the subsequent seizure causes some retrograde amnesia for immediately preceding events. The patient then goes rigid and becomes unconscious, falling down heavily if standing, often sustaining injury. During this phase, respiration is arrested and central cyanosis may be witnessed. After a few moments, the rigidity is periodically relaxed, producing clonic jerks. Some patients do not have a clonic phase and the rigidity is replaced by a flaccid state of deep coma which can persist for some minutes. The patient then gradually regains consciousness, but is in a confused and disorientated state for half an hour or so after regaining consciousness. Full memory function may not be recovered for some hours. During the attack urinary incontinence may occur, as may tongue-biting. (A severely bitten, bleeding tongue after an attack of loss of consciousness is pathognomonic of a generalised seizure.) After a generalised seizure the patient usually feels terrible, may have a headache, and will want to sleep. Witnesses of a seizure are usually frightened by the events, often believing the person to be dying, and may not give a clear account; this is in itself a helpful diagnostic pointer since syncope seldom produces such fear in onlookers.

Patients may have no tonic or clonic phase, and may not become cyanosed or bite their tongue. However, post-ictal confusion or headache and a period of subsequent malaise and/or confusion are usually seen, and this is useful in differentiating seizures from faints. Psychogenic non-epileptic attacks ('pseudo-seizures') may be accompanied by dramatic flailing of the limbs and arching of the back; however, these usually are not followed by the same degree of post-ictal confusion, and never cause cyanosis.

Complex partial seizures

Partial seizures may cause episodes of altered consciousness without the patient collapsing to the ground, especially if arising from the temporal or, less frequently, the frontal lobe. These may be referred to as 'blackouts'. The patient stops what he or she is doing and stares blankly, often making rhythmic smacking movements of the lips or displaying other automatisms, such as picking at their clothes. After a few minutes the patient returns to consciousness but may be initially muddled and feel drowsy. Immediately before such an attack the patient may report alterations of mood, memory and perception such as undue familiarity (déjà vu) or unreality (jamais vu), complex hallucinations of sound, smell, taste, vision, emotional changes (fear, sexual arousal), or visceral sensations (nausea, epigastric discomfort). If these changes of memory or perception occur without subsequent alteration in awareness the seizure is said to be a simple partial seizure.

Absence seizures

A type of minor seizure which resembles a complex partial seizure occurs in the generalised absence epilepsy of childhood, and is known as 'petit mal'. The attacks in petit mal are usually briefer and very much more frequent (20 or 30/day) than complex partial seizures and are not associated with post-ictal confusion. Absence attacks are caused by a generalised discharge which does not spread out of the hemispheres and so does not cause loss of posture.

Partial motor seizures

Epileptic activity arising in the precentral gyrus causes partial motor seizures affecting the contralateral face, arm, trunk or leg. Seizures are characterised by rhythmical jerking or sustained spasm of the affected parts. They may remain localised to one part, or may spread to involve the whole side. Some attacks begin in one part (e.g. mouth, thumb, great toe) and spread gradually; this is Jacksonian epilepsy. Attacks vary in duration from a few seconds to several hours. More prolonged episodes may leave paresis of the involved limb lasting for several hours after the seizure ceases (Todd's palsy).

Partial sensory seizures

Seizures arising in the sensory cortex cause unpleasant tingling or 'electric' sensations in the contralateral face and limbs. A spreading pattern like a Jacksonian seizure may occur, the abnormal sensation spreading much faster over the body (in seconds) than the 'march' of a migrainous focal sensory attack, which spreads over 10–15 minutes.

Versive seizures

A frontal epileptic focus may involve the frontal eye field, causing forced deviation of the eyes to the opposite side. This type of attack often becomes generalised to a tonic clonic seizure.

Partial visual seizures

Occipital epileptic foci cause simple visual hallucination such as balls of light or patterns of colour. Formed visual hallucinations of faces or scenes arise more anteriorly in the temporal lobes.

Factors precipitating seizures

Sometimes specific trigger factors can be identified. Some are listed in the information box.

TRIGGER FACTORS FOR SEIZURES

- Sleep deprivation
- Alcohol (particularly withdrawal)
- Recreational drug abuse
- Physical and mental exhaustion
- Flickering lights, including TV and computer screens (primary generalised epilepsies only)
- Intercurrent infections and metabolic disturbances
- Uncommonly: loud noises, music, reading, hot baths

EPILEPSY

Epilepsy means a tendency to have seizures and is a symptom of brain disease rather than a disease itself. A single seizure is not epilepsy but an indication for investigation. Medication should await evidence of a tendency to recurrent seizures. However, the recurrence rate after a first seizure approaches 70% during the first year and most recurrent attacks occur within a month or two of the first. Further seizures are less likely if a trigger factor is definable and avoidable (e.g. sleep deprivation, alcohol withdrawal etc.). There is a group of disorders whose only or main symptom is epilepsy, whilst in other disorders epilepsy is just one of the manifestations. The annual incidence of new cases of epilepsy after infancy is 20–70/100 000. Whilst the lifetime risk of having a single seizure is about 2%, the prevalence of epilepsy in European countries is about 0.5%, suggesting that many people have one or two seizures in their life without acquiring a diagnosis of epilepsy.

Types of epilepsy

The classification of epilepsy is best achieved by separately considering the clinical events (the seizures), the abnormal electrophysiology, the anatomical site of seizure genesis and the pathological cause of the problem (see the information box).

CLASSIFICATION OF EPILEPSY

Seizure type
- Simple partial
- Complex partial
- Absence
- Tonic clonic
- Tonic
- Atonic
- Myoclonic

Electrophysiology
- Focal spikes/sharp waves
- Generalised spike and wave

Anatomical site
- Cortex
  - Temporal
  - Frontal
  - Parietal
  - Occipital
- Generalised (diencephalon)
- Multifocal

Pathological cause

Primary generalised epilepsies

The primary or idiopathic epilepsies are a group of disorders which make up some 10% of all epilepsies, including some 40% of those with tonic clonic seizures. Onset is almost always in childhood or adolescence. No structural abnormality is present and there is often a substantial genetic predisposition. Some, like childhood absence epilepsy, are relatively uncommon, whilst others, like juvenile myoclonic epilepsy, are common (5–10% of all patients with epilepsy). Table 14.6 lists the more common varieties of primary generalised epilepsy, along with their clinical features and management.

Secondary generalised epilepsy

Generalised epilepsy may arise from spread of partial seizures due to structural disease or be secondary to drugs or metabolic disorders (see the information box). Epilepsy presenting in adult life is almost always secondary generalised, even if there is no clear history of a partial seizure before the onset of a major attack (an 'aura').

Partial epilepsy

Partial seizures may arise from any disease of the cerebral cortex, congenital or acquired, and frequently generalise. With the exception of a few idiopathic partial epilepsies of benign outcome in childhood, the presence of partial

CAUSES OF SECONDARY GENERALISED EPILEPSY

Secondary generalisation from partial seizures
(See next information box for causes of partial epilepsy)

Genetic
- Inborn errors of metabolism
- Storage diseases

Drugs
- Antibiotics: penicillin, isoniazid, metronidazole
- Antimalarials: chloroquine, mefloquine
- Cyclosporin
- Cardiac anti-arrhythmics: lignocaine, disopyramide
- Psychotropic agents: phenothiazines, tricyclics, lithium
- Amphetamines (withdrawal)

Alcohol (especially withdrawal)

Cerebral birth injury

Hydrocephalus

Cerebral anoxia

Metabolic disease
- Hypocalcaemia
- Hyponatraemia
- Hypomagnesaemia
- Hypoglycaemia
- Renal failure
- Liver failure

Infection
- Meningitis
- Post-infectious encephalopathy

Inflammatory disease
- Multiple sclerosis (uncommon)
- Systemic lupus erythematosus (SLE)

Diffuse degenerative disease
- Alzheimer's disease
- Creutzfeldt–Jakob disease

Table 14.6 Primary generalised epilepsies

	Incidence	Age of onset	Type of seizure	EEG features	Provoking factors	Treatment	Prognosis
Childhood absence epilepsy	6–8/100 000	4–8 yrs	Frequent brief absences	3/sec spike and wave	Hyperventilation, fatigue	Ethosuximide Valproate	40% develop tonic clonic seizures, 80% remit in adulthood
Juvenile absence epilepsy	1–2/100 000	10–15 yrs	Less frequent absences than childhood absence	Poly-spike and wave	Hyperventilation, sleep deprivation	Valproate	80% develop tonic clonic seizures, 80% seizure-free in adulthood
Juvenile myoclonic epilepsy	25–50/ 100 000	15–20 yrs	GTCS, absences, morning myoclonus	Poly-spike and wave, photosensitivity	Sleep deprivation, alcohol withdrawal	Valproate	90% remit with valproate but relapse on AED withdrawal
GTCS on awakening	Common	10–25 yrs	GTCS, sometimes myoclonus	Spike and wave on waking and at sleep onset	Sleep deprivation	Valproate	65% controlled with AEDs but relapse off treatment

(GTCS = generalised tonic clonic seizures; AED = anti-epilepsy drug)

CAUSES OF PARTIAL SEIZURES
Idiopathic
• Benign rolandic epilepsy of childhood • Benign occipital epilepsy of childhood
Focal structural lesions
• Genetic Tuberous sclerosis, neurofibromatosis, von Hippel–Lindau syndrome • Infantile hemiplegia • Dysembryonic Cortical dysgenesis, Sturge–Weber syndrome • Mesial temporal sclerosis (associated with febrile convulsions) • Cerebrovascular disease Intracerebral haemorrhage, cerebral embolus, arteriovenous malformation • Tumours • Trauma (including neurosurgery) • Infection Cerebral abscess (pyogenic), toxoplasmosis, cysticercosis, subdural empyema, encephalitis, HIV • Inflammatory disease Sarcoidosis, vasculitis

seizures signifies the presence of focal cerebral pathology. Common causes are listed in the information box.

Investigations

After a single seizure cerebral imaging with CT or MRI is advisable, although the yield of structural lesions is low unless there are focal features to the seizure or there are focal signs. Similarly, toxic and metabolic causes (see the information box) should be considered. EEG is only necessary when more than one seizure has occurred and the type of epilepsy needs to be established to guide therapy. The increasing sophistication of imaging techniques now allows the identification of the cause of epilepsy in an increasing number of patients, especially those with partial seizures. These patients warrant intensive investigation, especially if seizures arise for the first time in adult life. Investigations should be pursued more vigorously if the epilepsy is intractable to treatment. The investigations which may be undertaken in a patient with suspected epilepsy are shown in the information box.

Electroencephalography (EEG)

The EEG (see p. 927) may help to establish and characterise the type of epilepsy (i.e. primary generalised or partial with or without secondary generalisation). Inter-ictal records are abnormal in only about 50% of patients so the EEG is not a sensitive test for the presence of epilepsy. However, epileptiform changes (sharp waves or spikes) are fairly specific (falsely positive in only 1/1000). The sensitivity can be increased to about 85% by prolonging recording time, and including a period of natural or drug-induced sleep. Ambulatory EEG recording or video/EEG monitoring may provide helpful information when attacks are frequent.

INVESTIGATION OF SUSPECTED EPILEPSY
Epileptic nature of attacks?
• Ambulatory EEG • Video telemetry
Type of epilepsy?
• Standard EEG • Sleep EEG • EEG with special electrodes (foramen ovale, subdural)
Structural lesion?
• CT • MRI head
Metabolic disorder?
• Blood urea and electrolytes • Liver function tests • Blood glucose • Serum calcium, magnesium
Inflammatory or infective disorder?
• Blood count, erythrocyte sedimentation rate (ESR), C-reactive protein (CRP) • Chest radiograph • Serology for syphilis, HIV, collagen disease • CSF

Brain imaging

Imaging does not help establish a diagnosis of epilepsy but is useful in defining or excluding a structural cause; indications are summarised in the information box. Imaging is not required if a confident diagnosis of primary generalised epilepsy can be made with an EEG.

INDICATIONS FOR BRAIN IMAGING IN EPILEPSY
• Epilepsy onset after the age of 20 years • Seizures with local features clinically • EEG shows a focal seizure source • Control of seizures is difficult or deteriorates

CT is often sufficient to exclude a major structural cause of epilepsy. MRI of the brain may be indicated if CT shows no abnormality but a subtle structural change is still suspected, as in the case of patients with partial seizures (with or without secondary generalisation) which are resistant to therapy.

Management

It is important to explain the nature and cause of seizures to patients and their relatives, as is the instruction of relatives in the first aid management of major seizures. Many people with epilepsy feel stigmatised by society and may become unnecessarily isolated from work and social life. It should be emphasised that any brain can develop a seizure, that epilepsy is a common disorder which affects just under 1% of the population, and that good or complete control of seizures can be expected in more than 80% of patients.

Immediate care of seizures

Little can or need be done for a person during the time a major seizure is occurring except first aid and commonsense manoeuvres to limit damage or secondary complications (see the information box).

IMMEDIATE CARE OF SEIZURES

First aid (by relatives and witnesses)

- Move person away from danger (fire, water, machinery, furniture)
- After convulsions cease, turn into 'recovery' position (semi-prone)
- Ensure airway is clear
- Do **NOT** insert anything in mouth (tongue-biting occurs at seizure onset and cannot be prevented by observers)
- If convulsions continue for more than 5 minutes or recur without person regaining consciousness, summon urgent medical attention
- Person may be drowsy and confused for some 30–60 minutes and should not be left alone until fully recovered

Immediate medical care

- Ensure airway is clear
- Give oxygen to offset cerebral hypoxia
- Give intravenous anticonvulsant (e.g. diazepam 10 mg) **ONLY** if convulsions are continuous or repeated (if so, manage as for status epilepticus)
- Take blood for anticonvulsant levels (if known epileptic)

Restrictions

Until good control of seizures has been established, work or recreation above ground level, with dangerous machinery or near open fires or water should be avoided. Patients should take only a shallow bath, and then when a relative is in the house, and should not lock the bathroom door. Cycling should be discouraged until at least 6 months' freedom from seizures has been achieved. Recreations requiring prolonged proximity to water (e.g. swimming, fishing or boating) should always be in the company of someone who is aware of the chance of a seizure occurring. Any activity where loss of awareness might be very dangerous (e.g. mountaineering) should be discouraged.

In the UK, legal restrictions regarding vehicle driving apply to patients with epilepsy, defined as more than one seizure over the age of 5 years (see the information box). The patient should inform the licensing authorities about the onset of seizures. It is also wise for patients to notify their motor insurance company.

UK DRIVING REGULATIONS

Single seizure

- Cease driving for 1 year, then Driver and Vehicle Licensing Authority will restore a full licence (i.e. until age of 70 years)

Epilepsy

- Free from all types of seizure for 1 year, or from seizures exclusively during sleep for a period of 3 years (licence will require renewal every 3 years thereafter until there have been 10 seizure-free years)

Withdrawal of anticonvulsants

- Cease driving during withdrawal and for 6 months thereafter

Vocational drivers (heavy goods and public service vehicles)

- No licence permitted if any seizure has occurred since the age of 5 years, until off medication and seizure-free for more than 10 years, provided no potentially epileptogenic brain lesion present

Anticonvulsant drug therapy

Drug treatment should be considered after more than one seizure has occurred and the patient agrees that seizure control is worth while. Quite a range of anti-epilepsy drugs (AEDs) are available (see Table 14.7, p. 946). The mode of action is either to increase the inhibitory neurotransmission in the brain or to alter neuronal sodium channels in such a way as to prevent the abnormally rapid transmission of impulses. Of patients whose epilepsy is controllable, only a single drug is necessary in 80%, providing the choice of agent is appropriate and the dosage correct. The combination of more than two drugs is seldom necessary. Dose regimens should be kept as simple as possible to promote compliance. Some useful guidelines are listed in the information box.

Choice of drug. With the exception of absence attacks and juvenile myoclonic epilepsy, there is no hard evidence indicating that one drug is superior to another in the treatment of epilepsy. In general, the first line of treatment should be one of the established first-line drugs (see Table

GUIDELINES FOR ANTICONVULSANT THERAPY

- Start with one first-line drug (see Table 14.8, p. 947)
- Start with low dose; gradually increase to effective control of seizures or side-effects (use drug levels if appropriate)
- Check compliance (use minimum division of doses)
- If first drug fails (seizures continue or side-effects), start second-line drug whilst gradually withdrawing first
- Try three agents singly before using combinations (beware interactions)
- Do not use more than two drugs in combination
- If above fails, consider whether occult structural or metabolic lesion present

Table 14.7 Anticonvulsant drugs

	Seizure type	Dose range (mg/day)	Doses per day	Therapeutic range (μmol/l)	Dose-related side-effects	Idiosyncratic side-effects	Long-term side-effects	Interactions
Carbamazepine	Partial secondary GTCS	200–2000	2–3	30–50	Drowsiness, ataxia, nystagmus, diplopia, hyponatraemia	Rashes, thrombocytopenia, other blood dyscrasias	None	Other AEDs, warfarin, CCP, steroids, antimalarials, cimetidine
Clobazam	Partial (adjunctive)	20–30	1	Not applicable	Sedation, irritability		Anticonvulsant effect wears off after a few weeks	Other AEDs
Clonazepam	Partial (adjunctive), myoclonus	1–8	2	Not applicable	Sedation, irritability	Blood dyscrasias	Anticonvulsant effect wears off after a few weeks	Other AEDs
Ethosuximide	Childhood absence	500–1500	2	200–700	Dizziness, insomnia, ataxia	Rashes, blood dyscrasias		Other AEDs, antidepressants
Gabapentin	Partial	300–2400	3	Not applicable	Drowsiness, ataxia		Not yet known	Antacids
Lamotrigine	Partial secondary GTCS	25–500	1–2	Not applicable	Drowsiness, ataxia, diplopia, confusion	Rashes, blood dyscrasias	Not yet known	Carbamazepine, valproate
Phenobarbitone	Partial secondary GTCS	60–180	1	50–150	Drowsiness, ataxia, nystagmus, diplopia	Rashes, depression (adults), excitement (children), megaloblastic anaemia, SLE	Folate deficiency, osteomalacia, neuropathy	Other AEDs, anticoagulants, calcium channel blockers, digoxin, steroids, CCF theophylline, thyroxine, antidepressants, antimalarials
Phenytoin	Partial secondary GTCS	150–350	1	40–80	Drowsiness, ataxia, nystagmus, diplopia, tremor, dystonia, asterixis	Rashes, blood dyscrasias, liver damage, SLE	Gum hypertrophy, facial dysmorphism, hirsutism, folate deficiency, osteomalacia, neuropathy	Other AEDs, warfarin, amiodarone and other anti-arrhythmics, antimalarials, steroids, CCP, cimetidine, oral hypoglycaemics, theophylline, thyroxine
Primidone	Partial secondary GTCS	250–1000	1–2	50–150*	Drowsiness, ataxia, nystagmus, diplopia	Rashes, depression (adults), excitement (children), megaloblastic anaemia, SLE	As for phenobarbitone*	As for phenobarbitone*
Sodium valproate	Primary and secondary GTCS, absences, myoclonus	400–2500	1–2	Not applicable	Drowsiness, nausea, ataxia, nystagmus, diplopia, tremor	Alopecia, rashes, blood dyscrasias, liver damage, pancreatitis	Weight gain	Other AEDs, anticoagulants, antimalarials, cimetidine
Topiramate	Partial secondary GTCS	200–600	1–2	Not applicable	Drowsiness, nausea, ataxia, confusion	Nephrolithiasis, depression, taste alteration, diarrhoea, weight loss	Not yet known	Other AEDs, CCP
Vigabatrin	Partial secondary GTCS, infantile spasms	2000–6000	1–2	Not applicable	Drowsiness, nausea, ataxia, confusion	Aggression, alopecia, skin rash, increase in seizures, retinal atrophy	Not yet known	

* Primidone is converted in the liver to phenobarbitone. (GTCS = generalised tonic clonic seizures; AEDs = anti-epileptic drugs; CCP = combined contraceptive pill; SLE = systemic lupus erythematosus; CCF = congestive cardiac failure)

Table 14.8 Guidelines for the choice of AED

Epilepsy type	First-line	Second-line	Third-line
Partial and/or secondary GTCS	Carbamazepine Valproate Phenytoin	Lamotrigine Topiramate	Gabapentin Clobazam Primidone Phenobarbitone Vigabatrin
Primary GTCS	Valproate	Carbamazepine Lamotrigine Topiramate	Phenytoin Gabapentin Primidone Phenobarbitone
Absence	Ethosuximide	Valproate	Lamotrigine Clonazepam
Myoclonic	Valproate	Clonazepam	Phenobarbitone

N.B. Preferably one drug, or no more than two drugs, should be used at one time.
(GTCS = generalised tonic clonic seizures)

14.8), with the more recently introduced drugs as second choice. Phenytoin and carbamazepine are not ideal agents for a young woman wishing to use oral contraception, because the drugs induce liver enzymes. Carbamazepine or sodium valproate are preferable to phenytoin as first-line drugs, because of the side-effect profile of the latter and its complicated pharmacokinetics.

Anticonvulsant drug blood levels. The levels of AEDs in blood can be a useful guide to the appropriate dose for a patient but only in the case of some drugs. In some drugs like valproate there is no relationship between the drug levels and anticonvulsant efficacy, and levels should only be used to check compliance. Plasma level monitoring is particularly useful for phenytoin and carbamazepine. It is important to recognise that quoted 'therapeutic' ranges are approximations and need not be adhered to rigidly if the patient is otherwise well.

Prognosis

Overall, generalised seizures are more readily controlled than partial seizures. The presence of a structural lesion makes complete control of the epilepsy less likely. The overall prognosis for epilepsy is shown in the information box.

Withdrawal of anticonvulsant therapy

After complete control of seizures for 2–4 years, withdrawal of medication may be considered. Childhood-onset epilepsy, particularly classical absence seizures, carries the best prognosis for successful drug withdrawal. Other generalised epilepsies, such as juvenile myoclonic epilepsy, have marked liability to recur after AED withdrawal. Seizures which begin in adult life, particularly those with partial features, are also likely to recur, especially if there is an identified structural lesion. Overall, the recurrence rate of seizures after drug withdrawal is about 40%. Some adult patients tend to opt for continuation of therapy because they feel that the threat of further attacks (especially regarding driving) outweighs the complications of continuing with medication. The EEG is a poor predictor of seizure recurrence but if the record is still very abnormal, drug withdrawal is unwise. Withdrawal should be undertaken slowly, reducing the drug dose gradually over 6–12 months.

EPILEPSY: OUTCOME AFTER 20 YEARS

- 50% seizure-free, without drugs, for last 5 years
- 20% seizure-free for last 5 years but continue to take medication
- 30% seizures continue in spite of anti-epileptic therapy

Status epilepticus

Status epilepticus exists when a series of seizures occurs without the patient regaining awareness between attacks. Most commonly this refers to recurrent tonic clonic seizures (major status) and is a life-threatening medical emergency. Partial motor status is obvious clinically, but complex partial status and absence status may be difficult to diagnose, because the patient may merely present in a dazed, confused state. Status is never the presenting feature of idiopathic epilepsy but may be precipitated by abrupt withdrawal of anticonvulsant drugs, the presence of a major structural lesion or acute metabolic disturbance, and tends to be more common with frontal epileptic foci. Management is summarised in the information box. It

MANAGEMENT OF STATUS EPILEPTICUS

- Immediate care (see the information box, p. 945)
- Secure i.v. access
- Draw blood for glucose and electrolytes and save for future analysis (drugs etc.)
- Give diazepam 10 mg i.v. (or rectally)—repeat once only after 15 min; or lorazepam 4 mg i.v.
- Transfer to intensive care area, monitoring neurological condition, blood pressure, respiration and blood gases
- Commence longer-term anticonvulsant medication with one of:
  —Sodium valproate: 10 mg/kg i.v. over 3–5 minutes and then 800–2000 mg/day
  —Phenytoin: give loading dose of 15 mg/kg, infuse at < 50 mg/min, then 300 mg/day
  —Carbamazepine: 400 mg by nasogastric tube then 400–1200 mg/day
- If seizures continue, use chlormethiazole 0.8% i.v. solution, 40–400 ml at 5–15 ml/min to stop seizures and then 0.5–1 ml/min
- If seizures still refractory, use thiopentone (with intubation and ventilation) 100–250 mg bolus over 20 sec, then 50 mg boluses every 2–3 min until seizures controlled. Then infusion of 3–5 mg/kg/hour as necessary
- Investigate cause

should be remembered that psychogenic or non-epileptic attacks commonly masquerade as 'status epilepticus', so electrophysiological confirmation of the seizures should be obtained as early as possible.

Epilepsy, pregnancy and oral contraception

Hepatic enzyme induction caused by carbamazepine, phenytoin and barbiturates accelerates metabolism of the oral contraceptives, causing breakthrough bleeding and contraceptive failure. The safest policy is to use an alternative contraceptive method, but it is sometimes possible to overcome the problem by giving a higher oestrogen dose preparation. Sodium valproate has little interaction with oral contraception.

Epilepsy may worsen during pregnancy, particularly during the third trimester when plasma anticonvulsant levels tend to fall. More frequent monitoring of blood levels during pregnancy is therefore advisable. All the major anticonvulsant drugs have been associated with an increased incidence of fetal congenital abnormalities (cleft lip, spina bifida, cardiac defects). The risk is difficult to quantify, especially with the more recently introduced AEDs, but is greatest during the first trimester and in patients on multiple drug therapy. It is seldom possible to withdraw or change therapy before conception, but lamotrigine may be less teratogenic than the other agents. Folic acid (5 mg daily) taken 2 months before conception may reduce the risk of some fetal abnormalities. Occasionally, in a well-controlled patient, anticonvulsants can be withdrawn before conception, but if seizures have occurred in the preceding year this is unwise as the risk to the fetus from uncontrolled maternal major seizures is probably greater than the teratogenic effects. (Partial seizures probably carry little risk.)

A DIAGNOSTIC APPROACH TO THE PATIENT WITH TRANSIENT AMNESIA

Loss of memory for a period of time may be due to a transient toxic confusional state, a psychological fugue state, the post-ictal period after a seizure or the syndrome known as transient global amnesia. The latter two especially require careful distinction by analysis of the history. A period of amnesia often follows a seizure, either a complex partial or generalised seizure, and this may cause diagnostic confusion if the seizure was not witnessed—for example, if it occurred in sleep.

TRANSIENT GLOBAL AMNESIA

This is a syndrome affecting predominantly middle-aged patients in which there is an abrupt, discrete and reversible loss of short-term memory function for a period of some hours. During this time patients know who they are and can perform motor acts normally, but act in a bemused way, repeatedly asking the same questions. After 4–6 hours memory functions and behaviour return to normal but the patient is left with a period of time for which he or she has complete amnesia. There are none of the phenomena associated with seizures and, unlike epileptic amnesia, transient global amnesia tends not to recur. There are no associated cerebrovascular risk factors, making a vascular aetiology unlikely. Transient global amnesia is thought to be due to a benign process similar to that causing a migraine aura, occurring in the hippocampus. The patient has no physical signs and further investigation may not be needed if epilepsy can be excluded.

SLEEPINESS AND SLEEP DISORDERS

Disturbances of sleep are common. Apart from insomnia, patients may complain of excessive day-time sleepiness, disturbed behaviour of night-time sleep (sleep walking and talking, or night terrors) or disturbing subjective experiences during sleep (nightmares, hypnagogic hallucinations or sleep paralysis). A careful history will allow certain patterns of sleep disturbance to be identified.

Normal sleep is controlled by the reticular activating system in the upper brain stem and diencephalon. During overnight sleep, a series of repeated cycles of EEG patterns can be recorded. As drowsiness occurs, alpha rhythm disappears and the EEG gradually becomes dominated by deepening slow-wave activity. After 60–80 minutes this slow-wave pattern is replaced by a short spell of low-amplitude EEG background on which are superimposed rapid eye movements (REM). After a few minutes of REM sleep, another slow-wave spell starts and the cycle repeats several times throughout the night. The REM periods tend to become longer as the sleep period progresses. Dreaming takes place during REM sleep, which is accompanied by muscle relaxation, penile erection and loss of tendon reflexes. REM sleep seems to be the most important part of the sleep cycle for refreshing cognitive processes. Deprivation of REM sleep causes tiredness, irritability and impaired judgement.

SLEEP TALKING AND SLEEP WALKING

Automatic behaviour which is not recalled may take place during light sleep. Such phenomena are innocuous and common in normal children. Sleep walking is uncommon in adults but has no pathological significance.

NIGHT TERRORS

These occur as sudden arousals from deep slow-wave sleep. They are more common in children, but may affect adults. The sufferer wakes in a state of agitation, screaming and fearful. Occasionally, violent behaviour occurs. The agitation may last many minutes. Such events may be confused with nocturnal seizures, particularly those arising from the frontal lobe, or their post-ictal effects.

NIGHTMARES

These are frightening dreams from which the sufferer wakes in a state of fear or agitation. Most normal people have experienced such phenomena and they are not of any significance in terms of organic disease.

DAY-TIME SOMNOLENCE

Excessive sleepiness in the day is most commonly due to poor night-time sleep, which may in turn be due to sleep apnoea (see p. 319). More commonly, sleepiness is due to under-stimulation, fatigue and/or fitful night-time sleeping. In this case sleepiness particularly occurs after meals and during dull monotonous activities, such as long car journeys. Such banal causes of day-time sleepiness need to be distinguished from narcolepsy.

NARCOLEPSY

This disorder has strong human leucocyte antigen (HLA) association with DRW2 and is sometimes familial. Recurrent bouts of irresistible sleep are experienced, during which the EEG often shows direct entry into REM sleep. Sufferers tend to fall asleep when eating or talking, not just when under-stimulated. The periods of sleep are usually short and the person can be woken relatively easily. He or she usually feels refreshed after waking. In addition, patients with narcolepsy will report at least one other of the 'narcolepsy tetrad' (see the information box). These four symptoms may occur together or in combinations in the same patient; most often, sleep attacks and cataplexy occur together.

THE NARCOLEPSY TETRAD
Sleep attacks
• Brief, frequent and unlike normal somnolence *with*
Cataplexy
• Sudden loss of muscle tone set off by surprise, laughter, strong emotion etc. *and/or*
Hypnagogic hallucinations
• Frightening hallucinations experienced during sleep onset or waking; can occur in normal people *and/or*
Sleep paralysis
• Brief paralysis on waking; can occur in normal people

Management

Narcoleptic attacks are treated by stimulant drugs such as dexamphetamine (5–10 mg 8-hourly). Cataplexy responds to clomipramine (25–50 mg 8-hourly).

DISORDERS OF MOVEMENT

Lesions in various parts of the motor system produce distinctive patterns of motor deficit. These can be in the form of the negative symptoms of weakness, lack of coordination, lack of stability and stiffness, or positive symptoms such as tremor, dystonia, chorea, athetosis, hemiballismus, tics and myoclonus. When the lower limbs are affected, characteristic patterns of gait disorder may result.

THE MOTOR SYSTEM

A programme of movement which has been formulated by the pre-motor cortex is converted into a series of muscle movements in the motor cortex and then transmitted to the spinal cord in the pyramidal tract (see Fig. 14.10 on p. 950). This passes through the internal capsule and the ventral brain stem before decussating in the medulla to enter the lateral columns of the spinal cord. The pyramidal tract 'upper motor neurons' end by synapsing with the anterior horn cells of the spinal cord grey matter, which form the 'lower motor neurons'.

Movement of a body part necessitates changes in posture and alteration in the tone of many muscles, some quite distant from the part being moved. The motor system consists of a hierarchy of control mechanisms which maintain body posture and baseline muscle tone upon which a specific movement is superimposed. The lowest order of this hierarchy comprises the mechanisms housed in the grey matter of the spinal cord which control the muscle tone response to stretch and the reflex withdrawal response to noxious stimuli. The afferent side of the stretch reflex consists of the muscle spindles which detect lengthening of the muscle with this stretch initiating a monosynaptic reflex leading to muscle contraction. The sensitivity of the stretch reflex is modulated by descending input from the brain stem and cerebral hemispheres.

Polysynaptic connections in the spinal cord grey matter control more complex reflex actions of flexion and extension of the limbs which form the basic building blocks of coordinated actions but which require control from above to function usefully. Above the spinal cord, circuits between the basal ganglia and the motor cortex constituting the extrapyramidal system control background muscle tone

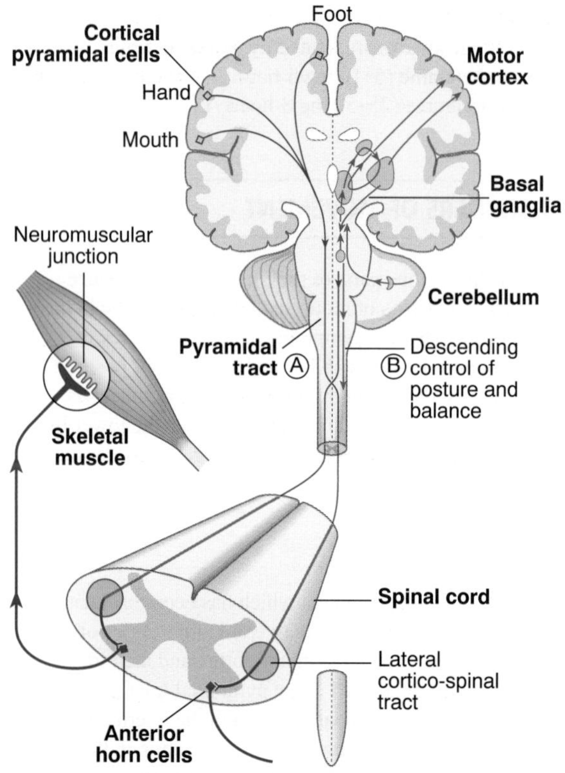

Fig. 14.10 The motor system. Neurons from the motor cortex descend as the pyramidal tract in the internal capsule and cerebral peduncle to the ventral brain stem, where most cross low in the medulla (A). In the spinal cord the upper motor neurons form the cortico-spinal tract in the lateral column before synapsing with the lower motor neurons in the anterior horns. The activity in the motor cortex is modulated by influences from the basal ganglia and cerebellum (B). Pathways descending from these structures control posture and balance (see also Fig. 14.11).

and body posture, and gate the initiation of movement (see Figs 14.10 and 14.11).

Accurately targeted and coordinated movements require the functioning of the cerebellum, which acts as an on-line guidance computer to fine-tune goal-directed movements initiated by the motor cortex. In addition, the cerebellum, through its reciprocal connections with the thalamus and cortex, participates in the planning and learning of skilled movements.

Pathophysiology

Lower motor neuron lesions

Groups of muscle fibres innervated by a single anterior horn cell (lower motor neuron) form a motor unit. Loss of function of lower motor neurons will cause the loss of contraction in their units' muscle fibres and the muscle will be weak and flaccid. Denervated muscle fibres atrophy in

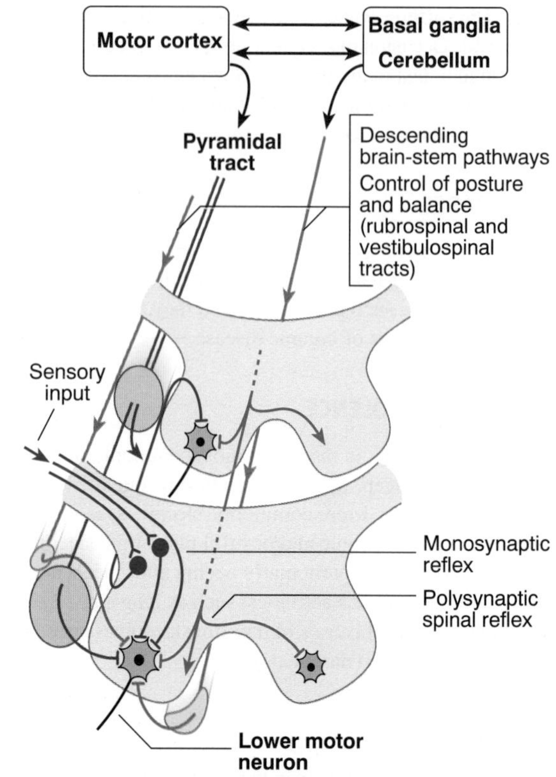

Fig. 14.11 Hierarchies of motor control. In addition to direct descending pathways from the cerebral motor cortex, motor neurons in the anterior horn are influenced by descending pathways controlling balance and posture as well as monosynaptic and polysynaptic spinal reflex pathways.

time, causing wasting of the muscle, and depolarise spontaneously, causing fibrillations which, except in the tongue, are only perceptible on an EMG. Re-innervation from neighbouring intact motor neurons may occur but the neuromuscular junctions of the enlarged motor units are unstable and depolarise spontaneously, causing fasciculations (twitches which are visible to the naked eye). Fasciculations therefore imply chronic partial denervation.

Upper motor neuron (pyramidal) lesions

When the spinal cord is disconnected from the modulating influence of the higher motor hierarchies, the anterior horn motor neurons are under the uninhibited influence of the spinal reflex mechanisms. Their innervated muscles will have an exaggerated response to stretch. The limbs show reflex patterns of movement, like flexion withdrawal to noxious stimuli and spasms of extension. An upper motor neuron lesion therefore manifests clinically with brisk tendon stretch reflexes, 'spastic' increase in tone greater in the extensors of the lower limbs and the flexors of the upper limbs, and extensor plantar responses. Spastic increase in tone can be seen on clinical examination to vary with both the degree and speed of stretch; this is the 'clasp-knife' phenomenon. Spasticity takes some time to develop and may not be present for weeks after the onset of an upper motor neuron lesion. Spasticity will be exacerbated by increased sensory input into the reflex arc, as may be caused by a bed sore or urinary tract infection in a patient with a spinal cord lesion.

Extrapyramidal lesions

Lesions of the extrapyramidal system produce an increase in tone, which is not an exaggerated response to stretch but is continuous throughout the range of movement (rigidity). Involuntary movements are also a feature of extrapyramidal lesions (see below) and a tremor combined with rigidity produces typical 'cogwheel' rigidity. Rapid movements are slowed and clumsy (bradykinesia). Extrapyramidal lesions also cause postural instability, precipitating falls.

Cerebellar lesions

A lesion in a cerebellar hemisphere causes lack of coordination on the same side of the body. The initial part of movement is normal but as the target is approached the accuracy of the movement deteriorates, producing an 'intention tremor'. The distances of targets are misjudged (dysmetria), resulting in 'past-pointing'. The ability to produce rapid, accurate, alternating movements is similarly impaired, causing 'dysdiadochokinesis'.

The central vermis of the cerebellum is concerned with the coordination of gait and posture. Disorders therefore produce a characteristic ataxic gait (see below).

A DIAGNOSTIC APPROACH TO THE PATIENT WITH LIMB WEAKNESS

Establishing the diagnosis in a patient with weakness requires application of basic anatomy, physiology and some pathology to the interpretation of the history and clinical findings (see Fig. 14.12 below and Table 14.9 on p. 952). Points to consider are shown in the information box.

Weakness in only some muscles in a limb suggests a problem in the peripheral nerve(s) or motor root(s).

ASSESSMENT OF WEAKNESS

- Does it affect a few muscles, a limb, both lower limbs (paraparesis) or both limbs on one side (hemiparesis)?
- Upper or lower motor neuron lesion?
- Evolution of the weakness: sudden and improving, gradually worsening over days or weeks, or evolving over months or years?

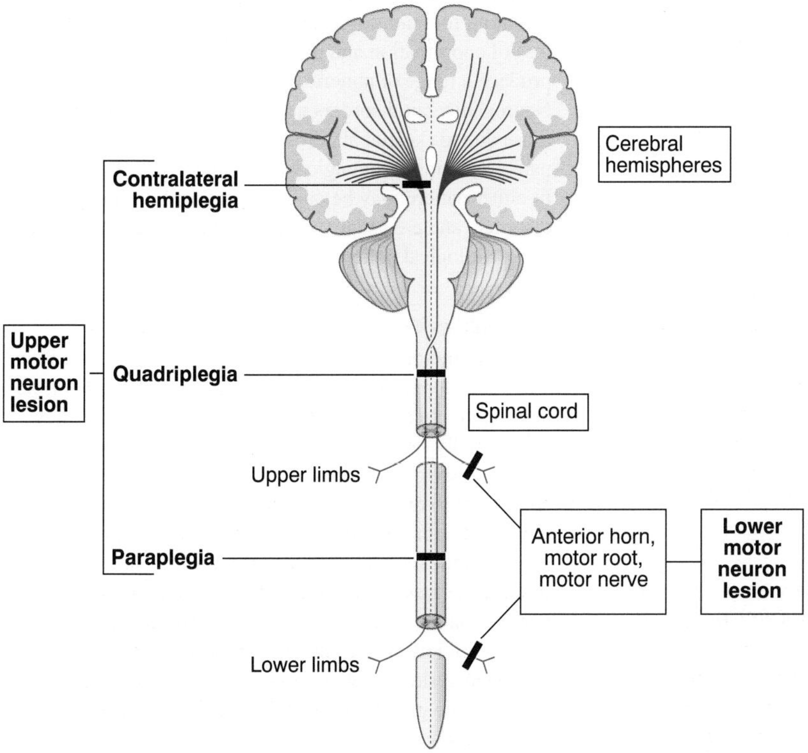

Fig. 14.12 Patterns of motor loss according to the anatomical site of the lesion.

Table 14.9 Physical signs in different types of motor deficit

Clinical sign	Upper motor (pyramidal) lesion	Lower motor lesion	Extrapyramidal lesion	Cerebellar lesion
Power	Weak	Weak	No weakness	No weakness
Wasting	None	Yes, after interval	None	None
Fasciculation	None	Yes, after interval	None	None
Tone	Spastic increase (after interval)	Flaccid from onset	Rigidity (cogwheel)	Normal/reduced
Reflexes	Increased	Reduced/absent	Normal	Normal
Plantar response	Extensor	Flexor	Flexor	Flexor
Coordination	Reduced by weakness	Reduced by weakness	Normal (but slowed)	Impaired

Weakness of the whole of one limb may be due to problems in the brachial or lumbosacral plexuses, or to a central lesion. Weakness in both lower limbs (paraparesis) and all four limbs (tetraparesis) suggests either a spinal cord lesion or a diffuse peripheral nerve problem such as Guillain–Barré syndrome. In such cases the condition of the reflexes is the most discriminating sign. The reflexes are absent in the Guillain–Barré syndrome (or other lower motor nerve lesions) and brisk in spinal cord (upper motor neuron) lesions. The paraparesis or tetraparesis of spinal cord lesions may be associated with a specific pattern of sensory loss (see p. 955) which gives a clue to the site of the lesion in the spinal cord.

Patients with a bradykinetic limb often complain of weakness. Therefore, if there are no reflex changes, wasting or sensory changes when a patient is complaining of weakness in a limb, then extrapyramidal signs of (cogwheel) rigidity and bradykinesia should be sought. Patients with Parkinson's disease usually present with symptoms in one limb which may be described as weak and clumsy, especially for fine manipulations. Often the typical rest tremor is a clue to the diagnosis.

LIMB WEAKNESS—ASSESSING THE CAUSE
Vascular lesions
• Sudden onset (over minutes) followed by a stable period and gradual recovery
Neoplastic lesions
• Deficit is gradual in onset and progressive over weeks or months. There may be signs caused by the mass effect of the lesion
Inflammatory lesions
• May be fairly acute of onset (over a few days), persist for a time and then improve (e.g. in multiple sclerosis)
Degenerative disorders
• May evolve over months or years (e.g. motor neuron disease or cervical spondylotic myelopathy)

Weakness down one side of the body (hemiparesis) is almost always due to a cerebral hemisphere lesion, although it could be caused by spinal cord or brain-stem lesions. The lesion is of upper motor neuron type, and the site and often the size of the lesion can be deduced by the concurrence of other signs and symptoms, such as higher cerebral function abnormalities or sensory change.

The evolution of a motor deficit over time suggests the likely underlying pathology (see the information box).

GAIT DISORDERS

As well as being an important element of assessing a patient's disability, seeing a patient walk can be very revealing for neurological diagnosis. Patterns of weakness, loss of coordination and proprioceptive sensory loss produce a range of abnormal neurological gaits. Neurogenic gait disorders need to be distinguished from those due to skeletal abnormalities, usually characterised by pain producing an antalgic gait, or limp. Gaits that do not fit either pattern may be due to 'functional' or non-organic disorders and are usually incompatible with any anatomical or physiological deficit.

Pyramidal gait

An upper motor neuron (pyramidal) lesion causes a gait in which the upper limb is held in flexion and the lower limb kept relatively extended. The pyramidal tract lesion slows the normally rapid ankle dorsiflexion needed to keep the toes from striking the ground as the leg swings through. In an attempt to overcome this, the leg is swung out at the hip (circumduction), but the affected foot still scuffs along the ground at the toes. The shoe on the affected side may be worn at the toes as evidence of this type of gait. In a hemiplegia the asymmetry between the affected and normal sides is obvious in walking. In a paraparesis both lower limbs move slowly, swung from the hips and dragged stiffly on the ground in extension, an effect that can often be heard as well as seen.

Foot drop
In normal walking, toe strike follows heel strike during the gait cycle. Weakness of ankle dorsiflexion disrupts this pattern. The result is a less controlled descent of the foot making a slapping noise. If the distal weakness is more severe the foot will have to be lifted higher at the knee to allow room for the inadequately dorsiflexed foot to swing through, producing a high stepping gait.

Waddling gait of proximal muscle weakness
During walking, alternate placement of the body's weight through each leg requires careful control of the hips by the gluteal muscles. In proximal muscle weakness, usually caused by muscle disease, the hips are not properly fixed by these muscles and trunk movements are exaggerated, producing a rolling or waddling gait.

Cerebellar ataxia
Patients with lesions of the central parts of the cerebellum (the vermis) walk with a characteristic broad-based gait, 'like a drunken sailor' (cerebellar function is particularly sensitive to alcohol). Patients with acute vestibular disturbances walk in a similar broad-based fashion, though the accompanying vertigo distinguishes them from those with cerebellar lesions. Less severe degrees of cerebellar ataxia can be detected by asking the patient to walk heel to toe; patients with vermis lesions are unable to do this.

Gait apraxia
In an apraxic gait there is normal power in the legs, and no abnormal cerebellar signs or proprioception loss, yet the patient cannot formulate the motor act of walking. This is a higher cerebral dysfunction in which the feet appear stuck to the floor and the patient cannot walk, even though movement is normal on the examination couch. Gait apraxia occurs in bilateral hemisphere disease such as normal pressure hydrocephalus and diffuse frontal lobe disease.

Marche à petits pas
Patients with multiple small-vessel cerebrovascular disease walk with small slow steps with instability. This looks different from the festinant gait of Parkinson's disease (see below) in that it does not have the variable pace and freezing. There are usually signs of bilateral upper motor neuron disease (bilateral extensor plantar responses and brisk jaw jerk).

Sensory ataxia
Loss of joint position sense makes walking unreliable, especially in poor light. The feet tend to be placed on the ground with greater emphasis, presumably in an attempt to increase what proprioceptive input is available. This results in a 'stamping' gait which is often combined with foot drop when caused by a peripheral neuropathy, but can occur in disorders of the dorsal columns in the spinal cord.

Extrapyramidal gait
Patients with Parkinson's disease and other extrapyramidal diseases have difficulty initiating walking and difficulty controlling the pace of their gait. The patient may get stuck whilst trying to start walking or when walking through doorways ('freezing'), but once started may then have problems controlling the speed of walking and have trouble stopping. This produces the festinant gait: initial stuttering steps which quickly increase in frequency while decreasing in length.

INVOLUNTARY MOVEMENTS

Abnormal movements usually imply a disorder in the basal ganglia, in which there is disinhibition of the activity of intrinsic rhythm generators or a disorder of postural control. Some, like tremor, are commonplace. Others, like chorea, athetosis and dystonia, have become more common as a result of pharmacological treatment of Parkinson's disease and psychiatric disease.

TREMOR

A tremor is a rhythmic oscillating movement of a limb or part of a limb, or of the head. Tremors are usefully divided into those occurring at rest and those seen only when a limb is in action. The other characteristic by which tremors can be classified is their frequency.

Rest tremor
This is pathognomonic of Parkinson's disease (see p. 988). The tremor is characteristically 'pill-rolling', and usually presents asymmetrically. However, patients with Parkinson's disease may have an abnormal action tremor as well. Tremor of the head in the upright position ('titubation') is not a rest tremor since this is a postural tremor, disappearing when the head is supported.

Action tremor
This is more frequently seen than rest tremor and potential causes are more numerous (see the information box). A physiological tremor (frequency between 8–12 Hz) can be

CAUSES OF TREMOR ON ACTION

- Exaggerated physiological tremor (see the information box on p. 954)
- Wilson's disease
- Essential tremor (may be familial)
- Parkinson's disease
- Postural tremor
  - Multiple sclerosis
  - Other lesions in cerebellar outflow/red nucleus
- Intention tremor
  - Cerebellar disease

CAUSES OF EXAGGERATED PHYSIOLOGICAL TREMOR

- Anxiety
- Fatigue
- Endocrine
  (e.g. Thyrotoxicosis, Cushing's disease, phaeochromocytoma, hypoglycaemia)
- Drugs
  (e.g. β-adrenoceptor agonists, theophylline, caffeine, lithium, dopamine agonists, sodium valproate, tricyclics, phenothiazines, amphetamines)
- Toxins
  (e.g. Mercury, lead, arsenic)
- Alcohol withdrawal

identified in the limbs of normal subjects and exaggeration of this physiological tremor occurs in anxiety and other situations, listed in the information box.

Essential tremor is distinct from a physiological tremor, although resembling it superficially. This tremor is slower than a physiological action tremor and may become quite disabling. The condition is often familial and in some families the tremor is most obvious during certain specific actions such as writing, and here there is an overlap with focal dystonias (see below). Characteristic of essential tremor is that alcohol suppresses it, sometimes to the extent that the patient becomes addicted. Centrally acting β-adrenoceptor antagonists such as propranolol are often effective in treatment.

An 'intention tremor' is the characteristic oscillation at the end of a movement which occurs in cerebellar disease, due to the breakdown of feedback control of targeted movements. Asterixis, the 'flapping' tremor seen in metabolic disturbances (see the information box), is the result of intermittent failure of the parietal mechanisms required to maintain a posture. Thus, when a patient is asked to hold out the arms with the hands extended at the wrists, this posture is periodically dropped, allowing the hands to transiently drop before the posture is taken up again. Occasionally, unilateral asterixis can be seen in an acute parietal vascular lesion.

CAUSES OF ASTERIXIS

- Renal failure
- Liver failure
- Hypercapnia
- Drug toxicity (e.g. phenytoin)
- Acute focal parietal or thalamic lesions

A more dramatic action tremor occurs with lesions in the superior cerebellar peduncle (the site of the cerebellar outflow towards the red nucleus). This 'peduncular' or 'rubral' tremor is a violent, large-amplitude postural tremor which worsens as a target is approached. This is common in advanced multiple sclerosis and may be a source of considerable disability. Stereotactic thalamotomy can reduce the tremor, although the overall functional result is often disappointing.

CHOREA, ATHETOSIS, BALLISM AND DYSTONIA

Non-rhythmic involuntary movements may be combinations of fragments of purposeful movements and abnormal postures. All of these abnormal movements represent disorders of the balance of activity in the complex basal ganglia circuitry. Jerky, small-amplitude, purposeless involuntary movements are termed 'chorea' (the Greek for 'dance'). In the limbs they resemble fidgety movements, and in the face, grimaces, and suggest disease in the caudate nucleus (as in Huntington's disease) or excessive activity in the striatum due to dopaminergic drugs used to treat Parkinson's disease. There are a range of other causes (see the information box). More dramatic ballistic movements of the limbs usually occur unilaterally (hemiballismus) in vascular lesions of the subthalamic structures. Slower writhing movements of the limbs are called athetosis. These are often combined with chorea (and have a similar list of causes) and are then termed 'choreo-athetoid' movements.

CAUSES OF CHOREA

Hereditary
- Huntington's disease
- Wilson's disease
- Neuroacanthocytosis
- Porphyria
- Paroxysmal choreoathetosis

Cerebral birth injury (including kernicterus)

Cerebral trauma

Drugs
- L-dopa
- Dopamine agonists
- Phenothiazines
- Tricyclics

Endocrine
- Pregnancy
- Oral contraceptive
- Thyrotoxicosis
- Hypoparathyroidism
- Hypoglycaemia

Infective/inflammatory
- Rheumatic fever (Sydenham's chorea)
- Systemic lupus erythematosus
- Henoch–Schönlein purpura
- Creutzfeldt–Jakob disease

Vascular
- Lacunar infarction
- Arteriovenous malformation

The term 'dystonia' is used to describe the movement disorder in which a limb (or the head) involuntarily takes up an abnormal posture. This may be generalised in various diseases of the basal ganglia or may be focal or segmental, as in spasmodic torticollis when the head involuntarily turns to one side. Other segmental dystonias may cause abnormal disabling postures of a limb to be taken up during certain specific actions, such as in writer's cramp or numerous other occupational 'cramps'. These segmental dystonias can be treated by the administration of botulinum toxin to a few of the responsible muscles, which seems to overcome the abnormal distribution of muscle activity for a period of time.

MYOCLONUS

Myoclonus refers to brief, isolated, random, non-purposeful jerks of muscle groups in the limbs. Myoclonic jerks occur normally at the onset of sleep (hypnic jerks). Similarly, a myoclonic jerk is a component of the normal startle response which may be exaggerated in some rare (mostly genetic) disorders. Unlike the movement disorders discussed so far, myoclonus may occur in disorders of the cerebral cortex, when groups of pyramidal cells fire spontaneously. Such myoclonus occurs in some forms of epilepsy in which the jerks are fragments of seizure activity. Alternatively, myoclonus can arise from subcortical structures or, more rarely, from diseased segments of the spinal cord. Myoclonus, especially of cortical origin, often responds to clonazepam, sodium valproate or piracetam.

TICS

Tics are repetitive semi-purposeful movements such as blinking, winking, grinning or screwing up of the eyes. They are distinguished from other involuntary movements by the ability of the patient to suppress their occurrence, at least for a short time. An isolated tic may be no more than a mild embarrassment, but may become frequent at certain times in childhood and then disappear. The uncommon syndrome of Gilles de la Tourette consists of a tendency to multiple tics and odd vocalisations, with obsessive behavioural abnormalities. The pathogenic basis is not understood, but there may be some response to major anti-dopaminergic tranquillising medication.

SENSORY DISTURBANCES

Sensory symptoms are very common but do not always denote nervous system disorder. For example, tingling in the fingers of both hands and around the mouth commonly suggests hyperventilation (see p. 314) or, very rarely, hypocalcaemia (see p. 578). The accuracy of patients in describing sensory disturbances is very variable and skill is needed in sifting through the history to make anatomical and pathophysiological sense of the complaints. Damage to the afferent nervous pathways conveying sensations of touch and pain produces either the negative sensation of numbness or positive symptoms, such as paraesthesia and pain. When there is dysfunction of the cerebral mechanisms of somatic sensation there may be distortion of the patient's perception of the wholeness or actual presence of the relevant part of the body.

A DIAGNOSTIC APPROACH TO THE PATIENT WITH SENSORY SYMPTOMS

In the history, the most useful features are the anatomical distribution and mode of onset of numbness, paraesthesia or pain. Certain patterns of onset of sensory symptoms can be recognised. For example, in a migraine attack the aura may consist of a front of tingling paraesthesia followed by numbness which takes 20–30 minutes to spread over one half of the body, splitting the tongue. Sensory loss due to a vascular lesion, on the other hand, will occur over the whole territory of the lesion more or less instantaneously. The rare, unpleasant paraesthesia of sensory epilepsy 'shoots' down one side of the body in seconds. The numbness and paraesthesia of spinal cord lesions often ascend one or both lower limbs to a level on the trunk over hours or days.

Examination of the sensory system needs to be approached with care since it is easy to produce confusing false positive results because of the inescapably subjective nature of sensory testing. However, the distribution of sensory loss and associated deficits in motor and/or cranial nerve function may enable a diagnostically helpful pattern of sensory loss to be identified.

Patterns of sensory disturbance (see Fig. 14.13, p. 956)

Peripheral nerve lesions

In peripheral nerve lesions the symptoms are usually of sensory loss and simple paraesthesia (pins and needles). Single peripheral nerve lesions will, as expected, cause disturbance in the sensory distribution of that nerve. In diffuse neuropathies the longest neurons are first affected, giving the characteristic 'glove and stocking' distribution. If the smaller nerve fibres are preferentially affected (e.g. in alcoholic neuropathy) temperature and pin-prick (pain) are lost, whilst modalities served by the larger sensory nerves (vibration and joint position) may be spared. On the other hand, the latter are particularly affected if the neuropathy is demyelinating in character (e.g. Guillain–Barré syndrome).

Nerve roots

Pain is more often a feature of lesions of nerve roots within the spine or of the limb plexuses. Pain is often felt in the muscles innervated by a root, i.e. the myotome rather than the dermatome. The site of nerve root lesions may be deduced from the dermatomal pattern of sensory loss, although this is often smaller than would be expected because of the overlap of sensory 'territories'.

Spinal cord lesions

Somatic sensory information from the limbs ascends the nervous system in two anatomically discrete systems, differential involvement of which is often of diagnostic assistance (see Fig. 14.14, p. 957). Fibres from proprioceptive organs and those mediating well-localised touch (including vibration) enter the spinal cord at the

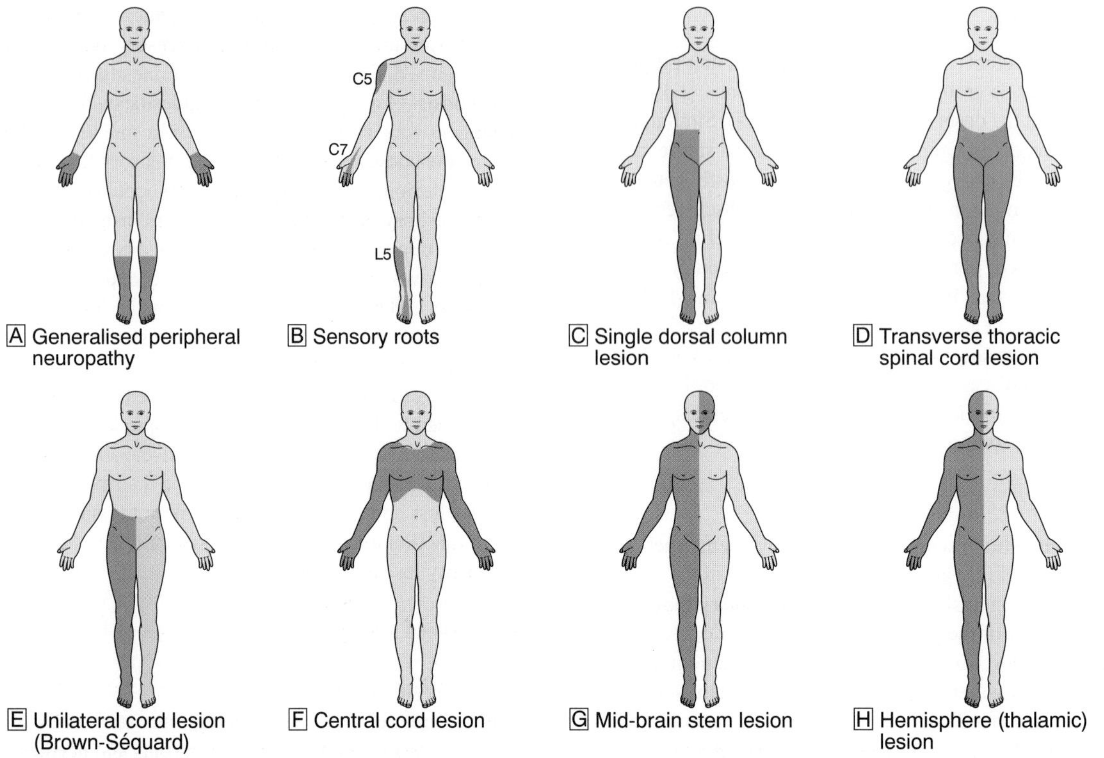

Fig. 14.13 Patterns of sensory loss. A Generalised peripheral neuropathy. B Sensory roots. C Single dorsal column lesion (proprioception and some touch loss). D Transverse thoracic spinal cord lesion. E Unilateral cord lesion (Brown-Séquard): ipsilateral dorsal column (and motor) deficit and contralateral spinothalamic deficit. F Central cord lesion: 'cape' distribution of spinothalamic loss. G Mid-brain stem lesion: ipsilateral facial sensory loss and contralateral loss on body below the vertex. H Hemisphere (thalamic) lesion: contralateral loss on one side of face and body.

posterior horn and pass without synapsing into the ipsilateral posterior columns. Fibres conveying pain and temperature sensory information synapse with second-order neurons which cross the midline in the spinal cord before ascending in the contralateral anterolateral spinothalamic tract to the brain stem.

Transverse lesions of the spinal cord produce loss of all modalities below that segmental level, although the level obtained clinically may vary by two or three segments. Very often at the top of the area of sensory loss there is a band of paraesthesia or hyperaesthesia. If the transverse lesion is vascular in origin (e.g. due to anterior spinal artery thrombosis) the posterior one-third of the spinal cord (and therefore the dorsal column modalities) may be spared.

Lesions damaging one side of the spinal cord will produce sensory loss for spinothalamic modalities (pain and temperature) on the opposite side and for dorsal column modalities (joint position and vibration) on the same side as the lesion. This is the pattern seen in the Brown-Séquard syndrome (see p. 1001).

Lesions in the centre of the spinal cord (e.g. syringomyelia, see p. 1005) spare the dorsal columns but affect the spinothalamic fibres crossing the cord from both sides over the length of the lesion. The sensory loss is therefore dissociated and suspended, often with reflex loss if afferent fibres of the reflex arc within the cord are affected.

There may be a lesion in the dorsal column alone, particularly in multiple sclerosis. This produces a characteristic unpleasant tight feeling over the limb involved and loss of proprioception which may severely affect the function of the limb without any loss of pin-prick or temperature sensation.

Brain-stem lesions

The second-order neurons of the dorsal column sensory system cross the midline in the medulla to ascend through the brain stem. Here they lie just medial to the (already crossed) spinothalamic pathway. Brain-stem lesions therefore can cause sensory loss affecting all modalities of the contralateral side of the body. Sensory loss on the face due to brain-stem lesions is dependent upon the anatomy of

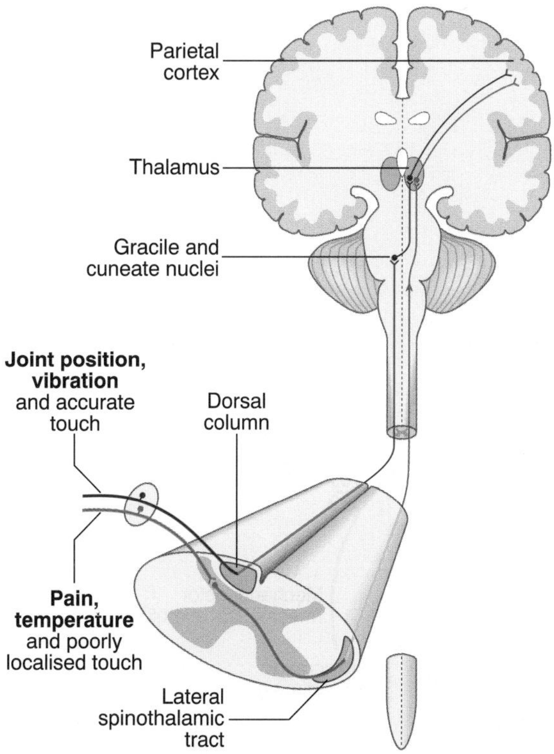

Fig. 14.14 The main somatic sensory pathways.

the trigeminal fibres within the brain stem. Fibres from the back of the face (near the ears) descend within the brain stem to the upper part of the spinal cord before synapsing, the second-order neurons crossing the midline and then ascending with the spinothalamic fibres. Fibres conveying sensation from progressively more forward areas of the face descend a shorter distance in the brain stem. Thus sensory loss in the face from low brain-stem lesions is in a 'balaclava helmet' distribution as the descending trigeminal fibres are affected.

Hemisphere lesions

Both the dorsal column and spinothalamic tracts end in the thalamus, relaying thence to the parietal cortex through the internal capsule. All modalities of sensation can therefore be affected by lesions in the hemispheres. In the thalamus discrete lesions (as may occur in small lacunar strokes) can cause loss of sensation over the whole contralateral half of the body. Lesions in the sensory cortex have to be very small (and therefore affect only a restricted area of the body) to avoid affecting the motor tracts deeper in the hemispheres. With substantial lesions of the parietal cortex (as with large strokes) there is severe loss of proprioception and even conscious awareness of the existence of the affected limb(s). The resulting loss of function in the limb may be impossible to distinguish from paralysis.

Pain

Pain is a complex percept which is only partly related to activity in nociceptor neurons (see Fig. 14.15, p. 958). In the posterior horn of the spinal cord the second-order neuron of the spinothalamic tract is subject to modulation by a number of influences in addition to its synapse with the fibres from nociceptors. Branches from the larger mechanoceptor fibres destined for the posterior column also synapse with the second-order spinothalamic neurons and with interneurons of the grey matter of the posterior horn. The nociceptor neurons release, in addition to excitatory transmitters, other neurotransmitters (such as substance P) which influence the excitability of the spinothalamic neurons. Neurons in the posterior horn are also subject to modulation by fibres descending from the peri-aqueductal grey matter of the mid-brain and raphe nuclei of the medulla. Neurons of this 'descending analgesia system' are activated by endogenous opiate (endorphin) peptides. The spinal cord's posterior horn is therefore much more than a way-station in the transmission of nociceptive sensory information; it is a complex organ for gating and modulating information of painful stimuli before this ascends in the spinothalamic tract. In the diencephalon the perception of pain is further influenced by the rich interconnections of the thalamus with the limbic system.

Neuropathic pain

Pain is of two main types: nociceptive pain, arising from a pathological process in a body part, and neuropathic pain, caused by dysfunction of the pain perception apparatus itself. Neuropathic pain has distinctive features and is described as a very unpleasant persistent burning paraesthetic sensation. There is always increased sensitivity to touch so that light brushing touches cause exquisite pain (hyperpathia). Painful stimuli appear to come from a larger area than that touched and spontaneous bursts of pain may occur. The perception of pain may be elicited by stimuli from other modalities (e.g. loud sounds) and is considerably affected by emotional influences. The most common syndromes of neuropathic pain are seen where there is partial damage to peripheral nerves ('causalgia'), to the trigeminal nerve (post-herpetic neuralgia) or to the thalamus. Treatment of these syndromes is very difficult. Drugs which modulate various parts of the nociceptive system, such as carbamazepine, tricyclics or phenothiazines, may help but usually only partially. Neurosurgical attempts to interrupt various pain pathways sometimes succeed but often increase the sensory deficit and may worsen the situation. Implantation of electrical stimulators has occasionally proved successful.

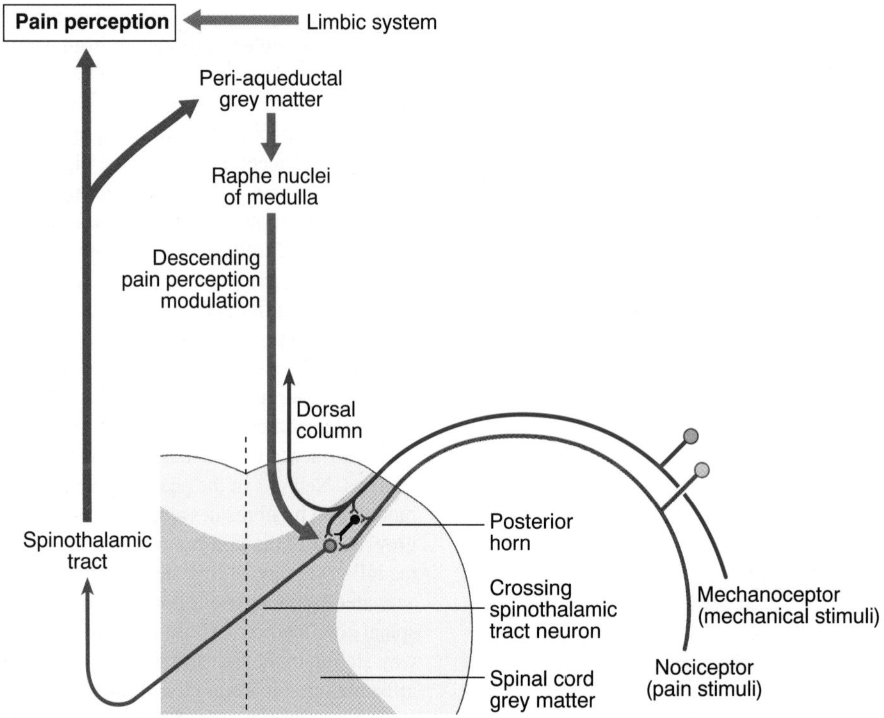

Fig. 14.15 The pain perception system.

COMA AND BRAIN DEATH

COMA

Persistent loss of consciousness or coma indicates disorder of the arousal mechanisms in the brain stem and diencephalon and indicates bilateral hemisphere or brain-stem disease. There are many causes of coma (see the information box). The history of the mode of onset of coma and of any precipitating event is crucial to establishing the cause and this should be obtained from family or other witnesses. As with any medical emergency, the top priority is assessment and stabilisation of the vital functions. Neurological examination may reveal important findings, e.g. evidence of head injury, papilloedema, meningism or eye movement disorder. In the majority of cases, however, there are no focal neurological signs since drug overdose and metabolic disturbance are the most common causes of unexplained coma requiring hospital admission.

CAUSES OF COMA

Metabolic disturbance
- Drug overdose
- Diabetes mellitus
  - Hypoglycaemia
  - Ketoacidosis
  - Hyperosmolar coma
- Hyponatraemia
- Uraemia
- Hepatic failure
- Respiratory failure
- Hypothermia

Trauma
- Cerebral contusion
- Extradural haematoma
- Subdural haematoma

Cerebrovascular disease
- Subarachnoid haemorrhage
- Intracerebral haemorrhage
- Brain-stem infarction/ haemorrhage
- Cerebral venous sinus thrombosis

Infections
- Meningitis
- Encephalitis
- Cerebral abscess

Others
- Epilepsy
- Tumour
- Thiamine deficiency

Assessment of conscious level

This is an essential component of the neurological examination. Terms such as ‘stuporose’, ‘semi-conscious’ and ‘obtunded’ are ill defined and a clear description of the patient’s level of arousal and response to stimuli is more helpful. Systematic assessment of the unconscious patient by the application of the Glasgow Coma Scale provides a grading of coma by using a numerical scale which allows serial comparison and may provide prognostic information, particularly in traumatic coma (see the information box).

GLASGOW COMA SCALE	
Eye-opening (E)	
• Spontaneous	4
• To speech	3
• To pain	2
• Nil	1
Best motor response (M)	
• Obeys	6
• Localises	5
• Withdraws	4
• Abnormal flexion	3
• Extensor response	2
• Nil	1
Verbal response (V)	
• Orientated	5
• Confused conversation	4
• Inappropriate words	3
• Incomprehensible sounds	2
• Nil	1
Coma score = E + M + V	
• Minimum	3
• Maximum	15

BRAIN DEATH

The widespread availability of mechanical ventilators has resulted in the survival of patients with severe and irreversible brain damage but functioning cardiovascular systems. Diagnostic criteria for brain death have been established in order that those patients without functioning brains who have no chance of recovery may be identified and ventilation discontinued.

The diagnosis of brain death depends on meeting a set of preconditions (see the information box), all of which must coexist, and then applying a series of clinical tests (see the information box top right), all of which must be fulfilled.

PRECONDITIONS FOR CONSIDERING A DIAGNOSIS OF BRAIN DEATH

- The patient is deeply comatosed
  (a) There must be no suspicion that coma is due to depressant drugs, e.g. narcotics, hypnotics, tranquillisers
  (b) Hypothermia has been excluded—rectal temperature must exceed 35°C
  (c) There is no profound abnormality of serum electrolytes, acid-base balance or blood glucose concentrations, and any metabolic or endocrine cause of coma has been excluded
- The patient is maintained on a ventilator because spontaneous respiration had been inadequate or had ceased. Drugs, including neuromuscular blocking agents, must have been excluded as a cause of the respiratory failure
- The diagnosis of the disorder leading to brain death has been firmly established. There must be no doubt that the patient is suffering from irremediable structural brain damage

TESTS FOR CONFIRMING BRAIN DEATH

ALL BRAIN-STEM REFLEXES ARE ABSENT

- The pupils are fixed and unreactive to light
- The corneal reflexes are absent
- The vestibulo-ocular reflexes are absent—there is no eye movement following the injection of 20 ml of ice-cold water into each external auditory meatus in turn
- There are no motor responses to adequate stimulation within the cranial nerve distribution
- There is no gag reflex and no reflex response to a suction catheter in the trachea
- No respiratory movement occurs when the patient is disconnected from the ventilator long enough to allow the carbon dioxide tension to rise above the threshold for stimulating respiration ($PaCO_2$ must reach 6.7 kPa)

The diagnosis of brain death should be made by two experienced doctors, one of whom should be a consultant and the other a consultant or specialist registrar. The tests are usually repeated after an interval of 6–24 hours, depending on the clinical circumstances, before brain death is finally confirmed

DISTURBANCES OF HIGHER CORTICAL FUNCTION

Many areas of cerebral cortex have a specialised function (e.g. the primary motor areas, language areas etc.). Focal lesions of the cerebral hemispheres can therefore cause disturbance of these individual functions, e.g. aphasia. Alternatively, diffuse or multifocal damage affects many areas, causing more global disturbance of higher cerebral function. Depending on speed of onset, and whether consciousness is impaired, global disturbances are broadly divided into dementias and acute confusional states. In order to understand these syndromes of higher cerebral dysfunction, it is helpful to have an understanding of the individual specialised areas of cerebral cortical function.

FOCAL DEFICITS

It is easiest to consider the individual cortical functions lobe by lobe, and the areas discussed are shown in Figure 14.16, page 960. Many of the functions are lateralised, and the side to which they are lateralised depends on which of the two hemispheres is dominant. This is the one in which language function is represented. In right-handed individuals this is almost always the left hemisphere, while in left-handers either hemisphere may be dominant, with about equal frequency.

Frontal lobes

These are concerned with executive function, movement and behaviour. Well-defined functional areas in the frontal lobe include the primary motor cortex in the pre-rolandic gyrus, and Broca's speech area just anterior to the inferior

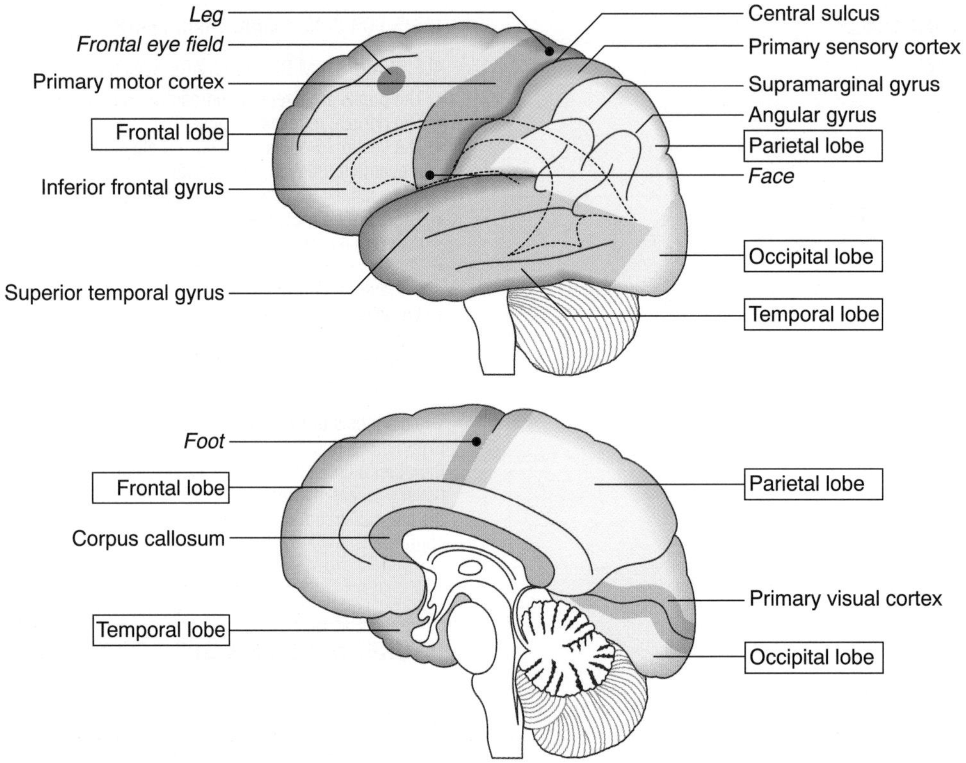

Fig. 14.16 The anatomy of the cerebral cortex.

end of this gyrus. The frontal eye fields lie higher up anterior to the primary motor cortex. There is also a supplementary motor area on the medial surface which is involved in higher-order motor control, and a micturition centre in the mesial frontal lobe involved in the maintenance of urinary continence. The positive and negative features of damage to these areas are listed in Table 14.10.

More diffuse damage to the frontal lobe results in behavioural disturbance. Personality can be affected in two broad directions. Patients with medial frontal lesions become increasingly withdrawn, unresponsive and mute (abulic), and this is often associated with urinary incontinence, gait apraxia, and the type of increase in tone known as gegenhalten. Those with lateral convexity lesions of the frontal lobes become disinhibited, sometimes to the point of grandiosity, or exhibit irresponsible behaviour (e.g. with financial affairs). Memory is substantially intact, and there may be focal physical signs such as a grasp reflex, palmomental response, or pout. As the frontal lobe overlies the olfactory bulb and tracts, structural lesions such as tumours in the inferior frontal lobes may be associated with anosmia.

Parietal lobe

The parietal lobes are concerned with the integration of sensory perception. The dominant parietal lobe contains part of the area which is involved in language, which is discussed below. Closely allied to the speech area are regions dealing with numerical function. The primary sensory cortex lies in the post-rolandic gyrus. Much of the remainder is devoted to 'association' cortex, damage to which gives rise to sensory (including visual) inattention and disorders of spatial perception and hence the disruption of spatially orientated behaviour leading to apraxia. Apraxia is the inability to perform complex, organised activity in the presence of a normal basic motor, sensory and cerebellar system (i.e. after weakness, numbness and ataxia have been excluded as causes). Such complex activities include dressing, the use of tools and finding one's way around geographically. As discussed below in the section on vision, parietal lobe lesions may also involve the optic radiations deep to the cortex, giving rise to homonymous inferior quadrantanopias of the contralateral visual space.

Temporal lobe

Well-defined functional areas in the temporal lobes include the primary auditory cortex and primary vestibular cortex. On the medial side lies the olfactory cortex, and the

Table 14.10 Cortical lobar functions

Lobe	Function	Effects of damage: Cognitive/behavioural	Effects of damage: Associated physical signs	Positive phenomena
Frontal	Personality Emotional control Social behaviour Contralateral motor control Language Micturition	Disinhibition Lack of initiation Antisocial behaviour Impaired memory Expressive dysphasia Incontinence	Impaired smell Contralateral hemiparesis Frontal release signs	Aversive seizures Focal motor seizures (Jacksonian march) Continuous partial seizures (epilepsia partialis continua)
Parietal: dominant	Language Calculation	Dysphasia Dyscalculia Dyslexia Apraxia Agnosia	Contralateral hemisensory loss Astereognosis Agraphaesthesia Contralateral homonymous lower quadrantanopia Asymmetry of optokinetic nystagmus (OKN)	Focal sensory seizures
Parietal: non-dominant	Spatial orientation Constructional skills	Neglect of non-dominant side Spatial disorientation Constructional apraxia Dressing apraxia	Contralateral hemisensory loss Astereognosis Agraphaesthesia Contralateral homonymous lower quadrantanopia Asymmetry of OKN	Focal sensory seizures
Temporal: dominant	Auditory perception Language Verbal memory Smell Balance	Receptive aphasia Dyslexia Impaired verbal memory	Contralateral homonymous upper quadrantanopia	Complex hallucinations (smell, sound, vision, memory)
Temporal: non-dominant	Auditory perception Melody/pitch perception Non-verbal memory Smell Balance	Impaired non-verbal memory Impaired musical skills (tonal perception)	Contralateral homonymous upper quadrantanopia	Complex hallucinations (smell, sound, vision, memory)
Occipital	Visual processing	Visual inattention Visual loss Visual agnosia	Homonymous hemianopia (± macular sparing)	Simple visual hallucinations (e.g. phosphenes, zigzag lines)

parahippocampal cortex which is involved in memory function. The temporal lobe contains many structures associated with the limbic system, including the hippocampus and the amygdala. Damage to these areas causes memory disturbance, and may also cause personality change.

The dominant temporal lobe shares the specialised language areas with the parietal lobe, and is particularly involved in verbal comprehension. Music processing occurs in both temporal lobes, rhythm being processed on the dominant side, and melody/pitch more on the non-dominant side. Temporal lobe lesions may be associated with contralateral homonymous superior quadrantanopias.

Occipital lobe

The occipital lobe is principally concerned with visual processing. The contralateral visual hemifield is represented in the primary visual (striate) cortex, and areas more anterior to this are involved in the processing of specific visual submodalities such as colour, movement or depth, and the analysis of more complex visual patterns such as faces.

DEMENTIA

Dementia is a clinical syndrome characterised by a loss of previously acquired intellectual function in the absence of impairment of arousal. There are many different potential causes of dementia (see Table 14.11, p. 962) but cerebral atrophy, usually due to Alzheimer's disease, and diffuse vascular disease are the most common.

When a patient presents with disturbance of personality or memory dysfunction, the first step is to exclude a focal lesion by determining that there is cognitive disturbance in more than one area. A careful history is, of course, essential and it is important to interview not just the patient, but a close family member. Simple bedside tests such as the mini-mental test are useful in assessing the cognitive deficit, but more formal help from clinical psychology may be required. General history and examination may give further clues to aetiology.

Many of the primary degenerative diseases which cause dementia have characteristic features which may allow a specific diagnosis during life. Creutzfeldt–Jakob disease is

Table 14.11 Causes of dementia

Type	Common	Unusual	Rare
Vascular	Diffuse small-vessel disease	Amyloid angiopathy Multiple emboli	Cerebral vasculitis
Degenerative/inherited	Alzheimer's disease	Huntington's disease Wilson's disease Pick's disease Cortical Lewy body disease Others (e.g. cortico-basal degeneration)	
Neoplastic	Secondary deposits	Primary cerebral tumour	Paraneoplastic syndrome (limbic encephalitis)
Traumatic	Chronic subdural haematoma	Post-head injury	Punch-drunk syndrome
Hydrocephalus		Communicating/non-communicating 'Normal pressure' hydrocephalus	
Toxic/nutritional	Alcohol	Thiamine deficiency B_{12} deficiency	Anoxia/carbon monoxide poisoning Heavy metal poisoning
Infective		Syphilis HIV	Post-encephalitic
Prion diseases		Creutzfeldt–Jakob disease	Kuru Gerstmann–Sträussler–Scheinker disease

usually relatively rapidly progressive (over months), is associated with myoclonus, and there may be characteristic abnormalities on EEG. Of the more slowly progressive dementias, Pick's disease presents with rather focal (temporal or frontal lobe) dysfunction often affecting language function early, and Lewy body dementia may present with visual disturbance. However, it is often difficult to distinguish these dementias from each other or from Alzheimer's disease during life. The distinction of senile from pre-senile dementia is unhelpful. However, rarer causes of dementia should be more actively sought in younger patients and those with short histories.

Investigations

The aim is to discover a treatable cause, if present, and to try to give an idea of prognosis if not, using a fairly standard set of investigations (see the information box). Imaging of the brain is important to exclude potentially treatable structural lesions such as hydrocephalus, cerebral tumour or chronic subdural haematoma, though often the only abnormality seen is generalised atrophy. If the initial tests fail to yield an answer, more invasive tests such as lumbar puncture or even brain biopsy may be indicated. If all investigations are negative, it is worth considering that the memory disturbance may be a manifestation of depressive illness (pseudo-dementia) and here formal neuropsychological evaluation is helpful.

INVESTIGATION OF DEMENTIA

In most patients	In selected patients
• Imaging of head (CT and/or MRI) • Blood tests Full blood count, ESR Urea and electrolytes, glucose Calcium, liver function tests Thyroid function tests Protein electrophoresis Vitamin B_{12} Venereal disease reference laboratory (VDRL) test ANA, anti-dsDNA • Chest radiograph • EEG	• Lumbar puncture • HIV serology • Brain biopsy

Management

This is directed at removing correctable causes, and at providing support for patient and carers if no specific treatment exists. Anticholinergic drugs, such as donepezil, have recently been introduced which appear to improve cognitive function to some extent in Alzheimer's disease. How useful these will be remains to be seen.

ACUTE CONFUSIONAL STATE

This is also known as delirium, and is seen much more commonly than dementia. Unlike dementia, there is global impairment of mental function associated with disturbance of arousal. This usually takes the form of drowsiness with disorientation, perceptual disturbances and muddled thinking. Patients typically fluctuate, confusion being worse at night, and there may be associated emotional disturbance (e.g. anxiety, irritability or depression) or psychomotor changes (e.g. agitation, restlessness or retardation).

Acute confusional states may be the result of acute

Table 14.12 Causes of acute confusional state

Type	Common	Unusual
Infective	Chest infection Urinary infection Septicaemia Viral illness Meningitis Encephalitis	Cerebral abscess Subdural empyema AIDS
Metabolic/ endocrine	Hypoxia (respiratory failure) Cardiac failure Acute (internal) haemorrhage Hyper-/hypoglycaemia Hyper-/hypocalcaemia Hyponatraemia Liver failure, renal failure	Carbon monoxide poisoning Hypo-/hyperthyroidism Adrenal disease Porphyria
Vascular	Acute cerebral haemorrhage/ infarction Subarachnoid haemorrhage	Vasculitis (e.g. SLE) Cortical venous thrombosis
Toxic	Alcohol intoxication/withdrawal Drugs (therapeutic/illicit)	
Neoplastic	Secondary deposits	Primary cerebral tumour Paraneoplastic syndrome
Trauma		Head injury (cerebral contusions) Subdural haematoma
Other	Post-ictal state	Acute hydrocephalus Complex partial status epilepticus

decompensation of any of the causes of dementia listed in Table 14.11. However, there are many other possible causes of acute confusion (see Table 14.12).

Diagnosis

The diagnosis of an acute confusional state involves careful history-taking. Patients are usually disorientated, often in both time and place, and therefore their account may not be helpful. As with dementia, it is vital to take a history from a witness (either a relative or a nurse). Examination may yield other clues to the cause (e.g. pyrexia, or focal chest or neurological signs). It is important to exclude a fluent aphasia, since patients with this speech disorder often appear confused despite having a focal cortical lesion. Often, however, the cause is not immediately obvious, and a wide screen of tests must be performed (see Table 14.13).

Management

The management of acute confusional states involves identifying the cause and correcting it if possible. Confused patients should be nursed in a well-lit room. During the period of confusion, drugs are best avoided, as they may serve simply to heighten the confusion, though occasionally sedative drugs such as chlorpromazine (25–100 mg 8-hourly) or haloperidol (2.5–10 mg 8-hourly) may be required. In delirium tremens (alcohol withdrawal), the treatment is a tapered course of chlormethiazole or chlordiazepoxide to accompany high-dose intravenous thiamin (see p. 521).

Table 14.13 Investigation of acute confusional state

	First-line	Other useful tests
Blood tests	Full blood count, ESR Urea and electrolytes, glucose Calcium, magnesium Liver function tests Thyroid function tests	Cardiac enzymes Protein electrophoresis Vitamin B_{12}, copper studies Syphilis serology ANA, anti-dsDNA Paraneoplastic markers, prostate-specific antigen
CNS investigations	Head imaging (CT and/or MRI)	Lumbar puncture EEG
Other	Arterial blood gases ECG Infection screen (blood cultures, chest radio-graph, urine culture)	Viral screen, as appropriate (e.g. HIV) Urinary porphyrins

SPEECH, SWALLOWING AND BRAIN-STEM FUNCTION

SPEECH

Speech is the process whereby vocal sounds are used to convey meaning between individuals. A large volume of the cerebral cortex is involved in this complex cognitive process, mostly in the dominant hemisphere. The decoding of speech sounds (phonemes) is a function of the upper part of the posterior temporal lobe. The perception of these sounds as meaningful language, as well as the formulation of the language required for the expression of ideas and concepts, occurs predominantly in the lower parts of the anterior parietal lobe (the angular and supramarginal gyri). The temporal speech comprehension region is referred to as Wernicke's area. Other parts of the temporal lobe contribute to language processing in areas specialising in verbal memory, where lexicons of meaningful words are 'stored'. The language information so generated then passes anteriorly via the arcuate fasciculus to Broca's area in the posterior end of the inferior frontal gyrus on the dominant side. The motor commands generated in Broca's area pass to the cranial nerve nuclei in the pons and medulla, as well as to the anterior horn cells in the spinal cord. The cerebellum has an important coordinating function. Nerve impulses then travel to the lips, tongue, palate, pharynx, larynx and respiratory muscles via the facial nerve and cranial nerves 9, 10 and 12, and result in the series of ordered sounds known as speech (see Fig. 14.17, p. 964).

These ordered sounds are detected by a listener in whom

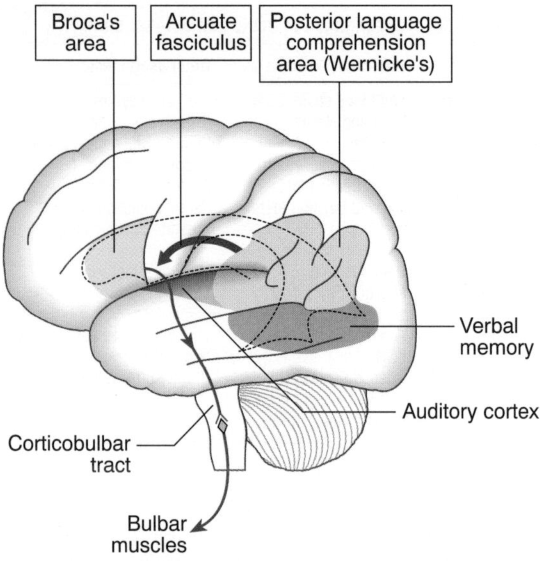

Fig. 14.17 Areas of the cerebral cortex involved in the generation of spoken language.

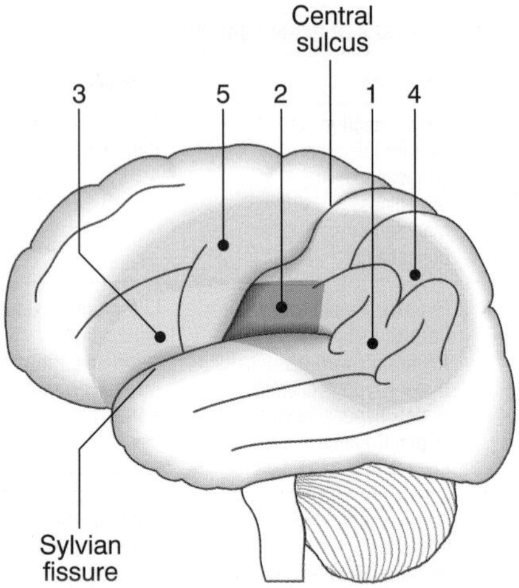

Fig. 14.18 Classification of aphasia, according to the site of the lesion and type of language deficit. All have naming difficulty (anomia). Fluent aphasias arise from lesions posterior to the central fissure; repetition is affected by lesions around the sylvian fissure. (1) Wernicke aphasia: fluent aphasia with poor comprehension and poor repetition. (2) Conduction aphasia: fluent aphasia with good comprehension and poor repetition. (3) Broca aphasia: non-fluent aphasia with good comprehension and poor repetition. (4) Transcortical sensory aphasia: fluent aphasia with good comprehension and good repetition. (5) Transcortical motor aphasia: non-fluent aphasia with good comprehension and good repetition. **N.B.** Large lesions affecting all regions 1–5 cause global aphasia.

nerve impulses are passed from the ears to the auditory cortex in the temporal lobe and hence to the speech comprehension areas. Parts of the non-dominant parietal lobe appear to contribute to non-verbal aspects of language in the recognition of meaningful intonation patterns of spoken words.

Aphasia

Aphasia is a disorder of the language content of speech. It can occur with lesions over a wide area of the dominant hemisphere. The term aphasia, rather than dysphasia, is now used to designate any degree of spoken language deficit. Aphasia is detected by the patient's inability to produce the correct word (anomia). When patients are asked to name objects or parts of objects, if anomia is present either no word will be produced or the wrong word or a nonsense word produced (paraphasia). Aphasia can be classified according to whether the speech output is 'fluent', in which a normal or increased number of (the wrong) words is produced, or 'non-fluent' if the verbal output is reduced. Patients with lesions anterior to the central fissure have non-fluent aphasia whilst those with lesions posterior to the central fissure in the speech areas have a fluent aphasia (and are often mistakenly thought to be 'confused'). By testing patients for the comprehension of words and their ability to repeat, their aphasia can be further classified into distinct syndromes of aphasia which have localising and prognostic implications (see Fig. 14.18).

If a patient is found to have difficulty with speech comprehension there is likely to be a lesion in the superior part of the posterior temporal lobe and/or the adjoining part of the parietal lobe. Patients with lesions around the sylvian (lateral) fissure will have difficulty with repetition, whilst those with lesions away from the sylvian fissure can repeat and may do so compulsively. Patients with large lesions over much of the speech area are not testable in such a refined manner, having no language production, and are said to have 'global aphasia'. Some patients with patchy lesions in the speech areas may not be easily classified according to the above scheme and are said to have anomic aphasia. Patients with fluent aphasia tend not to have an associated hemiparesis since the pyramidal tract is not involved, whilst those with the more anteriorly placed lesions causing non-fluent aphasia often do have a hemiparesis.

Dysphonia and dysarthria

Speech can be disturbed in a number of ways. At a simple level, the vocal cords may fail to generate sound properly, and this results in hoarse or whispered speech (dysphonia). If the muscles or nerves controlling the mouth, tongue, pharynx and lips are not functioning correctly, poorly articulated speech will result (dysarthria). There is no problem with choice of words, but the speech may or may not be intelligible, depending on severity. Cerebellar or brain-stem disease, lower cranial nerve lesions, myasthenia

Table 14.14 Causes of dysarthria

Type	Site	Characteristics	Associated features
Myopathic	Muscles of speech	Indistinct, poor articulation	Weakness of face, tongue and neck
Myasthenic	Motor end plate	Indistinct with fatigue and dysphonia Fluctuating severity	Ptosis, diplopia, facial and neck weakness
Bulbar	Brain stem	Indistinct, slurred, often nasal	Dysphagia, diplopia, ataxia
'Scanning'	Cerebellum	Slurring, impaired timing and cadence, 'sing-song' quality	Ataxia of limbs and gait tremor of head/limbs
Spastic	Pyramidal tracts	Indistinct, breathy, mumbling	Poor rapid tongue movements; increased reflexes and jaw jerk
Parkinsonian	Basal ganglia	Indistinct, rapid, stammering, quiet	Tremor, rigidity, slow shuffling gait
Dystonic	Basal ganglia	Strained, slow	Dystonia, athetosis

or muscle disease may all result in dysarthria. The quality of the speech tends to differ somewhat depending on the cause (see Table 14.14).

SWALLOWING

Swallowing is a complex activity involving the co-ordinated action of lips, tongue, soft palate, pharynx and larynx, which are innervated by the facial nerve and cranial nerves 9, 10, 11 and 12. This mechanism is potentially vulnerable to damage to many different areas of the nervous system, resulting in dysphagia which is usually accompanied by dysarthria. Structural causes of dysphagia are considered on page 612. Acute onset of dysphagia may occur as a result of brain-stem stroke, a rapidly developing neuropathy such as the Guillain–Barré syndrome or diphtheria. The upper motor neuron innervation of the cranial nerves responsible for swallowing is bilateral, so persistent dysphagia is unusual with a unilateral upper motor lesion. However, dysphagia may occur in the early stages of such a lesion if it is very acute, such as a hemisphere stroke. Dysphagia developing subacutely may be seen in myasthenia gravis, motor neuron disease, polymyositis, basal meningitis and inflammatory brain-stem disease. More slowly developing dysphagia suggests a myopathy or, possibly, a brain-stem or skull-base tumour.

BULBAR AND PSEUDOBULBAR PALSY

The lower cranial nerves, 9, 10, 11 and 12, are frequently affected bilaterally, producing dysphagia and dysarthria. The term 'bulbar palsy' is used if this results from lower motor neuron lesions, either at nuclear or fascicular level within the medulla, or from bilateral lesions of the lower cranial nerves outside the brain stem. The tongue is wasted and fasciculating and the palate moves very little. A 'pseudobulbar palsy' arises from an upper motor neuron lesion of the bulbar muscles from lesions of the corticobulbar pathways in the pyramidal tracts. Here the tongue is small and bunched, and moves slowly, and the jaw jerk is brisk. Causes of bulbar and pseudobulbar palsies are shown in Table 14.15.

BRAIN-STEM FUNCTION

Many different functional areas are tightly packed into the brain stem (see Fig. 14.19, p. 966). Long motor and sensory tracts course through its length, and are punctuated by individual brain-stem nuclei and cranial nerves, along with their respective interconnections and connections to the cerebrum and cerebellum. Thus, damage to even a small area of the brain stem potentially causes major disturbance of several systems. As the anatomy of the brain stem is very precisely organised, it is usually possible to localise the site of a lesion on the basis of careful history and examination to determine exactly which tracts/nuclei are affected. Lesions can occur singly, multiply or diffusely, but the

Table 14.15 Causes of bulbar and pseudobulbar palsy

	Pseudobulbar	Bulbar
Genetic		Kennedy's disease (X-linked bulbospinal neuronopathy)
Vascular	Bilateral hemisphere (lacunar) infarction	Medullary infarction
Degenerative	Motor neuron disease	Motor neuron disease Syringobulbia
Inflammatory/ infective	Multiple sclerosis Cerebral vasculitis	Myasthenia Guillain–Barré Poliomyelitis Lyme disease Vasculitis
Neoplastic	High brain-stem tumours	Brain-stem glioma Malignant meningitis

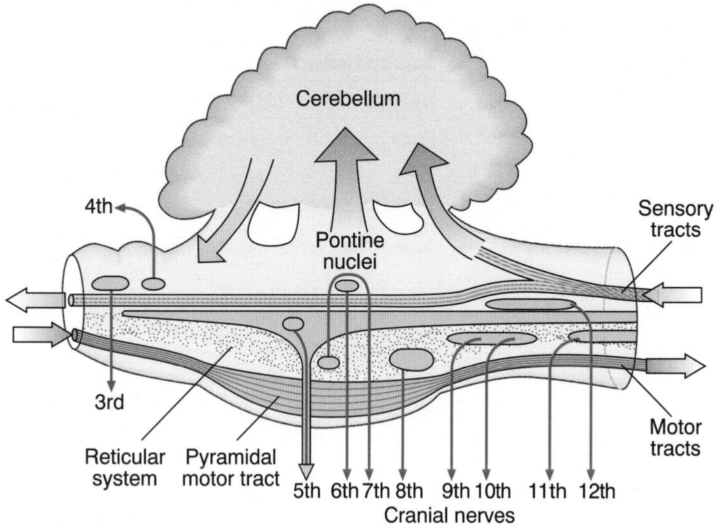

Fig. 14.19 Anatomy of the brain stem.

standard neurological approach is to try to explain all of a patient's problems in the minimum number of lesions (ideally just one).

An example would be a patient presenting with sudden onset of upper motor neuron features affecting the right face, arm and leg in association with a left 3rd nerve palsy. The lesion would have to be in the left cerebral peduncle in the brain stem where the pathology is likely to have been a small stroke, as the onset was sudden. This combination of signs is known as Weber's syndrome, and this is one of several well-described brain-stem stroke syndromes which are listed in Table 14.16.

Table 14.16 Major brain-stem stroke syndromes

Name of syndrome	Site of lesions	Clinical features
Weber	Anterior cerebral peduncle (mid-brain)	Ipsilateral 3rd palsy Contralateral upper motor neuron 7th palsy Contralateral hemiplegia
Claude	Cerebral peduncle involving red nucleus	Ipsilateral 3rd palsy Contralateral cerebellar signs
Parinaud	Dorsal mid-brain (tectum)	Vertical gaze palsy Convergence disorders Convergence retraction nystagmus Pupillary and lid disorders
Millard–Gubler	Ponto-medullary junction	Ipsilateral 6th palsy Ipsilateral lower motor neuron 7th palsy Contralateral hemiplegia
Wallenberg	Lateral medulla	Ipsilateral 5th, 9th, 10th, 11th palsy Ipsilateral Horner's syndrome Ipsilateral cerebellar signs Contralateral spino-thalamic sensory loss Vestibular disturbance

LOWER CRANIAL NERVE LESIONS

Bilateral lesions of cranial nerves 9, 10, 11 and 12 present as bulbar and pseudobulbar palsies and are discussed above (see Table 14.15). Cranial nerves 9, 10 and 11 may be affected together on one side as they pass through the jugular foramen at the skull base. The hypoglossal (12th) nerve exits the skull in its own foramen and lies close to the 9th, 10th and 11th nerves just outside the skull. All four lower cranial nerves are here anatomically related to the carotid artery and the ascending sympathetic innervation to the eye. Lesions affecting the lower cranial nerves at the skull base include tumours and dissection of the carotid artery (see Table 14.17).

DISTURBANCES OF THE VISUAL SYSTEM

Disturbances of vision are common and often related to problems with the eye rather than disorder of the nervous system. A common reason for presentation is loss of vision, but patients may also present with positive visual symptoms (e.g. hallucinations). The movements of the two eyes may be disturbed and give rise to double vision (diplopia) or blurred vision. Alternatively, patients may present with disordered appearance of their visual apparatus, and this can include the eyelids, the globe, the eye movements, the pupils or the appearance of the optic disc on fundoscopy (e.g. papilloedema).

Table 14.17 Syndromes of the lower cranial nerve lesions outside the brain stem

Syndrome	Cranial nerves involved	Site of lesion	Cause
Vernet	9, 10 and 11	Jugular foramen (inside skull)	Metastases, neurinoma, meningioma, epidermoid, carotid body tumour
Collet–Sicard	9, 10, 11 and 12	Jugular foramen just outside the skull, near foramen lacerum	Metastases, neurinoma, meningioma, epidermoid, carotid body tumour
Villaret	9, 10, 11 and 12 and Horner's	Posterior retropharyngeal space, near carotid artery	Carotid dissection, metastases, neurinoma, meningioma, epidermoid, carotid body tumour
Isolated 12th	12	Skull base (hypoglossal canal)	Metastases, neurinoma, meningioma, epidermoid

VISUAL LOSS

The visual pathway from the retina to the occipital cortex is topographically organised, so the pattern of visual field loss allows precise localisation of the site of the lesion. Fibres from ganglion cells in the retina pass to the optic disc and then backwards through the lamina cribrosa to the optic nerve. Nasal optic nerve fibres (subserving the temporal visual field because the image on the retina is inverted) cross at the chiasm, but temporal fibres do not. Hence all fibres in the optic tract and further posteriorly subserve both eyes' representation of contralateral visual space. From the lateral geniculate nucleus, lower fibres pass through the temporal lobes on their way to the primary visual area in the occipital cortex, while the upper fibres pass through the parietal lobe. Patterns of visual field loss are explained by this anatomy, as seen in Figure 14.20, and associated clinical manifestations are described in Table 14.18, page 968.

It is not uncommon for patients to present with transient visual loss. Visual loss lasting from 1–20 minutes is likely to have a vascular cause. This can affect one eye (amaurosis fugax) or one visual field. Whether the field loss was uniocular (carotid circulation) or a homonymous hemianopia (vertebro-basilar circulation) is crucial to further management, and this must be distinguished by careful history (e.g. did the patient try shutting separate eyes?). Transient visual loss lasting 20–30 minutes suggests migraine, especially if accompanied by headache and/or positive visual phenomena.

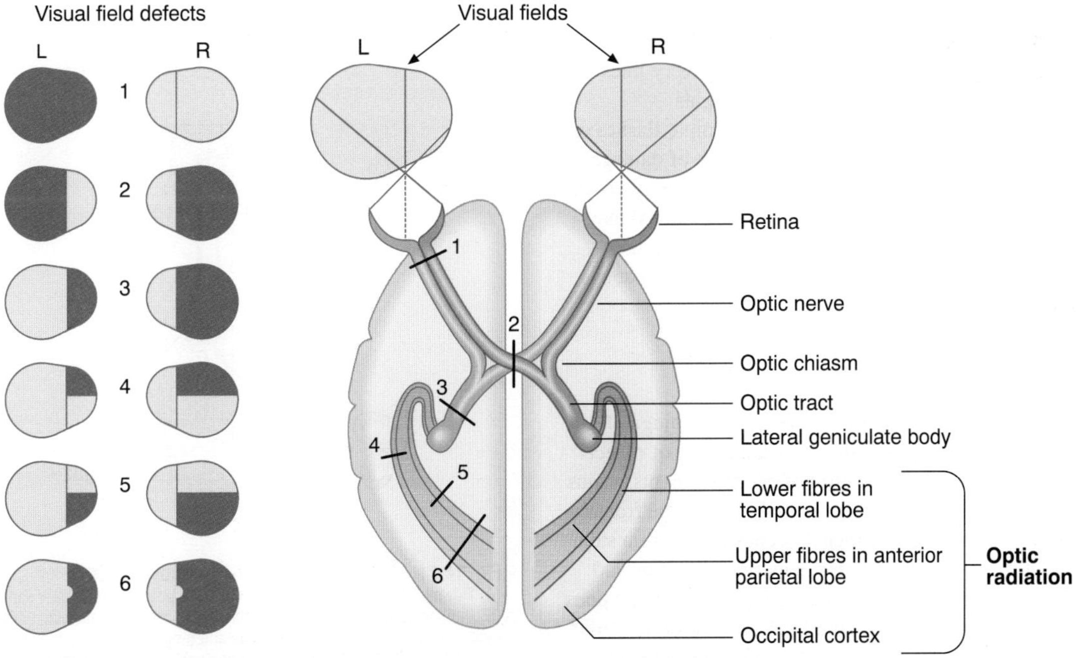

Fig. 14.20 Visual pathways and visual field defects.

Table 14.18 Clinical manifestations of visual field loss

Site	Common causes	Complaint	Visual field loss	Associated physical signs
Retina/optic disc	Vascular disease (including vasculitis) Glaucoma Inflammation	Partial/complete visual loss depending on site	Altitudinal field defect Arcuate scotoma	Reduced acuity Visual distortion (macula) Abnormal retinal appearance
Optic nerve	Optic neuritis Sarcoidosis Tumour Leber's hereditary optic neuropathy	Partial/complete loss of vision in one eye Often painful Central vision particularly affected	Central scotoma Paracentral scotoma Uniocular blindness	Reduced acuity Reduced colour vision Relative afferent pupillary defect Optic atrophy (late)
Optic chiasm	Pituitary tumours Craniopharyngioma Sarcoidosis	May be none Rarely diplopia ('hemifield slide')	Bitemporal hemianopia	Pituitary function abnormalities
Optic tract	Tumour Inflammatory disease	Disturbed vision to one side of midline	Incongruous contralateral homonymous hemianopia	
Temporal lobe	Stroke Tumour Inflammatory disease	Disturbed vision to one side of midline	Contralateral homonymous upper quadrantanopia	Memory/language disorders
Parietal lobe	Stroke Tumour Inflammatory disease	Disturbed vision to one side of midline Bumping into things	Contralateral homonymous lower quadrantanopia	Contralateral sensory disturbance Asymmetry of optokinetic nystagmus
Occipital lobe	Stroke Tumour Inflammatory disease	Disturbed vision to one side of midline Difficulty reading Bumping into things	Homonymous hemianopia (may be macula-sparing)	Damage to other structures supplied by posterior cerebral circulation

POSITIVE VISUAL SYMPTOMS

The most common cause of a positive visual disturbance is migraine, in which patients may see zigzag silvery lines (fortification spectra) or flashing coloured lights (teichopsia) which precede the headache. Simple flashes of light (phosphenes) can also be seen as a result of damage to the retina (e.g. detachment), or damage to the primary visual cortex. More complex visual percepts (hallucinations) may be caused by drugs, or may be due to structural damage resulting in epilepsy or 'release phenomena' (hallucinations which occur in a blind visual field).

EYE MOVEMENT DISORDERS

Under normal circumstances, the eyes move conjugately, though horizontal vergence allows visual fusion of objects at different distances. The control of eye movements begins in the cerebral hemispheres, particularly within the frontal eye fields, and the pathway then descends to the brain stem with input from the visual cortex, superior colliculus and cerebellum. Horizontal and vertical gaze centres in the pons and mid-brain, respectively, coordinate output to the ocular motor nerve nuclei (3, 4 and 6), which are connected to each other by the medial longitudinal fasciculus (MLF) (see Fig. 14.21). The MLF is particularly important in yoking

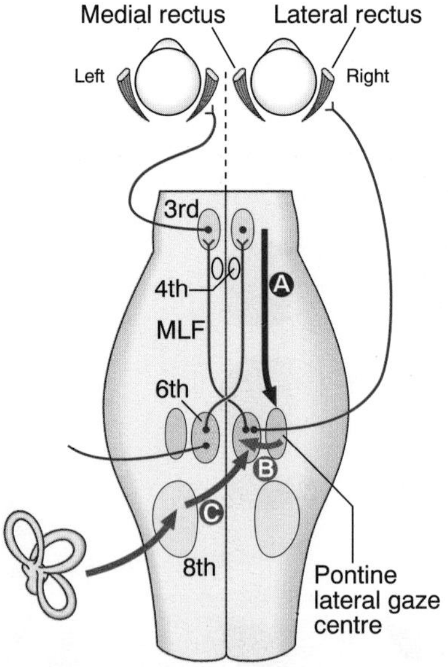

Fig. 14.21 Control of conjugate eye movements.
(A) Downward projections from the cortex to pontine lateral gaze centre. (B) Pontine gaze centre projects to the 6th cranial nerve nucleus, which innervates the ipsilateral lateral rectus and projects to the contralateral 3rd nerve nucleus (and hence medial rectus) via the medial longitudinal fasciculus (MLF). (C) Tonic inputs from the vestibular apparatus via the vestibular nuclei project to the contralateral 6th nerve nucleus.

the horizontal movements of the two eyes. The extraocular muscles are then supplied by the oculomotor (3rd), trochlear (4th) and abducens (6th) nerves.

Diplopia

This arises when eye movement is impaired so that the image of an object is not projected to homologous points on the two retinae. Impairment may result from central disorders, or from disturbance of the ocular motor nerves, muscles or the neuromuscular junction. The pattern of double vision, along with any associated features, usually allows localisation of the lesion whilst the mode of onset and subsequent behaviour (e.g. fatigability) suggest the aetiology.

The trochlear (4th) nerve innervates the superior oblique muscle, and the lateral rectus is innervated by the abducens (6th) nerve. The oculomotor (3rd) nerve innervates the remainder of the extraocular muscles along with the levator palpebrae superioris, and the ciliary body (pupil constriction, and accommodation). Causes of oculomotor nerve palsies are given in Table 14.19.

Complete oculomotor nerve lesions cause ptosis and a dilated pupil, and the eye tends to rest in a 'down and out' position due to unopposed tonic activity of the unaffected lateral rectus and superior oblique muscles. The pupil is often spared in ischaemic lesions (e.g. in diabetes), and its involvement requires that compressive lesions such as aneurysm be excluded. Trochlear nerve palsy presents with vertical diplopia (especially noticeable going downstairs), and the patient may have a head tilt and double vision when looking down to the side opposite the lesion. Abducens nerve palsy causes horizontal double vision when trying to look towards the side of the lesion. In diplopia of any cause, the image projected furthest away from primary position arises from the paretic eye, and this can often be determined by alternate eye cover.

Myasthenia gravis can cause diplopia by affecting any or all of the extraocular muscles. It is often associated with ptosis, and the hallmark is fatigability. Similarly, diseases of the extraocular muscles themselves can cause diplopia. Such diseases include thyroid eye disease, myopathies and orbital myositis.

Central lesions can also give rise to diplopia. Brain-stem lesions affecting the 3rd, 4th or 6th nerves or nuclei will cause diplopia, as will lesions of the MLF. The hallmark of an MLF lesion is an internuclear ophthalmoplegia (INO). The lateral gaze centre in the pons sends fibres to the ipsilateral 6th nerve nucleus. The nucleus contains two populations of neurons. Half the cells send their axons directly into the 6th nerve to supply the lateral rectus, while the remaining half send their fibres into the contralateral MLF and up to the contralateral 3rd nerve nucleus, where they synapse with neurons destined for the medial rectus (see Fig. 14.21). Hence, damage to the 6th nerve nucleus itself will prevent both eyes from moving ipsilaterally (gaze palsy), and a lesion of the MLF will interfere with adduction of the ipsilateral eye (INO). An INO may be partial or complete, and may be associated with nystagmus of the contralateral, abducting eye.

Table 14.19 Common causes of damage to cranial nerves 3, 4 and 6

Site	Common pathology	Nerve(s) involved	Associated features
Brain stem	Infarction Haemorrhage Demyelination Intrinsic tumour	3 (mid-brain) 6 (ponto-medullary junction)	Contralateral pyramidal signs Ipsilateral LMN 7 palsy (ponto-medullary junction) Other brain-stem/cerebellar signs
Intrameningeal course	Meningitis (infective/malignant)	3, 4 and/or 6	Meningism, features of primary disease
	Raised intracranial pressure	6 3 (uncal herniation)	Papilloedema Features of space-occupying lesion
	Aneurysms	3 (posterior communicating artery) 6 (basilar artery)	Pain Features of subarachnoid haemorrhage
	Cerebello-pontine angle tumour	6	8, 7, 5 lesions Ipsilateral cerebellar signs
	Trauma	3, 4 and/or 6	Other features of trauma
Cavernous sinus **Superior orbital fissure**	Infection/thrombosis Carotid artery aneurysm Caroticocavernous fistula Tumour (e.g. sphenoid wing meningioma) Granuloma	3, 4 and/or 6	May be 5 involvement also Pupil may be fixed, mid-position (sympathetic near carotid) May be proptosis, chemosis
Orbit	Vascular (e.g. diabetes, vasculitis) Infections Tumour Granuloma Trauma	3, 4 and/or 6	Pain Pupil often spared in vascular 3 palsy

Nystagmus

If the eye movement control systems are defective, the eyes may drift off target and it becomes necessary to perform recurrent corrections to return fixation to the object of interest. This results in a repetitive to-and-fro movement (drift-correction-drift etc.) which is known as nystagmus. Usually the drifts are slower than the corrections (slow and quick phases, respectively). The direction of the fast phase is usually designated as the direction of the nystagmus, because it is easier to see, although the abnormality is the slower drift of the eyes off target. Nystagmus may be horizontal, vertical or torsional, and is usually conjugate, i.e. the two eyes usually move together. Nystagmus is seen as a physiological phenomenon in response to sustained vestibular stimulation or movement of the visual world (optokinetic nystagmus). There are, however, many different causes of pathological nystagmus, the most common being disorders of the vestibular system (peripheral and central components) and brain-stem/cerebellar lesions.

In lesions of the vestibular system (most commonly peripheral labyrinthine lesions), damage to one side will allow the tonic output from the healthy, contralateral side to cause the eyes to drift towards the side of the lesion. This causes recurrent compensatory fast movements away from the side of the lesion; hence unidirectional nystagmus to the opposite side is seen, often with a torsional element. The nystagmus of peripheral labyrinthine lesions disappears (fatigues) quite quickly and is always accompanied by vertigo and quite often nausea and vomiting. Central vestibular nystagmus is more persistent.

The brain stem and the cerebellum are involved in maintaining eccentric positions of gaze. Lesions will therefore allow the eyes to drift back in towards primary position (gaze-evoked nystagmus). This produces nystagmus whose fast component beats in the direction of gaze. This is the most common type of 'central' nystagmus and is not usually accompanied by vertigo, but there may be other signs of brain-stem dysfunction. Brain-stem disease may also cause vertical nystagmus.

Unilateral cerebellar lesions may result in nystagmus when looking in the direction of the lesion (gaze-evoked nystagmus), where the fast phases are directed towards the side of the lesion. Cerebellar hemisphere lesions also cause 'ocular dysmetria', an overshoot of target-directed fast-eye movements (saccades) resembling 'past-pointing' in limbs.

Nystagmus also occurs as a result of toxicity (especially drugs) and nutritional deficiency (thiamine deficiency). The severity is variable, and it may or may not result in visual degradation, though it may be associated with a sensation of movement of the visual world (oscillopsia). Nystagmus may occur as a congenital phenomenon, in which case the nystagmus is often quasi-sinusoidal ('pendular') rather than having alternating fast and slow phases ('jerk').

EYELID, GLOBE AND PUPIL DISORDERS

Various disorders may cause drooping or ptosis of the eyelid, and these are listed in Table 14.20.

In some circumstances the globe is pushed forward in the orbit, either unilaterally (proptosis) or bilaterally (exophthalmos). By far the most common cause of both is thyroid eye disease, but other causes include orbital tumours or granulomas, cavernous sinus disease, or inflammatory orbital disease ('pseudotumour').

DISORDERS OF THE PUPIL

Pupillary response to light is achieved by a combination of parasympathetic and sympathetic activity. Parasympathetic fibres originate in the Edinger–Westphal subnucleus of the 3rd nerve, and pass with the 3rd nerve to synapse in the ciliary ganglion before supplying the constrictor pupillae of

Table 14.20 Causes of ptosis

Mechanism	Causes	Associated clinical features
3rd nerve palsy	Isolated palsy (see Table 14.19) Central/supranuclear lesion	Ptosis is usually complete Extraocular muscle palsy (eye 'down and out') Depending on site of lesion, other cranial nerve palsies (e.g. 4, 5 and 6), or contralateral upper motor neuron signs
Sympathetic lesion (Horner's syndrome) (see Fig. 14.22)	Central (hypothalamus/brain stem) Peripheral (lung apex, carotid artery pathology) Idiopathic	Ptosis is partial Lack of sweating on affected side Depending on site of lesion, brain-stem signs, or signs of apical lung/brachial plexus disease, or ipsilateral carotid artery stroke
Myopathic	Myasthenia gravis Dystrophia myotonica Progressive external ophthalmoplegia	Extraocular muscle palsies More widespread muscle weakness, with fatigability in myasthenia Other characteristic features of individual diseases
Other	Pseudo-ptosis (e.g. blepharospasm) Local orbital/lid disease Age-related levator dehiscence	Eyebrows depressed rather than raised May be local orbital abnormality

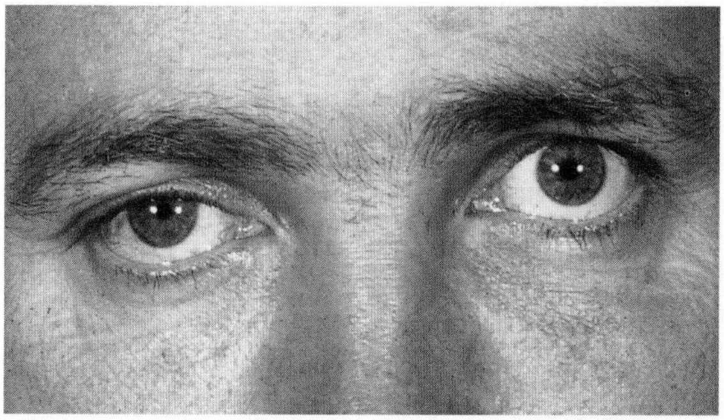

Fig. 14.22 Right-sided Horner's syndrome due to paravertebral metastasis at T1.

the iris. Sympathetic fibres originate in the hypothalamus, pass down the brain stem and cervical spinal cord to emerge at T1, return back up to the eye in association with the internal carotid artery and supply the dilator pupillae. Lesions in the sympathetic pathway cause Horner's syndrome (see Fig. 14.22). The pupils also constrict as part of the near reflex (in association with accommodation and convergence.

Lesions of the oculomotor nerve, ciliary ganglion and sympathetic supply produce characteristic 'efferent' disorders of pupillary function. 'Afferent' defects occur as a result of damage to an optic nerve, impairing the direct response of a pupil to light, although leaving the consensual response from stimulation of the normal eye intact.

Structural damage to the iris itself can also result in pupillary abnormalities. A summary is given in Table 14.21.

OPTIC DISC DISORDERS

Optic disc swelling

There are several causes of swelling of the optic disc, but the term 'papilloedema' is reserved for swelling in association with raised intracranial pressure. In raised intracranial pressure from any cause, axoplasmic flow from retinal ganglion cells is held up at the cribriform plate. This results in swollen nerve fibres, which in turn cause capillary and venous congestion, producing papilloedema. The first sign is the cessation of normal venous pulsation seen at the disc, and the disc margins then become red (hyperaemic). The margins become indistinct, and the whole disc is raised up, often with haemorrhages in the retina (see Fig. 14.23, p. 972).

Other causes of optic disc swelling are listed in the information box on page 972. Some normal variations of disc appearance can look like pathological disc swelling (pseudo-papilloedema).

Optic atrophy

Loss of nerve fibres causes the optic disc to appear pale, as the choroid becomes visible (see Fig. 14.24, p. 972). A pale disc (optic atrophy) follows optic nerve damage, and causes include previous optic neuritis, or ischaemic damage, long-standing papilloedema, optic nerve compression, trauma and degenerative conditions (e.g. Friedreich's ataxia).

Table 14.21 Pupillary disorders

Disorders	Cause	Ophthalmological features	Associated features
3rd nerve palsy	See Table 14.19, page 969	Dilated pupil Extraocular muscle palsy (eye is typically 'down and out') Complete ptosis	Other features of cause of 3rd palsy (see Table 14.19, p. 969)
Horner's syndrome (see Fig. 14.22)	Lesion to sympathetic supply	Small pupil Partial ptosis Iris heterochromia (if congenital)	Ipsilateral failure of sweating (anhidrosis)
Holmes–Adie syndrome (Adie pupil)	Lesion of ciliary ganglion (usually idiopathic)	Dilated pupil Light-near dissociation Vermiform movement of iris during contraction Disturbance of accommodation	Generalised areflexia
Argyll Robertson pupil	Dorsal mid-brain lesion (usually syphilis)	Small, irregular pupils Light-near dissociation (accommodate but do not react to light)	Other features of tabes dorsalis
Local pupillary damage	Trauma/inflammatory disease	Irregular pupils, often with adhesions to lens (synechiae) Variable degree of reactivity	Other features of trauma/underlying inflammatory disease (e.g. cataract, blindness etc.)
Relative afferent pupillary defect (Marcus Gunn pupil)	Damage to optic nerve (see Table 14.18, p. 968)	Pupils symmetrical, but degree of dilatation depends on which eye stimulated	Decreased visual acuity/colour vision Central scotoma Papilloedema/optic disc pallor

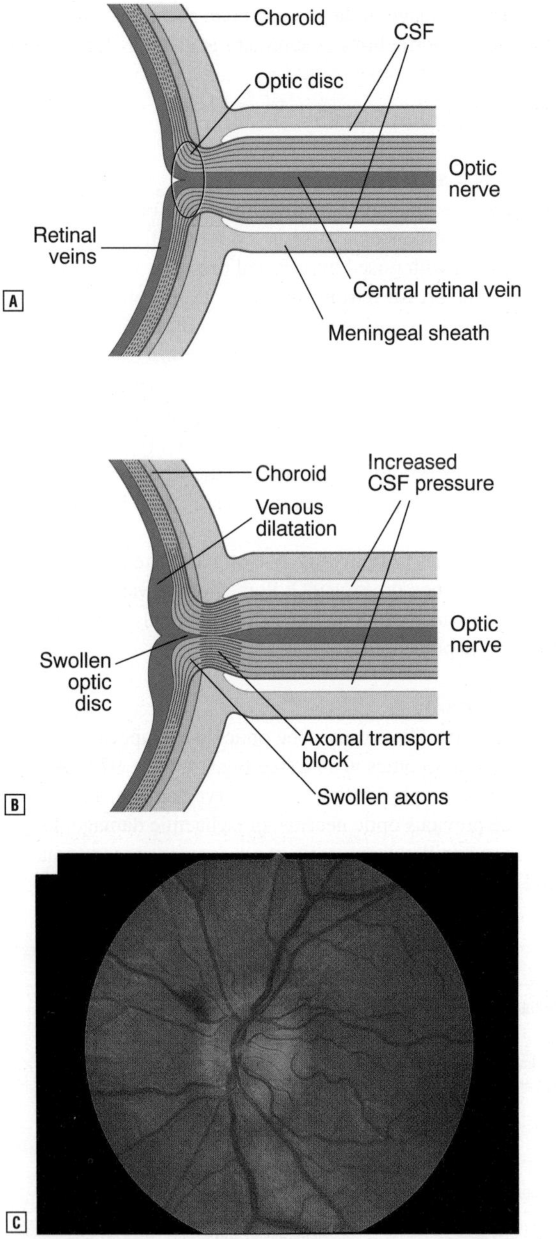

Fig. 14.23 Mechanism of optic disc oedema (papilloedema). [A] Normal. [B] Disc oedema (e.g. due to cerebral tumour). [C] Fundus photograph of the left eye showing optic disc oedema with a small haemorrhage on the nasal side of the disc.

COMMON CAUSES OF OPTIC DISC SWELLING
Raised intracranial pressure
• Cerebral mass lesion (tumour, abscess) • Hydrocephalus, haemorrhage, haematoma • Idiopathic intracranial hypertension
Obstruction of ocular venous drainage
• Central retinal vein occlusion • Cavernous sinus thrombosis
Systemic disorders affecting retinal vessels
• Hypertension • Vasculitis • Hypercapnia
Optic nerve damage
• Demyelination (optic neuritis/papillitis) • Leber's hereditary optic neuropathy • Ischaemia • Toxins (e.g. methanol) • Infiltration of optic disc • Sarcoidosis • Glioma • Lymphoma

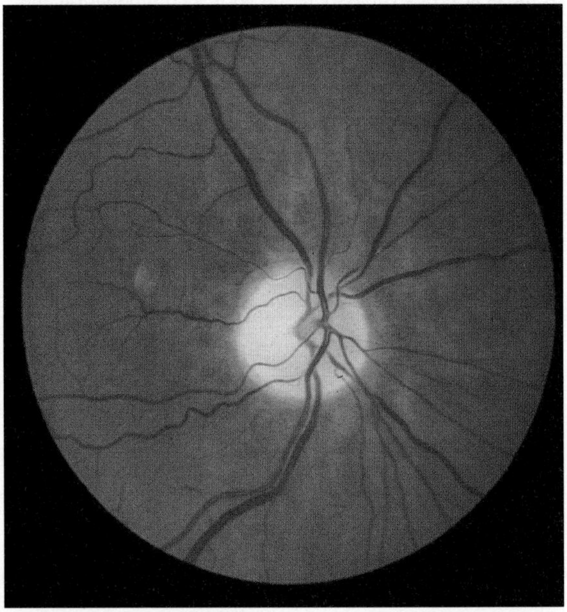

Fig. 14.24 Fundus photograph of the left eye of a patient with familial optic atrophy. Note marked pallor of optic disc.

SPHINCTER DISTURBANCE

BLADDER

The bladder is analogous to skeletal muscle in that neural control can be divided into upper and lower 'motor neuron' components. The parasagittal part of the frontal lobe contains a micturition centre. Connections pass from this area via a further micturition centre in the pons down into the spinal cord, where they are spread out in the lateral columns bilaterally. The sympathetic supply to the bladder leaves the upper lumbar spinal cord to synapse in the inferior hypogastric plexus, while the parasympathetic supply leaves from S2–4. In addition, a further somatic supply to the external (voluntary) sphincter arises from S2–4, travelling via the pudendal nerves. Stimulation of sympathetic fibres causes relaxation of the detrusor muscle and contraction of the internal sphincter, while stimulation of the parasympathetic fibres causes the reverse effects.

Afferent fibres from the bladder wall pass via the pelvic and hypogastric nerves. Distension of the bladder evokes reflex detrusor contraction (analogous to the muscle stretch reflex). Reciprocal changes in sympathetic activation and relaxation of the external sphincter aid this process. Normally unwanted bladder emptying is prevented by descending control from the medial frontal cortex via the spinal cord.

Damage to the 'lower motor neuron' component, i.e. the pelvic and pudendal nerves, gives rise to a flaccid bladder with overflow incontinence, often accompanied by loss of pudendal sensation. Such damage may be due to disease of the conus medullaris or sacral nerve roots, either within the dura (as in inflammatory or carcinomatous meningitis), or as they pass through the sacrum (trauma or malignancy), or due to damage to the nerves themselves in the pelvis (infection, haematoma, trauma or malignancy).

Damage to the pons or spinal cord results in an 'upper motor neuron' pattern of bladder dysfunction due to uncontrolled overactivity of the parasympathetic supply. The bladder is small, and highly sensitive to being stretched (analogous to spasticity). This results in frequency, urgency and urge incontinence. In lesions of the spinal cord, the phenomenon of detrusor-sphincter dyssynergia may develop in addition; the bladder itself is 'spastic', but the external sphincter does not relax at the same time as the detrusor contracts. This manifests as both urgency and an inability to pass water, which is distressing and painful, and which may last some minutes before partial emptying of the bladder is achieved. There is often a post-micturition residuum of urine which is prone to infection. More severe lesions of the spinal cord, as in spinal cord compression or trauma, can result in urinary retention; this will be painless, as bladder sensation, normally carried in the lateral spinothalamic tracts, will be cut off.

Damage to the mesial frontal lobes gives rise to loss of awareness of bladder fullness, and consequent incontinence. Coexisting cognitive impairment may result in inappropriate micturition. These features are seen typically in hydrocephalus, frontal tumours, dementia and bifrontal subdural haematomas.

When faced with a patient who has bladder symptoms, it is important to try to localise the lesion on the basis of history and examination. Clinical features are summarised in Table 14.22.

Management of bladder disturbance involves identifying the cause and correcting it if possible. A flaccid bladder can be stimulated with alpha-adrenoceptor-blocking drugs such as prazosin or indoramin, but spastic bladders are much more common in neurological disease. Unwanted detrusor activity (and hence urgency) can be lessened by anticholinergic drugs such as oxybutynin or imipramine. This will not solve the problem of detrusor-sphincter dyssynergia, however, and it may be necessary to teach the patient how to perform intermittent clean self-catheterisation; by emptying the bladder regularly, urinary frequency is reduced, as is the likelihood of infection. Long-term catheterisation (urethral or suprapubic) may be necessary, but this is avoided if at all possible as it is associated with infection as well as with technical problems such as blockage.

RECTUM

The rectum has an excitatory cholinergic input from the parasympathetic sacral outflow, and inhibitory sympathetic supply similar to the bladder. Continence depends largely

Table 14.22 Neurogenic bladder: clinical features and treatment

	Site of lesion	Result	Treatment
Atonic ('lower motor neuron')	Lesions of sacral segments of cord (conus medullaris) Lesions of sacral roots and nerves	Loss of detrusor contraction Difficulty initiating micturition Bladder distension with overflow	Alpha-adrenoceptor blockers Prazosin (500 μg 12-hourly) Indoramin (20 mg 12-hourly) Catheterisation
Hypertonic ('upper motor neuron')	Pyramidal tract lesion in spinal cord or brain stem	Urgency with urge incontinence Bladder sphincter incoordination (dyssynergia) Incomplete bladder emptying	Anticholinergics Oxybutynin (5 mg 8–12-hourly) Imipramine (25 mg 12-hourly) Flavoxate (200 mg 8-hourly) Baclofen (15–100 mg/day) Intermittent self-catheterisation
Cortical	Post-central Pre-central Frontal	Loss of awareness of bladder fullness Difficulty initiating micturition Inappropriate micturition Loss of social control	Intermittent catheterisation Intermittent catheterisation Catheterisation

on skeletal muscle contraction in the puborectalis and pelvic floor muscles supplied by the pudendal nerves, as well as the internal and external anal sphincters. Damage to the autonomic components causes constipation. Lesions affecting the conus medullaris, the somatic S2–4 roots and the pudendal nerves cause faecal incontinence.

PENILE ERECTION AND EJACULATION

These related functions are under autonomic control via the pelvic nerves (parasympathetic, S2–4) and hypogastric nerves (sympathetic, L1–2). Descending influences from the cerebrum are important for psychogenic erection, but erection can occur as a purely reflex phenomenon in response to genital stimulation. Erection is largely parasympathetic, and is impaired by drugs which have anticholinergic effects and also by some antihypertensive and antidepressant agents. Sympathetic activity is important for ejaculation, and may be inhibited by alpha-adrenoceptor antagonists.

FURTHER INFORMATION ON MAJOR MANIFESTATIONS OF NERVOUS SYSTEM DISEASE

Bradley W G, Daroff R B, Fenichel G M, Marsden C D 1996 Neurology in clinical practice (vol. I): Principles of diagnosis and management, 2nd edn. Butterworth–Heinemann, Boston
Duncan J S, Shorvan S D, Fish D R 1995 Clinical epilepsy. Churchill Livingstone, Edinburgh
Lance J W 1993 Mechanisms and management of headache, 5th edn. Butterworth–Heinemann, London
Plum F, Posner J B 1980 The diagnosis of stupor and coma, 3rd edn. F A Davis, Philadelphia

CEREBROVASCULAR DISEASE

Diseases of the cerebral blood vessels are the third most common cause of death in the developed world after cancer and ischaemic heart disease, and are responsible for a large proportion of physical disability, becoming more frequent with increasing age. The annual incidence of acute cerebrovascular disease in the over-45 age group in the UK is about 350 per 100 000.

Cerebrovascular disease can cause death and disability by ischaemia from occlusion of blood vessels (producing cerebral ischaemia and infarction) or haemorrhage through their rupture.

Clinical features of cerebrovascular disease

Cerebral arterial disease most commonly presents as an acute focal stroke, but ischaemic cerebral arterial disease may present, particularly in the elderly, with a gradual decline in intellectual function (dementia) with or without sensorimotor limb deficits or gait disorder. Haemorrhage from the major cerebral arteries of the circle of Willis into the subarachnoid space usually presents with a sudden, severe headache, vomiting and neck stiffness, with or without signs of focal brain damage (see p. 978). Disease of the cerebral venous circulation is rare and presents with characteristic clinical features which are usually distinct from those caused by cerebral arterial disease.

ACUTE FOCAL STROKE

Acute focal stroke is characterised by the sudden appearance of a focal deficit of brain function, most commonly a hemiplegia with or without signs of focal higher cerebral dysfunction (such as aphasia), hemisensory loss, visual field defect or brain-stem deficit. Provided that a clear history of such a sudden focal deficit is available, the chances of the brain lesion being anything other than vascular is 1% or less, but care needs to be taken to exclude other differential diagnoses, especially if the history is not clearly of a sudden deficit (see the information box).

DIFFERENTIAL DIAGNOSIS OF ACUTE STROKE

- Primary cerebral tumours
- Metastatic cerebral tumours
- Subdural haematoma
- Cerebral abscess
- Todd's paresis (after epileptic seizure)
- Demyelination
- Hypoglycaemia
- Encephalitis
- Hysterical conversion

Clinical classification of focal stroke

A stroke is defined as:

- completed if the focal deficit is persistent and not worsening
- transient if the deficit recovers within 24 hours
- evolving if the focal deficit continues to worsen after about 6 hours from onset.

Transient stroke

Since transient strokes are almost always ischaemic, the term 'transient ischaemic attack' (TIA) is often used, although occasionally small intracerebral haemorrhages present with a transient stroke deficit. Transient strokes are a major risk factor for disabling stroke, implying a 13-fold increased risk of stroke in the next year. The management of a patient with a transient stroke is therefore directed at secondary prevention of future disabling stroke. Many transient strokes last only for a few minutes, whilst some stroke deficits persist for some days before recovery. These minor completed strokes are managed in the same way as shorter-duration deficits.

Completed stroke

Of patients presenting with a persistent acute focal stroke, 85% have sustained a cerebral infarction and the remainder an intracerebral haemorrhage. It is not possible to distinguish between these reliably at the bedside. Headache may accompany the onset of both haemorrhagic and ischaemic strokes, although the combination of headache with vomiting at the onset strongly suggests that the stroke is primarily haemorrhagic. A history of hypertension and/or raised blood pressure is common in both types of stroke lesion, although other risk factors for atherosclerosis are more likely to be found with ischaemic strokes.

Evolving stroke

The majority of persistent stroke deficits have completed within 6 hours, many within minutes, but some evolve in a stuttering fashion over days. It is this small group of patients with evolving deficits which should be viewed with diagnostic suspicion in case a mass lesion has been misdiagnosed. However, the lesion is often due to progressive occlusion of a cerebral artery (either a major extracranial vessel or a small perforating artery).

The size of the deficit

The site of the lesion (in terms of which arterial territory is involved) and its size, which will have a bearing upon the management, can be determined by assessing the patient's neurological deficit in a fairly simple way. This involves assessing the patient for the presence of a motor deficit (hemiplegia), higher cerebral function deficit (e.g. aphasia or parietal deficit) or a hemianopia. In addition, the presence of simple sensory loss or a brain-stem deficit (e.g. an eye movement abnormality or vertigo) should be noted. Permutations of these deficits can define several syndromes of stroke, as in Figure 14.25.

Clinical assessment of the patient with a stroke should also include attention to the general examination, particularly the heart and peripheral arterial system (see the information box).

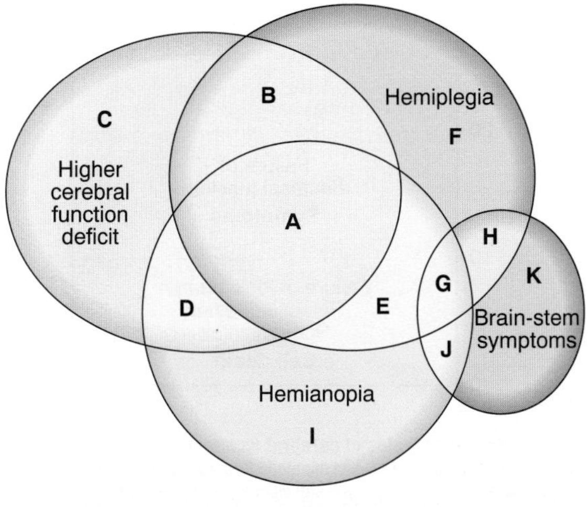

Fig. 14.25 Syndromes of acute stroke. (A) Total anterior circulation syndrome—TACS. (B, C, D and E) Partial anterior circulation syndromes—PACS. (F) Pure motor stroke—lacunar syndrome. (G, H, I, J and K) Posterior circulation syndromes—POCS.

POINTS FOR SPECIAL ATTENTION ON EXAMINATION OF A STROKE PATIENT
Eyes
• Diabetic changes • Hypertensive changes • Retinal emboli
Cardiovascular system
• Blood pressure (hypertension, hypotension) • Heart rhythm (atrial fibrillation) • Murmurs (sources of embolism) • Jugular venous pressure (heart failure, hypovolaemia) • Peripheral pulses and bruits (generalised arteriopathy)
Respiratory system
• Pulmonary oedema • Respiratory infection
Abdomen
• Urinary retention

CEREBRAL INFARCTION

Cerebral infarction is mostly due to thromboembolic disease secondary to atherosclerosis in the major extracranial arteries (carotid artery and aortic arch). About 20% of infarctions are consequent upon embolism from the heart, and a further 20% are due to occlusion of the small lenticulostriate perforating vessels by intrinsic disease (lipohyalinosis),

STROKE RISK FACTORS	
Irreversible	**Modifiable**
• Age • Gender (M > F, except in the very young and very old) • Race (Afro-Caribbean > Asian > European) • Heredity	• Hypertension • Heart disease (heart failure, atrial fibrillation) • Diabetes • Hyperlipidaemia • Smoking • Excess alcohol consumption • Polycythaemia • Oral contraceptives

producing so-called 'lacunar' infarctions. The risk factors for ischaemic stroke reflect the risk factors for these underlying vascular diseases (see the information box, p. 975).

Pathophysiology

Cerebral infarction is a process which takes some hours to complete, even though the patient's deficit may be maximal close to the onset of the causative vascular occlusion. After the occlusion of a cerebral artery, perfusion of its territory may be restored by the opening of anastomotic channels from other arterial territories. Furthermore, a reduction in perfusion pressure leads to other homeostatic changes to maintain oxygenation to the brain (see Fig. 14.26). These compensatory changes can prevent even occlusion of a carotid artery from having any clinically apparent effect.

When these homeostatic mechanisms fail, the process of ischaemia starts; this ultimately leads to infarction. As the cerebral blood flow descends, various neuronal functions fail at various thresholds (see Fig. 14.27). Once flow falls below the threshold for the maintenance of electrical activity, neurological deficit appears. At this level of blood flow the neurons are still viable; if the flow increases again function returns and the patient will have had a transient ischaemic attack. However, if the flow falls further a level is reached at which the process of cell death starts. Hypoxia leads to an inadequate supply of ATP, which in turn leads to loss of function of membrane pumps, thereby allowing influx of sodium and water into the cell (cytotoxic oedema) and the release of the excitatory neurotransmitter glutamate into the extracellular fluid. Glutamate opens membrane channels, allowing the influx of calcium and more sodium into the neurons. Calcium entering the neurons activates intracellular enzymes which complete the destructive process. The infarction process is worsened by the anaerobic production of lactic acid (see Fig. 14.28) and consequent fall in tissue pH.

The final result of the occlusion of a cerebral blood vessel therefore depends upon the competence of the

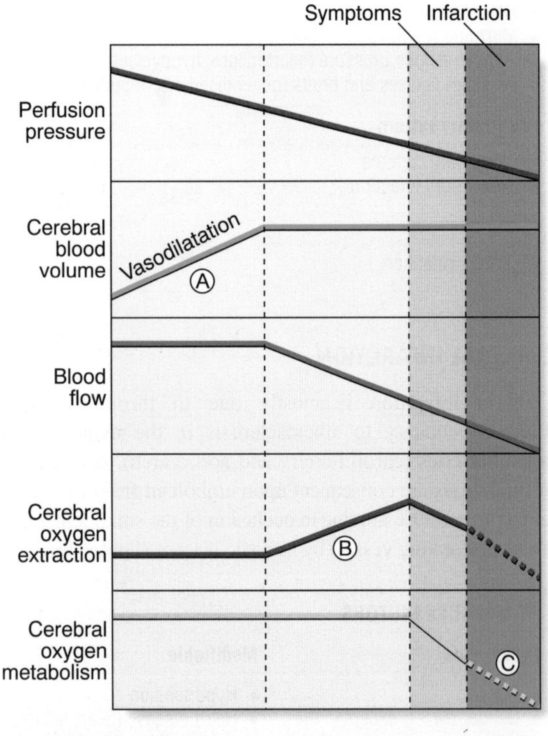

Fig. 14.26 Homeostatic responses to falling perfusion pressure in the brain following arterial occlusion. Vasodilatation initially maintains cerebral blood flow (A), but after maximal vasodilatation further falls in perfusion pressure lead to a decline in blood flow. An increase in tissue oxygen extraction, however, maintains the cerebral metabolic rate for oxygen (B). Still further falls in perfusion, and therefore blood flow, cannot be compensated; cerebral oxygen availability falls and symptoms appear, then infarction (C).

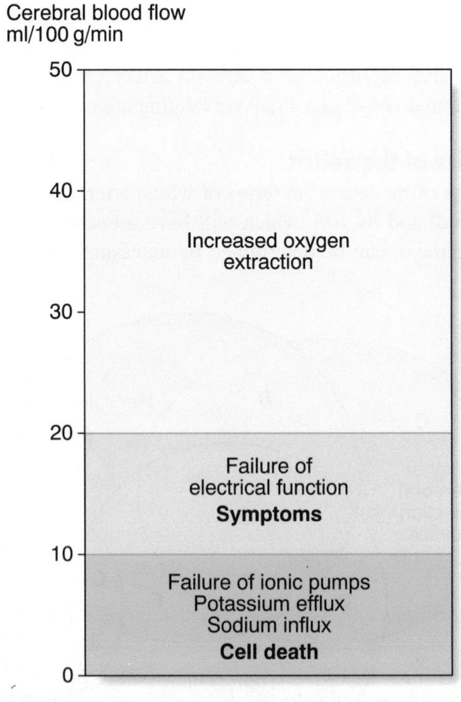

Fig. 14.27 Thresholds of cerebral ischaemia. Symptoms of cerebral ischaemia appear when the blood flow has fallen to less than half of normal and energy supply is insufficient to sustain neuronal electrical function. Full recovery can occur unless this level of flow is sustained for long periods. Further blood flow reduction below the next threshold causes failure of cell ionic pumps and starts the ischaemic cascade, leading to cell death. Brain tissue can sustain such depths of blood flow reduction only for brief periods without infarction.

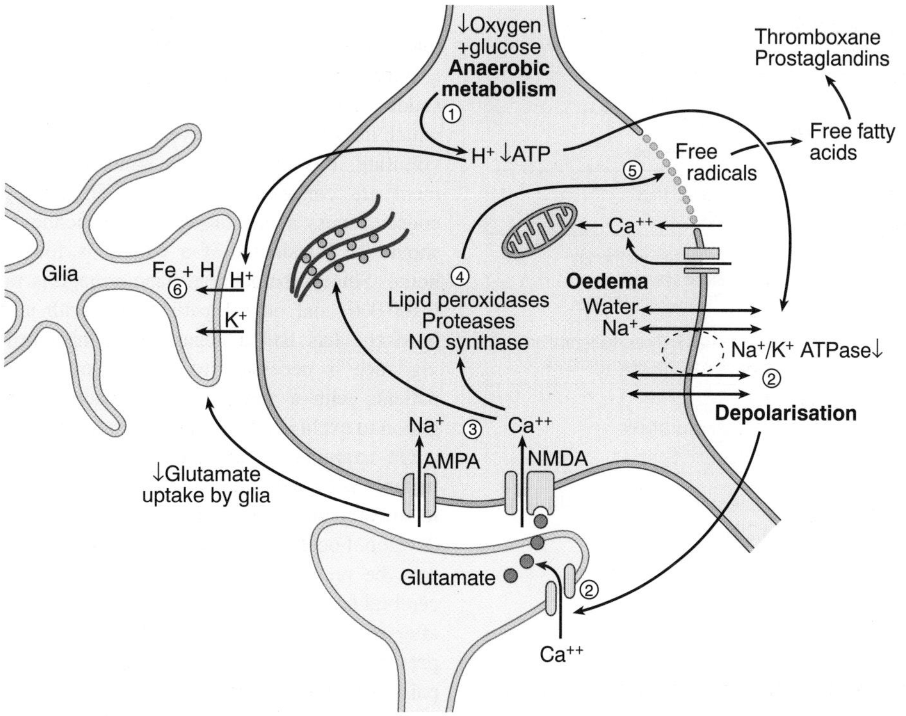

Fig. 14.28 The process of neuronal ischaemia and infarction. (1) Reduction of blood flow reduces supply of oxygen and hence ATP. H^+ is produced by anaerobic metabolism of available glucose. (2) Energy-dependent membrane ionic pumps fail, leading to cytotoxic oedema and membrane depolarisation, allowing calcium entry and releasing glutamate. (3) Calcium enters cells via glutamate-gated channels and (4) activates destructive intracellular enzymes, (5) destroying intracellular organelles and cell membrane, with release of free radicals. Free fatty acid release activates pro-coagulant pathways which exacerbate local ischaemia. (6) Glial cells take up H^+, can no longer take up extracellular glutamate and also suffer cell death, leading to liquefactive necrosis of whole arterial territory.

circulatory homeostatic mechanisms, and the severity and duration of the reduction in blood flow. If ischaemic damage has occurred to the vascular endothelium, restoration of blood flow may cause haemorrhage into the infarcted area. This is particularly likely to occur following embolic occlusion when the embolus is lysed by the blood's thrombolytic mechanisms.

Radiologically, a cerebral infarct can be seen as a lesion which comprises brain tissue that is ischaemic and swollen but recoverable (the ischaemic penumbra), and dead brain tissue that is already undergoing autolysis. The infarct swells with time and is at its maximal size a couple of days after the stroke onset. At this stage it may be big enough to exert some mass effect both clinically and radiologically. As the weeks go by the oedema subsides and the infarcted area is replaced by a sharply defined fluid-filled cavity.

INTRACEREBRAL HAEMORRHAGE

Of the 15% of acute cerebrovascular disease that is caused by haemorrhage, about half occurs through the rupture of a blood vessel within the brain parenchyma (primary intracerebral haemorrhage), resulting in an acute focal stroke. In addition, a patient with a subarachnoid haemorrhage may present with an acute focal stroke if the artery ruptures into the brain substance as well as into the subarachnoid space. Haemorrhage frequently occurs into an area of brain infarction (see above) and such haemorrhagic infarctions may be difficult to distinguish from primary intracerebral haemorrhage. The causes and risk factors of primary intracerebral haemorrhage are listed in Table 14.23, page 978.

Pathophysiology

The explosive entry of blood into the brain parenchyma during a primary intracerebral haemorrhage causes immediate cessation of function in that area as neurons are structurally disrupted and white matter fibre tracts are split apart. A rim of cerebral oedema forms around the resulting blood clot, which, with the haematoma, acts like a mass lesion. If big enough this can cause shift of the intracranial contents, producing transtentorial coning and sometimes rapid death. If the patient survives, the haematoma is

Table 14.23 Causes of intracerebral haemorrhage and associated risk factors

Disease	Risk factors
Charcot–Bouchard microaneurysms	Age Hypertension
Amyloid angiopathy	Familial (rare) Age
Impaired blood clotting	Anticoagulant therapy Blood dyscrasia Thrombolytic therapy
Vascular anomaly	Arteriovenous malformation Cavernous haemangioma
Substance abuse	Alcohol Amphetamines Cocaine

gradually absorbed, leaving a haemosiderin-lined slit in the brain parenchyma (see Fig. 14.29).

SUBARACHNOID HAEMORRHAGE

Clinical features

About three-quarters of those presenting with a subarachnoid haemorrhage are under 65 years and many are in their fourth decade. Women are more frequently affected than men and this difference increases with advancing age.

Subarachnoid haemorrhage typically presents with a sudden severe 'thunderclap' headache (usually occipital) which lasts for hours (or even days), often accompanied by vomiting. Physical exertion, straining and sexual excitement are common antecedents. There may be loss of consciousness at the onset, so subarachnoid haemorrhage should be considered if a patient is found comatose at home. Since subarachnoid haemorrhage is rare (incidence 6:100 000) and only 1 patient in 8 with a sudden severe headache has had a subarachnoid haemorrhage, clinical vigilance is necessary to avoid a missed diagnosis. All patients with a sudden severe headache require investigation to exclude a subarachnoid haemorrhage.

On examination the patient is usually distressed and irritable with photophobia. There may be neck stiffness due to subarachnoid blood but this takes some 6 hours to develop. Focal hemisphere signs (hemiparesis, aphasia etc.) may be present at onset if there is an associated intracerebral haematoma. Alternatively, these signs may develop after some days due to arterial vasospasm induced by the presence of blood in the subarachnoid space. A 3rd nerve palsy may be present due to local pressure from an aneurysm of the posterior communicating artery, though this is rare.

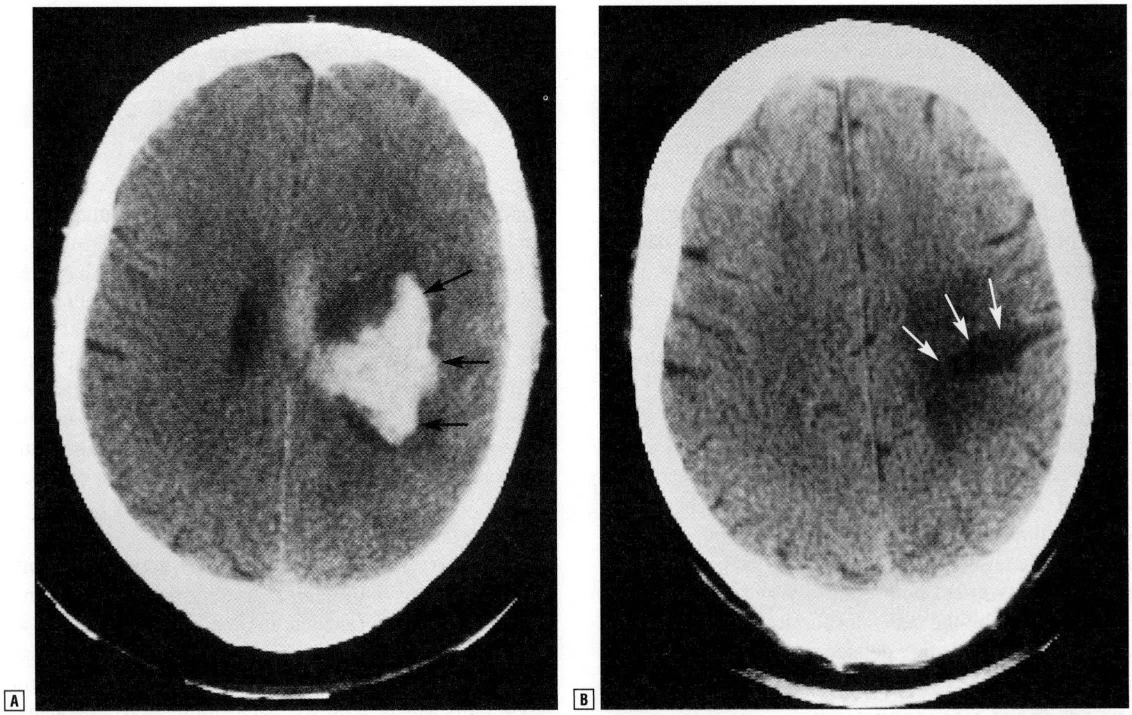

Fig. 14.29 CT scans of intracerebral haemorrhage. A Acute intracerebral haematoma (arrows). B Resolved lesion leaving a slit-shaped defect (arrows).

Fundoscopy may reveal a subhyaloid haemorrhage, which represents blood tracking along the subarachnoid space.

Pathology

Of all subarachnoid haemorrhages, 85% are caused by 'berry' aneurysms bulging out from the bifurcations of the cerebral arteries, particularly in the region of the circle of Willis. These develop during life from defects in the media of the arterial wall and rarely present before the age of 20. There is an increased risk in association with polycystic kidney disease and congenital collagen defects (e.g. Ehlers–Danlos syndrome). Of the remainder, 5% are due to rarities including arteriovenous malformations, and 10% are non-aneurysmal haemorrhages. The cause of these is not known, but they give rise to a very characteristic pattern on CT of peri-mesencephalic blood. Such haemorrhages are known to have a benign outcome in terms of mortality and recurrence.

Investigation of acute stroke

Investigation of a patient presenting with an acute stroke should be planned with a view to confirming the vascular nature of the lesion, the pathological type of vascular lesion, the underlying vascular disease, and the risk factors present (see Table 14.24). Whether the answer to these questions is important depends upon the type of stroke.

Transient stroke

Most transient strokes are due to transient cerebral ischaemia but CT occasionally reveals a small intracerebral haemorrhage. Which arterial territory was involved can be determined from the history of the attack. Approximately 80% occur in the carotid territory. Vertebro-basilar attacks are recognisable from a history of transient hemianopia or brain-stem features such as diplopia or vertigo. If these are not present a transient hemiplegia can be assumed to arise from carotid territory ischaemia.

Most transient strokes are caused by atherosclerotic thromboembolic disease of the major extracranial vessels. The risk of a disabling stroke or death after a transient ischaemic stroke can be reduced by 20–30% with aspirin (75–150 mg daily). If patients have a major stenosis (more than 70%) of their carotid artery, carotid endarterectomy is of proven benefit. However, only 20% of patients presenting with a carotid territory transient ischaemic attack will have a major carotid stenosis. These patients need to be identified with a non-invasive method of vascular imaging (MRA or ultrasound) before using the more invasive (and therefore risky) contrast angiography which is necessary to delineate the lesion for the surgeon. A suggested scheme for the management of transient stroke is shown in Figure 14.30.

Rarely, a cardiac source of embolism is thought to be the cause of a transient stroke. In this case anticoagulation with warfarin is necessary. In most transient strokes, however, anticoagulation has no net benefit since as many haemorrhagic strokes are caused as ischaemic ones prevented.

Table 14.24 Investigation of a patient with acute stroke

Diagnostic question	Investigation
Is it a vascular lesion?	CT/MRI scan
Is it ischaemic or haemorrhagic?	CT scan
Is it a subarachnoid haemorrhage?	CT scan Lumbar puncture
What is the underlying vascular disease?	ECG Cardiac ultrasound Magnetic resonance angiography (MRA) Doppler ultrasound Contrast angiography
What are the risk factors?	Blood count Cholesterol Clotting/thrombophilia screen Blood glucose

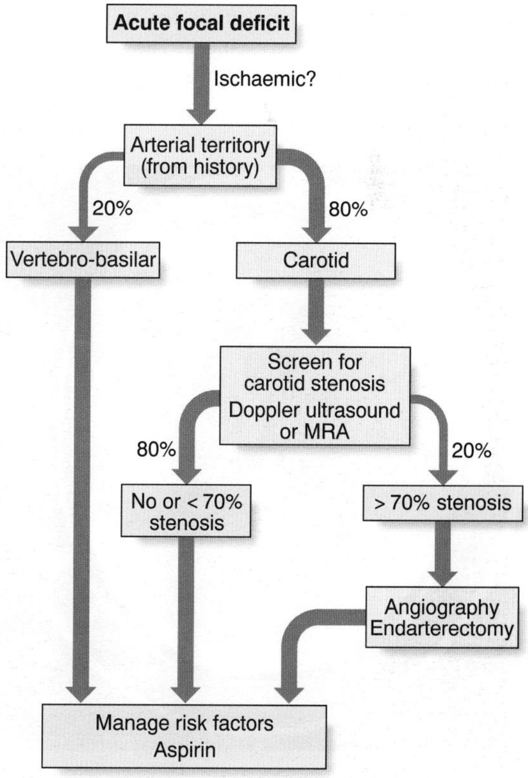

Fig. 14.30 Flow diagram depicting the management of a transient stroke.

Evolving stroke

Worsening of the focal deficit for more than 6 hours occurs in about 10% of patients with acute stroke. This should not be confused with a global deterioration of a patient's general condition, in particular level of arousal, which can occur some time after a large stroke due to the mass effect of a large swollen infarct. If the focal deficit worsens, the likely cause is progression of the vascular lesion causing the stroke but the possibility of a non-vascular lesion, such as a tumour, must be considered. Carotid or basilar stenosis can present with a progressive deficit, but this is unusual. About 30% of lacunar strokes evolve over a matter of days. These are recognisable by the presenting syndromes (see Fig. 14.25, p. 975) which suggest the small size of the brain lesion.

If haemorrhagic stroke has been excluded by imaging, attempts are sometimes made to halt progression of a stroke caused by carotid or basilar stenosis by anticoagulation with heparin. This is, however, of unproved value, as is the use of thrombolytic agents.

Completed stroke

A CT scan is necessary if a subarachnoid haemorrhage is suspected or there is doubt about the vascular nature of the lesion underlying the patient's presentation. In addition, if anticoagulant or thrombolytic drugs are to be given, a haemorrhagic lesion must be excluded. The scan will often reveal clues as to the nature of the arterial lesion. For example, the scan may show a small deep lacunar infarct in a perforating artery, or a more peripheral infarct in the territory of a leptomeningeal artery (see Fig. 14.31). In a haemorrhagic lesion, the presence of a haematoma in the sylvian fissure with subarachnoid blood suggests a ruptured middle cerebral artery aneurysm.

After a completed ischaemic stroke it may be 12 hours or more before an area of low density appears on CT, and very small (lacunar) infarcts may not appear at all. By the second week after an infarct the unenhanced CT may appear normal, even with substantial infarction. This is because invasion of the infarcted area by macrophages and new blood vessels renders it isodense. However, contrast enhancement usually shows at least the rim of the lesion (see Fig. 14.32).

Other investigations

Lumbar puncture to examine the CSF is only indicated if a subarachnoid haemorrhage is suspected but has not been seen on a CT scan. In this case it is best to wait 12 hours since it takes this long for xanthochromia to appear. After an acute focal stroke other investigations necessary to exclude disorders which may be important in immediate management and in secondary prevention are listed in Table 14.24, page 979. In younger patients without risk factors for stroke investigations for the rarer causes are indicated (see the information box).

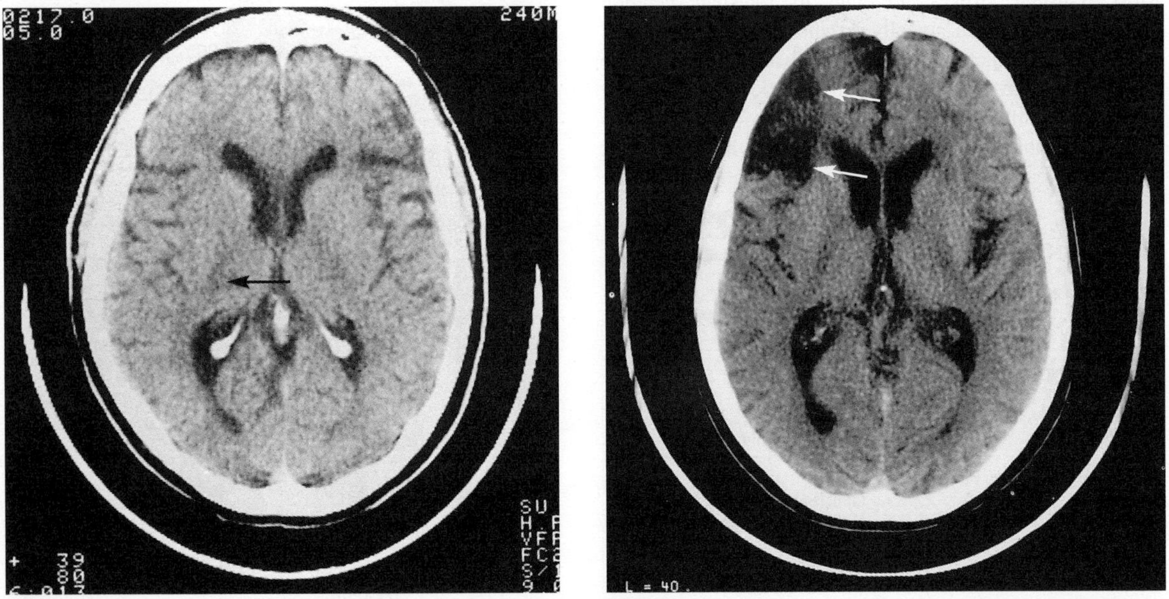

A B

Fig. 14.31 CT scans of lacunar and peripheral infarction. A Lacunar infarction caused by occlusion of a deep perforating artery (arrow). B Peripheral infarction from occlusion of a middle cerebral artery branch (arrows).

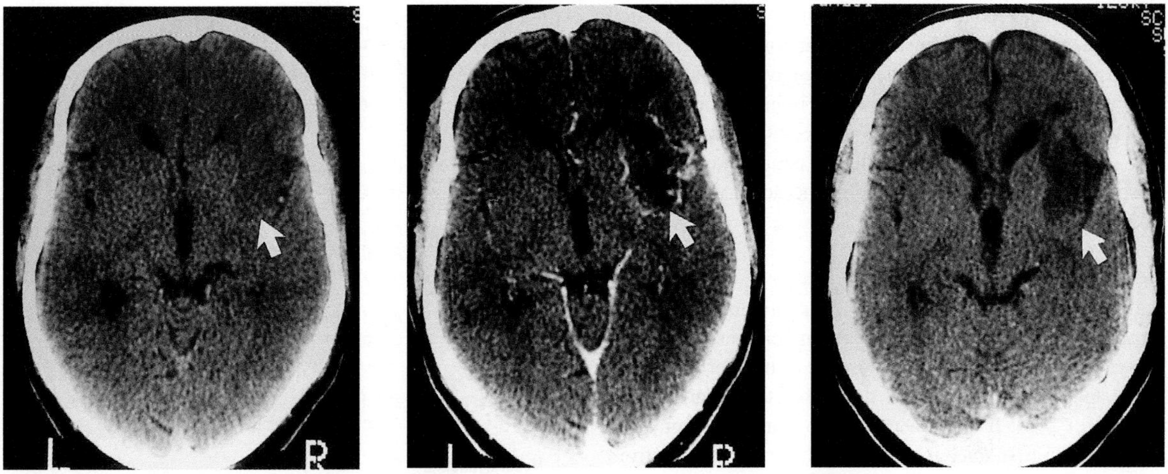

A B C

Fig. 14.32 CT scans showing progressive changes of cerebral infarction due to middle cerebral artery branch occlusion. A Within 6 hours of the stroke little change is seen on the scan except some effacement of sylvian fissure (arrow). B At 3 weeks an enhanced scan shows a low-density lesion with enhancement at the periphery (arrow). C After 2 months there is resolution of the swelling in the lesion and a more clearly defined low density denoting the established infarct (arrow).

CAUSES OF ACUTE STROKE IN YOUNG PATIENTS

- Embolism from heart
  Atrial fibrillation, post-myocardial infarction
- Hyperlipidaemia
- Carotid dissection
- Thrombophilia
  Protein S and C deficiency, antithrombin III deficiency
- Homocystinuria
- Anticardiolipin syndrome
- Vasculitis
  SLE, PAN
- Mitochondrial cytopathy
- Primary intracerebral haemorrhage
  Arteriovenous malformation (AVM), drug abuse, coagulopathy
- Subarachnoid haemorrhage
  Berry aneurysm, AVM, carotid dissection

Management of completed stroke

After a completed stroke, management is aimed at minimising the volume of brain that is irreversibly infarcted, preventing complications, reducing the patient's disability and handicap through rehabilitation, and preventing recurrent episodes. Patients with subarachnoid haemorrhage should be referred urgently to a neurosurgical centre, since these patients require investigation for, and surgical treatment of, the berry aneurysm which may be the cause.

Blood pressure

The blood pressure is usually acutely raised after a stroke and, unless acute end-organ damage is present, should not be lowered in the acute stage since it will always return towards the patient's normal level within 24–48 hours. Survival of the ischaemic penumbra may depend upon the raised perfusion pressure. The blood pressure tends to stay higher for longer with cerebral haematomas than with cerebral infarcts but, in terms of preventing further haemorrhage, there is no value in reducing this pressure until at least some days after the stroke. After 10 days gentle reduction of blood pressure may be contemplated as part of a secondary preventive strategy for ischaemic stroke.

Hydration and oxygenation

Adequate hydration and arterial oxygenation are important to preserve as much as possible of ischaemic but recoverable brain. After a stroke a patient may have difficulty in protecting the airway and therefore difficulty in safely maintaining adequate nutrition and hydration orally. In this case, intravenous hydration may be necessary in the first few hours and thereafter; if a patient's swallowing fails to recover, hydration should be maintained by nasogastric tube or gastrostomy.

Blood glucose

A raised blood sugar after a stroke increases infarct size and adversely affects functional outcome. This is probably because hyperglycaemia exacerbates the anaerobic production of lactic acid in the ischaemic penumbra. Hence, blood sugar should be normalised with insulin.

Increasing blood flow to the ischaemic penumbra

In the acute phase surgical revascularisation of a cerebral

infarct seems to have no practical value since more deficit is often caused by consequent haemorrhage into the ischaemic brain. Thrombolytic agents have similar effects, but may be useful if given within 3 hours of onset of an ischaemic stroke when the CT does not show extensive low density despite a significant neurological deficit. Vasodilator drugs have no place in the acute management of stroke.

Anticoagulation and aspirin

Anticoagulation after an acute stroke is only indicated if the cause is embolism from the heart. In this case, provided imaging has demonstrated the absence of haemorrhage, oral anticoagulation with warfarin should be started (aiming for an INR of 2–3). It is not necessary to start anticoagulation with heparin first since in the acute phase any benefit from this in preventing further embolism is offset by the increased risk of haemorrhagic conversion of the infarct. Aspirin (300 mg daily) should be started immediately after an ischaemic stroke, and carries a far lower risk of haemorrhagic complications.

Nursing care and rehabilitation

Many patients after a stroke are, at least initially, physically dependent, and require expert nursing care to avoid complications (see Table 14.25). Bladder and bowel care need special consideration. Nursing care may be better provided in specialised stroke units, which have been shown to reduce patient mortality and accelerate functional recovery. Consideration of a patient's rehabilitation needs should commence at the same time as the acute medical management (see above).

Prognosis and secondary prevention

About 75% of patients survive the acute stage of focal stroke due to cerebral infarction or primary intracerebral haemorrhage. The immediate mortality of aneurysmal subarachnoid haemorrhage is 50% with a recurrence rate of 50% in the first 6 months and 3% annually thereafter. Secondary prevention requires appropriate neurosurgical management. Half to three-quarters of those surviving an acute stroke achieve functional independence, mostly within the first 3 months. After a completed focal stroke there is an annual recurrence rate of 8–11%. Secondary prevention of stroke involves attention to those risk factors which are reversible and, in the case of ischaemic stroke, the use of aspirin. If the residual deficit after an ischaemic stroke is minimal, that patient should be managed in the same way as for a transient stroke.

CEREBRAL VENOUS DISEASE

Thrombosis of cerebral veins and venous sinuses is uncommon. The causes are listed in the information box.

Table 14.25 Complications of acute stroke

Complication	Prevention	Treatment
Pneumonia	Nurse semi-erect Physiotherapy	Antibiotics Oxygen
Dehydration	Check swallowing Nasogastric tube	Careful rehydration
Hyponatraemia	Check causes (e.g. diuretics) Avoid excess water replacement	Water deprivation
Hypoxaemia	Avoid and treat chest complications Treat heart failure	Oxygen
Seizures	Maintain cerebral oxygenation Avoid metabolic disturbance	Anticonvulsants
Hyperglycaemia	Treat diabetes	Insulin if necessary
Deep venous thrombosis/ pulmonary embolism	TED stockings Subcutaneous heparin	Anticoagulation (check if haemorrhagic stroke)
Frozen shoulder and subluxation	Physiotherapy Correct handling	Physiotherapy Local steroid injections
Pressure sores	Frequent turning Monitor pressure areas Avoid urinary contamination	Nursing care Special mattress
Urinary infection	Use penile sheath Avoid catheterisation if possible	Antibiotics
Constipation	Appropriate aperients and diet	Appropriate aperients

CAUSES OF CEREBRAL VENOUS THROMBOSIS

Predisposing causes	Local causes
• Dehydration	• Paranasal sinusitis
• Pregnancy	• Meningitis, subdural empyema
• Behçet's disease	• Penetrating head and eye wounds
• Thrombophilia	• Facial skin infection
• Hypotension	• Otitis media, mastoiditis
• Oral contraceptives	• Skull fracture

Cerebral venous occlusion causes an increase in intracranial pressure and patchy ischaemia, which is often haemorrhagic. The clinical features vary according to the part of the cerebral venous system involved (see below).

Cortical vein thrombosis

This may present with focal cortical deficits (aphasia, hemiparesis etc.) and epilepsy (focal or generalised), according to the area involved. The deficit may enlarge if spreading thrombophlebitis occurs.

Cerebral venous sinus thrombosis

The clinical features of cerebral venous sinus thrombosis depend on the sinus involved (see the information box).

CLINICAL FEATURES OF CEREBRAL VENOUS SINUS THROMBOSIS
Cavernous sinus
• Proptosis, ptosis, headache, external and internal ophthalmoplegia, papilloedema, reduced sensation in trigeminal first division • Often bilateral, patient ill and febrile
Superior sagittal sinus
• Headache, papilloedema, seizures • May involve veins of both hemispheres, causing advancing motor and sensory focal deficits
Transverse sinus
• Hemiparesis, seizures, papilloedema • May spread to jugular foramen to involve cranial nerves 9, 10 and 11

FURTHER INFORMATION ON CEREBROVASCULAR DISEASE

Bogousslavsky J, Caplan L 1995 Stroke syndromes. Cambridge University Press, Cambridge

Drug and Therapeutics Bulletin 1998 Management soon after a stroke 36: 7

Fisher M 1995 Stroke therapy. Butterworth–Heinemann, Boston

Sandercock P A G 1998 Transient ischaemic attacks: new treatments, new questions. Quarterly Journal of Medicine 91: 377–379

Warlow C P, Dennis M S, van Gijn J et al 1996 Stroke: a practical guide to management. Blackwell, Oxford

INFLAMMATORY DISEASES

MULTIPLE SCLEROSIS

In multiple sclerosis, one of the most common neurological causes of long-term disability, the myelin-producing oligodendrocytes of the central nervous system are the target of recurrent cell-mediated autoimmune attack. In the UK the prevalence is 80 per 100 000 of the population, with an annual incidence of around 5 per 100 000. The lifetime risk of developing multiple sclerosis is about 1 in 800. The incidence is higher in temperate climates and in people of European extraction and the disease is more common in women (male:female ratio of 1:1.5).

Aetiology

Epidemiological evidence suggests an environmental influence on causation. The incidence varies with latitude, being low in Equatorial areas and higher in the temperate zones of both hemispheres. A genetic influence is suggested by a 10-fold increase in risk in first-degree relatives and from twin studies in which there is higher concordance for multiple sclerosis in monozygotic twins compared to dizygotic twins. HLA tissue-typing has demonstrated an increased prevalence of haplotypes A3, B7, Dw2 and DR2 in affected patients in the UK, but different haplotypes are associated in other countries. An immune mechanism is suggested by increased levels of activated T lymphocytes in the CSF, and increased immunoglobulin synthesis within the central nervous system. There are increased levels of antibody to some viruses, including measles virus, in the CSF, but this may be an epiphenomenon. The relative importance of environmental, genetic and immunological factors is unresolved. Multiple sclerosis is likely to be multifactorial in origin.

Pathology

An attack of central nervous system inflammation in multiple sclerosis starts with the entry through the blood–brain barrier of activated T lymphocytes. These recognise myelin-derived antigens on the surface of the nervous system's antigen-presenting cells, the microglia, and undergo clonal proliferation. The resulting inflammatory cascade releases cytokines and initiates destruction of the oligodendrocyte-myelin unit by macrophages. Histologically, the characteristic lesion is a plaque of inflammatory demyelination occurring most commonly in the periventricular regions of the brain, the optic nerves and subpial regions of the spinal cord (see Fig. 14.33, p. 984). Initially, this is a circumscribed area of disintegration of the myelin sheath accompanied by infiltration by activated lymphocytes and macrophages, often with conspicuous perivascular inflammation. After an acute attack gliosis follows, leaving a shrunken grey scar.

Much of the initial acute clinical deficit is caused by the effect of inflammatory cytokines upon transmission of the nervous impulse rather than structural disruption of the myelin, which explains the rapid recovery of some deficits and probably the efficacy of steroids in ameliorating the acute deficit. However, the myelin loss which results from an attack reduces the safety factor for impulse propagation or causes complete conduction block, which lowers the efficiency of central nervous system functions. In established multiple sclerosis there is progressive axonal loss, probably due to direct damage to axonal integrity by the inflammatory mediators released in acute attacks (including nitrous oxide), and this is the cause of the phase of the disease where there is progressive and persistent disability (see Fig. 14.34, p. 984).

Clinical features

A diagnosis of multiple sclerosis requires the demonstration of lesions in more than one anatomical site at more than one time for which there is no other explanation. Around 80% of patients have a relapsing and remitting clinical

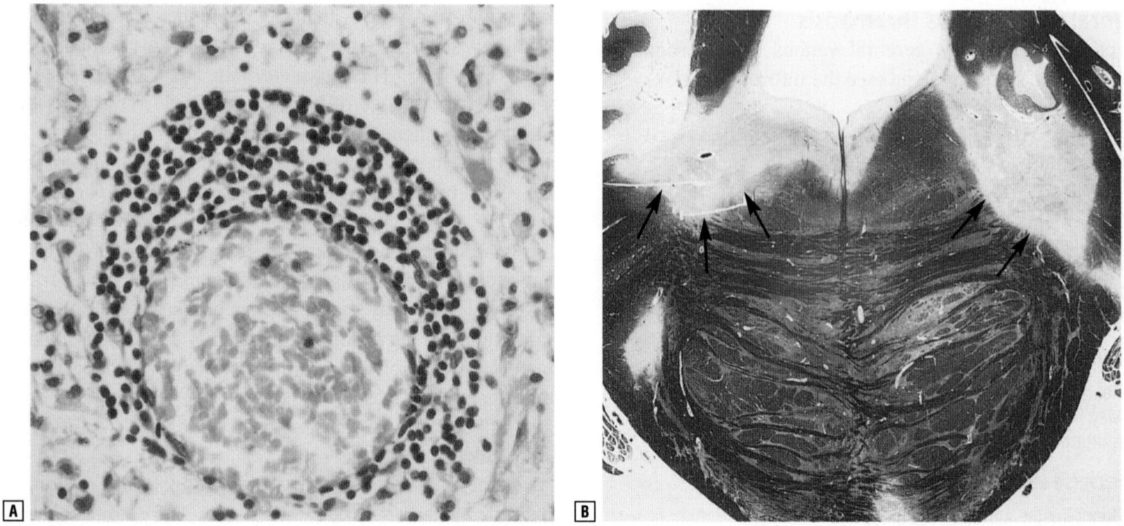

Fig. 14.33 Multiple sclerosis. A Photomicrograph from demyelinating plaque showing perivascular cuffing of blood vessel by lymphocytes. B Section through pons showing demyelinating plaques in white matter (arrows) (Weigert–Pal).

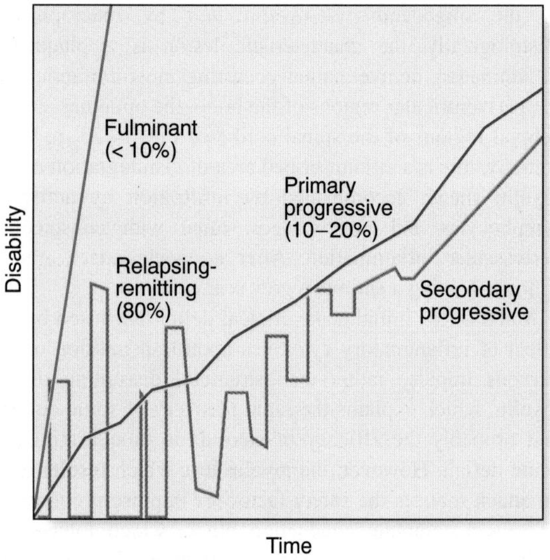

Fig. 14.34 The progression of disability in fulminant, relapsing-remitting and progressive multiple sclerosis.

course of episodic dysfunction of the central nervous system with variable recovery. Of the remaining 20%, most follow a slowly progressive clinical course, with a tiny minority who have a fulminant variety leading to early death (see Fig. 14.34). The peak age of onset is in the fourth decade, onset before puberty or after the age of 60 years being rare. There are a number of clinical symptoms and syndromes characteristic of multiple sclerosis, some of which may occur at presentation while others may develop in the course of the illness (see the information boxes).

Demyelinating lesions cause symptoms and signs which usually come on subacutely over days or weeks, and resolve over weeks or months. After a variable interval there may be a recurrence, often within 2 years. Frequent relapses with incomplete recovery indicate a poor prognosis, and in many patients a phase of secondary progression supersedes

COMMON PRESENTATIONS OF MULTIPLE SCLEROSIS

- Optic neuritis
- Relapsing and remitting sensory symptoms
- Subacute painless spinal cord lesion
- Acute brain-stem syndrome
- Subacute loss of function of upper limb
- 6th cranial nerve palsy

SYMPTOMS AND SYNDROMES SUGGESTIVE OF CNS DEMYELINATION

- Optic neuritis (afferent pupillary defect)
- Tingling in spine or limbs on neck flexion (Lhermitte's phenomenon)
- Dorsal column loss in one limb
- Progressive non-compressive paraparesis
- Partial Brown-Séquard syndrome
- Internuclear ophthalmoplegia with ataxia
- Focal brain-stem lesions
- Postural ('rubral') tremor
- Trigeminal neuralgia under the age of 50
- Recurrent facial palsy

the phase of relapse and remission. In a minority of patients there may be an interval of years or even decades between attacks, and in some, particularly if optic neuritis is the initial manifestation, there is no recurrence. Some presentations, such as optic neuritis with purely sensory relapses, have a good prognosis.

The physical signs observed in multiple sclerosis depend on the anatomical site of demyelination. Combinations of spinal cord and brain-stem signs are common, maybe with evidence of previous optic neuritis in the form of an afferent pupillary deficit. Significant intellectual impairment is unusual until late in the disease, when loss of frontal functions and impairment of memory are common.

Investigations

There is no specific test for multiple sclerosis and the results of investigation are taken in conjunction with the clinical picture in making a diagnosis of varying probability (see the information box below). The clinical diagnosis of multiple sclerosis can be supported by investigations which aim to exclude other conditions, provide evidence for an inflammatory disorder, and identify multiple sites of neurological involvement (see the information box right).

Following the first clinical event, investigations may help in confirming the disseminated nature of the disease. Visual evoked potentials can detect clinically silent lesions in up to 70% of patients, but auditory and somatosensory evoked potentials are seldom of diagnostic value. The CSF may show a lymphocytic pleocytosis in the acute phase and oligoclonal bands of IgG in 70–90% of patients between attacks. Oligoclonal bands are not specific to multiple sclerosis but denote intrathecal inflammation and occur in a range of other disorders. MRI is the most sensitive technique for imaging lesions in both brain and spinal cord (see Fig. 14.6C, p. 931) and in excluding other causes of the neurological deficit. However, the MRI appearances in multiple sclerosis may be difficult to distinguish from those of cerebrovascular disease or cerebral vasculitis. Diagnosis depends on the clinical history and examination, taken in combination with the investigative findings. It is important to exclude other potentially treatable alternative conditions such as infections, vitamin B_{12} deficiency and spinal cord compression.

CLINICAL DIAGNOSTIC CRITERIA FOR MULTIPLE SCLEROSIS

Clinically definite, requires all of

- Age < 60 years
- History or signs of deficits in two or more anatomical sites in CNS
- On CNS examination abnormal signs are present which indicate white matter involvement
- CNS involvement in one of two patterns
  Relapsing and remitting: two or more episodes lasting at least 24 hours and > 1 month apart
  Progressive: slow and/or stepwise progression over at least 6 months
- No other explanation of symptoms

Clinically probable

- Relapsing and remitting symptoms with one neurological sign commonly associated with MS *or*
- Documented single episode with partial or complete recovery, with signs of multifocal white matter disease *and* no other explanation

Clinically possible

- Relapsing and remitting symptoms without documented or objective signs to establish more than one anatomical site of CNS involvement
- No other explanation

INVESTIGATIONS IN A PATIENT SUSPECTED OF HAVING MULTIPLE SCLEROSIS

- Exclude other structural disease and identify plaques of demyelination
  Imaging (MRI, myelography)
- Demonstrate other sites of involvement
  Visual evoked potentials
  Other evoked potentials
- Demonstrate inflammatory nature of lesion(s)
  CSF examination (cell count, protein electrophoresis)
- Exclude other conditions
  Chest radiograph, serum angiotensin-converting enzyme (ACE), serum B_{12}, antinuclear antibodies

Management

The management of multiple sclerosis involves the treatment of the acute relapse, prevention of future relapse, treatment of complications, and management of the patient's disability.

Acute relapse

In a function-threatening relapse, high-dose intravenous steroids (methylprednisolone 1 g daily for 3 days) are indicated to shorten the duration of the relapse but do not affect long-term outcome. Pulsed intravenous steroids also have some effect in reducing spasticity. Prolonged administration of steroids does not alter the long-term outcome and is therefore avoided. Pulses of intravenous steroids can be given up to 3–4 times in a year but their administration should be restricted to those with significant function-threatening deficits.

Preventing relapses

Immunosuppressive agents including azathioprine have a marginal effect in reducing relapses and improving long-term outcome. In relapsing and remitting multiple sclerosis subcutaneous or intramuscular β-interferon reduces the number of relapses by some 30%, with a small effect on long-term disability. The effects of other immune modulation therapies are currently being evaluated

Table 14.26 Treatment of complications of multiple sclerosis

Complication	Treatment
Spasticity	Physiotherapy Oral baclofen 15–100 mg* Diazepam 2–15 mg* Dantrolene 25–400 mg* Tizanidine 8–32 mg Intrathecal baclofen Local injection of botulinum toxin Chemical neurectomy
Ataxia	Isoniazid 600–1200 mg* Clonazepam 2–8 mg*
Dysaesthesia	Carbamazepine 200–1800 mg* Phenytoin 200–400 mg Amitriptyline 50 mg
Bladder symptoms	See Table 14.22, page 973

* In divided doses.

and may have some use in the future. Special diets including a gluten-free diet, linoleic acid supplements or hyperbaric oxygen therapy are of no proven benefit.

Complications

The treatment of the complications of multiple sclerosis is summarised in Table 14.26. Of prime importance are a careful explanation of the nature of the disease and its outcome and the support of patients and their relatives when disability occurs. A frank discussion of the diagnosis and prognosis is necessary and may dispel fears, which are often ill-founded. Periods of physiotherapy may improve functional capacity in those patients who become disabled, and assessment by the occupational therapist will provide guidance in the provision of aids within the home and in reducing handicap.

The care of the bladder is particularly important. Infections should be treated with an appropriate antibiotic. Incontinence, urgency and frequency may be treated pharmacologically, by external drainage or by urinary catheter, which may be passed intermittently by the patient rather than left permanently in-dwelling. The choice of treatment is difficult and urodynamic assessment may be necessary in patients with troublesome symptoms. Sexual dysfunction is a source of anxiety in many patients and may be relieved by skilled counselling and, if necessary, prosthetic aids.

Prognosis

The outlook is difficult to predict with confidence in any individual patient, especially early in the disease. Furthermore, the ability to diagnose disease at an earlier stage means that older studies may not reliably reflect the outcome of those diagnosed with modern techniques. About 15% of those having one attack of demyelination do not suffer any more events, whilst those with relapsing and remitting multiple sclerosis have, on average, 1–2 relapses every 2 years. Approximately 5% of patients die within 5 years of onset, whilst others have a very benign outcome. Overall, after 10 years about one-third of patients are disabled to the point of needing help with walking, whilst after 15 years about 50% have this degree of disability.

ACUTE DISSEMINATED ENCEPHALOMYELITIS

This is an acute monophasic demyelinating condition in which there are areas of perivenous demyelination widely disseminated throughout the brain and spinal cord. The illness may occur apparently spontaneously but often occurs a week or so after a viral infection, especially measles and chickenpox, or following vaccination, suggesting that it is immunologically mediated.

Clinical features

Headache, vomiting, pyrexia, confusion and meningism may be presenting features, often with focal or multifocal brain and spinal cord signs. Seizures or coma may occur. Flaccid paralysis with extensor plantar responses are common and cerebellar signs may be present, particularly when the disorder follows chickenpox.

Investigations

MRI shows multiple high-signal areas in a pattern similar to that of multiple sclerosis, although often with larger areas of abnormality. The CSF may be normal or show a small increase in mononuclear cells and protein. The differential diagnosis from a first severe attack of what turns out to be multiple sclerosis may be difficult.

Management

The disease may be fatal in the acute stages but is otherwise self-limiting. Treatment with high-dose intravenous methylprednisolone, using the same regimen as for a relapse of multiple sclerosis, is recommended.

ACUTE TRANSVERSE MYELITIS

Transverse myelitis is an acute monophasic inflammatory demyelinating disorder affecting the spinal cord over a variable number of segments. Patients may be of any age and present with a subacute paraparesis with a sensory level, often with severe pain in the neck or back at the onset. MRI is needed to distinguish this from a compressive lesion of the spinal cord. CSF examination shows cellular pleocytosis, often with polymorphs at the onset. Treatment is with high-dose intravenous methylprednisolone. The outcome is variable; in some cases, near-complete recovery occurs despite a severe initial deficit. A small proportion of patients who present with acute transverse myelitis go on to develop multiple sclerosis in later years.

FURTHER INFORMATION ON INFLAMMATORY DISEASES

ffrench-Constant C 1994 Pathogenesis of multiple sclerosis. Lancet 343: 271–278
Matthews W B, Compston A, Allen I V, Martin C N 1991 McAlpine's multiple sclerosis, 2nd edn. Churchill Livingstone, Edinburgh
Thompson A J, Polman C, Hohlfield R 1997 Multiple sclerosis: clinical challenges and controversies. Martin Dunitz, London

DEGENERATIVE DISEASES

Many diseases cause degeneration in different parts of the nervous system without an identifiable external cause. Genetic factors are known to be involved in several, but the cause is still unknown for the majority. Clinical features depend on which structures are affected. Degeneration of the cerebral cortex causes dementia, the most common type being Alzheimer's disease. Degeneration of the basal ganglia results in movement disorder, which may manifest as either too little or too much movement, depending on the structures involved. Examples of these conditions are Parkinson's disease and Huntington's disease. Cerebellar degeneration usually causes ataxia. Degeneration can also occur in the spinal cord or peripheral nerves, giving rise to motor, sensory or autonomic disturbance.

DEGENERATIVE CAUSES OF DEMENTIA

As many as 5% of the population over 65 years of age suffer from a dementing illness. Over the age of 80, this rises to over 20%. Dementia therefore has major implications for health resources.

ALZHEIMER'S DISEASE

This is the most common cause of dementia, occurring mostly in patients over 45 years. Genetic factors are important, particularly if the age of onset is under 65 years, and the familial disease may account for some 15% of cases, though genetic abnormalities on several different chromosomes have been described, particularly chromosomes 1, 14 and 21. The inheritance of one of the alleles of apolipoprotein ε (apo ε), ε_4, is associated with a four-fold increase in the risk of developing the disease.

Pathology

Macroscopically, the brain is atrophic, particularly the cerebral cortex and hippocampus. Histology reveals the presence of senile plaques and neurofibrillary tangles in the cerebral cortex. Histochemical staining demonstrates

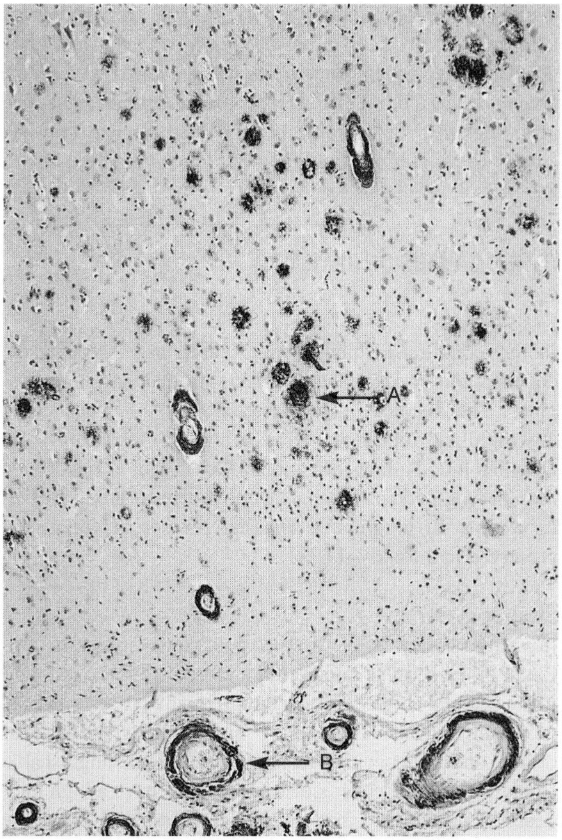

Fig. 14.35 Alzheimer's disease. Section of neocortex stained with polyclonal antibody against βA4 peptide showing amyloid deposits in plaques in brain substance (arrow A) and in blood vessel walls (arrow B).

significant quantities of amyloid in plaques (see Fig. 14.35). Many different neurotransmitter abnormalities have been described, in particular impairment of cholinergic transmission, though noradrenaline, 5-HT, glutamate and substance P are also involved (see Table 14.1, p. 926).

Clinical features

Patients present with gradual impairment of memory in association with disorders of other cortical function, as discussed above. Both short-term and long-term memory are affected, but defects in the former are usually more obvious. Other typical features are apraxia, visuo-spatial impairment and aphasia. In the early stages, patients may deny that there is anything wrong (anosognosia), and depression is common. Occasionally patients become aggressive, and the clinical features are made acutely worse by coexistent intercurrent illness.

Investigations and management

Investigation is aimed at excluding other treatable causes of dementia (see the information box, p. 962), as histological confirmation of the diagnosis usually occurs only after death. There is no known treatment, though recently donepezil, an inhibitor of cerebral acetylcholinesterase, has been shown to be of some benefit. Management consists largely of providing a familiar environment for the patient, and providing support for the carers.

OTHER CAUSES OF DEMENTIA

Pick's disease

In this condition, which is much rarer than Alzheimer's, degeneration predominantly affects frontal and temporal lobes. The histology is characterised by the presence of argyrophilic cytoplasmic inclusion bodies (Pick bodies) and chromatolytic ballooned neurons (Pick cells). Patients may present with personality change due to frontal lobe involvement or with progressive aphasia. Memory is relatively preserved in the early stages.

Lewy body dementia

In diffuse Lewy body disease, pathology similar to that found in the substantia nigra in Parkinson's disease is found in the cerebral cortex. This condition usually presents as cognitive impairment in the context of an extrapyramidal syndrome, and the cognitive features may be indistinguishable from those of Alzheimer's disease. Patients have a high incidence of visual hallucinations, and are particularly sensitive to this side-effect of antiparkinsonian medication. There is no specific treatment for this condition or Pick's disease.

PARKINSON'S DISEASE AND AKINETIC-RIGID SYNDROMES

There are a number of degenerative diseases affecting the basal ganglia, which present with differing combinations of slowness of movement (bradykinesia), increased tone (rigidity), tremor and loss of postural reflexes. The most common cause of these parkinsonian, or akinetic-rigid syndromes, is idiopathic Parkinson's disease.

IDIOPATHIC PARKINSON'S DISEASE

This condition has an annual incidence of about 0.2/1000, and a prevalence of 1.5/1000 in the UK. Whilst 10% of the patients are under 45 years at presentation, the incidence and prevalence both increase with age, the latter rising to over 1% in those over 60. Sex incidence is about equal. It is less common in cigarette smokers.

Aetiology

The cause is unknown, and no strong genetic factors have been identified, though recent work on twins has suggested that the genetic influence may be greater than previously thought. The discovery that methyl-phenyl-tetrahydropyridine (MPTP) caused severe parkinsonism in young drug abusers suggests that the idiopathic disease might be due to an environmental toxin; many candidate toxins have been studied, but there is no strong evidence in favour of any of them.

Pathology

There is depletion of the pigmented dopaminergic neurons in the substantia nigra, hyaline material (Lewy bodies) in nigral cells, atrophic changes in the substantia nigra and depletion of neurons in the locus coeruleus. Reduced dopaminergic output from the substantia nigra to the globus pallidus leads to reduced inhibitory effects on the subthalamic nucleus, neurons in which become more active than usual in inhibiting activation of the cortex. This in turn results in bradykinesia.

Clinical features

The classical syndrome of tremor, rigidity and bradykinesia

PHYSICAL ABNORMALITIES IN PARKINSONISM
General
• Expressionless face • Greasy skin • Soft, rapid, indistinct speech • Flexed posture • Impaired postural reflexes
Gait
• Slow to start walking • Shortened stride • Rapid, small steps, tendency to run (festination) • Reduced arm swing • Impaired balance on turning
Tremor
• Resting 4–6 Hz Usually first in fingers/thumb Coarse, complex movements, flexion/extension of fingers Abduction/adduction of thumb Supination/pronation of forearm May affect arms, legs, feet, jaw, tongue Intermittent, present at rest and when distracted Diminished on action • Postural 8–10 Hz Less obvious, faster, finer amplitude Present on action or posture, persists with movement
Rigidity
• Cogwheel type, mostly upper limbs • Plastic (lead pipe) type, mostly legs
Bradykinesia
• Slowness in initiating or repeating movements • Impaired fine movements, especially of fingers

may be absent initially, when non-specific symptoms of tiredness, aching limbs, mental slowness, depression and small handwriting (micrographia) may be noticed.

The presentation is almost always unilateral, a rest tremor in an upper limb being a common presenting feature. The tremor may also affect the legs, mouth and tongue. It may remain the predominant symptom for some years. Bradykinesia may develop gradually. Most patients have difficulty with rapid fine movements, and this manifests itself as slowness of gait and difficulty with tasks such as fastening buttons, shaving or writing. Rigidity, or increased muscular tone, causes stiffness and a flexed posture. Postural righting reflexes are impaired early on in the disease, but falls tend not to occur until later on. As the disease advances, speech becomes softer and indistinct. There are a number of abnormalities on neurological examination, and these are listed in the information box.

Although parkinsonian features are initially unilateral, gradual bilateral involvement is the rule. Muscle strength and reflexes remain normal, and plantar responses are flexor. There is a paucity of facial expression (hypomimia) and the blink reflex may be exaggerated and fail to habituate (glabellar tap sign). Eye movements are normal to standard clinical testing, provided one allows for the normal limitation of upward gaze with age. Sensation is normal and intellectual faculties are not affected initially. As the disease progresses, about one-third of patients develop cognitive impairment.

Investigations

The diagnosis is made clinically, as there is no diagnostic test for Parkinson's disease. Sometimes it is necessary to investigate patients to exclude other causes of parkinsonism if there are any unusual features. Patients presenting before the age of 50 are usually tested for Wilson's disease, and CT may be needed if there are any features suggestive of pyramidal, cerebellar or autonomic involvement, or the diagnosis is otherwise in doubt.

Management

Drug therapy

L-dopa combined with a peripheral-acting dopa-decarboxylase inhibitor provides the mainstay of treatment in Parkinson's disease but should only be started to help overcome a significant disability. Other agents include anticholinergic drugs, dopamine receptor agonists, selegiline and amantadine (see Fig. 14.36).

L-dopa. Although the number of dopamine-releasing terminals in the striatum is diminished in Parkinson's disease, remaining neurons can be driven to produce more

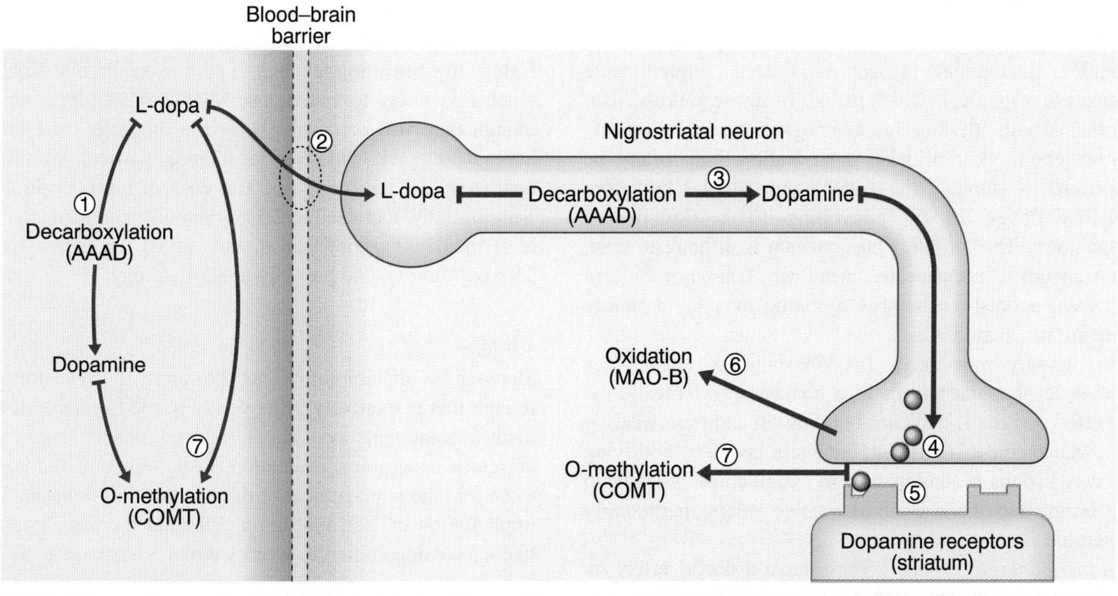

Fig. 14.36 Mechanisms of drug action in Parkinson's disease. (1) Decarboxylase inhibitors (carbidopa and benserazide) reduce side-effects by reducing peripheral conversion of L-dopa to dopamine by aromatic amino acid decarboxylase (AAAD). (2) Active transport of L-dopa into the brain may be inhibited by competition from dietary amino acids after a high-protein meal. (3) In the nigrostriatal neurons L-dopa is converted into dopamine. (4) Amantadine enhances the release of dopamine at the nerve terminal. (5) Dopamine agonists act directly on striatal receptors. (6) The monoamine oxidase type B (MAO-B) inhibitor selegiline increases the availability of neuronal dopamine by reducing its metabolism outside the neuron. (7) The catechol-O-methyl-transferase (COMT) inhibitors tolcapone and entacapone prolong the availability of dopamine by inhibiting the metabolism of dopamine and L-dopa outside the neuron.

dopamine by administering its precursor L-dopa. If L-dopa is administered orally, however, more than 90% is decarboxylated to dopamine peripherally in the gastrointestinal tract and blood vessels, and only a small proportion reaches the brain. This peripheral conversion of L-dopa is responsible for the high incidence of side-effects if used alone. The problem is largely overcome by giving a decarboxylase inhibitor which does not cross the blood–brain barrier along with the L-dopa. Two peripheral decarboxylase inhibitors, carbidopa and benserazide, are available as combination preparations with L-dopa.

The initiation of L-dopa therapy should be delayed until there is significant disability, since there is concern regarding long-term side-effects. L-dopa is particularly effective at improving bradykinesia and rigidity. Tremor is also helped but rather unpredictably. The initial dose is 50 mg 8- or 12-hourly, increased if necessary. The total L-dopa dose may be increased to over 1000 mg/day, but should be kept as low as possible. Side-effects include postural hypotension and nausea and vomiting, which may be offset by the use of a peripheral dopamine antagonist such as domperidone. Other dose-related side-effects are involuntary movements, particularly orofacial dyskinesias, limb and axial dystonias, and occasionally depression, hallucinations and delusions.

Late deterioration despite L-dopa therapy occurs after 3–5 years in one-third to one-half of patients. Usually this manifests as fluctuation in response. The simplest form of this is end-of-dose deterioration due to progression of the disease and loss of capacity to store dopamine. More complex fluctuations present as sudden, unpredictable changes in response, in which periods of severe parkinsonism alternate with dyskinesia and agitation (the 'on-off' phenomenon). End-of-dose deterioration can often be improved by dividing the L-dopa into smaller but more frequent doses, or by converting to a slow-release preparation. The 'on-off' phenomenon is difficult to treat, but sometimes subcutaneous injections of apomorphine (a dopamine agonist) are helpful to 'rescue' the patient rapidly from an 'off' period.

Involuntary movements (dyskinesia) may occur as a peak-dose phenomenon, or as a biphasic phenomenon (as the effects of the L-dopa are building up and then wearing off). Management is difficult, but again involves modifying the way L-dopa is administered to obtain constant levels in the brain, and the use of alternative drugs, particularly dopamine agonists.

Anticholinergic agents. These have a useful effect on tremor and rigidity, but do not help bradykinesia. They can be prescribed early in the disease before bradykinesia is a problem, but should be avoided in elderly patients in whom they cause confusion and hallucinations. Other side-effects include dry mouth, blurred vision, difficulty with micturition and constipation. Many anticholinergics are available—for example, benzhexol (1–4 mg 8-hourly) and orphenadrine (50–100 mg 8-hourly).

Amantadine. This has a mild, usually short-lived effect on bradykinesia, but may be used early in the disease before more potent treatment is needed. The dose is 100 mg 8-hourly or 12-hourly. Side-effects include livedo reticularis, peripheral oedema, confusion and seizures.

Selegiline. Selegiline has a mild therapeutic effect in its own right and there is some evidence, albeit controversial, that it slows the progression of the disease. However, there has been some doubt as to its safety. The usual dose is 5–10 mg in the morning.

COMT inhibitors. Tolcapone (100–200 mg 8-hourly) and entacapone (200 mg with each dose of L-dopa) reduce motor fluctuations when used with L-dopa. This allows the L-dopa dose to be reduced and given less frequently.

Dopamine receptor agonists. There are an increasing number of these drugs available which all have slightly different activity at the various dopamine receptors. Apomorphine given on its own causes marked vomiting and has to be administered parenterally. The vomiting can be overcome by the concomitant use of domperidone, and parenteral administration achieved through continuous subcutaneous infusion from a portable pump, or direct injection as needed. Dealing with the drug thus requires considerable nursing support, but, used correctly, it can be very useful.

More easily administered drugs include bromocriptine, lysuride, pergolide, cabergoline and ropinirole, which can all be taken orally. These drugs are less powerful than L-dopa in controlling features of parkinsonism, but they are much less likely to cause dose fluctuations or dyskinesia, though they will certainly exacerbate the latter once these have developed. Side-effects include nausea, vomiting, confusion and hallucination. The dose of bromocriptine is 1 mg initially, increased to 2.5 mg 8-hourly, and thereafter up to 30 mg/day. Pergolide dose starts at 50 μg, increased to 250 μg 8-hourly, and possibly to 3000 μg/day.

Surgery

Stereotactic thalamotomy can be used to treat tremor, though this is relatively infrequently needed because of the medical treatments available. Other stereotactic lesions are currently undergoing evaluation, in particular pallidotomy to help in the management of drug-induced dyskinesia. The implantation of fetal mid-brain cells into the basal ganglia to enhance dopaminergic activity remains experimental.

Physiotherapy and speech therapy

Patients at all stages of Parkinson's disease benefit from physiotherapy, which helps reduce rigidity and corrects abnormal posture. Speech therapy may help in cases where dysarthria and dysphonia interfere with communication.

Prognosis

The outlook for patients with Parkinson's disease is variable, and depends partly on the age of onset. If symptoms start in middle life, the disease is usually slowly progressive and likely to shorten lifespan because of the complications of immobility and tendency to fall. Onset after 70 is unlikely to shorten life or become severe.

OTHER AKINETIC-RIGID SYNDROMES

There are several degenerative conditions which can mimic idiopathic Parkinson's disease, particularly in the early stages. These conditions are relatively uncommon, but about 10% of those thought to have idiopathic Parkinson's disease have one of these variants.

Multiple systems atrophy (MSA)

This is a sporadic condition seen in middle-aged and elderly patients. Features of parkinsonism, often without tremor, are combined with varying degrees of autonomic failure, cerebellar involvement and pyramidal tract degeneration. The combination of parkinsonism with autonomic failure was called the Shy–Drager syndrome, but this term is declining in use. The degeneration is more widespread than in idiopathic Parkinson's disease, and the response to L-dopa and other antiparkinsonian drugs is often disappointing, probably because of degeneration of post-synaptic neurons in the basal ganglia. Autonomic features include postural hypotension, sphincter disturbance, and sometimes respiratory stridor; diagnosis is often assisted by performing tests of autonomic function. Management of postural hypotension includes physical measures such as head-up sleeping position and compressive stockings, and drugs such as fludrocortisone and adrenergic stimulants. Falls are much more common than in idiopathic Parkinson's disease, and life expectancy is considerably reduced.

Progressive supranuclear palsy

Like MSA, this sporadic condition presents in middle-aged patients, and is due to more widespread degeneration in the brain than is seen in idiopathic Parkinson's disease. The clinical features include parkinsonism, though posture is usually extended rather than flexed, and tremor is usually minimal. In addition, there must be a supranuclear paralysis of eye movements, usually downgaze, for the diagnosis to be made. Other features include pyramidal signs and cognitive impairment. As in MSA, the response to antiparkinsonian drugs is disappointing, and life expectancy is reduced.

HUNTINGTON'S DISEASE

This is an inherited disorder with autosomal dominant transmission, affecting both males and females, usually starting in adult life. It is due to expansion of a trinucleotide repeat on chromosome 4 (see p. 41), and frequently demonstrates anticipation, i.e. a younger age of onset in subsequent generations. Slightly different features of the disease occur, depending on whether the abnormal gene is inherited from father or mother.

Clinical features

Symptoms usually begin in middle adult life, with the development of chorea which gradually worsens. This is accompanied by cognitive impairment which often manifests initially as psychiatric symptoms, but later becomes frank dementia. In juvenile onset disease, there may be parkinsonian features with rigidity. Seizures may occur late in the disease.

Investigations

The diagnosis is made clinically, but this is supported by the finding of atrophy of the caudate nucleus on CT or MRI. DNA analysis can be used to confirm the diagnosis and provide pre-symptomatic testing.

Management

At present this is symptomatic only. The chorea may respond to tetrabenazine or dopamine antagonists such as sulpiride. Long-term psychological support and eventually institutional care are often needed as dementia progresses; depressive symptoms may be helped by antidepressant medication. Genetic counselling of relatives is important.

HEREDITARY ATAXIAS

This is a group of inherited disorders in which degenerative changes occur to varying extents in the cerebellum, brain stem, pyramidal tracts, spinocerebellar tracts and optic nerves. Onset may be in childhood or early adult life, and different disorders demonstrate recessive or dominant inheritance. Recently, the genetic abnormalities responsible for a few types of spinocerebellar ataxia (types 1–7) have been shown to be due to abnormal numbers of trinucleotide repeats in various genes, and these can now be detected by DNA analysis, allowing diagnostic confirmation, pre-diagnostic testing and genetic counselling. Clinically, various combinations of cerebellar, pyramidal, sensory, extrapyramidal and cognitive features may occur. Patterns of involvement of several conditions are given in Table 14.27, page 992.

MOTOR NEURON DISEASE

This is a progressive disorder of unknown cause, in which

Table 14.27 Types of hereditary ataxia

Type	Inheritance	Onset	Clinical features
Friedreich's ataxia	Autosomal recessive	8–16 years	Ataxia, nystagmus, dysarthria, spasticity, areflexia, proprioceptive impairment, diabetes mellitus, optic atrophy, cardiac abnormalities. Usually chairbound by age 20
Ataxia telangiectasia	Autosomal recessive	Childhood	Progressive ataxia, athetosis, telangiectasia on conjunctivae, impaired DNA repair, immunodeficiency, tendency to malignancies
Olivopontocerebellar atrophy	Autosomal dominant	Adult life	Slowly progressive ataxia, spasticity, dysarthria, extrapyramidal features, optic atrophy, deafness, pyramidal signs
Hereditary spastic paraplegia	Autosomal dominant	Adult life	Slowly progressive spasticity affecting legs > arms, extensor plantar responses, sensory signs minimal or absent

there is degeneration of motor neurons in the spinal cord and cranial nerve nuclei and pyramidal neurons in the motor cortex. About 5% of cases are familial, showing autosomal dominant inheritance. In many such families, the genetic defect lies on chromosome 21, the enzyme involved being a superoxide dismutase (SOD1). For the remaining 95%, possible causes include viral infection, trauma, exposure to toxins and electric shock, but no sound evidence exists to support any of these. The prevalence of the disease is about 5/100 000.

Clinical features

Patients present with a combination of lower and upper motor neuron signs without sensory involvement. The presence of brisk reflexes in wasted fasciculating limb muscles is typical. Common presenting features are listed in the information boxes.

CLINICAL FEATURES OF MOTOR NEURON DISEASE

Age of onset

- Usually after age 50 years
- Very uncommon before 30 years
- Males more common than females

Symptoms

- Limb muscle weakness, cramps, occasionally fasciculation
- Disturbance of speech/swallowing (dysarthria/dysphagia)

Signs

- Wasting and fasciculation of muscles
- Weakness of muscles of limbs, tongue, face and palate
- Pyramidal tract involvement causes spasticity, exaggerated tendon reflexes, extensor plantar responses
- External ocular muscles and sphincters usually remain intact
- No objective sensory deficit
- No intellectual impairment in most cases

Course

- Symptoms often begin focally in one part and spread gradually but relentlessly to become widespread

PATTERNS OF INVOLVEMENT OF MOTOR NEURON DISEASE

Progressive muscular atrophy

- Predominantly spinal motor neurons affected
- Weakness and wasting of distal limb muscles at first
- Fasciculation in muscles
- Tendon reflexes may be absent

Progressive bulbar palsy

- Early involvement of tongue, palate and pharyngeal muscles
- Dysarthria/dysphagia
- Wasting and fasciculation of tongue
- May be pyramidal signs as well

Amyotrophic lateral sclerosis

- Combination of distal and proximal muscle-wasting and weakness, fasciculation
- Spasticity, exaggerated reflexes, extensor plantars
- Bulbar and pseudobulbar palsy follow eventually
- Pyramidal tract features may predominate

Investigations

In many patients the clinical features are highly suggestive but alternative diagnoses need to be carefully excluded. In particular, potentially treatable disorders such as diabetic amyotrophy, spinal disorders and multifocal motor neuronopathy should be excluded. Electromyography helps to confirm the presence of fasciculation and denervation, and is particularly helpful when pyramidal features predominate. Sensory nerve conduction and motor conduction studies are normal but there is evidence of loss of axons. Spinal imaging and brain scanning may be necessary to exclude focal spinal or cerebral disease. CSF examination is usually normal, though a slight elevation in protein concentration may be found.

Management

No treatment significantly alters the progress of this disease, though glutamate antagonists (e.g. riluzole) and agents such as nerve growth factor show promise. Psychological and physical support, with help from occupational and speech therapists and physiotherapists, is essential to keep the patient's quality of life as good as possible. Mechanical aids such as splints, walking aids, wheelchairs and communication devices all help to reduce handicap. Feeding by percutaneous gastrostomy may be necessary if bulbar palsy is marked. Sometimes non-invasive ventilatory support may help distress from weak respiratory muscles although maintenance ventilation is usually not requested. Relief of distress in the terminal stages usually requires the use of opiates and sedative drugs.

Prognosis

Motor neuron disease is progressive; the mean time from diagnosis to death is 1 year, with most patients dying within 3–5 years of the onset of symptoms. Younger patients and those with early bulbar symptoms tend to show a more rapid course. Death is usually from respiratory infection and failure, and the complications of immobility.

SPINAL MUSCULAR ATROPHIES

This is a group of genetically determined disorders affecting spinal motor and cranial motor neurons, characterised by proximal and distal wasting, fasciculation and weakness of muscles. Involvement is usually symmetrical, but occasional localised forms occur. With the exception of the infantile form, progression is slow and the prognosis better than for motor neuron disease (see Table 14.28).

FURTHER INFORMATION ON DEGENERATIVE DISEASES

Bradley W G, Daroff R B, Fenichel G M, Marsden C D 1996 Neurology in clinical practice (vol. II): The neurological disorders, 2nd edn. Butterworth–Heinemann, Boston

Harding A E 1984 The hereditary ataxias and related disorders. Churchill Livingstone, Edinburgh

Quinn N P (ed) 1998 Parkinsonism. Baillière's Clinical Neurology 6: 1–218

Williams A C (ed) 1994 Motor neuron disease. Chapman & Hall, London

DISEASES OF NERVE AND MUSCLE

DISEASES OF PERIPHERAL NERVES

Peripheral nerves may be damaged by diffuse processes affecting all nerves to a greater or lesser extent (peripheral neuropathies), or individual nerves may be affected by local pathology including trauma, compression and entrapment. Alternatively, several individual nerves may be affected by multifocal pathology (mononeuritis multiplex), or there may be focal pathology in nerve plexuses.

ACQUIRED PERIPHERAL NEUROPATHIES

There are numerous causes of peripheral neuropathy (see Table 14.29, p. 994). The diagnostic possibilities are limited in an individual patient by the clinical features (motor, sensory, autonomic or mixed) and whether axons or myelin are predominantly affected (determined electrophysiologically).

Clinical features

The first manifestations are usually at the distal ends of the longest nerves. Distal paraesthesia is a frequent symptom, usually first affecting the feet and then the hands, and subsequently progressing proximally up the limbs. This is often associated with diminution of superficial sensation in a 'glove and stocking' distribution. There may be distal weakness, usually with diminished or absent tendon reflexes, and possibly autonomic disturbance. In hereditary neuropathies there may be a positive family history.

Investigations

A careful clinical history is essential, including details of family history, drug intake and potential exposure to toxins. Screening tests are listed in the information box, page 994. Nerve conduction studies confirm the presence of a neuropathy and indicate whether axons or myelin are primarily affected. In some cases, nerve biopsy may be indicated, particularly if an inflammatory aetiology is suspected.

Table 14.28 Types of spinal muscular atrophy

Type	Onset	Inheritance	Features	Prognosis
Werdnig–Hoffmann	Infancy	Autosomal recessive	Severe muscle-wasting/weakness	Poor
Kugelberg–Welander	Childhood, adolescence	Autosomal recessive	Proximal weakness and wasting. EMG shows denervation	Slowly progressive disability
Distal forms	Early adult life	Autosomal dominant	Distal weakness and wasting of hands and feet	Good, seldom disabling
Bulbospinal	Adult life, males only	X-linked	Facial and bulbar weakness, proximal limb weakness	Good

Table 14.29 Causes of peripheral neuropathy

Type	Common	Unusual	Rare
Metabolic/endocrine	Diabetes mellitus Chronic renal failure	Paraproteinaemia Cryoglobulinaemia Amyloidosis Hypothyroidism Liver failure	Porphyria
Toxic	Alcohol	Drugs (isoniazid, phenytoin, vincristine)	Heavy metals Organic solvents
Inflammatory	Acute (Guillain–Barré syndrome)	Chronic inflammatory demyelinating polyneuropathy Connective tissue disease (e.g. SLE, polyarteritis nodosa, Sjögren's syndrome) Infective (leprosy)	Multifocal neuropathy with conduction block
Genetic		Hereditary motor and sensory neuropathies (Charcot–Marie–Tooth) Friedreich's ataxia	Other hereditary neuropathies
Deficiency states		Vitamin B_{12} deficiency Thiamine deficiency Folate deficiency	Vitamin A, E deficiency Pyridoxine deficiency
Others		Malignant disease Critical illness neuropathy	

INVESTIGATION OF PERIPHERAL NEUROPATHY

Haematology
- Full blood count
- Erythrocyte sedimentation rate
- B_{12}
- Folate

Biochemistry
- Urea, electrolytes, calcium
- Creatinine
- Liver function tests
- Blood glucose ± tolerance test
- Thyroxine and thyroid-stimulating hormone (TSH)
- Plasma protein electrophoresis
- Serum lipids, lipoproteins
- Cryoglobulins
- Vitamin assays (e.g. vitamin E)
- Phytanic acid (Refsum's disease)
- Toxic metal and drug screen
- Urinary porphyrins
- Urinary Bence Jones protein

Immunology
- VDRL
- Serum autoantibodies (antinuclear factor, double-stranded DNA, rheumatoid factor, extractable nuclear antigens)
- Antiganglioside antibodies
- Antineuronal antibodies

Genetic testing
- Some hereditary neuropathies
- Friedreich's ataxia

Nerve conduction/EMG
- Axonal or demyelinating

Nerve biopsy
- Inflammatory
- Vasculitis

Exclusion of malignancy and systemic disorders
- Faecal occult blood
- Prostate-specific antigen
- Chest radiography/CT
- Mammogram
- Abdominal imaging

Management

In about one-third of patients, a treatable cause is identified. Toxins and offending drugs should be removed, and metabolic abnormalities or deficiency states corrected. Inflammatory neuropathies can often be treated with immunosuppressive agents or intravenous immunoglobulin. However, in many patients (about another third), a cause is identified for which there is no specific treatment and, in the remainder, no specific cause is found. Particularly if there is no specific therapy available (e.g. hereditary neuropathies), advice from physiotherapists and occupational therapists is important in helping patients to maintain their functional capacity.

GUILLAIN–BARRÉ SYNDROME

Also known as acute inflammatory or post-infective demyelinating polyneuropathy, this develops 1–4 weeks after respiratory infection or diarrhoea in 70% of patients, but can follow surgery or immunisation. Pathologically there is demyelination of spinal roots or peripheral nerves, which is immunologically mediated.

Clinical features

The characteristic clinical feature is rapidly progressive muscle weakness, often ascending from lower to upper limbs and more marked proximally than distally. Distal paraesthesia and limb pains often precede the weakness. Facial or bulbar weakness commonly develops, and respiratory weakness requiring ventilatory support occurs in 20% of cases. In most patients muscle weakness progresses for 1–3 weeks, but rapid deterioration with respiratory failure can develop within hours. The most striking findings on examination are diffuse weakness with widespread loss of reflexes. An unusual variant described by Miller Fisher comprises the triad of ophthalmoplegia, ataxia and areflexia.

Investigations

The protein content of the CSF is raised at some stage of the illness, but may be normal in the first 10 days. There is usually no rise in CSF cell number and a lymphocytosis > 50/mm^3 suggests an alternative diagnosis. Electrophysiological studies are often normal in the early stages, but show typical changes after a week or so, with multifocal motor slowing and proximal slowing. Investigation to identify an underlying cause, such as cytomegalovirus, *Mycoplasma* or *Campylobacter*, requires a chest radiograph, stool culture and appropriate immunological blood tests. Antibodies to the ganglioside GQ_{1b} are found in the Miller Fisher variant described above. Acute porphyria (see p. 540) can be excluded by urinary porphyrin estimation, and serum lead should be measured if there are only motor signs.

Management

During the phase of deterioration, regular monitoring of respiratory function (vital capacity and blood gases) is required, as respiratory failure may develop with little warning and require ventilatory support. Intubation and ventilation are often required because of bulbar incompetence leading to inhalation. General management to protect the airway and prevent pressure sores and venous thrombosis is essential. Steroid therapy is ineffective, but plasma exchange and intravenous immunoglobulin therapy shorten the duration of ventilation and improve prognosis, provided treatment is started within 14 days of the onset of symptoms.

Prognosis

Overall, 80% of patients recover completely within 3–6 months, 4% die, and the remainder suffer residual neurological disability which can be severe.

ENTRAPMENT NEUROPATHIES

These conditions often have a characteristic clinical history and physical signs (see Table 14.30).

Management

Lateral popliteal nerve palsies and radial nerve palsies are commonly due to local trauma, and complete recovery over 6–8 weeks can be expected without intervention. Meralgia

Table 14.30 Symptoms and signs in common entrapment neuropathies

Nerve	Symptoms	Muscle weakness/wasting	Area of sensory loss
Median (at wrist) (carpal tunnel syndrome)	Pain and paraesthesia on palmar aspect of hands and fingers, waking the patient from sleep. Pain may extend to arm and shoulder	Abductor pollicis brevis	Lateral palm and thumb, index, middle and half ring finger
Ulnar (at elbow)	Paraesthesia on medial border of hand, wasting and weakness of hand muscles	All small hand muscles, excluding abductor pollicis brevis	Medial palm and little finger, and half ring finger
Radial	Weakness of extension of wrist and fingers, often precipitated by sleeping in abnormal posture, e.g. arm over back of chair	Wrist and finger extensors, supinator	Dorsum of thumb
Peroneal	Foot drop, trauma to head of fibula	Dorsiflexion and eversion of foot	Nil or dorsum of foot
Lateral cutaneous nerve of the thigh (meralgia paraesthetica)	Tingling and dysaesthesia on lateral border of the thigh	Nil	Lateral border of thigh

paraesthetica often develops in relation to weight loss or gain and may respond to dietary advice and reassurance. Carpal tunnel syndrome and ulnar nerve palsy may remit if patients avoid activities involving repetitive wrist movement or pressure on the elbows, and may respond to nocturnal splinting of joints. Precipitating causes including diabetes mellitus and hypothyroidism should be excluded. In some patients decompression of the carpal tunnel or transposition of the ulnar nerve may be necessary. Electrophysiological investigation is advisable pre-operatively to confirm both diagnosis and site of compression.

MONONEURITIS MULTIPLEX

In this condition, multifocal peripheral or spinal nerve lesions occur serially or concurrently. Pathologically, the nerves are rendered susceptible to mechanical compression by ischaemia of the peripheral nerves due to vasculopathy of the vasa nervorum or infiltration of the nerves. Common causes are diabetes mellitus, leprosy, polyarteritis nodosa and rheumatoid arthritis.

BRACHIAL PLEXUS LESIONS

Trauma is the most common cause of damage to the brachial plexus, and frequently involves traction between the head and shoulder, or excessive abduction of the arm. Other causes include neoplasia in the cervical lymph nodes or pulmonary apex, compression at the thoracic outlet, radiotherapy and inflammatory/vascular disease (e.g. neuralgic amyotrophy—see below).

Clinical features

The clinical signs depend on the anatomical site of damage (see Table 14.31). There may be associated vascular symptoms and signs in the thoracic outlet syndrome.

Neuralgic amyotrophy presents with severe pain over one shoulder and sometimes follows infection, inoculation or operation. Within days, paralysis develops in the painful muscles (most commonly deltoid, the spinati and serratus anterior), and is rapidly followed by muscle-wasting. Occasionally, there is more extensive involvement of the muscles of the upper arm and there may be sensory loss over the deltoid. Pain usually subsides within 1–2 weeks and complete recovery of paralysis and wasting can be expected in 3–6 months without treatment.

Management

Surgical treatment may be indicated for congenital anomalies such as cervical rib or for traumatic lesions where grafts of nerve or muscle may aid regeneration. In this situation, regular passive movements of the affected limb prevent contractures while nerve fibres are regenerating. The prognosis for recovery in traumatic lesions is dependent on the site and severity of neuronal damage, which may be assessed electrophysiologically.

DISEASES AFFECTING THE CRANIAL NERVES

Cranial nerves may be affected as part of a generalised peripheral neuropathy, but are often involved singly or in groups by intracranial disease. Intracranial disease such as cerebral tumour may involve a cranial nerve directly (e.g. acoustic neuroma, see p. 1020) or may cause secondary dysfunction by stretching or compressing it against other structures (e.g. 3rd nerve palsy due to tentorial herniation of the medial temporal lobe). Diseases of most of the individual cranial nerves have already been discussed elsewhere (see pp. 965–972).

IDIOPATHIC FACIAL NERVE PALSY (BELL'S PALSY)

This is a common condition affecting all ages and both sexes. The cause is unknown, but the site of damage is probably the portion of the facial nerve lying within the facial canal. The onset is subacute, with symptoms usually developing over a few hours. Pain around the ear may precede loss of movement on one side of the face, initially noticed either by the patient or by family. Patients may describe the face as being numb, but there is no objective loss of sensation (except possibly taste, due to involvement of the chorda tympani). Hyperacusis occurs if the nerve to stapedius is involved, and there may also be loss of salivation and tear secretion.

Examination reveals only a lower motor neuron facial nerve palsy on one side. Vesicles in the ear or on the palate indicate that the facial palsy is due to herpes zoster

Table 14.31 Physical signs in brachial plexus lesions

Site	Root	Affected muscles	Sensory loss
Upper plexus (Erb–Duchenne)	C5/6	Biceps, deltoid, spinati, rhomboids, brachioradialis (triceps, serratus anterior)	Patch over deltoid
Lower plexus (Dejerine–Klumpke)	C8/T1	All small hand muscles, claw hand (ulnar wrist flexors)	Ulnar border hand/forearm
Thoracic outlet syndrome	C8/T1	Small hand muscles, ulnar forearm	Ulnar border hand/forearm (upper arm)

infection rather than Bell's palsy (see p. 1012). A reduction in the amplitude of the facial muscle action potential on EMG after the first week predicts a slow/poor recovery.

There is no proven medical treatment, though a course of steroids such as prednisolone 40 mg daily for a week may speed recovery. To prevent exposure of the cornea, artificial tear drops and ointment are applied to the eye, and the eye is taped shut overnight. About 70–80% of patients recover spontaneously within 2–12 weeks, but elderly patients with complete facial palsy have a poorer prognosis. Aberrant re-innervation may occur during the course of recovery, giving rise to unwanted facial movements (e.g. eye closure when the mouth is moved), or 'crocodile tears' (tearing during salivation).

CLONIC FACIAL (HEMIFACIAL) SPASM

This disorder usually presents after middle age. Symptoms start with intermittent twitching around one eye which spreads ipsilaterally over months to years to affect other parts of the face. The spasms of twitching are intermittent, often exacerbated by talking or eating, or when the patient is under stress. The cause is thought to be an aberrant loop of artery irritating the facial nerve as it emerges from the pons. It is important to image the facial nerve to exclude a structural lesion, especially in a young patient. Drug treatment is not effective, but injections of botulinum toxin into affected muscles can help, although these have to be repeated every 3 months or so. Occasionally, microvascular decompression is necessary, but this involves a posterior craniotomy.

DISORDERS OF THE NEUROMUSCULAR JUNCTION

MYASTHENIA GRAVIS

This condition is characterised by progressive inability to sustain a maintained or repeated contraction of striated muscle (fatigability).

Aetiology and pathology

Acetylcholine receptors in the post-junctional membrane of neuromuscular junctions are blocked or lysed by a complement-mediated autoimmune reaction between receptor protein and anti-acetylcholine receptor antibody. About 15% of patients (mainly those with late onset) have a thymoma, and the majority of the remainder have one of a number of thymic abnormalities, the most characteristic of which is thymic hyperplasia. There is an increased incidence of other autoimmune diseases (see p. 35), and the disease is linked with certain HLA haplotypes, the strongest associations in a north European population being with B8 and DRw3. Nothing is known about factors which trigger the disease itself, but penicillamine can cause an antibody-mediated myasthenic syndrome which may persist even after drug withdrawal. Some drugs, especially aminoglycosides and ciprofloxacin, may exacerbate the neuromuscular blockade and should be avoided in patients with myasthenia.

Clinical features

The disease usually presents between the ages of 15 and 50 years with women affected more often than men. It tends to run a relapsing and remitting course, especially during the early years.

The cardinal symptom is abnormal fatigable weakness of the muscles (which is different from a sensation of muscle fatigue). Although movement is initially strong, it rapidly weakens. Worsening of symptoms towards the end of the day or following exercise is characteristic. There are no sensory signs or signs of involvement of the central nervous system although weakness of the oculomotor muscles may mimic a central eye movement disorder.

The first symptoms are usually intermittent ptosis or diplopia, but weakness of chewing, swallowing, speaking, or of limb movement also occurs. Any limb muscle may be affected, most commonly those of the shoulder girdle; the patient is unable to undertake work above shoulder level, such as combing hair, without frequent rests. Respiratory muscles may be involved, and respiratory failure is a not uncommon cause of death. Aspiration may occur if the cough is ineffectual. Sudden weakness from a cholinergic or myasthenic crisis (see below) may require ventilatory support.

Investigations

The intravenous injection of the short-acting anticholinesterase, edrophonium bromide, is a valuable diagnostic aid (the Tensilon test); 2 mg is injected initially, with a further 8 mg given half a minute later if there are no undesirable side-effects. Improvement in muscle power occurs within 30 seconds and usually persists for 2–3 minutes. EMG with repetitive stimulation may show the characteristic decremental response. Anti-acetylcholine receptor antibody is found in over 80% of cases, though less frequently in purely ocular myasthenia. Positive antiskeletal muscle antibodies suggest the presence of thymoma but all patients should have a thoracic CT to exclude this condition, which may not be visible on plain radiographic examination. Screening for other autoimmune disorders, particularly thyroid disease, is important.

Management

The principles of treatment are:

1. to maximise the activity of acetylcholine at remaining receptors in the neuromuscular junctions and
2. to limit or abolish the immunological attack on motor end plates.

IMMUNOLOGICAL TREATMENT OF MYASTHENIA
Thymectomy
• Should be performed as soon as feasible in any patient with myasthenia not confined to extraocular muscles, unless the disease has been established for more than 7 years
Plasma exchange
• Removing antibody from the blood may produce marked improvement but, as this is usually brief, such therapy is normally reserved for myasthenic crisis or for pre-operative preparation
Intravenous immunoglobulin
• An alternative to plasma exchange in the treatment of severe myasthenia
Corticosteroid treatment
• Improvement is commonly preceded by marked exacerbation of myasthenic symptoms and treatment should be initiated in hospital. It is usually necessary to continue treatment for months or years, often resulting in adverse effects
Other immunosuppressant treatment
• Treatment with azathioprine 2.5 mg/kg daily is of value in reducing the dosage of steroids necessary and may allow steroids to be withdrawn. The effect of treatment on clinical disease is often delayed for several months

The duration of action of acetylcholine is greatly prolonged by inhibiting its hydrolysing enzyme, acetylcholinesterase. The most commonly used anticholinesterase drug is pyridostigmine, which is given orally in a dosage of 30–120 mg, usually 6-hourly. Muscarinic side-effects, including diarrhoea and colic, may be controlled by propantheline (15 mg as required). Over-dosage of anti-cholinesterase drugs may cause a cholinergic crisis due to depolarisation block of motor end plates, with muscle fasciculation, paralysis, pallor, sweating, excessive salivation and small pupils. This may be distinguished from severe weakness due to exacerbation of myasthenia (myasthenic crisis) by the clinical features and, if necessary, by the injection of a small dose of edrophonium.

The immunological treatment of myasthenia is outlined in the information box. Thymectomy in the early stages of the disease leads to a much better overall prognosis, whether a thymoma is present or not.

Prognosis

Prognosis is variable. Remissions sometimes occur spontaneously. When myasthenia is confined to the eye muscles, the prognosis is excellent and disability slight. Young female patients with generalised disease have high remission rates after thymectomy, whilst older patients are less likely to have a remission despite treatment. Rapid progression of the disease more than 5 years after its onset is uncommon.

OTHER MYASTHENIC SYNDROMES

There are other conditions which present with muscle weakness due to impaired transmission across the neuromuscular junction. The most common of these is the Lambert–Eaton myasthenic syndrome (LEMS), in which transmitter release is impaired, often in association with antibodies to pre-junctional voltage-gated calcium channels. Patients may have autonomic dysfunction (and a dry mouth) in addition to muscle weakness, but the cardinal clinical sign is absence of tendon reflexes, which can return immediately after sustained contraction of the relevant muscle. The condition is associated with underlying malignancy in a high percentage of cases, and investigation must be directed towards detecting such a cause. The condition is diagnosed electrophysiologically by the presence of post-tetanic potentiation of motor response to nerve stimulation at a frequency of 20–50/s.

DISEASES OF MUSCLE

Voluntary muscle is subject to a range of disorders which result in a limited spectrum of symptoms and physical signs. Diagnosis depends upon consideration of the clinical picture along with the results of EMG studies and muscle biopsy. In some muscular dystrophies, e.g. Duchenne dystrophy and dystrophia myotonica, a specific genetic abnormality has been identified. Screening tests are given in the information box.

MUSCULAR DYSTROPHY

Several inherited disorders are characterised by progressive degeneration of groups of muscles without involvement of the nervous system.

Clinical features

Wasting and weakness are usually symmetrical, there is no fasciculation and no sensory loss and, except in dystrophia myotonica, tendon reflexes are preserved until a late stage. Differential diagnosis is based on the age at onset, the distribution of affected muscles, and the pattern of inheritance (see Table 14.32).

Investigations

The diagnosis of muscular dystrophy can be confirmed by EMG and muscle biopsy. Creatine kinase is markedly elevated in Duchenne muscular dystrophy, but is normal or only moderately elevated in the other types.

Dystrophia myotonica may be diagnosed by the distribution of muscle weakness and other features including myotonia (slow relaxation of muscle), cataracts, ptosis, frontal baldness and gonadal atrophy. It is caused by expansion of a trinucleotide repeat of chromosome 19.

INVESTIGATION OF MUSCLE DISEASE
Haematology
• Full blood count • ESR
Biochemistry
• Urea, electrolytes • Calcium, phosphate • Creatine kinase • Lactate dehydrogenase • Liver function tests • Thyroxine and TSH • Plasma and urinary corticosteroids • Urinary calcium • Ischaemic lactate test
Immunology
• Antinuclear factor • Double-stranded DNA • Acetylcholine receptor • Voltage-gated calcium channel (Lambert–Eaton)
Genetic testing
• Some muscular dystrophies • Mitochondrial DNA
Nerve conduction study/EMG
• Exclude denervation • Metabolic or structural disease
Muscle biopsy
• Histology (light and electron microscopy) • Histochemistry • Tissue enzyme assay (e.g. myophosphorylase, phosphofructokinase, acid maltase, carnitine-palmityl transferase)
Exclusion of malignancy and systemic disorders
• Faecal occult blood • Chest radiograph/CT • Mammogram • Abdominal imaging

Management

There is no specific therapy for these conditions, although advice from the physiotherapist and occupational therapist may help the patient to cope with disability. Genetic counselling is important. The genetic defects of Duchenne dystrophy and facioscapulohumeral dystrophy have been mapped to chromosomes Xp21 and 4q35, respectively. DNA analysis may allow early diagnosis and prenatal testing in these conditions, as in dystrophia myotonica.

Prognosis

Most patients with Duchenne dystrophy die within 10 years of diagnosis, while the lifespan in limb girdle and facioscapulohumeral dystrophies is normal. Premature death due to respiratory or cardiac failure in early middle age is the usual outcome in dystrophia myotonica, although patients are affected very variably (c.f. the phenomenon of anticipation in trinucleotide repeat disorders, p. 41).

METABOLIC AND ENDOCRINE MYOPATHY

Muscle weakness may develop in a range of metabolic and endocrine disorders and is usually reversible. The causes are listed in the information box.

METABOLIC AND ENDOCRINE CAUSES OF MUSCLE WEAKNESS	
Acute muscle weakness	**Proximal myopathy**
• Hypokalaemia • Hyperkalaemia • Hypocalcaemia • Hypercalcaemia	• Hyperthyroidism • Hypothyroidism • Cushing's syndrome • Addison's disease

Clinical features

The weakness is often acute and generalised in metabolic disorders, while a proximal myopathy predominantly affecting the pelvic girdle is a feature of some endocrine disorders. This may develop without other manifestations of hormonal disturbance. Hypo- and hyperkalaemia may occur in the familial periodic paralyses, which are inherited conditions characterised by attacks of profound weakness lasting for several hours, often precipitated by eating or exertion.

Muscle pain on exercise is the characteristic feature of myophosphorylase deficiency (McArdle's syndrome) and a number of other rare recessively inherited disorders of metabolism (see the information box, p. 1000).

INFLAMMATORY MYOPATHY OR POLYMYOSITIS

See page 860.

Table 14.32 Diagnostic features in muscular dystrophy

Dystrophy	Inheritance	Age at onset (yrs)	Muscles affected
Duchenne	X-linked recessive	3–10	Proximal legs and arms, then general
Limb girdle	Autosomal recessive	10–30	Pelvic girdle, shoulder girdle or both
Facioscapulohumeral	Autosomal dominant	10–40	Facial, shoulder girdle, serratus anterior
Dystrophia myotonica	Autosomal dominant	Any age	Temporalis, facial, sternomastoid, distal limbs, myotonia

RARE DISORDERS OF MUSCLE METABOLISM
Myophosphorylase deficiency (McArdle's syndrome)
• Muscle pain on exercise • Increased glycogen in muscle • Failure of blood lactate to rise on exercise • Reduced myophosphorylase (muscle biopsy)
Phosphofructokinase deficiency
• Similar to above, but reduced phosphofructokinase (muscle biopsy)
Carnitine-palmityl transferase (CPT) deficiency
• Muscle pain after prolonged exercise • Increased lipid in muscle on biopsy • Reduced CPT (muscle biopsy)

CONGENITAL MYOPATHY

This is rare and presents in infancy with muscular weakness and limpness. Serum enzymes may be normal or slightly elevated and the EMG is usually myopathic. The syndrome may be caused by a number of specific conditions which have a variable inheritance, and are defined by the type of structural abnormality present in skeletal muscle fibres. Most patients have a slowly progressive disease and there is no specific therapy.

TOXIC MYOPATHY

A wide variety of drugs may cause disorders of muscle, including carbenoxolone, thiazide diuretics and steroids. Alcohol may cause a spectrum of muscle disease varying from a mild, proximal weakness to severe muscle necrosis. Avoidance of the offending agent usually results in recovery of muscle function.

FURTHER INFORMATION ON DISEASES OF NERVE AND MUSCLE

Dyck P J, Thomas P K, Griffin J W et al (eds) 1993 Peripheral neuropathy. W B Saunders, Philadelphia

Sanders D B (ed) 1994 Neurologic clinics: myasthenia gravis and myasthenic syndromes. W B Saunders, Philadelphia

Walton J, Karpati G, Hilton-Jones D (eds) 1994 Disorders of voluntary muscle. Churchill Livingstone, Edinburgh

DISORDERS OF THE SPINE AND SPINAL CORD

The spinal cord and spinal roots may be affected by intrinsic disease or by disorders of the surrounding meninges or bones. The clinical presentation of these depends on the anatomical level at which the cord or roots are affected and the nature of the pathology. It is important to recognise when emergency surgical intervention is necessary and plan the investigations to identify such patients.

COMPRESSION OF THE SPINAL CORD

Acute spinal cord compression is one of the most common neurological emergencies encountered in clinical practice and the common causes are listed in Table 14.33.

A space-occupying lesion within the spinal canal may damage nerve tissue either directly (by pressure) or indirectly (by interfering with blood supply). Oedema from venous obstruction impairs neuronal function, and ischaemia from arterial obstruction may lead to necrosis of the spinal cord. The early stages of damage are reversible, but severely damaged neurons do not recover; hence the importance of early diagnosis and treatment.

Clinical features

The onset of symptoms of spinal cord compression is usually slow (over weeks), but can be acute with trauma or metastases, especially if there is associated arterial occlusion. The symptoms are shown in the first information box.

Pain and sensory symptoms occur early, while weakness and sphincter dysfunction are usually late manifestations.

The signs vary according to the level of the cord compression and the structures involved. There may be tenderness to percussion over the spine if there is vertebral disease, and this may be associated with a local kyphosis. Involvement of the roots at the level of the compression may give dermatomal sensory impairment and corresponding lower motor signs. Interruption of fibres in the spinal cord causes sensory loss (see p. 955) and upper motor neuron signs below the level of the lesion, and there is often disturbance of sphincter function.

The distribution of these signs varies with the level of the lesion, as shown in the second information box.

Table 14.33 Causes of spinal cord compression

Site	Frequency	Causes
Vertebral (extradural)	80%	Trauma Intervertebral disc Metastatic carcinoma (e.g. breast, prostate, bronchus) Myeloma Tuberculosis
Meninges (Intradural extramedullary)	15%	Tumours (e.g. meningioma, neurofibroma, ependymoma, metastasis, lymphoma, leukaemia) Epidural abscess
Spinal cord (Intradural intramedullary)	5%	Tumours (e.g. glioma, ependymoma, metastasis)

SYMPTOMS OF SPINAL CORD COMPRESSION
Pain
• Localised over the spine or in a root distribution, which may be aggravated by coughing, sneezing or straining
Sensory
• Paraesthesia, numbness or cold sensations, especially in the lower limbs, which spread proximally, often to a level on the trunk
Motor
• Weakness, heaviness or stiffness of the limbs, most commonly the legs
Sphincters
• Urgency or hesitancy of micturition, leading eventually to urinary retention

SIGNS OF SPINAL CORD COMPRESSION
Cervical, above C5
• Upper motor neuron signs and sensory loss in all four limbs
Cervical, C5 to T1
• Lower motor neuron signs and segmental sensory loss in the arms, and upper motor neuron signs in the legs
Thoracic cord
• Spastic paraplegia with a sensory level on the trunk
Conus medullaris
• Lesions at the end of the spinal cord cause loss of sensation in the sacral area and extensor plantar responses
Cauda equina
• The spinal cord ends at approximately the T12/L1 spinal level and spinal lesions below this level can only cause lower motor neuron signs by affecting the cauda equina

The Brown-Séquard syndrome (see Fig. 14.13E, p. 956) results if damage is confined to one side of the cord; the findings are explained by the anatomy of the sensory tracts (see Figure 14.14, p. 957). On the side of the lesion there is a band of hyperaesthesia with loss of proprioceptive sense and upper motor neuron signs below it. On the other side there is loss of spinothalamic sensation (pain and temperature). With compressive lesions there is usually a band of pain at the level of the lesion in the distribution of the nerve roots subject to compression.

Investigations

Patients with a short history of a progressive spinal cord syndrome should be investigated urgently. Investigations necessary are listed in the information box.

Plain radiographs may show bony destruction and soft-tissue abnormalities and are an essential initial investigation (see Fig. 14.37, p. 1002). Routine investigations, including chest radiograph, may provide evidence of systemic disease. MRI of the spine is the investigation of choice (see Fig. 14.38, p. 1002), but myelography also localises the lesion and, with CT in suitable cases, defines the extent of compression and associated soft-tissue abnormality (see Fig. 14.39, p. 1003). CSF should be taken for analysis at the time of myelography. In cases of spinal block this shows a normal cell count with a very elevated protein causing yellow discoloration of the fluid (Froin's syndrome). Acute deterioration may develop after myelography and it is preferable to alert the neurosurgeons before such procedures are undertaken.

INVESTIGATION OF ACUTE SPINAL CORD SYNDROME
• Plain radiographs of spine • Chest radiographs • MRI of spine or myelography • CSF • Serum B_{12}

Management

The treatment and prognosis depend on the nature of the underlying lesion. Benign tumours should be surgically excised, and a good functional recovery can be expected unless a marked neurological deficit has developed before diagnosis. Extradural compression due to malignancy is the most common cause of spinal cord compression and has a poor prognosis, although useful function can be regained if treatment is initiated within 24 hours of the onset of severe weakness or sphincter dysfunction. Surgical decompression may be appropriate in some patients, but has a similar outcome to radiotherapy. Needle biopsy is required prior to radiotherapy to establish the histological nature of the tumour. Traumatic lesions of the vertebral column require specialised treatment in a neurosurgical centre.

CERVICAL SPONDYLOSIS

In the cervical spine, some degree of degenerative change is a normal radiological finding in the middle-aged and elderly. Degeneration of the intervertebral discs and secondary osteoarthrosis (cervical spondylosis) is often asymptomatic, but may be associated with neurological dysfunction. The C5/6, C6/7 and C4/5 vertebral levels and C6, C7 and C5 roots, respectively, are most commonly affected (see Fig. 14.40, p. 1003).

CERVICAL SPONDYLOTIC RADICULOPATHY

Compression of a nerve root occurs when a disc prolapses laterally. This may develop acutely, or more gradually due to osteophytic encroachment of the intervertebral foramina.

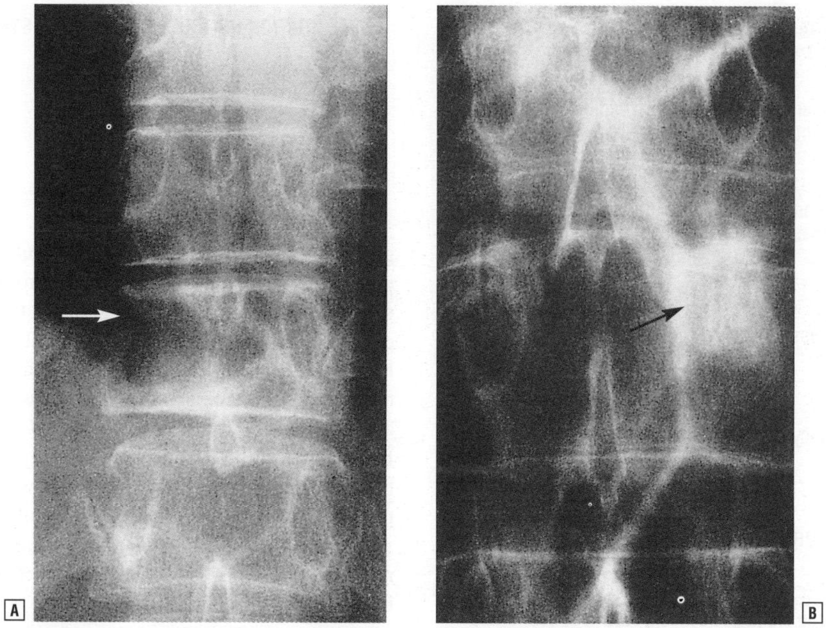

Fig. 14.37 Plain radiographs of the spine. [A] Loss of vertebral pedicle (arrow) by bony erosion of an osteolytic metastasis. [B] An osteosclerotic metastasis (arrow).

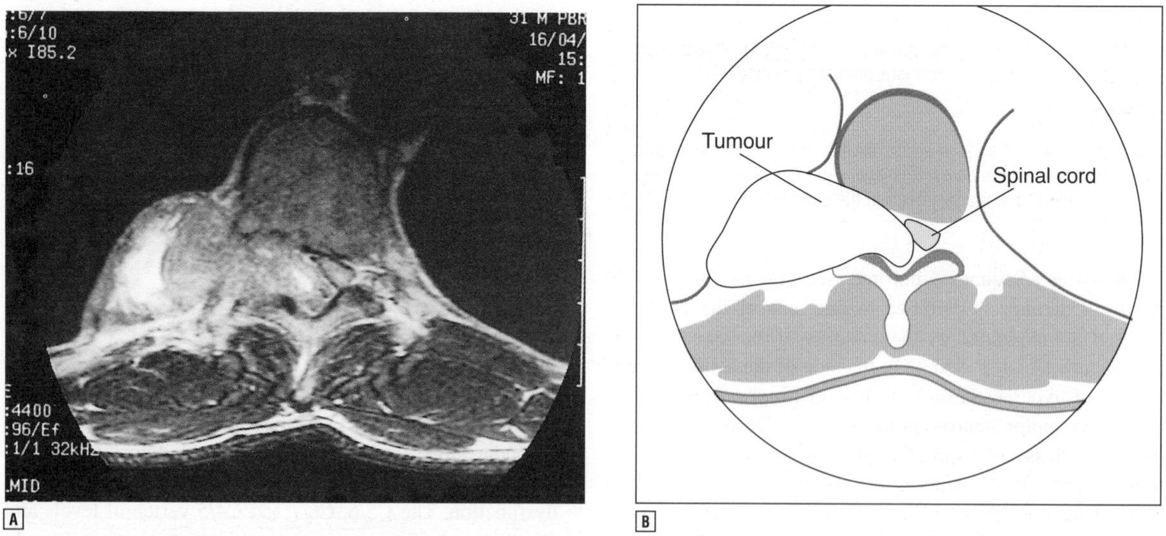

Fig. 14.38 Axial MRI of thoracic spine. [A] A meningioma is compressing the spinal cord and emerging in a 'dumbbell' fashion through the vertebral foramen into the paraspinal space. [B] Line diagram illustrating major structures.

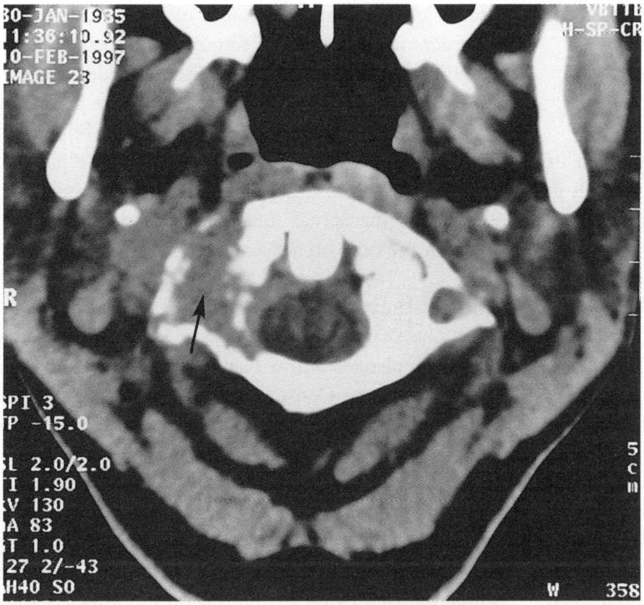

Fig. 14.39 CT myelogram of cervical spine at the level of C2 showing bony erosion of vertebra by a metastasis (arrow).

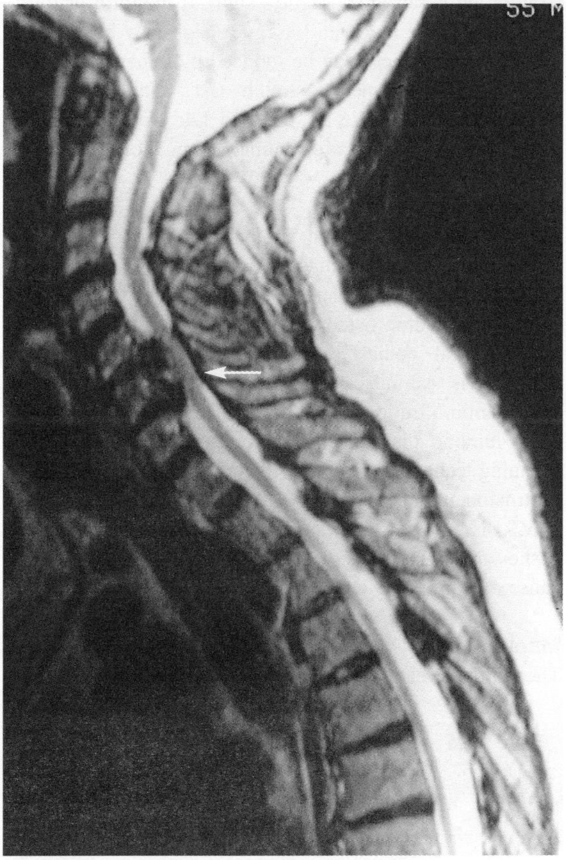

Fig. 14.40 MRI showing cervical cord compression (arrow) in cervical spondylosis.

Clinical features

The patient complains of pain in the neck which may radiate in the distribution of the affected nerve root. The neck is held rigidly and neck movements may exacerbate pain. Paraesthesia and sensory loss may be found in the affected segment and there may be lower motor neuron signs, including weakness, wasting and reflex impairment (see Table 14.34).

Investigations

Plain radiographs, including lateral and oblique views, should be obtained to confirm the presence of degenerative changes and to exclude other conditions, including destructive lesions. If surgery is contemplated, MRI is appropriate. Electrophysiological studies rarely add to the clinical examination, but may be necessary if there is doubt about the differential diagnosis between root and peripheral nerve lesions.

Management

Conservative treatment with analgesics and a cervical collar results in resolution of symptoms in the great

Table 14.34 Physical signs in cervical root compression

Root	Muscle weakness	Sensory loss	Reflex
C5	Biceps, deltoid, spinati	Upper lateral arm	Biceps
C6	Brachioradialis	Lower lateral arm, thumb, index finger	Supinator
C7	Triceps, finger and wrist extensors	Middle finger	Triceps

majority of patients, but a few require surgery in the form of foraminotomy or disc excision.

CERVICAL SPONDYLOTIC MYELOPATHY

Dorsomedial herniation of a disc and the development of transverse bony bars or posterior osteophytes may result in pressure on the spinal cord or the anterior spinal artery which supplies the anterior two-thirds of the cord (see Fig. 14.40, p. 1003).

Clinical features

The onset of symptoms is usually insidious and painless, but acute deterioration may occur after trauma, especially hyperextension injury. Upper motor neuron signs develop in the limbs, with spasticity of the legs usually appearing before the arms are involved. Sensory loss in the upper limbs is common, producing tingling numbness and proprioception loss in the hands, with progressive clumsiness. Sensory manifestations in the legs are much less common. The neurological deficit usually progresses gradually and disturbance of micturition is a very late feature.

Investigations

Plain radiographs confirm the presence of degenerative changes, and MRI or myelography may be indicated if surgical treatment is being considered. MRI may also show areas of high signal within the spinal cord at the level of compression. Imaging of the cervical spine should be considered if there is diagnostic doubt or if surgery is contemplated.

Management

Surgical procedures, including laminectomy and anterior discectomy, may arrest progression of disability but may not result in neurological improvement. The judgement as to whether surgery should be undertaken may be difficult. Manipulation of the cervical spine is of no proven benefit and may precipitate acute neurological deterioration.

Prognosis

The prognosis of cervical myelopathy is variable. In many patients the condition stabilises or even improves without intervention, but if progressive disability does develop, surgical decompression should be considered.

LUMBAR DISC HERNIATION

Low back pain ('lumbago') is the most common medical cause of inability to work in Western countries (see p. 815). In the great majority of patients it is due to abnormalities of joints and ligaments in the lumbar spine rather than herniation of an intervertebral disc. Pain in the distribution of the lumbar or sacral roots ('sciatica') is often due to disc protrusion, but can be a feature of other rare but important disorders including spinal tumour, malignant disease in the pelvis and tuberculosis of the vertebral bodies.

Acute lumbar disc herniation is often precipitated by trauma, usually by lifting heavy weights while the spine is flexed. The nucleus pulposus may bulge or rupture through the annulus fibrosus, giving rise to pressure on nerve endings in the spinal ligaments, changes in the vertebral joints or pressure on nerve roots.

Clinical features

The onset may be sudden or gradual. Alternatively, repeated episodes of low back pain may precede sciatica by months or years. Constant aching pain is felt in the lumbar region and may radiate to the buttock, thigh, calf and foot. Pain is exacerbated by coughing or straining and may be relieved by lying flat.

The altered mechanics of the lumbar spine result in loss of lumbar lordosis and there may be spasm of the paraspinal musculature. Root pressure is suggested by limitation of flexion of the hip on the affected side if the straight leg is raised (Lasègue's sign). If the third or fourth lumbar roots are involved Lasègue's sign may be negative, but pain in the back may be induced by hyperextension of the hip (femoral nerve stretch test). The roots most frequently affected are S1, L5 and L4; the signs of root pressure at these levels are summarised in Table 14.35.

Investigations

Plain radiographs of the lumbar spine may show no abnormality in acute disc herniation or there may be narrowing of the disc space. There may be degenerative changes, including osteophyte formation at the margins of the vertebral bodies in chronic low back pain. Plain radiographs can also exclude other conditions such as malignant infiltration of a vertebral body.

In lumbar disc disease CT, especially using spiral scanning techniques, can provide helpful images of the disc protrusion and/or narrowing of the exit foramina.

MRI is the investigation of choice if available, since soft tissues are well imaged, enabling the diagnosis of other causes of lumbar radicular syndromes.

Management

The initial treatment in all patients is bed rest on a

Table 14.35 Physical signs in lumbar root compression

Disc level	Root	Sensory loss	Weakness	Reflex loss
L3/L4	L4	Inner calf	Inversion of foot	Knee
L4/L5	L5	Outer calf and dorsum of foot	Dorsiflexion of hallux/toes	Hamstring
L5/S1	S1	Sole and lateral foot	Plantar flexion	Ankle

firm mattress, if necessary supported by wooden boards. Provided rest is absolute, pain and neurological signs, if present, resolve in over 95% of patients. On recovery the patient should be instructed in back-strengthening exercises and advised to avoid physical manoeuvres likely to strain the lumbar spine. Injections of local anaesthetic or steroids may be a useful adjunct to bed rest if symptoms are due to ligamentous injury or joint dysfunction.

Surgery may have to be considered if there is no response to conservative treatment or if progressive neurological deficits develop. Central disc prolapse with bilateral symptoms and signs and disturbance of sphincter function requires urgent surgical decompression.

LUMBAR CANAL STENOSIS

This is due to a congenital narrowing of the lumbar spinal canal, exacerbated by the degenerative changes which commonly occur with age.

Clinical features

The patients, who are usually elderly, characteristically develop exercise-induced weakness and paraesthesia in the legs (cauda equina claudication). These symptoms progress, exacerbated by continued exertion, often to the point that the patient can no longer walk, but are quickly relieved by a short period of rest. Physical examination at rest shows preservation of peripheral pulses with absent ankle reflexes. Weakness or sensory loss may only be apparent if the patient is examined immediately after exercise.

Investigations

Plain radiographs of the lumbar spine show narrowing of the lumbar canal, which may be confirmed by myelography, CT or MRI.

Management

Extensive lumbar laminectomy often results in complete relief of symptoms and recovery of normal exercise tolerance.

SYRINGOMYELIA

In this condition a fluid-filled cavity or cavities develops near the centre of the spinal cord (see Fig. 14.41). The expanding cavity disrupts second-order spinothalamic neurons (see Fig. 14.14, p. 957), may extend laterally to damage the anterior horn cells, and may compress the long fibre tracts.

Aetiology

Many patients have some obstruction to the flow of CSF at the foramen magnum. In some this is associated with congenital herniation of the cerebellar tonsils (Chiari type I malformation), and in others with basal arachnoiditis. It is assumed that the disturbed CSF dynamics cause the development of the syrinx but the mechanism is not clear. Rarely, a syrinx develops following spinal cord trauma. Similar cavities may appear in the medulla, producing brain-stem dysfunction (syringobulbia).

Clinical features

Patients usually present in the third or fourth decade, and symptoms are of insidious onset and slowly progressive. Pain in the neck or shoulder is common and patients may seek advice because of sensory loss in the upper limbs. The most characteristic physical sign is dissociated sensory loss (impaired pain and temperature sensation with preservation of dorsal column modalities), which has an upper and lower level in a mantle or hemicape distribution (see Fig. 14.13F, p. 956). Loss of protective sensory function leads to trophic lesions such as painless burns or ulcers on the hands, and sometimes painless, deranged joints (Charcot joints) in the upper limbs. Wasting of the small hand muscles is a common early feature and loss of one or more reflexes in the arm is usual. Upper motor neuron signs develop in the

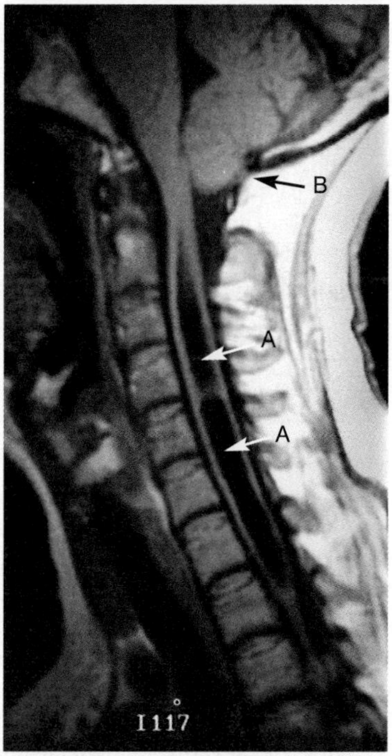

Fig 14.41 MRI scan showing syrinx (arrows A), with herniation of cerebellar tonsils (arrow B).

legs as the condition progresses. Kyphoscoliosis, pes cavus and spina bifida are common associations. Syringobulbia leads to dysarthria, palatal palsy, Horner's syndrome, nystagmus and sensory loss on the face.

Investigations

Plain radiographs may demonstrate congenital anomalies around the foramen magnum or expansion of the cervical canal. The most sensitive and least invasive investigation is MRI (see Fig. 14.41, p. 1005).

Management

Surgical decompression of the foramen magnum or the syrinx itself may arrest progression of the neurological deficit and often alleviates pain. The results of surgery are, however, often disappointing and in some patients the condition continues to progress slowly over long periods.

FURTHER INFORMATION ON DISORDERS OF THE SPINE AND SPINAL CORD

Critchley E, Eisen A (eds) 1997 Spinal cord disease: basic science, diagnosis and management. Springer-Verlag, London

INFECTIONS OF THE NERVOUS SYSTEM

The clinical features of nervous system infections depend upon the location of the infection (in the meninges or in the brain/spinal cord parenchyma), the causative organism (virus, bacteria or parasite) and whether the infection is acute or chronic. The major infections of the nervous system are listed in the information box. The frequency of these varies somewhat geographically.

MENINGITIS

Acute infection of the meninges presents with the characteristic combination of pyrexia, headache and meningism. Meningism consists of stiffness of the neck and irritability of the meninges with positive Kernig's and/or Brudzinski's signs, and can occur in other situations of meningeal irritation such as after subarachnoid haemorrhage. (With the hip joint flexed, extension at the knee causes spasm in the hamstring muscles—Kernig's sign; flexion of the neck causes flexion of the thighs and knees—Brudzinski's sign.) The severity of these features varies somewhat according to the causative organism, as does the presence of other features such as skin rashes. The abnormalities in the CSF (see Table 14.36) are very helpful in distinguishing the cause of meningitis. Causes of meningitis are listed in the information box below.

INFECTIONS OF THE NERVOUS SYSTEM*

Bacterial infections
- Meningitis
- Suppurative encephalitis
- Brain abscess
- Tuberculosis
- Paravertebral (epidural) abscess
- Neurosyphilis
- Leprosy (peripheral nerves)
- Diphtheria (peripheral nerves)
- Tetanus (motor cells)

Viral infections
- Meningitis
- Encephalitis
- Transverse myelitis
- Poliomyelitis
- Rabies
- Human immunodeficiency virus (HIV) infection

Slow virus/prion infections
- Creutzfeldt–Jakob disease
- Kuru
- Subacute sclerosing panencephalitis
- Progressive multifocal leucoencephalopathy

Protozoal infections
- Malaria
- Toxoplasmosis (in immunosuppressed)
- Trypanosomiasis
- Amoebic abscess

Helminthic infections
- Schistosomiasis (spinal cord)
- Cysticercosis
- Hydatid disease
- Strongyloidiasis

Fungal infections
- Cryptococcal meningitis (in immunosuppressed)
- *Candida* meningitis or brain abscess

* A number of these infections are not detailed in this chapter. They can be found in Chapter 2.

VIRAL MENINGITIS

Viral infection is the most common cause of meningitis, and usually results in a benign and self-limiting illness requiring no specific therapy. It is usually a much less serious illness than bacterial meningitis unless there is associated encephalitis, which is rare. A number of viruses can cause meningitis (see the information box), the most common being echoviruses and the mumps virus.

CAUSES OF MENINGITIS

Bacteria (see Table 14.37)

Viruses
- Enteroviruses (echo, Coxsackie, polio)
- Mumps
- Influenza
- Herpes simplex
- Varicella zoster
- Epstein–Barr
- HIV
- Lymphocytic choriomeningitis

Protozoa and other parasites
- *Toxoplasma*
- Amoeba
- Cysticercus

Fungi
- *Cryptococcus neoformans*
- Candidiasis
- *Histoplasma*
- *Blastomyces*
- *Coccidioides*
- *Brucella*
- *Sporothrix*

Table 14.36 Cerebrospinal fluid indices in meningitis

Condition	Cell type	Cell count	Glucose	Protein	Gram stain
Normal	Lymphocytes	< 5 per mm^3	> 60% of blood glucose	To 0.45 g/l	–
Viral	Lymphocytes	10–2000	Normal	Normal	–
Bacterial	Polymorphs	1000–5000	Low	Normal/elevated	+
Tuberculous	Polymorphs/lymphocytes/mixed	50–5000	Low	Elevated	Often –
Fungal	Lymphocytes	50–500	Low	Elevated	±
Malignant	Lymphocytes	0–100	Low	Normal/elevated	–

Clinical features

The condition occurs mainly in children or young adults, with acute onset of headache and irritability and the rapid development of meningeal irritation. In viral meningitis the headache is usually a more severe feature than the meningism. There may be a high pyrexia, but focal neurological signs do not occur since there is seldom parenchymal involvement of the brain.

Investigations

The CSF contains an excess of lymphocytes, but glucose and protein levels are normal.

Management

There is no specific treatment and the condition is usually benign and self-limiting. The patient should be treated symptomatically in a quiet environment. Recovery usually occurs within days, although a lymphocytic pleocytosis may persist in the CSF.

Meningitis may also occur as a complication of a viral infection primarily involving other organs: for example, in mumps, measles, infectious mononucleosis, herpes zoster and hepatitis. Complete recovery without specific therapy is the rule.

BACTERIAL MENINGITIS

Many bacteria can cause meningitis but some do so more frequently than others (see Table 14.37). Bacterial meningitis is usually secondary to a bacteraemic illness, although infection may result from direct spread from an adjacent focus of infection in the ear, skull fracture or sinus. Bacterial meningitis has become less common but the mortality and morbidity remain significant despite the availability of an increasing range of antibiotics. An important factor in determining prognosis is early diagnosis and the prompt initiation of appropriate therapy.

The meningococcus *(Neisseria meningitidis)* is the most common cause of bacterial meningitis in Britain. Spread is by air-borne route and epidemics occur, particularly in cramped living conditions or when the climate is hot and dry, e.g. areas of Africa. The organism invades through the nasopharynx, producing septicaemia which is usually

Table 14.37 Bacterial meningitis

Age of onset	Common	Less common
Neonate	Gram-negative bacilli (*E. coli, Proteus* etc.) Group B streptococci	*Listeria monocytogenes*
Pre-school child	*Haemophilus influenzae* *Neisseria meningitidis* *Streptococcus pneumoniae*	*Mycobacterium tuberculosis*
Older child and adult	*Neisseria meningitidis* *Streptococcus pneumoniae*	*Listeria monocytogenes* *Mycobacterium tuberculosis* *Cryptococcus neoformans* (in immunosuppressed) *Staphylococcus aureus* (skull fracture) *Haemophilus influenzae*

associated with pyogenic meningitis. Complications of meningococcal septicaemia are listed in the information box. Chronic meningococcaemia is a rare condition in which the patient can be unwell for weeks or even months with recurrent fever, sweating, joint pains and transient rash. It usually occurs in the middle-aged and elderly.

In pneumococcal and *Haemophilus* infections there may be an associated otitis media. Pneumococcal meningitis may be associated with pneumonia and occurs especially in older patients and alcoholics, as well as in patients without functioning spleens. *Listeria monocytogenes* has recently emerged as an increasing cause of meningitis and rhombencephalitis (brain-stem encephalitis) in the immunosuppressed, diabetics, alcoholics and pregnant women. It can also cause meningitis in the neonatal period.

COMPLICATIONS OF MENINGOCOCCAL SEPTICAEMIA

- Meningitis
- Rash (morbilliform, petechial or purpuric—see p. 63)
- Shock
- Intravascular coagulation
- Renal failure
- Peripheral gangrene
- Arthritis (septic or reactive)
- Pericarditis (septic or reactive)

Pathology

The pia-arachnoid is congested and infiltrated with inflammatory cells. A thin layer of pus forms and this may later organise to form adhesions. These may cause obstruction to the free flow of CSF leading to hydrocephalus, or they may damage the cranial nerves at the base of the brain. The CSF pressure rises rapidly, the protein content increases, and there is a cellular reaction which varies in type and severity according to the nature of the inflammation and the causative organism. An obliterative endarteritis of the leptomeningeal arteries passing through the meningeal exudate may produce secondary cerebral infarction. Pneumococcal meningitis is often associated with a very purulent CSF and a high mortality, especially in older adults.

Clinical features

Headache, drowsiness, fever and neck stiffness are the usual presenting features. In severe bacterial meningitis the patient may be comatose and later there may be focal neurological signs. Meningococcal meningitis may present very rapidly, with abrupt onset of obtundation due to cerebral oedema, probably as a result of endotoxin and/or cytokine release. There may be a petechial skin rash and circulatory collapse.

Investigations

If the patient is drowsy with focal neurological signs it may be wise to obtain a CT to exclude a mass lesion (such as a cerebral abscess) before lumbar puncture, but this should not delay treatment of a presumptive meningitis.

In bacterial meningitis the CSF is cloudy (turbid) due to the presence of many neutrophils (often > 1000 cells/mm^3), the protein content is significantly elevated and the glucose reduced. Gram film, culture or polymerase chain reaction (PCR) may allow identification of the organism. Blood cultures may be positive.

Management

Intravenous penicillin should be given immediately bacterial meningitis is suspected. The antibiotic regimen may be modified after CSF examination, depending on the infecting organism. Guidance as to the preferred antibiotic is given in Table 14.38 if the organism is known and in the information box if the organism has not been identified.

The dose of the various antibiotics which must be given intravenously depends on the age and weight of the patient.

Prevention of meningococcal infection

Household and other close contacts of patients with meningococcal infections, especially children, should be given 2 days of oral rifampicin (age 3–12 months 5 mg/kg 12-hourly, > 1 yr 10 mg/kg 12-hourly, adults 600 mg 12-hourly). In adults a single dose of 500 mg of ciprofloxacin is an alternative. Vaccines are available for the prevention of disease caused by meningococci of groups A and C, but not group B which is the most common serogroup isolated in many countries including Britain.

Table 14.38 Chemotherapy of bacterial meningitis

	Drug of choice	Alternative agents
Meningococcal	Benzylpenicillin	Chloramphenicol Cefotaxime
Pneumococcal	Cefotaxime*	Chloramphenicol
H. influenzae	Cefotaxime	Chloramphenicol
Neonatal		
Gram-negative bacilli	Cefotaxime	Gentamicin + ampicillin
Group B streptococci	Gentamicin + ampicillin	Chloramphenicol
L. monocytogenes	Gentamicin + ampicillin	Co-trimoxazole Rifampicin
C. neoformans	Amphotericin + flucytosine	Fluconazole
M. tuberculosis	See page 352	

* Penicillin-resistant pneumococci now common world-wide.

TREATMENT OF PYOGENIC MENINGITIS OF UNKNOWN CAUSE

Neonate
- Ampicillin with cefotaxime or gentamicin

Infant
- Ampicillin with cefotaxime

Pre-school child
- Cefotaxime

Older child and young adult
- Penicillin G and cefotaxime

Older patient (> 50 years)
- Ampicillin with cefotaxime

TUBERCULOUS MENINGITIS

Pathology

This occurs most commonly shortly after a primary infection in childhood or as part of miliary tuberculosis. The usual local source of infection is a caseous focus in the meninges or brain substance adjacent to the CSF pathway.

The brain is covered by a greenish, gelatinous exudate, especially around the base, and numerous scattered tubercles are found on the meninges.

Clinical features

The clinical features are listed in the information box.

CLINICAL FEATURES OF TUBERCULOUS MENINGITIS	
Symptoms	**Signs**
• Headache • Vomiting • Low-grade fever • Lassitude • Depression • Confusion • Behaviour changes	• Meningism (may be absent) • Oculomotor palsies • Papilloedema • Depression of conscious level • Focal hemisphere signs

Investigations

The CSF is under increased pressure. It is usually clear but, when allowed to stand, a fine clot ('spider web') may form. The fluid contains up to 500 cells/mm^3, predominantly lymphocytes. There is a rise in protein and a marked fall in glucose. Detection of the tubercle bacillus in a smear of the centrifuged deposit from the CSF may be difficult. The CSF should be cultured but as this result will not be known for up to 6 weeks, treatment must be started without waiting for confirmation. Brain imaging may show hydrocephalus, brisk meningeal enhancement on enhanced CT, and/or an intracranial tuberculoma.

Management

As soon as the diagnosis is made or strongly suspected, chemotherapy should be started using one of the regimens including pyrazinamide described on page 353. The use of steroids in addition to antituberculous therapy is controversial but may be indicated to treat raised intracranial pressure. Surgical ventricular drainage may be needed if obstructive hydrocephalus develops. Skilled nursing is essential during the acute phase of the illness and measures must be taken to maintain adequate hydration and nutrition.

Prognosis

Untreated tuberculous meningitis is fatal in a few weeks but complete recovery is the rule if treatment is started before the appearance of focal signs or stupor. When treatment is started at a later stage the recovery rate is 60% or less and the survivors may be mentally deficient, epileptic, deaf or blind, or show some other permanent neurological deficit.

OTHER FORMS OF MENINGITIS

Fungal meningitis (cryptococcosis) (see p. 147)

This usually occurs in patients who are immunosuppressed and is a recognised complication of HIV infection (see p. 98). The CSF findings are similar to those of tuberculous meningitis, but the diagnosis can be confirmed by microscopy or specific serological tests.

In some areas meningitis may be caused by spirochaetes (leptospirosis—see p. 137, Lyme disease—see p. 138, and syphilis—see p. 184), rickettsiae (typhus fever, p. 115) or protozoa (amoebiasis, p. 153).

PARENCHYMAL VIRAL INFECTIONS

Infection of the substance of the nervous system will produce symptoms of focal dysfunction (focal deficits and/or seizures) with general signs of infection depending upon the acuteness of the infection and the type of organism.

VIRAL ENCEPHALITIS

A range of viruses can cause encephalitis but only a minority of patients have a history of recent viral infection. In Europe, the most common cause of viral encephalitis is herpes simplex, which probably reaches the brain via the olfactory nerves. The development of effective therapy for some forms of encephalitis has enhanced the importance of clinical diagnosis and virological examination of the CSF. In some parts of the world viruses which are transmitted by mosquitoes and ticks (arboviruses) are an important cause of encephalitis. Acute encephalitic illness may occur in HIV infection, occasionally at the time of infection, but more commonly as a manifestation of AIDS.

Pathology

Inflammation can occur in the cortex, white matter, basal ganglia and brain stem, and the distribution of lesions varies with the type of virus. In herpes simplex encephalitis the temporal lobes are usually primarily affected. Inclusion bodies may be present in the neurons and glial cells and there is an infiltration of polymorphonuclear cells in the perivascular space. There is neuronal degeneration and diffuse glial proliferation, often associated with cerebral oedema.

Clinical features

Viral encephalitis presents with acute onset of headache, with fever, focal neurological signs (aphasia and/or hemiplegia) and seizures. Disturbance of consciousness ranging from drowsiness to deep coma supervenes early and may advance dramatically. Meningism occurs in many patients. Rabies presents a distinct clinical picture and is described on page 1010.

Investigations

CSF examination should be preceded by CT, which will exclude a mass lesion, and which, in herpes simplex encephalitis, may show low-density lesions in the temporal lobes. The cerebrospinal fluid usually contains excess lymphocytes, but polymorphonuclear cells may predominate in the early stages. Occasionally, the CSF is normal. The protein content may be elevated, but the glucose is normal. The EEG is usually abnormal in the early stages, especially in herpes simplex encephalitis, with characteristic periodic slow-wave activity in the temporal lobes. Virological investigations of the CSF may eventually reveal the causative organism but the initiation of treatment should not await this.

Management

Anticonvulsant treatment is often necessary (see p. 945) and raised intracranial pressure is treated with dexamethasone 8 mg 12-hourly. Herpes simplex encephalitis responds to aciclovir 10 mg/kg intravenously 8-hourly. This should be given early to all patients suspected of suffering from viral encephalitis.

Even with optimum treatment, mortality is 10–30% and a significant proportion of survivors have residual epilepsy or cognitive impairment.

BRAIN-STEM ENCEPHALITIS

This presents with ataxia, dysarthria, diplopia or other cranial nerve palsies. The CSF is lymphocytic, with a normal glucose. The causative agent is presumed to be viral. However, *Listeria monocytogenes* may cause a similar syndrome with meningitis (and often a polymorphonuclear CSF pleocytosis) and requires specific treatment with ampicillin 500 mg 6-hourly.

RABIES

Rabies is caused by a rhabdovirus which infects the central nervous tissue and salivary glands of a wide range of mammals, and is usually conveyed by saliva through bites or licks on abrasions or on intact mucous membranes. Humans are most frequently infected from dogs. In Europe the maintenance host is the fox and in recent years the zoonosis has spread from Poland westwards through Germany and France (see Table 14.39).

Table 14.39 Sources of infection in rabies

Area	Source	Transmission
World-wide	Dogs, other canines, cats Cattle etc. (to farmers) Other mammals Humans (undiagnosed)	Bite, lick Hand into mouth Bite, lick Corneal graft
North America	Skunks and raccoons	Bite, lick
Central and South America	Vampire bats Cave-dwelling bats	Bite Salivary aerosols

The incubation period, during which the virus is spreading centripetally along axons to the brain, varies in humans from a minimum of 9 days to many months but is usually between 4 and 8 weeks. Severe bites, especially if on the head or neck, are associated with short incubation periods.

Clinical features

Only a proportion of people bitten by a rabid animal develop the disease, but once manifest it is almost invariably fatal. At the onset there may be fever, and paraesthesia at the site of the bite. A prodromal period of from 1 to 10 days, during which the patient is increasingly anxious, leads to the characteristic fear of water, 'hydrophobia'. Although the patient is thirsty, attempts at drinking provoke violent contractions of the diaphragm and other inspiratory muscles and, thereafter, even the sight or sound of water may precipitate distressing spasms and attacks of panic. Delusions and hallucination may develop, accompanied by spitting, biting and mania, with lucid intervals in which the patient is acutely anxious. Cranial nerve lesions develop and terminal hyperpyrexia is common. Death ensues, within a week of the onset of symptoms.

In a small proportion of cases there is an ascending paralysis without mental excitement and these patients survive on average 12 days.

Investigations

During life the diagnosis is usually made on clinical grounds but rapid immunofluorescent techniques can detect antigen in corneal impression smears or skin biopsies.

Management

A few patients with rabies have survived. All received some post-exposure prophylaxis, and needed intensive care with facilities to control cardiac and respiratory failure. Otherwise, only palliative treatment is possible once symptoms have appeared. The patient should be heavily sedated with diazepam 10 mg 4–6-hourly, supplemented by chlorpromazine 50–100 mg if necessary. Nutrition and fluids should be given intravenously or through a gastrostomy.

Prevention

Pre-exposure prophylaxis is required by those who by profession handle potentially infected animals, those who work with rabies virus in laboratories and those who live at special risk in rabies-endemic areas. Protection is afforded by two intradermal injections of 0.1 ml human diploid cell strain vaccine, or two intramuscular injections of 1 ml, given 4 weeks apart, followed by yearly boosters.

Post-exposure prophylaxis

The wounds should be thoroughly cleaned, preferably with a quaternary ammonium detergent or soap; damaged tissues should be excised and the wound left unsutured. Rabies can usually be prevented if treatment is started within a day or two of biting. Delayed treatment may still be of value. For maximum protection hyperimmune serum and vaccine are required.

The safest antirabies antiserum is human rabies immune globulin; the dose is 20 i.u./kg body weight. Half is infiltrated around the bite and half is given intramuscularly at a different site from the vaccine. The dose of hyperimmune animal serum is 40 i.u./kg; hypersensitivity reactions, including anaphylaxis, are common.

The safest vaccine, free of complications, is human diploid cell strain vaccine; 1.0 ml is given intramuscularly on days 0, 3, 7, 14, 30 and 90. In developing countries, where human rabies globulin may not be obtainable, 0.1 ml of vaccine should be given intradermally into eight sites on day 1, with single boosters on days 7 and 28. Where human products are not available and when risk of rabies is slight (licks on the skin, or minor bites of covered arms or legs) it may be justifiable to delay starting treatment for up to 5 days while observing the biting animal or awaiting examination of its brain rather than use the older vaccine.

The biting animal should be confined, if possible. If it is healthy after 5 days, it does not have rabies and treatment is stopped. If it dies or is killed, the brain is examined by immunofluorescence for Negri bodies. If positive, treatment is continued.

Control of spread

Human rabies is an infrequent disease even in endemic areas. Its fearful manifestations, however, justify stringent attempts being made to limit its spread and prevent its importation into uninfected countries such as Britain. Measures to control rabies are listed in the information box.

CONTROL OF RABIES

- License and vaccinate domestic dogs
- Kill stray dogs
- Monitor reservoir hosts
- Control and quarantine imported animals
- Vaccinate at-risk animals and humans

POLIOMYELITIS

Aetiology and pathology

The disease is caused by one of three polioviruses, which are a subdivision of the enteroviruses group. It is much less common in developed countries following the widespread use of oral vaccines but is still a major problem in the developing world. Infection usually occurs through the nasopharynx.

The virus causes a lymphocytic meningitis and infects the grey matter of the spinal cord, brain stem and cortex. There is a particular propensity to damage anterior horn cells, especially in the lumbar segments.

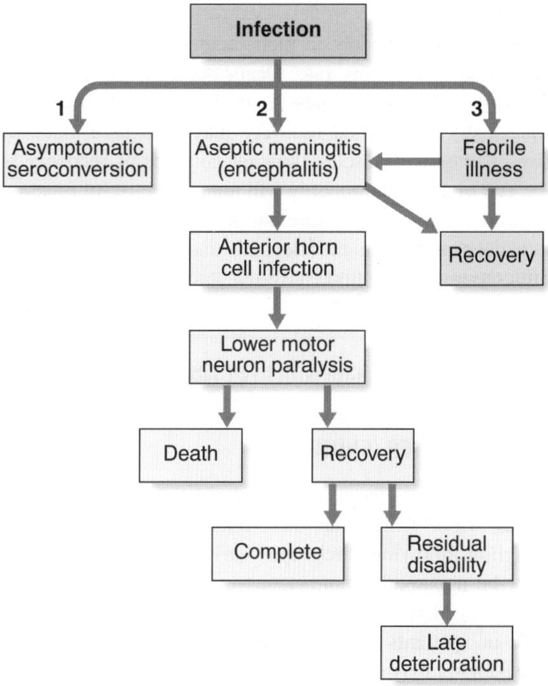

Fig. 14.42 Poliomyelitis. Possible consequences of infection.

Clinical features

The incubation period is 7–14 days. Figure 14.42 illustrates the various features of the infection. Many patients recover fully after the initial phase of a few days of mild fever and headache. In others, after a week of well-being, there is recurrence of pyrexia, headache and meningism. Weakness may start later in one muscle group and can progress to widespread paresis. Respiratory failure may supervene if intercostal muscles are paralysed or the medullary motor nuclei are involved.

Investigations

The CSF shows a lymphocytic pleocytosis, a rise in protein and a normal sugar content. Poliomyelitis virus may be cultured from CSF and stool.

Management

In the early stages bed rest is imperative because exercise appears to worsen the paralysis or precipitate it. At the onset of respiratory difficulties a tracheostomy and ventilation are required. Subsequent treatment is by physiotherapy and orthopaedic measures.

Prognosis

Epidemics vary widely in their incidence of non-paralytic cases and in mortality rate. Death occurs from respiratory paralysis. Muscle weakness is maximal at the end of the first week and gradual recovery may then take place for several months. Muscles showing no signs of recovery by the end of a month probably will not regain useful function. Second attacks are very rare but occasionally patients show late deterioration in muscle bulk and power many years after the initial infection.

Prevention

This is by immunisation with live (Sabin) vaccine.

HERPES ZOSTER (SHINGLES)

Herpes zoster is the result of reactivation of the varicella zoster virus which has lain dormant in a nerve root ganglion following chickenpox earlier in life. Reactivation may be apparently spontaneous (as usually occurs in the middle-aged or elderly) or be due to immunosuppression (as in patients with malignant disease or AIDS). Chickenpox may be contracted from a patient with shingles but not the reverse.

Clinical features

The first symptom is usually severe and continuous pain in the distribution of the affected nerve root. After 3 or 4 days the skin in the affected area becomes reddened and vesicles appear, which dry up over 5 or 6 days leaving small scars. The pain of zoster usually subsides as the eruption fades, but may be followed by neuralgia (see p. 938).

Any dorsal root ganglion may be infected, most commonly those supplying the trunk where two or three adjacent dermatomes on one side are often involved. Segmental muscle wasting may occur from involvement of the motor root. Infection of the trigeminal ganglion usually involves the ophthalmic division when vesicles may appear on the cornea and may lead to corneal ulceration. Infection of the geniculate ganglion presents with vesicles in the auricle and less often on the palate with ipsilateral facial paralysis and impairment of taste (Ramsay Hunt syndrome), which can be mistaken for a Bell's palsy (see p. 996). The virus occasionally causes myelitis or encephalitis.

Management

Oral aciclovir 800 mg 4–5-hourly is useful if started early. In immunocompromised patients, or when infection is severe, systemic aciclovir in a dose of 5 mg/kg 8-hourly is indicated. Idoxuridine may be applied to the skin in a 5% solution in the early stages of the evolution of the rash and 0.1% drops are used for corneal infections. The treatment of post-herpetic neuralgia is difficult. Analgesics are often unhelpful, but amitriptyline 25–100 mg daily and trans-cutaneous nerve stimulation are sometimes effective.

SUBACUTE SCLEROSING PANENCEPHALITIS

This is a rare, chronic, progressive and eventually fatal neurological disease caused by the measles virus, presumably as a result of an inability of the nervous system to eradicate the virus. It occurs in children and adolescents, usually many years after the primary virus infection. The onset is insidious, with intellectual deterioration, apathy and clumsiness followed by myoclonic jerks, rigidity and dementia.

The CSF may show a mild lymphocytic pleocytosis and the EEG is distinctive, with periodic bursts of triphasic waves. Although there is persistent measles-specific IgG in serum and CSF, antiviral therapy is ineffective and death ensues within years.

PROGRESSIVE MULTIFOCAL LEUCOENCEPHALOPATHY

This was originally described as a rare complication of lymphoma, leukaemia or carcinomatosis. It occurs now more frequently as a feature of AIDS. It is an infection of the brain oligodendrocytes by human polyomavirus JC, which causes widespread demyelination of the white matter of the cerebral hemispheres. Clinical signs include dementia, hemiparesis and aphasia which progress rapidly, usually leading to death within weeks or months. Areas of low density in the white matter are seen on CT but MRI is more sensitive, showing diffuse high signal on T2-weighted images.

PARENCHYMAL BACTERIAL INFECTIONS

CEREBRAL ABSCESS

Bacteria may enter the cerebral substance through penetrating injury, direct spread from sinuses or the middle ear, or through haematogenous spread from septicaemia associated with, for example, subacute bacterial endocarditis or pulmonary abscess. The site of abscess formation and likely causative organism are related to the source of infection (see Table 14.40).

Initial infection leads to local suppuration followed by loculation of pus within a surrounding wall of gliosis, which in a chronic abscess may form a tough capsule. Multiple abscesses occur, particularly with haematogenous spread.

Clinical features

Cerebral abscess may present acutely with fever, headache, meningism and drowsiness, but more commonly presents over days or weeks as a cerebral mass lesion with little or

Table 14.40 Site, source and organism in cerebral abscess

Site of abscess	Source of infection	Likely organism
Frontal	Frontal sinusitis	Streptococcus
Temporal	Otitis media	Streptococcus *Bacteroides* *Proteus*
Cerebellar	Otitis media	Streptococcus *Bacteroides* *Proteus*
Parietal	Embolic	Streptococcus *Bacteroides* *Proteus*
Any site	Trauma	Staphylococcus

no evidence of infection. Seizures, raised intracranial pressure and focal hemisphere signs occur alone or in combination, and distinction from a cerebral tumour may be impossible on clinical grounds.

Investigations

Lumbar puncture is potentially hazardous in the presence of raised intracranial pressure and CT should always precede lumbar puncture. CT shows single or multiple low-density areas, which enhance peripherally with contrast to provide a ring appearance with central low density and surrounding cerebral oedema (see Fig. 14.43). There may be an elevated blood white cell count and ESR in patients with active local infection.

Management

Antimicrobial therapy is indicated once the diagnosis is made and the likely source of infection should guide the choice of antibiotic (see Table 14.40). Surgical treatment by burr-hole aspiration or excision may be necessary, especially where the presence of a capsule may lead to a persistent focus of infection. Anticonvulsants are often necessary, as epilepsy frequently develops acutely or in the recovery phase.

Prognosis

The mortality rate remains at 10–20% despite an improvement in available surgical and medical treatments, and in some patients this is related to delay in diagnosis and initiation of treatment.

SUBDURAL EMPYEMA

This is a rare complication of frontal sinusitis, osteomyelitis of the skull vault, or middle ear disease. A collection of pus in the subdural space spreads over the surface of the hemisphere, causing underlying cortical oedema or thrombophlebitis. Patients present with severe pain in the face or head, pyrexia and often a history of preceding paranasal sinus or ear infection. The patient then becomes

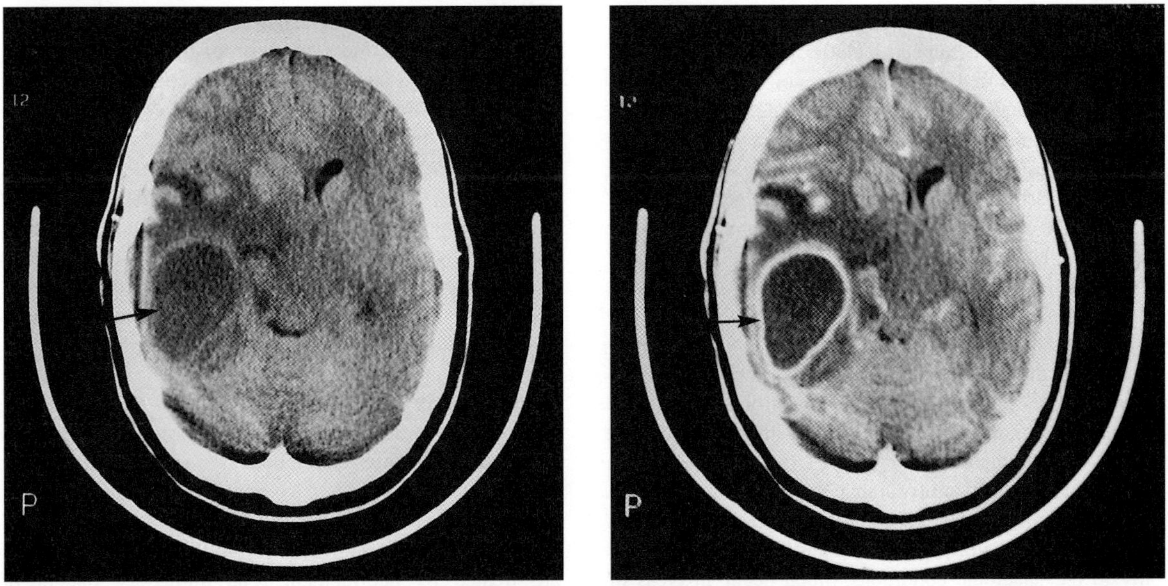

A B

Fig. 14.43 Right temporal cerebral abscess (arrows), with surrounding oedema and midline shift to the left. A Unenhanced CT image. B Contrast-enhanced CT image.

drowsy with seizures and focal signs such as a progressive hemiparesis.

The diagnosis rests on a strong clinical suspicion in patients with a local focus of infection and careful assessment of a head CT. This may show a subdural collection with underlying cerebral oedema but may be normal to cursory examination unless contrast is given and the films examined very carefully for evidence of intracranial shift.

Management requires aspiration of pus via a burr-hole and appropriate parenteral antibiotics. Any local source of infection must be treated to prevent reinfection.

SPINAL EPIDURAL ABSCESS

The characteristic clinical features are pain in a root distribution and progressive transverse spinal cord syndrome with paraparesis, sensory impairment and sphincter dysfunction. Infection is usually haematogenous, but a primary source of infection is easily overlooked.

Plain radiographs of the spine may show osteomyelitis, but such changes are often late. MRI or myelography should precede urgent neurosurgical intervention. Decompressive laminectomy with draining of the abscess relieves the pressure on the dura. This, together with appropriate antibiotics, may prevent complete and irreversible paraplegia. Organisms may be cultured from the pus or blood.

TETANUS

This disease results from infection with *Clostridium tetani*, which exists as a commensal in the gut of humans and domestic animals and is found in the soil. Infection enters the body through wounds, often trivial, such as those caused by a splinter, a nail in the boot or a garden fork or following septic infection such as a dirty abrasion. Tetanus is rare in Britain and occurs mostly in gardeners and farmers. By contrast, the disease is common in many developing countries where dust contains spores derived from animal and human excreta. If childbirth takes place in an unhygienic environment *Tetanus neonatorum* may result from infection of the umbilical stump, or the mother may develop the disease. Tetanus is still one of the major killers of adults, children and neonates in the tropics where the mortality rate can be nearly 100% in the newborn and around 40% in others.

In circumstances unfavourable to the growth of the organism, spores are formed and these may remain dormant for years in the soil. Spores germinate and bacilli multiply only in the anaerobic conditions which occur in areas of tissue necrosis or if the oxygen tension is low as a result of the presence of other organisms, particularly aerobic ones. The bacilli remain localised but produce an exotoxin with an affinity for motor nerve endings and motor nerve cells. The anterior horn cells are affected after the exotoxin has passed into the blood stream and their involvement results in rigidity and convulsions. Symptoms first appear from 2 days to several weeks after injury—the shorter the incubation period, the more severe the attacks and the outcome may well be fatal with an incubation period of only a few days.

Clinical features

Much the most important early symptom is trismus—spasm of the masseter muscles which causes difficulty in opening the mouth and in masticating, hence the name 'lockjaw'. This tonic rigidity spreads to involve the muscles of the face, neck and trunk. Contraction of the frontalis and the muscles at the angles of the mouth gives rise to the 'risus sardonicus'. There is rigidity of the muscles at the neck and trunk of varying degree. The back is usually slightly arched and there is a board-like abdominal wall.

In the more severe cases violent spasms lasting for a few seconds to 3–4 minutes occur spontaneously, or may be induced by stimuli such as moving the patient or making a noise. These convulsions are painful, exhausting and of very serious significance, especially if they appear soon after the onset of symptoms. They gradually increase in frequency and severity for about 1 week and the patient may die from exhaustion, asphyxia or aspiration pneumonia. In less severe illness convulsions may not commence for about a week after the first sign of rigidity and in very mild infections they may never appear. Autonomic involvement may cause cardiovascular complications such as hypertension.

Rarely, the only manifestation of the disease may be 'local tetanus'—stiffness or spasm of the muscles near the infected wound—and the prognosis is good if treatment is commenced at this stage.

Investigations

The diagnosis is made on clinical grounds. It is rarely possible to isolate the infecting organism from the original locus of entry. Spasm of the masseters due to dental abscess, septic throat or other causes is painful, in contradistinction to tetanus. Conditions which can mimic tetanus include hysteria and phenothiazine overdosage.

Management

This should be begun as soon as possible. The essentials are shown in the information box.

Prevention

Active immunisation must be given. Contaminated injuries are treated by débridement. The immediate danger of tetanus can be greatly reduced by the injection of 1200 mg of penicillin followed by a 7-day course of oral penicillin. For those who are allergic to penicillin, erythromycin should be used. When the risk of tetanus is judged to be

TREATMENT OF TETANUS
Neutralise absorbed toxin
• I.v. injection of 3000 i.u. of antitoxin
Prevent further toxin production
• Débridement of wound • Benzylpenicillin 600 mg 6-hourly i.v. (metronidazole if allergic to penicillin)
Control spasms
• Nurse in a quiet room • Avoid unnecessary stimuli • I.v. diazepam—if spasms continue paralyse patient and ventilate
General measures
• Maintain hydration and nutrition • Treat secondary infections

present, an injection of 250 units of human tetanus antitoxin should be given and an intramuscular injection of toxoid which should be repeated 1 month and 6 months later. For those already protected only a booster dose of toxoid is required.

LYME DISEASE

See page 138.

NEUROSYPHILIS

Neurosyphilis may present as an acute or chronic process and may involve singly or in combination the meninges, blood vessels and parenchyma of the brain and spinal cord. The clinical manifestations are diverse and, although the condition is now rare, early diagnosis and treatment remain important.

Clinical features

The clinical and pathological features of the three most common presentations are summarised in Table 14.41.

Neurological examination reveals signs appropriate to the anatomical localisation of lesions. Pupillary abnormalities, described by Argyll Robertson, may accompany any neurosyphilitic syndrome. The pupils are small and irregular, and react to convergence but not directly to light. Delusions of grandeur suggest general paresis of the insane, but more commonly there is simply progressive dementia. The combination of physical signs in tabes dorsalis is characteristic. Argyll Robertson pupils are found in 90% of patients and there is depression of tendon reflexes, hypotonia, distal impairment of deep pain sensation in the legs resulting in perforating painless ulcers and Charcot joints, and impairment of pin-prick sensation over the nose, perineum and distal lower limbs.

The clinical syndromes outlined above may occur in combination giving rise to mixed pictures, which may mimic many other neurological disorders.

Investigations

Routine screening for syphilis is warranted in the great majority of neurological patients. Serological tests (see p. 186) are positive in the serum in most patients, but CSF examination is essential if neurological involvement is suspected. Active disease is suggested by an elevated cell count, usually lymphocytic, and the protein content may be elevated to 0.5–1.0 g/l with an increased gamma-globulin fraction. Serological tests in the CSF are usually positive, but progressive disease can occur with negative CSF serology.

Management

The essential part of the treatment of neurosyphilis of all types is the injection of procaine penicillin 600 mg–1.2 g daily for 3 weeks (see p. 185). Further courses of penicillin must be given if symptoms are not relieved, or the condition continues to advance, or the CSF continues to show signs of active disease. The cell count returns to normal within 3 months of completion of treatment, but the elevated protein takes longer to subside, and some serological tests may never revert to normal. Evidence of clinical progression at any time is an indication for renewed treatment.

PRION DISEASES: TRANSMISSIBLE SPONGIFORM ENCEPHALOPATHIES

A number of neurological diseases develop many months or even years after infection with a transmissible agent which

Table 14.41 Clinical and pathological features of neurosyphilis

Type	Pathology	Clinical features
Meningovascular (5 years)*	Endarteritis obliterans Meningeal exudate Granuloma (gumma)	Stroke Cranial nerve palsies Seizures/mass lesion
General paralysis of the insane (5–15 years)*	Degeneration in cerebral cortex/cerebral atrophy Thickened meninges	Dementia Tremor Bilateral upper motor signs
Tabes dorsalis (5–20 years)*	Degeneration of sensory neurons Wasting of dorsal columns Optic atrophy	Lightning pains Sensory ataxia Visual failure Abdominal crises Incontinence Trophic changes

* Interval from primary infection

has properties distinct from conventional viruses or bacteria. There is a characteristic pathology with neuronal loss, spongiform change and gliosis, with deposition of characteristic prion protein. This is a glycoprotein which accumulates in amyloid-like plaques. Similar spongiform encephalopathy can occur in inherited conditions (e.g. the Gerstmann–Sträussler–Scheinker syndrome). An infective spongiform encephalopathy has long been described in sheep (scrapie), and more recently in cows (bovine spongiform encephalopathy or BSE), mink and other animals. The nature of the infection in these conditions is not clear. The prion protein is host-derived and it may be that the infective agent induces a spreading conformational change in native prion protein, causing a toxic deposition of an insoluble isomer of the protein.

KURU

This occurred only in members of a cannibalistic New Guinea tribe and was probably transmitted by eating the brains of dead tribal members. There is a progressive ataxia and dementia with spongiform degeneration of grey matter, most marked in the cerebellum.

CREUTZFELDT–JAKOB DISEASE (CJD)

This usually occurs sporadically in middle-aged to elderly patients, with an annual incidence in the UK of one in a million. There is a rapidly progressive dementia, with myoclonus and a characteristic EEG pattern. Death occurs after 8 or 9 months. CJD is transmissible experimentally to chimpanzees and rarely from person to person—for example, by the administration of cadaver-derived human growth hormone. In the latter case the disorder presents more like kuru, with a progressive ataxia leading eventually to dementia but with less dramatic EEG changes.

New-variant CJD

A new variant of CJD has been described in a few younger patients in the UK, presenting initially with psychiatric and cognitive changes with ataxia, progressing to dementia. The brain pathology is distinct, with very florid plaques containing prion proteins. This disease has been speculatively linked with ingestion of beef from cows suffering from BSE.

FURTHER INFORMATION ON INFECTIONS OF THE NERVOUS SYSTEM

Prusiner S B, Hsiao K K 1994 Human prion diseases. Annals of Neurology 35: 385–395

Tyler K L, Martin J B 1993 Infectious diseases of the central nervous system. F A Davis, Philadelphia

INTRACRANIAL MASS LESIONS AND RAISED INTRACRANIAL PRESSURE

Mass lesions in the head may be neoplastic, infective, inflammatory or of other types (see the information box). Tuberculoma is a common intracranial mass lesion in developing countries, whilst in developed countries cerebral neoplasms are most frequent. The clinical features relate to the site of the mass, its nature and its rate of expansion. Symptoms and signs are produced by a number of mechanisms listed in the second information box.

INTRACRANIAL MASS LESIONS

- Cerebral neoplasm (benign and malignant)
- Cerebral abscess
- Embryonic dysplastic lesions (e.g. craniopharyngiomas and hamartomas)
- Arachnoid cyst
- Colloid cyst (in the ventricles)
- Tuberculoma
- Sarcoid mass
- Cysticercosis
- Echinococcosis (as hydatid cysts)
- Schistosomiasis

CLINICAL FEATURES OF INTRACRANIAL MASS LESIONS

- Local effects on adjacent brain tissue (e.g. Seizures, focal signs)
- Raised intracranial pressure
- False localising signs

RAISED INTRACRANIAL PRESSURE

Raised intracranial pressure may be caused by mass lesions (especially tumours), cerebral oedema, obstruction to CSF circulation (causing hydrocephalus), or impaired CSF absorption (as in idiopathic intracranial hypertension—see p. 1022—and cerebral venous obstruction).

Clinical features

The major features of raised intracranial pressure are shown in the information box. Impairment of conscious level is related to the level of intracranial pressure. Cerebral mass lesions occupy space within the rigid skull but compensatory mechanisms involving alteration in the volume of fluid in CSF spaces and venous sinuses may delay the development of raised pressure. Slow-growing mass lesions may thereby attain a large size before causing a rise in intracranial pressure. Raised pressure develops early in rapidly expanding masses (e.g. highly malignant tumours or abscesses), especially if the cerebrospinal circulation is obstructed. Papilloedema may not develop in raised intracranial pressure of very recent onset, particularly if this is from

CLINICAL FEATURES OF RAISED INTRACRANIAL PRESSURE

- Headache (see p. 936)
- Impairment of conscious level
- Papilloedema
- Vomiting, bradycardia, arterial hypertension

acute obstruction of CSF pathways. Vomiting, bradycardia and arterial hypertension develop as late features of raised intracranial pressure and usually parallel the other clinical signs. However, sudden vomiting may be an early feature of tumours of the cerebellum, especially in children.

Management

The management of raised intracranial pressure is largely dictated by its specific cause, as described later.

'CONING' AND FALSE LOCALISING SIGNS

The rise in intracranial pressure from a mass lesion is not usually uniform within the cerebral substance and alterations in pressure relationships within the skull may lead to displacement of parts of the brain between its various compartments. Downward displacement of the temporal lobes through the tentorium due to a large hemisphere mass may cause 'temporal coning' (see Fig. 14.44). This may stretch the 3rd and/or 6th cranial nerves, or cause pressure on the contralateral cerebral peduncle (resulting in ipsilateral upper motor neuron signs). Downward movement of the cerebellar tonsils through the foramen magnum may compress the medulla—'tonsillar coning' (see Fig. 14.45). This coning may result in brain-stem haemorrhage and/or acute obstruction of the CSF pathways. As coning progresses, the patient may adopt a decerebrate posture and death almost invariably ensues. These uneven pressure disturbances cause impairment of consciousness and may be accelerated if the pressure dynamics are suddenly disturbed by lumbar puncture.

INTRACRANIAL NEOPLASMS

Cerebral tumours account for 2% of deaths at all ages. The majority are metastatic tumours from malignancies outside the nervous system. Benign or malignant neoplasms of the central nervous system tissue account for the remainder of

FALSE LOCALISING SIGNS OF A MASS LESION

- Pupillary dilatation (ipsilateral to lesion)
- 6th cranial nerve lesion (unilateral or bilateral)
- Hemiparesis (ipsilateral to lesion)
- Bilateral extensor plantar responses

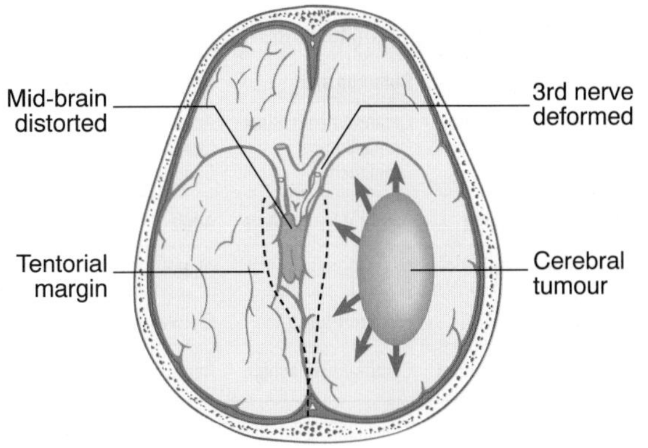

Fig. 14.44 Cerebral tumour displacing medial temporal lobe and causing pressure on the mid-brain and 3rd cranial nerve.

cerebral tumours. Meningiomas account for about one-fifth of intracranial tumours.

Pathology

Metastases from extracranial primary tumours are usually located in the white matter of the cerebral or cerebellar hemispheres, and common sources are bronchus, breast and gastrointestinal tract. Primary intracerebral tumours are classified by their cell of origin and degree of malignancy, and vary in incidence by age and localisation (see Tables 14.42 and 14.43). Even when malignant they do not metastasise outside the nervous system.

Clinical features

Headache

Headache is not an invariable manifestation of cerebral tumour. If present, it may have the characteristics suggesting raised intracranial pressure (see p. 936), or be caused by

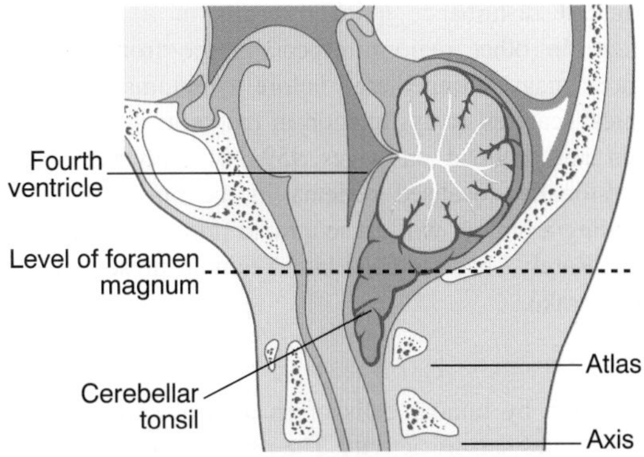

Fig. 14.45 Tonsillar cone. Downward displacement of the cerebellar tonsils below the level of the foramen magnum.

Table 14.42 Primary malignant intracranial tumours

Histological type	Common site	Age
Glioma (astrocytoma)	Cerebral hemisphere Cerebellum Brain stem	Adult Childhood/adult Childhood/young adult
Oligodendroglioma	Cerebral hemisphere	Adult
Medulloblastoma	Posterior fossa	Childhood
Ependymoma	Posterior fossa	Childhood/adolescence
Microglioma (cerebral lymphoma)	Cerebral hemisphere	Adult

Table 14.43 Primary benign intracranial tumours

Histological type	Common site	Age
Meningioma	Cortical dura Parasagittal Sphenoid ridge Suprasellar Olfactory groove	Adult
Neurofibroma	Acoustic neuroma	Adult
Craniopharyngioma	Suprasellar	Childhood/adolescence
Pituitary adenoma	Pituitary fossa	Adult
Colloid cyst	3rd ventricle	Any age

traction on the pain-sensitive intracranial structures (see p. 935). The localisation of the headache is often difficult to correlate with the site of the tumour, although posterior fossa tumours often cause pain in the occiput or neck.

Local effects

In general the focal deficits produced by a cerebral tumour are of slow onset and progressive. Tumours may present at an early stage in some areas, such as the brain stem, where structural disturbance quickly results in a neurological deficit. In other regions, especially the frontal lobe, a tumour may be quite large before symptoms occur. The clinical features of dysfunction in the various lobes of the brain are outlined on pages 959–961 (see Fig. 14.16). Occasionally, localised oedema in the brain tissue surrounding a tumour will cause a rapid progression of symptoms. Rarely, haemorrhage into a tumour presents like an acute stroke.

Seizures

Infiltration by tumour cells of an area of cerebral cortex often excites seizure activity. The resulting seizures may be generalised or partial in nature, and the development of focal seizures in adult life should always suggest the possibility of a tumour.

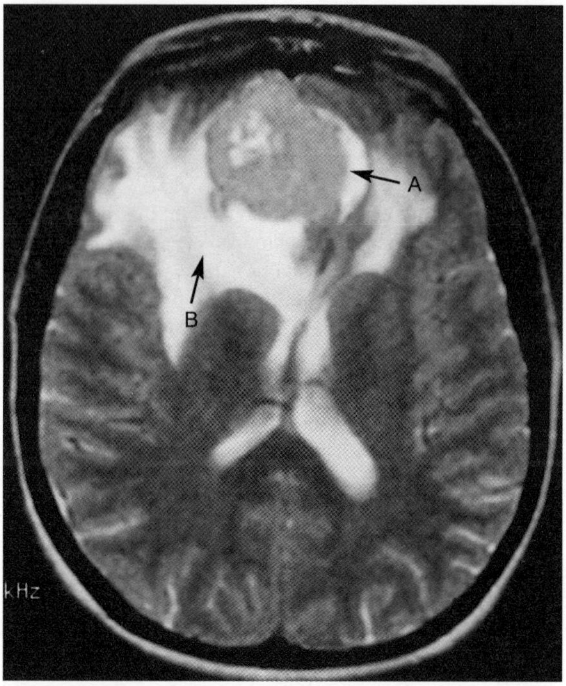

Fig. 14.46 MRI showing meningioma in frontal lobe (arrow A) with associated oedema (arrow B).

Investigations

CT or MRI of the head is the definitive investigation, allowing accurate localisation of the tumour and providing some guidance as to the likely histological type (see Fig. 14.46). Distortion of intracranial structures and the size of the ventricular system can be assessed and may provide accurate evaluation of the extent of the tumour. Plain skull radiographs are rarely of diagnostic value except in pituitary tumours. Chest radiography is an important investigation and may provide evidence of a primary pulmonary tumour or other systemic malignancy. MRI is of particular value in the investigation of tumours of the posterior fossa and brain stem (see Fig. 14.47). MRI has largely replaced angiography in delineating the nature and extent of tumours prior to surgery.

Management

Medical

Relief of raised intracranial pressure is often required when surgery is not possible or when life is threatened before investigation has revealed the diagnosis. Dexamethasone, 8 mg 12-hourly, either orally or by injection, is used to lower intracranial pressure by resolving the reactive oedema around a tumour. A striking improvement in conscious level is often produced and focal disabilities may regress. In severe and acutely raised intracranial pressure 16–20 mg of dexamethasone may be given intravenously or 200 ml of a 20% solution of mannitol may be infused.

Prolactin- or growth hormone-secreting pituitary tumours may respond to treatment with the dopamine agonists bromocriptine, cabergoline or quinagolide.

Surgical

Surgery is the mainstay of treatment, although only partial excision may be possible if the tumour is inaccessible or if its exposure is likely to cause unacceptable brain damage. Biopsy by a direct or stereotactic technique should be considered even if the tumour cannot be removed, since the histological diagnosis has important implications for management and prognosis.

Meningiomas and acoustic neuromas offer the best prospects for complete removal without unacceptable damage to surrounding structures. Meningiomas rarely recur, although those of the sphenoid ridge can often be only partially excised. Pituitary adenomas can often be extirpated by a trans-sphenoidal route, thus avoiding the necessity for a craniotomy.

Radiotherapy and chemotherapy

Radiotherapy and chemotherapy have only a marginal effect on survival in cerebral metastases and malignant gliomas in adults. Ependymomas, some pineal tumours and low-grade gliomas in children and young adults are often radiosensitive. A combination of radiotherapy and chemotherapy has greatly improved the prognosis in medulloblastoma. Radiotherapy also reduces the risk of recurrence of pituitary adenoma after surgery. Radiotherapy may also be helpful as an adjunct to operative treatment in those meningiomas whose anatomical site precludes complete excision or whose histology suggests an increased tendency to recurrence.

Prognosis

Gliomas can rarely be completely excised as infiltration may spread beyond the radiologically evident boundaries of the tumour. Recurrence is common, even if the mass of the tumour is apparently completely removed. Partial excision ('debulking') may be useful in alleviating raised intracranial pressure, but survival in highly malignant gliomas is poor even if such a decompressive procedure is attempted. Prognosis is related to histological grade; the better grades (I–II) may survive many years, whilst only 20% of patients with grade IV gliomas (glioblastoma multiforme) survive 1 year.

The prognosis in benign tumours is good, provided complete surgical excision can be achieved. Ependymomas

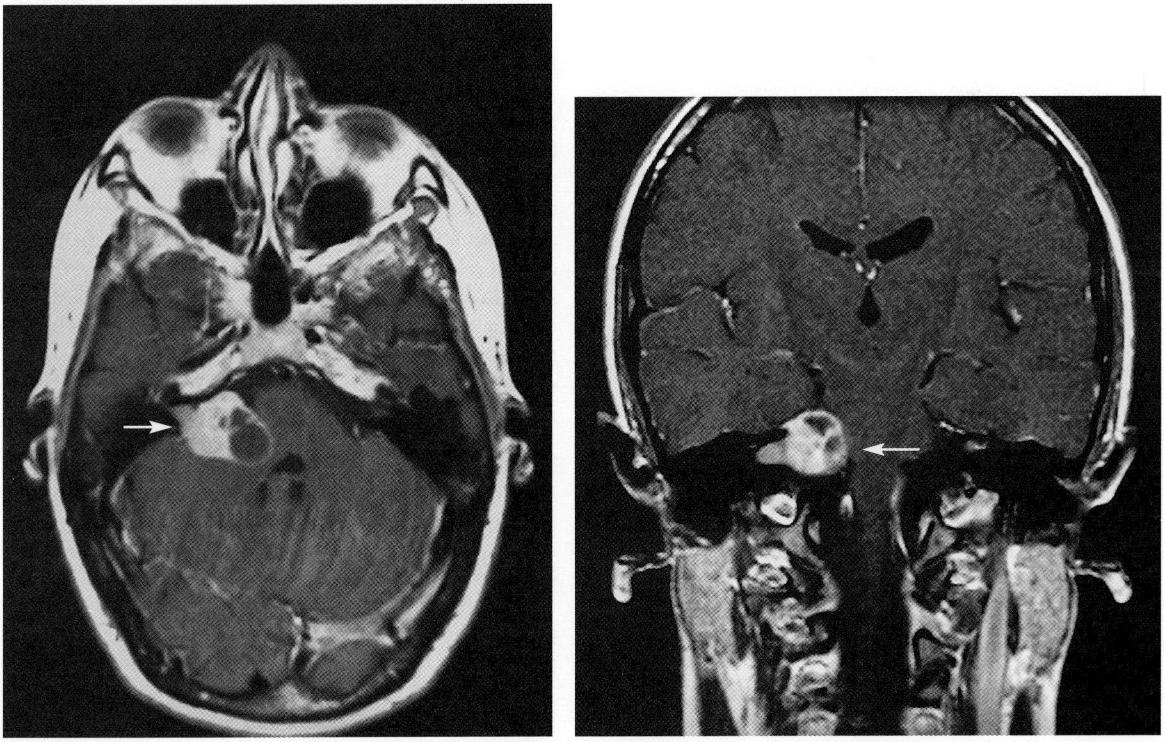

A B

Fig. 14.47 MRI of an acoustic neuroma (arrows) in the posterior fossa compressing the brain stem. A Axial image. B Coronal image.

and medulloblastomas may be excised with minimal residual disability, but may recur with seeding of the tumour via the CSF. Oligodendrogliomas are often slow-growing and relatively benign in the early stages, but may transform to a more malignant form and behave as gliomas.

NEUROFIBROMATOSIS

This is a disorder of autosomal dominant inheritance due to an abnormal gene on chromosome 17 (q11.2, type 1 neurofibromatosis, NF1) or 22 (q12.2, type 2 neurofibromatosis, NF2). Multiple fibromatous tumours develop from the neurilemmal sheaths of peripheral and cranial nerves. Most of the lesions are benign but sarcomatous change may occur. In NF1 (von Recklinghausen's disease) there are characteristic cutaneous manifestations and other extracranial manifestations (see the information box).

TYPES OF NEUROFIBROMATOSIS
Type 1 Peripheral form > 70% of cases
• Multiple cutaneous neurofibromas, 'soft' papillomas, café-au-lait patches, axillary freckling, iris fibromas, plexiform neurofibromas, spinal neurofibromas, aqueduct stenosis, scoliosis, endocrine tumours
Type 2 Central form
• Few or no cutaneous lesions, bilateral acoustic neuromas, cerebral and optic nerve gliomas, meningiomas, spinal neurofibromas

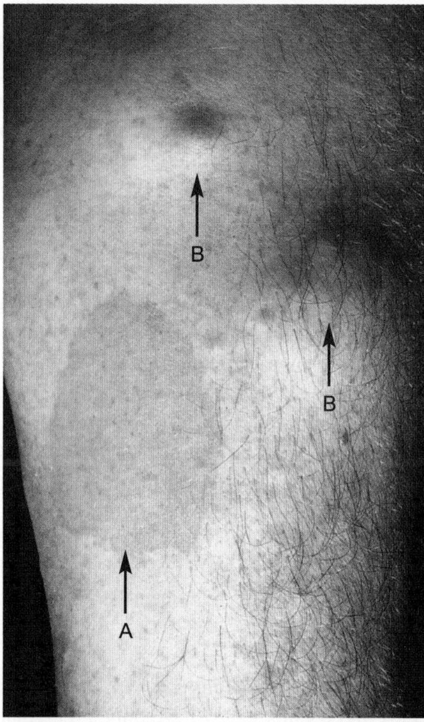

Fig. 14.48 A café-au-lait spot (arrow A) and subcutaneous nodules (arrows B) on the forearm of a patient with neurofibromatosis type 1.

Patients with NF1 are easily recognised because of the cutaneous lesions (see Fig. 14.48) which increase in number throughout life. Investigation and treatment are only indicated if there are symptoms of cerebral or spinal involvement, or if malignant change is suspected.

Patients with NF2 present with acoustic neuromas, often bilateral, and/or other central neoplasms, and have fewer, if any, cutaneous lesions. A family history of cerebral or spinal tumours should be noted with care, since relatives of patients with NF2 may require screening for acoustic neuromas.

ACOUSTIC NEUROMA

This is a benign tumour of Schwann cells of the 8th cranial nerve, which may arise in isolation or as part of NF2 (see above). As an isolated finding, an acoustic neuroma occurs after the third decade and is more frequent in females. The tumour commonly arises near the nerve's entry into the medulla or in the internal auditory meatus, usually on the vestibular division. Such schwannomas of the 8th nerve make up 80–90% of tumours at the cerebello-pontine angle.

Clinical features

These depend somewhat on the site of the tumour along the acoustic or vestibular nerve. (Similar tumours arise rarely from the trigeminal nerve.) Hearing loss is almost invariable, although may not be the presenting feature. Vertigo and sensory symptoms in the face are also common symptoms at presentation. Distortion of the brain stem and/or cerebellar peduncle may cause ataxia and/or cerebellar signs in the limbs. Distortion of the fourth ventricle and cerebral aqueduct may cause hydrocephalus, which may be the presenting feature (see p. 1022). Facial weakness of any severe degree is unusual at presentation, but facial palsy may follow surgical removal of the tumour.

Investigations

MRI is the investigation of choice (see Fig. 14.47), CT being less useful in this region of the posterior fossa.

Management

This involves surgical removal and if this is complete the prognosis is excellent. Deafness and facial weakness, if not present before surgery, usually result from the operation.

VON HIPPEL–LINDAU DISEASE

This is a dominantly inherited disease due to a defective gene on chromosome 3p25–26, characterised by the combination of retinal and intracranial (typically cerebellar) haemangiomas and haemangioblastomas. There may be associated extracranial hamartomatous lesions, which may undergo malignant change. About 10% of posterior fossa tumours are cerebellar haemangioblastomas. Von Hippel–Lindau disease needs to be considered in patients with such lesions, so that screening for other lesions and, if necessary, of family members can be instituted.

PARANEOPLASTIC NEUROLOGICAL DISEASE

Neurological disease may occur with systemic malignant tumours in the absence of metastases. Mild degrees of myopathy and neuropathy are quite frequent with the common malignancies. Much rarer are certain disabling, and often fatal, paraneoplastic syndromes which often have an inflammatory basis, with associated autoantibodies which cross-react with neural and tumour antigens (see Table 14.44). In the case of the Lambert–Eaton myasthenic syndrome the autoantibodies have a functional effect on neuromuscular transmission (see p. 998).

Pathology

The neoplasms with which these syndromes are particularly associated include small-cell carcinoma of the lung, ovarian tumours, and lymphomas. In addition to the presence of autoantibodies, there is usually a lymphocytic infiltrate of the neural tissue affected.

Clinical features

These are summarised in Table 14.44; in most instances the neurological disease progresses quite rapidly over a few months. In 50% of patients with a paraneoplastic syndrome the neurological disease precedes clinical presentation of the primary neoplasm. Paraneoplastic disease should be considered in the diagnosis of any unusual progressive neurological syndrome.

Investigations

See Table 14.44. The presence of characteristic autoantibodies in the context of a suspicious clinical picture may be diagnostic. The causative tumour may be very small and therefore CT of the chest or abdomen is often necessary to find it. The CSF often shows an increased protein and lymphocyte count with oligoclonal bands.

Table 14.44 Paraneoplastic syndromes

Syndrome	Clinical features	Antibody	Associated tumours	Investigations
Retinal degeneration	Painless progressive visual loss	Anti-retinal	Small-cell carcinoma of lung	Chest radiograph, CT chest Electroretinogram
Opsoclonus-myoclonus	Arrhythmic chaotic rapid eye movements	Anti-Ri	Ovarian, lung Neuroblastoma (in children)	Chest radiograph, CT chest Pelvic ultrasound or CT
Sensory neuropathy	Limb pain, paraesthesia Distal numbness	Anti-Hu	Small-cell carcinoma of lung Hodgkin's disease	Chest radiograph, CT chest Nerve conduction studies
Limbic encephalitis	Memory loss, progressive dementia, seizures	Anti-Hu	Small-cell carcinoma of lung Hodgkin's disease	Chest radiograph, CT chest MRI (head) CSF (pleocytosis, raised protein)
Myelitis	Progressive spinal cord lesion (usually cervical cord)	Anti-Hu	Small-cell carcinoma of lung	Chest radiograph, CT chest MRI (cord, head)
Cerebellar degeneration	Progressive ataxia, nystagmus (down-beating), vertigo	Anti-Yo Anti-Hu	Small-cell carcinoma of lung Ovarian Hodgkin's disease	Chest radiograph, CT chest Pelvic ultrasound or CT CSF (raised protein, oligoclonal bands)
Subacute motor neuronopathy	Subacute, patchy progressive, usually lower limb weakness and wasting	Anti-Hu	Hodgkin's disease Small-cell carcinoma of lung	Chest radiograph, CT chest Nerve conduction studies/EMG
Sensorimotor peripheral neuropathy	Mild, non-disabling peripheral; limb numbness and paraesthesia	Not known	Small-cell carcinoma of lung Breast Other carcinoma	Chest radiograph, CT chest Nerve conduction studies/EMG
Lambert–Eaton myasthenic syndrome	Weakness of proximal limb muscles, fatigue with exertion after initial improvement, areflexia	Anti-Ca^{++} channel	Small-cell carcinoma of lung	Chest radiograph, CT chest EMG
Dermatomyositis/ Polymyositis	Proximal limb weakness and pain, heliotrope skin rash, Grotten's papules on knuckles	Anti-Jo-1	Lung, breast, ovary	Chest radiograph, CT chest Creatine kinase (CK) EMG, muscle biopsy
Guillain–Barré	Ascending weakness, distal paraesthesia	Not known	Hodgkin's disease	Nerve conduction studies/EMG

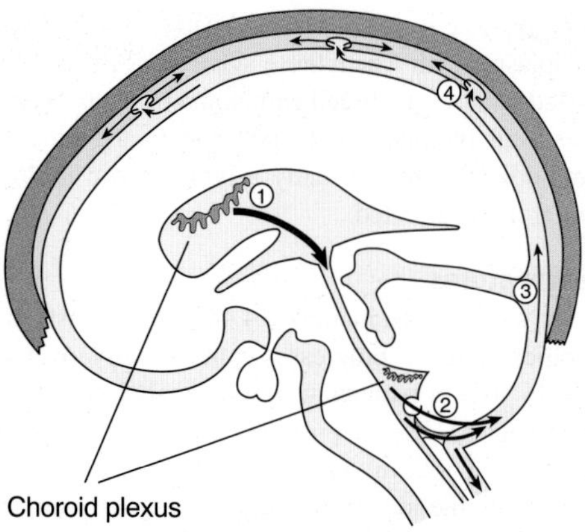

Fig. 14.49 The circulation of cerebrospinal fluid. (1) CSF is synthesised in the choroid plexus of the ventricles, and flows from the lateral and third ventricles through the aqueduct to the fourth ventricle. (2) At the foramina of Luschka and Magendie it exits the brain, flowing over the hemispheres (3) and down around the spinal cord and roots in the subarachnoid space. (4) It is then absorbed into the dural venous sinuses via the arachnoid villi.

Management

This is directed at the primary tumour. Occasionally, successful therapy of the tumour is associated with improvement of the paraneoplastic syndrome. Some improvement may occur following intravenous immunoglobulin.

HYDROCEPHALUS

Hydrocephalus (dilatation of the ventricular system) may be due to obstruction of the CSF circulation (see Fig. 14.49). Hydrocephalus is said to be 'communicating' if the obstruction is outside the ventricular system (usually in the basal cisterns). Obstruction within the ventricles is most common in the narrow channels of the third ventricle and aqueduct, and may be caused by tumour or a congenital anomaly such as aqueduct stenosis (see Fig. 14.50). Causes of hydrocephalus are given in the information box.

Diversion of the CSF by means of a shunt procedure between the ventricular system and the peritoneal cavity or right atrium may result in prompt relief of symptoms in obstructive or communicating hydrocephalus.

NORMAL PRESSURE HYDROCEPHALUS

In this condition the dilatation of the ventricular system is caused by intermittent rises in CSF pressure, which occur particularly at night. It occurs predominantly in old age and is suggested by the combination of gait apraxia (see p. 953) and dementia, with urinary incontinence as an early feature.

CAUSES OF HYDROCEPHALUS

Communicating (obstruction outside ventricular system)

- Bacterial meningitis (esp. tuberculous)
- Sarcoidosis
- Subarachnoid haemorrhage
- Head injury
- Idiopathic ('normal pressure')

Non-communicating (obstruction within ventricular system)

- Tumours
- Colloid cyst
- Arnold–Chiari malformation
- Aqueduct stenosis
- Cerebellar abscess
- Cerebellar or brain-stem haematoma

This cause of dilatation of the ventricles needs to be distinguished from that occurring in cerebral atrophy, where the cortical sulci are also dilated. The result of shunting procedures for normal pressure hydrocephalus is unpredictable.

IDIOPATHIC INTRACRANIAL HYPERTENSION

This condition, previously known as benign intracranial hypertension, usually occurs in obese young women. Raised intracranial pressure develops without a space-occupying lesion, ventricular dilatation or impairment of consciousness. The aetiology is uncertain but there may be a diffuse defect of CSF reabsorption by the arachnoid villi. The condition can be precipitated by drugs, including tetracycline, the oral contraceptive pill and withdrawal of corticosteroid therapy.

Clinical features

Characteristically, there is a headache, sometimes with transient diplopia and visual obscurations, but few other symptoms. There are usually no signs other than papilloedema, which may be discovered incidentally at a routine visit to an optician.

Investigations

The CT is normal, with normal-sized or small ventricles. Once this has been demonstrated, a lumbar puncture is safe and will allow confirmation of the raised CSF pressure and form part of treatment. MR angiography or cerebral venography will exclude cerebral venous occlusion. True papilloedema may need to be distinguished from other causes of disc swelling by fluorescein angiography.

Management

Withdrawal of CSF to obtain a normal pressure is often

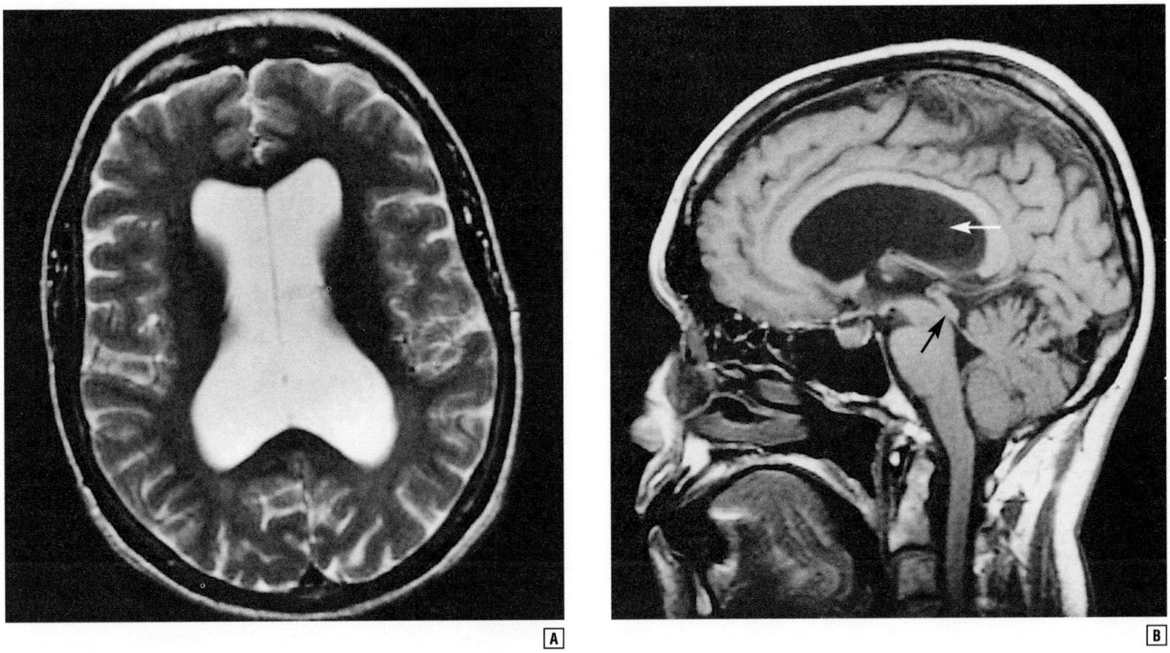

Fig. 14.50 MRI of hydrocephalus due to aqueduct stenosis. A Axial image: note the dilated lateral ventricles. B Sagittal image: note the dilated ventricles (top arrow) and narrowed aqueduct (bottom arrow).

successful, although this may need to be repeated a number of times. Any precipitating medication should be withdrawn and a reducing diet instigated, if indicated. The carbonic anhydrase inhibitor, acetazolamide, may help to prevent recurrence. Patients failing to respond, in whom chronic papilloedema threatens vision, may require optic nerve sheath fenestration or a lumbo-peritoneal shunt.

FURTHER INFORMATION ON INTRACRANIAL MASS LESIONS AND RAISED INTRACRANIAL PRESSURE

Posner J B 1995 Neurologic complications of cancer. F A Davis, Philadelphia
Thomas D G T, Graham D I (eds) 1995 Malignant brain tumours. Springer-Verlag, London

Principles of critical care medicine 15

D.F. TREACHER • N.A. BOON

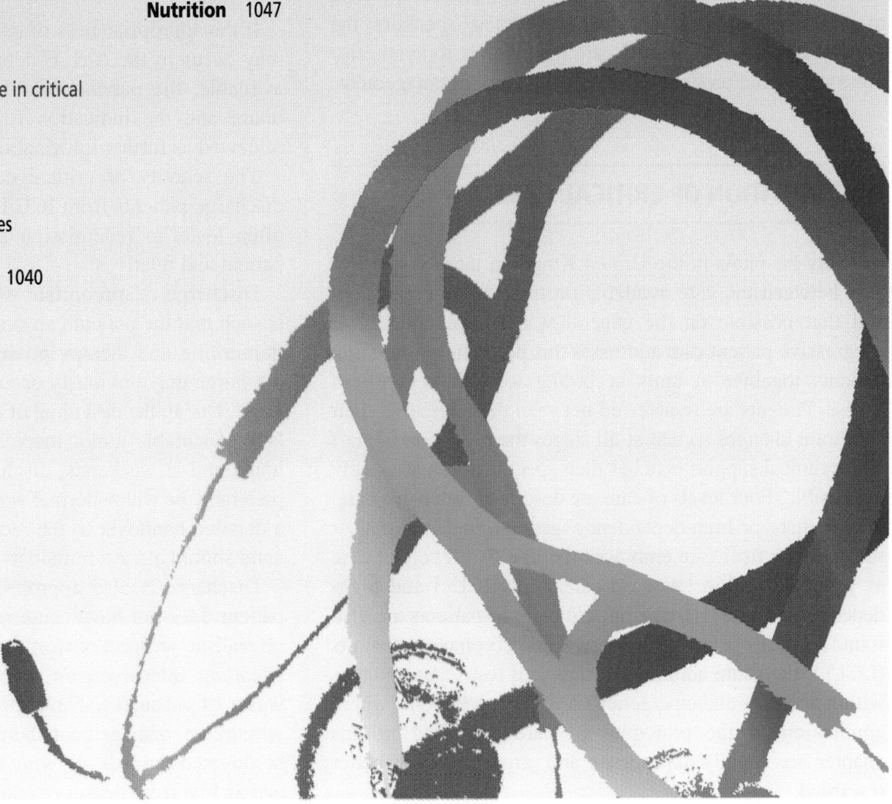

PROVISION OF CRITICAL CARE

BASIC PRINCIPLES

Hospital inpatients are usually grouped together by major specialty, according to specific organ dysfunction; however, this approach is not appropriate for the initial management of the critically ill patient because there is often no established diagnosis, the history is often patchy or incomplete, and examination is frequently inconclusive. Moreover, the physical signs on which classical diagnosis depends may disappear as the patient approaches death.

A different approach is required, based upon:

- analysis of the deranged physiology
- prompt resuscitation adhering to advanced life support guidelines (see p. 235) and the principles of cardiorespiratory management explained in this chapter
- careful monitoring of the patient's condition and response to treatment
- establishing the complete diagnosis in stages as further history, results of investigations and the effects of treatment become available.

Multiple expert opinions (surgeons, physicians, microbiologists etc.) are frequently appropriate but each will tend to adopt the 'parochial' perspective of 'their' specialty; the joy and challenge of critical care medicine is to synthesise these views and produce an integrated plan of management.

ORGANISATION OF CRITICAL CARE

In many hospitals in the United Kingdom there is a major gulf between the care available on the intensive care unit and that possible on the general wards. The concept of progressive patient care addresses this problem by grouping patients together in units according to their severity of illness. Patients are transferred between these areas as their condition changes so that at all stages the provision of staff and technical support matches their specific needs as closely as possible. Four levels of care are described: intensive care, intermediate or high-dependency, general, and minimal or self-care. Critical care embraces the first two levels of care as practised within intensive care units (ICUs) and high-dependency units (HDUs), but critically ill patients are also found in post-operative recovery areas, coronary care units (CCUs), the acute admission wards and resuscitation areas within accident and emergency (A & E) departments where application of the principles of care described in this chapter are equally appropriate and, arguably, even better rewarded.

ADMISSION AND DISCHARGE GUIDELINES

Rigid rules to cover admission to and discharge from ICU/HDU are destined to fail because every case must be evaluated on its own merits. None the less, broad guidelines are required to avoid causing unnecessary suffering and loss of valuable resources by admitting patients who have nothing to gain from intensive care because they are either too well or have no realistic prospect of recovery. Potential organ donors are an obvious exception, in whom admission for continued active management is appropriate despite the hopeless prognosis. The existence of an empty bed does not justify admission.

FACTORS IN THE ASSESSMENT OF A POSSIBLE ICU ADMISSION

- Primary diagnosis and other active medical problems
- Prognosis of underlying condition
- Severity of physiological disturbance—is recovery still possible?
- Availability of the required treatment/technology
- Life expectancy and anticipated quality of life post-discharge
- Wishes of the patient and/or relatives

N.B. Age alone should not be a contraindication to admission.

If the appropriateness of admission remains uncertain, as may occur in the A & E department when little history is available, the patient should be given the benefit of the doubt and the indication for continued active treatment reviewed as further information becomes available.

The scarcity of critical care beds creates pressure to discharge patients from ICU/HDU but premature discharge often leads to readmission and further suffering for the patient and relatives.

Discharge is appropriate when the physiological reserve is such that the patient can survive independent of the close monitoring and therapy possible on intensive care; such a discharge may obviously occur earlier if the hospital has an HDU. Due to the deskilling of the general wards and frequent lack of suitable junior medical and nursing support out of hours and at weekends, discharges from ICU/HDU should preferably be within normal working hours and should include a detailed handover to the receiving team. The critical care team should always remain available for advice.

Discharge is also appropriate when it is clear that the patient does not have acute reversible disease and there is no realistic prospect of worth-while recovery because in these situations intensive care becomes futile, and an inhumane waste of resources. Nevertheless, when active support is withdrawn, management should remain positive and should be directed towards allowing the patient to die with dignity and as free from distress as possible.

Communication with the patient, whenever possible, with the family, with the referring clinicians and between members of the critical care team is crucial. Failure in this area damages working relations, causes stress and unrealistic expectations, and leads to subsequent unhappiness, anger and litigation.

SCORING SYSTEMS IN CRITICAL CARE

Admission and discharge criteria vary between units so it is important to define the characteristics of the patients admitted (case mix) in order to assess the effects of the care provided on the outcome achieved. Figure 15.1 illustrates how outcome is determined by case mix, and by the care and organisation of the unit.

Two systems are widely used to measure severity of illness:

- 'APACHE' II—Acute Physiology Assessment and Chronic Health Evaluation
- 'SAPS' 2—Simplified Acute Physiology Score.

These scores include assessment of certain admission characteristics (e.g. age and pre-existing organ dysfunction) and a variety of routine physiological measurements (e.g. temperature, blood pressure, Glasgow coma score—see p. 959) that reflect the response of the patient to his or her illness. Predicted mortality figures by diagnosis have been calculated from large databases generated from a range of ICUs. This allows a particular unit to evaluate its performance compared to the reference ICUs, by calculating standardised mortality ratios (SMRs) for each diagnostic group:

$$SMR = \text{observed mortality} \div \text{predicted mortality}$$

A value of unity indicates the same performance as the reference ICUs while a value < 1 indicates a better than predicted outcome. A unit may have a high SMR in a certain diagnostic category and this would prompt investigation into how such patients were managed, with the intention of identifying aspects of care that could be changed and demonstrating improved outcome on re-evaluation.

When combined with the admission diagnosis, scoring systems have been shown to correlate well with the risk of hospital death. Such outcome predictions can never be 100% accurate and should be viewed as only one of many factors that the clinician considers when deciding whether or not further intervention is appropriate.

The outcome measure most widely used is survival but the timing of this assessment must be specified. Discharge policy potentially influences ICU/HDU mortality and therefore survival to hospital discharge, to 28 days and to 6 months is usually quoted. Quality of life is also an important outcome measure but its measurement and interpretation are difficult, not least because with emergency admissions no objective pre-morbid assessment is available.

USES OF CRITICAL CARE SCORING SYSTEMS

- Comparison of the performance of different units
- Assessment of new therapies
- Assessment of changes in unit policies and management guidelines
- Measurement of the cost-effectiveness of care

COST OF INTENSIVE CARE

Measuring the costs of intensive care is complex. The most widely used system in the UK is the Therapeutic Intervention

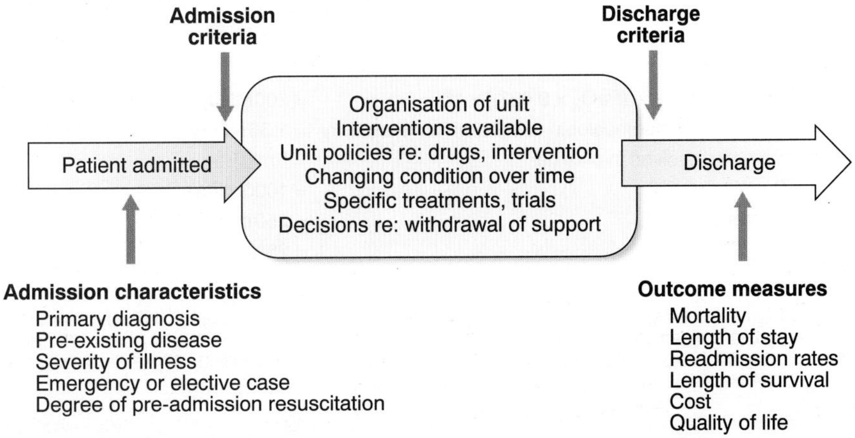

Fig. 15.1 The interaction of factors that may influence admission, discharge and outcome in critically ill patients.

Scoring System (TISS), which scores interventions and nursing activities for each day of admission and has been shown to correlate reasonably well with detailed measurements of staff, equipment and drug costs incurred within the unit. Since it focuses on nurse-based interventions, TISS is also used as an index of nurse dependency.

Current estimates of the daily cost of intensive care in the UK vary from £800 to £1600, with high-dependency care approximately 50% and general ward care 20% of these costs. In the UK approximately 6% of gross domestic product (GDP) is spent on health care and only 1% of total expenditure is spent on critical care.

OXYGEN DELIVERY

The major function of the heart, lungs and circulation is the provision of oxygen and other nutrients to the various tissues of the body. During this process carbon dioxide and the other waste products of metabolism are removed. The rate of this supply and removal should match the specific metabolic requirements of the individual tissues. This requires adequate oxygen uptake in the lungs, global matching of delivery and consumption, and regional control of the circulation. Failure to supply sufficient oxygen to meet the

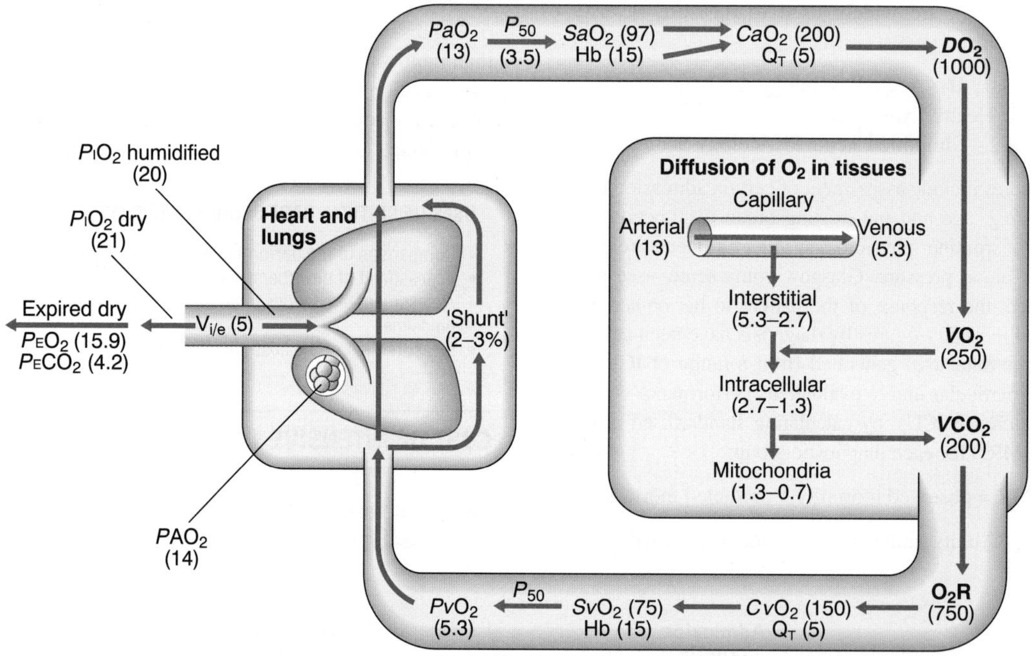

Calculations

$CaO_2 = [Hb \times SaO_2 \times k + (PaO_2 \times 0.023)] \times 10$ = 200 ml O_2/litre

k = coefficient of haemoglobin oxygen-binding capacity = 1.36 ml O_2/gram of 100% saturated Hb

$PaO_2 \times 0.23$ = oxygen dissolved in plasma = 3 ml/litre

$DO_2 = Q_T \times CaO_2$ = 1000 ml/min

$VO_2 = Q_T (CaO_2 - CvO_2)$ = 250 ml/min

$OER = VO_2/DO_2 \times 100$ = 25%

Fig. 15.2 Transport of oxygen from inspired gas to the cell demonstrating the 'oxygen cascade', with equations for calculation of arterial oxygen content, global oxygen delivery, consumption and extraction. Values in parentheses for a normal 70 kg individual (body surface area: 1.67 m^2) breathing air (FiO_2: 0.21) at standard atmospheric pressure P_B: 101 kPa). Partial pressures of O_2, CO_2 in kPa; saturation in %; contents (CaO_2, CvO_2) in ml/litre; Hb in g/100 ml; blood/gas flows (Q_T, $V_{i/e}$) in litre/min; oxygen transport (DO_2, O_2R), VO_2 and VCO_2 in ml/min.

CaO_2 = arterial O_2 content; O_2R = oxygen return; PiO_2 = inspired PO_2; SO_2 = oxygen saturation (%);
CvO_2 = mixed venous O_2 content; PaO_2 = arterial PO_2; PO_2 = oxygen partial pressure (kPa); SvO_2 = mixed venous SO_2;
DO_2 = oxygen delivery; PAO_2 = alveolar PO_2; PvO_2 = venous PO_2; VCO_2 = CO_2 production;
Hb = haemoglobin; $PECO_2$ = mixed expired PCO_2; Q_T = cardiac output; $V_{i/e}$ = minute volume: inspired/expired;
OER = oxygen extraction ratio PEO_2 = mixed expired PO_2; SaO_2 = arterial SO_2; VO_2 = oxygen consumption;

Table 15.1 The effects of progressive increments in inspired oxygen concentration and then transfusion on the oxygen content of arterial blood in an anaemic, hypoxaemic patient

	FiO_2	PaO_2 (kPa)	SaO_2 (%)	Hb (g/100 ml)	Dissolved O_2 (ml/100 ml)	CaO_2 (ml/%)	CaO_2 (% change)
Air	0.21	6	75	8	0.14	8.3	–
35% O_2	0.35	9.5	93	8	0.22	10.3	+ 24
60% O_2	0.60	16.5	98	8	0.38	11.0	+ 7
Transfusion	0.60	16.5	98	12	0.38	16.4	+ 48

(FiO_2 = inspired oxygen concentration; PaO_2 = arterial oxygen partial pressure; SaO_2 = arterial oxygen saturation; Hb = haemoglobin; CaO_2 = oxygen content of arterial blood)

metabolic requirements of the tissues is the cardinal feature of shock.

OXYGEN TRANSPORT

The transport of oxygen from the atmosphere to the mitochondria within individual cells is illustrated in Figure 15.2. The important points to note are:

- The majority of oxygen is carried in the blood attached to haemoglobin, with only a small amount dissolved in the plasma.
- The arterial oxygen saturation of haemoglobin (SaO_2) and the haemoglobin concentration are the major determinants of the oxygen content of arterial blood (see Table 15.1) and, together with cardiac output, global oxygen delivery (DO_2).
- The regional distribution of oxygen is vital. If skin and muscle receive high blood flows but the splanchnic bed does not, the gut will become hypoxic even if overall oxygen delivery is high.
- The movement of oxygen from capillary to cell occurs by diffusion and depends on the oxygen gradient, the diffusion distance and the ability of the cell to take up and use oxygen. Therefore microcirculatory, tissue diffusion and cellular factors, as well as global oxygen delivery, influence the oxygen status of the cell.
- Supranormal levels of oxygen delivery cannot compensate for diffusion problems between capillary and cell, nor for metabolic failure within the cell.

OXYGENATION OF THE BLOOD

The oxyhaemoglobin dissociation curve (see Fig. 15.3) describes the relationship between the saturation of haemoglobin (SO_2) and the partial pressure (PO_2) of oxygen in the blood. Its position and the effect of various physicochemical factors are defined by the PO_2 at which 50% of the haemoglobin is saturated (P_{50}), which is normally 26 mmHg (3.5 kPa).

A shift in this relationship will influence the uptake and release of oxygen by the Hb molecule; for example, if the curve moves to the right, the haemoglobin saturation will be lower for any given oxygen tension and therefore less oxygen will be taken up in the lungs but more will be released to the tissues. This means that there will be increased unloading of oxygen in the tissues as capillary PCO_2 rises, a phenomenon known as the Bohr effect.

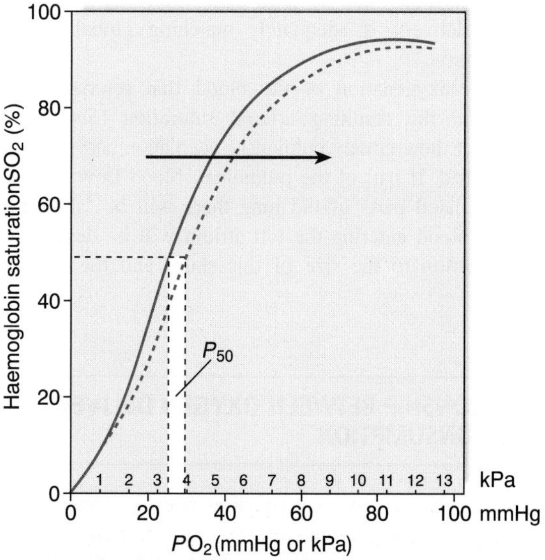

Fig. 15.3 The relationship between oxygen tension (PO_2) and percentage saturation of haemoglobin with oxygen (SO_2). The dotted line illustrates the rightward shift of the curve (i.e. P_{50} increases) caused by increases in temperature, $PaCO_2$, metabolic acidosis and 2,3,diphosphoglycerate (DPG).

The optimum haemoglobin concentration in a critically ill patient is usually between 10 and 11 g/dl and represents a balance between maximising the oxygen content of the blood and avoiding regional microcirculatory problems due to increased viscosity.

OXYGEN CONSUMPTION

The sum of the oxygen consumed by the various organs represents the global oxygen consumption (VO_2) and is approximately 250 ml/min for an adult of 70 kg undertaking normal daily activities. VO_2 may be derived from measurement of cardiac output and arterial and mixed venous oxygen saturations, as shown in Figure 15.2, but can also be calculated from measurements of inspired and mixed-expired oxygen and CO_2 concentrations.

The oxygen saturation in the pulmonary artery, otherwise known as the mixed venous oxygen saturation (SvO_2), represents a measure of the oxygen not consumed by the tissues (DO_2–VO_2). The saturation of venous blood from different organs varies considerably; for example, the hepatic venous saturation is usually 30–40% but the renal venous saturation often exceeds 80%, reflecting the great difference in the metabolic requirements of these organs. The SvO_2 will be influenced by changes both in oxygen delivery (DO_2) and consumption (VO_2) and, provided the microcirculation and the mechanisms for cellular oxygen uptake are intact, can be used to monitor whether global oxygen delivery is adequately matching global oxygen consumption.

The re-oxygenation of the blood that returns to the lungs and the resulting arterial saturation (SaO_2) will depend on how closely pulmonary ventilation and perfusion are matched. If part of the pulmonary blood flow perfuses non-ventilated parts of the lung there will be 'shunting', and the blood entering the left atrium will be desaturated in proportion to the size of this shunt and the level of SvO_2.

RELATIONSHIP BETWEEN OXYGEN DELIVERY AND CONSUMPTION

Normally, tissue oxygen extraction rises as consumption increases or supply diminishes (see Fig. 15.4) but when the maximum oxygen extraction ratio (usually 60–70%) is reached, any further increase in oxygen consumption or decline in oxygen delivery will cause tissue hypoxia leading to anaerobic metabolism and the production of lactic acid. In this situation the appropriate treatment is to increase oxygen delivery by increasing the intravascular

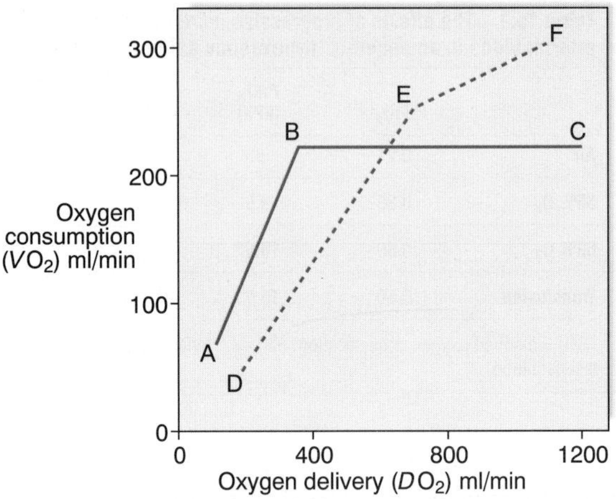

Fig. 15.4 The effects of changing oxygen delivery on consumption. The solid line (ABC) represents the normal relationship and the dotted line (DEF) the altered relationship believed to exist in sepsis.

volume, relieving obstruction in the circulation (e.g. thrombolysis in pulmonary embolism), or augmenting cardiac function.

In sepsis the slope of maximum oxygen extraction ratio falls (see Fig. 15.4), reflecting the reduced ability of tissues to extract oxygen, but the curve does not plateau and oxygen consumption continues to increase even at 'supranormal' levels of oxygen delivery. This concept has encouraged some physicians to treat septic shock using vigorous volume loading (i.v. fluid) and inotropic support, usually with dobutamine, with the aim of achieving very high oxygen deliveries (> 600 ml/min/m^2) in the belief that this strategy will increase oxygen consumption, relieve tissue hypoxia, prevent multi-organ failure and improve prognosis. Unfortunately, several major studies have failed to demonstrate any benefit from this approach and such aggressive volume loading is frequently detrimental.

FACTORS THAT MAY INCREASE METABOLIC RATE IN CRITICALLY ILL PATIENTS

- Fever (10–15% increase in VO_2 for every 1°C rise)
- Sepsis
- Trauma
- Burns
- Surgery
- Sympathetic activation (pain, agitation, shivering)
- Interventions (e.g. nursing procedures, physiotherapy, visitors)
- Drugs (e.g. β-adrenoceptor agonists, amphetamines, tricyclics)

N.B. Sedatives, analgesics and muscle relaxants will reduce metabolic rate

In the later stages of severe sepsis the essential problem is at the level of the microcirculation; hence oxygen uptake and utilisation are impaired due to failure of the regional distribution of flow within the organs and direct cellular toxicity despite apparently adequate global oxygen delivery. Tissue oxygenation can be improved and aerobic metabolism sustained by reducing demand, i.e. metabolic rate (see the information box).

MAJOR MANIFESTATIONS OF CRITICAL ILLNESS

SHOCK

Shock is a loosely defined term used to describe the clinical syndrome that develops when oxygen delivery is inadequate to meet the metabolic requirements of the tissues due to some form of acute circulatory failure.

There are numerous causes and these can be classified into five broad categories:

1. *Hypovolaemic shock.* May be due to any condition provoking a major reduction in blood volume, e.g. internal or external haemorrhage, severe burns, dehydration (e.g. diabetic ketoacidosis).

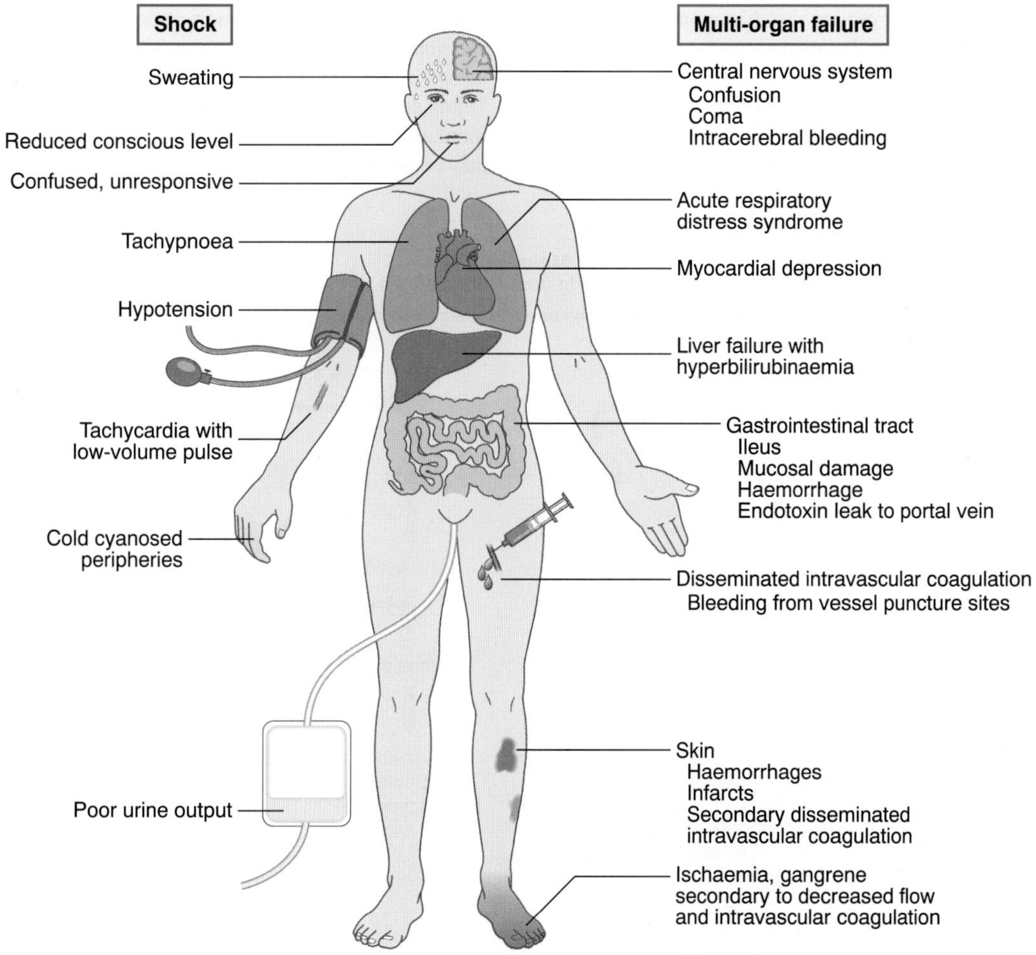

Fig. 15.5 Some features of shock. The early signs of shock are shown on the left and the organs affected in multi-organ failure are shown on the right.

GENERAL FEATURES OF SHOCK

- Hypotension (systolic BP < 100 mmHg)
- Tachycardia (> 100/min)
- Cold, clammy skin
- Rapid, shallow respiration
- Drowsiness, confusion, irritability
- Oliguria (urine output < 30 ml/hour)
- Elevated or reduced central venous pressure (see text)
- Multi-organ failure (see Fig. 15. 5)

2. *Cardiogenic shock.* May be caused by any form of severe heart failure, e.g. myocardial infarction, acute mitral regurgitation.
3. *Obstructive shock.* Due to some form of obstruction within the circulation, e.g. major pulmonary embolism, cardiac tamponade.
4. *Anaphylactic shock.* Due to inappropriate vasodilatation triggered by an allergen such as a bee sting.
5. *Septic shock.* Due to capillary damage, arteriovenous shunting and inappropriate vasodilatation caused by severe infection or inflammation.

Clinical features and complications

Although these depend to some extent on the underlying cause, a range of clinical features and complications are common to most cases (see the information box and Fig. 15.5).

The first three types of the syndrome produce the 'popular' image of shock, with cold peripheries, weak central pulses and evidence of a low cardiac output. In contrast, anaphylaxis and severe sepsis are usually associated with warm peripheries, bounding pulses and features of a high cardiac output.

The central venous pressure (jugular venous pressure or JVP) is typically reduced in hypovolaemic and anaphylactic shock, elevated in cardiogenic and obstructive shock, and may be low, normal or high in septic shock. This is an important distinction and direct measurement of the central venous pressure or pulmonary artery wedge pressure (see below) may be very helpful if the physical signs are difficult to interpret. Figure 15.6 indicates how the likely diagnosis may be established by careful analysis of the central venous pressure, peripheral perfusion (temperature), pulse volume and haematocrit.

Many of the potential complications of shock can cause additional tissue damage. For example, declining myocardial contractility may set up a vicious cycle of falling cardiac output and deteriorating tissue perfusion. Similarly, alveolar oedema and progressive lung damage may cause increasing hypoxia and generalised ischaemia.

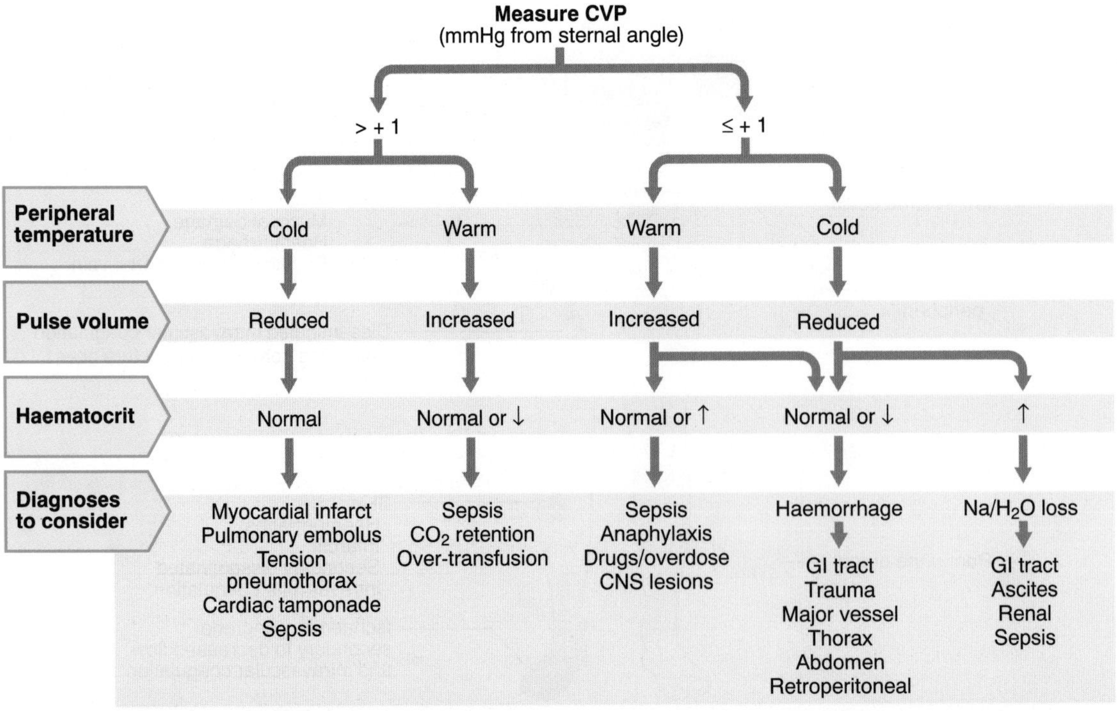

Fig. 15.6 A guide to the initial analysis and diagnosis of circulatory shock.

INITIAL MANAGEMENT OF SHOCK
• Measure blood gases • Correct hypoxaemia • Consider intubation if: $PaCO_2$ > 6.5 kPa Respiratory rate > 25/min Impaired consciousness • Correct acidaemia with i.v. sodium bicarbonate if: pH < 7.25 when $PaCO_2$ < 6 kPa (i.e. base excess > –8) • Measure CVP (off ventilator) Give volume challenge (100 ml normal saline or colloid) if CVP < +1 Consider pulmonary-artery catheter if CVP > +1

Secondary infections may occur because destruction of the intestinal mucosa allows bacterial toxins and even organisms to enter the portal venous circulation and multi-organ failure often supervenes.

Initial management

The key steps in the early management of shock are listed in the information box. In hypovolaemic shock the main priority is to resuscitate the patient by administering appropriate intravenous fluids at a rate dictated by the circulatory response to the infusion, while trying to identify and treat the source of fluid loss.

The management of cardiogenic shock and of tamponade is described in Chapter 3 (see pp. 207–210) and the management of pulmonary embolism is described on page 380.

SEPSIS

Sepsis is a major problem in critical care; at any one time over half of intensive care unit patients will be treated with antibiotics and in half of these cases the infections will have been acquired after admission to the unit.

As few as 10% of ICU patients with a clinical diagnosis of 'septic' shock will have positive blood cultures, due to the effects of prior antibiotic treatment and the fact that the 'septic' state is not always caused by microorganisms. The appropriate terminology used to describe the critically ill patient with an inflammatory response is defined in the information box; the term 'septicaemia' should now be abandoned.

Pathophysiology of septic shock

The characteristic features of sepsis are mediated by the host's immunological response, which involves the release of cytokines (e.g. tumour necrosis factor, endotoxin, interleukins, platelet activation factor) and activation of white blood cells, endothelial cells, platelets, the complement cascade and the coagulation pathways. The activated white cells, particularly polymorphs and macrophages, adhere to and damage the vascular endothelium, allowing fluid and cells to pass into the interstitial spaces, disrupting function and leading to organ failure. Nitric oxide (NO) is released by these mediators and contributes to the myocardial depression, vasodilatation and microcirculatory chaos that are characteristic of septic shock.

TERMINOLOGY USED TO DESCRIBE THE INFLAMMATORY STATE
Infection
• Invasion of normally sterile host tissue by microorganisms
Bacteraemia
• Viable bacteria in the blood
Systemic inflammatory response syndrome (SIRS)
• This term encompasses the inflammatory response to both infective and non-infective conditions such as pancreatitis, trauma, cardiopulmonary bypass, vasculitis etc. and is defined by the presence of: Temperature > 38°C or < 36°C Heart rate > 90/min Respiratory rate > 20/min $PaCO_2$ < 32 mmHg or ventilated White blood cell count > 12 000 or < 4000/mm^3
Sepsis
• SIRS caused by infection
Septic shock
• Sepsis associated with features of shock (hypotension and evidence of abnormal organ perfusion)
Multiple organ dysfunction syndrome (MODS)
• Development of impaired organ function in critically ill patients with SIRS. **Multiple organ failure (MOF)** may ensue

Presentation of sepsis

Infection may be the primary admission diagnosis, e.g. severe community-acquired pneumonia, or may be acquired on the ICU (nosocomial infection). The likely causative microorganism will depend on this distinction, which will therefore direct the initial choice of antibiotics.

The haemodynamic changes in septic shock are very variable and are not specific for the Gram status of the infecting organism. Severe sepsis may present as

RISK FACTORS FOR NOSOCOMIAL INFECTION
• Mechanical ventilation • Trauma • Invasion with catheters, e.g. i.v., urinary, nasogastric tubes • Stress ulcer prophylaxis with H_2-antagonists • Prolonged length of stay

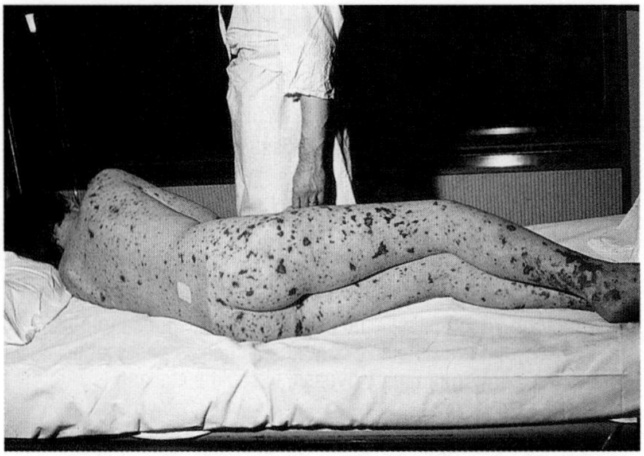

Fig. 15.7 The characteristic rash of meningococcal sepsis.

unexplained hypotension and can even simulate a major pulmonary embolus or myocardial infarction.

Examination may reveal an obvious focus of infection, such as erythema around an intravenous line, and may provide clues about the likely infecting organism, such as the characteristic rash in meningococcal sepsis (see Fig. 15.7). The common sites of infection in critically ill patients and some of the appropriate investigations to consider are listed in Table 15.2.

Investigations of septic shock

The most important objective is to identify and treat the underlying cause.

The initial investigations should include:

- cultures of blood, sputum, intravascular lines, urine and any wound discharges
- coagulation profile, plasma lactate, arterial blood gases, urinalysis, chest radiograph and electrocardiogram (ECG).

Specific investigations will be driven by the history and examination. For example, erect/decubitus abdominal radiographs, ultrasound and CT scanning might be considered in cases of suspected intra-abdominal sepsis (see Table 15.2).

Management of septic shock

Antibiotics

Prompt administration of appropriate antibiotics with a spectrum wide enough to cover probable causative organisms, based on an analysis of the likely site of infection, any previous antibiotic therapy and the known resistance patterns on the unit, is essential.

Haemodynamic management

The early stages of septic shock are often dominated by hypotension with relative volume depletion due to marked arteriolar and particularly venular dilatation. Sufficient i.v. fluid should be given to ensure that the intravascular volume is not the limiting factor in determining global oxygen delivery. However, excessive fluid replacement in pursuit of 'supranormal' goals is not beneficial (see pp. 1030–1031).

Table 15.2 Sites of infection in critically ill patients

Sites of infection	Investigations and comments
Major	
Intravenous lines (particularly central)	These should always be suspected; if the patient develops evidence of sepsis and the lines have not been changed for > 4 days, they must be replaced
Lungs	The risk of nosocomial pneumonia is high in intubated patients. When the patient has been on the ICU for > 3–4 days the nasopharynx becomes colonised with Gram-negative organisms, particularly if he or she has received antibiotics, which migrate to the lower respiratory tract. The use of H_2-antagonists promotes this overgrowth and increases the risk of pneumonia
Abdomen	Intra-abdominal abscesses or necrotic gut must be considered in patients who have had abdominal surgery. Pancreatitis or acute cholecystitis may develop as a complication of critical illness. Ultrasound, computed tomography (CT) scan, aspiration of collections of fluid/pus and laparotomy are the relevant investigations
Urinary tract	A catheter specimen of urine should always be taken in cases of unexplained sepsis but the lower urinary tract is a relatively unusual cause of severe sepsis
Other	
Heart valves	Transthoracic or transoesophageal echocardiogram
Meninges	Lumbar puncture but check coagulation and platelet count first
Joints and bones	Radiograph, gallium or technetium white cell scan
Nasal sinuses, ears, retropharyngeal space	Clinical examination, plain radiograph, CT scan
Genitourinary tract (particularly post-partum)	Per vaginam examination, ultrasound
Gastrointestinal tract	Per rectum examination, stool culture, *Clostridium difficile* toxin, sigmoidoscopy

In contrast to other forms of shock, the major defect in established septic shock is an inability of tissues to take up oxygen in spite of supranormal global oxygen delivery. This effective bypassing of the tissues is characterised by reduced arteriovenous oxygen difference, a low oxygen extraction ratio, a raised plasma lactate and a paradoxically high mixed venous oxygen saturation (SvO_2).

Myocardial function is usually impaired, with a flat left ventricular stroke function curve (see Fig. 3.17, p. 211 and Fig. 3.19, p. 214), so that increases in filling pressures produce relatively small increments in ventricular work. The marked reduction in systemic vascular resistance (SVR) results in a high cardiac output but a low blood pressure.

The choice of the most appropriate vasoactive drug to use should be based on a full analysis of the circulation and knowledge of the different inotropic, dilating or constricting properties of these drugs (see Table 15.4, p. 1042). For example, a constrictor may be necessary to increase SVR and blood pressure, while an inotrope may be necessary to maintain cardiac output and prevent regional ischaemia.

Specific therapies

Steroids have no role in established sepsis and attempts at intervening in the inflammatory cascade using anticytokine and other novel drug therapies have produced disappointing results in several large multicentre trials.

SPECIFIC FORMS OF ORGAN FAILURE IN CRITICAL ILLNESS

MULTIPLE ORGAN FAILURE (MOF)

All forms of shock require early identification and treatment because, if inadequate regional tissue perfusion and cellular dysoxia persist, multiple organ failure will develop (see Fig. 15.5, p. 1031). The mortality of MOF is high and increases with the number of organs that have failed, the duration of organ failure and the patient's age. Failure of four or more organs is associated with a mortality of more than 90%.

CONDITIONS PREDISPOSING TO ARDS

Direct injury	Indirect injury
• Aspiration of gastric contents • Toxic gases • Smoke injury • Blunt chest trauma • Near-drowning	• Sepsis • Necrotic tissue (particularly bowel) • Multiple trauma • Pancreatitis • Cardiopulmonary bypass • Severe burns • Drugs (heroin, barbiturates, thiazides) • Major blood transfusion reaction • Anaphylaxis (wasp, bee, snake venom) • Fat embolism • Obstetric crises (amniotic fluid embolus, eclampsia)

ACUTE RESPIRATORY DISTRESS SYNDROME (ARDS)

This term describes acute, diffuse, inflammatory lung injury that may be caused by direct (e.g. inhaled) or indirect (e.g. blood-borne) insults (see the information box). The condition is characterised by hypoxaemia, reduced pulmonary compliance, pulmonary hypertension and diffuse infiltrates on the chest radiograph (see Fig. 15.8) in the presence of a normal, or only slightly elevated, left atrial or 'wedge' pressure and is often part of the multiple organ dysfunction syndrome (MODS).

The history and chest examination typically reveal shortness of breath, tachypnoea, central cyanosis and lung crepitations but the symptoms and signs are in no way diagnostic and share many features with other serious pulmonary conditions.

Pathology

Neutrophils activated by cytokines and monocytes adhere to the pulmonary endothelium, release free radicals and proteolytic enzymes and, together with an array of inflam-

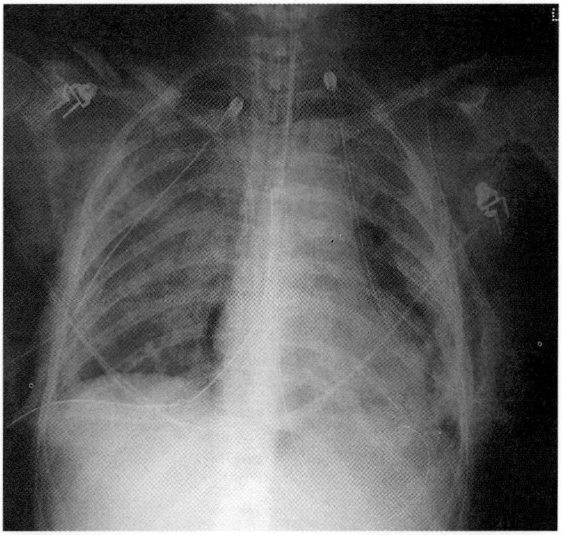

Fig. 15.8 Chest radiograph in acute respiratory distress syndrome (ARDS). This 22-year-old woman was involved in a road traffic accident. Note bilateral lung infiltrates, pneumomediastinum, pneumothoraces with bilateral chest drains, surgical emphysema, and fractures of the ribs, right clavicle and left scapula.

matory mediators, promote cell damage. Proteins, fluid and cells leak into the interstitial and alveolar spaces where they coalesce to form hyaline membranes. All this occurs at normal levels of left atrial pressure, hence the description 'non-cardiogenic pulmonary oedema'. Destruction of surfactant-producing cells leads to widespread alveolar collapse and a fall in functional residual capacity and pulmonary compliance with ventilation/perfusion (V/Q) mismatch and hypoxaemia. Local activation of the coagulation cascade causes thrombosis and obstruction in the pulmonary capillaries, which, together with regional hypoxic vasoconstriction, increases pulmonary vascular resistance, resulting in the development of pulmonary hypertension.

Management

Early and effective treatment of the precipitating cause is the key to successful management of ARDS. In the early stages supplementary oxygen and physiotherapy may suffice, but if the condition progresses, non-invasive or full invasive mechanical ventilation may be necessary. High airway pressures are often required to achieve adequate tidal volumes during mechanical ventilation and this increases the risk of barotrauma to the lung (pneumothorax, pneumomediastinum, development of lung cysts) and adverse circulatory effects (see the information box).

Exuberant fluid loading is harmful. The circulatory goal should therefore be to maintain the left atrial pressure as low as possible in order to minimise alveolar flooding without compromising perfusion to other organs. The strategy may be summarised as maintaining adequate oxygen delivery to sustain the other organs while resting, recruiting and repairing the lung.

There is no evidence to support the use of steroids in ARDS. Inhaled nitric oxide may improve gas exchange by selectively increasing perfusion to the ventilated areas of lung but no survival benefit has been demonstrated.

PRINCIPLES OF MECHANICAL VENTILATION IN ARDS

- Optimum ventilator settings are:
  - Pressure-controlled
  - Long inspiratory-to-expiratory time
  - Positive end-expiratory pressure (PEEP)
- Allow $PaCO_2$ to rise (permissive hypercapnia) and tolerate lower oxygen saturations than normal (e.g. 88–90%)
- Avoid:
  - Tidal volume of more than 10 ml/kg
  - Airway pressure of more than 40 cm H_2O
  - FiO_2 of more than 0.8
- Remember that high intrathoracic pressures compromise circulatory function so oxygen delivery may actually fall in spite of improved oxygenation
- Management must be a balance between improving gas exchange, minimising the risk of subsequent pulmonary fibrosis due to lung injury, and avoiding adverse circulatory effects

Nursing the patient in the prone position is another strategy that may cause a dramatic improvement in gas exchange in some cases, although the mechanism of this benefit remains unclear.

Prognosis

Mortality is determined by the precipitating condition but is generally high (> 50%). The cause of death is usually multiple organ failure but severe secondary (nosocomial) pneumonias and progressive pulmonary fibrosis also contribute to mortality. If the patient survives to leave the ICU, there is usually considerable resolution of the chest radiograph changes and significant symptomatic improvement over the subsequent months.

DISSEMINATED INTRAVASCULAR COAGULATION (DIC)

This is also known as consumptive coagulopathy and is one of the acquired disorders of haemostasis (see p. 794); it is common in critically ill patients and often heralds the onset of multi-organ failure. The condition is characterised by an increase in prothrombin time, partial thromboplastin time and fibrin degradation products and a fall in platelets and fibrinogen. The clinically dominant feature may be either widespread bleeding from vascular access points, the GI tract, bronchial tree and surgical wound sites or widespread microvascular and even macrovascular thrombosis. Treatment is supportive with infusions of fresh frozen plasma, platelets and low-dose heparin.

ACUTE RENAL FAILURE

A fall in urine output is often an early sign of systemic problems in a critically ill patient and, conversely, restoration of good renal function, as reflected by acid-base balance, urine flow, plasma potassium and creatinine, can be a useful indicator of successful resuscitation. Although diuretics do have a role in treating the avid salt and water retention that may occur in critical illness, they are essentially renal poisons and the resulting urine flow should not be interpreted as evidence that renal perfusion and intravascular volume are adequate.

The osmotic diuretic mannitol is a physiological method of producing a diuresis and is particularly valuable when the kidneys are exposed to toxins such as intravenous contrast media or myoglobin (rhabdomyolysis).

Low-dose dopamine is often prescribed to improve renal blood flow and specifically to protect the kidneys when multiple organ failure threatens. The evidence that this approach improves outcome is scanty but in low doses dopamine does have a modest inotropic, natriuretic and global systemic dilator effect, all of which may be beneficial in incipient multi-organ failure.

The renal lesion in multi-organ failure is almost always acute tubular necrosis (see p. 447) and, provided the underlying problem can be treated and a normal pre-renal environment restored, function will return between 5 days and several weeks later. Properly managed haemofiltration (see p. 438) effectively replaces renal function in critically ill patients, who may still die but not from renal failure or its treatment. Mortality figures of over 50% are still reported in such patients, although with modern haemofiltration techniques and intensive care support this has fallen to below 40% in certain units.

HEPATIC FAILURE AND THE GASTROINTESTINAL TRACT

The gastrointestinal tract and liver play a central role in the development of the sepsis syndrome and the evolution of multiple organ failure in critical illness, even when the primary diagnosis is not related to the abdomen.

The gut has a very rapid cell turnover rate and even fasting alone produces marked changes in mucosal structure and function. In critical illness the gut mucosal barrier is often severely damaged by a combination of fasting, catabolic stress and reduced splanchnic blood flow; this allows intraluminal toxins, particularly endotoxin, and bacteria to enter the portal circulation. For this reason the gut has been called the 'motor' or the 'undrained abscess' of multiple organ failure.

The normal liver is well equipped to deal with minor episodes of toxic spill from the gut but in critical illness the load may become excessive and the liver itself is often compromised by poor perfusion; if the hepatic defences are overwhelmed, the lungs and other organs will be exposed to the toxins from the gut and multi-organ failure may ensue.

The measurement and possible manipulation of regional blood flow to vital organs such as the gut is a major challenge in critical care. Gastric tonometry measures intramucosal PCO_2, which reflects the adequacy of gut perfusion, and is one of the first clinically applicable techniques for assessing regional blood flow.

MONITORING

GENERAL PRINCIPLES

On entering an ICU, relatives, students and even clinicians may be intimidated by the numerous tubes and cables attaching each patient to a battery of 'alarming' machines (see Fig. 15.9). Much of the bedside nurse's time is spent observing, recording and reacting to the information displayed by these monitors, particularly the ECG, CVP, arterial BP, temperature and ventilator data. The trends observed over time, interpreted in relation to changes in therapy, are an important guide to the patient's progress.

The critically ill patient should be monitored according to the following principles:

- Regular clinical examination should never be neglected.
- Simple physical signs such as respiratory rate, the appearance of the patient, restlessness, conscious level and indices of poor peripheral perfusion (pale, cold skin, delayed capillary refill in the nail bed) are just as

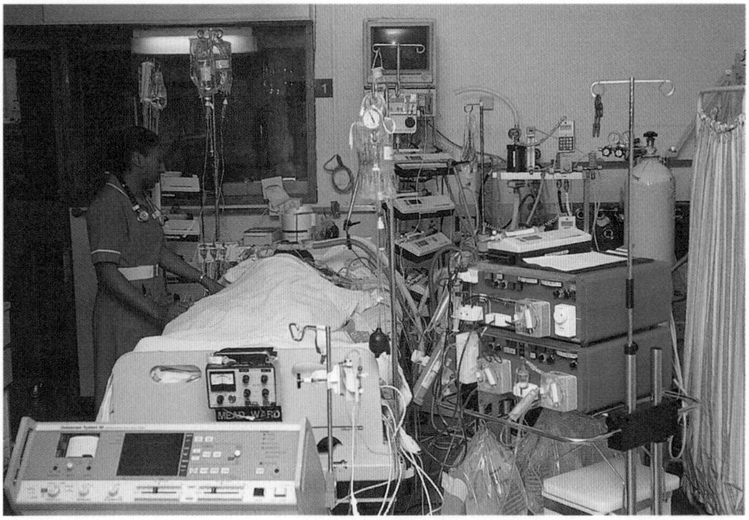

Fig. 15.9 A patient with multi-organ failure supported by haemodynamic monitoring, cardiac pacing, a counterpulsation aortic balloon pump, haemofiltration and nitric oxide therapy.

important as a set of blood gases or numbers impressively displayed on expensive monitors.
- If there is conflict between clinical assessment and the information on a monitor, the monitor should be presumed to be wrong until all potential sources of error have been checked and eliminated. For example, CVP measurement is often erroneous because the line is blocked, the system has not been re-zeroed after a change in the patient's position, the tip of the cannula is lying in the right ventricle, or another infusion has been attached to the same central line.
- Changes and trends are more important than any single absolute number.
- Many monitors have alarms which will activate if certain maximum and minimum values are breached. This is a crucial safety feature and may, for example, help to identify the fact that a patient has become disconnected from the ventilator. Despite the understandable desire to avoid extra noise, the alarm limits should always be set to define physiologically 'safe' limits for the variable being monitored.
- Sophisticated monitoring systems are often invasive and pose certain hazards (see the information box). Always ask 'Is it necessary?', and cease monitoring as soon as possible.

SPECIFIC MONITORING TECHNIQUES

MONITORING THE CIRCULATION

ECG

Standard monitors display a single-lead ECG, record rate and identify rhythm changes. More sophisticated machines can monitor ST segment shift, which may be useful in patients with ischaemic heart disease.

Blood pressure

This may be measured intermittently using an automated sphygmomanometer but in critically ill patients continuous intra-arterial monitoring, using a line placed in the radial artery, is preferable. It is important to appreciate that when there is vasoconstriction with a high systemic vascular resistance (SVR), the mean arterial pressure may be normal or high even though the cardiac output is low. Conversely, if the SVR is low (e.g. sepsis), the mean arterial pressure may be low in spite of a high cardiac output.

Central venous pressure (CVP)

CVP is monitored using a catheter placed in either the internal jugular or subclavian vein to measure right atrial pressure. This is a useful means of assessing the circulating blood volume and determining the appropriate rate of intravenous fluid replacement. In severe hypovolaemia the right atrial pressure may be sustained by peripheral venoconstriction and transfusion may initially produce little or no change in the CVP (see p. 1040).

Pulmonary artery wedge or occlusion pressure (PAWP/PAOP)

In most situations the central venous pressure is an adequate guide to the filling pressures of both sides of the heart; however, this may not be the case in critically ill patients, particularly those with pulmonary vascular disease or right ventricular dysfunction. In these situations it may therefore be advisable to monitor the PAWP (see Fig. 15.10). These catheters can also be used to measure cardiac output and other haemodynamic variables such as the systemic vascular resistance. The mean PAWP normally lies between 6 and 12 mmHg but in left heart failure it may be grossly elevated and is often more than 35 mmHg. Provided the pulmonary capillary membranes are intact, the optimum PAWP in acute circulatory failure is generally 12–15 mmHg because this will ensure good left ventricular filling without risking pulmonary oedema.

COMPLICATIONS AND PITFALLS OF CENTRAL VENOUS AND PULMONARY ARTERY (PA) CANNULATION
At insertion
• Pneumothorax—more likely with subclavian than internal jugular approach • Haematoma from accidental arterial puncture • Air embolism • Arrhythmia • Damage to thoracic duct with left internal jugular approach • Knotting of catheter* • Pulmonary artery rupture*
In situ
• Sepsis • Thrombosis • Pulmonary infarct* • Erroneous information • Inappropriate response to information
* Risk associated specifically with PA catheterisation.

Cardiac output

The most widely used method for cardiac output measurement is the thermodilution technique. A bolus of cold 5% dextrose is injected into a central vein which, after mixing with the total venous return in the right ventricle, will cause a fall in temperature in the pulmonary artery that is measured by a thermistor at the end of a PA catheter. The flow or cardiac output is derived from the volume of injectate used and the temperature gradient between the

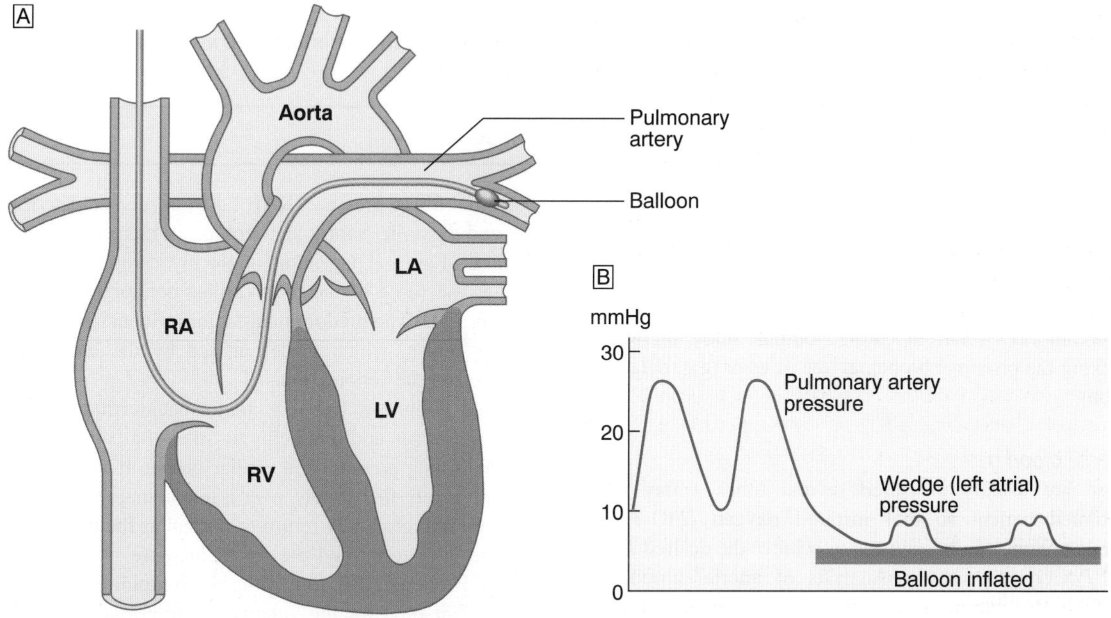

Fig. 15.10 A pulmonary artery catheter. A There is a small balloon at the tip of the catheter and pressure can be measured through the central lumen. The catheter is inserted via a subclavian or femoral vein and advanced through the right heart until its tip lies in the pulmonary artery. When the balloon is deflated the pulmonary artery pressure can be recorded. B Advancing the catheter while inflating the balloon will 'wedge' the catheter in the pulmonary artery. In this position blood cannot flow past the balloon so the tip of the catheter will now record the pressure transmitted from the pulmonary veins and left atrium. This is known as the pulmonary artery wedge pressure or pulmonary artery occlusion pressure and provides an indirect measure of the left atrial pressure.

injectate and the baseline PA temperature, and is inversely proportional to the area under the temperature–time curve. Although generally viewed as the 'gold standard' for clinical measurement of cardiac output, the error is at least 10%.

Some pulmonary artery catheters provide continuous monitoring of cardiac output, mixed venous oxygen saturation and assessment of RV ejection fraction.

Interaction between ventilator and intravascular pressure measurements

The raised intrathoracic pressure associated with positive pressure ventilation may lead to marked swings in atrial pressures and blood pressure in time with respiration. CVP measurements off the ventilator should be used to guide fluid management because these values provide the most accurate measure of ventricular end-diastolic transmural pressure.

Urinary flow

This is a sensitive measure of renal perfusion, provided that the kidneys are not damaged (e.g. acute tubular necrosis) or affected by drugs (e.g. diuretics), and can be monitored accurately if a urinary catheter is in place. It is normally measured hourly and the lower limit of normal is 0.5 ml/hour/kg body weight.

Fluid balance

Assessing fluid balance in critically ill patients is a difficult but important discipline. Weighing the patient daily can be helpful but it is extremely difficult to obtain accurate measurements in bed-bound patients and assessment is usually based on fluid balance charts which record:

- inputs: oral, nasogastric and intravenous, classified as crystalloid and colloid
- outputs: urine, nasogastric, fistulae, vomiting and diarrhoea.

The insensible loss from skin, respiration etc. is normally 500–1000 ml/day but can exceed 2 litres/day in a pyrexial patient with open wounds.

Peripheral/skin temperature

This is usually measured over the dorsum of the foot and reflects cutaneous blood flow. The gradient between peripheral and central/core temperature (rectal, oesophageal or possibly tympanic) is a more sophisticated measure of peripheral perfusion.

MONITORING RESPIRATORY FUNCTION

Oxygen saturation (SpO_2)

This is measured by a probe that is usually attached to a finger or earlobe and uses spectrophotometric analysis to determine the relative proportions of saturated and desaturated haemoglobin. The technique is unreliable if peripheral perfusion is poor and may produce erroneous results in the presence of nail polish, excessive movement or ambient light. In general, oxygenation is satisfactory if SpO_2 is greater than 90%. Sudden falls in SpO_2 may be caused by pneumothorax, a fall in cardiac output, thick secretions blocking the proximal bronchial tree or error (e.g. detached probe).

Arterial blood gases

These are usually measured several times a day in a ventilated patient so that inspired oxygen ($F\text{I}O_2$) and minute volume can be adjusted to achieve the desired PaO_2 and $PaCO_2$ respectively. Analysis of arterial blood gas results is also a useful means of monitoring disturbances of acid-base balance (see Ch. 5).

Lung function

In ventilated patients lung function is monitored by:

- alveolar-arterial PO_2 gradient and oxygenation index ($PaO_2/F\text{I}O_2$), which are measures of gas exchange
- arterial and end-tidal CO_2, which are measures of alveolar ventilation
- tidal volume (V_T), respiratory rate (f), minute volume ($V_T \times f$), airway pressure and compliance, which are measures of the adequacy of ventilation, 'stiffness' of lungs and the required work of breathing.

Capnography

The CO_2 concentration in inspired gas is zero but in expired gas rises progressively during expiration to reach a plateau which represents the alveolar or end-tidal CO_2. An infrared sensor inserted between the ventilator tubing and the endotracheal tube can be used to measure this cyclical change in CO_2 concentration and produce a capnogram. Provided there is no marked variation in the spatial and temporal distribution of ventilation, the end-tidal CO_2 closely mirrors $PaCO_2$ and can be used to assess the overall adequacy of alveolar ventilation. In addition, the volume and flow signals from a ventilator can be used to calculate CO_2 production.

CIRCULATORY MANAGEMENT

Cardiac output (Q_T) is the product of stroke volume and heart rate ($Q_T = SV \times HR$). Three factors determine stroke volume: 'preload', 'afterload' and myocardial contractility.

PRELOAD

The atrial filling pressure (RAP, LAP) or preload determines the end-diastolic ventricular volume which, according to Starling's Law and depending on the myocardial contractility, defines the force of the next cardiac contraction (see Fig. 3.17, p. 211). The predominant factor influencing preload is venous return, which is determined by the intravascular volume and the venous 'tone'.

When volume is lost (e.g. major haemorrhage), venous 'tone' increases and this helps to offset the consequent fall in atrial filling pressure and cardiac output. If the equivalent volume is returned slowly, over a few hours, the right atrial pressure will gradually return to normal as the intravascular volume is restored and the reflex increase in venous tone abates. However, if fluid is infused too rapidly there will be insufficient time for the venous and arteriolar tone to fall and pulmonary oedema may occur, even though the intravascular volume has only been restored to the pre-morbid level.

If the preload is low, volume loading (i.v. fluids) is the most appropriate means of improving cardiac output and oxygen delivery and should be the priority in circulatory resuscitation.

When the preload is high, due to excessive intravascular volume, impaired myocardial contractility or increased afterload, it is advisable to remove volume from the circulation (diuretics, venesection, haemofiltration) or increase the capacity of the vascular bed using venodilator therapy (glyceryl trinitrate, morphine).

AFTERLOAD

The tension in the ventricular myocardium during systole, or afterload, is determined by the resistance to ventricular outflow, which is a function of the peripheral arteriolar resistance. If the considerable assumption is made that flow in the circulation is linear and non-pulsatile, the resistance against which each ventricle works may be calculated as the pressure drop across the resistance bed divided by the flow:

$$\text{Systemic vascular resistance (SVR)} = (\text{MAP} - \text{RAP}) / Q_T$$
$$\text{Pulmonary vascular resistance (PVR)} = (\text{PAP} - \text{LAP}) / Q_T$$

If the pressures are measured in mmHg and flow in litres/min, these calculations give the resistances in simple or 'Wood' units; multiplication by 80 converts to SI units. For a normal 70 kg adult:

$$SVR = (90 - 0)/5 \times 80 = 1440 \text{ dyn.sec.cm}^{-5}$$
$$PVR = (10 - 5)/5 \times 80 = 80 \text{ dyn.sec.cm}^{-5}$$

Understanding the reciprocal relationship between pressure, flow and resistance is crucial for appropriate circulatory management. High resistances produce lower flows at higher pressures for a given amount of ventricular work. Therefore, a systemic vasodilator such as sodium nitroprusside will allow the same cardiac output to be maintained for less ventricular work but with reduced arterial blood pressure.

MYOCARDIAL CONTRACTILITY

This determines the work that the ventricle performs under given loading conditions or, put another way, the stroke volume that the ventricle will generate against a given afterload for a particular level of preload.

The relationship between stroke work and filling pressure is shown in Figure 3.17, page 211. The ventricular stroke work is the external work performed by the ventricle with each beat and is calculated from the stroke volume (SV) and the pre- and afterload pressures:

$$\text{Ventricular stroke work (VSW)} = SV \times (\text{afterload} - \text{preload})$$
$$\text{e.g. LVSW} = SV \times (MAP - LAP) \text{ ml.mmHg}$$

Using the data for a normal adult shown in Table 15.3, and multiplying by 0.0136 to convert to SI units of gram.metres, LVSW and RVSW are 80 and 10 g.m respectively.

Consideration of ventricular work is important because it is desirable to maintain satisfactory perfusion and oxygen delivery to all organs at maximum cardiac efficiency and therefore minimise myocardial ischaemia (see the information box, p. 248). Myocardial contractility is frequently reduced in critically ill patients due to either pre-existing cardiac disease (usually ischaemic heart disease) or the disease process itself (particularly sepsis).

If the cardiac output is inadequate and myocardial contractility is poor, as defined by a flattened stroke work/filling pressure equation, the available treatment options are:

- *Reduce afterload*. This can be achieved by using an arteriolar dilator (e.g. ACE inhibitor) which may be

Table 15.3 Typical circulatory measurements in a normal adult and in various cardiorespiratory conditions that may cause circulatory 'shock'

Clinical condition	RAP/ CVP (mmHg)	LAP/ PAWP (mmHg)	PAP (mmHg)	MAP (mmHg)	Heart rate /min	Cardiac output (l/min)	SVR*	PVR*	Venous compliance (ml/mmHg)	CaO_2 (ml/100 ml)	DO_2 (ml/min)
Normal	0	5	10	90	70	5	18	1	300	20	1000
Major haemorrhage	–6	–2	5	75	120	3	27	2.3	40	16	480
Left heart failure	2	14	18	90	100	3.7	24	1	80	18	670
Severe cardiac tamponade	10	12	15	60	110	2	25	1.5	40	20	400
Major pulmonary embolism	6	0	30	75	110	2.5	28	12	40	16	400
Exacerbation of COAD	5	4	36	76	100	6	12	5	150	18	960
Septic shock											
Pre-volume load	–3	2	8	49	130	4.5	12	1.3	340	15	675
Post-volume load	3	9	17	54	120	7.5	7	1.1	200	14	1050

* Multiply by 80 to give SI units: dyn.sec.cm^{-5}. To adjust for the size of the patient, the measurements of flow and resistance are frequently indexed by dividing by the patient's body surface area.
(RAP/LAP = right/left atrial pressure; CVP = central venous pressure; PAWP = pulmonary artery wedge pressure; PAP/MAP = pulmonary artery/mean arterial pressure; SVR/PVR = systemic/pulmonary vascular resistance; CaO_2 = arterial oxygen content; DO_2 = global oxygen delivery; COAD = chronic obstructive airways disease)
Note These values are merely examples. The severity of the condition and pre-existing cardiorespiratory disease will affect the precise figures obtained in individual cases. Note that unlike the other conditions the oxygen delivery is high in septic shock after volume loading. When the circulatory abnormalities have been defined in this way, appropriate management may be planned.
Pressures quoted referenced to zero at sternal angle in semi-recumbent patient. Add vertical distance from mid-axilla to sternal angle (approx. 5–7 mmHg) if mid-axilla used as reference point.

Table 15.4 Circulatory effects of commonly used vasoactive drug infusions

Drug	Cardiac contractility	HR	BP	Cardiac output	Splanchnic blood flow	SVR	PVR
Dopamine							
(< 5 μg/kg/min)	+	0/+	0/+	+	0/+	0/+	0/+
(> 5 μg/kg/min)	++	+	+	++	0	+	+
Adrenaline	++	+	++	+++	–	+	+
Noradrenaline	0/+	0	++	–	– –	++	++
Isoprenaline	+	++	+/0	+	0/+	0/–	–
Dobutamine	+	+	+/0	++	0	–	–
Dopexamine	+	+	0	+	+	–	–
Glyceryl trinitrate	0	+	–	+	+	–	–
Nitroprusside	0	+	– –	+	+	– –	–
Prostacyclin	0	+	– –	+	+	–	– –

+ = increases; 0 = no change; – = decreases.
These effects are guidelines only. The exact response will depend on the circulatory state of the patient and the dose of the drug.

limited by the consequent fall in systemic pressure. A counterpulsation balloon pump offers the ideal physiological treatment because it both reduces LV afterload and increases diastolic pressure and flow; this is particularly valuable in treating myocardial ischaemia.

- *Increase preload.* However, if there is significant impairment of myocardial contractility, the increase in stroke volume generated by increasing filling pressure will be small and there is a risk of precipitating pulmonary oedema.
- *Improve myocardial contractility.* Table 15.4 lists some of the characteristics of the commonly used inotropic agents.
- *Control heart rate and rhythm.* The optimum heart rate is usually between 90 and 110 per minute.

RESPIRATORY MANAGEMENT

Management of respiratory problems in the critically ill should include the following:

1. *Oxygen therapy.* If there is significant oxygen desaturation when breathing air ($SaO_2 < 94\%$), supplementary oxygen should be administered via a face mask or nasal cannulae at whatever FIO_2 is necessary to correct the problem. Certain patients with chronic obstructive pulmonary disease require controlled oxygen therapy to avoid carbon dioxide retention and many require mechanical respiratory support.
2. *Attempts to reduce the work of breathing.* This is an important issue when considering the need for mechanical ventilatory support and the timing of its withdrawal. The work of breathing normally consumes less than 5% of total oxygen consumption but in a catabolic critically ill patient this figure may exceed 30%.

   A patient who cannot sustain the required work of breathing will display the symptoms and signs of acute respiratory distress and will require mechanical ventilation unless the underlying problem can be successfully and promptly treated.

   Work of breathing may be reduced by:
   - improving compliance (clear secretions, treat oedema, recruit collapsed lung)
   - reducing airway resistance (bronchodilator therapy)
   - minimising metabolic rate (see the information box, p. 1030).

   Pulmonary oedema reduces lung compliance and increases the work of breathing; this means that the heart must generate a greater cardiac output in order to supply sufficient oxygen to the respiratory muscles and explains why mechanical ventilation may be beneficial in patients with heart failure but normal lungs.
3. *Prompt identification and treatment of pulmonary or other infection.*
4. *Optimisation of functional residual capacity.* Functional residual capacity may be low (lung collapse, pneumonia, oedema, pleural effusion, ARDS) or high (asthma, chronic obstructive pulmonary disease, bronchiolitis) and it is advisable to select ventilatory strategies that will tend to correct any such abnormality because this will help to improve pulmonary compliance and reduce the work of breathing.

MECHANICAL VENTILATION (ARTIFICIAL VENTILATION)

The partial or complete replacement of a patient's own inspiratory muscle function by external mechanical support can improve gas exchange and reduce the work of breathing. Over 60% of appropriate ICU admissions require mechanical ventilation, and the accompanying information boxes list the major indications for mechanical ventilation and explain some of the common abbreviations and terminology.

The different types of ventilatory support are illustrated in Figure 15.11 and the pressure and flow-time curves for some modes of ventilation are shown in Figure 15.12.

Modern ventilators provide considerable flexibility, allowing the clinician to change from mandatory, full-support modes to partial-support modes that allow the ventilator to be matched to the patient's demands, thereby avoiding the hazards of paralysis and deep sedation and allowing the patient to be conscious yet comfortable.

COMMON INDICATIONS FOR MECHANICAL VENTILATION
Post-operative
• e.g. After major abdominal or cardiac surgery
Respiratory
• ARDS • Pneumonia • COPD • Acute severe asthma • Aspiration • Smoke inhalation, burns
Circulatory
• Following cardiac arrest • Pulmonary oedema • Low cardiac output
Neurological
• Status epilepticus • Drug overdose • Respiratory muscle failure (e.g. Guillain–Barré, poliomyelitis, myasthenia gravis) • Head injury—to avoid hypoxaemia, hypercapnia and coughing and to reduce intracranial pressure • Bulbar abnormalities causing risk of aspiration (e.g. cerebrovascular accident, myasthenia gravis)
Multiple trauma
Additional considerations
• Metabolic factors Metabolic rate (ventilatory requirements rise as metabolic rate increases) Nutritional reserve (low potassium or phosphate reduces respiratory muscle power) • Condition of the abdomen Distension due to surgery or tense ascites causes both discomfort and splinting of the diaphragm, compromising spontaneous respiratory effort and promoting bilateral basal lung collapse

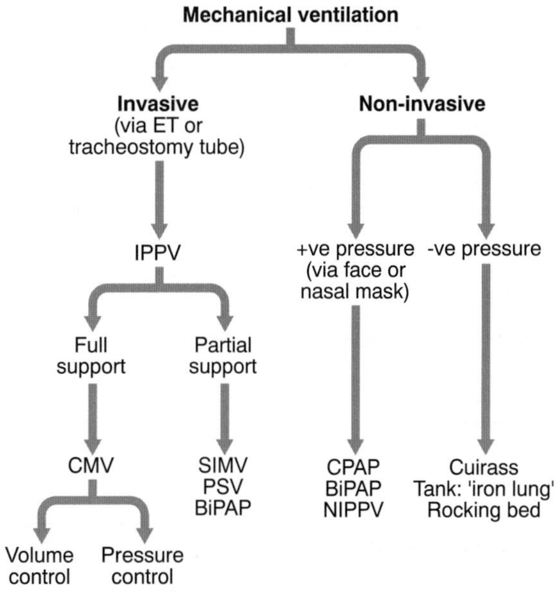

Fig. 15.11 Different types of invasive and non-invasive ventilatory support. (See the information box on p. 1044 for abbreviations.)

GENERAL CONSIDERATIONS IN THE MANAGEMENT OF THE VENTILATED/INTUBATED PATIENT

1. Beware the restless patient and try to establish the cause of the problem before simply administering sedation. Possibilities include pneumothorax, hypercapnia due to inadequate ventilation, inadequate analgesia, onset of sepsis, cardiac decompensation (pulmonary oedema, dysrhythmia, infarction) and proximal airway obstruction, e.g. secretions.
2. Patients who are breathing spontaneously adjust their ventilation to compensate for metabolic derangements; this cannot occur in patients who are ventilated using mandatory modes so the clinician must either correct the underlying metabolic abnormality or make appropriate changes to the ventilator settings. For example, a patient with severe diabetic ketoacidosis will hyperventilate to compensate for the metabolic acidosis; if mechanical ventilation is instituted there will be a potentially catastrophic fall in pH unless the acidosis is corrected by administering sodium bicarbonate or a high minute volume (artificial hyperventilation) is delivered.

MODES AND TERMS USED IN ARTIFICIAL RESPIRATORY SUPPORT
IPPV/CMV—Intermittent Positive Pressure Ventilation/Controlled Mechanical Ventilation
• Mandatory mode with preset ventilatory parameters • May be either volume or pressure controlled • Does not allow spontaneous breathing • Appropriate for initial control of patients with little respiratory drive, severe lung injury, gas trapping or circulatory instability
PEEP—Positive End-Expiratory Pressure
• Positive airway pressure applied throughout the respiratory cycle during mandatory invasive ventilation • Increases functional residual capacity by recruiting areas of collapsed/atelectatic or oedematous lung and improves oxygenation • High airway pressures increase risk of barotrauma (pneumothorax, pneumomediastinum, development of lung cysts)
SIMV—Synchronised Intermittent Mandatory Ventilation
• Delivers a set number of mechanically imposed breaths of predetermined tidal volume and therefore achieves a predetermined minimum mandatory minute volume (MMV) • Allows spontaneous breathing that is pressure-supported • Useful in settling a patient on the ventilator with minimum sedation and when weaning
PSV—Pressure Support Ventilation
• Breaths are initiated or triggered by the patient but pressure support is provided to augment the patient's own respiration • May be used with SIMV and then alone when weaning
CPAP—Continuous Positive Airway Pressure
• Same objective as PEEP but applied to a spontaneously breathing patient via an endotracheal tube or tightly fitting face or nasal mask • Provided by a flow generator connected to a wall oxygen supply that entrains air to achieve the desired FiO_2 between 30 and 100% • Positive pressure is typically set at 5–10 cm H_2O. Airway pressure and therefore the risk of barotrauma is less than with PEEP • Appropriate for patients with low functional residual capacity but should be avoided in patients with bronchospasm and those at risk of gas trapping • Discourages coughing and clearance of lung secretions • The tight-fitting mask is uncomfortable and may increase the risk of aspiration
BiPAP—BIlevel Positive Airway Pressure
• Delivers two levels of pressure in phase with respiration. The higher pressure provides inspiratory support and augments tidal volume; the lower pressure is applied during expiration and increases functional residual capacity • May be applied via face or nasal mask • May be set in spontaneous or mandatory mode • Permits gradual transition from mandatory ventilation and is ideal for weaning
NIPPV—Non-invasive Intermittent Positive Pressure Ventilation
• Provides pressure support (typically 25 cm H_2O) at onset of inspiration which ceases at the onset of expiration • May be applied via a face or nasal mask • Benefits patients with an acute exacerbation of chronic obstructive pulmonary disease or primary alveolar hypoventilation who are tiring and cannot generate sufficient work of breathing • Oxygen can be added but it is difficult to achieve an $FiO_2 > 0.4$ • A lot of time has to be spent reassuring the patient and matching the timing and trigger sensitivity to his or her respiratory pattern
NINPV—Non-Invasive Negative Pressure Ventilation
• Operates by producing negative pressures within an external shell (cuirass), tank or iron lung that encases all or part of the thorax • Developed following the polio epidemics of the 1950s and now largely superseded by NIPPV

3. Ventilator alarms should be set to detect:
   - minimum acceptable minute volume to identify inadvertent disconnection
   - maximum acceptable airway pressure to prevent barotrauma.
4. Humidify and warm inspired gas to prevent inspissation of secretions.
5. Arrange regular positioning, physiotherapy and suctioning to clear secretions and prevent both proximal airway obstruction and distal alveolar collapse.
6. Obtain a chest radiograph to check the position of the endotracheal tube following intubation (the appropriate position is 4 cm above the carina).
7. Bronchoscopy should be readily available to:
   - investigate upper airways obstruction (plugging of the proximal bronchial tree by inspissated mucus is the most common cause)

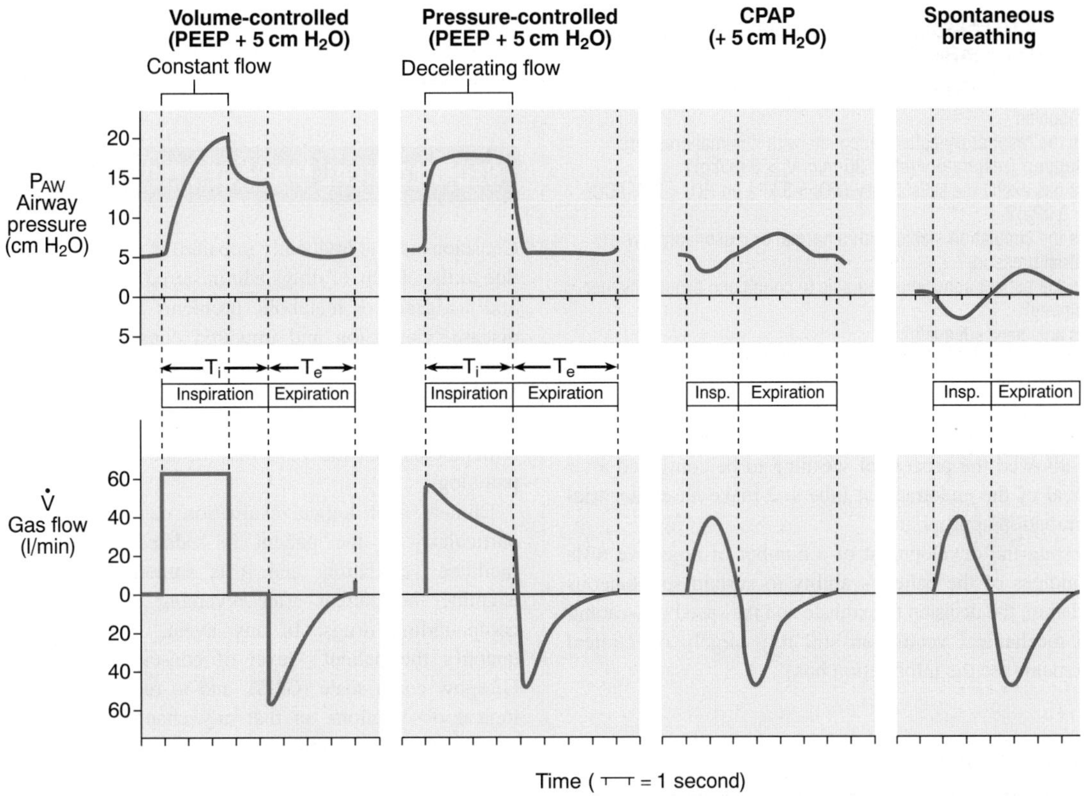

Fig. 15.12 Pressure-time and flow-time curves in mechanical and spontaneous ventilation. In volume-controlled mode, the gas flow is constant until the preset tidal volume is achieved and the airway pressure varies, but in pressure-controlled mode the pressure is constant throughout the inspiratory phase and gas flow varies. The inspiratory time (T_i) is the entire period before the expiratory phase (T_e) starts; in volume-controlled mode it includes the period of gas flow during which the preset tidal volume is achieved, and an end-inspiratory 'pause' time during which there is no flow. In the mandatory modes both the lungs and chest wall/diaphragm are displaced by work from the ventilator and this results in higher airway pressures than in spontaneous breathing when the respiratory muscles contract to produce negative intrathoracic pressure which causes the lungs to inflate at lower airway pressures. Continuous positive airway pressure (CPAP) allows a spontaneous respiratory pattern but with a 'background' pressure raised above atmospheric (positive pressure) throughout the respiratory cycle, i.e. T_i and T_e.

- assist in cases of difficult intubation or tracheostomy tube change
- obtain bronchoalveolar lavage specimens for microbiology
- identify the cause of haemoptysis (not always easy)
- exclude tracheobronchial disruption after thoracic trauma.

WEANING FROM RESPIRATORY SUPPORT

This is the process of progressively reducing and eventually removing all external ventilatory support and associated apparatus. The majority of patients require mechanical ventilatory support for only a few days and do not need weaning. In these patients simple trials of breathing via the endotracheal tube will usually indicate whether the patient can be successfully extubated or not.

In contrast, patients who have required long-term ventilatory support may initially be unable to sustain even a modest degree of respiratory work because their respiratory muscles have become weak. These patients therefore require weaning until respiratory muscle strength improves to the point that all support can be discontinued. This often involves graduation to partial support modes and then non-invasive modes of ventilatory support.

Synchronised intermittent mandatory ventilation (SIMV), pressure support ventilation (PSV), bilevel positive airway pressure (BiPAP) and continuous positive airway pressure (CPAP) are the weaning techniques used to allow the gradual withdrawal of mechanical support (see the information

FACTORS TO CONSIDER IN DECIDING WHETHER OR NOT TO EXTUBATE A VENTILATED PATIENT

- Has the original indication for mechanical ventilation resolved?
- Is the respiratory pattern adequate with minimal pressure support (respiratory rate < 30/min; V_T > 6 ml/kg)?
- Is gas exchange satisfactory (PO_2 > 8 kPa on FiO_2 < 0.4; PCO_2 < 6 kPa)?
- Is the circulation stable, with a normal or reasonably low left atrial pressure?
- Is the patient conscious and able to cough and protect his/her airway?
- Is analgesia adequate?
- Are any metabolic problems well controlled?

boxes). The techniques for non-invasive respiratory support have allowed the process of weaning to be continued after removal of the endotracheal tube and make an earlier trial of extubation appropriate.

Despite the development of a number of objective tests and indices of the patient's ability to sustain spontaneous ventilation, the decision to extubate and the speed of weaning from mechanical ventilation still rely largely on clinical judgement (see the information box).

TRACHEOSTOMY

Patients may be ventilated using modern endotracheal tubes with low pressure cuffs for long periods but the risk of long-term damage to the vocal cords and/or tracheal stenosis means that tracheostomy is usually advisable after 2 weeks or as soon as it is evident that the patient will require prolonged intubation.

A mini-tracheostomy employs a much smaller tube (5–6 mm in diameter) inserted through the cricothyroid membrane, through which a small suction catheter can be passed, and may be useful in patients who have difficulty clearing secretions due to an impaired level of consciousness or weak cough.

TRACHEOSTOMY

Advantages

- Comfort
- Improved mouth care/oral hygiene
- Reduced sedation
- Earlier weaning
- Patient may speak with the cuff deflated or with a special speaking tube inserted

Disadvantages

- Patient must be transferred to an operating theatre
- Haemorrhage
- Infection, particularly *Pseudomonas*, may develop around the stoma

N.B. The technique of percutaneous tracheostomy, performed at the bedside, obviates many of these problems and has encouraged early use of tracheostomy in intubated patients.

NEUROLOGICAL MANAGEMENT

Consciousness is frequently impaired in critically ill patients due to the effects of drugs administered to provide sedation and analgesia, or metabolic problems caused by systemic disease. Confusion and impaired consciousness are also features of sepsis, particularly in the elderly. Moreover, meningitis, cerebral oedema, infarction and haemorrhage may all complicate critical illness and it must be remembered that the CNS may be the site of the primary pathology.

Clinical neurological evaluation can be very difficult, particularly if the patient is sedated or paralysed to facilitate ventilation, and it is sometimes advisable to examine the patient after reversing the effects of the compounding drugs. In any event, it is important to quantify the patient's level of consciousness, using the Glasgow coma scale (GCS), and to record formal neurological observations so that any change in the patient's condition can be identified promptly. If there is evidence of a focal neurological deficit, a CT scan of the brain should be performed followed by a lumbar puncture, provided that raised intracranial pressure has been excluded and severe coagulopathy excluded or treated.

The causes of coma are listed on page 958.

HEAD INJURY

Neurological observations should be recorded frequently (at least hourly) in patients with significant head injuries so that any change, particularly the development of focal neurology, can be identified early. The response to painful stimuli is important; no response or extension of all limbs (decorticate posturing) is associated with severe cortical injury and, unless there is rapid improvement, a very poor prognosis. A flexor response is encouraging and indicates that a good outcome is still possible.

The outcome after severe head injury (GCS < 8) is disappointing; approximately 50% of patients either die or are left in a persistent vegetative state and only one-third recover with little or no residual disability.

RAISED INTRACRANIAL PRESSURE (ICP)

This is a common development in critically ill patients and

is most frequently seen after traumatic head injury or global anoxic insult following cardiac arrest; it may also complicate metabolic disorders, particularly advanced liver failure, and primary cerebral pathologies such as infarction, haemorrhage and tumour.

Rising intracranial pressure may damage the cerebral cortex and can eventually lead to extrusion of the brain stem through the foramen magnum ('coning'), leading to brain-stem death.

Intracranial pressure may be measured via pressure transducers inserted directly into the brain tissue or held in place on the dura. The normal pressure is minus 2 to plus 15 mmHg and sustained pressures of more than 30 mmHg are associated with a very poor prognosis.

Patients with cerebral oedema, particularly following head injury, should be managed according to the following principles:

1. Avoid hypoxaemia and hypotension.
2. Maintain cerebral perfusion pressure (the difference between mean systemic arterial pressure and intracranial pressure) above 65 mmHg.
3. The following strategies may be employed to keep intracranial pressure below 20 mmHg:
   - Use sedation, analgesia and occasionally paralysis to prevent coughing.
   - Nurse with 30° head-up tilt and avoid excessive flexion of the head or pressure around the neck to ensure good cerebral venous pressure drainage.
   - Epileptiform activity must be controlled with appropriate anticonvulsant therapy and an EEG may be necessary to ensure this is achieved.
   - Maintain strict glycaemic control with blood glucose between 4 and 8 mmol/l.
   - Aim for a core body temperature of between 36 and 37°C.
   - Use i.v. normal saline to maintain sodium above 140 mmol/l and avoid either dehydration or fluid overload.
   - Use hyperventilation to reduce the PCO_2 to 30 mmHg (4 kPa) for 24 hours only.

BRAIN DEATH

The preconditions for considering brain-stem death and the criteria for establishing the diagnosis are listed on page 959.

The purpose of declaring formal brain death is to demonstrate that it is futile to continue supporting life with mechanical ventilation, and to meet the legal requirements for organ donation. All intensive care units have a responsibility to identify those patients who meet brain-stem death criteria and to approach the relatives to ask consent for organ donation. This can be a very difficult task but it is easier if the patient was known to carry an organ donor card. In the UK, each region has a team of transplant coordinators who can help with the process and will provide information and advise about the necessary tests.

NUTRITION

In critical illness some degree of negative energy and nitrogen balance is inevitable due to the metabolic milieu that results from the associated inflammatory response. Normal energy expenditure and nitrogen losses in a 70 kg adult are 1500–2000 kCal and 8–12 g respectively; however, these figures may rise to over 3000 kCal and 20 g in the severely catabolic critically ill patient. Some of the problems and complications that may stem from the resulting malnutrition are illustrated in Figure 15.13, which helps to emphasise that adequate nutrition is an essential means of damage limitation in critical illness.

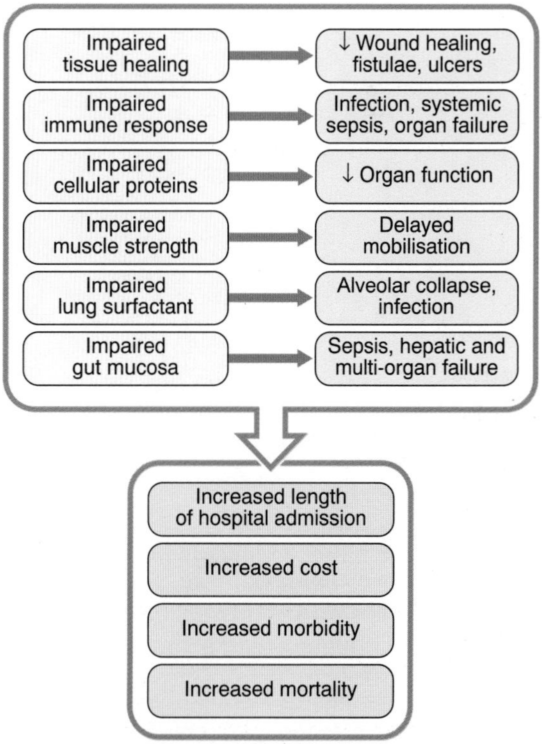

Fig. 15.13 Consequences of malnutrition in critical illness.

Enteral nutrition is always the optimum strategy, and total parenteral nutrition (TPN) should only be started if all attempts to implement enteral feeding have failed (less than 5% of all ICU patients). Appropriate indications for commencing parenteral nutrition include a high gastro-intestinal fistula or perforation, major resection of small bowel and distal bowel obstruction.

The recognition that at least 50% of the energy consumed during normal gut mucosal cell metabolism is derived from glutamine, which is predominantly absorbed from the gut lumen, has led to considerable interest in the potential protective effects of glutamine supplementation and explains the value of establishing enteral feeding as early as possible in the course of critical illness.

FURTHER INFORMATION ON PRINCIPLES OF CRITICAL CARE MEDICINE

Bradley R D, Treacher D F 1996 Intensive care. In: Weatherall D J, Ledingham J G G, Warrell D A (eds) Oxford Textbook of Medicine. Oxford University Press, Oxford

Bradley R D 1977 Studies in acute heart failure. Edward Arnold, London

Goldhill D R, Withington P S 1997 Textbook of intensive care. Chapman & Hall, London

Principles of oncological and palliative care

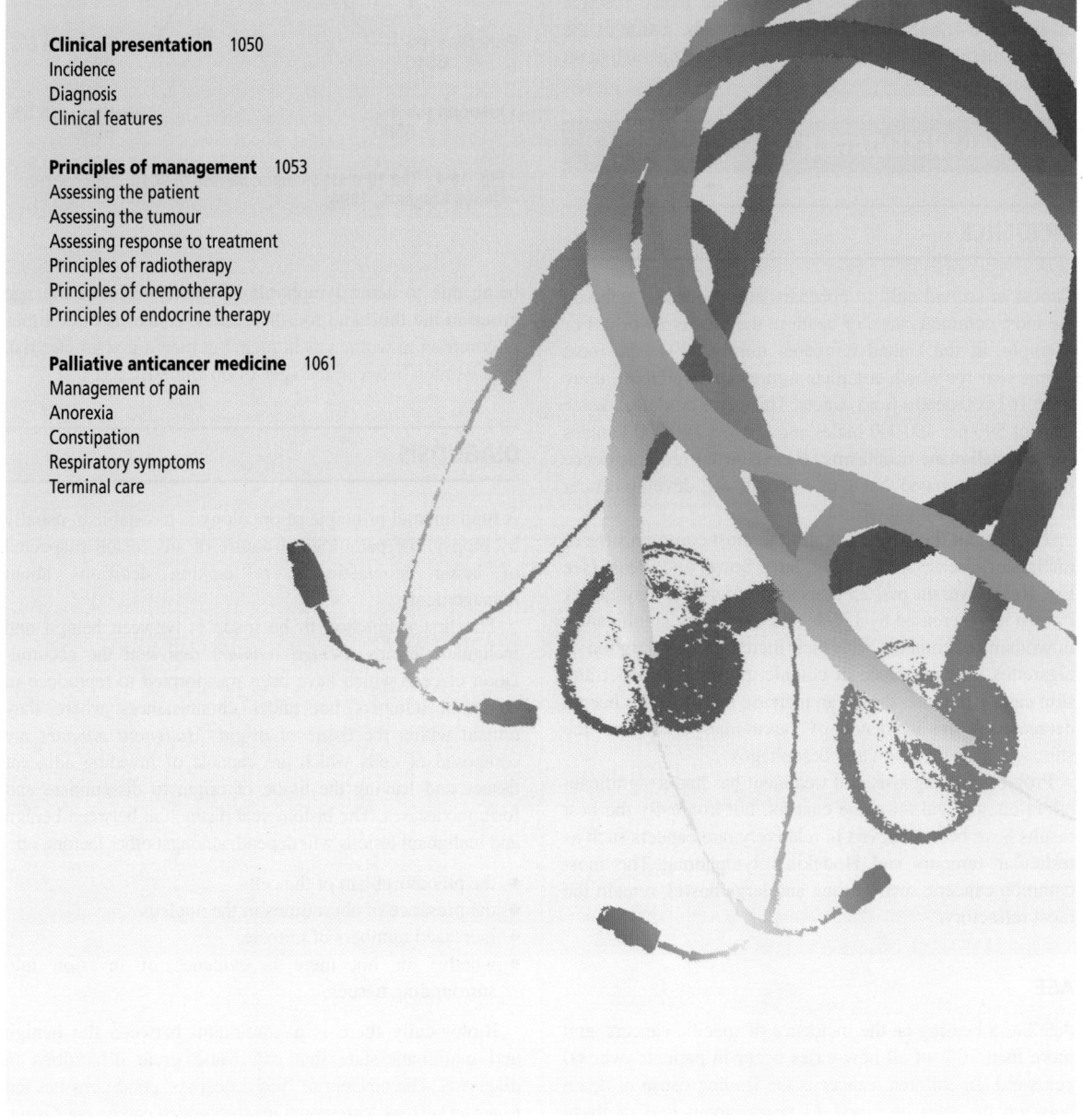

16

J.F. SMYTH

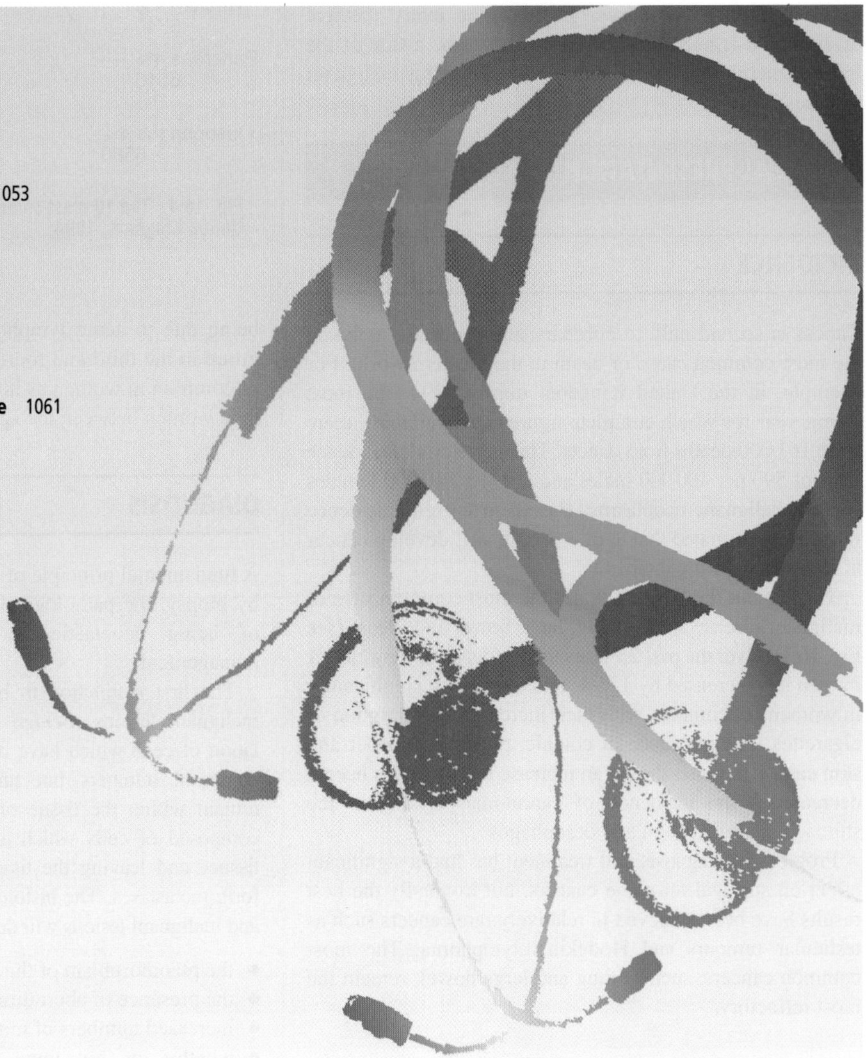

'Oncology' is the study of tumours. 'Neoplasia' means abnormal new growth, which may be benign or malignant. 'Cancer' is a term that is used to describe a wide variety of malignant diseases, the management of which requires several medical disciplines. Traditionally, physicians have played a lesser role than surgeons or radiotherapists in the treatment of these diseases but the development of cytotoxic drugs and major advances in palliative care have resulted in the greater involvement of physicians in the overall management of malignancy. The use of cytotoxic drugs, and of medicines to control the symptoms of advanced malignancy, requires specialised knowledge and experience but since cancer impinges on every medical discipline, it is necessary for all doctors to be aware of the basic principles of investigating and managing malignant diseases.

CLINICAL PRESENTATION

INCIDENCE

Cancer is second only to coronary artery disease as being the most common cause of death in the Western world. For example, in the United Kingdom during 1994 (the most recent year for which complete figures are available), there were 161 000 deaths from cancer. This gives crude incidence rates of 590 per 100 000 males and 566 per 100 000 females for all malignant neoplasms. Based on current incidence rates, it is estimated that 1 in 3 people will develop cancer at some time during their life.

Throughout the Western world the most common sites of malignant disease are the lung, large bowel and breast (see Fig. 16.1). Over the past 25 years the incidence of lung cancer in men has increased by 125%, and even more significantly in women concomitant with their increased consumption of cigarettes. The incidence of colonic, prostatic, bladder and skin cancer has also shown an increase but there has been a decrease in the incidence of carcinomas arising in the stomach, uterus, rectum and oesophagus.

Progress in diagnosis and treatment has had a significant effect on survival for some cancers, but ironically the best results have been achieved in relatively rare cancers such as testicular tumours and Hodgkin's lymphoma. The most common cancers, such as lung and large bowel, remain the most refractory.

AGE

Age has a bearing on the incidence of specific cancers, and more than 70% of all new cases occur in patients over 60 years old. In children, cancer is the leading cause of death between the ages of 3 and 13 years, about half of these being due to acute lymphoblastic leukaemia. For the age group in the third and fourth decades, cancer is three times as common in women as in men, but men are at greater risk than women between the ages of 60 and 80.

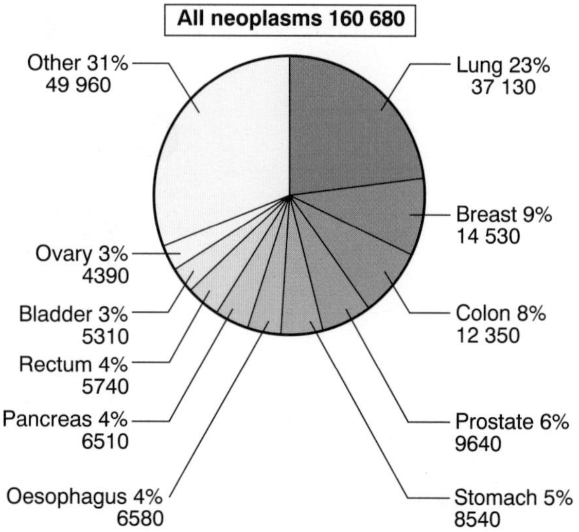

Fig. 16.1 The 10 most common causes of death from cancer, United Kingdom, 1994.

DIAGNOSIS

A fundamental principle of oncology is to establish, usually by biopsy, the pathological nature of any lesion suspected of being neoplastic before making decisions about management.

The first distinction to be made is between benign and malignant lesions. *Benign tumours* represent the accumulation of cells which have been transformed to reproduce in abnormal numbers but under circumstances where they remain within the tissue of origin. *Malignant tumours* are composed of cells which are capable of invading adjacent tissues and leaving the tissue of origin to disseminate and form metastases. The histological distinction between benign and malignant lesions will depend, amongst other factors, on:

- the pleomorphism of the cells
- the presence of aberrations in the nucleus
- increased numbers of mitoses
- whether or not there is evidence of invasion into surrounding tissues.

Biologically there is a continuum between the benign and malignant state that can cause great difficulties in diagnosis. The concept of 'pre-cancerous' conditions has led to terms such as 'carcinoma in situ', which can be confusing.

Table 16.1 Classification of cancers

Type	Tissue or cell of origin	Examples
Carcinoma	Endoderm or ectoderm	Epithelial lining of gut (e.g. adenocarcinoma of colon) or bronchus (e.g. squamous cell or small-cell carcinoma of bronchus)
Sarcoma	Mesoderm	Osteosarcoma Fibrosarcoma
Leukaemia	White blood cell	Acute lymphoblastic leukaemia
Lymphoma	Monocyte, macrophage	Hodgkin's disease

To be preferred is the term 'intraepithelial neoplasia', which recognises the continuum between dysplasia or atypical hyperplasia and 'carcinoma in situ'. A grading system is frequently used with intraepithelial neoplasia to indicate increasing degrees of severity, e.g. for cervical cancer CIN-1, CIN-2 and CIN-3, where CIN-1 represents minimal morphological change and CIN-3 the carcinoma in situ state where the entire epithelium from basement membrane to the surface is composed of malignant cells.

Cancers are classified into four major groups (see Table 16.1). Within a given tissue there may be major differences in the cell type from which the tumour has arisen. Thus, for example, bronchogenic carcinomas are classified histologically into four major groups: squamous carcinomas, adenocarcinomas, and small-cell and large-cell undifferentiated carcinomas.

Such distinctions are essential to clinical management since the choice between surgery, radiotherapy and chemotherapy will depend on whether the lesion is benign or malignant, and whether or not the particular histological subtype is sensitive to radiotherapy or chemotherapy. As regards the latter, there is a great variation in the sensitivity of different tumours to different cytotoxic drugs, and therefore appropriate therapy can be prescribed only when the tumour tissue has been accurately classified.

Although there is evidence to support the concept that many human tumours arise from the transformation of a single cell, i.e. are clonal in origin, it is not unusual to find a mixed histological picture; for example, in the testis, teratomas and seminomatous tissue may occur together, and in the lung, squamous and small-cell undifferentiated tumours may present in the same biopsy specimen.

In addition to defining whether the tumour is benign or malignant and from which cell type it arises, it is useful to define the degree of differentiation or anaplasia of the cancer cell since, for many tumour types, this has been shown to correlate with prognosis and response to treatment.

CYTOLOGY

Whilst most histology is performed on tissue that is obtained by surgical biopsy, in certain circumstances it is possible to achieve excellent classification from cytology alone. Thus, for example, sputum may be examined for malignant bronchogenic cells, pleural or peritoneal effusions may provide suitable cells for diagnostic purposes, and smears can be prepared from the uterine cervix. Increasing use is being made of needle aspiration for cytological diagnosis. A fine-gauge needle can be inserted into breast lumps, subcutaneous deposits, and intrathoracic or hepatic lesions, and a smear for cytological evaluation can be made from the aspirated material. In experienced hands, this technique has many advantages over the more conventional surgical biopsy technique, mainly because of speed and simplicity.

IMMUNOHISTOCHEMISTRY

The production of polyclonal and, more recently, monoclonal antibodies has made a very significant contribution to the further identification and classification of histological and cytological preparations of tumour tissues. Highly specific antibodies raised against tumour antigens can be labelled with fluorescein or used in immunohistochemical techniques to detect tumour cell products such as enzymes, hormones or receptors. This technique can be used for the more confident distinction between benign and malignant tissues, and to differentiate between histological subtypes of similar tumours; for example, in a histologically undifferentiated bronchogenic tumour a monoclonal antibody that stains positively for mucin, used in conjunction with one that detects keratin, may help distinguish an adenocarcinoma from a squamous carcinoma. Similarly, immunophenotyping (as it is called) of lymphomas and leukaemias can greatly enhance the distinction between morphologically related subtypes. Such categorisation is important in predicting the natural history of an individual patient's illness and in selecting the most appropriate therapy.

TUMOUR MARKERS

The presence of viable tumour tissue in the body may be detectable by the presence in the blood of biochemical products known as 'tumour markers'. These are normal metabolic constituents that are found either in abnormal amounts or at an inappropriate time of life—for example, fetal proteins being re-expressed in adult life.

Tumour markers of this type can be helpful in a number of different clinical situations. In theory they might be useful for screening whole populations for undetected cancers but in practice this has not proved useful. The predictive value of a screening test depends on the sensitivity of the test, its specificity and the prevalence of the particular disease. Sensitivity refers to the number of times a test is positive for patients known to have the disease, i.e. true positives, and specificity refers to the incidence of true negatives, i.e. that the test should prove negative in people known to be free of the disease. Unfortunately, sensitivity is inversely related to specificity. For example, it is known that some gastrointestinal tumours contain carcinoembryonic antigen (CEA), a substance that is present in the gut during fetal life but which is not found in normal adult gastrointestinal tissues. Radioimmunoassays of CEA in blood have shown an overall 67% positivity in patients with colorectal carcinoma but the test is also positive in alcoholic cirrhosis (70%), emphysema (57%) and diabetes mellitus (38%), amongst many other diseases. Screening the population at large for subclinical carcinomas of the colon with this method would therefore fail because of lack of specificity.

However, the presence of a tumour marker can be of clinical value in monitoring the progress of individual patients known to have a given malignancy. For example, testicular teratomas not infrequently secrete another oncofetal protein—alpha-fetoprotein (AFP). Figure 16.2 illustrates a typical case where, during the months following surgical resection of the primary tumour, a rising level of AFP was associated with (and preceded) the clinical appearance of metastases. The successful use of chemotherapy was associated with a disappearance of the abnormal tumour marker.

Table 16.2 illustrates some of the tumour markers currently in use to aid in prognosis and/or follow the effects of treatment.

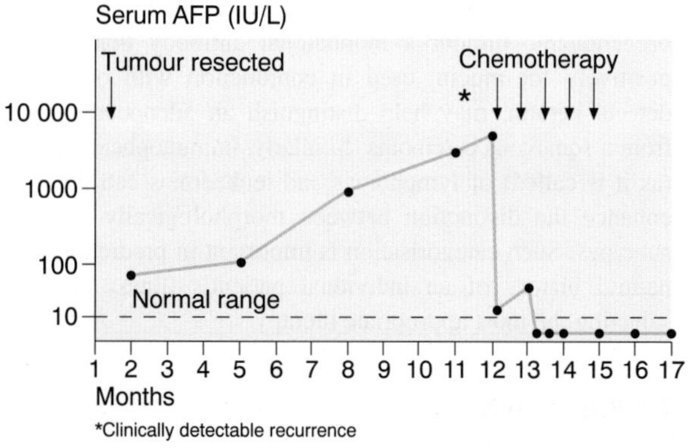

Fig. 16.2 Serum alpha-fetoprotein (AFP) levels in a young man with testicular teratoma. The levels of AFP fluctuate with disease state and can be used to monitor the effects of the treatment.

Table 16.2 Serum tumour markers

Cancer	Marker
Testicular (germ cell)	Alpha-fetoprotein (AFP) β-human chorionic gonadotrophin (β-HCG)
Choriocarcinoma	β-HCG
Ovary	Ca-125
Prostate	Prostate specific antigen (PSA)
Hepatocellular carcinoma	AFP
Colorectal	CEA

CLINICAL FEATURES

Malignant diseases manifest themselves in a variety of ways resulting from general or localised effects. Some of these are illustrated in Figure 16.3. The presence of an abnormal accumulation of cells may, by virtue of its physical bulk alone, produce clinical symptoms and signs. Thus, for example, painless swellings in the breast or in muscle may indicate an underlying carcinoma or sarcoma respectively. Lymphomas usually present as painless enlargements of lymph nodes or spleen. Intracranial space-occupying lesions may cause focal manifestations, fits, headaches, vomiting and papilloedema. Tumours in the distal colon may partially obstruct the lumen of the bowel with a resulting change in bowel habit. Bronchogenic tumours may cause cough or shortness of breath resulting from partial or complete occlusion of an airway.

HAEMORRHAGE

Malignant tumours not infrequently present as haemorrhage from an eroded epithelial surface. For example, bronchogenic

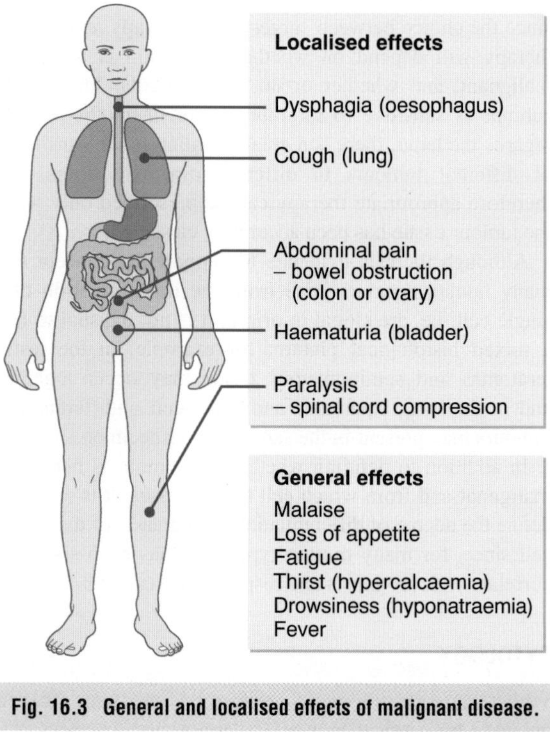

Fig. 16.3 General and localised effects of malignant disease.

carcinomas may present with haemoptysis, gastric carcinomas with iron deficiency anaemia or, occasionally, haematemesis, colonic carcinoma with bleeding per rectum, and renal and bladder carcinomas with haematuria.

PAIN

This is often thought to be an inevitable accompaniment of malignant disease but in fact it is not a common symptom, especially at presentation of most cancers. When pain does occur, it usually reflects either nerve compression or distension of an organ. The most common peripheral nerve compressions are due to involvement of the brachial plexus (carcinomas of the lung or breast), the sacral plexus (carcinomas of the rectum or cervix) or the paraspinal nerves (carcinomas of the pancreas). Metastatic tumours in the liver may cause pain as a result of distension and stretching of its capsule. Bone pain resulting from primary, or more commonly, secondary deposits usually occurs in the weight-bearing bones, and results from compression secondary to weakening of the structural component of the bone. Pathological fractures may arise as a consequence. Patients may present with referred pain, most frequently in the shoulder, hip or knee, as when a nerve root is involved directly or by metastases.

CACHEXIA

This is a profound state of general ill health—anorexia, weight loss and altered metabolism. It is a clinical feature of many malignant diseases presenting at an advanced stage, especially carcinomas of the gastrointestinal tract, lung, ovary and testis. Cachexia is not, however, a universal phenomenon; it is rare in breast cancer and in tumours of the central nervous system, and uncommon in leukaemia and lymphomas.

Cachexia may arise as a direct result of malnutrition from a tumour in the gastrointestinal tract. Malabsorption may arise rarely as a consequence of tumour replacing the absorptive epithelia but more commonly from reduced exocrine function (from carcinomas of the pancreas), or loss of bile from carcinomas of the upper gastrointestinal tract that obstruct biliary outflow. Loss of taste and the malaise that accompanies many malignant diseases may contribute to poor food intake but all of these factors in promoting malnutrition do not of themselves fully explain the cachexia of malignancy. Although many patients will have a negative nitrogen balance, others who are in positive balance may show caloric deficit. It has been shown that in the cachexia accompanying malignant disease, caloric expenditure remains high, with an elevated basal metabolic rate despite reduced dietary intake (the reverse of the situation that follows starvation); this indicates that the phenomenon results from a profound systemic derangement of host metabolism, the pathogenesis of which remains unclear.

PARANEOPLASTIC FEATURES

In addition to generalised clinical features that are commonly associated with the presentation of a malignant disease, there are a variety of syndromes for which the term 'paraneoplastic' has been used. These syndromes include many that arise as a result of the secretion into the blood of tumour products (usually polypeptide hormones) which produce clinical symptoms and signs as a consequence of their action on target organs remote from the primary tumour.

A number of neurological paraneoplastic syndromes have been described for which the tumour product remains unknown. These include peripheral neuropathies, a myasthenia-like syndrome and subacute cerebellar degeneration. Whilst all of these syndromes may improve with successful treatment of the primary tumour, complete resolution is rare.

Dermatomyositis and polymyositis (see p. 860) present as gradually progressive muscle weakness predominantly affecting the proximal musculature, coming on over a period of months. Whilst these disorders are not universally associated with malignancy, patients suffering from them have a greatly increased risk of an underlying neoplasm compared with the general public, and malignancies of the breast, lung and gastrointestinal and genitourinary tracts should be considered.

Acanthosis nigricans (see p. 919), a rare condition characterised by the appearance of black velvety verrucose lesions in the flexures around the neck, axillae and groin, is particularly seen in patients with carcinomas of the stomach.

PRINCIPLES OF MANAGEMENT

In order to plan optimal management for an individual patient the doctor must:

- have an understanding of the therapeutic options for the particular disease in question
- assess the patient to decide which options are appropriate (e.g. is it a realistic aim to cure the patient or should treatment be focused on palliation of symptoms?)
- (related to the point above) assess the tumour, particularly to define whether or not it has metastasised.

ASSESSING THE PATIENT

As a general rule, patients should be informed that they have a malignant disease prior to starting treatment but not necessarily of the exact prognosis.

The first interview with a patient suspected of having a malignant disease should be performed in a quiet and unhurried manner. In addition to a routine history of symptoms and previous illnesses, it is important to ascertain whether patients already know that they have a malignant disease and what this means to them. The patient will be helped very considerably by positive assurance that symptoms can almost always be improved, even if the underlying disease cannot be eradicated.

The essence of good oncologic management is to develop good communication between doctor and patient. First and foremost, this requires that the doctor learns to *listen* to the patient. Detailed studies of patients' attitudes to the diagnosis of cancer have identified common trends in behaviour. Initial shock is replaced by disbelief (sometimes even denial), leading on to a mixture of anxiety and depression, usually followed by a measure of acceptance. The doctor must be sensitive to the patient's needs, which will vary during the difficult transition from shock to acceptance, and must be prepared to discuss the effect of each phase on the individual patient. A common failing on the part of doctors who are not prepared to engage in this challenging dialogue is to use distancing or avoidance techniques (consciously or unconsciously) that create a barrier for the patient and may greatly undermine the value of subsequent treatment. Examples of such avoidance behaviour include ignoring distressing comments offered by the patient in favour of paying attention selectively to less emotional—usually physical—factors; offering inappropriate reassurance to patients about the outcome of treatment—e.g. rapid relief of pain—and the use of statements such as 'you should not worry about …', denying the patient further participation in discussion.

PERFORMANCE STATUS

In addition to the anatomical assessment of tumour extent evaluated by staging procedures (see below), it is important to assess the overall degree of functional impairment that the disease is causing the patient at the time of diagnosis. A variety of 'performance status' scales have been devised, such as the Eastern Cooperative Oncology Group (ECOG) scale shown in the information box. These have been found useful in assessing prognosis and also the efficacy and toxicity of treatment.

EASTERN COOPERATIVE ONCOLOGY GROUP PERFORMANCE STATUS SCALE

- **0** Fully active, able to carry on all usual activities without restriction and without the aid of analgesics
- **1** Restricted in strenuous activity but ambulatory and able to carry out light work or pursue a sedentary occupation. This group also contains patients who are fully active, as in grade 0, but only with the aid of analgesics
- **2** Ambulatory and capable of all self-care but unable to work. Up and about more than 50% of waking hours
- **3** Capable of only limited self-care, confined to bed or chair more than 50% of waking hours
- **4** Completely disabled, unable to carry out any self-care and confined totally to bed or chair

ASSESSING THE TUMOUR

Tumours that have not metastasised are amenable to local forms of treatment (e.g. surgery or radiotherapy), whilst tumours that have already disseminated require systemic treatment with chemotherapy or hormonal therapy. It is frequently necessary to use a combination of these measures, particularly if aiming for complete eradication of the tumour. Radiotherapy and chemotherapy both act by causing damage to DNA. This will occur not only in tumour cells but in any normal host cells that are exposed to treatment. Hence the doses of either form of treatment are limited by the tolerance of normal tissues, rather than by the 'sensitivity' of the cancer cells. Some host toxicity is inevitable and for this reason it is important to decide whether or not cure is feasible in order to minimise treatment-related toxicity in circumstances where an aggressive therapeutic approach would be inappropriate.

STAGING

It is usually necessary to perform specialised investigations to determine the extent of dissemination of the tumour prior to selecting treatment—the process of 'staging' the tumour. Staging investigations take time and the delay causes anxiety for the patient.

Staging is important both for the selection of appropriate treatment, and to provide information about prognosis. Usually advancing stage indicates a worse prognosis, even if the tumour has not yet metastasised. Inadequate or inaccurate staging may lead to under- or over-treatment, resulting in failure to cure or unnecessary toxicity respectively.

The internationally recognised staging system is known as the TNM classification and is shown in the information box. It is a clinical staging system but if supplemented by the pathological examination of biopsied or resected specimens the suffix 'p' is added.

The TNM system is increasingly being used for the majority of malignant diseases, particularly to facilitate comparisons of the results of treatments in different international centres. For certain diseases it has proved useful to define staging systems which differ from the TNM classification, as, for example, the Ann Arbor staging for Hodgkin's lymphoma and Dukes classification for carcinomas of the rectum.

TNM CLASSIFICATION	
T*	Extent of primary tumour
N*	Extent of regional lymph node involvement
M	Presence or absence of metastases
Extent of disease	
• T0	Excised tumour
• T1 • T2 • T3	Increases in primary tumour size
Increased involvement of nodes	
• N1 • N2 • N3	Increasing involvement
Presence of metastases	
• M0	Not present
• M1	Present
* Exact criteria of size and region of nodal involvement have been defined for each anatomical site.	

The investigations required to define the T, N or M status of a tumour vary for different diseases. Examples are shown in the information box below.

INVESTIGATIONS TO DEFINE TNM STATUS

Tumour

- Palpation
- Inspection including endoscopy (e.g. bronchoscopy, cystoscopy)
- Radiology (conventional, computed tomography (CT), magnetic resonance imaging)
- Cytology/aspiration/biopsy

Nodes

- Palpation
- Aspiration
- Biopsy
- Radiology (CT scanning)

Metastases

- Biochemical screening (e.g. liver function tests)
- Radionuclide scans (e.g. liver, brain, bone)
- Ultrasound of liver
- Radiology (e.g. chest radiograph, CT scan of liver, brain, thorax)
- Laparoscopy
- Laparotomy

ASSESSING RESPONSE TO TREATMENT

With presently available therapies most methods of cancer treatment are associated with significant morbidity. It is thus essential to evaluate the response to therapy as accurately as possible and use properly defined criteria for evaluating response, so as to make valid comparisons between different treatments. The concept of 'survival time', especially the traditional use of '5-year survival', places too much emphasis on cure. Since palliation is a much more common objective in management planning, more subtle criteria are required than crude survival figures.

The terms universally accepted for evaluating treatment are defined as shown in the information box.

TERMS FOR EVALUATING TREATMENT

Objective response

- Any response that fulfils the criteria of complete or partial response

Complete response

- Complete disappearance of all known disease in the absence of any new lesions appearing

Partial response

- A reduction in size by at least 50% of the tumour in the absence of any new lesions appearing

No response

- No change, or an increase of less than 25% or decrease of no greater than 25% in the size of the tumour in the absence of new lesions

Progressive disease

- Increase in the size of the tumour by at least 25% or the development of any new lesions

The term 'complete response' may or may not indicate true eradication of the tumour and for any given disease these terms can only reflect the ability to detect viable tumour.

PRINCIPLES OF RADIOTHERAPY

It is important that physicians should be familiar with an outline of the procedures involved when their patients are referred for this form of treatment.

Radiotherapy involves the exposure of a defined area of the body to a source of ionising radiation under carefully controlled conditions. Treatment planning involves accurate localisation of the tumour and prescription of multiple daily fractions of irradiation for a specified period of time. The biological effect of radiation depends on the amount of energy absorbed per unit mass. The unit of absorbed dose is the gray (Gy) and is equivalent to 1 joule per kilogram.

Ionising radiation damages cells by interaction with nuclear DNA, thus preventing the normal reproduction of that cell. As with cytotoxic drugs there is only a relative selectivity in this process, and normal (non-malignant) cells are readily damaged by radiation. For this reason radiotherapy planning must take into account the exact anatomical distribution of the tumour in order to minimise the exposure of normal tissues, whilst at the same time ensuring that all of the diseased tissues are included in the treated area. Great care is taken to ensure that the patient can be accurately and reproducibly repositioned whilst radiotherapy is being undertaken.

Patients are usually treated in the supine position although the prone position may be more suitable for some abdominal and pelvic tumours. In order to immobilise the area to be treated, moulds, casts and shells are constructed for the individual patient.

With the patient comfortably positioned and the treatment area immobilised, the tumour is localised by a variety of techniques such as the placement of radio-opaque seeds in the tumour or the use of contrast media as in conventional radiography. Increasingly, computed tomography (CT) is being used to assist in planning radiotherapeutic treatment, especially since CT can provide information about tumour margins in the transverse plane in which most radiotherapy is administered.

EQUIPMENT

Radiotherapy localisation is usually carried out on specialised equipment known as a simulator, which is designed to allow isocentric rotation and thus to simulate the exact axis distance of the treatment machine.

To maximise the absorbed dose within the tumour area and minimise the dose to normal tissues, treatment is given through multiple portals—for example, as a four-field box technique for the pelvis—or through fields at right angles to each other with wedge filters to even the dose distribution where the beams overlap.

TELETHERAPY

Most radiotherapy is performed with 'teletherapy' techniques, i.e. a beam of photons is used to irradiate the tumour from outside the patient. Alternatively for specific sites, 'brachytherapy' is used, whereby a source of radiation is implanted in a body cavity or within the tumour itself. Teletherapy techniques include the use of low-energy ortho- or kilovoltage sources and the more widely used megavoltage sources. Low-energy radiation (50–100 kVp range) is useful for treating carcinomas of the skin and lip, and orthovoltage (250–300 kVp) machines are sometimes used for the palliative treatment of bone metastases and lesions of the chest wall. However, orthovoltage machines are unsuitable for the treatment of more deep-seated tumours.

^{60}Cobalt machines and linear accelerators are the most widely used teletherapy equipment. ^{60}Cobalt machines provide a less well-defined beam of radiation than a linear accelerator. In addition to producing X-rays, the high-energy linear accelerators can be used to produce accelerated electrons. The latter are charged particles which are absorbed within a finite range of tissue and can be useful in the treatment of superficial lesions where it is desirable to spare underlying tissues. Thus, for example, electrons may be employed (with advantage) for the treatment of some lesions of the head and neck, lymph nodes near the spinal cord, and lesions of the chest wall such as occur in breast carcinoma.

FRACTIONATION OF DOSE

Radiotherapy is most frequently prescribed in daily fractions of 2 gray (Gy) for 5 days a week where, depending on the tumour type and management plan, treatment may continue for 3–6 weeks. This fractionation of dose is used in order to increase the tumoricidal effect without increasing normal tissue damage. Many patients, particularly those treated with target volumes greater than 500 cm^3, will experience some malaise and fatigue. Nausea and anorexia are common and vomiting is a frequent problem if it is necessary to irradiate very large volumes, particularly in the upper abdomen. Acute skin reaction usually consists of mild erythema, best treated by keeping the skin dry. Oral and pharyngeal mucosal reactions are common if the area receives high radiation doses. Particular attention to oral hygiene is required and close inspection for candidiasis is essential.

Radiation effects on the bone marrow may occur. Minor decreases in lymphocyte count are common and a frequent check on the peripheral blood must be made throughout treatment. Maintenance of haemoglobin is important since hypoxia may render the tumour less sensitive to radiation damage. Irradiation of the gastrointestinal tract may result in temporary dysphagia, diarrhoea, tenesmus or production of mucus per rectum.

PRINCIPLES OF CHEMOTHERAPY

During the 1940s research into the action of mustard gas showed that sulphur and nitrogen mustard could destroy dividing cells in lymph nodes and the bone marrow. The potential therapeutic benefit was explored in treating some lymphomas with nitrogen mustard, which was then developed as the first clinically useful cytotoxic drug. Study of the effects of altering folic acid metabolism in leukaemic cells resulted in the second cytotoxic drug of therapeutic value—the antifolate, methotrexate. Thereafter, many naturally occurring substances were tested, resulting in some 35 effective antineoplastic drugs.

CLASSIFICATION OF ANTICANCER DRUGS

Anticancer drugs are divided into six main groups (see Table 16.3). The site of action of each group is shown in Figure 16.4.

Table 16.3 Classification of anticancer drugs

Group	Examples
1. **Antimetabolites** (metabolism of substance in parenthesis is interrupted)	Methotrexate (folic acid) 6-mercaptopurine (hypoxanthine) 6-thioguanine (guanine) 5-fluorouracil (uracil) Cytosine arabinoside (cytidine)
2. **Alkylating agents**	Nitrogen mustard Cyclophosphamide Chlorambucil Busulphan Melphalan Iphosphamide
3. **Plant alkaloids**	Vinblastine Vincristine Vindesine VP-16-213 VM 26
4. **Antibiotics**	Doxorubicin Daunorubicin Actinomycin D Bleomycin Mitomycin C
5. **Taxanes**	Taxol Taxotere
6. **Miscellaneous synthetic compounds**	DTIC Cisplatinum Procarbazine Hexamethylmelamine Hydroxyurea Mitozantrone

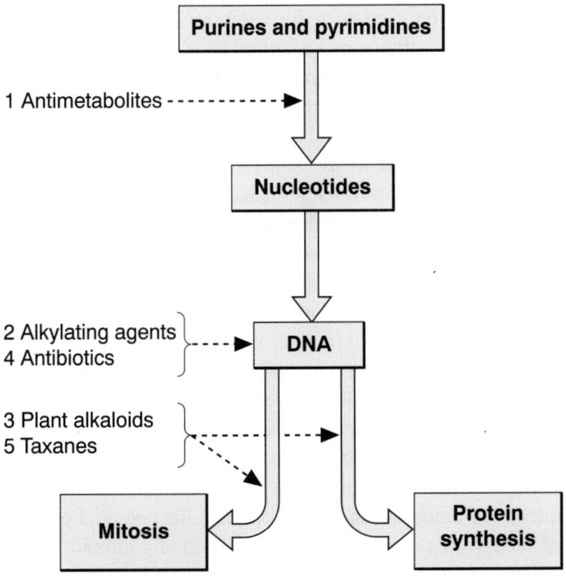

Fig. 16.4 Anticancer drugs: site of action of major groups.

Antimetabolites

Methotrexate acts to inhibit folate metabolism by preventing the cell from replenishing its source of reduced folates necessary for purine and pyrimidine synthesis (see p. 759). The term 'antimetabolite' is used for this group of drugs.

Alkylating agents

Nitrogen mustard is thought to destroy cells by the process of alkylation—the addition of an alkyl group to constituents of DNA, thus interfering with replication and transcription of messenger RNA.

Plant alkaloids

These inhibit cell division by binding to tubulin and disrupting the mitotic spindle.

Antibiotics

The compounds grouped together as antibiotics include doxorubicin and actinomycin, which act by intercalating between base pairs and DNA, and bleomycin, which causes breaks in both single- and double-stranded DNA.

Taxanes

These naturally derived products act by stabilising the mitotic spindle.

THERAPEUTIC INDEX

Unfortunately none of these biochemical events is confined to the metabolism of malignant cells. Systemic exposure to these cellular poisons therefore must inevitably result in some damage to normal host tissues, particularly to those which rely on rapid cell division, such as the bone marrow and gastrointestinal tract. In addition to their relative lack of selectivity, anticancer drugs are very potent because they act at low concentrations. Together with a tendency towards steep dose-response curves, these factors all account for the narrow 'therapeutic index' of cytotoxic drugs (see Fig. 16.5).

The narrow therapeutic index of antineoplastic drugs means that the greatest care is required in their administration. Whenever anticancer drugs are used, it is necessary to monitor the peripheral blood count and be aware of any functional disturbances such as dysphagia or diarrhoea. Since the maximum dose of any cytotoxic drug that can be prescribed on any one occasion is governed by its toxicity to normal cells, only partial tumour shrinkage results from any single treatment. It is therefore necessary to administer these drugs repeatedly, the total duration of treatment varying from a few months to several years. To prevent damage to host tissues, intermittent administration is necessary to allow host tissue to recover between treatments. Damage to bone marrow results in depression of the blood counts 10–14 days later. Thus many cytotoxic drug regimens are given on 21-day cycles to preserve bone marrow integrity.

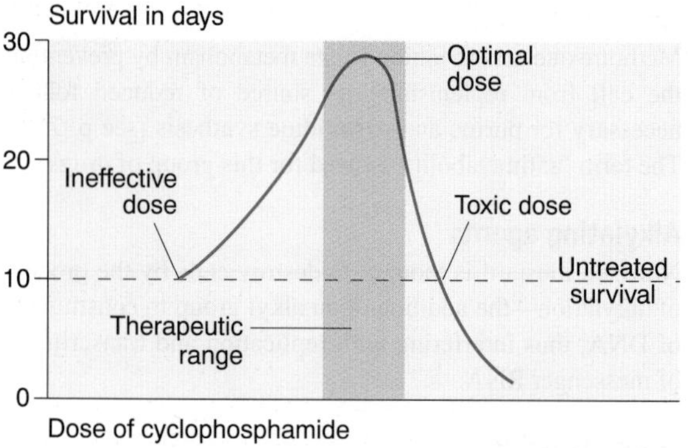

Fig. 16.5 Dose-response curve for cyclophosphamide in mice bearing the L1210 leukaemia. Too low a dose is ineffective but beyond a narrow therapeutic range too high a dose kills the animals from haematological toxicity.

Drug resistance

The problem of drug resistance continues to be the subject of major attention for cancer research workers. Distinction is made between 'intrinsic' and 'acquired' drug resistance. The former is typified by malignant melanoma or renal cell cancer, where currently available drugs have little or no effect on cancer growth. Conversely, 'acquired' resistance is exemplified by small-cell lung cancer—a disease that is initially highly sensitive to a range of cytotoxic drugs, but where drug-resistant clones of cells eventually emerge and the disease recurs. Many biological factors contribute to the development of acquired drug resistance but one major process that has been revealed involves the enhanced production of a glycoprotein termed p180. This normally occurring transmembrane protein can be produced in greatly enhanced quantity by genetic amplification as a cancer cell reacts to the presence of a perceived poison (a cytotoxic drug). The p180 protein acts as a transport pump which extrudes drug from within the cell, thereby rescuing itself from cytotoxic damage. This form of drug resistance is seen in response to several classes of anticancer drug, e.g. doxorubicin, the vinca alkaloids and the epipodophylotoxins. Research is now focused on finding ways to block the amplification of p180 and thereby prevent the emergence of this type of drug resistance.

COMBINATION CHEMOTHERAPY

The theory behind combination chemotherapy is that simultaneous disruption of the metabolism of a tumour cell at more than one site may have far more profound effects on the cell than a single metabolic lesion. Thus, for example, in Hodgkin's disease, a treatment with the four-drug combination of nitrogen mustard, vincristine, procarbazine and prednisolone yields complete remissions in more than 80% of patients, whereas when these same drugs were used singly they produced remissions in only 15–20% of cases. Similarly, combination chemotherapy for acute leukaemia has increased the remission rate from 20% to 90%.

Combination chemotherapy is valuable in many other malignant diseases including carcinomas of the breast, ovary, lung and testis, and several of the childhood tumours. The five general principles governing its use are listed in the information box.

GENERAL PRINCIPLES OF COMBINATION CHEMOTHERAPY

- Each drug in the combination should have been demonstrated to have some activity on its own against the tumour type for which the combination is being used
- Drugs with a similar mechanism of action should not be combined
- As far as is possible the major dose-limiting toxicity of each drug should differ from that of the other components of the combination
- Since it is rarely possible to avoid some overlap in toxicity to host tissues, it is usually necessary to reduce the dose of each of the component drugs compared with the optimal dose which would be used if the drugs were prescribed individually
- There should be no known adverse interaction between the drugs

MULTIMODALITY TREATMENT

Since in many situations cytotoxic drugs are capable of shrinking only a proportion of the tumour, increasing attention has been paid to the use of chemotherapy in conjunction with surgery or radiotherapy. Thus chemotherapy can be used to reduce tumour bulk prior to local therapy with surgery or radiotherapy—as, for example, in treating head and neck tumours—or drug treatment can be introduced after primary resection or irradiation to prevent the growth of subclinical micrometastases. The latter is frequently referred to as 'adjuvant' chemotherapy, and is now widely used for treating breast carcinomas, lymphomas, and several tumours in children.

Caution must be exercised to prevent additive damage to host tissues, particularly to bone marrow if radiotherapy and chemotherapy are used together, but the principle of combining local and systemic therapy has many potential advantages, since as a general principle small tumours are much more susceptible to chemotherapy than large ones. This is explained in part by the fact that drugs penetrate small tumours more effectively but also by the fact that the emergence of drug resistance may be related to the frequency of mutations in the tumour, and the potential number of such events increases with the growth of a tumour.

One major difficulty with adjuvant chemotherapy is to decide for how long it should be continued. In obvious advanced tumours, it is possible to measure tumour shrinkage and continue treatment for as long as benefit lasts. Conversely, drug resistance is detectable and thus further inappropriate chemotherapy can be avoided. However, in the 'adjuvant' setting where there is no measurable tumour, it is not possible to be certain in the short term whether or not treatment is proving effective. Clinical trials have demonstrated that, for curable tumours in children, it is necessary to continue chemotherapy for 1–2 years. For lymphomas and carcinomas in adults, the optimum duration of adjuvant chemotherapy is less certain.

Of the common tumours, breast cancer has been researched in the greatest detail and it is now accepted that adjuvant chemotherapy results in significant prolongation both of disease-free and overall survival, especially for pre-menopausal women where tumours do not contain oestrogen receptors (see below). The most widely used adjuvant treatment is a combination of cyclophosphamide, methotrexate and 5-fluorouracil (CMF), administered for 6 months after primary surgery.

CONTRIBUTION OF CHEMOTHERAPY TO MANAGEMENT OF VARIOUS MALIGNANT DISEASES

Tumours for which chemotherapy can be curative

- Acute lymphoblastic leukaemia in children
- Burkitt's lymphoma
- Hodgkin's lymphoma
- Wilms tumour
- Rhabdomyosarcoma
- Testicular teratoma
- Choriocarcinoma
- Diffuse histiocytic lymphoma
- Ewing's sarcoma

Tumours highly sensitive to chemotherapy—remissions prolong life

- Breast carcinoma
- Ovarian carcinoma
- Small-cell anaplastic lung carcinoma
- Non-Hodgkin's lymphoma
- Chronic lymphocytic leukaemia
- Acute myeloid leukaemia
- Medulloblastoma

Tumours sensitive to chemotherapy—life sometimes prolonged

- Gastric carcinoma
- Pancreatic carcinoma
- Myeloma
- Colorectal carcinoma
- Bladder carcinoma
- Anaplastic thyroid carcinoma

Tumours refractory to available chemotherapy

- Squamous cell lung carcinoma
- Soft tissue sarcoma
- Carcinoma of the oesophagus
- Melanoma

It is possible to rank many malignant diseases into groups comprising those for which chemotherapy contributes to cure, those for which effective control prolongs useful life and those for which benefit is less certain or unproven. These are listed in the information box.

SIDE-EFFECTS OF CHEMOTHERAPY

Due to the relatively poor selectivity of presently available anticancer drugs, it is impossible to avoid some damage to normal host tissues, resulting in a variety of side-effects. Table 16.4 illustrates one representative study of side-effects. Nevertheless, when properly administered and monitored, many cytotoxic drugs can be given without producing symptomatic side-effects. For example, the effect on the bone marrow should not cause significant symptoms, provided adequate time is allowed between cycles of treatment and the blood count is monitored prior to subsequent treatment.

Mouth ulceration and diarrhoea result from necrosis of the rapidly dividing epithelial cells lining the gut. Appropriate timing of chemotherapy can prevent this but sometimes it is necessary to adjust the dose of the drug if an individual is particularly sensitive.

Nausea and vomiting

For many patients the worst side-effect of chemotherapy (and sometimes radiotherapy) is emesis—nausea and/or vomiting. The events leading to nausea and vomiting almost certainly include a direct central nervous system response to many cytotoxic drugs. Recent research has identified the importance of receptors for 5-hydroxytryptamine (5-HT, serotonin) in the small bowel and in the brain, which are triggered by the presence of some chemotherapeutic drugs, e.g. cisplatinum. Stimulation of these receptors results in a release of 5-HT in the brain, which in

Table 16.4 Rank order of the distressing side-effects of chemotherapy

Symptom	Rank
Being sick (vomiting)	1
Feeling sick (nausea)	2
Loss of hair	3
Thought of coming for treatment	4
Length of time treatment takes at clinic	5
Having to have a needle	6
Shortness of breath	7
Constantly tired	8
Difficulty sleeping	9
Affects family or partner	10
Affects work/home duties	11
Trouble finding somewhere to park	12
Feeling anxious or tense	13
Feeling low, miserable (depression)	14
Loss of weight	15

turn triggers the vomiting centre and causes emesis. Development of highly selective 5-HT_3 receptor antagonists has resulted in a new generation of effective antiemetics. For the cytotoxic drugs which are known to cause nausea and vomiting, it is necessary to prescribe antiemetics prior to and following administration of the cytotoxic drug.

Not all cytotoxic drugs cause emesis, and individuals vary considerably in the degree to which they experience the problem. As illustrated in the information box, cisplatinum and other platinum-containing compounds are the most emetogenic of all cytotoxic drugs and hence prophylaxis is necessary. Nausea may persist for 5–7 days after starting therapy, and therefore antiemetic treatment must be continued for this period. For most patients given platinum the combination of ondansetron or granisetron and dexamethasone affords the best antiemetic treatment (see Table 16.5).

Cytotoxic drugs such as the alkylating agents cyclophosphamide, iphosphamide and nitrogen mustard cause emesis of less severity and shorter duration. Antiemetic therapy should, however, be administered, and as with platinum therapy it is important to administer the antiemetic prior to the cytotoxic treatment, since prevention is very much more successful than trying to stop nausea and/or vomiting once they have started. For these alkylating agents and for the widely used anthracycline doxorubicin, dexamethasone, metoclopramide, lorazepam, prochlorperazine or domperidone is usually successful in abolishing emesis. Recommended doses of these antiemetics are given in Table 16.5. There is increasing use of antiemetics in combinations of two or more drugs.

COMMON CYTOTOXIC DRUGS IN RANK ORDER OF EMETIC POTENTIAL

Increasing emetic potential	Drug
Most ↑	Cisplatinum
	Dacarbazine
	Dactinomycin
	Cyclophosphamide
	Carmustine
	Lomustine
	Doxorubicin
	Cytarabine
	Procarbazine
Increasing emetic potential	Etoposide
	Mitomycin C
	Methotrexate
	5-fluorouracil
	Hydroxyurea
	Bleomycin
	Vinblastine
	Vincristine
Least	Chlorambucil

Alopecia

Alopecia is associated with the administration of some cytotoxic drugs, particularly doxorubicin and cyclophosphamide. If such drugs are prescribed, it is important to warn the patient in advance and, if appropriate, to arrange for a wig to be fitted. Alopecia is almost always reversible on cessation of therapy.

Psychological effects

The psychological effect of chemotherapy over a period of many months is one of which the physician must be aware. If properly counselled, many patients tolerate being informed of their diagnosis and also their early treatment remarkably well, only to become anxious and depressed as treatment continues, even though their tumour may be obviously responding. Awareness of this is essential and constant reassurance and support are necessary.

Altered growth

The chronic toxicity of cancer chemotherapy is important now that increasing numbers of patients are surviving for longer periods. Data from the follow-up of children cured of malignant disease have shown that physical growth can be stunted by the use of combinations of cytotoxic drugs with radiation but there is conflicting evidence as to whether or not these agents cause significant intellectual impairment.

Impaired fertility

This is preserved for the majority of pre-pubertal children treated with cytotoxic drugs but for adults fertility may be lost. This is particularly the case for men. For women the problem is more variable, depending on their premorbid menstrual pattern and the length of time prior to the expected menopause. Many patients suffering from malignant diseases may be subfertile at the time of diagnosis and

Table 16.5 Commonly used antiemetic regimens

Cytotoxic drug	Antiemetic	Dose regimen
Cisplatinum	Ondansetron Dexamethasone	8 mg i.v. 12-hourly or 8-hourly 16 mg in 20 ml normal saline given i.v. over 10–15 minutes at time of cisplatinum administration
Cyclophosphamide, iphosphamide	Dexamethasone	As above
Nitrogen mustard, DTIC	Lorazepam	2–4 mg i.v. 4-hourly
Doxorubicin	Domperidone	10–20 mg orally or by suppository 4–8-hourly

amenorrhoea is common for the months during which women are receiving treatment. Nevertheless, this is not a universal finding and since cytotoxic drugs are potentially teratogenic, patients of both sexes should be advised to use contraceptive measures whilst they are receiving chemotherapy.

It is now established that children who receive curative treatment for cancer may successfully produce children of their own in adult life. The number of successful pregnancies in this situation is only approximately half that of the normal population, but the frequency of congenital malformations amongst second-generation children is no greater than that expected in the rest of the population.

Second malignancy

Cytotoxic drugs may be associated with the eventual development of a second malignancy in a small proportion of patients. The cases have usually been of acute myelomonocytic leukaemia developing 5–10 years following the use of alkylating agents. In a study of over 5000 cases of ovarian cancer treated with alkylating agents, it was shown that the risk of developing acute leukaemia was 36 times that of the normal population. However, only certain classes of anticancer drug are associated with this rare phenomenon, which has arisen only as a result of developing therapies which may cure the primary tumour.

PRINCIPLES OF ENDOCRINE THERAPY

Tumours which develop in organs that are known to be under hormonal control sometimes retain hormonal dependency. This can be used therapeutically either by withdrawing the source of the hormone, by prescribing an antihormone or by the administration of another hormone. Carcinomas of the breast, prostate, endometrium and thyroid are the diseases currently amenable to endocrine therapy. The therapeutic use of adrenal corticosteroids is exceptional in that these compounds influence non-endocrine-related tumours, e.g. the lymphomas and leukaemias.

The biological effect of hormones such as oestrogen and progesterone is dependent on the hormone binding to a cytoplasmic receptor protein that transports the hormone to the nucleus, where it interacts with DNA to modulate gene expression. Oestrogen receptors can be assayed in biopsies of breast tumours or lymph nodes containing metastases. It has been found that for about 65% of patients whose tumours possess a significant amount of this receptor protein, removal of the source of oestrogen will be therapeutically useful, whilst for those in whom this protein is absent, hormonal therapy is usually of no benefit. The presence of progesterone receptor further increases the likelihood of hormone sensitivity. The development of techniques to predict hormone sensitivity has had a major influence on the management of patients with breast carcinomas. If oestrogen receptor activity is present, then pre-menopausal patients may benefit from oophorectomy, and both pre- and post-menopausal patients may respond to the administration of tamoxifen, a compound that blocks oestrogen binding.

FURTHER INFORMATION ON CLINICAL PRESENTATION AND PRINCIPLES OF MANAGEMENT

Cavalli F, Hansen H, Kaye S 1997 Textbook of medical oncology. Martin Dunitz, London
De Vita V T, Hellman S, Rosenburg S A 1993 Cancer: principles and practice of oncology, 4th edn. J P Lippincott, Philadelphia
Franks L M, Teich N M 1991 Introduction to the cellular and molecular biology of cancer. Oxford University Press, Oxford
Kirkwood J M, Lotze M T, Yasko J M 1994 Current cancer therapeutics. Current Medicine, Philadelphia
Peckham M J (ed) 1995 Oxford textbook of oncology. Oxford University Press, Oxford
Tobias J S 1992 Clinical practice of radiotherapy. Lancet 339: 159–163
Withers H R 1992 Biological basis of radiation therapy. Lancet 339: 156–159

PALLIATIVE ANTICANCER MEDICINE

Patients with advanced cancer frequently present with a complex mixture of symptoms—physical and psychological—for example, pain, anorexia, nausea, constipation, dyspnoea and restlessness. Whenever possible, the underlying cause should be treated, but if this is not feasible then a clear symptomatic management plan should be established.

MANAGEMENT OF PAIN

Pain is relatively rare as a presenting symptom of early or localised malignant disease, but patients often associate the diagnosis of cancer as leading inevitably to severe and intractable pain, and many need reassurance that such a situation is both rare and preventable. However, advanced cancer is frequently associated with some degree of pain and its management forms an essential part of palliative medicine.

ACCURATE DEFINITION OF THE SITE AND CAUSE OF PAIN

This is essential before deciding on therapy; for example, bone pain as caused by myeloma or metastases from tumours such as breast cancer often has two components—a background of diffuse aching pain unrelated to activity, and localised intensive pain triggered by touch or weight-bearing. Abdominal colic is typically of sudden, intermittent type, whereas headache arising from raised intracranial pressure tends to be more constant. Musculoskeletal and joint pains are usually localised, as are the consequences of nerve entrapment such as can result from tumour infiltration (for example, of the brachial plexus), or collapsed vertebrae secondary to bone metastases.

ASSESSMENT OF THE SEVERITY OF PAIN

This should be recorded in the patients' notes so that the results of analgesic therapy can be *regularly reviewed.* Several grading systems are used, such as the one shown in the information box.

SCALE FOR GRADING PAIN

- Grade 1: Pain relieved by occasional mild analgesics
- Grade 2: Pain requiring regular mild analgesics
- Grade 3: Pain requiring regular medium-strength analgesics
- Grade 4: Pain requiring regular strong analgesics
- Grade 5: Pain not controlled by regular strong analgesics

Only 10–15% of patients with cancer fall into the category of grade 4 or 5. It cannot be over-emphasised that successful pain control requires not only the selection of the analgesic most appropriate to the particular cause of painful stimulus, but the *regular* administration of therapy to constantly suppress pain and prevent its re-emergence.

As indicated in the above grading of pain, analgesics can be classified as mild, medium or strong in terms of their effect. Examples of doses of mild and medium-strength analgesics are given in Table 16.6.

RELIEF OF PAIN

Mild analgesics

Widely used mild analgesics include paracetamol, aspirin, dextropropoxyphene and flurbiprofen. Non-steroidal anti-inflammatory drugs (NSAIDs) such as flurbiprofen are particularly useful for pain arising in bone—a frequent site of metastases.

Table 16.6 Mild and medium-strength analgesics

Analgesic	Dose	Side-effects
Mild		
Paracetamol	1 g 4-hourly	Hepatotoxic (rare)
Aspirin (with codeine)	300–600 mg (with 8–16 mg codeine) 4-hourly	Gastritis
Dextropropoxyphene	65–130 mg 6-hourly	Constipation, sedation
NSAIDs	See *British National Formulary* for details	Gastritis
Medium-strength		
Dihydrocodeine	30–60 mg 4-hourly	Constipation, sedation
Dipipanone (with cyclizine)	10 mg / 30 mg } 6-hourly	Sedation

Medium-strength analgesics

Dihydrocodeine and dipipanone are useful as medium-strength analgesics. Dihydrocodeine is the most commonly used of these and is well tolerated apart from causing constipation. Co-proxamol (dextropropoxyphene and paracetamol) is equally effective and may be preferred since constipation is less of a problem. Dipipanone is stronger than dihydrocodeine and provides useful analgesia for grade 3 symptoms.

Strong analgesics

Dextromoramide, morphine and diamorphine are the most widely used potent analgesics. Dextromoramide is limited by short duration of action (approximately 2 hours) but for the same reason is valuable for 'breakthrough' pain that may occur occasionally when a patient is on long-term opiates. Morphine and diamorphine play an essential role in the management of severe chronic pain, but these substances are all too often prescribed in suboptimal ways. Two common mistakes are overcautious prescription for fear of inducing addiction, and prescribing 'cocktails' containing substances such as cocaine and chlorpromazine (e.g. Brompton's mixture). Addiction is irrelevant in the management of severe pain in advanced malignancy, and the stimulant or sedative effects of cocaine or chlorpromazine can induce confusion, anxiety and emotional distress.

There is little to choose between morphine and diamorphine, but the availability of slow-release oral morphine is useful for ambulant patients, and the greater solubility of diamorphine can be useful in reducing the volume of parenteral injection. Slow-release preparations of morphine are available that contain morphine in different strengths (10, 30, 60 and 100 mg), and are formulated to provide slow release for up to 12 hours. For these and standard formulations of morphine and diamorphine the dose must be titrated to the needs of the individual patient. For oral administration of standard preparations the dose must be repeated every 4 hours and dosage will vary from 20–100 mg or more. Intravenous administration of high doses may be appropriate for hospitalised patients, but the introduction of highly accurate slow-release pumps has enabled opiates to be given by continuous subcutaneous administration. The two major advantages of this are that these portable devices allow patients to remain ambulant, and that even very large doses can be given without causing significant central nervous system depression resulting in lethargy and confusion.

Constipation is an inevitable consequence of prolonged administration of opiates, and patients requiring these should always be given regular laxatives at the same time. Stool softeners such as dioctyl sodium sulphosuccinate and compounds that stimulate peristalsis such as bisacodyl are appropriate to ease constipation.

Localised techniques for pain relief

In addition to systemic analgesics, there are a number of localised techniques that may prove useful for the management of severe, intractable pain. These include:

- the injection of anaesthetics
- neurosurgical ablation
- transcutaneous electrical nerve stimulation (TENS).

The principal advantage of such techniques is to spare the systemic effects of strong analgesics (drowsiness, constipation etc.) but this has to be balanced with the morbidity of the procedure.

The use of *anaesthetics* includes a wide range of procedures where techniques now exist to target most major divisions of the nervous system. A relatively widely used technique is that of spinal opioid administration including epidural, intrathecal or subarachnoid administration of opioids. Spinal opioids are particularly appropriate for patients with deep constant somatic pain, but intermittent somatic pain (for example, that caused by a pathological fracture) may also respond.

Neurosurgical procedures have become less widely used with improvements in analgesic medication, and ablative procedures should only be used when pharmacological pain therapies have failed. Ablative procedures include peripheral neurectomy, sympathectomy, cordotomy and hypophysectomy.

TENS is used in several forms—for example, continuous, pulsed or acupuncture-like. The types of pain for which TENS may have particular use include predominantly nociceptive pain—for example, pain from metastatic bone disease or abdominal pain from hepatomegaly—and neuropathic pain due to compression of a nerve—for example, a lumbar nerve compressed by a retroperitoneal tumour.

ANOREXIA

Cancer-induced cachexia—anorexia, weight loss and altered carbohydrate, lipid and protein metabolism—is a source of major distress to patients and their families. Unless the malignant disease is successfully treated, reversal of cachexia is very difficult. Appetite stimulants have a role for some patients but are not routinely recommended, since the effects are short-lived and apparent weight gain may also reflect fluid retention. Prednisolone (10 mg daily) or progestogen megestrol acetate (160–320 mg daily) are the most widely used medicines for this purpose.

CONSTIPATION

Reduced food and fluid intake, relative immobility and the use of analgesics all contribute to the problem of constipation, from which many patients suffer. Opiates are a particular problem for patients with advanced cancer and all patients needing this type of analgesic should receive a stool softener (e.g. lactulose) and a bowel stimulant such as senna or bisacodyl. Preparations containing both a stool softener and a stimulant are now available (e.g. co-danthramer).

RESPIRATORY SYMPTOMS

Cough, dyspnoea and inability to clear tracheal secretions cause distress and exacerbate fatigue in debilitated patients. As with all symptom control, primary concern should be given to treating any known underlying cause. Cough and dyspnoea may resolve with appropriate treatment of a chest infection or improvement in heart failure. Physiotherapy may be useful in assisting expectoration of sputum. Methadone or morphine suppresses the cough reflex and may be particularly helpful when taken in the evening to restrict nocturnal coughing. The inability to clear secretions from the main airways ('death rattle') may be helped by using subcutaneous hyoscine hydrobromide (400 μg 4-hourly) and this is compatible with addition to diamorphine if the latter is being used in a syringe-driver.

TERMINAL CARE

An essential component of oncological medicine is the management of patients in the terminal phase of their illness. Psychological support is the most important aspect but this can be provided only if positive measures are taken to relieve pain, to ensure adequate and appropriate nutrition, and to treat specific symptoms such as cough, pruritus and nausea. Successful symptomatic treatment allows patients to prepare themselves mentally for death, and the relief of physical distress will also help the patient's family to cope with impending bereavement.

An individual patient's reaction to the inevitability of death from a malignant disease depends on a host of interrelated variables including his or her cultural and religious background, age, education, the duration of the illness and the reactions of dependants. Nevertheless, certain common patterns of behaviour are recognisable. A period of initial disbelief and denial is often replaced by a period of depression which is almost universal but many patients, with or without medical intervention, enter a final phase of peacefully accepting the inevitability of death.

When to tell patients that they have a terminal illness is a matter of experience. Death does not necessarily represent a failure of treatment and it is essential that those caring for the terminally ill do not avoid discussion of the processes of terminal illness. Such avoidance can only enhance the patient's sense of loneliness and isolation.

It is not always appropriate to present all of the facts to a patient, most especially on a single occasion, and time must be spent to determine patients' awareness of their situation, and their expectations. Non-committal, even ambiguous statements about the future may be appropriate but the patient should never be told what is known to be untrue.

Preparation for death is not the sole responsibility of the medical profession and, especially for patients dying in hospital, it is important to make provision for the adequate access of relatives, friends and other professionals such as the clergy when patients request their support. Religious belief does not necessarily make death any easier and even for patients who hold such beliefs it should not be forgotten that fear of the unknown is something shared by patients and all those who are caring for them.

The most important principle of managing terminal illness is to provide adequate time for talking with the patient. In a busy world this is difficult and it is sometimes easier to use the lack of time as an excuse for avoiding demanding consultations that drain the doctor's emotional resources. Nevertheless, to develop the ability to listen to patients and to learn from them how best to provide psychological support during terminal illness can be one of the most rewarding experiences in medicine.

FURTHER INFORMATION ON PALLIATIVE ANTICANCER MEDICINE

Doyle D, Hanks G, Macdonald N 1993 Oxford textbook of palliative medicine. Oxford University Press, Oxford

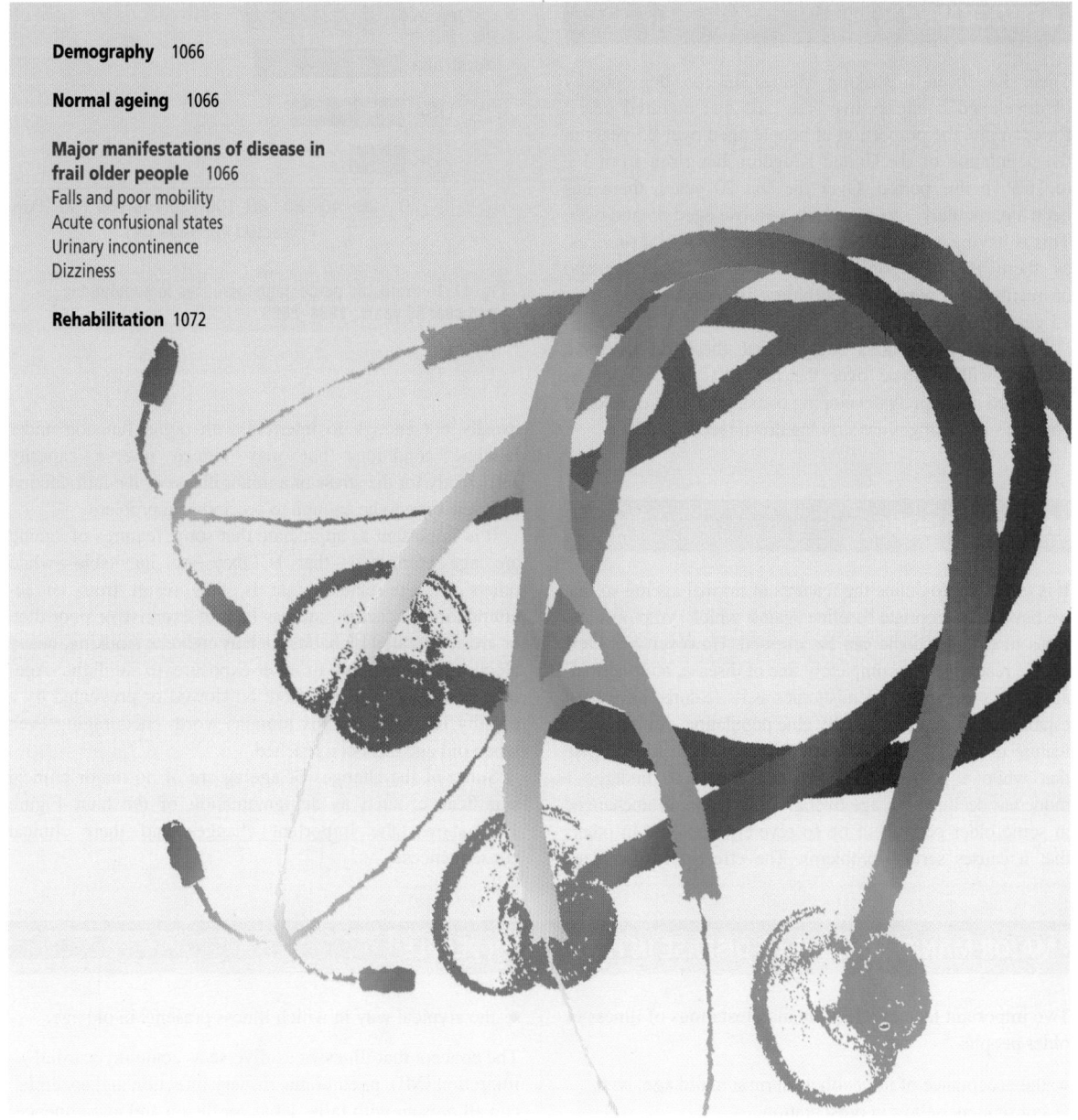

Principles of geriatric medicine 17

N.R. COLLEDGE

Geriatric medicine encompasses much of the knowledge and clinical skills of the organ-based specialties, and applies these to a particularly complex group: the frail elderly. What defines this group is the frequent presence of multiple pathology and the atypical way in which illness can present with confusion, falls, and loss of mobility and day-to-day functioning. Older people are also particularly prone to adverse drug reactions, partly because of polypharmacy and partly because of age-related changes in response to drugs and their elimination (see p. 1106).

DEMOGRAPHY

There has been a striking change in the demography of developed countries over the past one hundred years; for example, the proportion of people aged over 65 years in the population of the United Kingdom has risen from 5% to 16% in this period. Over the last 20 years, there has been a particularly steep increase in those aged 85 and over. This is having a major impact on health and social services, as there is an exponential increase in disability, and in mental and physical morbidity in people aged over 75 years.

Population projections suggest that these demographic changes will continue over the next 20 years in underdeveloped and rapidly developing countries, but in developed countries the changes are slowing down (see Fig. 17.1).

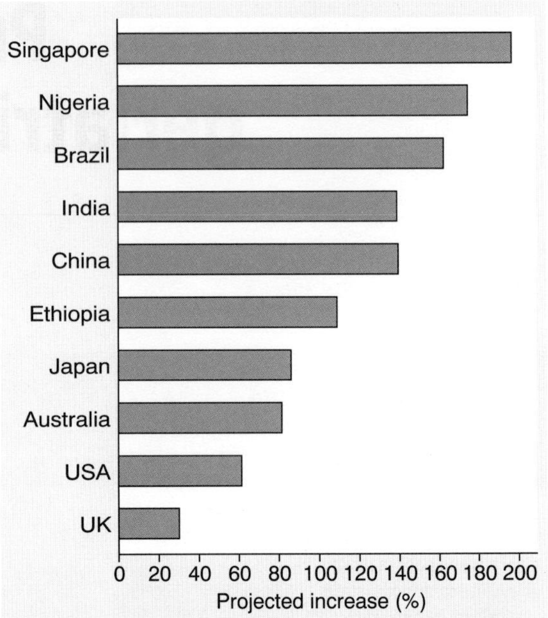

Fig. 17.1 Projected percentage increases in populations aged over 65 years, 1994–2020.

NORMAL AGEING

It is important to define the features of normal ageing so that we have an appropriate baseline against which symptoms and signs in elderly people can be assessed. However, very few people reach old age completely free of disease, and 'normal' ageing is something of a misnomer as its features have been established from a biologically élite population. An important feature of ageing is the increase in variation in function, so that while a particular feature may appear to undergo a moderate decline with age overall, it may remain unchanged in some older people but be so severely impaired in others that it causes serious problems. The effects of ageing are usually not enough to interfere with organ function under baseline conditions but may reduce reserve capacity sufficiently for the stress of a minor illness or the introduction of a new drug to be enough to precipitate a problem.

It is important to appreciate that some features of ageing are age-determined—that is, they are inevitable—while others are age-related—that is, they result from an accumulation of factors such as lack of exercise or poor diet, or are accelerated by habits such as cigarette smoking, heavy alcohol consumption or over-exposure to sunlight. Age-related changes can therefore be slowed or prevented by a healthy lifestyle and this remains worth encouraging even when old age has been reached.

Some of the changes of ageing are of no major clinical significance, such as depigmentation of the hair. Figure 17.2 shows the important changes and their clinical consequences.

MAJOR MANIFESTATIONS OF DISEASE IN FRAIL OLDER PEOPLE

Two important factors affect the manifestations of illness in older people:

- the acceptance of ill health as normal in old age, with consequent delays in presentation
- the atypical way in which illness presents in old age.

The concept that illnesses as diverse as acute myocardial infarction (MI), pneumonia, urinary infection and anaemia can all present with falls, acute confusion and incontinence

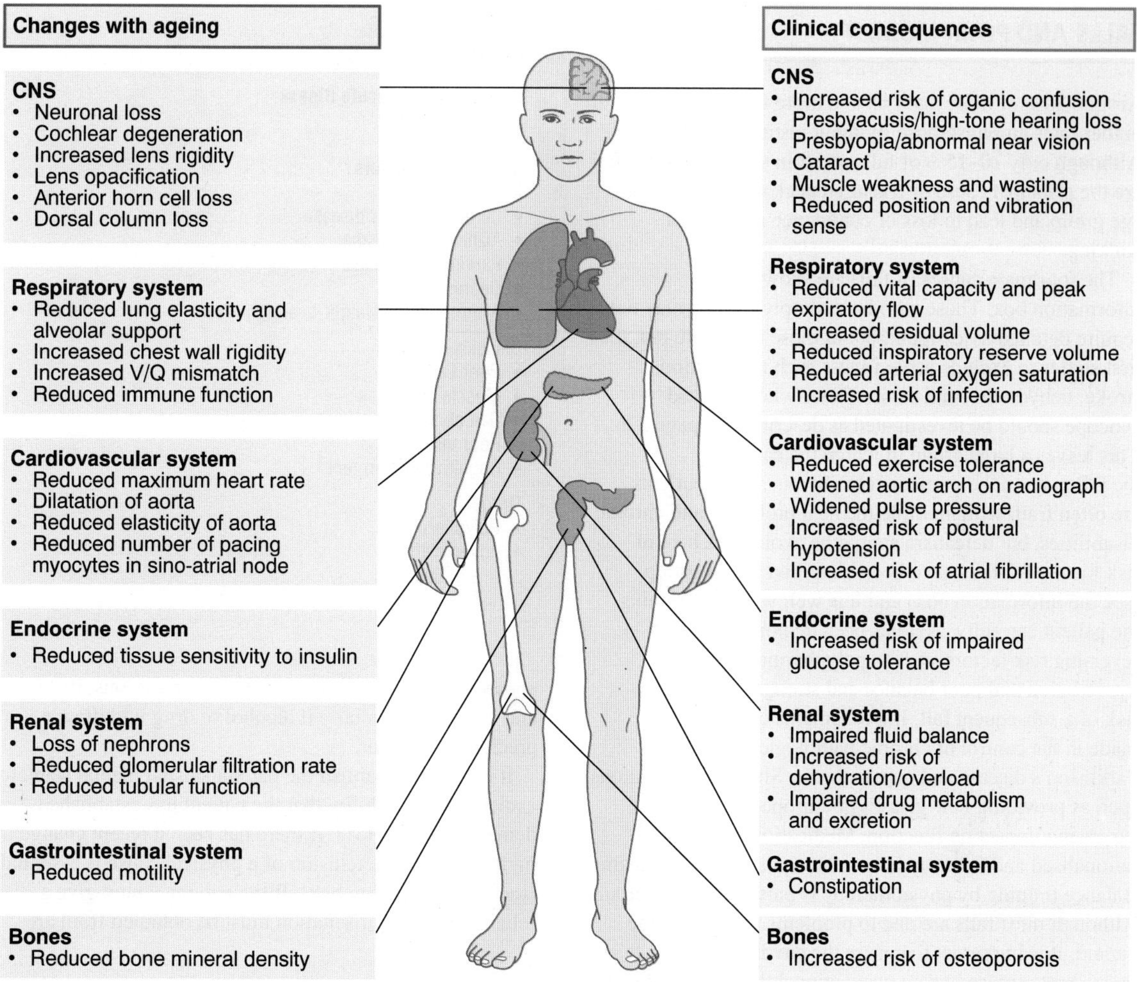

Changes with ageing
CNS
• Neuronal loss
• Cochlear degeneration
• Increased lens rigidity
• Lens opacification
• Anterior horn cell loss
• Dorsal column loss
Respiratory system
• Reduced lung elasticity and alveolar support
• Increased chest wall rigidity
• Increased V/Q mismatch
• Reduced immune function
Cardiovascular system
• Reduced maximum heart rate
• Dilatation of aorta
• Reduced elasticity of aorta
• Reduced number of pacing myocytes in sino-atrial node
Endocrine system
• Reduced tissue sensitivity to insulin
Renal system
• Loss of nephrons
• Reduced glomerular filtration rate
• Reduced tubular function
Gastrointestinal system
• Reduced motility
Bones
• Reduced bone mineral density
Clinical consequences
CNS
• Increased risk of organic confusion
• Presbyacusis/high-tone hearing loss
• Presbyopia/abnormal near vision
• Cataract
• Muscle weakness and wasting
• Reduced position and vibration sense
Respiratory system
• Reduced vital capacity and peak expiratory flow
• Increased residual volume
• Reduced inspiratory reserve volume
• Reduced arterial oxygen saturation
• Increased risk of infection
Cardiovascular system
• Reduced exercise tolerance
• Widened aortic arch on radiograph
• Widened pulse pressure
• Increased risk of postural hypotension
• Increased risk of atrial fibrillation
Endocrine system
• Increased risk of impaired glucose tolerance
Renal system
• Impaired fluid balance
• Increased risk of dehydration/overload
• Impaired drug metabolism and excretion
Gastrointestinal system
• Constipation
Bones
• Increased risk of osteoporosis

Fig. 17.2 Features and consequences of normal ageing.

rather than more specific signs and symptoms, is one of the fundamental elements of geriatric medicine. It means that a wide base of knowledge of adult medicine is required as disease in any organ system, and often many systems, has to be managed.

The reasons for these atypical presentations are not always easy to explain but may reflect the effects of normal ageing, poor nutrition, intercurrent drug treatment and the presence of multiple pathology. The latter is particularly important, as often a number of causes may be contributing to a single problem; a patient may fall because of osteoarthritis of the knees, postural hypotension due to diuretic therapy for hypertension and poor vision due to cataracts. All will have to be addressed in order to prevent further falls.

When assessing an elderly patient with falls, confusion or incontinence, it is very difficult to know whether an acute illness has been the precipitant until it is established if the patient's present state is a change from his or her usual level of function. For example, it is unlikely that investigation for an acute MI or pneumonia will be relevant in a patient whose mobility has been deteriorating over several months, whereas if there has been a sudden loss of mobility, investigations for acute illness would indeed be appropriate.

The following sections describe the common presentations of illness in old age. It is vital to recognise that these are not diagnoses and that a cause or causes should always be sought. Patients often present with a full house of confusion, incontinence, falls and loss of mobility. These manifestations often share underlying causes and may precipitate each other. For the sake of clarity, each is described separately here.

FALLS AND POOR MOBILITY

Around 30% of those aged 65 and more fall each year, with higher rates amongst those living in institutional care. Although only 10–15% of falls result in serious injury, they are the principal cause of fractured neck of femur in this age group and lead to loss of confidence and fear of walking.

The four main causes of falls are shown in the information box. Those who have simply tripped may not require detailed assessment, but in those who have not, the first step is to exclude acute illness such as infection, stroke, dehydration and so on. Those who have had syncope should be investigated as described on page 226. This leaves a large group in whom the cause of the fall may not be immediately obvious. Such patients are often frail, with multiple medical problems and chronic disabilities, but defeatism should be avoided. A host of risk factors for falls have been identified in this group (see the information box) and it is well worth examining the patient carefully, as it has been demonstrated that reversing risk factors such as polypharmacy, postural hypotension and poor balance and strength reduces the risk of a subsequent fall. Improvements can often be made in the control of chronic pathologies such as Parkinson's disease and osteoarthritis. Simple interventions such as providing new glasses or chiropody can have a surprising impact on function. Medication can often be rationalised and this may help reduce postural hypotension. Balance training by physiotherapy is particularly important. Although most falls are due to problems intrinsic to the patient, it is important to ensure the environment is safe and this is best assessed by an occupational therapist visiting the patient's home. Personal alarms can be provided so that patients can summon help, should they fall again.

Poor mobility shares many of the causes of falls. If its onset is recent, it may be due to an acute illness, but in most cases, one or several of the risk factors shown are present and mobility will improve with appropriate intervention.

CAUSES OF FALLS

Simple trip or accident

Collapse due to acute illness

Syncope

Multiple risk factors

Disease
- Cerebrovascular disease
- Alzheimer's disease
- Parkinson's disease
- Depression
- Arthropathy of weight-bearing joints

Disabilities
- Poor balance
- Muscle weakness
- Gait abnormalities
- Poor vision
- Cognitive impairment

Drugs
- Polypharmacy
- Adverse effects
  e.g. Sedation
  Postural hypotension

ACUTE CONFUSIONAL STATES

Acute confusional states cause a global impairment in mental function with varying degrees of impaired conscious level and memory disturbance, especially for recent events, which leads to disorientation in time and place. Perceptual disturbances take place and may lead to visual or tactile hallucinations, and thought disturbance causes slowing of responses and the development of paranoid ideas. Slowing of motor and mental activity may lead to apparent apathy, although many appear anxious, irritable and agitated, especially if alcohol or drug withdrawal is a precipitating factor.

It is vital to establish the patient's usual mental state, to exclude the possibility that the patient has established dementia (see p. 961). If there has been a recent change in mental state, the exclusion of a physical cause is essential (see the information box). If the patient cannot give a reliable history, information must be obtained from an

CAUSES OF ACUTE CONFUSION

Infection
- Chest
- Urinary

Metabolic disturbances
- Uraemia
- Hyponatraemia
- Hypoglycaemia
- Hypo-/hypercalcaemia
- B_{12} deficiency
- Hypo-/hyperthyroidism
- Hepatic failure
- Hypothermia

Hypoxia
- Pneumonia
- Exacerbation of chronic obstructive pulmonary disease (COPD)
- Pulmonary oedema
- Pulmonary embolism

Toxic states
- Drugs, e.g. digoxin, opiate, L-dopa
- Drug withdrawal
- Alcohol withdrawal
- Drug interactions

Other cerebral pathology
- Stroke/transient ischaemic attack
- Subarachnoid haemorrhage
- Chronic subdural haematoma
- Tumour
- Epilepsy/post-ictal state
- Normal pressure hydrocephalus

Hypotension
- Acute myocardial infarction
- Sudden blood loss, e.g. gastrointestinal bleed
- Gram-negative septicaemia

alternative source, such as the general practitioner or relatives, and should include past history and medication. A full examination is required, particularly for signs of infection or focal neurological abnormalities.

Initial investigations include blood chemistry to exclude metabolic disturbance, an infection screen, e.g. chest radiograph, urine and blood cultures, and a full blood count and electrocardiography. If these simple investigations fail to reveal an obvious cause, or focal neurological deficits are present, computed tomography should be performed. This should also be considered if the patient fails to improve despite appropriate initial treatment for identified non-neurological illness.

Management is essentially that of the underlying cause, but supportive measures may also be necessary. The patient should be nursed in a well-lit room and intravenous fluids may be required to correct fluid and electrolyte imbalance. Sedative drugs should not be prescribed unless the patient is highly disruptive; thioridazine 10–25 mg or droperidol 2.5–10 mg can be given acutely, but in alcohol withdrawal a benzodiazepine (e.g. diazepam 10–20 mg 6-hourly) is the drug of choice.

URINARY INCONTINENCE

Urinary incontinence is defined as an involuntary loss of urine sufficiently severe to cause a social or hygiene problem. It occurs in all age groups but becomes most prevalent in old age, affecting about 15% of women and 10% of men aged over 65 years. While age-dependent changes in the lower urinary tract predispose older people to incontinence, it is not an inevitable consequence of ageing, and always requires investigation.

Incontinence frequently occurs transiently in the context of an acute illness or hospitalisation. Contributory factors are shown in Table 17.1, and when these are reversed, continence is usually restored. As the table shows, there are three principal aetiological categories for persistent incontinence: stress incontinence, urge incontinence, and retention and overflow incontinence. Figure 17.3 shows a flow chart for assessing an incontinent patient.

Stress incontinence

Stress incontinence occurs most commonly in females. Urine leaks when abdominal pressure rises, e.g. during coughing, laughing or carrying heavy weights. Perineal examination may reveal leakage of urine when the patient is asked to cough, and may also reveal a prolapse or atrophic vaginitis. Continence can be improved by pelvic floor exercises and oestrogen replacement if appropriate. The insertion of a ring pessary may be sufficient to control prolapse, but if symptoms are severe, surgical intervention such as pelvic floor repair may be necessary.

Table 17.1 Causes of urinary incontinence

Type	Cause
Transient	Restricted mobility Acute confusional state Urinary tract infection Severe constipation Drugs, e.g. diuretics, sedatives Hyperglycaemia Hypercalcaemia
Persistent	
Stress	Laxity of pelvic floor musculature Secondary to childbirth Atrophic vaginitis Prolapse
Urge	Detrusor instability Frontal cortex abnormalities Cerebrovascular disease Alzheimer's disease
Retention and overflow	Outflow obstruction Prostatic hypertrophy or tumour Pelvic tumour Urethral stricture Neurological disease Peripheral neuropathy Cauda equina disease Spinal cord disease

Urge incontinence

Patients with urge incontinence are unable to inhibit leakage of urine when they feel the urge to micturate. This is most commonly due to detrusor instability in which spontaneous bladder contractions are resistant to cortical inhibitory stimuli. This can be diagnosed by urodynamic testing, which provides information about the dynamic filling pressures within the bladder. In practice, this is an invasive and time-consuming procedure and so the diagnosis is more often one of exclusion. In motivated patients, symptoms can be improved by bladder retraining. The patient is instructed initially to empty his or her bladder frequently and then at progressively longer intervals over a period of a few weeks. The anticholinergic drug oxybutynin (2.5–5 mg 12-hourly) acts as a bladder relaxant and may also be useful.

Retention and overflow incontinence

Overflow incontinence occurs when urinary retention progresses to the point at which the bladder can no longer expand and the pressure within the bladder exceeds outlet pressure. It may be caused by outflow tract obstruction or abnormalities of neurological control (see Table 17.1). Abdominal examination may reveal a palpable bladder suggesting urinary retention, and a pelvic mass which may be causing obstruction. Rectal examination is important to assess prostatic size and character, faecal loading and anal tone. A full CNS examination is also required. Ultrasound examination confirms a high post-micturition volume (> 100 ml) indicative of urinary retention, and there

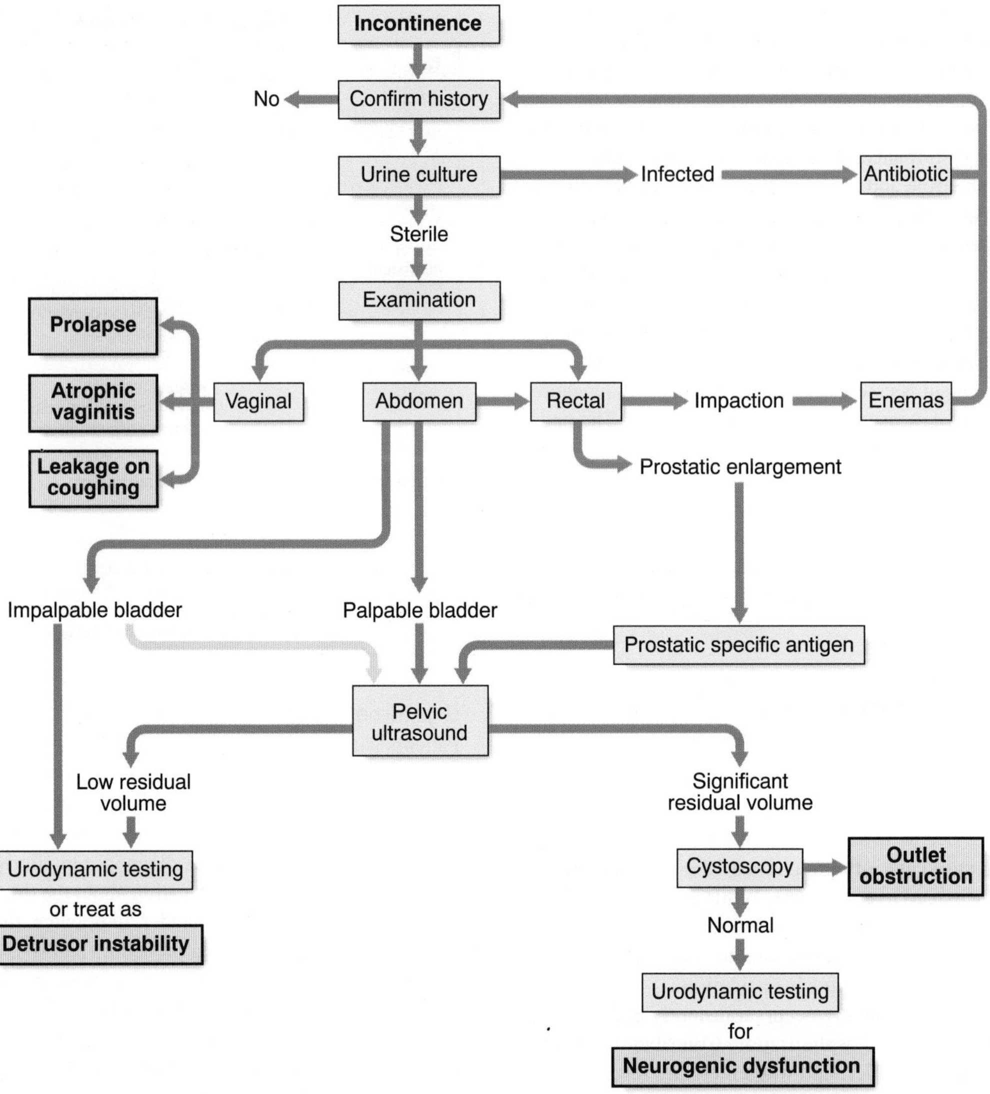

Fig. 17.3 Assessing urinary incontinence.

may also be evidence of secondary hydroureter or hydronephrosis. Cystoscopy is required to identify outlet obstruction, and if this is excluded, urodynamics may then help identify the nature of any underlying neurological abnormality.

Treatment of an obstructive lesion is surgical. In those with a neurological cause, intermittent self-catheterisation is the best long-term management, but for the very frail, a long-term catheter may be necessary. The only other indications for long-term catheterisation are when the perineal skin is at risk of breakdown or quality of life is impaired by intractable incontinence. In the UK incontinence pads are provided free by the National Health Service.

DIZZINESS

Dizziness is a very common presenting symptom in the elderly, affecting at least 30% of those aged over 65 in community surveys. It is an excellent example of the importance of a problem-based rather than an organ-based approach in medicine in old age, as it can be caused by disease in many different systems. Acute dizziness is relatively straightforward; common causes include acute shock, acute posterior fossa stroke or vestibular neuronitis. However, older people more commonly present with recurrent dizzy spells. They often find it difficult to describe the sensation they experience, so assessment can be very frustrating. Common symptoms include either lightheadedness suggestive of presyncope, vertigo suggestive of inner ear disease or unsteadiness suggestive of an underlying balance problem, although more than one of these may be present. Figure 17.4 demonstrates a means of assessing these patients and the most common underlying diagnoses in this age group. Chapter 3 (p. 225) describes the investigation of presyncope and blackouts in more detail. Vertigo with tinnitus and hearing loss suggests vestibulocochlear pathology. Anxiety and poor vision are frequent concomitants of dizziness but rarely the only cause. Lightheadedness and unsteadiness on head and neck movement associated with restricted neck movement suggest cervical spondylosis. Postural hypotension is defined as a drop in blood pressure of 20 mmHg systolic or 10 mmHg diastolic pressure on standing from supine, and causes dizziness on rising from sitting or lying. It is frequently exacerbated by drugs such as antihypertensives and diuretics. Cerebrovascular disease causes unsteadiness and is described in detail in Chapter 14 (p. 974). Chronic hyperventilation can cause lightheadedness.

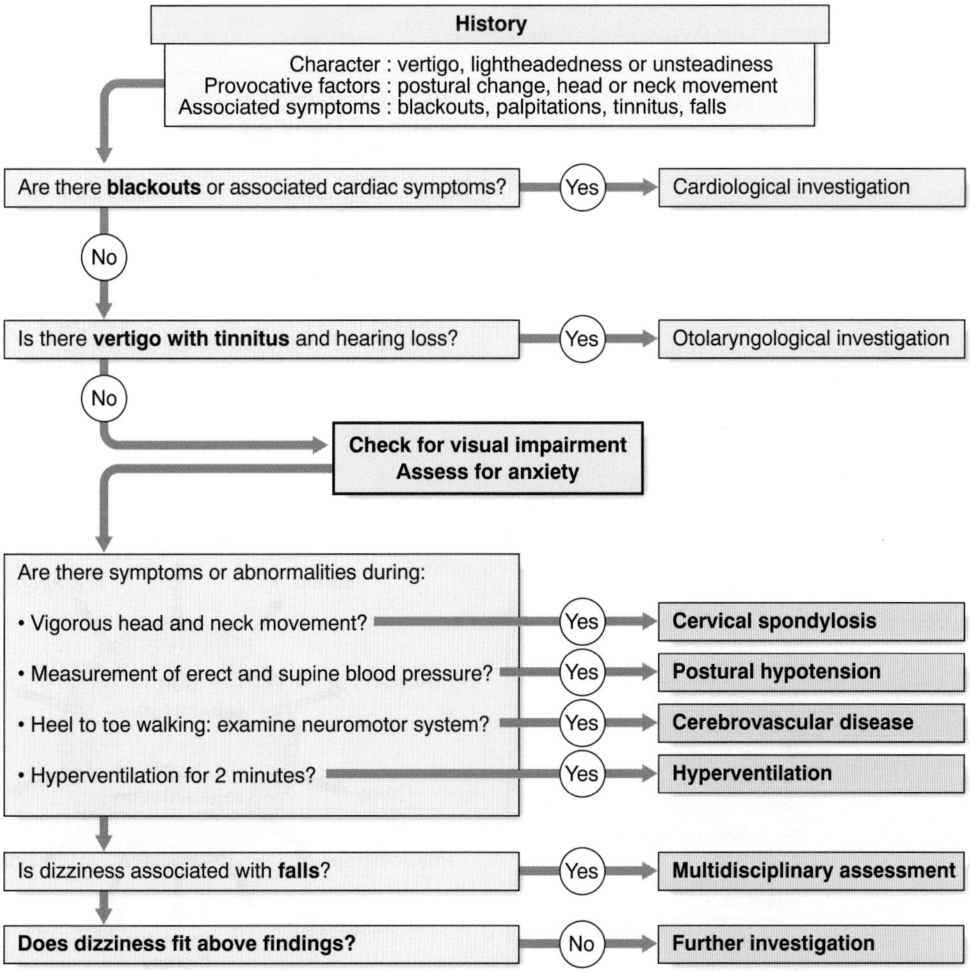

Fig. 17.4 Assessing dizziness in elderly people.

If the patient is falling as a result of dizziness, a full assessment by the rehabilitation team is essential (see below). If symptoms and signs do not fit the algorithm, further investigation, such as CT or magnetic resonance scanning and electronystagmography, may be necessary.

REHABILITATION

Rehabilitation is concerned with reducing the impact of disability. This is particularly important in geriatric medicine as the prevalence of disability is strongly related to age, and acute illness in older people is often associated with loss of day-to-day function. It involves several professional disciplines (see Table 17.2) and the patient is an active participant in the process. It should address not only patients' physical function but also their psychological and social functioning. The purpose of rehabilitation is to promote independence by special or general therapeutic techniques and by optimising the environment. A key element is the process of assessment and this must take place at four different levels:

- *pathology*, i.e. the underlying disease, e.g. stroke, osteoarthritis
- *impairment*, i.e. the resultant loss of function, e.g. hemiparesis, visual impairment
- *disability*, i.e. the resultant loss of activity, e.g. walking, dressing
- *handicap*, i.e. the resultant loss of social function, e.g. going shopping, driving, sporting activities.

Such an assessment allows planning of the essential components of an individual patient's rehabilitation and setting of appropriate goals. The process of assessment should be ongoing and reviewed regularly amongst all members of the rehabilitation team, and with the patient and his or her carer so that any changes in the treatment programme can be agreed.

The techniques involved in rehabilitation can be divided into 'hard' and 'soft' interventions which often overlap (see Fig. 17.5). The emphasis required will be different depending on the patient's disabilities and psychological status. A positive attitude, with team-working and involvement of the patient and carer, is essential to successful rehabilitation. There is good evidence that these methods improve functional outcome and reduce mortality after a stroke (see p. 974).

Table 17.2 Roles of the rehabilitation team

Team member	Role
Physiotherapist	Promotion of balance, mobility and upper limb function
Occupational therapist	Promotion of activities of day-to-day living, e.g. dressing, cooking Assessment of home environment
Speech and language therapist	Management of speech and swallowing disorders
Dietitian	Management of nutrition
Social worker	Organisation of home support services or institutional care
Nurse	Reinforcement of rehabilitation programme Encouragement to regain independence Communication with relatives and other professionals
Doctor	Management of medical problems Coordinator of rehabilitation programme

FURTHER INFORMATION ON PRINCIPLES OF GERIATRIC MEDICINE

Bennett G C J, Ebrahim S 1995 The essentials of health care in old age, 2nd edn. Edward Arnold, London

Colledge N R, Barr-Hamilton R M, Lewis S J, Sellar R J, Wilson J A 1996 Evaluation of investigations to diagnose the cause of dizziness in elderly people. British Medical Journal 313: 788–792

Tinetti M E, Baker D I, McAvay G et al 1994 A multifactorial intervention to reduce the risk of falling among elderly people living in the community. New England Journal of Medicine 331: 821–827

Young J 1996 Rehabilitation and older people. British Medical Journal 313: 677–681

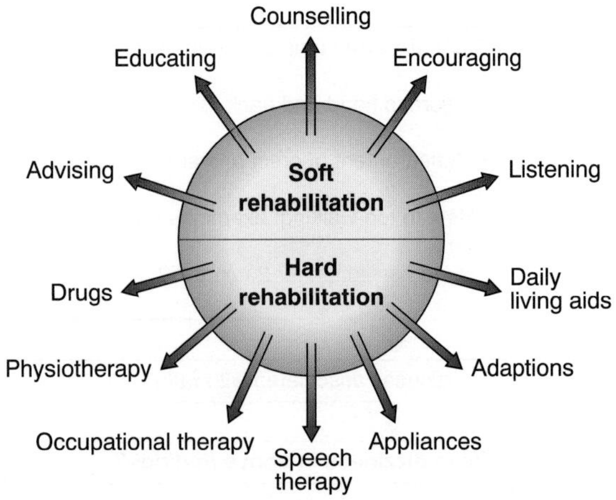

Fig. 17.5 Common rehabilitation interventions.

Principles of medical psychiatry 18

G.G. LLOYD

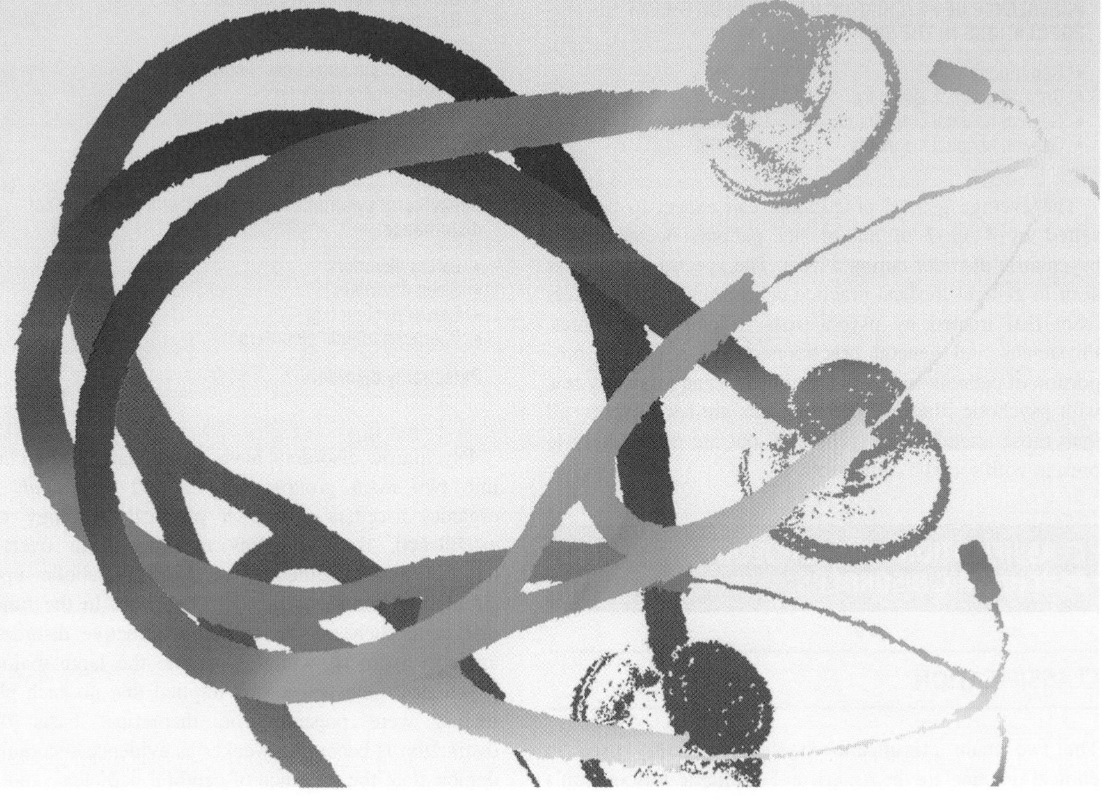

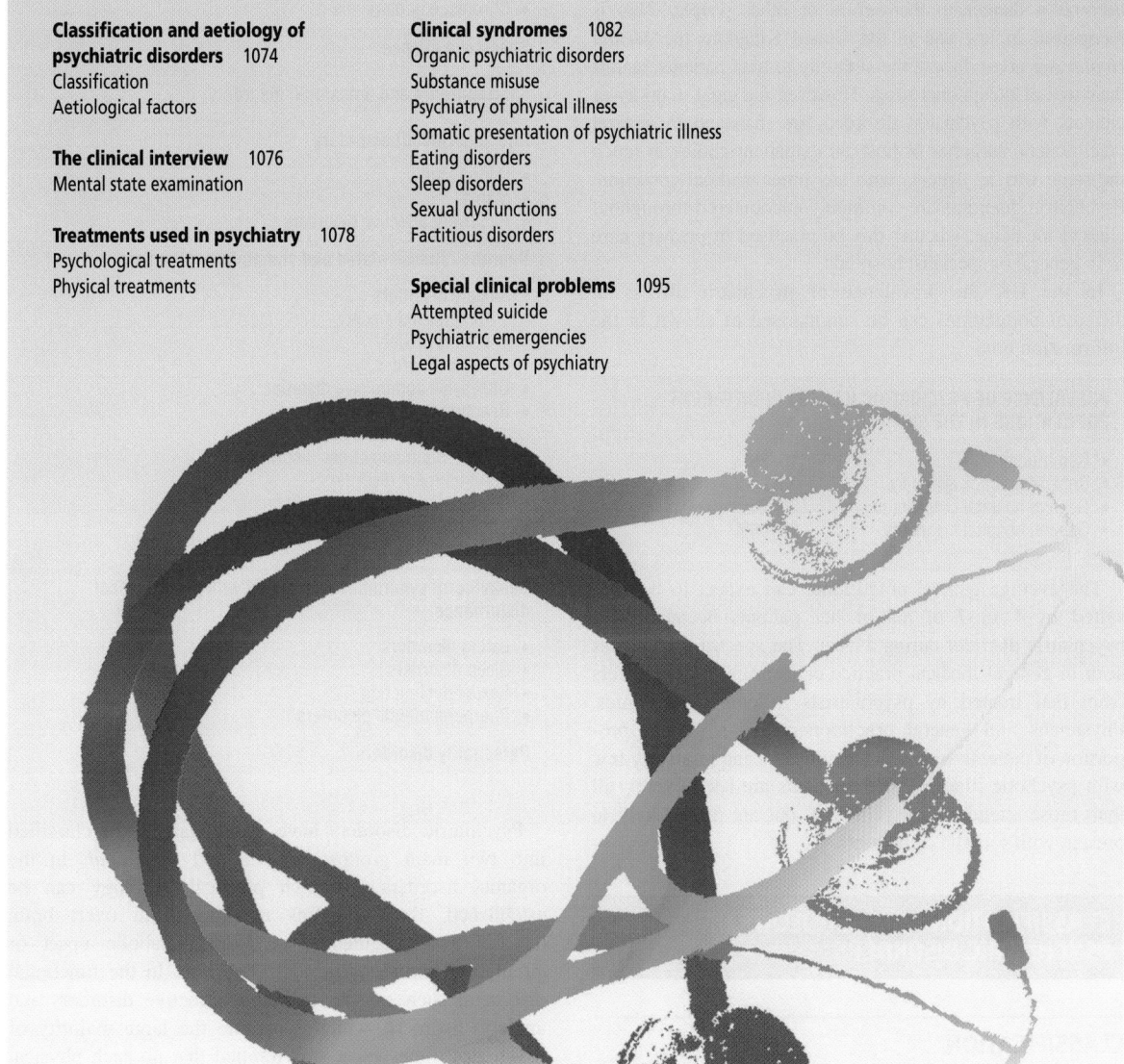

Diagnosis in psychiatry is mainly based on recognised patterns of subjective symptoms which are volunteered by the patient or elicited during a clinical interview. With the exception of the organic psychiatric disorders there are no objective markers of disease, such as radiological or laboratory abnormalities, by which diagnosis can be confirmed. In this context psychiatry differs from other branches of medicine where diseases have come to be classified in terms of their aetiology, such as an infective agent, biochemical abnormality or structural lesion. The symptoms of psychiatric disorders involve abnormalities of behaviour, mood, perception, thinking and intellectual function. Some of these abnormalities impair judgement or contact with reality so that patients become a danger to themselves or other people. This is recognised in law and in the United Kingdom the *Mental Health Act* gives doctors the authority to treat patients against their will in exceptional cases. However, the great majority of patients with psychiatric disorders are managed in general practitioners' surgeries or hospital outpatient clinics in much the same way as patients with any other medical condition. Psychiatric disorders are commonly encountered throughout clinical medicine, whether this be practised in primary care or in general or specialist hospitals.

In the UK the prevalence of psychiatric illness in different populations can be summarised as shown in the information box.

PREVALENCE OF PSYCHIATRIC ILLNESS IN DIFFERENT POPULATIONS IN THE UK	
• Community	15–20%
• General practice attenders	30%
• General hospital outpatients	20–30%
• General hospital inpatients	25–40%

The average general practitioner can expect to be consulted by 1 in 7 of his or her patients because of a psychiatric disorder during 1 year. The spectrum of illness seen in general medical practice or in primary care differs from that treated by psychiatrists in outpatient clinics. Physicians and general practitioners see a greater proportion of patients with neurotic illnesses and relatively few with psychotic illnesses; their patients are less severely ill than those attending a psychiatrist, but are more likely to present with somatic complaints.

CLASSIFICATION AND AETIOLOGY OF PSYCHIATRIC DISORDERS

CLASSIFICATION

The two main classification systems currently used in clinical practice are the American Psychiatric Association's Diagnostic and Statistical Manual (4th edition), usually abbreviated to DSM-IV, and the World Health Organization's International Classification of Disease (10th edition), known as ICD-10. The two systems are very similar but ICD-10 is the more widely accepted outside the United States. The classification of clinical syndromes used in this chapter will be based on ICD-10, an outline of which is shown in the information box.

CLASSIFICATION OF PSYCHIATRIC DISORDERS

Organic

- Acute, e.g. delirium
- Chronic, e.g. dementia

Substance misuse

Schizophrenia and delusional disorders

Affective (mood) disorders

- Depression
- Mania
- Recurrent affective disorders

Neurotic, stress-related and somatoform disorders

- Anxiety disorders
  - Generalised anxiety
  - Phobic anxiety
  - Panic disorder
- Obsessive compulsive disorder
- Reaction to severe stress
  - Acute stress disorder
  - Post-traumatic stress disorder
  - Adjustment disorder
- Dissociative (conversion) disorder
- Somatoform disorder
- Neurasthenia

Behavioural syndromes associated with physiological disturbance

- Eating disorders
- Sleep disorders
- Sexual dysfunction
- Puerperal mental disorders

Personality disorders

Psychiatric disorders have traditionally been classified into two main groups: *organic* and *functional*. In the organic disorders a known physical aetiology can be established, the symptoms resulting from overt brain disease, as in dementia, or from metabolic upset or circulating toxins, as in acute delirium. In the functional disorders, such as schizophrenia, affective disorders and anxiety disorders, which constitute the large majority of psychiatric illnesses, it was implied that no such physical factors were present. The theoretical basis of this distinction is becoming weaker as evidence accumulates to demonstrate the presence of cerebral pathology and neurotransmitter disturbance at synaptic level in schizophrenia and the affective disorders. However, the term 'organic' is still useful in practice; it has been retained by ICD-10 and will be used here to describe certain disorders.

Another traditional distinction which has become eroded is the separation of the functional disorders into *psychotic* or *neurotic*, depending on the presence of certain 'psychotic' symptoms. These are abnormal beliefs (delusions), abnormal perceptions (hallucinations and illusions) and certain disturbances in the pattern of thinking. Neurotic symptoms, in contrast, are mainly exaggerations of emotions such as anxiety and depression which are universally experienced. Psychotic illnesses were often regarded as being associated with lack of insight, while patients with neurotic disorders were considered to have insight into their condition. Although this is true as a generalisation there are important caveats. Many psychotic patients recognise the nature of their symptoms, while some neurotic patients are strikingly lacking in understanding. Insight varies from time to time and its presence is not an all-or-none phenomenon, rather a matter of degree. Nor is it true to say that all psychotic illnesses are severe while neurotic illnesses are mild.

This chapter does not aim at a comprehensive account of psychiatric disorders but concentrates on those areas of psychiatry which are most relevant to physicians and general practitioners.

AETIOLOGICAL FACTORS

The causes of most psychiatric disorders are unknown, yet there is considerable information concerning the range of factors which are regarded as important aetiologically. Causation is nearly always multifactorial and the aetiological factors should be regarded as having *predisposing*, *precipitating* or *maintaining effects*. The classification of these factors is shown in the information box.

CLASSIFICATION OF AETIOLOGICAL FACTORS IN PSYCHIATRIC DISORDERS
Predisposing
• Increase susceptibility to psychiatric disorder • Established in utero or in childhood • Operate throughout patient's lifetime (e.g. genetic factors, congenital defects, chronic physical illness, disturbed family background)
Precipitating
• Trigger an episode of illness • Determine its time of onset (e.g. stressful life events, acute physical illness)
Maintaining
• Delay recovery from illness (e.g. lack of social support, chronic physical illness)

Genetic factors

There is a genetic contribution to several psychiatric disorders, including schizophrenia and affective illness. The evidence is derived from various observations:

- a higher prevalence of the disorder among first-degree relatives than in the general population
- a higher concordance rate in monozygotic than in dizygotic twins, even if the monozygotic twins have been reared apart
- a higher prevalence rate for children of mentally ill parents who are brought up by healthy adoptive parents.

Some disorders are due to single gene transmission. These include Huntington's chorea (autosomal dominant, see p. 991) and some uncommon causes of mental retardation (e.g. fragile X syndrome). However, for the majority of psychiatric disorders in which heredity undoubtedly plays a role, no single gene has been isolated and it is assumed that several genes have an influence on the development of the condition.

Family background

Many patients with psychiatric disorders report an unhappy childhood background and it seems likely that a traumatic upbringing predisposes to future mental illness. Important factors are loss of a parent in childhood, either due to death or separation, parental disharmony and physical, especially sexual, abuse. In later life the family environment can adversely influence the course of an illness if parents are emotionally over-involved and express critical or hostile attitudes towards the patient.

Physical illness

Chronic physical ill health predisposes to psychiatric disorder. There is an especially well-established link between brain injury and subsequent schizophrenic and depressive illness. Physical illness of acute onset can give rise to psychiatric disorder due either to its effect on cerebral anatomy and physiology or to its emotional significance and implications for the patient's future well-being.

Stressful life events

A wide range of stressful life events can precipitate episodes of illness in vulnerable people. These events usually involve a sense of loss and include death of a close relative, marital breakdown, redundancy, retirement and major financial crisis.

Social factors

Many psychiatrically ill patients are socially isolated. The lack of a network of people with whom they can interact socially often appears to be a contributory factor in their illness. Particularly important is the lack of a close, confiding relationship. Social deprivation is associated with various conditions such as attempted suicide, alcoholism and drug dependence.

FURTHER INFORMATION ON CLASSIFICATION AND AETIOLOGY OF PSYCHIATRIC DISORDERS

American Psychiatric Association 1994 Diagnostic and statistical manual of mental disorders, 4th edn. American Psychiatric Association, Washington

World Health Organization 1992 The ICD-10 classification of mental and behavioural disorders. WHO, Geneva

THE CLINICAL INTERVIEW

Many of the areas explored during a psychiatric interview (see the information box) need to be included in an assessment conducted by a general practitioner or hospital specialist, particularly if the patient presents with emotional complaints or has somatic symptoms which do not appear to have a physical basis. A physical examination, with particular attention to the neurological system, is an essential component of any psychiatric assessment.

Wherever the interview is conducted, interviewers should introduce themselves to a newly referred patient and explain the purpose of the interview. Patients should be allowed to describe their problems in their own words but the doctor must be in charge and guide the course of the interview by appropriate prompting and interjections. If possible the doctor should ask to see a reliable informant who should be interviewed separately. There are several aims to be borne in mind during the interview (see the information box).

AIMS OF INTERVIEW

- Establish rapport with patient
- Elicit symptoms and history
- Examine mental state
- Facilitate cathartic effect by allowing patient to ventilate symptoms and associated problems

MENTAL STATE EXAMINATION

Several aspects of the patient's current mental state will have become apparent while the history is being recorded. However, it is always necessary to proceed to ask about current symptoms. The sequence of questions should be flexible, depending on which aspects of the mental state

TOPICS COVERED DURING INTERVIEW

Reason for referral
- Why the patient has been referred and by whom

Presenting complaints
- The patient should be asked to describe briefly the symptoms for which help is requested

History of present illness
- The patient should then be asked to describe the course of the illness from the time when symptoms were first noticed. The interviewer needs to ask direct questions to determine the nature, duration and severity of symptoms and factors associated with them

Family history
- Description of parents and siblings, the patient's relationship with them and a record of mental illness in relatives

Personal history
- Birth history, major events in childhood, developmental milestones, schooling, higher education, occupational history, sexual development, relationships, marriage, children, current social circumstances and forensic problems

Previous medical and psychiatric history
- An enquiry into previous health, accidents and operations; use of alcohol, tobacco and other drugs. Direct questions may be needed concerning previous psychiatric history since this may not be volunteered; for example, 'Have you ever been treated for depression or nerves?' or 'Have you ever suffered a nervous breakdown?'

Previous personality
- This refers to the characteristic patterns of behaviour and thinking which determine a person's adjustment to the environment—including attitudes, moral values, interests, quality of relationships with other people and reactions to stress. Personality attributes are usually developed by adolescence and are then stable throughout the person's life, and should be assessed independently of symptoms of psychiatric illness. However, certain personality types predispose to illness; an individual's personality will also influence the nature of the symptoms if psychiatric illness develops, and the emotional reaction if physical illness occurs. Several questionnaires are available for quantifying personality, the best known in the UK being the Eysenck Personality Questionnaire which measures extraversion, neuroticism and psychoticism as dimensions. For clinical purposes the most useful information can be obtained from a personality description given by one or more reliable informants who have known the patient well for many years

seem most important. These aspects are listed in the information box.

ASPECTS OF MENTAL STATE TO BE EXAMINED

- General appearance and behaviour
- Speech
- Mood
- Thought content
- Abnormal beliefs
- Abnormal perceptions
- Cognitive function

GENERAL APPEARANCE AND BEHAVIOUR

Describe succinctly the patient's appearance, dress and general tidiness. Is there a normal relationship with the examiner or is there avoidance of eye contact or uncooperative behaviour? Note any abnormalities of alertness and motor behaviour. For example, is there restlessness or retardation? Does the patient pace repeatedly up and down the interview room?

SPEECH

Speed and fluency of speech should be noted. Is there retardation of speech or difficulty finding words? Does the patient speak excessively rapidly so that it appears speech is generated under pressure and it is difficult to interrupt the flow? Are there rapid changes in the topic of the conversation? Is it difficult to follow the patient's train of thought?

MOOD

Does the patient appear agitated, depressed or elated? This can be judged by facial expression, mannerisms, posture and other motor movements. The patient's subjective mood should be elicited by asking for a description of current spirits. Some patients find it difficult to describe their mood in terms of anxiety or depression; questions which help elicit their mood include inquiries as to whether they have lost the ability to enjoy themselves or derive pleasure from life (anhedonia) or whether they have lost interest in themselves and those around them. People who are depressed should be asked about feelings of low self-esteem, guilt and worthlessness. It is also important to determine how they see their future. They should be asked about suicidal ideas; for example, 'Do you ever feel that life is not worth living?' Patients who reply positively need to be asked whether they have suicidal thoughts and active plans for putting an end to their lives.

Elated patients should be asked about feelings of grandiosity and general well-being. Manic patients may be irritable with the examiner who does not share their view of themselves. However, irritability is seen in other disorders of mood, not only mania.

THOUGHT CONTENT

Patients should be asked about their main preoccupations. This is best done simply by asking them to describe what is on their mind at present or what are their main worries. It can then be elicited whether the preoccupations are appropriate to the circumstances or whether they are indicative of psychological disorder. Is there evidence of phobic symptoms? A phobia is defined as an abnormal fear of an object or situation, the fear being sufficiently intense to lead to avoidance of the particular stimulus. Are there any obsessional symptoms? These are defined as thoughts, impulses or actions which enter the patient's mind repeatedly against his/her resistance but which nevertheless are recognised as his/her own thoughts. They are often associated with behavioural rituals such as repeated hand washing or checking.

ABNORMAL BELIEFS

It is necessary to establish whether the patient has any delusional beliefs. These are abnormal beliefs which are held with conviction and which cannot be argued away, but which are out of keeping with the patient's social, cultural and educational background. They may be paranoid, grandiose or depressive in nature. Leading questions are often necessary to elicit delusional beliefs: for example, whether the patient believes anything unusual is going on or, if paranoid delusions are suspected, whether there are beliefs that people have malevolent intent.

Primary delusions arise suddenly, often on the basis of a normal perception which is interpreted by the patient in a morbid manner. Thus the patient may see special significance in a particular arrangement of furniture in the room and conclude that there is a conspiracy organised by a secret political agency. Primary delusions of this type are characteristic of schizophrenia.

Secondary delusions are those which occur due to some other psychological disorder such as a mood disturbance, in which case they are congruent with the prevailing mood. They are commonly encountered in severe depression, when they tend to involve gloomy themes of guilt, wickedness and punishment. When the mood is abnormally elated, as in mania, the delusions are typically grandiose.

ABNORMAL PERCEPTIONS

The patient may report unusual sensory experiences but more often these have to be elicited by direct questions such as 'Have you had any strange experiences recently?' or 'Do you ever hear people talking about you even though there is no one near you at the time?'. The main abnormalities of perception are depersonalisation, illusions and hallucinations.

Depersonalisation refers to an unpleasant subjective feeling in which the patient's body is perceived as if it is changed, lifeless or unreal. It is often accompanied by a sensation that the external world seems changed in that it appears grey, unreal or two-dimensional; this phenomenon is known as derealisation.

Illusions are abnormal perceptions of normal external stimuli. They occur most commonly in the auditory and visual modalities. Sounds appear distorted, muffled or louder than usual. Objects may be seen as larger (macropsia) or smaller (micropsia) than normal, distorted in shape or more vividly coloured.

Hallucinations are sensory perceptions which occur in the absence of external stimuli. They can also occur in any sensory modality. It is important to establish whether the patient perceives the sensation as emanating from within the mind or from the outside world. It is also important to establish the degree of insight into the experience. Hallucinations which arise from within the patient's mind and whose origins the patient recognises are known as pseudohallucinations. Auditory hallucinations are characteristic of schizophrenia and affective psychoses. Visual, olfactory, gustatory and tactile hallucinations usually indicate organic mental disorder.

COGNITIVE FUNCTION

Intellectual abilities need to be assessed, particularly with regard to the possibility of mental handicap or dementia. They can be gauged from the history of the patient's educational background and attainments but can also be assessed during the interview from the patient's fluency, vocabulary and grasp of the interviewer's questions.

The level of consciousness should be noted. Does the patient remain alert throughout the interview or is there a tendency to drift off and lose the ability to concentrate on what is being asked? Concentration can be assessed more thoroughly by asking the patient to perform a simple repetitive task, such as subtracting 7 from 100 serially or repeating the months of the year backwards. Memory should be assessed under several headings. Recall of recent and distant events is determined by the patient's ability to describe details of personal history, dating back to childhood. It is also important to determine the ability to recall events occurring during the last few days and weeks. Registration is determined by presenting the patient with simple new information such as a name and address and then asking for this to be repeated immediately. The ability to consolidate and recall the information is checked by asking for the information to be repeated 5 minutes later, during which time the patient's attention should be diverted to other tasks. Memory is also assessed by checking on orientation. Does the patient know his/her exact location (orientation in place) and what day, date, month and year it is now (orientation in time)? Orientation in person refers to the patient's ability to describe details of personal identity—that is, name, date of birth, marital status, address and other intimate details. Loss of personal orientation does not usually occur in organic brain disorders but is a feature of psychogenic amnesia. The patient should be asked to describe recent current events; this gives an indication of general intelligence and interest in external events. The Mini-Mental State Examination (MMSE) is a useful screening questionnaire to detect cognitive impairment.

FURTHER INFORMATION ON THE CLINICAL INTERVIEW

Institute of Psychiatry, London 1987 Notes on eliciting and recording clinical information, 2nd edn. Oxford University Press, Oxford
Leff J P, Isaacs A D 1990 Psychiatric examination in clinical practice, 3rd edn. Blackwell, Oxford

TREATMENTS USED IN PSYCHIATRY

Some of the treatment approaches in psychiatry are unfamiliar in other branches of medicine so they will be summarised here. The doctor is often the coordinating member of a multidisciplinary team and needs to liaise closely with other professionals such as nurses, occupational therapists, social workers and psychologists, any one of whom may be responsible for a particular aspect of treatment.

PSYCHOLOGICAL TREATMENTS

PSYCHOTHERAPY

This is based on a continuing relationship between patient and doctor in which the patient confides his or her symptoms and the doctor uses his or her understanding of the patient in a therapeutic manner. There are two main types: supportive and interpretive.

Supportive psychotherapy

Supportive psychotherapy underlies all other treatments in psychiatry. Indeed, it is a crucial element in treatment throughout clinical medicine, much more so than many doctors realise. It involves a process of empathic listening during which the doctor encourages patients to describe their symptoms, express their feelings and reflect on associated problems in their lives. A single interview conducted sympathetically often has a healthy cathartic effect, but usually the doctor has to see patients at regular intervals over a long period and be prepared for them to become dependent. The doctor should give an explanation of symptoms, advice, practical guidance and reassurance when indicated. Supportive psychotherapy does not aim at any fundamental psychological change but when successful it fosters a therapeutic alliance and improves compliance with other forms of treatment. In patients with incurable and chronic conditions it forms a vital source of emotional support over many years.

Interpretive psychotherapy

Interpretive psychotherapy, in contrast, attempts a radical restructuring of the patient's psychological conflicts and behaviour. It is based on one of the several schools of psychoanalytic theory and should only be conducted by professionals with special training. At the basis of all types of interpretive psychotherapy lies the assumption that the presenting symptoms result from unacceptable memories or conflicts which have been repressed so that they exist only in the patient's unconscious mind. Treatment aims at bringing these memories or conflicts into patients' consciousness by allowing them to associate freely or to describe the content of dreams which the therapist can interpret, and help them understand and modify their behaviour as a result. An important element in treatment is an analysis of the transference, a term which refers to the patients' attitudes and feelings towards the doctor. The transference is thought to reflect the patients' feelings towards other people during their development, particularly their parents. Patients suitable for this type of treatment have to be highly motivated and are usually suffering from anxiety, depression or certain types of personality disorder, especially when these conditions are associated with disturbed interpersonal relationships. Treatment is contraindicated for those who have psychotic symptoms, paranoid traits, alcohol or drug abuse or who act in an antisocial manner. Interpretive psychotherapy is conducted during regular sessions of an hour's duration at least once a week and lasts for several months or even years. It can be conducted on an individual or group basis; its principles are also applied in marital and family therapy.

BEHAVIOUR THERAPY

Behaviour therapy is derived from the psychological principles of learning theory which state that many psychiatric disorders result from maladaptive patterns of learned behaviour. Treatment is aimed specifically at relief of symptoms. It is not thought necessary to modify or even understand aetiological factors from the patients' previous experiences. A behavioural analysis is essential before treatment is planned. This involves a detailed account of the symptoms, their severity, frequency and duration, together with an assessment of factors which trigger and maintain them. Several types of behaviour therapy have been evolved, as described below.

Systematic desensitisation

This is used in the treatment of phobias and other anxiety-related disorders. Its key elements are listed in the information box.

KEY ELEMENTS OF SYSTEMATIC DESENSITISATION

- Training the patient to relax
- Constructing a hierarchy of anxiety-provoking situations
- Introducing the patient, while fully relaxed, to anxiety-provoking stimuli from the hierarchy, working from the least to the most distressing. This can be done in the imagination or in real life

Flooding

This is also used in the treatment of phobias. It involves introducing the patient to the most stressful stimulus from the start and maintaining contact with the stimulus until anxiety subsides to normal levels. It is based on observations that anxiety eventually diminishes if avoidance of the anxiety-provoking stimulus is prevented. To allow this to occur, each session should last at least 1 hour and sometimes considerably longer.

Response prevention

This is used to treat the compulsive rituals which are characteristic of obsessional neurosis. The patient is exposed to stimuli which induce compulsive behaviour (e.g. checking or hand washing) but is prevented from carrying out the rituals.

Modelling

In this technique a therapist demonstrates normal behaviour in the presence of the stimulus. It is a useful supplement to response prevention. It is also used as a basis for social skills training.

Operant conditioning

This uses a system of positive and negative reinforcements to alter particular aspects of behaviour. Positive reinforcements (or rewards) are given following desired behaviour, while negative reinforcements (or punishments) are used following undesired behaviour. Operant conditioning forms the basis of token economy systems used to reduce behavioural problems in chronic schizophrenia and mental handicap.

Bell and pad training

This is used in the treatment of enuresis. A special pad is placed under the patient's bed sheet. It contains an electrical circuit which is completed when wetted by urine, thereby sounding an alarm bell which wakes the patient.

Micturition is interrupted and the patient gets up to complete emptying his or her bladder. After repeated training the patient learns to respond to sensations of bladder distension and wakens before micturition occurs.

COGNITIVE THERAPY

This approach is based on the assumption that some psychiatric disorders are due to a negative pattern of thinking which is an enduring characteristic. In depression a negative triad has been described, the three components of which are:

- devaluation of the self
- negative view of current life experiences
- negative view of the future.

Cognitive therapy is a problem-orientated approach which aims at modifying patterns of thinking in a positive way; it is assumed that improvements in mood and behaviour will follow. The treatment has been used for depression, anxiety and eating disorders. The therapist has to identify the negative thoughts and help the patient see the connection between them and his or her mood or behaviour. The patient is encouraged to monitor the negative thoughts and to analyse them logically by examining the evidence on which they are based. The final step is to substitute positive patterns of thinking which are more in keeping with reality.

PHYSICAL TREATMENTS

DRUGS

Drugs used to treat psychiatric disorders are known collectively as psychotropics. They are classified according to their main mode of action (see Table 18.1).

Table 18.1 Classification of psychotropic drugs

Action	Main groups	Clinical use
Antipsychotic	Phenothiazines Butyrophenones Thioxanthenes Diphenylbutylpiperidines Substituted benzamides Dibenzodiazepine Benzisoxazole Thienobenzodiazepine	Schizophrenia Mania Acute confusion
Antidepressant	Tricyclics and related drugs	Depressive illness Obsessive compulsive disorder
	Monoamine oxidase inhibitors	Depressive illness Phobic disorders
	Amine precursors	Depressive illness (in combination)
	Noradrenergic and 5-HT re-uptake inhibitors	Depressive illness
Mood-stabilising	Lithium	Prophylaxis of manic depression Acute mania
	Carbamazepine	Prophylaxis of manic depression
Anti-anxiety	Benzodiazepines	Anxiety disorders Insomnia Alcohol withdrawal
	β-adrenoceptor blockers	Anxiety (somatic symptoms)
	Azapirone	Anxiety disorders

Antipsychotics

The essential mechanism of many of these drugs, which are also known as neuroleptics, is their ability to block central dopamine receptors. This has been thought to explain their antipsychotic effect. Antipsychotics are used to treat acute schizophrenia and mania and to prevent relapse in chronic schizophrenia. They are also useful in the management of disturbed behaviour due to acute confusional states. In low doses they are used to treat anxiety.

The drugs have many unwanted side-effects so the indications for their use should be reviewed regularly. Weight gain due to increased appetite is common and may cause the patient to refuse further treatment. Side-effects related to dopamine blockade include parkinsonism, akathisia (an unpleasant, irresistible motor restlessness), acute dystonia (muscular spasm), tardive dyskinesia (persistent movements predominantly affecting the tongue and other facial muscles), gynaecomastia and galactorrhoea. The drugs also possess anticholinergic properties which cause dry mouth, blurred vision, constipation, urinary retention and impotence. In the elderly, postural hypotension and hypothermia can occur. Hypersensitivity reactions include cholestatic jaundice, blood dyscrasias and photosensitive dermatitis. Ocular complications which can occur in long-term treatment are opacities in the cornea and lens; pigmentary retinopathy has been described with thioridazine.

Clozapine, risperidone and olanzapine have a much lower incidence of extrapyramidal side-effects, probably because of their strong blocking effect on 5-hydroxytryptamine (5-HT, serotonin) receptors and relatively weaker dopamine (D_2) blockade. Neutropenia occurs in 3% of patients treated with clozapine and several fatalities have occurred from agranulocytosis. Its use is currently restricted to schizophrenic patients who have not responded to other antipsychotic drugs and who are specially registered with a haematological monitoring service. The drug must be stopped if neutropenia develops; the neutrophil count then reverts to normal levels. Other troublesome side-effects of clozapine include hypersalivation, weight gain and seizures.

Commonly used antipsychotics are shown in Table 18.2.

Antidepressants

Commonly used antidepressants are shown in Table 18.3.

Table 18.2 Antipsychotic drugs

Group	Drug	Usual dose
Phenothiazines	Chlorpromazine Thioridazine Trifluoperazine Fluphenazine	100–1500 mg daily 50–800 mg daily 5–30 mg daily 20–100 mg fortnightly
Butyrophenones	Haloperidol	5–30 mg daily
Thioxanthenes	Flupenthixol	40–200 mg fortnightly
Diphenylbutyl-piperidines	Pimozide	4–30 mg daily
Substituted benzamides	Sulpiride	600–1800 mg daily
Dibenzodiazepine	Clozapine	25–900 mg daily
Benzisoxazole	Risperidone	2–16 mg daily
Thienobenzodiazepine	Olanzapine	5–20 mg daily

Table 18.3 Antidepressant drugs

Group	Drug	Usual dose
Tricyclics	Amitriptyline Imipramine Dothiepin Clomipramine	75–150 mg daily 75–150 mg daily 75–150 mg daily 75–150 mg daily
5-HT re-uptake inhibitors	Fluoxetine Fluvoxamine Sertraline Paroxetine	20 mg daily 100–200 mg daily 50–100 mg daily 20–50 mg daily
Monoamine oxidase inhibitors	Phenelzine Tranylcypromine Moclobemide	60–90 mg daily 20–40 mg daily 300–600 mg daily
Noradrenergic and 5-HT re-uptake inhibitors	Venlafaxine	75–375 mg daily

Tricyclic antidepressants

These have been the drugs of first choice in the treatment of depressive illness. They inhibit the re-uptake of amines (noradrenaline and 5-HT) at synaptic clefts and this action has been used to support the hypothesis that affective disorders result from a deficiency of these amines which serve as neurotransmitters in the central nervous system. There is a delay of 2–3 weeks between the start of treatment and the onset of therapeutic effect. Side-effects can be particularly troublesome during this period; they include anticholinergic effects, postural hypotension and cardiotoxicity.

The recently introduced drugs, fluoxetine, fluvoxamine, paroxetine and sertraline, are selective inhibitors of 5-HT re-uptake. They are less cardiotoxic, less sedative and have fewer anticholinergic effects than tricyclics but can cause headache, nausea and anorexia. Their antidepressant effects are equivalent to those of tricyclics but they are generally better tolerated. At present their high cost limits their use to patients for whom tricyclics are not effective or for whom they are contraindicated because of side-effects.

Monoamine oxidase inhibitors (MAOIs)

These increase the availability of neurotransmitters at synaptic clefts by inhibiting metabolism of noradrenaline and 5-HT. They are less effective than tricyclics for severe depressive illness but are equally effective for milder illness, particularly when depression is associated with anxiety and phobic symptoms. They also have a place in the management of primary phobic disorders.

Monoamine oxidase inhibitors have acquired notoriety because of their interaction with various drugs such as amphetamines and opiates, and foods rich in tyramine such as cheese, pickled herrings, degraded protein and red wine. Amines accumulate in the systemic circulation causing a hypertensive crisis and fatalities have occurred from cerebral haemorrhage. These interactions have resulted in considerable anxiety about prescribing the drugs. However, they are relatively safe if the offending foods are avoided, and MAOIs are not used as often as they should be. Patients taking MAOIs should be given a card listing all the substances to be avoided. Moclobemide is a reversible and selective inhibitor of monoamine oxidase, subtype A. It causes minimal potentiation of the pressor response to dietary tyramine so the need for dietary precautions is considerably reduced.

Mood-stabilising drugs

Lithium carbonate

This drug, which inhibits neurotransmitter-stimulated phosphoinositide hydrolysis, is the main drug used in the prophylaxis of affective disorders. It should be given to patients who have had two or more episodes of illness requiring drug therapy within 2 years. It is more effective in bipolar illness (mania and depression) than in unipolar illness. Lithium is also used for acute mania and in combination with a tricyclic or an MAOI for resistant depression. It has a narrow therapeutic range so regular blood monitoring is required to maintain a serum level of 0.5–1.0 mmol/l. This is usually achieved with a daily dose of 800–1200 mg.

Toxic effects include nausea, vomiting, tremor and convulsions. With long-term treatment, weight gain, hypothyroidism, nephrogenic diabetes insipidus and renal failure can occur. Thyroid and renal function should be checked before treatment is started and every 6 months thereafter. Lithium has a significant teratogenic effect and should never be prescribed during the first trimester of pregnancy.

Carbamazepine

Carbamazepine, an established anticonvulsant drug, has been used successfully as prophylaxis in manic depression for patients who have not responded to lithium. The dose is 400–1200 mg daily although it is usual to start with a lower dose and increase it gradually. Common side-effects are drowsiness, ataxia, headache, rashes, nausea and vomiting.

Table 18.4 Anti-anxiety drugs

Group	Drug	Usual dose
Benzodiazepines	Diazepam Chlordiazepoxide Nitrazepam Temazepam	2–30 mg daily 5–30 mg daily 5–10 mg daily 10–20 mg at night
β-adrenoceptor blockers	Propranolol	20–80 mg daily
Azapirone	Buspirone	10–45 mg daily

Anti-anxiety drugs

Examples of commonly used anti-anxiety drugs are shown in Table 18.4.

Benzodiazepines

These agents have been used widely for the treatment of insomnia and anxiety-related disorders but they have been shown to cause dependence and withdrawal symptoms in many patients who have taken them for 6 weeks or more. These symptoms occur especially with short-acting benzodiazepines and if medication is stopped abruptly. They are listed in the information box.

BENZODIAZEPINE WITHDRAWAL SYMPTOMS

- Anxiety
- Heightened sensory perception
- Hallucinations
- Epileptic seizures
- Ataxia
- Paranoid delusions

In view of problems of dependence, psychological methods of anxiety management should be considered first in the treatment of anxiety but if benzodiazepines are prescribed they should be given in short courses, no more than 3 weeks, to help with limited periods of stress, and the dose should be tailed off gradually thereafter. They have superseded chlormethiazole in the management of alcohol withdrawal. Buspirone, which is unrelated to any other psychotropic drug, is claimed not to have withdrawal effects nor does it have sedative or muscle relaxant properties. Its mode of action is slow, over 3 or 4 weeks, and this is obviously a disadvantage when a quick response is required.

β-adrenoceptor blockers

β-adrenoceptor antagonists such as propranolol have a limited role in the treatment of anxiety where somatic symptoms are prominent.

ELECTROCONVULSIVE THERAPY (ECT)

Electroconvulsive therapy has been used in psychiatry for more than 50 years. It involves the administration of high-voltage, brief, direct-current impulses to the head while the patient is anaesthetised and paralysed by muscle relaxants. Electrodes can be placed either bilaterally, or unilaterally over the non-dominant hemisphere. Bilateral ECT is more effective but unilateral ECT causes less short-term memory impairment. The main use of ECT is for depressive illness but it is sometimes used in mania and acute schizophrenia. Up to 12 applications may be needed to produce optimal results.

There has been a decline in the use of ECT following the introduction of psychotropic drugs but it remains the most effective treatment for severe depression with psychotic symptoms. ECT is safe and side-effects are few. Headache and a brief period of confusion often occur during the immediate post-ictal period. There may be amnesia for events occurring a few hours before (retrograde) and after (anterograde) ECT. Permanent anterograde amnesia has been claimed to occur but is infrequent.

PSYCHOSURGERY

This treatment has been rendered virtually obsolete by modern drug therapy. It is now carried out for a small number of patients with severe, resistant depression or obsessional disorder and should only be undertaken at specialised centres. The operation involves a stereotactic technique to interrupt the frontolimbic pathways bilaterally.

FURTHER INFORMATION ON TREATMENTS USED IN PSYCHIATRY

Andrews G 1993 The essential psychotherapies. British Journal of Psychiatry 161: 447–451
Henry J A 1992 The safety of antidepressants. British Journal of Psychiatry 160: 439–441
Silverstone T, Turner P 1995 Drug treatment in psychiatry, 5th edn. Routledge, London

CLINICAL SYNDROMES

ORGANIC PSYCHIATRIC DISORDERS

This group of disorders results from pathological lesions within the brain or acting on the brain from a focus elsewhere in the body. The most common syndromes are delirium (see p. 962), dementia (see p. 961) and organic mood disorders (see p. 1089).

SUBSTANCE MISUSE

ALCOHOLISM

Alcohol consumption in the UK has risen greatly during the last four decades and this has been accompanied by increases in the social, psychological and physical problems due to alcohol. The term 'alcoholism' is now used in a broad sense to describe a pattern of drinking which is harmful to the individual or to his or her family. The more restricted term, 'alcohol dependence', has the criteria listed in the information box.

CRITERIA OF ALCOHOL DEPENDENCE

- Narrowing of the drinking repertoire
- Priority of drinking over other activities
- Tolerance of effects of alcohol
- Repeated withdrawal symptoms
- Relief of withdrawal symptoms by further drinking
- Subjective compulsion to drink
- Reinstatement of drinking behaviour after abstinence

National statistics indicate that morbidity related to alcohol closely correlates with mean per capita consumption. Men are more likely to have alcohol-related problems than women, although the gap is closing. Approximately *one-quarter* of male patients in general hospital medical wards have a current or previous alcohol problem.

Aetiology

Although genetic factors make a small contribution to the development of alcohol abuse, cultural factors are much more important. Alcohol problems are rare among Muslims and Jews and common in countries which have large alcohol-producing industries—for example, France, Italy and Portugal. In the United Kingdom problems are more common among the Scots and Irish. Availability of alcohol is important, as shown by high rates among those employed in the drink trade. Doctors previously held a high position in the occupational league table but are now only just above the average. There is a close correlation between consumption and the price of alcohol relative to average earnings. The cheaper the relative price, the higher the consumption, with the effect that a larger proportion of the population will develop alcohol-related problems.

No consistent predisposing personality profile has been identified. The majority of alcoholics do not have an underlying psychiatric illness but in a few it appears that heavy drinking has developed in an attempt to relieve the unpleasant symptoms of an anxiety state, depression or schizophrenia.

Problems caused by alcohol

Many patients' alcohol problems are not detected by their doctors. A high index of suspicion is important, particularly in cases where there are repeated consultations for vague symptoms or minor accidents. If in doubt, a drinking history should be taken in which the patient is asked to describe a typical week's drinking. Consumption should be quantified in terms of units of alcohol; one unit contains approximately 9 g of alcohol and is the equivalent of half a pint of beer, a single measure of spirits or a glass of table wine. Current opinion suggests that drinking becomes hazardous at levels above 21 units weekly for men and 14 units weekly for women. Conversely, there is some evidence which suggests that regular, modest consumption of alcohol may have a protective effect against the development of coronary artery disease. Laboratory tests are useful in confirming alcohol abuse. Mean corpuscular volume (MCV) or gamma-glutamyl transpeptidase (gamma GT) is raised in approximately 50% of problem drinkers. Although the low sensitivity of these tests makes them unsuitable for population screening, they are useful for monitoring treatment response in individual cases where their values were elevated originally.

Social problems

These include absenteeism from work, unemployment, marital tensions, child abuse, financial difficulties and problems with the law, including violence and traffic offences.

Psychological problems

Depression. This is common and is usually reactive to the numerous social problems which heavy drinking creates. Alcohol also has a direct depressant effect. Attempted suicide and completed suicide are much more common in alcoholics than in the rest of society.

Morbid jealousy. This is a syndrome characterised by delusions of sexual infidelity. It is usually seen in alcoholics of sensitive or paranoid disposition whose sexual relationship has deteriorated because of impotence or rejection by the partner. The alcoholic suspects and accuses his or her partner of having a relationship with another person and goes to extreme lengths to obtain corroborative evidence, such as repeatedly searching the partner's personal possessions or employing a private detective to follow him or her. Accusations lead to violence and sometimes murder. Morbid jealousy can also occur in schizophrenia, depressive illness and paranoid personality disorder.

Withdrawal symptoms. These indicate physical dependence. The earliest manifestation is a subjective sensation of tension on waking in the morning. This may be accompanied by a tremor which makes it difficult to shave or hold a cup of tea. Another alcoholic drink relieves these symptoms, thus establishing a pattern of morning drinking. Less common but more serious withdrawal symptoms are epilepsy and delirium tremens, the latter having the features of a severe confusional state characterised by impaired consciousness, visual hallucinations, memory disturbance and seizures. Alcoholic hallucinosis also occurs following relative or absolute withdrawal. Its essential features are auditory hallucinations occurring in clear consciousness; the hallucinations take the form of derogatory or persecutory voices which discuss the individual in the third person or comment directly to him or her. They are similar to the auditory hallucinations reported by schizophrenics.

Vitamin deficiencies. These occur in alcoholics who have a severely impoverished diet. The most important is thiamine (B_1) deficiency, which leads to the acute phenomena of Wernicke's encephalopathy or the chronic features of Korsakoff's syndrome.

Wernicke's encephalopathy often has an abrupt onset; mental state examination reveals drowsiness, disorientation in time and place and an impaired ability to recall recent events or to register new information. Physical examination reveals a horizontal nystagmus, evidence of external ocular palsies, ataxia and peripheral neuropathy. This syndrome results from damage to the mammillary bodies, dorsomedial nuclei of the thalamus and adjacent areas of grey matter. In those who die in the acute stage, microscopic examination of the brain shows hyperaemia, petechial haemorrhages and astrocytic proliferation. Wernicke's encephalopathy in Western countries is nearly always due to poor nutrition associated with chronic alcoholism; other causes are prolonged vomiting, diarrhoea and severe starvation.

Immediate treatment with thiamine 50 mg intravenously is essential to minimise permanent damage. Fluid replacement may also be required and intramuscular thiamine should be given daily until an adequate diet can be resumed. It is usual to give this with other vitamins in the form of Parentrovite, which is available as paired ampoules for injection, either as intravenous high potency, intramuscular high potency or intramuscular maintenance. One of the ampoules contains thiamine, riboflavin and pyridoxine and the other nicotinamide and ascorbic acid. Two to four pairs of high-potency intravenous ampoules are given 4–8-hourly for 2 days, followed by high-potency intramuscular injections daily for 5–7 days.

When recovery is incomplete a chronic amnesic syndrome develops, this being known as *Korsakoff's psychosis*. Characteristically, the patient is fully conscious but has a profound impairment of memory recall and new learning ability. A striking feature is a tendency to confabulate, which has been defined as a falsification of memory in clear consciousness. For example, if the patient is asked to describe his or her activities during the previous week he or she will reply by reporting events which have taken place many years previously. Confabulation probably results from an inability to distinguish the temporal sequence of past events. Other cognitive functions remain intact in the Korsakoff syndrome but memory disturbance is often so profound that the patient is incapable of living independently and institutional care is required.

Direct toxic effects on the brain

These cause the familiar features of drunkenness. In very heavy drinkers there are periods of amnesia (alcoholic blackouts) for events which occurred during bouts of intoxication. When alcoholism has been established for several years, cortical atrophy can occur and the clinical picture of dementia develops.

Indirect effects on behaviour. These can result from head injury, hypoglycaemia and portasystemic encephalopathy.

Physical problems

These are protean and can affect virtually any organ in the body, giving rise to the comment that alcohol has replaced syphilis as the great mimic of disease. The diseases are grouped together in Figure 18.1 and are discussed in detail in their respective sections.

Management

Straightforward advice about the harmful effects of alcohol and safe levels of consumption is often all that is needed. In more serious cases patients may have to be advised to alter leisure activities or change jobs if these are contributing to the problem. Supportive psychotherapy is often crucial in helping the patient effect the necessary changes in lifestyle. Interpretive psychotherapy, either individual or group, can help patients who have recurrent relapses. Treatment of this type is available at specialised centres and is also provided by voluntary organisations such as Alcoholics Anonymous (AA).

Drug therapy also has a valuable role in treatment. Benzodiazepines are the drugs of choice for withdrawal symptoms and can be given safely in large doses (e.g. diazepam 20 mg 6-hourly), provided they are tailed off over a period of 5–7 days as symptoms subside. It is usual to give high-dose vitamins during withdrawal treatment because of the possibility of thiamine deficiency. Only rarely are antidepressants required; the depressive symptoms, if present, usually resolve with abstinence. Phenothiazines (e.g. chlorpromazine 100 mg 8-hourly) are required for alcoholic hallucinosis. Disulfiram (200–400 mg daily) can be given as a deterrent to patients who have difficulty resisting sudden impulses to drink after becoming abstinent. The drug blocks the metabolism of alcohol, causing acetaldehyde to accumulate in the body. When alcohol is consumed by someone taking the drug there follows an unpleasant reaction consisting of headache, flushing, nausea and laboured breathing. Knowledge that this reaction will occur can provide an insurance against drinking and even remove craving. Disulfiram should always be seen as an

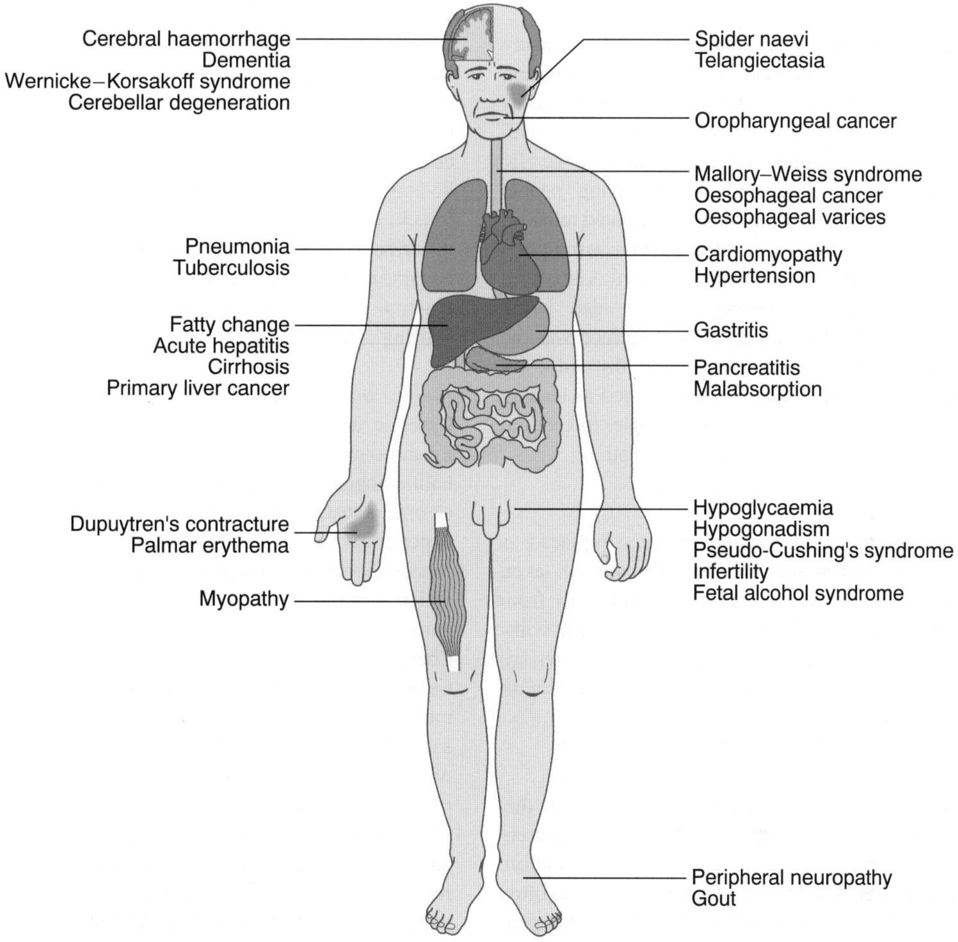

Fig. 18.1 Physical effects of alcohol abuse.

adjunct to other treatments, especially supportive psychotherapy. Acamprosate has recently been introduced to maintain abstinence by reducing craving for alcohol.

DRUG MISUSE

Dependence on illegal and prescribed drugs has become a major problem in Western countries during the last two decades. In the UK there are now 50 000–100 000 opiate addicts and 2% of the population regularly take benzodiazepines. Many of the aetiological factors which apply to alcohol abuse are also relevant to drug dependence. The main factors are cultural pressures, particularly within a peer group, and availability of a drug. In the case of some drugs availability has been increased by medical overprescribing but there has also been a relative decline in price.

Benzodiazepines

More people are dependent on benzodiazepines than on any other group of drugs. They are effective anti-anxiety drugs if given in short courses but tolerance occurs after 6 weeks of daily consumption. Withdrawal symptoms can then occur if the drug is stopped abruptly. These include anxiety, increased sensory perception, epileptic fits and psychotic experiences. Withdrawal symptoms are particularly likely to occur with short-acting drugs such as lorazepam. Benzodiazepine dependence nearly always occurs because the drugs have been prescribed for the wrong reasons or because repeat prescriptions have been issued for several months. However, there is also a vogue for intravenous benzodiazepines, notably temazepam, among some adolescent groups who have never been given medical prescriptions for the drug.

Cannabis

Cannabis, derived from the plant *Cannabis sativa*, is usually smoked mixed with tobacco. It quickly produces a sensation of relaxation and well-being; psychological dependence is common but tolerance and withdrawal symptoms are unusual. It is probably the most common illegal drug taken in the UK and is often the only drug with which young people experiment. The extent of its use cannot be estimated reliably.

A toxic confusional state occurs after heavy consumption and acute psychotic episodes are well recognised. Long-term consequences of regular consumption are also being appreciated. One of the first effects to be described was the 'amotivational syndrome', characterised by apathy and slothfulness. Chronic consumption has been described as leading to a schizophrenic syndrome or, in some people, to cerebral atrophy but these claims have not been confirmed.

Barbiturates

These are now rarely prescribed, having been replaced as hypnotics by benzodiazepines. However, they are still taken by some people who manage to obtain them indirectly from doctors. They soon cause dependence, and sudden withdrawal is very likely to cause epileptic fits. Barbiturates are dangerous in overdose because of their depressant effect on respiration.

Opiates

Morphine, heroin and codeine are the main drugs in this group, with heroin having become especially prominent recently. Taken orally, intravenously or by inhalation, heroin gives a rapid, intensely pleasurable experience, often accompanied by heightened sexual arousal. Physical dependence occurs within a few weeks of regular high-dose injection, with the result that the dose is escalated and the addict's life becomes increasingly centred around obtaining and taking the drug. Intravenous users are prone to bacterial infections, hepatitis B and human immunodeficiency virus (HIV) infection through needle contamination. Accidental overdose is common. The withdrawal syndrome, which can start within 12 hours in some people, can present with intense craving, rhinorrhoea, lacrimation, yawning, perspiration, shivering, piloerection, vomiting, diarrhoea and abdominal cramps. Examination shows a tachycardia, hypertension, mydriasis and facial flushing.

Amphetamines

These have a stimulating central effect and are taken to produce increased energy, elevated mood and greater capacity for concentration. There is also a suppression of appetite which accounts for their use in obesity. Amphetamines are taken orally or intravenously. Physical dependence is unusual but withdrawal of the drug results in rebound depression, anxiety and fatigue. Chronic ingestion can cause a syndrome identical to paranoid schizophrenia.

Cocaine

Cocaine is becoming increasingly popular, taken either intravenously or by sniffing or 'snorting' the powder into the nostrils through a tube. Absorption occurs through the nasal mucous membranes and gives a rapid stimulating effect similar to amphetamine. Cocaine hydrochloride may be converted by a simple chemical process into freebase or 'crack' cocaine which can be smoked, giving a rapid onset of effect similar to intravenous use. A toxic psychosis occurs with high levels of consumption, and tactile hallucinations (formication) may be prominent. Chronic cocaine sniffing can cause ulceration of the nasal mucosa.

Hallucinogenic drugs

Lysergic acid diethylamide (LSD) and psilocybin (magic mushroom) are currently the most commonly used hallucinogens. Perceptual changes occur within 40 minutes of oral ingestion. Vision is affected most often; the subject experiences heightened visual awareness of objects, especially colours. Images may be distorted in shape or size and true hallucinations occur. These can be terrifying in nature, the experience then being referred to as a 'bad trip'. There may also be distorted perception of time, sounds and tactile sensations. Flashback experiences can occur several months after the last dose; during these the psychotic experiences of LSD are experienced again with their original intensity. A chronic psychotic illness has also been reported after regular LSD use.

Ecstasy, the popular name for a synthetic amphetamine analogue, has become fashionable among young people for recreational use at dance parties or 'raves'. It has both stimulant and hallucinogenic properties, thus producing feelings of euphoria and emotional intimacy together with distorted sensory perceptions. There is no evidence that it is addictive but there are several reports of physical complications. Fatalities have occurred from cardiac arrhythmias, hyperthermia, disseminated intravascular coagulation, acute renal failure and cerebral haemorrhage. Paranoid psychoses have also been reported.

Organic solvents

The inhalation of organic solvents (glue sniffing) has become popular in some adolescent groups. These substances produce acute intoxication characterised by euphoria, excitement, dizziness and a floating sensation. Further inhalation leads to loss of consciousness; death can occur from the direct toxic effect of the solvent or from asphyxiation if the substance is inhaled from a plastic bag.

Management of drug abuse

The first step in management is usually aimed at helping the patient withdraw from the drug. When there are signs of severe physical dependence withdrawal is best undertaken in hospital and this also enables physical complications, such as infections, to be treated. Decreasing doses of the relevant drug are given over a period of 1–3 weeks, the dose being titrated against objective withdrawal symptoms. Oral methadone is used for opiate dependence. In some cases complete withdrawal is not successful and the patient functions better if maintained on regular doses of oral methadone as an outpatient. This decision should only be undertaken by a specialist and the long-term supervision requires the patient to attend a specially designated drug treatment centre. The withdrawal period may need to be extended to several months for some drugs—for example, benzodiazepines. A regimen for managing benzodiazepine withdrawal is shown in the information box.

MANAGING BENZODIAZEPINE WITHDRAWAL

1. Reduce daily dose by one-eighth every fortnight
2. For patients taking a drug other than diazepam and who cannot reduce it, switch to equivalent dose of diazepam preferably taken at night
3. Reduce diazepam by 2 or 2.5 mg every fortnight
4. If withdrawal symptoms occur, maintain the dose until symptoms improve
5. Reduce dose further in fortnightly steps until drug stopped completely
6. Provide regular counselling
7. Avoid other drugs (e.g. β antagonists, antidepressants) unless specifically indicated
8. It is better to reduce too slowly than too quickly. Successful withdrawal may take a year or more

Long-term support is necessary if patients are to remain drug-free. Many doctors can achieve good results if they strike up a rapport with the patient. Complicated or relapsing patients should be referred to specialist centres. Support can also be provided by self-help groups and voluntary bodies such as Narcotics Anonymous.

PSYCHIATRY OF PHYSICAL ILLNESS

Most people who become physically ill experience some degree of psychological upset which is usually brief and not distressing. During illness it is acknowledged that changes in lifestyle have to be made in accordance with the degree of disability and demands of treatment. These are usually temporary but chronic illness requires long-term readjustment.

In some cases the emotional impact of illness is sufficiently profound to precipitate psychiatric disorders which need special attention from the physician or psychiatrist. Several factors influence this development, including the patient's personality, social circumstances, the type of treatment required and the nature of the physical illness. Psychiatric disorders have been observed to be most commonly associated with cancer, haematological malignancy, chest disease and ischaemic heart disease. In recent years special attention has been given to the psychological problems associated with AIDS, particularly the need for counselling before and after HIV testing and the management of depression and confusional states as the disease becomes more advanced.

ADJUSTMENT DISORDER

This is the most common psychological response to physical illness. The predominant symptoms are depression or anxiety, or a mixture of the two, but these are not sufficiently intense to justify the diagnosis of an affective or anxiety disorder. These symptoms develop within a month of the onset of physical illness and their duration and severity reflect the course of the underlying physical condition, resolution tending to occur with physical recovery.

Grief reactions are a particular type of adjustment disorder. A bereaved person usually experiences a brief period of emotional numbing, followed by a period of distress lasting several weeks, during which sorrow, tearfulness, sleep disturbance, loss of interest and a sense of futility are common. Perceptual distortions may occur, including misinterpreting sounds as the dead person's voice or sensing the deceased's presence. The distinction between normal and abnormal grief is an arbitrary one. Considerable importance is given to the intensity and duration of symptoms and associated social dysfunction. Symptoms which are considered to indicate abnormal grief are suicidal ideas, denial of the loss, guilt and identification with the dead person by adopting some of his/her symptoms.

Adjustment disorders in general do not usually require psychotropic medication; patients can be helped by supportive measures, particularly reassurance, explanation and advice. Skilled psychotherapy is, however, required for patients with abnormal grief reactions.

ACUTE STRESS REACTION

Following an exceptionally stressful event some people with no previous psychiatric history develop a characteristic pattern of symptoms which include a sense of bewilderment, anxiety, anger, depression, overactivity and withdrawal. The symptoms are transient; they start to subside within a few hours and have usually completely resolved within 3 days of their onset. Precipitating events include major accidents, military action, criminal assault and rape.

GENERALISED ANXIETY DISORDER

Anxiety is a universal human experience which only assumes medical significance if it is disproportionate to external events or if it persists long after precipitating factors have been resolved. Symptoms of anxiety can be conveniently divided into two groups, psychological and somatic, as shown in the information box.

SYMPTOMS OF ANXIETY DISORDER

Psychological	Somatic
• Apprehension • Fear of impending disaster • Irritability • Depersonalisation	• Tremor • Sweating • Palpitations • Chest pain • Breathlessness • Headache • Dizziness • Diarrhoea • Frequency of micturition • Initial insomnia • Poor concentration

These symptoms can complicate the presentation of the underlying physical illness but it is important to remember that several physical conditions can initially manifest themselves with anxiety before other symptoms and signs develop.

PHYSICAL ILLNESSES WHICH MIMIC ANXIETY DISORDER

- Hyperthyroidism
- Phaeochromocytoma
- Hypoglycaemia
- Paroxysmal arrhythmias
- Alcohol withdrawal
- Temporal lobe epilepsy

Anxiety is a common emotion during the early stages of illness but it usually subsides, as in an adjustment disorder. Persistent anxiety is distressing, interferes with the course of the physical disorder and requires specific treatment.

PHOBIC ANXIETY DISORDER

A phobia is an abnormal fear of a particular object or situation which leads to avoidance of the provoking stimulus. Conditioned phobic responses can develop to venepuncture, hypodermic injections, chemotherapy or radiotherapy. Phobic symptoms may be so severe that the patient abandons further treatment.

Management of the anxiety disorders

Psychological approach

Explanation and reassurance are essential in the management of all forms of anxiety. The nature of the symptoms should be explained and the patient reassured that they form part of a recognised illness. Reassurance is also needed to allay fears of physical illness if this can be given after appropriate examination and investigation. Specific relaxation techniques should be taught to those who do not respond to reassurance, and are always required for patients with panic attacks. For phobic disorders relaxation should be accompanied by graded exposure (desensitisation) or flooding.

Drugs

Drugs have a limited role. Benzodiazepines are prescribed less often than previously because of the risk of dependence but they are useful in treating anxiety when symptoms can be expected to last no more than a few weeks. Diazepam can be given in doses of 2–10 mg 8-hourly but should be reduced and tailed off after 3 weeks or dependence may occur. A β-adrenoceptor blocking drug, such as propranolol 20–80 mg daily, can help when the peripheral somatic symptoms of anxiety are prominent. Antidepressant drugs, either a tricyclic (amitriptyline 50–150 mg at night) or MAOI (phenelzine 15 mg 6-hourly), are the most effective drugs in managing anxiety and should be used for generalised anxiety when symptoms do not respond to psychological approaches. They can be given in conjunction with behaviour therapy for phobic disorders and appear to be very effective for panic attacks.

POST-TRAUMATIC STRESS DISORDER (PTSD)

This is a delayed and protracted response to a stressful event of an exceptionally threatening or catastrophic nature, outside the range of everyday human experience, which would be likely to cause distress in almost everyone. The events include natural disasters, terrorist activity, serious accidents and witnessing violent deaths. There is usually a delay ranging from a few weeks to several months between the traumatic event and the onset of symptoms. Typical symptoms are recurrent intrusive memories (flashbacks) of the traumatic event, sleep disturbance, nightmares, autonomic arousal, emotional blunting and avoidance of any situation which evokes memories of the trauma. Anxiety and depression are associated features and excessive use of alcohol or drugs may complicate the clinical picture. The condition runs a fluctuating course, and most people recover within 2 years, although in a small proportion the symptoms become chronic.

Management

Current opinion favours a preventive approach in the management of this disorder by arranging immediate counselling for those who have survived a major catastrophe, with the aim of preventing the development of symptoms of PTSD. Counselling can be of various types but the essentials are to provide support, direct advice and the opportunity for catharsis by reliving the trauma. In established PTSD structured psychological approaches, particularly cognitive therapy, are used, often in conjunction with antidepressant medication.

DEPRESSIVE DISORDER

Depressive symptoms sometimes persist after physical recovery has occurred. They usually result from the patient's awareness of the implications of the illness and the need to alter future aspirations and lifestyle. As with anxiety, the symptoms of depression can be divided into psychological and somatic (see the information box) but anorexia, weight loss, fatigue and other somatic symptoms cannot be given their usual diagnostic importance because they may all be directly related to organic pathology. Greater significance should be attached to psychological symptoms, particularly loss of interest and anhedonia. Depression can prolong functional disability, thereby delaying return to work and resumption of leisure activities. It may contribute to a lifestyle of invalidism and incapacity. Such a development is likely if there are factors in the patient's environment which encourage disability. For example, the patient may, with varying degrees of insight, wish to avoid returning to an unsatisfactory job, gain attention from an unsympathetic partner or exaggerate symptoms if financial compensation is involved.

SYMPTOMS OF DEPRESSIVE DISORDER

Psychological	Somatic
• Depressed mood	• Reduced appetite
• Reduced self-esteem	• Weight change
• Pessimism	• Disturbed sleep
• Guilt	• Fatigue
• Loss of interest	• Loss of libido
• Loss of enjoyment (anhedonia)	• Bowel disturbance
• Suicidal thinking	• Retardation
	• Poor concentration

Management

The persistent nature of the symptoms requires active treatment. Psychotherapy and cognitive therapy are both useful and have been shown to be effective. Antidepressant drugs can be used in combination with psychological approaches. Tricyclic antidepressants are poorly tolerated by physically ill people and are contraindicated in the presence of heart disease, glaucoma and prostatism because of their anticholinergic properties. Paroxetine (or other 5-HT re-uptake inhibitors) and venlafaxine are the drugs of choice.

Depression or mania may be the presenting symptoms of various underlying physical illnesses. In these cases the psychological symptoms result from disturbances of neurotransmitter function or interruption of anatomical pathways in the brain. Physical examination is essential in patients presenting with a new episode of psychiatric illness, and suspicion of underlying physical pathology should be aroused, particularly in the circumstances listed in the information box.

POINTERS TO AN ORGANIC CAUSE FOR PSYCHIATRIC DISORDER

- Late age of onset of psychiatric illness
- No previous history of psychiatric illness
- No family history of psychiatric illness
- No apparent psychological precipitant

These symptomatic psychiatric disorders can occur in the conditions listed in the information box below.

ORGANIC CAUSES OF AFFECTIVE DISORDERS

Neurological
- Cerebrovascular disease
- Cerebral tumour
- Multiple sclerosis
- Parkinson's disease
- Huntington's chorea
- Alzheimer's disease
- Epilepsy

Endocrine
- Hypothyroidism
- Hyperthyroidism
- Cushing's syndrome
- Addison's disease
- Hyperparathyroidism

Infections
- Glandular fever
- Herpes simplex
- Brucellosis
- Typhoid
- Toxoplasmosis

Connective tissue disease
- Systemic lupus erythematosus

Malignant disease

Drugs
- Reserpine, phenothiazines
- Methyldopa, oral contraceptives
- Corticosteroids, phenylbutazone

SOMATIC PRESENTATION OF PSYCHIATRIC ILLNESS

Somatic symptoms such as fatigue, dizziness, headache and other pains are commonly experienced during periods of emotional stress. This becomes a medical problem when the symptoms are attributed to physical illness for which the patient requests medical attention. Many patients with psychiatric illness present in this manner to their general practitioner or hospital specialist. This phenomenon, known as somatisation, results in considerable misdiagnosis because the somatic presentation misleads the doctor into suspecting physical illness and distracts attention from underlying psychiatric problems. Not only does the patient have somatic symptoms but sometimes there is also a concern about a specific physical illness such as cancer, heart disease, AIDS or myalgic encephalomyelitis.

Among patients attending general hospital medical clinics at least one-fifth have no significant organic disease to account for their symptoms but have a psychiatric illness which is only detected when specific questions are asked.

Most have a depressive illness or one of the anxiety disorders (generalised anxiety, panic attacks or phobic disorder). The symptoms may have an abrupt onset, in which case the history is short and a good response can be expected to conventional treatment. In a small proportion there is a longer history of complaints and disability; these patients are often diagnosed as having hypochondriasis, Briquet's syndrome (somatisation disorder) or dissociative disorder and are less easy to treat.

PSYCHIATRIC DISORDERS IN SOMATISING PATIENTS

Acute	Chronic
• Adjustment disorder	• Somatisation disorder
• Phobic anxiety disorder	• Hypochondriacal disorder
• Panic disorder	• Somatoform autonomic dysfunction
• Generalised anxiety disorder	• Somatoform pain disorder
• Dissociative disorder	• Neurasthenia

Aetiology

The presenting somatic complaints are often amplifications of normal physiological sensations or muscular aches. During episodes of depression or anxiety these sensations are exaggerated, and interpreted in a morbid manner, thus becoming the focus for medical complaint. A family history or previous personal history of a particular physical illness may influence the location of symptoms as well as their interpretation. Many patients selectively emphasise somatic symptoms when they visit their doctor because they believe there is more medical interest in physical illness. Their pattern of somatisation is subsequently reinforced if special investigations are arranged, particularly if these yield equivocal results.

DISSOCIATIVE (CONVERSION) DISORDER

This is one of the most controversial concepts in psychiatry. It has, at least temporarily, replaced the previously used term 'hysteria' in the ICD-10 classification but many clinicians still prefer to retain 'hysteria' as a diagnostic category. Controversy has occurred because of the high rate of organic disease in patients previously diagnosed as having hysteria and also because of the multiple uses of the term, which has been used to describe symptoms, a personality type, an epidemic phenomenon and clinical syndromes.

'Dissociative disorder' is best used to define a syndrome characterised by a loss or distortion of neurological function not fully explained by organic disease.

Aetiology

The condition is considered to result from unconscious psychological processes, implying that the patient lacks insight into the nature of the symptoms. In psychoanalytic terms, dissociative disorder has been seen as a maladaptive way of coping with an unresolved psychological conflict—that is, by becoming ill. The patient thus derives primary gain by relieving the conflict, and secondary gain by obtaining sympathy and attention from others or by avoiding everyday responsibilities. Dissociative disorder is more commonly diagnosed in women and children, groups who often lack an effective means of verbal communication because of an inferior social position.

The role of organic neurological disease is unclear. Although, by definition, the symptoms of hysteria are not themselves caused by organic disease, there is coexisting disease of the nervous system in up to 50% of cases. Organic disease may facilitate dissociative mechanisms and provide a model for symptoms, thus, for example, explaining the occurrence of pseudoseizures in patients with epilepsy.

Clinical features

The most common symptoms of dissociative disorder mimic lesions in the motor or sensory nervous system and in classic cases there is apparent unconcern (belle indifférence) even in the face of gross physical disability. However, this should not be relied upon for diagnostic purposes. The presentations of dissociative disorder are given in the information box.

COMMON PRESENTATIONS OF DISSOCIATIVE DISORDER

- Gait disturbance
- Loss of function in limbs
- Aphonia
- Pseudoseizures
- Sensory loss
- Blindness

Dissociative disorder can also involve higher mental functions, especially memory and general intelligence.

Dissociative amnesia usually develops acutely. The memory loss is patchy and inconsistent; a characteristic feature is a loss of personal identity so that the patient is unable to recall his or her name, address or other personal and family details. Memory loss of this degree does not occur in organic disease unless there is gross dementia. Dissociative amnesia is occasionally accompanied by a tendency to travel aimlessly many miles from familiar surroundings; this is known as a hysterical fugue. When global intelligence is affected, the cognitive deficits are variable and the patient's behaviour is not in keeping with the apparent degree of dementia.

Management

A full physical and psychiatric assessment should be completed to determine whether other disorders are present.

Once the doctor is satisfied that relevant organic disease has been excluded, no further investigations should be undertaken and therapeutic effort should be directed towards restoring optimal function. Many patients resist the idea that their symptoms are not entirely somatic. Confrontation is best avoided and initial management should concentrate on simple explanation and reassurance that the symptoms conform to a recognised pattern and will get better with treatment. This involves identifying those factors which appear to have precipitated the symptoms and helping the patient to cope with them more adaptively. Secondary reinforcing factors in the patient's social network must be corrected and physical treatment—for example, physiotherapy—should be arranged to provide an acceptable framework for recovery. Little is to be gained by debating how much insight the patient really has into his or her condition. Acute symptoms respond well to treatment. In resistant cases recovery can be helped by abreaction under the influence of hypnosis or small intravenous doses of a short-acting benzodiazepine. During abreaction the patient is encouraged to describe, in a cathartic manner, the emotional trauma which provoked the symptoms while the doctor makes use of the patient's enhanced suggestibility to predict symptom relief.

SOMATOFORM DISORDERS

The essential feature of this group of disorders is repeated medical consultation for physical symptoms which have no adequate physical basis. In most cases a psychiatric assessment will show that the physical symptoms bear a close relationship with stressful life events or emotional conflicts. Unfortunately, the degree of psychological understanding which the patient achieves is often minimal and a physician's attempts to discuss the possibility of psychological causation are firmly resisted. Several syndromes are described within this group; there is considerable overlap between them, both in aetiology and clinical presentation, and they also have similarities with dissociative disorder.

Somatisation disorder

This syndrome runs a chronic and fluctuating course over many years. Symptoms start in early adult life, are more frequent in women and may be referred to any part of the body. Common complaints include pain, vomiting, nausea, headache, dizziness, menstrual irregularities and sexual dysfunction. By the time the patient is referred to a psychiatrist there is usually a multitude of negative investigations and unhelpful operations, particularly hysterectomy and cholecystectomy.

Hypochondriacal disorder

This refers to a morbid preoccupation with the possibility of having a serious physical illness. Hypochondriacal symptoms commonly occur in anxiety and depressive disorders but occasionally they are primary and persist for many years. In a small proportion of cases conviction of disease reaches delusional intensity, the best-known example being the conviction of parasitic infestation ('delusional parasitosis'), which leads patients to consult dermatologists. Pimozide (2–12 mg daily) has been claimed to be effective for this syndrome. A preoccupation with bodily disfigurement (body dysmorphic disorder) leads to inappropriate requests for cosmetic surgery.

Somatoform autonomic dysfunction

Symptoms are referred to organs which are largely under autonomic control. The most common examples involve the cardiovascular system (cardiac neurosis), respiratory system (psychogenic hyperventilation) and gut (psychogenic vomiting and irritable bowel syndrome).

Somatoform pain disorder

The cardinal feature is severe, persistent pain which cannot be explained by a physical illness or physiological disturbance. Sufficient emotional conflicts or psychosocial problems are evident to conclude that these are the main causal influences on the pain. Patients with this disorder usually make great demands for emotional support from their families and for treatment from the medical profession.

Management of somatoform disorders

Similar principles apply as in the management of dissociative disorders. Physical examination and investigations should be arranged according to the pattern of symptoms and once organic disease has been excluded requests for further investigations should be resisted if there is sufficient positive evidence to make a psychiatric diagnosis. Most of the somatoform disorders are chronic so complete recovery must not be expected. Treatment involves a multidisciplinary team approach and aims to minimise the rewards of the sick role and to encourage healthy behaviour. The attitudes of close relatives may need to be modified to effect these changes because they may have adopted an over-protective role, unwittingly reinforcing the patient's disability.

Antidepressant drugs have a limited role in treating depressive episodes when they arise; they are also useful in some cases of psychogenic pain.

NEURASTHENIA

Also known as chronic fatigue syndrome, this condition is characterised by excessive fatigue after minimal physical or mental exertion, poor concentration, dizziness and muscular aches. There may be various autonomic symptoms affecting the cardiovascular or gastrointestinal systems. The sleep pattern is altered, with frequent waking or hypersomnia.

This pattern of symptoms may follow a viral infection such as infectious mononucleosis, influenza or hepatitis; the term 'myalgic encephalomyelitis' is used by those who favour a viral aetiology. However, in most cases there is no convincing evidence of viral infection, either from the history or antibody titres. There is a considerable overlap with the symptoms of an affective disorder and many psychiatrists regard neurasthenia as a variant of depression.

Current approaches to treatment favour an active programme of rehabilitation combined with cognitive therapy and antidepressant medication without sedative effects.

EATING DISORDERS

ANOREXIA NERVOSA

This disorder, which sometimes causes extreme emaciation, typically develops during adolescence and predominantly affects girls. Only 5–10% of cases occur in males; occasionally the condition develops in older women. There is a higher prevalence in the upper social classes and the patients are often hard-working, perfectionist and ambitious. Theories about aetiology are speculative. Current social pressures to maintain a slim figure are thought to have caused a recent increased incidence. Some girls have a history of obesity and embark on an extreme course of dieting after being teased about their fatness. Anorexia has also been regarded as an attempt to remain pre-pubertal by girls who have fears of sexual maturation. In other cases anorexia appears a non-specific response to family crises which often involve the parental relationship. Hormonal changes have been suggested as aetiologically important. However, the endocrine abnormalities nearly always revert to normal following restoration of weight and are probably secondary to the effects of weight loss.

Clinical features

These are listed in the information box.

In boys, loss of sexual interest replaces amenorrhoea as a diagnostic criterion. Other features include a striking indifference to the weight loss and a denial of problems. Emaciation may be disguised by wearing loosely fitting clothes and hiding heavy objects in the clothing when weight is checked on scales. Subjects are often physically overactive; they may use laxatives or induce vomiting secretly after meals. Although they avoid carbohydrates and fats they are often preoccupied with food and enjoy making elaborate meals for their families. Other physical signs include a downy, lanugo hair on the trunk and limbs, hypotension, bradycardia and peripheral cyanosis. Psychosexual immaturity is often prominent.

ESSENTIAL DIAGNOSTIC CRITERIA FOR ANOREXIA NERVOSA

- Weight loss of at least 25% of original body weight (or weight 25% below norm for age and height)
- Avoidance of high-calorie foods
- Distortion of body image so that the patient regards herself as fat even when grossly underweight
- Amenorrhoea for at least 3 months

Management

The first objective is to restore normal body weight, which is most likely to be achieved if a trusting relationship can be established with the patient from the first interview. Treatment can be conducted on an outpatient or day patient basis unless there is a risk of suicide or serious physical complications. Inpatient treatment should then be arranged. By educating the patient about the dangers of starvation it should be possible to establish the need for weight gain and to agree on a target weight which should be reached slowly in a controlled manner. If inpatient treatment becomes necessary the patient should be supervised during meals and for 1 hour subsequently to ensure vomiting does not occur. A series of target weights should be set and the patient is allowed increasing privileges and independence as each target is achieved. The final target should be within the normal range for the patient's age and height. Psychotherapy is an essential part of management. Individual therapy allows the patient to acquire insight into her condition and associated problems. Family therapy is also necessary to help resolve tensions which are nearly always evident by the time the patient presents for treatment.

The short-term prognosis is good if this programme is followed but the long-term outlook is less favourable. Approximately 20% make a full recovery, 20% remain chronically ill and 60% have recurring episodes of anorexia. Death occurs from suicide or physical complications in 5% of cases.

BULIMIA NERVOSA

This disorder was described in the late 1970s and is related to anorexia nervosa. It is almost exclusively confined to women and the age of onset is slightly older than for anorexia. Prevalence has been estimated at 1% of women in their early twenties.

Clinical features

These are listed in the information box.

DIAGNOSTIC CRITERIA FOR BULIMIA NERVOSA

- Recurrent bouts of binge-eating
- Lack of self-control over eating during binges
- Self-induced vomiting, purgation or dieting after binges
- Weight maintained within normal limits

The binges occur at least twice weekly and involve rich foods such as cakes, chocolates and dairy products; over 20 000 calories may be consumed during the day of a binge. Despite this intake weight is usually maintained within the normal range and menstruation is often regular. Physical complications from vomiting and purgation include erosion of dental enamel, hypokalaemia and metabolic alkalosis. Electrolyte and fluid disturbances can cause cardiac arrhythmias or renal damage. A bilateral enlargement of the parotid glands is seen in some patients.

Management

Most treatment can be undertaken on an outpatient basis. Cognitive behaviour therapy is the currently preferred approach, the central component being self-monitoring of eating behaviour. The patient is asked to keep a full eating diary, together with a record of emotions and circumstances associated with binges. A series of tasks are set which are directed at helping the patient cope more appropriately with provoking stimuli, thereby reducing the frequency and severity of binges. Treatment may need to be continued for several months; short-term results are encouraging but the long-term prognosis of the condition is not known.

OBESITY

This is the most common form of eating disorder but it is rarely seen as a presenting problem in psychiatric practice. It is defined in terms of a high body mass index (BMI), i.e. weight in kilograms divided by the square of height in metres. The normal range of BMI is 20–25 (see p. 526) and on these figures one-third of the British population is obese. Obesity results from excessive intake of food and insufficient exercise, but constitutional and cultural factors are important in its aetiology and maintenance. There is no consistent association between obesity and psychiatric illness or personality traits but many obese people find the condition highly embarrassing. The management of patients with mild to moderate (BMI 25–40) and gross (BMI over 40) obesity is discussed on pages 528–531.

SLEEP DISORDERS

Sleep has a restorative function and is important for conservation of energy and growth. It comprises two distinct physiological states: rapid eye movement (REM) sleep and non-REM sleep. Non-REM sleep consists of four stages, two of which are known as 'slow wave' or deep sleep because they are associated with low-frequency, synchronised waves on the electroencephalogram. REM sleep develops after progression through the various stages of non-REM sleep, usually within 90 minutes. It is the stage in which most dreaming occurs. During a night's sleep there is a cycle of non-REM and REM sleep, with the episodes of REM becoming relatively longer.

INSOMNIA

Insomnia is a condition of inadequate quantity or quality of sleep. It may be a symptom of a depressive illness, anxiety disorder or other psychiatric condition. More commonly it arises at a time of increased life stress; some people then become preoccupied with lack of sleep and fear trying to get to sleep. This establishes a vicious circle which perpetuates the problem.

When insomnia results from a definite psychiatric illness treatment should be directed towards the underlying condition. Counselling, cognitive therapy, psychotherapy and medication all have their place. Sleep disturbance is a particularly distressing symptom of depressive illness, in which case an antidepressant drug with marked sedative properties (e.g. amitriptyline, dothiepin) should be prescribed to be taken at night.

Hypnotic drugs are useful for short-term treatment of insomnia due to acute stress: for example, bereavement or separation. They should not be taken for longer than 3 weeks. Benzodiazepines such as temazepam (10–20 mg) are most commonly used. It is claimed that tolerance and dependence are less likely to develop with some of the newer hypnotics—for example, zopiclone.

Drugs are not appropriate when insomnia is a chronic condition. In such cases much can be achieved by giving advice about regular exercise and avoiding heavy meals, alcohol and caffeine-containing drinks during the evening. Behavioural techniques such as relaxation exercises and various cognitive strategies to cope with intrusive thoughts are generally helpful.

PARASOMNIAS

The two most important are sleepwalking and night terrors, both of which occur during slow-wave sleep. During sleepwalking vision and coordination remain intact but serious accidents can occur. It is important that these patients sleep in a protected environment.

Night terrors start with a frightening scream which is associated with sweating, increased heart and respiratory rates and a scared expression. The patient is usually unable to recall the episodes (unlike nightmares). It is claimed that parasomnias resolve with improved sleep hygiene, particularly reduced consumption of alcohol and caffeine.

SEXUAL DYSFUNCTIONS

These complaints include low sexual interest and various difficulties experienced during intercourse which reduce mutual satisfaction. Sexual dysfunction can occur transiently as a symptom of an anxiety disorder or depressive illness or it may be a manifestation of a relationship problem. Physical health has an important influence and needs careful assessment. Sexual interest and performance are impaired during any debilitating illness. Endocrine, cardiovascular and neurological disorders should be especially considered; for example, impotence may be a presenting feature of hypogonadism, diabetes, peripheral vascular disease or multiple sclerosis. Finally, an alcohol and drug history should be taken. Any drug which has a depressant effect on the central nervous system can impair sexual function, as also can drugs which act on the peripheral autonomic system (e.g. alpha-methyldopa, phenothiazines, tricyclic antidepressants).

IMPOTENCE

This involves complete or partial erectile failure with normal sexual desire. It is often transient and improves with reassurance. If persistent it can be helped by a behavioural programme in which the partner's cooperation is essential. Successful results have also been obtained by injecting papaverine into the corpora cavernosa and this treatment is now preferred in many clinics. Drugs taken orally are also available, e.g. sildenafil.

PREMATURE EJACULATION

This is defined as ejaculation prior to penetration or, if penetration occurs, before the partner can achieve orgasm. It is often associated with high levels of anxiety, which appear to perpetuate the condition. Successful treatment is based on behavioural techniques derived from the work of Masters and Johnson.

VAGINISMUS

Vaginismus is due to spasm of the pelvic muscles which prevents full penetration. It results from intense fear of penetration, and a conditioned reflex is established resulting in pelvic spasm even at the thought of intercourse. Treatment consists of instructing the patient in relaxation exercises followed by insertion of vaginal dilators of increasing size, initially by the doctor, then the patient and finally the partner.

FEMALE ORGASMIC DYSFUNCTION

Most cases result from ignorance of sexual technique. Counselling is usually effective in overcoming the problem. Approximately 10% of women appear physiologically incapable of orgasm due to absence of the bulbocavernosus reflex.

SEXUAL DEVIATIONS

Sexual deviations involve obtaining sexual arousal from inanimate objects or unwilling partners. Examples include exhibitionism (genital exposure in public), fetishism (arousal from female clothing), transvestism (arousal by dressing in clothes of the opposite sex) and paedophilia (sexual arousal with children).

TRANSSEXUALISM

This rare condition results from a disturbance of gender identity. The patient, usually a man, is convinced he should have been born female and strongly identifies with feminine psychology. He wishes to live his life as a woman and may request medical help to do so. Transsexuals should be referred to special clinics where hormone therapy may be given to enable suitable patients to develop the secondary sexual characteristics of the opposite sex. Surgical treatment can be undertaken to reassign external genitalia if the patient can successfully adopt the lifestyle of the opposite sex for at least 12 months.

FACTITIOUS DISORDERS

This term is used in connection with individuals who, in the absence of a distinct psychiatric or physical disorder, repeatedly induce the signs or symptoms of disease. The behaviour is consistent and deliberate. It is often difficult to understand the underlying motives other than as an attempt to gain access to the role of patient and to fool doctors.

One pattern is seen predominantly in young women who usually work in nursing or one of the other professions allied to medicine. These patients surreptitiously fabricate the signs of disease: for example, by regularly taking hormone preparations or by inducing anaemia by repeated bleeding. Other presentations include chronic ulcerating skin lesions (dermatitis artefacta), pyrexia of unknown origin and hypoglycaemia.

Another form of factitious disorder, Münchausen's syndrome, is seen in patients who present with dramatic symptoms of a medical emergency such as myocardial infarction or intra-abdominal catastrophe. The patient fabricates a convincing history which persuades an unsuspecting doctor to undertake complicated investigations or exploratory surgery. If suspicions are aroused it may be possible to trace the patient's history showing that he or she has presented similarly at several other hospitals, often changing his or her name several times during the course of these travels. When confronted with the fraudulent nature of the symptoms the patients discharge themselves angrily, only to present again at another hospital shortly afterwards. This condition is named after the German Baron von

Münchhausen, who was legendary for his inventive lying. Treatment is strikingly ineffective but it is important to recognise the syndrome to avoid unnecessary investigations.

Management

By their nature, personality disorders cannot be cured but some individuals can be helped to make necessary changes so that their behaviour is less distressing to themselves or other people. Various psychological treatments have been used and success has been claimed for behaviour therapy and interpretive psychotherapy. Some experts believe group therapy is especially helpful.

It is important to remember that people with personality disorders can develop other psychiatric illnesses, the features of which are coloured by underlying personality. These illnesses respond to conventional treatment but often remain undetected.

In a minority of patients a depressed mood persists for weeks or months after physical recovery and is accompanied by the characteristic symptoms of loss of interest, low self-esteem, sleep disturbance and weight change. The diagnosis of a secondary depressive illness is then warranted and treatment with antidepressant medication is required. Physically ill patients tolerate antidepressant drugs poorly. Lower doses than usual should be used initially and if side-effects to tricyclics are troublesome one of the newer drugs like fluoxetine (20–80 mg daily) can be given. Close collaboration between physician and psychiatrist is essential for optimal management. Nowhere is this more important than in the care of the elderly, who are prone to multiple problems, physical, psychological and social.

Depression can prolong functional disability following physical illness, thereby delaying return to work and resumption of leisure activities. In other cases recovery is delayed even though there is no evidence of depression. These patients remain incapacitated and adopt a lifestyle of invalidism or abnormal illness behaviour. The explanation can be found by examining the patient's social environment, when various factors prolonging the disability may be uncovered.

FURTHER INFORMATION ON CLINICAL SYNDROMES

Bancroft J 1989 Human sexuality and its problems, 2nd edn. Churchill Livingstone, Edinburgh

Bass C, Benjamin S 1993 The management of chronic somatisation. British Journal of Psychiatry 162: 472–480

British Medical Association 1997 Misuse of drugs. Harwood, Amsterdam

Lishman W A 1997 Organic psychiatry, 3rd edn. Blackwell, Oxford

Lishman W A 1990 Alcohol and the brain. British Journal of Psychiatry 156: 635–644

Shapiro C M 1992 ABC of sleep disorders. British Medical Journal Publishing Group, London

Sharp C W, Freeman C P L 1993 The medical complications of anorexia nervosa. British Journal of Psychiatry 162: 452–462

SPECIAL CLINICAL PROBLEMS

ATTEMPTED SUICIDE

There was a steady increase in hospital admissions for suicide attempts from the early 1960s so that by the end of the 1970s there were over 100 000 admissions annually in the UK. Since then there has been a slight decrease but attempted suicide is still one of the most common reasons for acute medical admission. The term 'attempted suicide' is potentially misleading in that the majority of patients are not unequivocally trying to kill themselves. However, alternative terms such as 'parasuicide' and 'deliberate, non-fatal self-harm' have not been widely accepted and 'attempted suicide' can be retained provided it is realised that it does not inevitably involve fatal intent.

Most suicide attempts involve overdose, either of prescribed or non-prescribed drugs. Less common methods include wrist slashing, asphyxiation, drowning, hanging, jumping from a height or in front of a moving vehicle, and using firearms. Methods which carry a high chance of being fatal are more likely to be associated with serious psychiatric illness.

Suicide attempts are more common in women than in men and in young adults than in the elderly. In contrast, completed suicide is more common in men and in the elderly, although there has recently been an increased rate of suicide in young adults. There is a higher incidence of suicide attempts among the lower socio-economic groups, particularly those living in crowded, socially deprived urban areas. Patients often have a deprived family background due to early loss of a parent through death or separation. There are also links with alcohol abuse, child abuse, unemployment and recently broken relationships.

A thorough psychiatric and social assessment must be carried out in all cases. In most hospitals this involves an interview with a psychiatrist. This need not always be the case because it is now recognised that junior physicians, nurses and social workers can assess these patients competently if properly trained and supervised. The assessment should be undertaken after emergency medical

ASSESSMENT OF PATIENTS AFTER ATTEMPTED SUICIDE

- Explanation of attempt
- Degree of suicide intent
- Presence of psychiatric illness
- Current suicidal risk
- Previous suicide attempts
- Family and personal history
- Social support available to patient
- Patient's usual ability to cope with stress
- Further management

treatment has been completed. In patients who have taken drug overdoses it is important that sufficient time has elapsed to allow the toxic effects of the drug to wear off. Topics to be covered when assessing a patient are listed in the information box.

The patient should be asked about events occurring immediately before the act and whether the attempt had been planned beforehand. In some cases there will be clear evidence that suicide was intended; the patient may have recently made a will, disposed of treasured possessions, gone to considerable effort to avoid discovery or left an explicit suicide note. All these help explain the motivation behind the attempt. The interviewer needs to assess the severity of any current symptoms of psychiatric illness and to assess what personal and social supports would be available if the patient were to leave hospital.

The majority of patients have depressive and anxiety symptoms which are reactive to an acute life crisis superimposed on a background of chronic social and personal difficulties. They do not require psychotropic medication or specialised psychiatric treatment. They need emotional support and practical advice to help them cope with the crisis which has precipitated the attempt. A social worker may be the most appropriate person to provide this help. Admission to a psychiatric ward is necessary for patients who have a major psychiatric illness, who remain intent on suicide or who require temporary respite from intolerable domestic circumstances. Admission should also be arranged when further information is needed to clarify the patient's mental state.

Approximately 20% make a repeat attempt during the following 12 months and 1% succeed in killing themselves. Factors which are known to be associated with an increased risk of suicide after a suicide attempt are listed in the information box.

RISK FACTORS FOR SUICIDE AFTER A SUICIDE ATTEMPT

- Psychiatric illness (depressive illness, schizophrenia)
- Age over 45
- Male sex
- Living alone
- Unemployed
- Recently bereaved, divorced or separated
- Chronic physical ill health
- Drug or alcohol abuse
- Violent method used (e.g. hanging, jumping)
- Suicide note written
- History of previous attempts

PSYCHIATRIC EMERGENCIES

These can occur in the community or in hospital wards but one of the most common locations where doctors encounter psychiatric emergencies is in the accident and emergency department of a general hospital. They require urgent action because the patient's behaviour is potentially dangerous to himself or herself or other people; the behaviour disturbance may be aggression, extreme overactivity or suicidal activity.

Rapid assessment is required. Two main decisions need to be taken. First, is the behaviour disturbance due to psychiatric illness? If not, the patient may have to be dealt with by the police. If the patient is psychiatrically ill, the second decision is whether it is an organic or functional illness. A full history and mental state examination will be out of the question. As much information as possible should be obtained from informants. This should include enquiries about recent mood change, paranoid ideas or other psychiatric symptoms. There may be a history of previous psychiatric illness, recent physical illness, head injury or drug abuse. When assessing the patient's mental state the key elements are evidence of cognitive impairment, paranoid delusions, and aggressive or suicidal intent. It is also important to understand any triggering events which have precipitated the emergency.

Many aggressive and overactive patients are frightened because their behaviour is determined by paranoid experiences. They can be calmed by a confident, non-threatening approach. It is helpful if they feel the doctor understands what has brought on their distress. If there is a high risk of violence, the patient must be restrained. This should not be attempted until sufficient staff are present to overpower the patient safely. The police need to be involved if the patient is armed or causing actual physical harm. Once restraints have been imposed it is likely that sedation will be required. Haloperidol is the drug of choice. It can be given intramuscularly at an initial dose of 10–20 mg; this can be repeated if necessary until the patient is calmed. A decision can then be taken about the next stage in management, depending on the nature of the underlying psychiatric disorder.

LEGAL ASPECTS OF PSYCHIATRY

Psychiatry has closer links with the law than most other branches of medicine because psychiatric illness sometimes impairs judgement to the extent that the patients are not considered fully responsible for their actions. A doctor may therefore be required to prepare a report if a patient is considered psychiatrically ill and has been charged with committing an offence. This may need to concentrate on whether the patient is able to understand the charge, fit to plead, able to instruct a lawyer, able to follow proceedings in court and able to understand the verdict. The report should describe the patient's background and mental state at the time of the assessment and give an opinion of the patient's mental state at the time the offence was committed. A summary should comment on the patient's criminal responsibility and make recommendations for future management if it is thought more appropriate for the patient to be treated in a medical context rather than to be sent to prison. This may involve a probation order conditional on regular psychiatric outpatient attendance.

All doctors in clinical practice need to be familiar with the legal aspects of admitting psychiatrically ill patients to hospital against their will or detaining them in hospital after admission. It should be reiterated here that these regulations apply only to a small minority, less than 10% of psychiatric inpatients.

All countries have specific laws to deal with the treatment of mental illness but only the British ones can be dealt with in detail here.

The law in England and Wales is governed by the *Mental Health Act*, 1983. This is principally concerned with the grounds for detaining patients in hospital or placing them under guardianship. Application for compulsory admission to hospital can only be made when the patient, who is suffering from mental disorder, is not willing to be admitted voluntarily and ought to be detained in the interests of his or her own health or safety or with a view to the protection of other persons. The definition of mental disorder includes mental illness, mental impairment and psychopathic disorder, the latter resulting in abnormally aggressive or

Table 18.5 Important provisions of the *Mental Health Act*, 1983 (England and Wales)

Purpose	Section	Duration	Signatures required	Appeal
Emergency admission	4	72 hours	One doctor plus relative or social worker	None
Assessment and treatment	2	28 days	Two doctors (one approved) plus nearest relative or social worker	To Tribunal within 14 days of admission
Treatment	3	6 months	Two doctors (one approved) plus nearest relative or social worker	To Tribunal within first 6 months and once during each subsequent period for which detention renewed
Emergency detention of patient in hospital	5 (2)	72 hours	Doctor in charge	None
Emergency detention of patient in hospital	5 (4)	6 hours	Nurse (REM status)	None
Assessment of persons in public places thought to be mentally ill and in need of safety	136	72 hours	Police officer	None

Table 18.6 Important provisions of the *Mental Health (Scotland) Act*, 1984

Purpose	Section	Duration	Signatures required	Appeal
Emergency admission	24	72 hours	One doctor; consent of relative or mental health officer, if practicable	None
Short-term detention and treatment	26	28 days (further to Section 24 or 25 (i))	Approved doctor in addition to recommendation under Section 24 or 25 (i); consent of nearest relative or mental health officer, if practicable	To Sheriff or Mental Welfare Commission
Non-urgent admission	18	6 months	Two doctors (one approved); nearest relative or mental health officer; Sheriff's approval	To Mental Welfare Commission; to Sheriff if detention extended after 6 months
Emergency detention of patient in hospital	25 (i)	72 hours	Doctor in charge	None
Emergency detention of patient in hospital	25 (ii)	2 hours	Nurse (RMN status)	
Detention of person in public place thought to be mentally ill and in need of safety	118	72 hours	Police officer	None

seriously irresponsible conduct. Significant changes were introduced to improve patients' rights by allowing appeal against detention under certain sections of the Act. Appeals are heard by a Mental Health Review Tribunal. This consists of three members: a circuit judge or equivalent who acts as president of the tribunal, a medical representative and a lay representative. Table 18.5 summarises the most important sections of the Act with which doctors need to be familiar.

Similar legislation for Scotland was passed by the *Mental Health (Scotland) Act*, 1984. Reasons for hospital admission and detention are similar to those for England and Wales, except that psychopathic disorder is not included. Appeals in Scotland can be made to the Mental Welfare Commission or to the Sheriff. The most important sections of this Act for medical practice are summarised in Table 18.6.

FURTHER INFORMATION ON SPECIAL CLINICAL PROBLEMS

Appleby L 1992 Suicide in psychiatric patients: risk and prevention. British Journal of Psychiatry 161: 749–758

Gelder M, Gath D, Mayou R 1994 Concise Oxford textbook of psychiatry. Oxford University Press, Oxford

Goldberg D, Benjamin S, Creed F 1994 Psychiatry in medical practice, 2nd edn. Tavistock, London

Hawton K, Fagg J, Platt S, Hawkins M 1993 Factors associated with suicide after parasuicide in young people. British Medical Journal 306: 1641–1644

Lloyd G G 1993 Acute behaviour disturbances. Journal of Neurology, Neurosurgery and Psychiatry 56: 1149–1156

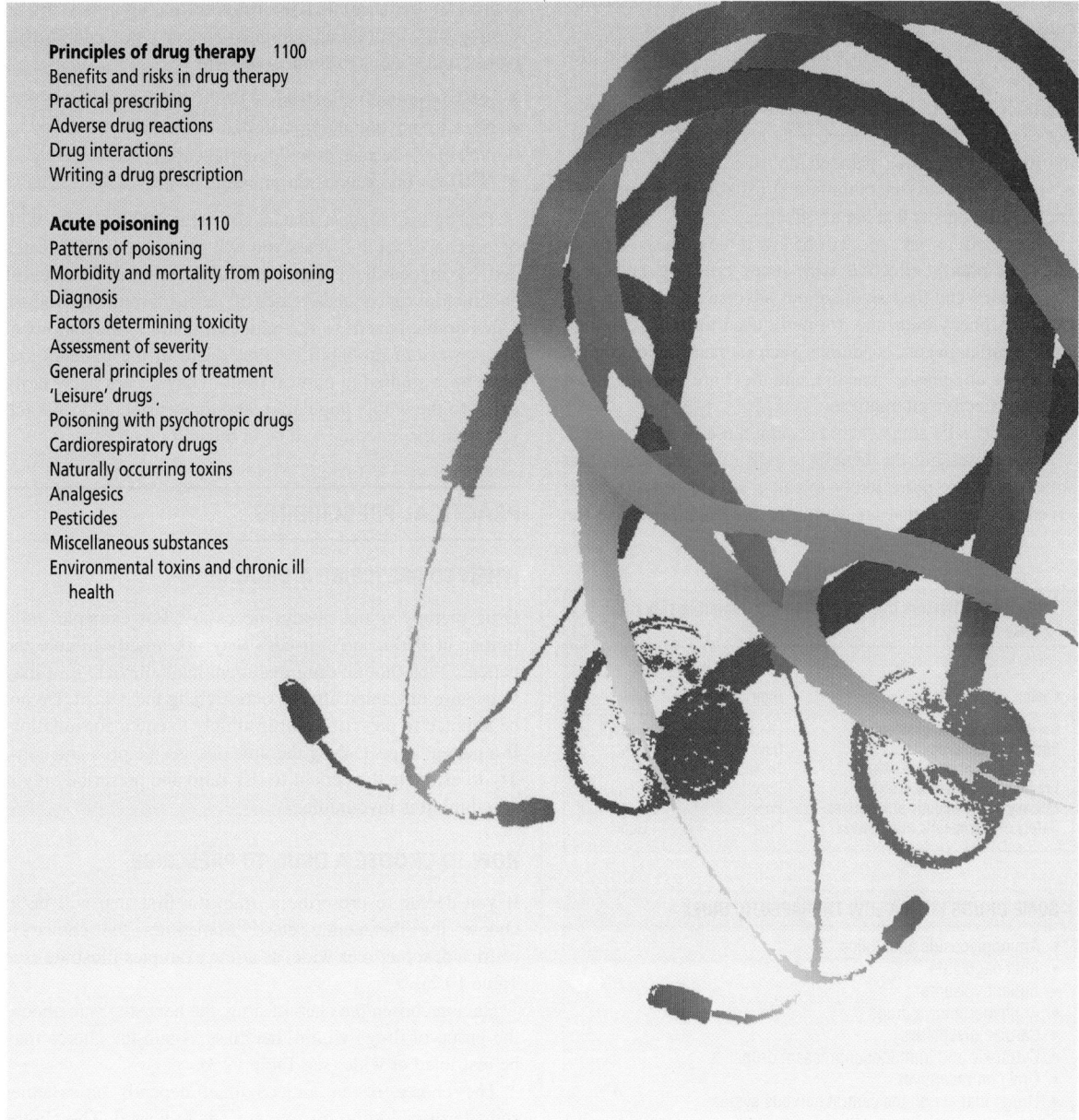

Principles of drug therapy and management of poisoning

19

J.K. ARONSON • A.T. PROUDFOOT

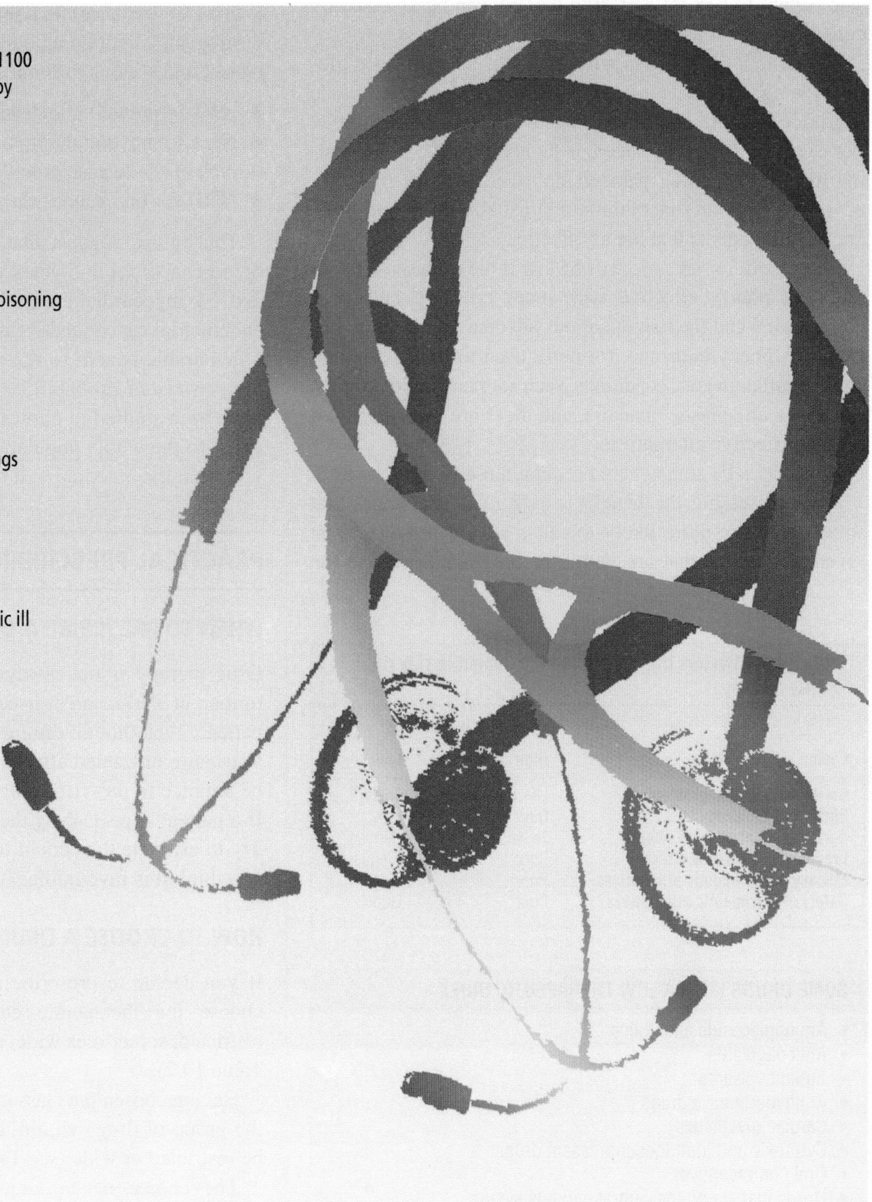

PRINCIPLES OF DRUG THERAPY

The purpose of drug therapy is to cure or ameliorate disease or alleviate symptoms. However, all drugs have adverse effects to a greater or lesser extent. Before prescribing, the potential benefits should be weighed against the risks.

BENEFITS AND RISKS IN DRUG THERAPY

The benefit to risk ratio of drug therapy can be assessed by considering various factors (see Table 19.1).

The benefit to risk ratio will be high if the disease is life-threatening, the drug highly effective and the only one available, and the risk of serious adverse effects negligible. For example, N-acetylcysteine is highly effective in preventing liver damage after paracetamol overdose (see p. 1119), adverse effects are uncommon and usually mild, and there are no other agents that are as effective.

The benefit to risk ratio will be low if the disease is trivial, the drug poorly effective with more effective and safer competitors, and the risk of serious adverse effects high. For example, phenylbutazone, formerly used to treat acute and chronic inflammatory conditions, such as rheumatoid arthritis, can cause an aplastic anaemia, and there are now safer and equally effective alternatives.

Most cases lie somewhere between these two extremes.

When assessing the benefit to risk ratio remember that some drugs are more likely to cause adverse effects when given in dosages that are within or only a little above the usual therapeutic range; these drugs are said to have a low therapeutic index (see the information box).

Table 19.1 Factors that determine the benefit to risk ratio in drug therapy

	Benefit to risk ratio	
Factor	**High**	**Low**
Seriousness of the problem	Life-threatening	Trivial
Efficacy of the drug	High	Low
Seriousness of adverse effects	Trivial	Serious
Frequency of adverse effects	Rare	Frequent
Efficacy of therapeutic alternatives	Poor	Good
Safety of therapeutic alternatives	Poor	Good

SOME DRUGS WITH A LOW THERAPEUTIC INDEX

- Aminoglycoside antibiotics
- Anticoagulants
- Anticonvulsants
- Antihypertensive drugs
- Cardiac glycosides
- Cytotoxic and immunosuppressant drugs
- Oral contraceptives
- Drugs that act on the central nervous system

Benefit is often expressed as the so-called number needed to treat (NNT), which is the number of patients that you would need to treat in order to prevent one clinical event (for example, a stroke or a pregnancy). The other side of the coin, the number needed to harm (NNH), can be similarly calculated. However, the benefit to risk ratio is not a simple ratio of these two numbers, since quality of benefit and severity of risk also need to be considered, but knowing the numbers can help. Consider, for instance, tamoxifen, which prolongs survival in breast cancer (by anti-oestrogenic action) and reduces the risk of myocardial infarction (by an oestrogenic effect on blood lipids) but can cause endometrial cancer and venous thromboembolism:

- NNT to prevent one death = 17
- NNT to prevent one myocardial infarction = 29
- NNH for one case of endometrial cancer = 143
- NNH for one venous thromboembolism = 130

The figures suggest that if you treat 1000 women with breast cancer for 2–5 years you will prevent about 60 deaths and 34 myocardial infarctions, at the cost of 7 cases of endometrial cancer and 7 cases of venous thromboembolism, a favourable benefit to risk ratio. Of course, calculations of this sort yield probabilities that relate to the patients that have been studied in clinical trials. They do not necessarily apply to the whole population and they certainly do not tell you what the outcome will be in the individual case.

PRACTICAL PRESCRIBING

WHEN TO PRESCRIBE A DRUG

Drug therapy is not always necessary. For example, mild tremor in Parkinson's disease may not unduly trouble the patient; even though drug treatment may alleviate it, it may also cause unwanted effects, outweighing the benefit. Do not be tempted to prescribe a drug simply to end a consultation. If a patient expects drug therapy, discuss the pros and cons. Try to estimate the benefit to risk ratio and prescribe only if you think it is favourable.

HOW TO CHOOSE A DRUG TO PRESCRIBE

If you decide to prescribe a drug, the first step will be to choose the therapeutic class. Sometimes the choice is restricted, sometimes wide, as a few examples illustrate (see Table 19.2).

Having chosen the class of drug, the next step is to choose the group of drugs within that class. Again the choice may be restricted or wide (see Table 19.3).

The choice of an anticoagulant depends on whether short-term or long-term treatment is indicated. The choice of a diuretic in the treatment of cardiac failure depends on the severity of the problem, whether acute or chronic therapy is indicated, the convenience of the timing of the diuresis, and potassium balance. The choice of an antibiotic depends on the sensitivities of the infecting organism, the site of infection and contraindications, as some examples show (see Table 19.4).

Drug interactions can also affect therapy, as in the case of antibiotics (see Table 19.5).

Table 19.2 Examples of choosing a therapeutic class of drug

Indication	Therapeutic class
Infection	Antibiotic
Depression	Antidepressant
Acute attack of asthma	Bronchodilators
Diabetes mellitus	Oral hypoglycaemic drugs Insulin
Congestive cardiac failure	Diuretics Angiotensin-converting enzyme (ACE) inhibitors Vasodilators
Hypertension	Diuretics ACE inhibitors β-adrenoceptor antagonists Calcium antagonists

Table 19.3 Examples of choosing a group of drugs from within a class

Therapeutic class	Therapeutic group
Anticoagulants	Coumarins/warfarin Heparins
Diuretics	Thiazides Loop diuretics Potassium-sparing diuretics
Antibiotics	Penicillins Cephalosporins Tetracyclines Aminoglycosides Macrolides Quinolones

Table 19.4 Examples of contraindications to antibiotics

Antibiotic	Example of contraindication
Cephalosporins	Allergy
Penicillins	Allergy
Quinolones	Pregnancy and children (teratogenic in animals)
Tetracyclines	Children (affects growing bones and teeth) Renal impairment (e.g. reduced renal function with age)
Trimethoprim	Pregnancy (teratogenic)

The last step is to choose a particular drug from within the class. In some cases the choice is unimportant. For example, all thiazide diuretics have equal efficacy and adverse effects. In contrast, the choice of a specific penicillin is important and will depend on the type of organism (see Table 19.6).

How to make a rational choice

Many factors dictate the choice of a particular drug:

- *Absorption*. Bumetanide is better absorbed than frusemide; it may be effective in congestive cardiac failure if oral frusemide has failed; alternatively use intravenous frusemide.
- *Distribution*. Some antibiotics are well distributed to a particular tissue; for example, tetracyclines are concentrated in the bile, and lincomycin and clindamycin in bones.
- *Metabolism*. In severe liver disease (for example, hepatic cirrhosis) try to avoid drugs that are extensively metabolised: for example, opiate analgesics.
- *Excretion*. In renal failure try to avoid drugs that are extensively excreted; for example, avoid the aminoglycoside antibiotics in patients with renal impairment if alternative antibiotics are suitable.
- *Efficacy*. The sulphonylureas are more efficacious hypoglycaemic drugs than the biguanides.
- *Features of the disease*. Choose an antibiotic to match the known or suspected sensitivity of the infective organism; for example, ampicillin for a patient with a community-

Table 19.5 Examples of drug interactions with antibiotics

Antibiotic	Interacting drug	Mechanism	Effect
Gentamicin	Frusemide	Additive	Ototoxicity
Chloramphenicol	Warfarin	Inhibition of metabolism	Potentiation of anticoagulation
Metronidazole	Alcohol	Inhibition of aldehyde dehydrogenase	'Disulfiram reaction'
Metronidazole	Warfarin	Inhibition of metabolism	Potentiation of anticoagulation
Rifampicin	Oestrogens (oral contraceptives)	Induction of metabolism	Reduced contraceptive effect
Rifampicin	Warfarin	Induction of metabolism	Reduced effect of warfarin
Tetracycline	Antacids	Chelation	Reduced effect of tetracycline
Tetracycline	Warfarin	Altered clotting factor activity	Potentiation of anticoagulation

Table 19.6 Examples of choosing a particular drug from within a group

Therapeutic group	Drug
Thiazide diuretics	Bendrofluazide Chlorothiazide Cyclopenthiazide Hydrochlorothiazide Hydroflumethiazide Polythiazide
Penicillins	Benzylpenicillin Penicillin V (phenoxymethylpenicillin) Amoxycillin Co-amoxiclav (amoxycillin + clavulanic acid) Ampicillin Flucloxacillin Azlocillin Ticarcillin

acquired bronchopneumonia, since the likeliest organisms will be the pneumococcus *(Streptococcus pneumoniae)* or *Haemophilus influenzae*; sputum culture, with identification of the organism and its sensitivity to different antibiotics, will help.

- *Severity of disease*. Mild pain will generally respond to aspirin or paracetamol; more severe pain may require more potent analgesics, such as codeine phosphate or even morphine. Moderate hypertension often responds to a single drug, such as a thiazide diuretic or a β-adrenoceptor antagonist; more severe hypertension may require a combination.
- *Coexisting diseases*. In hypertension coexisting left ventricular failure would prompt the use of a diuretic combined with an ACE inhibitor; coexisting angina pectoris without heart failure would prompt the use of a β-adrenoceptor antagonist.
- *Avoiding adverse effects*. In asthma avoid β-adrenoceptor antagonists. In penicillin hypersensitivity choose an alternative drug (for example, a cephalosporin in bronchopneumonia).
- *Avoiding adverse drug interactions*. Avoid aspirin and other non-steroidal anti-inflammatory drugs, which can cause gastrointestinal bleeding, in patients taking warfarin. Avoid tetracyclines, sulphonamides and chloramphenicol in patients taking warfarin, since they inhibit its metabolism.
- *Patient compliance*. Atenolol, which can be taken once daily, is often prescribed instead of short-acting β-blockers, in the hope that minimising the frequency of drug administration will improve compliance.
- *Cost*. At the time of writing lansoprazole is cheaper than omeprazole and is equally effective and safe. There are many other examples.

CHOOSING THE ROUTE OF ADMINISTRATION

There are several reasons for choosing a particular route of administration, as some examples illustrate (see Table 19.7).

Table 19.7 Reasons for choosing a particular route of administration

Reason	Example
Only one route possible	Dopamine (intravenous) Glibenclamide (oral)
Compliance	Phenothiazines and thioxanthenes (intramuscular depot injections, in schizophrenia)
Poor absorption	Frusemide (intravenous, in heart failure)
Vomiting	Phenothiazines (rectal) Sumatriptan (sublingual)
Avoiding first-pass metabolism	Glyceryl trinitrate (sublingual)
Rapid action	Glyceryl trinitrate (sublingual) Sumatriptan (sublingual)
Direct access to the site of action	Bronchodilators (inhalation, in asthma) Corticosteroids (rectal, in ulcerative colitis)
Ease of access	Diazepam in status epilepticus (rectal rather than intravenous) Subcutaneous fluids (hypodermoclysis)
Slow release	Insulin (subcutaneous)

CHOOSING A FORMULATION

Oral formulations include tablets, capsules, granules, elixirs and suspensions. Drugs for injection come as lyophilised powders for reconstitution before injection, or as solutions ready for injection; solutions come in single-dose ampoules, single-dose or multiple-dose vials, and half-litre or litre bottles for infusion.

Some examples show how the choice of formulation can be important.

Potassium salts are available as modified-release formulations, as effervescent tablets that dissolve in water for drinking, or as elixirs immediately ready to drink. Patient preference may dictate the choice, but it would be logical to choose a soluble formulation in a patient with gastrointestinal hurry, in whom the modified-release formulation might pass through the gut unabsorbed.

Lithium salts and theophylline come in several different ordinary and modified-release formulations, each with different absorption characteristics. A formulation that produces adequate plasma lithium or theophylline concentrations in one patient may not be suitable for another, and it is sometimes worth changing the formulation if plasma concentrations are suboptimal.

Iron salts are available as tablets for twice- or thrice-daily administration or as modified-release formulations for once-daily administration. Patient compliance is better and adverse effects fewer with the modified-release formulations, but the iron is more erratically absorbed. It is usual to start with an ordinary formulation of iron and change to a modified-release formulation if adverse effects are intolerable.

CHOOSING A DOSAGE REGIMEN

The dose of the drug, and the frequency and timing of its administration constitute the dosage regimen. Each prescription should be treated as an experiment in which you try to find the regimen that produces the best therapeutic effect with minimal adverse effects, according to some simple principles:

- Start with a dosage at the lower end of the recommended dosage range. Exceptions to this rule include corticosteroids and carbimazole, which are begun in high dosages and then reduced to maintenance dosages, and drugs for which a loading dose may be required (for example, digoxin, warfarin and amiodarone).
- Increase the dosage slowly, monitoring the therapeutic effect at regular intervals and looking for adverse effects.
- If adverse effects occur, reduce the dosage or try another drug; in some cases lower dosages may be possible by combining drugs (for example, azathioprine reduces corticosteroid dosage requirements in immunosuppression).
- Think of drug interactions and avoid potentially dangerous combinations.
- Remember that pharmacokinetic and pharmacodynamic variability can alter dosage requirements, as discussed below.
- Take particular care with drugs that have a low therapeutic index.

Pharmacokinetic variability

Because absorption, distribution and elimination of drugs vary from patient to patient, flexibility in dosages is necessary. The examples in Table 19.8 show how to respond to differences in pharmacokinetics.

Table 19.8 Therapeutic approaches to pharmacokinetic problems

Pharmacokinetic problem	Therapeutic approach
Poor absorption	Increase the dose Choose another route of administration Use another drug
Altered tissue distribution	One-off doses may have to be altered Usually does not affect chronic therapy, unless distribution to the target tissue is altered
Altered protein binding	Usually does not affect long-term doses (but does alter steady-state total plasma drug concentration)
Reduced renal elimination	Reduce dosage (use creatinine clearance as a guide)
Reduced hepatic elimination	Low-clearance drugs: reduce oral and intravenous doses High-clearance drugs: reduce oral (but not intravenous) doses

Pharmacodynamic variability

Pharmacological responses are usually governed by the dose-response curve. An example is seen in Figure 19.1, which shows the effect of two loop diuretics, bumetanide and frusemide, on urinary sodium excretion. The two diuretics have different potencies, which can be dealt with by using different dosages; however, they both have the same efficacy, so that comparable dosages should produce the same diuretic effect.

Variability in dose-responsiveness dictates flexibility in prescribing. If a therapeutic effect does not occur with the first dosage chosen, an effect may be produced by making small increases within the therapeutic dosage range. Of course, increasing the dosage will also increase the risk of dose-related adverse effects. Certain diseases can alter a dose-response curve (for example, there is resistance to digoxin in hyperthyroidism) and the pharmacodynamics of a drug can be affected by another drug.

CHOOSING THE FREQUENCY OF DRUG ADMINISTRATION

Patient compliance is improved if drugs are given only once or twice daily, rather than three or four times. In general, therefore, try to choose drugs that can be given no more than twice daily. A modified-release formulation may be useful in this respect. There are some special examples of frequency of drug administration (see Table 19.9).

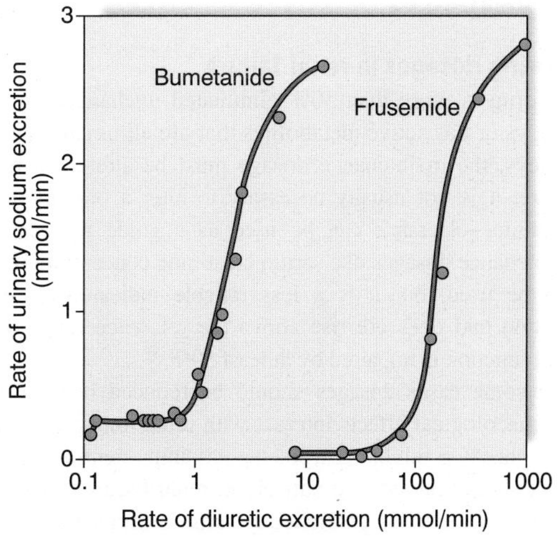

Fig. 19.1 Dose-response curve for bumetanide and frusemide. The two drugs have different potencies but the same efficacy.

Table 19.9 Some special examples of frequency and timing of drug administration

Drug	Recommended frequency or timing	Reason
Frusemide	Once in the morning	Kidney refractory to a second dose within 6 hrs; night-time diuresis undesirable
Corticosteroids	Once in the morning	Minimises effects on adrenal function
Salmeterol	Once at night	Prevents early morning symptoms
Antidepressants	Once at night	Allows adverse effects to occur during sleep
Digoxin	Once at night	So that blood samples for plasma concentration measurement can be taken 12 hrs later
Spironolactone	Twice daily	Minimises gastrointestinal disturbance
Long-acting nitrates	No later than 2000 hrs	To avoid tolerance
Tetracyclines	2 hrs before or after food	Divalent and trivalent cations chelate tetracyclines
Opiates	In anticipation of pain	Better relief in chronic pain
Glyceryl trinitrate	When required	According to symptoms
L-dopa	When required	Dictated by the duration of action (often wears off quickly during long-term therapy)

CHOOSING THE TIME OF DRUG ADMINISTRATION

For many drugs the time of administration is unimportant, but there are occasionally pharmacokinetic or therapeutic reasons for giving drugs at particular times (see Table 19.9). Meal times do not usually affect drug administration, since although food may reduce the *rate* of absorption of a drug it generally does not reduce its *extent* of absorption; tetracyclines are an exception—their absorption is greatly reduced by divalent and trivalent cations, and they should not be taken with food or antacids. Food may sometimes help reduce adverse gastrointestinal effects; for instance, the effects of aspirin on the stomach may be reduced by taking it with food.

ALTERING DRUG DOSAGES IN SPECIAL CIRCUMSTANCES

Altering dosages in renal failure

If a drug is more than 50% eliminated unchanged by the kidneys or has active metabolites that are eliminated by the kidneys, the maintenance dosage must be altered in renal failure; it is not usually necessary to alter a one-off dose. Creatinine clearance can be used as a guide to reducing maintenance dosages; the serum creatinine concentration can also be used, but it is a less reliable indicator of renal function and does not rise above the reference range until renal function is impaired by at least 50%.

In some cases dosages should be reduced because the pharmacological effects interact with renal impairment (for example, ACE inhibitors worsen potassium retention). Some drugs should be avoided entirely in renal failure, for either pharmacokinetic or pharmacodynamic reasons (see Table 19.10).

Diuretics are relatively ineffective in severe renal impairment, partly because they cannot gain access to their site of action, the luminal epithelium. Thiazide diuretics should therefore not be used and high dosages of loop diuretics may be required for efficacy. Potassium-sparing diuretics should not be used, because of the increased risk of hyperkalaemia.

Altering dosages in hepatic failure

The liver has a large functional capacity, and chronic hepatic impairment usually has to be considerable before it affects

Table 19.10 Some drugs whose dosages are affected by renal failure

	Creatinine clearance	Serum creatinine
Mild renal impairment	20–50 ml/min	150–300 μmol/l
Aminoglycosides		
Chlorpropamide		
Digoxin		
Fibrates		
Lithium		
Zidovudine		
Moderate renal impairment	10–20 ml/min	300–700 μmol/l
Some β-blockers (e.g. atenolol, sotalol)		
Opioid analgesics		
Severe renal impairment	< 10 ml/min	> 700 μmol/l
Azathioprine		
Cephalosporins		
Cimetidine		
Isoniazid		
Penicillins		
Sulphonylurea hypoglycaemic drugs (gliclazide, glipizide, gliquidone)		
Drugs to avoid in severe renal failure		
Chloramphenicol		
Chloroquine		
Fibrates		
Lithium—even in moderate renal failure		
Mesalazine—even in mild renal failure		
Metformin—even in mild renal failure		
Methotrexate—even in moderate renal failure		
Non-steroidal anti-inflammatory drugs—even in mild renal failure		
Sulphonylurea hypoglycaemic drugs (chlorpropamide, glibenclamide)		
Tetracyclines (except doxycycline and minocycline)—even in mild renal failure		

drug dosages. However, hepatic drug clearance may be reduced in acute hepatitis, in hepatic congestion due to cardiac failure, and if there is intrahepatic arteriovenous shunting. In chronic liver disease, jaundice, ascites, a prolonged prothrombin time, hypoalbuminaemia, malnutrition and encephalopathy all make clinically important impairment of drug metabolism more likely.

In contrast to renal failure there is no easy way of calculating changes in dosage in patients with impaired hepatic function, because there are no good tests of hepatic drug-metabolising capacity, even by a single metabolic route, or of biliary excretion. Dosages of drugs that are metabolised by the liver should therefore be altered according to the therapeutic response, and with careful clinical monitoring for signs of adverse effects.

If a drug has a high rate of hepatic clearance (see the information box) it will be mostly cleared during its first passage through the liver (the so-called 'first-pass' effect). In such cases hepatic impairment increases the amount of drug that escapes metabolism in the liver after oral administration, reducing oral dosage requirements but not altering intravenous dosage requirements. For example, chlormethiazole is normally extensively metabolised presystemically by the liver, and this is reduced by chronic liver disease such as alcoholic cirrhosis. When treating a chronic alcoholic with oral chlormethiazole take care to ensure that overdose, with the risk of respiratory depression, does not occur.

SOME DRUGS OF LOW AND HIGH HEPATIC CLEARANCE RATES

Low	High
• Aspirin	• Chlormethiazole
• Codeine	• Ergotamine
• Diazepam	• Glyceryl trinitrate
• Isoniazid	• Labetalol
• Nortriptyline	• Lignocaine
• Paracetamol	• Morphine
• Phenobarbitone	• Pethidine
• Phenytoin	• Propranolol
• Procainamide	• Simvastatin
• Quinidine	
• Theophylline	
• Tolbutamide	
• Warfarin	

The pharmacological effects of some drugs are altered in liver disease, with increased risks of adverse effects (see Table 19.11).

Altering dosages in elderly people

Dosage regimens of some drugs are different in old people. Adverse drug reactions are 2–3 times more common in old people. Polypharmacy is common and the scope for drug interactions is large; the error rate in taking drugs is about 60% in patients over 60 years of age, and the rate of error increases markedly if more than three drugs are prescribed.

Table 19.11 Some drugs whose actions are increased in liver disease

Drug	Adverse effect
Oral anticoagulants	Increased anticoagulation (reduced clotting factor synthesis)
Metformin	Lactic acidosis
Chloramphenicol	Bone-marrow suppression
Non-steroidal anti-inflammatory drugs	Gastrointestinal bleeding
Sulphonylureas	Hypoglycaemia

Many old people find it difficult to swallow tablets, and the more frail and the more ill they are, the more difficult it becomes. For example, many potassium tablets are large and can be difficult to swallow. Tablets or capsules can adhere to the oesophageal mucosa, and to avoid hold-up tablets should be swilled down with at least 60 ml of water. Elixirs may be preferable, but not all drugs are available as elixirs, and they may have their own problems. For example, the taste of a potassium elixir may not be acceptable.

Drug distribution may be altered in old people. Dosages should be adjusted for body weight, particularly for drugs with a low therapeutic index.

Old people have an increased proportion of body fat, and lipid-soluble drugs tend to accumulate to a greater extent than in younger patients.

The metabolism of some drugs is reduced in old people—for example, propranolol, lignocaine, chlormethiazole, nifedipine, theophylline, phenobarbitone and paracetamol. Dosages of these drugs should therefore be reduced.

Renal function falls with age and drugs that are mainly excreted in the urine, or that have active metabolites that are excreted, may require dosage reductions (see above).

Some drugs are best avoided in old people. For example, tetracyclines accumulate when renal function is poor, causing nausea and vomiting, which in turn cause dehydration and further deterioration in renal function.

Drug sensitivity may be altered (usually increased) in old age. Old people are more sensitive to the effects of digoxin, probably because of increased sensitivity of their Na^+/K^+ ATPase. This, combined with their increased susceptibility to potassium loss due to diuretics and their reduced renal function, makes them more liable to digoxin toxicity. In contrast, there is reduced sensitivity of β-adrenoceptors in old people, and this may reduce some of the pharmacological effects of β-adrenoceptor agonists and antagonists. Altered sensitivity to drugs in old people may be due to altered physiological responses. For example, reduced baroreceptor function can lead to increased hypotension after the administration of antihypertensive drugs. Other examples include increased sensitivity to the anticoagulant effects of warfarin and increased responsiveness of the brain to centrally active drugs—for example, hypnotics, sedatives, tranquillisers, antidepressants and neuroleptic drugs.

In general, when prescribing drugs for old people try to use as few drugs as possible, start with low dosages, and increase the dosages carefully only if required. Choose easily swallowed formulations, and keep therapy as simple as possible (for example, with once-daily drugs and formulations).

WHEN TO STOP DRUG TREATMENT

A single dose of aspirin may be enough to treat a headache, or a single dose of diamorphine may be sufficient to treat the pain of myocardial infarction. In contrast, life-long therapy is usually required for the treatment of diabetes mellitus, essential hypertension, hypothyroidism and pernicious anaemia.

However, there may be difficulty with treatments of intermediate duration. For example, it is still not clear for how long treatment with warfarin should be continued in the treatment of deep venous thrombosis and pulmonary embolism (see p. 380). The duration of treatment of infections with antibiotics varies from infection to infection, and depends on the infecting organism, the site of infection, and the response to treatment. For example, uncomplicated urinary tract infection with cystitis usually requires treatment for only a few days, pyelonephritis requires treatment for 1–2 weeks, and acute prostatitis 4–6 weeks. When you start a drug treatment it is wise to plan the likely duration of therapy. You should also review long-term treatment at regular intervals to assess whether continued treatment is required. A hospital admission is often an opportunity for revising drug therapy, and it is not uncommon for drugs to be withdrawn in the interim or even permanently following an acute severe illness.

ADVERSE DRUG REACTIONS

An adverse drug effect may be due to either a toxic effect or a side-effect. A toxic effect is an adverse effect that arises through an exaggeration of the same pharmacological effect that is responsible for the therapeutic effect of the drug—for example, hypokalaemia due to diuretic therapy—and is therefore dose-related. A side-effect is an adverse effect that arises through some pharmacological action other than that which produces the therapeutic effect; such effects may be dose-related (for example, anticholinergic effects of tricyclic antidepressants) or not dose-related (for example, a rash associated with an antibiotic). The term 'adverse effects' covers all types of unwanted effects. A classification is given in the information box.

CLASSIFICATION OF ADVERSE DRUG EFFECTS

- Dose-related
- Non-dose-related
- Long-term and withdrawal effects
- Delayed effects

Table 19.12 Examples of adverse effects classified by cause

Mechanism	Example
1. Dose-related effects	
Pharmaceutical variation	Changing modified-release formulations (e.g. lithium)
Pharmacokinetic variation	
Pharmacogenetic variation	Succinylcholine apnoea
Hepatic disease	Sedation due to chlormethiazole
Renal disease	Digoxin toxicity
Pharmacodynamic variation	
Hepatic disease	Encephalopathy due to opioid analgesics
Altered fluid and electrolyte balance	Digoxin toxicity due to hypokalaemia
2. Non-dose-related effects	
Immunological reactions	Penicillin allergy
Pseudoallergic reactions	Aspirin 'allergy'
Pharmacogenetic variation	Drug-induced porphyria
3. Long-term effects	
Adaptive changes	Tardive dyskinesia
Rebound phenomena	Opiate withdrawal syndrome
Dose- and time-related effects	Amiodarone (lung and liver damage)
4. Delayed effects	
Carcinogenesis	Cancer chemotherapy
Effects concerned with reproduction	
Impaired fertility	Sulphasalazine; cytotoxic drugs
Teratogenesis (first trimester)	Alcohol; tetracyclines; valproate
Adverse effects on the fetus during the later stages of pregnancy	Aminoglycosides; aspirin; warfarin
Drugs in breast milk	Lithium; phenytoin; tetracyclines

Examples of important adverse drug effects are given in Table 19.12, classified by cause.

Dose-related toxic effects can be avoided by using dosages at the lower end of the recommended range and increasing cautiously, monitoring carefully for therapeutic and adverse effects. Dose-related side-effects may not be avoidable; if they occur despite careful dosage adjustment it may be necessary to use a different drug. Adverse effects that are due to long-term therapy cannot necessarily be avoided; careful monitoring will help to minimise their impact. Delayed effects can be minimised by reducing the length of exposure to a drug or avoided by not using drugs that are known to have delayed effects.

DRUG INTERACTIONS

A drug interaction occurs when the effects of one drug (the object drug) are altered (increased or decreased) by the effects

Table 19.13 Classification of drug interactions by mechanism

	Example		
Mechanism	**Object drug**	**Precipitant drug**	**Result**
Pharmaceutical	Sodium bicarbonate	Calcium gluconate	Precipitation of calcium carbonate
Pharmacokinetic			
Reduced absorption	Tetracyclines	Calcium, aluminium, magnesium salts	Reduced tetracycline absorption
Reduced protein-binding	Phenytoin	Aspirin	Reduced phenytoin plasma concentration with same therapeutic effect
Reduced metabolism (mixed-function oxidase)	Warfarin	Chloramphenicol	Warfarin toxicity
Reduced metabolism (other enzymes)	Azathioprine	Allopurinol	Azathioprine toxicity
Increased metabolism	Warfarin	Carbamazepine	Warfarin resistance
Reduced renal elimination	Digoxin	Amiodarone	Digoxin toxicity
Pharmacodynamic			
Direct antagonism	Opiates	Naloxone	Reversal of opiate effects
Direct potentiation	Alcohol	Antidepressants	Increased sedation
Indirect potentiation	Anti-arrhythmic drugs	Diuretics (hypokalaemia)	Pro-arrhythmia

of another drug (the precipitant drug). Although a drug interaction usually results in an adverse effect, in some cases it may prove beneficial—for example, the pharmacodynamic synergy between diuretics and ACE inhibitors in the treatment of hypertension. The classification of drug interactions by mechanism is shown in Table 19.13.

PHARMACEUTICAL INTERACTIONS

Pharmaceutical interactions are physico-chemical interactions, either of a drug with an intravenous infusion solution or of two drugs in the same solution, resulting in the loss of activity of the drugs involved. Pharmaceutical interactions are too numerous to remember in detail, but they can be simply avoided by:

- giving intravenous drugs by bolus injection if possible or via an infusion burette
- by using only dextrose or saline for drug infusion
- by not mixing drugs in the same infusion solution, unless the mixture is known to be safe (e.g. potassium chloride with insulin).

PHARMACOKINETIC INTERACTIONS

Pharmacokinetic interactions occur when the absorption, distribution or elimination (metabolism or excretion) of the object drug is altered by the precipitant drug.

Absorption interactions

Absorption interactions are usually not important. Exceptions include impaired absorption of tetracyclines by chelation with divalent and trivalent cations. Metoclopramide increases the rate of gastric emptying and this hastens the absorption of analgesics in the treatment of an acute attack of migraine, a beneficial effect.

Protein-binding displacement

Protein-binding displacement causes an increase in the circulating concentration of unbound drug. However, this is only important if the object drug is highly protein-bound (greater than 90%) and is not widely distributed to body tissues. In practice, this limits important interactions of this type to warfarin and phenytoin. When these drugs are displaced their clearance rate increases in proportion to the degree of displacement and so at steady state the total concentration of drug in the plasma falls to a new equilibrium value, and the unbound concentration is the same as it was before the precipitant drug was introduced, in spite of an increase in the unbound fraction. This means that provided the patient can 'weather' the increase, if any, in unbound concentration of the object drug for as long as it takes to reach the new steady state, such an interaction will not be of clinical importance.

Metabolism interactions

Drug interactions involving metabolism occur when the metabolism of an object drug is either inhibited or increased by a precipitant drug. There are two phases of drug metabolism. Phase I metabolic reactions (for example, hydroxylation, deamination, dealkylation, sulphoxidation) are carried out by isoenzymes of the mixed-function oxidase system and are subject to interactions. Phase II reactions are conjugations (for example, acetylation, methylation, glucuronidation, sulphatation), which are not affected by interactions.

Induction of drug metabolism

Induction of the metabolism of a drug reduces the amount of drug in the body, and therefore reduces its effects. This can result, for example, in pregnancy despite what would otherwise have been adequate oral contraception.

Inhibition of drug metabolism

Inhibition of drug metabolism occurs through inhibition of either the mixed-function oxidase reactions or other specific metabolic pathways.

Examples of the former include the inhibition of warfarin metabolism by chloramphenicol, cimetidine, metronidazole and quinolones, inhibition of phenytoin metabolism by isoniazid, and inhibition of theophylline metabolism by quinolone and macrolide antibiotics (for example, erythromycin).

Examples of the latter include the inhibition by allopurinol of the metabolism of azathioprine and 6-mercaptopurine by xanthine oxidase and of dietary amines by monoamine oxidase inhibitors.

Excretion interactions

Competition for renal tubular secretion reduces drug excretion. For example, probenecid inhibits the tubular secretion of penicillin, increasing the blood concentration of penicillin and prolonging its therapeutic effects, a beneficial interaction. Amiodarone, quinidine and verapamil inhibit the tubular secretion of digoxin by inhibiting the transport protein P glycoprotein, increasing plasma digoxin concentrations and causing toxicity. Salicylates inhibit the active secretion of methotrexate.

PHARMACODYNAMIC INTERACTIONS

In pharmacodynamic interactions the effect of a drug is altered at its site of action. Such interactions may be either direct or indirect.

Direct pharmacodynamic interactions

Direct pharmacodynamic interactions occur when two drugs either act on the same site (antagonism or synergism) or act on two different sites with a similar end result. For example, naloxone reverses the effects of opiates and vitamin K reverses the effects of warfarin (beneficial antagonistic interactions). The anticoagulant effects of warfarin are increased in direct synergistic interactions with anabolic steroids and tetracyclines. Any drug that has a depressant action on central nervous function can potentiate the effect of another such drug, whether or not the two drugs have effects on the same receptors; for example, alcohol potentiates the action of any other centrally acting drug.

Indirect pharmacodynamic interactions

In indirect pharmacodynamic interactions a pharmacological, therapeutic or toxic effect of the precipitant drug in some way alters the therapeutic or toxic effect of the object drug, but the two effects are not themselves related and do not themselves interact.

The effects of anticoagulants can be increased by three indirect effects: reduced platelet aggregation (for example, by salicylates, dipyridamole, ticlopidine and non-steroidal anti-inflammatory drugs) or thrombocytopenia; gastrointestinal ulceration (for example, non-steroidal anti-inflammatory drugs); and increased fibrinolysis (for example, metformin).

Alterations in fluid and electrolyte balance by diuretics increase the effects of cardiac glycosides and class I anti-arrhythmic drugs (for example, lignocaine, quinidine, procainamide and phenytoin).

AVOIDING ADVERSE DRUG INTERACTIONS

The simple way of avoiding adverse drug interactions is to avoid combinations that are known to be dangerous. If that is not possible, the dosage of the object drug should be reduced in advance of starting the precipitant drug and the precipitant drug should be introduced slowly. When a theoretical interaction is anticipated on the basis of the known properties of two drugs, even if it has not been previously described, careful monitoring will help recognise adverse effects early.

WRITING A DRUG PRESCRIPTION

A prescription should be a precise, accurate, clear and readable set of instructions, sufficient for a nurse to administer a drug accurately in hospital, or for a pharmacist to provide a patient with both the correct drug and the instructions on how to take it (see Fig. 19.2).

INFORMATION TO BE GIVEN ON A PRESCRIPTION OUTSIDE HOSPITAL

- The date
- The patient's name, initials and address
- The age of a child under 12
- The name of the drug, preferably in capitals (use generic names when possible)—see Ch. 20
- The formulation to be prescribed
- The strength of the formulation
- The dose
- The frequency of administration
- The route of administration
- The doctor's name, address and signature

WRITING DRUG DOSES

- Quantities of 1 gram or more should be written in grams. For example, write 2 g.
- Quantities less than 1 gram but more than 1 milligram should be written in milligrams. For example, write 100 mg, not 0.1 g.
- Quantities less than 1 milligram should be written in micrograms or nanograms as appropriate. Do not abbreviate micrograms or nanograms. For example,

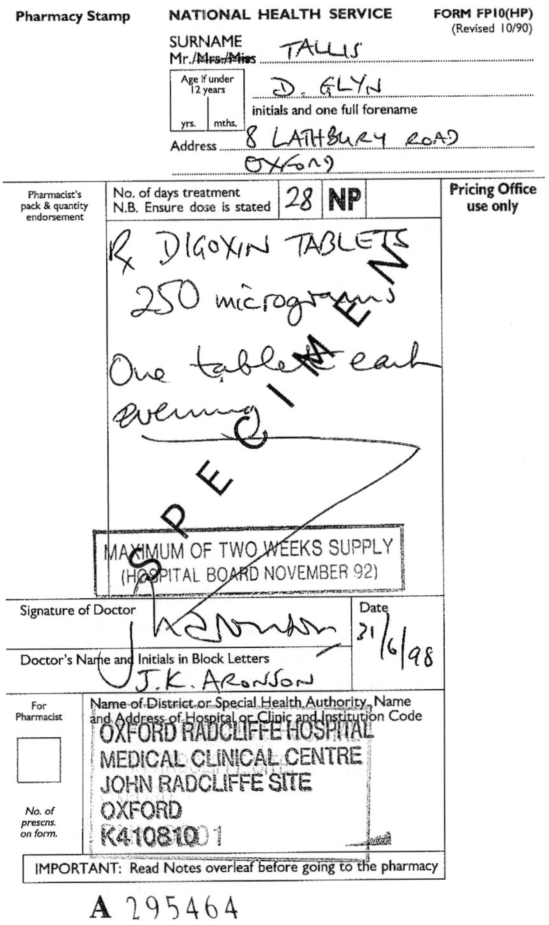
Pharmacy Stamp NATIONAL HEALTH SERVICE FORM FP10(HP) (Revised 10/90)
SURNAME Mr./Mrs./Miss TALLIS
Age if under 12 years yrs. mths. D. GLYN
initials and one full forename
Address 8 LATHBURY ROAD OXFORD
Pharmacist's pack & quantity endorsement
No. of days treatment N.B. Ensure dose is stated 28 NP
Pricing Office use only
Rx DIGOXIN TABLETS
250 micrograms
One tablet each evening
SPECIMEN
MAXIMUM OF TWO WEEKS SUPPLY (HOSPITAL BOARD NOVEMBER 92)
Signature of Doctor
Date 31/6/98
Doctor's Name and Initials in Block Letters J.K. ARONSON
For Pharmacist
Name of District or Special Health Authority. Name and Address of Hospital or Clinic and Institution Code
OXFORD RADCLIFFE HOSPITAL
MEDICAL CLINICAL CENTRE
JOHN RADCLIFFE SITE
OXFORD
K4108101
No. of prescns. on form.
IMPORTANT: Read Notes overleaf before going to the pharmacy
A 295464

Fig. 19.2 An example of a prescription for a prescription-only medicine (digoxin).

write 100 micrograms, not 0.1 mg, 100 µg, 100 mcg or 100 ug.

- If a decimal point cannot be avoided for values less than 1, write a zero before it. For example, write 0.5 ml, not .5 ml.
- For liquid medicines given orally the dose should be stated as the number of milligrams in either 5 ml or 10 ml of solution.

PRESCRIBING CONTROLLED DRUGS

Because of the problems of drug addiction and misuse of drugs, drugs likely to be abused are the subject, in the United Kingdom, of the *Misuse of Drugs Act* (1971), the *Misuse of Drugs (Notification of and Supply to Addicts) Regulations* (1973) and the *Misuse of Drugs Regulations* (1985). A sample prescription for a controlled drug is shown in Figure 19.3.

REQUIREMENTS FOR PRESCRIPTIONS FOR CONTROLLED DRUGS

Prescriptions for controlled drugs must:

- be completely written in the prescriber's handwriting in ink
- be signed and dated by the prescriber
- specify the prescriber's address
- specify the name and address of the patient
- state the form and strength (if appropriate) of the drug
- state the total quantity of the drug or the number of dose units to be dispensed in both words and figures
- state the exact size of each dose in both words and figures

ABBREVIATIONS

Some abbreviations that are used in prescribing are listed in Table 19.14. Other abbreviations should be avoided and instructions should be written in plain English.

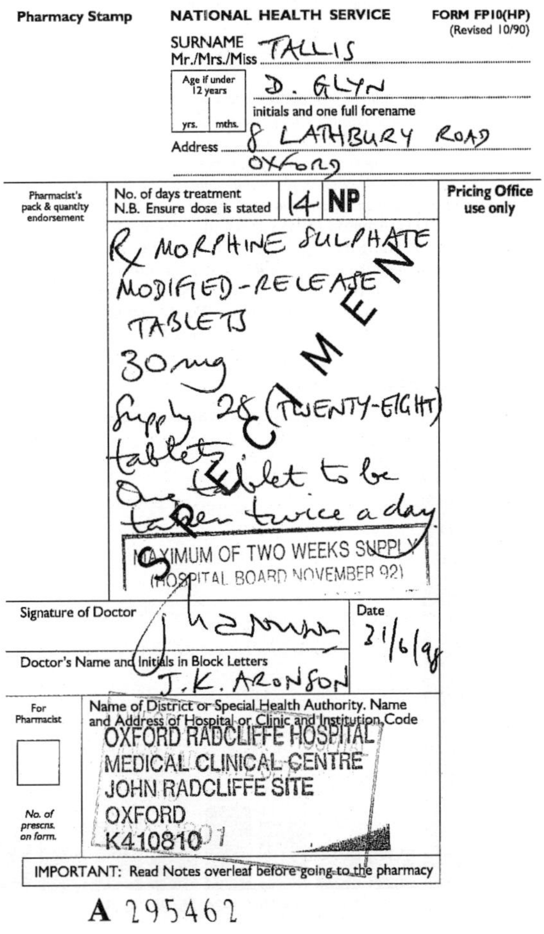
Pharmacy Stamp NATIONAL HEALTH SERVICE FORM FP10(HP) (Revised 10/90)
SURNAME Mr./Mrs./Miss TALLIS
Age if under 12 years yrs. mths. D. GLYN
initials and one full forename
Address 8 LATHBURY ROAD OXFORD
Pharmacist's pack & quantity endorsement
No. of days treatment N.B. Ensure dose is stated 14 NP
Pricing Office use only
Rx MORPHINE SULPHATE MODIFIED-RELEASE TABLETS
30 mg
Supply 28 (TWENTY-EIGHT) tablets
One tablet to be taken twice a day
SPECIMEN
MAXIMUM OF TWO WEEKS SUPPLY (HOSPITAL BOARD NOVEMBER 92)
Signature of Doctor
Date 31/6/98
Doctor's Name and Initials in Block Letters J.K. ARONSON
For Pharmacist
Name of District or Special Health Authority. Name and Address of Hospital or Clinic and Institution Code
OXFORD RADCLIFFE HOSPITAL
MEDICAL CLINICAL CENTRE
JOHN RADCLIFFE SITE
OXFORD
K4108101
No. of prescns. on form.
IMPORTANT: Read Notes overleaf before going to the pharmacy
A 295462

Fig. 19.3 An example of a prescription for a controlled drug (morphine).

Table 19.14 Acceptable abbreviations in prescriptions

Abbreviation	Latin meaning	English translation
b.d. or b.i.d.	Bis in die	Twice daily
gutt.	Guttae	Drops
i.m.	–	Intramuscular(ly)
i.v.	–	Intravenous(ly)
o.d.	Omni die	(Once) every day
o.m.	Omni mane[1]	(Once) every morning
o.n.	Omni nocte[1]	(Once) every night
p.o.	Per os	By mouth
PR	Per rectum	By the anal route
p.r.n.	Pro re nata	Whenever required
PV	Per vaginam	By the vaginal route
q.d.s.	Quater die sumendum[2]	Four times daily
s.c.	–	Subcutaneous(ly)
stat.	Statim	Immediately
t.d.s.	Ter die sumendum[2]	Three times daily

[1] Sometimes written simply as mane or nocte.
[2] .t.i.d. or q.i.d. (ter or quater in die) are sometimes used instead.

FURTHER INFORMATION ON PRINCIPLES OF DRUG THERAPY

British National Formulary. New edition every 6 months. British Medical Association and the Pharmaceutical Society of Great Britain, London. *Guide to currently available formulations, with notes on dosages, uses, adverse effects and interactions; chapters on prescribing, especially in renal failure, in liver disease, in pregnancy and during breastfeeding, and appendices on drug interactions and intravenous additives*

Grahame-Smith D G, Aronson J K 1992 Oxford textbook of clinical pharmacology and drug therapy. Oxford University Press, Oxford. *Contains a more detailed account of the principles outlined here*

Sackett D L, Richardson W S, Rosenberg W, Haynes R B 1997 Evidence-based medicine: how to practise and teach EBM. Churchill Livingstone, Edinburgh. *A useful introduction to evidence-based medicine*

ACUTE POISONING

Acute poisoning is a common problem in all developed, and many developing, countries of the world. In the UK it accounts for 15–20% of all medical emergency admissions to hospital. This chapter deals with the clinical features, diagnosis and treatment of acute poisoning and makes brief reference to chronic poisoning and long-term illness alleged to be due to exposure to low levels of toxins. Food poisoning is discussed on page 124.

PATTERNS OF POISONING

A classification of acute poisoning is shown in the information box.

The age distribution of acute poisoning in the UK is shown in Figure 19.4. It is biphasic and typical of most developed countries, with the largest peak in children under the age of 5 years, where poisoning is almost always accidental, and a lower, much broader peak mainly covering the age group 12–35 years and tailing off into old age. Poisoning in the latter is usually self-inflicted and includes unexpected adverse effects from the leisure use (misuse) of drugs and plants.

The main groups of substances involved in poisoning episodes differ between children and adults, as shown in Figure 19.5. Drugs are clearly important at all ages and at

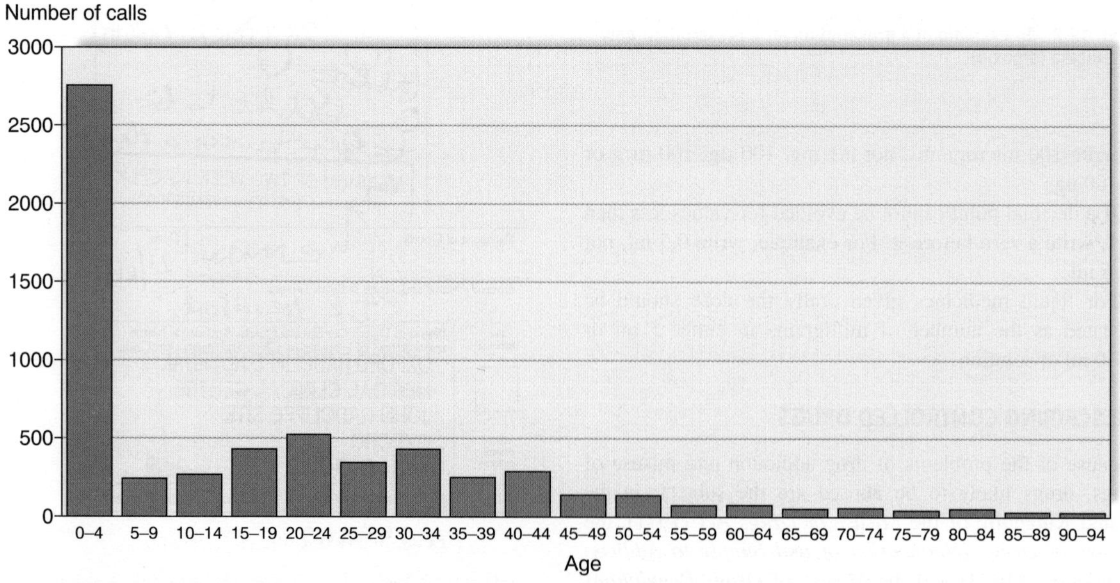

Fig. 19.4 Age distribution of poisoned patients. Based on 7247 calls to the Scottish Poisons Information Bureau in 1996.

CLASSIFICATION OF POISONING

Accidental

- Most common in children under the age of 5 years. Uncommon in adults but may occur as the result of occupational exposure

Non-accidental

- Deliberate poisoning of a child by one of its parents. Sometimes referred to as Münchausen's syndrome by proxy

Misadventure

- Accidental poisoning of a patient by medical or nursing staff—usually the result of errors in the calculation or administration of doses

Deliberate self-poisoning

- This is the most common form of poisoning in individuals over the age of 15 years but is not uncommon in even younger patients. It is a form of parasuicide (see p. 1095)

Homicidal

- Rare

least 30% of self-poisoning episodes involve more than one drug, excluding alcohol which will be taken in addition to drugs by about 60% of males and 40% of females. The pattern of drugs taken in overdose reflects fashions in prescribing and recreational use and what can be purchased by the public over the counter at chemists and other outlets. More than 60% of adults ingest drugs that have been prescribed for themselves or a close relative. It is not surprising, therefore, that the major pharmacological groups involved in acute poisoning at the present time are benzodiazepines, serotonin-specific re-uptake inhibitors, tricyclic antidepressants, anticonvulsants and analgesics, including non-steroidal anti-inflammatory drugs, salicylates, opioids and, above all, paracetamol (acetaminophen).

MORBIDITY AND MORTALITY FROM POISONING

Estimates of the morbidity from acute poisoning are largely based on patients who reach hospitals. However, many experience so few consequences that they do not seek medical advice or are treated at home by friends or their general practitioners. In developed countries about 20% of children will develop features after exposure to poisons but only in about 1% will they be serious. Most incidents are 'scares' rather than true poisonings. As a result, symptomless children reaching emergency departments are commonly discharged. The morbidity from poisoning in adults is generally greater than in children and is life-threatening in a significantly higher proportion. Those in whom it is relatively minor are admitted to hospital so that the psychiatric and social factors precipitating the episode can be more accurately assessed after the effects of the poisons have worn off.

There are almost 4500 deaths from poisoning each year in the UK, with more than 80% of them occurring outside hospital. The major agents are carbon monoxide (by far the most important), benzodiazepines, tricyclic antidepressants, paracetamol and opioid co-formulations and salicylate. In hospital the mortality from poisoning is less than 1% overall and should be less than 2% in severely ill patients.

Inevitably, the pattern of poisoning and the subsequent morbidity and mortality are very different in other parts of the world. Snake bite causes several thousand deaths every year in India, East Asia and Africa, and elsewhere insecticides such as organophosphate compounds and metal phosphides and the herbicide paraquat are important.

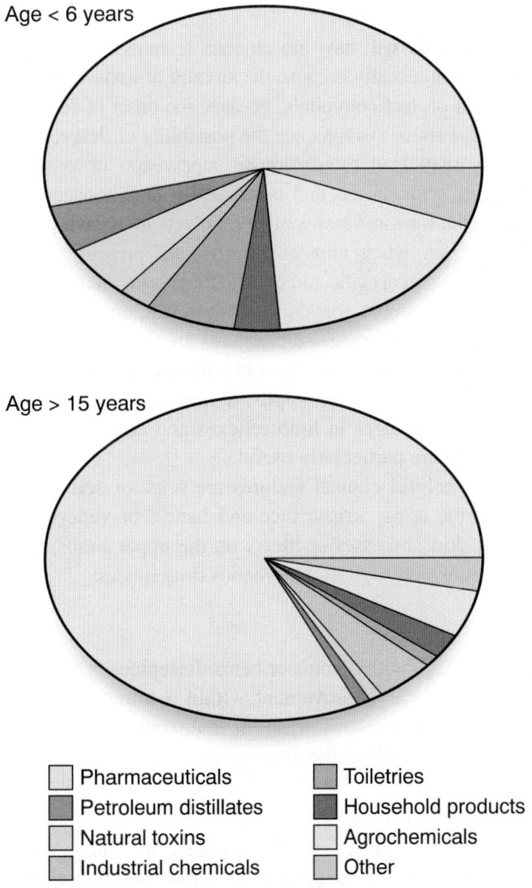

Fig. 19.5 The main groups of substances involved in acute poisoning in children (aged < 6 years) and adults (> 15 years).

DIAGNOSIS

Clinical assessment

A diagnosis of poisoning is made on the basis of one or more factors including the history given by the patient, circumstantial evidence, the findings on examination, diagnostic trials of antidotes, the results of laboratory investigations and the evolution of the illness.

History and circumstantial evidence

A diagnosis of acute poisoning is most commonly made on the basis of the history given by the patient or a witness. In other cases, particularly when the patient is unconscious, it may be suspected from the circumstances under which he or she was found. It is helpful to remember that acute drug overdosage is the most common cause of coma in the 15–35 age group. Hypoglycaemia must be excluded at an early stage.

Symptoms and signs

Many patients will have no obvious features of toxicity on presentation, usually because the amount of toxin involved is too small or, less commonly, because the onset of features is delayed. Failure to appreciate the possibility of delayed-onset toxicity may lead to inadequate supervision or premature discharge with serious and occasionally fatal consequences; the mechanisms and toxins often involved are shown in Table 19.15. Even when clinical features are present they are commonly non-specific and of little diagnostic value. In some cases—for example, tricyclic antidepressant, opioid analgesic and salicylate overdose—the features are sufficiently characteristic to support the history of ingestion. Neurological signs, such as the size of the pupils, abnormal eye movements, nystagmus, changes in limb reflexes and abnormal plantar responses, are particularly useful.

Other helpful clinical features are scars of self-inflicted cuts to the arms, wrists, face and hands, or venepuncture marks, skin abscesses or ulcers on the upper limbs, groins and feet, which suggest intravenous drug misuse.

Trials of antidotes

If overdosage with opioids or benzodiazepines is suspected, obvious clinical improvement within a minute or two of giving an intravenous dose of naloxone or flumazenil respectively confirms the diagnosis.

Clinical progress

Most patients who are unconscious as the result of poisoning can be expected to show significant clinical improvement within 12 hours. Failure to do so should prompt review of the diagnosis. Do not miss intracranial haemorrhage.

Table 19.15 Mechanisms of delayed toxicity

Mechanism	Toxins
Delayed absorption of the poison	Ingestion of sustained-release drug formulations, particularly theophylline and lithium salts Dermal exposure, e.g. to organophosphate insecticides
Delayed distribution of the poison to tissues	Lithium salts
Need for metabolic activation of the poison	Paracetamol, methanol, ethylene glycol
Competition for the enzymes that activate the poison	Simultaneous ingestion of ethanol with methanol or ethylene glycol
Inhibition of the enzymes that activate the poison	Ingestion of ethanol or cimetidine with paracetamol
Slow development of the target organ response to the poison	Monoamine oxidase inhibitors, irritant gases such as chlorine

Tablet identification

Some tablets and capsules are readily recognisable, while others can be identified from the codes stamped on them. Hospital drug information pharmacists and poisons information services in the UK commonly undertake this using a computerised database, 'Tic-Tac'.

Laboratory screening for poisons

Screening for unidentified or unsuspected poisons is of limited value. The single most important exception is paracetamol, for which screening should be carried out routinely in the circumstances listed on page 1120. A 5 ml sample of blood is adequate for this purpose. When screening for other toxins it is better to send the laboratory a 50 ml sample of vomitus, gastric aspirate or urine taken in the first few hours following ingestion, since the concentration of toxic substances or related metabolites in these is almost always much higher than in the blood. Discussion with the laboratory staff and a list of the agents used in the recent treatment of the patient are prerequisites.

FACTORS DETERMINING TOXICITY

The toxicity that a chemical causes depends on its inherent properties (physico-chemical as well as pharmacological), the quantity or concentration involved, the route of absorption and factors specific to the individual who is exposed. While many poisons pass through the gut and respiratory mucosae, skin and conjunctiva without causing damage, others with irritant or corrosive actions inflict varying degrees of local

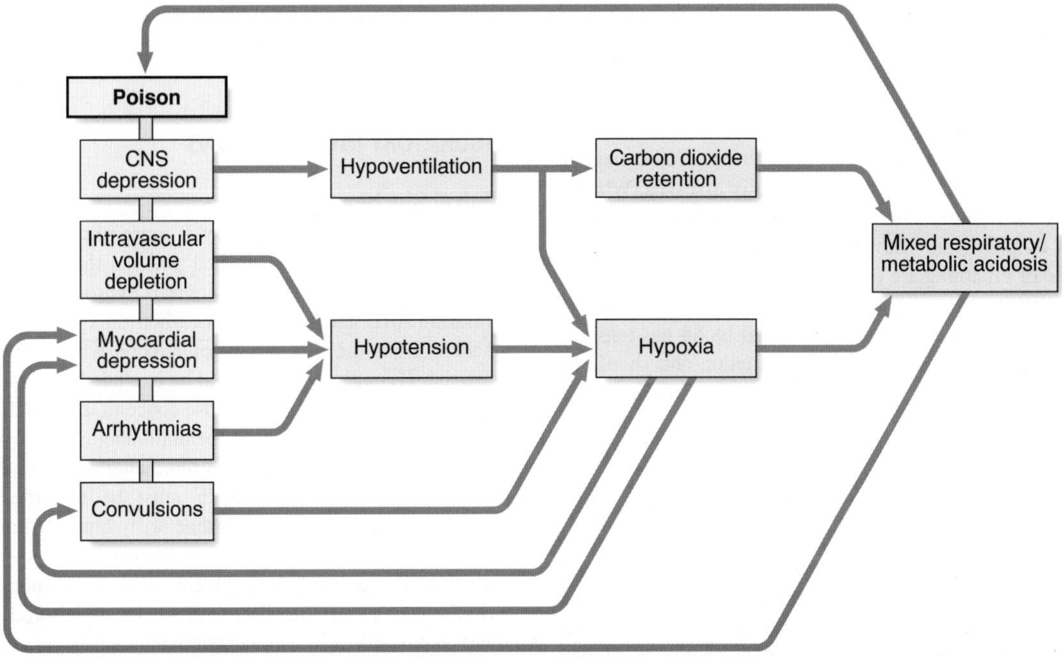

Fig. 19.6 The main ways in which a toxic substance may cause organ damage with resultant functional disturbance.

inflammation or destruction. Absorption of the poison may then elicit systemic responses that are organ-specific or non-specific. These, in turn, can compound toxicity by impairing oxygen delivery to tissues—for example, by depressing respiration or causing hypotension, arrhythmias, seizures or acidosis or a combination of these (see Fig. 19.6). The rate at which features of toxicity develop depends on a number of factors, principal amongst which is the route of exposure, which determines the speed of absorption. Thus virtually immediate effects can be expected after intravenous injection, while those after inhalation, ingestion and dermal exposure (in descending order) can be expected to develop more slowly. Most potential poisons are ingested and at least some toxic features, if they are going to develop, would be expected by about 4 hours. The possibility that the onset of features might be delayed is not widely appreciated; possible mechanisms and scenarios are listed in Table 19.15.

Fortunately, in the case of drugs the primary toxic effects are usually completely reversed with elimination of the drug. Even massive hepatic necrosis induced by paracetamol will reverse completely if the patient survives. However, quinine and chemicals such as iron salts and strong acids and alkalis may leave permanent organ damage.

ASSESSMENT OF SEVERITY

With some important exceptions, the severity of poisoning is best assessed clinically. This initial evaluation is of paramount importance, not only for establishing the baseline from which progress may be appraised, but also for deciding upon the treatment required. Initial physical examination and laboratory investigations, therefore, should be directed to determining the magnitude of disturbance of vital functions and although it must be rapid, it must also be sufficiently comprehensive to detect any coincident disease which may influence the treatment given.

CLINICAL EXAMINATION

Neurological assessment

Massive overdosage with drugs and some other poisons may produce complex neurological abnormalities. Estimation of the level of consciousness is the most important component of evaluating hypnotic, sedative and psychotropic drug overdoses and the Glasgow coma scale (see p. 959) is commonly applied to poisoned patients. With the exception of unequal pupils, unilateral neurological signs virtually exclude a diagnosis of poisoning as a cause of coma unless they can be explained on the basis of pre-existing disease.

Respiration

A clear airway is the first requirement for adequate respiration; it must therefore be carefully assessed. While a reduced respiratory rate (bradypnoea) is one of the hallmarks of poisoning with opioid analgesics, alterations in the rate of breathing are of little diagnostic help; neither do they assist in attempting to decide if adequate gas exchange is taking place. Measurement of arterial blood gas tensions is the optimum way of assessing ventilation and should be performed as soon as possible if there is any suspicion that it is insufficient.

Cardiovascular function

Clinical assessment of the circulation in acute poisoning is often difficult since the typical features of shock may not be apparent in the presence of central nervous depression and hypothermia. In practice it is reasonable to assume that hypotension exists if the systolic blood pressure falls below 90 mmHg in patients over the age of 40 and below 80 mmHg in younger patients. Consideration of possible causes (listed in the information box) is necessary before determining management.

CAUSES OF HYPOTENSION IN ACUTE POISONING

- Volume depletion from vomiting, diarrhoea, gastrointestinal haemorrhage
- Relative volume depletion from dilatation of the venous bed
- Myocardial depression—tricyclic antidepressants, β-adrenoceptor blockers
- Severe brady- and tachyarrhythmias
- Metabolic acidosis

Other features

Hypothermia due to a combination of central nervous system depression and low environmental temperatures is commonly present in patients who take overdoses of drugs which render them unconscious and may contribute to shock, acidosis and hypoxia. Usually the rectal temperature is in the range 30–36°C. Hypothermia of less than 30°C is rare but is potentially life-threatening, since at this level body temperature tends to fall progressively unless active reheating is undertaken.

Conversely, hyperthermia can be a feature of poisoning with central nervous system stimulants such as theophylline, amphetamines and cocaine and may be associated with convulsions, rhabdomyolysis, hyperkalaemia and acute renal failure.

Skin blisters, predominantly over pressure areas, may be found in patients who have lain unconscious for some hours. Rhabdomyolysis and, rarely, radial and common peroneal nerve palsies are also potential complications in such circumstances.

LABORATORY INVESTIGATIONS

Clinical biochemistry

In general, clinical biochemistry is more important for the management of acutely poisoned patients than is analysis for toxins. Measurement of arterial hydrogen ion concentration (pH) and oxygen and carbon dioxide tensions is mandatory for the assessment of anyone who is severely poisoned. Hypoglycaemia should be excluded in those who are unconscious and blood glucose concentrations will have to be monitored in overdoses of antidiabetic drugs. Some poisons cause dramatic and very rapid alterations in plasma potassium concentrations which must be identified and treated to lessen the risk of cardiac arrhythmias. Similarly, plasma calcium concentrations may be reduced in poisoning with fluorides and ethylene glycol, again predisposing to arrhythmias. Liver function should be monitored after significant overdosage with hepatotoxins such as paracetamol but measurement of the prothrombin time or international normalised ratio (INR) can usually be done more quickly than biochemical tests and is of greater clinical relevance.

Quantitative laboratory toxin analyses

Measurement of the concentration of some drugs and chemicals in plasma or serum is essential for assessment of the severity of poisoning and determining the need for treatment (see the information box). For most others it is not practicable and seldom useful to try to obtain laboratory confirmation of the toxin or toxins involved because the results seldom influence treatment; occasionally they may be of value for medico-legal purposes, however.

TOXINS FOR WHICH EMERGENCY CONCENTRATIONS ARE REQUIRED

- Paracetamol
- Salicylate
- Iron
- Lithium
- Theophylline
- Methanol
- Ethylene glycol

GENERAL PRINCIPLES OF TREATMENT

Treatment of the great majority of poisoned patients involves the application of intensive care principles (see Ch. 15), coupled with careful clinical assessment and knowledge of the effects of the poison or poisons involved.

BE PREPARED

Most developed countries provide round-the-clock poisons information services from which doctors can obtain details of the active ingredients of products and the features and time course of intoxication with them. Many also provide advice on the management of specific patients. The centres in the United Kingdom National Poisons Information Service are given in Appendix I at the end of this chapter.

EMERGENCY MEASURES

The resuscitation of severely poisoned patients is no different from that of other ill patients. Once the patient is stabilised consideration should then be given to the need for preventing absorption of the poison and the use of antidotes and elimination techniques.

Prevention of absorption of the poison

Inhaled poisons

Individuals who have inhaled toxic fumes must be removed to fresh air as quickly as possible but rescuers should take care not to expose themselves to toxic gases. Soiled clothing may be a source of continuing exposure to some volatile toxins and should be removed and placed in a suitable container.

Skin decontamination

Occasionally, particularly in occupational accidents, poisoning results from absorption of chemicals spilled on to the skin or clothing. Where possible, the victims themselves should remove their clothes, putting them into an appropriate receptacle. They should then wash off any poison, paying particular attention to skin folds, the ears, hair and under the nails. Soap and large volumes of warm water are all that are required. When carers have to undertake this task they must take appropriate steps to avoid contaminating themselves.

Gut decontamination

Gut decontamination is the term currently in vogue to encompass measures intended to reduce the absorption of toxins from the gastrointestinal tract. The use of gut decontamination seems logical and for decades patients have been made to vomit (most commonly and safely by giving syrup of ipecacuanha orally) or have been subjected to gastric aspiration and lavage. In the UK induced emesis became mainly, but not exclusively, identified with children and gastric lavage with adults. However, critical review of the amounts of toxins recovered by these procedures and evaluation of their effects on the subsequent course of poisoning have shown that they are of little value. Nor are they without adverse consequences and whether or not they should be used clearly depends on the balance of benefits and risks. In young children, in particular, the morbidity from so-called 'poisonings' is so low that it is widely considered insufficient to justify the protracted vomiting, irritability, drowsiness and other symptoms that frequently accompany treatment with syrup of ipecac. The same undesirable effects occur in adults and the combined view of the European Association of Poisons Centres and Clinical Toxicologists and the American Academy of Clinical Toxicology is that syrup of ipecacuanha no longer has a role in the management of poisoning. Similarly, it is recommended that the use of gastric lavage, a long over-used treatment, should be considered only in those individuals who have ingested a potentially toxic dose of an agent within the preceding 1–2 hours.

Reduced use of gastric emptying to limit absorption of toxins is being replaced by greater reliance on the use of oral activated charcoal, alone or as an adjunct to gastric lavage. Charcoal binds many potential toxins, so reducing their absorption; the notable exceptions are listed in the information box. The earlier charcoal is given after the poison has been swallowed, the more effective it will be; it is unlikely to be of value if more than 2 hours have elapsed unless the poison (usually a drug) has been formulated in such a way as to delay its release. The effective ratio of charcoal to amount of poison to be adsorbed is estimated to be of the order of 10:1. It is therefore most useful when the poison ingested is toxic in small doses. In practice, patient compliance is likely to be the most important factor limiting the value of oral activated charcoal. Its colour, gritty texture and taste make it unacceptable to many.

IMPORTANT TOXINS THAT DO NOT ADSORB TO ACTIVATED CHARCOAL

- Iron salts
- Lithium salts
- Methanol
- Ethylene glycol
- Acids and alkalis
- Petroleum distillates

Antidotes

Specific antidotes are available for only a very small number of poisons (see Table 19.16). Some of them cause significant side-effects and should be used only where poisoning is serious and life-threatening. Their use is described in the sections on relevant poisons.

Table 19.16 The antidotes in most common use in clinical toxicology

Antidote	Toxin
Acetylcysteine	Paracetamol
Naloxone	Opioid analgesics
Flumazenil	Benzodiazepines
Desferrioxamine	Iron

Techniques to increase the elimination of poisons

The more gravely ill the patient, the greater the amount of toxin that must have been absorbed and the more pertinent it is to consider whether active measures to enhance elimination of the poison might be of value. Poisons information services (see Appendix I) will advise on their appropriate use.

Invasive techniques

The most invasive techniques available include peritoneal dialysis, haemodialysis, haemoperfusion and plasmapheresis but fortunately they are seldom indicated or required. Forced diuresis should also be regarded as invasive; its value is heavily outweighed by its risks and it should no longer be used. Alkalinisation of the urine still has a role in the management of salicylate overdose but can be achieved with modest fluid loads.

Gut dialysis. The comparatively recent appreciation that administration of repeated doses of activated charcoal by mouth enhances the elimination of some drugs from the circulation has been a major advance in clinical toxicology (see the information box). This has been termed gut dialysis because of the mechanism by which it works. First, the charcoal binds the drugs avidly, ensuring that their concentration in the fluid in the gut lumen is negligible. Second, the mucosa covering the villi of the small intestine is very thin and presents a vast surface area with a rich capillary circulation. The combination of these two factors establishes a concentration gradient which allows drug to move from the capillaries into the gut lumen; in effect, the mucosa is acting as a dialysis membrane. The usual dose of charcoal in this case is 50 g initially, then 25 g 4-hourly, until the patient is improved or charcoal appears in the faeces.

DRUGS WHOSE ELIMINATION MAY BE ENHANCED BY REPEAT DOSE ORAL ACTIVATED CHARCOAL

- Salicylate
- Carbamazepine
- Dapsone
- Digoxin
- Barbiturates
- Phenytoin
- Quinine
- Theophylline

Additional supportive therapy

In poisoning with psychotropic drugs metabolic acidosis should be corrected with intravenous sodium bicarbonate only after carbon dioxide retention and hypoxia have been rectified as far as possible. Acidosis complicating methanol and ethylene glycol poisoning should be corrected immediately. Fluid and electrolyte balance is achieved by correction of acidosis and appropriate replacement therapy. Single short-lived seizures should not automatically be treated with anticonvulsants, but if they are prolonged or occurring at short intervals intravenous diazepam (see p. 940) is indicated to avoid increasing hypoxia and acidosis and possibly inducing arrhythmias.

'LEISURE' DRUGS

A number of drugs that have little or no use in medical practice, 'designer drugs', volatile substances and some naturally occurring substances, are taken not because of medical need but for the pleasurable feelings they produce. Some stimulate and/or depress the central nervous system while others distort perception. Inability to cope with the consequences and accidental overdosage are not uncommon and may result in referral to hospital.

AMPHETAMINES AND COCAINE

While amphetamines ('speed') are usually ingested, they may also be injected. Cocaine can also be injected but is more commonly smoked or snorted (sniffed up the nostrils as an aqueous solution). Ecstasy, a major source of public concern in contemporary Britain, is also an amphetamine derivative. In general, the features of toxicity of these compounds are similar although differences occur.

Clinical features

Excitement, restlessness, mydriasis, tachycardia, hypertension, hyperventilation and tremor are common. Amphetamines may induce hallucinations and paranoid behaviour. Both amphetamines and cocaine cause convulsions, hypotension and ventricular arrhythmias but these occur much less frequently. Rare complications include rhabdomyolysis, hyperpyrexia, arteritis, intracranial haemorrhage, myocardial infarction and dissection of the aorta. Ecstasy has caused severe hyponatraemia and acute liver necrosis.

Management

Few patients require more than supportive care. Droperidol (5–15 mg) or haloperidol (5–10 mg) by slow intravenous injection may be given for severe agitation.

OPIOID ANALGESICS

Dihydrocodeine, buprenorphine, dipipanone, pentazocine, pethidine, methadone, morphine and heroin, the more potent of the opioid analgesics, induce dependence and feature prominently in the illicit drug scene. Methadone is of particular toxicological relevance because of its widespread availability secondary to its use in community drug detoxification projects and its long half-life.

Clinical features

All of the opioids produce similar effects but the severity of toxicity depends on the potency of the drug taken. Coma, pinpoint pupils and a reduced respiratory rate are the hallmarks of serious poisoning with respiratory depression, often with non-cardiogenic pulmonary oedema, the usual mode of death. Since most overdoses of these drugs occur in dependent individuals, evidence of the routes of misuse may be found.

Management

Severe opioid poisoning requires the same emergency measures as any other agent causing life-threatening CNS depression. However, the need for airway, ventilatory and other support may be obviated by giving naloxone, a true pharmacological antagonist of the opioid analgesics. Its effects are usually obvious within a minute or two of administration of an intravenous bolus but are short-lasting because of its half-life of about 1 hour. Repeat doses may therefore be necessary. Opioid-dependent patients may respond to naloxone with an acute withdrawal syndrome but it is seldom severe and concern about it should not inhibit the use of a potentially life-saving antidote. The effects of opioids in non-dependent adults can usually be reversed completely by 0.8–1.2 mg of naloxone. Partial reversal only is generally recommended for misusers of these drugs because of the behavioural problems that complete reversal commonly induces. In these cases naloxone should be given by slow intravenous injection to the stage where airway care and breathing are not causes for concern but full consciousness is not restored.

CANNABIS AND LYSERGIC ACID DIETHYLAMIDE (LSD)

Poisoning with these substances is uncommon in hospital practice and is unlikely to be serious. Occasionally the distortion of perception and hallucinations that may be induced are more than some individuals can handle so that behavioural problems result. Most can be 'talked down' but others may require sedation.

'MAGIC' MUSHROOMS

In the autumn adolescents in the UK commonly scour public parks, golf courses and other green areas searching for what they term 'magic' mushrooms. These are commonly *Psilocybe semilanceate* and *Panaeolus foenisecii* which contain the hallucinogens psilocybin and psilocin. Although mushrooms cannot be classified as drugs of abuse, they are consumed for the same reasons and it is appropriate to consider them here. The number of mushrooms required to obtain the desired effect varies and 80 or more may be eaten at one time. Apart from behavioural changes ranging from extreme apathy to agitation, acute gastroenteritis may result. Psychiatric symptoms which continue for weeks have been reported.

VOLATILE SUBSTANCES

Inhalation of volatile substances is common, causes hypoxaemia, induces destructive behaviour, impairs consciousness and sensitises the heart to circulating catecholamines leading to arrhythmias and death. Suffocation, falls from heights and burns are other potential complications. Treatment other than supportive care is not usually required though sedation may occasionally be necessary.

POISONING WITH PSYCHOTROPIC DRUGS

BARBITURATES

These drugs are still commonly available in developing countries but not in developed ones, where concern about the high number of deaths they caused and the arrival of benzodiazepines led to their disappearance. Drowsiness and coma develop rapidly and may persist for 1–2 days in severe cases. The pupils do not show specific changes, muscle tone and limb reflexes are reduced, and respiratory depression and hypotension may be severe. Hypothermia is common and skin blisters occur in 6% of patients. Supportive care is the mainstay of management. Gastric lavage may be considered if the patient presents within 1–2 hours of ingestion of a toxic amount and provided the airway can be protected. Repeat dose oral activated charcoal should be given. In the unlikely event of deterioration or failure to respond, haemodialysis should be considered for phenobarbitone poisoning and charcoal haemoperfusion for shorter-acting barbiturates.

TRICYCLIC ANTIDEPRESSANTS

Overdosage of tricyclic and related antidepressant drugs is becoming less common as they have been supplanted by the serotonin-specific re-uptake inhibitors (SSRIs). Despite this, poisoning with them remains an important part of clinical toxicology and carries considerable morbidity and mortality. Many of their toxic effects are the result of their anticholinergic actions.

Clinical features

The main toxic effects of this group of drugs are given in the information box. They usually appear 1–2 hours after ingestion and settle within 18–24 hours.

FEATURES OF POISONING WITH TRICYCLIC ANTIDEPRESSANTS	
Common	**Uncommon**
• Impairment of consciousness • Dilated pupils • Sinus tachycardia • Dry mouth • Urinary retention • QRS prolongation • Agitation and delirium	• Convulsions • Skin blisters • Broad-complex tachycardia • Bradycardia

Management

Supportive measures should be implemented where necessary and seizures controlled if they are prolonged or recurring frequently. In general, it is advisable to avoid the use of anti-arrhythmic drugs if at all possible. However, on occasions one may be compelled to treat ventricular tachycardia. In these cases lignocaine is the agent of choice, not least because of its short half-life. Magnesium infusions are indicated in the torsades de pointes variety (see p. 234). Diazepam or other sedation may be required during the recovery period to control agitation and delirium.

BENZODIAZEPINES

The benzodiazepines are commonly involved in drug overdoses. When taken alone, they rarely cause deaths. They are more important because they potentiate the effects of other central nervous system depressants including ethanol. Conversely, their inclusion in an overdose may be beneficial when the co-ingestant causes convulsions (e.g. tricyclic antidepressants).

Clinical features

The toxic effects are usually surprisingly mild even after ingestion of large doses. Drowsiness, ataxia and nystagmus are the usual features. Coma, hypotension and respiratory depression are less common. Recovery is usually rapid.

Management

Most patients require no treatment. Supportive measures are all that is required in the remainder. In unusually severe poisoning the benzodiazepine antagonist, flumazenil, may be given. The dose is 0.2 mg over 15 seconds then 0.1 mg at 60-second intervals. Most patients will respond to a total of 3 mg. The use of flumazenil may precipitate acute withdrawal symptoms and seizures in benzodiazepine-dependent individuals.

SEROTONIN-SPECIFIC RE-UPTAKE INHIBITORS (SSRIs)

SSRIs are rapidly replacing tricyclic compounds as the antidepressant drugs most commonly encountered in overdosage. They include fluoxetine, fluvoxamine and venlafaxine, although others may be expected soon. Serious toxicity is uncommon. The usual features include nausea, tremor, anxiety and tachycardia.

LITHIUM SALTS

Clinical lithium toxicity is most commonly the result of excessive therapeutic doses. In contrast, acute massive overdose or overdose superimposed on therapeutic doses may be associated with few, if any, features despite markedly raised serum lithium concentrations. The difference is explained by the slow rate at which lithium appears to cross cell membranes.

Clinical features

Nausea, vomiting and diarrhoea occur early, while neurological features including apathy, sluggishness, coarse tremor, hypertonicity, vertigo, dysarthria, muscular rigidity and twitching, ataxia and convulsions develop later. Hypernatraemia, hypokalaemia and ECG changes, including first-degree AV block and prolongation of QRS and QT intervals, may be present.

Management

Supportive measures should be implemented as necessary, renal function assessed and the serum lithium concentration measured urgently. (Ensure that the blood sample is not put in a lithium heparin container.) Gastric lavage is indicated if a potentially toxic dose has been ingested within the preceding 2 hours. Activated charcoal and forced diuresis are of no value. Patients with neurological features require haemodialysis but clinical improvement can be expected to lag well behind reduction of serum lithium concentrations. Asymptomatic patients with high lithium concentrations should be monitored closely and lithium concentrations should be measured twice daily until they are clearly shown to be falling. Dialysis is very unlikely to be required.

CARDIORESPIRATORY DRUGS

It is relatively uncommon to encounter cardiorespiratory drugs in acute overdosage, probably because they are usually prescribed for an older age group that is seldom involved in deliberate self-poisoning. However, serious morbidity and deaths can occur. The features of poisoning with the main cardiovascular agents are given in Table 19.17. Most antibiotic and bronchodilator overdoses cause few, if any,

Table 19.17 Features of poisoning with cardiovascular drugs

Drug group	Features of poisoning	Comment
β-adrenoceptor blockers	Bradycardia, hypotension	Convulsions with propranolol, ventricular tachyarrhythmias with sotalol
Calcium channel blockers	AV block, hypotension, hyper- and hypokalaemia, hyperglycaemia	Calcium gluconate is of little value
ACE inhibitors	Hypotension, tachycardia	
Cardiac glycosides	Nausea, vomiting, bradycardia, hypotension, hyperkalaemia	Therapeutic overdose much more serious than acute overdose An antidote is available
Nitrates	Hypotension, tachycardia	Serious toxicity is uncommon because of extensive first-pass metabolism

problems but theophylline overdoses must be handled with the utmost care.

THEOPHYLLINE

Most UK doctors are not aware that many theophylline formulations are of the delayed or sustained-release variety. They may therefore be lulled into a false sense of security by the absence of features in the first few hours after overdosage with these agents. Toxicity may only become apparent 12 or more hours later and can be severe and life-threatening, as shown in the information box.

CLINICAL FEATURES OF THEOPHYLLINE OVERDOSE

- Nausea and vomiting (often severe), abdominal pain, haematemesis and diarrhoea
- Thirst, polyuria, hypokalaemia, hyperventilation and agitation; common
- Cardiac arrhythmias, hypotension, metabolic acidosis and convulsions; indicate severe poisoning with a poor prognosis, particularly in the elderly

NATURALLY OCCURRING TOXINS

MUSHROOMS

Fortunately, serious poisoning with mushrooms is uncommon in Britain, probably because a relatively small number of fungi in this country are poisonous and the British do not share the enthusiasm of continental Europeans for mushroom collecting. Ingestion of relatively non-toxic species for the distortion of perception and hallucinations they induce is most common. This is considered under 'leisure' drugs.

Identification of harmful species of fungi is not easy and dangerous mushrooms often grow side by side with edible varieties. The speed with which symptoms develop after ingestion of fungi is an important indicator of their toxicity. Those that cause an acute gastrointestinal illness within about 4 hours of ingestion are seldom reasons for major concern. In contrast, the mushrooms which produce features only 6–12 hours and occasionally as long as 24 hours after being eaten are much more toxic and include the death cap mushroom *(Amanita phalloides)*, which may cause acute liver necrosis and failure, and *Cortinarius* species, which induce renal failure.

ANALGESICS

PARACETAMOL (ACETAMINOPHEN)

Paracetamol is the single most commonly encountered agent in acute poisoning in both adults and children in the UK and is now involved in up to 40% of all self-poisonings. While it is remarkably safe in therapeutic doses, paracetamol is potentially lethal in overdose. Acute hepatocellular and, less commonly, renal tubular necrosis may occur after the ingestion of a single dose of as little as 10–15 g (20–30 tablets) in adults and 150 mg/kg in children. Paracetamol poisoning is now the most common cause of acute liver failure in the UK. The liver is damaged by a highly reactive metabolite of paracetamol (N-acetyl-p-benzoquinonimine—NAPQI). Hepatic glutathione inactivates this metabolite but in massive paracetamol overdosage is rapidly depleted, allowing NAPQI to bind to cell proteins. Administration of N-acetylcysteine (NAC) and methionine restores the levels of glutathione and prevents or reduces liver damage. Clinical evidence suggests that patients who chronically ingest ethanol in excess of safe limits, are on treatment with drugs which induce microsomal oxidase (anticonvulsants, rifampicin) or are malnourished (anorexia nervosa, starvation) are at increased risk of paracetamol-induced liver damage.

Clinical features

Nausea and vomiting, the only early features of poisoning, usually settle after 24 hours. If they persist and are accompanied by right hypochondrial pain, it is likely that liver necrosis is developing. Liver function test abnormalities are maximal about 72–96 hours after ingestion and plasma alanine aminotransferase (ALT) activities of 10 000 iu/litre and higher are common. Marked prolongation of the prothrombin time (PT) also occurs secondary to the inability of the liver to synthesise clotting factors. Hypoglycaemia may occur at any time. Liver damage progresses to hepatic encephalopathy and cerebral oedema in a small minority of patients in whom mortality is high. Hypotension, metabolic acidosis, renal failure, pancreatitis and thrombocytopenia may complicate the late stages.

Management

Predicting those at risk of liver damage

The single most useful predictor of which patients will go on to develop severe and potentially fatal liver damage is the plasma paracetamol concentration related to the number of hours since ingestion. Emergency measurement of the plasma paracetamol concentration is therefore essential in every case of disclosed paracetamol overdose, every ingestion of unidentified white tablets and all patients who are unconscious as the result of a drug overdose. A total of 60% of patients whose values related to time fall above the 'normal' paracetamol 'treatment line' (see Fig. 19.7) are at risk of developing 'severe' liver damage. However, it is important to appreciate that 'severe' liver damage was defined as an ALT activity of 1000 i.u./litre or higher; the line does not predict life or death. The lower line of Figure 19.7 should be used in the assessment of patients considered to be at increased risk. Factors increasing the risk of hepatotoxicity after paracetamol overdose include regular alcohol consumption in excess of recommended limits; long-term treatment with carbamazepine, phenytoin, phenobarbitone and rifampicin; and malnutrition (as in anorexia nervosa, AIDS and starvation). Paracetamol concentrations in samples taken earlier than 4 hours from ingestion cannot be interpreted and extrapolation of the line beyond 15 hours is unjustified because of the lack of data from untreated patients.

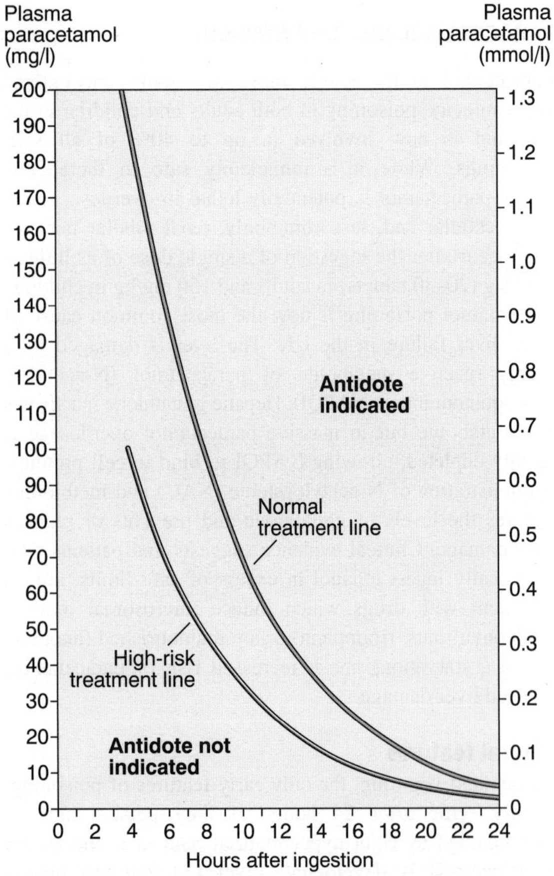

Fig. 19.7 Lines used to predict hepatotoxicity and guide the use of antidotes in acute paracetamol poisoning.

Further measures

Management depends on the time interval from ingestion (see the information box). Intravenous NAC is the preferred antidote for patients in whom specific treatment is indicated (see Fig. 19.7). The dosage regimen is given in

MANAGEMENT OF PARACETAMOL POISONING ACCORDING TO THE TIME SINCE INGESTION
Less than 4 hours
• Gastric lavage should be performed if the patient presents within 1–2 hours of ingestion of >125 mg/kg body weight • Give activated charcoal if the patient presents within 1–2 hours of ingestion • Wait till 4 hours post-ingestion then take a blood sample for measurement of the plasma paracetamol concentration • Identify risk factors • Give an antidote if indicated from the relevant prognostic line (see Fig. 19.7)
4–8 hours
• Gastric lavage and activated charcoal are of no value • Take a blood sample for measurement of the plasma paracetamol concentration • Identify risk factors • Give an antidote if indicated from the relevant prognostic line (see Fig. 19.7)
Longer than 8 hours
• Start NAC immediately • Take a blood sample for measurement of the plasma paracetamol concentration • Identify risk factors • Stop or continue the antidote as indicated by the relevant prognostic line (see Fig. 19.7)
Longer than 15 hours
• Start NAC immediately • Contact the poisons information service for advice

Table 19.18 N-acetylcysteine doses for intravenous infusion

Dose	N-acetylcysteine (mg/kg body weight)	Volume of 5% dextrose for dilution	Duration of infusion
1	150	200 ml	15 min
2	50	500 ml	4 hrs
3	50	500 ml	8 hrs
4	50	500 ml	8 hrs

Table 19.18. Oral methionine is an alternative but vomiting may impair its absorption and therefore its efficacy. In addition, it has not been shown to be effective more than 12 hours following the overdose. The dose is 2.5 g orally 4-hourly for 4 doses.

Monitoring

Patients who do not require treatment with antidotes or who had the antidote started within 10 hours of ingestion do not need to have their liver and renal function monitored. Others should have standard liver and renal function tests performed at least daily, remembering that the plasma creatinine is the preferred measure of renal function in the presence of liver damage. The single most useful indicator of the severity of liver necrosis and the need for intervention is the prothrombin time (PT). This should be measured daily and more often in patients who are deteriorating. Bedside monitoring for hypoglycaemia is important in those with liver damage. Patients may be discharged as soon as they are asymptomatic and liver function is clearly reverting to normal.

Management of patients with liver damage

Patients with liver damage should be monitored as outlined above. Administration of clotting factors should be avoided if at all possible since they invalidate the usefulness of the PT as the best indicator of liver function. Similarly, sedative drugs should only be used as a last resort. NAC administration may confer benefits at this stage. Liver transplantation (see p. 704) is potentially life-saving for patients with fulminant hepatic failure. If a patient's PT in seconds exceeds the number of hours from the overdose the advice of a specialist liver centre should be sought at an early stage to determine the desirability of transfer for assessment for transplantation. Those who develop severe liver damage and recover do not suffer long-term sequelae.

Adverse reactions to NAC

Adverse reactions to NAC occur in up to 15% of patients given it. They include nausea, vomiting, flushing, urticarial rashes and, less frequently, hypotension and wheezing. They usually occur within an hour of starting treatment and most settle within minutes of stopping the infusion. It is then often possible to restart NAC at the rate in dose 3 in Table 19.18. Occasionally, it may be necessary to give antihistamines and rarely corticosteroids. Methionine can be used if there are serious doubts about the advisability of restarting NAC.

SALICYLATES

Although the incidence of acute salicylate overdose has fallen in recent years it continues to be an important cause of poisoning. Aspirin (acetylsalicylic acid) is the most important salicylate.

Clinical features

Tinnitus and impaired hearing are the hallmarks of salicylism and are usually associated with nausea, vomiting, sweating and vasodilatation. Hyperventilation may be apparent. Impairment of consciousness indicates severe poisoning. A mixed acid-base upset due to a combination of respiratory alkalosis and metabolic acidosis is usual. In adults the former tends to predominate, resulting in blood hydrogen ion concentration being normal or low (pH normal or high).

Management

Emergency measurement of the plasma salicylate concentration is essential in assessing the severity of the poisoning. A concentration of 500 mg/litre (3.6 mmol/litre) in adults indicates moderate toxicity. Impaired consciousness and concentrations in excess of 700 mg/litre (5.1 mmol/litre) indicate severe poisoning with a mortality of about 5%. In these cases arterial blood gas analysis should be carried out urgently; acidaemia is a further poor prognostic finding.

Gastric lavage should be undertaken in patients who present within 1–2 hours of ingestion of a potentially toxic dose. Those who are only mildly poisoned (salicylate concentration < 300 mg/litre or 2.2 mmol/litre) do not require treatment other than being encouraged to drink freely. In more serious poisoning, repeat dose oral activated charcoal (see p. 1116) should be given and the need for active measures to enhance the elimination of absorbed salicylate should be considered. Forced diuresis is no longer advised but alkalinisation of the urine increases the excretion of salicylate. This is achieved by giving 1.5 litres 1.26% sodium bicarbonate intravenously over 3 hours and ensuring adequate potassium replacement if necessary. Haemodialysis is a very effective method of removing salicylate from the body and should be considered in all patients with impaired consciousness, pulmonary oedema and salicylate concentrations of 700 mg/litre (5.1 mmol/litre) or more.

OPIOID ANALGESICS

The features of poisoning with the opioid analgesics are considered under 'leisure' drugs. While codeine is very unlikely to cause serious toxicity when taken in overdose, dihydrocodeine and dextropropoxyphene in large doses can be lethal and are important because they are commonly co-formulated with paracetamol. Patients may then require specific treatment for both opioid and paracetamol intoxication.

NON-STEROIDAL ANTI-INFLAMMATORY DRUGS

The toxic effects of the individual members of this varied group of compounds are relatively similar. Ibuprofen and mefenamic acid are the most commonly encountered. The former causes few effects while the latter in overdose commonly causes convulsions. Gastric lavage (see p. 1115) should be considered but most patients will not require specific treatment. Convulsions should be controlled (see p. 945).

PESTICIDES

ORGANOPHOSPHORUS (OP) INSECTICIDES

These insecticides are very toxic and one of the most important causes of poisoning deaths world-wide. They inhibit cholinesterases in the brain and at synapses and neuromuscular junctions, and the symptoms of poisoning with them are largely due to the presence of excess acetylcholine at these structures.

Clinical features

Constricted pupils, sweating, salivation, nausea, vomiting, diarrhoea, urgency of bowel and bladder emptying and fasciculation are common. Muscle weakness, bronchospasm, bronchorrhoea and pulmonary oedema contribute to respiratory failure, the usual cause of death, although the direct effect of OPs on the brain is the main cause. Coma, convulsions, bradycardia and arrhythmias also occur.

Management

Decontamination measures according to the route of exposure and supportive measures, including care of the airway, ensuring adequate ventilation and oxygenation and control of convulsions, are vital. Atropine (2 mg intravenously) should be given at 10–30-minute intervals until full atropinisation is achieved. Oximes such as pralidoxime and obidoxime reactivate cholinesterase and improve muscle power and consciousness. The former should be given by slow intravenous injection in a dose of 30 mg/kg body weight. Administration of oximes may require reduction in the doses of atropine.

PARAQUAT DICHLORIDE

The liquid formulations of this herbicide supplied to farmers and horticulturists are exceedingly toxic. A granular preparation is available for amateur use.

Clinical features

Local features develop over several hours and are determined by the concentration of the pesticide in contact with the tissues. Contact with the eyes results in severe inflammation and possibly corneal ulceration while skin contamination may lead to acute irritation and blistering, and occasionally ulceration. Epistaxis and pharyngitis are possible after inhalation. Paraquat poisoning is most commonly the result of ingestion, which causes a burning sensation in the mouth and abdomen, nausea and vomiting. Ulceration of the lips, tongue and pharynx develop later.

Only ingestion is likely to cause systemic features. Large doses cause convulsions, shock, metabolic acidosis, pulmonary oedema and death within a few hours. Lesser amounts lead to multi-organ failure over a period of days though renal and hepatic damage is often relatively slight. However, over the course of a week or sometimes longer, a relentless proliferative alveolitis develops, causing death from respiratory failure.

Management

Gastric lavage should be carried out if the appropriate criteria (see p. 1115) are met. Fuller's earth (250 ml of a 30% solution) or activated charcoal should be left in the stomach and further doses given 2–4-hourly for the following 48 hours. However, it is extremely doubtful that they alter outcomes. Administration of cathartics may be necessary to prevent the adsorbent material causing intestinal obstruction. Supportive and symptomatic measures are implemented as clinically indicated but there is currently no effective treatment for this form of poisoning. Contact the poisons information service for the most up-to-date management.

MISCELLANEOUS SUBSTANCES

CHLOROQUINE

Acute overdosage with chloroquine is fortunately uncommon but ingestion of more than 5 g is potentially lethal.

Clinical features

Features are likely to develop within an hour of ingestion. Nausea, vomiting, drowsiness, dysarthria, breathlessness, hypotension and hypokalaemia precede convulsions, coma, QRS widening, ventricular dysrhythmias and acute pulmonary oedema. Cardiac arrest within 3 hours is not unusual.

Management

Supportive measures, including repeated doses of oral charcoal, are of vital importance. Correction of hypokalaemia may lead to serious hyperkalaemia as chloroquine is eliminated and it is best not undertaken unless cardiac dysrhythmias are present. Intravenous diazepam reduces mortality but doses of up to 2 mg/kg body weight may be required. Severely poisoned patients should therefore be intubated and ventilated at an early stage. Adrenaline (0.25 µg/kg increasing by 0.25 µg/kg/min until a systolic blood pressure of at least 100 mmHg is obtained) also reduces mortality.

IRON SALTS

Iron salts, particularly those prescribed for adults, remain an important cause of mortality in children. Severe poisoning in adults is uncommon. The elemental iron content of the salt is more important than the amount of the salt itself.

Clinical features

The course of acute iron overdose is traditionally divided into four stages:

- The initial features are those of direct gut irritation and damage and include epigastric pain, nausea, vomiting and grey-black diarrhoea. The vomit and stools may be blood-stained. Shock and coma are rare.
- The abatement of these symptoms after a few hours marks the start of the second phase and, in most cases, the end of toxicity.
- The third stage is characterised by the onset or recurrence of hypotension and evidence of the onset of acute liver necrosis and its complications. Most deaths occur in this stage.
- Features of high intestinal obstruction occur in the fourth phase 2–6 weeks after ingestion and are due to stricture formation.

Management

Supportive measures for shock, coma and acidosis are essential and patients with these features should be given desferrioxamine as a matter of urgency. The dose is 15 mg/kg body weight per hour up to a maximum of 80 mg/kg in 24 hours. Gastric lavage should be performed if the overdose was ingested within 2 hours of presentation. Activated charcoal is of no value. Selection of other cases for treatment with desferrioxamine is difficult. With the exceptions of shock and coma, clinical features are poor indicators of the severity of iron poisoning. Acidosis may be helpful since it is an indicator of cell health. Emergency measurement of the serum iron concentration is generally advised and patients with levels above 5 mg/litre (90 µmol/litre) should be given the antidote.

CARBON MONOXIDE

Carbon monoxide poisoning usually results from the inhalation of smoke or car exhaust, or from incomplete combustion of fuel gases due to faulty heaters or flues, and is a major cause of completed suicide. Carbon monoxide has an affinity for haemoglobin about 300 times that of oxygen and combines with haemoglobin to form carboxyhaemoglobin, thus reducing the oxygen-carrying capacity of the blood. It may also combine with myoglobin and have effects on cytochrome oxidases.

Features of acute poisoning

The most dangerous effects are on the central nervous system and myocardium. Agitation, headache, confusion and coma may occur. Carboxyhaemoglobin is said to impart a pink colour to the skin and mucous membranes but it is unusual in life. Pallor is more common. Skin bullae and rhabdomyolysis may develop if coma is prolonged and cardiac arrhythmias, hypotension and myocardial infarction have been reported. Irreparable central nervous system damage is a hazard, with loss of intellect, personality change, parkinsonism and cerebral infarction. Cerebral oedema secondary to capillary leakage may be delayed for hours or days after exposure. Significant poisoning in pregnancy may lead to fetal death and abortion.

Delayed neuropsychiatric sequelae

About 10% of patients who have seemingly made a complete recovery from acute poisoning are said to develop a variety of disabling neurological, behavioural and psychiatric features, commonly after an interval of 2–4 weeks. The basis for these has not been defined and their existence remains controversial. There is no specific treatment for delayed neuropsychiatric sequelae. Most patients recover spontaneously within a year.

Management

Remove the patient to fresh air and administer 100% oxygen as soon as available. Cardiorespiratory resuscitation (see p. 235) should be instituted if necessary and the patient transferred to hospital. Supportive measures for the airway, ventilation, hypotension, hypothermia and the skin are dictated by clinical need. Cerebral oedema can be anticipated in all severe poisonings; intravenous infusion of mannitol (1 g/kg as a 20% solution over 15 minutes followed by 500 ml dextrose 5% over the next 4 hours) may be of benefit. Though hyperbaric oxygen therapy is entirely logical to increase the rate of dissociation of carboxyhaemoglobin, its effectiveness in reducing mortality and acute and long-term morbidity remains controversial. This is a developing subject and the possibility of using it in seriously poisoned patients, particularly those who are or have been unconscious or have carboxyhaemoglobin concentrations exceeding 40%, should be discussed with the poisons information service.

CORROSIVE AND IRRITANT SUBSTANCES

Direct contact of many household products and chemicals irritates and inflames tissues to varying degrees. Domestic bleaches and disinfectants, detergents for automatic dishwashers, solutions of plant oils and denture cleaning materials are amongst the most commonly ingested but rarely cause more than superficial, minor damage which resolves rapidly. Others, particularly the strong acids (hydrochloric, nitric and sulphuric) and alkalis (sodium and potassium hydroxide), are frankly corrosive and can cause long-term morbidity and death.

Clinical features

A feeling of burning in the mouth, throat and abdomen are common and associated with salivation, nausea and vomiting. The vomitus may be blood-stained. Dysphonia and stridor may develop if the larynx becomes contaminated. Shock, perforation of the gut and hepatic or renal damage are potential complications.

Management

The extent of management depends on the agent involved. Gastric emptying by any means is contraindicated and there is no merit in spending time looking for substances to neutralise the pH of the poison. In the worst cases analgesics, fluid or blood replacement and correction of acid-base abnormalities may all be required. Upper GI endoscopy by an experienced operator is required to determine the extent of the injury and thus to determine optimum management and the duration of hospital care. Surgical advice should be sought at an early stage if patients have sustained severe injuries. Exploratory laparotomy, with or without immediate corrective procedures, may be indicated.

PETROLEUM DISTILLATES

Petroleum distillates are long-chain hydrocarbons such as those found in petrol, paraffin, turpentine substitute and numerous household polishes and cleaning agents and as solvents for some pesticides. Their characteristic feature is the ability of small amounts to spread in a thin film over a wide area. Ingestion is the usual route of exposure but their gastrointestinal toxicity is low and does not require treatment. The major concern with these substances is that of aspiration into the lungs, which may result in cough, breathlessness and a lipoid pneumonia. Do not attempt to empty the stomach. Antibiotics may be required if aspiration has occurred.

ALCOHOLS AND GLYCOLS

The features of inebriation with ethanol (ethyl alcohol) are well known and include ataxia, dysarthria and impaired consciousness. Ethanol also potentiates the CNS effects of other psychotropic agents. Occasionally, hypoglycaemia may be a complication, especially in children. Supportive measures are all that is necessary. Poisoning with methanol and ethylene glycol, common ingredients of antifreezes and vehicle windscreen washes, is much more serious and potentially fatal. Both cause severe metabolic acidosis but while methanol intoxication may result in pulmonary oedema and permanent blindness, ethylene glycol causes severe hypocalcaemia and its complications. Diagnosis of poisoning with these chemicals requires a high degree of suspicion and they should be borne very much in mind for every ill patient who has a severe and unexplained acidosis. Correction of the acidosis and haemodialysis may be required in addition to appropriate supportive care and administration of ethanol to slow metabolism of methanol and ethylene glycol to their toxic metabolites.

ENVIRONMENTAL TOXINS AND CHRONIC ILL HEALTH

In affluent countries, it is virtually impossible to avoid contact with chemicals. They are in our diet, clothes, household items and offices. We benefit from their presence in so far as they lighten the burdens of daily living and add to the quality of our lives. They help ensure that we have access to plentiful and extraordinarily varied foods. Indeed, it is improbable that the brightly coloured, shiny and largely unmarked fruit and vegetables found on supermarket shelves irrespective of the time of the year could be achieved without them. Inevitably, the advantages are obtained at a price and so sophisticated are the techniques of analytical chemists that they can accurately measure even minute concentrations of residues in food, water, soil and air. The thought of them never crosses the minds of most shoppers. For some the very low levels provide reassurance that the products are safe; for others they are a source of concern—some of it justified, much of it not. All too often their very presence is regarded with suspicion or as evidence of toxicity.

As with all human activities, advantages must be balanced against the adverse consequences. The concepts of hazard, risk and risk management have therefore been developed. A hazard is an adverse effect of a substance or action while risk is the likelihood of that hazard occurring. Risk management is the process or processes by which the occurrence of a hazard can be reduced.

In recent years it has become increasingly common for patients to allege that their chronic and often severe symptoms are the result of exposure to low levels of toxins. Although many chemicals stand implicated, pesticides, especially organophosphate insecticides, head the list. The health effects include constant tiredness, often to the point of exhaustion, insomnia, irritability, mood swings, depression, inability to concentrate, memory impairment and somatic features such as muscle aches and difficulty in walking. The impact on work and family life can be catastrophic. As a result, a number of new 'diseases' have appeared, prominent amongst which are environmental illness, multiple chemical sensitivity, Gulf War illness and sheep dip poisoning.

Despite the utter conviction with which patients believe in the cause of their illness, diagnostic criteria for these conditions have not been established and there is considerable symptom overlap between them and with non-toxic conditions such as chronic fatigue, myalgic encephalomyelitis (ME) and fibromyalgia. There is no test that is diagnostic for any of them and detailed clinical examination and batteries of investigations usually fail to identify any abnormality despite the often profound nature of the symptoms. Although sophisticated neurobehavioural and nerve conduction studies have shown abnormalities, they are subtle and difficult to accept as providing a causal basis for such incapacitating symptoms. Indeed, the American Medical Association has declined to acknowledge multiple chemical sensitivity as a disease entity.

Several consequences may arise. First, the diagnostic category into which individuals place themselves or are placed is largely determined by their perception of the cause of their illness. Second, the doctor's suspicion of a major psychological component usually communicates itself to the patient sooner or later, arousing hostility, disbelief and accusations of lack of sympathy. Third, conventional therapeutics invariably prove hopelessly unsuccessful, causing patients to seek what relief they can find, sometimes at considerable financial cost, with alternative medicine and with their fellow sufferers. Patients with illnesses of this sort are difficult to manage in the light of present knowledge. That they have symptoms is not in doubt but it is far from clear that the causes they claim are correct. This area of medicine can be expected to develop over the forthcoming years and referral to a clinical toxicologist may be appropriate until the position is clarified.

FURTHER INFORMATION ON ACUTE POISONING

Proudfoot A T 1993 Acute poisoning: diagnosis and management, 2nd edn. Butterworth-Heinemann, London

Weatherall J D (ed) 1996 Oxford textbook of medicine. Section 8: Chemical and physical injuries and environmental and occupational diseases. Oxford University Press, Oxford

The above should be read in conjunction with guidelines on gut decontamination as published in Clinical Toxicology 1997 35(7)

APPENDIX I

POISONS INFORMATION CENTRES—24-HOUR SERVICE (UK AND REPUBLIC OF IRELAND)

London	0171 635 9191	0171 955 5095
Birmingham	0121 554 3801	
Edinburgh	0131 536 1000	
Leeds	01132 430715	01132 432799
Cardiff	01222 709901	
Newcastle	0191 232 5131	
Belfast	01232 240503	
Dublin	003531 379964	003531 379966

TOXBASE on-line poisons information service is available to users within the National Health Service throughout the UK.

Appendices 20

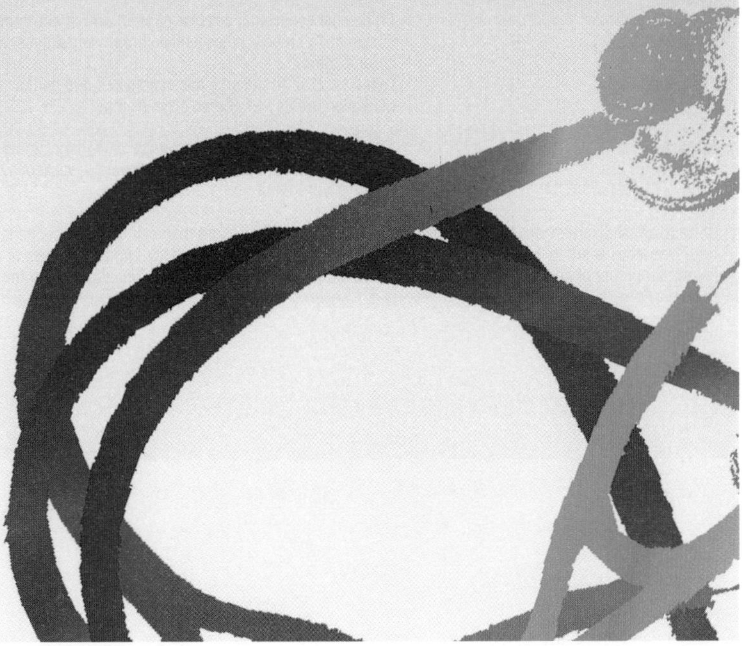

GENETIC DISEASES

The following tables illustrate examples of the types of disease discussed in Chapter 1.

Sites of genes are given by chromosomal location: chromosome number, p (short arm) or q (long arm), and band (e.g. q13).

For further details, Victor McCusick's Online Inheritance in Man (OMIM) is recommended at

http://www.ncbi.nlm.nih.gov/Omim/searchomim.html

Table 20.1 Examples of chromosomal disorders

Chromosomes	Result
2n (46, XX)	Normal female
2n (46, XY)	Normal male *(male karyotype illustrated below for simplicity)*
NUMERICAL ABNORMALITIES	
Triploidy (3n), **tetraploidy** (4n)	Spontaneous abortion
Parthenogenesis (2n from same parent)	Spontaneous abortion (can be compatible with life in chimera)
Aneuploidy (2n + specific chromosome)	
Trisomy 21 (47, XY,+21)	Down's syndrome (characteristic facies, IQ usually < 50, congenital heart disease, reduced life expectancy)
Trisomy 18 (47, XY,+18)	Edwards' syndrome (characteristic skull and facies, frequent malformations of heart, kidney and other organs)
Trisomy 13 (47, XY,+13)	Patau's syndrome (cleft lip and palate, polydactyly, small head, frequent congenital heart disease)
Sex chromosome aneuploidies	
Phenotypically male	
47, XXY	Klinefelter's syndrome (infertility, gynaecomastia, small testes)
47, XYY	XYY male (usually asymptomatic, often tall)
Phenotypically female	
47, XXX	Trisomy X (usually asymptomatic, 20% mentally handicapped)
45, XO	Turner's syndrome (short stature, webbed neck, primary amenorrhoea)
STRUCTURAL CHROMOSOME ABERRATIONS	
Inherited	
46, XY,del(5p)	Cri du chat syndrome, deletion of short arm of chromosome 5
45, XY,t(14;21)	Fusion of 14 and 21, no essential chromosomal material lost. (NORMAL, but balanced carrier of abnormal chromosome)
46, XY,t(14;21)	Fused 14;21 chromosome has segregated into gamete with normal chromosome 21, and fertilisation has generated trisomy 21 (Down's syndrome)
Acquired	*Occur in over 50% of haematological malignancies; also common in other neoplastic cells*
46, XY,t(9,22)	Philadelphia chromosome (chronic myeloid leukaemia)
46, XY,t(2,8) or t(8,14) or t(8,22)	Burkitt's lymphoma

Chromosomal disorders are extremely common and probably affect more than half of all conceptions. However, most spontaneously miscarry, so that the live-born frequency is about 0.6%, of which one-third are clinically serious. There are two broad types of chromosome aberration: numerical, where there is an incorrect number of chromosomes in somatic cells; and structural, where there is an alteration in the structure of one or more chromosomes.

Table 20.2 Examples of diseases inherited as autosomal dominant traits

A. ONE MAJOR GENE

Chromosome	Gene	Disease
1p	*Uroporphyrinogen decarboxylase*	**Porphyria cutanea tarda**
2q	*PAX3*	**Waardenburg's syndrome 1**
3p	*VHL*	**Von Hippel–Lindau syndrome**
4p	*Huntingtin*	**Huntington's disease**
4p	*FGFR3*	**Achondroplasia**
4p	*FGFR3*	**Crouzon's syndrome**
5q	*APC*	**Polyposis coli**
5q	*SMN1*	**Spinal muscular atrophy types 1, 2, 3**
7q	*Elastin*	**Cutis laxa**
8p	*Ankyrin*	**Congenital spherocytosis**
9q	*Frataxin*	**Friedreich's ataxia**
10q	*FGFR2*	**Apert's syndrome**
11p	$p57^{KIP2}$	**Beckwith-Wiederman syndrome**
12p	*VWF*	**Von Willebrand's disease (also recessive)**
13q	*RB*	**Retinoblastoma**
15q	*Fibrillin1*	**Marfan's syndrome**
16p	*Marenostrin*	**Familial Mediterranean fever**
17p	*p53*	**Li–Fraumeni syndrome**
17q	*SLC4A1*	**Distal renal tubular acidosis**
19p	*LDL receptor*	**Familial hypercholesterolaemia**
19q	*DM kinase*	**Myotonic dystrophy**

Table 20.2 Examples of diseases inherited as autosomal dominant traits *(contd)*

B. TWO OR MORE MAJOR GENES

Chromosome	Gene
Alzheimer's disease *(early onset)*	
1q	*Presenelin II*
14q	*Presenelin I*
19q	*Apolipoprotein E (ApoE)* *(not strictly dominant as dose-related effects)*
21q	*Amyloid precursor protein (APP)*
Mitochondrial DNA	
Breast carcinoma (familial, early onset)	
17q	*BRCA1*
13q	*BRCA2*
Numerous other genes also implicated	
Charcot–Marie–Tooth (HMSN)	
1q	*Myelin protein* (HMSN 1B)
17p	*Myelin protein 22* (HMSN 1A)
Also X-linked and recessive forms	
Ehlers–Danlos syndrome	
Numerous collagen genes, e.g. *COL1A1 (7q)*, *COL1A2 (7q)*, *COL3A1 (2q)*, *COL5A1 (9q)*	
Epidermolysis bullosa	
Numerous collagen and keratin genes	
Hereditary elliptocytosis	
1q	*α-spectrin*
14q	*β-spectrin*
Hirschsprung's disease	
Complex disorder which may be inherited as an autosomal dominant (mutations in RET proto-oncogene, 10q), recessive (endothelin 3B receptor on 13q) or polygenic trait	
Hypertrophic cardiomyopathy	
14q	*Cardiac myosin heavy chain*
1q	*Troponin-T*
15q	*α-tropomyosin*
11p	*Cardiac myosin-binding protein C*
and others	
Multiple endocrine neoplasia (MEN)	
10q	*RET proto-oncogene* (MEN IIA)
11q	*Menin* (MEN I)
Neurofibromatosis	
17q	*Neurofibromin* (NF1)
22q	*Merlin* (NF2)
Osteogenesis imperfecta	
Numerous collagen genes, e.g. *COL1A1 (7q)*, *COL1A2 (7q)*, *COL4A1 (2q)*	
Polycystic kidney disease (PKD)	
16p	*PKD1*
4q	*PKD2*
Rendu–Osler–Weber syndrome (HHT)	
9q	*Endoglin* (HHT1)
12q	*ALK1* (HHT2)
Retinitis pigmentosa types	
> 18 genes, including *rhodopsin (3q)* and *peripherin (6p)*	
Tuberose sclerosis (TS)	
9q	*Hamartin* (TS1)
16p	*Tuberin* (TS2)
Wilms' tumour	
11p	WT1
11p	WT2

Table 20.3 Examples of autosomal recessive disorders

Chromosome	Gene	Disease
1q	*Factor H*	Haemolytic-uraemic syndrome
1q	*Glucocerebrosidase*	Gaucher's disease
3q	*Homogen β1,2 diox.*	Alkaptonuria
4q	*Mic TG transfer prot.*	Abetalipoproteinaemia
7q	*CFTR*	Cystic fibrosis
10q	*Phytanoyl-CoA hydroxylase*	Refsum's disease
11p	*β globin*	Sickle-cell anaemia
11p	*β globin*	Beta-thalassaemia
11q	*ATM*	Ataxia-telangiectasia
11q	*Tyrosinase*	Albinism *(also 9p, 15q)*
12q	*Phenylal. hydrox.*	Phenylketonuria
13q	*ATP7B (Copper transporter)*	Wilson's disease
14q	*α_1-protease inhibitor*	α_1-protease (antitrypsin) deficiency
15q	Hexosaminidase A	Tay–Sachs disease
19q	*Br-chain-α-keto DH*	Maple syrup urine disease *(also 1p, 6p)*
20q	*Adenosine deaminase (ADA)*	Adenosine deaminase (ADA) deficiency
21q	*β_2-integrin ITGB2*	Leucocyte adhesion deficiency (LAD)
21q	*Cystathionine β-synthetase*	Homocystinuria
Multiple		Xeroderma pigmentosum
Multiple	*Peroxins*	Zellweger's syndrome

Table 20.3 A selection of autosomal recessive disorders *(contd)*

Chromosome	Gene	Disease
Mucopolysaccharidoses		
4p	*α-L-iduronidase*	Hurler's syndrome (type I)
17q	*Heparan sulphatase*	Sanfilippo's (type III)
16q	*Galactose-6-sulphatase*	Morquio's (IVA)
3p	*β-galactosidase*	Morquio's (IVB)
5q	*Aryl sulphatase*	Maroteaux–Lamy (VI)
7q	*β-glucuronidase*	Sly's (VII)
(N.B. Hunter's syndrome, (type II) X-linked: no type V or VIII)		
Glycogen storage diseases (N.B. type VIII X-linked)		
17q	*Glucose-6-phosphatase*	Type I (von Gierke's syndrome)
17q	*α-1,4 glucosidase*	Type II (Pompes, acid maltase deficiency)
1p	*Glycogen debrancher*	Type III (Forbe's deficiency)
3p	*Glycogen brancher*	Type IV (Andersen's)
11q	*Myophosphorylase*	Type V (McArdle's)
14q	*Hepatic phosphorylase*	Type VI (Hers')
12q	*Phosphofructokinase*	Type VII (Tauri)
(N.B. Type VIII X-linked)		

(ATP7B (copper transporter) = ATPase binding copper transporter; Br-chain-α-keto DH = branched-chain-α-keto acid dehydrogenase; phenylal. hydrox. = phenylalanine hydroxylase; CFTR = cystic fibrosis conductance regulator; homogen β1,2 diox. = homogentisate β1,2 dioxygenase; mic TG transfer prot. = microsomal triglyceride transfer protein)

Many recessive diseases are due to inherited defects in genes encoding enzymes. These present as recessive disease when 50% activity provides sufficient function for an individual to be clinically normal (although subtle defects may be demonstrated biochemically, or under periods of metabolic stress). Activity must be impaired from both alleles to generate disease.

Table 20.4 Examples of X-linked disorders

Site	Gene	Disease
Recessive (most)		
Xp22	*Microsomal steroid sulphatase*	X-linked ichthyosis
Xp22	*Liver phosphorylase kinase*	Glycogen storage disease type VIII
Xp21	*Dystrophin*	Duchenne's muscular dystrophy
Xp21	*Dystrophin*	Becker's muscular dystrophy
Xp21	*CLCN5*	Dent's disease/type I nephrolithiasis
Xq13	*IL-2 receptor γ chain*	X-linked severe combined immunodeficiency
Xq13	*IL-2 receptor γ chain*	Agammaglobulinaemia (Swiss type)
Xq13	*Connexin 32*	Charcot–Marie–Tooth (HMSN) X-linked
Xq13	*Ribosomal protein S4*	Turner's syndrome
Xq21	*Bruton tyrosine kinase*	Bruton agammaglobulinaemia
Xq22	*COL4A5*	Alport's syndrome
Xq22	*α-galactosidase*	Fabry's disease
Xq22	*Double cortin*	X-linked lissencephaly
Xq25	*Lymphoproliferative syndrome*	Progressive X-linked lymphoproliferative syndrome
Xq27	*Factor IX*	Haemophilia B
Xq27	*FRAXQ27*RFA*	Fragile X syndrome
Xq28	*Factor VIII*	Haemophilia A
Xq28	*Arginine vasopressin receptor*	Nephrogenic diabetes insipidus
Xq28	*Glucose-6-phosphate dehydrogenase*	G6PD deficiency/haemolytic anaemia
Xq28	*Iduronate sulphatase*	Mucopolysaccharidosis type II (Hunter's)
Dominant (rare)		
Xp22	*PEX*	Vitamin D-resistant rickets

Table 20.5 Imprinted genes implicated in human disease

Chromosome	Gene(s)	Disease example
6q26	*IGF2R*	Tumour suppressor—inactivated by inappropriate imprinting
11p13	*WT1*	Wilms' tumour: *WT1* gene mutated in 10–15% of cases
11p15	*p57KIP2* *HASH2, INS2* *IGF2, H19*	Beckwith–Wiederman syndrome: General 'over-growth', advanced ageing and increased childhood tumours. Probably due to mutations in p57KIP2
	WT2	Wilms' tumour
15q11–13	*SNRPN* *Necdin* *and* *others*	Prader–Willi syndrome: Obesity, hypogonadism and varying degrees of mental retardation. Lack of paternal contribution (due to deletion of paternal 15q11–q13, or inheritance of both chromosome 15q11–q13 regions from the mother). Currently thought to be a contiguous gene syndrome, due to loss of at least SNRPN and necdin
	Ubiquitin protein ligase E3A (UBE3A)	Angelman syndrome (AS): Severe mental retardation, ataxia, epilepsy and inappropriate laughing bouts due to mutations in the *UBE3A* gene inherited from the patient's mother. The neurological phenotype results because most tissues express both maternal and paternal alleles of *UBE3A*, whereas the brain expresses predominantly the maternal allele
X chromosome		Duchenne's muscular dystrophy: If, by chance, a sufficient number of the X chromosomes containing the normal gene are inactivated in muscle, even heterozygotes may have symptoms. Conversely, if a higher proportion of the disease-gene-carrying chromosome is inactivated, a carrier female may test negative on biochemical screening for elevated creatinine kinase levels

Table 20.6 Diseases associated with triplet and other repeat sequences

		No. of repeats				
	Repeat	**Normal**	**Mutant**	**Gene**	**Gene location**	**Inheritance**
A. Coding repeat expansion						
Huntington's disease	[CAG]	6–34	> 35	*Huntingtin*	4p16	Autosomal dominant
Spinocerebellar ataxia (type 1)	[CAG]	6–39	> 40	*Ataxin*	6p22–23	Autosomal dominant
Spinocerebellar ataxia (types 2,3,6,7)	[CAG]			Various	Various	Autosomal dominant
Dentatorubral-pallidoluysian atrophy	[CAG]	7–25	> 49	*Atrophin*	12p12–13	Autosomal dominant
Machado–Joseph disease	[CAG]	12–40	> 67	*MJD*	14q32	Autosomal dominant
Spinobulbar muscular atrophy	[CAG]	11–34	> 40	*Androgen receptor*	Xq11–12	X-linked recessive
B. Non-coding repeat expansion						
Myotonic dystrophy	[CTG]	5–37	> 50	*DMPK* - 3'UTR	19q13	Autosomal dominant
Friedreich's ataxia	[GAA]	7–22	> 200	*Frataxin* - intronic	9q13	Autosomal dominant
Progressive myoclonic epilepsy	$[---]_{4-6}$	2–3	> 25	*Cystatin B* - 5'UTR	21q	Autosomal recessive
Fragile X mental retardation	[CGG]	5–52	> 200	*FMR1* - 5'UTR	Xq27	X-linked dominant
Fragile X E mild mental retardation	[GCC]	6–35	> 200	*FMR2*	Xq28	X-linked, probably recessive

The triplet repeat diseases fall into two major groups: those with disease resulting from expansion of [CAG]n repeats in coding DNA, resulting in polyglutamine tracts, and those with non-coding repeats. The latter tend to be longer. Parents usually display 'pre-mutation' allele lengths that are just above the normal range, and may encroach on a stability threshold for trinucleotides of approximately 144–156 bp. (UTR = untranslated region)

Table 20.7 Clinical disease states associated with mitochondrial DNA abnormalities

Disease	Other features	Types of mutation detected
A. Mitochondrial myopathies		
e.g. Mitochondrial encephalomyopathy, lactic acidosis and stroke-like episodes		Point mutation in tRNA (Leu-URR) gene
Chronic progressive external ophthalmoplegia (CPEO)	Ophthalmoplegia	Deletions in > 50%; point mutations also detected
Kearns–Sayre syndrome	Ophthalmoplegia, heart block	Rearrangement, long deletions in 45–75%
Overlap syndromes characteristically display features such as external ophthalmoplegia, optic atrophy, bilateral sensorineural deafness, muscle wasting, peripheral neuropathy, early strokes and diabetes. Identical deletions are reported in CPEO and Kearns–Sayre syndrome		
B. Disease characterised by non-myopathic features		
Leber's optic atrophy		Specific missense mutations affecting genes encoding complexes I, III and IV of the respiratory chain
C. Other diseases in which mitochondrial DNA abnormalities have been observed		
Senescence Alzheimer's Diabetes Parkinson's disease		Not all are likely to be genuinely causative or modifying disease outcome. Some reports have reflected incidental age-related changes and erroneous amplification of nuclear pseudogenes
D. Diseases due to nuclear-encoded mitochondrial proteins		
Friedreich's ataxia	Cardiomyopathy, blindness, deafness, diabetes	Chromosomal mutations in *frataxin* on 9q *See also Tables 20.2 and 20.6*

INCUBATION PERIODS, IMMUNISATION SCHEDULES AND NOTIFIABLE DISEASES

Table 20.8 Incubation periods of important infections

Infection	Incubation period: Maximum range	Incubation period: Normal range
Short incubation periods (< 7 days)		
Anthrax	2–5 days	
Bacillary dysentery	1–7 days	
Cholera	Hours–5 days	2–3 hours
Diphtheria	2–5 days	
Gonorrhoea	2–5 days	
Meningococcaemia	2–10 days	3–4 days
Scarlet fever	1–3 days	
Intermediate incubation periods (7–21 days)		
Amoebiasis	14 days–months	21 days
Chickenpox	14–21 days	
Lassa fever	7–14 days	
Malaria	8 days–months	
Measles	7–14 days	10 days
Mumps	12–21 days	18 days
Poliomyelitis	3–21 days	7–10 days
Psittacosis	4–14 days	10 days
Rubella	14–21 days	18 days
Trypanosoma rhodesiense infection	14–21 days	
Typhoid fever	7–21 days	
Typhus fever	7–14 days	12 days
Whooping cough	7–10 days	7 days
Long incubation periods (> 21 days)		
Brucellosis	Days–months	
Filariasis	3 months–years	
Hepatitis A	2–6 weeks	4 weeks
Hepatitis B	6 weeks–6 months	12 weeks
Leishmaniasis		
Cutaneous	1 week–months	
Visceral	2 weeks–2 years	2–4 months
Leprosy	Years	2–5 years
Rabies	Variable	2–8 weeks
Schistosomiasis	Weeks–years	
Trypanosoma gambiense infection	Weeks–years	
Tuberculosis	Months–years	

Table 20.9 Notifiable infectious diseases in Britain

Under the Public Health (Control of Diseases) Act 1984

- Cholera
- Food poisoning
- Plague
- Relapsing fever
- Smallpox
- Typhus

Under the Public Health (Infectious Diseases) Regulations 1988

- Acute encephalitis
- Acute poliomyelitis
- Anthrax
- Diphtheria
- Dysentery (amoebic or bacillary)
- Leprosy
- Leptospirosis
- Malaria
- Measles
- Meningitis
- Meningococcal septicaemia (without meningitis)
- Mumps
- Ophthalmia neonatorum
- Paratyphoid fever
- Rabies
- Rubella
- Scarlet fever
- Tetanus
- Tuberculosis
- Typhoid fever
- Viral haemorrhagic fever

Table 20.10 Periods of infectivity in childhood infectious diseases

Disease	Infectious period
Chickenpox	5 days before rash to 6 days after last crop
Diphtheria	2–3 weeks (shorter with antibiotic therapy)
Measles	From onset of prodromal symptoms to 4 days after onset of rash
Mumps	3 days before salivary swelling to 7 days after
Rubella	7 days before onset of rash to 4 days after
Scarlet fever	10–21 days after onset of rash (shortened to 1 day by penicillin)
Whooping cough	7 days after exposure to 3 weeks after onset of symptoms (shortened to 7 days by antibiotics)

Table 20.11 Immunisation schedule recommended in the United Kingdom

Age	Visits	Vaccine	Intervals
3–12 months	3	Three simultaneous administrations of DTP + OPV and *Haemophilus influenzae* type B	4 weeks (ideal start at 3 months of age) 4–6 months
12–24 months	1	MMR vaccination	
1st year at school	1	Booster DT + OPV	
10–13 years	1	BCG for the tuberculin-negative	
Girls: 11–13 years	1	Rubella vaccination	
15–19 years or on leaving school	1	Td + OPV	

(DTP = diphtheria, tetanus, pertussis ('triple') vaccine; OPV = oral poliomyelitis vaccine; DT = diphtheria, tetanus vaccine; Td = tetanus, low-dose diphtheria toxoid; MMR = measles, mumps and rubella vaccine)

Table 20.12 Immunisation schedule recommended by WHO for developing countries*

Age	Vaccine
Birth or first contact	BCG
6, 10, 14 weeks	DPT and OPV
9 months	Measles
12 months	Yellow fever (in endemic areas)
18–24 months	DPT and OPV
5 years	DT and OPV

* MMR and hepatitis B are being introduced to schedules in many areas, also meningococcal vaccine in epidemic seasons.
(DTP = diphtheria, tetanus, pertussis ('triple') vaccine; OPV = oral poliomyelitis vaccine; DT = diphtheria, tetanus vaccine; MMR = measles, mumps and rubella vaccine)

Table 20.13 Indications for prophylactic immunoglobulins

Human normal immunoglobulin (pooled immunoglobulin)

- Virus A hepatitis (travellers* and debilitated children)
- Measles (child with heart or lung disease)

Human specific immunoglobulin

- Virus B hepatitis (needlestick injuries, sexual partner)
- Tetanus (susceptible injured patients)
- Rabies (post-exposure protection)
- Chickenpox (immunosuppressed children)
- Respiratory syncytial virus infection (high-risk infants, e.g. premature—investigational use)

* If not protected by active immunisation.

Table 20.14 Indications for chemoprophylaxis

Infection to be prevented	Indication for prophylaxis	Antimicrobial agent indicated	Adult dose
Diphtheria	Susceptible contacts	Erythromycin	500 mg 6-hourly for 5 days
Meningococcal infection	Susceptible contacts	Rifampicin Ciprofloxacin	600 mg 12-hourly for 2 days 500 mg as single dose
Whooping cough	Susceptible contacts	Erythromycin	500 mg 6-hourly for 7 days
Tuberculosis	Susceptible contacts	Isoniazid	300 mg daily for 6 months
Rheumatic fever	Following rheumatic fever	Penicillin	250 mg 12-hourly
Endocarditis	Heart valve lesion	Amoxycillin *or* Erythromycin	See page 286
Tetanus	Wound or injury	Erythromycin	500 mg 6-hourly for 7 days
Gas gangrene	Wound or injury	Penicillin *or* Metronidazole	600 mg 6-hourly for 5 days 500 mg 8-hourly for 5 days
Abdominal/pelvic sepsis	Colonic or gynaecological surgery	Gentamicin *or* Cephalosporin + metronidazole (single dose)	
Malaria	Travel to malarious countries	Depends on country (see page 148)	

NOTES ON INTERNATIONAL SYSTEM OF UNITS (SI UNITS)

Examples of basic SI units

Length	metre (m)
Mass	kilogram (kg)
Amount of substance	mole (mol)
Energy	joule (J)
Pressure	pascal (Pa)

Examples of decimal multiples and submultiples of SI units

Factor	*Name*	*Symbol*
10^6	mega-	M
10^3	kilo-	k
10^{-1}	deci-	d
10^{-2}	centi-	c
10^{-3}	milli-	m
10^{-6}	micro-	µ
10^{-9}	nano-	n
10^{-12}	pico-	p
10^{-15}	femto-	f

Volume

The basic SI unit of volume is the cubic metre (1000 litres). Because of its convenience, the litre is used as the unit of volume in laboratory work.

Mass concentration

Mass concentration (e.g. g/l, µg/l) is used for all protein measurements, for substances which do not have a sufficiently well-defined composition and for serum vitamin B_{12} and folate measurements.

SI units are not employed for enzymes, nor usually for immunoglobulins.

BIOCHEMICAL AND HAEMATOLOGICAL VALUES

Reference ranges are largely those used in the Department of Clinical Biochemistry, Royal Infirmary, University of Edinburgh and the Department of Haematology, the Western General Hospital NHS Trust, Edinburgh, UK. These can vary from laboratory to laboratory, depending on the assay method used and other factors; this is especially the case for the enzyme assays. Although the SI *system* of units is widely used in the UK, *units* of measurement can vary and lead to laboratory differences.

No details are given of the collection requirements which may be critical to obtaining a meaningful result.

Unless otherwise stated, reference ranges apply to adults; *values in children may be different.*

Table 20.15 Arterial blood analysis

Analysis	Reference range	Units
Bicarbonate	21–27.5	mmol/l
Hydrogen ion	36–44	nmol/l
$PaCO_2$	4.4–6.1	kPa
PaO_2	12–15	kPa
Oxygen saturation	Normally > 97	%

Table 20.16 Cerebrospinal fluid

Analysis	Reference range	Units
Cells	Up to 5 (all mononuclear)	cells/mm^3
Chloride	120–170	mmol/l
Glucose	2.5–4.0	mmol/l
IgG index*	< 0.65	
Total protein	100–400	mg/l

* A crude index of increase in IgG attributable to intrathecal synthesis.

Table 20.17 Reference values in venous serum for the more common analytes in adults

Analysis	Reference range	Units
α_1-antitrypsin	1.7–3.2	g/l
Alanine amino-transferase (ALT)	10–40	U/l
Albumin	36–47	g/l
Alkaline phosphatase	40–125	U/l
Amylase	50–300	U/l
Aspartate amino-transferase (AST)	10–35	U/l
Bilirubin (total)	2–17	µmol/l
Caeruloplasmin	150–600	mg/l
Calcium	2.12–2.62	mmol/l
Carboxyhaemoglobin	Not normally detectable Up to 1.5% in non-smokers	%
Chloride	95–107	mmol/l
Cholesterol (total)	[See note 1]	
HDL-cholesterol		
Male	0.5–1.6	mmol/l
Female	0.6–1.9	mmol/l
Copper	13–24	µmol/l
Creatinine	55–120	µmol/l
Creatine kinase (MB isoenzyme)	Normally < 6% of total CK	
Creatine kinase (total)		
Male	30–200	U/l
Female	30–150	U/l
Ethanol	Not normally detectable 65–87 (marked intoxication) 87–109 (stupor) > 109 (coma)	mmol/l
Ferritin		
Male	17–300	µg/l
Female	14–150	µg/l
Gamma-glutamyl transferase (GGT)		
Male	10–55	U/l
Female	5–35	U/l
Glucose (fasting)[2]	3.6–5.8	mmol/l
Glycated haemoglobin (HbA_1)	5.0–6.5	%
Immunoglobulin A	0.5–4.0	g/l
Immunoglobulin G	5.0–13.0	g/l

Table 20.17 Reference values in venous serum for the more common analytes in adults *(contd)*

Analysis	Reference range	Units
Immunoglobulin M		
Male	0.3–2.2	g/l
Female	0.4–2.5	g/l
Iron		
Male	14–32	µmol/l
Female	10–28	µmol/l
Iron-binding capacity	45–72	µmol/l
Lactate	0.4–1.4	mmol/l
Lactate dehydrogenase (total)	230–460	U/l
Lead[3]	< 1.7	µmol/l
Magnesium	0.75–1.0	mmol/l
Osmolality	280–290	mmol/kg
Phosphate (fasting)	0.8–1.4	mmol/l
Potassium (plasma)	3.3–4.7	mmol/l
Potassium (serum)	3.6–5.1	mmol/l
Protein (total)	60–80	g/l
Sodium	132–144	mmol/l
Total CO_2	24–30	mmol/l
Transferrin	2.0–4.0	g/l
Triglycerides (fasting)	0.6–1.7	mmol/l
Urate		
Male	0.12–0.42	mmol/l
Female	0.12–0.36	mmol/l
Urea	2.5–6.6	mmol/l
Zinc	11–22	µmol/l

[1] Cholesterol (total) ideally < 5.2 mmol/l
mild increase 5.2–6.5 mmol/l
moderate increase 6.5–7.8 mmol/l
severe increase > 7.8 mmol/l
(as defined by the European Atherosclerosis Society).

[2] Values quoted for venous plasma or serum. Diagnostic criteria for 75 g oral glucose tolerance test (venous plasma) are detailed in Table 7.5, page 481.

[3] Up to 1.2 µmol/l in children.

Table 20.18 Reference values for the more common analytes in urine

Analysis	Reference range	Units
Albumin	[See note 1]	
Calcium	1.2–3.7 (low calcium diet) Up to 12 (normal diet)	mmol/24 hrs
Copper	Up to 0.6	μmol/24 hrs
Cortisol	9–50	μmol/mol creatinine
Creatinine	10–20	mmol/24 hrs
5-hydroxyindole-3-acetic acid (5-HIAA)	< 60	μmol/24 hrs
Metadrenalines		
Normetadrenaline	0.4–3.4	μmol/24 hrs
Metadrenaline	0.3–1.7	μmol/24 hrs
Oxalate		
Male	80–490	mmol/24 hrs
Female	40–320	mmol/24 hrs
Phosphate	15–50	mmol/24 hrs
Potassium[2]	25–100	mmol/24 hrs
Protein	Up to 0.3	g/l
Sodium	100–200	mmol/24 hrs
Urate	1.2–3.0	mmol/24 hrs
Urea	170–600	mmol/24 hrs

[1] Albumin/creatinine ratio (ACR) and urinary albumin excretion rate (AER) are used to detect microalbuminuria, i.e. excessive albumin excretion in patients with diabetes mellitus, which is of predictive value in identifying patients at risk of progression to diabetic nephropathy. The test should only be carried out in the absence of overt proteinuria (dipstix negative).

ACR

Reference range:	< 3.5 mg albumin/mmol creatinine
'Borderline':	3.5–10 mg albumin/mmol creatinine
Positive test:	> 10 mg albumin/mmol creatinine

AER

Reference range:	< 20 μg albumin/min
Microalbuminuria:	20–200 μg albumin/min

[2] The urinary output of electrolytes such as sodium and potassium is normally a reflection of intake. This can vary widely, especially on a cultural, world-wide basis. The values quoted are more appropriate to a 'Western' diet.

Table 20.19 Hormones in serum

Hormone	Reference range	Units
Adrenocorticotrophic hormone (ACTH) (plasma)	7–51 (07:00–10:00 h)	ng/l
Cortisol	150–550 (at 08:00 h) < 200 (at 22:00 h)	nmol/l
Follicle-stimulating hormone (FSH)		
Male	1.5–9.0	U/l
Female*	3.0–15 (early follicular) Up to 20 (mid-cycle) > 30 (post-menopausal)	U/l
Gastrin (plasma)	Up to 120	ng/l
Growth hormone (GH)	Very variable, usually less than 2, but may be up to 50 with stress	mU/l
Insulin	Highly variable and interpretable only in relation to plasma glucose and body habitus	mU/l
Luteinising hormone (LH)		
Female*	2.5–9.0 (early follicular) Up to 90 (mid-cycle) > 20 (post-menopausal)	U/l
Male	1.5–9.0	U/l
Oestradiol-17β		
Female	110–180 (early follicular) 550–1650 (mid-cycle) 370–770 (luteal) < 150 (post-menopausal)	pmol/l
Male	< 200	pmol/l
Parathyroid hormone (PTH)	10–65	ng/l
Progesterone		
Male	< 2.0	nmol/l
Female	< 2.0 (follicular) > 15 (mid-luteal) < 2.0 (post-menopausal)	nmol/l
Prolactin (PRL)	60–390	mU/l
Testosterone		
Male	10–30	nmol/l
Female	0.4–2.8	nmol/l
Thyroid-stimulating hormone (TSH)	0.15–3.5	mU/l
Thyroxine (free) (free T_4)	10–27	pmol/l
Tri-iodothyronine (T_3)	1.0–2.6	nmol/l
TSH receptor antibodies (TRAb)	< 7	U/l

* Luteal phase values similar to follicular phase.

Notes

1. A number of hormones are unstable, and collection details are critical to obtaining a meaningful result. Refer to local hospital handbook.
2. Values in the table are only a guideline; hormone levels can often only be meaningfully understood in relation to factors such as sex (e.g. testosterone), age (e.g. FSH in women), time of day (e.g. cortisol) or regulatory factors (e.g. insulin and glucose, PTH and [Ca^{++}]). Also, reference ranges may be critically method-dependent.

Table 20.20 Haematological values

	Units
Bleeding time (Ivy)	Less than 8 mins
Body fluid (total)	50% (obese)–70% (lean) of body weight
Intracellular	30–40% of body weight
Extracellular	20–30% of body weight
Blood volume	
Male	75 ± 10 ml/kg
Female	70 ± 10 ml/kg
Coagulation screen	
Prothrombin time	12–14 s
Activated partial thromboplastin time	30–40 s
Erythrocyte sedimentation rate*	
Adult male	0–5 mm/hr
Adult female	0–7 mm/hr
Fibrinogen	1.5–4.0 g/l
Folate	
Serum	1.9–9.0 µg/l
Red cell	150–500 ng/l
Haemoglobin	
Male	130–180 g/l
Female	115–165 g/l
Haptoglobin	0.3–2.0 g/l
Leucocytes (adults)	4.0–11.0 × 10^9/l
Differential white cell count	
Neutrophil granulocytes	2.0–7.5 × 10^9/l
Lymphocytes	1.5–4.0 × 10^9/l
Monocytes	0.2–0.8 × 10^9/l
Eosinophil granulocytes	0.04–0.4 × 10^9/l
Basophil granulocytes	0.01–0.1 × 10^9/l
Mean corpuscular haemoglobin (MCH)	27–35 pg
Mean corpuscular haemoglobin concentration (MCHC)	31–35 g/dl
Mean corpuscular volume (MCV)	76–98 fl
Packed cell volume (PCV) or haematocrit	
Male	0.40–0.54
Female	0.37–0.47
Platelets	150–400 × 10^9/l
Red cell count	
Male	4.5–6.5 × 10^{12}/l
Female	3.8–5.8 × 10^{12}/l
Red cell lifespan (mean)	120 days
Red cell lifespan $T_{\frac{1}{2}}$ (^{51}Cr)	25–35 days
Reticulocytes (adults)	10–100 × 10^9/l
Vitamin B_{12}	250–900 ng/l

* Higher values in older patients are not necessarily abnormal.

DRUG NOMENCLATURE

Drugs have different kinds of name:

- *the chemical name*, whose form generally follows the rules issued by the International Union of Pure and Applied Chemistry (IUPAC).
- *the approved (official or generic) name*. This is usually the International Non-proprietary Name (INN), recommended (rINN) or proposed (pINN) by the World Health Organization (WHO), but may be some locally approved name (for example, the British Approved Name—BAN, or United States Adopted Name—USAN).
- *the proprietary name* (brand name or trade name), given to it by a pharmaceutical manufacturer.

For example:

- *chemical name*: 6-[[amino(4-hydroxyphenyl)acetyl]-amino]-3,3-dimethyl-7-oxo-4-thia-1-azabicyclo[3.2.0]heptane-2-carboxylic acid
- *International Non-proprietary Name*: amoxicillin; British Approved Name: amoxycillin
- *proprietary names*: Almodan®, Amix®, Amoram®, Amoxil®, Galenamox®, Rimoxallin®.

Since the chemical name is generally, as in this case, unsuitable for routine prescribing, either the approved name or proprietary name is used. Which should one choose? For some drugs the question is trivial, since only one proprietary formulation exists—for example, losartan is currently available in the UK only as Cozaar®.

However, several proprietary formulations of the same chemical entity may become available when the patent expires on a drug with a previously unique proprietary name. For instance, amoxycillin was first marketed as Amoxil®. When the patent expired the number of proprietary brands (see above) multiplied. This can cause prescribing and dispensing problems. For example, in the UK, whether the prescriber writes 'losartan BP' or 'Cozaar', the patient will receive Cozaar®. However, if the prescriber writes 'amoxycillin BP' the pharmacist may dispense any proprietary formulation, provided that it conforms to the description laid out in the BP *(British Pharmacopoeia)*, and will generally dispense the cheapest available.

By writing the proprietary name, the prescriber can ensure that a particular formulation of a drug is prescribed. However, in the UK, hospital pharmacies often stock only one formulation, and even if the hospital doctor writes 'Amoxil' on an inpatient prescription chart, the pharmacist may dispense some other approved formulation for which the hospital will have negotiated an economic deal with the supplier.

There are advantages and disadvantages to the prescribing of drugs by their generic as opposed to their proprietary names. The advantages include:

- *awareness of one's prescription*. Since the name of the compound often tells you to what class it belongs, usually by virtue of its suffix; e.g. -statin (HMG-CoA reductase inhibitors), -olol (β-blockers, although beware stanozolol), -floxacin (quinolone antibiotics).
- *drug stocks*. If you prescribe, say, 'Almodan' rather than 'amoxicillin' and an outside pharmacy stocks only Amoxil®, the pharmacist cannot legally dispense the prescription without first consulting the doctor; clearly this can cause inconvenience to all concerned and might result in delayed treatment.
- *expense*. It is generally cheaper to prescribe by the approved name, since the pharmacist will dispense the cheapest variant held in stock.

Disadvantages of prescribing by approved name include:

- *remembering names*. Proprietary names are chosen by pharmaceutical companies because they are catchy, usually easier to remember than the corresponding generic name, and shorter and easier to spell. (Compare, for example, 'Librium' with 'chlordiazepoxide'.) Furthermore, a single proprietary name will do when the formulation may, in fact, contain two or more drugs. (Compare, for example, 'Fefol' with 'ferrous sulphate plus folic acid'.) However, in recent years there has been a move in the UK to counteract this problem, by giving single approved names to some common combinations of drugs; for example, the combination of dihydrocodeine with paracetamol (acetaminophen) is known as co-dydramol.
- *quality of product*. For a few drugs a change in tablet excipients has large effects on the absorption of the drug from the formulation; important examples include lithium salts and theophylline, which should always be prescribed by brand name.
- *continuity of treatment*. Patients not infrequently become confused if the drug they are being given changes its form with every prescription; continuity can be achieved by prescribing the same proprietary formulation every time.

In hospital it is usually better to prescribe by approved name, since the pharmacy will dispense whatever formulation is held in stock. The proprietary name can be used when a combination product is prescribed for which no single approved name exists (for example 'Fefol'). In general practice it is usually best to prescribe by approved name also. Many practitioners prefer to prescribe by proprietary name and in some cases (for example, lithium salts and theophylline) should do so. However, doctors who make the effort to prescribe when possible by approved name will generally find it as easy as prescribing by proprietary name.

Recently, the Medicines Control Agency has decided that the UK should be brought into conformity with European law with regard to the use of approved names (directives 65/65 and 92/27/EEC). This means that British Approved Names will be replaced by International Non-proprietary Names when the two are different; for example, we shall start to call amoxycillin amoxicillin. This will happen immediately, apart from some important exceptions for which a transition period of at least 5 years has been proposed but for which dual naming will be used for the moment (e.g. on drug labels). These exceptions are listed in Table 20.21.

Table 20.21 Drug names for which dual naming (BAN and INN) will be used for the time being

British approved name (BAN)	International non-proprietary name (rINN)
Acrosoxacin	Rosoxacin
Adrenaline	Epinephrine
Amethocaine	Tetracaine
Bendrofluazide	Bendroflumethiazide
Benzhexol	Trihexyphenidyl
Chlorpheniramine	Chlorphenamine
Dicyclomine	Dicycloverine
Dothiepin	Dosulepin
Eformoterol	Formoterol
Flurandrolone	Fludroxycortide
Frusemide	Furosemide
Hydroxyurea	Hydroxycarbamide
Lignocaine	Lidocaine
Methotrimeprazine	Levomepromazine
Methylene blue	Methylthioninium chloride
Mitozantrone	Mitoxantrone
Mustine	Chlormethine
Nicoumalone	Acenocoumarol
Noradrenaline	Norepinephrine
Oxpentifylline	Pentoxifylline
Procaine penicillin	Procaine benzylpenicillin
Salcatonin	Calcitonin (salmon)
Stilboestrol	Diethylstilbestrol
Thymoxamine	Moxisylyte
Thyroxine sodium	Levothyroxine sodium
Trimeprazine	Alimemazine

This section on nomenclature has been adapted from text in Grahame-Smith DG, Aronson JK 1999 The Oxford Textbook of Clinical Pharmacology and Drug Therapy. Oxford Unitersity Press, Oxford, 3rd edition.

STANDARD REFERENCE BOOKS FOR DRUG NAMES

Association of the British Pharmaceutical Industry Compendium of data sheets and summaries of product characteristics. Datapharm, London, 1998–9 (new edition each year)

Joint Formulary Committee British National Formulary. British Medical Association and Royal Pharmaceutical Society of Great Britain, London. Published twice a year

FURTHER INFORMATION ON DRUG NOMENCLATURE

Aronson J K 1995 Confusion over similar drug names: problems and solutions. Drug Safety 12: 155–160

Medicines Control Agency 1997 BANs to INNS. Mail 103: 2–3

THERAPEUTIC DRUG CONCENTRATIONS

Table 20.22 Usual therapeutic and toxic plasma concentrations of commonly measured drugs

		Concentration below which a therapeutic effect is unlikely		Concentration above which a toxic effect is more likely	
Drug	**Optimal sampling time**	**Mass units**	**Molar units**	**Mass units**	**Molar units**
Aspirin (salicylate)					
Analgesic	Just before next dose	20 µg/ml	0.15 µmol/l	300 µg/ml	2.2 µmol/l
Anti-inflammatory	Just before next dose	150 µg/ml	1.1 µmol/l	300 µg/ml	2.2 µmol/l
Carbamazepine	Just before next dose	4 µg/ml	17 µmol/l	10 µg/ml	42 µmol/l
Cardiac glycosides					
Digitoxin	Just before next dose	15 ng/ml	20 nmol/l	30 ng/ml	39 nmol/l
Digoxin	11 hrs after last dose	0.8 ng/ml	1.0 nmol/l	2 ng/ml	2.6 nmol/l
Cyclosporin*	Just before next dose	125 ng/ml	104 nmol/l	200 ng/ml	166 nmol/l
Lithium	12 hrs after last dose	—	0.4 mmol/l	—	1.0 mmol/l
Phenytoin	Just before next dose	10 µg/ml	40 µmol/l	20 µg/ml	80 µmol/l
Theophylline	Just before next dose	10 µg/ml	55 µmol/l	20 µg/ml	110 µmol/l

* Measured in whole blood by specific radioimmunoassay or h.p.l.c.

Notes

1. Care should be taken in comparing results between different laboratories (particularly with cyclosporin).
2. The concentration below which a therapeutic effect is unlikely and the concentration above which a toxic effect is more likely together constitute a target range within which satisfactory therapy is likely to be achieved; however, dosages should be adjusted according to the clinical response not the concentration, which should only be used as a guide.
3. Note the units used when interpreting results. The data in the table are all in SI units, but laboratories may report in mass units or molar units.
4. Remember that pharmacokinetics differ from individual to individual; for within-patient comparisons always use the same time after the last dose.
5. Remember that pharmacodynamics differ from individual to individual and that different individuals respond differently to the same concentration of drug; other factors that can alter the individual response should be considered.
6. For paracetamol see Figure 19.7, page 1120.
7. For aminoglycosides consult your laboratory.

Picture and table credits

We are grateful to the following individuals and organisations for the loan of illustrations:

Chapter 1

Fig. 1.39C Dr G.M.F. Wallace

Chapter 2

Illustrative material supplied by Dr R. Davidson and the EM and Histopathology Unit, London School of Hygiene and Tropical Medicine; Figs 2.12, 2.14, 2.18, 2.19 Audio-Visual Department, St Mary's Hospital, London; Fig. 2.23 Institute of Ophthalmology, Moorfields Eye Hospital, London; Fig. 2.27 Reproduced by permission of the World Health Organization; Fig. 2.38 Professor K. Vickerman; Figs 2.53, 2.55 Dr P. Hay, St George's Hospital, London

Chapter 3

Figs 3.20A and B Dr B. Cullen

Chapter 4

Figs 4.6, 4.7 Dr J. Reid; Fig. 4.10 Professor N.J. Douglas; Fig. 4.12B British Lung Foundation; Fig. 4.15B Dr A. Greening; Fig. 4.31C Dr C. Flower, Addenbrooke's Hospital, Cambridge

Chapter 6

Illustrative material supplied by Dr I. Beggs and Dr J. Reid; Figs 6.1C and E, 6.21A, C, D and E Dr J.G. Simpson, Aberdeen Royal Infirmary; Figs 6.3A and B, 6.4A, B and C, 6.5, 6.6B, 6.8, 6.24A and B, 6.27 Dr A.P. Bayliss and Dr P. Thorpe, Aberdeen Royal Infirmary; Fig. 6.6A Dr D. Fowler, Leeds General Infirmary; Figs 6.7, 6.31 Dr P. Robinson, St James's University Hospital, Leeds; Fig. 6.11 Dr G.M. Iadarola and Dr F. Quarello, G Bosco Hospital, Turin (from http://www.sin-italia.org/imago/sediment/sed.htm); Fig. 6.17 Data from the Scottish Renal Registry; Fig. 6.19B and C Dr Jill Collar, St Mary's Hospital, London; Figs 6.21F, G and H Dr R. Herriot

Chapter 7

Fig. 7.18 Dr A.W. Patrick and Dr I.W. Campbell; Fig. 7.24 Dr R.G. Whitehead; Fig. 7.25 Institute of Ophthalmology

Chapter 12

Fig. 12.9 Dr I. Beggs

Chapter 14

Figs 14.23C, 14.24 Dr B. Cullen; Figs 14.6A, B and C, 14.7A, B and C, 14.8A, B, C and D, Dr D. Collie

The following figures are reproduced with publishers' permission as listed:

Chapter 1

Fig. 1.26 Janeway and Travers 1997 Immunobiology 3rd edn, Current Biology Ltd/Garland Publishing Inc.
Fig. 1.33C Wyatt et al 1998 The antigenic structure of the HIV gp120 envelope glycoprotein. Nature 393: 705–711, with permission of the publishers and authors. Copyright 1998 Macmillan Magazines Ltd; Fig. 1.34 Dr M. Mikkelsen, from Brock D J H, Rodeck C H, Ferguson-Smith M A 1992 Prenatal diagnosis and screening. Churchill Livingstone, Edinburgh

Chapter 2

Fig. 2.4 Reproduced from Halstead S B 1997 Dengue and Monath T P 1997 Yellow fever. Medicine 25: 1. By kind permission of the Medicine Publishing Company and Dr T P Monath; Fig. 2.8 Hu D J et al 1996 The emerging diversity of HIV. Journal of the American Medical Association 275: 210–216; Fig. 2.9 Perelson A S, Neumann A U, Markowitz M et al 1996 HIV-1 dynamics in vitro: virion clearance rate, infected cell lifespan and viral generation time. Science 271: 1592; Fig. 2.28 Bryceson A D M, Pfaltzgraff R E 1990 Leprosy, 3rd edn. Churchill Livingstone, Edinburgh; Figs 2.37, 2.39A Knight R 1982 Parasitic disease in man. Churchill Livingstone, Edinburgh; Fig. 2.44 Cook G C (Ed.) 1995 Manson's tropical diseases, 20th edn. W B Saunders, London: 1415; Fig. 2.49 Gibbons L M 1986 SEM Guide to the morphology of nematode parasites of vertebrates. Commonwealth Agricultural Bureau International, Farnham Royal, Slough; Table 2.36 Knight R 1982 Parasitic disease in man. Churchill Livingstone, Edinburgh

Chapter 3

Fig. 3.8 Hampton J R 1994 The ECG made easy, 4th edn. Churchill Livingstone, Edinburgh; Fig. 3.21 British

Hypertension Society; Figs 3.40, 3.41 European Resuscitation Council 1998 Guidelines for basic life support and Guidelines for adult advanced life support. Resuscitation 37: 67–90; Fig. 3.73 inset Savin J A, Hunter J A A, Hepburn N C 1997 Skin signs in clinical medicine. Mosby-Wolfe, London

Chapter 4

Fig. 4.14 1997 BTS guidelines for management of COPD. Thorax: 52, suppl. 5. By permission of the BMJ Publishing Group; Fig. 4.15C Reproduced with permission from Brewis R A L et al 1995 Respiratory medicine, 2nd edn. Baillière Tindall, London; Fig. 4.37 Johnson N McL 1986 Respiratory medicine. Blackwell Science, Oxford; Fig. 4.44 Hampton J R 1992 The ECG in practice, 2nd edn. Churchill Livingstone, Edinburgh

Chapter 5

Fig. 5.10 Flenley D 1971 Lancet 1: 1921

Chapter 6

Fig. 6.18 Beutler J J, Koomans H A 1997 Malignant hypertension: still a challenge. Nephrology Dialysis Transplantation 12: 2019–2023. Photograph courtesy of Prof P J Slootweg, University Hospital, Utrecht. By permission of Oxford University Press; Table 6.13 Adapted from Boulton Jones J M et al 1982 Diagnosis and management of renal and urinary diseases. Blackwell Science, Oxford

Chapter 7

Fig. 7.3 De Fronzo R A et al 1992 Pathogenesis of NIDDM. A balanced overview. Diabetes Care 15: 319, Fig. 2; Fig. 7.11 Nutrition Subcommittee of British Diabetic Association 1992 Dietary recommendations for people with diabetes: an update for the 1990s. Diabetic Medicine 9: 196, Fig. 1. Copyright John Wiley & Sons Ltd, reproduced with permission; Fig. 7.26 World Health Organization 1976 Report of a joint WHO/USAID meeting, vitamin A deficiency and xerophthalmia (WHO technical report series no. 5 W); Fig. 7.33 Gaw A 1995 Clinical biochemistry: 120. Churchill Livingstone, Edinburgh; Table 7.17 Frisancho A R 1981 American Journal of Clinical Nutrition 34: 2540–2545, and Bishop C W et al 1981 American Journal of Clinical Nutrition 34: 2530–2539

Chapter 8

Fig. 8.14 Toft A et al 1978 Thyroid function after surgical treatment of thyrotoxicosis: a report of 100 cases treated with propranolol before operation. New England Journal of Medicine 298: 643–647; Table 8.13 Ross E J, Linch D C 1982 Cushing's syndrome—killing disease: discriminatory signs and symptoms aiding early diagnosis. Lancet 1: 726–728

Chapter 9

Figs 9.32A and B Hayes P, Simpson K 1995 Gastroenterology and liver disease. Churchill Livingstone, Edinburgh

Chapter 10

Figs 10.13, 10.22 Hayes P, Simpson K 1995 Gastroenterology and liver disease. Churchill Livingstone, Edinburgh; Fig. 10.23 Hayes P C, Bell D 1996 Clinical signs. Churchill Livingstone, Edinburgh; Fig. 10.28 Shearman D J C, Finlayson N D C 1989 Diseases of the gastrointestinal tract and liver, 2nd edn. Churchill Livingstone, Edinburgh

Chapter 11

Fig. 11.15 Hoffbrand A V, Pettit J E 1992 Essential haematology, 3rd edn. Blackwell Science, Edinburgh; Tables 11.7, 11.8 Ludlam C 1990 Clinical haematology. Churchill Livingstone, Edinburgh

Chapter 12

Fig. 12.19 Stockwell R A 1991 Cartilage failure in osteoarthritis: relevance of normal structure and function—a review. Clinical Anatomy 4: 161–191; Information box, p. 852 Southwood T R, Woo P 1995 Juvenile chronic arthritis. Baillière's Clinical Rheumatology 9: 331–353; Fig. 12.26A and B Maddison P J, Isenberg D A, Woo P, Glass D N 1993 Oxford textbook of rheumatology. Oxford University Press, Oxford

Chapter 13

Fig. 13.6 Munro J, Edwards C R W (eds) 1995 MacLeod's clinical examination. Churchill Livingstone, Edinburgh

Chapter 16

Fig. 16.1 Cancer Research Campaign 1995 Factsheet 3.1; Table 16.4 Coates A, Abraham S, Kaye S B et al 1983 On the receiving end: patient perception of the side-effects of cancer chemotherapy. European Journal of Cancer and Clinical Oncology 19/2: 203–208

Chapter 17

Fig. 17.4 Colledge N R, Barr-Hamilton R M, Lewis S J et al 1996 Evaluation of investigations to diagnose the cause of dizziness in elderly people. British Medical Journal 313: 788–792. By permission of the BMJ Publishing Group; Fig. 17.5 Young J 1996 Rehabilitation and older people. British Medical Journal 313: 677–681. By permission of the BMJ Publishing Group

Chapter 19

Fig. 19.1 Brater D C, Chennavasin P, Day B et al 1983 Bumetanide and furosemide. Clinical Pharmacology and Therapeutics 34: 207–213, reproduced with permission of Mosby Inc, St Louis, Missouri; and Chennavasin P, Seiwell R, Brater D C 1980 Pharmacokinetic-dynamic analysis of the indomethacin-furosemide interaction in man. Journal of Pharmacology and Experimental Therapeutics 215: 77–81, with permission of the American Association for Pharmacology and Experimental Therapeutics; Figs 19.2, 19.3 Crown copyright; reproduced with the permission of the Controller of Her Majesty's Stationery Office

Index

Page numbers in bold indicate a major reference

A

B

C

D

E

F

G

H

I

M

N

O

P

Q

R

S

T

U

V

W

X

Y

Z